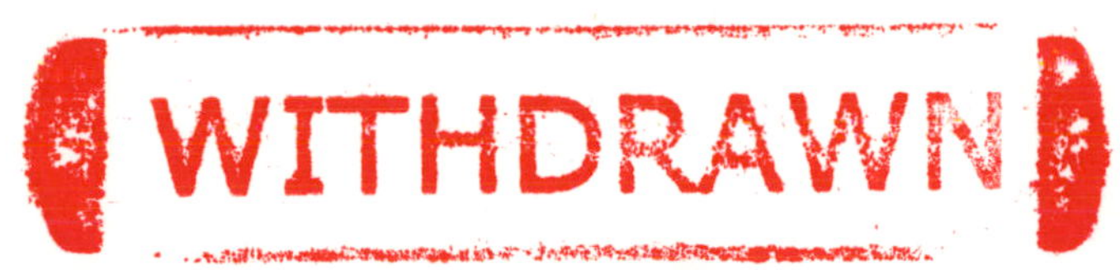
WITHDRAWN

Bacterial Infections of Humans

Epidemiology and Control

THIRD EDITION

Bacterial Infections of Humans

Epidemiology and Control

THIRD EDITION

Edited by

Alfred S. Evans

Late of Yale University School of Medicine
New Haven, Connecticut

and

Philip S. Brachman

The Rollins School of Public Health of Emory University
Atlanta, Georgia

PLENUM MEDICAL BOOK COMPANY
New York and London

Library of Congress Cataloging-in-Publication Data

On file

ISBN 0-306-45320-7 (Hardbound)
ISBN 0-306-45323-1 (Paperback)

233 Spring Street, New York, N.Y. 10013

Plenum Medical Book Company is an imprint of Plenum Publishing Corporation

http://www.plenum.com

10 9 8 7 6 5 4 3 2 1

Printed in the United States of America

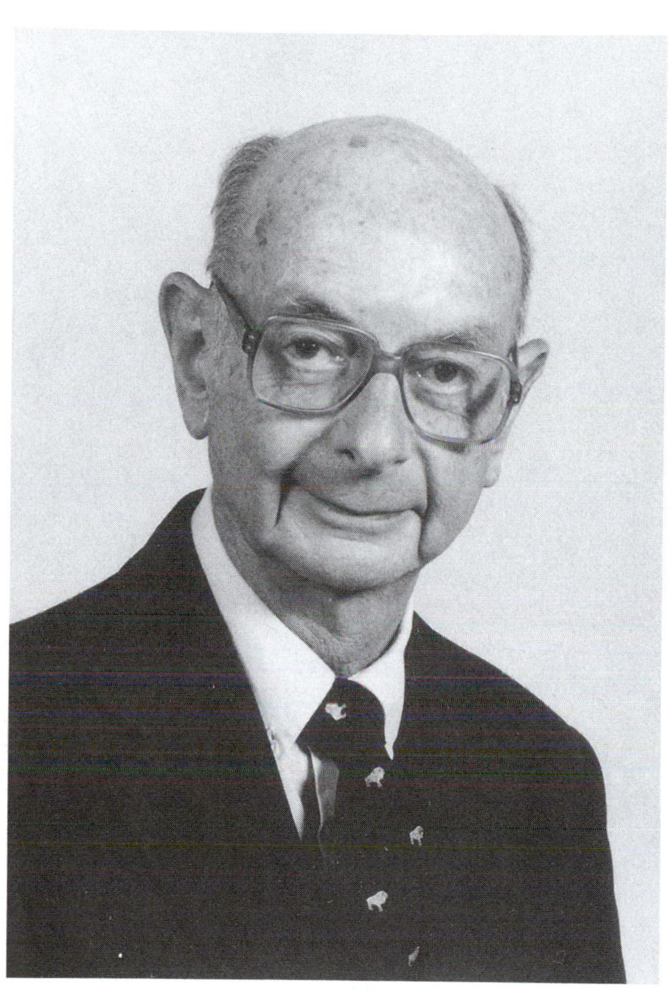

Alfred S. Evans
1917–1996

Contributors

E. Russell Alexander, Seattle–King County Department of Public Health, Seattle, Washington 98104

Ban Mishu Allos, Division of Infectious Diseases, Vanderbilt University School of Medicine, Nashville, Tennessee 37232

Frederick J. Angulo, Foodborne and Diarrheal Diseases Branch, Division of Bacterial and Mycotic Diseases, National Center for Infectious Diseases, Centers for Disease Control and Prevention, Atlanta, Georgia 30333

Donald Armstrong, Department of Medicine, Memorial Sloan-Kettering Cancer Center, New York, New York 10021

Gregory L. Armstrong, Epidemiology and Emergency Response Program, Food Safety and Inspection Service, US Department of Agriculture, Washington, DC 20250

Robert S. Baltimore, Departments of Pediatrics and Epidemiology and Public Health, Yale University School of Medicine, New Haven, Connecticut 06520-8064

Michael L. Bennish, Department of Pediatrics and Medicine, Tupper Research Institute, Division of Geographic Medicine and Infectious Diseases, New England Medical Center, Boston, Massachusetts 02111

Philip S. Brachman, The Rollins School of Public Health of Emory University, Atlanta, Georgia 30322

Robert F. Breiman, Respiratory Diseases Branch, Division of Bacterial and Mycotic Diseases, National Center for Infectious Diseases, Centers for Disease Control and Prevention, Atlanta, Georgia 30333

Jay C. Butler, Respiratory Diseases Branch, Division of Bacterial and Mycotic Diseases, National Center for Infectious Diseases, Centers for Disease Control and Prevention, Atlanta, Georgia 30333

Willard Cates, Jr., Family Health International, Research Triangle Park, North Carolina 27709

David L. Cohn, Denver Disease Control Service, University of Colorado Health Sciences Center, Denver, Colorado 80204

George W. Comstock, School of Hygiene and Public Health, The Johns Hopkins University, Baltimore, Maryland 21742-2067

James DeMaio, Division of Infectious Diseases, Johns Hopkins Hospital, Baltimore, Maryland 21205

Louise M. Dembry, Department of Hospital Epidemiology and Infection Control, Yale University School of Medicine, Yale–New Haven Hospital, New Haven, Connecticut 06504

David T. Dennis, Division of Vector-Borne Diseases, National Center for Infectious Diseases, Centers for Disease Control and Prevention, Public Health Service, US Department of Health and Human Services, Fort Collins, Colorado 80522

J. Stephen Dumler, Department of Pathology, Johns Hopkins Medical Institution, Baltimore, Maryland 21287

Herbert L. DuPont, Center for Infectious Diseases, The University of Texas at Houston, and St. Luke's Episcopal Hospital, Houston, Texas 77225

Alfred S. Evans,† Department of Epidemiology and Public Health, Yale University School of Medicine, New Haven, Connecticut 06510

Solly Faine, Department of Microbiology, Monash University, Clayton Vic. 3168, Australia

Paul Fiset, Department of Microbiology and Immunology, University of Maryland School of Medicine, Baltimore, Maryland 21201

Hjordis M. Foy, Department of Epidemiology, School of Public Health and Community Medicine, University of Washington, Seattle, Washington 98195-7236

Bruce G. Gellin, Division of Microbiology and Infectious Diseases, National Institute of Allergy and Infectious Diseases, National Institutes of Health, Bethesda, Maryland 20892

Dale N. Gerding, Chicago Health Care System, Lakeside Division, Department of Medicine, University Medical School, Chicago, Illinois 60611

Barry M. Gray, Division of Medical Education, Spartanburg Regional Medical Center, Spartanburg, South Carolina 29303

Wendell H. Hall, Infectious Disease Section, Veterans Affairs Medical Center, and Departments of Medicine and Microbiology, University of Minnesota, Minneapolis, Minnesota 55455

Iain R. B. Hardy,† National Immunization Program, Centers for Disease Control and Prevention, Atlanta, Georgia 30333

Craig Hedberg, Minnesota Department of Health, Minneapolis, Minnesota 55440-9441

Walter J. Hierholzer, Jr., Department of Hospital Epidemiology and Infection Control, Yale University School of Medicine, Yale–New Haven Hospital, New Haven, Connecticut 06504

Jill Hollingsworth, Epidemiology and Emergency Response Program, Food Safety and Inspection Service, US Department of Agriculture, Washington, DC 20250

Richard B. Hornick, Medical Education Administration, Orlando Regional Medical Center, Orlando, Florida 32806

Robert R. Jacobson, Gillis W. Long Hansen's Disease Center, Carville, Louisiana 70721

Stuart Johnson, Chicago Health Care System, Lakeside Division, Department of Medicine, University Medical School, Chicago, Illinois 60611

Georg Kapperud, National Institute of Public Health, 0403 Oslo, Norway; and Norwegian College of Veterinary Medicine, 0033 Oslo, Norway

Arnold F. Kaufmann, National Center for Infectious Diseases, Centers for Disease Control and Prevention, Atlanta, Georgia 30333

Gerald T. Keusch, Department of Medicine, Tupper Research Institute, Division of Geographic Medicine and Infectious Diseases, New England Medical Center, Boston, Massachusetts 02111

Myron M. Levine, Center for Vaccine Development, University of Maryland School of Medicine, Baltimore, Maryland 21201

John J. Mathewson, Center for Infectious Diseases, The University of Texas at Houston, Houston, Texas 77225

John E. McGowan, Jr., The Rollins School of Public Health of Emory University, Atlanta, Georgia 30322

Kristine A. Moore, Minnesota Department of Health, Minneapolis, Minnesota 55440-9441

J. Glenn Morris, Jr., Epidemiology and Emergency Response Program, Food Safety and Inspection Service, US Department of Agriculture, Washington, DC 20250; and Division of Infectious

†*Deceased.*

Diseases, Department of Medicine, University of Maryland School of Medicine, and Veterans Affairs Medical Center, Baltimore, Maryland 21201

Edward A. Mortimer, Jr., Department of Epidemiology and Biostatistics, Case Western Reserve University School of Medicine, Cleveland, Ohio 44106-4945

Robert R. Muder, Infectious Diseases Division, Department of Medicine, University of Pittsburgh School of Medicine, Pittsburgh, Pennsylvania 15213

Richard J. O'Brien, Division of Tuberculosis Elimination, National Center for HIV, STD, and TB Prevention, Centers for Disease Control and Prevention, Atlanta, Georgia 30333

Walter A. Orenstein, National Immunization Program, Centers for Disease Control and Prevention, Atlanta, Georgia 30333

Michael Osterholm, Minnesota Department of Health, Minneapolis, Minnesota 55440-9441

Julie Parsonnet, Department of Health Research and Policy, Stanford University School of Medicine, Stanford, California 94305-5405

Andrew T. Pavia, Department of Medicine, Division of Pediatric Infectious Diseases, University of Utah Medical Center, Salt Lake City, Utah 84132

Peter L. Perine, Center for AIDS and STS, Department of Epidemiology, School of Public Health and Community Medicine, University of Washington, Seattle, Washington 98195

Jack D. Poland, Division of Vector-Borne Diseases, National Center for Infectious Diseases, Centers for Disease Control and Prevention, Public Health Service, US Department of Health and Human Services, Fort Collins, Colorado 80522

Arthur L. Reingold, Division of Public Health Biology and Epidemiology, University of California, Berkeley, California 94720-7360

Frederick L. Ruben, Infectious Diseases Division, Department of Medicine, University of Pittsburgh School of Medicine, Pittsburgh, Pennsylvania 15213

Julias Schachter, Department of Laboratory Medicine, University of California, San Francisco, California 94110.

George P. Schmid, Division of STD Prevention, National Center for HIV, STD, and TB Prevention, Centers for Disease Control and Prevention, Atlanta, Georgia 30333

Eugene D. Shapiro, Departments of Pediatrics and Epidemiology and Public Health, Yale University School of Medicine, New Haven, Connecticut 06520-8064

Sally Bryna Slome, Kaiser Permanente Medical Center, Oakland, California 94611

Karen L. Smith, Department of Medicine, Stanford University School of Medicine, Stanford, California 94305-5405

Michael E. St. Louis, Division of STD Prevention, National Center for HIV, STD, and TB Prevention, Centers for Disease Control and Prevention, Atlanta, Georgia 30333

Roland W. Sutter, National Immunization Program, Centers for Disease Control and Prevention, Atlanta, Georgia 30333

Robert V. Tauxe, Foodborne and Diarrheal Diseases Branch, Division of Bacterial and Mycotic Diseases, National Center for Infectious Diseases, Centers for Disease Control and Prevention, Atlanta, Georgia 30333

David N. Taylor, Division of Communicable Disease and Epidemiology, Walter Reed Army Institute of Research, Washington, DC 20307

Fred C. Tenover, Nosocomial Pathogens Laboratory Branch, Hospital Infections Program, National Center for Infectious Diseases, Centers for Disease Control and Prevention, Atlanta, Georgia 30333

Constance M. Vadheim, UCLA Center for Vaccine Research, Harbor–UCLA Medical Center, UCLA School of Medicine, Torrance, California 90509

Joel I. Ward, UCLA Center for Vaccine Research, Harbor–UCLA Medical Center, UCLA School of Medicine, Torrance, California 90509

Steven G. F. Wassilak, National Immunization Program, Centers for Disease Control and Prevention, Atlanta, Georgia 30333

Theodore E. Woodward, Department of Medicine, University of Maryland School of Medicine, Baltimore, Maryland 21201

Leo J. Yoder, Gillis W. Long Hansen's Disease Center, Carville, Louisiana 70721

Edward J. Young, Medical Service, Veterans Affairs Medical Center, and Departments of Medicine, Microbiology, and Immunology, Baylor College of Medicine, Houston, Texas 77030

Jonathan Zenilman, Division of Infectious Diseases, Johns Hopkins Hospital, Baltimore, Maryland 21205

Marcus J. Zervos, Division of Infectious Diseases, William Beaumont Hospital, Royal Oak, Michigan 48072

Preface

In Memoriam of Alfred S. Evans

This third edition of *Bacterial Infections of Humans* is dedicated to Alfred Spring Evans, who died on January 21, 1996, 2½ years after a diagnosis of cancer. Al was the senior editor of this textbook, which he founded with Harry Feldman in 1982.

Al was a clinician, epidemiologist, educator, catalyst for biomedical research, historian, author, speaker, seeker of the truth, sincere friend of students, sports enthusiast, traveler, and truly a man of all seasons. He was a devoted husband to Brigette Klug Evans, father of three children, and grandfather of four.

Al was born in Buffalo, New York, on August 21, 1917, to Ellen Spring and John H. Evans, M.D., one of the United States's first anesthesiologists and an early researcher in the field of oxygen therapy. He received his undergraduate training at the University of Michigan; was awarded an M.D. degree in 1943 from the University of Buffalo; interned in Pittsburgh, Pennsylvania; and performed his medical residency at the Goldwater Hospital in New York City. He was in the United States Army from 1944 to 1946, assigned as a public health officer to a base in Okinawa, Japan. It was there that he met Drs. Albert Sabin and John R. Paul, who came to Okinawa to test a new Japanese encephalitis vaccine. Al was invited by Dr. Paul to come to Yale University to work on the identification of the cause of infectious mononucleosis. He accepted this invitation and became an associate professor of medicine in the Department of Medicine from 1946 to 1950. He was then called back to active duty in the Army and acted as chief of the Hepatitis Research Laboratory in Munich, Germany. It was there that he met his future wife.

In 1952, he joined the University of Wisconsin Medical School faculty and was professor and chairman of the Department of Preventive Medicine. In 1959 he also became director of the state Laboratory of Hygiene. He took a sabbatical leave in 1960 to study for his M.P.H. degree, which he received from the University of Michigan in 1961. In 1966 he accepted the position of John Rodman Paul Professor of Epidemiology at Yale University. Additionally, he became the director of the WHO's Serum Reference Bank at Yale. He remained active as a teacher and researcher until 1988 when he became an emeritus professor. He retired from Yale in 1994.

Al was dedicated to teaching both undergraduate and graduate students, and his expertise included a full range of topics in preventive medicine, public health, epidemiology (both applied and clinical), infectious diseases, and other related subjects. He was one of the founders and the first director of the Graduate Summer Session in Epidemiology, which was first held in the summer of 1965 at the University of Wisconsin. He remained on its faculty when it was held at the University of Minnesota from 1967 to 1987, and then at the University of Michigan School of Public Health from 1988 through the summer of 1994. During his 29 years of association with the Graduate Summer Session, he was not only a lecturer, primarily in epidemiology and infectious diseases, but was also an active participant on the Planning Committee and was the unofficial social chairman for the 3-week session.

Al was a popular lecturer who used expected and unexpected visual aids and injected humor throughout his lectures. He enjoyed teaching, and his students were eager recipients, greatly stimulated by his teaching, who frequently acknowledged his excellence with words, deeds, and appropriate awards, such as the Bedpan Award for Clinical Teaching given at the University of Wisconsin in 1952. As a teacher he constantly looked for new methods of presenting information to students. He was dedicated to the method of problem-oriented sessions and developed his own infectious disease case studies, which he would incorporate into his lectures. Additionally, he was a popular guest lecturer at universities and institutions in the United States and throughout the world. He was never too busy for his students and provided ongoing consultation concerning their training and careers.

His research ranged over broad fields of infectious disease as well as public health and epidemiology, with an emphasis on the Epstein–Barr virus and the relationships between cancer and infectious agents. He was the author or coauthor of more than 230 scientific, peer-viewed publications covering a broad area of topics, including such titles as "Sneezes, Wheezes, and Other Diseases" (1961), "Farm Injuries" (1958 and 1961), and "The Instant-Distant Infection" (1966). He was a medical historian, writing essays on John Evans, Austin Flint, and Max von Pettenkofer. He constantly promoted the incorporation of presentations on medical or public health history in the programs of various societies and training programs. He was an active supporter of Yale's historic Beaumont Medical Club.

Al firmly believed in the importance of accuracy in investigations, whether in the laboratory or in the field. His initial involvement in a field investigation incorporated comprehensive descriptive epidemiology that, when appropriate, was followed by methodical and carefully conceived analytic epidemiological methods. He was innovative in the use of observational field studies, which is reflected in his studies of the Epstein–Barr virus. Al constantly promoted the development and use of serum banks, as reflected by the WHO Serum Reference Bank at Yale. There are numerous examples of how this facility made significant contributions to Al's studies of infectious mononucleosis, other infectious diseases, and, more recently, HIV/AIDS. He made significant contributions to the concepts of disease causation and researched and reworked Koch's postulates. In this regard, he acknowledged the important contributions that Jakob Henle made to the topic and renamed Koch's postulates the Henle–Koch postulates.

He was author or coauthor of five well-received textbooks: *Viral Infections of Humans* (which in 1977 received The American Medical Writers' Association award for the best book written for physicians), *Bacterial Infections of Humans*, *Methods in Observational Epidemiology*, *Causation and Disease: A Chronological Journey*, and *Symposium on Latency and Masking in Viral and Rickettsial Infections*. He was also an editor of the *Yale Journal of Biology and Medicine*. He was a consultant to the WHO, the Pan American Health Organization, the United States Public Health Service, and the National Aeronautics and Space Agency and worked specifically with the space program in establishing the infection quarantine programs for the Apollo 13 space mission. He frequently consulted with numerous Ministries of Health in other countries, including Czechoslovakia, Kuwait, France, Spain, Taiwan, the Philippines, and Vietnam.

Al remained current with the medical literature, applied new technology in his own research, and brought appropriate new information into his lectures and writings. He constantly acquainted his colleagues and students with pertinent new written information culled from the current medical literature.

He belonged to and was an avid supporter of a number of societies, including the American Epidemiological Society, for which he served as secretary-treasurer (1968–1972) and president (1973); The American College of Epidemiology, of which he was one of the cofounders and later served as president (1990); The Society of Epidemiologic Research; The Infectious Disease Society of America; The Society of Medical Consultants to the Armed Forces, for which he served as president (1983); and the American Public Health Association (where he was president of the Epidemiology Section). He was also a fellow of the American Association for the Advancement of Science.

Al received numerous prestigious awards and lectureships, including the Thomas Parron Lecturer and Award, University of Pittsburgh (1977); the Thomas Francis Lectureship, University of Michigan

School of Public Health (1986); the Abraham Lilienfeld Lectureship, American College of Epidemiology (1986); the First Harry Feldman Memorial Lectureship, American Epidemiological Society (1987); the John R. Seal Award, The Society of Medical Consultants to the Armed Forces (1987); the W.B. Harrington Lecture and Award, University of Buffalo (1988); the Abraham Lilienfeld Award, Epidemiology Section, American Public Health Association (1990); and the Kass Lecturer, The Infectious Disease Society of America (1995). He was a renowned poet, but never published any of his works. He enjoyed reciting them in the classroom, in private discussions, and at social events.

During his life, he set standards to which others will aspire. The world is richer for the activities of Alfred Spring Evans, and we will all be better scientists and humanitarians because of his contributions.

The contents of this book were written by experts in the specific topics of each chapter, many of whom Al knew personally. Al reviewed more than half of the chapters for this third edition prior to his death. The quality of the chapters reflects the multiple contributions that Alfred Spring Evans made to each of our professional lives.

Contents

II. Acute Bacterial Infections

Chapter 6

Botulism

Frederick J. Angulo and Michael E. St. Louis

Chapter 7

Brucellosis

Edward J. Young and Wendell H. Hall

Chapter 8

***Campylobacter* Infections**

Ban Mishu Allos and David N. Taylor

PART I

Introduction and Concepts

Introduction

Philip S. Brachman

As Alfred S. Evans and Harry A. Feldman indicated in the preface to the first edition of *Bacterial Infections of Humans: Epidemiology and Control*, the aim of the text was to bridge "the gap between texts on basic microbiology and those on clinical infectious diseases. . . ." The purpose of the text was and remains to discuss "the pathogenesis of infection and disease both within the community and within the individual." This is done in the context "that a variety of factors in both the external and internal environment, and in the nature of the infectious agent, influence exposure, the development of infection, and the pattern of host response. An understanding of the epidemiology and pathogenesis of these processes forms the basis for approaches to control and prevention."

The format for the third edition has not changed from the previous editions. All of the chapters have been updated by the authors, and new chapters—"The Epidemiology of Bacterial Resistance to Antimicrobial Agents," "*Clostridium difficile*," and "*Helicobacter pylori*"—have been added. Each of the chapters has been organized following the same outline. The first three chapters discuss general concepts, and the remaining chapters in alphabetical order discuss specific infections or clinical syndromes. There may be some overlap and repetitious discussions, but this serves to make each chapter independent of other chapters. Additionally, there are some bacterial infections that are not discussed in this edition due to their very recent emergence to prominence. There are a number of excellent textbooks on infectious diseases to which the reader can refer concerning these infections.

As in the previous edition, we are including summaries of each chapter that review the advances in our knowledge concerning the particular topic or disease since the second edition. Additionally, the three new chapters are reviewed.

Philip S. Brachman • The Rollins School of Public Health of Emory University, Atlanta, Georgia 30322.

I. Introduction and Concepts

Chapter 1: Epidemiological concepts. This introductory chapter has been updated and new data and ideas have been incorporated. The section on immune response has been rewritten.

Chapter 2: Public Health Surveillance. This chapter has been revised and updated, with new examples provided. New technology supporting public health surveillance is discussed, such as the use of the computer and the improved methods of laboratory identification including molecular tools and new serological tests. New special surveillance programs are discussed such as for emerging–reemerging infections.

Chapter 3: The epidemiology of bacterial resistance to antimicrobial agents. Many new mechanisms of resistance have been described in bacteria during the last 4–5 years. These include novel mechanisms of vancomycin resistance in enterococci, cefotaxime and ceftriaxone resistance in pneumococci, fluoroquinolone resistance in *Neisseria gonorrhoeae*, and extended-spectrum β-lactam resistance in *Klebsiella pnemoniae*, to name a few examples. In some cases, such as the emergence of β-lactamase-producing enterococci, the resistance mechanism is not new but rather represents the spread of a well-known resistance gene, one previously recognized in staphylococci, to a new host. The genetic mechanisms that allow organisms to increase their complement of resistance genes has also expanded with the recognition of integrons. These genetic elements serve as a backbone into which resistance gene "cassettes" can insert with relative ease. Plasmids and transposons continue to allow the movement of multiple resistance genes among unrelated organisms as widespread antimicrobial use in humans, animals, fish, and plants provides a selective environment that encourages the development and spread of resistant microorganisms.

II. Acute Bacterial Infections

Chapter 4: Anthrax. A proven human case of anthrax has not been reported in the United States since 1988. However, cases continue to be reported from other countries. An epidemic of inhalation anthrax was reported from Russia related to a biological warfare research laboratory. Newer methods of identification of the organism include antigen and toxin assays and use of polymerase chain reaction technology and DNA probes. Some new data are presented related to the aerosolized dose for inhalation anthrax and immunity in humans.

Chapter 5: Bacterial foodborne disease. Reports over the last 5 years have solidified our understanding of the epidemiology of foodborne *Staphylococcus aureus*, *Bacillus cereus*, and *Clostridium perfringens*. Methods for detecting these organisms and their toxins have improved with the development of polymerase chain reaction (PCR) technology and more discriminatory subtyping methods. Because outbreaks due to *Vibrio parahaemolyticus* have continued to be rare in the United States and Europe, we have chosen to place greater emphasis in this edition on other pathogenic vibrios such as *V. vulnificus* and non-epidemic *V. cholerae*. We have also included sections on two related genera, *Aeromonas* and *Plesiomonas*, which, despite lingering doubts as to their roles as pathogens, have attracted increasing interest among public health experts.

Chapter 6: Botulism. Although botulism continues to be a rare disease in the United States, patients with botulism often require intensive care and prolonged hospitalization. Most cases of foodborne botulism are still caused by consumption of home-canned foods; however, active surveillance is necessary to provide early warning of commercial products containing botulism neurotoxin. Recent outbreaks caused by cheese sauce and potato chip dip illustrate the potential for foods other than home-canned foods to cause serious illness.

Chapter 7: Brucellosis. Although the number of cases of human brucellosis in the United States remains around 100 per year, less than 50% were actually reported to the Centers for Disease Control and Prevention (CDC) in 1990–1991. In addition, the epidemiology of brucellosis in states bordering Mexico has shifted in recent years. Previously, the majority of cases occurred in Caucasian men engaged in the livestock industry and the principal mechanism of transmission was direct exposure to infected animals. Currently, cases occur primarily in Hispanics of both sexes, with the vehicle of transmission being ingestion of unpasteurized goat's milk cheese. The role of wild animals in the epidemiology of brucellosis in domestic animals remains controversial. Nevertheless, *Brucella suis* infection in feral swine is emerging as a threat to human health, especially among hunters who may be unaware of the risk of contracting the disease.

Advances in microbiological techniques have resulted in an improved ability to isolate brucellae from clinical specimens. Rapid isolation techniques, including lysis concentration, can shorten the time of recovery of brucellae from weeks to days. Current studies include the use of the PCR in identifying brucellae. Caution is advised in the use of some rapid identification systems, since not all have the profiles to detect *Brucella*. Advances in nucleotide sequencing and hybridization have provided evidence that the genus *Brucella* is in fact a single species. Nevertheless, the traditional classification based on preferred animal hosts remains useful for epidemiological and clinical purposes.

Although the serum agglutination test (SAT) and 2-mercaptoethanol (2ME) agglutination remain the standards against which other serological tests are compared, the *Brucella* enzyme immunosorbent assay (ELISA) shows promise to be a more sensitive test for antibodies.

Chapter 8: *Campylobacter* infections. Campylobacters remain one of the most commonly recognized bacterial causes of diarrhea worldwide. Although diarrheal illnesses resulting from *Campylobacter* infections produce substantial morbidity and mortality, there is increasing appreciation of the impact of later sequelae of infection such as Guillain–Barré syndrome (GBS). GBS is a demyelinating disease of peripheral nerves that results in ascending paralysis and can lead to respiratory muscle compromise and death. *Campylobacter jejuni* infections may trigger GBS; indeed, as many as 40% of GBS cases are preceded by *C. jejuni* infection. Furthermore, *C. jejuni*-associated GBS may be more severe with a greater likelihood of irreversible neurologic deficits.

The use of antibiotic-free filtration techniques for isolating campylobacters from stools has implicated increasing numbers of "atypical" or unusual *Campylobacter* species as human pathogens. These organisms are most frequently identified in immunocompromised persons. Because of the more serious consequences that *Campylobacter* infections pose in persons with HIV/AIDS or other immune deficiency states, these people should be cautioned against eating or drinking foods that are known to carry a high probability of being contaminated with campylobacters. Newer antimicrobial agents initially believed to be useful in treatment of campylobacters (e.g., fluoroquinolones) are now ineffective against many campylobacters that have quickly become resistant to these agents. Thus, erythromycin remains the treatment of choice when antibiotic therapy is indicated in *Campylobacter* infections.

Chapter 9: Chancroid. In the past decade, immigration, illegal drug use (principally crack cocaine), and the HIV epidemic have brought unprecedented interest to chancroid. Previously a disease of low incidence in industrialized countries, immigration from the developing world, where chancroid is common, brought infected individuals into scattered locations; prostitution (particularly in the United States, fueled by illegal drugs) created small epidemics. In the industrialized world chancroid has been associated with enhanced transmission of HIV, and in the developing world chancroid plays an important role in the spread of HIV infection. As a result of the burgeoning interest in chancroid, new diagnostic and serological tests have been developed and the control of chancroid has become of vital interest.

Chapter 10: Chlamydial infections. The emergence of *Chlamydia pneumoniae* as an important human pathogen has been striking. From initial observations associating the organism with mild pneumonia, information has developed showing the organism causes a broad variety of respiratory tract diseases. *C. pneumoniae* is clearly one of the more common and important pathogens, as serological studies find a worldwide distribution with seroprevalence rates as high as 60% or more in most countries that have been studied. Recent studies have shown an association of this infection with coronary artery disease, with the organism being demonstrated in the lesions. Much research is focused on elucidating the role of this infection in the disease because chlamydial infections are treatable.

Major advances in *C. trachomatis* include the introduction of single-dose therapy (1 g oral azithromycin), which is more than 95% effective in curing uncomplicated lower genital tract infections. This development, together with the introduction of highly sensitive and specific diagnostic tests based on amplified DNA technology (ligase chain reaction, PCR), promises to provide tools that could be the basis of effective public health programs to control what is our most common and most costly bacterial sexually transmitted disease. That urine specimens can be used with these tests means noninvasive screening tests are added to the tools available to the public health establishment.

Chapter 11: Cholera. Cholera has increased in incidence and in geographic spread in the last decade. The 7th pandemic, which began in 1961, continues unabated in Asia and Africa and, since 1991, in Latin America. In 1993, more countries reported cholera to the World Health Organization (WHO) than ever before. A new strain of *Vibrio cholerae*, serotype 0139 Bengal, appeared in India in 1992, and since has spread through much of Asia, causing new epidemics among populations that had already experienced the 7th pandemic. As has been the case historically for cholera, the most affected countries are those in the mid-Industrial Revolution. Steady progress in improving rehydration treatment has decreased the case-fatality rate, but prevention lags behind. Although there has been considerable progress, no vaccine yet provides sufficiently durable and substantial protection to make it useful as a public health tool. Epidemic cholera is transmitted through a number of foodborne and waterborne routes, so that prevention depends on providing disinfected water and on preparing food safely. New and simple technologies are being tested for disinfecting water and storing it safely at the household level. Cholera continues to be an important stimulus to bring the "sanitary revolution" to the developing world.

Chapter 12: *Clostridium difficile*. *C. difficile* is the etiologic agent of *C. difficile*-associated diarrhea (CDAD) and pseudomembranous colitis (PMC) and is the most frequently identified cause of nosocomial diarrhea. *C. difficile* is unique in its propensity to cause disease only in animals or humans who have received antimicrobial or antineoplastic treatment. Diagnosis of CDAD is made in patients with diarrhea by detection of *C. difficile* cytotoxin (toxin B) or enterotoxin (toxin A) in stool, by culture of a toxigenic strain of *C. difficile* from stool, or by visualization of pseudomembranes in the colon at endoscopy. Epidemiologically the organism is a spore former and is known to contaminate the environment, inanimate objects, and hands of hospital personnel. Asymptomatic colonization with *C. difficile* is frequent in hospitalized patients and may serve as a reservoir for transmission. Most effective control measures have been barrier precautions, particularly use of gloves in handling body substances, use of disposable devices such as rectal thermometers, and restriction of use of certain antimicrobial agents such as clindamycin. Control of outbreaks in institutions has been frustratingly difficult and reports of hospital infections continue to increase despite utilization of known control measures.

Chapter 13: Diphtheria. In most of the world, the incidence of diphtheria has fallen to low levels as a result of widespread immunization with diphtheria toxoid. In most industrialized countries, it appears that toxigenic strains of *Corynebacterium diphtheriae* have been virtually eliminated. However, whereas in the prevaccine era most adults were immune to diphtheria because of natural exposure to the organism, currently up to 50% or more of adults in developed countries lack protective levels of diphtheria antitoxin. If these low levels of population immunity are not improved, there is potential for diphtheria to reemerge as a public health problem in countries where it has been well controlled for decades. This danger has been illustrated by a rapidly expanding epidemic of diphtheria that began in Russia in 1990, and by late 1995, it had spread to all 15 New Independent States of the former Soviet Union. In 1994, over 47,000 cases and 1,700 deaths from diphtheria were reported from the New Independent States. As with other recently reported outbreaks, a majority of cases have been among persons aged 15 years or older. In addition to continuing to strive to achieve high levels of immunization coverage among children, more attention to maintaining adult immunity by regular booster doses of diphtheria toxoid is needed.

Chapter 14: *Escherichia coli* diarrhea. Since the last edition, additional studies of diarrheagenic *E. coli* have been carried out. Molecular biological techniques have been more routinely employed for detection of diarrheagenic *E. coli* strains. Several new colonization factor antigens important in the adherence of enterotoxigenic *E. coli* strains to the small intestine have been described. An oral cholera vaccine has been evaluated for prevention of enterotoxigenic *E. coli* diarrhea. The genetics of adherence of enteropathogenic *E. coli* have been further clarified. Better description of enterohemorrhagic *E. coli* strains have allowed development of routine screening tests and transmission of this organism based on recently described outbreaks is now better understood.

Chapter 15: Gonococcal infections. The 1990s have witnessed a surge in our understanding of the gonococcus. Novel epidemiological models, such as the core group hypothesis, have allowed public health authorities to better utilize scarce resources. Basic science has helped clarify gonococcal virulence factors and the host response to infection. New diagnostic techniques, such as the PCR, have been added to the traditional techniques of Gram's stain and culture. Most recently, the complex interaction of HIV and *N. gonorrhoeae* has been partially elucidated.

Despite these advances, the incidence of infection remains high in selected populations, particularly the urban poor. The development of drug resistance has posed a major new threat to effective patient care. The success of future control measures will require a concerted effort on the part of primary health care providers and public health authorities.

Chapter 16: *Haemophilus influenzae*. Since the last edition, we have seen the virtual elimination of invasive *H. influenzae* type b (Hib) disease in the United States and in most developed countries. This is a major public health triumph of immunization, although it is not widely appreciated. Since 1991, the decline of Hib disease is a consequence of the routine immunization of infants with Hib conjugate vaccines. Prior to 1990, an estimated 25,000 persons developed invasive Hib disease (bacteremia and meningitis) each year in the United States, and it was estimated that the cumulative incidence of disease was one episode in every 200 children during the first 5 years of life. In populations adopting universal Hib immunization, there has been a greater than a 95% decrease in disease incidence.

A second change since the last edition has been the realization that Hib is an important cause of morbidity and mortality worldwide. In areas of Africa, Oceania, and South America, *H. influenzae* appears to rank as the leading cause of bacterial meningitis. Reported rates of Hib meningitis in children from the Gambia are comparable to those seen in the United States during the prevaccine era. In the Gambia, Hib was also shown to be a leading cause of serious pneumonias, and the use of Hib vaccine significantly reduced this morbidity and mortality. Pneumonia caused by *H. influenzae* has been shown to be a significant cause of childhood morbidity and mortality in several developing countries. Therefore, the next decade should bring increased use of Hib conjugate vaccines worldwide with a consequent decrease in the global burden of meningitis, sepsis, pneumonia, septic arthritis, and epiglottitis, as well as a savings in health care expenditures.

Another important trend since the last edition has been the increasing prevalence of antibiotic resistance. Resistance to a wide variety of antibiotics has been described. Of greatest importance is resistance to ampicillin, as this drug has been the primary antibiotic used for therapy of invasive Hib disease. Since 1970, ampicillin resistance has become widespread, ranging between 5 and 50% of isolates in various parts of the world. Although chloramphenicol-resistant strains are rare in the United States, they are increasingly prevalent in some areas of the world, and strains resistant to both ampicillin and chloramphenicol have been reported. Currently, third-generation cephalosporins, in particular ceftriaxone and cefotaxime, are the mainstays of antibiotic therapy for invasive disease. Concerns about the potential for the development of resistance to these highly effective agents further emphasizes the need for means to prevent disease.

Last, the development of polysaccharide vaccines against *S. pneumoniae*, *N. meningitidis*, and group B streptococcus are all based on the Hib conjugate vaccine technology and experience.

Chapter 17: *Helicobacter pylori* infections. *H. pylori* is a corkscrew-shaped, gram-negative bacteria that infects the gastric mucosa of humans. At least half of the world's population is chronically infected. Although the vast majority of these infections are clinically silent, *H. pylori* infection is now recognized as a major cause of peptic ulcer disease. There is also strong evidence linking infection with development of gastric adenocarcinoma and some evidence for an association with gastric lymphoma. Despite numerous studies, the mode of transmission of *H. pylori* remains an area of extensive research.

Chapter 18: Legionellosis. At least 39 species of *Legionella* have now been identified, yet *L. pneumophila* continues to be the most common cause of legionellosis in humans. Understanding the factors associated with virulence, such as expression of the macrophage infectivity potentiator (Mip) gene, is rapidly expanding. A number of methods for subtyping of *Legionella* isolates have been developed and the benefits and limitations of subtyping data in epidemiological investigations are discussed. Recent data on the incidence of legionellosis among patients with community-acquired pneumonia indicate that less than 5% of cases that occur are diagnosed and reported to public health officials. Although outbreaks of Legionnaires' disease receive much attention in the media, most cases are sporadic (i.e., not occurring as part of an epidemic). The underrecognition of nosocomial cases and infection acquired during travel is stressed. Cooling towers and potable water systems continue to be recognized as sources of the organism in outbreaks, but other aerosol-producing devices, such as a supermarket mister, a decorative fountain, and a whirlpool on a cruise ship, have been recently reported. The difficulty of diagnosing legionellosis on the basis of clinical findings and the importance of laboratory diagnosis are emphasized. Maintaining water systems at temperatures that do not favor growth of *Legionella*, use of appropriate biocides, and engineering practices that diminish aerosol production and transmission are the foundation of prevention.

Chapter 19: Leprosy. A number of major advances have occurred in leprosy. The WHO's short-term therapy has proven to be highly successful and this has led to a WHO-sponsored campaign to eliminate leprosy as a public health problem by the year 2000 (prevalence $<$ 1/10,000). As a result, prevalence of the disease has dramatically fallen and control improved nearly everywhere. Methods for rapid drug screening for activity against *Mycobacterium leprae* have been developed. These and other efforts have resulted in several new drugs that are strongly bactericidal for the bacillus, increasing the possibility of shortening therapy still further. New techniques such as PCR offer the hope of improved early diagnosis of the disease and better epidemiological studies and recent trials have demonstrated that BCG offers significant protection against all types of leprosy. We now clearly have the technology to fully control leprosy if not eliminate it.

Chapter 20: Leptospirosis. Formal acceptance of genetic taxonomy has led to the recognition of several genospecies in the genus *Leptospira*. Some serovars are classified in more than one species. Major advances in molecular understanding of leptospires include description of the genome and its unique organization and cloning of heat-shock protein and the *rfb* gene of the surface lipopolysaccharide antigens. Increasingly, PCR is being applied to direct diagnosis on specimens, as well as to identification of isolated strains, with the aid of batteries of monoclonal antibodies to facilitate and simplify serological classification. Waterborne epidemics, especially in children in various parts of the United States, emphasize dangers of jumping into and swimming in natural fresh water pools. Genital carriage and transmission is important in some domesticated animals that are sources of infection for humans.

Chapter 21: *Listeria monocytogenes* infections. Although not a common opportunistic infection among patients infected with HIV, listeriosis has recently been shown to be at least 100 times as frequent in AIDS patients than in the general population. Over the past decade, there has been nearly a 50% reduction in listeriosis infection and death with statistically significant decreases in both nonperinatal and perinatal disease. It is likely that multi-faceted prevention efforts by industry, food regulatory agencies, public health efforts, and from the widely disseminated consumer guidelines have been responsible for this decline.

Though not of assistance to the clinician faced with a patient with febrile gastroenteritis, the investigation of recent epidemics have shown promise in the use of a serological test for antilisteriolysin O to assist in clarifying such an epidemic and to help in further defining the epidemiology of this infection. Because of concern of *Listeria* contamination in the food industry, a variety of rapid diagnostic techniques have been developed for its detection in food and environmental samples. These have included DNA probes based on the listeriolysin O gene sequence or species-specific rDNA sequences, monoclonal antibodies to cell surface antigens and PCR. Since just three principal serotypes cause most human disease, this subtyping system has been of limited use in epidemic investigations and stimulated the development of more discriminatory subtyping techniques, including multilocus enzyme electrophoresis, restriction fragment-length polymorphism (RFLP), ribosomal DNA fingerprinting (ribotyping), and PCR-based randomly amplified polymorphic DNA (RAPD) patterns.

The investigations of epidemics of invasive listeriosis have regularly identified a variety of contaminated food products as the source of infection; however, recent investigations of point-source foodborne epidemics has convincingly documented that such an exposure can cause a typical syndrome of gastroenteritis with fever occasionally accompanied by vomiting, nausea, and abdominal pain, indistinguishable from other common forms of food poisoning. Importantly, such an illness may be the prodrome of a more severe invasive infection, especially in groups known to develop the invasive forms of this infection marked by sepsis and meningitis.

Sterile-site cultures remain the gold standard for diagnosis of invasive infection, but with the recent description of listeria gastroenteritis, stool cultures that specify the search for *Listeria monocytogenes* may be of value if there is suspicion of this organism. However, routine stool culture medium in most clinical microbiology laboratories will not isolate this organism.

Chapter 22: Lyme disease. Lyme disease, caused by the spirochete *Borrelia borgdorferi*, is considered the most common tick-borne disease in the United States. Cases have been reported from 44 states and at least 21 countries on four continents. Current findings suggest that *B. borgdorferi* spirochetes can sequester themselves in selected anatomical sites and persist for years in host tissue. The persistence of spirochetes now appears to be the most likely mechanism for pathogenesis of acute and chronic manifestations of Lyme disease. Improvements have recently been made in the diagnosis of Lyme disease. Currently, two-step serological testing is recommended, with the use of an initial sensitive screening assay [such as enzyme immunoassay (EIA) or indirect fluorescent antibody (IFA)] followed by a confirmatory test such as the Western immunoblot. Consistent application of this process will improve standardization of laboratory diagnosis. Polymerase-chain-reaction-based tests have also been developed and may become standardized in the future for use in reference laboratories. A vaccine against the outer-surface protein A (OspA) has been found to be safe and immunogenic in humans. Phase 2 and 3 safety studies and trials are now underway. A human vaccine against Lyme disease may be available in the future.

Chapter 23: Meningococcal infections. New reports of unusual transmissions have added to our knowledge of the epidemiology of meningococcal infections. Epidemics in classrooms and laboratory-associated infections have been reported in the past few years. Refinements in typing of meningococci have allowed investigators to follow the transmission of unique strains from person-to-person and to trace the origins of strains responsible for large epidemics in different countries. Spread of organisms from the Indian subcontinent to Arab countries to Africa have been reported. While susceptibility to meningococcal infections had previously been traced to a deficiency of the terminal components of the complement cascade, newer studies have shown that a substantial proportion of adults with sporadic meningococal infections have such deficiencies and screening laboratory tests for such individuals has been advocated. Finally, occasional strains of meningococcal resistant to penicillin have been reported. It will be important to monitor laboratory reports in future years to see if this is to become a major worldwide problem as it has been with pneumococci.

Chapter 24: *Mycoplasma pneumoniae* and other human mycoplasmas. Improved methods for detecting mycoplasmas, especially the PCR, have led to the detection of *M. pneumoniae* and *M. hominis* at extrapulmonary and extragenital sites, respectively. Using PCR, *M. pneumoniae* may be isolated for a longer period after illness than with conventional culture methods.

The many reports of finding *M. pneumoniae* in cerebrospinal fluid in patients with various neurological syndromes suggest that *M. pneumoniae* is an important agent in neurological disease, especially in children. *M. hominis* infections in various peripheral sites have occurred in immunosuppressed patients and after transplantation. The susceptibility of antibody-deficient patients to *M. pneumoniae* infection has been further elucidated. Vaccine development for *M. pneumoniae* has taken new avenues and studies in chimpanzees suggest that immunization for this infection may be feasible.

Newer macrolides and quinolones may be more effective in treatment of *M. pneumoniae* infection than the older antibiotics, but properly conduced randomized trials of such antibiotics are lacking.

Chapter 25: Nosocomial bacterial infections. Recent changes in health care delivery have produced a shift in practice patterns. Many patients who previously received care in the acute-care setting now receive care in outpatient, long-term care and rehabilitation facilities. Methods for surveillance, prevention, and control of nosocomial bacterial infections need to be developed and applied in these settings just as they have been in the acute-care setting. Over the past decade, hospitals have been admitting more high-risk and immunosuppressed patients.

They have also had to care for more patients with resistant microorganisms, some of which are untreatable with currently available antibiotics, and they have been challenged to control the spread of these organisms to other high-risk immunosuppressed patients.

The CDC recommended a new isolation system in 1996, which is expected to simplify and improve the efficacy of isolation precautions. Recommendations for the prevention and control of spread of vancomycin resistance have been published separately. In addition, new guidelines for the prevention of intravascular device-related infections (1996) and prevention of nosocomial pneumonia (1994) have been published. These guidelines were developed for use by acute-care hospitals and will need to be evaluated for their applicability to other settings.

Chapter 26: Pertussis. Several new developments in the epidemiology and control of pertussis are discussed. From the epidemiological standpoint, these include the apparent slight increase in incidence of the disease in the United States and additional evidence that infected adults with waning immunity and mild or unrecognized disease are an important source of transmission. Developments that should enhance control of the disease include better diagnostic methods, both serologically and by use of the PCR, to identify *Bordetella pertussis* in respiratory secretions when less sensitive methods such as culture and fluorescent antibody testing fail. Additionally, there has been further progress in understanding the relationships of various components of the organism to infection, disease, and immunity. A major step has been the vindication of pertussis vaccine in relation to most, if not all, allegations of causation of death and neurological disability, thus reassuring providers and the public. Field trials of acellular pertussis vaccines have demonstrated that they are not only less unpleasantly reactive but also display efficacy in infants comparable to that of the whole cell preparation.

Chapter 27: Plague. The worldwide occurrence of plague has continued with little change over the past decade, with a mean of about 1200 cases reported annually to the WHO by approximately 15 countries; significant recent outbreak activity has been reported from Peru, several eastern and southern African states, Madagascar, India, Myanmar, and Vietnam. The reports of concurrent bubonic and pneumonic plague outbreaks in two states in west central India in 1994 and concern about possible spread of the disease to major Indian cities caused international alarm and severe economic repercussions for India. Reference diagnostic laboratory testing capability has been enhanced by the availability of recombinant fraction 1 (F1) antigen, PCR tests to amplify *Yersinia pestis* DNA, and the use of monoclonal antibodies to identify specific *Y. pestis* antigens. Recombinant F1 and V antigens have been found to be experimentally immunoprotective in mice. Computerized geographic information services data and enhanced satellite imagery data permit rapid mapping of the landscape epidemiological features of plague.

Chapter 28: Pneumococcal infections. The most notable change in the behavior of the pneumococcus is the rapid development of resistance to penicillin and other antibiotics. While the problem of resistance was noted previously, it was uncommon and limited geographically. In the past 5 years, resistance has been seen worldwide and resistant strains have been encountered in substantial numbers. The rate of intermediate and high-level resistance may exceed 20%. This has forced clinicians to reevaluate appropriate antibiotic therapy for pneumococcal infections, but the occurrence of multi-antibiotic-resistant strains makes it difficult to find nontoxic single agents that can be used effectively.

There have been a number of recent studies that have focused on populations with exceptional risk for pneumococcal infections. Studies show increased risk in HIV-1-infected individuals, in North Americans, in prison inmates, and children, especially in developing countries.

While the pneumococcal vaccine was first licensed in 1977, this is still an underutilized vaccine. Recent case–control studies have demonstrated the efficacy of this vaccine in the elderly, but immunosuppressed individuals have considerably less protection. New-generation conjugate pneumococcal vaccines are currently in large-scale testing and are likely to provide protection for the very young and possibly increased protection for all high-risk individuals.

Chapter 29: Q fever. The information concerning the skin testing procedure has been revised and the treatment recommendations are updated.

Chapter 30: Rocky Mountain spotted fever. Laboratory confirmatory techniques have improved, with better identification of rickettsial nucleic acids in blood or tissues with PCR, amplification and detection of specific antibody using indirect florescent antibody, and specific ELISA procedures. A new technique for very early diagnosis of Mediterranean spotted fever (similar to Rocky Mountain spotted fever) utilizes antiendothelial cell monoclonal antibodies to attract rickettsia from blood specimens and identification by immunofluorescence.

The specific mechanisms responsible for the rickettsial vasculitis and ultimate clinical manifestations are better understood. An effective Rocky Mountain spotted fever vaccine is not available, but therapy with specific antibiotics is very effective when treatment is initiated before the later stages, when marked vascular alterations have occurred.

Chapter 31: Salmonellosis: Nontyphoidal. The steady increase in salmonellosis since the 1970s has leveled off in the last decade, with approximately 40,000 reported isolates a year. One serotype, *Salmonella* serotype Enteritidis, continues to increase, accounting for 26% of all salmonellosis in 1994. This serotype is widespread in the nation's egg-laying flocks and can contaminate the contents of normal-looking eggs. Specific control measures are being implemented by the industry to detect infected flocks and prevent infection from occurring in the rest. Antimicrobial resistance continues to increase, so that in 1990, 31% of *Salmonella* isolated from humans were resistant to at least one antimicrobial, including ampicillin and gentamicin. The incidence of *Salmonella* bacteremia parallels the AIDS epidemic and represents an important and largely preventable opportunistic infection among persons infected with HIV. Although most salmonellosis comes from foods, a growing number of infections are associated with pet lizards, particularly iguanas. Successful control of salmonellosis is possible. The continuing challenge for public health is to understand the specific routes of transmission well enough to interrupt them.

Chapter 32: Shigellosis. Since the second edition, there has been enormous progress in understanding the basis of virulence in *Shigella* and in identifying both the genes (including those involved in regulation) and gene products involved. Cell invasion is recognized to be an increasingly complex process, involving multiple interactions of the organism and host cell, often usurping host proteins to serve the needs of the organism. The expression of microbial virulence is also regulated in a complex manner by host processes such as phosphorylation. The host inflammatory response, orchestrated by cytokines induced during invasion, clearly participates in pathogenesis as well as host defenses. New enterotoxins have been discovered of, as yet, uncertain relevance, while Shiga toxin, a previously known cytotoxin produced by *S. dysenteriae* 1 and its related family of Shiga-like toxins in *E. coli*, is now clearly implicated in the injury of endothelial cells, leading to the microangiopathic lesions of hemolytic–uremic syndrome. New molecular methods to characterize strains have been developed that will permit improved epidemiological investigations and tracking of isolates. Trends in prevalence of *Shigella* species continue, with diminishing isolations of *S. flexneri* and increasing *S. sonnei* in developed countries and continued dominance of *S. flexneri* along with endemic and sometimes epidemic *S. dysenteriae* 1 in developing countries. Everywhere, increasing antimicrobial resistance has been a problem. Where available, new 4-fluoroquinolones and third-generation cephalosporins remain generally effective.

Chapter 33: Staphylococcal infections. Since the second edition, several major features of staphylococcal disease have taken place: (1) Coagulase-negative staphylococci are increasing in importance. The incidence of disease from coagulase-negative staphylococci seems to parallel technological and biomechanical advances in patient care. In many instances, coagulase-negative staphylococcal disease is because of these advances, such as biosynthetic prostheses, catheters, and shunts. (2) The second new feature of staphylococcal disease is the widespread occurrence of methicillin-resistant *Staphylococcus aureus*. This is now very common in the United States as it is throughout the world. Previously it was present primarily in Europe. (3) A third area of great interest is the identification of the carrier state of *S. aureus* in patients such as those on chronic ambulatory peritoneal dialysis. Carriage of staphylococci in these patients increases the likelihood that they will develop staphylococcal disease. Interventions designed to eradicate the carrier state have led to significant reductions in disease incidence. (4) Another advance or new feature of staphylococcal disease are the newer techniques for identifying strains of both *S. aureus* and coagulase-negative staphylococci. The old phage-typing systems, although still used, are being replaced by molecular techniques that are far more sensitive and superior to phage-typing techniques for determining the similarity between strains and the spread of epidemics. (5) A final feature is the concern that staphylococci, like enterococci, particularly *Enterococcus faecium*, have the potential for becoming resistant to vancomycin. At the time this chapter is written, there are no alternative drugs to vancomycin. If *S. aureus* develops resistance to vancomycin, we will be left with a situation where we have no antibiotics to treat this infection, which is a state similar to the preantibiotic era.

Chapter 34: Streptococcal infections. Major developments since the second edition include changes in the epidemiology, advances in genetics and molecular microbiology, and progress toward new modes of prevention of various streptococcal disease. There has been an apparent increase in the incidence of serious invasive group A streptococcal infections and the emergence of "streptococcal toxic shock" as a distinct clinical entity. There has been a dramatic increase and geographical spread of pneumococci that are resistant to penicillin and other antibiotics. Enterococci resistant to vancomycin have emerged as a significant cause of nosocomial infections. Strategies for prevention of neonatal group B streptococcal infection have evolved from a handful of clinical trials into a set of guidelines for intrapartum antibiotic prophylaxis. Vaccine development now includes pneumococcal polysaccharide–protein conjugates that have proved immunogenic in infants and children. Similar group B streptococcal polysaccharide–protein conjugate vaccines have been successful in animal models. Advances at the molecular level have included complete genome sequencing of representative group A streptococci and pneumococci. Molecular methodologies are being developed for identifying, classifying, and tracking strains and particular clones, further opening the field of "molecular epidemiology" to various streptococcal species.

Chapter 35: Syphilis. At the end of the 20th century, syphilis remains nearly as much of an epidemiological enigma as it did in the early 1900s. Over the last decade, we have seen a resurgence of syphilis among the most disenfranchised heterosexual populations in the United States, fueled by the epidemic of crack cocaine and the exchange of sex for drugs. Rates in southern states and rural areas remain high, despite the availability of primary and secondary prevention programs. Innovative approaches to address the continuing high levels of infectious syphilis are urgently needed. More accessible clinical services, wider population-based partner notification programs, targeted use of prophylactic penicillin treatment, greater community involvement in syphilis control, and improved training of clinicians in the techniques of diagnosing and managing syphilis patients will be necessary to further decrease syphilis levels in the United States.

Chapter 36: Nonvenereal treponematoses. Yaws and endemic syphilis persist in the rural populations of west and central Africa and may be increasing in prevalence as economic conditions in these regions deteriorate. Yaws has shown remarkable resilience on Kar Kar Island in Papua New Guinea where two selective mass penicillin treatment campaigns have failed to prevent new yaws infections. There is little evidence that pathogenic treponemies have acquired resistance to penicillins, and their persistence may have more to do with reinfection within the months following penicillin treatment than with antibiotic resistance.

Chapter 37: Tetanus. Tetanus in the United States continues to be a disease primarily of older adults who are also at highest risk for tetanus mortality. To decrease this remaining tetanus burden, in 1994, the Advisory Committee on Immunization Practices and other advisory committees recommended that for patients aged 50 years and older, health care providers should review adult vaccination status, administer tetanus and diphtheria toxoid as indicated, and determine whether a patient has one or more risk factors that indicate the need to receive pneumococcal and annual influenza vaccination. In developing countries where the major tetanus disease burden continues to be borne by neonates, improvements in maternal vaccination coverage rates have led to decreases in the incidence of neonatal tetanus. However, the tetanus toxoid coverage was still below 50% among pregnant women globally in 1993, and the global target of neonatal tetanus elimination (defined as <1 case per 1000 live births) was not attained in 1995 nor in 1996. The most promising approach toward achievement of neonatal tetanus elimination has been to target additional efforts, including mass vaccination campaigns, to high-risk areas that continue to report cases. This strategy, augmented by the continued efforts to vaccinate an ever-increasing proportion of women of child-bearing age and to train birth attendants to foster clean deliveries, should further decrease the global neonatal tetanus burden and holds the promise of accomplishing neonatal tetanus elimination in the next several years.

Chapter 38: Toxic shock syndrome. Since the second edition, most of the advances in our understanding of toxic shock syndrome (TSS) relate to improved understanding of the biological properties of toxic shock syndrome toxin (TSST-1), which has proven to be an extremely potent and interesting macromolecule. In addition, we now have a better understanding of how tampons and their components influence the production of TSST-1 *in vitro*, with possible implications for how TSS cases, due to *S. aureus* infections at a variety of body sites, continue to occur at a low incidence rate in the United States.

Chapter 39: Tuberculosis. We have seen major changes in tuberculosis since the second edition. At that time, the unprecedented period of no decline in the tuberculosis case rates in the United States from 1984 to 1988 was the only available clue to the resurgence of tuberculosis occurring throughout most of the world. Fueled by increasing numbers of persons at high risk of developing tuberculosis—the HIV infected, refugees, drug addicts, the homeless, and the poor—tuberculosis was helped in its comeback by concomitant decreases in tuberculosis control funds.

Little new information has been learned during this period about the epidemiology of tuberculosis, owing to decreased funds and interest. However, some previously underappreciated factors have been widely recognized. The spreading HIV epidemic has called attention to the fact that immunosuppression causes loss of tuberculin sensitivity, greatly speeds up the progress to disease after infection, and is associated with unusual clinical presentations. At long last, the problems of treatment failure and multidrug resistance have been successfully attacked by greatly increased emphasis on directly observed administration of short-course treatment regimens. Widespread application of this knowledge has been stimulated by the WHO and its proclamation of tuberculosis as the leading infectious killer of adults. Epidemiologists will be challenged to evaluate control programs and to search for new ways in which tuberculosis can be successfully attacked.

Chapter 40: Nontuberculous mycobacterial disease. Major advances have recently been made in the diagnosis, treatment, and prevention of nontuberculous mycobacterial diseases. The use of molecular diagnostic techniques, such as the use of DNA probes for speciation and nucleic acid amplification for identification, now permit rapid diagnosis of infection. With both antiretroviral therapy and improved treatment of opportunistic infections in AIDS patients, disseminated disease due to *Mycobacterium avium* complex (MAC) has become one of the most important causes of HIV-related morbidity and mortality among AIDS patients in North America and Europe. At the same time, the introduction of clarithromycin has significantly improved response to the therapy of MAC disease. Finally, the use of rifabutin chemoprophylaxis has been shown to delay the onset of MAC disease and improve survival of AIDS patients.

Chapter 41: Tularemia. The pathogenesis of tularemic infections has been further defined as new virulence factors of *F. tularemisis* have been identified. Their ability to survive inside cells is aided by the assimilation of iron from the host cell. Other proteins, e.g., molecular chaperones, are induced and these may protect the environment for survival of the bacteria. A new therapeutic advance has been the demonstration of the efficacy of ciprofloxacin in a small series of patients.

Chapter 42: Typhoid fever. The most important event in the area of the epidemiology of typhoid fever has been the spread throughout Asia and northeast Africa of strains of *Salmonella typhi* harboring a plasmid encoding resistance to the three antimicrobial agents (chloramphenicol, trimethoprim–sulfamethoxazole, and amoxicillin) that were the mainstays of oral therapy just a few years ago. Since the control of typhoid fever in developing countries has in large part been the consequence of early antimicrobial therapy based on clinical diagnosis, the inability to treat with these drugs has had important consequences. For example, the frequency of occurrence of cases with complications and fatalities has increased and the cost of treatment has risen notably.

The spread of multiresistant strains of *S. typhi* has invigorated interest in the possible use of typhoid vaccines as interventions to assist in the control of typhoid fever in developing countries. Two well-tolerated vaccines—oral Ty21a and parenteral Vi polysaccharide—are available that are known to be effective in school-age children. However, so far, no developing countries have undertaken school-based immunization programs with Ty21a or Vi parenteral vaccines. Rather, several countries facing this typhoid public health threat have expressed interest in a vaccine that could be administered to infants through the Expanded Programme on Immunization and that would confer long-term immunity through childhood and adolescence. Candidate vaccines that might serve the pursuit of this strategy are in early clinical development. They include Vi–conjugate vaccines and newly engineered strains of *S. typhi*, such as CVC 908-*htrA*, that are given as live oral vaccines.

Chapter 43: *Yersinia enterocolitica* infections. *Y. enterocolitica* encompasses a spectrum of phenotypic variants, of which only a few have been conclusively associated with human or animal disease. During the past decade, there appears to have been a real and generalized increase in incidence. Considerable progress has been made in our understanding of the reservoirs and routes of transmission for *Y. enterocolitica*. There is strong indirect evidence that the swine constitutes an important reservoir for human infection with *Y. enterocolitica* serogroups O:3 and O:9. Two case–control studies of endemic yersiniosis have supported the role of pork as a vehicle for *Y. enterocolitica* infection. Other studies have indicated that *Y. enterocolitica* is more common in pork products than previously documented. Thus, preventive measures that reduce contamination and improve hygiene during all stages of pork processing are essential to reduce infection with serogroups O:3 and O:9. Changes in slaughtering procedures, including technological improvements, may be required to reduce contamination during these activities. Until recently, the most frequently reported serogroups in the United States were O:8 followed by O:5,27. In recent years, serogroup O:3 has been on the increase in this country. It has been suggested that the epidemiology of yersiniosis in the United States has evolved into a pattern similar to the picture in Europe, where serogroup O:3 predominates. Since few laboratories in the United States routinely screen clinical specimens for *Y. enterocolitica*, it is likely to be underdiagnosed and underrecognized by clinicians. Great strides have been made in our understanding, at the molecular level, of the mechanisms by which *Y. enterocolitica* causes disease. One recently explored avenue of investigation relates to the genetic determinants of virulence.

CHAPTER 1

Epidemiological Concepts

Alfred S. Evans†

1. Introduction

Epidemiology is the study of the distribution and determinants of health-related states, conditions, or events in specified populations and the application of the results of this study to the control of health problems.[(1)] It is a quantitative science concerned in infectious diseases with the circumstances under which disease processes occur, the factors that affect their incidence and the host response to the infectious agent, and the use of this knowledge for control and prevention.[(2)] It includes the pathogenesis of disease in both the community and the individual. For infectious diseases, one must study the circumstances under which both *infection* and *disease* occur, for these may be different. Infection is the consequence of an encounter of a potentially pathogenic microorganism with a susceptible human host through an appropriate portal of entry, and usually involves a demonstrable host response to the agent. Exposure is the key factor, and the sources of infection lie mostly outside the individual human host, within the environment, or in other infected hosts. Disease represents one of the possible consequences of infection, and the factors important in its development are mostly intrinsic to the host, although the dosage and virulence of the infecting microbe play a role. These intrinsic factors include the age at the time of infection, the portal of entry, the presence or absence of immunity, the vigor of the primary defense system, the efficiency and nature of humoral and cell-mediated immune responses, the genetic makeup of the host, the state of nutrition, the presence of other diseases, and psychosocial influences. These factors that result in the occurrence of clinical illness among those infected have been called the "clinical illness promotion factors,"[(3)] and many of them remain unknown. The host responses can include death, the classic clinical features of the disease, mild or atypical forms, subclinical and inapparent infections, and the carrier state, which may exist in the absence of a detectable host response. While the clinician is primarily concerned with disease, the epidemiologist is interested in both infection and disease. Infection without disease is a common phenomenon, so that a study limited to clinical illness alone would give an incomplete epidemiological picture and would be a poor basis for control and prevention.[(4)] A full understanding involves the pathogenesis of the process leading to clinical disease both in the community and in the individual.

The concepts of epidemiology in bacterial infections are very similar to those of viral infections as expounded in the companion volume, *Viral Infections of Humans*,[(5)] so there will be overlap and repetition in this volume. Some of the differences between viral and bacterial infection include the intracellular position of all viruses, their smaller size, the requirement of living tissues for viral multiplication, the ease with which many viruses are spread by respiratory routes or by insect vectors, the relatively high order of immunity following viral infection, the usefulness of serological tests for the diagnosis of most viral infections, and the failure of viral infections to respond to antibiotic therapy. Highly sensitive and specific molecular methods are being increasingly employed to define the agent and the host response to it.[(6–8)]

Many concepts and methods of epidemiology apply to both infectious and noninfectious diseases, and there should be no essential dichotomy between the two.[(9)] In general, epidemiology can be regarded as the development, pathogenesis, and expression of infection and disease in a community in much the same way as clinical

Alfred S. Evans • Department of Epidemiology and Public Health, Yale University School of Medicine, New Haven, Connecticut 06510.

†Deceased.

Dr. D. Scott Schmid, National Center for Infectious Diseases, Centers for Disease Control and Prevention, Atlanta, Georgia, assisted in revising Section 10, Immune Response, after Dr. Evans' death.

medicine is concerned with the development, pathogenesis, and expression in the individual. This book will attempt to cover both these aspects. While the "epidemiology of infectious diseases" has disappeared from the curriculum of many schools of medicine and public health in developed countries, the current epidemic of the acquired immunodeficiency syndrome (AIDS) has reawakened interest in the subject. In addition, the emergence of new diseases such as Legionnaires' disease, Lyme disease, the toxic shock syndrome and the development of antibiotic–resistant pneumococci and tubercle bacilli, the appearance of erythrogenic streptococci ("flesh-eating" streptococci) and a new cholera strain termed 0139, foodborne outbreaks of *Escherichia coli* O157:H7, and a large waterborne outbreak of cryptosporidiosis are among the "emerging infections" that continue to pose challenges to epidemiologists[10] and for which the Centers for Disease Control and Prevention (CDC) are developing preventive strategies.[11] It is becoming apparent that in developed countries, the continuing, and in some instances the increasing, importance of infectious diseases is causing concern among public health authorities.

In developing countries, infectious diseases are still a major cause of morbidity and mortality, and efforts are in progress to develop training programs in epidemiology and in surveillance in such areas. The Field Epidemiology Training Program of the CDC is a fine example of this effort. Several recent texts address the problems of surveillance.[12–16]

2. Definitions and Methods

2.1. Definitions

A working understanding of the terms commonly used in epidemiology and infectious diseases may be helpful to the student, microbiologist, and clinician unfamiliar with them. They are derived from those in *A Dictionary of Epidemiology*,[1] *Viral Infections of Humans*,[5] and from the American Public Health Association handbook entitled *Control of Communicable Diseases Manual*.[17]

Attack rate or case ratio: This ratio expresses incidence rates in population groups during specified time periods or under special circumstances such as in an epidemic. It is often expressed as a percent (cases per 100). The *secondary attack rate* is the proportion of persons who develop infection within an appropriate incubation period after exposure to a primary case divided by the number exposed. The groups so exposed are frequently family members or persons located in an institution.

Carrier: A carrier is a person, animal, or arthropod who harbors a specific infectious agent in the absence of clinical illness with or without a detectable immune response. The carrier state may reflect carriage of the organism in the incubation period before clinical symptoms appear, during an apparent or inapparent infection (healthy or asymptomatic carrier), or following recovery from illness; it may be of short or long duration (chronic carrier), and it may be intermittent or continuous. Carriers may spread the infectious agent to others.

Case fatality rate: Number of deaths of a specific disease divided by the number of cases × 100.

Cell-mediated immunity: This term has been used previously to designate immune mechanisms largely dependent on lymphocyte activity and in contrast to "humoral immunity." As T lymphocytes are now recognized as playing an important role in both, the term *T-cell immunity* is being more widely used.

Chemoprophylaxis: Administration of a chemical or antibiotic to prevent infection or to prevent the development of disease in a person already infected.

Colonization: Multiplication of an organism on a body surface (e.g., skin, epithelium, mucus membrane) without evoking a tissue or immune response.

Communicable period: Time during which a person (or animal) is infectious for another person, animal, or arthropod.

Endemic: This term denotes the constant or usual presence of an infection or disease in a community. A high degree of endemicity is termed *hyperendemic*, and one with a particularly high level of infection beginning early in life and affecting most of the population is called *holoendemic*.

Epidemic: An epidemic or outbreak is said to exist when an unusual number of cases of a disease occur in a given time period and geographic area as compared with the previous experience with that disease in that area. For diseases already present in the community, it is necessary to know the number of existing cases (prevalence) as well as new cases (incidence) to determine whether an increase has occurred. The definition of increases or excess cases is arbitrary and will vary from disease to disease. See Section 3 for further discussion.

Host: A person, animal (including birds), or arthropod in which infectious agents subsist or infect under natural conditions. In this book the term will most often refer to the "human host" unless otherwise stated.

Immunity: The specific resistance to an infectious agent resulting from humoral and local antibodies and from cell-mediated responses constitutes immunity. Immunity may be acquired through natural infection, by active immunization, by transfer of immune factors via the placenta, or by passive immunization with antibodies from another person or animal. The immune state is relative and not absolute, is governed largely through genetic control, and may be altered by disease- or drug-induced immunosuppression.

Immunodeficiency: A state representing impairment of the immune system of the host that affects its ability to respond to a foreign antigen. This may result from an inherited defect, or an acquired one such as a result of the disease itself, or of immunosuppressive drugs or an infectious agent that depresses the immune system. The human immunodeficiency viruses (HIV-1 and HIV-2) are the major examples of the latter.

Incidence rate: The number of new events (specific infection or disease) occurring in a given time period in a given population as the numerator and the number of susceptible persons in that population exposed to the agent as the denominator. This is usually stated as cases (or infections) per 100, 1000, or 100,000. This rate may be adjusted for an age- or sex-specific numerator and denominator or any other characteristic of interest. Laboratory procedures may be required for numerator data on new infections, as measured by isolation of the agent or by antibody rises, or by both. They may also be required to identify those actually at risk in the denominator, i.e., those lacking antibody; other means of refining the denominator would be by eliminating adults in calculating rates of childhood diseases or eliminating those with a valid history of having had the disease.

Incubation period: The incubation period is the interval between exposure and the appearance of the first detectable sign or symptom of the illness. Ill-defined exposure to a source of infection or exposure to persons without apparent illness may obscure the starting point of the incubation period, and vague, premonitory, or prodromal signs of illness may obscure its termination point. The best estimate is often derived from single exposures of short duration to a clinical case or established source of infection (e.g., air, food, water, arthropod vector) and the development of the first characteristic or classic features of the disease. Experimental infections in volunteers give well-defined incubation periods, but these may not always be the same as under natural conditions. See Section 7 for further discussion.

Index case: This is the index or primary case of an illness in a family, group, institution, or community that may serve as a source of infection to others.

Infection: Infection represents the deposition, colonization, and multiplication of a microorganism in a host and is usually accompanied by an immune response. Infection may occur with or without clinical illness.

Isolation: This is a term applied to the separation of infected persons in such places and/or under such conditions as to prevent contact or airborne transmission of the infectious agent to others during the period of communicability. Infection control practice in hospitals as recommended by the CDC has divided isolation into two tiers of isolation precautions. The first tier is known as *standard precautions* and the second tier are *transmission-based precautions*. Hand washing remains a prime preventive measure in regards to nosocomial infections.

Morbidity rate: An incidence rate in which the numerator includes all persons clinically ill in a defined time and population and the denominator is the population involved or a subunit thereof, usually expressed as the number of cases per 100,000 persons at risk.

Mortality rate: The same as morbidity rate except the numerator consists of deaths. This may be the total number of deaths in a population group (crude mortality rate, usually expressed as deaths per 1000) or deaths from a specific disease (disease-specific mortality, usually expressed as deaths per 100,000).

Nosocomial infections: This term refers to infections that develop after entry into a hospital or other health care institution and that are not present or incubating at the time of admission or the residual of an infection acquired during a previous admission.

Pathogenicity: The ability of an infectious agent to produce disease in a susceptible host. Some nonpathogenic agents can become pathogenic in an immunocompromised host such as persons infected with HIV.

Prevalence rate: The ratio of the number of persons in a defined population who are affected with the disease at any one time as the numerator and the exposed population at that point as the denominator. If this is based on the frequency of cases at a moment in time, then the term *point prevalence* is used. If it reflects the proportion of persons affected over a longer period, then the term *period prevalence* is employed. Most infectious diseases are acute and short-lived, so that prevalence rates are not commonly used. The use of prevalence rates is more relevant to more protracted illnesses such as subacute bacterial endocarditis, tuberculosis, and leprosy, or to reflect carrier states that may persist for months or years. Prevalence rates reflect incidence times duration of disease. In seroepidemiological usage, the term *prevalence* denotes the presence of antigen, antibody, or another component in the blood.

Quarantine: The restriction of persons or animals exposed to an infected source during the incubation period for that disease to observe if the disease develops in order that other persons will not be exposed to the infectious agent during that period.

Reservoir: A person, animal, soil, or other environment in which an infectious agent normally exists and multiplies and which can be a source of infection to other hosts.

Surveillance: As concerns public health, surveillance is the systematic collection of data pertaining to the occurrences of specific diseases or health-related conditions, the analysis and interpretation of these data, and the dissemination of consolidated and processed information to contributors to the program and other interested persons for purposes of control and/or prevention (see Chapter 2 for detailed discussion and Cutts *et al.*[12] for a World Health Organization definition, as used in the Expanded Programme in Immunization). *Serological surveillance* is the identification of current and past infection through measurement of antibody or of antigen in serum from representative samples of the population or other target groups.

Susceptibility: A state in which a person or animal is capable of being infected with a microorganism. The lack of specific protective antibody usually indicates susceptibility to that agent, although reactivation or reinfection to some agents may occur in the presence of antibody.

Transmission: The mechanism by which an infectious agent is spread to another host (see Section 5).

Virulence: A measure of the degree of pathogenicity of an infectious agent as reflected by the severity of the disease produced and its ability to invade the tissues of the host.

Zoonosis: An infection or infectious disease transmissible under natural conditions from animals to man. It may be *endemic* (enzootic) or *epidemic* (epizootic).

2.2. Methods

Epidemiology can be divided into descriptive, analytical, experimental, and serological epidemiology. The major analytic methods in use are the cohort (prospective) and case–control (retrospective). This section will briefly present these concepts. For more detailed descriptions, textbooks and recent articles of epidemiology are recommended.[18–21] A textbook on epidemiological methods that includes discussion and examples in infectious disease[18] is recommended before undertaking an epidemiological study. An excellent brief book on all aspects of epidemiological studies has been published by the World Health Organization (WHO).[22]

2.2.1. Types of Epidemiological Studies. Epidemiological studies may be descriptive or analytical. Descriptive studies are based on available data sources and describe the patterns of disease in population groups according to time, place, and person factors. Epidemic investigations begin with a descriptive study. These data often suggest clues to the etiology of the condition or to the risk factors involved. Analytical studies are then designed to test the hypotheses of causation developed from the descriptive studies and usually require new data to do so. Three common analytical methods are employed in pursuing epidemiological studies.

2.2.1a. Cohort Study. This is the most definitive and expensive type of study and is based on identifying a group or groups of persons (cohorts) who are followed over time for the development of disease (or infection) in the presence or absence of suspected risk factors that are measured at the start of the study. These studies are usually carried out by identifying a cohort or usually two or more cohorts at the present time and then following them longitudinally over time. One cohort will be the group exposed to a risk factor or there may be several cohorts, each with a different degree of exposure. There usually is another cohort of unexposed persons who are followed in the same way. The cohorts are followed until the effect of the exposure occurs or the study is terminated for another reasons. If the occurrence of disease is the expected outcome, persons immune to the disease at the beginning of the study would not be included in a study cohort. This has been called a *prospective cohort study* or simply a *prospective study*. In infectious disease epidemiology, it may be possible to identify the persons in the cohort who are susceptible or immune at the start of the study by measuring the presence or absence of antibody in the initial serum specimens. Serial serum samples are then taken in which the appearance of antibody indicates the approximate time at which infection occurs. The occurrence of clinical disease at the same time provides information of the clinical–subclinical ratio. If the appropriate serum samples are taken and frozen, the actual testing can be delayed to the end of the study.

An alternative method of conducting a cohort study is to identify a group of persons at some time in the past who were presumably free of the disease under investigation at that time, as indicated by examining existing records. The cohort is then followed to the present, or even beyond, by measuring the occurrence of infection (by serological tests) or disease in that defined population. This approach is called a *historical cohort study* or a *retrospective cohort study*. Because the case–control study is also retrospective in terms of the time when the observations are made, it must be distinguished from the historical cohort study.

In a cohort study the statistical methods involve the calculation of the relative risk of the prevalence in the ill individuals as compared with the controls. This can be

Table 1. Matrix for Calculating Relative Risk Ratios

Characteristic or factor	Number of persons		
	With disease	Without disease	Total
Present	a	b	$a + b$
Absent	c	d	$c + d$
Total	$a + c$	$b + d$	

calculated using the format of a fourfold matrix as depicted in Table 1. If the frequency, $a/a + b$, of the characteristic in persons with the disease (a) in this total group ($a + b$) is statistically significantly greater than the frequency of the characteristic in those without the disease ($c/c + d$), then an association may exist between the characteristic and the disease. For further details of the mathematical and epidemiological techniques and the biases involved in the selection of cases and controls, readers are referred to recent texts such as *Methods in Observational Epidemiology*.[18]

2.2.1b. Case–Control Study. This has been called a retrospective study because it studies persons already ill with the disease and compares their characteristics with a control group without the disease for the presence or absence of certain possible risk factors. When a significant difference in the prevalence of a characteristic or risk factor is found, then the possibility of a causal association is suspected. Further studies using the cohort method are then often carried out to add strength to the association. The case–control study is usually the first type made because it is based on existing data, can be completed in a relatively short time, and is the least expensive. However, it cannot define the true incidence of the disease in relation to the various factors because the denominator at risk is not known.

A variation of the case–control study, and one encompassing the concept of a cohort study, is termed the *nested case–control study*. In this a large cohort is studied either prospectively or retrospectively for the occurrence of a specific disease, then these cases are matched by age and sex with persons in the original cohort who did not develop the disease. Various attributes of the two groups defined at the start of the study can then be compared. This method is very useful for diseases or conditions of low frequency in which analysis of the entire cohort would be an overwhelming task. An example of this is a recent study of Hodgkin's disease in relation to elevated levels of antibody to Epstein–Barr virus (EBV).[23] In this analysis, 240,000 persons whose sera had been collected and stored in four serum banks were followed for 5 years through cancer registries or hospital records for the development of Hodgkin's disease. Forty-three cases were identified in this manner and the EBV and other antibody levels were determined in sera from the group and compared with results from matched controls bled at the same time. A significant increase in certain EBV antibodies over those of controls were found 3–5 year preceding the diagnosis of Hodgkin's disease.

Biases may occur in case–control studies in the selection of cases, in the selection of controls, and in the elucidation of data by interview or records concerning the characteristics in question in both cases and controls. The selection of cases should ensure that they are representative of all patients with that disease. Ideally, this would assume that all patients with the disease seek medical attention, that the correct diagnosis is made and substantiated, that all medical facilities are canvassed, and that all cases are detected. In practice, these criteria are seldom met, and patients, for example, from a single hospital may be the only ones studied. This introduces a bias, since certain patients may be excluded from a given hospital because of such factors as age (e.g., no pediatric wards), socioeconomic level, or military or civilian status; the patient or physician may select a given hospital because of nearness, religious affiliation, the physician's privileges, nature of payment, or other considerations. These patients are not representative of all patients with the disease. The presence or absence of the characteristic under study may also influence the selection process for either the case or the control group or both, giving spurious associations.

Biases also are common in the selection of controls. Usually, controls should be selected from the same population group from which the patients are drawn and should be closely comparable to the cases in all known characteristics (age, sex, socioeconomic level, ethnic groups) except the one under study. Random selection from a large group may equalize those differences, but usually groups matched for certain variables or individuals matched carefully for paired comparisons are selected. However, if the two groups are matched too closely, the association between the cause and its effect may be masked. In a hospital setting, ill patients with diseases other than those under study are sometimes chosen. Bias may occur if some of these patients have diseases that are influenced by the characteristic in question. To limit this, patients with noninfectious diseases are often chosen in an infectious disease study. In a community setting, healthy controls may be advantageous. In matching, only those variables known to affect the disease should be selected. Each matching factor included, while controlling the results, eliminates the possibility of evaluating that factor itself.

To avoid bias regarding the presence or absence of a characteristic in the procurement of data by interview or from records, those charged with data collection should not know which is case or control, and the ascertainment should be uniform or standard. Once the data have been obtained, the odds ratio associated with a given characteristic is calculated from Table 1 by the cross-product of $a \times d$ divided by $b \times c$. This estimate is based on the assumption that the frequency of the disease in the population is relatively small and that cases and controls are representative of their respective ill and non-ill populations for that disease. Examples of case–control studies for an infectious disease would include the influence of some characteristic such as genetic makeup (HLA type), smoking, preexisting disease, or socioeconomic level as a risk factor in a given disease. It should be emphasized that a particular risk factor might operate at different levels or at several levels: it might affect exposure and infection, the severity of illness after infection has occurred, the duration of disease, the development of complications, or the case-fatality rate.

The advantages of case–control studies as compared with cohort studies (see Table 2) include the relatively small numbers of subjects needed, their relatively high efficiency, the shorter time to complete the study, and their suitability for diseases of low incidence. Their disadvantages include difficulty in finding the needed information about the characteristic in question, or the inaccuracy of the information; bias in obtaining data; and bias in the selection of cases and controls. The appropriate selection of the control groups is probably the most difficult task.

2.2.1c. Cross–Sectional or Prevalence Study. This third type of investigation examines the occurrence of disease and of suspected risk factors in population groups at a point in time or over a relatively short period of time. Prevalence rates among those with and without the exposure are determined and compared. This approach is usually limited to diseases of slow onset and long duration for which medical care is often not sought until the disease has progressed to a relatively advanced stage. Thus, the risk factors present at the start of the disease may be difficult to identify. This method is used for certain chronic diseases, such as osteoarthritis, chronic bronchitis, and some mental disorders,[24] but it may also be useful in certain infectious diseases such as those occurring in a hospital setting.

The reader should review more detailed descriptions of epidemiological methods such as found in Refs. 18–22 before undertaking any type of epidemiological study, as

Table 2. Some Features of Cohort and Case–Control Studies

Features	Cohort	Case–control
Approach	Identify the subsequent incidence of disease in persons with or without given characteristic(s)	Identify the presence or absence of characteristic(s) in persons with or without a given disease
Starting point	Persons with or without certain characteristics	Ill persons and controls (healthy or with other disease)
Measurement	Incidence of infection or disease or both	Prevalence of characteristic
Type of observation	Serial, longitudinal surveillance of entire group for development of infection or disease or both	Single analysis by interview, records, or a laboratory test of the characteristic in persons with and without disease
Advantages and disadvantages		
Incidence	Can be measured directly	Not measurable directly
Risk	Direct assessment	Indirect assessment
Disease spectrum	Can be measured from infection to mild and severe disease in relation to characteristic(s) and to other diseases	Not measureable; a clinical case is the starting point
Factor(s) or characteristic(s)	Defined before disease develops	Factor(s) defined after disease develops
Bias	Little, usually, since information is recorded before the outcome is known, but problems in ascertainment, diagnosis, and follow-up may create bias	Bias may be present in interviewer, in patient, and in control; data from records may be incomplete
Attrition	Individuals may be lost to observation or refuse to be studied	Cases and controls may die prior to completion of study
Time	Often long period of observation	Can be short
Efficiency	Low except for diseases of high incidence	Comparatively high
Sample size	Large, depending on incidence of the infection or disease	Relatively small

well as consult with a statistician in the planning stage to ensure the validity of the procedures and the adequacy of the number of subjects involved. See Section 5 for discussion of methods in epidemic investigation.

2.2.2. Experimental Epidemiology. In infectious diseases, this represents planned experiments designed to control the influence of extraneous factors, among those exposed or not exposed to an etiologic factor, preventive measure, or environmental manipulation by the investigator. One example is the planned introduction of an infectious agent in a controlled fashion into a group of animals or volunteers and the analysis of the spread of infection and disease within these groups as compared to a nonexposed group. Such studies offer the most scientifically controlled method of epidemiological study. Unfortunately, many bacterial species or agents may not induce infection or disease in animal models. Certain susceptible animals (marmosets, chimpanzees) may not be available for study or are too expensive. Volunteers are very difficult to utilize in today's ethical, legal, and social environment, and there are good reasons for these restrictions.

2.2.3. Serological Epidemiology. The systematic testing of blood samples from a defined sample of a target population for the presence of antibodies, antigens, genetic markers, specific cell-mediated immunity, and other biological characteristics is called a *serological* or *immunological survey*. It constitutes an important epidemiological tool. Serological techniques can: (1) identify the past and current prevalence of an infectious agent in a community; (2) identify the incidence of infection by seroconversion or a rise in titer in samples obtained at two different times; (3) reveal the ratio of subclinical to clinical infections, when combined with clinical data; and (4) determine the need for immunization programs and evaluate their effectiveness as to the presence, level, and quality of antibody produced; its duration; and the degree of protection against disease. Serological techniques are useful in defining the incidence, clinical importance, and spectrum of illness of a new agent such as *Legionella pneumophila*. The presence of antibody or antitoxin to diphtheria, pertussis, and tetanus, as determined in a serological study, is a good reflection of the level of immunization and public health practice in a community. This is especially true of tetanus, since antitoxin is acquired almost solely through immunization and rarely, if at all, through natural infection. The use of serological surveys in areas where medical care, diagnostic facilities, and reporting practices are inadequate may provide information essential for the control and evaluation of immunization programs. The uses, advantages, and disadvantages of serological surveillance and seroepidemiology for viral infections are presented in Chapter 2 of the companion book[5] to this volume.

Seroepidemiology is more widely applicable to viral than to bacterial diseases because of the wider occurrence of demonstrable antibodies in viral than in bacterial infections and because of the better means to measure them. Nevertheless, these techniques have proved useful in variable degrees for brucellosis, cholera, diphtheria, legionellosis, leptospirosis, *Mycoplasma pneumoniae* infections, pertussis, Q fever, Rocky Mountain spotted fever, syphilis, tetanus, tularemia, and typhoid fever. Specific mention of their applicability will be found in the relevant chapters of this book. The development of monoclonal antibodies and of diagnostic techniques, such as the enzyme-linked immunosorbent assay (ELISA) and the radioimmunoassay (RIA), permit highly specific, sensitive, and rapid serological diagnoses. Development of sensitive and simple DNA probes and the ability to amplify DNA by the polymerase chain reaction (PCR) provide tools not only for diagnostic microbiology, but also for the identification of antigens in stored paraffin or frozen sections.[6]

3. Epidemics and Their Investigation

Detailed descriptions of the concepts and methods of epidemic investigation can be found in a number of articles and book chapters.[24–26] An excellent recent article discussing the use of the case–control method in epidemic investigation gives a thorough review of the subject and an extensive table of examples.[27] This section will only deal with the highlights of epidemic investigation.

3.1. Pathogenesis of an Outbreak

Three essential requirements for an outbreak of an infectious disease are: (1) the presence or introduction of an infectious agent by an infected human, animal, bird, or arthropod vector, or its occurrence in air, water, food, soil, or other environmental source, or its presence in or on a fomite; (2) an adequate number of susceptibles; and (3) an effective means of transmission between the two. Five circumstances in which epidemics occur can be mentioned: first, when a new group of susceptibles is introduced into a setting where a disease is endemic; second, when a new source of infection is introduced into an area from which the microbial agent has been absent and many susceptibles are therefore present, as in the return of visitors from a foreign country, or the arrival of new immigrants, or the contamination of food, water, or other source of exposure by an agent not normally present; third, when effective contact is made between a preexisting infection of low endemicity with susceptible persons as a result of changes in social, behavioral, sexual, or cultural practices. Crowding as in a prison camp or institution or exposure of a new portal of entry are examples. A fourth possibility is an increased susceptibility to infection or disease or both through immunosuppression or other factors that influence the host response, such as a preceding viral infection, nutritional disorder, treatment with immunosuppressive drugs, or presence of a chronic disease. The devastating effect of HIV on the immune system has resulted in a worldwide epidemic of enormous and increasing proportions. A fifth circumstance might be the increase in the virulence or dosage of a microbial agent. This may have accounted for the massive outbreak of waterborne *Cryptosporidium* infection that occurred in Milwaukee, Wisconsin in March–April 1993, which involved 404,000 infected persons of whom 4,400 required hospitalization.[28]

Epidemics or outbreaks are often classified from the standpoint of the source of infection. A common-source or common-vehicle outbreak may result from exposure of a group of persons to a single source of infection. This could be an exposure to a common source occurring at a single point in time, as in most foodborne outbreaks (point epidemics), and characterized by a sharply defined and limited epidemic curve, often within the incubation period of the disease. It could be exposure on a continued or extended basis, as would be the case from a contaminated water supply or air source (airborne), and would result in an extended epidemic curve. In the latter setting, variations in the epidemic curve could result from differences in the dosage and time of occurrence of the microbial contaminant in the common vehicle or in the amount consumed, or they could result from changes in the frequency of exposure of the persons at risk to infection. The secondary spread of certain infectious agents from human to human in a common-source outbreak will also alter the epidemic curve, often producing a group of scattered cases after the initial epidemic wave subsides; these are called *secondary cases* and can lead to *tertiary cases*.

A second type of epidemic spread called *propagated* or *progressive* is due to multiplication and spread of an agent from one host to another. This is also called *contact spread* and may be direct, indirect, or by droplets (see Section 7). This is most often human-to-human spread, but could involve animal or arthropod intermediates. Here, the epidemic curve depends on the number of susceptibles, the degree of contact with an infected host, the incubation period of the disease, the mechanism of transmission, the portal of entry, and the infectiousness of the causative agent. In either common-source or propagated outbreaks, the epidemic decreases or stops when (1) the number of susceptibles effectively exposed to the source is diminished by natural attrition, by immunization, by antibiotic prophylactics, or by actual development of the disease itself; (2) the source of infection is eliminated; or (3) the means of transmission is interrupted.

3.2. Investigation of an Outbreak

The general strategy in the investigation of an outbreak includes establishing whether an epidemic actually exists, determining its extent, identifying the circumstances under which it occurred (e.g., time, place, person), evaluating its probable mode of spread, and initiating the steps to be taken for its control. Notification to appropriate health authorities should be made and help in epidemic investigation sought, if needed, from appropriate national or state disease control agencies; written reports should be prepared and distributed. News releases should be prepared to inform but not unnecessarily alarm the public. The epidemiologist, clinician, and laboratory experts all have roles in the analysis and management of an epidemic. The specific steps in epidemic investigations are presented in Table 3.

Table 3. Steps in the Investigation of an Epidemic

1. Determine that an epidemic or outbreak actually exists by comparing with previous data on the disease.
2. Establish an etiologic diagnosis if possible; if not, define the condition epidemiologically and clinically. Collect materials for isolation and serological test, and data from sick and well exposed persons.
3. Investigate the extent of the outbreak by a quick survey of hospitals, physicians, and other sources and its basic epidemiological characteristics in terms of time, place, person, probable method of spread, and the spectrum of clinical illness. Prepare a spot map of cases and an epidemic curve. Call in outside help if needed.
4. Formulate a working hypothesis of the source and manner of spread as a basis for further study.
5. Test the hypothesis by determining infection and illness rates in persons exposed or not exposed to putative source(s) of infection by questionnaire, interview, and laboratory tests. Try to isolate the agent from the putative source(s).
6. Extend epidemiological and laboratory studies to other possible cases or to persons exposed but not ill.
7. Analyze the data and consider possible interpretations.
8. On the basis of the analysis, initiate both short- and long-term control measures.
9. Report the outbreak to appropriate public health officials.
10. Inform physicians, other health officials, and the public of the nature of the outbreak and the ways to control it.

3.2.1. Determination of the Presence of an Epidemic. An epidemic or outbreak is usually defined as a substantial increase in the number of cases of a disease in a given period of time for that particular geographic area; e.g., an increase in the number of deaths from influenza and pneumonia that exceeds by 2 standard deviations the average experience for that week over the past 5 years is said to indicate an influenza outbreak.

A clinical diagnosis confirmed by laboratory findings is most important in determining whether a specific disease has exceeded the number of previously recorded cases. Unfortunately, a laboratory-proved diagnosis may be difficult or impossible to establish, especially early in an epidemic.

A clinical and epidemiological definition including the key features of the disease may be needed as a guide to reporting and for disease recognition until the etiologic agent is identified and appropriate methods are developed for isolation of the agent and/or its serological identification. Recent examples of the use of this type of definition are Legionnaires' disease, toxic shock syndrome, and AIDS. Even when the causative agent is known and laboratory tools for diagnosis are available, the disease may not be reportable, thus making comparison with past experiences impossible. On a practical level, any apparent concentration in time or geographic area of an acute illness of marked severity or with unique clinical features involving the respiratory, gastrointestinal, skin, or central nervous system, deserves evaluation. In the absence of a specific diagnosis, a simple working definition of a case should be established on the basis of available clinical and epidemiological data. It should be concise and clear-cut. The number of such cases should then be determined by a quick telephone or record survey of hospitals, clinics, and appropriate practicing physicians in the area. If the epidemic seems to be widespread, as with influenza, a random telephone survey of homes may give an estimate of the attack rate. The rate of absenteeism from key industries and schools may also help define the magnitude of the outbreak.

3.2.2. Determination of the Circumstances under Which the Outbreak Occurred. This often involves two phases: a preliminary assessment based on available data and a more intensive investigation when the situation is better defined.

3.2.2a. Preliminary Assessment. This is usually based on existing clinical records. In addition to the key clinical features, the age, sex, race, occupation, home and work addresses, unusual behavioral or cultural characteristics, date of onset, recent travel, and functions attended by others in the group in the recent past should be recorded. A time graph is drawn of the epidemic cases by date (and maybe time) of onset, from which the incubation period may be estimable. The time from the onset of the first cases to the peak may give a clue to this, as will unique or single exposures to the presumed source of infection. A spot map (place) may reveal clustering of cases or a relationship to a common source in the environment (food, water, air, anthropod). The data are analyzed to identify the persons at highest risk or some common denominator of risk and to postulate the most likely means of transmission. Early identification of a common-source outbreak is most important for instituting control measures. This might be a single (point) exposure, as in a food outbreak, or a continued exposure, as in a contaminated water supply. Person-to-person spread, airborne transmission, arthropod-borne spread, and zoonotic disease, especially of domestic animals, should be considered.

Appropriate materials for laboratory investigation should be collected early in the outbreak, such as throat washings, stool specimens or rectal swabs, blood for culture, and an acute-phase serum sample. A public health or hospital laboratory should be consulted in this endeavor. Since antibody to an infectious agent may already be present in many persons already ill in an outbreak, it may be desirable for baseline antibody levels to collect serum from other unexposed persons or from those incubating the disease, such as other family members or neighbors. A higher geometric mean antibody titer to a specific agent in ill compared to unexposed persons implicates that agent in the epidemic. Appropriate samples from the environment (water, food) or from possible vectors (mosquitoes, lice) should also be collected for isolating the agent.

On the basis of this preliminary assessment, a hypothesis of transmission may be formulated and recommendations for immediate control and isolation techniques made. Surveillance plans for identifying added cases may be drawn up, the appropriate environmental data assembled (water, milk, food, air), and questionnaires prepared for cases and controls (if a case–control study is to be conducted) in a fashion permitting easy analysis (marginal punch cards, computer). Standardized forms for foodborne outbreaks are available from state health departments and the CDC.

3.2.2b. Intensive Study. This analysis should confirm or negate the hypothesis. The questionnaires prepared for this phase should include all possible circumstances under which the epidemic occurred and be administered to those ill, those exposed but not ill, and a comparable group neither exposed nor ill. Sera and other materials should be collected from these groups for antigen and antibody tests. The completed questionnaires may then be analyzed for comparison of attack rates (illness rate) in the three groups and as related to various risk factors. Antibody analysis of sera taken at the time of the outbreak and of those taken 2–3 weeks later may not only confirm the diagnosis but also identify the occurrence of infection in persons who were exposed but did not become ill. It may be possible to identify the specific nature of an ongoing outbreak by comparing the geometric mean antibody titer of those patients who are acutely ill with that of other patients already convalescing or by comparing the titer of those not exposed with that of those who are ill. More intensive study of the environment, of insect vectors, and of animal reservoirs may be needed. The analysis should include hypotheses to find the one that best fits the available data.

On the basis of this appraisal, control measures, including immunization programs, and other preventive measures should be initiated. Irrespective of whether the causative agent can be identified or not, the key element is the interruption of the chain of transmission. A written analysis of the epidemic should be given to the appropriate authorities. If no causative agent can be identified, then the acute and convalescent sera and material for antigen identification should be frozen for later study when new etiologic agents or laboratory techniques are discovered. A good example of the benefit of this procedure is its use in retroactively identifying several outbreaks of Legionnaires' disease that had occurred prior to the outbreak in 1976 in Philadelphia, from which the organism was first isolated.[(29)]

3.3. Example of Investigating a Foodborne Outbreak

An outbreak of illness characterized by diarrhea, abdominal cramps, and little or no fever involved 366 college students on February 24, 1966, in a new dormitory complex at the University of Wisconsin.[(30)] A quick assessment indicated that illness was confined to students who ate in three of six dining halls that served food from a common kitchen to 3000 students. No other dormitories were involved, and the cases were sharply limited in time. The epidemic curve shown in Fig. 1 indicates a peak incubation of 14 h. Stool specimens were obtained both from ill and healthy students and from food handlers. Samples of leftover items of food were not available; however, refrigerated samples of routinely collected food items were found for testing. Food menus for the preceding evening revealed that the three dining halls in which ill students had eaten offered a choice of fish or roast beef with gravy, whereas the other three dining halls had a choice of hamburger or fish; the other food items were common to all six dining halls. On the basis of this preliminary assessment, the hypothesis was formulated that this was a foodborne outbreak due to an agent with an average incubation period of about 14 h (range 10–20 h) that was present in or introduced into one or more of the food items served exclusively in the three dining halls where students became ill. The laboratory was notified of this as a guide to its tests. For more intensive investigation, questionnaires concerning foods eaten, time of onset, and the clinical symptoms were distributed to both sick and well students who ate in the three dining halls. They were returned by 366 ill and 740 well students, representing all the ill and two thirds of the well students. The clinical data indicated that the illness lasted less than 24 h and was characterized mainly by diarrhea; about half the ill students complained of abdominal cramps. Nausea, vomiting, and fever were rare. The average incubation period was too long for a staphylococcal toxin, and the clinical features would be unusual for *Salmonella* or *Shigella*.

An analysis of food items is given in Table 4. The evidence incriminating a food is usually based on the greatest difference in percentage ill between those who ate and those who did not eat a given food. In this outbreak, 69.9% of those who ate beef with gravy became ill compared to 4.9% who did not eat this item who became ill; furthermore, no one who ate beef without gravy became ill, thus clearly incriminating the gravy as the likely source. The gravy as well as other foods available were negative on aerobic and anaerobic culture. Mouse-inoculation tests for toxin in the gravy were also negative; however, it was not known whether the gravy sample tested was from the incriminated meal or was set aside from a fresh gravy preparation. Laboratory analysis of fecal samples yielded the answer. Stool specimens from 19 of 20 ill students were positive for heat-resistant *Clostridium perfringens*, as was 1 of 24 stools from food handlers; no stools from 13 healthy students who had not eaten beef with gravy were positive. The organisms were isolated in thioglycollate broth after being heated 1 h in a boiling water bath. It was learned later that approximately 27 gallons of bone beef stock had been kept overnight in the refrigerator in 9-gallon plastic bags, mixed with 7 gallons of fresh beef stock the next day, heated to a rolling boil, and served separately from the roast beef. Apparently, the inadequate heating of a heat-resistant preformed toxin in a very large volume of fluid had failed to destroy it. The control measures instituted were to prohibit future use of leftover gravy stock and to heat all items in smaller containers. *C. perfringens* food poisoning has an incuba-

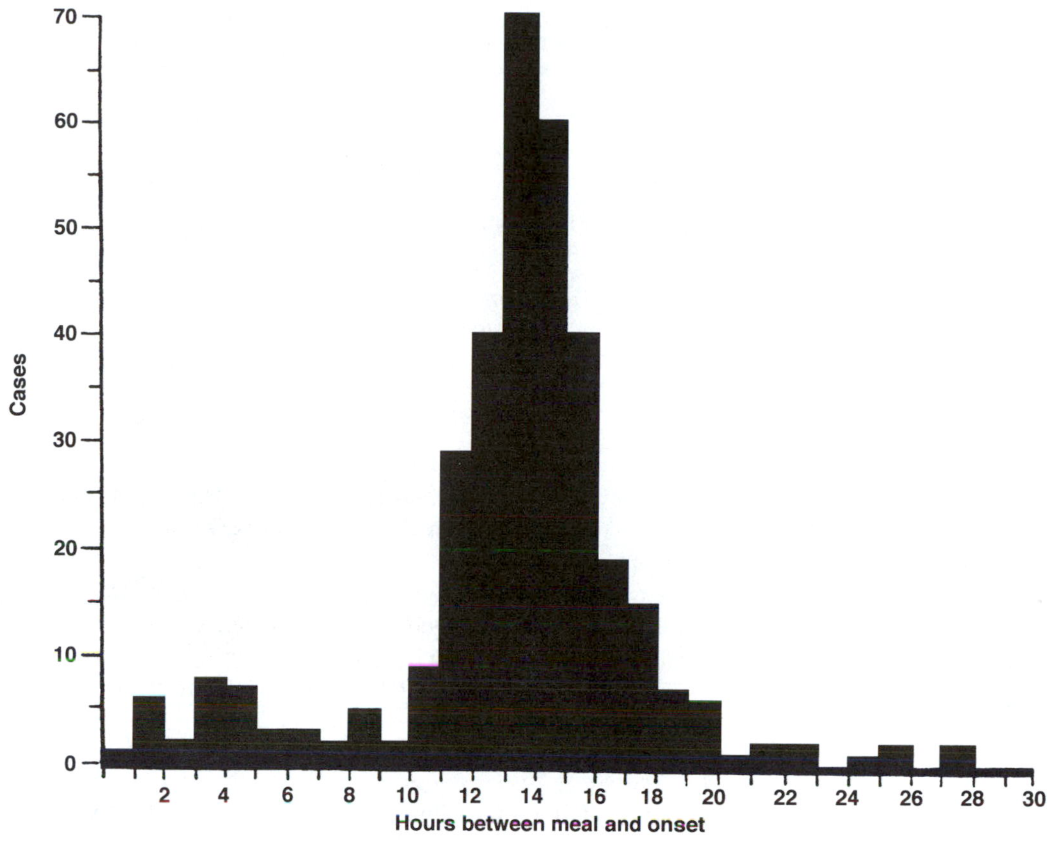

Figure 1. Epidemic curve of outbreak of *Clostridium perfringens* in a food outbreak involving 366 students at the University of Wisconsin. From Helstad *et al.*[30]

tion period of 8–22 h with a peak of 10–14 h, closely fitting the outbreak described.

4. Agent

This book deals with microorganisms classified under "Lower protists (Prokaryotic): Bacteria." This grouping includes also: the *Chlamydiae* (*Bedsoniae*) and the *Rickettsiae*, which are somewhat smaller than bacteria and are intracellular parasites.[31] Viruses, while classed as microorganisms, are sharply differentiated from all other cellular forms of life; they consist of a nucleic acid molecule, either DNA or RNA, that is enclosed in a protein coat, or capsid. The principal groups of bacteria are presented in Table 5, which is derived from an "informal classification" presented by Jawetz *et al.*[31] in their excellent *Review of Medical Microbiology*, to which readers are referred for discussions of microbiology, immunology, and host–parasite relationships. The new, beautifully illustrated book, *Medical Microbiology*, by Mims *et al.*[32] is also highly recommended.

The characteristics of microorganisms of epidemiological importance include those concerned with transmission through the environment, the development of infection, and the production of clinical disease. Table 6 summarizes some of these characteristics of bacteria, which include species pathogenic for humans.

4.1. Characteristics of Organisms that Are Involved in Spread through the Environment

For the spread of infection, a sufficient number of organisms must enter and survive transport through the environment to reach another susceptible host. Resistance to heat, UV light, drying, and chemical agents is important for survival of bacteria in nature. Some organisms such as *Vibro cholerae* and *Legionella pneumophila* can survive for months in water, even in distilled water; others, such as *Bacillus anthracis*, attain survival through highly resistant

Table 4. Analysis of Attack Rate for Different Foods Eaten in a College Outbreak of Diarrhea[a]

	Ate food			Did not eat food			
		Ill			Ill		Difference between ill and non-ill
Food item	Number	Number	Percent	Number	Number	Percent	(percent)
Fish	391	16	4.1	715	340	47.6	—
Hamburger	188	15	8.0	918	351	38.2	—
Beef							
With gravy	479	335	69.9	627	31	4.9	65.0
Without gravy	48	0	0	1058	366	34.6	—

[a]Derived from Helstad *et al.*[30]

spores. Organisms capable of actual multiplication within the environment in soil, plants, food products, milk, and elsewhere have an advantage for survival. The capacity to infect a nonhuman host such as animals or birds, or to be transferred through an insect vector such as the *Rickettsiae*, offers alternative pathways for the persistence and spread of microorganisms.

4.2. Characteristics of Organisms that Are Involved in Production of Infection

Once bacteria have survived transport through the environment or intermediate host to reach a susceptible human host, several features of the bacteria are important in the initiation and development of infection. One is the

Table 5. Key to Principle Groups of Bacteria Including Species Pathogenic for Humans[a]

Characteristics	Genera
I. Flexible, thin-walled cells with motility conferred by gliding mechanism (gliding bacteria)	
II. Same as I but with motility conferred by axial filament (spirochetes)	*Treponema*, *Borrelia*, *Leptospira*
III. Rigid, thick-walled cells, immotile or motility conferred by flagella	
Mycelial (actinomycetes)	*Mycobacterium*, *Actinomyces*, *Nocardia*, *Streptomyces*
Simple unicellular	
Obligate intracellular parasites	*Rickettsia*, *Coxiella*, *Chlamydia*
Free-living	
Gram-positive	
Cocci	*Streptococcus*, *Staphylococcus*
Nonsporulating rods	*Corynebacterium*, *Listeria*, *Erysipelothrix*
Sporulating rods	
Obligate aerobes	*Bacillus*
Obligate anaerobes	*Clostridium*
Gram-negative	
Cocci	*Neisseria*
Nonenteric rods	
Spiral forms	*Spirillum*
Straight rods	*Pasteurella*, *Brucella*, *Yersinia*, *Francisella*, *Haemophilus*, *Bordetella*, *Legionella*
Enteric rods	
Facultative anaerobes	*Escherichia* (and related coliforms), *Salmonella*, *Shigella*, *Klebsiella*, *Proteus*, *Vibrio*
Obligate aerobes	*Pseudomonas*
Obligate anaerobes	*Bacteroides*, Fusobacterium
IV. Lacking cell walls (mycoplasmas)	*Mycoplasma*

[a]Derived from Jawetz *et al.*[31]

Table 6. Bacterial Characteristics of Epidemiological Importance[a]

Epidemiological aspects	Bacterial characteristics
1. Features involved in *spread* through the environment	Number of organisms released by infected host
	Resistance to physical of environment (e.g., heat, UV, moisture)
	Ability to multiply within environment
	Ability to infect intermediate host or insect vector
2. Features involved in initiation and development of *infection*	Host range of organisms
	Genetic makeup and antigenic diversity
	Infectivity of organism
	Pathogenicity of organism
	Number of organisms entering host and the portal of entry
	Enzymes involved in spread through tissues
3. Features involved in production of *clinical disease*	Most characteristics under (2)
	Virulence of organism
	Invasiveness of organism
	Production of endo- and exotoxins
	Immunopathologic potential

[a]Host attributes are considered in Table 7.

infectiousness, expressed as the ratio: number infected/number susceptible and exposed. A second is *pathogenicity*, a term used to denote the potential for an infectious organism to induce disease. It can be expressed quantitatively as: number with disease/number infected. The determinants of pathogenicity include mobile genetic elements such as plasmids, bacteriophages, and transposons.[(33)] The pathogenic process is complex and represents sequence of events in which many components are involved.[(34)] The adherence of organisms to host surfaces is a highly specific and essential step for subsequent events to develop. Epithelial surfaces provide appropriate sites for many bacteria. *Mycoplasma pneumoniae* and *Haemophilus influenzae* find attachment sites in the respiratory epithelium, *Neisseria gonorrhea* in the urethral epithelium, and many enteric organisms (*Vibrio cholerae*, *Escherichia coli*, *Salmonella typhosa*, *Shigella flexneri*) in intestinal or colonic epithelium. Pathogenic organisms must possess characteristics that protect them against such host defenses as mucus and phagocytic cells. These protective features of the bacteria themselves include polysaccharide capsules (pneumococci, *Klebsiella*, *Haemophilus*), hyaluronic acid capsules and M proteins (β-hemolytic streptococci), and a surface polypeptide (*B. anthracis*). Toxins and certain extracellular enzymes may be important in the establishment of infection and in spread through tissues. The latter include collagenase (*C. perfringens*), coagulase (staphylococci), hyaluronidases (staphylococci, streptococci, clostridia, pneumococci), streptokinase or fibrinolysin (hemolytic streptococci), hemolysins and leukocydins (streptococci, staphylococci, clostridia, gram-negative rods), and proteases (*Neisseria*, streptococci) that can hydrolyze immunoglobulins, such as secretory IgA.[(34)] These surface properties and enzyme production contribute to the invasiveness of an organism.

4.3. Characteristics of Organisms that Are Involved in Production of Disease

Disease is a rare consequence of infection. Usually, the presence of microorganisms on various surfaces of the body, their colonization on or in diverse epithelial cells, and their multiplication are unattended by signs of clinical disease. As with most viruses, infection without disease is a common outcome. However, since infection is a necessary basis for disease (excepting ingestion of preformed toxin), the attributes of organisms that are involved in infection are also important in clinical illness (see Section 4.2 and Table 6). The term *virulence* is used as a quantitative expression of the disease-producing potential of a pathogenic organism. Molecular studies of the determinants of virulence include how agents enter epithelial cells, a property that may be carried in different ways. In enterovasive *E. coli* it may be on a large plasmid, whereas for *Yersinia pseudotuberculosis* it is by a small DNA segment of the bacterial chromosome.[(35)] This property may be exchanged between bacteria, making noninvasive bacteria invasive.

Some organisms may lose apparent virulence if their structural identity is too close to the host's carbohydrates (for which the term *camouflage strategy* has been suggested). The factors that result in disease in an infected person are also determined by the host, as discussed in Section 6. Those that relate to the organism are invasiveness, the production of toxins, and the induction of an immune response that usually is beneficial but sometimes is detrimental to the host.

Invasiveness does not always correlate with disease and a widely disseminated organism does not always induce illness, but the wide distribution of a pathogen and its contact with many cells provide the potential amplification of any detrimental host response. That wide dissemination and a large number of organisms, even in the bloodstream, do not inevitably lead to toxemia is exemplified by the minimal host response evoked by large numbers of *Mycobacterium leprae* bacilli in the blood in lepromatous leprosy.

Organisms that produce endotoxins or exotoxins are likely to produce disease, since most are toxic to cells and evoke inflammatory responses. The exotoxins liberated by many gram-positive bacteria cause local cell and tissue injury; some damage phagocytic cells and thereby facilitate the spread of the organism. Examples include *Clostridium welchii, botulinum, tetanus, Corynebacterium diphtheriae, Shigella dysenteriae, Vibrio cholerae, B. anthracis, Bordetella pertussis, Streptococcus pyogenes*, and *Staphylococcus aureus.*[36] Some exotoxins are directly responsible for the characteristic clinical features of the disease, some are antiphagocytic, and some promote spread in tissues. They cause little or no fever in the host. Endotoxins are an integral part of the cell wall of gram-negative organisms. They are liberated in soluble form both during bacterial growth and presumably during death and disintegration of the organism. Endotoxins are strong immunologic adjuvants. They may produce fever in man and many other vertebrates; the pyrogenic action is mediated by a product synthesized by monocytes ("endogenous pyrogen") that acts on the thermoregulatory center in the hypothalamus. Other endogenous agents, such as prostaglandins and catecholamines, may also play a role. The lipopolysaccharide (LPS) is the most important component of endotoxin and is composed of a core polysaccharide common to many gram-negative bacteria, an O-specific polysaccharide conferring virulence and serological specificity, and a lipid A portion, mainly responsible for toxicity.[35] The effects of endotoxins appear to be mediated through leukotrienes, prostaglandins, and cachectin/TNF. Cachectin, which is identical to tumor necrosis factor,[37] is indistinguishable functionally from lymphotoxin, a product of activated T cells. This protein is produced by macrophages and by T cells in response to bacteria, viruses, and parasites and also occurs during cancers, resulting, in order of increasing dosage, in the following sequence of events: inflammation, cytotoxicity, cachexia, organ failure, irreversible shock, and death. There is a synergism between it and interleukin-1 in this phenomenon. Monoclonal antibody to cachectin/TNF can inhibit these responses and glucosteroids can also prevent endotoxin deaths. The gene for cachectin has been identified, and when put into hamster ovarian cells and then into nude mice results in cachexia. Despite these deleterious effects, cachectin/TNF in small doses appears to be beneficial in serving as a growth factor for macrophages and as a tissue remodeler, a role for which it may have been designed in nature. It is not clear whether all these effects are mediated directly by cachectin/TNF or through mediators released by them. With large doses of endotoxins, there is also an effect that produces vascular collapse and death. Unlike exotoxins, endotoxins are heat-stable and are not fully convertible to protective toxoids. Endotoxins are normally released by many gram-negative bacteria in the intestines of healthy individuals, presumably absorbed in small amounts, and degraded by the Kuppfer cells. This occurs without pathological consequences on a continual basis and has a beneficial effect in stimulating the development of the immune system in the immature individual.[33]

Exotoxins are excreted by living cells, are quite unstable to heat, and consist of polypeptides of molecular weights from 10,000 to 900,000. They are highly antigenic and result in high titers of antitoxin that can neutralize the toxin. This antigenic property is useful in immunization with toxins rendered nontoxic by formalin, heat, and other methods. Different toxins produce disease via different mechanisms.[31] *Corynebacterium diphtheriae* toxin results in inhibition of protein synthesis and necrosis of epithelium, heart muscle, kidney, and nerve tissues. The toxin of *Clostridium tetani* reaches the central nervous system by retrograde axon transport where it increases reflex excitation in neurons of the spinal cord by blocking an inhibitor mediator. *Clostridium botulinum* exerts its effect on the nervous system by blocking the release of acetylcholine at synapses and neuromuscular junction. Gut organisms, such as *Clostridium difficile*, produce a necrotizing toxin that leads to antibiotic-associated colitis, and that of *S. aureus* stimulates neural receptors from which impulses are transmitted to medullary centers controlling gut motility. *Vibrio cholerae* toxin binds to ganglioside receptors on the villi of the small intestine, leading to a large increase in adenylate cyclase and AMP concentrations and the resulting massive hypersecretion of chloride and water and the impairment of absorption of sodium that characterizes the severe diarrhea and acidosis of cholera. Other toxins, such as that of hemolytic lysogenic streptococci, result in the punctate maculopapular rash of scarlet fever.

The production of clinical disease through immunopathologic mechanisms is more important for viral than for bacterial infections, but there are some examples of the latter. In streptococcal infections, antibodies may develop against an unknown component of the organism that is antigenically similar to heart muscle, leading to myocarditis. Immune complexes may also form, deposit in the kidney, and result in glomerulonephritis. In infections due to *Mycoplasma pneumoniae*, the production of "heterophile" antibodies against human O erythrocytes (cold agglutinins) occasionally leads to acute hemolytic anemia. In primary infections by *Mycobacterium tuberculosis*, the pathological picture is dominated by a vigorous and persistent cell-mediated immune response to the invading organism. The inflammatory, pathological, and immunologic processes of the host culminating in disease may be detrimental both to the host and to the microorganism. A successful parasite is one that leads to the least host response. For a more detailed discussions of microbial virulence factors, readers are referred to recent texts on infectious diseases and microbiology[32,38] and to recent articles.[34,39]

5. Environment

The external environment provides the setting in which the agent and host usually interact and is the usual means of transmission between the two. The effects of the environment on the organism itself are discussed in Section 4.1. The environment also contain the physical and biological mechanisms required for spread. The former includes air, water, and food and the latter animal, bird, and insect vectors. For some bacterial infections, the primary host is not man but some other living creature in the environment. This includes anthrax, brucellosis, leptospirosis, Lyme disease, Q fever, bubonic plague, Rocky Mountain spotted fever, salmonellosis, and tularemia. For infections involving insect transmission such as louse-borne typhus, Rocky Mountain spotted fever, and bubonic plague, the humidity, temperature, vegetation, and other factors in the environment may play a central role in limiting the occurrence of the infection to well-defined geographic areas favorable to the vector. Through climatic factors, the environment exerts an influence on exposure of the host to microorganisms. Warm weather and tropical climates result in recreational and occupational exposures to water, sewage, swimming pools, wild animals, and insects; they promote spread of skin infections in unclothed persons with abrasions on their skin. Certain organisms grow or survive better in warmer environments, especially enteric organisms. Intestinal infections flourish under such conditions. Inadequate refrigeration leads to foodborne outbreaks. Epidemics of Legionnaires' disease appear to depend on a chain of warm weather events. These include appropriate temperature and humidity for the organism to grow in soil or water, the contamination of a water-cooling tower or air conditioner, and airborne carriage or propulsion of the organism to susceptible humans, frequently in an enclosed environment (e.g., hotel, hospital, institution, club); July and August are good months for this. The colder winter months, as well as school seasons in temperate climates of the Northern Hemisphere, bring individuals into close contact in a closed environment, facilitating spread of infections by the respiratory route. This includes bacterial infections of the central nervous system such as the meningococcus, *H. influenzae*, and pneumococcus organisms as well as true respiratory infections such as pertussis, bacterial and mycoplasmal pneumonias, tuberculosis, diphtheria, and streptococcal pharyngitis–tonsillitis. The peak period of different diseases varies from one season to another. For example, pertussis and *M. pneumoniae* infections tend to occur most commonly in the fall and streptococcal infections in the spring. In addition, longer-term temporal trends in infection and disease occur within the same environment (as discussed in Chapter 2, Section 8.2). These changes reflect the complex interplay of agent, host, and environment. New strains of the organism, environmental alterations, varying behavioral patterns of the host, and the degree of immunization practice may change the pattern from one season to another.

The particular environmental setting—the macro- or microenvironment—also influences disease occurrence and its clinical patterns. In hospitals, certain types of skin, wound, and urinary infections are common, and their severity may be enhanced in persons who are already ill with another disease or are receiving immunosuppressive therapy. Antibiotic-resistant organisms are frequent in this setting. In prisons and in institutions for the mentally retarded or ill, low levels of personal hygiene and crowding contribute to the spread of respiratory, intestinal, and skin infections. Exposure in meat-packing and slaughterhouses or tanneries, or travel to developing countries, involves the risk of infection by various bacterial agents within that environment. With regard to children, the day-care center is posing an increasing hazard for them, as well as their parents for certain infectious diseases, especially respiratory and intestinal infections.[40] However, for young children infection is much more common than disease. For example, among 10,860 case contacts of an index case of *H. influenzae* type b infection in day-care centers, none of whom had received rifampin chemoprophylaxis, no clinical disease developed over an average 60-day observation period, although the carrier state was common.[41] Thus, rifampin prophylaxis of contacts may be unnecessary in these settings, although some other investigators disagree with this. For HIV infection, the environments of the brothel, the bar, and the bathhouse have provided ready transmission of this and other sexually transmitted infections, as has the "shooting gallery" of intravenous drug abusers. Travel to or residence in developing countries may result in exposure not only to specific tropical infections such as malaria, schistosomiasis, and cholera, but also to many common respiratory and intestinal infections that the traveler might not encounter in a more hygienic setting. Even the homebody working in the garden or walking in the woods near home in endemic areas may be exposed to the bite of the deer tick or related species and become infected with *Borrelia burgdorferi*, the cause of Lyme disease.

6. Host

The occurrence of infection depends on exposure to a source of infection and on the susceptibility of the host. The development of disease in an infected person depends largely on factors intrinsic to the host, although some properties of the organism itself influence this. Some of the host factors are presented in Table 7.

They have been called the "clinical illness-promotion factors."[(3)] Exposure to a pathogenic organism depends on characteristics of the human host that result in contact with sources of infection within the environment or that promote person-to-person spread. The behavioral pattern of the individual at different ages brings varying types of exposure in different seasons, cultures, and geographic areas. Personal habits such as intravenous drug usage or sexual promiscuity are also determinants of exposure. The family unit comprises an important setting for exposure and spread of infectious agents. The genetic background, nutritional habits, cultural and behavioral patterns, and level of hygiene within families create common patterns of exposure. The number and age of family members and the degree of crowding within the home also affect the transmissibility of infection. Hospitalization or institutionalization brings new exposures in closed environments. Heightened person-to-person contact and a mixture of susceptibles with infected or infectious individuals (carriers) underlie the increased risk of military recruits, children in day-care centers, and residents of institutions. Streptococcal, meningococcal, *M. pneumoniae*, *H. influenzae* type b, and enteric infections are common in such settings.

Occupational risks involve special types of exposures in certain occupations. The worker in the abattoir or slaughterhouse, meat-packing industry, or even at the butcher block is at risk to brucellosis, tularemia, and various parasitic infections. The sewage and sugarcane worker and the swine handler are exposed to leptospirosis, the tannery worker to anthrax, and the hunter to tularemia. The hospital worker is at increased risk to a variety of infectious agents, of which HIV is currently of greatest concern, although the risk is extremely small if universal hospital infection regulations are strictly followed. Hepatitis B infection is also of concern, and HBV vaccine should be given to all hospital staff exposed to blood or blood products.

Race does not usually influence infection if exposure is equal, but the response to infection may vary, such as the increased severity of tuberculosis in blacks. However, the separation of ethnic origin from other cultural, socioeconomic, behavioral, and genetic differences is often impossible. Recreational pursuits and hobbies influence

Table 7. Host Factors that Influence Exposure, Infection, and Disease

Factors that influence exposure	
Behavioral factors related to age, drug usage, alcohol consumption	Military service
Familial exposure	Occupation
Hospitalization, especially intensive care	Recreation, sports, hobbies
Hygienic habits	Sexual activity: hetero- and homosexual, type and number of partners
Institutionalization: nurseries, day care center, homes for the elderly and mentally retarded, prisons and other closed environments	Socioeconomic level
	Travel, especially to developing countries
Factors that influence infection, and occurrence and severity of disease	
Age at the time of infection	Entry portal of organism and presence of trauma at site of implantation
Alcoholism	Genetic makeup, especially influences on the immune response
Anatomic defect	Immune state at time of infection
Antibiotic resistance	Immunodeficiency: natural, drug-induced, or viral (HIV)
Antibiotics in tissues	Mechanism of disease production: inflammatory, immunopathologic, or toxic
Coexisting diseases, especially chronic	Nutritional status
Dosage: amount and virulence of organism to which person is exposed	Receptors for organism on cells needed for attachment or entry of organism
Double infection	
Duration of exposure to organism	

exposures in both internal and external environments. The homemaker who prepares home preserves improperly may expose the ingestor to botulism; the home gardener or farmer is at risk to tetanus or Lyme disease, and the outdoorsman to various infections of wild animals. The influence of gender on occupational exposures has become of little importance, since women have entered almost all work areas including military life and many hazardous occupations. On the other hand, pregnancy is attended by special qualitative risks to infection, more commonly viral than bacterial, to which the male is not heir. Streptococcal B infections and syphilis are of special concern to the pregnant woman and her baby. Differences between the sexes in the portal of entry of microorganisms may result in different patterns of infection and disease, as is true in male homosexuals practicing passive rectal intercourse, in which the risk of infection with HIV is greatly increased. Genital lesions and discharges from sexually transmitted infections may also increase this risk in both sexes.

The socioeconomic level of the individual or the community affects the frequency, nature, and age at the time of infection. In developing countries and lower socioeconomic settings, infectious diseases, especially respiratory and enteric, constitute a leading cause of illness and death. The socioeconomic status influences infection and disease through a complex interaction of hygienic practices, environmental contamination, nutritional status, crowding, and exposure to animal and insect vectors.

Travel is an increasingly important risk factor because it may bring individuals into new settings, especially tropical or developing countries. Enteric infections are common hazards, especially toxogenic *E. coli*, *Campylobacter*, amebiasis, shigellosis, typhoid fever, salmonellosis, yersiniosis, and giardiasis. Enterotoxigenic *E. coli* (ETEC) is the most common cause and was found in 42% of diarrheal episodes in Latin America, 36% in Africa, and 25% in Asia. Other causes are various *Shigella* and *Salmonella* species. *Campylobacter jejuni*, *Vibrio cholera*, *E. histoliticia*, *Giardia lamblia*, rotaviruses, and Norwalk-like viruses.[42] Mixed infections also occur. Bismuth subsalicate had reduced the incidence of traveler's diarrhea by 65% in one study,[43] and its use is suggested for periods of up to 6 weeks.

Once infection has occurred, a number of factors influence whether clinical disease will develop and determine its severity (Table 7, part 2). Most of these factors are intrinsic to the host, although the dosage, virulence, and antibiotic resistance of the infecting organism play a role (see Section 4), as does the portal of entry. Entry sites that are close to vital organs or that permit easy access to invasion of the bloodstream may result in more severe and complicated infections. Among the host factors, age at the time of infection is an important determinant of the frequency of clinical illness and its clinical features and severity. The presence of chronic diseases or other infections are risk factors. HIV infection greatly enhances the risk of opportunistic infections, of the reactivation of latent agents, and of malignancy.

Transmission of infection to the fetus *in utero* may result in fetal death or congenital abnormalities as with *Treponema pallidum*. Infections of the newborn such as those due to *Streptococcus B*, *Clostridium botulinum*, and *Chlamydia trachomatis* may be severe and fatal. As is true in many viral infections, bacterial infections in childhood are often subclinical and less well localized than in the adult. The concept of "streptococcosis" illustrates this (see Chapter 34). In the newborn infant, respiratory involvement from group A infections is uncommon, although group B streptococci may cause sepsis and meningitis. In the age group 6 months to 3 years, group A infections have insidious development and mild symptoms. In the older infant and preschool child, a nonspecific streptococcal group A illness may be characterized by low-grade fever, irritability, and nasal discharge, sometimes accompanied by anorexia and vomiting. Clinical diagnosis is difficult. In the school-age child, upper respiratory infections due to group A predominate, and over half are manifested by the classic features of acute streptococcal pharyngotonsillitis: sore throat, often with tonsillar exudate, pharyngeal edema, dysphagia, enlargement of the anterior cervical nodes, and systemic symptoms (fever, chills, malaise). Another 20% may have milder and less localized illness, and 20% more may have either mild or no illness.

In general, the highest mortality from infection occurs very early in life, when immune defense mechanisms are immature, and in old age when they may be deteriorating. The clinical response to infection may also be more severe in conditions that alter or depress immune defenses. These include infection with HIV, organ transplantation, immunosuppressive drugs, preexisting chronic disease, especially of the specific target organ of the infection; occurrence of a viral, parasitic, or other bacterial infection preceding or accompanying the current illness; and the prior use of alcohol or tobacco. The vigor and efficiency of the immune response may alter the host either favorably by control of the infection or unfavorably by certain immunopathologic processes. Genetic traits influence both susceptibility and disease. Their role in regulating the immune response is an important but often ill-defined one in relation to the occurrence and severity of the clinical disease. In tuberculosis, clinical illness among those infected has occurred more commonly in monozygotic twins and zygotic twins, even when other factors are controlled.[44] The nutritional level also affects host resistance. Malnutrition (especially severe protein deficiency) adversely affects phagocytosis and other primary defense mechanisms, the development of the thymus, and the efficacy of cell-mediated immunity against infections such as tuberculosis. In general, antibody formation is not impaired. The precise role of nutrition and vitamins in infection and disease is not well understood. Immunity is also influenced by vaccination, whether active or passive.

In summary, host factors may be divided into three major stages: (1) those that lead to exposure, (2) those that lead to infection among those effectively exposed, and (3) those that lead to clinical disease among those infected. The concepts of a clinical illness promotion factor that leads to clinical illness[3] and of other, protective factors that result in subclinical or inapparent illness have been discussed.[4] Many of them remain unknown and they remain an important challenge to epidemiologists, microbiologists, immunologists, and geneticists.

7. Routes of Transmission

The major routes of transmission of bacterial infections are listed in Table 8 in general order of their importance. Many organisms have several routes. The sequence of spread usually involves the exit of the organism from the infected host; transport through the environment via air, water, food, insect, or animal, with or without bacterial multiplication; and the entry of a sufficient number of viable organisms into an appropriate portal of a susceptible host to initiate infection. For most infectious agents, specific receptors on the cell surface are needed to permit attachment and multiplication of the organism. Table 8 is loosely divided into human, animal–insect, and inanimate sources of infection in order to follow infection from its source to a human host, but the arrangement is sometimes artificial for those infections that exist primarily in other species or for those organisms that can multiply or survive in the natural environment.

7.1. Respiratory or Airborne

Organisms infecting the respiratory tract are either airborne via droplet nuclei or transmitted via droplets that are not considered true airborne transmission (see Section 7.2). The sources of the organisms carried by the air (droplet nuclei) include animate sources, the respiratory tract or oropharynx of infected persons, or from infected lesions of the skin, or from inanimate sources such as from water-cooling towers, as with *Legionella* organisms. Their success in reaching a susceptible host depends on the number of organisms present, the particle size, the force with which they are propelled into the environment, the resistance to drying, the temperature and humidity of the air, the presence of air currents, and the distance to the host. Some infections may be carried great distances from their sources, e.g., Q fever, tuberculosis, or Legionnaires' disease. As with viruses, respiratory-transmitted bacterial infections are difficult to control. The size of the particles in the aerosol influences its dispersion distance and the site in the respiratory passages at which the particles are trapped. Particles larger than approximately 5 μm in diameter are usually filtered out in the nose, while those up to 5 μm in diameter are deposited on sites along the upper and lower respiratory tract.

7.2. Contact

Contact transmission can be either direct, indirect, or by droplets, which due to particle size are not truly airborne. Direct contact transmission means the agent is transmitted from an infected person or animal directly to a susceptible host; indirect contact transmission means the agent moves from the source to the susceptible host by means of an inanimate object. Droplets are infected particles more than 5 μm in diameter that only travel up to approximately 3 feet through the air before they infect a susceptible host or fall to a horizontal surface. Direct contact spread includes genital or sexually transmitted diseases, some gastrointestinal or fecal–oral spread diseases, and some other diseases such as tularemia resulting from contact with an infected animal.

Bacterial infections of the skin are transmitted usually person to person from an infected lesion or via squamae. They are commonly due to staphylococcus or streptococcus or a mixture of the two. They are manifested as boils, carbuncles, impetigo, and erysipelas. They are particularly common in warm and tropical climates and in settings of poor hygiene. Yaws, a nonvenereal, contagious disease of the skin and bones due to *Treponema pertenue*, is endemic in many tropical areas and is similarly transmitted; effective eradication programs with penicillin sponsored by the WHO have been carried out in many countries. Diphtheritic skin infections may also occur, especially in tropical climates, and may contaminate wounds.

Table 8. Transmission of Bacterial Infection[a]

Route of exit	Route of transmission	Examples	Factors	Route of entry
1. Human source				
1.1. Respiratory	Respiratory droplets or droplet nuclei	Bacterial pneumonias	Close contact or airborne	Respiratory
	RS and fomites	Diphtheria	Carriers	Respiratory, skin
	Nasal discharges	Leprosy	Household contact	? Skin, repiratory
	RS → droplets	Meningococcus	Crowding, military recruits, carriers	Respiratory
	RS → air, fomites	Pertussis	Direct contact	Respiratory
	RS → air	Plague (pneumonic)	Pneumonic case	Respiratory
	RS → droplets	Streptococcal	Close contact, carrier	Respiratory
	RS → droplet nuclei	Tuberculosis	Household contact	Respiratory
1.2. Skin squames	Respiratoy, direct contact	Nosocomial bacterial infections	Hospitalization, surgery	Nose, repiratory, skin
	Direct contact	Impetigo due to staph and/or strep	Low socioeconomic level, tropics	Skin
	Close contact	Skin diphtheria	War wounds	Skin
		Yaws	Endemic foci	Skin
1.3. Gastrointestinal				
Enteric fevers	Stool → water	Cholera	Water, food, carrier	Mouth
	Stool → food	Salmonellosis	Food, animal contact	Mouth
	Stool → man	Shigellosis	Man-to-man only	Mouth
	Stool → water, food	Typhoid fever	Also food, flies	Mouth
Food poisoning	Food	Staph, *C. perfringens*, *Salmonella*, strep, *Vibrio parahemolyticus*	Inadequate refrigeration or cooking	
		Botulism	Home canning	Mouth
1.4. Urine	Water (swimming)	Leptospirosis	Infected animals	Skin
	Water	Typhoid fever	Poor sanitation	Oral
1.5. Genital	Sexual contact (hetero- or homosexual)	Chancroid	Mostly tropics	Urethra
		Chlamydia	Also carriers	Urethra, rectum
		Gonorrhea	Also carriers	Urethra, rectum
		Syphilis	Moist surfaces	Urethra, placenta
1.6. Placental	Congenital	Syphilis	Up to 4th month of pregnancy	Blood
1.7. Umbilical	Direct contact	Neonatal tetanus	Poor birth hygiene	Cord
2. Animal sources	Infected animal	Anthrax	Tanning	Skin, respiratory
		Tularemia	Skinning, dressing	Skin, eyes
	Bite of tick	Rocky Mt. spotted fever, Lyme disease	Outdoor exposure	Skin
	Rat flea	Bubonic plague	Infected rat	Skin
	Infected placenta via air	Q fever	Cows	Respiratory
3. Inanimate sources	Soil, air, water, food	Tetanus	Wound, childbirth	Skin
		Legionnaires' disease	Warmth, humidity, water coolers, air conditioners, potable water supplies	Respiratory

[a]This table is representative only and does not include all organisms. RS, respiratory secretions.

7.3. Genital or Sexually Transmitted

The term *venereally transmitted* is now being limited to the five classic infections clearly transmitted by sexual intercourse (gonorrhea, syphilis, chancroid, lymphogranuloma venereum, and granuloma inguinale). The newer term, *sexually transmitted diseases* (STD), is broader, applies to both hetero- and homosexual activity, and encompasses all infections transmitted person to person during sexual activity. In recent years, *Chlamydia trachomatis* has been identified in this group as the cause of almost half of nongonorrheal urethritis (see Section 11.2.6 and Chapter 9), and *Ureaplasma* is under evaluation; enteric infections are of increasing importance in male homosexuals. The presence of ulcers due to STDs enhances the spread of HIV, especially a penile lesion from syphilis or herpes simplex.

7.4. Gastrointestinal or Fecal–Oral

The fecal–oral route of transmission is a close rival in frequency to respiratory spread and there are many sources of infection. A first group is called enteric fevers. Bacterial organisms from ill persons or carriers exit via the gastrointestinal tract to the external milieu for transmission via water, food, or direct contact to another individual. They constitute a major group of bacterial infections. The mouth is the common portal of entry. Some enteric infections involve only a human-to-human cycle, such as cholera, typhoid fever, and shigellosis. Others, such as salmonellosis, *Campylobacter* infections, and yersiniosis, also involve animal hosts. A variety of mechanisms may transmit the organism from the infectious stool to a susceptible person. Cholera is commonly transmitted by water, and on occasion by food (such as undercooked seafood like oysters and clams). Shigellosis is spread by the fecal route from patients or carriers and also be food, water, or flies. Typhoid fever is transmitted by food or water contaminated by the feces or urine from a patient or carrier and sometimes through contaminated shellfish or canned goods. *Salmonella* organisms are widely disseminated in nature and infect many domestic animals and birds, providing many potential sources of contamination of food and, less commonly, of water. *Campylobacter fetus* subsp. *jejuni* and *Yersinia enterocolitica* also infect many animals, including domestic ones such as puppies, and can infect exposed humans through direct contact or through water, milk, or food. For shigellosis, exposure to an infected human during the acute illness or shortly thereafter is the main source of infection; here, direct or indirect fecal–oral contact is usually more important than water or food. There is no extrahuman reservoir of infection.

A second group of gastrointestinal infections is called food poisoning. Here, contamination of food may occur from the feces of an infected person or carrier (food handler), but other sources of the organism are also common. The animal food source may be infected (i.e., *Salmonella* in chickens), or the organism may be present on the skin of the food handler (staphylococcus, streptococcus), in the environment (staphylococcus), in the soil (*C. perfringens*, *C. botulinum*), or in raw seafood (*V. parahemolyticus*).

The transmission of enteric fevers and food poisoning is largely preventable. A good source of water, proper chlorination or boiling, frequent hand washing, appropriate refrigeration of foods, and thorough cooking are effective ways of interrupting the chain of infection. However, in developing countries and low socioeconomic settings, neither the means nor the education to carry them out may be available. Some may be prevented by immunization. Transmission of enteric infections by homosexual activity is a newly recognized and important problem in this group, and infection in HIV-infected patients may result not only from a wide variety of usual pathogens such as *E. coli*, but also from organisms usually regarded as commensal and nonpathogenic such as the parasitic infection *Cryptosporidium*. However, this organism caused a massive outbreak related to the public water supply of the city of Milwaukee in normal hosts.[28] This organism and other related ones are able to pass through usual water filters and are highly resistant to the usual levels of control. Increased surveillance of their occurrence in wells and public water systems is currently being carried out in several states under the auspices of the CDC.

7.5. Urinary

Urinary spread of infection is not common, but may occur in typhoid fever from an infected person and in leptospirosis from many animal hosts. Water is the common vehicle of transmission.

7.6. Perinatal

These infections occur at the time of childbirth. In *congenital infections*, the organism is transmitted *vertically* from an infected mother via the placenta to the fetus. Congenital syphilis, rubella, and toxoplasmosis are examples of this. Infections may occur *horizontally* from an infected cervix to the baby as it passes through the birth canal, as in gonococcal ophthalmia and chlamydial infections. Infections may also be acquired immediately after birth, as exemplified by tetanus neonatorum due to contamination of the newly cut umbilical cord by soil or a contaminated substance applied to the umbilical stump.

7.7. Insect Vectors

Rocky Mountain spotted fever is transmitted by the bite of the tick, which may remain infective for a long time, and the infection is maintained in nature by transovarian and transstadial passage. A mite has been implicated as the means of transmission of rickettsialpox from infected house mice. The transmission of bubonic (sylvatic) plague is through the rat flea (mostly *Xenopsylla cheopis*) from infected wild rodents. *Borrelia burgdorferi*, the cause of Lyme disease, is transmitted by small ixoid ticks, such as the deer tick, *Ixodes dammini*.

8. Pathogenesis

A section on pathogenesis is included in every chapter of this volume that deals with specific infections. Only a few concepts will be presented here. An excellent book by Mims,[35] entitled *The Pathogenesis of Infectious Diseases*, should be consulted for details, as well as more recent articles by him[36] and others.[33,34] Recent texts of medical microbiology[32] and infectious diseases[38] also contain excellent discussions.

8.1. Localized or Superficial Infections

Many bacterial infections produce diseases through the cells with which they first come in contact in skin or epithelial surfaces and remain limited to that area. Tissue damage results from the direct action of the bacteria, microbial toxins, indirect injury, inflammation, or immunopathologic processes. Most bacteria have specific attachment sites on epithelial surfaces (see Section 4.2). Examples of localized infections include diphtheria and streptococcal infections of the throat, gonococcal infections of the conjunctiva or urethra, cholera, and most *Salmonella* infections of the intestine. Many gram-negative bacteria have a limited capacity to invade tissues and tend to remain localized; some are able to invade only in debilitated, malnourished, or immunocompromised patients. Host antibacterial forces limit the spread of many bacteria. At the subepithelial level, three important defense mechanisms are called into play: (1) tissue fluids, (2) the lymphatic system leading to the lymph nodes, and (3) phagocytic cells (macrophages) in tissues and polymorphonuclear cells in the blood. Each of these mechanisms depends on the inflammatory response for its action,[35] as manifested by four cardinal signs: *warmth* and *redness* due to vasodilatation, *swelling* (vasodilatation and exudate), and *pain* (tissue distention, pain mediators). Polymorphonuclear cells enter, as well as macrophages and lymphocytes; exudation occurs. Tissue fluids provide plasma proteins, including immunoglobulins, such as IgG, complement, and properdin. The primary mediators of inflammation include histamine, 5-hydroxytryptamine, and kinins. Prostaglandins E and F are thought to play a role in the termination of the response. Microorganisms in peripheral lymphatics are rapidly carried to lymph nodes, where they are exposed to macrophages lining the sinus that act as a bacterial filter. Here, too, polymorphs, serum factors accumulating during inflammation, and the initiation of the immune response limit the infection. The phagocytic cells play a key role in the interaction with microorganisms, ingesting and killing bacterial invaders. Among the chemotractant factors for phagocytosis are platelet activating factors, leukotriene B4, C5a, and certain formyl peptides.[33] The details are fully described by Mims,[32,36] as are the ways in which some bacteria are able to resist or interfere with phagocytic activity. Organisms that escape must still face one or two encounters with the macrophages, as well as other immune mechanisms, before successfully reaching the venous system.

8.2. Systemic Infections

Organisms that escape phagocytic cells and the other local defense mechanisms can spread through the tissues and, more distantly, via the lymphatics and the bloodstream. Some viruses (herpes, HIV, poxviruses, measles), some rickettsiae (*R. rickettsii*, *R. prowazekii*), and some bacteria (*Mycobacterium tuberculosis*, *M. leprae*, *Listeria monocytogenes*, *Brucella* spp., and *Legionella pneumophila*) actually multiply in macrophages. The toxins, enzymes, and surface components of bacteria that protect them against phagocytic destruction and promote invasiveness have been mentioned in Section 4. It is not clear what exact role the proteinases, collagenases, lipases, and nucleases produced by bacteria play in the pathogenesis of infection or which ones are related to nutritional and bacterial metabolism.

Lymphatic spread may occur from the lymph node, which serves not only as a focus of phagocytic and immune forces but also, if these fail, as a focus of dissemination. These results occur when the lymph flow rate is high from inflammation of tissues or from exercise of muscles, when the number of bacterial particles exceeds the filtration rate or the defense mechanisms of the node or both, and when phagocytic activity is impaired. In some instances, certain organisms such as *Pasteurella pestis* and brucellosis actually multiply in the lymph node and spread via efferent lymph channels. In other instances, vigorous inflammatory responses localize the infection, and the node becomes a graveyard of dead and damaged bacteria and of tissue cells.

Bloodstream or *hematogenous spread* is the most effective mechanism for the dissemination of an infection throughout the body. Bacteria may exist free in the plasma (pneumococci, *B. anthracis*, *Leptospira*), intracellularly in monocytes (*Listeria*, tubercle and leprosy bacilli, *Brucella*), or in association with polymorphonuclear cells (many pyogenic bacteria). The *bacteremia* may be transient and with little or no systemic response, as follows dental extraction in a healthy person; even a continuous bacteremia may exist with few toxic signs, as in leprosy where the organism exists in large numbers inside blood monocytes. On the other hand, severe systemic manifestations may accompany the presence of large numbers of organisms in the blood such as the pneumococcus, meningococcus, or group A *Streptococcus pyogenes*. This is called a *septicemia*. Bacteria may succeed in setting up foci of infection in areas where the blood flow is slow enough, or they may establish multiplication in sites previously damaged by disease or injury, such as *Streptococcus viridans* on abnormal heart valves producing subacute bacterial endocarditis; or staphylococci in the traumatized long bones of children may lead to osteomyelitis. Depending on the site of the infection, the liver and lung may receive many organisms during bacterial invasion of the bloodstream. The lung, liver, spleen, and bone marrow may also serve as important foci of dissemination of organisms, as in brucellosis, leptospirosis, and typhoid fever. Rashes accompany the dissemination of many viral and some bacterial infections to the skin. They may result from localization and growth of the organism in small blood vessels, producing thrombosis, infarction, and hemorrhage as in the rickettsial diseases, Rocky Mountain spotted fever, and typhus, as well as the petechial and purpuric lesions of meningococcemia. Immunopathologic processes involving sensitized lymphocytes, antibodies, and immune complexes play a role in many rashes, especially viral. A bacterial toxin may induce the rash as in scarlet fever. Some organisms such as *Treponema pallidum* in secondary syphilis extravasate from blood vessels and multiply in extravascular tissues. This results in highly infectious lesions that discharge to the exterior. Dissemination of *T. pallidum* to the blood–fetal junction in the placenta during pregnancy may result in infection of the fetus; slow blood flow in the placenta may contribute to this possibility.

Central nervous system (CNS) and meningeal involvement can occur by bloodstream carriage of the organism to the blood–cerebrospinal fluid junctions in the meninges or choroid plexus; from there, passive transport occurs into the flow of fluid from ventricles to subarachnoid spaces and throughout the CNS. Examples of bacteria that traverse this barrier and produce meningitis are the meningococcus, tubercle bacillus, *L. monocytogenes*, and *H. influenzae*. Actual spread along peripheral nerves has been shown for rabies and herpesviruses and is the means of centripetal passage of tetanus toxin.[45]

9. Incubation Period

The period of time from exposure to a source of infection to the first signs or symptoms of clinical illness is called the incubation period (IP). It varies with (1) the nature and dosage of the organism; (2) the portal of entry; (3) the type of the infection (localized or systemic); (4) the mechanism responsible for tissue injury (invasion, toxin, immunopathologic process); (5) the immune status of the host, being prolonged in the presence of partial immunity; and (6) other unknown factors individual to the host. The IP has many uses in epidemiology: (1) it helps define the etiologic agent in an epidemic; (2) it helps differentiate common-source from propagated epidemics and to identify the reservoir and/or source of the agent; (3) it delineates the period for which a person exposed to an infection is at risk to development of disease; (4) it assists in identifying the period of infectiousness; (5) it provides a guide to the possible effectiveness of active or passive immunization; and (6) it gives clues to the pathogenesis of the disease.

The IPs of common bacterial diseases are given in Fig. 2. Signs and symptoms due to preformed toxins or associated with food poisoning usually occur within 36 h after ingestion, sometimes as soon as 2–4 h, as in diarrhea due to *Bacillus cereus* or staphylococcal contamination of food. Traveler's diarrhea due to toxigenic *E. coli* has an IP of 12–72 h. Pontiac fever, the term used to describe an acute febrile disease without pneumonia recognized first in the Pontiac, Michigan, health department clinic and due to *Legionella pneumophila*, has a peak IP of 36 h, as compared to a peak IP of 5 days for Legionnaires' disease (pneumonia). It is not known whether this difference is due to a larger number of organisms inhaled in Pontiac fever (unlikely because of the comparative mildness of the disease), to dead organisms, or to some other factor.

Diseases due to direct involvement of epithelial surfaces have relatively short IPs, often under a week, such as streptococcal sore throat, bacterial pneumonias, shigellosis, cholera, gonorrhea, and chancroid. This is not invariably true, since diphtheria and pertussis both tend to have an IP of over a week, sometimes up to 3 weeks, and *M. pneumoniae* pneumonia has an IP of 2–3 weeks. These organisms may be less pathogenic. Diseases with longer

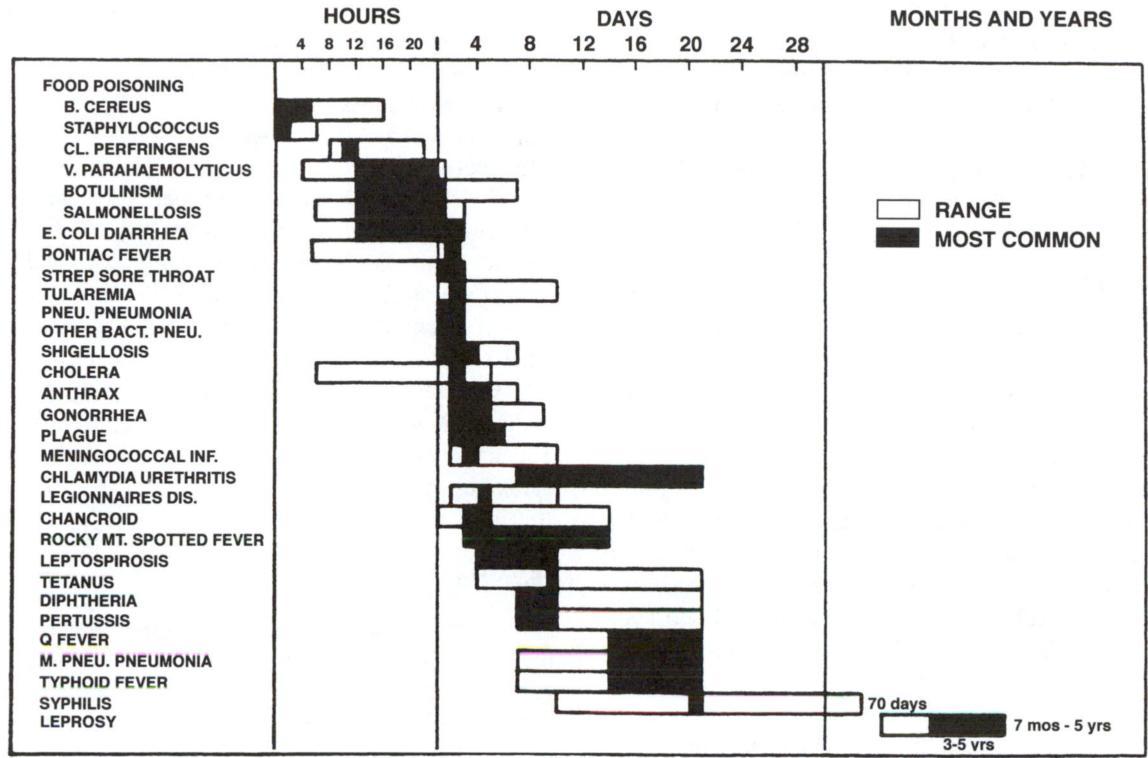

Figure 2. Incubation periods of common bacterial diseases. Derived from *Control of Communicable Diseases in Man*.[17]

incubation periods in the range of 2–3 weeks include systemic infections such as typhoid fever and brucellosis. The IP of syphilis most commonly is 3 weeks, although it may be as short as 10 days. Leprosy has an extremely long IP of 7 months to over 5 years.

10. Immune Response

A concomitant requirement for the evolution of multicellular life-forms was the development of methods for assuring the integrity of self. In the absence of the ability to recognize and cull out foreign cells, multicellularity could not have succeeded as a strategy. The mammalian immune system is probably the most sophisticated antimicrobial defense in nature and represents the culmination of a billion-plus years of evolutionary refinement to the methodology of discriminating self from nonself.

Defense against microorganisms takes place at several levels in mammals. The term *innate immunity* refers to various features of an animal that confer natural resistance to invasion by microbes. These include physical barriers such as the skin and mucous membranes, chemical barriers (e.g., skin pH, lysozyme in saliva and tears), and the symbiotic bacterial flora of an animal that discourage colonization by pathogenic microbes.

Nonspecific immunity involves those processes in the immune response that do not react to specific individual foreign bodies and materials (antigens), but react to all foreign antigens with more or less equal vigor. The nonspecific immune system includes phagocytic cells, such as macrophages and polymorphonuclear neutrophils, the complement system, natural killer cells, cytokines such as the interferons and tumor necrosis factors, eosinophils, and basophils.

The third component of mammalian immunity is *antigen-specific immunity* or *adaptive immunity*. It is this component that appears to be unique among the vertebrates. Orchestrated by the lymphocytes, antigen-specific immunity recognizes foreign antigen in a highly specific fashion, expanding and activating only that subset of lymphocytes that can directly recognize and engage that precise antigen and no other. One of the most remarkable features of the antigen-specific immune system is the breadth of its capacity: The mature human immune system has been estimated to have the ability to respond discreetly to as many as a billion different antigens.

What follows is a very cursory overview of the components of the human immune system. For readers interested in more in-depth coverage, consult the general textbooks by Paul[46] or Kuby.[47]

10.1. Nonspecific Immunity

Nonspecific immunity plays numerous critical roles in the immune system. Many of the cells involved in nonspecific immunity participate in inflammatory responses and include macrophages, neutrophils, eosinophils, basophils, and mast cells. Overt tissue injury, whether caused by physical insult or invasion by a pathogen, stimulates the release of chemotactic factors that promote the migration and accumulation of various inflammatory cells at the damage site. Macrophages and neutrophils, particularly when activated by T-cell cytokines such as interferon-γ (IFN-γ), interleukin-4 (IL-4), and granulocyte–monocyte colony–stimulating factor (GM-CSF), are aggressively phagocytic cells. In the earliest phases of an infection, these cells serve to destroy bacteria and viruses and to mop up any debris, such as dead cells. Eosinophils are poorly phagocytic but are prominent in parasitic lesions, where they may be triggered to release a potent cocktail of enzymes and chemicals that destroy infecting parasites. Basophils and mast cells also have roles in immunity to parasites, but more as facilitators for the accumulation of other cells into a lesion.

Complement is a conglomeration of interacting proteins present in the bloodstreams of all vertebrates that have several important roles in nonspecific immunity. Various components of activated complement can promote and regulate inflammation, enhance phagocytosis through improved binding between the phagocyte and its target, and directly mediate cytotoxicity against cells and microbes. Several cleavage products of the complement activation cascade (C3a, C5a) have chemotactic and vasodilatory activity. A cleavage product of complement component C3, termed C3b, binds to specific receptors on macrophages and has lectinlike binding affinity for many bacteria, thus promoting opsonization. Complement activation culminates with the production of cannuluslike pores that self-insert into cell membranes (including those of bacteria), leading to colloid osmotic lysis.

Natural killer (NK) cells are a population of large granular lymphocytes that lack a receptor for specific antigen. They have a role in the immune surveillance of tumor cells, and are capable of destroying their target cells by inducing apoptosis or programmed cell death.

Nonspecific immunity often serves to delay the progression of infection until the adaptive arms of the immune system have time to respond more specifically and effectively. Nonspecific immune mechanism are also frequently enhanced through the formation of partnerships with components of adaptive immunity. For example, specific antibodies may bind through specialized receptors to the surface of phagocytic cells, thus conferring antigen specificity to cells that otherwise have none. Cytokines secreted through the antigen-driven activation of T cells may enhance the level of activity of phagocytic cells or direct them to migrate to the site where they are needed. The activity of NK cells may also be enhanced by T-cell cytokines, particularly IL-2.

10.2. Humoral Immunity

There are two compartments of the immune system that are capable of responding specifically to foreign antigens. Humoral immunity, mediated by antibody molecules, is generated by B lymphocytes. Mature B lymphocytes bear specific receptors for antigen on their surface; the receptor on each circulating naive B lymphocyte is different from that of all others, and each lymphocyte has one and only one specificity for an antigen. The receptor on the B lymphocyte is the immunoglobulin, or antibody, molecule itself, and upon activation, copies of this antibody are actively secreted. Since only those B lymphocytes that bind specifically with the antigens of a given bacterium or virus will be activated, the population of secreted antibodies that results is also specific for the invading pathogen.

With one limited exception, B-cell activation is absolutely dependent on the participation of T lymphocytes, which provide helper activity in the form of cytokines. T-cell cytokines are required for the activation of the B cell, for its differentiation into a plasma cell (the antibody secreting cell), and for its proliferation (required to maximize the production of specific antibody). T-cell-derived cytokines also direct the class of antibody molecule that a B cell will ultimately produce.

Five distinct classes or *isotypes* of antibody molecules are found in the mammalian immune system, each of which has distinct roles in antimicrobial defense:

1. *IgM* has at least two important roles in humoral immunity. In monomeric form, it is expressed on the surface of all mature, naive B lymphocytes and serves as the receptor for antigen on those cells. In the circulation,

IgM occurs as a pentamer, with five identical subunit antibodies bound together by a protein called J chain. IgM is the predominant antibody produced during the first exposure to an antigen. In serum, pentameric IgM has the highest binding avidity of any of the isotypes of immunoglobulin. It is extremely efficient at agglutinating bacteria and is an excellent opsonin, promoting phagocytosis by macrophages and neutrophils. In addition, IgM is the most effective antibody at activating complement.

2. *IgG* is the most abundant immunoglobulin in serum, making up 75% of the total serum antibody. It is the predominant antibody produced in a secondary, or anamnestic immune response. Four distinct subclasses of IgG are recognized. All four subclasses of IgG can activate the complement cascade, although with widely different efficiencies. In addition, specific receptors for the constant region of all four IgG subclasses have been identified on a variety of cell types, including macrophages, mast cells, neutrophils, and lymphocytes. The combination of antibody with these other cell types either confers opsonic capacity or leads (in the presence of specific antigen) to the release of mediators. On lymphocytes, the binding of immunoglobulin molecules to such receptors appears to have regulatory functions, such as switching off the secretion of antibody. IgG is the only immunoglobulin that is capable of crossing the placenta, a process that is mediated by a specific receptor for IgG located on placental cells. In addition to its other activities, IgG is the most important neutralizing antibody in the serum, by virtue of its relative abundance.

3. *IgA* is the principal antibody found in local secretions. IgA antibody can be found in tears, saliva, milk, sweat, lungs, nasal passages, the urogenital tract, and the gut. IgA plays a crucial role in the defense of mucosal surfaces, neutralizing bacteria and viruses at local mucosa before they have an opportunity to invade. The presence of large quantities of IgA antibody in milk and colostrum enables the efficient transfer of maternal humoral immunity to newborn infants. IgA is incapable of fixing complement. It serves primarily as an agglutinating and neutralizing antibody.

IgA in local secretions occurs as a dimer, bound by J chain. IgA transport to local mucosa is mediated by a molecule called the secretory piece, produced by cells adjacent to mucosal sites. IgA associates with the secretory piece on the cell surface and is endocytosed, transported across the cytoplasm, and deposited at local mucosa.

4. *IgE* makes up less than 0.01% of the total serum antibody. IgE is best recognized for its role in mediating immediate-type hypersensitivity, caused by the degranulation of mast cells and basophils in various mucosal tissues. IgE has an important role in the response against parasites. The purpose of the release of vasoactive substances when IgE bound to the surface of a mast cell or basophil encounters antigen is to enhance the accessibility of neutrophils and eosinophils, serum IgG, and complement to the site of parasitic infection.

5. *IgD* has no direct role in mediating defense against infectious diseases. It is present, together with monomeric IgM, on the surface of all naive B lymphocytes and appears to have a role in primary B lymphocyte activation.

10.3. Cell-Mediated Immunity

The second compartment of antigen-specific immunity is cell-mediated immunity (CMI). It is mediated by T lymphocytes. T cells are superficially indistinguishable from B cells. The T-cell receptor for antigen is structurally similar to the B-cell receptor, and yet the two cell types recognize specific antigen in fundamentally different ways. B cells recognize intact antigen and respond with the production of molecules that bear an exact copy of the surface receptor's binding site. T cells have no capacity for recognizing intact antigen. To engage a T-cell receptor, antigen first must be processed into small peptides, which are then inserted into the binding cleft of a major histocompatibility (MHC) antigen. The MHC antigens are a highly polymorphic family of dual polypeptide proteins, at least some of which are expressed on nearly every cell type in the body. Because there are at least several hundred allelic variants of MHC antigens, and because no human being can express more than 12 different variants (up to two each of six different subclasses), the likelihood of two randomly selected individuals expressing the same panel of MHC antigens is remote in the extreme. Thus, the MHC antigens expressed by an individual to a very large extent define the property of self. This is particularly true for T cells. During the process of maturation in the thymus, nascent T cells undergo a rigorous selection process, and only cells displaying an antigen receptor that has a weak binding affinity for one or more self-MHC antigens are permitted to complete their differentiation into mature T cells. Cells with no affinity for self and cells with too strong an affinity, i.e., strong enough to activate a T cell on its own, are destroyed. When a foreign peptide is inserted into the cleft of an MHC molecule, its affinity is altered. A small number of T cells, perhaps one in half a million, will bind to this altered MHC with a high enough affinity to activate. Thus, T cells are able to recognize and respond to minute changes in the normal display of self, as represented by an individuals unique collection of MHC molecules.

There are two general effector mechanisms for CMI. The first, cytotoxic T-cell-mediated lysis, is mediated primarily by the subset of T cells that express the protein CD8 on their surfaces. These T cells are restricted to their recognition of foreign peptide on the surface of a class I MHC molecule, which are present on most of the body's cells. Once activated, these cells recognize their specific combination of foreign peptide and MHC on a target cell and have two methods for dispatching the target. The first involves the deposition of perforin pores, which bear a striking resemblance to the terminal complement complex, onto the surface of the cell. The second approach is to induce apoptosis in the target, directing the cell to essentially commit suicide. Both processes result in the destruction of the target cell. Cytotoxic T lymphocytes (CTL), by virtue of their ability to discern the presence of foreign peptides from microbial pathogens inside of a cell, are ideally suited for the elimination of intracellular parasites such as viruses. They are also considered to have an important role in the elimination of tumor cells.

Another CMI mechanism is mediated primarily by the other main subpopulation of T cells, those that express the protein CD4 on their surface. These T cells are restricted in their recognition of foreign peptides on class II MHC molecules. Class II MHC antigens are normally expressed on only a few populations of cells in the body, chiefly B cells, macrophages, and dendritic cells. All of these cell types are capable antigen-presenting cells, since $CD4^+$ T cells also have the central role in the regulation of T-cell responses, the limited expression of class II antigens in the body is thought to reflect a safety restraint aimed at limiting the responsiveness of immune cells. In addition to providing helper activity to both B and T cells, $CD4^+$ T cells are typically recruited to the site of tissue damage and infection, where they coordinate and amplify the effectiveness of both specific and nonspecific arms of the immune system.

10.4. Cellular Interaction in Immune Responses

The immune system is arrayed with an arsenal of weapons capable of causing colossal destruction of tissues if left unchecked. While it provides an invaluable service in the defense against microbial invasion and the spontaneous development of neoplastic cells, extremely tight controls are required to ensure that its activities do not escalate to the point where they become deleterious to the host. As such, the level of intercellular interaction in the immune system is extraordinarily high. As mentioned previously, B-cell responses are generally not possible in the absence of T-cell help. If specific cytokines, such as IL-2 for proliferation, are not made available to the antigen-stimulated B cell, a suboptimal response will result. The generation of T-cell help, in turn, is absolutely dependent on the presence of a suitable antigen-presenting-cell-bearing peptide on a class II MHC antigen. Thus, the participation of at least three different cell types is required to mount an effective immunoglobulin response to antigen. Similarly, a CTL response requires the participation of both a helper T cell and an antigen-presenting T cell for the activation of both T-cell help and the naive CTL.

These cellular interactions take place in at least two ways. Transmembrane surface proteins on both participating cell types may come into direct physical contact, potentially sending an activation signal across the cytoplasmic membrane into both cells. An alternative unidirectional signaling method is to produce soluble hormonelike proteins known as cytokines, that bind to a specific ligand on their target cell and send an activation signal across the membrane. A large number of cytokines has been identified and characterized, and each cytokine typically has more than one activity, often depending on the type of cell it engages.

Cellular interactions are not limited to the activation of immune responses. When a threat to bodily integrity has been eliminated, there is no continued need for a response. The action of down-regulating immune responses is termed *immune suppression*. T cells are also the critical regulators for immune suppression. Many of these functions of immune regulation appear to be performed by discreet subpopulations of specialized T cells. At last count, there are at least several functionally distinct subsets of helper T cells, a similar number of suppressor T cells, and so forth. In addition, functionality among T cells does not appear to be set in stone. There are circumstances in which $CD4^+$ T cells perform cytotoxic function and population of $CD8^+$ T cells that serve various regulatory functions. Thus, the complexity of interaction among cells in the human immune system is quite high, and a meaningful discussion of the current, admittedly limited, level of understanding of those interactions is beyond the scope of this overview. Suffice it to say that, under ordinary circumstances, these interactions serve as a system of controls that ensure the immune system will mount a transient, surgical strike against any disease threat.

Occasionally, elements of the interregulatory network break down, sometimes leading to autoimmune disease, a condition in which the immune system causes damage to various host tissues. Such diseases include type

I diabetes, rheumatoid arthritis, and systemic lupus erythematosus. Autoimmune diseases run the gamut from chronic disabling conditions to life-threatening diseases.

10.5 The Generation of Diversity in Antigen Recognition

The immune system presents a great enigma that was a matter of pure philosophical speculation until only two decades ago. Namely, how does the body go about the business of preparing a population of cells, each of which bears a distinct receptor for one of as many as a billion different antigens, none of which it has ever seen before? The two extremes of the philosophical argument went as follows: (1) One's genetic material contains the information required to encode all one billion different specificities for foreign antigen, and selects from that collection of genes in a random fashion; and (2) the genetic material encodes for only a few antigen receptor genes and the rest of the diversity results from extraordinarily high rates of mutation. The interesting feature of these two "obvious" solutions to the enigma is that neither of them came terribly close to the truth.

Immunoglobulin genes and T-cell receptor genes are arranged in clusters of subsegments, as shown in the illustration of an immunoglobulin heavy chain gene map (Fig. 3). The immunoglobulin genes and T-cell receptor genes are assembled from randomly selected segments into a single functional gene. The construction of variable region (which encodes the antigen binding site) of a heavy chain gene, for example, would involve the co-alignment of one of approximately 1000 V gene segments, with one of four J-segment genes and one of 12 D-segment genes. This results in $1000 \times 4 \times 12 = 48{,}000$ possible heavy chain variable gene segments. The various segments are aligned through intrachain recombination events. Recombinational diversity for the immunoglobulin light chains is somewhat more limited, providing for approximately 1,000 different light chain variable genes. Since every functional antibody molecule is made up of two identical light chains and two identical heavy chains, the number of different combinations becomes $1{,}000 \times 48{,}000$ or 480,000. Added to that is the fact that the junction sites between V, J, and D segments vary, leading to junctional diversity due to single base substitutions and even short frame shifts. Finally, the mutation rate in the immunoglobulin gene cluster is approximately fivefold that of normal mutation rates. All of this is estimated to provide potential for diversity in the antibody population on the order of a billion different specificities. The T-cell receptors rearrange similarly.

11. Patterns of Host Response

The clinician usually deals with persons already ill with an infectious disease severe enough for them to seek medical care. The epidemiologist must study not only those clinically ill but also the full range of host responses that follow infection. These can vary quantitatively from

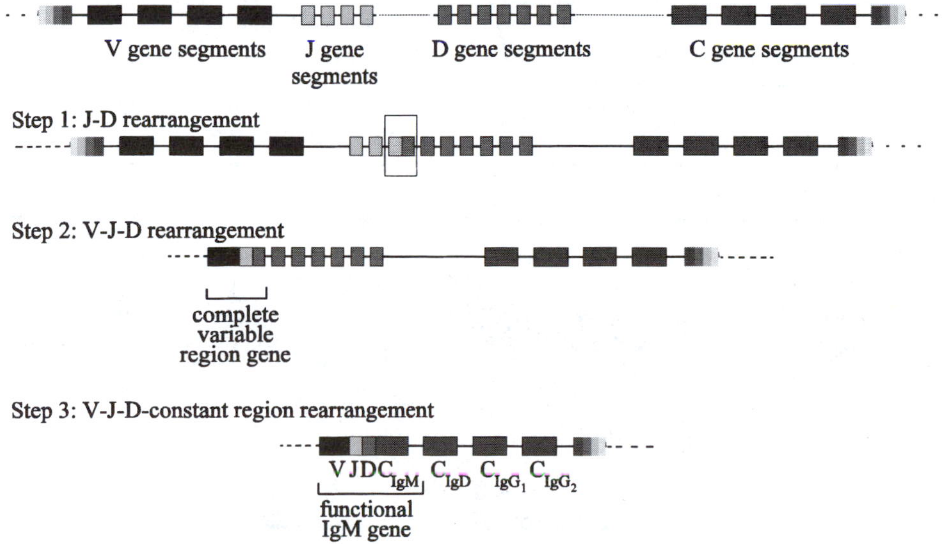

Figure 3. Immunoglobulin heavy chain gene cluster.

inapparent infection to severe illness to death in what is called a *biological gradient.* They can also vary qualitatively in different signs and symptoms that make up different clinical syndromes. The detection of persons with inapparent or subclinical infection requires laboratory tests to detect the presence of antibody or antigen.

11.1. Biological Gradient

When a susceptible host is exposed to a source of infection, a wide range of quantitative responses may occur.[4] These are often depicted as an iceberg, as shown in Fig. 4, with the largest number of responses occurring subclinically, below the waterline of clinical recognition. The right side of Fig. 4 represents the responses of the host. These range subclinically from exposure without successful attachment or multiplication of the bacterial organism, to colonization without tissue injury, to infection that evokes a host immune response but no clinical disease. The existence of these inapparent events can be recognized only by laboratory means such as isolation of the organism or measurement of the immune response. In viral infections, the ratio of inapparent–apparent (subclinical–clinical) infection has been determined through prospective studies correlating the number with an antibody response to the number clinically ill. The occurrence of inapparent infections is also suggested in persons with antibody but no history of clinical disease. Some information has also come from the rate of secondary infection in families with an index case and from volunteer studies. This type of information is not available for many bacterial infections because serological techniques are not as useful and/or widely employed in measuring infection rates, but a few examples may be cited. In leptospirosis, serological tests of persons heavily exposed (veterinarians, abattoir workers) but without known illness have shown an antibody prevalence of 16%. This suggests that only 16 of 100 exposed persons have been infected as manifested by an antibody response. There are no data for leptospirosis indicating the subclinical–clinical ratio, but of those clinically ill, 90% or so have an acute, self-limited illness without jaundice and with good prognosis; the overall case-fatality rate in 791 cases reported to the CDC from 1965 to 1974 was 7.7% (see Chapter 20). In tuberculosis, it was estimated that of the 50,000 clinical cases reported in 1963, 80% came from the 24 million infected in previous years and 20% from persons infected the same year (see Chapter 39).

In summary, a wide range of quantitative and qualitative responses can occur on exposure to a pathogenic organism. The determinants of this pattern lie both in the pathogenicity and virulence of the infecting organism (see

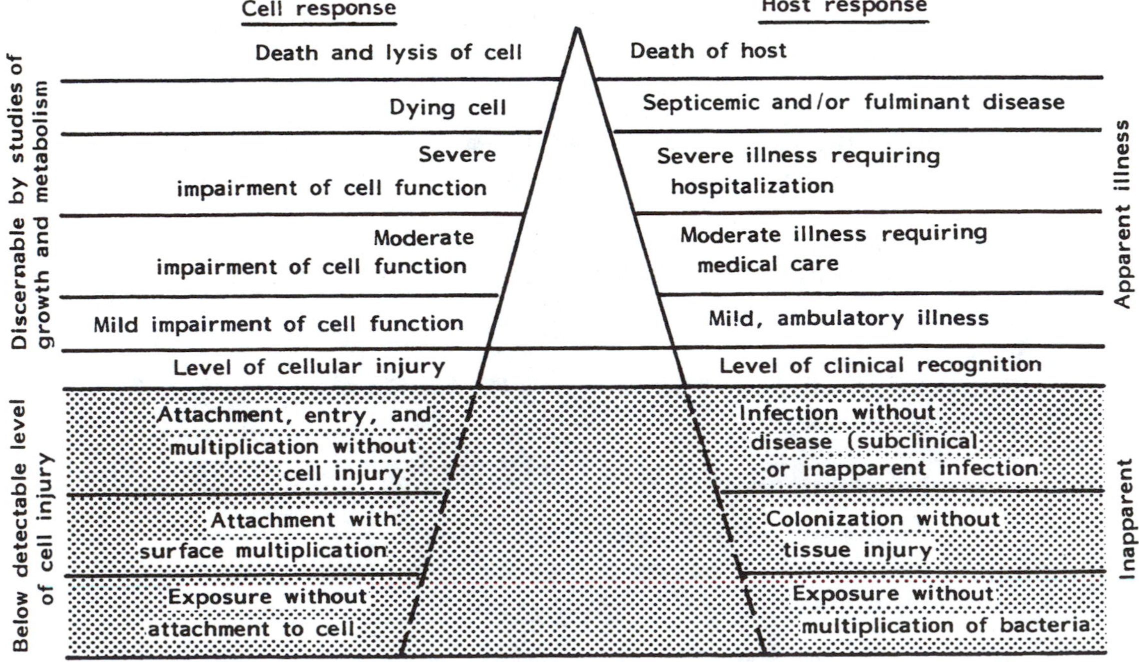

Figure 4. Biological spectrum of response to bacterial infection at the cellular level (left) and of the intact host (right).

Section 4) and in the age, genetic makeup, immune response, portal of entry, and other characteristics of the host (see Section 6).

The left side of Fig. 4 is a simplistic expression of the response to bacterial infection at the cellular level. Cell injury may result from enzymes and other metabolic products of bacteria, from toxins produced by them, from entry and multiplication of the organisms intracellularly, as with *M. tuberculosis*, *M. leprae*, *B. abortus*, or as a consequence of the phagocytic and immunologic defense mechanisms induced by the infection. Epidemiologically, the message is that most organisms do not result in cell dysfunction or death and that the healthy person lives in symbiosis with millions of bacteria.

11.2. Clinical Syndromes

The host can show qualitative as well as quantitative differences in response to the same bacterial infection. These qualitative responses are manifested by different clinical syndromes, the patterns of which depend on the portal of entry of the organism, age of the host at the time of infection, immune status, and other factors. This variation is not as great with bacterial infections as with viral infections. Many bacterial infections such as anthrax, cholera, diphtheria, leprosy, pertussis, tetanus, tularemia, and typhoid fever present with fairly characteristic clinical features that vary quantitatively, but not qualitatively, from host to host, and a diagnosis can often be made on clinical grounds alone. Others, such as streptococcal infections, leptospirosis, syphilis, tuberculosis, and Lyme disease, may involve different tissues and organs in different persons, resulting in different clinical presentations, often depending on the site of infection and the age group involved. On the other hand, there are many clinical syndromes of diverse cause in which etiologic diagnosis is difficult on clinical grounds alone. It is here that epidemiological probabilities will help clinical judgment. Infections of mucosal and serosal surfaces fall into this category because of the limited spectrum of local responses that can result. These can involve the meninges, respiratory tract, intestinal tract, urinary system, and urethra. Invasion of the bloodstream (septicemia) by different bacteria also invokes a common group of signs and symptoms that may be difficult to differentiate etiologically.

This section will present some of the common causes of these clinical syndromes that may vary with the age of the person at the time of infection. Knowing the most common causes in a given age group may help to establish a tentative diagnosis and to initiate proper treatment.

11.2.1. Infections of the CNS. Meningitis is a common clinical syndrome caused by bacteria, viruses, fungi, and protozoa. The clues that suggest bacterial infections are polymorphonuclear leukocytosis in blood and cerebrospinal fluid (CSF) (500–20,000/mm^3), low CSF glucose concentrations (usually <35 mg/100 ml or CSF–serum ratio ≤ 0.5), elevated CSF protein (80–500 mg/100 ml), and in about 75%, the presence of bacteria in the Gram-stained smear of a centrifuged sample of CSF. These findings characterize purulent meningitis, but may be altered by treatment with antibiotics so that they resemble nonpurulent bacterial infections, such as *M. tuberculosis* and leptospirosis, or viral meningitis. The etiologic agents that produce meningitis in different age groups will vary some by geographic area, year, and socioeconomic level.

The age-specific incidence per 100,000 of various types of meningitis by age group is presented in Table 9 from an excellent review article on the diagnosis and management of meningitis by Klein *et al.*,[48] which incor-

Table 9. Annual Age-Specific Incidence of Meningitis, United States, 1978 to 1981[a]

Age	*Neisseria meningitidis*	*Haemophilus influenzae*	*Streptococcus pneumoniae*	Group B *streptococcus*	*Listeria monocytogenes*	Total meningitis
<1 mo	2.0	6.7	3.5	44.6	7.6	99.5
1–2 mo	9.1	18.6	5.7	10.0	1.3	56.7
3–5 mo	11.5	52.0	11.6	1.4	0.1	83.3
6–8 mo	10.6	65.1	8.0	0.3	0	88.4
9–11 mo	7.9	48.1	4.7	0	0.1	63.3
1–2 yr	3.8	19.0	1.5			25.3
3–4 yr	1.8	3.9	0.5			6.8
5–9 yr	0.7	0.7	0.3			2.0
10–19 yr	0.6	0.1	0.1			1.0

[a]Results are reported as numbers of children with meningitis per 100,000 population. Data were provided by C. V. Broome, Centers for Disease Control, Atlanta, and by Schlech *et al.*[49] From Ref. 48.

porates data from the CDC and a National Surveillance Study by Schlech *et al.*[49] The overall incidence of meningitis is highest in the newborn, drops in the first 2 months of life, and then rises to high levels between 3 and 8 months of life. Based on a National Surveillance Study of 18,642 cases reported from 1973 to 1981, *H. influenzae* accounted overall for 48.3% of the cases, *N. meningitis* for 19.3%, and *S. pneumoniae* for 13.3%, totaling 81%.[49] Rates in males exceeded females (3.3 vs. 2.6 per 100,000). By age, the most common causes were as follows: in the newborn, group B streptococcus and *E. coli*; in infants, *H. influenzae* type b and *N. meningitidis*; in toddlers, similar to the newborn; and in schoolchildren and adolescents, *S. pneumoniae*, *N. meningitidis*, and *H. influenzae* are the major pathogens in the decreased number of cases in that age group. An analysis of 493 episodes in 1993 of bacterial meningitis in hospitalized adults over 16 years of age in a Boston hospital from 1962–1988 revealed that 40% were of nosocomial origin with a mortality of 35%.[50] The risk factors included age ⩾ 60 years, obtunded mental state on admission, and seizures within the first 24 h. Gram-negative bacilli (other than *H. influenzae*) caused 33% of these episodes. Of 296 community-acquired meningitis cases, *S. pneumoniae* accounted for 37%, *N. meningitides* for 13%, and *Listeriae monocytogenes* for 10%. Only 4% of all episodes were due to *H. influenzae*.[50]

The characteristics of the organisms involved and the patterns of disease can be found in the individual chapters of this book. Suffice it to mention here that in the newborn, most cases of group B streptococci are due to subtype III, and that infection usually arises from vaginal and rectal infections of the mother that can lead to a 40–70% infection rate in the newborn; the K1 antigen of *E. coli* is involved in 75% of neonatal meningitis, and *L. monocytogenes* is becoming increasingly important in meningitis in this age group in several areas of the country.[48] In children beyond the newborn period, head trauma may precede the onset of meningitis and organisms may then enter through the cribiform plate or the paranasal sinuses. Meningitis may also follow neurosurgical procedures or osteomyelitis of the skull or vertebral column.

Acute bacterial meningitis is a medical emergency, and it is most important to establish the identity of the infecting organisms as quickly as possible as a guide to antibiotic therapy. However, until this is done, a Gram-stained smear of the CSF should provide a reasonable basis for initial chemotherapy.

11.2.2. Acute Respiratory Infections. These represent the commonest causes of morbidity in the developed world. Their importance as a cause of both morbidity and mortality in developing countries has now been recognized, and major programs of control have been initiated under the auspices of the WHO. In developing countries, it is estimated that over 4.5 million children under the age of 5 years die annually of acute respiratory tract infections (ARI), which represents some 30% of the 14 million deaths in this age group yearly.[51–54] The commonest causes are *S. pneumoniae* (see chapter 34) and *H. influenzae* (see Chapter 16). A study of respiratory infections in children age 0–59 months in several different developing countries revealed rates of 12.7–16.8 new episodes of ARI per 100 child-weeks at risk and 0.2–3.4 for lower respiratory tract infections.[55] Case management intervention strategies using community health workers have helped reduce the mortality, but many gaps remain in our understanding of the etiology, epidemiology, and pathogenesis of these conditions.

Fewer than 10% of acute upper respiratory infections (AURIs) are due to bacteria in either developed or developing countries, although in the latter, infections with *Bordetella pertussis* (see Chapter 26) and *M. pneumoniae* (see Chapter 24) are important in certain settings. The syndrome of epiglottis in children aged 6 months to 2 years (up to age 6), however, is due to a bacterial pathogen, *H. influenzae* type b in about 90% of cases worldwide. This is often a serious and fulminant infection with a high mortality. A vaccine is now available.

The viruses involved in AURIs in both developing and developed countries are respiratory syncytial virus (RSV) in children under 3 years of age, parainfluenza in older children, and coronaviruses, rhinoviruses, and influenza in all ages.

The syndrome of acute pharyngitis and tonsillitis is due to streptococcal infections, mostly group A, in about one fourth to one third of cases, another one third are due to various viruses, and the remainder are of unidentified cause, although chlamydial infections may play a role in some of these.[56,57] Streptococcal infections can lead to acute rheumatic fever; this disease had been disappearing rapidly in developed countries until very recently when a recrudescence was reported in several areas of the United States. A very invasive streptococcal group A infection producing a toxic shocklike syndrome has recently been described in several parts of the world[58,59] (see Chapter 38). In developing countries, some 1.2 episodes of rheumatic fever are said to occur for every 1000 untreated streptococcal infections, but this, too, seems to be decreasing.[52] *Corynebacterium diphtheriae* (see Chapter 13) is also a cause of exudative tonsillitis in some Third World countries, and a recent outbreak occurred in Sweden involving 17 cases and 3 deaths despite very high immunization coverage.[60]

Acute lower respiratory infections are due mostly to viruses in young children, except for infants, to *M. pneumoniae* and viruses in young adults and to bacterial pathogens in older adults and the elderly. Prospective studies in community settings of developed countries suggest that five agents—RSV, parainfluenza virus, influenza virus, adenovirus, and *M. pneumoniae*—account for some 80% of acute lower respiratory infections in these population groups.[52]

Common respiratory syndromes in young children such as croup, laryngotracheitis, and bronchiolitis are usually due to viruses, especially RSV and parainfluenza viruses. Diphtheria may also cause a croup syndrome when the toxic membrane involves the larynx. Acute bronchitis is most often due to a variety of viral infections, but bacteria such as *M. pneumoniae*, *Bordetella pertussis*, and *Chlamydia trachomatis* (TWAR strain) may also produce this syndrome. Chronic bronchitis, on the other hand, is largely associated with nontypable *H. influenzae* and pneumococci (*S. pneumoniae*).

Pneumonia is the sixth most common cause of death in the United States and has varied causes at varied ages. In infancy (under 6 months), about 30% are now recognized as chlamydial and present as a gradually developing nontoxic illness with cough, pulmonary congestion, rales, and patchy infiltrates on X ray (see Chapter 10). Chlamydial genital infection of the mother carries a 10–20% risk of pneumonia in her infant. In another study of 205 infants under 3 months old hospitalized with pneumonitis, Brasfield *et al.*[61] identified a causal agent in 70%. *C. trachomatis* was found in 36%, RSV in 23%, cytomegalovirus in 20%, *Pneumocystis carinii* in 17%, and *Ureaplasma urealyticum* in 16%. In older children, the causes of pneumonitis and pneumonia are roughly one fourth viral, one third unknown cause, and the rest bacterial. More careful bacteriological culturing techniques have identified a bacterial etiology in 15–50% of this age group: pneumococci (*S. pneumoniae*) are the most common organism, and *H. influenzae* next most common; rarely, *Staphylococcus aureus* and group A streptococci are involved.

A review of the bacteriological aspirates in children with pneumonia from many countries revealed a bacterial agent in 62% of 1029 cases: *H. influenzae* and *S. pneumoniae* accounted for 54% of all isolates, while *S. aureus* was responsible for 17%.[52] Viral infections were associated with 17–40% of pneumonia in hospitalized children in several developing countries.[52] The true role of *Chlamydia* and *M. pneumoniae* infections in childhood respiratory infections in developing countries has not been well studied yet because of technical problems with the laboratory diagnosis, but it seems likely they may play as important a role as in developed countries. Community studies of *M. pneumoniae* pneumonia have shown the highest incidence in school-age children, with a decline after puberty and with the lowest rates in the over 40-year-old age group, possible reflecting immunity. However, some 25–50% of pneumonia in young adults, such as college students, is due to this organism, and infection rates are high in military recruits (see Chapter 24). In a long-term study of some 15,000 episodes of pneumonia in a group health plan in Seattle, about 45% were tested for *M. pneumoniae* by isolation and serological tests, and 15% were found to be due to this agent, with the highest rate in children.[62] A new chlamydial strain, designated as TWAR (for Taiwan acute respiratory), has been shown to be an important pathogen in acute respiratory infections such as pneumonia, bronchitis, sinusitis, as well as mild upper respiratory infections.[63,64] In a retrospective examination of 200 patients from a group cooperative study,[62] 8% were due to this organism, which is a rate of 1 per 1000 per year and with the highest incidence in the elderly. Only about 2% of patients with *M. pneumoniae* require hospitalization, and infection with *Chlamydia pneumoniae* is usually mild or asymptomatic. The secondary intrafamilial infection rate is high after an index case of *M. pneumoniae* is introduced and involves about 84% of children and 41% of adults.

In adults, especially older adults, most pneumonias are bacterial in origin. In the past, *S. pneumoniae* caused 50–90% of community-acquired pneumonias, but in recent years this has decreased to some 16–60%, still the dominant organism.[65–67] In an excellent prospective study of 359 community-acquired cases of pneumonia admitted to three Pittsburgh hospitals in 1986–1987, the most frequent etiologic agents were: *S. pneumoniae* (15.3%), *H. influenzae* (10.9%), *Legionella* spp (6.7%), *C. pneumoniae* (TWAR) (6.1%), and gram-negative organisms (6%).[65] In 32.9%, the etiology was indeterminate. No distinctive clinical picture was diagnostic for any etiologic agent. The underlying illnesses were immunosuppression (36.3%), chronic obstructive pulmonary disease (32.4%), and malignancy (28.4%). The median age was 62 years. The mortality was 13.7% and was highest for *S. aureus*. For most cases, erythromycin therapy would be effective. In recent years, gram-negative organisms are of increasing importance, perhaps causing 7–18% of pneumonia, and of special importance in the elderly. Some 30–40% of community-acquired pneumonias are of unknown etiology, due perhaps to 30% of persons unable to produce sputum for culture, or one third who have received antibiotics before hospitalization, or in about one fourth the organisms are difficult to isolate, such as *M. pneumoniae*,

C. pneumoniae, *Coxiella burnetti*, and *Legionella* species, as well as viruses. Even invasive diagnostic techniques in three studies left 43% of unknown etiology, 8% were polymicrobial, and 49% were due to a wide variety of pathogens that varied according to geographic region.[67] Antibiotic-resistant organisms and toxic streptococcus are emerging pathogens in pneumonias, and *M. pneumoniae* is appearing as a pathogen in the elderly.[68]

11.2.3. Acute Otitis Media. This is a common infection of children, with a peak age of 6–18 months. It occurs seasonally throughout the year, but is highest in fall and winter.

Family aggregation is common for recurrent disease. Accurate diagnosis is dependent on cultures taken by aspiration from the middle ear. A recent review of etiology by Klein[69] reports that a bacterial antigen was isolated from two thirds of such aspirations: *S. pneumoniae* was the leading cause in 25–50%, then nontypable *H. influenzae* in 15–30%, *Moraxella catarrhalis* in 3–20%, group A streptococci and staphylococcus in 2–3%, and viruses alone or with bacteria in about 33%. *M. pneumoniae* was uncommon in middle-ear infections in most children. In children under 6 months, *C. trachomatis* with acute respiratory infections was found to be associated with middle-ear infections. It is important to emphasize that the etiology cannot be diagnosed by the clinical picture alone and that culture of aspirated material from the middle ear is needed.

11.2.4. Intestinal Infections and Intoxications. These may be divided into foodborne poisons and intestinal infections.

11.2.4a. Bacterial Food Poisoning. While this section is concerned with bacterial causes, it is important to emphasize that Norwalk and Norwalk-like viruses are probably one of the major causes of both food- and waterborne outbreaks worldwide[70] Bacterial food poisoning is dealt with in more detail in Chapter 5. In an analysis of 2841 outbreaks of known etiology from 1973–1987 reported to the CDC and which involved 124,824 persons, 66% were caused by bacterial pathogens, 25% were due to chemicals, 5% to parasites, and 5% to viruses. The major contribution of bacterial etiology to the 124,824 cases were: *Salmonella* (45% of total), involving 55,864 cases in 790 outbreaks; *S. aureus* (14% of total), involving 17,248 cases in 367 outbreaks; *Shigella* (12% of total), involving 14,399 cases in 104 outbreaks; and *Clostridium perfringes* (10% of total), with 12,234 cases in 190 outbreaks. *Clostridium botulinum* was reported in 231 outbreaks (8%) and affected 494 persons.[71] It should be emphasized that food outbreaks are greatly underreported.

11.2.4b. Intestinal Infections. The causes of enteric infections vary with age and geographic area. They are perhaps the most common cause of morbidity worldwide, rivaling acute respiratory infections. In this book, they are dealt with under *Campylobacter* (Chapter 8), cholera (Chapter 11), *Clostridium difficile* (Chapter 12), *E. coli* (Chapter 14), *Helicobacter pylori* (Chapter 17), salmonellosis (Chapter 31), shigellosis (Chapter 32), typhoid fever (Chapter 42), and yersiniosis (Chapter 43).

The magnitude, special settings, and etiology of diarrhea in both developing and developed countries have recently been reviewed.[72] The incidence in developed countries is estimated as 1 to 3 illnesses per person per year and 5 to 18 illnesses per children per year in tropical, developing countries. An estimated 12,600 deaths per day occur in children in some of these developing areas of Asia, Africa, and Latin America. In all countries the peak incidence is in young children, usually under age 3 years and often earlier in developing countries. The causes involve bacteria, viruses, and parasites, and sophisticated laboratory techniques are required to diagnose some of them, thus making definitions of etiologic patterns difficult in areas without modern laboratory facilities.

In children, viruses play a predominant role in some seasons, and the rotaviruses may cause about half the cases of acute diarrhea in children under age 3 years on a worldwide basis. In older children and adults, Norwalk-like agents are important, and intestinal adenoviruses are increasingly being recognized in young children. Among the bacterial pathogens, enterotoxic *E. coli* is probably the most common, with its production of both the choleralike LT toxin or the ST toxin.[72]

In travelers, *E. coli* (ETEC) is also the most common cause and is found in 42% of diarrheal episodes in Latin America, 36% in Africa, and 16% in Asia.[42] The enterotoxigenic form has been found in 15–30% of illnesses in the community or in hospitals, especially in tropical, developing settings, and are also common in adults in these areas.[72] *Campylobacter jejuni* is perhaps the most common cause of inflammatory diarrhea in developed countries and *H. pylori* is increasingly recognized as a cause of gastritis, peptic ulcer disease, and probably of gastric carcinoma.[73,74] The organism can be eliminated in 80–90% of infections by treatment with bismuth and antibiotics, and such therapy is routinely recommended for gastric ulcers.[75]

Diarrhea is increased in incidence in certain special settings. The importance of nosocomial diarrhea is being increasingly recognized. It accounted for 17% of all nosocomial infections in a children's hospital in Buffalo[76] and 42% in an adult intensive care unit in a London hospital.[77] The etiology of nosocomial diarrhea as reported to the CDC from 1980–1984 was *C. difficile* in 45.1% and *Salmonella* species in 11.8%.[72] In extended care facilities for the elderly, diarrhea is also an important problem, where about one third of patients experience a significant episode each year, and *C. difficile* is a common cause. Outbreaks of diarrhea in child care centers are also common, and frequent causes include rotavirus, *Shigella*, *C. jejuni*, *C. difficile*, *G. lamblia*, and *Cryptosporidium*. High attack rates are seen with rotavirus and some bacterial infections. Finally, some 50–60% of patients infected with HIV in the United States have diarrhea at the onset of illness, and initial diarrhea is seen in over 90% of AIDS patients in Africa and Haiti.[78] A wide variety of organisms may be involved, of which *Cryptosporidium* is the most frequent, accounting for 3–21% in AIDS patients in the United States and 50% in Africa and Haiti.[78] This organism may also produce diarrhea in normal persons and its contamination of a public water supply in Milwaukee resulted in a massive outbreak involving over 403,000 persons.[28]

As mentioned above, *Campylobacter* enteritis is an increasingly recognized cause of intestinal infections in the United States, Great Britain, and Australia, accounting for some 5–14% of the cases in several large series (see Chapter 8). The clinical disease is characterized by watery diarrhea with mucus, blood, or pus, often cramping abdominal pain and fever, and sometimes gross blood in the stools of children. *Yersinia enterocolitica* is another recently recognized cause of acute diarrhea attended by some cramps, fever, and occasionally a rash; the incubation period is 1–3 days. There may be associated mesenteric adenitis, arthritis, and erythema (see Chapter 43).

The prevention of traveler's diarrhea is important because some 40% of travelers from developed countries with temperate climates will develop diarrhea, as reviewed by DuPont and associates.[43,79,80] The use of bismuth subsalicylate has proved useful in the short term and antibiotic prophylaxis and treatment is recommended for longer exposures. The following recommendations are quoted from DuPont *et al.*[79]

> In most cases a bacterial pathogen is responsible for the illness. The antimicrobial agents with the greatest activity against these organisms are cotrimoxazole (trimethoprim/sulfamethoxazole) during the summer months in the interior of Mexico (a region where this agent has been studied extensively), and the fluoroquinolones for other places or other times, until data become available to indicate the appropriateness of cotrimoxazole here as well. Persons at risk should take along with them a drug to treat symptoms of travelers' diarrhea, and an appropriate antimicrobial agent. At the passage of the third unformed stool, it is recommended that travelers treat themselves with fluids and salt (flavored mineral water augmented with saltine crackers is sufficient in most cases), symptomatic treatment and antibacterial therapy. Of these, the antimicrobial is the most important component, which is given either as a single large dose or once or twice daily for 3 days. Perhaps optimal therapy for afebrile nondysenteric patients is loperamide in combination with the antibacterial drug. In the face of fever or dysentery, the antimicrobial should be used alone. In special situations where food and beverage restrictions cannot be followed and where the itinerary cannot tolerate even the slightest alterations because of illness, chemoprophylaxis can be considered. The most effective preventive medication in this case is the antimicrobial also used for therapy, taken in half the therapeutic dosage daily while in the area of risk. However, the majority of travelers should not use this approach.

11.2.5. Acute Urinary Tract Infections. In various studies of acute urinary tract infections (UTI) of inpatients and outpatients, *E. coli* is by far the most common organism in both settings, accounting for up to 80% of initial urinary infections in outpatients.[81] In a more recent compilation of etiologic agents in hospitalized cases, Andriole[82] found 35.8% due to *E. coli*, 16.4% due to *P. mirabili*, 16.3% due to *Enterobacter aerogenes*, 10.1% due to *K. pneumoniae*, and less than 6% each due to other causes. Over 80% are associated with use of urethral catheters. The spectrum of urinary infections varies and each syndrome has its own unique epidemiology, natural history, and clinical manifestations.[83] The major risk factors include the newborn (particularly the premature), prepubertal girls, young boys, sexually active young women, elderly males, and elderly females. Risk factors that contribute to lower tract infection in women include sexual intercourse, diaphragm–spermicide use, and voiding behavior.[84] UTI is the most common infectious disease of the elderly and is especially prevalent in debilitated, institutionalized older individuals. Unlike UTI in younger women, which tends to be related to frequency of sexual intercourse and is uncomplicated, in the elderly it is more difficult to treat and its pathogenesis is related to abnormal bladder function, bladder outlet obstruction, vaginal and urethral atrophy, use of long-term indwelling catheters, and puddling related to bed rest. The spectrum of organisms causing infection relates to the ecology of the patients' environments; those residing in nursing homes, and especially with permanent indwelling catheters, tend to have a greater variety of pathogenic organisms, many of which may be relatively antibiotic resistant.[85]

The immediate diagnosis of UTI is based on relatively simple techniques. The presence of pyuria and bacteriuria, the two most important indicators of UTIs, are most accurately determined by standard techniques. In quantitating pyuria, the finding of 10 leukocytes/mm^3 of urine by either hemocytometry or direct microscopy correlates highly with symptomatic, culture-proven UTIs.[86]

11.2.6. Sexually Transmitted Diseases. The term *sexually transmitted diseases* (STD) encompasses the five classic venereal diseases (gonorrhea, syphilis, chancroid, lymphogranuloma venereum, granuloma inguinale), plus other major ones such as HIV-1, HIV-2, human T-cell lymphotropic virus type I (HTLV-I), herpes simplex 1 and 2, papillomaviruses, hepatitis A and B, *Chlamydia trachomatis*, *Candida albicans*, and *Trichomonas vaginalis*. The number of cases and rates per 100,000 of major bacterial causes of STDs reported to state health departments in 1988 and in 1992 are given in Table 10. While *C. trachomaits* infections are among the most prevalent of all sexually transmitted diseases, problems in diagnosis, lack of public health laws, and other problems have made surveillance of this disease incomplete, and therefore it is not included in Table 10. Reflecting increasing recognition and reporting of this infection, the rates per 100,000 have risen from 3.2 in 1984 to 182.6 in 1992 when 36 states reported to the CDC.[87] In large cities with more than 200,000 population the rates were 296.8 in 1992. An estimated 4 million cases occur annually, many of which cause pelvic inflammatory disease with serious sequelae such as ectopic pregnancy and infertility.

It is important to emphasize that many of these STDs occur in synergy with HIV infection and that the transmission of both are enhanced in the presence of the other. Overall, the trends in recent years show that reported rates for gonorrhea have declined 19%, with rates decreasing from 250 per 100,000 in 1991 to 202 per 100,000 in 1992, and with declines in primary and secondary syphilis rates from 17.3 to 13.7 in the same period. This decline may reflect the adoption of safer sexual practices. The proportion of adolescent women aged 15–19 years who reported having sexual intercourse, however, increased from 29% in 1970 to 52% in 1988.[88] The rates of gonorrhea and syphilis in the adolescent age group are three times that of the general population, and thus are a major target for education and control. The risk for STD is also much higher in blacks than in whites, with rates for primary and secondary syphilis being 60-fold higher and for gonorrhea 40-fold higher; for Hispanics the increases are five- and threefold higher, respectively.

Adequate surveillance data are not available for several sexually transmitted diseases. Some information of trends are seen in the office practice of certain physicians based on the National Disease and Therapeutic Index as analyzed in graphs in a CDC report.[87] For human papillomavirus genital warts, physician visits in this survey have risen from about 45,000 in 1966 to 200,000 in 1992. Trichomonal infections have declined slowly over this period, starting with 500,000 in 1966, but other vaginal infections have increased sharply from about 120,000 to 3,000,000.

Many of the newer agents of STD account for as many as or more infections seen in STD clinics or by private physicians than are accounted for by the classic causes. These infections are most common in the 15- to 30-year age group—the time of greatest sexual activity, especially extramarital. They are more commonly diagnosed in men, both because men tend to have more sexual partners than do women (except prostitutes) and because the lesions are more apparent in men. Multiple infections are common in both sexes, and gonorrhea and syphilis should be excluded by appropriate examination in every patient seen with an STD. The changing nature of and the increase in these infections have several causes, including the use of measures other than the condom for contraception, changing practices in heterosexual and homosexual activities, especially involving genital–oral and genital–anal contact, the importation of infection from Southeast Asia, and increased public confidence in the availability and effectiveness of antibiotic therapy.

The increasing importance of *Chlamydia* infections deserves further emphasis. Chlamydial genital infections include urethritis, acute epididymitis in men, and pelvic inflammatory disease in women; these are discussed in Chapter 10. Overall, about half the cases of urethritis in men are nongonococcal, and among male college students, this rises to 80–90%. *C. trachomatis* (immunotypes D through K) is responsible for 30–50% of symptomatic cases of nongonococcal urethritis (NGU), and is more

Table 10. Reported Cases and Rates per 100,000 of Classical Sexually Transmitted Diseases Reported to State Health Departments in the Civilian Population, United States—1988 and in 1992[a]

	Number of cases		Rate per 100,000	
Disease	1988	1992	1988	1992
Gonorrhea	738,160	501,409	300.3	201.6
Syphilis (all stages)	104,546	112,541	45.5	45.3
Chancroid	4,891	1,886	2.0	0.8
Lymphogranuloma venereum	194	302	0.1	0.1
Granuloma inguinale	11	6	0.0	0.0

[a]Derived from Table 1, in Ref. 87.

common in white than in black men and in higher than in lower socioeconomic levels. Its incubation period is longer than that of gonorrhea, and symptoms of urethritis in males may appear 1–2 weeks or longer after penicillin or spectinomycin treatment for gonorrhea, involving one third to two thirds of these men. Oral therapy of NGU with tetracycline or erythromycin hastens recovery. There is no clinical counterpart of NGU in women who develop *Chlamydia* infections of the cervix with or without cervicitis, but this organism may be involved in up to 30% of pelvic inflammatory diseases in females.[89] The other agents of NGU in men are uncertain, although *Ureaplasma urealyticum* is considered the cause of 10–20% of NGU cases. If laboratory facilities are not available for the diagnosis of *Chlamydia* infections in persons with NGU, both the case and the sexual partner should be treated with appropriate broad-spectrum antibiotic therapy (usually tetracycline or doxycycline) as though they had it. For detailed information on STD infections, see Chapter 9 on chancroid, Chapter 10 on *Chlamydia* infections, Chapter 15 on gonococcal infections, and Chapter 35 on syphilis. Viral causes are discussed in the companion book on viruses.[5]

11.2.7. Hospital (Nosocomial) Infections. These are infections acquired after a admission to a hospital and are discussed in detail in Chapter 25. More than 2 million patients annually in the United States develop nosocomial infections. In the largest study to date, 5.7% of 159,526 patients in 338 hospitals developed a nosocomial infection.[90] Each such patient stayed an average of 4 extra days in the hospital, paying an extra $2100 for each infection. Some 19,027 deaths were directly attributable to a nosocomial infection and it was a contributory factor in 58,092. In reports to the CDC's National Nosocomial Infections Surveillance program in 1991–1992, which involves 149 hospitals, urinary tract infections were the most common site (33.1%), followed by pneumonias (15.5%), surgical site infections (14.9%), and primary bloodstream infections (13.1%), and this order was similar irrespective of the size of the hospital. Among 71,411 isolates from all sites, *E. coli* and *S. aureus* were the most common (12% each), followed by coagulase-negative staphylococcus (11%), *Enterococcus* spp. (10%), *Pseudomonas aeruginosa* (9%), *Enterobacter* spp. (6%), and all other organisms 5% or less.[90] Unfortunately, the major nosocomial pathogens either are naturally resistant to clinically useful antibiotics or are potentially able to develop resistance. This includes both gram-positive organisms (*S. aureus*, *Enterococcus* spp.), and gram-negative organisms (*K. pneumoniae*, *P. aeruginosa*, and *Enterobacter* spp.).

12. Diagnosis of Bacterial Infections

Identification of the causal agent is essential to establish the etiology of a bacterial infection and as a guide to selecting appropriate antibiotic therapy. It depends primarily on: (1) microscopic examination of exudates, body fluid, or tissues after staining (Gram's stain, acid-fast), or by dark-field examination or immunofluorescent-labeled antibody tests, or by the newer techniques for antigen identification such as counterimmunoelectrophoresis and latex agglutination, as used in respiratory infections; (2) appropriate bacteriological culture techniques; (3) a variety of new techniques to identify the antigen and a particular antigenic strain, many based on molecular methods; and (4) serological tests. Serological tests are not as commonly employed as in viral infections because of the ease and rapidity with which the diagnosis can often be established by smear and culture for most bacterial infections. For slow-growing or difficult-to-culture organisms such as *Legionella pneumophila*, the spirochetes, and the rickettsiae, serological tests play an important role in diagnosis. Animal inoculation may be required to identify fastidious organisms and the toxins of certain bacteria, and skin tests may be useful to diagnose infections that show delayed hypersensitivity.

This section will briefly review some of these techniques, but for more definitive information, see textbooks on laboratory methods,[91,92] medical microbiology,[32] or clinical infectious diseases.[38] An informative pamphlet on the services available from the CDC for the diagnosis of diseases of public health importance is available that indicates specimen collection, tests done, shipment instructions, and federal regulations on interstate shipment of etiologic agents.[93] All such specimens with proper justification and a completed request form must be submitted to the National Center for Infectious Diseases of the CDC in Atlanta by or through the state health laboratory with the knowledge and consent of the state laboratory director or designee.

An important decision for the physician is the differentiation of bacterial from viral infections on first examination in order to decide on the necessity of antibiotic therapy and as a guide to laboratory tests. This may not always be possible, but the presence of bacterial infections is suggested by the vigor and acuteness of the clinical onset, leukocytosis, and the presence of purulent lesions with polymorphonuclear cells. Nonpurulent responses to bacteria are seen in such diseases as brucellosis, tuberculosis, and typhoid fever. The presence of more than 10 white blood cells/mm^3 of urine by either hemocytometry or direct microscopy is indicative of an acute bacterial urinary infection,[86] as is the presence of white blood cells in the stool of a bacterial pathogen involved in diarrhea, or of polymorphonuclear leukocytes (not lymphocytes) in spinal fluid of a bacterial meningitis.

12.1. Collection of Specimens

The selection of the appropriate site from which to obtain the specimen, its collection prior to antibiotic therapy, and its transport to the laboratory in a manner to preserve the viability of any organisms present are three essential ingredients of successful diagnostic microbiology. The specimen should be taken from the site of the infection or from the body fluid most likely to contain organisms from the infected site. The collection should be made with sterile swabs and collecting units. Cotton applicator swabs are commonly used, but since cotton may be toxic to certain bacteria, a synthetic material such as calcium alginate is preferable. An adequate sample must be obtained to prepare smears and cultures and for special isolation purposes (viruses, fungi). Swabs may be inadequate for this purpose, and the fluid itself, or a washing of it (e.g., throat, nasal, lesion), may be needed for quantitative measurement, as in urine, to determine the number of organisms present. A syringe aspirate is desirable for anaerobic cultures of purulent lesions. Since most large laboratories have special sections for bacterial, viral, fungal, parasitic, and treponemal diagnostic techniques, separate specimens for each microbiological group considered as a possible etiologic agent in a given infection should be collected. Special techniques may be needed to avoid contamination by normal flora in needle or surgical aspirations from a lesion or from a transtracheal or transurethral site.

To preserve viability, material from patients may be: (1) inoculated into appropriate transport media directly at the bedside, for which purpose kits are now commercially available; (2) carried to the laboratory for immediate inoculation; or (3) preserved in a transport medium that maintains viability, prevents desiccation, and limits overgrowth of other organisms; media containing agar and charcoal are commonly employed (Stuart's transport medium or Arnie's modification thereof). If transport media are used, smears should be prepared separately at the time of collection with a separate swab because the agar in the transport medium makes this difficult. If viruses are suspected, a separate specimen should be collected and immediately frozen in dry ice for transport to the laboratory. Blood samples should be collected aseptically in amounts of 10–15 ml. If shipment to a laboratory is needed, the serum should be separated aseptically and forwarded preferably in the frozen state, but this will vary, depending on the infection. Infections of certain sites or with certain organisms may require special collection or transport methods or both; these are described in the appropriate individual chapters in this book or in books on bacteriological diagnosis.

12.2. Requests for Testing

There must be good communication between the physician or epidemiologist and the microbiologist. In the face of an outbreak, the epidemiologist is urged to consult with the laboratory prior to the investigation or have a laboratory specialist accompany the investigator to make the proper specimen collection and method of transporting it to the laboratory. The wide array of specialized laboratory techniques and culture media available makes it necessary that the laboratory be provided information on a clinical and epidemiological assessment of the etiologic possibilities. The age, sex, clinical diagnosis (or at least the organ system involved), previous antibiotic therapy, and other pertinent patient information plus the site, time, and date of collection and method of transport to the laboratory of the specimen are helpful data to the laboratory worker in pursuit of the correct techniques to be employed. In return, the clinical microbiologist must provide periodic reports to help the physician in selecting appropriate therapy until the organism is fully identified and its antibiotic sensitivity determined.

12.3. Tests Employed

The details of laboratory methods are beyond the scope of this section, but a few comments will be made; specific techniques are mentioned in each chapter. The importance of a properly obtained and thoroughly examined Gram's stain of the exudate or body fluid cannot be overemphasized as a guide to initial therapy. For example, the etiology of some 85% of acute purulent meningitis cases and of many bacterial pneumonias can be identified by smear, especially if capsular swelling occurs in the presence of specific antisera. Simple microscopic examination of an unstained, uncentrifuged specimen of urine that shows bacteria indicates a quantitative bacterial count of 10^4–10^5/ml, and the morphology may point to the proper etiology. The examination of bacteria in fresh preparations or on culture, after staining with specific, immunofluorescent-labeled antisera, provides specific diagnosis of group A hemolytic streptococci, plague bacillus, and *E. coli*; it has also been useful in identifying the organism in acute meningitis, in cervical gonorrhea, and in primary syphilis.

The rapid detection of antigen in body fluids such as respiratory secretions and in urine is now being accomplished by immunofluorescence, counterimmunoelectrophoresis, enzyme immunoassays, DNA probe hybridization, and latex agglutination. Commercial kits are becoming rapidly available for many of these techniques.[94] A number of molecular techniques are now being used for both phenotypic and genotypic identification of organisms and are well reviewed in a recent article.[95] Those used for epidemiological studies of *phenotypic variants* include antibiotic resistance patterns (antibiograms), biotyping, bacteriocin production, serotyping, outer membrane protein analysis, phage typing, immunoblotting, and multilocus enzyme electrophoresis. The limitations of these techniques are that they do not take genetic exchange or mutations into account, are nonspecific, and are not widely applicable. Independent isolates of the same strain may vary in their phenotype. *Genotypic typing* methods are used to identify the genetic composition of the organism by study of chromosomal, plasmid, or transposon DNA. The techniques include plasmid profile analysis, restriction endonuclease analysis, ribotyping, pulsed field electrophoresis, polymerase chain reaction digests, arbitrarily primed polymerase chain reactions, and nucleotide sequence analysis. Variations in the reproducibility and discriminatory power of the two general methods differ; in general, those that involve genotypic methods are better. Their application permits identification of specific patterns of transmission of an organism, differentiation between reinfection and reactivation, and recognition of the geographic distribution of a particular strain. The epidemiology of antibiotic resistance involves (1) R plasmid spread (inter- and intraspecies), (2) strain (clonal) dissemination, and (3) transposition of R genes into R plasmids or chromosomes. These many techniques now provide the epidemiologist the means for the rapid identification of many organisms, including the specific strain involved, so that transmission patterns can be followed. Of special interest are the so-called emerging infections, which in the United States include *E. coli* O157:H7 disease, cryptosporidiosis, coccidioidomycosis, multidrug-resistant pneumococcal disease, vancomycin-resistant enterococcal infections, and Hantavirus infections. Special surveillance and diagnostic centers have been established to monitor these infections.[96]

The culture media used will depend on the organisms suspected and whether they are aerobic or anaerobic. Blood agar plates and broth cultures are widely used as a starting point. See individual chapters for specialized media for specific organisms. A useful table indicating the bacteria found by common culture media (and the media used), by type of specimen (urine, respiratory secretions, genital, etc.), and the specialized media needed to detect organisms missed by these standard procedures is available in the appendix of a recent microbiology text.[32]

Once the organism is isolated its antibiotic sensitivity is usually determined and is useful not only in the selection of the proper antibiotic but also in "fingerprinting" the organism for epidemiological tracing. However, this is not necessary for some organisms that are known to be uniformly sensitive to certain antibiotics or that are uniformly resistant to all but one or two antibiotics. *In vitro* antibiotic testing is not always relevant to a particular infection, especially if the infection is due to mixed organisms. It often does not provide quantitative data or express the effect of an antibiotic on different points in the growth cycle of the organism, and the testing procedure may not include the antibiotic best suited to the clinical situation. The tests must be made on organisms obtained before antibiotic therapy is initiated. Despite these limitations, *in vitro* antibiotic testing is widely employed and is especially useful for organisms prone to develop antibiotic resistance such as staphylococci, enterobacteria, and *M. tuberculosis*.

The *in vitro* tests commonly employed are the disk-diffusion techniques in agar and dilution-sensitivity tests on agar plates or in tubes with nutrient broth. The disk procedure is simpler and more rapid, but the zone of inhibition cannot be directly correlated with the concentration of the antibiotic needed to inhibit growth of the organism *in vivo*. Antibiotic resistance to two antibiotics by disk diffusion does not exclude *in vivo* effectiveness of the combination; disk diffusion cannot be used for combinations of antibiotics.

The dilution tests provide quantitative data, permitting estimation of the minimum inhibitory concentration of the antibiotic as well as the minimum lethal concentration necessary for killing, which may differ from the minimum inhibitory concentration. The techniques used for dilution tests, however, may vary from laboratory to laboratory; the results are dependent on the size of the inoculum and the broth medium employed. Many laboratories now use automated broth microdilution susceptibility testing, which is rapid and has some economical and procedural advantages over both disk-diffusion and broth macrodilution methods.

As indicated earlier, serological tests have limited

Table 11. Some Serological Tests Used in Bacteriological Diagnosis

Disease	Test antigen	Test(s)[a]	Comment
Brucellosis	Organism	Agglutination	Four strains
Legionellosis	Organism	IF	Twenty serotypes
Leptospirosis	Organism	Microagglutination, CF, hemolytic, IFA	Crossings occur; many types
Lyme disease	Organism	ELISA IgG, IgM	Needs standardization
Mycoplasma pneumonia	Organism	IF, TRI, CF	
	O rbc	Cold agglutinins	60% positive
Q fever	Organism	CF, agglutination	
Rickettsialpox	Organism	CF	
Rocky Mountain spotted fever	Soluble antigen	CF	
	Proteus strains	Weil Felix	Ox19+++, Ox2+++
		Agglutination	OxKO
Streptococcosis	Extracellular products	Antistreptolysin O, DNase	Confirm past infection
Syphilis	Nontreponemal	VDRL flocculation test	Presumptive
	Treponemal	Rapid reagent tests	Presumptive
		TPI, CF, FTA-ABS	Specific
Yaws	Same as syphilis	Same as syphilis	Cannot differentiate from syphilis
Tularemia	Organism	Agglutination	Often 1:640 or more
Typhoid fever	O antigen	Widal-agglutination	≤4-fold increase

[a]IF, immunofluorescence; CF, complement fixation; IFA, indirect fluorescent antibody; TRI, tetrazolium-reduction inhibition; VDRL, Veneral Disease Research Laboratory; TPI, treponemal immobilization; FTA-ABS, fluorescent-treponemal-anitbody absorption.

application for many bacterial infections. However, they are useful for a number of treponemal, leptospiral, and rickettsial infections. Some of the key tests are indicated in Table 11. Chlamydial infections, including the TWAR strain, are being increasingly recognized as a cause of a variety of clinical syndromes, especially of the respiratory and genital tracts, and microimmunofluorescence tests are available for both IgG and IgM antibodies as well as a genus-specific complement fixation test. Certain levels of titers of antibody are needed to be indicative of recent infection and differentiation between *C. trachomatis* and *C. psittaci* is not possible.

As with viral diagnostic tests, acute and convalescent serum samples should be collected for all bacterial serological tests and the sera tested simultaneously; a fourfold or greater rise in titer is indicative of recent infection. Remember that there is only one time to take the acute-phase sample—in early illness.

For legionellosis, the IgG immunofluoresence titer must reach 1:128 or higher to be significant because of nonspecificity at lower dilutions; similarly, only cold agglutinin titers of 1:64 or higher are regarded as diagnostic of *M. pneumoniae* infection, and even then only about 60% of hospitalized *M. pneumonia* patients are positive, depending on the severity of the infection. The presence of specific IgM antibody is often diagnostic of an acute infection, if demonstrable, as for *Borrelia burgdorferi*, the cause of Lyme disease, but the laboratory diagnosis of this infection is subject to wide variation and standardization of procedures is badly needed. For rickettsial infections, both the organism itself and *Proteus* antigens are useful in serological diagnosis. In streptococcal infections, an increase occurs in a group of antienzyme tests but is too late to be useful diagnostically; a high titer is said to place the person at greater risk of developing rheumatic fever. In syphilis, a great variety of serological tests have been used, employing both nontreponemal and treponemal antigens. The VDRL test is most widely employed as an initial test and is highly sensitive and well standardized but lacks high specificity. The diagnosis can be confirmed by the fluorescent-treponemal-antibody absorption (FTA-Abs) or hemagglutination (MHA-TP) tests, which are highly specific and available at most state and a few large private laboratories, as well as at the CDC. The *Treponema pallida* immobilization test (TPI) test is a highly specific test but requires maintenance of a mobile, live treponemal antigen; it is available at the CDC. Yaws (*T. pertenue*) shares identical reactivities with *T. pallidum* and cannot be differentiated serologically. Typhoid fever results in increases to the H, O, and other antigens of the organism; an increase in O-antigen titer in the absence of recent immunization is indicative of recent infection. Skin tests may also be useful in diagnosis by demonstration of hypersensitivity to various bacterial antigens. They are commonly employed in tuberculosis, leprosy, nontuberculous mycobacteriosis, brucellosis, and tularemia.

12.4. Interpretation of Tests

The isolation of a bacterial organism from an ill person does not always represent a causal relationship. The organism could reflect: (1) part of the normal flora; (2) a healthy carrier state; (3) contamination during the collection process; (4) a transient microorganism contaminating a body surface; (5) a dual or multiple infection, in which the organism isolated is not the one causing the clinical illness; (6) a laboratory error or mix-up; or (7) the true cause of the illness. The factors that point toward a causal relationship are: (1) isolation in pure culture or of only one organism; (2) the presence of large numbers of the same organism; (3) the presence of the organism in direct smear from a lesion; (4) procurement from a site normally free of bacteria; (5) repeated isolation of the same organism; (6) demonstration of an immune response; and (7) history of possible recent exposure to the organism in an ill person, in travel, in occupation, or otherwise. The response of the patient to an antibiotic to which the organism is sensitive provides suggestive evidence that the organism caused the disease; but because other organisms are also sensitive to the same antibiotic, this cannot weigh too heavily. Clinical and laboratory judgment plus knowledge of the qualitative and quantitative behavior of human pathogens constitute the best grounds for deciding a causal relationship. It should be remembered that some organisms not usually regarded as pathogenic may cause disease in patients with naturally occurring or drug-induced defects in their immune defenses, or in patients infected with HIV.

On the other hand, the failure to isolate an organism does not exclude a bacterial etiology. Such "false-negatives" could result from: (1) prior antibiotic therapy; (2) failure to obtain a specimen from the proper site; (3) collection at the wrong time; (4) a loss of viability during transport to the laboratory; (5) use of inappropriate media, temperature, gaseous environment, or other conditions for growth of the organism; or (6) failure to hold the culture media for a sufficiently long time, as with certain *Brucella* species. For organisms difficult or impossible to culture, molecular tools such as the polymerase chain reaction are providing important techniques for direct diagnosis, but extremely careful laboratory procedures are needed to avoid cross-contamination and false-positive results.[(6)]

Serological tests are also subject to misinterpretation. False-positive rises can result from cross-reacting antigens, nonspecific inhibitors, double infection with the other organism causing the illness, and antibody response to vaccination rather than to natural infection. False-negatives, i.e., failure to demonstrate an increase in titer, can occur when the serum specimen is taken too late in illness, two samples are taken too close together to demonstrate a titer rise, the organism is a poor immunogen, the wrong antigen is used in the test, some inhibitor or non-specificity (as in immunofluorescence tests) obscures a true rise, or the wrong type of test is used for the timing of the serum specimens. Serological tests are also not available for many bacterial infections. One of the common problems is the interpretation of a high IgG antibody titer in a single specimen. The demonstration of IgM-specific antibody is strong but not absolute evidence of a recent infection; it could result from reactivation. The presence of antibody to a rare infection, or to one not usually present in that area as in a returned traveler, or the history of some recent unusual exposure such as in hunting, a new occupation, or a visit from overseas friends also adds weight to the recency of that infection. Such problems are more common in viral and parasitic infections.

13. Proof of Causation

The classic postulates were suggested by Jakob Henle in 1840,[(97)] some 40 years before bacteria were discovered, and then further developed by his pupil, Robert Koch, in 1884 and 1890, after he had isolated *M. tuberculosis*,[(98,99)] as well as by Edwin Klebs.[(100)] A recent book has reviewed the development and subsequent changes in these postulates.[(101)] The postulates are presented in Table 12. While fulfillment of these postulates provides strong evidence of a causal association, the failure to fulfill them does not exclude this relationship. Even at the time of presentation in 1890, Koch himself recognized some of these limitations, especially the inability to reproduce some diseases in experimental animals. At that time, this was true of cholera, typhoid fever, diphtheria, leprosy, and

Table 12. Henle–Koch Postulates[a]

1. Parasite occurs in every case of the disease in question and under circumstances that can account for the pathological changes and clinical cause of the disease
2. Occurs in no other disease as fortuitous and nonpathogenic parasite
3. After being fully isolated from the body and repeatedly grown in pure culture, can induce the disease anew

[a]From Koch.[(98,99)]

relapsing fever, for which Koch felt it necessary to fulfill only the first two postulates. Since then, many other limitations have been recognized,[102] as our knowledge of microbiology, epidemiology, and pathogenesis has increased. These include recognition of the asymptomatic carrier state, which would invalidate the second postulate if an individual were carrier of organism A and his disease was caused by organism B. The concepts of multiple causation, of inapparent infection, and of the biological gradient of disease are also limitations. The postulates are not generally applicable to viral and parasitic diseases or for organisms that cannot be grown in culture or induce an immune response. Criteria are also needed for chronic diseases. In an effort to cover these various possibilities, a "unified" set of postulates based mainly on epidemiological criteria have been proposed.[103] It is clear that all postulates and guidelines of causation are limited by the technology available to prove them and by our knowledge of disease mechanisms at the time. The need for establishing guidelines for causation is ever present in the field of bacteriology, where the causal relationship between parasite and disease must be established for newly recognized diseases such as Lyme disease, Legionnaires' disease, Pittsburgh pneumonia, chlamydial pneumonia and urethritis, infant botulism, enterotoxic *E. coli* diarrhea, *Helicobacter pylori* and gastric ulcer and carcinoma, toxic shock syndrome, and streptococcal B infections in infancy. New causes for old diseases, new diseases from old causes, and new diseases with new causes keep appearing as our techniques for their isolation and identification improve.

14. Control and Prevention

The three major principles of control of infectious diseases are: (1) eliminate or contain the sources of infection; (2) interrupt the chain of transmission; and (3) protect the host against infection or disease or both. Additionally, the environment may contribute to the occurrence of disease by its effect on any of the above three areas.

14.1. Environmental Control

The provision of clean and safe air, water, milk, and food; the proper management of sewage and garbage; and the control of insect vectors of disease are regarded as not only essential to health but also a legal right in most countries. The extent to which they are attained depends on the economy, energy resources, political will, and educational level of the country.

14.1.1. Air. While many infectious agents are airborne on droplet nuclei or particles from infected hosts or environmental sources to susceptible subjects, effective control of this means of transmission has been most difficult to achieve. In open environments, it has been impossible to attain, and even in closed environments attempts to sterilize the air by UV light filtration, propylene glycol, and other chemical aerosols have met with very limited success. At best, control of the air currents generated by air conditioners, water coolers, and fans will help slow down spread of organisms such as *L. pneumophila*, *M. tuberculosis*, and staphylococci. For patient isolation, laminar-flow units have been effective if properly used. The pollution of air by automobiles and industrial sources does not carry a direct risk of infection, but may depress host defense mechanisms so that disease develops, as in persons with chronic pulmonary diseases.

14.1.2. Water. Improvement in our water supplies has been one of the major factors in the environmental control of infectious diseases, especially of enteric infections such as *Campylobacter*, yersiniosis, cholera, typhoid fever, amebiasis, bacillary dysentery, as well as waterborne viruses like Norwalk viruses. The details of water purification and treatment can be found elsewhere, but involve removal of extraneous materials by filtration, settling, and coagulation, the replenishment of oxygen by aeration, and disinfection by chlorination. Bacteriological and chemical standards for the purity of water have been established and are reinforced by governmental and legal regulations. The presence of *E. coli* in defined numbers per milliliter* is taken as an index of fecal contamination of water. However, its absence does not guarantee water safety, since organisms such as hepatitis A and E viruses may escape filtration and chlorination procedures, and more recently *Cryptosporidium* cysts escaped a filtration system in a public water supply in Milwaukee, causing a massive outbreak of diarrhea involving over 403,000 persons.[28] This organism is also resistant to tolerable levels of chlorine. For the traveler, treatment of water with chlorine-release tablets or a drop of Lugal's iodine solution per quart of water 30 min prior to use or by boiling for 5 min (portable heating units can be purchased) will decrease the likelihood of acquiring bacterial intestinal infections in developing countries. Small millipore filter kits are also available for the traveler and are said to remove bacteria, *Giardia lamblia*, and even some viruses.

*Usually, water is not acceptable for drinking if coliform bacteria exceed 4/100 ml in more than 5% of water samples per month using the membrane-filter technique; samples should be taken at points representative of the distribution system.[104]

Should these methods not be available, one can allow the water to run until very hot, collect it, and then use it for drinking water. Bottled water, wine, and beer or other bottled or canned beverages are usually safe.

14.1.3. Sewage and Garbage. Sewage water carries fecal material, industrial and chemical products, and other waste products. It must be safely conveyed without human hazard to septic tanks or to reprocessing, filtration, and activated sludge treatment centers, but has not posed a problem of infectious disease unless cross-contamination with water pipes occurs. The dumping of untreated sewage into streams, rivers, and the open sea is detrimental to fish and marine life and esthetically distasteful, and impairs recreational use of such waters. It might result in transmission of certain intestinal pathogens via raw seafood to humans, such as the hepatitis A or E viruses, cholera, or *Cryptosporidium* in water itself. Clams and oysters have been responsible for many outbreaks of this sort, and thorough cooking is needed to kill organisms such as cholera or hepatitis viruses.

The proper disposal of the large amount of garbage, refuse, and other solid waste products produced by our modern society is an increasing challenge to proper land use and modern technology. Direct discharge into the sewage system after grinding and flushing is one method; compactors of garbage and waste material are now available even for home use. If stored and carried elsewhere for disposal, this must be done in closed, stable containers that protect against rats, flies, and other predators. The separation and recycling of certain reusable products such as glass, bottles, paper, and cans is to be encouraged. Large incinerators for burning garbage and refuse provide a safe but energy-expensive procedure. Landfill sites in communities are increasingly scarce, costly as land values increase, and objected to on esthetic grounds. Disposal of radioactive and other toxic wastes generated by medical, industrial, and energy uses in oceans raises international concern about the long-term food and energy potential of oceans, and land or tank disposal, especially of nuclear wastes, is unacceptable to most communities. The increasing uses of pesticides, and domestic and wild animal wastes in streams or rivers that may wash down into public water supplies, pose an increasing threat.

14.1.4. Milk and Food. Milk and food must be protected against contamination at their source, during transport and storage, and in their preparation for consumption. Cows must be free from tuberculosis, brucellosis, and Q fever. The milk must be collected under clean conditions, preferably by automated machines that avoid human contamination, and its quality in the raw state and after pasteurization must meet bacteriological standards.* Common pasteurization procedures are heating to 65°C (149°F) for 30 min or the high-temperature or flash method at 72°C (162°F) for 15 sec. The heat inactivation of the enzyme alkaline phosphatase, normally present in milk, provides the basis for the phosphatase test to ensure proper pasteurization. Before and promptly after pasteurization, milk must be stored and transported at 5–10°C (41–50°F) to storage areas or the consumer. The pasteurization process, even if performed correctly, may not decontaminate some intracellular organisms and those that are cold-tolerant, such as *Listeria*. Milk and other food products may contain antibiotics used in treatment of cattle or for growth promotion and pose a hazard to highly sensitive persons.

Our food supplies must also be properly grown, cultivated, stored, and prepared. In developing and tropical areas, vegetables such as lettuce and other products grown in soil enriched by human excreta pose a serious hazard for intestinal infections, and these foods should be avoided by wary travelers. Our modern supermarkets are now selling foodstuffs of all types that have been rapidly imported from other countries and that may carry pathogens. In the summer months, 75% of many fruits and vegetables are harvested outside the country and delivered within days to grocery stores and restaurants in the United States.[105] Salad bars, now present in most restaurants, provide fruits and vegetables that may have originated in Mexico, Central America, or tropical or semitropical climes and are a major source of food poisoning.[106] The fast-food chain, particularly those serving undercooked hamburgers, have been the source of food outbreaks, particularly due to *E. coli* O157:H7 infection in the United States[107]; this organism has also led to an epidemic in a child care center. Foodborne outbreaks have also been due to shigellosis on a commercial airline,[108] and to *Salmonella* in a multistate outbreak due in contaminated cheese.[109] These developments have led to a changing epidemiology of foodborne disease and to new approaches to prevention.[110,111] Human handling during preparation may result in contamination by many bacteria, especially staphylococci, *Salmonella*, and *Shigella*. Thorough cooking immediately prior to eating will reduce the hazard of infection but may fail to inactivate preformed heat-stable toxins such as *C. perfringens*. Proper refrigeration or freezing of food has been as important as water and sewage management in the reduction of intestinal diseases. It prevents the multiplication of most bacteria, and freezing often destroys some parasites such as *Toxo-*

*Under 200,000 bacteria/ml by standard plate count before pasteurization and under 30,000 bacteria/ml after pasteurization.

plasma gondii and *Trichinella spiralis*. However, most organisms or toxins already present at the time of refrigeration or freezing will be preserved in the process and can multiply after thawing and reaching the proper temperature.

14.1.5. Animals and Insect Vectors. Animals provide the source of infection for many of the diseases discussed in this book, such as anthrax, brucellosis, *Campylobacter* infection, leptospirosis, plague, salmonellosis, tularemia, and yersiniosis. The types of exposure differ: some are occupational (anthrax) or avocational (tularemia), some result from common environmental exposures (leptospirosis, salmonellosis), some from close contact with domestic animals (*Campylobacter*) or from contamination of water sources (*Campylobacter*, yersiniosis) by animals. Knowledge of these potential sources of infection and of appropriate specific measures to avoid or minimize exposure are needed.

Insect vectors may play a passive or active role in transmission of bacterial infections. Passive transfer of the organisms of cholera, salmonellosis, and typhoid fever by flies and other insects may occur but does not seem to be of much epidemiological significance. Good food sanitation, proper storage, and screens are useful to prevent such transfer. The active transport of infection involves multiplication in the insect host. Rickettsial infections are commonly transmitted by insect vectors: *Rickettsia rickettsii* of Rocky Mountain spotted fever by wood, dog, and Lone Star ticks; *R. akari* of rickettsialpox by the mouse mite; and *R. prowazekii* of typhus fevers by the body louse (louse-borne typhus) or rat flea (murine typhus). *Borrelia burgdorferi*, the spirochete that causes Lyme disease, is transmitted by ticks of the *Ixodid* genus, such as *I. dammini*, the deer tick in eastern and midwestrn states, and by *I. pacifus* in western states. Ticks may also transmit ehrlichiosis (Sennetsu fever) and babesiosis, and cases have been recognized in the eastern United States.

The control of many of these insect vectors is very difficult, since they exist widely in nature and in many domestic gardens and lawns in endemic areas. Careful protection of the body, especially wearing long pants and high stockings along with an antitick insecticide in summer months in outside work are important in prevention of tick bites. Intensive searching of the body, as well as domestic pets, after potential exposure is important in preventing Lyme infection, since the tick must remain on the skin some 24 h before it can transmit the organism. Attention should also be directed at the control or avoidance of the dog, rat, mouse, deer, or other animal hosts on which the ticks usually reside. The body louse is controlled by good personal and clothing hygiene and by delousing procedures (heat and chemical treatment).

14.2. Host Factors

The human host may be protected against infection and disease by quarantine or isolation from the sources of infection, by good personal hygiene (especially hand washing), by specific immunization, and by chemoprophylaxis.

14.2.1. Quarantine and Isolation. Quarantine, which began around 1348 as a 40-day period of keeping suspected plague victims aboard ships or in house quarantine in Venice, has now been rendered largely obsolete by air travel. The WHO now evokes quarantine measures only for plague, yellow fever, and cholera. We rely on surveillance techniques, as discussed in Chapter 2 and by Teutsch,[16] to provide constant monitoring and analysis of infectious diseases and of other conditions of public health importance. The emergence of new and antibiotic-resistant infectious agents[10] has alerted us to the deficiencies in our current surveillance system in the United States,[112] as well as in Europe.[15] A prevention and surveillance strategy has been developed by the CDC for these emerging infections.[96]

Isolation requirements and techniques have also undergone redefinition and reassessment (see Chapter 25 and recent books for details).[113,114] Varying isolation standards in hospitals have been developed for various groups of diseases and often depend on state laws or hospital regulations. Infectious diseases in hospitals have been grouped according to the degree of isolation recommended. Standard precautions are recommended for all patients regardless of their diagnosis. Specific precautions, "transmission-based precautions," are recommended for specific situations. Hand washing remains as a recommendation following any patient contact.

Standard precautions are now legally mandated based on the assumption that the blood and certain body fluids (amniotic fluid, pericardial fluid, peritoneal fluid, pleural fluid, cerebrospinal fluid, semen, vaginal secretions, and any body fluid visibly contaminated with blood) are potentially infected, irrespective of the patient from which it is derived. With this in mind, the CDC has issued recommendations for the prevention of transmission of HIV, hepatitis B, and other blood-borne pathogens in medical care settings.[115] These standard precautions are to be applied to all patients, including those coming into emergency rooms, where there is often risk of such exposures and the status of the patient is usually unknown. The approach also applies to outpatient settings that involve handling of blood or body fluids. Standard precautions specifically involve the use of gloves whenever contact with blood or other such body fluids is anticipated and other barrier techniques (masks, gowns, and protective eyewear) whenever splashes of such fluids are expected. This would apply to the use of gloves when touching blood and body fluids, mucous membranes, or soiled articles or surfaces, and when doing venipunctures or inserting intravenous lines, and to the use of masks in operative or invasive procedures. The decision to initiate routine HIV testing or testing of high-risk patients and of high-risk hospital personnel engaged in invasive or other procedures is left to physicians or individual institutions. If such testing is carried out, the CDC outlines the principles of informed consent and confidentiality involved.(116)

14.2.2. Hygiene. High standards of cleanliness of the individual, the family, the food prepared, and the community contribute to the prevention of infectious diseases. The simple measure of thorough and frequent hand washing is of the highest importance in protecting the individual against pathogens and in interrupting the spread of organisms to others. It plays an essential role in controlling the spread of infection in hospitals and institutions, in restaurants, and in food processing both in industries and in the home. The promotion, distribution, and proper use of soap and water for personal hygiene in developing countries need greater emphasis. Its use should decrease enteric and respiratory infections.

14.2.3. Immunization. The specific protection of the individual against infection and disease is the key to modern preventive practice. It may be either passive protection by the transfer of a specific antibody (or antitoxin) from another person or animal immune to it, or active immunization through induction of antibody by the organism itself or an antigenic derivative of it. An ideal vaccine closely simulates the protection from natural infection, i.e., it produces good humoral, cellular, and local immunity of long duration. Preferably, it should be better than the short-lived or incomplete immunity found in certain infections such as cholera or shigellosis. It should be in a form of administration and at a cost acceptable to the public. The cost of the vaccine and any side effects should be less than those of the natural disease prevented by it. These ideals are most closely met by well-attenuated live vaccines or antigenic derivatives thereof. The live bacterial vaccines include bacille Calmette–Guérin (BCG) for tuberculosis, a recently developed and licensed oral vaccine (using strain Ty21a) for typhoid fever, and tularemia vaccine. BCG is sparsely used in the United States, and controversy exists about its efficacy (see below). Tularemia vaccine is used in rather small, high-risk groups. Most bacterial vaccines are formalin-, acetone-, or phenol-killed organisms or an antigenic derivative such as the capsular polysaccharides of the meningococcus and pneumococcus (23 types), the toxoids of diphtheria and tetanus, or the protein antigens of *B. anthracis*.

Newer or improved vaccine preparations for many bacterial diseases are under development, testing, or licensure such as those for cholera, *H. influenzae* type b conjugate (now licensed and used) pertussis, shigellosis, and typhoid fever. The use of conjugated polysaccharide vaccines improves their antigenicity, permitting them to be used in young children.

Someday, timed-release biodegradable polymers may permit pulsed release of vaccines, such as tetanus, thus permitting a single shot to be effective, and avoid the loss now occurring in women and children who do not return to complete the multiple doses required for most killed vaccines. The Institute of Medicine of the US National Academy of Sciences has published a comprehensive evaluation of vaccine priorities for both developed and developing countries based on their feasibility, cost, need, effectiveness, acceptability, side reactions, and other factors.(117)

In developing countries, the WHO's Expanded Program in Immunization is making an enormous effort to vaccinate the young children of the world against six targeted diseases using diphtheria–pertussis–tetanus (DPT), polio, measles, and BCG vaccines, as well as hepatitis B and yellow fever vaccine in some regions. Important progress is being made, and the worldwide coverage in 1996 was approximately 70%. Other organizations are now joining in this effort, as part of a "Child Survival Program," and there is a focus on "growth, oral rehydration therapy, breast feeding, and immunization" (GOBI). The Children's Vaccine Initiative, the organization that manages the technological transition toward new vaccines, has outlined the desired characteristics of such vaccines and has stated that they should be capable of being given orally in the first year of life. In the United States, the recommendation by states that all children be immunized before being allowed into school has greatly expanded coverage in this country. Of the nine diseases against which children are routinely vaccinated, the reported number for five of these and for congenital rubella syndrome were at or near the lowest levels ever.(118) The reported number of these five diseases in 1996 were: diphtheria (2 cases), measles (508 cases), poliomyelitis (wild virus—0 cases), rubella (238 cases), and tetanus (36 cases). Only seven cases of congenital rubella syndrome were reported. Measles is a good example of the progress made. After an outbreak of measles between 1989 and 1991 that involved more than 50,000 cases and 11,000 hospitalizations, reported cases declined from 9643 cases in 1991 to only 281 in 1993.[118,119] Rapid progress is being made in the reduction of meningitis caused by type b *H. influenzae* due to the widespread use of Hib vaccines.

In a survey in 1987, however, serious vaccine deficiencies were found in adults.[120] For example, serosurveys indicated that 49–66% of persons 60 years or over lacked reliable protective levels of circulating antitoxin against tetanus, and 41–84% lacked adequate protection against diphtheria. Tetanus is a completely preventable disease, and persons over 50 account for 70% of reported cases; thus, special emphasis must be placed on this age group for tetanus boosters, or an initial series if not previously vaccinated. Pneumococcal vaccine is also badly underutilized as indicated by the fact that less than 10% of the higher-risk groups have been vaccinated. A similar lack of protection of our adult population exists against many viral diseases, especially influenza, measles, mumps, rubella, and hepatitis B, as well as pneumonia. Today, some 50,000 to 70,000 adults die each year of influenza, pneumococcal infections, and hepatitis B, with a cost to society of these and other vaccine-preventable diseases of adults exceeding 10 billion dollars each year.[121] Detailed recommendations have been issued to improve this situation[121] and a call for action issued by the CDC.[122]

Recommendations for the immunization of persons with altered immunocompetence, such as AIDS, have been made by the Advisory Committee on Immunization Practice (ACIP). In general, live viral or bacterial vaccines are contraindicated in persons with severe immunodeficiency due to any cause, including HIV-infected persons. However, evaluation and testing for HIV infection of asymptomatic persons are not necessary before administering measles–mumps–rubella (MMR) vaccine, since no documented serious adverse reactions have been noted in either asymptomatic or symptomatic persons infected with HIV. Thus, MMR vaccine is recommended for both adults and children when otherwise indicated, regardless of HIV status. Enhanced, inactivated poliomyelitis vaccine is preferred in HIV-infected persons, as is pneumococcal vaccine of these persons over age 2 years. HIV-infected children under 2 years should receive Hib vaccine according to the routine schedules. Both HIV-infected children may have suboptimal immune responses to such vaccines. Recent studies suggest, however, that the benefits of measles, mumps, and rubella vaccines outweigh the risks to children with AIDS, at least in developing countries. It should be noted that in developing countries where the risks of exposure are higher, greater use of live vaccines is recommended. The WHO thus recommends use of standard Expanded Programme on Immunization (EPI) vaccines in persons with symptomatic or asymptomatic HIV infections,[123] but suggests that inactivated poliomyelitis vaccine (IPV) be considered as an alternative to oral polio vaccine (OPV). Some complications have arisen with BCG vaccine in such immunosuppressed children, and its use should be suspended in unimmunized individuals with symptomatic AIDS in countries where the other targeted diseases remain serious risks; in asymptomatic HIV-infected individuals in areas where the risk of tuberculosis is high, BCG is recommended at birth or soon thereafter. Guidelines should be consulted for updated recommendations, as data are often incomplete. Separate needles are required to avoid the possibility of parenteral transmission of HIV (and hepatitis B virus). The jet gun should not be used in immunization programs, except in an epidemic emergency, until further data are available on the possible risks associated with its use.

Table 13[124] gives the current recommended schedule for active vaccination of infants and children. Standards for pediatric immunization have also been issued by the same committee.[125] Information for international travelers,[126] as well as the uses and limitations of each vaccine, will be found in the appropriate chapters of this book. A brief summary follows.

14.2.3a. Anthrax. No confirmed cases reported in the United States since 1988. The vaccine is distributed only by the Division of Biologics, Michigan Department of Public Health, and is intended only for high-risk occupational exposures, such as persons working with imported goat hair, wool, and hides (sheep and goats) and laboratory workers regularly exposed to this organism. The vaccine is a killed cell-free culture filtrate prepared from the protective antigen. A recent review of anthrax is available.[127] (See also Chapter 4.)

14.2.3b. Botulism. There are three forms: classical, infant, and wound; a total of 119 cases were reported in 1996. Passive immunization is available consisting of horse serum with anti-A, B, and E toxins and used for persons strongly suspected of botulism or when disease is first diagnosed. Trivalent antitoxin is available from the CDC in Atlanta. There is a 10–15% risk of adverse reactions (anaphylaxis, serum sickness). Botulism toxoid is also available and effective, but because of the rarity of the intoxication, it is recommended only for laboratory workers and others working directly with the toxin. It can be obtained from the CDC. (See also Chapter 6.)

14.2.3c. Cholera. The available inactivated vaccine offers rather poor protection (about 50%) over a short

Table 13. Recommended Childhood Immunization Schedule, United States, 1997 [a]

Vaccine	Birth	1 mo	2 mos	4 mos	6 mos	12 mos	15 mos	18 mos	4–6 yrs	11–12 yrs	14–16 yrs
	Age										
Hepatitis B[b,c]	Hep B-1										
			Hep B-2		Hep B-3					Hep B[c]	
Diphtheria, and tetanus toxoids and acellular pertussis[d]			DTap or DTP	DTap or DTP	DTap or DTP		DTap or DTP		DTap or DTP	Td	
Haemophilus influenzae type b[e]			Hib	Hib	Hib	Hib					
Poliovirus[f]			Polio[f]	Polio			Polio		Polio		
Measles, mumps, rubella[g]						MMR			MMR	or MMR	
Varicella virus[h]							Var			Var	

[a]This schedule indicates the recommended age for routine administration of currently licensed childhood vaccines. Some combination vaccines are available and may be used whenever administration of all components of the vaccine is indicated. Providers should consult the manufacturers' package inserts for detailed recommendations. Vaccines are listed under the routinely recommended ages. Bars indicate range of acceptable ages for vaccination. Shaded bars indicate catch-up vaccination: at 11–12 years, hepatitis B vaccine should be administered to children not previously vaccinated, and varicella virus vaccine should be administered to unvaccinated children who lack a reliable history of chickenpox. Use of trade names and commerical sources is for identification only and does not imply endorsement by the Public Health Service or the U.S. Department of Health and Human Services. Source: Advisory Committee on Immunization Practices (ACIP), American Academy of Pediatrics (AAP), and American Academy of Family Physicians (AAFP).

[b]**Infants born to hepatitis B surface antigen (HBsAg)-negative mothers** should receive 2.5 μg of Merck vaccine (Recombivax HB®) or 10 μg of SmithKline Beecham (SB) vaccine (Energix-B®). The second dose should be administered >1 month after the first dose. **Infants born to HBsAg-positive mothers** should receive 0.5 mL hepatitis B immune globulin (HBIG) within 12 hours of birth and either 5 μg of Merck vaccine (Recombivax HB®) or 10 μg of SB vaccine (Engerix-B®) at a separate site. The second dose is recommended at age 1–2 months and the third dose at age 6 months. **Infants born to mothers whose HBsAg status is unknown** should receive either 5 μg of Merck vaccine (Recombivax HB®) or 10 μg of SB vaccine (Engerix-B®) within 12 hours of birth. The second dose of vaccine is recommended at age 1 month and the third dose at age 6 months. Blood should be drawn at the time of delivery to determine the mother's HBsAg status; if it is positive, the infant should receive HBIG as soon as possible (no later than age 1 week). The dosage and timing of subsequent vaccine doses should be based on the mother's HBsAg status.

[c]Children and adolescents who have not been vaccinated against hepatitis B during infancy may begin the series during any childhood visit. Those who have not previously received three doses of hepatitis B vaccine should initiate or complete the series at age 11–12 years. The second dose should be administered at least 1 month after the first dose, and the third dose should be administered at least 4 months after the first dose and at least 2 months after the second dose.

[d]Diphtheria and tetanus toxoids and acellular pertussis vaccine (DTaP) is the preferred vaccine for all doses in the vaccination series, including completion of the series in children who have received one or more doses of whole-cell diphtheria and tetanus toxoids and pertussis vaccine (DTP). Whole-cell DPT is an acceptable alternative to DTaP. The fourth dose of DTaP may be administered as early as 12 months of age provided 6 months have elapsed since the third dose and if the child is considered unlikely to return at age 15–18 months. Tetanus and diphtheria toxoids (Td), absorbed, for adult use, is recommended at age 11–12 years if at least 5 years have elapsed since the last dose of DTP, DTaP, or diphtheria and tetanus toxoids. Subsequent routine Td boosters are recommended every 10 years.

[e]Three *H. influenzae* type b (Hib) conjugate vaccines are licensed for infant use. If PRP-OMP (PedvaxHIB® [Merck]) is administered at ages 2 and 4 months, a dose at age 6 months is not required. After completing the primary series, any Hib conjugate vaccine may be used as a booster.

[f]Two poliovirus vaccines are currently licensed in the United States: inactivated poliovirus vaccine (IPV) and oral poliovirus vaccine (OPV). The following schedules are all acceptable by ACIP, AAP, and AAFP, and parents and providers may choose among them: 1) IPV at ages 2 and 4 months and OPV at age 12–18 months and at age 4–6 years; 2) IPV at ages 2, 4, and 12–18 months and at age 4–6 years; and 3) OPV at ages 2, 4, and 6–18 months and at age 4–6 years. ACIP routinely recommends schedule 1. IPV is the only poliovirus vaccine recommended for immunocompromised persons and their household contacts.

[g]The second dose of measles-mumps-rubella vaccine is routinely recommended at age 4–6 years or at age 11–12 years but may be administered during any visit provided at least 1 month has elapsed since receipt of the first dose and that both doses are administered at or after age 12 months.

[h]Susceptible children may receive varicella vaccine (Var) during any visit after the first birthday, and unvaccinated persons who lack a reliable history of chickenpox should be vaccinated at age 11–12 years. Susceptible persons aged $\geqslant 13$ years should receive two doses at least 1 month apart.

period (3–6 months); the transmission of infection is not prevented. No country or territory currently requires immunization for entry.[(126)] However, local authorities may require it, and one dose satisfies such regulations and is valid for 6 months. For persons highly exposed in highly endemic areas, a three-dose primary series is given 1 week to 1 month apart and a booster dose every 6 months. The vaccine is probably not effective against the newly discovered *V. cholera* 039 strain. A number of oral cholera vaccines are under development and testing, some of which contain the *V. cholera* 039-Bengal strain.

14.2.3d. Diphtheria–Pertussis–Tetanus (DPT) Vaccine (see Table 13). Routine primary immunization with DPT vaccine is given at 2, 4, and 6 months with a fourth dose at 15 months and a booster at 4–6 years before entry into school.[(124)] Some 20% of adults or more may be unprotected against diphtheria and need either a full primary series or a booster dose of a preparation for adults or children >7 years old (Td). Booster doses of Td are suggested for all adults every 10 years.[121] Local Arthus-type reactions and sometimes systemic immune complex reactions (serum sickness) may occur in hyperimmunized adults. These may be attended by severe head, muscle, and joint aches and fever of about 24 h duration. Corticosteroids may be given orally over 3 to 5 days, for symptomatic relief. Diphtheria antitoxin should be given to asymptomatic, unimmunized contacts in whom close surveillance is not possible, plus penicillin (600,000 U of the benzathine form or, if sensitive, a 7-day course of erythromycin) and injection of diphtheria toxoid. If close surveillance is possible, the antitoxin can be omitted.

14.2.3e. Haemophilus influenzae Type b Vaccine (Hib). This infection is an important cause of meningitis in children, particularly those under the age of 5 years, and is now being recognized as important in older persons whose immunity has waned. Two forms of conjugated vaccines are available, and two in combination with DPT. They are given at 2, 4, and 6 months with DPT and OPV and again at 12–15 months when MMR is given. One preparation (PRP–OMP) is not given at 6 months (see Table 13 on routine active vaccination of infants and children). (See also Chapter 16.)

14.2.3f. Meningococcal Infections. Meningococcal infections can result in epidemics but, in US civilians, most commonly occur as single cases or localized clusters, with a third of the cases occurring in persons 20 years of age or over. Two polysaccharide vaccines are currently available in the United States: a bivalent A-C and a quadrivalent vaccine containing A, C, Y, and W-135 polysaccharides. A single dose of either is adequate to induce serospecific immunity.[32] Routine vaccination is not recommended in the United States because of the relatively low risk of infection and because a good group B antigen is not available. Vaccine usage is recommended as an adjunct to antibiotic chemoprophylaxis for household and other close contacts of persons with meningococcal disease due to serotypes A, C, Y, and W-135. The quadrivalent vaccine is recommended for travelers to endemic areas. The duration of protection is unclear. Side reactions are infrequent and mild, but the safety for pregnant women has not been established. Because of the high risk in military recruits, they have received meningococcal vaccine on entering the services since the early 1970s. Currently, they receive groups A, C, Y, and W-135. (See also Chapter 23.)

14.2.3g. Plague. The vaccine consists of formalin-inactivated organisms; its efficacy has not been critically evaluated. It should be given only to high-risk groups such as field and laboratory personnel exposed to the organism and possibly to workers in plague enzootic or endemic rural areas where avoidance of rodents, fleas, and wild rabbits is not feasible (agricultural advisors, Peace Corps volunteers, or military personnel on maneuvers).[24] The schedule consists of five injections, with dosage varying with age. In the face of continued exposure, single booster doses at about 6-month intervals are given for two doses, then at 1- to 2-year intervals. Local reactions are common, sterile abscesses are rare, and systemic reactions (fever, headache, and malaise) may occur on repeated injections. (See also Chapter 27.)

14.2.3h. Pneumococcal Infections. The estimated annual incidence of pneumococcal pneumonia in the United States is 68 to 260 cases per 100,000 population and of bacteremia is 7–25 per 100,000. Mortality is highest in patients with bacteremia, meningitis, underlying medical conditions, and those over 60 years of age. The currently available pneumococcal polysaccharide vaccine contains purified capsular materials from 23 types of *Streptococcus pneumoniae*, which together account for 87% of recent bacteremic pneumonia in the United States. The vaccine is particularly recommended for three groups: (1) adults with chronic diseases, especially of the cardiovascular or pulmonary systems; (2) adults with chronic illnesses specifically associated with an increased risk of pneumococcal infection or its complications (splenic dysfunction, Hodgkin's disease, multiple myeloma, cirrhosis, alcoholism, renal failure, CSF leaks, and in immunosuppressed patients); and (3) older adults, especially those 65 years of age and over, regardless of whether they are healthy or diseased. Vaccination is recommended for hospitalized patients in these high-risk groups before discharge. A single dose is recommended without a booster. Mild side reactions consisting of erythema and of pain at the site of injection occur in about half the recipients. Medicare helps pay the cost in these designated groups. Pneumococcal infections are also a problem in young children in developing countries, so that there is increasing interest in the use of the vaccine in these groups. (See also Chapter 28.)

14.2.3i. Tetanus. See DPT (see Section 14.2.3d) for routine immunization. For wound management, tetanus–diphtheria (Td) adult-type, or tetanus toxoid (TT) only, is used alone or in combination with tetanus immune globulin (TIG) in doses of 250 U (in separate site and syringe), depending on the severity of the wound and the history of prior immunization. Moderate to severe local and systemic reactions may occur in some hyperimmune adults receiving booster doses or for wound prophylaxis. (See also Chapter 37.)

14.2.3j. Tuberculosis. This disease remains the most important cause of death in the world due to an infectious agent. It is a major killer of individuals in persons aged 20 to 30 years. In 1994, the WHO declared this disease to be a public health emergency,[128] and it is believed to be "out of control" in many parts of the world. The WHO identified ten industrial countries in which cases of tuberculosis increased 5–33% in recent years. In the United States, an estimated 15 million persons are believed to be infected. The increase of infection in HIV-infected persons with the emergence of multidrug resistant strains in this group and in others who were inadequately treated is of special concern. Such resistant strains spread readily to others. About 4.5% of tuberculosis in the United States was associated with HIV infection, and a rise to 13.8% is anticipated by the year 2000. As Comstock[129] has pointed out, the patterns of change and reasons for it are multiple and complex both in the United States and other areas of the world. While HIV is widely blamed, there are many other factors such as migration, poverty, malnutrition, and decreased tuberculosis control efforts, and it is difficult to assess the relative importance of each in the trends observed. In 1991, 56% of active cases were reported among Hispanics and African Americans. The only vaccine available is BCG, and contradictory evidence exists as to its efficacy. An excellent brief review has recently summarized the evidence.[130] More people have received BCG vaccine than any other vaccine, yet it efficacy remains in doubt. It is a part of the routine WHO EPI program. For example, the WHO estimates that 85% of all children born in 1990 received BCG vaccine in their first year of life. Estimates of its efficacy range from 0 to 80% in different settings. Such great variation has been attributed to different vaccine strains, methodological differences, variation in the infecting organism in different countries, the genetic background of the exposed groups, and environmental interactions with other mycobacterial strains in the population. Indeed, a higher efficacy has been seen against leprosy than tuberculosis in some studies. One recent meta-analysis involving 14 trials and 12 observational studies concluded that BCG reduced the risk of tuberculosis by 50%,[131] despite great heterogeneity in the data. In another meta-analysis of results showing homogeneity, BCG was 86% effective against miliary tuberculosis and tuberculous meningitis; the preventive effect against pulmonary tuberculosis showed such heterogeneity that they did not calculate a summary measure.[132] It seems reasonable to believe that BCG is effective against the spread of tuberculosis within the body, such as miliary spread and spread to the meninges, but that its protection against infection varies greatly in different settings and with different vaccines. Comstock[129] has discussed the use of BCG and the CDC has outlined its use in control in a joint statement with the ACIP and the Advisory Committee on the Control of Tuberculosis.[133] General problems in the production standards for BCG and the need for recombinant technology in the development of a vaccine whose mechanism of action and efficacy can be better understood and evaluated have been recently presented.[134–136] BCG use is not routinely recommended in the United States because of the generally low incidence of disease and because BCG interferes with the interpetation of the tuberculin skin test. These recommendations may have to be modified for high-risk groups, in view of recent increases in incidence and resistant organisms. (See also Chapter 39.)

14.2.3k. Typhoid. Not recommended for routine use in the United States or for international travel except for areas where there is a recognized risk of exposure to *Salmonella typhi*. It is recommended for travelers who will have prolonged exposure to potentially contaminated food and water in smaller cities or villages in rural areas in Africa, Asia, and Central and South America. An oral, live attenuated vaccine is licensed containing the Ty21a strain. It is taken in an enteric-coated capsule on alternate days for four doses, with a booster dose every 5 years if exposure continues.[137] An inactivated parenteral vaccine is also available and soon a Vi capsular polysaccharide vaccine will be available. Few reactions are due to the oral vaccine, but local and systemic reactions lasting 1–2 days are common with the inactivated parenteral vaccine. (See also Chapter 42.)

14.2.4. Antibiotic Prophylaxis The success of preventing natural infection or disease or both with antibiotic prophylaxis depends on the sensitivity of the organism to the drug employed, whether single or multiple bacterial species are involved, the timing of administration in relation to infection, and the ability of the drug to reach effective concentrations in body sites before the organism is present. It has been employed in persons at high risk after known exposure in epidemics (meningococcus), in household contacts of cases (e.g., streptococcus, meningococcus, tuberculosis), and in sexual partners (gonococcus, syphilis), one of whom is infected. It has been employed after infection is diagnosed to prevent further spread or to limit complications (tuberculosis, rheumatic fever) or to limit the duration of the carrier state. The major limitations have been the development of antibiotic resistance, multiple organisms causing the disease, and poor patient compliance for long-term prophylaxis. Any mass prophylactic program aimed at a large group, especially a closed population, over a long term

Table 14. Prophylactic Uses of Antibiotics

Condition	Chapter (section) in this volume	Persons at risk	Antibiotic	Dose/time
Diphtheria	13(9)	Carriers of toxigenic strains	Penicillin or erythromycin	Full dose over 7–10 days
Gonorrhea	15(9)	Persons sexually exposed to infection	Penicillin	Full dosage as for treatment
Meningococcal meningitis	23(9)	Intimate contacts of cases or in closed outbreaks	Sulfadiazene for sensitive organisms	1 g adults or 0.5 g children q 12 h × 4 doses
			Rifampin	10 mg/kg per day for 4 days
Strep and rheumatic fever	34(9)	Rheumatic heart disease patients (prevention of rheumatic fever)	Penicillin (benzathine), i.m.	1.2 million U/mo
		Sometimes family contacts of strep cases	Penicillin, oral	200,000–250,000 U daily
Surgical infections	25(9.2.8)	Certain surgical patients[a]	Dependent on site of operation	
Syphilis	35(9)	Known exposures ("epidemiological treatment")	Penicillin	Same as treatment
Tuberculosis	39(9.3)	Recent skin test positives	INH	Adults 5 mg/kg per day for 12 mo
		Contacts of cases		
		Healed Tb patients; nevertreated Tb cases		

[a]C-V, C-section and vaginal hysterectomy, prophylactic hip, certain intestinal, biliary, CNS.

sets the stage for the development of resistance in the organism of interest as well as other circulating organisms. Antibiotic prophylaxis has met with debatable success when the bacterial sensitivity is not high, if the antibiotic is inhibitory but not bactericidal, if multiple organisms are involved (especially gram-negative), and if the risk of infection is relatively low, as in clean surgical operations. For greater detail, see books on clinical infectious diseases[(38)] or reviews on antibiotic usage,[(138)] as well as specific chapters in this book.

Table 14 lists some uses of antibiotic prophylaxis. The most successful are the prevention of recurrent streptococcal infections in persons with rheumatic heart disease and the prevention of disease in persons with infections due to *M. tuberculosis*, especially recent infections. Antibiotic prophylaxis with sulfadiazine for sulfa-sensitive organisms or rifampin for sulfa-resistant organisms is advocated for family or close contacts of patients with meningococcal meningitis or outbreaks in closed settings. These principles apply in large community outbreaks when sulfadiazine is given on a mass basis for sulfonamide-sensitive meningococci; of resistant strains in this situation, rifampin is not recommended because of the possibility of developing resistance to this drug.[(17)] "Epidemiological treatment" after known sexual exposure to gonorrhea or syphilis is effective, but requires a full therapeutic regimen. Prevention of infection during and after surgery is advocated in surgical procedures at high risk to infection such as total hip and knee replacement, colon–rectal surgery, and transurethreal resection of the prostate.[(139)] Patients whose immune status is compromised by steroids, irradiation, alkylating and antimetabolic agents, and other immunosuppressive drugs are at high risk to certain bacterial, fungal, and viral organisms, including some that are not normally pathogenic, but no antimicrobial prophylaxis has been effective. They may be placed in protective isolation (see Section 14.2.1) and closely watched and antibiotic therapy instituted if infection occurs. A possible exception to the ineffectiveness of antibiotics in preventing infections is the prophylactic use of isoniazid in immunosuppressed patients with inactive tuberculosis. Antibiotics or other prophylactic measures for prevention of traveler's diarrhea are recommended only for the long-term traveler in high-risk endemic areas[(80,106)]; for short-term visitors, bismuth subsalicylate has proved useful.[(43)]

15. References

1. Last, J. M. E., *A Dictionary of Epidemiology*, 2nd ed., Oxford University Press, New York, 1988.
2. Evans, A. S., Re: Definitions of epidemiology [letter], *Am. J. Epidemiol.* **109:**379–381 (1979).
3. Evans, A. S., The clinical illness promotion factor. A third ingredient, *Yale J. Biol. Med.* **55:**193–199 (1985).

4. Evans, A. S., Subclinical epidemiology. The First Harry A. Feldman Memorial Lecture, *Am. J. Epidemiol.* **125:**545–555 (1987).
5. Evans, A. S., and Kaslow, R. A. (eds.), *Viral Infections of Humans: Epidemiology and Control*, 4th ed., Plenum Medical, New York, 1997.
6. Eisenstein, B. L., The polymerase chain reaction: A new method of using molecular genetics for medical diagnosis, *N. Engl. J. Med.* **322:**178–183 (1990).
7. Centers for Disease Control and Prevention, *Reference and Disease Surveillance*, Centers for Disease Control and Prevention, Atlanta, 1994.
8. Tompkins, L. S., The use of molecular methods in infectious diseases, *N. Engl. J. Med.* **327:**1290–1297 (1992).
9. Kuller, L. H., Relationship between acute and chronic disease epidemiology, *Yale J. Biol. Med.* **60:**363–366 (1987).
10. Lederberg, J., Shope, R. E., and Oaks, S. C. J. (eds.), *Emerging Infections: Microbial Threats to Health in the United States*, National Academy Press, Washington, DC, 1992.
11. Centers for Disease Control, Addressing emerging infectious disease threats: A prevention strategy for the United States. Executive summary, *Morbid. Mortal. Week. Rep.* **43**(No. RR-5)**:** 1–18 (1994).
12. Cutts, F. T., Waldman, R. J., and Zoffman, H. M. D., Surveillance for the Expanded Programme on Immunization, *Bull. World Health Organ.* **71:**633–639 (1993).
13. Brogan, D., Flagge, E. W., Deming, M., and Wsalsman, R., Increasing accuracy of the Expanded Programme on Immunization's cluster survey design, *Ann. Epidemiol.* **4:**302–311 (1993).
14. Centers for Disease Control, Guidelines for evaluating surveillance systems, *Morbid. Mortal. Week. Rep.* **37:**S–5 (1988).
15. Desenclos, J.-C., Bijkerk, H., and Huisman, J. Variations in national infectious diseases surveillance in Europe, *Lancet*, **341:**1003–1006 (1993).
16. Teutsch, S. M., and Churchill, R. E. *Principles and Practice of Public Health Surveillance*, Oxford University Press, New York, 1994.
17. Benenson, A. S., *Control of Communicable Diseases Manual*, 16th ed., American Public Health Association, New York, 1995.
18. Kelsey, J. L., Thompson, W. D., and Evans, A. S. *Methods in Observational Epidemiology*, Oxford University Press, New York, 1989.
19. Hennekens, C. H., and Buring, J. E., *Epidemiology in Medicine*, Little, Brown, Boston, 1987.
20. Rothman, K. J., *Modern Epidemiology*, Little, Brown, Boston, 1986.
21. Lilienfeld, D. E., and Stolley, P., *Fundamentals of Epidemiology*, 3rd ed., Oxford University Press, New York, 1994.
22. Beaglehole, R., Bonita, R., and Kjellstrom, T., *Basic Epidemiology*, World Health Organization, Geneva, 1993.
23. Mueller, N., Evans, A. S., Harris, N. L., Comstock, G. W., Jellum, E., Magnus, K., Orientreich, N., Polk, B. F., and Vogelman, J., Hodgkin's disease and Epstein–Barr virus. Altered antibody patterns before diagnosis, *N. Engl. J. Med.* **320:**689–695 (1989).
24. Kelsey, J. L., Thompson, W. D., and Evans, A. S. (Eds.), Epidemic investigation, in: *Methods in Observational Epidemiology*, pp. 212–253, Oxford University Press, London, 1986.
25. Gregg, M. B., The principles of epidemic investigation, in: *Oxford Textbook of Public Health* (A. Chappie, W. W. Holland, R. Detels, and G. Knox, eds.), pp. 284–297, Oxford University Press, London, 1986.
26. Centers for Disease Control, Investigation of disease outbreaks, *Homestudy Course 3030-G, Manual 6*, p. 1–79 (1979).
27. Dwyer, D. M., Strickler, H., Goodman, R. A., and Armenian, H. A., Use of case–control studies in outbreak investigations, *Epidemiol. Rev.* **16:**109–123 (1994).
28. MacKensie, W. R., Hoxie, N. J., Proctor, M. E., *et al.*, A massive outbreak in Milwaukee of *Cryptosporidium* infection transmitted through the public water supply, *N. Engl. J. Med.* **331:**161–167 (1994).
29. Fraser, D. W., Tsai, T. R., Orenstein, W., Perkin, W. E., Beecham, H. J., Sharrar, R. G., Harris, J., Mallison, G. F., Martin, S. M., Shepard, C. C., Brachman, P. S., and the Field Investigation Team, Legionnaire's disease—Description of an epidemic of pneumonia, *N. Engl. J. Med.* **287:**1189–1197 (1977).
30. Helsted, A. G., Mandel, A. D., and Evans, A. S., Thermostable *Clostridium perfringens* as cause of food poisoning outbreak, *Public Health Rep.* **82:**157–161 (1967).
31. Jawetz, E., Melnick, J., and Adelberg, E. A. *Review of Medical Microbiology*, 17th ed., Lange, Los Altos, CA, 1987.
32. Mims, C. A., Playfair, J. H. L., Roitt, I. M., Wakelin, D., and Williams, R., *Medical Microbiology*, Mosby, St. Louis, 1993.
33. Urbaschek, B., and Urbaschek, R., Introduction and summary. Perspectives on bacterial pathogenesis and host defense, *Rev. Infect. Dis.* **9**(Suppl 5)**:**S431–S436 (1987).
34. Smith, H., Pathogenicity and the microbe *in vivo*. The 1989 Fred Griffin Lecture, J. Gen. Microbiol. **136:**377–393 (1990).
35. Mims, C. A., *The Pathogenesis of Infectious Disease*, 3rd ed., Grune & Stratton, New York, 1987.
36. Mims, C. A., The Zvonimir Dinter Memorial Lecture. New insights into the pathogenesis of viral infection, *Vet. Microbiol.* **33:**5–12 (1992).
37. Ruddle, N., Tumor necrosis factor and related cytotoxins, *Immunol. Today* **8:**129–130 (1987).
38. Mandell, G. L., Bennett, J. E., and Dolin, R. (eds.), *Principles and Practice of Infectious Diseases*, Churchill Livingstone, New York, 1995.
39. Mims, C. A., The origin of major human infections and the crucial role of person-to-person spread, *Epidemiol. Infect.* **106:**423–433 (1991).
40. Aronsen, S. S., and Osterholm, M., Infectious disease in child day care: Management and prevention. Summary of the symposium and recommendations, *Rev. Infect. Dis.* **8:**672–679 (1986).
41. Osterholm, M. T., Pierson, L. M., and White, K. E., Libby, T. A., Kuritsky, J. N., and McCollough, J. G., The risk of subsequent transmission of *Hemophilus influenzae* type B disease among children in a daycare center: Results of a two-year statewide prospective surveillance and contact survey, *N. Engl. J. Med.* **316:**1–5 (1987).
42. Black, R. E., Epidemiology of travelers' diarrhoea and relative importance of various pathogens, *Rev. Infect. Dis.* **12**(Suppl. 1)**:** S73–S79 (1990).
43. DuPont, H. L., Ericsson, C. D., Johnson, P. C., and Cabada, J., de la, Use of bismuth subsalicate for the prevention of travelers diarrhoea, *Rev. Clin. Infect. Dis.* **12**(Suppl. 1)**:**S54–S67 (1990).
44. Comstock, G., Tuberculosis in twins: A re-analysis of the Prohphit survey, *Am. Rev. Respir. Dis.* **117:**621–624 (1978).
45. Price, D. L., Tetanus toxoid: Direct evidence for retrograde intraaxonal transport, *Science* **188:**945–947 (1975).
46. Paul, W. E., *Fundamental Immunology*, 3rd ed., Raven Press, New York, 1993.
47. Kuby, J., *Immunology*, 2nd ed., W.H. Freeman, New York, 1994.

48. Klein, J. O., Feigin, R. D., and McCracken, G. H. J., Report on the task force on the diagnosis and management of meningitis, *Pediatrics* **78**(Suppl. Part 2):956–989 (1986).
49. Schlech, W. F., Ward, J. I., Band, J. D., Hightower, A., Graser, D., and Broome, C., Bacterial meningitis in the United States, 1978–1981. The National Bacterial Meningitis Surveillance Study, *J. Am. Med. Assoc.* **253:**1749–1754 (1985).
50. Durand, M. L., Calderwood, S. B., Weber, D. J., *et al.*, Acute bacterial meningitis in adults. A review of 493 episodes, *N. Engl. J. Med.* **328:**21–28 (1993).
51. Grant, J. P., *The state of the World's Children, 1990*, Oxford University Press, Oxford, 1990.
52. Berman, S., and McIntosh, G., Selective primary health care: Strategies for control of disease in the developing world: XXI. Acute respiratory infections, *Rev. Infect. Dis.* **7:**674–691 (1985).
53. Berman, S., Acute respiratory infections, *Infect. Dis. Clin. North Am.* **5:**319–336 (1991).
54. Berman, S., Epidemiology of acute respiratory infections in children of developing countries, *Rev. Infect. Dis.* **13**(Suppl. 6):S454–462 (1991).
55. Selwyn, B. J., Epidemiology of acute respiratory tract infection in young children: Comparison of findings from several developing countries, *Rev. Infect. Dis.* **12**(Suppl. 8):S870–S888 (1990).
56. Evans, A. S., and Dick, E. C., Acute pharyngitis and tonsillitis in University of Wisconsin students, *J. Am. Med. Assoc.* **190:**699–708 (1964).
57. Glezon, W. P., Clyde, W. A., Senior, J. J., Schaeffer, C. I., and Denny, F. W., Group A streptococcus, mycoplasmas, and viruses associated with acute pharyngitis, *J. Am. Med. Assoc.* **292:**455–460 (1967).
58. Stevens, D. L., Invasive group A streptococcus infections, *Clin. Infect. Dis.* **14:**2–11 (1992).
59. Stevens, D. L., Invasive group A streptococcal infections: The past, present and future, *Pediatr. Infect. Dis. J.* **13:**561–566 (1994).
60. Rappule, R., Perguni, M., and Falsen, E., Molecular epidemiology of the 1984–1986 outbreak of diphtheria in Sweden, *N. Engl. J. Med.* **318:**12–14 (1988).
61. Brasfield, D. S., Stagno, S., Whitley, R. J., Cloud, G., Cassell, G., and Teller, R. E., Infant pneumonitis associated with cytomegalovirus, *Chlamydia*, *Mycoplasma pneumoniae*, and ureaplasma. Follow up, *Pediatrics* **79:**76–83 (1982).
62. Foy, H. M., Kenny, G. E., Sepi, R., Ochs, H. D., and Allan, I. D., Long-term epidemiology of infections with *Mycoplasma pneumoniae*, *J. Infect. Dis.* **139:**681–687 (1979).
63. Grayston, J. T., Kuo, C. C., Wang, S. P., and Altman, J., A new *Chlamydia psittace* strain, TWAR, isolated in acute respiratory tract infections, *N. Engl. J. Med.* **315:**161–168 (1986).
64. Grayston, J. T., *Chlamydia pneumoniae* (TWAR), in: *Mandell, Douglas and Bennett's Principles and Practice of Infectious Diseases* (G. L. Mandell, J. E. Bennett, and R. Dolin, eds.), pp. 1696–1701, Churchill Livingstone, New York, 1995.
65. Fang, G. D., Fine, M., Orloff, J. S., SArisume, D., Yu, V. L., Kapoor, W., Grayston, J. T., Kohler, R. R., Yee, Y. C., Rih, D., and Vickers, R. M., New and emerging pathogens for community-acquired pneumonia with implication for therapy: A prospective multicenter study of 349 cases, *Medicine* **69:**307–316 (1990).
66. Marrie, T. J., Epidemiology of community acquired pneumonia in the elderly, *Semin. Respir. Infect.* **5:**260–268 (1990).
67. Marrie, T. J., Community-acquired pneumonia, *Clin. Infect. Dis.* **4:**501–515 (1994).
68. Marrie, T. J., New aspects of old pathogens of pneumonia, *Med. Clin. North Am.* **78:**987–995 (1994).
69. Klein, J. O., Otitis media, *Clin. Infect. Dis.* **19:**823–833 (1994).
70. Hedberg, C. W., and Osterholm, M. T., Outbreaks of food-borne and waterborne viral gastroenteritis, *Clin. Microbiol. Rev.* **6:**199–210 (1993).
71. Bean, N. H., and Griffin, P. M., Food-borne disease outbreaks in the United States, 1973–1987: Pathogens, vehicles and trends, *J. Food Protect.* **53:**804–817 (1990).
72. Guerrant, R. L., Hughes, J. M., Lima, N. L., and Crane, J., Diarrhea in developed and developing countries: Magnitude, special settings, and etiologies, *Rev. Infect. Dis.* **12**(Suppl. 1)**:**S41–S49 (1990).
73. Blaser, M. J., *Helicobacter pylori* and the pathogenesis of gastroduodenal inflammation, *J. Infect. Dis.* **161:**626–633 (1990).
74. Blaser, M. J., and Parsonnet, J., Parasitism by the slow bacterium *Helicobacter pylori* leads to altered gastric homeostasis and neoplasia, *J. Clin. Invest.* **94:**4–8 (1994).
75. National Institutes of Health, Summary of the NIH consensus. *Helicobacter pylori* in peptic ulcer disease, *Md. Med. J.* **43:**923–924 (1994).
76. Welliver, R. C., and McLaughlin, S., Unique epidemiology of nosocomial infection in a children's hospital, *Am. J. Dis. Child.* **138:**131–135 (1984).
77. Kelly, T. W. J., Patrick, M. R., and Hillman, K. M., Study of diarrhoea in critically ill patients, *Crit. Care Med.* **11:**7–9 (1983).
78. Gelb, A., and Millers, S., AIDS and gastroenterology, *Am. J. Gastroenterol.* **81:**619–622 (1986).
79. DuPont, H. L., Travellers' diarrhoea. Which antimicrobial? *Drugs* **45:**910–917 (1993).
80. DuPont, H. L., and Ericsson, C. D., Prevention and treatment of traveler's diarrhea [see comments], *N. Engl. J. Med.* **328:**1821–1827 (1993).
81. McAllister, T. A., Oercival, A., Alexander, J. G., Boyce, J. H. M. H., Dulake, C., and Wormald, P. J., Multicenter study of sensitivities of urinary tract pathogens, *Postgrad. Med. J.* **47**(Suppl.)**:** 7–40 (1971).
82. Andriole, V. T., Pyelonephritis, in: *Infectious Diseases* (P. D. Hoeprich, C. Jordan, and A. R. Ronald, eds.), pp. 602–612, Harper & Row, New York, 1994.
83. Johnson, C. C., Definitions, classification, and clinical presentation of urinary tract infections, *Med. Clin. North Am.* **75:**241–252 (1991).
84. Neu, H. C., Urinary tract infections, *Am. J. Med.* **92:**63S–70S (1992).
85. McCue, J. D., Urinary tract infections in the elderly, *Pharmacotherapy* **13:**51S–53S (1993).
86. Pappas, P. G., Laboratory in the diagnosis and management of urinary tract infections, *Med. Clin. North Am.* **75:**313–325 (1991).
87. Centers for Disease Control and Prevention, *Sexually Transmitted Disease Surveillance, 1992–1993*, Centers for Disease Control and Prevention, Atlanta, 1994.
88. Centers for Disease Control, Premarital sexual experience among adolescent women—United States, 1970–1988, *Morbid. Mortal. Week. Rep.* **39:**929–932 (1991).
89. Holmes, K. K., and Stamm, W. E., Chlamydial genital infections: A growing problem, *Hosp. Pract.* **14:**105–117 (1979).
90. Emori, T. G., and Gaynes, R. P., An overview of nosocomial infections, including the role of the microbiology laboratory, *Clin. Microbiol. Rev.* **6:**428–442 (1993).
91. Koneman, E. W., *Introduction to Diagnostic Microbiology*, Lippincott, Philadelphia, 1994.

92. Baron, E. J., Peterson, L. R., and Finegold, S. M., *Bailey and Scott's Diagnostic Microbiology*, 9th ed., Mosby, St. Louis, 1994.
93. Centers for Disease Control, *Reference and Disease Surveillance—1993*, Centers for Disease Control, Atlanta, 1993.
94. Woods, G. L., and Washington, J. A., The clinician and the microbiology laboratory, in: *Principles and Practice of Infectious Diseases* (G. L. Mandell, J. E. Bennett, and R. Dolin, eds.), pp. 169–199, Churchill Livingstone, New York, 1995.
95. Maslow, J. N., Mulligan, M. E., and Arbeit, R. D., Molecular epidemiology: Applications of contemporary techniques to the typing of microorganisms, *Clin. Infect. Dis.* **17:**153–164 (1993).
96. Centers for Disease Control and Prevention, *Addressing Emerging Infectious Disease Threats. A Prevention Strategy for the United States*, Department of Health and Human Services, Public Health Services, Atlanta, 1994.
97. Henle, J., *On Miasmata and Contagie*, Johns Hopkins Press, Baltimore, 1938 (translated and with an introduction by G. Rosen).
98. Koch, R., Ueber die Aetologie der Tuberculose, in: *Verhandlungen des Kongresses fur Inner Medicin. Erst Kongress*, Verlag von J.F. Bergmann, Weisbaden, 1882.
99. Koch, R., Ueber bacteriolgische Forschung, in: *Verh X Int. Med. Cong.*, August Hirschwald, Berlin, 1892.
100. Klebs, E., Ueber Tuberculose, *Deutsch Naturforschung Aertze* **50:**274 (1877).
101. Evans, A. S., *Causation and Disease. A Chronological Journey*, Plenum Medical, New York, 1993.
102. Evans, A. S., Limitations of Koch's postulates, *Lancet* **2:**1277–1278 (1977).
103. Evans, A. S., Evans postulates, in: *Dictionary of Epidemiology* (J. Last, ed.), p. 44, Oxford University Press, New York, 1988.
104. Maxy, K. G., Roseneau, M. J., and Last, J. M. (eds.), *Public Health and Preventive Medicine*, 12th ed., Appleton-Century-Crofts, New York, 1986.
105. Osterholm, M. T., Hedberg, C. W., and MacDonald, K. L., Prevention and treatment of traveler's diarrhea [letter; comment], *N. Engl. J. Med.* **329:**1584; discussion 1585 (1993).
106. Ericsson, C. D., and DuPont, H. L., Travelers' diarrhea: Approaches to prevention and treatment, *Clin. Infect. Dis.* **16:**616–624 (1993).
107. MacDonald, K. L., and Osterholm, M. T., The emergence of *Escherichia coli* O157:H7 infection in the United States. The changing epidemiology of foodborne disease [editorial; comment], *J. Am. Med. Assoc.* **269:**2264–2266 (1993).
108. Hedberg, C. W., Levine, W. C., White, K. E., *et al.*, An international foodborne outbreak of shigellosis associated with a commercial airline [see comments], *J. Am. Med. Assoc.* **268:**3208–3212 (1992).
109. Hedberg, C. W., Korlath, J. A., D'Aoust, J. Y., White, K. E., Schell, W. L., Miller, M. R., Cameron, D. N., MacDonald, K. L., and Osterholm, M. T., A multistate outbreak of *Salmonella javiana* and *Salmonella oranienburg* infections due to consumption of contaminated cheese [see comments], *J. Am. Med. Assoc.* **268:** 3203–3207 (1992).
110. Hedberg, C. W., MacDonald, K. L., and Osterholm, M. T., Changing epidemiology of food-borne disease: A Minnesota perspective, *Clin. Infect. Dis.* **18:**671–682 (1994).
111. Hedberg, C. W., and Osterholm, M. T., Food safety for the 1990s, *Minn. Med.* **76:**33–36 (1993).
112. Berkelman, R. L., Bryan, R. T., Osterholm, M. T., LeDuc, J. W., and Hughes, J. M., Infectious disease surveillance: A crumbling foundation, *Science* **264:**368–370 (1994).
113. Bennett, J. V., and Brachman, P. S. (eds.), *Hospital Infections*, Little, Brown, Boston, 1992.
114. Wenzel, R. P. (ed.), *Prevention and Control of Nosocomial Infections*, Williams and Wilkins, Baltimore, 1993.
115. Centers for Disease Control, Update: Universal precautions for prevention of human immunodeficiency virus, hepatitis B virus, and other blood-borne pathogens in the health-care setting, *Morbid. Mortal. Week. Rep.* **37:**377–388 (1988).
116. Centers for Disease Control, Public health guidelines for counseling and antibody testing to prevent HIV infection and AIDS, *Morbid. Mortal. Week. Rep.* **36:**509–515 (1987).
117. National Academy of Sciences, Institute of Medicine, *New Vaccine Development Establishment of Priorities*, National Academy of Sciences, Washington, 1985.
118. Centers for Disease Control, Reported vaccine-preventable diseases—United States, 1993, and the Childhood Immunization Initiative, *Morbid. Mortal. Week. Rep.* **43:**57–60 (1994).
119. Centers for Disease Control, Summary of notifiable diseases, United States, 1993, *Morbid. Mortal. Week. Rep.* **42:**73 (1994).
120. Centers for Disease Control, Summary of the second national community forum on adult immunization, *Morbid. Mortal. Week. Rep.* **36:**509–515 (1987).
121. National Vaccine Advisory Committee, *Adult Immunization*, National Vaccine Program, Washington, DC; 1994.
122. Centers for Disease Control, *Immunization of Adults. A Call to Action*, Public Health Service, Atlanta, 1994.
123. World Health Organization, Special program on AIDS and Expanded Programme in Immunization. Joint statement. Consultation on human immunodeficiency virus and routine childhood immunizations, *WHO Week. Epidemiol. Rec.* **62:**297–299 (1988).
124. Centers for Disease Control and Prevention, Recommended immunization schedule—United States, 1997. *Morbid. Mortal. Week. Rep.* **46:**35–40 (1997).
125. Centers for Disease Control and Prevention, Standards of pediatric immunization practices. Recommended by the National Vaccine Advisory Committee, *Morbid. Mortal. Week. Rep.* **42**(RR-5):1–13 (1993).
126. Centers for Disease Control and Prevention, *Health Information for International Travel*, HHS Publ. No. (CDC) 94-8280, 1994.
127. La Force, M. F., Anthrax, *Clin. Infect. Dis.* **19:**1009–1014 (1993).
128. World Health Organization, Tuberculosis Programme, *TB: A Global Emergency*, World Health Organization, Geneva, 1994.
129. Comstock, G. W., Variability of tuberculosis trends in a time of resurgence, *Clin. Infect. Dis.* **19:**1015–1022 (1994).
130. Fine, P. F., Bacille Calmette–Guérin vaccines: A rough guide, *Clin. Infect. Dis.* **20:**11–14 (1995).
131. Colditz, G. A., Brewer, T. F., Berkey, C. S., *et al.*, Efficacy of BCG vaccine in the protection against tuberculosis: A meta-analysis, *Int. J. Epidemiol.* **271:**698–702 (1994).
132. Rodrigues, I. C., Diwan, V. K., and Wheeler, J. G., Protective effect of BCG against tuberculous meningitis and miliary tuberculosis: A meta-analysis, *Int. J. Epidemiol.* **22:**1154–1158 (1993).
133. Centers for Disease Control, Use of BCG in the control of tuberculosis: A joint statement by the ACIP and the Advisory Committee for Elimination of Tuberculosis, *Morbid. Mortal. Week. Rep.* **37:**663–664, 669–675 (1988).
134. Groves, M. J., Pharmaceutical characterization of *Mycobacterium bovis* bacillus Calmette–Guérin (BCG) vaccine used for the treatment of superficial bladder cancer, *J. Pharm. Sci.* **82:** 555–562 (1993).
135. Stover, C. K., de la Cruz, V. F., Bansal, G. P., Hansaon, M. S.,

Fuerst, T. R., Jacobs, W. R., Jr., and Bloom, B. R., Use of recombinant BCG as a vaccine delivery vehicle, *Adv. Exp. Med. Biol.* **327:**175–182 (1992).

136. Lugosi, L., Theoretical and methodological aspects of BCG vaccine from the discovery of Calmette and Guérin to molecular biology. A review, *Tuber. Lung Dis.* **73:**252–261 (1992).
137. Centers for Disease Control, *Health Information of International Travel 1994*, Superintendent of Documents, Washington, 1994.
138. Beam, T. R., Gilbert, D. N., and Kunin, C., General guidelines for the clinical evaluation of anti-infective drug products, *Clin. Infect. Dis.* **15**(suppl. 1)**:**S1–S346 (1992).
139. Gorbach, W. I., Condon, R. E., Conte, J. E., Kaiser, A. B., Ledger, W. J., and Nichols, R. L., Evaluation of new anti-infective drugs for surgical prophylaxis, *J. Infect. Dis.* **15**(Suppl. 1)**:**S313–S338 (1992).

16. Suggested Reading

Benenson, A. S. (ed.), *Control of Communicable Diseases Manual*, 16th ed., American Public Health Association, Washington, DC, 1995.

Evans, A. S., and Kaslow, R. A. (eds.), *Viral Infections of Humans: Epidemiology and Control*, 4th ed., Plenum Medical, New York, 1997.

Feigin, R. D., and Cherry, J. D. (eds.), *Textbook of Pediatric Infectious Diseases*, 3rd ed., Saunders, Philadelphia, 1992.

Hennekens, C. H., and Buring, J. L., *Epidemiology in Medicine*, Little, Brown, Boston, 1987.,

Hoeprich, P. D., Jordan, M. C., and Roland, A. R. (eds.), *A Treatise on Infectious Diseases*, 5th ed., Harper & Row, New York, 1994.

Jawetz, E., Melnick, J. L., and Adelberg, E. A., *Review of Medical Microbiology*, 17th ed., Lange, Los Altos, CA, 1987.

Kelsey, J., Thompson, W. D., and Evans, A. S., *Methods in Observational Epidemiology*, Oxford University Press, London, 1986.

Mandell, G. L., Douglas, R. G., Jr., and Dolin, R. (eds.), *Principles and Practice of Infectious Diseases*, 4th ed., Volumes 1 and 2, Wiley, New York, 1995.

Mims, C. A., *The Pathogenesis of Infectious Disease*, 3rd ed., Academic Press/Grune & Stratton, New York, 1987.

Mims, C. A., Playfair, J. H. L., Roitt, I. M., Wakelin, D., and Williams, R. *Medical Microbiology*, Mosby, St. Louis, 1993.

CHAPTER 2

Public Health Surveillance

Philip S. Brachman

1. Introduction

The term *surveillance*, derived from the French word meaning "to watch over," may be defined as a system of close observation of all aspects of the occurrence and distribution of a given disease through the systematic collection, tabulation, analysis, and dissemination of all relevant data pertaining to that disease.[1] The preferred term is *public health surveillance*, which emphasizes the focus of surveillance as discussed in this chapter to develop data that results in a public health preventive action. This distinguishes public health surveillance from other types of surveillance.[2] Although the methodology of surveillance is basically descriptive, its function is more than merely collective and archival. Surveillance must be dynamic, current, purposeful, and result in a public health action. This action frequently results in the establishment of a new or the reinforcement of an existing public health policy. It is fundamental for the prompt and effective control and prevention of disease. Traditionally, surveillance was first applied to the acute communicable diseases in the mid-1800s.[3] Since then, the science of surveillance has been extended to cover a large number of infectious diseases,[1] a wide variety of noninfectious diseases, and also other health-related events such as environmental hazards, injuries, immunizations, the distribution of biological products, and health care delivery.

2. History

William Farr, of the General Registrar's Office of England and Wales, is credited with initiating disease surveillance in the mid-1800s. He collected, collated, and analyzed vital statistical data and distributed reports to appropriate health personnel as well as to the public.[3] The collection of national morbidity data was initiated in 1878, when Congress authorized the Public Health Service (PHS) to collect reports of the occurrence of the quarantinable diseases, that is, cholera, plague, smallpox, and yellow fever. In 1893, Congress passed an act stating that weekly health information should be collected from all state and municipal authorities. In 1902, in an attempt to develop uniformity, the Surgeon General of the PHS was directed to provide forms for collecting, compiling, and publishing surveillance data. In 1913, the state and territorial health authorities recommended that every state send weekly telegraphic summaries reporting the occurrence of selected diseases to the PHS. All states were reporting the occurrences of diseases by 1925. In 1949, when the National Office of Vital Statistics (NOVS) was established in the PHS, the communicable-disease-reporting function (morbidity reporting) was merged with the national mortality registration and reporting functions that were the primary responsibility of the NOVS. Until the early 1950s, the communicable disease reports were published weekly in the official journal *Public Health Reports*. When this journal became a monthly publication, the NOVS issued a separate weekly bulletin, the *Morbidity and Mortality Weekly Report* (MMWR), that was distributed to state health officers, state epidemiologists, county and city health officers, and others including persons who requested its receipt. In January 1961, the responsibility for receiving morbidity reports from the states and larger cities and the issuing of the MMWR was transferred from Washington, DC, to the Communicable Disease Center [now called the Centers for Disease Control and Prevention (CDC)] in Atlanta, Georgia.

In the United States, the application of the term *surveillance* to the watchfulness over a nationally important communicable disease (malaria) was begun in 1946

Philip S. Brachman • The Rollins School of Public Health of Emory University, Atlanta, Georgia 30322.

by the CDC[4] in part to monitor veterans who were returning from endemic areas. The application of critical epidemiological evaluation to the former rather crude reports revealed that malaria had ceased to be an indigenous disease. Endemic spread of infection had ceased some years before through control of the vector.

In 1955, following the outbreak of killed vaccine-related poliomyelitis (the so-called "Cutter Incident"), a national surveillance of poliomyelitis was directed by the Surgeon General as an essential step toward a solution for this national disaster.[5] In 1957, influenza was placed under surveillance because of the impending pandemic of Asian influenza for which a comprehensive national program of widespread immunization and education of doctors and hospitals to meet such a possible disaster was undertaken by the Surgeon General. The influenza surveillance program has continued, and one of its essential functions is to provide information to guide manufacturers in the preparation of influenza vaccine as concerns its antigenic composition and the amount of vaccine to produce. In 1961, because of the increasing public health concern with salmonellosis, a special *Salmonella* surveillance program was developed in conjunction with the states to better define the problem so that appropriate control and prevention measures could be instituted.

The CDC has published a series of reports that further define public health surveillance. These include an outline of a comprehensive program,[6] "Guidelines for Evaluating Surveillance Systems,"[7] and "Case Definitions for Public Health Surveillance."[8] More recently, concern has been expressed about the "crumbling foundation" of public health surveillance systems and the need to be concerned about surveillance for emerging infections.[9] There are several textbooks that have been published on public health surveillance (see Suggested Readings).

At present, the occurrence of 52 diseases is reported weekly and that of 7 other diseases is reported annually by state health departments to the CDC. Additionally, 7 other diseases are reported by either special case-reporting forms or line-listing forms submitted either monthly or annually. These reports are published in the MMWR and are summarized annually in the *MMWR Annual Summary*.[10] These lists are reviewed annually by the state and territorial epidemiologists and modified as indicated by the changing nature of the diseases and the occurrence of new diseases. Additionally, more intensive surveillance is maintained over selected diseases by means of special surveillance efforts to develop more specific data concerning these diseases. Selected chronic conditions are also under similar surveillance.

National disease surveillance programs are maintained by most countries in the world. The methods used to obtain reports, the diseases reported, the analyses, and the type and frequency of reports vary, but the value and importance of surveillance is universally recognized. A number of European countries have been working to improve national surveillance programs to develop a European reporting system.[11] Desenclos has discussed various methods for collecting surveillance data.[12] The World Health Organization (WHO) maintains surveillance on the quarantinable diseases (cholera, plague, and yellow fever) as well as other selected diseases. The most recent disease to come under worldwide surveillance is acquired immunodeficiency syndrome (AIDS). The WHO prepares weekly reports as well as other reports summarizing these data.

3. Use of Surveillance

A surveillance program can be designed to produce a variety of output data depending on the purpose of the program. It can portray the natural history of the disease, including a description of the occurrence of the disease by time, place, and person. Surveillance data should describe the background (sporadic, endemic, or ongoing) level of the disease, as well as changes in the occurrence of the disease as modified by nonrecurring events such as epidemics or a hyperendemic situation. Surveillance can be used to monitor changes in the agent, such as antibiotic resistance of gonococci, streptococcus, pneumococcus, and *Mycobacterium tuberculosis*.

Analysis of surveillance data can help to establish priorities for developing or allocating appropriate health resources for approaching a problem. Surveillance can also be used to confirm a hypothesis or indicate the need for further study or additional data. Analysis of surveillance data can lead to the development and/or institution of control and/or prevention measures such as chemotherapy, chemoprophylaxis, new resources or resource allocation (e.g., people, equipment, or monies), or additional training for persons involved in control and prevention activities. Surveillance can be used to evaluate the effectiveness of newly instituted control and/or prevention measures. Surveillance data are also important in forecasting or predicting the future pattern of the occurrence of a disease.

In this chapter, surveillance is discussed primarily as it involves bacterial infectious diseases. Surveillance techniques for other infectious diseases are similar, though there may be some variation in the data collection procedures.

4. Data Sources

The WHO in 1968 codified the term *surveillance* on a truly global basis.[(13)] The "elements" or distinguishable sources of data were identified; one or any combination of the ten can be used to support a disease-specific surveillance program. The sources used to develop the surveillance data depend on the disease itself, the methods used for identifying the disease, the goals of the program, the personnel and material resources available, the population involved, and the characteristics of the disease's occurrence. One source of data can be used regularly and other methods utilized as necessary to improve the sensitivity and/or specificity of the data depicting the occurrence of the disease.

4.1. Mortality Data

Mortality registration has been used the longest, but it is useful only for diseases that are associated with fatalities. If the case–fatality ratio is too low, mortality statistics may not provide an accurate assessment of the occurrence of the disease. If mortality rate data are accurate and if the proportion of deaths to cases is known from past studies, then the number of deaths can provide an estimate of the actual number of cases that have occurred.

Unfortunately, there is wide variation in the accuracy with which death certificates are filled out. Additionally, the disease under surveillance may have been a contributory cause of death and may not be noted on the death certificate. Also, there is a time lag in reporting deaths, so that a surveillance program based on mortality registration has an inherent delay of from weeks to months.

An example of the use of mortality data for surveillance is the collection of pneumonia and influenza weekly mortality reports from 121 American cities.[(14)] These data are used to describe weekly pneumonia and influenza activity. Another example occurred in the 1960s during an investigation of shigellosis in rural areas in Central America where there was no ongoing surveillance program.[(15)] The only available reports of any of the cases were listings of deaths that were routinely noted in "vital statistics" books maintained in the communities. By noting the recording of deaths and by knowing the case–fatality ratio, it was possible to develop information concerning the occurrence of cases of shigellosis.

4.2. Morbidity Data

The second source of surveillance data and the one most commonly used is that of morbidity or case reporting. This is a prompt, simple, and relatively accurate system that is dependent on the reporting of cases of the diseases under surveillance. Reporting the occurrence of disease is the responsibility of the patient's health care professional, usually a physician. He or she may delegate this responsibility to someone else such as a nurse, clerk, or administrator. Cases may be reported by the responsible person calling the health department or vice versa, or they may be reported each day or each week on a special form sent by mail. Copies of laboratory reports may also be submitted to the public health authorities. The techniques of reporting are described in greater detail in Section 6.

4.3. Individual Case Reports

Individual case investigation is more likely to be performed with rare diseases or unusual cases of a more common disease. For diseases of high frequency, investigating individual cases is usually neither practical nor necessary, but may be conducted as a check on the validity of morbidity or mortality reporting. As a disease decreases in incidence, individual case investigation may be of increasing importance to determine why the case occurred and to further direct control and prevention measures. As the occurrence of a disease decreases, leading toward prevention, elimination, or eradication status, then intensive investigation of each reported case is important. This was dramatically demonstrated in the smallpox eradication program[(13)] and is currently being practiced in the international poliomyelitis eradication program.[(16)] Additionally, as measles immunization activities are being intensified in the United States, individual case reporting is being emphasized.[(17)]

4.4. Epidemic Reporting

The fourth source of surveillance data is the reporting of epidemics. Frequently, there is quantitative improvement of reporting when clusters of cases occur. Thus, single cases of shigellosis or salmonellosis may not be individually reported, but if there is an epidemic, then all cases that are part of the epidemic may be reported.

4.5. Epidemic Field Investigation

Epidemic field investigations may uncover more cases of the disease than would have been reported without the investigation. In the epidemic of salmonellosis in Riverside, California, in 1965, several hundred cases were initially reported; however, following a field investigation, 16,000 cases were estimated to have occurred.[18] In 1987, an epidemic of *Salmonella typhimurium* gastroenteritis occurred in Chicago, Illinois, related to pasturized milk and 16,000 cases were cultured positive for the organism. However, community surveys suggested that between 170,000 and 200,000 cases occurred.[19] The decision to investigate an epidemic will be based on the specific disease, the seriousness of the outbreak, the extent of the problem, the anticipated need for more specific information concerning the occurrence of the epidemic, availability of resources, research potential, and possibly political pressures.

4.6. Laboratory Reporting

The laboratory is essential in identifying and confirming pathogens. Although many diseases can be adequately described clinically, there are others for which laboratory identification of the etiologic agent is essential for accuracy. For example, gastroenteritis may be caused by various organisms; it is frequently not possible to be certain of the etiology on the basis of clinical and epidemiological data alone, and thus it is necessary to incorporate laboratory testing before the etiologic agent can be identified. The accuracy of the *Salmonella* and *Shigella* surveillance programs in the United States is dependent on laboratory testing.

In addition to disease identification, the laboratory can also provide important information concerning specific characteristics of microorganisms. For example, the antigenic characteristics of influenza strains are important, since significant changes in the prevalent strain will necessitate changes in formulation of vaccine to be used before the next influenza season. Identifying the serotype of salmonellae isolated from different patients may be necessary in order to associate different isolates as part of a single outbreak. Careful attention to antibiotic sensitivity patterns can indicate a change in the epidemiological pattern of the disease or may be a forewarning of an impending upsurge in the occurrence of the disease. This has been seen in the increasing frequency with which antibiotic-resistant gonococci are being identified,[20] the spread of methicillin-resistant *Staphylococcus aureus*[21] within and between hospitals, and the increasing identification of vancomycin-resistant enterococci as well as of multiresistant *M. tuberculosis* (see Chapters 15, 33, 25, and 39). A variety of molecular tools are now available that provide highly specific identification of a strain or substrain of an organism. Methods for both phenotyping and genotyping are now used. New techniques such as the polymerase chain reaction (PCR), immunoblot electropheresis, and a variety of DNA and RNA probes have given high sensitivity and high specificity to the detection of organisms in various tissues and to the precise identification of the particular strain causing a given outbreak. Highly specific antibody identification is also now possible through commercially available monoclonal antibodies. These techniques make it possible to follow the spread of an organism in an outbreak and to differentiate between exogenous reinfection and endogenous reactivation.

The serology laboratory also contributes to surveillance by identifying and/or confirming the presence of a specific disease. Usually, two serum specimens are obtained from each individual, one during the acute phase and one during the convalescent phase of illness, to demonstrate a significant change (usually fourfold) in titer. However, if only a single serum specimen is obtained, the occurrence of a specific disease may be suggested if the antibody titer to that disease is elevated beyond a certain value or by the presence of IgM antibody. Also, if elevated titers are found in serum specimens from a group of patients who had similar illnesses, then these single specimens can be of assistance in making the diagnosis (see Chapter 1).

4.7. Hospital Reporting

The reporting of infectious diseases among hospitalized or outpatients is a valuable and important source of information. These infections may be truly hospital acquired (nosocomial) or community acquired. Community-acquired infections among patients admitted to a hospital reflect the occurrence of infectious diseases in the community. Infections that develop among hospitalized patients or outpatients may represent an endogenous or exogenous source of infection. If exogenous, the source may be another patient, hospital employee, rarely a visitor, or the hospital environment. An exogenous source may reflect a community problem. Endogenous infections reflect organisms from the patient who may have become colonized from a community source.

4.8. Surveys

Surveys can provide information concerning the prevalence of disease. Clinical surveys may include questions related to the occurrence of a disease, physical examination such as spleen surveys to identify patients with malaria, or diagnostic tests such as skin tests to determine the prevalence of histoplasmosis or tuberculosis. In some countries, blood smear surveys may be used in surveillance for malaria. Other types of surveys include household surveys, such as the National Health Interview Survey, which includes 55,000 households surveyed annually; cluster surveys, such as are used in evaluating immunization programs; and telephone surveys, which can be used to estimate the magnitude of an outbreak of a disease.

Serological tests for certain bacterial, rickettsial, and treponemal infections carried out on a representative sample of a population can provide prevalence data for different age, sex, and geographic segments of the group tested. Incidence data can be obtained by demonstrating the appearance or rise in antibody titer to a given infection in two serum specimens spaced in time such as the start and end of an epidemic, military service, or a college year; the occurrence of recent infection can also be demonstrated in a single specimen by determining the presence of specific IgM antibody for that infectious agent or by testing for an antibody type of short duration such as certain complement-fixing antibodies. The uses of seroepidemiology are presented in more detail in the companion book on viral infections.[(22)]

4.9. Animal Reservoir and Vector Distribution

Animal reservoir and vector distribution studies are important in maintaining surveillance of zoonotic and arthropod-borne diseases. Information about rabies in animal reservoirs in a specific geographic area can be important in making a decision concerning the need to treat a human exposed to an unidentified animal. The knowledge that tularemia is occurring in animals or that ticks infected with *Francisella tularensis* are present in an area would support reports of suspect cases of tularemia in humans. Similar studies are in progress to define the distribution of Lyme disease, which is caused by *Borrelia burgdorferi* whose vector is one of several Ixodid ticks. Knowledge about the occurrence of plague in prairie dogs or rodents can be important in evaluating data concerning possible cases of human plague.

4.10. Biologics and Drug Distribution

The utilization of biologics and drugs for treatment or prophylaxis of a disease may be used to monitor disease occurrence. For example, in an outbreak of diarrheal disease, the increasing sales of antidiarrhea medications by pharmacies serve to corroborate the occurrence of disease. Similarly, an increase in requests for immune serum globulin can be a clue to the occurrence of cases of viral hepatitis.

4.11. Demographic and Environmental Data

Demographic and environmental data are necessary in order to analyze disease occurrence data effectively. Such data may include age, sex, occupation, residence, or other personal information. Incidence rates cannot be determined until denominator data concerning the population are available. For example, when an increase in the number of isolations of *Salmonella eastbourne* was noted, an analysis of cases by age showed a significant number of cases among young children.[(23)] This fact was an important clue in leading the investigators to identify chocolate candy as the vehicle of infection. The ability of new molecular and electrophoretic techniques to identify the specific strain of organisms such as *Salmonella* has allowed outbreaks in different geographic areas to be interlinked and a common commercial source identified.[(24)]

4.12. News Media

Another useful source of surveillance information is public information gathered through the news media. It is not uncommon for the occurrence of a disease, and especially an epidemic, to be first noted by the news media. Additionally, the news media can perform an important role in alerting the public to the occurrence of a disease outbreak, and thus stimulate the reporting of cases that otherwise might not have been diagnosed or reported. In an outbreak of botulism associated with a restaurant in a western state, radio reports alerted a patron of the restaurant to the possibility of exposure after the patron had returned to his home several hundred miles from the restaurant.[(25)] At the time he heard the radio report, he was experiencing some symptoms. Accordingly, he sought medical assistance, botulism was diagnosed, he was successfully treated, and another case was reported.

5. Routine Surveillance

As previously indicated, routine surveillance of a specific disease will not include all the data sources discussed above. The methods that provide the most accurate information collected in a practical and efficient manner that satisfies the objectives of the surveillance program should be utilized. If more information is needed concerning occurrence of the disease, then additional sources of information can be incorporated into the surveillance system.

The need for completeness of reporting varies according to the incidence of the disease under surveillance. For those diseases that either normally do not occur in an area or occur at a very low incidence, it is essential, for control purposes, that all cases that occur be reported. Examples (in the United States) include plague, yellow fever, poliomyelitis, human rabies, measles, and hanta virus disease.

On the other hand, to maintain surveillance on diseases that commonly occur, it is not critical for all cases to be reported. In the United States, it is estimated that only 1% of cases of salmonellosis, for example, and 15–20% of cases of viral hepatitis are reported. The fact that all cases are not reported should not reduce the effectiveness of surveillance, since it is generally the trends of disease occurrence that are important in the implementation of control and prevention measures. Changes in the trend should reflect real changes in the occurrence of disease and not changes reflecting a variation in the methods of surveillance. If the methods of obtaining the surveillance data have not changed significantly during a period of time and the data collected are a representative sampling of the cases that have occurred, then these data should be suitable for determining the trend of the disease. However, a change in the methods used to collect the surveillance data, followed by a change in the reported occurrence of the disease, may be falsely interpreted as a change in the incidence of the disease. An example of this artifact could have occurred in the national *Shigella* surveillance program that was initiated in 1964, with routine reporting from 17 states. Several years later, the remaining states began reporting their isolates; the sudden increase in reported cases could have been misinterpreted if attention had not been given to the mechanics of the surveillance program.[26] Similar artifacts in surveillance data have occurred in the national AIDS surveillance program. As the definition of a case of AIDS has been modified to accommodate new knowledge concerning the clinical manifestations of the disease, the overall surveillance data have reflected these changes.[27]

Case reporting of certain diseases may be discontinued because effective control measures are not available. One such example is streptocococal infections, which may give the uninformed the wrong idea that these infections are no longer of importance.

To validate surveillance data, various methods have been used. These include: (1) active surveillance, that is, physicians in the reporting area can be called and asked if they reported all cases of the disease among the patients within a specific time period; (2) hospital records can be checked by means of a prevalence study to see that all notifiable diseases have been reported; and (3) laboratory reports from hospital and public health laboratories for a given disease can be compared to the cases reported to the health department.

6. Reporting

In general, detailed individual case data are not necessarily useful in surveillance programs. It is the analysis of collective data that provides meaningful information. If more specific case information is necessary, then individual cases can be traced back and additional data obtained.

The quality of a surveillance program is as good as the quality of the data collected. In morbidity reporting, an integral component is the person who has the responsibility for reporting the occurrence of the disease. Most frequently, this is the person who has medical responsibility for the patient, and usually that person is a physician. This responsibility may be delegated to someone else, such as the physician's nurse or, in a hospital, the house staff or the administrator. The increasing use of computers by hospitals and large health maintenance organizations (HMOs) for recording diagnoses and the development of linkage systems for such data provide new means of collecting and evaluating surveillance data. In reporting cases of any disease by any means, confidentiality of the patient must be respected and maintained.

Within a community, cases are reported to the local health authority, such as a city health department. At regular intervals, usually weekly, these cases will be reported to the state health department. In the United States, the weekly totals and selected individual case data will be reported to the CDC. Computers have been introduced into the surveillance system at various levels.[28] All state health departments report their data to the CDC via computers. The development of worldwide systems of communication such as the internet and world wide web has yielded a global method of making such data widely available. The MMWR and the *WHO Weekly Record* are available in these systems. Computer reporting by health care physicians has been initiated in France[29] and in China.[30]

6.1. Motivation

The diligence with which cases are reported reflects the motivation of the person responsible for reporting. Physicians frequently do not wish to assume this responsibility because of the constraints on their time and the low priority they give to reporting. There needs to be some motivation developed for reporting other than that related to disease-reporting laws. Motivation may result from being a participant in a public health project or from professional or personal gain. A report summarizing the surveillance data (see Section 9) may be motivational (as well as educational), so that the reporter does recognize that there is some action resulting from disease reporting. Motivation may also be derived from knowledge that surveillance data can support the development of effective control and prevention programs, with a decreased incidence in the occurrence of disease.

Reporting may be stimulated by the availability of an epidemiologist to provide assistance to the reporting physician on request. Another source of motivation may be that the reporting of surveillance data results in important clinical and therapeutic data being made available to the practitioner. For example, the increase in antibiotic-resistant strains of *Neisseria* gonococci reported through the CDC's surveillance program is important information for practicing physicians to have when they see a patient, make a clinical diagnosis of gonorrhea, and want to initiate therapy immediately. Another example is the increasing number of reports of antibiotic-resistant tuberculate bacillus, which is a significant problem to clinicians as well as to public health professionals. Also, the worldwide problem of resistant strains of the pneumococcus is another serious situation. These examples of the application of surveillance data to the practice of medicine can serve to motivate physicians to participate in surveillance activities. Disease reporting can also be stimulated by making specific therapeutic drugs available to the physician on notification of the occurrence of a specific disease. In some communities, reports of hepatitis A result in serum immune globulin being made available for prophylactic use. A report of a case of botulism may lead public health authorities to make trivalent botulinum antitoxin available. Reports of certain tropical parasitic diseases make it possible for physicians to obtain certain therapeutic drugs from the CDC not otherwise available. For example, the availability of a drug exclusively from the CDC in the early 1980s to treat cases of *Pneumocystis carinii* pneumonia led to recognition of the occurrence of a new disease, AIDS, in 1981.[31]

A reward system for reporting can be used. The reward can be publicity given to the reporting physicians by listing their names in the surveillance report or in a scientific paper summarizing the surveillance data. A monetary reward system has also been used, with an annual payment or a specific amount of money being given for each report submitted. This activity was not very successful, however, and is no longer being practiced.

Health officials must recognize the negative effect of a reporting mechanism that is too complex or that demands excessive expenditure of time on the part of the reporter. If reporting of cases brings adverse publicity to the patient, physician, hospital, or community, surveillance will be inhibited. Adverse publicity that leads to a loss of money or to legal action against the reporter or hospital also has a negative effect on the reporting of disease. Some countries choose not to report quarantinable diseases to the WHO because of the knowledge that publicity concerning the occurrence of those diseases may have an adverse effect on the movement of people and goods across their borders.

6.2. Ease of Reporting

To stimulate reporting, the mechanisms must be simple and yet compatible with an effective and sensitive surveillance system. There must be a relatively easy mechanism by which cases can be reported to the public health authorities. However, the information being requested must provide adequate data for developing a meaningful and practical control and prevention program. It is important to request only data that meet the objectives of the surveillance program. If superfluous data are requested and collected but not used, the reporter will question the surveillance effort, and support for the program will decline.

6.3. Case Definition

It is important in developing a surveillance program that specific case definitions be developed and publicized so that those persons participating can accurately report cases. The definition must be simple, acceptable, and understandable and not incorporate diagnostic criteria that are difficult to comprehend; if laboratory test results are part of the definition, the test must be readily available and inexpensive and not demand a great deal of the patient. It is also important to consider whether only confirmed cases should be reported or whether reporting should also include cases that are less definite as cases of the specific disease and are classified as presumptive or suspect cases of the disease; if so, the definitions of these categories must be acceptable and publicized. The CDC has developed and published a compilation of case definitions for public health surveillance that standardizes definitions for all the diseases reportable in the United States.[8]

6.4. Passive Reporting

Surveillance reporting may be passive or active. Passive surveillance is the routine reporting in which case reports are initiated by the reporter. Preprinted postcards or reporting forms and stamped envelopes routinely supplied to the reporter can be used to report the requested surveillance data. These cards can be mailed individually or at weekly or monthly intervals, summarizing all cases seen during that time interval; negative reports, i.e., the lack of occurrence of cases, can also be requested. Some states divide the reportable diseases into those commonly seen and those only rarely seen. The reporting official is asked to provide a negative report if no cases of the common diseases are seen and to fill out the form for a rare disease only when a case is actually seen. The reporting form can be a general form suitable for a number of diseases or a specific form used only for a single disease. Special forms can be developed if more detailed data are desired.

Reporting to the local public health office may be done by telephone. The report may be taken by a clerk during working hours or tape-recorded if phoned in outside working hours. The tape recording can be subsequently transcribed by a clerk, who can call the physician if more data are required. To stimulate reporting from throughout an area such as an entire state, a toll-free telephone system can be established. It has been demonstrated that the availability of an automatic telephone-answering service for use at any time has stimulated reporting of disease by physicians. The personal computer may also be used as mentioned above.

6.5. Active Reporting

An active surveillance system can be instituted to improve the opportunities to obtain surveillance data; it can be used for routine surveillance or be an integral part of a special surveillance program established to monitor a specific disease such as during an epidemic. In active surveillance, the reporter is contacted at regular intervals and specifically asked about the occurrence of the disease(s) under surveillance. Thus, there is an active attempt by public health officials to obtain disease occurrence information from the reporter. The introduction of an active surveillance system may greatly increase the number of reported cases of a given disease and may even simulate an epidemic. The users of the surveillance data must be thoroughly informed of such changes in surveillance methods and an interpretation of the increase discussed in an editorial comment. While this system increases the sensitivity of reporting, it also increases the cost of surveillance due to the time needed to make active contact with the reporter.(32)

6.6. Sentinel Physician Reporting

A sampling system that can incorporate either active or passive surveillance is known as a sentinel reporting system. Depending on the size of the community, the degree of reporting desired, and the disease(s) under surveillance, the sentinel physicians may be a sample drawn from all practicing physicians or from among certain specialists who are more likely to see cases of the disease under surveillance. If a patient with the disease under surveillance may be seen by any physician, then the sample should be drawn from among all practicing physicians; however, if a childhood disease is under surveillance, then pediatricians and family practitioners would be the group from which the sample is drawn. The same sentinel physicians can be requested to report regularly, or alternating sentinel physicians can be selected to report weekly or monthly. If the reporting physicians were selected randomly, then the reported cases may be extrapolated to project the total number of cases of the disease that occurred in the area covered by the physicians, weighing each physician's reported cases according to the size of his or her practice. This will allow a fairly accurate estimate of the total cases to be made. However, if the sentinel physicians were not randomly selected or if they were volunteers, the total number of cases can only be approximated from the number reported.

6.7. Laboratory Surveillance

Disease surveillance can also be maintained by regular monitoring of laboratory reports for the identification of etiologic organisms for diseases under surveillance. This system may be of secondary importance in that it serves to confirm a clinical diagnosis, or it may be of primary importance in identifying the etiology that was suspected by the clinician. For example, a case of pulmonary tuberculosis can be fairly accurately diagnosed on the basis of history and clinical evidence, including radiographs and a positive skin test. Identification of the organism in sputum confirms the diagnosis. However, with some diseases such as salmonellosis or shigellosis, accurate diagnosis is dependent on the laboratory identification of the etiologic agent. In diseases in which the laboratory plays a key role in identifying the etiologic agent, it is important to use the appropriate media necessary for this identification. For example, in maintaining surveillance for *Vibrio cholerae* in the United States, it is necessary to use special plating media such as thiosulfate–citrate–bile salt–sucrose (TCBS) agar if the organism is to be identified. Another example is the recognition of the importance of *Yersinia enterocolitica*. When 3 weeks of cold maintenance was required for culturing the organism, very few cases of diarrhea due to this organism were identified. With the introduction of a new culture medium (CIN) that eliminated cold storage, rapid identification became possible and cases are now being identified in routine laboratories. DNA/RNA probes and other microbiological molecular methods of diagnosis are becoming increasingly available and used.

6.8. Hospital Surveillance

Surveillance can also be maintained by using hospital records (inpatient or outpatient) to detect either hospital-acquired or community-acquired infections. The records can be abstracted by specially trained enumerators or by record-room personnel (see Section 7.7 for further discussion of hospital surveillance, as well as Chapter 25).

6.9. Absenteeism Surveillance

Other methods of obtaining surveillance information depend on the specific disease. For diseases with high morbidity, an effective surveillance program can be developed by noting absenteeism from schools or industry, depending on the ages of the involved population. All absenteeism during the period under surveillance may not reflect cases of the disease, so that further information may be needed, such as the rate of absenteeism due to other causes. Sickness benefit or insurance claims can also be utilized to develop surveillance data.

7. Special Surveillance

Special surveillance efforts can be established when the rate of occurrence of a disease increases either as part of the expected trend of that disease (periodic or seasonal increase) or as an unusual increase (epidemic). Special surveillance programs can also be developed in relation to the identification of a new disease entity; to provide disease data for research or investigation projects; to define the population among whom prevention measures should be instituted, such as vaccination; and also to evaluate control and prevention measures. Once the immediate need for a special surveillance system has been accomplished, either the system should be stopped or a regular surveillance program for that disease should be developed. In 1981, when the first cases of AIDS were reported, a special surveillance program was initiated. Once the national importance of surveillance data was identified, a regular surveillance program was established. All states now routinely report cases of AIDS to the CDC as part of the weekly surveillance program.

7.1. Influenza

Surveillance information concerning influenza is developed from the regular weekly reporting by 121 American cities of deaths from pneumonia and influenza. Reports of outbreaks of respiratory disease and reports of virus isolation from laboratories doing routine diagnostic work also provide surveillance data. To complement this system, at the beginning of the anticipated influenza season, additional surveillance activities are initiated to improve the knowledge concerning the occurrence of the disease.[33] Reports of absenteeism are solicited from selected industries and schools, since increased absenteeism may be one indication of increased influenza activity. Sentinel family practitioner volunteers from throughout the country report the percentage of patients they see in their practice with the clinical diagnosis of influenza. Virus laboratories are encouraged to process additional specimens from patients with symptoms of respiratory diseases, in order to increase the opportunity of isolating influenza viruses and subsequently to report the results to public health authorities. New rapid laboratory methods now facilitate recognition. These special surveillance activities are helpful in increasing the sensitivity of surveillance for influenza.

7.2. Gastroenteritis

During an outbreak of a gastrointestinal illness, such as salmonellosis, special surveillance efforts of a particularly high-risk group can be introduced to improve the information developed concerning the occurrence of the disease. This may include morbidity reporting, laboratory surveillance, case reporting, or field investigations. Only with these extra data may it be possible to recommend the most appropriate control and prevention measures.

7.3. Guillain–Barré Syndrome

During the swine flu vaccination program (1976), the reported occurrence of Guillain–Barré syndrome among vaccinated persons resulted in the development of a separate, active, surveillance effort involving special reports from neurologists.[34]

7.4. Reye's Syndrome

To develop information concerning the possible association of Reye's syndrome with influenza, special surveillance activities and reporting forms were established for use by pediatricians and neurologists, who were more likely than other physicians to see patients with Reye's syndrome.[35]

7.5. Infant Botulism

When the first reports of infant botulism were published, it was apparent that a previously unrecognized public health problem needed defining. Accordingly, a special attempt at developing surveillance data was initiated by alerting public health officials as well as pathologists, pediatricians, and laboratories to the disease entity.[36] A special reporting form was developed so that pertinent information could be obtained on each case. These special efforts resulted in the reporting of additional cases and the accumulation of important epidemiological data that have provided leads to the epidemiology of the disease. Cases of this disease are now reported as part of the routine surveillance program in the United States.

7.6. Legionnaires' Disease

When this disease was first identified, there were many unsolicited reports of possible cases. In an effort to standardize these data to define the clinical entity better and to develop more useful epidemiological data, a special surveillance reporting form was developed and a specific definition of a case of Legionnaires' disease was publicized.[37] This resulted in important, new data being uncovered concerning this newly described disease entity. Also, cases of this disease continue to be reported as part of the routine national surveillance program.

7.7. Hospital Infections

Because of the increasing problem of hospital-acquired infections (nosocomial infections), special surveillance efforts have been developed within hospitals to accumulate data that might be useful for instituting procedures to control and prevent nosocomial infections.[38] The development of infection control committees with many responsibilities, one of which is to supervise a nosocomial infection surveillance program, has been of prime importance to these surveillance programs. Special personnel are usually dedicated to this activity. Surveillance data can be collected by various techniques including individual reports from physicians or floor nurses, ward rounds by the infection control nurse, and regular review of the laboratory and pathology records. During ward rounds, the infection control nurse seeks clues to infection by asking physicians and nurses whether any of their patients have infections and noting which patients have elevated temperatures, are receiving chemotherapeutic agents, or are in isolation. The outpatient department and the employee health service can also be kept under surveillance, since infections noted in these areas may reflect infections among inpatients. All these sources of nosocomial infection surveillance data may not be incorporated into the routine surveillance program at the same time. Also, surveillance may be targeted at specific high-risk patients, areas, or procedures. As with general surveillance programs, the methods incorporated should reflect the specific needs of the program and available resources. Community-acquired infections may also be brought under surveillance as an addition to the hospital infection surveillance program. The surveillance and recognition of hospital infections are dealt with in greater detail in Chapter 25.

7.8. High-Risk Population

A special surveillance program can be developed to identify the high-risk populations who will derive the greatest benefit from a particular prevention measure. For example, this has been useful for both meningococcal and pneumococcal disease for which specific, effective vaccines have been developed and are now recommended for use among specific highly susceptible populations that were defined from analysis of surveillance data.

7.9. Emerging Infections

The recognition of AIDS in the United States in 1981 raised the question of whether our surveillance systems were adequate to recognize new agents such as Lassa, Ebola, and Marburg viruses, as well as other older agents that were mutating, such as influenza, or the occurrence of antibiotic resistance to common infectious agents such as the pneumococcus, tubercle bacillus, and enterococci. This led to a National Institutes of Health (NIH) conference in May 1989 that dealt with emerging viral infections, their development, surveillance issues, and means of recognition, which has been subsequently published in a book edited by Morese.[39] Beginning in June 1991, the Institute of Medicine of the National Academy of Sciences convened a 19-member committee to review the broader field of emerging infections in all of microbiology, not just limited to viruses. This report was published in 1992, and included emergent bacteria, viruses, protozoans, helminths, and fungi, of which a brief summary was provided of each.[40]

The CDC was quick to recognize the need for additional methods for surveillance and control of these infections.[41] The CDC has established centers for specialized surveillance of certain of these infections, currently five in number (November 1995), in various medical and public health schools across the United States. The role of the United States in emerging infections has been defined by Henderson.[42]

7.10. Serosurveillance

The use of serological testing on a regular basis may provide disease occurrence information not available by other less costly methods. A reproducible serological test and a responsive, approved laboratory are necessary ingredients for this activity. Serology may be useful in adding information to regular surveillance methods and reflects clinical and subclinical infection. Another example of the use of serology is seen in communities in which there is an interest in determining the incidence of human immunodeficiency virus (HIV) infections among pregnant women for which a serosurveillance program is developed in order to provide the necessary data.

Other special surveillance techniques can be incorporated to handle specific problems. For example, if there is concern regarding foodborne diseases, then in addition to the routine reporting of cases and outbreaks, surveillance of potentially contaminated foods can be instituted by utilizing laboratory culturing of foods routinely supplied by commercial sources. The importation of food items from abroad and their nationwide distribution has resulted in interlinked geographically distant outbreaks of the same infection. This requires closely collaborative surveillance activities in state health departments working through the CDC. Surveillance of human carriers of certain pathogenic organisms such as staphylococci or salmonella can be initiated if there is concern about the occurrence of disease transmitted by asymptomatic carriers.

8. Data Analysis

Once the data have been collected, they must be collated and analyzed at regular intervals. The analysis can be simple or complex depending on the needs of the surveillance program, time constraints, how the data are to be used, and the personnel and facilities available. In addition to analyzing data in the routine manner (cases per 100 population), other methods of quantitating disease occurrence data are being utilized for some diseases. These methods provide a more realistic appraisal of the impact of the disease's occurrence upon a population. Some of these methods include calculating years of potential life lost (such as in evaluating injuries), number of cases of a disease per exposure day (such as urinary tract infections per catheter day), and number of cases of a disease per procedure performed (bacteremias per cardiac catheterization). As surveillance becomes more complex and as more data are handled, computerization of the data may be desirable and necessary. As previously stated, surveillance data can be entered directly into the computer by the reporting office instead of being handled by one or more intermediate individuals. There are software programs available that can analyze the surveillance data and prepare figures summarizing these analyses. One such software program is Epi Info-6, which is used by the CDC to handle the data reported through the country's disease surveillance program, including preparing the data for publication in the MMWR.

Data analysis will usually suggest the best point for intervention. Occasionally, additional data may need to be gathered by additional surveillance activities or by special investigations.

8.1. Frequency of Review

The frequency, type, and complexity of the analyses are dependent on the use of the summary data. A routine surveillance program may require analyses at monthly or weekly intervals; in epidemic circumstances, it may be necessary to review the surveillance data at more frequent intervals, such as weekly or even daily. The data should be analyzed according to time, place, and person.

8.2. Time

When characterizing the data by time, there are four trends to consider. The first is the *secular* trend, which refers to the occurrence of the disease over a prolonged period of time, such as years. The secular trend of tetanus is one of gradually decreasing incidence (Fig. 1). The decreasing secular trend of an infectious disease is usually the result of specific and nonspecific immunity factors among the involved population.

The *periodic* trend, which is the second time trend to consider, refers to the temporary variations from the secular trend. For example, in considering pertussis, periodic increases in incidence approximately every 5 years can be seen on the background of the overall secular trend of decreasing incidence of the disease (Fig. 2). The periodic trends represent variations in the level of immunity (herd immunity) to the etiologic agent influenced by natural infection, variation in the immunity levels of the popula-

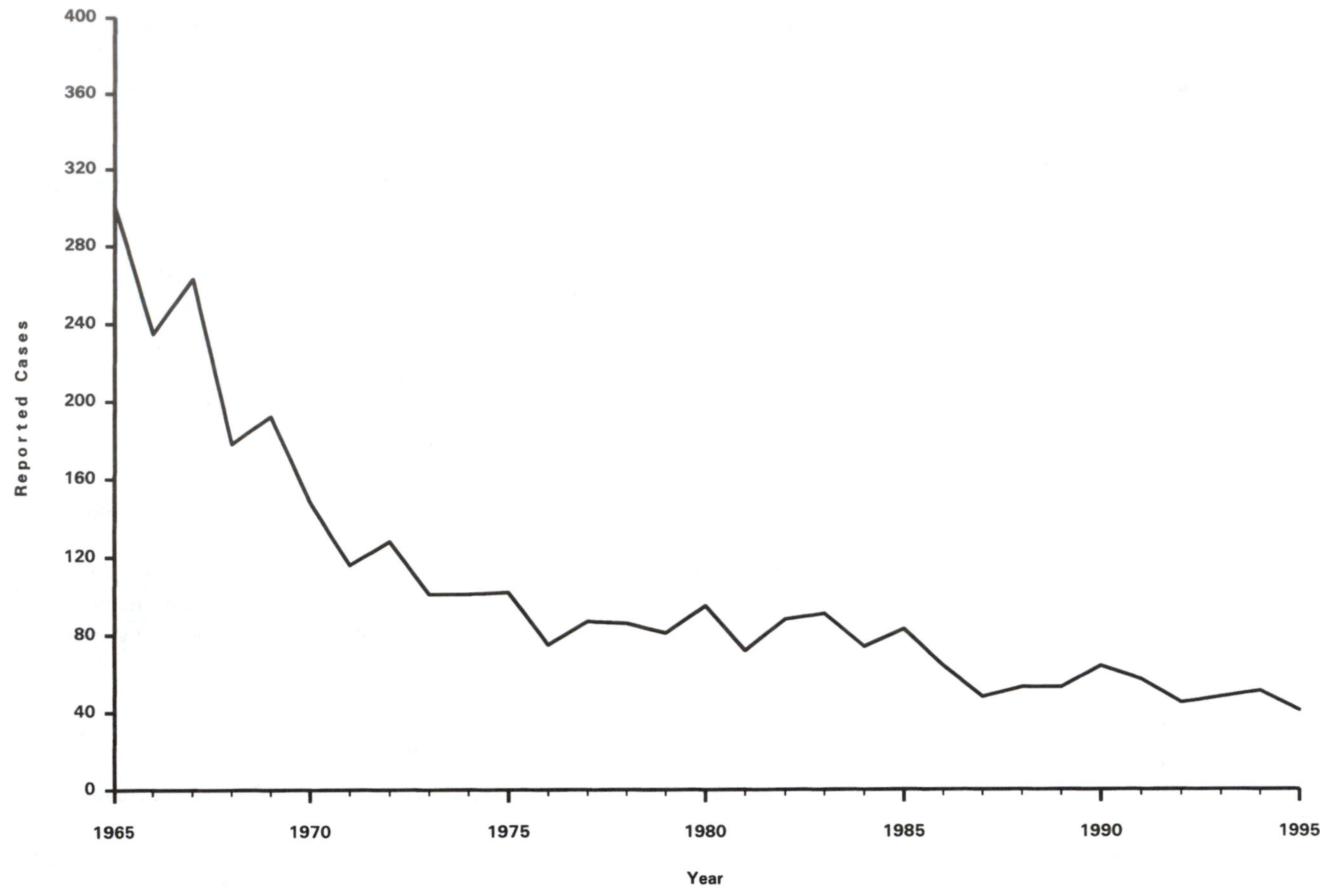

Figure 1. Tetanus: reported cases, United States, 1965–1995.

tion reflecting immunization, or migrating, or by changes in the antigenic composition of the agent.

The third trend is that of the *annual* variation, which frequently represents seasonal patterns. For example, foodborne diseases are associated with seasonal increases in the late summer and fall that may represent the influence of the ambient temperature on the ability of organisms to multiply in or on their reservoirs and sources, resulting in an increased concentration of organisms for potential contact with susceptible hosts. Additionally, the frequency of picnics and the lack of refrigeration add to the increased opportunity for small doses of agents to multiply to infectious doses. *Salmonella* surveillance data reflect annual trends (Fig. 3).

The fourth time trend is that of the *epidemic* occurrence of the disease. If not noted earlier, an epidemic may be discovered by analyzing surveillance data. This has been seen when cases related to a common source are scattered over several health jurisdictions. For example, a *Salmonella*-contaminated food may result in the occurrence of cases over the distribution route of the food; the individual cases may not serve to alert any one health jurisdiction, but the collection of multiple cases may be distinct enough to be identified as an epidemic. Thus, surveillance can serve as an early warning system for epidemics.

When surveillance data are analyzed for time trends, it is necessary to compare these data with data collected over past years, to accurately interpret the current pattern of the occurrence of disease. Otherwise, changes in the occurrence of the disease may not be definable as being either normal or unusual variations.

8.3. Place

When analyzing surveillance data by place, it is important to recognize that the place represented by surveillance data may represent the area where the patient

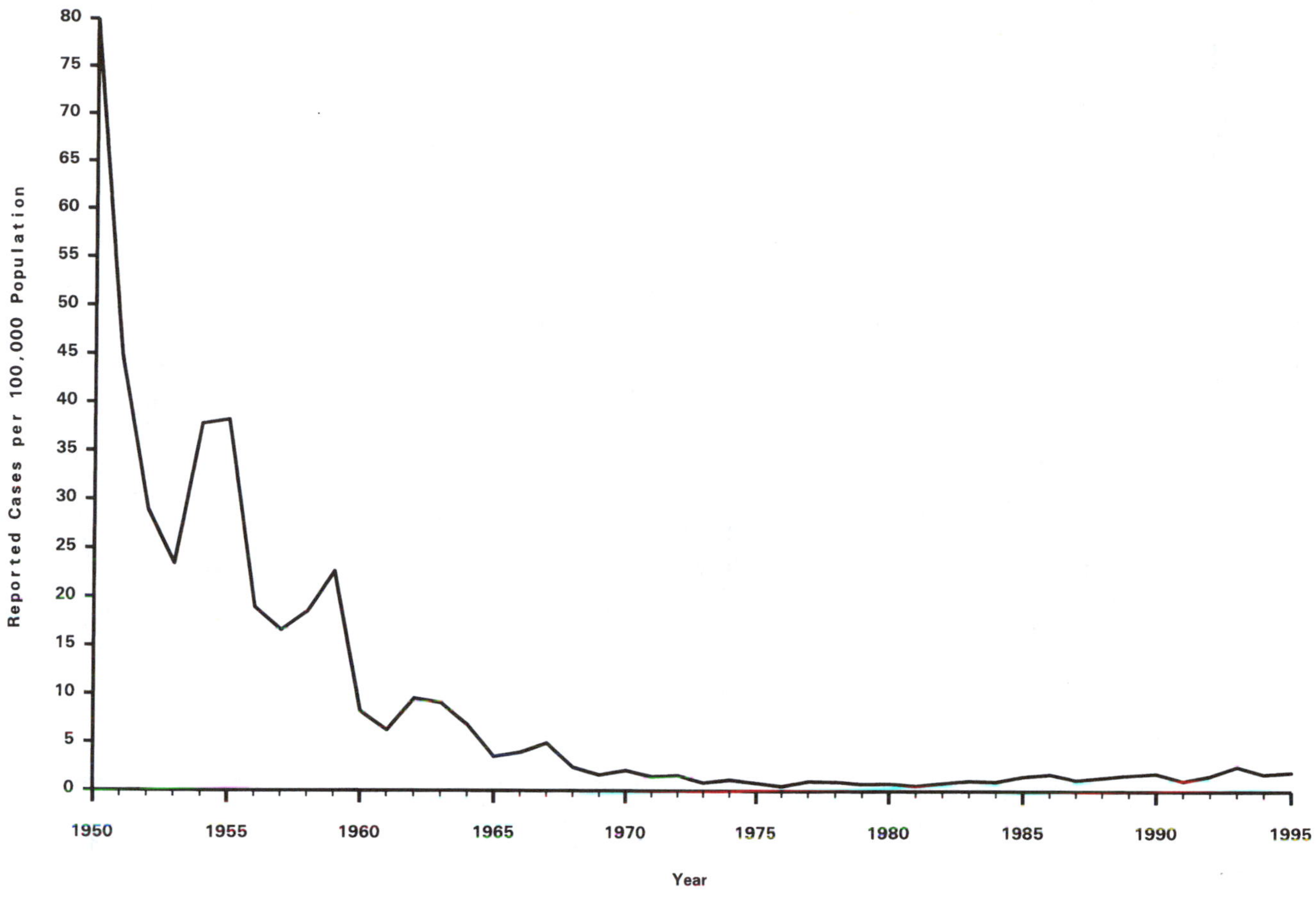

Figure 2. Pertussis: reported incidence rates per 100,000 population, United States, 1950–1995.

lives and not the area where the patient became infected. For epidemiological purposes, the important place(s) is where contact occurred between the patient and the infectious agent or the place where the source of infection became infected. The place of interest will be determined by whether there is interest in control of the current occurrence of the disease or in prevention of present and future cases. Control measures directed at the site where the host came into contact with the agent can lead to control of additional similar cases immediately related to the initial case, but may not prevent additional cases if there are other sources of the organism that susceptible individuals may have contact with. For example, if a food is contaminated with *Salmonella* in the factory where it is prepared and the exposure of the host occurs in a restaurant serving that food, then closing the restaurant will not prevent cases from occurring in association with another restaurant that also obtained contaminated food from the same factory. Prevention of future cases can be accomplished by eliminating the source of contamination, in this instance, at the food-processing plant.

8.4. Person

Person factors to be defined in analyzing surveillance data may include age, sex, nationality, level of immunity, nutrition, lifestyle (such as sexual practices and intravenous drug use), socioeconomic status, travel history, hobbies, personal habits, and occupation. The evaluation of these factors, frequently referred to as risk factors, is important in further describing the occurrence of disease. For example, age-specific attack rates can be important in determining where control and prevention measures should be directed. Occupation may give a clue as to where intervention measures need to be directed. For example, in evaluating cases of brucellosis, knowing that abattoir personnel who work on the kill floors are at a higher risk of developing disease than personnel in other

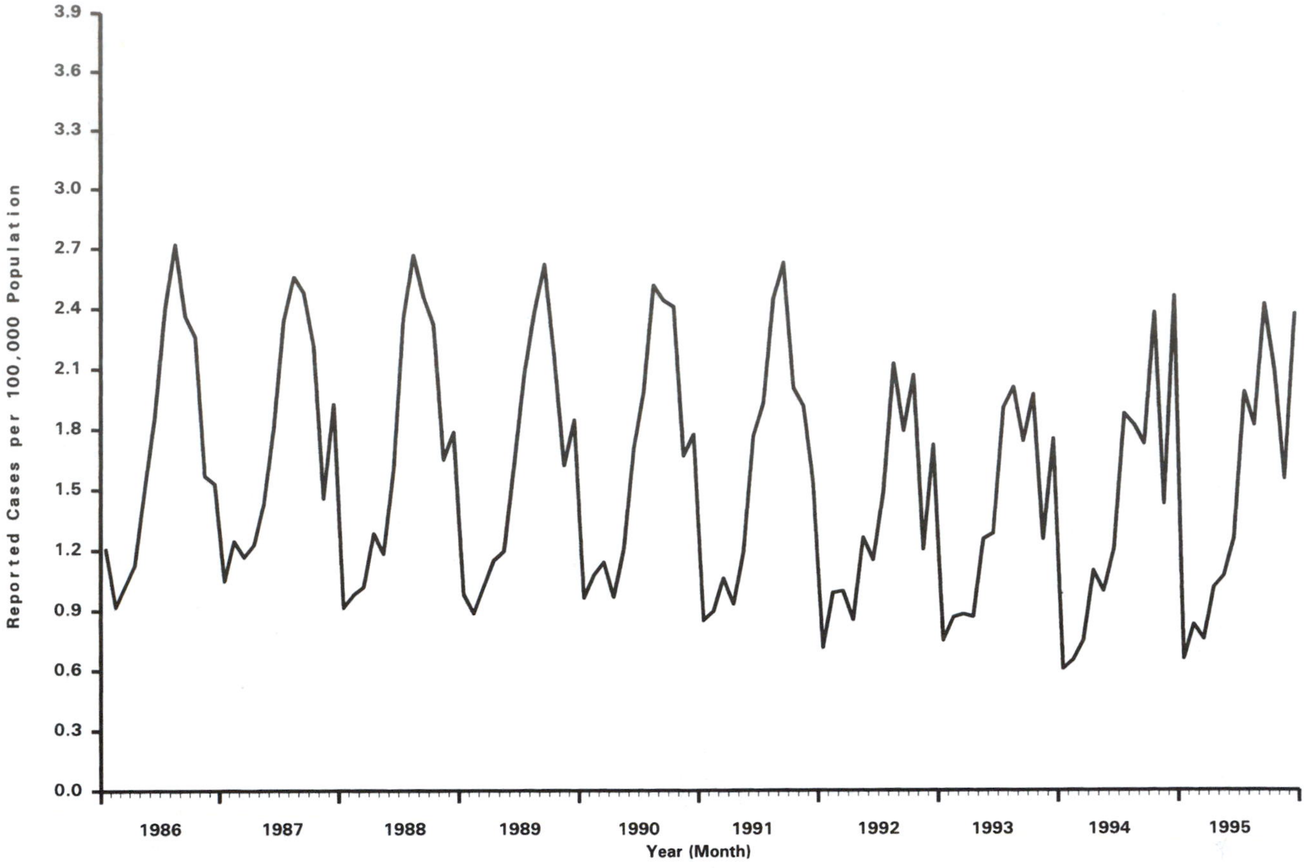

Figure 3. Salmonellosis (excluding typhoid fever): by month, United States, 1986—1995.

areas of the plant indicates where control measures need to be directed. The identification of those at highest risk for HIV is needed to direct initial control programs to these groups and to the specific methods of transmission within them.

9. Reports

Appropriate reports should be prepared and distributed to those individuals who participate in the surveillance program as well as those who have a responsibility for preventive action. The purpose of the surveillance report is to communicate with people, to disseminate information, to educate the reader, and to direct, stimulate, and motivate the persons responsible for action. Reports can also be useful in acknowledging contributors to the surveillance activity. The report should not only summarize the surveillance data but also provide an interpretation of the analyses. Control and prevention measures can be discussed. Surveillance reports can also serve to alert the reader to impending problems, newer methods of control and prevention, current investigations, and new information developed from research or field investigations.

Reports are usually prepared at regular intervals, such as weekly, monthly, quarterly, or annually. The frequency should reflect the interest in the data as well as the need for distribution of the data as related to control and prevention actions. During an epidemic, the immediate dissemination of data may be critical to stimulating reporting and to the institution of appropriate control measures; thus, daily or weekly reports may be indicated. It may be appropriate to distribute foodborne disease surveillance reports at weekly or monthly intervals during the summer and fall months due to the increased incidence of disease at these periods and then to reduce the frequency of reports during the remainder of the year. Special reports can be distributed as necessary; if rapid dissemination of the information is important, it can be distributed by express mail, telegram, telephone, fax, or computer. Rapid dissemination of information over a wide area may be of such critical importance that use of the public news media should be considered.

In the United States, almost all state health departments prepare and distribute at weekly or monthly intervals comprehensive surveillance reports that summarize their disease surveillance data. The national surveillance data are summarized by the CDC at varying intervals depending on the disease and its frequency. Those diseases reported weekly are summarized in the *MMWR*; other diseases are summarized in specialty surveillance reports that are distributed at regular intervals, from monthly to annually. Characteristic of many of the CDC surveillance reports and especially of the MMWR is the interpretation of surveillance data and editorial comments that are integral parts of the reports. These reports are available to anyone who would like to receive them. The MMWR is now available by computer through the CDC's world wide web server at http://www.cdc.gov/epo/mmwr/mmwr.html. World surveillance data are collected, summarized, and distributed by the WHO in a weekly and other reports.

10. Evaluation

Once a surveillance program has been developed and has been in operation for a period of time, it should be reviewed and evaluated. Even though the program is operational, it should not be assumed that it is effectively meeting the objectives of the surveillance activity. Thacker and Berkelman discuss evaluation(2) and the CDC has developed a guide for the evaluation of public health surveillance systems.(7)

11. Limitations of Surveillance

Surveillance of disease is dependent on a series of events that if not followed may prevent the case from being reported. The events include that the disease be severe enough; that medical attention is sought and if sought, must be available; laboratory diagnostic facilities may be necessary and should be available; the health care provider or his or her representative must report the case; and the respective health department must have adequate resources and direction to support the surveillance program. There needs to be consistency in the case definition, in the collection of data, and in the mechanism of reporting. Any alterations in these events may change the apparent pattern of disease. The consistency and stability of the occurrence of these events is vital to the development of reliable surveillance data. In addition to recognition of clinical cases, there may be many infected persons with mild or subclinical illnesses that are not noted in the routine surveillance system. For these cases to be noted, laboratory studies of the distribution of the organism or the antibody to it are required.

12. References

1. Langmuir, A. D., The surveillance of communicable diseases of national importance, *N. Engl. J. Med.* **268:**182–192 (1963).
2. Thacker, S. B., and Berkelman, R. L., Public health surveillance in the United States, *Epidemiol. Rev.* **10:**164–190 (1988).
3. Thacker, S. B., Historical development, in: *Principles and Practice of Public Health Surveillance* (S. M. Teutsch and R. E. Churchill, eds.), pp. 3–17, Oxford University Press, New York, 1994.
4. Andrews, J. M., Quinby, G. E., and Langmuir, A. D., Malaria eradication in the United States, *Am. J. Public Health* **40:**1045–1411 (1950).
5. Nathanson, N., and Langmuir, A. D., The Cutter incident, *Am. J. Hyg.* **78:**16–81 (1964).
6. Centers for Disease Control and Prevention, *Comprehensive Plan for Epidemiologic Surveillance*, CDC, Atlanta, GA, 1986.
7. Centers for Disease Control and Prevention, Guidelines for evaluating surveillance systems, *Morbid. Mortal. Week. Rep.* **37:**S–5 (1988).
8. Wharton, M., Chorba, T. L., Case definitions for infectious conditions under public health surveillance, *Morbid. Mortal. Week. Rep.* **46**(RR10)**:**1–55 (1997).
9. Berkelman, R. L., Bryan, R. T., Osterholm, M. T., *et al.*, Infectious disease surveillance: A crumbling foundation, *Science* **264:**368–370 (1994).
10. Centers for Disease Control, *Annual Summary, Morbid. Mortal. Week. Rep.* (1995).
11. Glesecke, J., Surveillance of infectious diseases in the European Union, *Lancet* **348:**1534 (1996).
12. Desenclos, J.-C., Bijkerk, H., and Huisman, J., Variations in national infectious diseases surveillance in Europe, *Lancet* **341:** 1003–1006 (1993).
13. World Health Organization, The surveillance of communicable diseases, *WHO Chronicle* **22**(10)**:**439–444 (1968).
14. Centers for Disease Control, *Influenza Surveillance Rep.* **91** (July 1977).
15. Gangarosa, E. J., Mata, L. J., Perera, D. R., Reller, L. B., and Morris, C. M., Shiga bacillus dysentery in Central America, in: *Uses of Epidemiology in Planning Health Services*, Proceedings of the Sixth International Scientific Meeting, International Epidemiological Association (A. M. Davies, ed.), pp. 259–267, Savremena Administracija, Belgrade, 1973.
16. de Quadros, C. A., Hersh, B. S., Olive, J. M., Andrus, J. K., Silveira, C. M., and Carrasc, P. A., Eradication of wild poliovirus from the Americas. Part 1. Acute flaccid paralysis surveillance, 1988–1994 *J. Infect. Dis.* **175**(Suppl. 1)**:**537–542 (1997).
17. Hinman, A. R., Brandling-Bennett, A. D., and Nieburg, P. I., The opportunity and obligation to eliminate measles from the United States, *J. Am. Med. Assoc.* **242:**1157–1162 (1979).
18. Riverside County Health Department, California State Department

of Public Health, Centers for Disease Control, National Center for Urban and Industrial Health, A waterborne epidemic of salmonellosis in Riverside, California, 1965—Epidemiologic aspects, *Am. J. Epidemiol.* **99:**33–48 (1970).

19. Ryan, C. A., Nickels, M. K., Hargrett-Bean, N. T., Potter, M. E., Endo, T., Mayer, L., Langkop, C. W., Gibson, C., McDonald, R. C., and Kenney, R. T., Massive outbreak of antimicrobial-resistant salmonellosis traced to pasteurized milk, *J. Am. Med. Assoc.* **258**(22)**:**3269–3274 (1987).
20. Centers for Disease Control, *Sexually Transmitted Disease Surveillance, 1992*, US Public Health Service, Atlanta, 1993.
21. Weinstein, R. A., Multiple drug-resistant pathogens: Epidemiology and control, in: *Hospital Infections*, 4th ed. (J. V. Bennett and P. S. Brachman, eds.), pp. 215–236, Little, Brown, Boston, 1998.
22. Evans, A. S., Surveillance and seroepidemiology, in: *Viral Infections of Humans: Epidemiology and Control*, 4th ed. (A. S. Evans, ed.), pp. 89–115, Plenum Medical, New York, 1997.
23. Craven, P. S., Baine, W. B., Mackel, D. C., Barker, W. H., Gangarosa, E. J., Goldfield, M., Rosenfeld, J., Altman, R., Lachapelle, G., Davies, J. W., and Swanson, R. C., International outbreak of *Salmonella eastbourne* infection traced to contaminated chocolate, *Lancet* **1:**788–793 (1975).
24. Threfall, E. J., Hampton, M. D., Ward, L. R., and Rowe, B., Application of pulsed-field gel electrophoresis to an international outbreak of *Salmonella agona*, *Emerging Infect. Dis.* **2:**130–132 (1996).
25. Centers for Disease Control, Botulism, *Morbid. Mortal. Week. Rep.* **25**(17)**:**137 (1976).
26. Centers for Disease Control, *Shigella Surveillance Rep.* **13:**2 (1966).
27. Centers for Disease Control and Prevention, Update: Trends in AIDS diagnosis and reporting under the expanded surveillance definition for adolescents and adults—United States, 1993, *Morbid. Mortal. Week. Rep.* **43:**825–831 (1994).
28. Graitcer, P. L., and Burton, A. H., The epidemiologic surveillance project: A computer-based system for disease surveillance, *Am. J. Prev. Med.* **3:**123–127 (1987).
29. Valleron, A. J., Bouvet, E., Garnerin, P., Menares, J., Heard, I., Letrait, S., and Lefaucheux, J., A computer network for the surveillance of communicable diseases: The French connection, *Am. J. Public Health* **76:**1289–1292 (1986).
30. Chumming, C., Disease surveillance in China. Proceedings of the 1992 International Symposium on Public Health Surveillance, *Morbid. Mortal. Week. Rep.* **41**(suppl.)**:**111–122 (1992).
31. Centers for Disease Control, AIDS, *Morbid. Mortal. Week. Rep.* **30:**250 (1981).
32. Vogt, R. L., La Rue, D., Klaucke, D. N., *et al.*, A controlled trial of disease surveillance strategies, *Am. J. Prev. Med.* **73:**795–797 (1983).
33. Centers for Disease Control, *National Influenza Immunization Program-13, Influenza Surveillance Manual* (July 1976).
34. Schonberger, L. B., Bregman, D. J., Sullivan-Bolyai, J. Z., Keenlyside, R. A., Ziegler, D. W., Retailliau, H. F., Eddins, D. L., and Bryan, J. A., Guillain–Barré syndrome following vaccination in the national influenza immunization program, United States, 1976–1977, *Am. J. Epidemiol.* **110:**105–123 (1979).
35. Nelson, D. B., Sullivan-Bolyai, J. Z., Marks, J. S., Morens, D. M., Schonberger, L. B., and the Ohio State Department of Health Reye's Syndrome Investigation Group, Reye's syndrome: An epidemiologic assessment based on national surveillance 1977–1978 and a population based study in Ohio 1973–1977, in: *Reye's Syndrome II* (J. F. Crocker, ed.), pp. 33–46, Grune & Stratton, New York, 1979.
36. Gunn, R. A., Epidemiologic characteristics of infant botulism in the United States, 1975–1978, *Rev. Infect. Dis.* **1:**642–646 (1979).
37. Storch, G., Baine, W. B., Fraser, D. W., Broome, C. V., Clegg, H. W., II, Cohen, B. D., Shepard, C. C., and Bennett, J. V., Sporadic community-acquired Legionnaires' disease in the United States, *Ann. Intern. Med.* **90:**596–600 (1979).
38. Haley, R. W., Aber, R. C., and Bennett, J. V., Surveillance of nosocomial infections, in: *Hospital Infections*, 2nd ed. (J. V. Bennett and P. S. Brachman, eds.), pp. 51–71, Little, Brown, Boston, 1986.
39. Morese, S. S. (ed.), *Emerging Viruses*, Oxford University Press, New York, 1993. 317.
40. Lederberg, J., Shope, R. E., and Oaks, S. C. J. (eds.), *Emerging Infections: Microbial Threats to Health in the United States*, National Academy Press, Washington, DC, 1992.
41. Centers for Disease Control and Prevention, Addressing emerging infectious disease threats: A prevention strategy for the United States, *Morbid. Mortal. Week. Rep.* **43:**1–46 (1994).
42. Henderson, D. A., Role of the United States in the global response to emerging infections, *J. Infect. Dis.* **170:**280–285 (1994).

13. Suggested Reading

Eylenbosch, W. J., and Noah, N. D. (eds.), *Surveillance in Health and Disease*, Oxford University Press, New York, 1988.

Halprin, W., and Baker, E. L., *Public Health Surveillance*, Van Nostrand Reinhold, New York, 1992.

Raska, K. National and international surveillances of communicable diseases, *WHO Chron.* **20:**315–321 (1966).

Teutsch, S. M., and Churchill, R. E. *Principles and Practice of Public Health Surveillance*, Oxford University Press, New York, 1994.

PART II

Acute Bacterial Infections

CHAPTER 3

The Epidemiology of Bacterial Resistance to Antimicrobial Agents

Fred C. Tenover and John E. McGowan, Jr.

1. Introduction

Infectious diseases have continually played a role in shaping human history. The plague pandemic of the 13th century claimed approximately 25% of the world's population. Dysentery decimated the forces of Napoleon, and tuberculosis, also known as "the white plague," condemned many of histories most influential leaders, writers, artists, and scientists to untimely deaths, often in their most productive years. Thus, it was assumed that with the introduction of antibiotics into clinical medicine during the 20th century, the conquest of infectious diseases was likely to be close at hand. Yet, a closer examination of the medical literature beginning in the 1940s reveals an ominous trend that would be repeated over and over again throughout the next several decades: The discovery of a new antibacterial agent was followed sooner or later by the recognition of bacterial resistance to the agent. How bacteria develop resistance to antimicrobial agents and how resistant microorganisms spread in hospitals, other health care settings, and communities will be the focus of this chapter.

Fred C. Tenover • Nosocomial Pathogens Laboratory Branch, Hospital Infections Program, National Center for Infectious Diseases, Centers for Disease Control and Prevention, Atlanta, Georgia 30333. **John E. McGowan, Jr.** • The Rollins School of Public Health of Emory University, Atlanta, Georgia 30322.

1.1. Historical Background

Even while the wonder drug penicillin was making headlines by providing dramatic cures for patients with puerperal sepsis, gonorrhea, and other illnesses, strains showing resistance to the drug were already becoming apparent. Both gram-negative and gram-positive bacteria were found to contain enzymes capable of hydrolyzing penicillin and destroying its antibacterial action.[1,2] Similarly, although the mechanisms of resistance were not understood in the 1940s and early 1950s, physicians treating patients with either of the new antituberculosis drugs, para-aminosalicylic acid or streptomycin, noted that after initial signs of improvement, some of their patients began to deteriorate clinically. The *Mycobacterium tuberculosis* strains recovered from the patients who failed therapy were now resistant *in vitro* to the antimicrobial agents they were given.[3] Today, there are no antimicrobial agents used in human medicine for which resistance has not been recognized.

The paradigm for antibacterial agents is that resistance follows use, and widespread use or misuse of a drug will eventually lead to its loss of effectiveness for treating human illness.[4] In some cases, resistance appears quickly. For example, resistance to the semisynthetic drug oxacillin developed in *Staphylococcus aureus* just a few years after its introduction.[5] However, for other drug–organism combinations, such as with vancomycin and *Enterococcus faecium*, almost 30 years passed between the introduction of the drug into human use and the emergence of resistance.(6) The reasons for the differences in time frames are unclear and probably multifactorial. Yet, the ability of bacteria to circumvent the killing action of antibiotics has clearly impeded our ability to treat individual patients and to control large outbreaks of infectious diseases.(7–9) Examples of emerging antimicrobial resistance problems that have developed during the last two decades are given in Figures 1 and 2.

2. Mechanisms of Resistance

2.1. Intrinsic Resistance

Some bacteria are intrinsically resistant to antimicrobial agents because they either lack the target site for that drug, the drug is unable to reach the site of action, or the organism contains a chromosomally encoded resistance mechanism. Most gram-negative organisms are resistant to vancomycin because this large, hydrophobic drug cannot penetrate the organism's cell membrane.(10) Thus, these organisms are intrinsically resistant due to a permeability factor. However, *Klebsiella pneumoniae* strains are resistant to ampicillin and other penicillins because these organisms contain a chromosomal β-lactamase that inactivates this and similar drugs. Thus, intrinsic resistance may be due to a number of different mechanisms.

2.2. Acquired Resistance

Bacteria that are by nature susceptible to an antimicrobial agent may become resistant by random chromosomal mutation or by the acquisition of new genetic material that encodes the proteins responsible for the resistance phenotype. Chromosomal mutations that occur within the genes that encode the target sites for antimicrobial agents may change the structure of the proteins enough to prevent binding of the drug. Streptomycin resistance in *M. tuberculosis* is a good example of this.(11) Furthermore, the accumulation of point mutations in several different key genes in *M. tuberculosis* under the selective pressure of inadequate antimicrobial therapy (often a result of patients not consistently taking their medications) probably resulted in the multidrug-resistant strains of tuberculosis that caused outbreaks in several large cities in the United States in the early 1990s.(12)

There are five major mechanisms by which bacteria develop resistance to antimicrobial agents through the acquisition of new DNA.(9) They include (1) destroying or inactivating the drug by modifying it chemically; (2) decreasing the permeability of the bacterial cell, thereby decreasing access of the drug to its target site; (3) altering the target site of the drug so that the antibiotic cannot bind; (4) providing an alternate metabolic pathway to the one a drug inhibits; and (5) pumping the antibiotic out of the cell before it can bind to its site of action (efflux). Examples of the various classes of drugs and the mechanisms of resis-

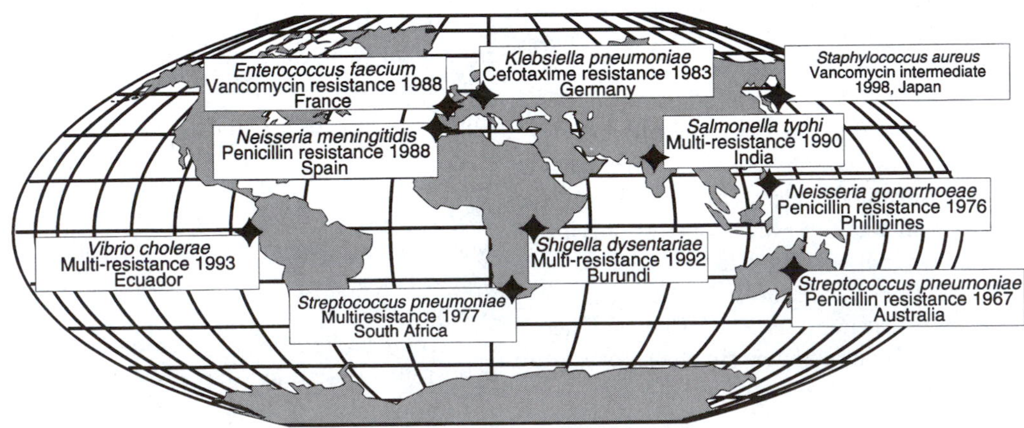

Figure 1. Global map showing emergence of a number of antimicrobial-resistant organisms. The location does not necessarily represent the first resistant isolate of a particular species to be isolated, but indicates the widespread nature and geographic diversity of the anitbiotic resistance problem. The *V. cholerae*, *S. dysenteriae*, and *S. typhi* strains were resistant to ampicillin, chloramphenicol, kanamycin, streptomycin tetracycline, sulfonamides, and trimethoprim/sulfamethoxazole. The *S. pneumoniae* strains from South Africa were resistant to penicilllin, chloramphenicol, tetracycline, and trimethoprim/sulfamethoxazole.

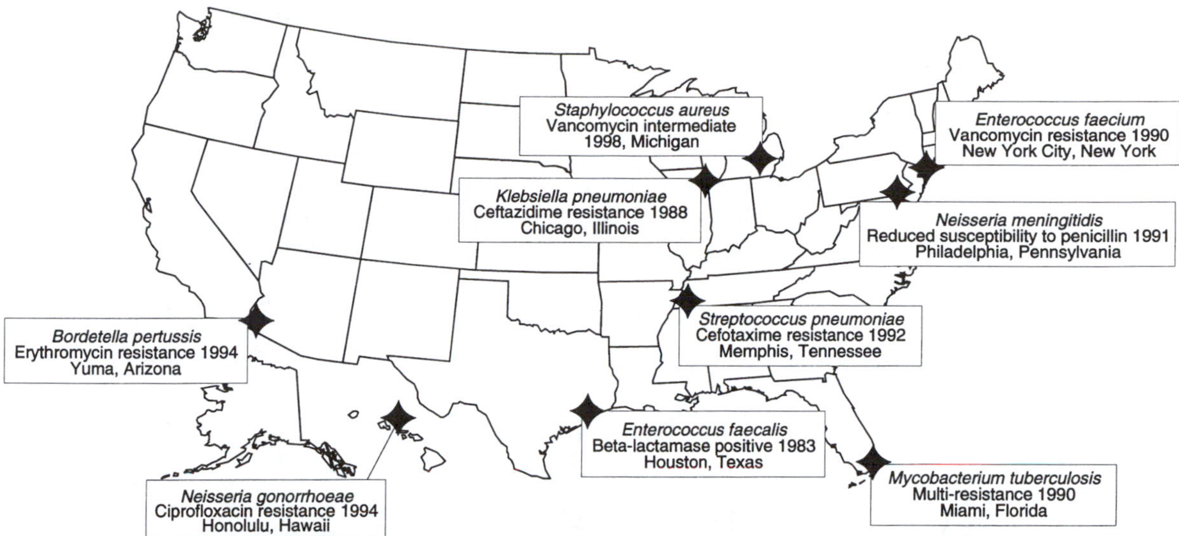

Figure 2. United States map showing emergence of a number of antimicrobial-resistant organisms. The location does not necessarily represent the first resistant isolate of a particular species to be isolated, but indicates the widespread nature and geographic diversity of the antibiotic resistance problem. The *M. tuberculosis* strain from Miami was resistant to isoniazid and rifampin, and was variably resistant to other antimycobacterial agents such as ethambutol and ethionamide.

tance associated with them are listed in Table 1 and are reviewed below.

2.3. Examples of Resistance Mechanisms for Various Classes of Antimicrobial Agents

2.3.1. β-Lactam Agents. Resistance to penicillins, cephalosporins, and other β-lactam antimicrobial agents most often results from the presence of enzymes in the bacterial cell (β-lactamases) that hydrolyze the β-lactam ring of the antibiotic, an action that detoxifies the drug.[13] There are at least 70 different types of β-lactamases that are found in bacteria and the number continues to grow. However, β-lactam resistance can also be mediated by changes in the site of action of the drugs, the penicillin-binding proteins (PBPs).[14] This occurs by remodeling of the genes that encode the PBPs through incorporation of foreign DNA acquired by the bacteria through transformation. These novel mosaic genes containing DNA from the host organism and DNA acquired from related organisms produce altered, albeit functional, PBPs. The latter mechanism is particularly important in the development of penicillin resistance in *Neisseria meningitidis* and *Streptococcus pneumoniae*.

2.3.2. Macrolides, Lincosamides, and Streptogramins. The macrolides, which include antibiotics such as erythromycin, clarithromycin, and azithromycin, are commonly administered oral drugs used for the treatment of many bacterial respiratory infections and superficial skin infections. Resistance is due either to inactivation of drug (mediated by erythromycin esterases), efflux of the drug out of the cell, or by modification of the site of action.[15,16] The latter mechanism, in which the 23S RNA of the 50S ribosome unit is methylated at a specific adenine residue, which prevents binding of the antibiotic to the ribosome, leads to high-level resistance to macrolides but also affects lincosamides (such as clindamycin) and streptogramins (such as pristinamycin), since all three classes of drugs act by binding to the same site on the bacterial ribosome. The so-called MLS-resistance phenotype (for macrolide–lincosamide–streptogramin) is typically observed in staphylococci and streptococci and is often plasmid mediated, but the genes encoding these enzymes also may be found on transposable elements.

2.3.3. Aminoglycosides. Aminoglycosides are commonly used in conjunction with β-lactam agents to treat serious bacterial infections, such as sepsis and endocarditis, because the two groups of drugs frequently act

Table 1. Examples of Bacterial Mechanisms of Antimicrobial Resistance

Antimicrobial class	Example	Mechanism	Organisms
Aminoglycosides	Gentamicin	Drug modification	*Enterobacteriaceae*
			Pseudomonas
			Enterococci
			Staphylococci
	Amikacin	Reduced permeability	*Pseudomonas*
β-lactam drugs	Penicillin	β-lactamase	Staphylococci
			Enterococci
			Enterobacteriaceae
			Pseudomonas
			Gonococci
β-lactam drugs	Penicillin	Altered cell wall	Pneumococci
			Meningococci
Fluoroquinolones	Ciprofloxacin	Altered DNA gyrase	Staphylococci
			Pseudomonas
			Enterobacteriaceae
Glycopeptides	Vancomycin	Altered DNA ligase	Enterococci
Macrolides	Erythromycin	RNA methylase	Staphylococci
			Pneumococci
			Streptococci
Tetracyclines	Doxycycline	Drug efflux	Streptococci
			Enterobacteriaceae
			Staphylococci
			Pseudomonas
Trimethoprim	Trimethoprim	Altered enzymes	*Enterobacteriaceae*
			Pseudomonas

[a]Adapted from Neu.[10]

synergistically. Resistance to aminoglycosides is typically mediated by enzymes that modify the drug so that uptake into the bacterial cell is impeded. However, efflux of drug out of the bacterial cell and permeability barriers to aminoglycosides are also recognized.[17] There are three types of aminoglycoside-modifying enzymes: those that acetylate, adenylate, or phosphorylate the drug. The number of genes encoding variants of these enzymes within each group is remarkably large and diverse. There is indirect evidence for two unique hypotheses on the origin of these resistance genes.[18] On the one hand, several of the genes are similar to those found in soil bacteria that produce antibiotics that protect the host organism from self-inhibition. The DNA encoding these genes may have been released into the soil through cell lysis and picked up by other bacteria, which in turn may have incorporated the DNA into a resident plasmid, allowing it to be mobilized to other bacterial species. An alternate hypothesis suggests that the proteins that modify the aminoglycosides have evolved from similar types of enzymes that have cellular "housekeeping" functions, such as phosphorylation of proteins to activate or inactivate enzymatic pathways.[18] These housekeeping enzymes became adapted over time to inactivation of aminoglycosides under the selective pressure of the presence of the antibiotics produced by other organisms in soil or in the hospital environment. Whether recruited from antibiotic-producing organisms or from other bacterial pathways, the array of aminoglycoside-resistance genes discovered to date is very diverse.

2.3.4. Tetracycline. Tetracyclines are oral drugs that are frequently used for treating patients with a wide variety of community-acquired infections, including skin infections, Rocky Mountain spotted fever, and chlamydia. Resistance is mediated both by actively pumping of the drug out of the bacterial cell before it can reach its site of action and by target site alteration.[19,20] Tetracycline-resistance genes are frequently located on plasmids and transposable elements, which enhances their ability to disseminate throughout diverse species of bacteria. There are over a dozen such resistance genes that are divided into several subgroups based on DNA sequence and mechanism. Tetracycline-resistance genes are frequently found on genetic elements with other resistance genes, such as those mediating resistance to chloramphenicol.

2.3.5. Trimethoprim and Sulfonamides. Trimethoprim and the sulfa drugs both inhibit the enzymatic pathway that synthesizes dihydrofolate.[21] Resistance is frequently the result of a plasmid-encoded enzyme that substitutes for a chromosomal enzyme normally inhibited by these drugs. Sulfonamides work through competitive inhibition of the enzyme dihydropteroate synthetase. The plasmid-coded enzyme is smaller and more heat sensitive and requires a thousand times as much sulfonamide to inhibit it as does the chromosomal enzyme. Similarly, some strains resistant to high levels of trimethoprim, an agent that inhibits dihydrofolate reductase, contain a plasmid-mediated gene coding for a new trimethoprim-resistant dihydrofolate reductase. In each of these instances, the plasmids provide a mechanism whereby products vital to the bacterial cell can be synthesized and the inhibiting effect of the drug is bypassed.

2.4. Key Factors in the Development of Resistant Microorganisms

There are three factors that appear to be critical in the continuing evolution of resistant microorganisms: mutations in common genes that extend their spectrum of resistance, transfer of resistance genes to new hosts, and increasing the selective pressures that enhance the development of spread of resistant organisms.[22,23] These three factors are interrelated.

The first factor—mutations in common resistance genes—can be observed in the progression of simple β-lactam hydrolyzing enzymes, i.e., penicillinases, to the extended-spectrum β-lactamases (ESBLs), which hydrolyze not only penicillin-type drugs and first-generation cephalosporins, but extended-spectrum cephalosporins (such as cefotaxime, ceftriaxone, and ceftazidime) and monobactams (such as aztreonam).[24] Such ESBL enzymes were first recognized in *K. pneumoniae* in Germany in 1982.[25] Mutations in the gene encoding the TEM-1 β-lactamase (named after the patient from whom the first ampicillin-resistant *Escherichia coli* was isolated) led to changes in three amino acids at key points in the enzyme. These changes enabled the active site of the enzyme to accommodate the much larger cephalosporins, which resulted in their inactivation. Further investigations of TEM β-lactamase mutants and of the mutants of a related β-lactamase, the SHV family of enzymes, have shown that even a single amino acid change can result in some ESBL activity.[26] Over 40 TEM and SHV mutants have now been recognized,[13] and the presence of such enzymes in the United States and Europe appears to be increasing.[27,28]

The second factor contributing to the development of novel resistance patterns is genetic exchange among bacteria, a process that may occur by transformation, conjugation, or bacteriophage-mediated transduction.[18,29] For example, conjugal transfer of the staphylococcal β-lactamase[30] and aminoglycoside-resistance genes[31] to enterococci led to development of multiply-resistant strains that have proven very difficult to treat, particularly when coupled with vancomycin resistance.[32] Vancomycin-resistant enterococci, in turn, have become a significant problem in the United States, particularly in hospital intensive care units.[33] Since vancomycin resistance is known to be transmissible, and since vancomycin-resistant strains of *S. aureus* have been achieved by mating *S. aureus* with highly vancomycin-resistant strains of enterococci *in vitro*,[34] the possibility exists that naturally occurring vancomycin-resistant clinical isolates of *S. aureus* may soon be recognized. Because hospital-acquired strains of *S. aureus* tend to be multiply resistant, the acquisition of vancomycin-resistance genes could make such strains virtually untreatable. The breadth of the genetic exchange network among microorganisms is only beginning to be understood.

The final factor in the evolution of resistance is the broadening of the selective pressure in hospital and community settings that facilitates the emergence of resistance. The term *selective pressure* refers to the environment created through the use of antibiotics that enhances the ability of an organism that becomes resistant by mutation or through acquisition of new DNA to survive and proliferate. The hospital has often been viewed as an important developing ground of resistant bacteria due to the extensive use of antimicrobial agents in this setting,[35] although resistance is not confined to hospital strains. The extensive use of antimicrobial agents among children for ear and respiratory infections[36,37] and the widespread use of antimicrobial agents in agriculture, animal husbandry, and aquaculture, in addition to human use,[3,38] have enhanced development of novel resistance patterns in a variety of pathogenic bacteria in the community setting as well as in the hospital.

2.5. Mechanisms of Gene Dissemination

A key factor in the spread of resistance is the movement of genetic elements independent of the spread of bacterial strains. Figure 3 shows the ways in which an organism may become multiply resistant to antimicrobial agents, which includes the accumulation of chromosomal mutations, acquisition of plasmids, acquisition of transposable elements, and insertion of resistance gene cassettes into integrons.

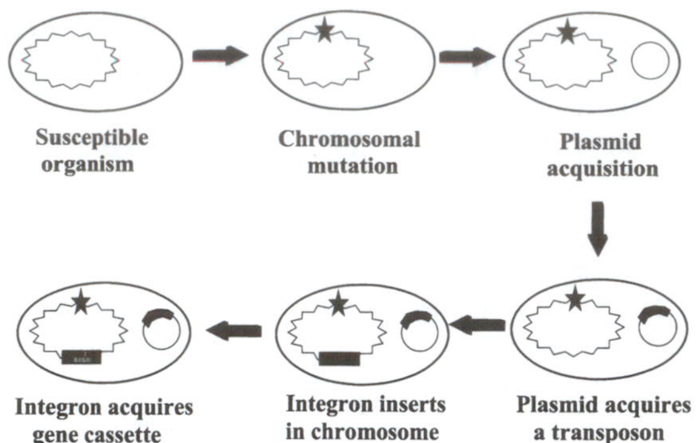

Figure 3. The evolution of multiple antimicrobial resistance in bacteria. The star indicates a chromosomal point mutation that leads to resistance. The circle indicates acquisition of new plasmid DNA containing a resistance gene. The curved, dark-hatched bar represents a transposon containing resistance genes that has been inserted into the plasmid. The black bar represents the insertion of an integron containing new resistance genes into the chromosomal DNA of the bacteria. The bar with vertical lines represents insertion of a new resistance gene cassette into the backbone of the integron.

Plasmids are extrachromosomal pieces of DNA that are not necessary for cell survival, but often give organisms a selective advantage to enhance survival. Plasmids may carry antimicrobial-resistance genes, and those plasmids may or may not be self-transmissible to other organisms via conjugations. Small, nontransmissible plasmids may still be mobilized to a bacterial recipient by larger conjugal plasmids present in the same cell. The transfer of resistance genes via plasmids was first noted in the 1950s by Japanese researchers who reported transfer of a multidrug-resistance phenotype from *Shigella* species to *E. coli*.(39) Plasmids have been reported to mediate resistance to as many as 12 antimicrobial agents,(40) and many plasmids are capable of being maintained by enteric bacilli, pseudomonads, vibrionaceae, and other gram-negative organisms.(29) One particular multiresistance plasmid, pLST1000, was isolated from gram-negative pathogens in several US cities and from isolates from Venezuela. The mode of intercontinental transmission was not apparent, but the stability of the plasmid over time was remarkable.(41)

As the phenomenon of plasmid transfer among microorganisms was emerging, another genetic element was recognized in gram-negative organisms—the transposon. This genetic element, which was capable of moving from replicon to replicon, such as plasmid to chromosome or vice versa, moved independently of the typical functions of generalized recombination. One family of transposons, those similar to Tn*21*, were found in a variety of multiply-resistant enteric organisms in the late 1970s and 1980s.(42) Later, a set of genetic elements with a very similar structure were discovered in gram-positive organisms, but these elements were conjugal, i.e., the elements were able to move from organism to organism via cell-to-cell contact.(43) These conjugal transposons were observed first in pneumococci(44) and later in *Bacteroides fragilis*.(45) Since pneumococci, in particular, do not maintain plasmids, conjugal transposons probably play a major role in the development of multiresistance in this species. Conjugal transposons apparently require cell-to-cell contact and probably transfer via formation of a circular intermediate form.(43) As many as five unique resistance genes have been reported to be present on conjugal transposons, and some, such as those encoding the *vanB* vancomycin-resistance gene in enterococci, seem to be extremely large, on the order of >200 kilobases.(46) Together with integrons, the elements into which resistance gene cassettes can enter with relative ease,(47) these elements serve to enhance the ability of resistance determinants to disseminate throughout bacterial populations at a rate much faster and more efficiently than could dissemination via plasmids alone.

3. Epidemiology of Antimicrobial Resistance

Studying the epidemiology of bacterial drug resistance has become more of a challenge over the past 20 years as organisms have developed multidrug resistance and the genes encoding resistance have apparently become more mobile. However, newer molecular strain typing techniques have enabled us to assemble a clearer picture of this process.(48)

The acquisition of a bacterial pathogen can occur in the hospital setting (Table 2) or in the community, although the two ecosystems are closely linked.(4,8,35,49) Those infections that occur in patients who have been a resident inside a hospital for more than 48 h are called nosocomial, or hospital acquired, while other infections are deemed to be community acquired.

3.1. Nosocomial Pathogens

During the 1960s and early 1970s, outbreaks of infection in hospitals caused by resistant bacteria likely represented the dissemination of a single resistant strain. Aminoglycoside-resistant strains of *S. aureus*(50,51) or multiply-resistant strains of *K. pneumoniae*(52) were reported in hospitals with increasing frequency. During the latter half of the 1970s and into the 1980s, the epidemio-

Table 2. Introduction and Spread of Antimicrobial Resistance into the Hospital Setting

Problem	Example
Introduction of new resistant organisms from outside sources	MRSA from nursing home patient
Mutation of susceptible endemic organisms that leads to a resistant phenotype	Ciprofloxacin-resistant *P. aeruginosa*
Acquisition of new DNA by susceptible endemic organisms that results in resistance	Vancomycin-resistant enterococci
Emergence of inducible resistance in organism that carry previously silent resistance genes	Ceftazidime-resistant *Enterobacter*
Selection of a resistant population of organisms from a heteroresistant population	Aminoglycoside-resistant *Acinetobater*
Spread of endemic resistant organism	*Serratia marcescens* in ICUs

Adapted from McGowan.(49)

logic picture began to change. Investigations of nosocomial outbreaks of infection often implicated not one, but multiple species of resistant gram-negative bacilli. Spread of a multiresistant strain of *Serratia marcescens*, for example, was followed by the appearance of *E. coli*, *Enterobacter cloacae*, and *Citrobacter freundii* strains with similar or identical antibiotic-resistance profiles.(40) Application of newly developed molecular techniques for plasmid analysis revealed that the initial phase of the outbreak involved dissemination of a single strain of *S. marcescens* that harbored a resistance plasmid. However, the same plasmid was then transmitted to other gram-negative bacilli, which subsequently were disseminated throughout the hospital in a second phase of the outbreak. Similar types of outbreaks involving spread of resistance plasmids to other species continue to occur.(28)

In the late 1970s, the discovery that transposable elements could mobilize as many as five resistance genes simultaneously in *Pseudomonas aeruginosa*(53) or in *Acinetobacter* species(54) showed that resistance genes could disseminate in nosocomial pathogens far more rapidly than originally hypothesized. The recognition of integrons(47) also shed light on why certain resistance gene combinations, including aminoglycoside-, sulfa-, and mercury-resistance genes, tended to be recognized together in bacterial strains, since these particular genes were commonly present in the backbone of integrons.

Two nosocomial pathogens continue to be of particular concern: methicillin-resistant *S. aureus* (MRSA) and vancomycin-resistant enterococci (VRE). In some hospitals, over 50% of the *S. aureus* isolated from inpatients are MRSA, and these strains often are resistant to all other drugs except vancomycin. Recently, strains of *S. aureus* with reduced susceptibility to vancomycin were isolated from patients in the United States and Japan(55a,55b) further complicating therapy.(55) MRSA have become endemic in many hospitals, which makes tracking of outbreaks more difficult. Once introduced into a hospital, this organism is very difficult to eradicate.(56) Problems with eradication are also true for vancomycin-resistant strains of *Enterococcus faecium*, which are often resistant to all other clinically approved drugs.(32,57) Vancomycin resistance in enterococci is often plasmid mediated and can be the result of several unique resistance determinants.(58) Recent guidelines from the Hospital Infection Control Practices Advisory Committee of the Centers for Disease Control and Prevention (CDC)(59) stress the need for prudent use of antimicrobial agents, the value of education programs on infection control for all hospital staff, and the requirements for adequate laboratory support of infection control. All are of critical importance if multiply-resistant organisms are to be contained and controlled in hospitals. It is imperative to reduce the selective pressure for the emergence of resistant microorganisms. Antibiotic use, particularly vancomycin and cephalosporins, is frequently a risk factor for developing VRE infections.(32)

Several species of multiresistant gram-negative organisms also continue to be significant pathogens in hospitals.(22) For example, *Enterobacteriaceae* resistant to aminoglycosides, β-lactams, chloramphenicol, and trimethoprim–sulfamethoxazole emerged in the late 1970s and have become endemic in a number of hospitals in the United States.(56) Many of these organisms now manifest resistance to the extended-spectrum cephalosporins as well. However, while strains of *K. pneumoniae* are resistant due to the production of ESBLs,(60) *Enterobacter* species are more likely to be have chromosomally encoded enzymes related to the AmpC family of β-lactamases.(61) Transmissible imipenem resistance was noted in *P. aeruginosa* in the late 1980s, but has yet to emerge as a major nosocomial problem.

3.2. Community-Acquired Pathogens

Development and spread of resistance in community-acquired bacteria has compromised many established therapeutic regimens for infectious diseases.(3,38) The increase in resistance has resulted from increased world travel where people are exposed to novel microorganisms that they bring back to the home country; greater reliance on foodstuffs, such as fruits and vegetables, from international sources that may be contaminated; and dramatic increases in worldwide antibiotic use. For example, in 1993, outbreaks of dysentery in Central Africa caused by *Shigella dysentariae* strains resistant to all major drug classes, except the fluoroquinolones, were reported.[63] These organisms contained a broad array of resistance genes, apparently assembled from a variety of enteric bacteria, and showed decreased susceptibility to the fluoroquinolones. If resistance to the fluoroquinolones developed, it would make these organisms essentially untreatable. Multiresistance in *Salmonella typhi*, the cause of typhoid fever, has also been noted, leaving the fluoroquinolones and sometimes mecillinam (amdinocillin) as the only options for treatment.[64] Thus, the quinolones have become key drugs for the treatment of several epidemic diarrheal diseases. However, widespread use of fluoroquinolones in hospitals for staphylococcal infections in the early 1990s led to the rapid and dramatic increase in resistance,[65] and this class of drugs has significantly reduced effectiveness in many hospitals for treating staphylococcal infections. A similar fate may be in store for *Shigella* and *Salmonella* strains.

Another important community-acquired pathogen, *S. pneumoniae*, is a major cause of meningitis, sepsis, pneumonia, and ear infections in the United States and around the globe.[66,67] Strains resistant to penicillin, tetracycline, chloramphenicol, and trimethoprim–sulfamethoxazole have now been isolated in the United States[68,69] and in several areas of the world[67,70] In the Atlanta area in 1994, 25% of pneumococcal isolates were no longer susceptible to penicillin and required alternate drugs for therapy of serious infections.[71] Other strains of pneumococci highly resistant to the extended-spectrum cephalosporins, the drugs of choice for treatment of penicillin-resistant strains, have emerged[72] and appear to be spreading. This has significantly impaired our ability to treat meningitis caused by these strains.[66] Pneumococci can spread particularly well among children in day care centers[36]; thus, the availability of more effective pneumococcal vaccines that are immunogenic in younger children (especially those ≤ 2 years of age) may play a significant role in controlling the spread of these resistant pathogens.[68] Another community-acquired pathogen that has engendered considerable interest due to its ability to acquire multiresistance is *Neisseria gonorrhoeae*, a sexually transmitted agent that has been epidemic in the world for almost three decades. High-level plasmid-mediated penicillin resistance emerged in *N. gonorrhoeae* in 1976.[73] The β-lactamase gene was similar to one found just one year previously in strains of *Haemophilus influenzae*.[74] The gene was likely transmitted to the gonococcus from *H. influenzae* or a related *Haemophilus* species by conjugation.[75] This was one of the first indications that the pathways of genetic exchange among microorganisms were much broader than originally perceived.[29] Penicillinase-producing *N. gonorrhoeae* are now common throughout the world and concern has shifted to the recent emergence of high-level fluoroquinolone resistance, which was first noted in 1994 in strains of gonococci from Hawaii.[76] Fluoroquinolones are key alternate therapeutics for gonorrhea, and the emergence of resistance threatens once again our ability to control this epidemic disease.

4. Surveillance of Resistant Microorganisms

Surveillance of resistant organisms occurs through established surveillance systems, outbreak investigations, and prospective studies.[4] The data, even from surveillance programs, are usually biased and incomplete, but nonetheless are critical for identifying trends in increasing resistance for organism/drug combinations.

4.1. Global Surveillance Programs

At present, a loosely knit network of microbiologists working in hospital, public health, and reference microbiology laboratories, and using a common software database known as WHONET, are gathering data on resistant bacteria in an effort to trace the spread of such organisms internationally. On a periodic basis, the data are provided via computer disk to the World Health Organization (WHO).[77] The goal of the program is to monitor changes in resistance patterns locally so that early intervention strategies to halt the spread of resistant strains can be implemented. However, the resistance data are also forwarded to the WHO, where national and regional trends can be assessed. In addition, several European surveillance networks, networks in Japan and Australia, and several new multicountry surveillance systems for targeted groups of bacteria, such as respiratory pathogens, are beginning to gather data on the incidence of resistant bacteria in various locales. Although most of these programs are just beginning to accumulate data, the levels of resistance seen in some regions of the world are astounding.

4.2. Surveillance Programs in the United States

At present, there are several for-profit antimicrobial-resistance surveillance programs and programs sponsored by pharmaceutical firms to monitor resistance in bacteria in the United States but only a single ongoing national program specifically designed for surveillance of resistant bacteria for public health purposes: the gonococcal isolate surveillance program (GISP) conducted by the CDC.[78] GISP monitors trends in minimum inhibitory concentrations in gonococcal isolates from 24 sentinel sites in the United States. In 1994, decreasing susceptibility to ciprofloxacin was noted among US isolates, indicating the need for more focused studies to identify the reasons for its emergence.

The National Nosocomial Infections Surveillance System (NNIS), which is also conducted by the CDC, consists of 240 hospitals that collect data on nosocomial infections in their hospitals and transmit the data to the CDC each month. The data set includes the identification of bacterial isolates that meet established criteria as a cause of a nosocomial infection and their antimicrobial-resistance patterns.[56] Although not specifically designed to monitor resistance, resistance patterns for specific organism/drug combinations are reviewed periodically to observe trends in certain organism/drug combinations. Other more loosely structured monitoring programs include laboratory surveillance of drug-resistant strains of *M. tuberculosis* by state health departments and, more recently, statewide monitoring of drug resistance in pneumococci in a few states. These systems, however, do not substitute for aggressive, local monitoring of bacterial resistance. Local monitoring of resistance patterns should be used to shape guidelines for empiric therapy for infections in a community. For example, local resistance rates for penicillin- and cefotaxime-resistant pneumococci should signal when vancomycin should be added to third-generation cephalosporins as empiric treatment of presumed bacterial meningitis.[68]

5. Conclusions

The epidemiology of antimicrobial resistance in bacteria has evolved from transmission of bacterial strains with a single resistance gene to the dissemination of large, complex genetic elements independent of a bacterial host. The newer mechanisms of gene dissemination, however, have not totally eclipsed the simple passage of resistant strains of MRSA from patient to patient via the hands of health care workers, or in contaminated water, in the case of resistant *Vibrio cholerae*.[79] As long as selective pressures exist, as fueled by misuse of antimicrobial agents in human and animal medicine, in agriculture, animal husbandry, and aquaculture, the problem of bacterial resistance to antibiotics will continue to grow.

6. Unresolved Problems

The unsolved problems of the resistance story are threefold: How to identify new targets for antimicrobial action for which resistance will be slow to develop; how to eliminate the spread of resistance genes located on plasmids and transposons to other organisms; and, most importantly, how to reduce the selective pressure in community and hospital settings that encourage the development and spread of antimicrobial-resistant microorganisms. Attention to each of these problems will help lessen the impact of antimicrobial resistance on human and animal health and prolong the effectiveness of the antimicrobial agents that we do have.

7. References

1. Abraham, E. P., Chain, E., An enzyme from bacteria able to destroy penicillin, *Nature* **146:**837–839 (1940).
2. Kirby, W. M. M., Extraction of a highly potent penicillin inactivator from penicillin resistant staphylococci, *Science* **99:**452–455 (1944).
3. Ryan, F., *The Forgotten Plague*, Little, Brown, Boston, 1993.
4. Cohen, M. L., Epidemiology of drug resistance: Implications for a post-antimicrobial era, *Science* **257:**1050–1055 (1992).
5. Barber, M., Methicillin-resistant staphylococci, *J. Clin. Pathol.* **14:**385–393 (1968).
6. Leclercq, R., Derlot, E., Duval, J., and Courvalin, P., Plasmid-mediated resistance to vancomycin and teicoplanin in *Enterococcus faecium*, *N. Engl. J. Med.* **319:**157–161 (1988).
7. Lederberg, J., Shope, R. E., and Oaks, S. C., Jr. (eds.), *Emerging Infections: Microbial Threats to Health in the United States*, National Academy Press, Washington, DC, 1992.
8. Murray, B. M., New aspects of antimicrobial resistance and the resulting therapeutic dilemmas, *J. Infect. Dis.* **163:**1185–1194 (1991).
9. Neu, H. C., The crisis in antibiotic resistance, *Science* **257:**1064–1073 (1992).
10. Neu, H. C., Overview of mechanisms of bacterial resistance, *Diagn. Microbiol. Infect. Dis.* **12:**109S–116S (1989).
11. Finken, M., Kirschner, P., Meier, A., Wreden, A., and Böttger, E. C., Molecular basis of streptomycin resistance in *Mycobacterium tuberculosis*: Alternations of the ribosomal protein A12 and point mutations within a functional 16S ribosomal RNA pseudoknot, *Mol. Microbiol.* **9:**1239–1246 (1993).
12. Edlin, B. R., Tokars, J. I., Grieco, M. H., Crawford, J. T., Williams, J., Sordilloo, E. M., Ong, K. R., Kilburn, J. O., Dooley, S. W., Castro, K. A., Jarvis, W. R., and Holmberg, S. D., An outbreak of multidrug resistant tuberculosis among hospitalized patients with acquired immunodeficiency syndrome, *N. Engl. J. Med.* **326:**1514–1521 (1992).
13. Bush, K., Jacoby, G. A., and Medeiros, A. A., A functional classification scheme for β-lactamases and its correlation with molecular structure, *Antimicrob. Agents Chemother.* **39:**1211–1233 (1995).
14. Spratt, B. G., Dowson, C. G., Zhang, Q. Y., Bowler, L. O., Brannigan, J. A., and Hutchisin, A., Mosaic genes, hybrid penicillin-binding proteins, and the origins of penicillin resistance in

Neisseria meningitidis and *Streptococcus pneumoniae*, in: *Perspectives on Cellular Regulation: From Bacteria to Cancer* (J. Campisi, D. Cunningham, M. Inouye, and M. Riley, eds.), pp. 73–83, Wiley-Liss, New York, 1991.

15. Arthur, M., Brisson-Noel, A., and Courvalin, P., Origin and evolution of genes specifying resistance to macrolide, lincosamide, and streptogramin antibiotics; data and hypotheses, *J. Antimicrob. Chemother.* **20:**783–802 (1987).
16. Eady, E. A., Ross, J. I., Tipper, J. L., *et al.*, Distribution of genes encoding erythromycin ribosomal methylases and an erythromycin efflux pump in epidemiologically distinct groups of staphylococci, *J. Antimicrob. Chemother.* **31:**211–217 (1993).
17. Shaw, K. J., Rather, P. N., Hare, R. S., *et al.*, Molecular genetics of aminoglycoside resistance genes and familial relationships of the aminoglycoside-modifying enzymes, *Microbiol. Rev.* **57:**138–163 (1993).
18. Davies, J., Inactivation of antibiotics and the dissemination of resistance genes, *Science* **264:**375–382 (1994).
19. Speer, B. S., Shoemaker, N. B., and Salyers, A. A., Bacterial resistance to tetracycline: Mechanisms, transfer, and clinical significance, *Clin. Microbiol. Rev.* **5:**387–399 (1992).
20. Levy, S. B., Evolution and spread of tetracycline resistance determinants, *J. Antimicrob. Chemother.* **24:**1–7 (1989).
21. Amyes, S. G. B., and Towner, K. J., Trimethoprim resistance; epidemiology and molecular aspects, *J. Med. Microbiol.* **31:**1–9 (1990).
22. Tenover, F. C., Novel and emerging mechanisms of antimicrobial resistance in nosocomial pathogens, *Am. J. Med.* **91**(Suppl. B): 76S–81S (1991).
23. Tompkins, L. S., Tenover, F., and Arvin, A., New technology in the clinical laboratory: What you always wanted to know but were afraid to ask, *J. Infect. Dis.* **170:**1068–1074 (1994).
24. Sougakoff, W., Goussard, S., Gerbaud, G., *et al.*, Plasmid-mediated resistance to third generation cephalosporins caused by point mutations in TEM-type penicillinase genes, *Rev. Infect. Dis.* **10:**879–884 (1988).
25. Knothe, H., Shah, P., Krcmery, V., *et al.*, Transferable resistance to cefotaxime, cefoxitin, cefamandole, and cefuroxime in clinical isolates of *Klebsiella pneumoniae* and *Serratia marcescens*, *Infection* **11:**315–317 (1983).
26. Philippon, A., Arlet, G., and Lagrange, P. H., Origin and impact of plasmid-mediated extended-spectrum beta-lactamases, *Eur. J. Clin. Microbiol. Infect. Dis.* **13**(Suppl. 1)**:**17–29 (1994).
27. Burwen, D. R., Banerjee, S. N., Gaynes, R. P., *et al.*, Ceftazidime resistance among selected nosocomial gram-negative bacilli in the United States, *J. Infect. Dis.* **170:**1622–1625 (1994).
28. Meyer, K. S., Urban, C., Eagan, J. A., *et al.*, Nosocomial outbreak of *Klebsiella* infection resistant to late-generation cephalosporins, *Ann. Intern. Med.* **119:**353–358 (1993).
29. DeFlaun, M. F., and Levy, S. B., Genes and their varied hosts, in: *Gene Transfer in the Environment* (S. B. Levy and R. V. Miller, eds.), pp. 1–32, McGraw-Hill, New York, 1991.
30. Murray, B. E., Mederski-Samoraj, B., Foster, S. K., *et al.*, *In vitro* studies of plasmid-mediated penicillinase from *Streptococcus faecalis* suggest a staphylococcal origin, *J. Clin. Invest.* **77:**289–293 (1986).
31. Kaufhold, A., Podbielski, A., Horaud, T., *et al.*, Identical genes confer high-level resistance to gentamicin upon *Enterococcus faecalis*, *Enterococcus faecium*, and *Staphylococcus aureus*, *Antimicrob. Agents Chemother.* **36:**1215–1218 (1992).
32. Montecalvo, M. A., Horowitz, H., Gedris, C., *et al.*, Outbreak of vancomycin-, ampicillin-, and aminoglycoside-resistant *Enterococcus faecium* bacteremia in an adult oncology unit, *Antimicrob. Agents Chemother.* **38:**1363–1367 (1994).
33. Centers for Disease Control and Prevention, Nosocomial enterococci resistant to vancomycin—United States, 1989–1993, *Morbid. Mortal. Week. Rep.* **42:**597–599 (1993).
34. Noble, W. C., Virani, Z., and Cree, R. G. A., Co-transfer of vancomycin and other resistance genes from *Enterococcus faecalis* NCTC 12201 to *Staphylococcus aureus*, *FEMS Microbiol. Lett.* **93:**195–198 (1992).
35. McGowan, J. E., Jr., Hall, E. C., and Parrott, P. L., Antimicrobial susceptibility in gram-negative bacteremia: Are nosocomial isolates really more resistant? *Antimicrob. Agents Chemother.* **33:** 1855–1859 (1989).
36. Infante-Rivard, C., and Fernandez, A., Otitis media in children: Frequency, risk factors, and research avenues, *Epidemiol. Rev.* **15:**444–465 (1993).
37. McCaig, L. F., and Hughes, J. M., Trends in antimicrobial drug prescribing among office-based physicians in the United States, *J. Am. Med. Assoc.* **273:**214–219 (1995).
38. American Society for Microbiology, *Report of the ASM Task Force on Antibiotic Resistance*, American Society for Microbiology, Washington, DC, 1995.
39. Akiba, T., Koyama, K., Ishiki, Y., *et al.*, On the mechanism of the development of multiple drug resistant clones of *Shigella*, *Jpn. J. Microbiol.* **4:**219–222 (1960).
40. Tompkins, L. S., Plorde, J. J., and Falkow, S., Molecular analysis of R-factors from multi-resistant nosocomial isolates, *J. Infect. Dis.* **141:**625–636 (1980).
41. O'Brien, T. F., del Pailr Pla, M., Mayer, K. H., *et al.*, Intercontinental spread of a new antibiotic resistance gene on an epidemic plasmid, *Science* **230:**87–88 (1985).
42. Grinstead, J., de la Cruz, F., and Schmitt, R., The Tn*21* subgroup of bacterial transposable elements, *Plasmid* **24:**163–189 (1990).
43. Clewell, D. B., and Gawron-Burke, C., Conjugative transposons and dissemination of antibiotic resistance in streptococci, *Annu. Rev. Microbiol.* **40:**635–659 (1986).
44. Shoemaker, N. B., Smith, M. D., and Guild, W. R., Organization and transfer of heterologous chloramphenicol and tetracycline resistance genes in *Pneumococcus*, *J. Bacteriol.* **139:**432–441 (1979).
45. Shoemaker, N. B., Barker, R. D., and Salyers, A., Cloning and characterization of a *Bacteroides* conjugal tetracycline–erythromycin resistance element by using a shuttle cosmid vector, *J. Bacteriol.* **171:**1294–1302 (1989).
46. Quintiliani, R., Jr., and Courvalin, P., Conjugal transfer of vancomycin resistance determinant vanB between enterococci involves the movement of large genetic elements from chromosome to chromosome, *FEMS Microbiol. Lett.* **119:**359–364 (1994).
47. Stokes, H. W., and Hall, R. M., A novel family of potentially mobile DNA elements encoding site-specific gene integration functions: Integrons, *Mol. Microbiol.* **3:**1669–1683 (1989).
48. Saminathan, B., and Matar, G. M., Molecular typing methods, in: *Diagnostic Molecular Microbiology. Principles and Applications* (D. H. Persing, T. Smith, F. C. Tenover, and T. White eds), pp. 25–50, American Society for Microbiology, Washington, DC, 1993.
49. McGowan, J. E., Jr., Antibiotic resistance in hospital bacteria: Current patterns, modes for appearance or spread, and economic impact, *Rev. Med. Microbiol.* **2:**161–169 (1991).
50. Jaffe, H. W., Sweeney, H. M., Weinstein, R. A., *et al.*, Structural and phenotypic varieties of gentamicin resistance plasmids in

hospital strains of *Staphylococcus aureus* and coagulase negative staphylococci, *Antimicrob. Agents Chemother.* **21:**773–779 (1982).

51. McGowan, J. E., Jr., Terry, P. M., Huang, T. S. R., *et al.*, Nosocomial infections with gentamicin-resistant *Staphylococcus aureus*: Plasmid analysis as an epidemiologic tool, *J. Infect. Dis.* **140:**864–872 (1979).
52. Sadowski, P. L., Peterson, B. C., Gerding, D. N., *et al.*, Physical characterization of ten R plasmids obtained from an outbreak of nosocomial *Klebsiella pneumoniae* infections, *Antimicrob. Agents Chemother.* **15:**616–624 (1979).
53. Rubens, C. E., McNeil, W. F., and Farrar, W. E., Jr., Transposable plasmid deoxyribonucleic acid sequence in *Pseudomonas aeruginosa* which mediates resistance to gentamicin and four other antimicrobial agents, *J. Bacteriol.* **139:**877–882 (1979).
54. Devaud, M., Kaiser, F. H., and Bächi, B., Transposon-mediated multiple antibiotic resistance in *Acinetobacter* strains, *Antimicrob. Agents Chemother.* **22:**323–329 (1982).
55. Panlilio, A., Culver, D. H., Gaynes, R. P., *et al.*, Methicillin-resistant *Staphylococcus aureus* in US hospitals, 1975–1991, *Infect. Control Hosp. Epidemiol.* **13:**582–586 (1992).

55a. Centers for Disease Control and Prevention. Reduced susceptibility of *Staphylococcus aureus* to vancomycin-Japan, 1996, *Morbid. Mortal. Week. Rep.* **46:**624 (1997).

55b. Centers for Disease Control and Prevention, *Staphylococcus aureus* with reduced susceptibility to vancomycin-United States, 1997, *Morbid. Mortal. Week. Rep.* **46:**765–766 (1997).

56. Emori, T. G., and Gaynes, R. P., An overview of nosocomial infections, including the role of the microbiology laboratory, *Clin. Microbiol. Rev.* **6:**428–442 (1993).
57. Handwerger, S., Raucher, B., Altarac, D., *et al.*, Nosocomial outbreak due to *Enterococcus faecium* highly resistant to vancomycin, penicillin, and gentamicin, *Clin. Infect. Dis.* **16:**750–755 (1993).
58. Arthur, M., and Courvalin, P., Genetics and mechanisms of glycopeptide resistance in enterococci, *Antimicrob. Agents Chemother.* **37:**1563–1571 (1993).
59. Hospital Infection Control Practices Advisory Committee (HICPAC), Recommendations for preventing the spread of vancomycin resistance, *Infect. Control Hosp. Epidemiol.* **16:**105–113 (1995).
60. Jacoby, G. A., and Medeiros, A. A., More extended spectrum beta-lactamases, *Antimicrob. Agents Chemother.* **35:**1697–1704 (1991).
61. Sanders, C. C., Chromosomal cephalosporinases responsible for multiple resistance to newer β-lactam antibiotics, *Annu. Rev. Microbiol.* **41:**573–593 (1987).
62. Watanabe, S., Iyobe, S., Inoue, M., *et al.*, Transferable imipenem resistance in *Pseudomonas aeruginosa*, *Antimicrob. Agents Chemother.* **35:**147–151 (1991).
63. Ries, A. A., Wells, J. G., Olivola, D., *et al.*, Epidemic *Shigella dysentariae* type I in Burundi: Pan-resistance and implications for prevention, *J. Infect. Dis.* **169:**1035–1041 (1994).
64. Threlfall, E. J., Ward, L. R., Rowe, B., *et al.*, Widespread occurrence of multiple drug-resistant *Salmonella typhi* in India, *Eur. J. Clin. Microbiol. Infect. Dis.* **11:**990–993 (1992).
65. Blumberg, H. M., Rimland, D., Carroll, D. J., *et al.*, Rapid development of ciprofloxacin resistance in methicillin-susceptible and -resistant *Staphylococcus aureus*, *J. Infect. Dis.* **163:**1279–1285 (1991).
66. Friedland, I. R., and McCracken, G. H., Jr., Management of infections caused by antibiotic resistant *Streptococcus pneumoniae*, *N. Engl. J. Med.* **331:**377–382 (1994).
67. Klugman, K., Pneumococcal resistance to antibiotics, *Clin. Microbiol. Rev.* **3:**171–196 (1990).
68. Centers for Disease Control and Prevention, Drug-resistant *Streptococcus pneumoniae*—Kentucky and Tennessee, 1993, *Morbid. Mortal. Week. Rep.* **43:**23–25 (1994).
69. McDougal, L. K., Facklam, R., Reeves, M., *et al.*, Analysis of multiply antimicrobial-resistant isolates of *Streptococcus pneumoniae* from the United States, *Antimicrob. Agents Chemother.* **36:**2177–2184 (1992).
70. Muñoz, R., Coffey, T. J., Daniels, M., *et al.*, Intercontinental spread of a multiresistant clone of serotype 23F *Streptococcus pneumoniae*, *J. Infect. Dis.* **164:**302–306 (1991).
71. Hofmann, J., Cetron, M. S., Farley, M. M., *et al.*, The prevalence of drug-resistant *Streptococcus pneumoniae* in Atlanta, *N. Engl. J. Med.* **333:**481–486 (1995).
72. Sloas, M. M., Barrett, F. F., Chesney, P. J., *et al.*, Cephalosporin treatment failure in penicillin- and cephalosporin-resistant *Streptococcus pneumoniae* meningitis, *Pediatr. Infect. Dis. J.* **11:**662–666 (1992).
73. Phillips, I., Beta-lactamase producing penicillin-resistant gonococcus, *Lancet* **2:**656–657 (1976).
74. Elwell, L. P, deGraaff, J., Seibert, D., *et al.*, Plasmid-linked ampicillin resistance in *Haemophilus influenzae* type b, *Infect. Immun.* **12:**404–410 (1975).
75. Sparling, P. F., Sox, T. E., Mohammed, W., *et al.*, Antibiotic resistance in the gonococcus: Diverse mechanisms of coping with a hostile environment, in: *Immunobiology of* Neisseria gonorrhoeae, pp. 44–52, American Society for Microbiology, Washington, DC, 1978.
76. Knapp, J. S., Ohye, R., Neal, S. W., *et al.*, Emerging *in vitro* resistance to quinolones in penicillinase-producing *Neisseria gonorrhoeae* strains in Hawaii, *Antimicrob. Agents Chemother.* **38:**2200–2203 (1994).
77. O'Brien, T. F., and the International Survey of Antibiotic Resistance Group, Resistance to antibiotics at medical centres in different parts of the world, *J. Antimicrob. Chemother.* **18**(C):243–253 (1986).
78. Schwarcz, S. K., Zenilman, J. M., Schnell, D., *et al.*, National surveillance of antimicrobial resistance in *Neisseria gonorrhoeae*, *J. Am. Med. Assoc.* **264:**1413–1417 (1990).
79. Weber, J. T., Mintz, E. D., Canizares, R., *et al.*, Epidemic cholera in Ecuador: Multidrug resistance and transmission by water and seafood, *Epidemiol. Infect.* **112:**1–11 (1994).

8. Suggested Reading

Neu, H. C., The crisis in antibiotic resistance, *Science* **257:**1064–1073 (1992).

Davies, J., Inactivation of antibiotics and the dissemination of resistance genes, *Science* **264:**375–382 (1994).

Levy, S. B., *The Antibiotic Paradox*, Plenum Press, New York, 1992.

CHAPTER 4

Anthrax

Philip S. Brachman and Arnold F. Kaufmann

1. Introduction

Anthrax, a zoonotic disease of herbivorous animals transmissible from animals to man, occurs primarily in three forms: cutaneous, inhalation, and gastrointestinal. Meningitis and septicemia occur but are secondary to one of the primary forms; occasionally, cases of anthrax meningitis are reported in which a primary focus is not identified. The etiologic agent is *Bacillus anthracis*, a gram-positive organism that in its spore form can persist in nature for prolonged periods, possibly years. The incidence of anthrax has decreased over the past 60 years, so that currently, human cases are seen only occasionally in the United States, where reporting is probably fairly accurate. Synonyms for anthrax include charbon, malignant pustule, Siberian ulcer, malignant edema, woolsorter's disease, and ragpicker's disease.

2. Historical Background

The earliest known description of anthrax is found in the book of Genesis; the fifth plague (1491 BC), which appears to have been anthrax, was described as killing the Egyptians' cattle. There are descriptions of anthrax involving both animals and humans in the early literature of the Hindus and Greeks. Virgil described anthrax during the Roman Empire (70–19 BC). In the 17th century, a pandemic referred to as "the black bane" swept through Europe, causing approximately 60,000 human deaths and many animal deaths. An association between human anthrax and contact with clothing made from wool and hides was reported.

In 1752, Moret more specifically characterized the disease in man, calling it "the malignant pustle." In 1780, Chabert described the disease in animals. The contagious nature of anthrax was noted in 1823 by Barthelemy. The first microscopic description of the organism was written by Delafond in 1838, and the organism was first described in infected animals in 1849 by Pollender. Pasteur discussed anthrax in some of his earlier writings on his germ theory of disease. In 1876, Koch used *B. anthracis* in developing his postulates concerning the relationships between bacteria and the diseases they cause. Greenfield developed an attenuated animal spore vaccine in 1880.[1–3] Pasteur, responding to a serious problem with anthrax in the French livestock industry, developed and field tested in sheep an attenuated spore vaccine in 1881. In 1939, Sterne reported his development of an animal vaccine that is a spore suspension of an avirulent, noncapsulated live strain.[4] This is the animal vaccine currently recommended for use.

Anthrax in the United States was first reported among animals in Louisiana in the early 1700s. Subsequently, sporadic animal cases have been reported from throughout the United States, and epizootics have been reported from the southern portion of the Great Plains states and the northeastern part of the country. The first human case was reported in a cattle tender in Kentucky in 1824.

Occupational anthrax occurred in the mid-1800s in England, where it was known as woolsorter's disease,[1] and in Germany, where it was known as ragpicker's disease. Ragpicker's disease occurred in individuals who handled rags that had been woven from contaminated animal fibers. The increasing problem of woolsorter's disease in England led to the development of a government inquiry committee that correctly identified the problem as being related to imported animal fibers contaminated with *B. anthracis*.[5] Subsequently, in 1921, a formaldehyde

Philip S. Brachman • The Rollins School of Public Health of Emory University, Atlanta, Georgia 30322. **Arnold F. Kaufmann** • National Center for Infectious Diseases, Centers for Disease Control and Prevention, Atlanta, Georgia 30333.

disinfecting station was built by the government in Liverpool.[6] All "dangerous" imported wools and goat hairs were first washed in formaldehyde baths, which successfully reduced contamination of the animal fibers with *B. anthracis*. The occurrence of inhalation anthrax was drastically reduced, so that only sporadic cases have been reported in England since 1922. The disinfecting station continued to operate until the mid-1970s, by which time the danger had been reduced to such a level that further disinfection with formaldehyde was not deemed necessary or economical.

In the United States, human anthrax cases have been reported from most of the states. Initially, cases were related to animal contact and reflected areas with enzootic and epizootic anthrax, primarily involving cattle and occasionally sheep and horses. As the United States became industrialized, human cases associated with the textile and tanning industries occurred with increasing frequency. In the early 1900s, these cases primarily occurred in the northeastern states. In the 1950s, cases began to occur in southeastern states, reflecting the movement of the industry.

In the 1920s, the annual number of cases reported in the United States ranged from 100 to 200 cases; in the 1950s, from 20 to 50 cases each year; in the 1970s, from 0 to 6 cases each year; in the 1980s, 4 cases were reported; and from 1990 through 1996, one case was reported in 1992. This decrease is the result of the use of a human cell-free anthrax vaccine among high-risk industrial groups, decreased utilization of imported potentially contaminated animal products, improved hygiene in industry, and improved animal husbandry. The incidence of animal anthrax has likewise decreased so that only occasional cases are reported and epizootics have not been reported for a number of years. This reduction is the result of improved animal husbandry and the appropriate utilization of animal anthrax vaccine.

3. Methodology

3.1. Sources of Mortality and Morbidity Data

In the United States, data on human anthrax are collected in individual states through the routine surveillance system. Usually, individual case data are obtained by use of special case-reporting forms and investigations. These data are then reported by means of the morbidity and mortality reporting system to the Centers for Disease Control and Prevention (CDC). Epidemic information and, at times, individual case data are reported to the CDC by telephone. Years ago, the reporting of anthrax was spotty; however, as health care providers have accepted their responsibilities to notify public health officials about the occurrence of reportable disease, overall surveillance has improved. Additionally, as the incidence of the disease has decreased and the use of the laboratory in assisting in diagnosing the disease has increased, reporting has become more complete.

Data concerning anthrax in animals are obtained through federal and state departments of agriculture or public health or both.

Worldwide data on anthrax are available from the World Health Organization (WHO) and the Food and Agriculture Organization. However, not all countries maintain adequate surveillance programs for infectious diseases, and thus all do not have data available on cases of human or animal anthrax. Reports of anthrax associated with rural areas, i.e., animal-associated cases, will be especially deficient because of the generally poorer reporting of diseases from rural areas. Another source of data is the scientific literature in which a report of a case or an epidemic of anthrax may be published, even though it was not officially reported to the country's central health authority. Additionally, reports of epidemics in the scientific literature may give the actual number of cases of the disease that occurred, whereas the number reported to the health authorities may only include those cases confirmed in the laboratory.

3.2. Surveys

Population surveys are not practical due to the low incidence of the disease. Serological surveys are not generally useful for obtaining information on anthrax, except in epidemic or epizootic investigations, because of limitations of the laboratory procedures. However, they may also be useful in ascertaining immunity levels in human and livestock populations.

3.3. Laboratory Diagnosis

3.3.1. Isolation and Identification. Swabs from lesions, vesicular fluid, or blood may be examined for the presence of *B. anthracis*.[7] *B. anthracis* is a gram-positive, nonmotile, hemolytic, spore-forming bacillus (1–1.3 × 3–10 μm) that grows on ordinary laboratory media at 37°C, producing round, grayish-white, convex colonies having comma-shaped outshootings with a ground-glass appearance that measure 2–5 mm in diameter. Colonies first appear approximately 8–12 hr after inoculation of the agar and show the typical characteristics 24–36 hr after inoculation. When an inoculated loop is drawn through the colony, tenacity is demonstrated; the disturbed part of the colony will be drawn perpendicular to the agar and will remain in this position, resembling beaten egg white. Microscopic examination (such as by Gram's stain) of growth from artificial media shows long parallel chains of organisms with square ends, referred to as "boxcars." Spore stains will reveal central or paracentral spores in *B. anthracis* organisms that have incubated at least 24 hr. Material from a fresh lesion will show shorter chains with single or two to four organisms in a row with slightly rounded ends. Direct fluorescent-antibody staining specific to either the cell wall or the capsule may also be used to identify the organisms from vesicular fluid cultures or from tissues.[8]

A bacteriophage designated gamma phage may be used to confirm the identification of *B. anthracis*.[9] Toxin production assays and DNA probes for presence of the pX01 and pX02 plasmids are newer identification methods available in some reference laboratories.[10] The DNA probe can be used to identify *B. anthracis* in nonviable specimens. Subcutaneous or intraperitoneal inoculation of guinea pigs, mice, or rabbits with agar-grown cells suspended in saline may be useful in differentiating *B. anthracis* from other gram-positive bacilli. *B. anthracis* will cause death from 24 to 72 hr after inoculation, and the animal will show evidence of general toxicity and multiple organ hemorrhages. Animals inoculated subcutaneously demonstrate subcutaneous gelatinous, hemorrhagic edema in addition to general toxemia. Broth-grown cultures must not be used because nonspecific death can result.

Tissue from autopsied patients should be cultured and microscopically examined.

3.3.2. Serological and Immunologic Diagnostic Methods. The virulence of *B. anthracis* is determined by the presence of three components: edema toxin, lethal toxin, and capsular material. To exert their effect within cells, both toxins require participation of a common transport protein, called protective antigen. The capsule material contains poly-D-glutamic acid, which helps protect the bacillus from ingestion by phagocytes. Production of the toxic factors is regulated by one plasmid (pX01) and that of the capsular material by a second plasmid (pX02).

An enzyme-linked immunosorbent assay (ELISA) has been developed to measure antibodies to the lethal and edema factors and the protective antigen. A fourfold rise in titer or a single titer of greater than 1:32 is indicative of current or recent infection or acquired immunity.[11,12] An electrophoretic-immunotransblot test that measures antibody to the protective antigen and the lethal factor is used to confirm ELISA results, or as the primary diagnostic test. Assays have been developed to detect the presence of the protective antigen component of the toxin in vesicular fluid as well as serum and cerebrospinal fluid (CSF).[11,13]

3.3.3. Pathology. Autopsy material, commonly from the mediastinal structures, lymph nodes, spleen, and liver, should be examined for organisms and pathological changes.[14] The most significant findings at autopsy are those seen in patients who have died of inhalation anthrax. The classic finding is that of hemorrhagic mediastinitis with enlarged, hemorrhagic lymphadenitis. There may be inflammation of the pleura and some pleural effusion. Acute splenitis may also be seen. Some patients may have hemorrhagic meningitis, and in one patient, hemorrhages were seen in the gastrointestinal tract.[15]

In deaths due to the abdominal form of gastrointestinal anthrax, there typically is hemorrhagic enteritis with congestion, thickening, and edema of the intestinal walls. Mucosal ulcers with necrosis may be seen in the terminal ileum and cecum. The regional lymph nodes are enlarged, edematous, and hemorrhagic with some necrosis. There may be acute splenitis. Peritonitis with ascitic fluid is present.

In some patients with significant cutaneous lesions on the head and neck or the oropharyngeal form of gastrointestinal anthrax, marked anterior cervical subcutaneous edema may compress the trachea at the thoracic inlet. Death in such patients is due to asphyxiation.

4. Biological Characteristics of the Organism

The resistance of the spore form of *B. anthracis* to physical and chemical agents is reflected in the persistence of the organism in the inanimate environment. Organisms have been demonstrated to persist for years in factories in which the environment became contaminated during the processing of contaminated imported materials of animal origin. Accordingly, they may serve as the source of infection for people who work in the area. Special efforts are required to decontaminate this environment; one method is to use paraformaldehyde vapor, which is successful in killing *B. anthracis* spores. In the laboratory, surfaces may be decontaminated with either 5% hypochlorite or 5% phenol (carbolic acid); instruments and other equipment may be autoclaved.

B. anthracis may also persist in certain types of soil for years.[16] Alluvial soil with a pH greater than 6.0 is best suited for survival of *B. anthracis*. Persistence of the organism in soil plus environmental conditions such as climatic variations, i.e., flooding or drought, triggering brief periods of bacterial growth thought to be associated with outbreaks of anthrax in animals grazing on contaminated pastures. Areas that are repeatedly the sites of animal anthrax are known as anthrax districts. One such area is the lower Mississippi River valley area, from which sporadic outbreaks of animal anthrax have been reported at irregular intervals for years.

5. Descriptive Epidemiology

5.1. Prevalence and Incidence

In 1958, Glassman,[17] using reports from the WHO, estimated the annual worldwide incidence of human anthrax to be from 20,000 to 100,000 cases. Data from the WHO[18] for 1981 reported 3200 cases from 43 countries, which undoubtedly is an underestimate. A review of reports from the WHO, Food and Agricultural Organization, and the Office Internationale des Epizooties for the 1990s provides some more recent data, but it is no more accurate than the previous estimates. In 1993, 1915 human cases were reported from 16 countries with 14 other countries reporting no cases, and in 1994, 694 cases were reported from 13 countries with another 17 countries reporting no cases. Animal anthrax remains an endemic problem in various Asiatic, African, South American, and Caribbean countries.[19] In countries with a significant animal anthrax problem, there is probably a related human anthrax problem. In China, for example, an average of 2115 human cases were reported annually in the period 1989–1993, primarily related to butchering and consuming infected livestock.[20] However, since the reporting of diseases from rural areas is sporadic, these data are not generally available. Industrial anthrax infections are related to the processing of animal products such as goat hair, wool, skins and hides, and dried bones. Industrial countries that process these materials will have industrially related cases at a rate inversely proportional to the level of development of appropriate hygienic measures directed at reducing the threat of anthrax.

In the United States, the annual number of cases of human anthrax decreased from an average of 127 for the years 1916–1925, to 44 cases for 1948–1957, to 9.6 cases for 1958–1967, to 2.4 cases for 1968–1977, and to 0.9 case for 1978–1987, and to 0.3 case for 1988–1996 (see Fig. 1).

Approximately 95% of anthrax cases in the United States are cutaneous and 5% are inhalation; confirmed cases of gastrointestinal anthrax have not been reported in the United States but have been reported in other countries. Some investigators report that from 5 to 10% of cases worldwide may be gastrointestinal cases, i.e., one such case to every 100 to 200 cutaneous cases. From 1955 through 1996, 235 cases of anthrax were reported in the United States; 224 cases were cutaneous (21 of which were at unknown sites) and 11 were inhalation. Of the 203 cutaneous cases for which the sites of infection were reported, the majority occurred on the exposed part of the body, with 51% on the arms, 27% on the head and neck, 5% on the trunk, and 3% on the legs (see Table 1).

It is estimated that approximately 20% of untreated cases of cutaneous anthrax will result in death. Of the 224 cutaneous cases that have been reported in the United States since 1955, 11 have been fatal. Inhalation anthrax is almost always fatal; since 1900, 16 of the 18 cases reported in the United States have resulted in death.

In the few reports available, the mortality from gastrointestinal anthrax has usually ranged from 25% to 60%. In 1989, a gastrointestinal anthrax epidemic in Tibet resulted in 507 cases, including 162 deaths (32%).[20]

5.2. Epidemic Behavior and Contagiousness

The first reports of inhalation anthrax (woolsorter's disease) in England in the late 1800s and early 1900s included clusters of cases associated with the sorting of certain lots of imported goat hair, frequently mohair.[21] In the United States, occasional epidemics occurred in industrial settings, epidemiologically related to the processing of batches of highly contaminated imported animal fibers, particularly goat hair. These epidemics were primarily of cutaneous anthrax.

The largest epidemic reported in the United States occurred in 1957, and involved employees in a goat-hair-processing plant.[22] Among the 600 employees over a 10-week period, there were nine cases of anthrax: four cases of cutaneous anthrax and five of inhalation anthrax. None of the patients with cutaneous anthrax died, but four of the five with inhalation anthrax died. Epidemiological investigations related the cases to a particular contaminated batch of goat hair imported from Pakistan.[23] More than 50% of samples from this particular batch were culture-positive for *B. anthracis*. A detailed examination of production records revealed that each of the patients had direct contact with this particular lot of goat hair during an appropriate period before the onset of disease.

An outbreak of human anthrax occurred in north central Russia (Sverdlovsk) in 1979, in which the source of infection was an accidental release of *B. anthracis* aerosol from a biological warfare research laboratory.[24] The exact number of cases is uncertain, but at least 77 persons developed inhalation anthrax subsequent to expo-

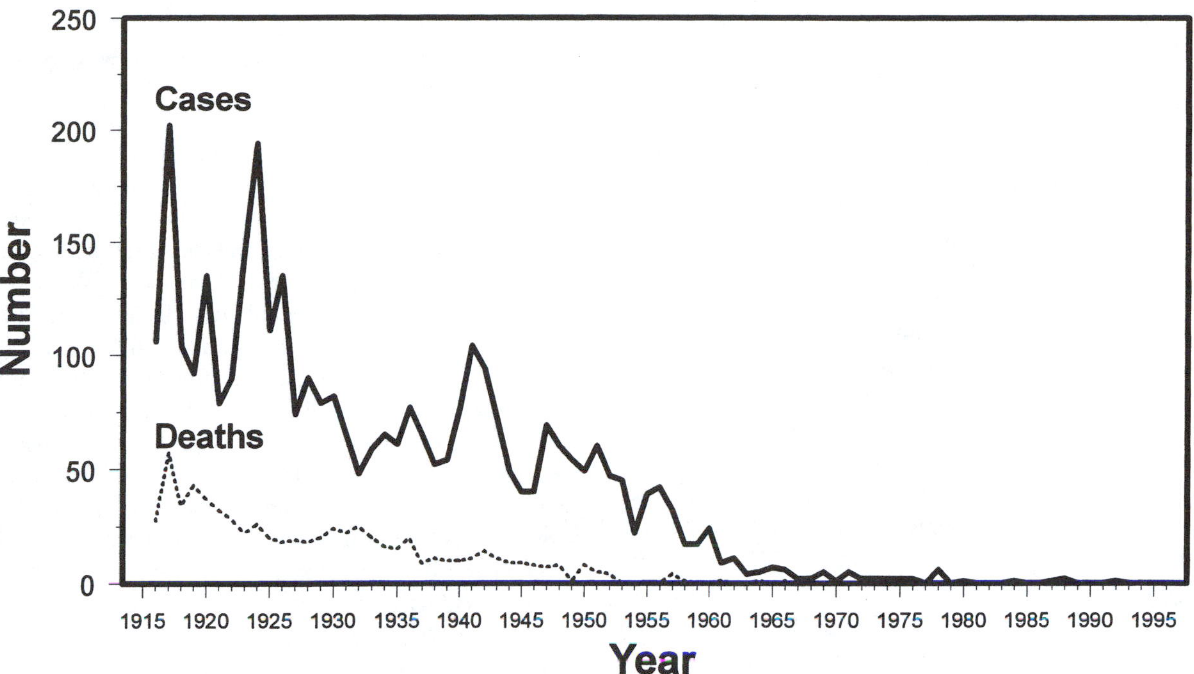

Figure 1. Anthrax in man in the United States, 1916–1996. Source: NOVS data.

sure in a narrow 4-km-long zone south of the laboratory. Deaths in sheep occurred up to 50 km from the laboratory as a result of the same accidental release. This incident was the largest inhalation anthrax epidemic reported to date.

Human-to-human transmission of anthrax rarely has been reported. A recent report on anthrax in China included information on 10 cases of person-to-person transmission in medical case staff.[20] However, data are not presented that confirm these cases as representing human-to-human transmission. Industrial infections result from exposure to the organisms in the industrial environment, from contact with organisms either in the materials actually being processed, or in the environment that has been contaminated by previously processed materials. Those employees who work in the earliest processing stages, in which the materials and the environment are more heavily contaminated with *B. anthracis*, are at greater risk of contracting anthrax than those who work with the materials at later stages in the manufacturing cycle. Occasional cases occur in persons who have direct or indirect contact with *B. anthracis* in a laboratory setting.

Agricultural cases occur in veterinarians and others who have direct contact with animals that have died of anthrax. There have been cases of human disease associated with epizootics of anthrax in cattle. The largest reported agricultural outbreak occurred in Zimbabwe with more than 10,000 cases reported between 1979 and 1985.[25] The peak number of cases, more than 6000, were reported to have occurred between October 1979 and March 1980. Endemic cases continue to occur in the involved area. The majority of patients had cutaneous infections located primarily on the exposed parts of the body; some gastrointestinal cases have been reported. Domestic cattle deaths were also noted. The humans were

Table 1. Sites of 235 Anthrax Infections, United States, 1955–1996

		Known cutaneous distribution	
Sites	Infections	Number	Percent
Cutaneous	203		
Arms		120	51
Head and neck		64	27
Trunk		11	5
Legs		8	3
Unknown	21		9
Inhalation	11		5

infected from contact with the diseased animals or by handling their carcasses during butchering or burial; the source of infection for the animals was not reported. Routine animal vaccination had not been practiced.

5.3. Geographic Distribution

Cases are distributed according to their association with an agricultural or industrial source of infection. From 1920 to 1954, more than 50% of all cases in the United States occurred in Pennsylvania, New York, New Jersey, Massachusetts, and New Hampshire, the location of industries that processed animal hair, hide, and bone.(26) Subsequently, industrial cases began to be reported from other states, such as North Carolina and South Carolina, as companies moved southward. In more recent years, cases have not shown a geographic localization, reflecting the decrease in industry-related cases and the low endemicity of agriculture-related cases.

Agricultural cases are distributed in rural areas associated with outbreaks in animals and primarily occur in the previously discussed anthrax districts. Some of these districts are located in Louisiana, Mississippi, and South Dakota.(16) Epizootics usually involve dairy cattle, but sheep and horses may also be involved.

5.4. Temporal Distribution

Industrial cases occur throughout the year without any seasonal pattern. Animal-related cases occur primarily in the spring and summer, the seasons when animal anthrax cases occur with the greatest frequency.

5.5. Age

The age distribution of cases reflects the age of the individuals who work in the involved industry or come in contact with infected carcasses. Primarily, these persons are 20–60 years of age. Occasional cases have been reported in children, one of whose parents worked in a factory in which *B. anthracis*-contaminated materials were processed; it has been hypothesized that *B. anthracis* organisms were transported into the home on the parent's clothing.

5.6. Sex

The predominance of males reflects the sex distribution of the people who work in the involved industries or have contact with infected carcasses.

5.7. Race

No distinctive racial patterns are found among persons with anthrax.

5.8. Occupation

Anthrax cases may be divided into two major categories: those associated with an industrial setting and those associated with an agricultural setting (see Table 2). However, some cases occur in people who live in urban areas in which the source of infection is unknown; in these cases, the source is assumed to be industrial. In addition, a few laboratory-associated cases have been reported.

Industrial cases occur in individuals who work in industries in which animal products, usually imported, are processed.(26,27) In the United States, this primarily involves workers in goat-hair- and wool-processing industries. Goat hair is imported primarily from Asiatic, Middle Eastern, and African countries in bales weighing 200–250 lb each. The hair is processed into yarn used in preparing interlinings for men's suit coats and also into a felt material used as underpads for carpets, insulation for pipes, saddle pads, and washers. The wools that have been implicated in cases of anthrax are imported from the same areas of the world and are primarily the coarser wools used in carpets as distinct from the finer wools used in clothing. Occasionally, however, anthrax has been associated with fine cashmere wool.

Anthrax has also been associated with the tanning industry and has resulted from contact with imported skins and hides. Cases have also been associated with the bone-meal-processing industry, in which dried bones are

Table 2. Source of Infection in 235 Cases of Human Anthrax, United States, 1955–1996

Source	Number
Industrial	
Goat hair	113
Wool	34
Goat skins	16
Meat	3
Bone	4
Unknown	12
Agricultural	
Animal	43
Vaccine (animal)	2
Unknown	8

imported for preparing bone meal for fertilizer, animal food supplements, or gelatin. The dried bones are usually gathered from animal grazing areas and are from animals that have died of unknown causes. However, bones may also be obtained from slaughtering or rendering plants.

There have been cases in which the source of infection has been domestic animal products. For example, in 1924, a number of persons developed cutaneous anthrax following their contact with hides from animals that died during an epizootic of anthrax.

Occasional cases have been reported among persons who have had contact with horsehair and pig bristles that are used in brushes, such as shaving brushes or hairbrushes. The number of cases associated with contaminated imported shaving brushes was significantly reduced in the 1920s by the enactment of laws requiring that these brushes be shown by culture to be free of *B. anthracis* organisms when imported into the country. In recent years, the use of animal fibers has decreased as synthetic materials have been used in increasing quantities. Accordingly, this risk of anthrax is negligible.

Agricultural cases have occurred in individuals who came into contact with sick or dead animals in rural areas. Primarily, these cases have involved cattle owners, veterinarians, and veterinary assistants who have had contact with animals, for example, while performing autopsies on infected carcasses. Another route of infection is by ingestion of raw or undercooked infected meat from an infected carcass. A few cases have resulted from the accidental self-injection of Pasteur-type animal spore vaccine into a finger or hand. No documented cases have resulted from the Sterne strain animal vaccine.

Agricultural cases have also occurred in individuals who used fertilizer or animal feed that contained contaminated bone meal. One particular epidemic related to feed supplement for pigs involved 846 cases in pigs, with some cases in persons who had contact with the pigs.[28]

Occasional cases have occurred in individuals who have had no known contact with industrial or agricultural sources. Usually, their cases are thought to have been caused by environmental contamination such as in the case of a housewife who lived near a tannery and died of inhalation anthrax. Another case occurred in an individual who every day walked by the receiving room door of a tannery where contaminated hides were processed.[29] It was shown that air could have flowed from the receiving area out into the street, where the individual could have inhaled an infecting dose of airborne *B. anthracis* organisms. At least 77 cases of inhalation anthrax occurred in Sverdlovsk, Russia in 1979, associated with the accidental release of an aerosol from a biological warfare research laboratory.

Several cases have occurred in persons whose contact has been in laboratories in which strains of *B. anthracis* have been handled.[30] Two of these cases were fatal inhalation cases.

5.9. Cases Related to Commercial Products

An occasional case has occurred in an individual after contact with a commercial product prepared from animal materials. Examples of cutaneous anthrax include contact with imported souvenir drums with drumheads made of goatskin[31] and a case in which the source of infection was most likely a newly purchased woolen coat. A fatal case of inhalation anthrax in a home weaver followed contact with imported yarn that contained animal fibers.[32]

5.10. Socioeconomic and Other Factors

Socioeconomic or other factors may contribute significantly to the risk of an anthrax infection. Among some people in certain societies, economic problems lead to individuals salvaging the meat, hair, or hides from carcasses of animals that died from anthrax, and thus increases their risk of developing an anthrax infection. Most gastrointestinal anthrax is related to butchering and consuming anthrax-infected animals by persons who cannot afford to waste a source of protein.

6. Mechanisms and Routes of Transmission

B. anthracis organisms are primarily transported by the contact or the airborne routes. Organisms can also be transmitted by a common vehicle, food (meat), though this is rare. Vectors (flies) have been reported to transmit organisms, although the actual relationship to subsequent disease has not been proven.

Contact spread is primarily by indirect contact, although direct contact and droplets may also be routes of transmission, and results in cutaneous lesions, most frequently on the exposed parts of the body. Direct contact spread occurs when a susceptible host has direct contact with an animal that is infected with *B. anthracis*, such as a veterinarian who autopsies an animal contaminated with the organism. Organisms may enter the body through a preexisting skin wound or may be accidentally injected by a sharp bone spicule or a knife.

Meat from an animal that died from anthrax is usually infected and can serve as a source of infection if eaten undercooked. Persons preparing the meat for consumption are at risk of cutaneous anthrax.

Indirect contact spread accounts for the majority of cutaneous industrial cases. The source of infection is either the animal products being processed or the environment that has been contaminated by animal products previously processed. Rarely, the finished product may be the source. By this route, organisms enter the skin through a preexisting wound, a new wound, or the mucous membranes (i.e., conjunctivae). Goat hair fibers may be flung from the manufacturing equipment like projectiles and enter the skin like needles, depositing *B. anthracis* organisms in the subcutaneous tissue.

Aerosols containing *B. anthracis* spores may be created by agitation of the hair or wool either when the bales are being opened and the fibers initially handled or as the fibers are being processed by the machinery. These aerosols may travel more than several feet, which represents airborne transmission. Particles less than 5 μm in diameter, if inhaled, may reach the terminal alveoli of the lungs and cause inhalation anthrax (see Section 7.1.2). The estimated human LD_{50} dose from inhaled small-particle aerosols has been estimated to be 8,000 to 10,000 spores.[24] Essentially all risk of infection occurs during exposure to the primary aerosol generated during processing. Inefficiency of small-particle aerosol deposition and resuspension minimizes any potential risk of significant secondary aerosol.[24]

The air in several goat-hair-processing plants has been sampled, and significant levels of airborne *B. anthracis* spores have been identified. For example, studies in a goat-hair-processing plant in the Northeast in 1958 demonstrated that "510 spores in particles 5 microns and less in size may be inhaled [by workers] in 8 hours without inducing infection."[33] In a similar mill in a southern state, 91 primates (cynomolgus monkeys) were exposed during a series of experiments to the air in the dustiest part of the mill.[34] They had an anthrax mortality rate of 10–25% from a calculated inhalation dose of 1000–5000 *B. anthracis* organisms accumulated over 3–5 days.

Animals become infected by ingestion of contaminated soil or feed. Some rural areas are associated with sporadic cases or outbreaks of animal anthrax. The soils in these areas are most frequently in the neutral pH range and are alluvial or loessal soils. Soil becomes contaminated from the discharges or carcasses of dead animals. Soil can also become contaminated from use of contaminated fertilizer or feed. It is reported that the spores may remain infectious in nature for many years, though this has never been scientifically proven. There is evidence to suggest that in some areas *B. anthracis* organisms can be considered as part of the endogenous soil flora. With certain climatic conditions, the spores germinate and multiply, resulting in an increase in the number of infectious organisms that could be ingested by susceptible grazing animals.

Insect vectors, such as horseflies, have been reported to transmit *B. anthracis* by means of mechanical transfer of *B. anthracis* organisms from contaminated foci to individuals or animals. Outbreaks of animal anthrax have been reported to result from transmission of *B. anthracis* by horseflies from an infected animal to a second animal. However, there is no scientific documentation, including field studies during an epizootic, that this potential method of transmission has any practical significance.

7. Pathogenesis and Immunity

7.1. Pathogenesis

7.1.1. Cutaneous Anthrax. The incubation period is from 3 to 10 days, most commonly 5 to 7 days. Spores deposited beneath the skin germinate, and the resulting vegetative forms multiply and produce a toxin. The local lesion results from the action of the toxin on the surrounding tissue, which causes tissue necrosis. This leads to the development of a scar at the site of the lesion. The toxin or organisms or both may be distributed throughout the body by the vascular system, causing systemic symptoms and signs of toxicity or bacteremia. Occasionally, organisms are picked up by the lymphatic system, resulting in lymphangitis and lymphadenopathy.

7.1.2. Inhalation Anthrax. The incubation period is usually stated to be 1 to 5 days (mean 3–4 days). However, in a recent epidemic of inhalation anthrax, the incubation period ranged from 4 to about 45 days (median 9–10 days).[24] The explanation for the prolonged incubation period is unknown, but may represent low-dose phenomenon or prophylactic use of antibiotics. *B. anthracis*-bearing particles less than 5 μm in size are inhaled and, if they reach the terminal alveoli, are deposited on the alveolar membranes, where they can be ingested by alveolar macrophages, carried across the membranes to the regional lymph nodes, and deposited. Spores will then germinate, multiply, and produce toxin. The toxin, in turn, destroys tissue and subsequently causes necrosis and hemorrhage. The classic picture at death is very distinctive. Examination of the mediastinal area reveals hemorrhagic mediastinitis with varied degrees of destruction of the normal architecture.[35] While the pathological changes are limited to the mediastinal area, there may be secondary involvement of the pulmonary tissue. Toxin may be distributed throughout the body, resulting in systemic symptoms and signs. Organisms may also be picked up by the vascular system, resulting in bacteremia and septicemia.

7.1.3. Gastrointestinal Anthrax. The incubation period is commonly 3 to 7 days. There are two clinical presentations following ingestion of *B. anthracis*-contaminated food: abdominal and oropharyngeal.

In the abdominal form, spores are ingested, absorbed through the intestinal mucosa, probably via M cells in the epithelium overlying Peyer's patches, and deposited in mucosal lymphoid tissue or regional lymph nodes; here, they germinate, and the vegetative cells multiply, producing toxin. An ulcerative lesion caused by the action of the toxin may develop within the mucosa of the gastrointestinal tract. The lesions are frequently described in the cecum and adjacent areas of the bowel. Some reports have described lesions in the large bowel, stomach, and rarely in the duodenum.[36] Alternatively, lymphadenitis or lymphadenopathy may occur. Hemorrhagic areas may develop within the mesentery as well as in the gastrointestinal tract.

In the oropharyngeal form, organisms are transported through the oral mucosa to the tonsils or cervical lymph nodes, where they germinate, multiply, and produce toxin. The result may be edema and tissue necrosis in the cervical area. There is a report from Thailand as well as several other countries of the development of an inflammatory lesion resembling a cutaneous lesion in the oral cavity involving the posterior wall, the hard palate, tongue, or the tonsils.[37]

7.2. Immunity

Apparently, once having had a cutaneous lesion, an individual develops some degree of immunity against another infection. There have been no well-confirmed second cases of cutaneous anthrax in individuals who have had a confirmed first case. There have been several reports of two cutaneous anthrax infections in the same individual, however, but in each of these reports, either one or both of the cases of anthrax have not been well documented.

Extensive serological studies have not been conducted. In one study, however, Norman *et al.*[38] studied 72 unvaccinated employees in a goat-hair-processing mill, none of whom had a history of an anthrax infection. Of the 72, 11 demonstrated a positive titer (precipitation-inhibition test), suggesting previous subclinical infection. Recovering cutaneous and gastrointestinal anthrax patients develop antibody to the toxin components as determined by ELISA and electrophoretic-immunotransblot (Western blot) testing.[39]

Detailed data concerning immunity following inhalation anthrax are not available because of the rarity of this form of the disease and the high fatality rate. In studies of the several persons who have recovered during the past 25 years, low levels of antibodies were detected following recovery from the clinical disease.

8. Patterns of Host Responses

8.1. Clinical Features

8.1.1. Cutaneous Anthrax. Typically, cutaneous anthrax occurs on the exposed parts of the body. Although a single cutaneous lesion is typical, some patients develop multiple discrete lesions. The lesion begins innocuously with a small papule that the patient may first notice because of pruritus. The papule develops after several days into a small vesicle or, occasionally, into several vesicles that then coalesce to form a ring. This area may be surrounded by a small ring of erythema and possibly some edema. The pruritus may continue, but there is no pain unless secondary infection or a significant degree of local edema is present. A small dark area can be seen beneath the center of the vesicle, or in the central area if a ring of vesicles has formed. Eventually, the vesicle or vesicular ring ruptures, discharging a clear fluid and revealing a depressed black necrotic central area known as an eschar. After 1–2 weeks, the lesion dries and the eschar begins to loosen and shortly thereafter separates, revealing a permanent scar.

The lesion is usually 1–3 cm in diameter and remains round and regular. Occasionally, a lesion may be larger and irregularly shaped. There may be regional lymphangitis and lymphadenopathy and some systemic symptoms such as a slight low-grade fever, malaise, and headache. Antibiotic therapy will not change the natural progression of the lesion itself; however, it will decrease or inhibit development of edema and systemic symptoms.

Occasionally, the cutaneous reaction is severe and is characterized by significant local and spreading edema associated with blebs, bullae, induration, chills, and fever. This type of reaction is referred to as malignant edema. Whether malignant edema results from increased pathogenicity or dosage of the organism or because of host factors is unknown.

Lesions in specific body sites occasionally result in

more severe local reactions. Several cases have been seen of anthrax involving tissue surrounding the eye in which extensive edema spread over the entire face and extended to the neck and upper thorax. In one such patient, edema involved his entire face and extended down to the upper part of the thorax. In this instance, the spread of the toxin resulted in an extensive cutaneous lesion with necrosis of both eyelids. Plastic surgery was necessary to repair the tissue damage of the eyelids and surrounding tissue.

Infrequently, meningitis may develop as a complication of cutaneous anthrax (see Section 8.1.4).

8.1.2. Inhalation Anthrax. This form shows a biphasic clinical pattern with a benign initial phase followed by an acute, severe second phase that is almost always fatal. The initial phase begins as a nonspecific illness consisting of malaise, fatigue, myalgia, mild fever, nonproductive cough, and, occasionally, a sensation of precordial oppression. Findings of the physical examination are essentially within normal limits except that rhonchi may be present. The illness may resemble a mild upper-respiratory-tract infection such as a cold or the "flu." After 2–4 days, the patient may show signs of improvement. However, there is then the sudden onset of severe respiratory distress with dyspnea, cyanosis, respiratory stridor, and profuse diaphoresis. In several cases, subcutaneous edema of the chest and neck has been described. The pulse, respiratory rate, and temperature become elevated. Physical examination reveals moist, crepitant rales over the lungs and possibly evidence of pleural effusion. Shock may develop. X-ray examination of the chest may reveal widening of the mediastinum and pleural effusion. Septicemia and meningitis may develop. Death occurs in most persons with inhalation anthrax within 24 hr after the onset of the acute phase.

8.1.3. Gastrointestinal Anthrax. There are two clinical presentations for disease resulting from ingestion of *B. anthracis*: abdominal and oropharyngeal. The symptoms of abdominal anthrax are initially nonspecific and include nausea, vomiting, anorexia, and fever. With progression of the disease, abdominal pain, hematemesis, and bloody diarrhea develop. Ascites may be present. Occasionally, the symptoms and signs resemble an acute surgical abdomen, which in some cases has resulted in surgery. With further progression, toxemia develops with shock, cyanosis, and death. The time from onset of symptoms to death has most frequently varied from 2 to 5 days. In oropharyngeal anthrax (also referred to as cervical anthrax), patients have experienced fever, submandibular edema, cervical lymphadenopathy, and anorexia. Some reports describe the presence of acute inflammatory lesions in the oral cavity and/or oropharynx. The mortality rate for gastrointestinal anthrax has been reported to vary from 25 to 60%.

8.1.4. Other Forms. Meningitis, seen in less than 5% of anthrax cases, may be a complication of any of the three forms of primary anthrax infection. Rarely, meningitis is reported without a known primary site of infection. Symptoms of meningeal anthrax develop one to several days after the onset of the primary lesion and are similar to those associated with hemorrhagic meningitis. Death, if it occurs, usually does so in 1 to 6 days after onset of disease. Septicemia is only rarely seen in patients with cutaneous lesions; it is more commonly seen in patients with inhalation and gastrointestinal anthrax.

8.2. Diagnosis

A source of exposure to the infectious agent is of importance in considering a diagnosis of anthrax. Only rarely have cases occurred for which the source of infection could not be identified.

Cutaneous anthrax should be suspected when an individual describes a painless, pruritic papule, usually on an exposed part of the body. Vesicular fluid should reveal *B. anthracis* organisms microscopically and on culture. The differential diagnosis should include contagious pustular dermatitis (ecthyma contagiosum or orf), milker's nodule, plague, staphylococcal disease, and tularemia.

The initial symptoms of inhalation anthrax are nonspecific and resemble those of an upper-respiratory-tract infection. Characteristically, with the sudden development of the acute phase, there is severe respiratory distress and radiographic examination of the chest should reveal widening of the mediastinum, a typical occurrence with inhalation anthrax. The acute phase resembles diseases that result in respiratory failure and shock.

In gastrointestinal anthrax, the patient presents with signs and symptoms of gastroenteritis. Organisms may be demonstrable in vomitus and feces from the infected individual. The differential diagnosis includes diseases that cause moderately severe gastroenteritis, such as shigellosis and *Yersinia* gastroenteritis. In the cervical form, the signs and symptoms might suggest pharyngitis, such as seen with streptococcal infections.

In anthrax meningitis, there should be a primary site of infection. CSF should contain *B. anthracis*. In septicemia, blood cultures should be positive for *B. anthracis*.

Several rapid diagnostic tests have been developed for specific diagnosis during the acute-phase illness. Toxin can be detected in clinical specimens using a capture ELISA or a chromatographic assay. Suitable specimens for toxin assay are vesicular fluid or lesion exudate in cutaneous cases, serum in gastrointestinal and inhalation cases, and CSF in meningitis cases.[13,40] Polymerase chain reaction detection of *B. anthracis*, whether living or dead, is possible utilizing primers targeting pX01 and pX02 plasmid DNA sequences.[10] Fluorescent antibody staining of clinical and autopsy specimens is an older approach that has been updated through use of monoclonal antibodies against cell wall and capsule components unique to *B. anthracis*.[8]

Serological tests currently being used in the United States include ELISA and electrophoretic-immunotransblot (EITB).[39] Both tests are based on detecting components of the anthrax toxin. The ELISA test is used primarily for screening and is less specific than the EITB. The EITB can be modified to demonstrate titer changes between acute and convalescent serum samples.

9. Control and Prevention

9.1. General Concepts

Restrictions on the importation of contaminated animal products would significantly decrease the risk of anthrax in the United States. Also, improving animal husbandry so that anthrax is no longer a significant infection among animals in countries from which the animal products are imported could reduce the rate of contamination of imported products. However, these improvements may be very difficult to accomplish. The next line of defense would be disinfecting the animal products either before they are imported or when they enter the United States. Washing with formaldehyde, as was done at the Liverpool Disinfection Station in England for many years, could be used; other methods that could be instituted are ethylene oxide treatment, irradiation, or autoclaving. However, because imported animal products enter the United States through a variety of ports, and due to complexities of these decontamination procedures, development of a central facility in which to process the imported materials would be very difficult.

In the United States, improvements in industrial hygiene have been of some benefit in reducing the exposure of the worker to infectious materials and aerosols. The most important are use of dust-collecting equipment during the initial processing cycle and institution of effective environmental cleanup procedures.

Employees should be educated about the disease and the recommendations for working in a contaminated environment and for reducing the risk of developing the disease. Medical consultation services should be available to the employees. Adequate cleanup facilities and clothes-changing areas should be available so that workers do not wear their contaminated clothes home.

It should be noted that the risk of industrial infection has been reduced significantly over the past years as the use of imported animal products has been reduced because of changing business conditions, the increased use of synthetic materials, and the use of human vaccine (see Section 9.3).

Gastrointestinal anthrax can be prevented by forbidding the sale of meat for consumption from sick animals or animals that have died from disease. Depending on the circumstances, it may be important to alert individuals who may come in contact with contaminated meat about the disease and about the need to cook all meats thoroughly.

All cases or suspected cases of anthrax should be reported to local public health officials so that appropriate epidemiological investigations can be conducted. Additional cases in humans or animals may be prevented by the prompt reporting and investigation of circumstances surrounding every case.

In the United States, agricultural anthrax is not a significant problem. This reflects the high standards of animal husbandry practiced in this country. Animals that graze in areas known as anthrax districts should be vaccinated annually with the Sterne strain animal vaccine. All animals suspected of dying from anthrax should be examined microbiologically; blood or tissue smears can be examined microscopically, and cultures can be set up from these same materials. All animals that have died with a confirmed diagnosis of anthrax should be thoroughly burned and the remaining bones and other materials buried deeply. Animals that die with a suspected diagnosis of anthrax should be cultured; this can be done by removing the dependent ear and culturing the cut end. The carcass should then be handled as outlined above. If incineration is not possible, then the carcass should be covered with lime and buried at least 6 ft deep to discourage its being uncovered by scavenging animals.

9.2. Antibiotic Prophylaxis and Chemotherapeutics

Prophylactic antibiotics or chemotherapeutic agents are not used for anthrax except in three situations. If an individual has been inoculated with a live Pasteur-type spore animal anthrax vaccine, prophylactic penicillin should be given. Additionally, prophylactic antibiotics should be considered if a person is known to have eaten contaminated meat. The third situation is when an individual has been exposed to a high-dose aerosol of *B. anthra-*

cis. In these instances, prophylaxis is given to kill any *B. anthracis* organisms that may have been inoculated, ingested, or inhaled, and thus prevent the production of toxin. Persons with gastrointestinal or aerosol exposure should receive a 30-day course of antibiotics and be concurrently immunized with the human anthrax vaccine.[41] When prophylactic antibiotics are given, the patient should be kept under surveillance for 10 days after initial therapy.

9.3. Immunization

There is an effective anthrax vaccine that was field-tested in employees of four different textile mills in the United States, which demonstrated an effectiveness of preventing cutaneous anthrax of 92.5%.[42,43] This vaccine should be used for all employees who may be exposed to contaminated materials or environment. Additionally, anyone who comes into a mill processing *B. anthracis*-contaminated materials should also be vaccinated. Currently, the vaccine is given parenterally with three doses given at 2-week intervals followed by three booster inoculations at 6-month intervals and then annual booster inoculations. Serological testing of vaccines has found a significant serological response to protective antigen beginning about 7 days after receipt of the second dose. Veterinarians, laboratory personnel, and other persons who, because of their occupation, have ongoing risk for contact with anthrax should also be immunized with the human anthrax vaccine. The human vaccine is available on a limited basis. Those interested should contact the Michigan Department of Public Health Division of Bio Products, 3500 N. Logan, Box 30035, Lansing, Michigan 48909.

10. References

1. Laforce, F. M., Woolsorters' disease, England, *Bull. N.Y. Acad. Med.* **54**:956–963 (1978).
2. Tigertt, W. D., Personal communication.
3. Wilson, G., The Brown Animal Sanatory Institution, *J. Hyg.* **82**:337–352 (1979).
4. Sterne, M., The use of anthrax vaccines prepared from avirulent (uncapsulated) variants of *Bacillus anthracis*, *Onderstepoort J. Vet. Sci. Anim. Ind.* **13**:307–312 (1939).
5. Anthrax Investigations Board (Bradford & District) First Annual Report (1906), pp. 3–4.
6. Wool disinfection and anthrax: A year's working of the model station, *Lancet* **2**:1295–1296 (1922).
7. Feeley, J. C., and Brachman, P. S., *Bacillus anthracis*, in: *Manual of Clinical Microbiology*, 2nd ed. (E. H. Lennette, E. H. Spaulding, and J. P. Truant, eds.), pp. 143–147, American Society for Microbiology, Washington, DC, 1974.
8. Ezzell, J. W., and Abshire, T. G., Encapsulation of *Bacillus anthracis* spores and spore identification. Proceedings of the International Workshop on Anthrax, *Salisbury Med. Bull.* **87**:42 (1996).
9. Brown, E. R., and Cherry, W. B., Specific identification of *Bacillus anthracis* by means of a variant bacteriophage, *J. Infect. Dis.* **96**: 34–39 (1955).
10. Ramisse, V., Patra, G., Vaude-Lautheir, V., Sylvestre, P., Therasse, J., and Guesdon, J.-L., Multiplex PCR assay for identification of *Bacillus anthracis* and differentiation from *Bacillus cereus* group bacteria. Proceedings of the International Workshop on Anthrax, *Salisbury Med. Bull.* **87**:51 (1996).
11. Ezzell, J. W., and Abshire, T. G., Immunological analysis of cell-associated antigens of *Bacillus anthracis*, *Infect. Immun.* **56**:349–356 (1988).
12. Little, S. F., and Knudson, G. B., Comparative efficacy of *Bacillus anthracis* live spore vaccine and protective antigen vaccine against anthrax in the guinea pig, *Infect. Immun.* **52**:509–512 (1986).
13. Ezzell, J. W., United States Army Medical Research Institute for Infectious Diseases, Frederick, Maryland, Personal communication, 1996.
14. Perl, D. P., and Dooley, J. R., Anthrax, in: *Pathology of Tropical and Extraordinary Diseases* (C. H. Binford and D. H. Connor, eds.), pp. 118–123, Armed Forces Institute of Pathology, Washington, DC, 1976.
15. Abramova, F. A., Grinberg, L. H., Yampolskaya, O. U., and Walker, D. H., Pathology of inhalation anthrax in 42 cases from the Sverdlovsk outbreak in 1979, *Proc. Natl. Acad. Sci. USA* **90**:2291–2294 (1993).
16. Fox, M., Kaufmann, A. F., Zendel, S. A., Kolb, R. C., Songy, C. G., Jr., Cangelosis, D. A., and Fuller, C. E., Anthrax in Louisiana, 1971: Epizootiologic study, *J. Am. Vet. Med. Assoc.* **163**:446–451 (1973).
17. Glassman, H. N., World incidence of anthrax in man, *Public Health Rep.* **73**:22–24 (1958).
18. *World Health Statistics Annual, 1980–1981. Infectious Diseases: Cases*, World Health Organization, Geneva, 1981.
19. Hugh-Jones, M. E., Personal communication, 1996.
20. Liang, X., Ma, F., and Li, A., Anthrax surveillance and control in China, presented at International Workshop on Anthrax, Winchester, UK, 1996.
21. Bell, J. H., Anthrax: Its relation to the wool industry, in: *Dangerous Trades* (T. Oliver, ed.), pp. 634–643, London Button, London, 1902.
22. Plotkin, S. A., Brachman, P. S., Utell, M., Bumford, F. H., and Atchison, M. M., An epidemic of inhalation anthrax: The first in the twentieth century. I. Clinical features, *Am. J. Med.* **29**:992–1001 (1960).
23. Brachman, P. S., Plotkin, S. A., Bumford, F. H., and Atchison, M. A., An epidemic of inhalation anthrax. II. Epidemiologic investigations, *Am. J. Hyg.* **72**:6–23 (1960).
24. Meselson, M., Guillemin, J., Hugh-Jones, M., Langmuir, A., Popova, I., Shelokov, A., and Yampolskaya, O., The Sverdlovsk anthrax outbreak of 1979, *Science* **266**:1202–1208 (1994).
25. Davies, J. C. A., A major epidemic of anthrax in Zimbabwe, *Cent. Afr. J. Med.* [Part 1] **28**:291–298 (1982), [Part 2] **29**:8–12 (1983), [Part 3] **31**:176–180 (1985).
26. Brachman, P. S., and Fekety, F. R., Industrial anthrax, *Ann. N.Y. Acad. Sci.* **70**:574–584 (1958).
27. Wolff, A. H., and Heimann, H., Industrial anthrax in the United States: An epidemiologic study, *Am. J. Hyg.* **53**:80–109 (1951).
28. Stein, C. D., and Stoner, M. G., Anthrax in livestock during the first

quarter of 1952 with special reference to outbreaks in swine in the mid-west, *Vet. Med.* **47:**274–279 (1952).
29. Brachman, P. S., Pagano, J. S., and Albrink, W. S., Two cases of fatal inhalation anthrax, one associated with sarcoidosis, *N. Engl. J. Med.* **265:**203–208 (1961).
30. Brachman, P. S., Inhalation anthrax, *Ann. N.Y. Acad. Sci.* **353:**83–93 (1980).
31. Centers for Disease Control, Cutaneous anthrax acquired from imported Haitian drums, Florida, *Morbid. Mortal. Week. Rep.* **23:**142, 147 (1974).
32. Suffin, S. C., Karnes, W. H., and Kaufmann, A. F., Inhalation anthrax in a home craftsman, *Hum. Pathol.* **9:**594–597 (1978).
33. Dahlgren, C. M., Buchanan, L. M., Decker, H. M., Freed, S. W., Phillips, C. R., and Brachman, P. S., *Bacillus anthracis* aerosols in a goat hair processing mill, *Am. J. Hyg.* **72:**24–31 (1960).
34. Brachman, P. S., Kaufmann, A. F., and Dalldorf, F. G., Industrial inhalation anthrax, *Bacteriol. Rev.* **30:**646–657 (1966).
35. Albrink, W. S., Brooks, S. M., Biron, R. E., and Kopel, M., Human inhalation anthrax, a report of three fatal cases, *Am. J. Pathol.* **36:**457–472 (1960).
36. Nalin, D. R., Sultana, B., Sahunja, R., Islam, A. K., Rahim, M. A., Islam, M., Costa, B. S., Mawla, N., and Greenough, W. B., Survival of a patient with intestinal anthrax, *Am. J. Med.* **62:**130–132 (1977).
37. Sirisanthana, T., Navacharoen, N., Tharavichitkul, P., Sirisanthana, V., and Brown, A. E., Outbreak of oral–oropharyngeal anthrax: An unusual manifestation of human infection with *Bacillus anthracis*, *Am. J. Trop. Med. Hyg.* **33:**144–150 (1984).
38. Norman, P. S., Ray, J. G., Brachman, P. S., Plotkin, S. A., and Pagano, J. S., Serological testings for anthrax antibodies in workers in a goat hair processing mill, *Am. J. Hyg.* **72:**32–37 (1960).
39. Sirisanthana, T., Nelson, K. E., Ezzell, J. W., and Abshire, T. G., Serological studies of patients with cutaneous and oral–oropharyngeal anthrax from northern Thailand, *Am. J. Trop. Med. Hyg.* **39:**575–581 (1988).
40. Burans, J. D., Keleher, A., O'Brien, T., Hager, J., Plummer, A., and Morgan, C., Rapid method for the diagnosis of *Bacillus anthracis* infection in clinical samples using a hand-held assay. Proceedings of the International Workshop on Anthrax, *Salisbury Med. Bull.* **87:**36–37 (1996).
41. Friedlander, A. M., Weldos, S. L., Pitt, M. L. M., Ezzell, J. W., Worsham, P. L., Rose, K. J., Ivins, B. E., Lowe, J. R., Howe, G. B., Mikesell, P., and Lawrence, W. B., Postexposure prophylaxis against experimental inhalation anthrax *J. Infect. Dis.* **167:**1239–1242 (1993).
42. Brachman, P. S., Gold, H., Plotkin, S. A., Fekety, F. R., Werrin, M., and Ingraham, N. R., Field evaluation of human anthrax vaccine, *Am. J. Public Health* **52:**632–645 (1962).
43. Wright, J. G., Green, T. W., and Kanode, R. G., Jr., Studies on immunity and anthrax. V. Immunizing activity of alum-precipitated protective antigen, *J. Immunol.* **73:**387–391 (1954).

11. Suggested Reading

Brachman, P. S., Anthrax, in: *Infectious Diseases*, 4th ed. (P. D. Hoeprich, ed.), pp. 1007–1013, Harper & Row, New York, 1989.

Dutz, W., and Kohout, E., Anthrax, *Pathol. Annu.* **6:**209–248 (1971).

Fox, M. D., Kaufmann, A. F., Zendel, S. A., Kolb, R. C., Songy, C. G., Jr., Cangelosis, D. A., and Fuller, C. E., Anthrax in Louisiana, 1971: Epizootiologic study *J. Am. Vet. Med. Assoc.* **163:**446–451 (1973).

LaForce, F. M., Anthrax, *Clin. Infect. Dis.* **19:**1009–1014 (1994).

Lincoln, R. E., Walker, J. S., Klein, F., and Haines, B. W., Anthrax, *Adv. Vet. Sci.* **9:**327–368 (1964).

Turnbull, P. C. B., Anthrax vaccines: past, present and future, *Vaccine* **9:**533–539 (1991).

Turnbull, P. C. B. (ed.), Proceedings of the International Workshop on Anthrax, *Salisbury Med. Bull.* **68:**(Suppl.)1–108 (1990).

Turnbull, P. C. B. (ed.), Proceedings of the International Workshop on Anthrax, *Salisbury Med. Bull.* **87:**(Suppl.)1–139 (1996).

Van Ness, G. B., Ecology of anthrax, *Science* **172:**1303–1307 (1971).

World Health Organization, Memoranda/Memorandums: Anthrax control and research, with special reference to national programme development in Africa: Memorandum from a WHO meeting, *Bull. WHO* **72:**13–22 (1994).

CHAPTER 5

Bacterial Foodborne Disease

Gregory L. Armstrong, Jill Hollingsworth, and J. Glenn Morris, Jr.

1. Introduction

Foodborne disease comprises a broad group of illnesses caused by the consumption of foods contaminated with toxic substances or pathogenic microorganisms. The agents responsible for foodborne illnesses can be divided into four general categories: chemical (e.g., mushroom or scombroid poisoning), parasitic (e.g., *Trichinella* or *Giardia*), viral (e.g., hepatitis A or Norwalk virus), and bacterial (e.g., *Salmonella* or *Campylobacter*). Only the bacterial will be considered in this chapter.

Because there are many foodborne bacterial pathogens, it is useful to categorize them further. Epidemiologically, one of the most useful methods is to divide these according to their reservoir (Table 1). *Campylobacter*, enterohemorrhagic *Escherichia coli* (called EHEC, the most common of which is *E. coli* O157:H7), nontyphoidal *Salmonella*, and *Yersinia* often live as commensals in the intestinal tracts of animals. They are transmitted to humans largely through beef (EHEC and *Salmonella*), pork (*Yersinia*), poultry (*Salmonella* and *Campylobacter*), and eggs (*Salmonella* serotype Enteritidis), *Brucella* is different from the others in this group in that it usually acts as a pathogen in animals; it is transmitted from the animal reservoir to humans via the consumption of milk as well as via other routes. Members of the family *Vibrionaceae*, including *Vibrio*, *Aeromonas*, and *Plesiomonas* species, all inhabit aquatic environments and are transferred to humans through seafood (*V. parahaemolyticus*, *Aeromonas*, and *Plesiomonas*) or through water (*V. cholerae* and *Plesiomonas*). Enterotoxigenic *E. coli* (ETEC), *Salmonella typhi*, *Shigella*, and *Staphylococcus* are species that are transmitted primarily from infected handlers through food. Finally, there is a group of organisms, including *Listeria*, *Clostridium perfringens*, *Clostridium botulinum*, and *Bacillus cereus*, that can be isolated from multiple environmental sources.

Alternatively, organisms can be classified according to the three main ways by which they produce illness: toxin production prior to consumption, toxin production *in vivo*, and invasion of the host (Table 2). Organisms in the first category, *C. botulinum*, *B. cereus* (emetic type illness), and *Staphylococcus*, produce toxins as they grow in food. Because these toxins are completely formed by the time the food is consumed, vomiting or diarrhea due to the latter two have a short incubation period (1–6 hr). As one might predict, the toxins produced by these organisms are generally resistant to stomach acid and to proteases found in the gastrointestinal tract. Organisms in the second category, *Aeromonas*, *B. cereus* (diarrheal type illness), *C. perfringens*, EHEC, ETEC, *Plesiomonas*, *V. cholerae*, and *V. parahaemolyticus*, produce toxins after ingestion as they multiply within the gastrointestinal tract. The incubation period for these illnesses is longer, generally 6 hr to several days, because of the time necessary to elaborate the toxins. The last category includes organisms that cause disease primarily by invading the host: *Brucella*, *Campylobacter*, *Listeria*, nontyphoidal *Salmonella*, *Salmonella typhi*, *Shigella*, *V. vulnificus*, and *Yersinia*. The incubation period for these organisms is even longer, lasting from 1 day to several weeks. These categories are not mutually exclusive. The pathogenesis of many foodborne pathogens is incompletely understood. Many of the invasive organisms also elaborate toxins that may be important in their ability to cause disease.

Most of the bacteria that cause foodborne illness are

Gregory L. Armstrong and Jill Hollingsworth • Epidemiology and Emergency Response Program, Food Safety and Inspection Service, US Department of Agriculture, Washington, DC 20250. **J. Glenn Morris, Jr.** • Epidemiology and Emergency Response Program, Food Safety and Inspection Service, US Department of Agriculture, Washington, DC 20250; and Division of Infectious Diseases, Department of Medicine, University of Maryland School of Medicine, and Veterans Affairs Medical Center, Baltimore, Maryland 21201.

Table 1. Foodborne Pathogens, Classified by Reservoir

Animal reservoir (vehicles include meat, poultry, eggs)	*Brucella* Nontyphoidal *Salmonella* *Campylobacter* *Yersinia* EHEC
Marine organims (vehicles include seafood and water)	*Vibrio* species *Aeromonas* *Plesiomonas*
Human reservoir (transmitted through food contaminated by infected or colonized food handlers)	ETEC *Staphylococcus* *Salmonella typhi* *Shigella*
Other environmental (can be found in soil, water, or a variety of foods)	*C. botulinum* *C. perfringens* *B. cereus* *Listeria*

discussed in separate chapters in this book (see Chapters 6, 7, 8, 11, 14, 21, 31, 32, 42, and 43). Because illness due to six organisms, *S. aureus*, *B. cereus*, *C. perfringens*, noncholera vibrios, *Aeromonas*, and *Plesiomonas*, is not discussed explicitly elsewhere, this chapter is devoted to these pathogens.

2. Historical Background

In the United States, formal surveillance for diarrheal illness began after World War I, when state and territorial health officers, concerned about high morbidity and mortality rates caused by typhoid fever and infantile diarrhea, recommended that cases of enteric fever by investigated and reported. In 1923, the United States Public Health Service published summaries of outbreaks of gastrointestinal illness attributed to milk. Outbreaks caused by all foods were added in 1938. These activities were instrumental in the enactment of public health measures that have decreased the incidence of enteric disease.

In 1961, the Communicable Disease Center [which later became the Centers for Disease Control and Prevention (CDC)] assumed responsibility for collecting and publishing reports on foodborne illness. The current system of surveillance of foodborne disease outbreaks began in 1966, by incorporating into an annual summary all reports of such outbreaks in the United States.

The National Notifiable Diseases Surveillance System has been collecting data on sporadic illness (i.e., illness not associated with an outbreak) since 1912. In that year the Public Health Service began recommending immediate telegraphic reporting of five infectious diseases and monthly reporting of ten others. Since then, the systems has expanded to include 52 infectious diseases and is currently administered by the CDC (see Section 3.2).

Table 2. Classification of Bacterial Foodborne Pathogens according to Pathogenesis

Organisms that cause disease by production of toxins in food prior to consumption	*B. cereus* (emetic type) *C. botulinum* *Staphylococcus*
Organisms that produce disease by production of toxins after ingestion	*Aeromonas* *B. cereus* (diarrheal type) *C. perfringens* EHEC ETEC *Plesiomonas* *V. cholerae* and *V. paraheaemolyticus*
Organisms that produce disease by invasion of the host	*Brucella* *Campylobacter* *Listeria* Nontyphoidal *Salmonella* *Salmonella typhi* *Shigella* *V. vulnificus* *Yersinia*

3. Methodology

3.1. Foodborne Disease Outbreak Surveillance

Much of our knowledge about the epidemiology of foodborne illness comes from the investigations of outbreaks. Such investigations are initiated by state and local health departments in response to requests by consumers or physicians or because of clustering of reported illnesses. On special request, the CDC will participate in an investigation, especially if an outbreak involves residents of multiple states. Reports of investigations are customarily forwarded to the CDC to be included in the yearly report. The database maintained by the CDC contains such information as the location, setting, etiologic agent, number of cases and deaths, vehicle, symptoms, incubation period, and factors thought to contribute to the outbreak.

The CDC has published guidelines for the confirmation of foodborne outbreaks (Table 3).[1] An outbreak is generally defined as an incident in which two or more individuals experience a similar illness after exposure to a common food. Prior to 1992, exceptions were made for cases of botulism or chemical-related illness, which were counted as outbreaks even if only one case occurred.

Table 3. Criteria for Confirmation of Foodborne Outbreaks Due to *B. cereus*, *C. perfringens*, *S. aureus*, *V. cholerae*, and *V. parahaemolyticus*[a]

Etiologic agent	Incubation period	Clinical syndrome	Confirmation
B. cereus			
Emetic type illness	1–6 hr	Vomiting, sometimes diarrhea	Isolation of organism from stools of ⩾ 2 ill persons and not from stools of controls OR Isolation of ⩾ 10^5 organisms/g from epidemiologically implicated food, provided specimen properly handled
Diarrheal illness	6–24 hr	Diarrhea, abdominal cramps, sometimes vomiting (fever is rare)	(Same as above)
C. perfringens	6–24 hr	Diarrhea, abdominal cramps (vomiting and fever are uncommon)	Isolation of ⩾ 10^6 organisms/g in stool of ⩾ 2 ill persons, provided specimen properly handled OR Demonstration of enterotoxin in stools of ⩾ 2 ill persons OR Isolation of ⩾ 10^5 organisms/g from epidemiologically implicated food, provided specimen properly handled
S. aureus	30 min to 8 hr; usually 2–4 hr	Vomiting and diarrhea	Isolation of organisms of same phage type in clinical specimens form ⩾ 2 ill persons OR Demonstration of enterotoxin in epidemiologically implicated food OR Isolation of ⩾ 10^5 organisms/g from epidemiologically implicated food, provided specimen properly handled
V. cholerae, nonepidemic	1–5 days	Watery diarrhea	Isolation of organisms of same serotype from stools of ⩾ 2 ill persons
V. parahaemolyticus	4–30 hr	Diarrhea	Isolation of Kanagawa-positive organisms from stools of ⩾ 2 ill persons OR Isolation of ⩾ 10^5 organisms/g from epidemiologically implicated food, provided specimen properly handled

[a]From CDC Surveillance Summaries.[1]

Since 1992, the definition has been revised such that any incident must involve at least two cases to be considered an outbreak. In order to confirm the etiology of an outbreak, specific criteria must be met. An outbreak of *B. cereus* emetic-type illness, for example, is considered confirmed if the organism is isolated from at least two cases but not from controls, or if the organism can be found in numbers greater than 10^5/g in the implicated food.

Summaries of the numbers of outbreaks and outbreak-related cases during a 10-year period are shown in Tables 4 and 5.[1–3] These numbers represent only a small, unrepresentative portion of the actual foodborne illness in the United States, because most outbreaks go unrecognized and because most foodborne illness is sporadic. Several factors determine the likelihood that any given outbreak will be recognized and investigated:

1. Size of the outbreak. Larger outbreaks are more likely to be recognized and investigated.
2. Severity of illness. Outbreaks of severe illness are more likely to be recognized and investigated. An outbreak of *C. perfringens* diarrhea, which causes relatively mild illness, will likely go unnoticed unless a large number of illnesses occur. Any outbreak of botulism, on the other hand, is likely to come to the attention of public health authorities. During the years from 1982 to 1991, the average size of *C. perfringens* outbreaks was 92 cases, whereas that of botulism outbreaks was just 2 cases (Table 5).
3. Incubation period. A short incubation period increases the likelihood that an outbreak will be recognized and a vehicle implicated. Illness due to *S. aureus*, for example, may be relatively easy to recognize as a common-source problem because of its short incubation period (usually 2–4 hr). An outbreak of listeriosis, however, may go undetected because its incubation period is several weeks (listeriosis was once known as "the graveyard of epidemiology" at the CDC because of the inherent difficulty of studying its transmission).

Table 4. Number of Outbreaks (and Outbreak-Related Cases), by Pathogen, in the United States[a]

	1982–1983	1984–1985	1986–1987	1988–1989	1990–1991
B. cereus	8 (200)	10 (65)	6 (196)	8 (112)	10 (296)
Campylobacter	10 (193)	13 (299)	7 (266)	12 (429)	9 (165)
C. botulinum	34 (76)	28 (49)	33 (45)	33 (73)	23 (47)
C. perfringens	27 (1542)	14 (1898)	5 (492)	7 (436)	21 (2453)
E. coli	5 (204)	3 (446)	1 (37)	3 (112)	5 (113)
Salmonella	127 (4483)	157 (24,139)	113 (4679)	211 (7907)	258 (10,436)
Shigella	11 (2109)	15 (711)	22 (7267)	12 (3838)	12 (946)
S. aureus	42 (1926)	25 (1574)	8 (350)	22 (769)	22 (703)
Streptococcus, grp A	2 (569)	3 (95)	3 (371)	1 (35)	1 (100)
V. cholerae	2 (899)	1 (2)	0 (0)	0 (0)	3 (32)
V. parahaemolyticus	3 (39)	0 (0)	3 (11)	0 (0)	4 (21)
V. vulnificus	0 (0)	0 (0)	0 (0)	0 (0)	1 (2)
Other bacteria	7 (343)	2 (161)	1 (69)	1 (2)	0 (0)
Total bacteria	278 (12,583)	271 (29,439)	202 (13,783)	310 (13,713)	369 (15,314)
Total viral	32 (5875)	14 (1021)	16 (1218)	20 (1166)	16 (566)
Total parasitic	5 (12)	20 (112)	12 (83)	8 (70)	8 (307)
Total chemical	92 (484)	100 (608)	87 (372)	66 (292)	58 (429)
Unknown etiology	754 (15,324)	633 (16,319)	537 (13,825)	552 (16,358)	610 (18,164)
Total	1161 (34,278)	1038 (47,499)	854 (29,281)	956 (31,599)	1061 (34,780)

[a]From CDC Surveillance Summaries.[1–3]

Table 5. Summary of Foodborne Outbreaks, Outbreak-Related Cases, and Outbreak-Related Deaths in the United States from 1982 to 1991[a]

	Total outbreaks	Percent of total	Total cases	Percent of all cases	Cases per outbreak	Total deaths	CFR
B. cereus	42	0.8%	869	0.5%	21	0	0%
Campylobacter	51	1.0%	1352	0.8%	27	3	0.22%
C. botulinum	151	3.0%	290	0.2%	2	23	7.93%
C. perfringens	74	1.5%	6821	3.8%	92	3	0.04%
E. coli	17	0.2%	912	0.5%	54	4	0.44%
Salmonella	866	17.1%	51,644	29.1%	60	81	0.16%
Shigella	72	1.4%	14,871	18.4%	207	2	0.01%
S. aureus	119	2.4%	5322	3.0%	45	1	0.02%
Streptococcus, grp A	10	0.2%	1170	0.7%	117	0	0%
V. cholerae	6	0.1%	933	0.5%	156	11	1.18%
V. parahaemolyticus	10	0.2%	71	0.04%	7	0	0%
V. vulnificus	1	0.02%	2	0.001%	2	1	50%
Other bacteria	11	0.2%	575	0.3%	57	75	13%
Total bacteria	1430	28.2%	84,832	47.8%	59	204	0.24%
Total viral	98	1.9%	9846	5.6%	100	7	0.07%
Total parasitic	53	1.0%	584	0.3%	11	2	0.34%
Total chemical	403	8.0%	2185	1.2%	5	5	0.23%
Unknown etiology	3086	60.9%	79,990	45.1%	26	4	<0.01%
All causes	5070	100%	177,437	100%	34	222	0.13%

[a]From CDC Surveillance Summaries.[1–3]

4. Setting. Outbreaks that occur in groups of persons that are clustered geographically are more likely to be recognized. Outbreaks occurring in schools or camps, for example, are more likely to be recognized than outbreaks occurring in the community.
5. Ease of diagnosis. The identification of certain organisms, such as vibrios or EHEC, requires special techniques that are not routinely performed when physicians request stool cultures. For this reason, outbreaks of these organisms often are not recognized.
6. Resources available to the local and state health departments. Even large outbreaks can go unrecognized if health departments are unable to devote resources to investigating them. A 1994 outbreak of *Salmonella* serotype Enteritidis involving tens of thousands of cases in over 30 states served to highlight this. Although this outbreak was huge by anyone's standards, the cases were widely dispersed geographically, and it was not immediately apparent that an outbreak was occurring. It was identified only because the Minnesota State Health Department had an aggressive program of serotyping *Salmonella* isolates sent to them, which allowed them to detect the sudden increase in one specific serotype.

The limitations of the data gathered through this system are obvious. Since the true numbers of outbreaks and cases are probably underestimated to a high degree by such a system, it cannot be used to estimate incidence. Also, because the degree of underreporting is not consistent from pathogen to pathogen, data from this system cannot be used to draw conclusions about the *relative* incidence of these illnesses. Trends are not always reliably noted by this system either; a decrease in the total number of foodborne outbreaks in the mid-1980s, for example, may have been due to the diversion of public health resources to combat the burgeoning acquired immunodeficiency syndrome (AIDS) epidemic.(5) Nonethelesss, information from this system has been invaluable in the identification and removal of contaminated products from the market, the determination of factors contributing to foodborne illness, the development of public health strategies to prevent foodborne illness, the evaluation of effectiveness of regulatory response, and the advancement of our understanding of the pathogenesis and clinical characteristics of foodborne illness.

3.2. Surveillance of Sporadic Diarrheal Illness

Data on sporadic diarrheal illness is largely obtained through passive surveillance systems. The National Notifiable Diseases Surveillance System (NNDSS) collects data on several illnesses that are sometimes foodborne: botulism, brucellosis, cholera, *E. coli* O157:H7, salmonellosis, shigellosis, and typhoid fever. The data collected are limited to numbers of cases and some demographic information. It is believed that these numbers are also subject to a very high degree of underreporting. In the case of salmonellosis, for example, it has been estimated that the true incidence in the United States is 20 to 90 times that reported to the CDC.(6) Because the NNDSS records both sporadic and outbreak-related illnesses, the numbers of cases registered by this system are typically much higher than those recorded by the outbreak surveillance system; in 1987, for example, the outbreak surveillance system reported 1846 cases of salmonellosis, whereas NNDSS reported 44,609 cases of this disease.(5) It is not known how many of the NNDSS cases were due to foodborne transmission. In addition to NNDSS, specific surveillance systems are operational and collect data on *Listeria*, *Vibrio* species, and *E. coli* O157:H7. These systems have included active surveillance components as well as case–control studies designed to determine the routes of transmission of such diseases.

It should be evident that all of the surveillance systems mentioned above have shortfalls and, even in the aggregate, fail to give an accurate assessment of the impact of foodborne illness in the United States. Because of this lack of adequate data, an active foodborne disease surveillance system was launched in 1995 by the CDC in cooperation with the US Department of Agriculture (USDA), Food and Drug Administration (FDA), and five state health departments. The goal of this system is to monitor foodborne diarrheal illness in the United States and to increase our understanding of the transmission of foodborne pathogens.

4. Etiologic Patterns

Despite their limitations, data from the foodborne outbreak surveillance system provide much information about outbreak-related disease. As shown in Tables 4 and 5, the single largest identified cause of morbidity, both in numbers of outbreaks and numbers of cases, is *Salmonella*. Following *Salmonella* in number of cases is *Shigella*, largely because of the large size of *Shigella* outbreaks, *C. perfringens*, and *S. aureus*. In number of outbreaks, *C. botulinum* ranks second, largely because even single cases of this disease were considered to be outbreaks. *S. aureus*, *C. perfringens*, and *Shigella* ranked third, fourth, and fifth.

A large portion of the outbreaks (45.1%) are of unknown etiology. In certain cases, etiologies may have been suspected by the investigators but not confirmed according to the CDC's requirements. It is possible that a large portion of these outbreaks are due to viruses, which are particularly difficult to diagnose. It is equally possible that there are other etiologic agents that have yet to be discovered. One study of outbreaks of unknown etiology reported to the CDC over a 15-year period showed that 35% of these had a median incubation period of 1 to 7 hr, which is consistent with *S. aureus* or *B. cereus* emetic-type illness.[(5)]

The mortality data from outbreak surveillance are shown in Table 5. For most of the pathogens on this chart, case fatality ratios are very low, with the majority of deaths occurring in the elderly or infirm. There are three notable exceptions to this: *C. botulinum*, *V. vulnificus*, and *Listeria*. Botulism is not nearly as deadly as it once was, largely because of improved medical technologies used to support patients during severe illness. *V. vulnificus* is generally a problem in immunocompromised hosts, especially those with liver disease, where it causes septicemia with a very high mortality rate. *Listeria* is also a problem in the immunocompromised patient as well as in infants and otherwise healthy pregnant women. *E. coli* O157:H7 should also be noted. Although the case fatality ratio for this organism is lower than that for such organisms as *Listeria*, many of the deaths occur in young children, in whom this infection can precipitate the hemolytic uremic syndrome.

It is important to note that etiologic patterns may vary throughout the world. These patterns are dependent on many factors, such as food preferences, physician and public awareness, and laboratory capabilities. Table 6 lists a comparison of five bacterial agents recognized in outbreaks in three areas of the world: the United States, England and Wales, and Japan.[(7)] In the United States, *S. aureus* and salmonellosis are the most common agents involved in foodborne outbreaks, representing over 50% of these outbreaks. In contrast, salmonellosis is implicated in over 90% of the recognized foodborne illness in England and Wales. *C. perfringens* is a frequently reported pathogen in both the United States and England. Japan, on the other hand, has very different etiologic patterns, probably related to many of the aforementioned factors. *V. parahaemolyticus* gastroenteritis, first described in that country, is the dominant pathogen in foodborne outbreaks and represents over 50% of the reported outbreaks. These associations generally reflect the different staples in diets around the world (i.e., higher seafood consumption in Japan, higher meat and poultry consumption in the United States). Clearly, some of these differences represent ascertainment bias; however, there is little doubt that different patterns exist in different regions of the world.

With this background, let us turn to a consideration of the specific agents *S. aureus*, *B. cereus*, *C. perfringens*, *Vibrio* species, *Aeromonas* and *Plesiomonas*.

5. *Staphylococcus aureus*

5.1. Historical Background

Although Dack modestly credited others for the discovery of staphylococcal food poisoning, he and his coworkers were the first to prove that this illness was due to toxin production by *S. aureus*.[(8)] They performed classic experiments in volunteers, demonstrating that culture filtrates of staphylococci isolated from a cream-filled sponge cake that had been the implicated vehicle in a foodborne outbreak could cause gastroenteritis.[(9)]

The work on the enterotoxins produced by *S. aureus* has been fundamental to our understanding of this syndrome. Dolman and Wilson[(10)] established that antibody to the enterotoxin could be made and, 15 years later, Surgalla *et al.*[(11)] showed that there was more than one immunologic type. Since these discoveries, Casman, Bergdoll, and others have characterized the physicochemical properties of these enterotoxins and have established that there are seven types: A, B, C_1, C_2, C_3, and D, and E.[(12)]

Table 6. Comparison among the United States, England and Wales, and Japan of the Most Common Foodborne Disease Outbreaks Reported from 1968 to 1972[a]

Organism or disease	United States		England and Wales		Japan	
	Number of outbreaks	Percentage of known etiology	Number of outbreaks	Percentage of known etiology	Number of outbreaks	Percentage of known etiology
S. aureus	208	29%	96	3%	891	29%
Salmonellosis	185	25%	3149	92%	414	13%
C. perfringens	102	14%	187	5%	—	—
V. parahaemolyticus	9	1%	1	<1%	1679	54%
B. cereus	6	<1%	6	<1%	—	—

[a]From Bryan.[(7)]

5.2. Microbiology

5.2.1. Biological Characteristics of the Organism. Staphylococci are gram-positive, nonencapsulated, nonmotile, non-spore-forming cocci that usually appear in grapelike clusters, hence the name. They are aerobic and facultatively anaerobic, may be β-hemolytic and catalase-positive, and ferment glucose. The genus *Staphylococcus* contains almost two dozen species that are traditionally divided into two groups on the basis of coagulase production. Coagulase-positive staphylococci are almost always *S. aureus*, although some strains of *S. intermedius* and *S. hyicus* also produce this enzyme.(12) All other species are coagulase-negative, the most important of which are *S. epidermidis* and *S. saprophyticus*.

S. aureus, the usual pathogen in foodborne disease, is capable of producing at least seven immunologically distinct enterotoxins, termed A, B, C_1, C_2, C_3, D, and E. Since there are strains of *S. aureus* that do not produce any of these but which are capable of causing emesis in monkeys, it is assumed that there are more staphylococcal enterotoxins that have yet to be identified. The known enterotoxins are all composed of single polypeptide chains with molecular weights of 28,366 to 34,700, which contain large numbers of lysine, aspartate, glutamate, and tyrosine residues. They are heat stable and resistant to a variety of proteases, including pepsin and trypsin.

The mechanism of action of staphylococcal enterotoxins is unknown. Since vagotomy and abdominal sympathectomy in monkeys renders them completely immune to the emetic effects of these toxins, their receptor or receptors are probably within the lumen of the gastrointestinal tract. Efforts to identify these receptors have proven fruitless.(12) The mechanism by which these toxins produce diarrhea is even less well understood; they fail to cause a reaction in rabbit ileal loop assays, though one group has been able to demonstrate fluid secretion in rat small intestine when challenged with staphylococcal enterotoxin B.(13)

A variety of other toxic substances are produced by *S. aureus* that are hemolytic, leukocytic, dermonecrotic, and lethal to animals. All *S. aureus*, by definition, produce a coagulase that causes coagulation of plasma; it is both free and bound to the cell wall. *S. aureus* also produces a fibrinolysin, hyaluronidase, deoxyribonuclease, and various lipases. Many of these substances are physiologically important for the other manifestations of staphylococcal infections, but are beyond the scope of this chapter; the reader is referred to Chapter 33 of this book for further information about these.

S. aureus is not the only species in this genus that is capable of producing staphylococcal enterotoxins. Strains of *S. intermedius*, *S. hyicus*, and *S. epidermidis* have been shown to produce these.(12) The latter has been implicated in a foodborne outbreak.(14)

5.2.2. Laboratory Diagnosis. The medium most frequently used to isolate staphylococci is an egg yolk–tellurite–glycine–pyruvate agar ("Baird-Parker agar"). Coagulase-positive staphylococci produce a zone of clearing in egg-yolk emulsion and reduce tellurite salt to tellurium, causing the staphylococci to form black colonies. Mannitol as the sole or major source of carbon in the medium, along with a high NaCl content, can also be used in a selective medium, although such conditions may inhibit the growth of heat-stressed staphyococci.(15)

Demonstration of staphylococcal enterotoxin is an important tool in outbreak investigations, since reheated food may contain toxin but no viable staphylococci. Several methods have been described, including enzyme-linked immunosorbent assay (ELISA),(16,17) enzyme immunoassay (EIA),(18) latex agglutination,(17) and immunoblot.(19) Any method should be capable of detecting concentrations of less than 1 ng/ml (as these methods are), since a dose of 100–200 ng of staphylococcal enterotoxin is sufficient to produce symptoms.(20) Oligonucleotide probes can also be used to demonstrate the presence of toxin genes in staphylococcal isolates.(21)

5.3. Descriptive Epidemiology

5.3.1. Prevalence and Incidence. Tables 4 and 5 summarize outbreak data from the United States from 1982 to 1991. In the United Kingdom, 10–15 outbreaks are investigated each year; these outbreaks, with an average of 15 cases each, are smaller than those in the United States.(22)

5.3.2. Epidemic Behavior and Contagiousness. Staphylococcal foodborne outbreaks are characterized by explosive onset between 30 min and 8 hr after consumption of a contaminated vehicle (usually 2–4 hr).(9,23) Attack rates are usually quite high, since very small quantities of enterotoxin can cause illness.(9) Secondary cases are not of concern in this type of food poisoning.

5.3.3. Geographic Distribution. There is no geographic clustering of cases, since outbreaks are related to food contamination from human staphylococcal carriers.

5.3.4. Temporal Distribution. Outbreaks from staphylococci can occur at any time of the year, but most outbreaks are reported during the warm weather months.(22,23) This is probably because higher ambient temperatures provide better conditions for bacteria to multiply when food handling errors occur.

5.3.5. Age, Sex, Race, and Occupation. There are no age, sexual, racial, or occupational characteristics that are peculiar to staphylococcal food poisoning.

5.3.6. Occurrence in Different Settings. Staphylococci are carried by so many people that almost any food-preparation setting can be involved. Most reported outbreaks are from large gatherings, i.e., schools, group picnics, clubs, and restaurants.

5.3.7. Foods Implicated in Outbreaks. For several years after the recognition of staphylococcal food poisoning, cream-filled baked goods were the leading source of this illness in the United States. In recent decades, other proteinaceous foods, especially meat and meat products, have predominated. In the United States and Great Britain, ham is now the most commonly implicated vehicle, which may be in part due to its relatively high salt context; *S. aureus* is very tolerant of salt, which increases its resistance to heat. Other vehicles have included potato salad, egg salad, cheese, and seafood. Milk has also been implicated as a vehicle. In one outbreak, the milk was allowed to sit at room temperature for 4 to 5 hr prior to pasteurization, during which the staphylococci produced enterotoxin that survived the heat treatment.[12] In other cases, milk was contaminated after pasteurization.[22]

5.4. Mechanisms and Routes of Transmission

The single most important source of staphylococcal contamination in foods are humans, where this organism can commonly be found on mucous membranes or the skin. Prevalence studies have found *S. aureus* on the mucous membranes of 25–65% of healthy individuals,[24] although these strains are often nontoxigenic.

In most outbreaks, food has been contaminated after processing by food workers who are carriers of enterotoxin-producing strains of staphylococci.[25] It was once observed that many of these workers had visible lesions on the hands or nose. This is an uncommon finding now, although it is true that *S. aureus* of the same phage type as that in the contaminated food can be found in food handlers in roughly two thirds of outbreaks.[23] These handlers are generally asymptomatic carriers.

Even though many animals and animal carcasses are contaminated before processing, this usually does not result in food poisoning. Competitive growth from other flora usually contains the slower-growing staphylococci. One exception to this is milk, which can be heavily contaminated with *S. aureus* when obtained from a mastitic animal.[12]

5.5. Pathogenesis and Immunity

5.5.1. Pathogenesis. There are three prerequisites for staphylococcal food poisoning to occur: (1) contamination of a food with enterotoxin-producing staphylococci; (2) a food that provides the necessary growth requirements for the organism; and (3) appropriate time and temperature for the organism to multiply. Enterotoxins A, B, C, D, and E have all been implicated in outbreaks of staphylococcal food poisoning in the United States and the United Kingdom. A majority of strains produce A either alone or in combination with other enterotoxins. Enterotoxin D is the second most common product. Of the less than 10% of strains that produce neither A nor D, many produce no known enterotoxin.[22,23] In one study of outbreak-related staphylococci, seven strains did not produce recognized enterotoxin; of these, five were tested, and all culture filtrates produced an emetic response in monkeys, suggestive of another as yet unidentified toxin.[26]

5.5.2. Immunity. It is not clear whether immunity develops in this illness. Although attack rates are not usually 100% in outbreaks, many individuals may not consume the enterotoxin or enough of the implicated vehicle. In outbreaks where small groups are involved in which everyone consumes the implicated food, attacks rates are very high (80–100%). Early attempts to "immunize" man or develop "tolerance" to toxin were not successful when broth filtrates of toxin-producing staphylococci were administered by mouth.[27]

Clearly, individuals have differing sensitivity to enterotoxin; in one investigation using volunteers, as little as 0.5 ml of a filtrate could cause illness in one person, whereas 13 ml administered to another individual caused no symptoms. Whether this is a case of immunity or physicochemical sensitivity of a receptor site is not clear. Whether immunity from one toxin confers cross-immunity to others has not been determined.

5.6. Patterns of Host Response

5.6.1. Clinical Features. The symptoms of staphylococcal food poisoning are primarily profuse vomiting, nausea, and abdominal cramps, often followed by diarrhea. In severe cases, blood may be observed in the vomitus or stool. Rarely, hypotension and marked prostration occur. Fatalities are unusual, and recovery is complete in 24 to 48 hr.[28] Fever is not a common accompaniment, but may be present if dehydration is severe.

5.6.2. Diagnosis. Staphylococcal food intoxication should be considered in anyone who presents with severe vomiting, nausea, cramps, and some diarrhea. A history of ingesting meats of high salt content may be helpful. Usually, the best epidemiological clue is the short incubation period (usually 2–4 hr). Of the bacterial foodborne diseases, only *B. cereus* emetic-type illness has a similar presenting illness with a short incubation period. This disease is so closely allied with fried rice as to allow an easy distinction.

6. *Bacillus cereus*

6.1. Historical Background

One of the first outbreaks implicating an aerobic spore-forming organism was described by Lubenau[29] in 1906, in which 300 inmates of a sanitorium developed a diarrheal illness from meatballs contaminated with an organism labeled *Bacillus peptonificans*. This isolate closely resembled what is today considered typical of *B. cereus*. During the several decades following this description, other European investigators cited similar aerobic spore-forming bacilli in food poisoning involving vanilla sauce, jellied meat dishes, and boiled beef. However, it was not until Hauge's[30] description of four separate Norwegian outbreaks in 1955 that *B. cereus* was conclusively implicated as a cause of diarrheal illness. These outbreaks, all linked to vanilla sauce containing large numbers of *B. cereus*, produced an illness characterized by profuse, watery diarrhea, abdominal pain, nausea, but rarely vomiting or fever. The incubation period averaged 10 to 12 hr, with illness resolving within 12 to 24 hr. Subsequent experiments in which Hauge and other volunteers ingested vanilla sauce inoculated with *B. cereus* substantiated the role of this organism.[30]

After Hauge's report, outbreaks of similar illness were described in northern and eastern Europe, particularly in the Netherlands and Hungary. The first well-documented outbreak of gastrointestinal disease in the United States was reported by Midura *et al.*[31] in 1970.

In 1974, another form of *B. cereus* illness was recognized that involved fried rice.[32] This illness was distinctly different from those previously described, in that the incubation period was shorter, ranging from 1 to 6 hr, and the illness was primarily vomiting (although some patients had diarrhea as well). Although this condition closely resembled staphylococcal food poisoning, *B. cereus* was recovered from the fried rice.

Since this report, it has become accepted that *B. cereus* is capable of producing two distinct foodborne syndromes. The emetic illness, usually associated with fried rice, is caused by ingestion of a preformed heat-stable toxin that is produced by the bacteria in the food. The diarrheal illness, associated with a large variety of foods, has a longer incubation period and is caused by a heat-labile toxin that is produced by the bacteria in the intestine.

6.2. Microbiology

6.2.1. Biological Characteristics of the Organism. *B. cereus* is a gram-positive, catalase-positive, aerobic spore-forming rod that is mobile by means of peritrichous flagella. Most strains are β-hemolytic. *B. cereus* is differentiated from *B. anthracis* on the basis of resistance to gamma phage, negative fluorescent-antibody test, lack of animal pathogenicity, and presence of β-hemolysis (see Chapter 4). For a detailed discussion of the biochemical properties of these organisms, the reader is referred to the review by Goepfert *et al.*[33]

Strains of *B. cereus* produce a wide variety of exotoxins, only two of which appear to be important in the pathogenesis of food poisoning: the "diarrheogenic enterotoxin" and the "emetic toxin." Spira and Goepfert[34] first studied the diarrheogenic enterotoxin, which causes fluid accumulation in rabbit ileal loops, alters vascular permeability in the skin of rabbits, and kills mice when injected intravenously. The enterotoxin does not bind tightly to the rabbit ileal-loop receptor site, since elution by washing with saline destroys its activity. Furthermore, homologous antiserum introduced into the loop 10 min after enterotoxin neutralizes its action. This toxin has a molecular weight of 48,000 Da and is highly sensitive to both heat (destroyed as 56°C in 5 min) and trypsin.[34]

The emetic toxin was first isolated from a strain implicated in an outbreak of vomiting-type illness. This toxin does not produce fluid accumulation in rabbit ileal loops and causes only vomiting when fed to rhesus monkeys. In contrast to the diarrheogenic enterotoxin, the emetic toxin is of low molecular weight (<10,000 Da) and is highly stable, resisting heat, extremes of pH, and exposure to trypsin.[35,36]

6.2.2. Laboratory Diagnosis. *B. cereus* can be cultured on blood agar, grown aerobically at 37°C. Some workers have employed a peptone-beef extract egg-yolk agar containing lithium chloride and polymyxin B as selective agents[37]; typical colonies are surrounded by an opaque zone due to the action of lecithinase. Others have utilized mannitol (which *B. cereus* cannot catabolize) in the egg yolk–polymyxin medium and have advocated incubation at 35–37°C for 24 hr.[38] To distinguish *B. cereus* from other *Bacillus* species, the sporangium of sporulating cells is examined for swelling (which is not characteristic of *B. cereus*) and for the presence of a parasporal body characteristic of *B. thuringiensis*. Fluorescent antibodies to spore coat antigens can be used to confirm the species.[39]

Enumeration of *B. cereus* can be performed either by direct plating or, if expected numbers are less than 1000/g, by most probable number methods.[35] The diarrheogenic toxin can be demonstrated by biological methods[35,40] or ELISA (Bioenterprises Party, Australia). However, even when sought, the enterotoxin is often not found because of the instability of this molecule, which is rapidly degraded by proteolytic enzymes.[41] There are as yet no commercially available kits for detecting emetic toxin.

6.3. Descriptive Epidemiology

6.3.1. Prevalence and Incidence. The incidence of *B. cereus* illness is unknown. As with many foodborne pathogens, disease due to this organism often goes undiagnosed and unreported. Outbreak surveillance data from 1982 to 1991 (Tables 4 and 5) show that this pathogen accounts for 2.1% of outbreaks of confirmed bacterial etiology in the United States. The average size of these outbreaks (21 cases) is relatively small, perhaps because the relatively short incubation period, especially in the emetic-type disease, increases the likelihood that small outbreaks will be recognized.

In Europe, *B. cereus* accounts for a larger portion of outbreaks, most of which are of the diarrheal type. In the Netherlands, for example, 18% of all foodborne outbreaks of confirmed etiology from 1985 to 1989 were due to this organism.[42] In Hungary, *B. cereus* was the third most common cause of foodborne illness from 1960 to 1968.[35] The relatively high incidence was attributed to a preference in the Hungarian population for well-spiced meat dishes. The spices used were found to contain large numbers of *Bacillus* spores. Poor postcooking storage procedures allowed the spores that survived cooking to germinate.

6.3.2. Epidemic Behavior and Contagiousness. In the original description by Hauge,[30] 82% of individuals who ate the incriminated meal were affected. Of the 19 who were not ill, 11 had not eaten the dessert (implicated vehicle), and 8 had eaten only a small quantity. Other reported outbreaks have indicated attack rates from 50 to 75%. In the reported vomiting-type outbreaks, virtually all individuals who consumed the contaminated fried rice became ill. There is minimal risk of secondary cases, since heavy contamination of the implicated vehicle is required.

The incubation period is 6 to 24 hr for diarrhea-type outbreaks and 1 to 6 hr for emetic-type outbreaks.

6.3.3. Geographic, Temporal, Age, Sex, Racial, and Occupational Distribution. *B. cereus* food poisoning has not shown any geographic or temporal distribution. There has been a suggestion by Bodnar[43] that affected children may become more severely ill than adults and require hospitalization. There does not appear to be any sexual, racial, or occupational predisposition.

6.3.4. Occurrence in Different Settings. Most reports of diarrheal illness have taken place in institutional settings (schools, hospitals, and others). This may be a reporting artifact, since foodborne outbreaks are more easily recognized in confined populations.

6.3.5. Other Factors. The clear-cut association between the vomiting syndrome and fried rice deserves emphasis. The first three reports of outbreaks of emetic-type *B. cereus* illness in the United States[44] and the report by Mortimer and McCann[32] of five outbreaks in Great Britain implicated fried rice as the vehicle. This association has been attributed to the method used to prepare this food in Chinese "takeout" restaurants (see below).

The diarrheal illness has been caused by a much larger variety of foods including boiled beef, sausage, chicken soup, macaroni and cheese, vanilla sauce, and puddings.

6.4. Mechanisms and Routes of Transmission

B. cereus is found in about 25–50% of many foodstuffs sampled, including cream, pudding, meat, spices, dry potatoes, dry milk, infant foods, spaghetti sauces, and rice.[37,42,45] Contamination of the food product generally occurs prior to cooking. If the food is prepared in such a manner that the temperature is maintained at 30–50°C, vegetative cell growth will occur. Spores can survive extreme temperatures, and when allowed to cool relatively slowly, they will germinate and multiply.[46] It is not known whether the ingested organisms multiply and make toxin *in vivo* or whether a preformed toxin is present in food.

The association of the emetic type illness with fried rice can be attributed to the method in which this food is prepared in Chinese restaurants. Rice is first boiled in bulk and then stored at room temperatures for periods as long as 3 days. Chefs in these institutions are usually reluctant to refrigerate the rice because this causes it to clump. The rice is then rapidly fried when needed with a mixture containing beaten eggs. The heat produced during this second cooking is insufficient to destroy the heat stable emetic toxin. Studies have found viable *B. cereus* in up to 93% of specimens boiled rice, though the number of organisms is usually less than 10^5/g.[45–47]

Human fecal carriage is not believed to play a role in transmission of *B. cereus*, though this organism can transiently colonize the intestinal tract for periods of up to 4 days.[48] The isolation rate of *B. cereus* in the stool of asymptomatic individuals can be as high as 40% and is thought to be due to the high prevalence of this species in foods.[49,50]

6.5. Pathogenesis and Immunity

6.5.1. Pathogenesis. *B. cereus* food poisoning is toxin-mediated in both the diarrheal form and the emetic form.[44] Whether the diarrheogenic, heat-labile enterotoxin is actually ingested or produced *in vivo* is not known; there are, however, several pieces of evidence to suggest that the latter mechanism may be operative. The incubation period in the diarrheal illness is longer than might be expected for preformed toxin, and a large inoculum (> 10%) is required to cause illness, suggesting a requirement for intestinal colonization.

The emetic illness is presumptively caused by preformed toxin that is heat-stable. The short incubation period and high attack rate provide support for this pathogenic mechanism.

6.5.2. Immunity. Our knowledge of immunity to either of these syndromes is largely uncharted. Antiserum to the diarrheogenic enterotoxin introduced into the rabbit ileal-loop model along with the toxin can prevent fluid accumulation; no careful studies in humans have been performed. There are many serotypes of *B. cereus*, but it is not known whether the various enterotoxins have immune cross-reactivity. The emetic toxin is poorly antigenic; when repeatedly challenged with this, rhesus monkeys develop no resistance to its action.[41]

6.6. Patterns of Host Response

6.6.1. Clinical Features. The initial report by Hauge[30] described the diarrheal illness of *B. cereus*, and his findings are consistent with what we know today. Illness is characterized by diarrhea (96%), abdominal cramps (75%), and vomiting (23%). Fever is uncommon. The duration of illness has ranged from 20 to 36 hr, with a median of 24 hr.[30,44]

The emetic form of the illness has the predominant symptoms of vomiting (100%) and abdominal cramps (100%). Diarrhea is present in only one third of affected individuals.[44] The duration of this illness has ranged from 8 to 10 hr, with a median of 9 hr. In both types of illness, the disease is usually mild and self-limited.

6.6.2. Diagnosis. The diagnosis of *B. cereus* food poisoning should be considered in any individual who has diarrhea without fever in association with lower abdominal cramps. The incubation period varies from 6 to 24 hr. The easiest way to make the diagnosis is by culture of the incriminated food product. The disease caused by *C. perfringens* is so similar to the diarrheal form of *B. cereus* that they cannot be differentiated clinically or epidemiologically; culture methods are required. The emetic form of the disease should be suspected in an individual presenting with nausea and vomiting 1 to 5 hr after consumption of a farinaceous food, especially fried rice. The clinical picture is indistinguishable from that of *S. aureus* food poisoning.

Because *B. cereus* can be found in many foodstuffs, this organism should only be considered significant if present in the incriminated food item in numbers of 10^5 or more per gram.[1] Similarly, since *B. cereus* can sometimes be found in the stools of healthy persons,[49,50] isolation of the organism from feces may not be suitable confirmation unless negative stool cultures are obtained from an appropriate control group. Demonstration of the presence of the enterotoxin supports the diagnosis.

Taylor and Gilbert[51] established a provisional serotyping schema by preparing agglutinating antisera against the flagellar (H) antigen of 18 strains isolated from various foodstuffs implicated in foodborne outbreaks around the world. This system has been expanded and is currently available through the Central Public Health Laboratory (London); a slightly different system is in use at the Tokyo Metropolitan Research Laboratory of Public Health in Japan. Of 200 outbreak-related *B. cereus* isolates from 11 different countries between 1971 and 1986, 91% were typable by the UK system.[35] Of these, 127 (64%) were H-type 1, a serotype found in 23% of cooked rice. Type 1 was also the most common serotype found in diarrheic outbreaks (4 of 20).[35] A phage typing system has been described and has been successfully implemented in Canada.[52]

7. *Clostridium perfringens*

7.1. Historical Background

C. perfringens was first recognized and confirmed in the United States as a foodborne pathogen in 1945 by

McClung,[53] who studied four outbreaks of diarrhea related to the consumption of chickens steamed 24 hr prior to consumption. *C. perfringens* was isolated from the cooked chickens. Prior to this discovery, workers in Europe had also recognized that gravy contaminated with anaerobic spore-forming bacilli, including *C. perfringens*, had caused gastrointestinal illness in children.[53,54]

Shortly after McClung's discovery, filtrates from strains of *C. perfringens* were administered by mouth to human subjects.[55] Cramps and diarrhea occurred in some individuals, but the incubation period was short: 45–80 min. Living cultures induced cramps and bloating in 4 hr and diarrhea several hours thereafter. Hobbs *et al.*[56] elegantly confirmed these results and outlined the epidemiological features of the disease in Great Britain in 1953.

The other major discovery in the late 1940s was the outbreak of a severe and often lethal intestinal disease labeled enteritis necroticans or "Darmbrand" that affected over 400 people in Germany[57]; this outbreak was similar to others described later in New Guinea and termed "pig bel"[58] (see Section 7.7). Both conditions were due to *C. perfringens*. The strains were originally designated *Clostridium welchii* type F but were later reclassified as *C. perfringens* type C.

Up to this time, all foodborne outbreaks were felt to be due to heat-resistant *C. perfringens*. Several investigators in the late 1960s confirmed that nonhemolytic and β-hemolytic, heat-sensitive strains could cause food poisoning.[59]

Investigations in the late 1960s and early 1970s provided convincing evidence that the pathogenesis of *C. perfringens* food poisoning is due to enterotoxin production while cells are sporulating. Furthermore, enterotoxin can be demonstrated in *C. perfringens* types A, C, and D. The toxins of types A and C are quite similar with regard to physicochemical properties.

7.2. Microbiology

7.2.1. Biological Characteristics of the Organism. Clostridia are gram-positive, spore-forming anaerobes. Although all species grow better under anaerobic conditions, *C. perfringens* is remarkably aerotolerant and may survive exposure to oxygen for as long as 72 hr. This organism has a characteristic "boxcar" appearance on Gram-stained slides and, unlike most *Clostridium* species, is nonmotile. The spores produced by this organism are oval, subterminal, and only rarely seen in clinical specimens.

C. perfringens produces 12 toxins that are active in tissues, as well as several enterotoxins. The species is divided into five types, A–E, on the basis of four major toxins, α, β, ε, and ι (see Table 7). Type A is the agent of classic *C. perfringens* food poisoning. Almost all strains of this type isolated from outbreaks produce α-toxin (a lecithinase) and a unique enterotoxin.[60,61]

This enterotoxin is a heat-labile protein with a molecular weight of approximately 35,000. It is produced during sporulation, but it is not, as once thought, an integral component of the spore coat.[60] The role of this toxin in producing diarrheal illness was confirmed by feeding cell-free filtrates to volunteers. Of 15 persons who consumed filtrates from toxin-producing strains, four developed diarrhea, whereas none of 16 persons fed filtrates from toxin-negative strains developed illness. The incubation period for illness in these volunteers was 2 to 2.5 hr. Similar results have been obtained in experimental animals.[62,63]

C. perfringens is ubiquitous in the environment. It can be found in almost any soil, where it performs its principal role in nature: the breakdown of organic waste. The organism is also a common component of the gastrointestinal tract of healthy humans and animals; surveys of asymptomatic individuals show that it can be isolated from almost any stool sample if enrichment techniques are used, but it is usually present at concentrations less than 10^4 CFU/g, except in the elderly, where it frequently exceeds 10^6 CFU/g. The lowest numbers are found in vegetarians, for unknown reasons. Because this organism is so common, enumeration of spores in the feces is recommended when attempting to confirm *C. perfringens* as the cause of a foodborne outbreak.

7.2.2. Laboratory Diagnosis. The recommended culture medium is the egg-yolk-free tryptose–sulfite–cycloserine agar. It allows sulfite-reducing clostridia to form black colonies and inhibits other facultative anaerobes.[64,65] Colonies can then be selected for nitrate production, motility, and liquefaction of gelatin.[64] Heat resistance is no longer considered a characteristic of food-poisoning strains, and this test is not necessary.

Three other characteristics are of use in the isolation

Table 7. Production of Major Toxins by Types of *C. perfringens*

Toxin	*C. perfringens* type A	B	C	D	E
α	+	+	+	+	+
β	−	+	+	−	−
ε	−	+	−	+	−
ι	−	−	−	−	+

of *C. perfringens*: a dual zone pattern of hemolysis on blood agar plates, opalescence (precipitation) on egg yolk media, and "stormy fermentation" in milk media. On blood agar, *C. perfringens* colonies are surrounded by a narrow inner ring of incomplete hemolysis, due to θ-toxin, and a much wider outer ring of complete hemolysis due to α-toxin. On egg yolk agar, colonies produce opalescence, termed the "Nagler reaction," which is due to the presence of α-toxin. Presumptive identification of *C. perfringens* can be achieved with an egg yolk agar plate, which is partly coated with *C. perfringens* α-antitoxin, which inhibits the opalescence. Stormy fermentation in milk media is characteristic of *C. perfringens*. Vigorous lactose fermentation produces both acid, which coagulates the casein in the milk medium, and large amounts of gas, which breaks apart the clot.[66]

None of these reactions are 100% sensitive or specific for *C. perfringens*. Other *Clostridium* species produce lecithinases that are inhibited by the α-antitoxin. Similarly, other species ferment lactose rapidly and produce stormy fermentation. Furthermore, many outbreak-related strains do not produce a double zone of hemolysis. Also, several lecithinase-negative strains have been isolated from outbreaks in the United Kingdom.[67]

ELISA tests have been developed to detect enterotoxin in fecal samples,[68] and a reversed passive latex agglutination test is available commercially (Oxoid). DNA probes can be used to test enterotoxigenicity of strains of *C. perfringens* isolated during outbreaks.[69]

7.3. Descriptive Epidemiology

7.3.1. Prevalence and Incidence. Almost all of our knowledge of the epidemiology of *C. perfringens* food poisoning comes from the study of outbreaks. Tables 4 and 5 summarize this data for the United States. Given that the diagnosis of *C. perfringens* food poisoning is difficult to confirm because of the ubiquity of the organism in foods and in stools, it is likely that a *C. perfringens* also accounts for at least some of the foodborne outbreaks for which an etiology is not found. In England and Wales, the number of outbreaks is considerably higher than in the United States, with 40–70 outbreaks and 1000–3000 cases reported annually.[70] This is probably a result of better detection, since the average number of cases per outbreak is considerably smaller (27).

Sporadic *C. perfringens* food poisoning is even less likely to be recognized, since definitive diagnosis in this setting is very difficult. Enterotoxin assays may change this in the future: One British study of stools submitted to a reference laboratory for culture found this toxin in 7% of samples.[68]

7.3.2. Epidemic Behavior and Contagiousness. Epidemics of *C. perfringens* are usually characterized by high attacks rates (usually >50%) with a large number of affected individuals; the median number of affected individuals per outbreak was 92 for the years 1982–1991 (see Table 5). There is no risk of secondary transmission.

The incubation period in most outbreaks varies between 8 and 14 hr (median 12 hr), but can be as short as 6 hr or as long as 24 hr.

7.3.3. Geographic, Age, Sex, Racial, and Occupational Distribution. Since the organism is widespread in nature, there is no geographic clustering associated with this organism. Outbreaks have been recorded throughout the United States, Europe, and Japan. No age, sex, racial, or occupational predilections are known.

7.3.4. Temporal Distribution. It has been stated for many years that outbreaks of *C. perfringens* are more common in the spring and fall in contrast to most other foodborne pathogens, which peak during the summer. However, no such trend has been noted in the United States in the past 10 years, with outbreaks occurring as frequently in the summer as during the other seasons.

7.3.5. Occurrence in Different Settings. Outbreaks due to this organism are most frequently reported from institutions or large gatherings. The pathogenesis of infection requires that a meat or fish dish be precooked and then reheated to be served. The association with large gatherings may be due to the practice of preparing food in advance for such events, or may be simply a reporting artifact, since only such groups may recognize the outbreak as food poisoning.

7.3.6. Nutritional Factors. Beef, turkey, and chicken are the most frequent vehicles of infection with *C. perfringens*; other foods implicated include gravy, stew, minestrone soup, bean burritos, rice pudding, and fried fish paste. *C. perfringens* is common in many foods: It can be recovered from 30–80% of raw or frozen meat and poultry,[71] though most strains found in food are non-enterotoxigenic.[72]

7.4. Mechanisms and Routes of Transmission

Most outbreaks involve meat-based meals that have been precooked in bulk, allowed to cool for several hours, and then inadequately reheated. The initial cooking is generally sufficient to kill the vegetative organisms but not the spores, which germinate when the temperature falls below 50°C. Unless this food is reheated to a very high temperature, it will contain many viable organisms.[73] In most outbreaks of *C. perfringens* food poisoning, the original source of the bacteria has been assumed to be the food itself.

7.5. Pathogenesis and Immunity

7.5.1. Pathogenesis. Symptoms in *C. perfringens* food poisoning are caused by *in vivo* production rather than by ingestion of preformed enterotoxin.[62,63,74] In volunteer experiments, this toxin is capable of producing the symptoms of food poisoning, but only when given in much higher amounts than are found in epidemiologically linked foods. In fact, by the time enough enterotoxin has accumulated in food to be detectable, the food is generally unpalatable.[75] The fact that the toxin is produced by the bacteria in the intestines accounts for a longer incubation period than that seen in illness such as *S. aureus* food poisoning, which is due to preformed toxin.

Relatively large numbers of organisms are required to produce illness. An early study showed that ingestion of 10^8 organisms was capable of producing illness in 50% of volunteers.[76] Other workers have estimated that five times that number may be necessary.

Once ingested, the organism proliferates in the intestine, sporulates, and produces its enterotoxin. This toxin has a number of effects in the intestine, including salt and water secretion into the lumen and increased intestinal motility.[77] In addition, the clostridial toxin inhibits glucose transport, damages the intestinal epithelium, and causes protein loss into the intestinal lumen. These effects are most prominent in the terminal ileum.[78,79]

7.5.2. Immunity. Immunity is not well understood. In one study, 65% of Americans and 84% of Brazilians had antienterotoxin activity in serum.[80] The significance of this finding is unknown. No outbreaks have been studied by these methods in which blood was available prior to the outbreaks so that antienterotoxin immunity could be assessed. In animal studies, enterotoxin antiserum can block the action of the toxin on ligated rabbit loops. It has been suggested, however, that the presence of antibody in serum has little or no effect on toxin activity in the intestine.[74,81]

7.6. Patterns of Host Response

7.6.1. Clinical Features. *C. perfringens* food poisoning is characterized by watery diarrhea and severe, crampy abdominal pain, usually without vomiting, beginning 8 to 24 hr after the incriminated meal. Fever, chills, headache, or other signs of infection usually are not present.

The illness is of short duration, 24 hr or less. Rare fatalities have been recorded in debilitated or hospitalized patients who are victims of clostridial food poisoning. Intestinal fecal impaction may be one contributing factor in the elderly.[82]

7.6.2. Diagnosis. The diagnosis of *C. perfringens* food poisoning should be considered in any diarrheal illness characterized by abdominal pain and moderate to severe diarrhea, *unaccompanied* by fever or chills. There are usually many other individuals involved in the outbreak, and the suspect food is beef or chicken that has been stewed, roasted, or boiled earlier and then allowed to sit without proper refrigeration.

B. cereus food poisoning can have a very similar presentation and can be ruled out only by bacteriological study. Enterotoxigenic *E. coli* can also present in this fashion (see Chapter 14), although low-grade fever may be present. Cholera has more profuse diarrhea, which helps differentiate it from clostridial intoxication. *Salmonella* infection has a longer incubation period and is sometimes accompanied by fever (Chapter 31). CDC criteria for confirmation of an outbreak of *C. perfringens* food poisoning are shown in Table 3. It should be noted when testing implicated foods that numbers of viable clostridia decline rapidly in refrigerated samples.

Several subtyping methods are of use in epidemiological studies. Serotyping[83] has proven useful in the United Kingdom but has been less successful in the United States, where many strains are untypeable. It is often advised to serotype more than one isolate from a fecal sample, since carriage of *C. perfringens* in the human gastrointestinal tract is normal. Bacteriocin typing,[84] plasmid typing,[85] and most recently ribotyping[86] have all been successfully applied to the investigations of *C. perfringens* outbreaks.

7.7. Enteritis Necroticans

Enteritis necroticans deserves to be considered separately from type A food poisoning because of its unique clinical features, epidemiology, and pathobiology. This illness is a much more severe, necrotizing disease of the small intestine with a high mortality. The incubation period is 24 hr, after which illness ensues with intense abdominal pain, bloody diarrhea, vomiting, and shock. The mortality rate is about 40% and is usually due to intestinal perforation.

In postwar Germany, where the illness was known as "Darmbrand," illness was linked to the consumption of underprocessed canned meat that contained *C. perfringens* type C spores. Women were disproportionately affected, particularly those aged 30 to 60 years. In 1947, the incidence was 11 in 100,000 and cases peaked in the summer.[57]

In Papua New Guinea, outbreaks of "pig-bel" have been clearly related to the consumption of pork during prolonged feasts. During such feasts, the pig is often improperly cooked, and large quantities of pork are consumed over 3 or 4 days. There is a clear male preponderance of cases, with attack rates being highest in boys less than 10 years of age. The incidence of pig-bel was as high as 500 in 100,000 on the island prior to the introduction of the β-toxoid vaccine (see below).[87]

Sporadic cases of enteritis necroticans have been described in several other countries, particularly in the developing world.[88] An outbreak of this illness occurred in a Khmer refugee camp in Thailand between 1985 and 1986; the incidence reached 440 in 100,000 in the 0- to 10-year-old age group, with a case fatality rate of 58%.[88]

The organism that causes enteritis necroticans is *C. perfringens* type C, which does not generally produce enterotoxin. Rather, β-toxin is felt to be the cause of this disease. This toxin is a 40-kDa protein that is extremely sensitive to proteases. It produces necrosis of the small intestine, especially at the level of the jejunum. But ingestion of β-toxin-producing bacteria is not sufficient in itself to produce enteritis necroticans. At least two other factors play a role in the pathogenesis of this disease: a low-protein diet and the presence of protease inhibitors. Both of these factors have the effect of decreasing the amount of trypsin in the intestine, and thereby permitting the toxin to act on the intestinal wall.[89]

Thus, in postwar Germany, epidemic malnutrition was an important enabling factor. In Papua New Guinea, the usual low-protein diet coupled with trypsin inhibitors in sweet potatoes (commonly eaten during pig feasts) or secreted by ascaris (present in 70–80% of the highland population) have been identified as factors in the pathogenesis of pig-bel.[58]

Antibodies to β-toxin are protective against enteritis necroticans. These antibodies, which are largely absent in European adults and Papuan children, are highly prevalent in Papuan adults; these antibodies may account for the lower incidence of pig-bel in the adult population of the island. A β-toxoid vaccine has been developed and is protective against this disease. The incidence of pig-bel in Papua New Guinea has declined dramatically since the introduction of this vaccine the early 1980s.[58]

8. "Noncholera" *Vibrio* Species

8.1. Historical Background

In the 1930s, cholera researchers realized that *Vibrio cholerae* isolates could be divided into two groups: those that agglutinated with serum from cholera patients (0 group 1) and those that failed to agglutinate. This latter group consisted primarily of environmental isolates that were thought to be nonpathogenic, although there was early speculation that some of these "nonagglutinating" or "noncholera" vibrios might be responsible for such syndromes as "paracholera." Firm evidence of the pathogenicity of these strains did not emerge until two decades later when the first outbreaks due to these organisms were identified and investigated. As these data accumulated, it became increasingly clear that many of the strains were so distinct from *V. cholerae* as to constitute separate species.[90]

Within the species *V. cholerae*, there are over 100 O groups, only two of which cause epidemic cholera: *V. cholerae* O1 and *V. cholerae* O139. Serotype O1 held a monopoly on this disease until 1992, when O139 emerged and rapidly spread in Asia (see Chapter 11). Other serotypes of *V. cholerae* ("nonepidemic" *V. cholera*) are different in that they generally cause only sporadic illness, rather than large-scale epidemics such as those for which O1 and O139 are infamous.

V. parahaemolyticus was the first noncholera *Vibrio* species to be recognized as an agent of foodborne illness. Fujino and co-workers[91] first isolated this organism from autopsy materials collected during an investigation of a food-poisoning outbreak. Over the subsequent decade, many other outbreaks in Japan incriminated a halophilic, hemolytic gram-negative organism similar to that described by Fujino. The vehicles in these outbreaks were usually raw fish, shellfish, and cucumbers in brine. The names *Pasteurella parahaemolytica*, *Pseudomonas enteritis*, and *Oceanomonas parahaemolytica* were all suggested before taxonomic studies firmly placed the organism within the genus *Vibrio*.

In addition to *V. parahaemolyticus*, several other *Vibrio* species are known to be enteropathogenic (see Table 8). *V. fluvialis*, *V. furnissii*, *V. hollisae*, and *V. minicus* have been well described as agents of sporadic gastroenteritis or of foodborne outbreaks. *V. vulnificus* can cause a syndrome of "primary septicemia" (septicemia without any other obvious source) associated with ingestion of the organism in shellfish; it may or may not cause gastroenteritis. Numerous other *Vibrio* species (there are over 3 dozen known *Vibrio* species) have been described but are not known to be pathogenic.[92]

8.2. Microbiology

8.2.1. Biological Characteristics of the Organisms. Vibrios are ubiquitous of microbes in aquatic environments. They are most common in marine and estuarine environments, though some species such as *V. cholerae* have been isolated from fresh water. In temperate climates, their numbers vary seasonally: In the sum-

Table 8. Clinical Syndromes Due to *Vibrio* Species

	Clinical presentation[a]		
	Gastroenteritis	Wound/ear infection	Primary septicemia
V. cholerae			
O1	++	(+)	
non-O1	++		+
V. mimicus	++	+	
V. parahaemolyticus	++	+	(+)
V. fluvialis	++	+	
V. furnissii	++		
V. hollisae	++		(+)
V. vulnificus	+	++	++
V. alginolyticus		++	
V. damsela		++	
V. cincinnatiensis			+
V. carchariae		+	
V. metschnikovii	?		?

[a]++, denotes the most common presentation; +, other clinical presentations; and (+) very rare presentations.

mer they can easily be isolated from water, suspended particulate matter, plankton, algae, sediment, fish, and shellfish; during the winter months, they decline markedly in number and are found primarily in sediments.[(92,93)] In studies in the Chesapeake Bay area, *V. vulnificus* constituted 12% of the total aerobic bacterial flora present in bay water, with peak counts in the range of 10^1–10^3/ml. Counts may be two orders of magnitude higher in filter-feedings mollusks, such as oysters. Virtually 100% of raw oysters harvested during warmer, summer months carry *V. vulnificus*. Studies conducted by the US FDA have identified nonepidemic *V. cholerae*, which is also a common environmental isolate, in 14% of oyster shell stock sampled.[(94)]

All *Vibrio* species are facultatively anaerobic, asporogenous, pleomorphic gram-negative rods. Most are highly motile with a single, polar flagellum and are catalase-positive on standard biochemical panels. One consequence of their marine habitat is that most vibrios are "halophilic," requiring salt (at least 1% NaCl) for growth; some will grow in salt concentrations as high as 12%. *V. cholerae* and *V. mimicus* are notable exceptions: Although they grow well in 1% NaCl and can tolerate salt concentrations as high as 6%, they are also able to grow in the absence of salt.

8.2.2. Laboratory Diagnosis. *Vibrio* species will grow on or in most nonselective culture media, including blood agar and commercially available blood culture media. For isolation from stool, use of a selective medium, thiosulfate, citrate, bile salts, and sucrose (TCBS agar), is generally necessary.[(92,95)] With the exception of some strains of *V. hollisae*, all pathogenic vibrios will grow on this medium, producing colonies that are yellow (sucrose fermenters such as *V. cholerae*) or blue-green (nonsucrose fermenters such as *V. parahaemolyticus* and most *V. vulnificus*). Because the routine use of TCBS is not considered cost effective in the United States, the Gulf Coast *Vibrio* Working Group (the state health departments of Florida, Alabama, Louisiana, and Texas) has recommended its use only in cases in which clinical or epidemiologial information indicate its use.

Confirmation of the genus and identification of the species can be accomplished using standard biochemical panels. Because many vibrios are halophilic, the addition of 1% NaCl to growth media is often necessary to prevent false-negative reactions. When examining environmental samples, especially water samples, concentration procedures or selective enrichment broths may be needed.[(95)] Direct identification from environmental samples may be facilitated by the use of specific DNA probes.

8.3. Descriptive Epidemiology

8.3.1. Prevalence and Incidence. Because TCBS media is not routinely used by most medical microbiology laboratories, *Vibrio* infections are probably underdiagnosed in the United States. A year-long study in 1989 conducted by the CDC and the Gulf Coast *Vibrio* Working Group has provided the best data to date on the epidemiology of *Vibrio* infections in North America (see Table 9).[(96)] The incidence of *Vibrio* infections varied from 0.2 to 0.7 in/100,000 and was highest in the shoreline counties of Alabama and Louisiana (1.8 and 1.3 in 100,000, respectively). Among patients with gastroenteritis, *V. parahaemolyticus* had the highest incidence (26 cases) followed by nonepidemic *V. cholerae* (18 cases). *V. hollisae*, *V. fluvialis*, *V. mimicus*, and *V. vulnificus* were identified less often (8, 7, 4, and 3 cases, respectively).

8.3.2. Epidemic Behavior and Contagiousness. Nonepidemic *V. cholerae*, unlike *V. cholerae* O1 and O139, usually causes only sporadic illness rather than widespread epidemics. Nonetheless, two foodborne outbreaks have been described: one on an airplane flight in Australia[(97)] and the other in a technical school in Czechoslovakia.[(98)] The incubation period in these cases varied from 5 to 40 hr, with attack rates exceeding 60%. A waterborne outbreak has also been described.[(99)]

V. parahaemolyticus, on the other hand, frequently occurs in outbreaks. In Japan, where consumption of raw seafood is relatively common, this organism accounts for 25–60% of all foodborne outbreaks. In the United States,

Table 9. Patients with Illness Associated with *Vibrio* Species Reported from Five Gulf Coast States[a,b]

		Syndromes		Complications	
	No.	Gastroenteritis	Primary septicemia or wound infections	Hospitalization	Death
Patients with one species isolated					
V. alginolyticus	7	0	5 (12)	3 (5)	0
V. cholerae					
Non-O1	28	18 (25)	10 (23)	20 (30)	3 (33)
O1 Non-toxigenic	1	1 (1)	0	0	0
V. damsela	1	0	1 (2)	0	0
V. fluvialis	7	7 (10)	0	3 (5)	0
V. hollisae	9	8 (11)	1 (2)	2 (3)	0
V. mimicus	4	4 (6)	0	2 (3)	0
V. parahaemolyticus	33	26 (37)	7 (16)	20 (30)	2 (22)
V. vulnificus	18	3 (4)	15 (35)	15 (23)	4 (44)
Not specified	2	0	2 (5)	0	0
Patients with two species isolated	6	4 (6)	2 (5)	1 (2)	0
Total	116	71 (100)	43 (100)	66 (100)	9 (100)

[a]Adopted from Levine *et al.*[96]
[b]Data are numbers; percentages are given in parentheses.

where foodborne outbreaks are usually attributed to raw oyster consumption or the mishandling of seafood, 10 outbreaks involving 71 cases were reported to the CDC from 1982 to 1991 (see Tables 4 and 5). Secondary cases after outbreaks of *V. parahaemolyticus* appear to be uncommon.

Gastrointestinal infections with other *Vibrio* species have a much lower incidence, generally occurring as sporadic cases. One large-scale outbreak of *V. fluvialis* occurred in India in 1981.[100]

The incubation period for nonepidemic *V. cholerae* in the few documented outbreaks has been from 12 hr to 5 days.[101] After experimental infection with one strain of this bacterium, volunteers developed gastroenteritis in a median of 10 hr (range, 5.5 to 96 hr). The incubation period for *V. parahaemolyticus* is similar, varying from 4 to 30 hr, with most illness occurring 12 to 24 hr after exposure.

8.3.3. Geographic and Temporal Distribution. As noted above, vibrios are common environmental isolates throughout the world. Human illness due to vibrios shares a similar distribution, although patterns of illness vary from region to region. In Japan, for example, *V. parahaemolyticus* accounts for a large portion of foodborne outbreaks. Dietary habits (i.e., the consumption of raw seafood) undoubtedly play a role here. In the United States, where *Vibrio* infections are much less common, outbreaks and sporadic cases are concentrated along the Atlantic, Gulf, and Pacific coastlines. Raw oyster consumption is the most common risk factor.[96] In developing countries, where *Vibrio* infections are more likely to go undetected, seafood consumption is less commonly implicated as a risk factor for infection. In Cancun, Mexico, where a 2-month survey found nonepidemic *V. cholerae* in 16% of 134 stool samples obtained from persons with diarrhea, home-prepared gelatin was the only statistically significant risk factor in a case control study.[102] Environmental investigation suggested other possible sources of infection: The organism was obtained from 86% of untreated well water samples, 92% of sewage samples, and 21% of seafood samples. A waterborne outbreak of nonepidemic *V. cholerae* occurred in the Sudan in 1968, due to contamination of surface water next to a well.[99]

The incidence of noncholera *Vibrio* infections varies with season, being highest in the summer and fall. This is most likely a consequence of the higher numbers of vibrios in aquatic environments as well as in fish and shellfish harvested during these months.

8.3.4. Age, Sex, Race, and Other Host Factors. Host factors appear to play little role in the acquisition of gastroenteritis from *Vibrio* species. Factors such as sex or race have not shown any consistent correlation with disease. The median age of persons diagnosed with *Vibrio* gastroenteritis varies with geographic location: In Cancun, Mexico, for example, children less than 1 year of age were at highest risk, whereas in Bangladesh and Thailand cases have tended to occur in older children and adults.[102–104] A survey of 14 sporadic infections in the United States found a median age of 45 years, which may reflect the older age of the population that consumes raw oysters.[105]

In contrast to this, host factors play a major role in the epidemiology of sepsis due to *Vibrio* species. Most patients with sepsis due to *V. vulnificus* and nonepidemic *V. cholerae*, for example, have an underlying chronic medical illness. Those with liver disease, such as alcoholic cirrhosis or hemochromatosis, are especially at risk. Although it has never been shown conclusively that these infections are acquired through the gastrointestinal tract, their strong association with raw oyster consumption has always been cited as evidence to support this assertion.[90]

8.4. Mechanisms and Routes of Transmission

Foodborne transmission has been by far the most important route of transmission of noncholera vibrios in studies of epidemic and sporadic illness. As noted above, waterborne outbreaks have occurred, but are rare and are limited to the developing world. Person-to-person transmission may occur, but evidence for this is scant.

In the United States and Japan, noncholera *Vibrio* gastroenteritis is acquired almost exclusively via the foodborne route. Seafood, especially raw seafood, is the most common vehicle implicated in outbreaks and in sporadic disease. During the Gulf Coast *Vibrio* Working Group study, 91% of patients with gastroenteritis or primary septicemia had eaten shellfish or finfish during the week prior to their illness.[96] Raw oyster consumption was the single-most important food-related risk factor: Of all the patients with gastroenteritis, 74% had eaten raw oysters. Other seafood such as crabs and shrimp have been implicated in outbreaks in the United States. In Japan, most outbreaks of *V. parahaemolyticus* have been due to saltwater fish or to foods contaminated by seawater.[106]

Food-handling practices frequently play a role in outbreaks of noncholera vibrios. Seafood naturally contaminated with vibrios and held at an improper temperature can become heavily contaminated. *V. parahaemolyticus*, for example, has a generation time of 12 min under optimal circumstances and can increase its numbers by 1000-fold in 2 hr.[107] Likewise, already contaminated seafood may be cooked to an inadequate time–temperature combination sufficient to kill the organism. Finally, even uncontaminated or properly cooked seafood may be washed with contaminated salt water after preparation. The latter mechanism has been described in several outbreaks of *V. parahaemolyticus* abroad cruise ships.[108]

Because secondary transmission after outbreaks of noncholera vibrios is unusual, person-to-person transmission is thought not to be important in the epidemiology of these organisms. Long-term carriage has not been documented, though asymptomatic infections may be relatively common. From a cohort of 479 physicians attending a meeting in New Orleans who agreed to submit stool samples, 51 stool samples were positive for noncholera vibrios (*V. parahaemolyticus*, nonepidemic *V. cholerae*, *V. vulnificus*, *V. fluvialis*, and *V. mimicus*), of which 36 had been collected from individuals reporting no recent diarrheal illness.[109] In a large study conducted in Iran in 1971, 1.6% of pilgrims returning from Mecca were estimated to be carriers of nonepidemic *V. cholerae* (compared with 0.015% of persons leaving for Mecca). Isolations of this organism from stool cultures obtained from the contacts of these pilgrims increased over the following 6 months and decreased thereafter. Of these contacts, 60% reported diarrheal illness.[110]

8.5. Pathogenesis and Immunity

8.5.1. Pathogenesis

8.5.1a. Nonepidemic V. cholerae. Given the relatively low incidence of this infection and the relatively high prevalence of these organisms in foods such as oysters, it is likely that virulence factors play a role in the epidemiology of these infections. Three enterotoxins—cholera toxin (CT), NAG-ST, and El Tor hemolysin—have been described. CT-producing species have been isolated most commonly in the Indian subcontinent and are associated with more severe disease.[111] NAG-ST is a heat-stable enterotoxin similar to that of *E. coli* and *Yersinia enterocolitica*. A NAG-ST-producing strain has been demonstrated to cause diarrhea in young, previously healthy volunteers, whereas an otherwise similar but NAG-ST-negative strain was unable to do so despite being able to colonize the gastrointestinal tract.[112] As with CT-producing strains, NAG-ST-positive strains account for only a small portion of all clinical nonepidemic *V. cholerae* isolates.[113,114] El Tor hemolysin, on the other hand, is present in all nonepidemic *V. cholerae* strains and is responsible for the hemolytic activity of this species. This hemolysin also has demonstrable enterotoxic activity and may be responsible for the enterotoxic activity of CT-negative strains. However, El Tor hemolysin alone is not sufficient to produce illness. Strains producing this hemolysin that are able to colonize the intestine do not necessarily produce diarrhea.[112] The production of a polysaccharide capsule has been found in some strains, including almost all strains isolated from blood cultures. This capsule confers resistance to serum bactericidal activity.[115]

8.5.1b. V. parahaemolyticus. The pathogenicity of *V. parahaemolyticus* isolates has traditionally been correlated with the production of the thermostable direct hemolysin (Vp-TDH), which is responsible for the β-hemolysis seen when these isolates are plated on Wagatsuma agar. Original studies in Japan showed that this phenomenon, named the Kanagawa phenomenon after the prefecture in Japan where it was discovered, was noted in 96% of clinical isolates but only 1% of environmental isolates.(106) Volunteer studies also demonstrated the importance of Vp-TDH: Kanagawa-positive strains produced diarrhea, whereas doses of up to 10^9 Kanagawa-negative strains failed to do so in 15 volunteers.(115) Furthermore, studies with isogenic mutants have shown that deletion of the Vp-TDH gene results in loss of enterotoxic activity in laboratory models (Ussing chamber and rabbit ileal loop assays).(116)

In recent years, it has become clear that the pathogenesis of *V. parahaemolyticus* is more complicated than originally thought. A second group of hemolysins, known as Vp-TDH-related hemolysins or Vp-TRH, can be found in certain clinical isolates, especially those that are Kanagawa-negative. These hemolysins are genetically related to Vp-TDH (they share around 70% sequence homology) but are more diverse (<2.8% divergence among most Vp-TDH vs. 16% between two subgroups of Vp-TRH).(117) A third virulence factor, urease production, has recently been identified, and may be especially important in isolates from the Pacific coast of North America. Urease positive strains that are Kanagawa-negative and lack Vp-TDH and Vp-TRH genes have shown enteropathic activity in a ligated rabbit ileal loop model.(118)

V. parahaemolyticus can cause a dysenterylike syndrome, indicating that they may also produce illness by invasion of the intestinal wall. Limited animal studies support this assertion.(119)

8.5.2. Immunity. Multiple serotypes of *V. parahaemolyticus* can be isolated from a patient's stools, and frequently more than one strain is isolated from an incriminated food.(120) It is not known whether infection results in immunity or whether such immunity is serotype- or species-specific. The fortuitous occurrence of two outbreaks of *V. parahaemolyticus* during a single Caribbean cruise demonstrates that it is possible for infection to occur more than once in a given individual within a relatively short period of time (6 days).(108)

8.6. Patterns of Host Response

8.6.1. Nonepidemic *V. cholerae*. Three distinct clinical syndromes—gastroenteritis, wound infections, and primary septicemia—are seen with this group of organisms, as well as with *V. parahaemolyticus* and *V. vulnificus*.

The severity of gastroenteritis produced by this organism varies from asymptomatic colonization to heavy, choleralike purges. In studies of sporadic illness where cases that have been identified retrospectively on the basis of stool cultures, illness has been relatively severe. Among 14 sporadic cases identified in a study in the United States, the median duration of illness was 6.4 days.(105) All of these patients had diarrhea, 71% had fever, but only 21% had nausea and vomiting. One quarter of these patients had bloody diarrhea. In a group of 19 sporadic cases in Bangladesh, the median stool volume was less than 1 liter, with a maximum of 8 liters; the median duration of illness was less than 24 hr, with a maximum of 2.5 days.(121) Experimental infections in normal volunteers and cases identified through outbreak investigations have shown less severe illness, with median durations of 12 to 24 hr and with diarrhea generally lasting less than 4 days.(101)

Septicemia with nonepidemic *V. cholerae* generally occurs in immunocompromised patients, particularly those with liver disease or hematologic malignancies. The case fatality rate among reported cases has been over 50%. Strains responsible for septicemia have been uniformly found to be heavily encapsulated.

Nonepidemic *V. cholerae* have been isolated from wounds, ears, sputum, urine, and cerebrospinal fluid. In many of these cases, a variety of other potential pathogens have also been isolated from the same site, making it uncertain that the nonepidemic *V. cholerae* was the true pathogen.(101)

8.6.2. *V. parahaemolyticus*. *V. parahaemolyticus* produces a spectrum of illness very similar to that of nonepidemic *V. cholerae*. Gastroenteritis is the most common syndrome, with diarrhea (98%), abdominal cramps (82%), nausea (71%), and fever (27%).(122) Bloody stools were noted in 35% of cases in the Gulf Coast *Vibrio* Working Group study,(96) as well as in cases in India and Bangladesh. In both the United States and Japan, illness tends to be mild, with a median duration of 3 days and a very low case-fatality rate. Outbreaks of severe gastrointestinal illness have been reported. Hypotension and shock occurred in three of five cases in one outbreak in Great Britain,(123) and there were 20 deaths among the 272 patients involved in the Japanese outbreak where *V. parahaemolyticus* was first identified.(124)

V. parahaemolyticus also causes infection in wounds exposed to seawater. Such infections can disseminate and cause sepsis. Primary septicemia has also been reported, but is not seen as commonly as with *V. vulnificus* or nonepidemic *V. cholerae*.

8.6.3. Other Pathogenic *Vibrio* Species. *V. fluvialis*, *V. furnissii*, *V. hollisae*, and *V. mimicus* all cause gastroenteritis. In the Gulf Coast study, *V. fluvialis* was particularly likely to produce bloody diarrhea (six of seven cases).[96]

The principal clinical manifestations of *V. vulnificus* include primary septicemia and wound infections. One third of patients with primary septicemia present in shock; 70–90% have characteristic bullous skin lesions. The mortality rate for persons with primary septicemia exceeds 50%. For patients who present in shock, mortality exceeds 90%. Survivors often have multiple organ system failure, requiring protracted hospitalization and rehabilitation. Wound infections range from mild, self-limited infections to severe, rapidly progressive myositis and fasciitis.[90]

9. *Aeromonas* Species

9.1. History

Microbiologists have studied aeromonads for over a century. Sanarelli was the first to observe these organisms, which he had isolated from a frog in 1891 and named *Bacillus hydrophilus*.[125] Although early studies showed that direct inoculation produced septicemia and death in animals, the role of these organisms as human pathogens was not recognized until the 1960s. Interest in aeromonads grew considerably with the first publication in 1968 of a review of 28 cases of human *Aeromonas* infections.[126] Although work since then has confirmed the pathogenicity of these organisms, doubt still remains as to the role of aeromonads in gastroenteritis. Even more confusion has been generated by taxonomy of this genus, which has undergone considerable changes in the past 20 years.

9.2. Microbiology

9.2.1. Biological Characteristics of the Organism. Aeromonads are facultatively anaerobic, gram-negative rods with single polar flagella. Species that are pathogenic in humans are oxidase-positive, catalase-positive, and reduce nitrate to nitrite. All ferment D-glucose and most will produce gas in doing so (hence their name). *Aeromonas* species can be divided into two groups: mesophiles, which grow well in a wide variety of temperatures (0 to 40°C), and psychrophiles, which grow only at lower temperatures (less than 35 to 37°C). Species in this latter group are not pathogenic in humans but can cause disease in cold-blooded vertebrates.[127]

The taxonomy of the *Aeromonas* genus, which until the mid-1970s was thought to consist of three species, has become complex, with more than 13 species now known to exist. The application of DNA hybridization techniques has led to the division of some phenotypic species (such as *A. sobria*) into two or more separate genomic species (*A. veronii*, *A. jandaei*, and *A. schubertii*, in this case).[128] Of *Aeromonas* species, three—*A. hydrophila*, *A. caviae*, and *A. veronii* biotype sobria—account for more than 85% of all clinical isolates from humans.[128–130] Another three—*A. jandaei*, *A. schubertii*, and *A. trota*—have also been implicated in human disease. Because of their phenotypic similarities, the genera *Aeromonas* and *Vibrio* have been placed into a single family (*Vibrionaceae*) along with one other genus, *Plesiomonas*. A growing body of genetic evidence suggests, on the other hand, that *Aeromonas* is so distinct from genera in other families including *Vibrionaceae* or *Enterobacteraceae* that it should constitute its own family, *Aeromonadaceae*.[131]

The ecology of aeromonads is similar to that of *Vibrio* species. They are autochthonous (free-living) organisms that can be isolated from freshwater, brackish water, and occasionally from seawater. Their numbers vary seasonally, being highest during the warmer months of May through November.

9.2.2. Laboratory Diagnosis. *Aeromonas* species are hardy organisms and will grow on a large variety of media, though they may be overlooked on certain semiselective media such as Hektoen enteric or MacConkey agars because some are sucrose-positive (most *Aeromonas* species) or lactose-positive (*A. caviae*). Blood agar has the advantage of allowing easy testing of colonies for oxidase and indole production and also permits the identification of hemolytic species (*A. hydrophila* and *A. veronii*).[132] The addition of ampicillin makes this medium more specific, but excludes 5–10% of *Aeromonas* species (including all *A. trota*) that are ampicillin-susceptible. Cefsulodin–irgasan–novobiocin (CIN) agar, which is commonly used for *Yersinia enterocolitica*, has also been shown to be useful for *Aeromonas*.[133] Selective enrichment on alkaline peptone water (pH 8.5) is useful for stools obtained after the acute phase of the illness, when numbers of viable organisms have usually dropped considerably.

Phenotypic species identification can be difficult in the case of *Aeromonas*: most commercially available kits are inadequate for this.[134] In outbreak investigations or for unusual clinical cases, genospecies identification should be attempted.[135] Serotyping may be useful in epidemiologic investigations.[136,137]

9.3. Descriptive Epidemiology

Perhaps the most debated topic in the epidemiology of *Aeromonas* species is whether these organisms are, in fact, true gastrointestinal pathogens. Despite more than three decades of research, definitive evidence in support of this has remained elusive. In support of their pathogenicity are several lines of evidence:

1. *Aeromonas* species are frequently isolated from stools of patients with diarrhea and, in some studies, have been the most frequently isolated potential pathogen.[125,138]
2. Several case–control studies have shown a significant association between the isolation of *Aeromonas* in stool and the presence of diarrhea. The most convincing of these has been an Australian study in which 10.8% of 1156 symptomatic children had enterotoxigenic aeromonads in their stool compared with 0.6% of age- and sex-matched controls.[139]
3. A number of case reports have described clinical resolution of *Aeromonas*-associated diarrhea with concomitant clearance of the organism from stools following treatment with antibiotics to which *Aeromonas* is susceptible.[140–143]
4. Serum IgM and IgG as well as fecal IgA antibodies against *Aeromonas* rise during the convalescent phase of *Aeromonas*-associated diarrhea.[144–146]
5. Several enterotoxins are elaborated by *Aeromonas* species (see below).

Despite this evidence, a number of findings shed doubt of the role of *Aeromonas* as a gastrointestinal pathogen:

1. Aeromonads can be found in up to 8% of asymptomatic individuals. Furthermore, although some studies have shown that *Aeromonas* is more common in stools of symptomatic patients, several studies have found *Aeromonas* to be equally common in asymptomatic individuals.[138]
2. Other potential pathogens are often found in stools testing positive for *Aeromonas*, suggesting that *Aeromonas* may simply be a nonpathogenic marker of diarrheal illness. Although most studies have found dual infection in only a small minority of cases, others have found this phenomenon in up to 50% of the stools from which *Aeromonas* was isolated.[147]
3. In contrast to other foodborne or waterborne pathogens such as *Plesiomonas shigelloides* or *Vibrio* species, no confirmed point source outbreaks of *Aeromonas* have been reported. In two reported day-care center outbreaks of *Aeromonas*-associated diarrhea, *Aeromonas* strains could only be isolated from a minority of the children and showed considerable phenotypic and genotypic heterogeneity.[148]
4. Volunteer studies using toxigenic *Aeromonas* strains, in which doses as high as 10^{10} CFU were given to volunteers, have been inconclusive. In one such study, only 2 of 57 volunteers developed diarrhea.[149]
5. A successful animal model of *Aeromonas* gastroenteritis has not been found.
6. Although the demonstrable immune response to *Aeromonas* that occurs after infection suggests pathogenicity, it does not prove this. Similar immune responses can be detected in volunteers after being challenged with nonpathogenic *V. cholera* strains that colonize the intestinal tract without causing illness.[112]

Whether or not *Aeromonas* is a true gastrointestinal pathogen, some generalizations can be made about its isolation in humans. Isolation from stool and from extraintestinal sites (predominantly blood and wounds) is more common in the warmer months of the year when aeromonads are present in higher numbers in the environment.[125] *Aeromonas*-associated diarrhea is more common in children, especially those less than 3 years old. The isolation rate of *Aeromonas* in studies of gastrointestinal pathogens ranges from less than 1% (Netherlands and France) to 50% (children in Peru). This rate is lowest in industrialized countries (such as France and the Netherlands) and is highest in developing countries (15% in Bali, 24%in the Ivory Coast), indicating that sanitary conditions may be one determining factor in the epidemiology of this infection. In the United States, surveys have found isolation rates of 2.5–75% in patients with diarrhea.

In California, where reporting of *Aeromonas* infections has been mandatory since 1988, a recent review showed the annual incidence to be 1.1 per 100,000 in all age groups combined and around 5 per 100,000 for children less than 2 years old.[150] The most common site of isolation was the gastrointestinal tract (85%), followed by wounds (9%).

9.4. Mechanisms and Routes of Transmission

The source of gastrointestinal *Aeromonas* infections has been difficult to elucidate because of the lack of confirmed outbreaks. *Aeromonas* was found in food samples taken from investigations of three separate outbreaks in the United Kingdom associated with the consumption of cooked prawns or oysters[151]; *Aeromonas* was also grown from a frozen specimen of oysters implicated in a large (472 cases) outbreak of diarrhea in Louisiana in 1982.[152] Unfortunately, stool specimens from the patients involved in these outbreaks were either not tested for *Aeromonas* or tested negative. In another oyster-associated outbreak in the United States and in one raw-fish-associated outbreak in Japan.[153] *Aeromonas* was isolated from both fecal and food specimens; unfortunately, no serotyping was performed on these isolates. Given the high prevalence of aeromonads in foods, such reports have to be viewed with skepticism.

Studies of sporadic *Aeromonas* infections have revealed different risk factors. One study in the United States found consumption of untreated well water to be associated with this infection[142]; a second study found both untreated well water and prior antibiotic therapy to be risk factors.[154]

9.5. Pathogenesis and Immunity

Two categories of virulence factors are believed to play a role in the pathogenesis of *Aeromonas*: colonization factors and exotoxin production. Flexible pili, which are morphologically distinct from the more numerous rigid pili, likely play a role in colonization. The subunit of these structures shares 91% amino acid sequence homology with subunits of a *V. cholerae* pili that has been implicated as a factor important for colonization by that species. *Aeromonas* isolates, especially those obtained from clinical specimens, secrete a number of exotoxins.[138,155] The best characterized of these is the "aerolysin," which is a β-hemolysin with enterotoxic activity.[156]

9.6. Patterns of Host Response

Gastroenteritis, the most frequent clinical syndrome attributed to *Aeromonas*, varies considerably in severity and is usually self-limited.[141,142,157–160] Watery diarrhea, with a median of eight bowel movements per day, is often associated with abdominal pain (60–70%), vomiting (20–40%), and fever (20–40%). The diarrhea is occasionally so severe that it resembles cholera, with up to 40 stools per day. A minority of patients with *Aeromonas* gastroenteritis will develop a dysenteric syndrome resembling shigellosis, with blood and mucus in the stools. Children with this form of illness often require hospitalization. There have also been descriptions of a third, much less common syndrome of subacute or chronic diarrhea lasting for more than 10 days and up to several years.[161] Reports of successful antibiotic treatment of patients with this syndrome lend support to the notion that *Aeromonas* is a true gastrointestinal pathogen.

Wound infections, the second most common clinical manifestation due to *Aeromonas*, usually (but not invariably) occur after exposure of open wounds to environmental water sources.[162,163] Cellulitis is the most common pattern and is readily treated with antibiotics. More severe infections can occur even in immunocompetent individuals, including myonecrosis with gas formation that is rapidly fatal without aggressive treatment.

In immunocompromised individuals, especially those with hepatobiliary disease, bacteremia has been described as well as other forms of invasive disease such as bacterial peritonitis. Other clinical syndromes reported in the literature include osteomyelitis, ocular infections, pelvic infections, and pneumonia.[125,164]

10. *Plesiomonas*

10.1. History

Plesiomonas was first described by Ferguson and Henderson[165] in 1947, who noted that the properties of this organism resembled those of *Shigella*. Originally named simply "C27," this species was later placed variously in the genera *Pseudomonas*, *Fergusonia*, *Scatamonas*, *Vibrio*, and *Aeromonas*, until 1962, when it was definitely placed into a genus by itself, *Plesiomonas*.[166] The name is derived from the Greek word for "neighbor" and was chosen because of the close relationship that was thought to exist between this genus and the genus *Aeromonas*.

10.2. Microbiology

10.2.1. Biological Characteristics of the Organism. *Plesiomonas shigelloides*, the only species in this genus, bears many similarities to *Aeromonas*. They are also facultative anaerobic, gram-negative rods that are positive for oxidase, catalase, and nitrite reduction. They are highly motile by means of two to five polar flagella. Although they ferment D-glucose, they do not produce gas in doing so. The species name, *shigelloides*, is due to its antigenic similarity to *Shigella* species, especially *S. sonnei*.[127] As with *Aeromonas*, controversy exists as to its taxonomy. Recent genetic studies, which indicate this organism is much closer to *Proteus* species than to any *Vibrionaceae*, have led to a proposal to move this genus into the family *Enterobacteraceae*.[167]

Plesiomonas shigelloides is primarily a freshwater organism, though it can also be found in estuaries and can occasionally be isolated from seawater. It can also be recovered from sediments, fish, shellfish, and occasionally in the feces of asymptomatic cold-blooded and warm-blooded animals.

10.2.2. Laboratory Diagnosis. Like *Aeromonas*, *Plesiomonas* will grow on a large variety of media including blood agar with ampicillin. In addition, inositol–brilliant green–bile salts agar is particularly useful, since this species, unlike most enteric organisms, can use inositol as a carbon source.[168] Selective enrichment in alkaline peptone water is also useful for *Plesiomonas* in certain situations. A serotyping system is available for epidemiological investigations.[169]

10.3. Descriptive Epidemiology

Whether *Plesiomonas shigelloides* is in fact a true enteropathogen has also remained in doubt. As with *Aeromonas* species, no animal model has proved successful and volunteer studies have failed to produce clinical illness. Moreover, there appears to be no secretory IgA response after natural *Plesiomonas* infections, as can be demonstrated with *Aeromonas*.[145] Nonetheless, as with *Aeromonas*, there is considerable evidence supporting the role of *Plesiomonas* as an enteropathogen. When asymptomatic controls have been studied, carriage rates have usually been low (<1%). In most reported cases of gastrointestinal disease. *Plesiomonas* has been the predominant organism in the stool. Other pathogens are generally not found when sought. Several case reports have noted clinical improvement and disappearance of *Plesiomonas* from stool cultures after treatment with antibiotics to which *Plesiomonas* is susceptible.[170,171] In further support of the enteropathogenic role of *Plesiomonas*, two outbreaks have been identified in which predominant serotypes (O17:H2 in one, O24:H5 in another) have been identified.[172]

The incidence of *Plesiomonas*-associated diarrhea is unknown. In a study of stool specimens submitted to a Canadian reference laboratory, the isolation rate was similar to that of *Aeromonas* (25 out of 17,820 specimens).[171]

10.4. Mechanisms and Routes of Transmission

Several possible *Plesiomonas*-related outbreaks have been reported, mostly from Japan. The most common vehicles implicated are raw or undercooked fish or shellfish. Chicken was also implicated in one outbreak and drinking water was implicated in two others.

Raw seafood has been also frequently implicated in sporadic *Plesiomonas* gastroenteritis, as has foreign travel.[170,171] In a case–control study of sporadic illness, published by the CDC, both of these factors were correlated with infection ($p<0.001$ for both); 21 of the 31 cases had one of both of these risk factors.[170]

10.5. Pathogenesis and Immunity

Little is known about virulence factors in *Plesiomonas*. No colonization factors such as pili have yet been described. A β-hemolysin has recently been found and is reported to be present in more than 90% of isolates.[173] This hemolysin may have enterotoxic activity similar to that of aerolysin and may be important in making iron available to the bacteria.

10.6. Patterns of Host Response

The clinical manifestations of enteric *Plesiomonas* infections are similar to those of *Aeromonas*.[170,171,174] Watery diarrhea is the most common form, with abdominal pain and sometimes with vomiting or fever. A majority of the patients in one review noted frank blood or mucus in their stool, although this may have been a result of the study's bias toward detecting more severe cases.[170] Prolonged diarrhea (up to 3 months) has been described; this responds well to appropriate antibiotic treatment.

Many forms of extraintestinal infection have been reported. Meningitis is the most common of these and is usually seen in neonates. Septicemia and bacterial peritonitis have been reported in adults, especially those with cirrhosis or who are otherwise immunocompromised. Septic arthritis, endophthalmitis, and cellulitis have been described.[174]

11. Control and Prevention

11.1. General Concepts

11.1.1. Food Safety Regulation in the United States. The USDA and Health and Human Services (HHS) are the two primary government departments charged with protecting the food supply. The Food Safety and Inspection Service (FSIS), USDA, regulates the safety of meat and poultry products largely through an inspection system that began in 1906 and relies heavily on the visual examination of carcasses. To update the inspection system, FSIS has initiated major changes, including a requirement that the meat and poultry industry produce food products using a system known as HACCP (hazard analysis and critical control points). The FDA, HHS, with jurisdiction over the majority of other food products not regulated by FSIS, also endorses the HACCP system. Legislation was enacted in December 1995 by the FDA requiring the use of HACCP in certain seafood processing operations.

The HACCP system provides a rational approach to the control of microbial hazards in food. First presented at the 1971 National Conference on Food Protection, the HACCP system consists of (1) identification and assessment of hazards associated with growing harvesting, processing, marketing, preparation, and use of a given raw material or food product; (2) determination of critical control points to control any identifiable hazard; and (3) establishment of systems to monitor critical control points.[175] Under the HACCP system, food products are monitored by industry and government personnel, including microbiological testing, visual examination, and other appropriate means to ensure safe food.

Some food products, like eggs, are covered by multiple jurisdictions. State, county, and local health departments have jurisdiction over food preparation facilities, such as restaurants, cafeterias, and other places where food is prepared for public consumption.

11.1.2. Methods to Further Reduce Foodborne Bacterial Disease

11.1.2a. Control of Pathogens in Animal Reservoirs. For zoonotic pathogens such as *Salmonella*, *Campylobacter*, and enterohemorrhagic *E. coli* that colonize the gastrointestinal tracts of animals without causing illness, eradication may be difficult. However, it may be possible to reduce the prevalence of these organisms on farms and in individual animals. As more is learned about the ecology of these organisms, better control measures can be instituted. For example, epidemiological studies have shown that *Campylobacter* may be introduced into chicken houses through contaminated water. Therefore, use of chlorinated water may decrease the prevalence of *Campylobacter*. Vaccination of chickens against *Campylobacter* may be another useful intervention.

Other foodborne pathogens have been successfully controlled or eliminated in animal reservoirs. A brucellosis eradication program by the USDA eliminated *Brucella melitensis* from sheep and has markedly decreased the prevalence of *B. abortis* in cattle. Other opportunities to control pathogens in animals include controlling breeding stock, using effective vaccines, and implementing other on-farm controls to decrease carriage of pathogens.

11.1.2b. Control of Pathogens during Food Production. A number of innovative approaches are currently being used to prevent or minimize contamination of meat, poultry, and seafood by pathogens. The major source of pathogens on meat and poultry is the gastrointestinal tract of animals, although environmental organisms can also be found on these foods. Table 10 shows results of a microbiological survey of raw meat products conducted by the USDA. For fish and other seafood, which frequently must be harvested under difficult conditions and at varying distances from processing, transport, and retail facilities, contamination may be from numerous sources, including the environment. In animal slaughter establishments, several methods are being used to reduce microbial contamination on carcass surfaces, including washing exterior surfaces of carcasses prior to slaughter, steam vacuuming of carcass surfaces during slaughter, and applying antimicrobial treatments to carcass surfaces immediately after slaughter. Meat, poultry, and seafood processors are constantly reviewing their operations to reduce processing errors that cause product contamination. The HACCP system, discussed in Section 11.1.1, will provide these industries with an effective means of minimizing potential hazards that could lead to pathogen contamination of food products.

11.1.2c. Improvement of Food-handling Practices. Food-handling errors frequently contribute to foodborne illness, allowing pathogens already present on foods to multiply to levels sufficient to cause illness. Such errors identified in outbreak investigations during a 15-year period included improper holding temperature (87%), poor personal hygiene (59%), inadequate cooking (56%), and contaminated equipment (47%).[5]

Pathogens on raw food products are the major source of foodborne illness. Persons handling and preparing raw food products, including the producer, processors, food service personnel, and the public, must have the knowledge necessary to control microbial hazards. The level of knowledge needed by each group depends on the role it plays in the overall process. In homes and food service establishments especially, it must be emphasized that improper food-handling practices, such as leaving foods in ovens at low temperatures or at room temperatures, or placing food in large containers prior to chilling, result in foodborne illness.[176]

Targeting specific education programs for persons at high risk should be a part of any consumer education program. For example, pregnant women should be ad-

Table 10. Prevalence of Various Pathogens Sampled at Slaughter Plants in the United States[a]

	Product sampled			
Pathogen	Steer/heifer carcasses (2089 samples)	Raw ground beef (563 samples)	Raw ground chicken (162 samples)	Raw ground turkey (165 samlpes)
C. perfringens	2.6%	18.8%	39%	27%
S. aureus	4.2%	30.5%	76%	49%
L. monocytogenes	4.1%	18.0%	35%	23%
C. jejuni/C. coli	4.0%	0.2%	60%	22%
E. coli O157:H7	0.2%	0%	0%	0%
Salmonella	1.0%	4.3%	38%	27%

vised of the potential risk of acquiring listeriosis from consuming certain soft cheeses. Persons with liver disease should be advised to avoid eating raw seafood. Immunocompromised persons, such as those undergoing cancer chemotherapy or those who have AIDS should be advised to avoid specific foods and take extra precautions in food handling and preparation.

Numerous publications are available from the FDA, FSIS, and other federal, state, and local government agencies on proper food handling. Educators, trainers, and organizations developing education and training materials for food workers and consumers may obtain information from the Foodborne Illness Education Information Center. The center, which is housed at the National Agriculture Library, USDA, in Beltsville, Maryland, was established jointly by the USDA and FDA as part of a national campaign to reduce the risk of foodborne illness.

11.2. Antibiotics and Chemotherapeutics

Antibiotics generally have no role in prevention of foodborne illness and in some cases may predispose individuals to infection with gastrointestinal pathogens. Occasionally, treatment of persons infected with such pathogens as *Shigella* may be warranted in order to prevent secondary transmission.

11.3. Immunizations

Immunizations, with few exceptions, have little role in the control of foodborne illness. Typhoid fever, which may be spread through the foodborne route, is readily preventable through vaccination (see chapter 42). New oral attenuated cholera vaccines show great promise, but are not widely available (see Chapter 11). Vaccination against β-toxin has proved successful in controlling pigbel in Papua New Guinea.

12. Unresolved Problems

The largest unresolved problem in this group of foodborne illnesses is determining the pathogens that make up the 45% of foodborne disease outbreaks with "unknown" etiology. While some of these outbreaks may be due to known pathogens, others surely await recognition. Also, the emergence of new pathogenic strains will continue to challenge the medical and public health communities; *E. coli* O157:H7 is an excellent example of this.

Underreporting of disease is another serious public health problem. Because most persons regard diarrhea as an inconvenience rater than a symptom of disease, the vast majority of diarrheal episodes do not result in visits to physicians, even though persons may be incapacitated for several days. For this reason, assessments of the impact of foodborne illness have always relied heavily on estimates and assumptions. One CDC study estimated that diarrhea causes 25 million illnesses and 10,000 deaths each year in the United States.(177) Another study attributed 80 million illnesses annually to foodborne diseases in the United States.(178) The CDC estimates that foodborne disease costs 19.5 billion dollars annually in lost productivity.(179) The CDC, FDA, and USDA are collecting data at five sentinel sites in the United States in an effort to obtain more precise estimates of numbers of cases, trends, and incidences of foodborne illness (see Section 3.2).

13. References

1. Bean, N. H., Goulding, J. S., Lao, C., and Angulo, F. J., Surveillance for food-borne disease outbreaks—United States, 1988–1992, *Morbid. Mortal. Week. Rep.* **45:**(ss–5) (1996).
2. MacDonald, K. L., and Griffin, P. M., Foodborne disease outbreaks, annual summary, 1982, *Morbid. Mortal. Week. Rep.* **35:**7SS–16SS (1986).
3. Bean, N. H., Griffin, P. M., Goulding, J. S., and Ivey, C. B., Foodborne disease outbreaks, 5-year summary, 1983–1987, *Morbid. Mortal. Week. Rep.* **39**(SS-1)**:**15–57 (1990).
5. Bean, N. H., and Griffin, P. M., Foodborne disease outbreaks in the United States, 1973–1987: Pathogens, vehicles, and trends, *J. Food Prot.* **53:**804–817 (1990).
6. Chalker, R. B., and Blaser, M. J., A review of human salmonellosis: III. Magnitude of *Salmonella* infection in the United States, *Rev. Infect. Dis.* **10:**111–124 (1988).
7. Bryan, F.L., Epidemiology of foodborne diseases, in: *Foodborne Infections and Intoxications* (H. Reimann and F. L. Bryan, eds.), pp. 3–69, Academic Press, New York, 1979.
8. Dack, G. M., Cary, W. E., Woolpert, O., and Wiggers, H., An outbreak of food poisoning proved to be due to a yellow hemolytic *Staphylococcus*, *J. Prev. Med.* **4:**167–175 (1930).
9. Dack, G. M., *Staphylococcus* food poisoning, in: *Food Poisoning* (G. M. Dack, ed.), pp. 109–158, University of Chicago Press, Chicago, 1956.
10. Dolman, C. E., and Wilson, R. J., Experiments with staphylococcal enterotoxin, *J. Immunol.* **35:**13–30 (1938).
11. Surgalla, M. J., Bergdoll, M. S., and Dack, G. M., Use of antigen–antibody reaction in agar to follow the progress of fractionation of antigenic mixtures: Application to purification of staphylococcal enterotoxin, *J. Immunol.* **72:**398–402 (1954).
12. Bergdoll, M. S., *Staphylococcus aureus*, in: *Foodborne Bacterial pathogens* (M. P. Doyle, ed.), pp. 463–523, Marcel Dekker, New York, 1989.
13. Sullivan, R., and Asano, T., Effects of staphylococcal enterotoxin B on intestinal transport in the rat, *Am. J. Physiol.* **222:**1793–1799 (1971).
14. Breckinridge, J. C., and Bergdoll, M. S., Outbreak of foodborne

gastroenteritis due to a coagulase-negative enterotoxin-producing staphylococcus, *N. Engl. J. Med.* **25:**541–543 (1971).

15. Baird, R. M., and Lee, W. H., Media used in the detection and enumeration of *Staphylococcus aureus*, *Int. J. Food Microbiol.* **26:**15–24 (1995).
16. Park, C. E., Akhtar, M., and Rayman, M. K., Nonspecific reactions of a commercial enzyme-linked immunosorbent assay kit (TECRA) for detection of staphylococcal enterotoxins in foods, *Appl. Environ. Microbiol.* **58:**2509–2512 (1992).
17. Wieneke, A. A., Comparison of four kits for the detection of staphylococcal enterotoxin in foods from outbreaks of food poisoning, *Int. J. Food Microbiol.* **14:**305–312 (1991).
18. Park, C. E., Akhtar, M., and Rayman, M. K., Evaluation of a commercial enzyme immunoassay kit (RIDASCREEN) for detection of staphylococcal enterotoxins A, B, C, D, and E in foods, *Appl. Environ. Microbiol.* **60:**677–681.
19. Orden, J. A., Goyache, J., Hernandez, J., *et al.*, Applicability of an immunoblot technique combined with a semiautomated electrophoresis system for detection of staphylococcal enterotoxins in food extracts, *Appl. Environ. Microbiol.* **58:**4083–4085 (1992).
20. Evenson, M. L., Hinds, W. M., Bernstein, R. S., and Bergdoll, M. S., Estimation of human dose of staphylococcal enterotoxin A from a large outbreak of staphylococcal food poisoning involving chocolate milk, *Int. J. Food Microbiol.* **7:**311–316 (1988).
21. Neill, R. J., Fanning, G. R., Delahoz, F., *et al.*, Oligonucleotide probes for detection and differentiation of *Staphylococcus aureus* strains containing genes for enterotoxins A, B, and C and toxic shock syndrome toxin 1, *J. Clin. Microbiol.* **28:**1514–1518 (1990).
22. Wieneke, A. A., Roberts, D., and Gilbert, R. J., Staphylococcal food poisoning in the United Kingdom, 1969–90, *Epidemiol. Infect.* **110:**519–531 (1993).
23. Holmberg, S. D., and Blake, P. A., Staphylococcal food poisoning in the United States, new facts and old misconceptions, *J. Am. Med. Assoc.* **251:**487–489 (1984).
24. Reagan, D. R., Doebbeling, B. N., Pfaller, M. A., *et al.*, Elimination of coincident *Staphylococcus aureus* nasal and hand carriage with intranasal application of mupirocin calcium ointment, *Ann. Intern. Med.* **114:**101–106 (1992).
25. Minor, T. E., and March, E. H., *Staphylococcus aureus* and staphylococcal food poisoning, *J. Milk Food Technol.* **35:**447–476 (1973).
26. Gilbert, R. J., Staphylococcal food poisoning and botulism, *Postgrad. Med. J.* **50:**603–611 (1974).
27. Dack, G. M., Jordan, E. O., and Woolpert, O., Attempts to immunize human volunteers with *Staphylococcus* filtrates that are toxic to man when swallowed, *J. Prev. Med.* **5:**151–159 (1931).
28. Weed, L. A., Michael, A. C., and Harger, R. A., Fatal staphylococcus intoxication from goat milk, *Am. J. Public Health* **33:** 1314–1318 (1943).
29. Lubenau, C., *Bacillus peptonificans* als Erreger einer Gastroenteritis-Epidemic, *Zentralb. Bacteriol. Parasitenkd. infectionskr. Hyg. Abt.* **40:**433–437 (1906).
30. Hauge, S., Food poisoning caused by aerobic spore-forming bacilli, *J. Appl. Bacteriol.* **18:**591–595 (1955).
31. Midura, T., Gerber, M., Wood, R., and Leonard, A. R., Outbreak of food poisoning caused by *Bacillus cereus*, *Public Health Rep.* **85:**45–48 (1970).
32. Mortimer, P. R., and McCann, G., Food poisoning episodes associated with *Bacillus cereus* in fried rice, *Lancet* **1:**1043–1045 (1974).
33. Goepfert, J. M., Spira, W. M., and Kim, H. U., *Bacillus cereus*: Food poisoning organism: A review, *J. Milk Food Technol.* **35:**213–227 (1972).
34. Spira, W. M., and Goepfert, J. M., Biological characteristics of an enterotoxin produced by *Bacillus cereus*, *Can. J. Microbiol.* **21:**1236–1246 (1975).
35. Kramer, J. M., and Gilbert, R. J., *Bacillus cereus*, in: *Foodborne Bacterial Pathogens* (M. P. Doyle, ed.), pp. 21–70, Marcel Dekker, New York, 1989.
36. Melling, J., Capel, B. J., Turnbull, P. C. B., and Gilbert, R. J., Identification of a novel enterotoxigenic activity associated with *Bacillus cereus*, *J. Clin. Pathol.* **29:**938–940 (1976).
37. Kim, H. U., and Goepfert, J. M., Occurrence of *Bacillus cereus* in selected dry food products, *J. Milk Food Technol.* **34:**12–15 (1971).
38. Mossel, D. A., Koopman, M. J., and Jongerius, E., Enumeration of *Bacillus cereus* in foods, *Appl. Microbiol.* **15:**650–653 (1967).
39. Kim, H. U., and Goepfert, J. M., Efficacy of a fluorescent-antibody procedure for identifying *Bacillus cereus* in foods, *Appl. Microbiol.* **24:** 708–713 (1972).
40. Jackson, S. G., Rapid screening test for enterotoxin-producing *Bacillus cereus*, *J. Clin. Microbiol.* **31:**972–974 (1993).
41. Turnbull, P., Kramer, J., Jorgensen, K., *et al.*, Properties and production characteristics of vomiting, diarrheal, and necrotizing toxins of *Bacillus cereus*, *Am. J. Nutr.* **32:**219–228 (1979).
42. Becker, H., Schaller, G., von Wiese, W., and Terplan, G., *Bacillus cereus* in infant foods and dried milk products, *Int. J. Food Microbiol.* **23:**1–15 (1994).
43. Bodnar, S., Uber durch *Bacillus cereus* verursachte Lebensmittelvergiftungen, *Z. Gesamte. Hyg.* **8:**368–372 (1962).
44. Terranova, W., and Blake, P. A., *Bacillus cereus* food poisoning, *N. Engl. J. Med.* **298:**143–144 (1978).
45. Gilbert, R. J., and Parry, J. M., Serotypes of *Bacillus cereus* from outbreaks of food poisoning and from routine foods, *J. Hyg.* **78:**69–74 (1977).
46. Gilbert, R. J., Stringer, M. F., and Peace, T. C., The survival and growth of *Bacillus cereus* in boiled and fried rice in relation to outbreaks of food poisoning, *J. Hyg.* **73:**433–444 (1974).
47. Bryan, F. L., Bartleson, C. A., and Christopherson, N., Hazard analyses, in reference to *Bacillus cereus*, of boiled and fried rice in Cantonese-style restaurants, *J. Food Prot.* **44:**500–512 (1981).
48. Turnbull, P. C., *Bacillus cereus* toxins, *Pharmacol. Ther.* **13:**453–505 (1981).
49. Turnbull, P. C., and Kramer, J. M., Intestinal carriage of *Bacillus cerreus*: Faecal isolation studies in three population groups, *J. Hyg.* **95:**629–638 (1985).
50. Ghosh, A. C., Prevalence of *Bacillus cereus* in the feces of healthy adults, *J. Hyg.* **80:**233–236 (1978).
51. Taylor, A., and Gilbert, R., *Bacillus cereus* food poisoning: A provisional serotyping scheme, *J. Med. Microbiol.* **8:**543–550 (1975).
52. Ahmed, R., Sankar-Mistry, P., Jackson, S., *et al.*, *Bacillus cereus* phage typing as an epidemiological tool in outbreaks of food poisoning, *J. Clin. Microbiol.* **33:**636–640 (1995).
53. McClung, L. S., Human food poisoning due to growth of *Clostridium perfringens* (*Cl. welchii*) in freshly cooked chicken: A preliminary note, *J. Bacteriol.* **50:**229–233 (1945).
54. Knox, K., and MacDonald, E. K., Outbreak of food poisoning in certain Leicester institutions, *Med. Off.* **69:**21–24 (1943).
55. Gravits, L., and Gilmore, J. D., Project I-756, Report No. 2, US Naval Medical Research Institute, Bethesda, MD, 1946.
56. Hobbs, B. C., Smith, M. E., Oakley, C. L., *et al.*, *Clostridium welchii* food poisoning, *J. Hyg.* **51:**75–101 (1953).

57. Zeissler, J., and Rassfeld-Sternberg, L., Enteritis necroticans due to *Clostridium welchii* type F, *Br. Med. J.* **1:**267–270 (1949).
58. Murrell, T. G., and Walker, P. D., The pigbel story of Papua New Guinea, *Trans. R. Soc. Trop. Med. Hyg.* **85:**119–122 (1991).
59. Sutton, R. G. A., and Hobbs, B. C., Food poisoning caused by heat-sensitive *Clostridium welchii*, *J. Hyg.* **66:**135–146 (1965).
60. Rood, J. I., and Cole, S. T., Molecular genetics and pathogenesis of *Clostridium perfringens*, *Microbiol. Rev.* **55:**621–648 (1991).
61. Hatheway, C. L., Toxigenic clostridia, *Clin. Microbiol. Rev.* **3:**66–98 (1990).
62. Duncan, C. L., and Strong, D. H., *Clostridium perfringens* type A food poisoning. I. Response of the rabbit ileum as an indication of enteropathogenicity of strains of *Clostridium perfringens* in monkeys, *Infect. Immun.* **3:**167–170 (1971).
63. Strong, D. H., Duncan, C. L., and Perna, G., *Clostridium perfringens* type A food poisoning, *Infect. Immun.* **3:**171–178 (1971).
64. Hauschild, A. H. W., Criteria and procedures for implicating *Clostridium perfringens* in foodborne outbreaks, *Can. J. Public Health* **66:**388–392 (1975).
65. Hauschild, A. H. W., and Hilsheimer, R., Evaluation and modifications of media for enumeration of *Clostridium perfringens*, *Appl. Microbiol.* **27:**78–82 (1974).
66. Mead, G. S., Selective and differential media for *Clostridium perfringens*, *Int. J. Food Microbiol.* **2:**89–98 (1985).
67. Brett, M. M., Outbreaks of food-poisoning associated with lecithinase-negative *Clostridium perfringens*, *J. Med. Microbiol.* **41:**405–407 (1994).
68. Brett, M. M., Rodhouse, J. C., Donovan, T. J., *et al.*, Detection of *Clostridium perfringens* and its enterotoxin in cases of sporadic diarrhoea, *J. Clin. Pathol.* **45:**609–611 (1992).
69. van Damme-Jongsten, M., Rodhouse, J., Gilbert, R. J., and Notermans, S., Synthetic DNA probes for detection of enterotoxigenic *Clostridium perfringens* strains isolated from outbreaks of food poisoning, *J. Clin. Microbiol.* **28:**131–133 (1990).
70. Berry, P. R., and Gilbert, R. J., *Clostridium perfringens* type A food poisoning, in: *Anaerobes in Human Disease* (B. I. Duerden and B. S. Drasar, eds.), Wiley-Liss, New York, 1991.
71. Labbe, R., *Clostridium perfringens*, in: *Foodborne Bacterial Pathogens* (M. P. Doyle, ed.), pp. 191–234, Marcel Dekker, New York, 1989.
72. Skjelkvale, R., Stringer, M. F., and Smart, J. L., Enterotoxin production by lecithinase-negative *C. perfringens* isolated from food poisoning outbreaks and other sources, *J. Appl. Bacteriol.* **47:**329–339 (1979).
73. Sutton, R. G. A., Kendall, M., and Hobbs, B. C., The effect of two methods of cooking and cooling on *Clostridium welchii* and other bacteria in meat, *J. Hyg.* **70:**415–424 (1972).
74. Skjelkvale, R., and Uemura, T., Experimental diarrhoea in human volunteers following oral administration of *Clostridium perfringens* enterotoxin, *J. Appl. Bacteriol.* **43:**281–286 (1977).
75. Genigeorgis, C., and Riemann, H., *Clostridium perfringens* toxicity, Presented to the 6th International Symposium of the World Association of Veterinary Food Hygienists, Elsinor, Denmark, 1973.
76. Dische, F. E., and Elek, S. D., Experimental food-poisoning by *Clostridium welchii*, *Lancet* **2:**71–74 (1957).
77. McClane, B. A., Hanna, P. C., and Wnek, A. P., *Clostridium perfringens* enterotoxin, *Microb. Pathog.* **4:**317–323 (1988).
78. McDonel, J. L., *In vivo* effects of *Clostridium perfringens* enteropathogenic factors on the rat ileum, *Infect. Immun.* **10:**1156–1162 (1974).
79. McDonel, J. L., and Duncan, C. L., Regional localization of activity of *Clostidium perfringens* type A enterotoxin in the rabbit ileum, jejunum, and duodenum, *J. Infect. Dis.* **136:**661–666 (1977).
80. Uemura, T., Genigeorgis, C., Riemann, H. P., and Franti, C. E., Antibody against *Clostridium perfringens* type A enterotoxin in human sera, *Infect. Immun.* **9:**470–471 (1974).
81. Naik, H. S., and Duncan, C. L., Detection of *Clostridium* enterotoxin in human fecal samples and anti-enterotoxin in sera, *J. Clin. Microbiol.* **7:**337–340 (1978).
82. Pollock, A. M., and Whitty, P. M., Outbreak of *Clostridium perfringes* food poisoning, *J. Hosp. Infect.* **17:**179–186.
83. Stringer, M. F., Turnbull, P. C. B., and Gilbert, R. J., Application of serological typing to the investigation of outbreaks of *Clostridium perfringens* food poisoning, 1970–1978, *J. Hyg.* **84:**443–456 (1980).
84. Scott, H. G., and Mahony, D. E., Further development of a bacteriocin typing system for *Clostridium perfringens*, *J. Appl. Bacteriol.* **53:**363–369 (1982).
85. Mahony, D. E., Clark, G. A., Stringer, M. F., *et al.*, Rapid extraction of plasmids from *Clostridium perfringens*, *Appl. Environ. Microbiol.* **51:**521–523 (1986).
86. Forsblom, B., Palmu, A., Hirvonen, P., and Jousimiessomer, H., Ribotyping of *Clostridium perfringens* isolates, *Clin. Infect. Dis.* **20:**S323–S324 (1995).
87. Murrell, T. G. C., Egerton, J. R., Rampling, A., *et al.*, The ecology and epidemiology of the pib-bel syndrome in man in New Guinea, *J. Hyg.* **64:**375–396 (1966).
88. Johnson, S., Echeverria, P., Taylor, D. N., *et al.*, Enteritis necroticans among Khmer children at an evacuation site in Thailand, *Lancet* **2:**496–500 (1987).
89. Lawrence, G., and Cooke, R., Experimental pigbel: The Production and pathology of necrotizing enteritis due to *Clostridium welchii* type C in the guinea-pig, *Br. J. Exp. Pathol.* **61:**261–271 (1980).
90. Morris, J. G., "Noncholera" *Vibrio* species, in: *Infections of the Gastrointestinal Tract* (M. J. Blaser, P. D. Smith, J. I. Ravdin, *et al.*, eds.), pp. 671–685, Raven Press, New York, 1995.
91. Fujino, T., Sakazaki, R., Tamura, K., Designation of the type strain of *Vibrio parahaemolyticus* and description of 200 strains of the species, *Int. J. Syst. Bacteriol.* **24:**447–499 (1974).
92. Janda, J. M., Powers, C., Bryant, R. G., and Abbott, S., Current perspectives on the epidemiology and pathogenesis of clinically significant *Vibrio* spp., *Clin. Microbiol. Rev.* **1:**245–267 (1988).
93. West, P. A., Brayton, P. R., Twilley, R. R., *et al.*, Numerical taxonomy of nitrogen-fixing "decarboxylase-negative" *Vibrio* species isolated from aquatic environments, *Int. J. Syst. Bacteriol.* **85:**198–205 (1935).
94. Twedt, R. M., Madeden, J. M., Hunt, J. M., *et al.*, Characterization of *Vibrio cholerae* isolated from oysters, *Appl. Environ. Microbiol.* **41:**1475–1478 (1981).
95. McLaughlin, J. C., *Vibrio*, in: *Manual of Clinical Microbiology*, 6th ed. (P. R. Murray, E. J. Baron, M. A. Pfaller, *et al.*, eds.), pp. 465–476, American Society for Microbiology, Washington, DC, 1995.
96. Levine, W. C., Griffin, P. M., and The Gulf Coast *Vibrio* Working Group, *Vibrio* infections on the Gulf Coast: Results of first year of regional surveillance, *J. Infect. Dis.* **167:**479–483 (1993).
97. Dakin, W. P. H., Howell, D. J., Sutton, R. G. A., *et al.*, Gastroenteritis due to non-agglutinable (non-cholera) vibrios, *Med. J. Aust.* **2:**487–490 (1974).

98. Aldova, E., Laznickova, K., Stepankova, E., and Lietava, J., Isolation of nonagglutinable vibrios from an enteritis outbreak in Czechoslovakia, *J. Infect. Dis.* **118:**25–31 (1968).
99. World Health Organization, Outbreak of gastroenteritis by non-agglutinable (NAG) vibrios, *WHO Week. Epidemiol. Rec.* **44:**10 (1969).
100. Thekdi, R. J., Lakhani, A. G., Rale, V. B., and Panse, M. V., An outbreak of food poisoning suspected to be caused by *Vibrio fluvialis*, *J. Diarrhoeal. Dis. Res.* **8:**163–165 (1990).
101. Morris, J. G., Non-O group 1 *Vibrio cholerae*: A look at the epidemiology of an occasional pathogen, *Epidemiol. Rev.* **12:** 179–191 (1990).
102. Finch, M. G., Valdespino, J. L., Wells, J. G., *et al.*, Non-O1 *Vibrio cholerae* infections in Cancun, Mexico, *Am. J. Trop. Med. Hyg.* **36:**393–397 (1987).
103. Black, R. E., Merson, M. H., and Brown, K. H., Epidemiological aspects of diarrhea associated with known enteropathogens in rural Bangladesh, in: *Diarrhea and Malnutrition* (L. C. Chen and N. S. Scrimshaw, eds.), pp. 73–86, Plenum, New York, 1983.
104. Taylor, D. N., Echeverria, P., Pitarangsi, C., *et al.*, Application of DNA hybridization techniques in the assessment of diarrheal disease among refugees in Thailand, *Am. J. Epidemiol.* **127:**179–187 (1988).
105. Morris, J. G., Wilson, R., Davis, B. R., *et al.*, Non-O group 1 *Vibrio cholerae* gastroenteritis in the United States, *Ann. Intern. Med.* **94:**656–658 (1981).
106. Sakazaki, R., Halophilic *Vibrio* infections, *Foodborne Infections and Intoxications* (H. Reimann, ed.), pp. 115–119, Academic Press, New York, 1969.
107. Katah, H., Studies on the growth rate of various food bacteria. I. On the generation time of *Vibrio parahaemolyticus*, *Jpn. J. Med. Bacteriol.* **20:**94–100 (1965).
108. Lawrence, D. N., Blake, P. A., Yashuk, J. C., *et al.*, *Vibrio parahaemolyticus* gastroenteritis outbreaks aboard two cruise ships, *Am. J. Epidemiol.* **109:**71–80 (1979).
109. Lowry, P. W., McFarland, L. M., Peltier, B. H., *et al.*, *Vibrio* gastroenteritis in Louisiana: A prospective study among attendees of a scientific congress in New Orleans, *J. Infect. Dis.* **160:**978–984 (1989).
110. Zafari, Y., Zafari, A. Z., Rahmanzadeh, S., and Fakhar, N., Diarrhea caused by non-agglutinable *Vibrio cholerae* (non-cholera *Vibrio*), *Lancet* **2:**429–430 (1973).
111. Datta-Roy, K., Banerjee, K., De, S. P., and Ghose, A. C., Comparative study of expression of hemagglutinins, hemolysins, and enterotoxins by clinical environmental isolates of non-O1 *Vibrio cholerae* in relation to their enteropathogenicity, *Appl. Environ. Microbiol.* **52:**875–879 (1986).
112. Morris, J. G., Takeda, T., Tall, B. D., *et al.*, Experimental non-O group 1 *Vibrio cholerae* gastroenteritis in humans, *J. Clin. Invest.* **85:**697–705 (1990).
113. Hoge, C. W., Sethabutr, O., Bodhidatta, L., *et al.*, Use of a synthetic oligonucleotide probe to detect strains of non-O1 *Vibrio cholerae* carrying the gene for heat stable enterotoxin (NAG-ST), *J. Clin. Microbiol.* **28:**1473–1476 (1990).
114. Gyobu, Y., Kodama, H., and Sato, S., Studies on the enteropathogenic mechanism of non-O1 *Vibrio cholerae*. III. Production of enteroreactive toxins, *Kansenshogaku Zasshi* **65:**781–787 (1991).
115. Sanyal, S. C., and Sen, P. C., Human volunteer study on the pathogenicity of *Vibrio parahaemolyticus*, in: *International Symposium of Vibrio parahaemolyticus* (T. Fujino and A. Sakaguchi, eds.), pp. 227–230, Saikon, Tokyo, 1974.
116. Nishibuchi, M., Fasano, A., Russell, R. G., and Kaper, J. B., Enterotoxigenicity of *Vibrio parahaemolyticus* with and without genes encoding thermostable direct hemolysin, *Infect. Immun.* **60:**3539–3545 (1992).
117. Nishibuchi, M., and Kaper, J. B., Thermostable direct hemolysin gene of *Vibrio parahaemolyticus*: A virulence gene acquired by a marine bacterium, *Infect. Immun.* **63:**2093–2099 (1995).
118. Kaysner, C. A., Abeyta, C., Jr., Trost, P. A., *et al.*, Urea hydrolysis can predict the potential pathogenicity of *Vibrio parahaemolyticus* strains isolated in the Pacific Northwest, *Appl. Environ. Microbiol.* **60:**3020–3022 (1994).
119. Calia, F. M., and Johnson, D. E., Bacteremia in suckling rabbits after oral challenge with *Vibrio parahaemolyticus*, *Infect. Immun.* **11:**1222–1225 (1975).
120. Sakazaki, R., Iwanami, S., and Tamura, K., Studies on the enteropathogenic, facultatively halophilic bacteria, *Vibrio parahaemolyticus*. III. Enteropathogenicity, *Jpn. J. Med. Sci. Biol.* **21:**325–331 (1968).
121. McIntyre, O. R., Feeley, J. C., Greenough, W. B., *et al.*, Diarrhea caused by non-cholera vibrios, *Am. J. Trop. Med. Hyg.* **14:**412–418 (1965).
122. Barker, W. H., *Vibrio parahaemolyticus* outbreaks in the United States, *Lancet* **1:**551–554 (1974).
123. Peffers, A. S. R., Bailey, J., Barrow, G. I., and Hobbs, B. C., *Vibrio parahaemolyticus* gastroenteritis and international air travel, *Lancet* **1:**143–145 (1973).
124. Fujino, T., Okuno, Y., Nahada, D., *et al.*, On the bacteriological examination of Shirasu-food poisoning, *Med. J. Osaka Univ.* **4:**299–304 (1953).
125. Janda, J. M., and Durrey, P. S., Mesophilic aeromonads in human disease: Current taxonomy, laboratory identification, and infectious disease spectrum, *Rev. Infect. Dis.* **10:**980–997 (1988).
126. von Graevenitz, A., and Mensch, A. H., The genus *Aeromonas* in human bacteriology: Report of 30 cases and review of the literature, *N. Engl. J. Med.* **278:**245–249 (1968).
127. Janda, J. M., Abbott, S. L., and Carnahan, A. M., *Aeromonas* and *Plesiomonas*, in: *Manual of Clinical Microbiology*, 9th ed. (P. R. Murray, E. J. Baron, M. A. Pfaller, *et al.*, eds.), pp. 477–482, American Society for Microbiology, Washington, DC, 1995.
128. Kuijper, E. J., Steigerwalt, A. G., Schoenmakers, B. S., *et al.*, Phenotypic characterization of DNA relatedness in human fecal isolates of *Aeromonas* species, *J. Clin. Microbiol.* **27(1):**132–138 (1989).
129. Altwegg, M., Steigerwalt, A. G., Altwegg-Bissig, R., *et al.*, Biochemical identification of *Aeromonas* genospecies isolated from humans, *J. Clin. Microbiol.* **28:**258–264 (1990).
130. Kokka, R. P., Janda, J. M., Oshiro, L. S., *et al.*, Biochemical and genetic characterization of autoagglutinating phenotypes of *Aeromonas* species associated with invasive and noninvasive disease, *J. Infect. Dis.* **163:**890–894 (1991).
131. Colwell, R. R., MacDonell, M. T., and De Ley, J., Proposal to recognize the family *Aeromonadaceae*, *J. Systematic Bacteriol.* **36:**473–477 (1986).
132. Kelly, M. T., Stroh, E. M. D., and Jessop, J., Comparison of blood agar, ampicillin blood agar, MacConkey–ampicillin–Tween agar, and modified cefsulodin–irgasan–novobiocin agar for isolation of *Aeromonas* spp. from stool specimens, *J. Clin. Microbiol.* **30:**1262–1266 (1988).

133. Altorfer, R., Altwegg, M., Zollinger-iten, J., and von Graevenitz, A., Growth of *Aeromonas* spp. on cefsulodin–irgasan–novobiocin agar selective for *Yersinia enterocolitica*, *J. Clin. Microbiol.* **22:**478–480 (1985).
134. Carnahan, A. M., Behram, S., and Joseph, S. W., Aerokey II: A flexible key for identifying clinical *Aeromonas* species, *J. Clin. Microbiol.* **29:**2843–2849 (1991).
135. Abbott, S. L., Cheung, W. K., Kroske-Bystrom, S., *et al.*, Identification of *Aeromonas* strains to the genospecies level in the clinical laboratory, *J. Clin. Microbiol.* **30:**1262–1266 (1992).
136. Shimada, T., and Kosako, Y., Comparison of two O-serogrouping systems for mesophilic *Aeromonas* spp., *J. Clin. Microbiol.* **29:**197–199 (1991).
137. Thomas, L. V., Gross, R. J., Cheasty, T., and Rowe, B., Extended serogrouping scheme for motile, mesophilic *Aeromonas* species, *J. Clin. Microbiol.* **28:**980–984 (1990).
138. Janda, J. M., Abbott, S. L., and Morris, J. G., *Aeromonas*, *Plesiomonas*, and *Edwardsiella*, in: *Infections of the Gastrointestinal Tract* (M. J. Blaser, P. D. Smith, J. I. Ravdin, *et al.*, eds.), pp. 905–917, Raven Press, New York, 1995.
139. Gracey, M., Burke, V., and Robinson, R., *Aeromonas*-associated gastroenteritis, *Lancet* **2:**1304–1306 (1982).
140. Trust, T. J., and Chipman, D. C., Clinical involvement of *Aeromonas hydrophila*, *Can. Med. Assoc. J.* **120:**942–946 (1979).
141. Holmberg, S. D., and Farmer, J. J., *Aeromonas hydrophyla* and *Plesiomonas shigelloides* as causes of intestinal infections, *Rev. Infect. Dis.* **6:**633–639 (1984).
142. Holmberg, S. D., Schell, W. K., Fanning, G. R., *et al.*, *Aeromonas* intestinal infections in the United States, *Ann. Intern. Med.* **105:**683–689 (1986).
143. Cohen, M. B., Etiology and mechanisms of acute infectious diarrhea in infants in the United States, *J. Pediatr.* **118:**S34–S39 (1991).
144. Kuijper, E. J., van Alphen, L., Peeters, M. F., and Brenner, D. J., Human serum antibody response to the presence of *Aeromonas* spp. in the intestinal tract, *J. Clin. Microbiol.* **28:**853–856 (1990).
145. Jiang, Z. D., Nelson, A. C., Mathewson, J. J., *et al.*, Intestinal secretory immune response to infection with *Aeromonas* species and *Plesiomonas shigelloides* among students from the United States in Mexico, *J. Infect. Dis.* **164:**979–982 (1991).
146. Kokka, R. P., Velji, A. M., Clark, R. B., *et al.*, Immune response to S layer-positive O:11 *Aeromonas* associated with intestinal and extraintestinal disease, *Immunol. Infect. Dis.* **2:**111–114 (1992).
147. Pazzaglia, G., Sack, R. B., Salazar, E., *et al.*, High frequency of coinfecting enteropathogens in *Aeromonas*-associated diarrhea of hospitalized Peruvian infants, *J. Clin. Microbiol.* **29:**1151–1156 (1991).
148. de la Morena, M. L., Van, R., Singh, K., *et al.*, Diarrhea associated with *Aeromonas* species in children in day care centers, *J. Infect. Dis.* **168:**215–218 (1993).
149. Morgan, D. R., Johnson, P. C., Dupont, H. L., *et al.*, Lack of correlation between known virulence properties of *Aermonas hydrophila* and enteropathogenicity for humans, *Infect. Immun.* **50:**62–65 (1985).
150. King, G. E., Werner, S. B., and Kizer, K. W., Epidemiology of *Aeromonas* infections in California, *Clin. Infect. Dis.* **15:**449–452 (1992).
151. Kirov, S. M., The public health significance of *Aeromonas* spp. in foods, *Int. J. Food Microbiol.* **20:**179–198 (1993).
152. Abeyta, C., Kaysner, C. A., Wekell, M. M., *et al.*, Recovery of *Aeromonas hydrophila* from oysters implicated in an outbreak of foodborne illness, *J. Food Prot.* **49:**643–646 (1986).
153. Kobayashi, K., and Ohnaka, T., Food poisoning due to newly recognized pathogens, *Asian Med. J.* **32:**1–12 (1989).
154. Moyer, N. P., Clinical significance of *Aeromonas* species isolated from patients with diarrhea, *J. Clin. Microbiol.* **25:**2044–2048 (1987).
155. Janda, J. M., Recent advances in the study of the taxonomy, pathogenicity, and infectious syndromes associated with the genus *Aeromonas*, *Clin. Microbiol. Rev.* **4:**397–410 (1991).
156. Asao, T., Kinoshita, Y., Kozaki, S., *et al.*, Purification and some properties of *Aeromonas hydrophila* hemolysin, *Infect. Immun.* **46:**122–127 (1984).
157. George, W. L., Nakata, M. M., Thompson, J., and White, M. L., *Aeromonas*-related diarrhea in adults, *Arch. Intern. Med.* **145:** 2207–2211 (1985).
158. Agger, W. A., McCormick, J. D., and Gurwith, M. J., Clinical and microbiological features of *Aeromonas hydrophila*-associated diarrhea, *J. Clin. Microbiol.* **21:**909–913 (1985).
159. Challapalli, M., Tess, B. R., Cunningham, D. G., *et al.*, *Aeromonas*-associated diarrhea in children, *Pediatr. Infect. Dis. J.* **7:**693–698 (1988).
160. San Joaquin, V. H., *Aeromonas*, *Yersinia*, and miscellaneous bacterial enteropathogens, *Pediatr. Ann.* **23:**544–548 (1994).
161. del Val, A., Moles, J. R., and Garrigues, V., Very prolonged diarrhea associated with *Aeromonas hydrophila*, *Am. J. Gastroenterol.* **85:**1535 (1990).
162. Voss, L. M., Rhodes, K. H., and Johnson, K. A., Musculoskeletal and soft tissue *Aeromonas* infection: An environmental disease, *Mayo Clin. Proc.* **67:**422–427 (1992).
163. Gold, W. L., and Sallit, I. E., *Aeromonas hydrophila* infections of the skin and soft tissue: Report of 11 cases and review, *Clin. Infect. Dis.* **16:**69–74 (1992).
164. Ko, W. C., and Chuang, Y. C., *Aeromonas* bacteremia: Review of 59 episodes, *Clin. Infect. Dis.* **20:**1298–1304 (1995).
165. Ferguson, W. W., and Henderson, N. D., Description of strain C27: A motile organism with the major antigen of *Shigella sonnei* phase I, *J. Bacteriol.* **54:**179–181 (1947).
166. Habs, H., and Schubert, R. H. W., Ueber die biochemischen Merk-male und die taxonomische Stellung von *Pseudomonas shigelloides*, *Zentralbl. Bakteriol. I.* **186:**316–327 (1962).
167. East, A. K., Allaway, D., and Collins, M. D., Analysis of DNA encoding 23S rRNA and 16S-23S rRNA intergenic spacer regions from *Plesiomonas shigelloides*, *FEMS Microbiol. Lett.* **74:**57–62 (1992).
168. von Graevenitz, A., and Bucher, C., Evaluation of differential and selective media for isolation of *Aeromonas* and *Plesiomonas* spp. from human feces, *J. Clin. Microbiol.* **17:**16–21 (1983).
169. Aldova, E., Serovars of *Plesiomonas shigelloides*, *Int. J. Med. Microbiol. Virol. Parasitol. Infect. Dis.* **281:**38–44 (1994).
170. Holmberg, S. D., Wachsmuth, I. K., Gickman-Brenner, F. W., *et al.*, *Plesiomonas* enteric infections in the United States, *Ann. Intern. Med.* **105:**690–694 (1986).
171. Kain, K. C., and Kelly, M. T., Clinical features, epidemiology, and treatment of *Plesiomonas shigelloides* diarrhea, *J. Clin. Microbiol.* **27:**998–1001 (1989).
172. Tsukamoto, T., Kinoshita, Y., Shimada, T., and Sakazaki, R., Two epidemics of diarrhoeal disease possibly caused by *Plesiomonas shigelloides*, *J. Hyg. Camb.* **80:**275–280 (1978).
173. Janda, J. M., and Abbott, S. L., Expression of hemolytic activity

by *Plesiomonas shigelloides*, *J. Clin. Microbiol.* **31:**1206–1208 (1993).

174. Brenden, R. A., Miller, M. A., and Janda, J. M., Clinical disease spectrum and pathogenic factors associated with *Plesiomonas shigelloides* infections in humans, *Rev. Infect. Dis.* **10:**303–316 (1988).
175. National Academy of Sciences, *An Evaluation of the Role of Microbiological Criteria for Foods and Food Ingredients*, National Academy Press, Washington, DC, 1985.
176. International Commission on Microbiological Specifications for Foods, Application of the hazard analysis critical control points (HACCP) system to ensure microbiological safety and quality, in *Micro-organisms in Foods*, pp. 129–136, Blackwell Scientific Publications, Boston, 1988.
177. Bennett, J. V., Holmberg, S. D., and Rogers, M. F., Infectious and parasitic disease, *Am. J. Prev. Med.* **3**(Suppl.)**:**102 (1987).
178. Archer, D. L., and Kvenberg, J. E., Incidence and cost of food-borne diarrheal disease in the United States, *J. Food Prot.* **48:**887–894 (1985).
179. Garthright, W. E., Archer, D. L., and Kvenberg, J. E., Estimates of incidence and costs of intestinal infectious diseases in the United States, *Public Health Rep.* **103:**107–116 (1988).
180. United States Department of Agriculture, *Nationwide Microbiologic Baseline Studies*, United States Department of Agriculture, Food Safety and Inspection Service, Science and Technology, Washington, DC, 1995.

14. Suggested Reading

Blaser, M. J., Smith, P. D., Ravdin, J. I., *et al.* (eds.), *Infections of the Gastrointestinal Tract*, Raven Press, New York, 1995.

Bryan, F. L., Outbreaks of food-borne disease, in: *Manual of Clinical Microbiology*, 6th ed. (P. R. Murray, E. J. Baron, M. A. Pfaller, *et al.*, eds.), pp. 209–227, American Society for Microbiology, Washington, DC, 1995.

Doyle, M. P., *Foodborne Bacterial Pathogens*, Marcel Dekker, New York, 1989.

CHAPTER 6

Botulism

Frederick J. Angulo and Michael E. St. Louis

1. Introduction

Botulism is a neuroparalytic illness resulting from the action of a potent toxin produced by the organism *Clostridium botulinum*. Foodborne botulism is rare, but it may kill rapidly, and contaminated products may expose many persons. Foodborne botulism therefore represents a medical and a public health emergency that places a premium on rapid, effective communication between clinicians and public health officials.

According to the mode of acquisition of the toxin, there are four distinct forms of botulism. Foodborne botulism results from the ingestion of food containing preformed toxin. Wound botulism is caused by organisms that multiply and produce toxin in a soil-contaminated wound. Infant botulism is due to the endogenous production of toxin by germinating spores of *C. botulinum* in the intestine of the infant. Child or adult botulism from intestinal colonization is represented by those cases in which no food vehicle can be identified, there is no evidence of wound botulism, and there is the possibility of intestinal colonization in a person older than 1 year of age.

The seven types of *C. botulinum* (A–G) are distinguished by the antigenic characteristics of the neurotoxins they produce. Types A, B, E, and, in rare cases, F cause disease in humans. Types C and D cause disease in birds and mammals. Type G, identified in 1970, has not yet been confirmed as a cause of illness in humans or animals. Important epidemiological features and some clinical characteristics distinguish the types of botulism that cause human illness. Rare cases of infant and adult botulism cases have been confirmed to be the result of intestinal colonization by non-*botulinum Clostridium* species that were able to produce botulinal neurotoxin.

Frederick J. Angulo • Foodborne and Diarrheal Diseases Branch, Division of Bacterial and Mycotic Diseases, National Center for Infectious Diseases, Centers for Disease Control and Prevention, Atlanta, Georgia 30333. **Michael E. St. Louis** • Division of STD Prevention, National Center for HIV, STD, and TB Prevention, Centers for Disease Control and Prevention, Atlanta, Georgia 30333.

2. Historical Background

In the late 18th century, a syndrome characterized by muscle weakness and respiratory failure linked to eating blood sausage was described and termed "sausage poisoning." Similar outbreaks related to sausage, other meats, and fish were reported in Germany, Scandinavia, and Russia. In time, the syndrome became known as "botulism" after "botulus," the Latin word for sausage.

In 1897, Van Ermengem detected the potent neurotoxin in a ham implicated in an outbreak of botulism in Belgium and isolated an organism that produced the toxin and grew only in the absence of oxygen. In a series of pioneering microbiological experiments, he determined: (1) that foodborne botulism is not an infection, but rather an intoxication caused by a toxin produced in the food by the bacterium; (2) that the bacterium will not produce toxin in food if the salt concentration is high enough; (3) that the toxin is heat-labile; (4) that the toxin when ingested with contaminated food is resistant to acid and proteolytic enzymes; and (5) that not all animal species are affected equally by ingested toxin.

In 1904, Landman first identified a nonmeat product (home-canned beans) as the cause of an outbreak of botulism. During and shortly after World War I, the practice of home-canning vegetables increased markedly, as did the number of cases of botulism. Meyer made major contributions to the understanding of botulism during these years, studying the distribution of spores in soil in the United States and Europe, characterizing the epidemiology of botulism transmitted by home-canned vegetable and fruits, and even identifying a new type of *C. botulinum*. In

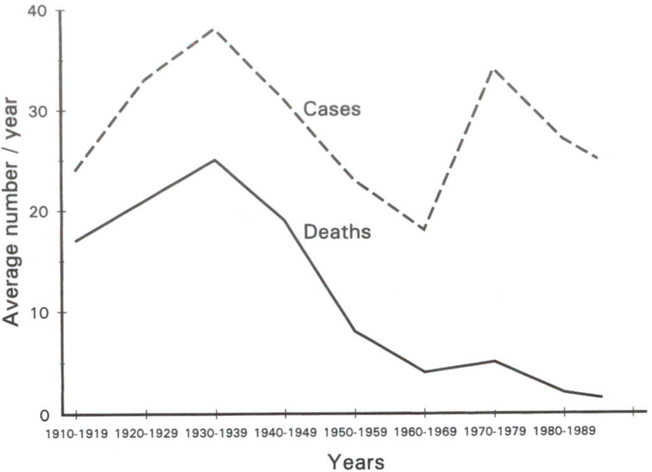

Figure 1. Average annual number of cases and deaths from foodborne botulism, United States, 1899–1994.

the mid-1940s, with the increased availability of refrigeration and the widespread application of improved preservation methods both in the home and by industry, the incidence of botulism began a decline that continued until recent years, when the occurrence of large restaurant-associated outbreaks caused the incidence to rise again (Fig. 1).

Although it had been noted earlier that the toxins of the Van Ermengem and the Landman strains were serologically distinct, it was in 1919 that the first two type designations (A and B) were established. The types were based on strains isolated in the United States and could not be directly related to the earlier European strains, since the latter were no longer available for study. *C. botulinum* types C and D were discovered in relation to outbreaks of botulism in domestic birds and animals. *C. botulinum* type E was first isolated in 1936, from fish implicated in a botulism outbreak. *C. botulinum* type F was first isolated and recognized as a cause of human botulism in 1960. In 1970, *C. botulinum* type G was isolated from soil in Argentina, but although there have been reports of isolation of the organism from human autopsy specimens, it has not yet been confirmed as a cause of botulism.(1) Neurotoxigenic strains of *Clostridium baratii*(2) and *C. butyricum*(3) have been implicated in type F and type E human botulism, respectively.

3. Methodology

3.1. Sources of Mortality and Morbidity Data

The Centers for Disease Control and Prevention (CDC) maintains surveillance of botulism in the United States. The sources of morbidity and mortality surveillance data include: (1) state, territorial, and local health departments (botulism is a reportable disease in all states); (2) state and territorial public health laboratories that contact CDC for laboratory support; (3) the US Food and Drug Administration, which becomes involved if the implicated food item is commercially produced or distributed; (4) the US Department of Agriculture, which becomes involved if the contaminated food item is derived from meat, poultry, or eggs; (5) clinicians who contact the CDC for consultation, laboratory support, or antitoxin; and (6) the manufacturers of antitoxin, who are sometimes contacted initially by a patient's physician.

The CDC provides epidemiological consultation and laboratory diagnostic services to state health departments in suspected botulism cases. In addition, because the CDC authorizes or monitors the release of all botulism antitoxin administered in the United States, nearly all diagnosed cases of adult botulism are eventually reported to the CDC. Underreporting of botulism results mainly when cases are misdiagnosed (as, for example, myasthenia gravis, Guillain–Barré syndrome, or stroke). Mild cases of botulism may escape diagnosis because of a lack of overt neurological findings, and even severe cases resulting in death may be diagnosed only after death, if at all.[4,5] Misdiagnosis of botulism is an important public health problem, because lack of recognition precludes epidemiological investigation and prevention of subsequent cases due to the same contaminated foods.[5,6]

3.2. Laboratory Diagnosis

Since botulism results from the action of a toxin, the most definitive laboratory confirmation of the disease is the demonstration of the toxin itself in clinical specimens (serum, feces, wound, or gastric aspirate) or foods.[7] Isolation of *C. botulinum* from foods or wounds supports the diagnosis of botulism but may not be definitive, as the organism may be present in foods or wounds without producing toxin. On the other hand, isolation of *C. botulinum* from human feces is very rare except in persons suspected of having botulism, and may be considered strong evidence supporting the diagnosis.[8] Because of the delays inherent in laboratory confirmation, the initial treatment decisions should be made on clinical grounds.

The mouse inoculation assay is currently the most sensitive, specific, and commonly used method for detecting botulinal toxin.[7,9] A standard volume of the test specimen (e.g., an aliquot of serum or extract of feces or food) is injected into the peritoneum of test mice and from this site is absorbed into the bloodstream. The same volume of test specimen is combined with selected monovalent (usually types A, B, and E) and/or polyvalent (ABE or ABCDEF) botulinal antitoxins and injected into the peritoneum of control mice. The presence of botulinal toxin is considered proven only if the mice that were inoculated with only the test specimen die while those protected by botulinal antitoxin suffer no ill effects. Failure of any of the antitoxins to protect mice demonstrates that some factor capable of killing mice was present in the specimen that was not neutralized by botulinal antitoxin; the mice deaths, therefore, cannot be attributed to botulism. Specific neutralization assays with one of the monovalent antitoxins establishes the specific type of toxin present. To increase the specificity of the laboratory diagnosis, experienced laboratory workers can recognize the clinical manifestations of botulism in the mouse. It is therefore important that this specialized assay be conducted in reference laboratories that perform the test frequently enough to maintain expertise.

By definition, the mouse inoculation assay can detect as little as one mouse lethal dose (the lowest dilution of the test specimen that kills 100% of injected mice) of botulinal toxin. One mouse lethal dose is equivalent to approximately 20 pg botulinal toxin. In one instance, an oral human lethal dose of type B toxin was calculated as 3500 mouse lethal doses,[10] and in another instance, the dose for type E toxin was calculated as 500,000 mouse lethal doses.[11] With the mouse assay, results may be evident within 24 hr, but final results (necessary for negative results, in particular) are not reported until 96 hr after inoculation. While the neutralization procedure ensures the specificity of the test, nonspecific toxicity may decrease the sensitivity of the assay by masking the presence of botulinal toxin.

Much effort has been made for the development of satisfactory *in vitro* assays for botulinal toxin. The status of studies on immunodiffusion, passive hemagglutination, immunofluorescence, radioimmunoassay, enzyme-linked immunosorbent assay (ELISA), and biosensors have been recently reviewed.[12] A very sensitive variant of the ELISA, the enzyme-linked clotting assay (ELCA) has been reported[13,14] and is currently being evaluated by a group of independent laboratories. Nevertheless, because of the extraordinary biological potency of botulinal toxins, the mouse inoculation assay remains substantially more sensitive and more specific than other tests yet developed and remains the method of choice. The mouse assay also allows the detection of any type of botulinal toxin rather than being limited to a particular antigenic type. Thus, only the mouse assay would be capable of demonstrating the action of a new type of botulinal toxin that is antigenically distinct from those currently recognized.

C. botulinum may be isolated using a spore-selection technique in enrichment culture.[15] Approximately 0.25 ml from a suspension of the clinical or environmental specimens is heated at 80°C for 10 min or treated with 100% ethanol to kill nonsporing organisms. The sample is then inoculated into chopped-meat enrichment medium and incubated anaerobically. Another 0.25-ml sample from the initial suspension is also directly inoculated into enrichment medium and incubated. Maximum toxin production occurs in 3–5 days in pure cultures; the time may be longer in specimen cultures. Toxicity tests are performed on the enrichment culture supernatant. The culture is also streaked on egg-yolk agar and the plates are incubated anaerobically for 48 hr. Colonies showing the lipase reaction (an iridescent sheen) are then chosen and injected into tubes of chopped-meat–dextrose–starch medium. After incubation for 4 days at 30°C, the identity of the pure culture can be established by toxicity and neutralization tests and conventional biochemical procedures.[15]

4. Biological Characteristics of the Organism

C. botulinum is not a single species but rather a group of culturally distinct organisms that are alike only in that they are clostridia and produce antigenically distinct neurotoxins with a similar pharmacological action. *C. botulinum* organisms are straight to slightly curved, gram-positive (in young cultures), motile, anaerobic rods, 0.5–2.0 μm in width by 1.6–22.0 μm in length, with oval, subterminal spores.[16] Certain strains of *C. sporogenes* are indistinguishable from some *C. botulinum* by culture and by DNA homology, but are nontoxigenic. Cases of human botulism due to other species of clostridia, *C. baratii*[2] and *C. butyricum*,[3,17] have further strained the taxonomic classification of botulism-causing organisms. The seven types of *C. botulinum* (A–G) are distinguished by immunologically distinct types of toxin. *C. botulinum* organisms have also been divided into group I (proteolytic; type A and some strains of types B and F), and group II (nonproteolytic; type E and some strains of types B and F), group III (types C and D, which are closely related to *C. novyi*), and group IV (type G for which the name *C. argentinense* has been proposed[18]).

The specific cultural and biochemical characteristics of *C. botulinum* are described elsewhere.[10,16] Because of the practical importance of temperature, salt concentration (water activity), and pH in the preservation of foods, the effects of these factors on the growth of *C. botulinum* have been thoroughly investigated. All strains of *C. botulinum* are mesophilic, although some nonproteolytic strains have been noted to grow at temperatures as low as 3°C.[19] The organism will generally not grow in an acid environment (pH <4.6) or in foods with a high salt content (water activity <.93). Temperature, pH, and salt content are interrelated factors; lowering the pH or raising the salt concentration increases the minimum temperature at which spores will germinate or vegetative cells will begin to grow.[20]

The ability of *C. botulinum* to cause food poisoning in humans is directly related to the production of heat-resistant spores that survive preservation methods that kill nonsporulating organisms.[21] The heat resistance of spores varies from type to type and even from strain to strain within each type; although some strains will not survive at 80°C, spores of many strains require temperatures above boiling to ensure destruction.[22,23] The thermal resistance of spores also increases with higher pH and lower salt content of the medium in which the spores are suspended.[24] In general, type A and proteolytic type B spores are more heat-resistant than type E and nonproteolytic type B spores. Spores are also susceptible to some types of radiation.[23,25,26] Nitrites are effective as well in preventing growth from spores that germinate[26] and are used commercially in semiprocessed meats.

C. botulinum types C and D have bacteriophages that are associated with toxigenicity. Nonlysogenic, nontoxigenic mutants have been obtained by "curing" them of their phages. These mutants can be made lysogenic and toxigenic again by infection with phages obtained from other lysogenic strains.[27] Hence, the ability of *C. botulinum* types C and D to produce toxin seems to depend on the presence of specific bacteriophages. No association between bacteriophages and toxigenicity has been found, however, for type A, B, E, and F strains of *C. botulinum*. The association between lysogenization by phage and toxin production has been noted with *Corynebacterium diphtheriae*. The genetic information for the production of neurotoxin by *Clostridium tetani*, however, appears to be located in a plasmid.[28]

Toxin is released from *C. botulinum* organisms only after lysis of the cells. The lytic enzymes responsible for this autolysis are located in the cell wall. More than one such bacteriolysin has been identified, and at least some appear to be group-specific.[29]

5. Descriptive Epidemiology

5.1. Foodborne Botulism

Botulism has been reported from all parts of the world, although the causative strains of *C. botulinum*, the characteristic food vehicles responsible for botulism, and even the resulting patterns of clinical illness may vary widely among regions. Botulism in continental Europe is almost exclusively type B disease and is predominantly caused by eating home-cured hams. The resulting illness is relatively mild and slowly progressive compared with botulism in the United States.[30] Most outbreaks in Canada and Japan are type E botulism associated with the consumption of preserved seafood.[31,32] In China, where home-fermented bean curd is the most common vehicle of botulism poisoning, the causative strains are a mixture of types A and B.[33] Illness is more severe and case-fatality ratios are substantially higher for type A than for type B botulism in the United States,[7,34] but are marginally higher for type B than for type A botulism in China.[33] In 1991, a large outbreak of type E botulism occurred in Egypt traced to consumption of faseikh, a fermented fish dish eaten since the time of the Pharaohs.[35]

In the United States between 1899 and 1994, 998 outbreaks of foodborne botulism involving 2422 persons were reported. The mean annual incidence of reported foodborne botulism in the United States in 1985 through 1994 was 0.1 cases per 1,000,000 persons. Generally, the northern and western states in the contiguous United States have had higher rates of foodborne botulism than the southern and eastern states. Alaska had the most cases (111) between 1985 and 1994 and had by far the highest rate of reported botulism (193.0 cases per 1,000,000 population).

Since botulism in adults most commonly results from eating improperly preserved home-canned (or home-bottled) foods, outbreaks usually occur in family groups and affect small groups of people. In recent years, however, novel vehicles of foodborne botulism have been reported. These differ in being "fresh" rather than preserved food, and include potato salad,[36,37] baked potatoes,[38] sautéed onions,[39] commercial potpies,[40] turkey loaves,[38] and beef stew.[38] In each case, these unpreserved foods were prepared by ordinary cooking procedures (which do not kill *C. botulinum* spores) and then stored for many hours to days under relatively anaerobic conditions (e.g., baked potatoes in foil, sautéed onions under melted butter) at temperatures warm enough to encourage the outgrowth of spores and production of toxin but not hot enough to destroy the heat-labile toxin. The foods were then eaten without having been thoroughly reheated.

Food that is commercially prepared or distributed may cause illness in a large number of persons who may be spread over a wide geographic area.[6,37] Since 1976, large outbreaks of botulism have increasingly occurred in association with foods served in restaurants; although such outbreaks constituted only 3% of botulism outbreaks in 1976 through 1994, then accounted for 32% of all cases of botulism.[41] Such large outbreaks of botulism often result in extraordinary economic costs as well as extensive morbidity.[42,43]

Although foodborne botulism affects all age groups, it occurs mainly in persons aged 30–60 years.[44,45] This age distribution may reflect that of persons who eat home-canned foods. Although it has been hypothesized that younger persons may be less susceptible to botulism, recent evidence indicates that the lower case-fatality ratios for the younger age groups are due to fewer complications during intensive respiratory support rather than to inherent resistance to the effects of botulinal toxin.[46] The disease occurs with nearly equal frequency in men and women. No clear time trend is evident in the incidence of foodborne botulism (Fig. 1).

Corresponding to the distribution of botulinal spores in soil samples,[47] between 1985 and 1994, 80% of botulism outbreaks that occurred in the western United States (excluding Alaska) were type A and 19% were type B, compared with outbreaks east of the Mississippi River, where 65% of outbreaks were due to type A and 30% were due to type B. In Alaska, approximately 89% of outbreaks were of type E botulism during this period; outbreaks in Alaska have uniformly been due to fermented or otherwise preserved fish or aquatic mammals.[48]

5.2. Infant Botulism

Since 1980, infant botulism is the most common form of botulism reported in the United States. It is epidemiologically distinct from foodborne botulism, representing the effect not of ingestion of toxin preformed in contaminated foods, but of colonization (infection) of the intestine by spores of *C. botulinum*, with subsequent *in vivo* toxin production.[49] Although infant botulism was first described in 1976,[50,51] earlier cases have been identified retrospectively, and its detection only in recent years probably reflects advances in diagnostic capabilities rather than the emergence of a new clinical syndrome. Cases have been reported in the United States, Australia, Argentina, Canada, Chile, Czechoslovakia, France, Great Britain, Italy, Japan, Spain, Sweden, Switzerland, and Taiwan.[52]

In the United States, 1273 cases were reported from 45 states to the CDC between 1976 and 1994 (Fig. 2). Since reporting began to stabilize in 1980, the average annual incidence of reported infant botulism in the United States has been approximately 1.9 in 100,000 live births. Since 1985, 46% of all infant botulism cases have been reported from California. The incidence is highest in Delaware, Hawaii, Utah, and California (9.0, 8.8, 6.3 and 5.7 per 100,000 live births, respectively), perhaps reflecting better diagnosis and reporting in those states.

The illness is confirmed by demonstrating botulinal toxin in and isolating *C. botulinum* from the infant's stool. Toxin may be detected in serum (13% of tested infants), more often in type A cases (36%) than in type B cases (2%).[53] In the United States, between 1985 and 1994, 47% of infant botulism cases were caused by *C. botulinum* type A and 53% by type B. Two US cases were associated with type F toxin and caused by *C. baratii*.[3] Two cases in Italy were associated with type E toxin and caused by *C. butyricum*.[17] Infant botulism is first seen most commonly in the second month of life and occurs somewhat earlier in cases of type B disease (median 9 weeks) than in cases of type A disease (median 11 weeks). There is no sex predilection and no apparent pattern of seasonal variation.

The characteristics of infant botulism cases have been clarified in recent years. Infants hospitalized with the disease tend to have had higher birthweights than other infants, and their mothers tend to be white, older, and better educated than mothers in the general population. Affected infants are also more commonly breast-fed[54,55]; breast-feeding is associated with an older age at onset in type B cases.[55] Clustering of cases of infant botulism has been noted in some suburban areas in the eastern United States and in small towns and rural areas of apparent high incidence of infant botulism in the West.[56–58]

Evidence of infant botulism was detected in several cases of sudden infant death syndrome (SIDS) in California.[59] The similar age distribution of infant botulism and

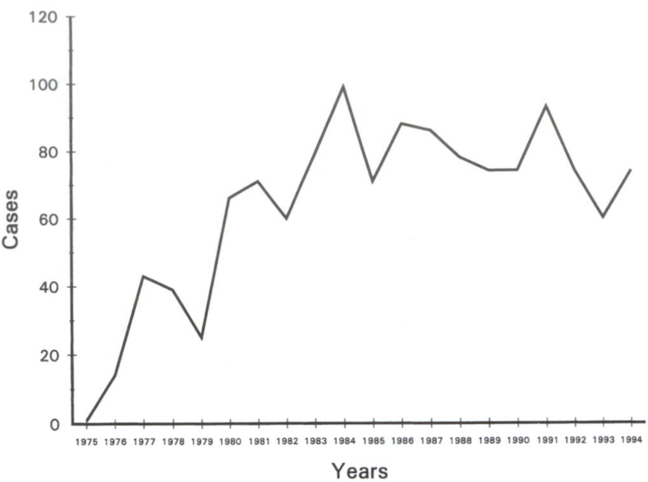

Figure 2. Cases of infant botulism reported to the Centers for Disease Control and Prevention, United States, 1976–1994.

SIDS contributed to the hypothesis that unrecognized infant botulism might be an important cause of SIDS. However, despite extensive investigations, no case of SIDS in the United States outside of California has yet been confirmed as a case of infant botulism. In addition, descriptive characteristics of SIDS patients, who tend to be black and have a history of low birthweight and less well educated mothers living in large cities, differ sharply from those of infant botulism patients.[(55)]

5.3. Wound Botulism

Wound botulism is a rare disease resulting from the growth of *C. botulinum* spores in a contaminated wound with *in vivo* toxin production.[(60)] Between 1943, when the syndrome was first recognized, and 1994, 67 cases of wound botulism were reported in the United States. Of 25 laboratory-confirmed cases in the United States, 17 were type A, 7 type B, and 1 a mixture of type A and type B organisms.[(9)] The median age of the patients was 21 years (range 6–44 years); 81% were male. The wounds were usually deep and contained avascular areas; many patients had compound fractures, and four had extensive crush injuries of the hand. The median incubation period in cases of trauma was 7 days (range 4–21 days).[(61)] Since 1980, several wound botulism cases have occurred in persons who used illicit drugs; these were associated either with needle puncture sites or with nasal or sinus lesions due to chronic cocaine sniffing.[(62)] In such cases, as in traditional wound botulism cases, the wounds may not be obvious or grossly infected.

5.4. Child or Adult Botulism from Intestinal Colonization

Isolated cases of botulism in which extensive investigation failed to implicate a specific food as the cause of the disease have been recorded by the CDC since 1978 as cases of "undetermined origin" rather than of foodborne botulism; through 1995, all of these cases have been in adults. Although there has been speculation on the matter since the 1920s, careful investigation has now demonstrated that some of these cases are caused by colonization of the gastrointestinal tract by *C. botulinum* and *C. baratii* with *in vivo* production of toxin, analogous to the pathogenesis of infant botulism.[(1,63)] Support for the diagnosis of botulism from intestinal colonization is provided by the demonstration of the prolonged excretion of toxin and *C. botulinum* in the stool and by the demonstration of spores of *C. botulinum* but not preformed toxin in suspect foods. In some cases of botulism strongly suspected of representing intestinal colonization, the patients had preceding gastrointestinal surgery or illnesses, such as inflammatory bowel disease, that may have predisposed them to enteric colonization.[(1)] No other specific risk factors have been identified.

6. Mechanisms and Routes of Transmission

6.1. Foodborne Botulism

Foodborne botulism is caused by consuming improperly preserved food in which spores of *C. botulinum* have germinated and organisms have grown and produced toxin. Home-processed foods accounted for 95% of foodborne botulism outbreaks in the continental United States in the past decade. Mass-processed commercial foods accounted for only 5% of outbreaks and 3% of cases. Even the large, restaurant-associated outbreaks of recent years have generally been caused by foods either home-canned in the restaurant[64] or otherwise improperly handled or stored,[6,39] rather than by defective commercially canned products.

Temperatures obtainable only with a pressure cooker are usually necessary to kill *C. botulinum* spores.[21,65] Boiling alone does not kill the spores of proteolytic strains, but does kill competing organisms and creates an anaerobic environment that will support the growth of *C. botulinum* once the spores germinate. The toxin itself is heat-labile; heating to 80°C for 10 min is sufficient to destroy the toxin. However, some home-canned foods are not cooked before being eaten, and those that are cooked may not be subjected to sufficient heat to destroy all the toxin present.

Although the epidemiological investigation of outbreaks has improved and the vehicles of botulism outbreaks have been more frequently identified in recent years, the proportional contribution of different types of food to cases of foodborne botulism has remained relatively stable (Table 1). Vegetables, especially those of more neutral pH such as asparagus, green beans, peppers, and mushrooms, are responsible for most type A and type B outbreaks. Spores may survive when either hot-pack or cold-pack canning methods are used[65]; cold-pack canning is acceptable only for certain fruits because of their high acidity or low water activity due to their high sugar content, which inhibit outgrowth of *C. botulinum* spores.

Table 1. Vehicles of Foodborne Botulism in the United States, 1899–1977 (1961 Cases), 1978–1985 (235 Cases), and 1986–1994 (227 Cases)

	Percent of total cases		
Vehicle (number of cases)	1899–1977 (1961)	1978–1985 (235)	1986–1994 (227)
Unknown	65.5	3.0	16.0
Identified	34.5	97.0	84.0
Vegetables	57.0	64.0	45.0
Fish/aquatic animals	15.6	19.3	45.0
Fruits	11.0	0.9	0
Condiments	8.7	10.1	4.7
Meat/dairy	7.5	5.7	3.7

Type E outbreaks are most often caused by products derived from fish and marine mammals. For example, many type E outbreaks in Alaska are associated with "muktuk" and "stink eggs," in which whale blubber or fish eggs are fermented in an anaerobic milieu, allowing the outgrowth of *C. botulinum* organisms.[48,66]

6.2. Infant Wound and Child or Adult Botulism from Intestinal Colonization

In contrast to foodborne botulism, which is an intoxication, infant, wound, and child or adult botulism from intestinal colonization result from infection with or colonization by *C. botulinum*. This organism is widely distributed in nature and can easily be ingested with foods[47,67] or contaminate a traumatic wound. The low frequency of *C. botulinum* infections despite the ubiquity of the organism in nature suggests that host factors are prominent in the epidemiology of these infectious forms of botulism.

Infant botulism results after colonization of the infant intestine.[49] In a prototypical case, type B organisms, but no toxin, were isolated from honey fed to an infant with infant botulism whose fecal specimens contained type B organisms and toxin. Family members who ate some of the same honey did not become ill. In several studies, more than 20% of affected infants had ingested honey before the onset of botulism.[55,68,69] In many cases, *C. botulinum* spores of the same type were cultured from honey in the same households.

However, since most infants with infant botulism have had no exposure to honey, the risk factors and vehicles of transmission of *C. botulinum* for the majority of cases remain unclear.[49,70] A survey of foods commonly fed to infants revealed *C. botulinum* in specimens of corn syrup as well as honey, but in no other tested category of foods.[67] In other studies, the same types of *C. botulinum* that caused disease were isolated from soil in an infant's yard and from vacuum cleaner dust; investigators have also frequently noted environmental conditions that might expose infants directly to environmental sources of *C. botulinum* spores, such as a shared crib, dusty or windy locales, nearby building construction, or outdoor activities.[56,58] These exposures have not, however, been evaluated by controlled studies. Infants hospitalized with botulism have also more typically been breast-fed than have control infants.[55,70–72] Breastfeeding is known to affect the fecal flora differently than formula feeding; in mice, the fecal flora have been shown to be an important susceptibility factor in challenge experiments with *C. botulinum* type A spores.[73]

Wound botulism, like tetanus, gas gangrene, and other clostridial diseases, can result from soil contamination of a wound.[61] Although the diagnosis of wound botulism may be frequently missed, the extreme rarity of wound botulism despite the wide distribution of the organism in the environment raises many questions regarding its pathogenesis: Are many wounds contaminated but few suitable for proliferation of the organism? Or is wound contamination with *C. botulinum* without signs of botulism truly uncommon? Data are scarce. Part of the problem is the difficulty in obtaining adequate anaerobic cultures and in differentiating *C. sporogenes* (a common wound isolate) from *C. botulinum*. In addition, the factors involved in spore germination, growth, and toxin production in tissues or *in vivo* systems have not been well studied. In wound botulism associated with chronic drug abuse, it is unclear if drugs or needles are vehicles for transmission of spores or are instead only associated with host factors for colonization, such as depressed immunity or chronically inflamed mucous membrane or skin lesions.[62]

In cases of adult botulism in which intestinal colonization was proven or suspected, vehicles have included canned cream of coconut[63] and blackberry preserves,[74] in each of which *C. botulinum* organisms of the appropriate type were detected. In a case strongly suggestive of this syndrome, a healthy, 27-year-old asymptomatic consumer of blood sausage was shown to have intestinal carriage of *C. botulinum* 19 days after an outbreak attributed to the sausage, but did not develop clinical symptoms and botulinal toxemia until 47 days after the outbreak.[1] The limited data about enteric infectious botulism in adults do not suggest that the vehicles of transmission are categorically different from those of traditional foodborne botulism due to preformed toxin.

7. Pathogenesis and Immunity

Incubation periods for foodborne botulism are reported to be as short as 6 hr or as long as 10 days,[6] but generally the time between toxin ingestion and onset of symptoms ranges from 18 to 36 hr.[34] Among patients with foodborne botulism, incubation periods are shorter for patients with illness from type E toxin.[34] The incubation periods for wound botulism (4–14 days) are longer than those usually seen in cases of foodborne botulism, and presumably reflect the time required for the multiplication of *C. botulinum* in the wound and the release of toxin. The incubation period has not been determined for cases of infant botulism. It has been shown that those individuals with shorter incubation periods—apparently those who ingest and/or absorb larger amounts of toxin—have more severe disease and a graver prognosis.[75]

Botulinal toxin is absorbed into the bloodstream from the gastrointestinal tract or from a wound and is transported via lymphatics and blood to cholinergic neuromuscular junctions. Here the toxin is fixed at and then internalized into the presynaptic nerve endings. It subsequently blocks the release of the neurotransmitter acetylcholine by binding to its release site at the neuronal membrane.[76,77] Evidence suggests that this binding is irreversible[77]; hence, functional recovery occurs only with the regeneration of neuronal fibrils and the reestablishment of the neuromuscular junction. This may explain why muscular weakness persists in many individuals for weeks or more after toxin has been eliminated from the intestine and bloodstream and why in severely affected individuals recovery may take many months to years or may never be complete.[39,78]

Botulinal toxin affects acetylcholine release only at peripheral sites; the central nervous system is not affected. Whether this is because botulinal toxin does not cross the blood–brain barrier or because it does not bind to acetylcholine release sites in the central nervous system is not known. Both the autonomic and voluntary motor activities of the cranial nerves seem to be uniquely susceptible to the effects of botulinal toxin. The cranial nerves are nearly always affected earlier and to a greater degree than are the nerves to the peripheral and respiratory muscles. Certain cranial nerves seem to be more sensitive to one botulinal toxin type than to others. Pupillary paralysis, for example, is apparently more commonly noted in type A botulism than in type B botulism.[34,46,78] Correspondingly, distinctions in the effect of type A and B toxin on laboratory preparations of the neuromuscular junction have been observed.[79] Although the reason for this is not clear, molecular differences between toxin types that account for immunologic distinction might, through stearic interactions, also result in disparate binding capabilities at neuromuscular junctions.

Botulinal toxin is so potent that the lethal dose is far below that required to induce an antibody response. Hence, immunity from natural intoxication does not occur.[80] Whether continuous exposure to low levels of toxin produced by organisms that have colonized the intestine (infant botulism) or a wound (wound botulism) may lead to significant antibody production has not been determined.

Animal models of infant botulism have yielded insight into mechanisms of intestinal colonization and *in vivo* growth of *C. botulinum*. Successful intraintestinal colonization by *C. botulinum* spores inoculated into the stomachs of infant mice is strongly age-dependent, peaking at 7 to 13 days old, a period during which the enteric microbial flora are in transition.[81] Although normal adult mice are highly resistant to colonization, germ-free adult mice may develop botulism after ingesting as few as ten spores,[82] and antimicrobial treatment of normal adult mice dramatically lowers the dose of ingested spores necessary to yield intraluminal outgrowth and production of toxin.[83] In mice, therefore, enteric infection is limited to a narrow age range in infancy and to occurrence in adults who have undergone a manipulation of the normal intestinal microbial flora. It is possible that anatomic variations, stasis, or constipation due to mechanical or motility factors, or some combination of these contributes to the creation of an environment favorable to the growth of the organism.

Factors other than just the physical production of toxin in the gut may also contribute to the expression of clinical illness. *C. botulinum* organisms and toxin have been recovered from the feces of human infants more than 8 weeks after the onset of botulism, and the peak excretion of toxin may not occur until several weeks after the illness has already begun to resolve.

8. Patterns of Host Response

8.1. Clinical Features

The clinical syndrome of botulism, whether foodborne, infant, wound, or adult or child intestinal colonization, is dominated by the neurological symptoms and signs resulting from a toxin-induced blockade of the voluntary motor and autonomic cholinergic junctions and is essentially quite similar for each syndrome and toxin type.[46,49,61,72] The ingestion of other bacteria and their toxins in the improperly preserved food accounts for the abdominal pain, nausea and vomiting, and diarrhea that often precede or accompany the neurological symptoms of foodborne botulism. Dryness of the mouth, inability to focus to a near point (prompting the patient to complain of "blurred vision"), and diplopia are usually the earliest neurological complaints. If the disease is mild, no other symptoms may develop and the initial symptoms will gradually resolve. The person with mild botulism may not come to medical attention. In more severe cases, however, these initial symptoms may be followed by dysphonia, dysarthria, dysphagia, and peripheral-muscle weakness. If illness is severe, respiratory muscles are involved, leading to ventilatory failure and death unless supportive care is provided. Patients have required ventilatory support for up to 7 months before the return of muscular function, although a 2- to 8-week duration of ventilatory support is more common.[46] Death occurs in 5–10% of cases of foodborne botulism; early deaths result from a failure to recognize the severity of disease or from pulmonary or systemic infections, whereas deaths after 2 weeks are from the complications of long-term mechanical ventilatory management or respiratory malfunction.[46]

Perhaps because infants are not able to complain about the early effects of botulinal intoxication, the neurological dysfunction associated with infant botulism often seems to develop suddenly. The major manifestations are poor feeding, diminished suckling and crying ability, neck and peripheral weakness (the infants are often admitted as "floppy babies"), and ventilatory failure.[49,54,72] Constipation is also often seen in infants with botulism and, in some, has preceded by many days the onset of neurological abnormalities. Loss of facial expression, extraocular muscle paralysis, dilated pupils, and depression of deep tendon reflexes have been reported more frequently with type B than with type A infant botulism.[72] Treatment with aminoglycoside antimicrobial agents may potentiate neuromuscular weakness in infant botulism[84] and has been associated with an increased likelihood of needing mechanical ventilation.[49,72] The median length of hospital stay in cases of infant botulism is 27 days (range, 2–150 days).[49,72] Fewer than 2% of reported cases of infant botulism result in death.

8.2. Diagnosis

Botulism is probably substantially underdiagnosed. The diagnosis is not difficult when it is strongly suspected, as in the setting of a large outbreak. However, since cases of botulism most often occur singly, the diagnosis may pose a more perplexing problem. Findings from many outbreaks have suggested that early cases are commonly misdiagnosed and may be diagnosed only retrospectively after death, after the subsequent clustering of cases of botulismlike illness finally alerts public health personnel to the occurrence of an outbreak of botulism[4,5,80]; other cases are undoubtedly missed entirely. Entire outbreaks may even go undetected despite severe illness in patients; for example, one outbreak was recognized retrospectively only after a second cluster of cases occurred due to the same vehicle.[6]

Botulism should be suspected in any adult with a history of gastrointestinal, autonomic (e.g., dry mouth, difficulty focusing), and cranial nerve (diplopia, dysarthria, dysphagia) dysfunction or in any infant with poor feeding, diminished sucking and crying ability, neck and peripheral muscle weakness, and/or ventilatory distress.[7,85] The demonstration of bilateral cranial nerve findings and the documentation of neurological progression (peripheral muscle weakness, ventilatory compromise) increase the level of suspicion. The diagnosis is even more likely if an adult patient has recently eaten home-canned foods or if family members are similarly ill, or both. If the typical clinical syndrome is present and no food item can be pinpointed as a means of transmission, a contaminated wound should be sought. If the typical syndrome is seen and a wound is identified, the wound should be explored and specimens taken for culture and toxicity testing even if the wound appears clean.

The differential diagnosis includes myasthenia gravis, stroke, Guillain–Barré syndrome, bacterial and chemical food poisoning, tick paralysis, chemical intoxication (e.g., from carbon monoxide, barium carbonate, methyl chloride, methyl alcohol, organic phosphorus compound, or atropine), mushroom poisoning, medication reactions (e.g., from antibiotics such as neomycin, streptomycin, kanamycin, or gentamicin), poliomyelitis, diphtheria, and psychiatric illness. In infant botulism, sepsis (especially meningitis), electrolyte–mineral imbalance, metabolic encephalopathy, Reye's syndrome, Werdnig–Hoffman disease, congenital myopathy, and Leigh's disease should also be considered.

Routine laboratory studies are not helpful in confirming the clinical suspicion of botulism. Serum electrolytes, renal and liver function tests, complete blood tests, urinalysis, and electrocardiograms will all be normal unless secondary complications occur. A normal cerebrospinal fluid (CSF) examination helps differentiate botulism from Guillain–Barré syndrome, although a slightly elevated CSF protein level is occasionally seen with botulism.[46] Normal neuroradiological studies, such as computed tomographic scans or magnetic resonance imaging, help to rule out stroke, another condition commonly confused with botulism.[6,80]

Electromyography (EMG) may be helpful in distinguishing botulism from myasthenia gravis and Guillain–Barré syndrome, diseases that botulism often mimics closely. A characteristic EMG pattern observed in adult patients with botulism has been well described.[78,86,87] A low-amplitude response to a single stimulus, a decremental trend in amplitude of the elicited action potentials to repetitive low-frequency stimulation (2–5 Hz), and an incremental trend (facilitation) to rapid repetitive stimulation (20–50 Hz) may be seen. However, rapid repetitive stimulation is much more sensitive and specific for botulism than is low-frequency stimulation.[6] EMGs should be performed on clinically involved muscles; positive results may be obtained from only one muscle even though many are weak.

The most prominent EMG finding is infant botulism is the same as that in adults: an incremental response to rapid repetitive stimulation.[88] However, another EMG pattern has been described as characteristic of infant botulism.[89] This is the pattern of "brief duration, small amplitude, overly abundant (for the amount of power being exerted)" motor unit action potentials, termed "BSAP" by Engel.[90] Polyphasicity may also be part of this pattern. It is not unusual to find either a BAP pattern (if the motor unit potentials are only brief) or an SAP pattern (if the motor unit potentials are only small) in patients who have typical BSAP findings in other parts of a muscle or in other muscles.

Toxicity testing of serum specimens, culture of tissues debrided from a wound, and toxicity testing plus culture of stool specimens or epidemiologically incriminated foods or both are the best methods for confirming the diagnosis of botulism.[7,8] Cultures were positive for 51% of stool specimens and toxin testing was positive for 37% of sera and 23% of stool specimens collected from 309 persons with clinically diagnosed botulism reported to the CDC from 1975 to 1988; at least one laboratory test was positive for 65% of patients.[34] Collecting stool and sera samples early during the course of illness increases the likelihood of obtaining positive results. However, in any given situation, these tests may not be helpful; large outbreaks have occurred in which none[91] or a very low percentage[92] of specimens yielded positive results. In addition, laboratory results may not be reported until many hours or days after the specimens are received. The administration of antitoxin is the only specific therapy available for botulism, and evidence suggests that it is effective only if given very early in the course of neurological dysfunction.[75] Hence, the diagnosis of this illness cannot await the results of studies that may be long delayed and may be confirmatory only in some cases. The diagnosis should be made on the basis of the history and physical findings.

9. Prevention, Control, and Treatment

9.1. Prevention and Control

The prevention of foodborne botulism depends on destroying all *C. botulinum* spores in food as it is preserved or creating a milieu in the preserved foods that will not allow the growth of any organisms that survive preservation procedures. This requires careful home canning and commercial canning techniques. Several private and government agencies (e.g., the US Department of Agriculture) provide information on the proper methods of home canning. Although the heat resistance of *C. botulinum* spores is quite variable, cooking at 121°C (250°F) or higher is usually sufficient to destroy all spores.[21–23] These temperatures can be achieved only in a pressure cooker. Boiling alone may kill competitive organisms and create an anaerobic environment highly favorable to the growth of *C. botulinum*. Boiling is sufficient for fruits and certain vegetables because their high sugar content will not support the growth of *C. botulinum*.[20] Commercial chopped garlic bottled under oil has caused two outbreaks of botulism.[6,93] As a result, this food must now be acidified with phosphoric acid. Until recently, tomatoes were thought to be an extremely low-risk food because of their acidity. Recent cases of botulism, however, have been caused by contaminated foods that contained tomatoes (such as spaghetti sauce) and by tomato juice.[45] These cases have been attributed to the low-acidity tomatoes that are now being bred for increased "sweetness."

Home-canned foods that are contaminated with proteolytic *C. botulinum* organisms or concurrently contaminated with other anaerobic or aerobic organisms will spoil. Foods that look or smell spoiled should not be tasted. Foods contaminated by nonproteolytic strains of *C. botulinum* (and sometimes proteolytic strains as well) may not appear spoiled. Food items suspected of having transmitted botulism should be refrigerated and saved for culture and toxin testing. Although *C. botulinum* spores are resistant to heat, botulinal toxins are heat-labile and are readily destroyed by boiling. Thorough boiling of home-canned foods is an added safeguard against botulism.

Commercial canners use a variety of methods to prevent the growth of *C. botulinum*. Commercial canners routinely heat foods to 120°C for 3 min, and often acidify high-risk, low-acid foods such as peppers to inhibit the growth of *C. botulinum*. Semipreserved meat products (e.g., hot dogs and luncheon meats) have nitrites added for similar reasons. Systems for killing spores in foods by radiation are also under investigation. *C. botulinum* is a gas-producing organism, and its growth inside a can may produce enough gas to make the can bulge or swell. More common causes of bulging include overpacking by the manufacturer, gas caused by interaction of the contents and the metal container, or contamination by some other organisms due to a fractured seal. Nevertheless, swollen, bulging cans or cans with spoiled contents should be reported to local health authorities or to the FDA.

Physicians also have an important role in the control of botulism. All suspect cases of foodborne botulism should be reported immediately to local or state health authorities or directly to the CDC in Atlanta (telephone 404-639-2888); it is important that this be done quickly and efficiently, especially if the suspected vehicle is a commercial product. If the diagnosis is suspected, a search for other cases (initially by identifying persons who shared the implicated food) should be immediately undertaken.

Because the mechanism of transmission for infant botulism has not been totally defined, control measures are not available. Controlled epidemiological studies will be required to develop the necessary data. Since honey is the one identified source of *C. botulinum* spores for susceptible infants and since it is not essential for good infant nutrition, it is recommended that honey not be fed to infants under age 1 year.[49] The prevention of wound botulism depends on the thorough cleansing and debridement of wounds, especially those of any depth or that are contaminated by soil.

Although antibiotic prophylaxis will not protect against foodborne botulism, since this results from ingestion of preformed toxin, administration of an oral penicillin or a nonabsorbable antibiotic might prove useful in preventing the occurrence or shortening the course of infant botulism. On the other hand, antibiotic-induced lysis of *C. botulinum* organisms might result in the release and subsequent absorption of increased amounts of toxin, as is suggested by the higher rate of respiratory failure among infants with infant botulism who have been treated with aminoglycoside antibiotics.[72] Antibiotic prophylaxis for a contaminated wound is indicated for reasons other than the prevention of botulism and cannot substitute for thorough cleansing and debridement. Wound botulism has occurred in patients undergoing treatment with antibiotics that are effective against *C. botulinum in vitro* tests.

Botulinal toxoid is available and effective for active immunization.[94] However, because of the rarity of botulism in the general population and the side effects of immunization, toxoid administration is recommended only for laboratory personnel working directly with the organism and the toxin. The toxoid is available from the CDC.

9.2. Treatment

The mainstays of treatment of foodborne and wound botulism are as follows: (1) administration of botulinal antitoxin in an attempt to prevent neurological progression of a moderate, slowly progressive illness or to shorten the duration of ventilatory failure in those with a severe, rapidly progressive illness; (2) careful monitoring of respiratory vital capacity and aggressive respiratory care for those with ventilatory insufficiency; and (3) meticulous and intensive care for the duration of the often prolonged paralytic illness.

Antitoxin therapy is more effective if undertaken early in the course of illness.[75] This is not surprising when one considers that equine antitoxin neutralizes only toxin molecules yet unbound to nerve endings.[77] If passive immunization is indicated, trivalent equine antitoxin (anti-A, -B, and -E in combination) is recommended and is available free to patients from the CDC through state health departments. Most persons (more than 80%) with adult botulism in the United States are treated with antitoxin, while few infants have been given the product because of concerns that potential reactions with the equine-derived product might be more severe in infants.[49] Administration of one vial of trivalent botulism antitoxin by the intravenous route results in serum levels of type A, B, and E antibodies capable of neutralizing serum toxin concentrations manyfold in excess of those reported for botulism patients. Therefore, contrary to the package insert, administration of one vial of antitoxin intravenously is recommended and antitoxin need not be repeated, since the circulating antitoxins have a half-life of 5 to 8 days.[95] However, treatment is not without risk as approximately 9.0% of persons treated experience hypersensitivity reactions.[96] It is therefore extremely important that physicians recognize botulism as early in its course as possible, and yet not mistake other neurological syndromes for botulism.

10. Unresolved Problems

Much is now known concerning the epidemiological and clinical aspects of adult forms of botulism. The most prominent persisting problem may be the low index of suspicion for botulism among clinicians who are unlikely to diagnose even one case in a career. The development of laboratory tests more rapid than but equally as sensitive and specific as the mouse neutralization assay would be helpful in diagnosing and treating this illness, but this is unlikely to take place soon. The development of an antitoxin derived from human serum or by DNA hybridization techniques could provide an approach to antitoxin therapy that is safer (because less likely to cause hypersensitivity reactions than equine antitoxin) and perhaps less expensive. Although the clinical spectrum of illness and descriptive epidemiology of infant botulism have been well characterized in the few years since its discovery, specific risk factors and vehicles of transmission remain obscure for most cases. Controlled epidemiological studies are needed to further clarify ways of preventing this important source of childhood morbidity. The recent demonstration in some adults of a pathogenic mechanism similar to that of infant botulism blurs somewhat the distinction between adult and infant forms of the disease, and may initiate reconsideration of pathogenesis and treatment in both groups. Finally, the recent discovery of clostridia other than *C. botulinum* that may produce botulinal toxin has further aggravated the taxonomic inconsistencies in this group of organisms, and may finally precipitate a taxonomic reclassification of botulinogenic organisms.

11. References

1. McCroskey, L. M., and Hatheway, C. L., Laboratory findings in four cases of adult botulism suggest colonization of the intestinal tract, *J. Clin. Microbiol.* **26:**1052–1054 (1988).
2. Sonnabend, O., Sonnabend, O., Heinzle, R., *et al.*, Isolation of *Clostridium botulinum* type G and identification of type G botulinal toxin in humans: Report of five sudden unexpected deaths, *J. Infect. Dis.* **143:**22–27 (1981).
3. Hall, J. D., McCroskey, L. M., Pincomb, B. J., and Hatheway, C. L., Isolation of an organism resembling *Clostridium baratii* which produces type F botulinal toxin from an infant with botulism, *J. Clin. Microbiol.* **21:**654–655 (1985).
4. Badhey, H., Cleri, D. J., D'Amato, R. F., *et al.*, Two fatal cases of type E adult food-borne botulism with early symptoms and terminal neurologic signs, *J. Clin. Microbiol.* **23:**616–618 (1986).
5. Horwitz, M. A., Marr, J. S., Merson, M. H., *et al.*, A continuing common-source outbreak of botulism in a family, *Lancet* **1:**1–6 (1975).
6. St. Louis, M. E., Peck, S. H., Bowering, D., *et al.*, Botulism from chopped garlic: Delayed recognition of a major outbreak, *Ann. Intern. Med.* **108:**363–368 (1988).
7. Centers for Disease Control, *Botulism in the United States, 1899–1973: Handbook for Epidemiologists, Clinicians, and Laboratory Workers*. CDC, Atlanta, 1978.
8. Dowell, V. R., McCroskey, L. M., Hatheway, C. L., *et al.*, Coproexamination for botulinal toxin and *Clostridium botulinum*, *J. Am. Med. Assoc.* **238:**1829–1832 (1977).
9. Hatheway, C. L., Botulism, in: *Laboratory Diagnosis of Infectious Diseases: Principles and Practice*, Volume 1 (A. Balows, W. J. Hausler, Jr., and M. Ohashi, eds.), pp. 111–133, Springer-Verlag, Berlin, 1988.
10. Smith, L. D., and Sugiyama, H., *Botulism: The Organism, Its Toxins, the Disease*, 2nd ed., Charles C. Thomas, Springfield, IL, 1985.
11. Dolman, C. E., Darby, G. E., and Lane, R. F., Type E botulism due to salmon eggs, *Can. J. Public Health* **46:**135–141 (1955).
12. Hatheway, C. L., and Ferreira, J. L., Detection and identification

of *Clostridium botulinum* neurotoxins, *Adv. Exp. Med. Bio.* **391:**481–498 (1996).

13. Doelgast, G. J., Beard, G. A., Bottoms, J. D., *et al.*, Enzyme-linked immunosorbent assay and enzyme-linked coagulation assay for detection of *Clostridium botulinum* neurotoxins A, B, and E and solution phase complexes with dual-label antibodies, *J. Clin. Microbiol.* **35:**104–111 (1994).
14. Doelgast, G. J., Triscott, M. X., Beard, G. A., *et al.*, Sensitive enzyme-linked immunosorbent assay for detection of *Clostridium botulinum* neurotoxins A, B, and E using signal amplification via enzyme-linked coagulation assay, *J. Clin. Microbiol.* **31:**2402–2409 (1993).
15. Dowell, V. R., and Hawkins, T. M., *Laboratory Methods in Anaerobic Bacteriology: CDC Laboratory Manual*, CDC, Atlanta, 1974.
16. Cato, E. P., George, W. L., and Finegold, S. M., Genus *Clostridium*, in: *Bergey's Manual of Systematic Bacteriology*, Volume 2 (P. H. A. Sneath, N. S. Mair, and M. E. Sharpe, eds.), pp. 1141–1200, Williams & Wilkins, Baltimore, 1986.
17. Aureli, P., Fenicia, L., Pasolini, B., *et al.*, Two cases of type E infant botulism caused by neurotoxigenic *Clostridium butyricum* in Italy, *J. Infect. Dis.* **154:**207–211 (1986).
18. Suen, J. C., Hatheway, C. L., Steigerwalt, A. G., *et al.*, *Clostridium argentinense*, sp. nov: A genetically homogenous group composed of all strains of *Clostridium botulinum* toxin type G and some nontoxigenic strains previously identified as *Clostridium subterminale* or *Clostridium hastiforme*, *Int. J. Syst. Bacteriol.* **38:**375–382 (1988).
19. Roberts, T. A., and Hobbs, G., Low temperature growth characteristics of clostridia, *J. Appl. Bacteriol.* **31:**75–88 (1968).
20. Baird-Parker, A. C., and Freame, B., Combined effect of water activity, pH, and temperature on the growth of *Clostridium botulinum* from spores and vegetative cell inocula, *J. Appl. Bacteriol.* **30:**420–429 (1967).
21. Kim, J., and Foegeding, P. M., Principals of control, in: *Clostridium botulinum: Ecology and Control in Foods* (A. H. W. Hauschild and K. L. Dodds, eds.), pp. 121–176, Marcel Dekker, New York, 1992.
22. Ito, K. A., Seslar, D. J., Ercern, W. A., *et al.*, The thermal and chlorine resistance of *Clostridium botulinum* types A, B, and E spores, in: *Botulism 1966* (M. Ingram and T. A. Roberts, eds.), pp. 108–122, Chapman & Hall, London, 1967.
23. Roberts, T. A., and Ingram, M., The resistance of spores of *Clostridium botulinum* type E to heat and radiation, *J. Appl. Bacteriol.* **28:**125–137 (1965).
24. Zezones, H., and Hutchings, I. J., Thermal resistance of *Clostridium botulinum* (62A) spores as affected by fundamental food constituents, *Food Technol.* **19:**1003–1005 (1965).
25. El Bisi, H. M., Radiation death kinetics of *C. botulinum* spores at cryogenic temperatures, in: *Botulism 1966* (M. Ingram and T. A. Roberts, eds.), pp. 89–107, Chapman & Hall, London, 1967.
26. Pivnick, H., Johnston, M. A., Thacker, C., *et al.*, Effect of nitrite on destruction and germination of *Clostridium botulinum* and putrefactive anaerobes 3679 and 3679h in meat and in buffer, *Can. Inst. Food Technol. J.* **3:**103–109 (1970).
27. Eklund, M. W., Poysky, F. T., Reed, S. M., *et al.*, Bacteriophage and the toxigenicity of *Clostridium botulinum* type C, *Science* **172:**480–482 (1971).
28. Eisel, V., Jarausch, W., Goretsky, K., *et al.*, Tetanus toxin: Primary structure, expression in *E. coli*, and homology with botulinum toxins, *EMBO J.* **5:**2495–2502 (1986).
29. Mitsui, N., Kiritani, K., and Nishida, S., A lysin(s) in lysates of *Clostridium botulinum* A190 induced by ultra-violet ray or mitomycin C, *Jpn. J. Microbiol.* **17:**353–360 (1973).
30. Roblot, R., Fauchere, J. L., Devilleger, A., *et al.*, Retrospective study of 108 cases of botulism in Poiters, France, *J. Med. Microbiol.* **40:**379–384 (1994).
31. Hauschild, A. H. W., and Gauvreau, L., Food-borne botulism in Canada, 1971–84, *Can. Med. Assoc. J.* **133:**1141–1146 (1985).
32. Iida, H., Epidemiological and clinical observations of botulism outbreaks in Japan, in: *Proceedings of the First U.S.—Japan Conference on Toxic Microorganisms* (M. Herzberg, ed.), pp. 357–359, US Department of the Interior, Washington, DC, 1970.
33. Shih, Y., and Chao, S., Botulism in China, *Rev. Infect. Dis.* **8:**984–990 (1986).
34. Woodruff, B. A., Griffin, P. M., McCroskey, L. M., *et al.*, Clinical and laboratory comparison of botulism from toxin types A, B, and E in the United States, 1975–1988, *J. Infect. Dis.* **166:**1281–1286 (1992).
35. Weber, J. T., Hibbs, R. G., Darwish, A., *et al.*, A massive outbreak of type E botulism associated with traditional salted fish in Cairo, *J. Infect. Dis.* **167:**451–454 (1993).
36. Mann, J. M., Hatheway, C. L., and Gardiner, T. M., Laboratory diagnosis in a large outbreak of type A botulism. Confirmation of the value of coproexamination, *Am. J. Epidemiol.* **115:**598–605 (1982).
37. Seals, J. E., Snyder, J. D., Edell, T. A., *et al.*, Restaurant-associated type A botulism: Transmission by potato salad, *Am. J. Epidemiol.* **113:**436–444 (1981).
38. Centers for Disease Control, Botulism from fresh foods—California, *Morbid. Mortal. Week. Rep.* **34:**156–157 (1985).
39. MacDonald, K. L., Spengler, R. F., Hatheway, C. L., *et al.*, Type A botulism from sauteed onions, *J. Am. Med. Assoc.* **253:**1275–1278 (1985).
40. California Department of Health Services, Type A botulism associated with commercial pot pie, *California Morbidity*, December 30, 1976, p. 51.
41. MacDonald, K. L., Cohen, M. L., and Blake, P. A., The changing epidemiology of adult botulism in the United States, *Am. J. Epidemiol.* **124:**794–799 (1986).
42. Mann, J. M., Martin, S., Hoffman, R. E., *et al.*, Patient recovery from type A botulism: Morbidity assessment following a large outbreak, *Am. J. Public Health* **71:**266–269 (1981).
43. Mann, J. M., Lathrop, G. D., and Bannerman, J. A., Economic impact of a botulism outbreak. Importance of the legal component in food-borne disease, *J. Am. Med. Assoc.* **249:**1299–1301 (1983).
44. Gangarosa, E. J., Donadio, J. A., Armstrong, R. W., *et al.*, Botulism in the United States, 1899–1969, *Am. J. Epidemiol.* **93:**91–100 (1971).
45. Horwitz, M. A., Hughes, J. M., Merson, M. H., *et al.*, Foodborne botulism in the United States, 1970–1975, *J. Infect. Dis.* **136:**153–159 (1977).
46. Hughes, J. M., Blumenthal, J. R., Merson, M. H., *et al.*, Clinical features of types A and B food-borne botulism, *Ann. Intern. Med.* **95:**442–445 (1981).
47. Smith, L. D., The occurrence of *Clostridium botulinum* and *Clostridium tetani* in the soil of the United States, *Health Lab. Sci.* **15:**74–80 (1978).
48. Wainwright, R. B., Heyward, W. L., Middaugh, J. P., *et al.*, Food-borne botulism in Alaska, 1947–1985: Epidemiology and clinical findings, *J. Infect. Dis.* **157:**1158–1162 (1988).

49. Arnon, S. S., Infant botulism, in: *Textbook of Pediatric Infectious Diseases* (R. Feigen and J. Cherry, eds.), pp. 1095–1102, W.B. Saunders, Philadelphia, 1992.
50. Midura, T. F., Arnon, S. S., Infant botulism: Identification of *Clostridium botulinum* and its toxin in faeces, *Lancet* **2:**934–936 (1976).
51. Pickett, J., Berg, B., Chaplin, E., *et al.*, Syndrome of botulism in infancy, *N. Engl. J. Med.* **295:**770–772 (1976).
52. Dodds, K. L., Worldwide incidence and ecology of infant botulism, in: *Clostridium botulinum: Ecology and Control in Foods* (A. H. W. Hauschild and K. L. Dodds, eds.), Marcel Dekker, pp. 105–107, New York, 1993.
53. Hatheway, C. L., and McCroskey, L. M., Examination of feces and serum for diagnosis of infant botulism in 336 patients, *J. Clin. Microbiol.* **25:**2334–2338 (1987).
54. Long, S. S., Gajewski, J. L., Brown, L. W., *et al.*, Clinical, laboratory, and environmental features of infant botulism in southeastern Pennsylvania, *Pediatrics* **75:**935–941.
55. Morris, J. G., Snyder, J. D., Wilson, R., *et al.*, Infant botulism in the United States: An epidemiologic study of the cases occurring outside California, *Am. J. Public Health* **73:**1385–1388 (1983).
56. Istre, G. R., Compton, R., Novotny, T., *et al.*, Infant botulism: Three cases in a small town, *Am. J. Dis. Child.* **140:**1013–1014 (1986).
57. Long, S. S., Epidemiologic study of infant botulism in Pennsylvania, *Pediatrics* **75:**928–934 (1985).
58. Thompson, J. A., Glasgow, L. A., and Warpinski, J. R., Infant botulism: Clinical spectrum and epidemiology, *Pediatrics* **66:** 936–942 (1980).
59. Arnon, S. S., Midura, T. F., Damus, K., *et al.*, Intestinal infection and toxin production by *Clostridium botulinum* as one cause of sudden infant death syndrome, *Lancet* **1:**1273–1277 (1978).
60. Weber, J. T., Goodpasture, H. C., Alexander, H., *et al.*, Wound botulism in a patient with a tooth abscess: Case report and review, *Clin. Infect. Dis.* **16:**635–639 (1993).
61. Merson, M. H., and Dowell, V. R., Epidemiologic, clinical, and laboratory aspects of wound botulism, *N. Engl. J. Med.* **289:**1005–1010 (1973).
62. MacDonald, K. L., Rutherford, G. W., Friedman, S. M., *et al.*, Botulism and botulism-like illness in chronic drug abusers, *Ann. Intern. Med.* **102:**616–618 (1985).
63. Chia, J. K., Clark, J. B., Ryan, C. A., *et al.*, Botulism in an adult associated with foodborne intestinal infection with *Clostridium botulinum*, *N. Engl. J. Med.* **315:**239–241 (1986).
64. Health and Welfare Canada, Restaurant-associated botulism from in-house bottled mushrooms—British Columbia, *Can. Dis. Week. Rep.* **13:**35–36 (1987).
65. United States Department of Agriculture, *Home Canning of Fruits and Vegetables, Home and Garden Bulletin*, No. 8, USDA, Washington, DC, 1975.
66. Shaffer, N., Wainwright, R. B., and Middaugh, J. P., Botulism among Alaska natives: The role of changing food preparation and consumption practices, *West. J. Med.* **153:**390–393 (1990).
67. Kautter, D. A., Lilly, T., Solomon, H. M., *et al.*, *Clostridium botulinum* spores in infant foods: A survey, *J. Food Protect.* **45:**1028–1029 (1982).
68. Arnon, S. S., Midura, T. F., and Damus, K., Honey and other environmental risk factors for infant botulism, *J. Pediatr.* **94:**331–336 (1979).
69. Chin, J., Arnon, S. S., and Midura, T. F., Food and environmental aspects of infant botulism in California, *Rev. Infect. Dis.* **1:**693–696 (1979).
70. Spika, J. S., Shaffer, N., and Hargrett-Bean, N., Risk factors for infant botulism in the United States, *Am. J. Dis. Child.* **143:**828–832 (1989).
71. Arnon, S. S., Damus, K., Thompson, B., *et al.*, Protective role of human milk against sudden death from infant botulism *J. Pediatr.* **10:**568–573 (1982).
72. Wilson, R., Morris, J. G., Snyder, J. D., *et al.*, Clinical characteristics of infant botulism in the United States: A study of the non-California cases, *Pediatr. Infect. Dis.* **1:**148–150 (1982).
73. Wells, C. L., Sugiyama, H., and Bland, S. E., Resistance of mice with limited intestinal flora to enteric colonization by *Clostridium botulinum*, *J. Infect. Dis.* **146:**791–796 (1982).
74. Centers for Disease Control, Botulism—Kentucky, *Morbid. Mortal. Week. Rep.* **22:**417 (1973).
75. Tackett, C. O., Shandera, W. X., Mann, J. M., *et al.*, Equine antitoxin use and other factors that predict outcome in type A foodborne botulism, *Am. J. Med.* **76:**794–798 (1984).
76. Kao, I., Drachman, D. B., and Price, D. L., Botulism toxin: Mechanism of presynaptic blockade, *Science* **193:**1245–1258 (1976).
77. Sugiyama, H., *Clostridium botulinum* neurotoxin, *Microbiol. Rev.* **44:**419–448 (1980).
78. Cherington, M., Botulism: Ten-year experience, *Arch. Neurol.* **30:** 432–437 (1974).
79. Sellin, L. C., Thesleff, S., and Dasgupta, B. R., Different effects of types A and B botulinum toxin on transmitter release at the rat neuromuscular junction, *Acta Physiol. Scand.* **119:**127–133 (1983).
80. Koenig, G. M., Spickard, A., Cardella, M. A., *et al.*, Clinical and laboratory observations on type B botulism in man, *Medicine* **43:** 517–545 (1964).
81. Sugiyama, H., and Mills, D. C., Intraintestinal toxin in infant mice challenged with *Clostridium botulinum* spores, *Infect. Immun.* **21:**59–63 (1978).
82. Moberg, L. J., and Sugiyama, H., Microbial ecological basis of infant botulism as studied with germfree mice, *Infect. Immunol.* **25:**653–657 (1979).
83. Burr, D. H., and Sugiyama, H., Susceptibility to enteric botulinum colonization of antibiotic-treated adult mice, *Infect. Immun.* **36:** 103–106 (1982).
84. L'Hommedieu, C., Stough, R., and Brown, L., Potentiation of neuromuscular weakness in infant botulism by aminoglycosides, *J. Pediatr.* **95:**1065–1070 (1979).
85. Terranova, W. A., Palumbo, J. N., and Breman, J. G., Ocular findings in botulism type B, *J. Am. Med. Assoc.* **241:**475–477 (1979).
86. Cherington, M., and Ginsberg, S., Type B botulism: Neurophysiologic studies, *Neurology* **21:**43–46 (1971).
87. Kimura, J., *Electrodiagnosis in Diseases of Nerve and Muscle*, Davis, Philadelphia, 1983.
88. Clay, S. A., Ramseyer, J. D., Fishjman, L. S., *et al.*, Acute infantile motor unit disorder: Infant botulism, *Arch. Neurol.* **34:**236–243 (1977).
89. Cornblath, D. R., Sladsky, J. T., and Sumner, A. J., Clinical electrophysiology of infantile botulism, *Muscle Nerve* **6:**448–452 (1983).
90. Engel, W. K., Brief, small, abundant motor unit potentials, *Neurology* **25:**173–176 (1975).
91. Centers for Disease Control, Follow-up: Botulism associated with commercial cherry peppers, *Morbid. Mortal. Week. Rep.* **25:**148 (1976).
92. Terranova, W. A., Breman, J. G., Locey, R. P., *et al.*, Botulism type B: Epidemiologic aspects of an extensive outbreak, *Am. J. Epidemiol.* **108:**150–156 (1978).
93. Morse, D. L., Pickard, L. K., Guzewich, J. J., *et al.*, Garlic-in-oil

associated botulism: Episode leads to product modification, *Am. J. Public Health* **80:**1372–1374 (1990).

94. Cardella, M. A., Botulinum toxoids, in: *Botulism* (K. H. Lewis and K. Cassel, eds.), pp. 113–130, US Public Health Service, Cincinnati, 1964.
95. Hatheway, C. L., Snyder, J. D., Seals, J. D., *et al.*, Antitoxin levels in botulism patients treated with trivalent equine botulism antitoxin to toxin types A, B, and E, *J. Infect. Dis.* **150:**407–412 (1984).
96. Black, R. E., and Gunn, R. A., Hypersensitivity reactions associated with botulinal antitoxin, *Am. J. Med.* **69:**567–570 (1980).

13. Suggested Reading

Arnon, S. S., Infant botulism, in: *Textbook of Pediatric Infectious Diseases* (R. Feigen and J. Cherry, eds.), pp. 1095–1102, W. B. Saunders, Philadelphia, 1992.

Centers for Disease Control, *Botulism in the United States, 1899–1973: Handbook for Epidemiologists, Clinicians, and Laboratory Workers*, CDC, Atlanta, 1978.

Hatheway, C. L., Botulism, in: *Laboratory Diagnosis of Infectious Diseases: Principles and Practice*, Volume 1 (A. Balows, J. Hausler, Jr., M. Ohashi, and A. Turano, eds.), pp. 111–113, Springer-Verlag, Berlin, 1988.

Weber, J. T., Goodpasture, H. C., Alexander, H., *et al.*, Wound botulism in a patient with a tooth abscess: Case report and review, *Clin. Infect. Dis.* **16:**635–639 (1993).

Hatheway, C. L., Toxigenic clostridia, *Clin. Microbiol. Rev.* **3:**66–98.

State of Alaska Department of Health and Social Services, *Botulism in Alaska: A Guide for Physicians and Health Care Providers*, Alaska Printing, Anchorage, 1994.

CHAPTER 7

Brucellosis

Edward J. Young and Wendell H. Hall

1. Introduction

Brucellosis is an infectious disease of animals (zoonosis) that is transmissible to humans. Man is always an accidental host, playing no role in maintaining the disease in nature. In the United States, brucellosis has largely been controlled as a result of the Federal/State Cooperative Bovine Brucellosis Eradication Program.[1] Consequently, reports of human brucellosis have declined to about 100 cases per year.

Although there is a high degree of relatedness among *Brucella* species, the genus is traditionally classified into six nomen species based on their principal animal hosts: *B. abortus* (cattle), *B. melitensis* (goats and sheep), *B. suis* (swine), *B. canis* (dogs), *B. ovis* (sheep), and *B. neotomae* (desert wood rats). Human infection has not been reported with either *B. ovis* or *B. neotomae*. *Brucella*-infected animals can appear healthy, yet they shed organisms in large numbers in their milk and cyetic products. Pregnant animals suffer from placentitis, resulting in spontaneous abortions. Brucellosis in animals results in significant economic losses worldwide, as well as posing a threat to human health. Animals are the only source of brucellosis, and there are no known vectors. Brucellosis in humans is a protean disease characterized by fever and a host of nonspecific complaints, such as fatigue, anorexia, weight loss, malaise, body aches, and depression. Aside from fever and occasionally hepatosplenomegaly, there can be a paucity of abnormal physical findings.

2. Historical Background

Brucellosis has undoubtedly existed since man first domesticated animals; however, Jeffrey Allen Marston, a Royal Army Medical Corps (RAMC) Surgeon, is credited with the first clinical description of the disease in 1863 among troops invalided to Malta during the Crimean War. Marston called it Mediterranean or gastric remittent fever, and his last case history was a poignant depiction of his own suffering from brucellosis.[2] David Bruce, another RAMC surgeon, researched Malta fever among military personnel at the Station Hospital in Valletta. In 1887, he isolated a gram-negative coccobacillus that he termed *Micrococcus* (later *Brucella*) *melitensis* from spleen tissue of seven fatal cases. M. L. Hughes[3] published the classic monograph *Mediterranean, Malta or Undulant Fever* in 1897, describing the clinical and pathological features of brucellosis. In the same year, Wright and Semple successfully applied the method of serum agglutination for diagnosis, enabling clinicians to differentiate brucellosis from typhoid, malaria, and other fevers.

The impact of brucellosis on the British presence in Malta was so great that in 1904 the Mediterranean Fever Commission was established; between 1904 and 1907, the Commission published seven *Reports*, detailing the bacteriology, epidemiology, and pathogenesis of brucellosis.[4] A major breakthrough occurred in 1905, when Themistocles Zammit successfully incriminated the Maltese goat as the animal host of brucellosis. Zammit discovered that the blood of many apparently healthy goats agglutinated brucella organisms, and later he recovered the bacteria from their blood and milk. Fresh goat's milk was conclusively shown to be the source of human infection when the

Edward J. Young • Medical Service, Veterans Affairs Medical Center, and Departments of Medicine, Microbiology, and Immunology, Baylor College of Medicine, Houston, Texas 77030. **Wendell H. Hall** • Infectious Disease Section, Veterans Affairs Medical Center, and Departments of Medicine and Microbiology, University of Minnesota, Minneapolis, Minnesota 55455.

incidence of brucellosis declined dramatically following the substitution of tinned condensed milk for fresh goat's milk in the military mess. Further evidence for goat's milk as the source of human brucellosis derived from an outbreak of the disease on the *S.S. Joshua Nicholson*. This merchant vessel, trading between Egypt and Antwerp, anchored at Malta in August 1905, taking on board 65 milk goats bound for the United States. En route to Antwerp, practically the entire crew drank unboiled milk from the goats, and within weeks, all contracted brucellosis.

The Danish physician and veterinarian, L. F. Benhard Bang, isolated *Bacterium* (later *Brucella*) *abortus* in 1895 from placental tissue of cattle suffering from contagious abortion.[5] Using cultures of this organism, Bang successfully reproduced the disease in pregnant heifers. In 1918, Alice Evans published data showing the antigenic relatedness between *B. melitensis*, the causative organism of Malta fever, and *B. abortus*, the agent of contagious abortion in cattle (Bang's disease).[6] Subsequently, the genus was named *Brucella* to honor the work of David Bruce. Human infection with *B. abortus* was documented in 1924 by Orpen[7] in Great Britain, although studies by Morales-Otero using human volunteers in Puerto Rico showed that *B. abortus* was more easily transmitted via direct inoculation through breaks in the skin than by ingestion in milk.[8] Keefer[9] had reported a case of human brucellosis in Baltimore in 1924 thought to be due to *B. abortus*, however, the organism was later identified as *B. suis*.

A third species, *Brucella suis*, was discovered in 1914 by Jacob Traum from an aborted swine fetus.[10] In 1931, Hardy *et al.*[11] reported 300 cases of human brucellosis in Iowa, including 35 caused by *B. suis* among persons in close contact with infected pigs. *Brucella suis* has a more limited geographic distribution than either *B. abortus* or *B. melitensis*, and its biovars have different natural hosts. Biovars 1, 2, and 3 cause infections in swine, whereas biovar 4 is limited to reindeer and caribou populations of the sub-Arctic regions of Alaska, Canada, and Siberia. Biovar 5 is a rodent pathogen, and human infections have been associated with laboratory accidents with this organism.[12]

Brucella canis was first reported as the cause of abortions among kennel-bred beagle dogs in 1964 by the virologist Leland E. Carmichael.[13,14] Serological studies of kennel-bred and stray dogs of various breeds indicate that *B. canis* is widespread throughout the world.[15] Nevertheless, only a handful of human infections caused by *B. canis* have been documented,[16] and the majority have been laboratory acquired.

3. Methodology

3.1. Sources of Data

In the United States, human brucellosis is a notifiable disease, and morbidity and mortality data are reported annually by the Centers for Disease Control and Prevention (CDC)[17]; however, there is evidence to suggest that underreporting remains a problem. For example, a recent study by the Texas Department of Health indicated that less than 50% of human brucellosis cases diagnosed in Texas in 1990–1991 were reported.[18]

Worldwide information on human brucellosis is tabulated by the World Health Organization (WHO); however, since brucellosis is not a notifiable disease in many countries, the reliability of these data is variable. In addition, the lack of diagnostic facilities and reporting mechanisms, especially in developing nations, renders these data questionable. The WHO periodically publishes information provided by members of the Expert Committee on Brucellosis; however, the last report was published in 1986.[19] The occurrence of brucellosis in various animal species is reported in the FAO/WHO/OIE Animal Health Yearbook, but the reliability of these data is also variable.

3.2. Surveys

Serological surveys for brucellosis in cattle and swine are routinely performed under the guidelines of the Brucellosis Eradication Program[1] and states are rated according to the numbers of reactor animals in test herds and at sale barns. Periodically, the US Department of Agriculture sponsors meetings to disseminate information regarding the epidemiology of brucellosis,[20] and brucellosis rules and regulations are periodically published in the Federal Register.

3.3. Laboratory Diagnosis

3.3.1. Isolation and Identification of the Organism. A definitive diagnosis of brucellosis is made by recovering *Brucella* from blood, bone marrow, or other tissues. Since brucellae are facultative intracellular pathogens that rapidly localize within organs of the reticuloendothelial system, cultures of bone marrow are reported to have a higher yield than blood.[21] A variety of bacteriologic methods are used, including the double broth–agar technique of Castaneda; however, routine blood culture techniques are equally as good, as long as the cultures are maintained for at least 4 weeks. Rapid isolation techniques can shorten the time of recovery from weeks to days, and systems such as the BACT/ALERT have improved the yield of blood cultures in an inverse linear relationship between the initial concentration of bacteria and the time of detection.[22] Still further shortening of the recovery time has been obtained using the lysis-concentration technique.[23] The use of the polymerase chain reaction (PCR) employing synthetic oligonucleotide primers is now being actively pursued, but is not routinely available.[24]

The identification of *Brucella* spp. is based on a variety of tests, including (1) requirements for growth in an atmosphere of added CO_2, (2) production of H_2S, (3) growth on media containing various concentrations of dyes, such as thionine and basic fuchsin, (4) agglutination by monospecific antisera, (5) lysis by specific brucellaphages, and (6) metabolic tests (Table 1). Many clinical laboratories now employ rapid identification systems based on patterns of biochemical profiles. These systems should be used with caution, since all characteristics of *Brucella* spp. are not incorporated into all databases, and some *Brucella* spp. have been misidentified as *Moraxella* spp. or *Haemophilus* spp.[25,26] Regardless of the method used, handling of *Brucella* spp. is a risk for laboratory personnel, and the use of biohazard precautions is mandatory.

3.3.2. Serological and Immunologic Tests. In the absence of bacteriologic confirmation, the diagnosis of brucellosis can be made by demonstrating high or rising titers of specific antibodies in the serum. During the course of infection with *Brucella* spp., antibodies of various immunoglobulin classes are generated against surface and intracellular antigens. The major antigen employed in standard serological tests is smooth lipopolysaccharide (S-LPS) that is present in *B. abortus*, *B. melitensis*, and *B. suis*. Since *B. canis* is naturally rough and lacks S-LPS, a homospecific antigen is required to diagnose infection with this organism.[27] A variety of methods have been used in the serological diagnosis of brucellosis,[28] but the serum agglutination test (SAT) is the most widely used and remains the test against which others are compared.[29] Techniques for performing the SAT have been published.[19]

Following infection, immunoglobulin M (IgM) appears early and for a few days is the only antibody present. Later, a switch to immunoglobulin G (IgG) synthesis occurs, after which, this isotype predominates. Upon resolution of the infection, the titer of IgG usually declines first; however, low levels of IgM can remain in the serum for months to years.[30] The rapid decline in IgG antibodies is said to be prognostic of successful therapy,[31] whereas a persistent elevation or a continued rise in IgG presages a clinical relapse or chronic infection.[32] The SAT measures the total quantity of agglutinating antibodies directed against S-LPS of *Brucella* spp. The S-LPS molecules carry the A and M epitopes, which are present in different quantities in smooth *Brucella* biovars. Owing to cross-reactions with these epitopes, a standardized (and commercially available) antigen prepared from *B. abortus* strain 1119 can be used to detect antibodies against *B. abortus*, *B. melitensis*, and *B. suis*. Cross-reactions can also occur with antibodies directed against other gram-negative bacteria, including *Vibrio cholera*, *Francisella tularensis*, *Escherichia coli* serotypes 0:116 and 0:157, *Salmonella* serotypes of the Kauffman-White group N, *Pseudomonas maltophilia*, and *Yersinia enterocolitica* serotype 0:9. However, non-*Brucella* cross-reacting antibodies are generally present in low titer and rarely preclude the diagnosis. Although no single titer of *Brucella* antibodies if *always* diagnostic, the majority of patients with brucellosis have titers $\geqslant$1:160 by the SAT. When high titers of antibodies are present, a *prozone* can occur in which there is a failure of agglutination at low dilutions of serum. A false-negative result can be avoided by routinely diluting the serum $\geqslant$ 1:320. Rarely, the serum of a patient with bacteriologically proven brucellosis will fail to agglutinate even at high dilutions, owing to the presence of a "blocking" substance. So-called "blocking antibodies" have been detected in the sera of experimental animals after intensive and prolonged immunization.[33] Electrophoresis of serum reveals that maximum blocking is found in the IgA and IgG fractions. Clinically, the appearance of blocking substance is rare, but when the SAT results are negative and the diagnosis of brucellosis is suspected, it is warranted to perform a blocking antibody test or a Coombs test.

As already mentioned, the SAT does not differentiate between IgM and IgG agglutinins. Since IgM antibodies can persist in the serum for months to years after treatment, it is important to determine the relative contributions of IgM and IgG to the agglutination reaction. This is especially important when faced with patients with delayed convalescence or persistent complaints following therapy, since the persistence of IgG antibodies can signify chronic infection or relapse. A simple method to distinguish immunoglobulin isotypes is based on the reduction of disulfide bonds of the IgM pentamer by agents such as 2-mercaptoethanol (2-ME) or dithiothreitol (DTT).[31,34] Treatment of serum with 0.05 M 2-ME reduces the agglutinating activity of IgM without affecting that of the IgG. Hence, the SAT is used to measure the total quantity of agglutinins (IgM + IgG) and the 2ME or DTT tests measure the quantity of IgG agglutinins. This is often important to distinguish between active and previously treated infection.

Table 1. Differentiation of *Brucella* Species Pathogenic for Man[a]

Species and biotypes		CO_2 requirement	H_2S production	Growth on dyes[b]		Agglutination with monospecific sera[c]		Lysis by phage Tb at RTD[d]	Metabolic tests				Common host Reservior
				Thionin	Basic fuchsin	A	M		Glutamic acid	Ornithine	Ribose	Lysine	
B. melitensis	1	−	−	+	+	−	+	−	+	−	−	−	Sheep, goats
	2	−	−	+	+	+	−	−	+	−	−	−	Sheep, goats
	3	−	−	+	+	+	+	−	+	−	−	−	Sheep, goats
B. abortus	1	+	+	−	+	+	−	+	+	−	+	−	Cattle
	2	+	+	−	−	+	−	+	+	−	+	−	Cattle
	3	+	+	+	+	+	−	+	+	−	+	−	Cattle
	4	+	+	−	+	−	+	+	+	−	+	−	Cattle
	5	−	−	+	+	−	+	+	+	−	+	−	Cattle
	6	−	+	+	+	+	−	+	+	−	+	−	Cattle
	9	+	+	+	+	−	+	+	+	−	+	−	Cattle
B. suis	1	−	++	+	−	−	−	−	±	+	+	+	Pigs
	2	−	−	+	−	−	−	−	+	+	+	−	Pigs
	3	−	−	+	+	−	−	−	+	+	+	+	Pigs
	4	−	−	+	−	+	−	−	+	+	+	+	Reindeer, caribou
	5	−	−	+	−	+	−	−	+	+	+	+	Rodents
B. canis	1	−	−	+	−	−	−	−	+	+	+	+	Dogs

[a]Modified from Corbel.[39]
[b]Growth on Albimini or trypticase agar with added dyes: thianin 20 μg/ml; basic fuchsin 20 μg/ml.
[c]A, *B. abortus*; M, *B. melitensis*.
[d]Tbilisi (Tb) phage used at routine test dilution (RTD).

Among the newer serological techniques, the enzyme-linked immunosorbent assay (ELISA) is the most promising.[35] *Brucella* S-LPS is the antigen most frequently used, but salt-extracted proteins and outer membrane proteins have also been studied. Although ELISA appears to be more sensitive than agglutination, currently there is no standardization of reagents or end point determinations, making it difficult to compare results between laboratories.[29]

Although humoral antibodies are produced during the course of brucellosis, it is the development of cellular immunity that predominates in recovery.[36] A variety of tests have been devised to examine cellular immunity in humans and animals, but few, if any, are useful in clinical diagnosis. Tests include Huddleston's opsonophagocytic index, lymphocyte transformation, leukocyte migration, and skin tests,[37] using various antigens. Although useful in understanding the pathophysiology of brucellosis, these tests have little application in the clinical diagnostic laboratory. Skin tests are not recommended for the diagnosis of human brucellosis because there are no standardized preparations, they have the potential to alter the humoral immune response, and they do not identify patients with active infection.[38]

4. Biological Characteristics of the Organism

Brucella spp. are small gram-negative coccobacilli measuring about 0.6 μm long by 0.5 to 0.8 μm wide. They lack a capsule, endospores, flagellae, or native plasmids. The outer cell membrane resembles other gram-negative bacilli, with a dominant lipopolysaccharide (LPS) component. Most strains do not have an obligatory requirement for carbohydrates; however, the growth of *B. abortus* strains is enhanced by erythritol, which is used in preference to glucose as an energy source. Metabolism is oxidative and all strains are aerobic, although some require an atmosphere of 5 to 10% CO_2, especially for primary isolation[39] (Table 1).

Phylogenetically, *Brucella* spp. appear to have a common origin with free-living, soil-dwelling bacteria. Based on 5S and 16S ribosomal RNA sequences, *Brucella* is now included in the alpha-2 group of the family *Proteobacteriaceae*.[40,41] The genus *Brucella* was originally classified according to the principal animal hosts; however, on the basis of DNA analysis, measured by hybridization, Verger *et al.*[42] proposed that the genus is comprised of only one species: *B. melitensis*. Nevertheless, by current convention the original nomen species scheme is retained for epidemiological considerations.

Identifying *Brucella* spp. isolated from humans can provide clues to the likely source of infection and may reflect the prevalence of disease in animals. Furthermore, identification of biovars is of special importance with regard to *B. suis* strains. For example, most human infections due to *B. suis* are caused by biovars 1 and 3, which originate in swine. *B. suis* biovar 2 is found largely in wild rabbits in Europe and is a rare cause of human infection.[12] On the other hand, *B. suis* biovar 4 is limited to reindeer and caribou, and human infection with this organism generally relates to exposure to these animals or ingestion of their meat.[43] Identification at the biovar level is also important for detecting new variants within geographic regions.[44,45]

The principal virulence factor of *Brucella* spp. appears to be cell wall LPS. Strains containing S-LPS show greater virulence and are more resistant to serum bacteriolysis and intracellular killing by phagocytic cells. The immunodominant epitopes of S-LPS reside within the O-side chain and include the A and M antigens described by Wilson and Miles.[46] The structure of the A and M epitopes has been elucidated,[39] and similarities in structure explains the cross-reaction with other gram-negative bacteria.

Resistance to antimicrobial drugs has rarely been documented among *Brucella* spp,[47] and organisms recovered from patients who relapsed after a course of treatment have the same antimicrobial sensitivity patterns as pretreatment isolates.[48]

5. Descriptive Epidemiology

5.1. Prevalence and Incidence

In the United States, the incidence of human brucellosis declined after World War II from more than 6000 cases per year (4.5 cases per 100,000 population) in 1948 to approximately 100 cases per year (0.05 cases per 100,000 population) in 1993. The annual incidence reported to the CDC between 1965 and 1995 is shown in Fig. 1. Recent data suggest that cases of foodborne brucellosis caused by *B. melitensis* are increasing in the United States.[49] The overall decline in cases of human brucellosis is attributed to compulsory pasteurization of milk and to the control of the disease in dairy cattle.[1]

The situation worldwide is less encouraging, and in recent years infection predominantly caused by *B. melitensis* has reached epidemic proportions in some areas, notably the Middle East. To some degree this represents better awareness, surveillance, and case identification. For example, in Jordan, brucellosis was not a notifiable disease before 1981. When it was recognized to be a public

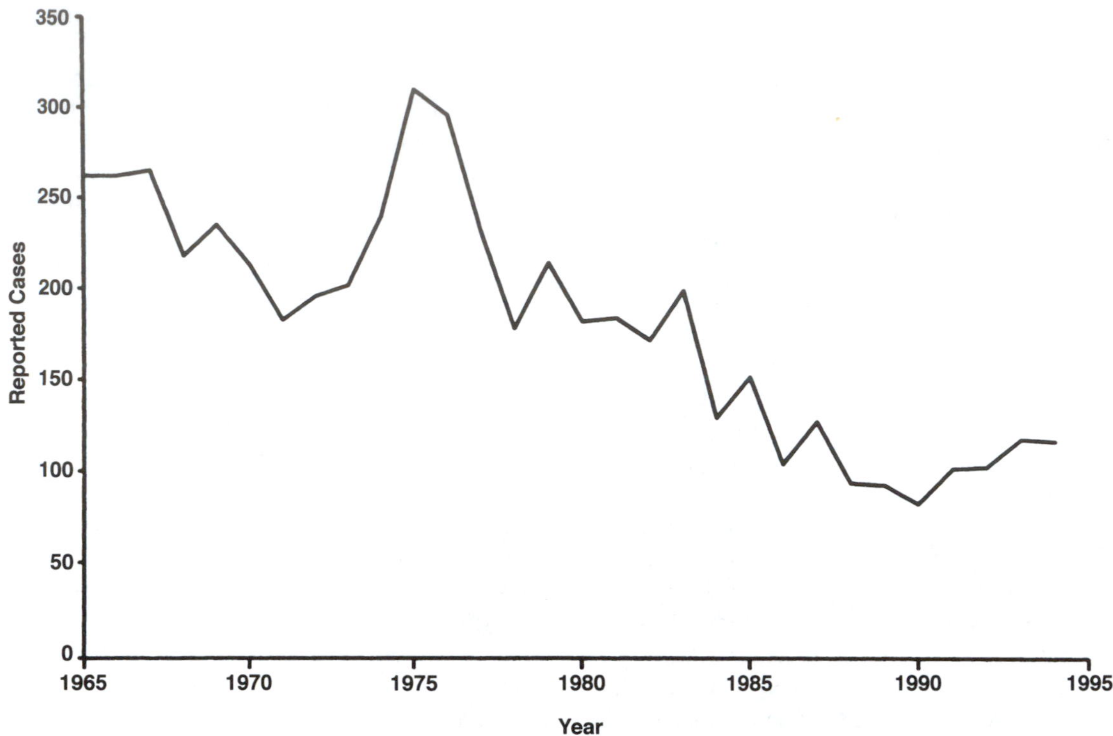

Figure 1. Brucellosis—by year, United States, 1965–1994. From Ref. 49.

health problem in 1985, the number of cases reported rose from less than 10 to more than 400 per year over the ensuing 3 years.[50] In Kuwait, between 1982 and 1985, the infection rate from *B. melitensis* rose from 5.1 to 68.9 per 100,000 population before steps were taken to combat the disease.[51]

5.1.2. High-Risk Categories. Traditionally brucellosis has been an occupational hazard for farmers, ranchers, veterinarians, abattoir workers, and laboratory personnel. In recent years, the epidemiology of human brucellosis has changed in some areas. For example, in Texas, between 1977 and 1986, the majority of patients with brucellosis were Caucasian men with documented exposure to cattle or swine in the course of their occupations. In contrast, between 1982 and 1986, the preponderance of cases occurred in Hispanics of both sexes, and the source of infection was not occupationally acquired but rather the ingestion of unpasteurized goat's milk products (e.g., cheese) originating in Mexico or other areas where *B. melitensis* is enzootic.[52] The shift from occupationally acquired brucellosis to foodborne transmission has also been reported in California.[53] Tourists visiting countries where brucellosis is enzootic are also at risk, especially if they partake of local "delicacies" such as goat's milk cheese.[54] With the speed of international travel, the symptoms of brucellosis may not become apparent until the tourist returns to the United States. Unless a history of foreign travel or unusual food consumption is elicited, brucellosis may not be considered.[55]

5.2. Epidemic Behavior and Contagiousness

Foodborne outbreaks caused by *B. melitensis* have been reported among individuals ingesting unpasteurized goat's milk cheese.[56] Such outbreaks often involve entire families, including children, without direct contact with animals. In contrast, infection with *B. abortus* is more often sporadic and usually involves direct contact with diseased animals. Traditionally, the majority of human infections caused by *B. suis* have occurred in abattoirs, where infected swine are slaughtered.[57] Abattoir-associated brucellosis continues to be a problem in the United States[58] and elsewhere[59]; however, sporadic cases of *B. suis* infection are also being recognized among hunters of feral swine.[60]

Brucellosis in humans is not as contagious as it is in animals, and human-to-human transmission is largely unknown. Nevertheless, brucellae have been recovered from banked human spermatozoa,[61] and in several cases, venereal transmission has been suggested.[62] Although the evidence is circumstantial, it may be prudent to advise individuals with brucellosis to refrain from unprotected sexual activity until the disease is resolved. A case of *B. melitenis* isolated from human milk also suggests that women with brucellosis should avoid breast-feeding until the disease is treated.[(63)]

Brucellosis is a recognized hazard for laboratory personnel working with *Brucella* spp-infected specimens.[(64)] Although infection with any species of *Brucella* can occur from laboratory accidents, in view of its greater virulence, *B. melitensis* accounts for the majority of cases. One might expect facilities with little experience to be involved more often[(65)]; however, most have occurred in laboratories with experienced personnel, using biohazard containment equipment.[(66)] Although brucellosis is not generally considered a nosocomial infection, hospital personnel caring for patients with brucellosis should practice blood-borne pathogen precautions.[(67)]

5.3. Geographic Distribution

Brucellosis is especially prevalent in the Mediterranean basin, Arabian peninsula, Indian subcontinent, and in parts of Mexico and Central and South America. No accurate overall estimate can be made of the prevalence of brucellosis worldwide, because adequate information is unavailable for many countries.[(12)]

In the United States, there has been a steady decline in brucellosis in cattle, and the widespread use of *B. abortus* strain 19 vaccine is credited with much of the success in brucellosis eradication. In 1992, only 415 herds were under quarantine for brucellosis, primarily in southern and south-central states. With the relative control of bovine brucellosis, there was a coincident decrease in disease in humans, and the epidemiology of brucellosis has shifted from primarily occupationally acquired infection to foodborne disease caused by *B. melitensis*.[(52,53)] Hence, states bordering Mexico are the geographic areas experiencing the largest number of cases relating to the importation of unpasteurized goat's milk cheese. For example, of the 120 cases of human brucellosis reported to the CDC in 1993, almost half came from Texas (34 cases) and California (19 cases).[(17)] In 1993, 27 cases were reported from North Carolina, which represented an outbreak of abattoir-associated infections at a swine-processing plant.[(58)]

5.4. Temporal Distribution

Although brucellosis can be contracted at any time of the year, depending on the circumstances of exposure, seasonal trends have been reported. In a series of cases from California, the onset of symptoms in bacteriologically confirmed cases occurred between February and May in 55.5%.[(53)] In a series from Texas, the onset of symptoms occurred in all months, with more than half between March and July.[(52)] In Saudi Arabia, cases were reported to peak in the spring and fall, when many people camp in the desert, increasing the likelihood of exposure to animals.[(68)] In the Southern Hemisphere, where the seasons are reversed, the disease occurs in the fall. In Peru, for example, outbreaks between 1939 and 1967 coincided with epizootics in goats. Years in which there was abundant rainfall were followed by increased parturition, more susceptible goats, and increased milk and cheese production.[(69)]

5.5. Age and Sex Distribution

Brucellosis can afflict persons at any age; however, most cases occur in men between 20 and 60 years who are likely to contract the disease from occupational exposure.[(70)] In countries where *B. melitensis* is enzootic, and with the trend toward foodborne transmission in the United States, increasingly brucellosis is seen in women, children, and the elderly.

Once considered rare in childhood, it is now recognized that in countries where *B. melitensis* is the predominant species, children less than 15 years of age account for up to 40% of cases.[(71)] This trend has also been noted in Texas and California,[(52,53)] where persons of Hispanic ancestry are at increased risk, perhaps reflecting the increase in immigration and food preferences of this population.

Regardless of the age of the patients, the spectrum of human brucellosis is variable, with clinical manifestations ranging from subclinical to chronic.[(70)] Although some authors have commented that children and teenagers are more likely than adults to present with gastrointestinal complaints,[(53)] this most likely represents the route of transmission, since such symptoms are also common among adults infected with *B. melitensis*.[(72)] Similar to adults, children can contract brucellosis by ingestion of contaminated food or by direct contact with diseased animals. The latter mode is especially common in cultures where newborn animals share a common living space with humans. On rare occasions, brucellosis has been reported during the neonatal period, raising the possibility of transplacental transmission or via breast milk.[(73)] When dealing with young children, clinicians should be alert to brucellosis as a cause of osteoarticular complaints[(74)] and as a cause of fever of undetermined origin.[(75)]

5.6. Brucellosis during Pregnancy

The relationship between brucellosis and abortion in humans is a frequent question and source of some controversy. The localization of brucellae within the reproductive organs of animals of both sexes is well known, and Keppie[76] hypothesized that erythritol in the placenta and other fetal tissues of pregnant cows is a growth stimulant for *B. abortus*. The absence of erythritol in human tissues was offered as an explanation for the lack of this localized form of brucellosis. Nevertheless, women who contract brucellosis during pregnancy are at some risk of abortion, but it is not clear that this risk is any greater than bacteremic infection with other pathogens. In one study, the rate of abortions was not higher among women with brucellosis than the expected rate in a population of healthy gravidas.[77] Khan and Kiel[78] recently reported a high abortion rate among women infected with *B. melitensis* in Saudi Arabia, but that antibiotic treatment given early in the course of illness prevented abortion.

5.7. Other Factors

Although there are no known racial or genetic differences in susceptibility to brucellosis in humans, genetic factors can be demonstrated in animals. Studies of genetic control of resistance to infection with *Brucella* spp. have been performed in mice, rabbits, swine, and cattle. Templeton and associates, at Texas A & M University, found that the frequency of natural resistance to *B. abortus* among cross-bred cattle was approximately 18%. Naturally resistant cows challenged with *B. abortus* did not abort and showed only a transient, short-lived rise in IgM antibodies. In addition, macrophages from resistant cows were better able to control the replication of brucellae *in vitro* than similar cells from susceptible animals.[79]

Poor nutrition and parasitic infestation is said to contribute to the severity of brucellosis. Although bacterial superinfection occurs with some intestinal parasites, concomitant brucellosis is rare.[80] The low pH of normal gastric juice appears to provide some protection against oral infection with *Brucella* spp., as evidenced by cases of brucellosis occurring in patients taking antacids or histamine-blocking drugs.[81]

6. Mechanisms and Routes of Transmission

Cutaneous inoculation occurs via minor cuts and abrasions of the unprotected skin. This is the usual route of transmission of *B. abortus* among farmers or veterinarians in the course of assisting aborting cattle during parturition. *Brucella abortus* can also be transmitted via unpasteurized cow's milk, but it appears to be less pathogenic by the gastrointestinal route than *B. melitensis*.[8] Veterinarians immunizing cattle with *B. abortus* strain 19 are at some risk of contracting brucellosis from accidental needle sticks or eye splashes with live-attenuated vaccine.[82]

The transmission of *B. melitensis* is predominantly via ingestion of unpasteurized milk or milk products from goats, sheep, and (in some areas of the world) camels, although direct contact with infected animals is not uncommon among goat and sheep herders.

The transmission of *B. suis*, other than biovar 4, has generally been associated with the slaughter of swine. Outbreaks of brucellosis in abattoirs usually occur in the kill areas where workers are exposed to aerosols of contaminated blood that can enter the respiratory tract or the conjunctival sac.[57,83] With the increased popularity of feral swine as a game animal, cases of *B. suis* infection have occurred among hunters who may be unaware of the risk of dressing the kill without taking precautions to prevent exposure to blood.[60]

6.1. Brucellosis in Wildlife

Although brucellosis occurs mainly among domestic animals, a variety of wildlife are susceptible, including elk, caribou, and bison. The role of wildlife as a source of brucellosis for domestic animals in nature continues to be debated,[84] despite evidence that under experimental conditions, bison-to-cattle transmission of *B. abortus* has been demonstrated.[85]

7. Pathogenesis and Immunity

The incubation period of brucellosis in humans is variable, depending on the infecting species, the route of transmission, and the size of the inoculum. However, the majority of patients become symptomatic within 1 to 4 weeks after infection. The onset of illness is acute in about one half the cases and insidious in the rest. Any species of *Brucella* is capable of producing serious infection; however, in general, *B. melitensis* and *B. suis* are more virulent than *B. abortus* or *B. canis*. Although the morbidity of brucellosis is considerable, with antibiotic treatment the mortality rate is less than 1%. The mortality rate of untreated brucellosis is difficult to determine from the literature of the preantibiotic era; however, it is clear that the species of *Brucella* causing infection and the localization of disease were important factors (see Ref. 86, pp. 411–417). Infections caused by *B. melitensis* and *B. suis* are generally more severe than infections caused by *B. abortus* or *B. canis*. In addition, *Brucella* endocarditis was often fatal prior to the advent of antimicrobial therapy and valve replacement surgery. We are aware of a recent case of infection due to *B. melitensis* in which death occurred from severe thrombocytopenia complicated by intracerebral hemorrhage.

The pathogenesis of human brucellosis may differ in some respects according to the method of transmission and the route of inoculation. Regardless, "natural antibodies" in human serum have some bactericidal activity against *Brucella* spp. This activity is greater against *B. abortus* than *B. melitensis* or *B. suis*, and is undetectable against *B. canis*.[87] In addition, chemotactic factors attract neutrophils to the site of inoculation, where brucellae, opsonized by complement, are phagocytized. *In vitro* studies using neutrophils from normal donors indicate that strains of *B. abortus* are destroyed more efficiently than strains of *B. melitensis*.[88] The mechanisms by which brucellae survive within neutrophils is poorly understood; however, virulent strains of *B. abortus* appear to contain a potent superoxide dismutase enzyme and nucleotidelike substances (5′-guanosine monophosphate and adenine) that suppress the myeloperoxide-H_2O_2-halide killing mechanism.[89,90] Brucellae that escape killing enter the lymphatics where they localize within organs of the reticuloendothelial system (RES). Brucellae replicate within macrophages until these cells are "activated" by specifically committed T lymphocytes. CD^{4+} T cells play a role either by activating CD^{8+} T cells or by secreting cytokines.[91] Among the cytokines implicated, interferon-γ (INF-γ) appears to be prominent in up-regulating the bactericidal action of macrophages.[92] Although humoral antibodies appear to play some role in resistance to brucellosis, cell-mediated immunity predominates.

8. Patterns of Host Response

The host response in brucellosis is somewhat dependent on the infecting species of *Brucella* and the tissue in which it is viewed. Characteristically, infection with *B. abortus* induces a granulomatous reaction, which can be demonstrated in the bone marrow, liver, spleen, and lymph nodes. Granulomas are detected in the bone marrow in up to 75% of cases[93]; however, they are often small and have indistinct borders. Occasionally there is an increase in histiocytes showing erythrophagocytosis.[94]

The liver is the best studied organ, and percutaneous liver biopsies from patients infected with *B. abortus* reveal characteristic noncaseating epithelioid granulomas indistinguishable from sarcoidosis.[95] In contrast, *B. melitensis* can induce a spectrum of hepatic lesions ranging from small to large aggregates of mononuclear cells that can expand into the liver parenchyma in a fashion resembling active hepatitis.[96] Occasionally, these aggregates contain epithelioid cells resembling granulomas. Infection with *B. suis* generally induces abscesses, which can calcify and can give rise to reactivation many years after initial infection.[97]

8.1. Clinical Features

The spectrum of human brucellosis ranges from subclinical to chronic. Whether the onset is acute or insidious, it is characterized by nonspecific complaints, such as fever, sweats, weakness, malaise, fatigue, headache, joint pains, and depression. When untreated, the fever pattern is undulating, but follows the usual diurnal variations. Physical findings can include mild lymph node enlargement and hepatosplenomegaly, but some patients have neither. Treatment with appropriate antimicrobial agents lessens the severity of disease and decreases the incidence of complications, some of which can be life threatening. Any organ or organ system can be involved; however, osteoarticular complications are the most frequent, occurring in up to 40% of cases in some series.[98] A variety of bone and joint manifestations have been reported, but sacroiliitis appears to be the most common.[99]

Other complications of brucellosis can involve respiratory, gastrointestinal, hepatobiliary, genitourinary, cardiovascular, and nervous systems.[70] Although morbidity is great, the mortality rate is 1% or less, most often associated with infective endocarditis.[100]

With treatment, most patients recover within weeks to months; however, as many as 15% relapse, depending on the agents used and the duration of therapy. Clinical relapse occurs within 3 to 6 months after stopping therapy and is usually not caused by the emergence of antibiotic-resistant strains.[48] The causes of relapse are multifactorial but discontinuation of antibiotics before completing a full 6-week course is an important consideration. Relapses of brucellosis are characterized by the reappearance of symptoms, often less severe than initially, and the reisolation of brucellae from blood or other tissues. The majority of patients with relapse can be treated successfully by repeating a full course of the same antibiotics.

The symptoms of brucellosis usually resolve within days to weeks of starting therapy. Some patients experience delayed convalescence with persisting complaints, despite a decline in IgM and IgG antibody titers. Rarely, chronic infection occurs, during which patients experience bouts of fever and other symptoms and the titer of IgG antibodies remains elevated. The cause is usually a focus of infection in the tissues, which requires surgical drainage and prolonged antibiotics.

8.2. Diagnosis

The diagnosis of brucellosis requires a high index of suspicion and knowledge about the disease. A detailed history is essential, including occupation, avocations, exposure to known animal hosts, ingestion of high-risk foods, and travel to enzootic areas. Routine laboratory tests are generally not helpful; however, the total white blood cells count is often normal or low, which is uncharacteristic of most infections.[101] Although patients with brucellosis develop cutaneous reactivity to *Brucella* antigens, skin tests are not helpful in making a diagnosis. A definitive diagnosis is made by recovering a *Brucella* sp. from blood, bone marrow, or other tissues. In the absence of bacteriologic confirmation, the diagnosis rests with the demonstration of high or rising titers of specific antibodies in the serum. The differential diagnosis includes many other infectious diseases, notably typhoid fever, tuberculosis, infectious mononucleosis, and tularemia, as well as noninfectious diseases, such as lymphoma and sarcoidosis.

9. Control and Prevention

9.1. General Concepts

Despite the availability of effective vaccines to prevent infection in animals, brucellosis remains enzootic in many parts of the world and transmission to humans continues, sometimes to epidemic proportions. What then hampers the control and eradication of this important zoonosis? In 1993, the International Task Force for Disease Eradication concluded that brucellosis would not be targeted for eradication worldwide because of "low political will.[102] In part, this reflects the high cost of brucellosis eradication programs, but it also indicates the failure of governments to recognize the public health implications of animal diseases. Epidemiological studies have shown that the persistence of brucellosis in animals, and man's risk of contracting the disease, are closely linked to (1) methods of animal husbandry, (2) standards of hygiene, and (3) habits and customs associated with the preparation of foods. It is imperative that livestock producers be educated about the dangers of brucellosis and of long-held customs and traditions in animal husbandry that contribute to the persistence of the disease. Veterinarians must be educated about the availability and effectiveness of *Brucella* vaccines, and abattoir workers, hunters, and laboratory personnel should be reminded of the precautions necessary when handling infected animals or contaminated carcasses. Travelers to countries where brucellosis is enzootic should be cautioned against eating local delicacies, such as goat's or camel's milk, cheeses, or candies, and foods should only be purchased from vendors who can attest to the safety of their wares. Physicians must be familiar with the clinical manifestations of brucellosis and the importance of reporting cases to public health authorities. Perhaps most important, lawmakers should be encouraged by the medical and veterinary professions to support programs designed to eliminate brucellosis in domestic animals.

9.2. Chemotherapy and Prophylaxis

A variety of antimicrobial agents are effective for treating brucellosis, and the subject has been recently reviewed by Hall.[103] Current recommendations for human brucellosis include doxycycline (100 mg twice daily by mouth for 6 weeks) plus streptomycin (1 g daily intramuscularly for the first 7 to 14 days). Alternatively, doxycycline (100 mg twice daily by mouth for 6 weeks) plus rifampin (600 to 900 mg per day by mouth for 6 weeks) yields generally comparable results. For young children and pregnant women, for whom tetracyclines are contraindicated, owing to the staining of deciduous teeth, trimethoprim–sulfamethoxazole (TMP/SMZ) (four tablets each containing 80 mg TMP/400 mg SMZ daily by mouth for a minimum of 21 days) has been recommended.

Treatment of brucellosis in animals is not economically feasible, nor is chemoprophylaxis of livestock. Accidental exposure to *Brucella* vaccines carries a risk of brucellosis, depending on the immune status of the victim and the amount of vaccine inoculated.[104] Vaccine sprayed into the eyes is a greater risk than needle sticks.[82] Individuals with antibodies to *Brucella* may have some immunity, but often exhibit a transient, self-limited allergic reaction. Although antibiotic prophylaxis has been recommended for humans accidentally exposed to *Brucella* vaccines,[105] there is no convincing evidence for the efficacy of this practice. Nevertheless, exposure to *B. melitensis* Rev-1 vaccine, and all cases of conjunctival inoculation, should be treated with effective antibiotics administered for at least 4 weeks.

9.3. Immunization

Vaccines for use in animals were used at one time to immunize humans at high risk of brucellosis in the Soviet Union and China. Such vaccines are not approved for human use in the United States, owing to the risk of vaccine-associated brucellosis. Killed *Brucella* vaccines and various antigenic preparations have been studied in humans, but they have not been proven to be effective.

10. Unresolved Problems

A need remains for an effective antigenic preparation to protect livestock, including swine, to replace live vaccines that induce humoral antibodies as well as protective immunity. In addition, there is a need for a simple, low-cost, sensitive and specific serological test to diagnose human brucellosis. The ELISA could be such a test if a standardized antigen could be found. Although effective antimicrobial agents exist, a need remains for an agent that can be administered orally, as monotherapy, for less than 4 to 6 weeks without the risk of relapse.

11. References

1. Brown, G., The history of the brucellosis eradication program in the United States, *Ann. Sclavo.* **19:**19–34 (1977).
2. Vassallo, D. J., The corps disease: Brucellosis and its historical association with the Royal Army Medical Corps, *J. R. Army Med. Corps* **138:**140–150 (1992).
3. Hughes, M. L., *Mediterranean, Malta, or Undulant Fever*, Macmillan, London, 1897.
4. Williams, E., The Mediterranean Fever Commission: Its origin and achievement, in: *Brucellosis: Clinical and Laboratory Aspects* (E. J. Young and M. J. Corbel, eds.), pp. 11–23, CRC Press, Boca Raton, FL, 1989.
5. Bang, B., The etiology of epizootic abortion, *J. Comp. Pathol. Ther.* **10:**125–149 (1897).
6. Evans, A. C., Further studies on *Bacterium abortus* and related bacteria. II. A comparison of *Bacterium abortus* with *Bacterium bronchisepticus* and with the organism which causes Malta fever, *J. Infect. Dis.* **22:**580–593 (1918).
7. Orpen, L. J. J., The connection between undulant (Malta) fever and contagious abortion, *Trans. R. Soc. Trop. Med. Hyg.* **22:**75–79 (1924).
8. Morales-Otero, P., Experimental infection of *Brucella abortus* in man: Preliminary report, *Puerto Rico J. Pub. Hlth. Trop. Med.* **5:**144–157 (1929).
9. Keefer, C. S., Report of a case of Malta fever originating in Baltimore, Maryland, *Bull. Johns Hopkins Hosp.* **35:**6–10 (1924).
10. Mohler, J. R., Infectious abortion in cattle, in: *Annual Report*, p. 30, US Bureau Animal Industry, 1913–1914.
11. Hardy, A. V., Jordan, C. F., Borts, I. H., and Hardy, G. C., Undulant fever with special reference to a study of *Brucella* infections in Iowa, *US Natl. Inst. Health Bull.* **158:**1–89 (1931).
12. Corbel, M. J., Brucellosis: Epidemiology and prevalence worldwide, in: *Brucellosis: Clinical and Laboratory Aspects* (E. J. Young and M. J. Corbel, eds.), pp. 25–40, CRC Press, Boca Raton, FL, 1989.
13. Carmichael, L. E., and Bruner, D. W., Characteristics of a newly recognized species of *Brucella* responsible for infectious canine abortions, *Cornell Vet.* **58:**579–592 (1968).
14. Hall, W. H., Epidemic brucellosis in beagles, *J. Infect. Dis.* **124:**615–617 (1971).
15. Brown, J., Blue, J. L., Wooley, R. E., and Dreesen, D. W., *Brucella canis* infectivity rates in stray and pet dog populations, *Am. J. Public Hlth.* **66:**889–992 (1976).
16. Swenson, R. M., Carmichael, L. E., and Cundy, K. R., Human infection with *Brucella canis*, *Ann. Intern. Med.* **76:**435–438 (1972).
17. Centers for Disease Control and Prevention, Summary of notifiable diseases, United Stats, 1994, *Morbid. Mortal. Week. Rep.* **43**(53):24 (1994).
18. Texas Department of Health, Underreporting of four infectious diseases by Texas hospitals, *Dis. Prevent. News* **53**(7):1–3 (1993).
19. *Joint FAO/WHO Expert Committee on Brucellosis, Sixth Report*, World Health Organization, Geneva, Switzerland, 1986.
20. US Department of Agriculture, Animal and Plant Health Inspection Services, Veterinary Services, Brucellosis Epidemiology Conference Proceedings, Memphis, TN, April 2–4, 1991.
21. Gotuzzo, E., Carrillo, C., Guerra, J., and Llosa, L., An evaluation of diagnostic methods for brucellosis: The value of bone marrow cultures, *J. Infect. Dis.* **153:**122–125 (1986).
22. Solomon, H. M., and Jackson, D., Rapid diagnosis of *Brucella melitensis* in blood: Some operational characteristics of the BACT/ALERT, *J. Clin. Microbiol.* **30:**222–224 (1992).
23. Navas, E., Guerrero, A., Cobo, J., and Llosa, E., Faster isolation of *Brucella* spp. from blood by isolator compared to Bactec NR, *Diagn. Microbiol. Infect. Dis.* **16:**78–81 (1993).
24. Bricker, B. J., and Halling, S. M., Differentiation of *Brucella abortus* bv. 1,2, and 4, *Brucella melitensis*, *Brucella ovis*, and *Brucella suis* bv. 1 by PCR, *J. Clin. Microbiol.* **32:**2660–2666, 1994.
25. Peiris, V., Faser, S., Fairhurst, M., Weston, D., and Kaczmarski, E., Laboratory diagnosis of brucella infection: Some pitfalls, *Lancet* **2:**1415–1416 (1992).
26. Barham, W. B., Church, P., Brown, J. E., and Paparello, S., Misidentification of *Brucella* species with use of rapid bacterial identification systems, *Clin. Infect. Dis.* **17:**1068–1069 (1993).
27. Polt, S. S., and Schaefer, J., A microagglutination test for human *Brucella canis* antibodies, *Am. J. Clin. Pathol.* **77:**740–744 (1982).
28. Diaz, R., and Moriyon, I., Laboratory techniques in the diagnosis of human brucellosis, in: *Brucellosis: Clinical and Laboratory Aspects* (E. J. Young and M. J. Corbel, eds.), pp. 73–83, CRC Press, Boca Raton, FL, 1989.
29. Young, E. J., Serologic diagnosis of human brucellosis: Analysis of 214 cases by agglutination tests and review of the literature, *Rev. Infect. Dis.* **13:**359–372 (1991).
30. Macdonald, A., and Elmslie, W. H., Serologic investigations in suspected brucellosis, *Lancet* **1:**380–382 (1967).
31. Buchanan, T. M., and Faber, L. C., 2-Mercaptoethanol brucella agglutination test: Usefulness for predicting recovery from brucellosis, *J. Clin. Microbiol.* **11:**691–693 (1980).
32. Pellicer, T., Ariza, J., Foz, A., Pallares, R., and Gudiol, F., Specific antibodies detected during relapse of human brucellosis, *J. Infect. Dis.* **157:**918–924 (1988).
33. Hall, W. H., Manion, R. E., and Zinneman, H. H., Blocking serum lysis of *Brucella abortus* by hyperimmune rabbit immunoglobulin A, *J. Immunol.* **107:**41–46 (1971).

34. Reddin, J. L., Anderson, R. K., Jenness, R., and Spink, W. W., Significance of 7S and macroglobulin brucella agglutinins in human brucellosis, *N. Engl. J. Med.* **272:**1263–1268 (1965).
35. Araj, G. F., Lulu, A. R., Mustafa, M. Y., and Khateeb, M. I., Evaluation of ELISA in the diagnosis of acute and chronic brucellosis, *J. Hyg.* **97:**457–469 (1986).
36. Serre, A., Immunology and pathophysiology of human brucellosis, in: *Brucellosis: Clinical and Laboratory Aspects* (E. J. Young and M. J. Corbel, eds.), pp. 85–95, CRC Press, Boca Raton, FL, 1989.
37. Bertrand, A., Serre, A., Janbon, F., and Vendrell, J. P., Aspects immunologiques de la brucellose: Etude evolutive et valeur pratique des diverse explorations biologiques, *Med. Mal. Infect.* **12:**582–587 (1982).
38. Bradstreet, P. C. M., Tannahill, A. S., Pollock, T. M., and Mogford, H. E., Intradermal test and serological tests in suspected *Brucella* infection in man, *Lancet* **1:**653 (1970).
39. Corbel, M. J., Microbiology of the genus *Brucella*, in: *Brucellosis: Clinical and Laboratory Aspects* (E. J. Young and M. J. Corbel, eds.), pp. 53–72, CRC Press, Boca Raton, FL, 1989.
40. Minnick, M. F., and Stiegler, G. L., Nucleotide sequences and comparison of the 5S ribosomal RNA genes of *Rochalimeae henselae*, *R. quintana*, and *Brucella abortus*, *Nucleic Acid Res.* **21:**2518 (1993).
41. Triplett, E. W., Breil, B. T., and Splitter, G. A., Expression of tfx and sensitivity to the rhizobial antibiotic trifolitoxin in a taxonomically distinct group of proteobacteria including the animal pathogen *Brucella abortus*, *Appl. Environ. Microbiol.* **60:**4163–4166 (1994).
42. Verger, J. M., Grimont, F., Grimont, P. A. D., and Grayson, M., *Brucella*, a monospecific genus as shown by deoxyribonucleic acid hybridization, *Int. J. Syst. Bacteriol.* **35:**292–295 (1985).
43. Chan, J., Baxter, C., and Wenman, W. M., Brucellosis in an Inuit child, probably related to caribou meat consumption, *Scand. J. Infect. Dis.* **21:**337–338 (1989).
44. Ewalt, D. R., and Forbes, L. B., Atypical isolates of *Brucella abortus* from Canada and the United States characterized as dye sensitive with M antigen dominant, *J. Clin. Microbiol.* **25:**698–701 (1994).
45. Banai, M., Mayer, I., and Cohen, A., Isolation, identification, and characterization in Israel of *Brucella melitensis* biovar 1 atypical strains susceptible to dyes and penicillin, indicating evolution of a new variant, *J. Clin. Microbiol.* **28:**1057–1059 (1990).
46. Wilson, G. S., and Miles, A. A., The serological differentiation of smooth strains of the *Brucella* group, *Br. J. Exp. Pathol.* **13:**1–13 (1932).
47. Hall, W. H., Modern chemotherapy for brucellosis in humans, *Rev. Infect. Dis.* **12:**1060–1099 (1990).
48. Ariza, J., Bosch, J., Gudiol, F., Linares, J., Fernandez Viladrich, P., and Martin, R., Relevance of *in vitro* antimicrobial susceptibility of *Brucella melitensis* to relapse rate in human brucellosis, *Antimicrob. Agents Chemother.* **30:**958–960 (1986).
49. Centers for Disease Control and Prevention, Summary of notifiable diseases, United States, 1994, *Morbid. Mortal. Week. Rep.* **43**(53):24 (1995).
50. Dajani, Y. F., Masoud, A. A., and Barakat, H. F., Epidemiology and diagnosis of brucellosis in Jordan, *Eastern Mediterranean Region Epidemiol. Bull.* **9:**13–22 (1988).
51. Lulu, A. R., Araj, G. F., Khateeb, M. I., Mustafa, M. Y., Yusuf, A. R., and Fenech, F. F., Human brucellosis in Kuwait: A prospective study of 400 cases, *Q. J. Med.* **66:**39–54 (1988).
52. Taylor, P. M., and Perdue, J. N., The changing epidemiology of human brucellosis in Texas, 1977–1986, *Am. J. Epidemiol.* **130:**160–165 (1989).
53. Chomel, B. B., DeBess, E. E., Mangiamele, D. M., Reilly, K. F., Farver, T. B., Sun, R. K., and Barrett, L. R., Changing trends in the epidemiology of human brucellosis in California from 1973 to 1992: A shift toward foodborne transmission, *J. Infect. Dis.* **170:**1216–1223 (1994).
54. Young, E. J., and Suvannoparrat, U., Brucellosis outbreak attributed to ingestion of unpasteurized goat cheese, *Arch. Intern. Med.* **135:**240–243 (1975).
55. Young, E. J., Brucellosis in travelers and brucella that travels, in: *Travel Medicine* (R. Steffen, H. O. Lobel, J. Haworth, and D. J. Bradley, eds.), pp. 375–377, Springer-Verlag, New York, 1989.
56. Thapar, M. K., and Young, E. J., Urban outbreak of goat cheese brucellosis, *Pediatr. Infect. Dis.* **5:**640–643 (1986).
57. Buchanan, T. M., Hendricks, S. L., Patton, C. M., and Feldman, R. A., Brucellosis in the United States, 1960–1972: An abattoir-associated disease. III. Epidemiology and evidence for acquired immunity, *Medicine* **53:**427–439 (1974).
58. Centers for Disease Control and Prevention, Brucellosis outbreak at a pork processing plant—North Carolina, 1992, *Morbid. Mortal. Week. Rep.* **43:**113–116 (1994).
59. Davos, D. E., Cargill, C. F., and Kyrkou, M. R., Brucellosis outbreak at a South Australian abattoir II. Epidemiological investigations, *Med. J. Aust.* **2:**657–660 (1981).
60. Robson, J. M., Harrison, M. W., Wood, R. N., Tilse, H. M., McKay, A. B., and Brodribb, T. R., Brucellosis: Re-emergence and changing epidemiology in Queensland, *Med. J. Aust.* **159:**153–158 (1993).
61. Vandercam, B., Zech, F., DeCooman, S., Bughin, C., Gigi, J., and Wauters, G., Isolation of *Brucella melitensis* from human sperm, *Eur. J. Clin. Microbiol. Infect. Dis.* **9:**303–304 (1990).
62. Rubin, B., Band, J. D., Wong, P., and Colville, J., Person-to-person transmission of *Brucella melitensis*, *Lancet* **1:**14–15 (1991).
63. Al-Mofada, S. M., Al-Eissa, Y. A., Saeed, E. S., and Kambal, A. M., Isolation of *Brucella melitensis* from human milk, *J. Infect.* **26:**346–347 (1993).
64. Gruner, E., Bernasconi, E., Galeazzi, R. L., Buhl, D., Heinzle, R., and Nadal, D., Brucellosis: An occupational hazard for medical laboratory personnel: Report of five cases, *Infection* **22:**33–40 (1994).
65. Staszkiewicz, J., Lewis, C. M., Colville, J., Zervos, M., and Band, J., Outbreak of *Brucella melitensis* among microbiology laboratory workers in a community hospital, *J. Clin. Microbiol.* **29:**287–289 (1991).
66. Miller, C. D., Songer, J. R., and Sullivan, J. F., A twenty-five year review of laboratory-acquired infections at the National Animal Disease Center, *Am. Ind. Hyg. Assoc. J.* **48:**271–275 (1987).
67. Kiel, F. W., and Khan, M. Y., Brucellosis among hospital employees in Saudi Arabia, *Infect. Control Hosp. Epidemiol.* **14:**268–272 (1993).
68. Al-Ballaa, S. R., Al-Balla, S. R., Al-Aska, A., Kambal, A., and Al-Hedaithy, M. A., Season variations of culture positive brucellosis at a major teaching hospital, *Ann. Saudi Med.* **14:**12–15 (1994).
69. Escalante, J. A., and Held, J. R., Brucellosis in Peru, *J. Am. Vet. Med. Assoc.* **155:**2146–2152 (1969).
70. Young, E. J., Human brucellosis, *Rev. Infect. Dis.* **5:**821–842 (1983).
71. Khuri-Bulos, N. A., Daoud, A. H., and Azab, S. M., Treatment of

childhood brucellosis: Results of a prospective trial on 113 children, *Pediatr. Infect. Dis.* **12**:377–381 (1993).

72. Al Aska, A. K., Gastrointestinal manifestations of brucellosis in Saudi Arabian patients, *Trop. Gastroenterol.* **10**:217–219 (1989).
73. Lubani, M. M., Dudin, K. I., Sharda, D. C., Abu Sinna, N. M., Al-Shab, T., Al-Refe'ai, A. A., Labani, S. M., and Nasrullah, A., Neonatal brucellosis, *Eur. J. Pediatr.* **147**:520–522 (1988).
74. Al-Eissa, Y. A., Kambal, A. M., Al-Nasser, M. N., Al-Habib, S. A., Al-Fawaz, I. M., and Al-Zamil, F. A., Childhood brucellosis: A study of 102 cases, *Pediatr. Infect. Dis. J.* **9**:74–79 (1990).
75. Chusid, M. J., Perzigian, R. W., Dunne, W. M., and Gecht, E. A., Brucellosis: An unusual cause of a child's fever of unknown origin, *Wis. Med. J.* **88**:11–13 (1989).
76. Keppie, J., Williams, A. E., Witt, K., and Smith, H., The role of erythritol in the tissue localization of the brucellae, *Br. J. Exp. Pathol.* **46**:104–108 (1965).
77. Criscuolo, E., and diCarlo, F. C., El aborto y ostras manifestaciones genecobstetricas en el curso de la brucelosis humana, *Rev. Fac. Cien.* (Med. Univ. Nac. Cordoba) *12*:321–323 (1954).
78. Khan, M. Y., and Kiel, F. W., Outcome of *Brucella melitensis* in pregnancy, *Intersci. Conf. Antimicrob. Agents Chemother.* Abs. No. 1370, p. 355, 1988.
79. Templeton, J. W., and Adams, L. G., Natural resistance to bovine brucellosis, in: *Advances in Brucellosis Research* (L. G. Adams, ed.), pp. 144–149, Texas A & M University Press, College Station, 1990.
80. Walus, M. A., and Young, E. J., Concomitant neurocysticercosis and brucellosis, *Am. J. Clin. Pathol.* **94**:790–792 (1990).
81. Steffen, R., Antacids—a risk factor in travelers brucellosis? *Scand. J. Infect. Dis.* **9**:311–312 (1977).
82. Young, E. J., *Brucella* antibodies in veterinarians exposed to strain 19, in: *Advances in Brucellosis Research* (L. G. Adams, ed.), p. 465, Texas A & M University Press, College Station, 1990.
83. Kaufmann, A. F., Fox, M. D., Boyce, J. M., Anderson, D. C., Potter, M. E., Martone, W. J., and Patton, C. M., Airborne spread of brucellosis, *Ann. NY Acad. Sci.* **353**:105–114 (1980).
84. McCorquodale, S. M., and DiGiacomo, R. F., The role of wild North American ungulates in the epidemiology of bovine brucellosis: A review, *J. Wildl. Dis.* **21**:351–357 (1985).
85. Davis, D. S., Role of wildlife in transmitting brucellosis, in: *Advances in Brucellosis Research* (L. G. Adams, ed.), pp. 373–385, Texas A & M University Press, College Station, 1990.
86. Spink, W. W., *The Nature of Brucellosis*, University of Minnesota Press, Minneapolis, 1956.
87. Hall, W. H., Studies of immunity to brucellosis and the bactericidal action of human blood against *Brucella*, Ph.D. thesis, University on Minnesota, Minneapolis, 1950.
88. Young, E. J., Borchert, M., Kretzer, F., and Musher, D. M., Phagocytosis and killing of *Brucella* by human polymorphonuclear leukocytes, *J. Infect. Dis.* **151**:682–690 (1985).
89. Tatum, F. M., Detilleux, P. G., Sacks, J. M., and Halling, S. M., Construction of Cu-Zn superoxide dismutase deletion mutants of *Brucella abortus*: Analysis of survival *in vitro* in epithelial and phagocytic cells and *in vivo* in mice, *Infect. Immun.* **60**:2863–2869 (1992).
90. Canning, P. C., Roth, A., and Deyoe, B. L., Release of 5′-guanosine-monophosphate and adenine by *Brucella abortus* and their role in intracellular survival of the bacteria, *J. Infect. Dis.* **154**:464–470 (1986).
91. Oliveira, S. C., Zhu, Y., and Splitter, G. A., Recombinant L7/L12 ribosomal protein and γ-irradiated *Brucella abortus* induce a T-helper 1 subset response from murine CD^{4+} T cells, *Immunology* **83**:659–664 (1994).
92. Zhan, Y., and Cheers, C., Endogenous gamma interferon mediates resistance to *Brucella abortus* infection, *Infect. Immun.* **61**:4899–4901 (1993).
93. Sundberg, D., and Spink, W. W., The histopathology of lesions in the bone marrow of patients having active brucellosis, *Blood* (Special Issue No. 1):7–32 (1947).
94. Martin-Moreno, S., Soto-Guzman, O., Bernaldo-de-Quiros, J., Reverte-Cejudo, D., and Bascones-Casas, C., Pancytopenia due to hemophagocytosis in patients with brucellosis: A report of four cases, *J. Infect. Dis.* **147**:445–449 (1983).
95. Spink, W. W., Hoffbauer, F. W., Walker, W. W., and Green, R. A., Histopathology of the liver in human brucellosis, *J. Lab. Clin. Med.* **34**:40–58 (1949).
96. Young, E. J., *Brucella melitensis* hepatitis: The absence of granulomas, *Ann. Intern. Med.* **91**:414–415 (1979).
97. Spink, W. W., Host–parasite relationship in human brucellosis with prolonged illness due to suppuration of the liver and spleen, *Am. J. Med. Sci.* **247**:129–136 (1964).
98. Mousa, A. R. M., Muhtaseb, S. A., Almudallal, D. S., Khodeir, S. M., and Marafie, A. A., Osteoarticular complications of brucellosis: A study of 169 cases, *Rev. Infect. Dis.* **9**:531–543 (1987).
99. Ariza, J., Pujol, M., Valverde, J., Nolla, J. M., Rufi, G., Viladrich, P. F., Corredoira, J. M., and Gudiol, F., Brucellar sacroiliitis: Findings in 63 episodes and current relevance, *Clin. Infect. Dis.* **16**:761–765 (1993).
100. Al-Harthi, S. S., The morbidity and mortality pattern of *Brucella* endocarditis, *Int. J. Cardiol.* **25**:321–324 (1989).
101. Crosby, E., Llosa, L., Quesada, M. M., Carrillo, C., and Gotuzzo, E., Hematologic changes in brucellosis, *J. Infect. Dis.* **150**:419–424 (1984).
102. Centers for Disease Control and Prevention, Recommendations of the International Task Force for Disease Eradication, *Morbid. Mortal. Week. Rep.* **42**:28 (1993).
103. Hall, W. H., Modern chemotherapy for brucellosis in humans, *Rev. Infect. Dis.* **12**:1060–1099 (1990).
104. Blasco, J. M., and Diaz, R., *Brucella melitensis* Rev-1 vaccine as a cause of human brucellosis, *Lancet* **1**:805 (1993).
105. Benenson, A. S. (ed.), *Control of Communicable Diseases in Man*, 15th ed., American Public Health Association, Washington, DC, 1990.

12. Suggested Reading

Madkour, M. M., *Brucellosis*, Butterworths, Boston, 1989.

Nielsen, K., and Duncan, J. R. (Eds.), *Animal Brucellosis*, CRC Press, Boca Raton, FL, 1990.

Spink, W. W., *The Nature of Brucellosis*, University of Minnesota Press, Minneapolis, 1956.

Young, E. J., and Corbel, M. J. (Eds.), *Brucellosis: Clinical and Laboratory Aspects*, CRC Press, Boca Raton, FL, 1989.

Young, E. J., Brucellosis, in: *Principles and Practice of Infectious Diseases*, 4th ed., (G. L. Mandell, J. E., Bennett, and R. Dolin, eds.), pp. 2053–2060, Churchill Livingstone, New York, 1994.

CHAPTER 8

Campylobacter Infections

Ban Mishu Allos and David N. Taylor

1. Introduction

Campylobacters are slender, spiral or curved, microaerophilic gram-negative rods that are one of the most commonly reported bacterial causes of diarrhea in the developing and developed world. Campylobacters also may cause systemic illness in humans and a number of diseases in wild and domestic animals. Because of morphological similarity with vibrios, these organisms were originally classified as *Vibrio fetus*.[1,2] *Campylobacter* (Greek for "curved rod") was proposed as a name of a new genus when it was found that these organisms differed in their biochemical characteristics from true members of the genus *Vibrio*. *C. jejuni* is now regarded as among the leading causes of diarrheal disease in humans. Worldwide, more than 80% of *Campylobacter* isolates implicated in human disease are *C. jejuni*; however, culture media commonly used to identify campylobacters may not support other potentially pathogenic *Campylobacter* species. Other *Campylobacter* or *Campylobacter*-like species that have been associated with human disease include *C. coli*, *C. fetus*, *C. laridis*, *Helicobacter fennelliae*, *H. cinaedi*, *C. hyointestinalis*, *C. upsaliensis*, *C. jejuni* subsp. *doyleii*, *C. sputorum*, *Arcobacter cryaerophila*, and *A. butzleri* (Table 1). *C. fetus* also causes systemic infections in immunocompromised hosts. *Helicobacter pylori* (formerly *C. pylori*) is associated with gastritis, peptic ulcer disease, and gastric cancer in humans, and unlike all other *Campylobacter*-like species does not now appear to have an animal host. Although morphologically similar, taxonomic studies do not place *H. pylori* in the same group with the other campylobacters.[3] For this reason and because it is associated with a separate clinical entity, *H. pylori* will not be discussed in this chapter.

Ban Mishu Allos • Division of Infectious Diseases, Vanderbilt University School of Medicine, Nashville, Tennessee 37232. **David N. Taylor** • Division of Communicable Disease and Epidemiology, Walter Reed Army Institute of Research, Washington, DC 20307.

2. Historical Background

The first identification of *Campylobacter* was in 1909, during an investigation of infectious abortion, when MacFadyean and Stockman,[4] two English veterinarians, isolated organisms from placentas and aborted fetuses of cattle that they called *Vibrio fetus*. Subsequently, similar organisms were found to cause infectious abortion in sheep.[4] *V. fetus* became known as a major cause of enzootic and epizootic abortion in cattle and sheep.[5] Over the next 30 years, these organisms were isolated from calves[6] and swine with diarrhea[7] and from fowl with hepatitis and diarrhea.[5] Although *V. fetus* was at first believed to cause diarrheal illness in these hosts, this association has not been clearly documented.

The first isolation of *V. fetus* from a human was in 1947 from the bloodstream of a pregnant woman who had an infectious abortion.[8] Over the next 30 years, there were occasional reports in the medical literature of isolation of these organisms from the bloodstream, cerebrospinal fluid, joint aspirates, endovascular tissue, and abscess cavities. Most of the hosts were debilitated by alcoholism, neoplasm, diabetes mellitus, cardiovascular disease, or old age.[9,10] *V. fetus* was thought to be an unusual cause of systemic illness in debilitated hosts, and it was thus considered to be an opportunistic organism. However, in 1957, Elizabeth King[11] at the Communicable Disease Center (CDC) recognized that not all the *V. fetus* organisms were the same; she identified two groups with distinct serological and biochemical characteristics. The majority of the isolates grew at 25 and 37°C, but the rest grew only at 37 and 42°C. She called this latter group

Table 1. Biochemical Characteristics of *Campylobacter* and Related Species[a]

									H_2S			Growth at			
Organism	Cat[b]	Nit red[c]	Ind ace[d]	Aryl sulf[e]	Pyrazin[f]	Hipp[g]	Nal[h]	Ceph[i]	Rapid[j]	Lead ace[k]	TSI[l]	25°C	37°C	42°C	H_2 required
C. jejuni bio 1[m]	+	+	+	−	+	+	S	R	−	++	−	−	+	+	−
C. jejuni bio 2	+	+	+	+	+	+	S	R	+	++	−	−	+	+	−
C. coli	+	+	+	−	+	−	S	R	−	++	−	−	+	+	−
C. fetus	+	+	−	−	−	−	R	S	−	+	−	+	+	−	−
C. upsaliensis	(+)	+	+	−	+	−	S	S	−	(+)	−	−	+	(+)	n
C. lari	+	+	−	−	+	−	R	R	+	+	−	−	+	+	−
C. hyointestinalis	+	+	−	−	−	−	R	S	−	5+	3+	(+)	+	+	n
H. fennelliae[o,p]	+	−	+	+	−	−	S	(S)	−	+	−	−	+	−	−
H. cinaedi[o]	+	+	−	−	−	−	S	(S)	−	(+)	−	−	+	−	−
C. jejuni s. *doylei*	(+)	−	+	−	+	(+)	S	(S)	−	−	−	−	+	(+)	n
A. cryaerophilis[q]	+	+	+	−	−	−	S	(R)	−	−	−	+	+	−	−
A. butzleri[q]	(+)	+	+	−	−	−	S	(R)	−	−	−	−	+	(+)	−
C. sputorum bio. *sputorum*	−	+	−	+	+	−	R	S	+	5+	3+	−	+	+	−
C. sputorum bio. *bubulis*	−	+	−	+	−	−	R	S	+	5+	3+	−	+	(+)	−
C. sputorum bio. *faecalis*	+	+	−	+	+	−	R	S	+	5+	3+	−	+	+	−
C. concisus	−	+	−	+	+	−	(R)	S	−	3+	(+)	−	+	(−)	+
C. mucosalis	−	+	−	−	−	−	R	S	−	5+	+	(−)	+	(−)	+
C. curvus	−	+	+	+	+	−	R	S	−	5+	+	−	+	+	+
C. rectus	−	+	+	+	+	−	S	R	−	3+	+	−	+	+	+

[a]+, Positive; (+), most strains positive; −, negative; (−), most strains negative; R, resistant; (R), most strains resistant; S, susceptible; (S), most strains susceptible.
[b]Catalase.
[c]Nitrate reduction.
[d]Indole acetate.
[e]Aryl sulfatase.
[f]Pyrazinamidase.
[g]Hippurate hydrolysis.
[h]Nalidixic acid resistance.
[i]Cephalothin resistance.
[j]Rapid H_2S. Method of Skirrow and Benjamin.[249]
[k]Lead acetate.
[l]Triple sugar iron.
[m]*C. jejuni* subsp. *jejuni* biotypes 1 and 2 refer to Skirrow's scheme. Susceptibilities are based on 30-μg disks.
[n]Some isolates grow much better in H_2-enhanced growth conditions.
[o]Spreading, noncolonial growth.
[p]Hypochlorite odor.
[q]Aerobic growth occurs at 30°C.

"related vibrios" and noted that although they were isolated from the bloodstream; in each case the patient had had a diarrheal illness. She postulated that the related vibrios caused acute diarrheal illness, but because they were slow growing and fastidious, they could not be isolated from fecal specimens.[11]

Based on King's and his own observations that the related vibrio was associated with diarrhea, Bokkenheuser[9] concluded that this organism was probably present in feces, but could not be detected with the available laboratory techniques. Cooper and Slee[12] in Australia isolated *V. fetus* (*C. jejuni*) from the stool of an immunocompromised patient with recurrent bacteremia and diarrhea by inoculating the patient's feces onto a horse blood agar plate containing cephalothin disks and incubating it overnight in a carbon dioxide-enriched atmosphere. In 1972, Dekeyser *et al.*[13] reported a positive stool culture for *Campylobacter* from a 22-year-old woman from whom *C. jejuni* had been isolated from the blood. The stool isolate was obtained by filtering fecal specimens through a 0.65-μm Millipore filter with a syringe. Using this filtration procedure, Butzler *et al.*[14] were able to isolate *Campylobacter* from 5.1% of 800 children in Brussels with diarrhea and only 1.3% of 1000 children without diarrhea.

Skirrow[15] showed that an agar medium containing antibiotics could be used instead of filtration as a primary isolation technique and that *C. jejuni* was as important a cause of diarrheal disease in England as Butzler *et al.*[14] had found it in Belgium. The use of antibiotic-containing selective media combined with simple methods for obtaining a microaerobic atmosphere have made isolation of *Campylobacter* a routine procedure and have opened up the study of *Campylobacter* infections on a worldwide scale. In 1973, Veron and Chatlain[16] reported that *V. fetus* and related vibrios had biochemical characteristics dissimilar to those of the Vibrionaceae, and a new genus, *Campylobacter*, was proposed. Under this scheme and later modification by Smibert,[5] King's related vibrios became *C. jejuni* and *C. coli*, and the opportunistic organisms became *C. fetus* subsp. *fetus*, respectively.[2,16]

New members of the genus *Campylobacter* and related genera are being identified with regularity. Some Campylobacters, particularly the hippurate-negative group, are not thermotolerant and are susceptible to antibiotics, such as cephalothin and colistin, that are incorporated into selective isolation media. These *Campylobacter* can be isolated at 37°C on media without antibiotics by inoculating a stool suspension directly on a 0.45-μm Millipore filter that has been placed directly on a blood agar plate.[17] Using these and other similar methods, increasing numbers of these organisms have been isolated from humans with gastrointestinal illness, suggesting that "atypical" campylobacters play a greater role in causing human disease than previously thought. Nevertheless, at present, *C. jejuni* remains the most important cause of diarrheal disease in this group, and the importance of these "related" campylobacters as human pathogens has not yet been fully defined.

3. Methodology

3.1. Sources of Mortality Data

Limited information is available concerning the importance of *Campylobacter* in fatal diarrheal disease; however, judging from the frequency of *Campylobacter* infection in patients ill enough to seek medical attention, the bacterium may be a major cause of mortality due to diarrheal disease. In developed countries in recent years, mortality due to diarrheal diseases has been low. Several deaths due to infection by *C. jejuni* have been reported, which have allowed for limited population-based estimates of mortality.[18] The uncommon human infections with *C. fetus* subsp. *fetus*, usually occurring in debilitated hosts, have sometimes been fatal.[9,19] Campylobacter infections occurring in persons with human immunodeficiency virus (HIV) infection or other immunodeficiencies may be associated with higher mortality rates. Guillain–Barré syndrome and the hemolytic–uremic syndrome are uncommon complications of *C. jejuni* infections that are also potentially fatal (Section 8.1).

3.2. Sources of Morbidity Data

Because campylobacters produce diarrheal illnesses that are usually indistinguishable from those caused by other viral and bacterial enteric pathogens, it is not possible to obtain data on morbidity in the absence of laboratory identification of the organism. Most data on morbidity in Europe and the United States come from hospital-based or community-based studies of *Campylobacter* infections.[20–22] Estimates of incidence in HIV-infected persons are made by studying patients in AIDS clinics.[23,24] Surveys from hospitals and clinics have also been conducted in developing countries. At the International Center for Diarrheal Disease Research in Bangladesh, surveillance is based on culturing 4% of patients who come to the center with acute diarrheal disease.[25] In England and Wales, 200 public health and hospital laboratories report *Campylobacter* isolations to the Communicable Disease Surveillance Center.[26] In the United States, *Campylobacter* isolations are routinely reported to the Centers for Disease Control and Prevention (CDC).[27,28] Outbreaks of *Campylobacter* infection are routinely reported to the CDC *Campylobacter* National Surveillance system.[28]

3.3. Serological Surveys

Serological surveys using one or several antigens common to the majority of *Campylobacter* strains have been performed among healthy populations in the United States, Bangladesh, and Thailand.[29–31] Surveys have been made to confirm the diagnosis in patients with diarrhea, to investigate outbreaks, to determine the etiology when multiple pathogens were isolated, to investigate occupational exposure and other high-risk groups,[32,33] and to investigate the association of *Campylobacter* with postinfection complications such as reactive arthritis and Guillain–Barré syndrome.[34,35]

3.4. Laboratory Diagnosis

Stools or rectal swabs, the usual specimens submitted to the laboratory for examination, are inoculated onto selective media to permit isolation of *Campylobacter*. A transport medium such as Cary–Blair should be used if a delay of more than 2 hr is anticipated before arrival of the specimen to the laboratory.[36] The three most commonly used selective media for isolation of *C. jejuni* or *C. coli* are Skirrow's,[15] Butzler's,[37] and Campy–BAP,[38] all with rich basal media enriched with sheep or horse blood and all containing antibiotics to inhibit the normal enteric flora. Skirrow's medium is the least inhibitory to the enteric flora; however, in most patients with *Campylobacter* enteritis, the titer of *Campylobacter* organisms per gram of stool ranges from 10^6 to 10^9,[39] a quantity easily detected with this medium. Butzler's media, Virion, which contains cefaperazone and is more inhibitory to competing flora, also appears to be very useful.[40] Blood-free media containing antibiotics have also been used successfully,[41] and several enrichment media have been found to support the growth of *Campylobacter*.[40] Enrichment methods are probably not necessary for detection of *Campylobacter* is diarrheal stools, but may be useful in detecting carriers. A combination of blood-free media such as cefoperazone deoxycholate agar and charcoal-based selective medium may achieve the highest yield of *C. jejuni* or *C. coli* from stool specimens.[42]

Many campylobacters that cause diarrhea are inhibited by cephalothin or colistin, which are present in selective media, or by incubation at 42°C.[17,43] In the United States, more than 99% of reported *Campylobacter* isolates are *C. jejuni*.[28] This predominance probably reflects the types of culture media routinely used for detection of campylobacters in this country. In studies where antibiotic-free media or filtration methods are used, the proportion of campylobacters that are non-*jejuni* species is over 20%. Both Campy–BAP and Butzler's media contain cephalosporins, which inhibit most strains of *C. fetus* subsp *fetus* and many of the "atypical" organisms; for this reason, the potential of these organisms to cause human disease may be underappreciated.[44,45] Steele demonstrated a 0.45-μm cellulose acetate membrane filter placed directly on an antibiotic-free blood agar plate could be used to isolate *Campylobacter* at 37°C.[17] *Campylobacter* in saline solution are able to pass through the filter while other fecal flora do not. A 0.65-μm filter may offer better isolation rates than the 0.45 μm, although the number of contaminating bacteria is also increased. Because the yield for detecting atypical campylobacters is so much higher with a filter and nonselective medium such as chocolate agar, this technique is now recommended for primary isolation of campylobacters from feces or rectal swabs.

Campylobacters require an atmosphere with an oxygen concentration of 5–10% for optimal growth. A microaerobic atmosphere may be produced by using *Campylobacter*-specific gas-generating kits[46] or by evacuating vacuum jars or bags and refilling with a mixture of 5% oxygen, 10% carbon dioxide, and 85% nitrogen. Campylobacters are capnophilic, although carbon dioxide is not essential for growth.[2] Incubation of plates in a candle jar may permit isolation from most positive specimens, but should best be used at 42°C.[46]

When using selective antibiotic media, optimal isolation of *C. jejuni* is obtained at an incubation temperature of 42°C; however, some *Campylobacter* species cannot be isolated at that temperature (Table 1). All organisms will grow at 37°C. When using the more selective media, the higher temperature for incubation is recommended. If the membrane filter method is employed, the optimum incubation temperature is 37°C.

After incubation of cultures under these conditions for 24–48 hr, colonies that are gray, mucoid, or wet-appearing, or discrete should be suspected of being *Campylobacter* and may be identified as such using standard biochemical tests[2] (Table 1). A rapid presumptive identification can be made by the following characteristics: (1) typical colonial morphology; (2) typical Gram's stain showing gram-negative curved rods; (3) indication of oxidase and catalase positivity; and (4) motility. *Campylobacter* can be isolated from body fluids or tissues that do not have a normal flora by using thioglycollate broth or biphasic media. Some commercial blood culture systems are superior to others for detection of bacteremia due to *Campylobacter* species.[47]

Direct examination of stools has been used as a rapid screening test for *Campylobacter* in developed countries.[48–50] These methods are usually specific, but are only about 50–75% sensitive. Staining with 1% aqueous basic fuchsin was reported to be the most sensitive method[49] Sensitivity was increased in the presence of fecal leukocytes.[50]

Serological diagnosis is possible in which antibodies to the homologous strain or to a common acid-extracted antigen are detected.[29] DNA probes for the diagnosis of *Campylobacter* are still in the experimental stage.[51] Specific oligonucleotide probes have been produced and will eventually be useful when nonradioactive means of detection become available.[52]

A biotyping scheme for *C. jejuni*, *C. coli*, and *C. laridis* strains has been developed that is based on hippurate hydrolysis, rapid H_2S production, and DNA hydrolysis.[53] A phage-typing system has also been developed for *C. jejuni* and *C. coli*.[54] The two most widely used serotyping systems for *C. jejuni* and *C. coli* are the Penner system, which identifies soluble, heat-stable (somatic, O) antigens by passive hemagglutination,[55] and the Lior system, which measures heat-labile (flagellar, H) antigens by slide agglutination.[56] There are over 90 reference serotypes defined by the Penner system and 112 by the Lior system. Both systems identify over 90% of *Campylobacter* isolated from humans and nonhuman sources.[57,58] The Lior system is easier to use and more rapid and consequently more applicable for use outside reference laboratories.[59] Strains of a single serotype in one system may belong to multiple serotypes in another system. These two systems may eventually be combined to produce a system similar to *Escherichia coli* serotyping based on both O and H antigen grouping.

4. Proof of Causation and Biological Characteristics of the Organism that Affect the Epidemiological Pattern

The evidence that *C. jejuni* is an etiologic agent for human diarrheal disease can be summarized as follows: (1) In developed countries, *Campylobacter* has been isolated from the stools of 3–14% of patients presenting at hospitals with diarrhea, but only rarely from stool samples of controls (Table 2). (2) Outbreaks of gastrointestinal illness have occurred among previously healthy populations in which no other pathogen has been found, and *Campylobacter* has been isolated from the stools of patients but not from controls (Section 6). (3) In natural settings and in experimental models, *Campylobacter* has caused diarrheal illness in avian species[60] and in mammals such as puppies[61] and nonhuman primates.[62] (4) In several patients who had diarrheal illness, *Campylobacter* was simultaneously isolated from stool and blood.[11–13] (5) Rising titers of specific serum antibody to the infecting organisms have been shown.[29,38] (6) Treatment of ill *Campylobacter*-infected patients with erythromycin, an agent to which most other recognized enteric pathogens do not respond, has been followed by rapid clearance of organisms and rapid remission of symptoms.[63] (7) Two volunteers ingested organisms in a glass of milk and developed a typical gastrointestinal illness after 3 days, and *Campylobacter* was isolated from their stools.[64] (8) Finally, two strains of *C. jejuni* isolated from persons with diarrhea were fed to 111 American adult volunteers

Table 2. Isolation of *Campylobacter* from Fecal Cultures from Patients with Diarrhea and from Healthy Controls in the Developed Countries, 1973–1986

			Patients with diarrhea				Healthy controls	
Reference	Location	Population	No. studied	% with *C. jejuni*	% with *Salmonella*	% with *Shigella*	No. studied	% with *C. jejuni*
Butzler[14]	Belgium	Children	800	5.1			1000	1.3
Skirrow[15]	England	All ages	803	7.1			194	0
Brunton[217]	Scotland	All ages	196	8.7	2.5	6.7	50	0
Bruce[218]	England	All ages	280	13.9	4.3	3.9	156	0.6
Kendall[21]	England	All ages	3,250	14.9	2.1	1.1		
Severin[219]	Netherlands	All ages	584	10.8	10.0		120	0
Lopez-Brea[220]	Spain	All ages	446	4.5	12.1	1.3		
Delorme[221]	France	All ages	100	9.0	0	1.0	330	0
Graf[222]	Switzerland	All ages	665	5.7	12.6	0.9	800	0
Velasco[223]	Spain	All ages	6,970	7.3	10.2	5.4		
Figura[224]	Italy	Children	643	9.0	9.6	0		
Cevenini[225]	Italy	Children	561	8.0	7.3	0		
Svedhem[22]	Sweden	All ages	2,550	10.9	7.2	3.5		
Walder[181]	Sweden	All ages	5,771	6.9	4.1	1.7	2000	0.25
Pitkanen[125]	Finland	Adults	775	7.1	NR	NR		
Lassen[85]	Norway	All ages	7,700	3.0	4.7	2.9		
Steingrimsson[89]	Iceland	All ages	4,019	1.7	4.1	0.2		
Blaser[97]	United States	All ages	2,670	4.6	3.4	2.9	157	0
Blaser[20]	United States	All ages	8,097	4.6	2.3	1.0		
Pien[226]	Hawaii	All ages	471	8.7	4.2	3.8		
Pai[227]	Canada	Children	1,004	4.3	5.1	1.4	176	0
Thompson[88]	Canada	All ages	146,842	3.8	7.9	0.2		
Burke[228]	Australia	Children	975	7.4	5.7	1.3	975	0.6
Kirubakaran[229]	Australia	Children	386	4.4	12.2	3.4	332	0
MacDonald	United States	All ages	6,485	3.0	1.7	0.6		
Skirrow[230]	England	All ages	1,873	5.5	3.4	0.8		

with sodium bicarbonate.[65] The minimum infective dose was 1000 organisms. With one strain (81-176), all became infected (i.e., *Campylobacter* was isolated from their stools) and 18 (46%) of 39 developed diarrhea with fecal leukocytes or fever after ingestion of 10^6 organisms. The findings thus fulfill the Henle–Koch postulates of causation (see Chapter 1, Section 13).

Campylobacters grow best at the body temperatures of warm-blooded hosts. *C. jejuni* has been identified as a part of the enteric flora in swine, dogs, cats, nonhuman primates, rodents, cattle, sheep, and other ruminants.[5] Optimal growth occurs at 42°C, the body temperature of fowl, and *C. jejuni* appears to be commensal in adult domestic fowl. *Campylobacter* appears to be an enteric pathogen for primates,[62] but its role as an enteric pathogen in other animal species is not well defined.

Viability of organisms under environmental conditions is temperature-dependent. *C. jejuni* will survive for weeks in water, feces, urine, and milk when kept at 4°C; however, at 25°C, viability persists for a few days or less.[39] *Campylobacter*, like *Salmonella*, is quite sensitive to low pH and will not survive longer than 5 min at a pH less than 2.3. At neutrality or alkaline pH, especially in bile, organisms may multiply and survive up to 3 months at 37°C.[39]

Of clinical isolates of *Campylobacter* in a Toronto study, 15% were resistant to tetracycline and 15% to ampicillin. [66] Erythromycin resistance is generally reported to be less than 10%, but may be much greater and clinically significant in other countries such as Thailand.[67] *C. coli* isolated from animals or humans are more resistant to both erythromycin and tetracycline.[67] Ampicillin resistance was associated with chromosomally mediated β-lactamase production. Tetracycline resistance is carried on a 45-kilobase (kb) transmissible plasmid.[68] Kanamycin resistance in *C. coli* may be mediated on the same plasmid and may be due to synthesis of 3′-aminoglycoside phosphotransferase type III.[69] This type of aminoglycoside resistance was previously found only in gram-positive cocci and suggests that *Campylobacter* could acquire resistance plasmids from unrelated bacterial species.[70] Strains are generally susceptible to chloramphenicol, gentamicin, furazolidone, nalidixic acid, and the newer nalidixic acid analogues such as norfloxacin and ciprofloxacin.[71,72]

5. Descriptive Epidemiology

5.1. Prevalence and Incidence

It is now well established that *C. jejuni* is an important cause of diarrheal illness in the developed world in all age groups. Prevalence of *disease* caused by *Campylobacter* is based on the rate of isolation of the organism from patients with diarrheal illness. Inferences drawn from such studies must be tempered by knowledge of the data artifacts implicit in laboratory-based culture surveys. Defining the presence of *infection* due to *Campylobacter* in a community includes prevalence of isolation of the bacterium from the stools of healthy persons and the presence of antibodies to *Campylobacter* among a representative population sample.

Campylobacter infections have been evaluated as part of surveys on the etiology of diarrheal disease among persons coming to the hospital or clinic. In the developed world, *Campylobacter* ranks among the most commonly isolated bacterial pathogens from persons with diarrheal disease and is uncommonly isolated from populations of healthy controls (Table 2). Studies in communities, cities, and states in the United States, England, and Israel show that the rate of reported *Campylobacter* isolations ranges from 1.4 to 100 per 100,000 population per year.[18,26,73,74] Rates of *Campylobacter* infections vary according to the age distribution and location of the study population. The rate of *Campylobacter* isolation in the United States reported to the CDC has been stable at 5 to 6 per 100,000 population since 1982.[75] Because many hospital laboratories still do not routinely culture diarrheal stools, this reported rate likely represents a gross underestimate of the true rate of *Campylobacter* infections.

Two prospective studies document the true incidence of campylobacters relative to salmonellae and shigellae. In the first, eight hospital microbiology laboratories routinely looked for campylobacters every time they cultured stools for other pathogens. *Campylobacter* was isolated twice as frequently as *Salmonella* and 4.5 times as frequently as *Shigella*.[20] In the second study, a Seattle health maintenance organization (HMO) cultured all diarrheal stools for the same three pathogens. Campylobacters were again isolated twice as frequently as salmonellae and seven times as frequently as shigellae.[76] Because the reported rate of *Salmonella* infections is 20 per 100,000 population, if clinical laboratories cultured diarrheal stools as often as they cultured them for salmonellae, the incidence of *Campylobacter* infections would be twice this rate—40 per 100,000 population.

Another reason for underreporting of *Campylobacter* infections is the mildness of many infections; patients might not find it necessary to seek medical care. In a community wide outbreak of *C. jejuni* infections caused by a contaminated water supply, only 1 of 18 symptomatic persons sought medical care.[77] In another outbreak at a summer camp, only 4 (10%) of 41 infected persons were sufficiently ill to seek medical attention.[78] These and other studies indicate that the true annual incidence of

Campylobacter infections in the United States is 1000 per 100,000 population.[79] Similarly, in England the reported rate of *Campylobacter* infections is only 20 per 100,000 population per year; however, studies at the level of community-based physicians also showed that the true annual incidence is 1,100 per 100,000 population.[21] The case-fatality rate for *Campylobacter* infections has been estimated at 0.05 per 1000 cases.[18]

In developing countries, *Campylobacter* infection is hyperendemic and asymptomatic infection may be frequent (Table 3). The case-to-infection ratio is probably quite high and varies inversely according to age, suggesting that immunity is an important factor.[80] Furthermore, adults naturally and experimentally infected with *C. jejuni* were less susceptible to illness if they had preexisting antibody titers to *Campylobacter*.[32,81] *Campylobacter* infections are an important cause of childhood morbidity from watery diarrhea in developing countries.

5.2. Epidemic Behavior

In addition to endemic infection, outbreaks of disease associated with *Campylobacter* regularly occur in developed countries. Outbreaks do not occur where *Campylobacter* infections are hyperendemic, such as in many areas of the developing world, probably because of a high prevalence of postexposure immunity.[30] Outbreak investigations have provided much of the information about specific vehicles for transmission of infection (Section 6).

Investigations of outbreaks have shown that asymp-

Table 3. Isolation of *Campylobacter* from Fecal Cultures from Patients with Diarrhea and from Healthy Controls in the Developing Countries

Reference	Location	Year	Population	Patients with diarrhea		Healthy controls	
				No. studied	% with *Campylobacter*	No. studied	% with *Campylobacter*
	Asia						
Ringertz[231]	Indonesia	1980	0–9 yr	144	10	7	29
Blaser[92]	Bangladesh	1980	Children	204	12	141	18
Rajan[232]	India	1982	All ages	305	15	—	—
Glass[93]	Bangladesh	1983	All ages	3038	14	333	7
Nair[233]	India	1983	All ages	116	10	—	—
Lim[234]	Malaysia	1984	All ages	—	4	—	2
Ho[168]	Hong Kong	1985	0–2 yr	1957	2	1841	2
Young[235]	China	1986	0–15 yr	48	19	105	9
Taylor[a(122)]	Thailand	1986	0–5 yr	1230	13	1230	11
Nath[237]	India	1993	Children	604	4	529	1
	Europe						
Popovic-Urovic[238]	Yugoslavia	1989	All ages	2080	16	—	—
	Africa						
Billingham[127]	Gambia	1981	All ages	287	14	383	4
De Mol[90]	Rwanda	1983	Children	271	14	203	3
Olusanya[239]	Nigeria	1983	5–39 yr	—	12	—	2
Georges[250]	Central African Republic	1984	0–15 yr	1197	11	748	7
Pazzaglia[236]	Egypt	1993	Children	880	17	1079	6
Zaki[240]	Egypt	1986	All ages	3135	2	702	1
Megraud[a]	Algeria	1987	0–15 yr	868	16	376	15
Bokkenheuser[9]	South Africa	1979	0–2 yr	78	35	63	16
Mauff[241]	South Africa	1981	All ages	2323	4	—	—
	South Africa	1981	0–2 white	—	5	—	—
	South Africa	1981	0–2 black	—	13	—	—
Mackenjee[242]	South Africa	1984	Hospital	126	21	128	5
	South Africa	1984	Outpatient	352	7	—	—
Lastovica[243]	South Africa	1986	Children	2951	10	—	—
	Latin America						
Hull[244]	Trinidad	1982	Children	60	12	—	2
Mata[245]	Costa Rica	1983	Children	233	8	—	—
Guerrant[246]	Brazil	1983	Children	40	8	—	—
Olarte[247]	Mexico	1983	Children	265	9	54	4
Figueroa[248]	Chile	1986	Children	35	6	—	—

[a]Presented at the IV International Conference on *Campylobacter* infections (1987).

tomatic infection may occur in those exposed to an implicated vehicle[78,82,83] and that the spectrum of illness produced may be broad. Secondary spread of infection does occur in close contacts such as family members. In follow-up studies in Israel, 20 (10%) of 200 family contacts were found to excrete *Campylobacter*.[84] However, in most sporadic cases the source is not known and it is difficult to distinguish co-primary from secondary infections.

5.3. Geographic Distribution

Campylobacter infections are present in all parts of the world, as documented by studies of diarrheal disease on all inhabited continents (Tables 2 and 3). Isolations have been made from patients in tropical, temperate, and Arctic climates. Travelers who have acquired *Campylobacter* infections in every region of the world represent a considerable proportion of the total cases in Scandinavian countries.[85,86] Similarly, persons from developed countries who are living in developing countries are also at risk for *Campylobacter* infection.[87] In northern climates such as Canada[88] and Iceland,[89] *Campylobacter* infections are reported more commonly among persons in rural areas. In Ontario, Canada, the annual case rate was 80 per 100,000 in urban or nonfarm areas and 350 to 400 per 100,000 in farm areas where cases were often associated with raw milk ingestion.[88] High isolation rates in rural areas of Africa have been attributed to close association with domestic animals.[90]

The prevalence of *Campylobacter* infection is higher in developing than in developed areas (Table 3). Studies of healthy children in rural South Africa,[91] rural Bangladesh,[92,93] Central African Republic,[80] and The Gambia[94] found that asymptomatic infection of young children was prevalent. In The Gambia, 7.6% of asymptomatic children 2–4 years old were infected, and in both South Africa and Bangladesh, 40% of healthy children 9–24 months old were culture-positive on a single determination. In a longitudinal study, *Campylobacter* infections were found in 41% of 127 children who were cultured biweekly from birth until 6 months of age.[80] As a consequence of continued and widespread exposure to campylobacters, in developing countries there is no difference in the isolation rate of *Campylobacter* from children with and without diarrhea. Furthermore, because infection and immunity are acquired early in life, *Campylobacter* infections are uncommon in adults in developing countries; no difference in isolation rates was observed among adults with and without diarrhea in Bangladesh.[95] After infection, the duration of excretion of *Campylobacter* is shorter (about 7 days) than it is among persons in developed countries. The high *Campylobacter* isolation rate among persons with diarrhea is caused by frequent transmission of organisms among the population rather than prolonged convalescent excretion.[96]

5.4. Temporal Distribution

In industrialized countries in temperate climates there is a definite increase in isolation rate during the hot summer months and a definite decrease during the cold winter months.[97,98] In Scandinavian countries there is another peak after winter holiday seasons resulting from infections in travelers.[85] In tropical, developing countries there is usually no seasonal variation.[93]

5.5. Age and Sex

In industrialized countries there is a bimodal age distribution. The largest peak occurs in children less than 5 years old and a second peak occurs in young adults 20 to 29 years old (Fig. 1A). Among hospitalized patients, a third peak is observed among persons 60 to 80 years old.[31,86] In *Campylobacter* infections among children and young adults, males usually predominate[27] (Fig. 1A), and among older persons the ratio is equal or in favor of females. In Colorado, for example, males predominate in all age groups under 40 and the greatest difference between sexes was in infants, where the male-to-female ratio was over 2:1.[99] In keeping with the second peak of isolation in young adults, *Campylobacter* is the predominant cause of diarrheal disease at American universities.[100] Eating undercooked chicken and close association with cats are recognized risk factors among university students.[100,101]

In developing countries, isolation rates are highest among children less than 1 year old and do not increase again in young adults (Fig. 1B). The highest isolation rate occurs in children 6 to 12 months old (Fig. 1B inset). In developing countries, one to two *Campylobacter* infections per year for children under 5 years of age would be a conservative estimate. Serological surveys among healthy persons have shown a peak in *Campylobacter* IgG antibodies in children aged 1 year in Thailand and ages 2 to 4 years in Bangladesh.[30] Infection, even in infants, is frequently not associated with disease in areas of hyperendemicity.[80]

5.6. Occupation

There have been reports of infection immediately after occupational contact with cattle and sheep or with beef, swine, or chicken carcasses.[33,102] At present, there

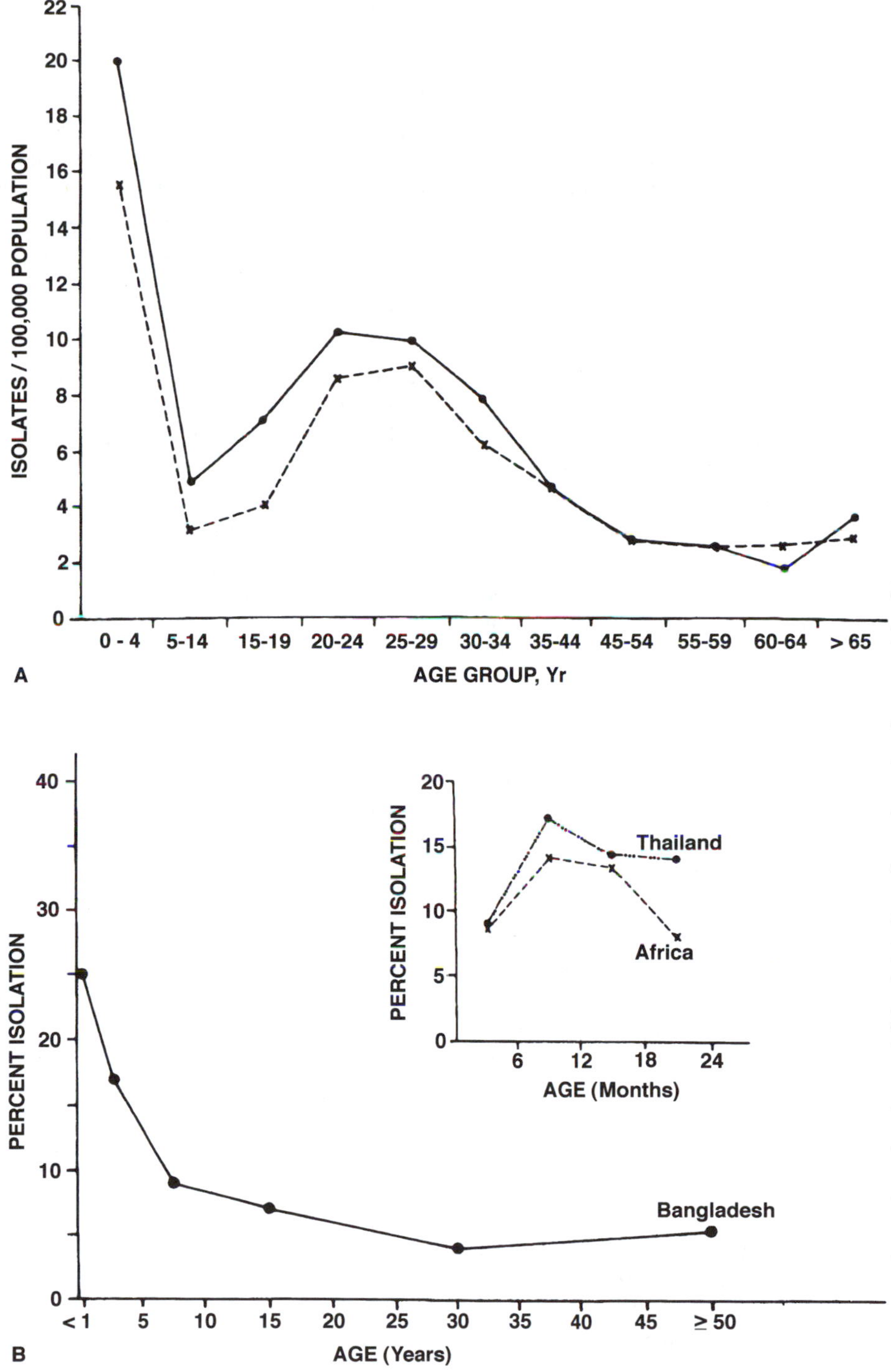

Figure 1. (A) Age-specific isolation rates of *Campylobacter* from persons with diarrhea in the United States in 1982. Solid line indicates males and dashed line indicates females.(73) (B) Age-specific isolation rates of *Campylobacter* from persons with diarrhea in Bangladesh in 1980.(93) Inset indicates the isolation rates from children less than 2 years old with diarrhea in the Central African Republic (Africa) in 1981–1982 and in Thailand in 1985.(96)

is no information to suggest that hospital personnel are at increased risk of infection.

5.7. Other Factors

Campylobacter infections may also be sexually transmitted in homosexual men.[103] Two species, *C. cinaedi* and *C. fennelliae* (now reclassified as *Helicobacter cinaedi* and *H. fennelliae*) have been isolated from homosexual men,[43,104] as have *C. fetus* subsp. *fetus*[101] and *C. hyointestinalis*.[71] Homosexuals who have been infected with multiple etiologic agents appear to be at an increased risk of these *Campylobacter* species of low virulence. Prolonged or unusually severe *C. jejuni* infections have been recognized in patients with hypogammaglobulinemia or acquired immunodeficiency syndrome (AIDS) (Section 8.1). Most patients infected with *C. fetus* subsp. *fetus* have been debilitated or compromised by chronic disease or were at the extremes of age.[44,106,107] Since most *C. fetus* subsp. *fetus* infections are detected by blood culture, it is possible that only the severe end of the spectrum of disease is recognized. When *C. fetus* subsp. *fetus* was isolated from stool in a milk-borne outbreak, it caused a diarrheal disease indistinguishable from *C. jejuni*.[45]

5.8. Atypical *Campylobacter* Species

In places where antibiotic-free media or filtration methods are used, the proportion of non-*jejuni* campylobacters is >20%. These organisms are increasingly recognized as human pathogens, perhaps in all populations but especially in immunocompromised persons (Table 1).[108–110]

C. fetus typically causes bacteremia or other extraintestinal infections in immunocompromised hosts.[111,112] This species also may cause uncomplicated diarrhea in immunocompetent persons. *C. fetus* infections may be transmitted to humans via raw milk or other raw or undercooked foods of bovine or ovine origin.[45] *C. upsaliensis* is a catalase-negative, thermotolerant *Campylobacter* that causes diarrhea in young children; the organism has also been isolated from blood.[45,113] *C. upsaliensis* was first isolated from dogs, which are the principal reservoirs for this organism. In some parts of the world, such as South Africa and the Netherlands, more than 10% of all *Campylobacter* isolated are *C. upsaliensis*.[110,114] *C. hyointestinalis*, a causal agent of proliferative enteritis in swine, also has been associated with watery, nonbloody diarrhea in young children.[15] *C. lari* (formerly *C. laridis*) is found in 25% of healthy seagulls; this *Campylobacter* can produce acute diarrheal illness in young children and has been isolated from the blood of immunocompromised persons.[30,116]

Helicobacter cinaedi and *H. fennelliae*, once called "*Campylobacter*-like organisms," are a cause of enteritis and proctocolitis in homosexual men and sometimes also may cause bacteremia.[117,118] Malnourished children in developing countries also are susceptible to infection with these organisms.[119] *H. cinaedi* is found commonly in stools of healthy hamsters.[120] *Arcobacter cryaerophila* and *A. butzleri* were moved from the *Campylobacter* genus in 1991; both organisms can cause gastroenteritis.[121,122] *C. jejuni* subsp *doylei* has been isolated from the stools of children with diarrhea.[123] The organism also has been isolated from blood, usually in children with gastrointestinal symptoms, suggesting an intestinal source of infection. H2-requiring Campylobacters (*C. concisus*, *C. rectus*, *C. curvus*, *C. mucosalis*) have been associated with periodontal disease.[124] Their role as gastrointestinal pathogens has not been established.

6. Mechanisms and Routes of Transmission

Transmission of *Campylobacter* appears similar to that for other known enteric pathogens, i.e., transmission by way of contaminated food and water or by oral contact with fecal material from infected animals or humans. This information comes from investigation of several large and small outbreaks and by inference from single cases. Increasing numbers of outbreaks are being reported in which contaminated water or food, especially uncooked food, has been implicated as the vehicle. A history of travel to developing countries is common in some groups of *Campylobacter*-positive patients[70,125]; consumption of contaminated food and water is considered the usual mode of transmission for travelers' diarrhea.

Since the animal species with which humans come into contact most frequently—including dogs, cats, cattle, sheep, goats, chickens, turkeys, swine, horses, and rodents[126]—have been shown to excrete *C. jejuni* in their feces, the potential reservoir for human infection is enormous. Serotypes of *Campylobacter* isolated from animals are essentially the same as those isolated from humans.

The best-documented mode of transmission of *Campylobacter* infection is the ingestion of unpasteurized milk. Unpasteurized milk has been the source of numerous epidemics and appears to be an important cause of endemic disease in rural areas in the United Kingdom, the United States, and Australia.[45,127–130] Although poultry consumption may cause most sporadic *Campylobacter* infections, most outbreaks are caused by drinking raw milk.[28] From 1972 to 1990, 20 raw milk associated outbreaks involving 458 people occurred among children and teenagers.[131] Fecal excretion of *Campylobacter* in milk cows and cattle is common and probably the usual source of contamination. *Campylobacter* infection of the bovine udder (mastitis) also may be a source of milk contamination. *Campylobacter* remain viable in refrigerated milk for 3 weeks and when ingested in milk may be protected from the effect of gastric acid.[39] As few as 500 *Campylobacter* cells are infective when given with milk.[64] Persons who regularly drink raw milk have elevated levels of antibodies to *Campylobacter* compared to age-matched persons who do not drink raw milk.[32] *C. fetus* subsp. *fetus* also has been associated with diarrheal disease after the ingestion of raw milk.[45] In the United Kingdom, pasteurized, bottled milk may be a source of *Campylobacter* infections because of contamination of the milk by birds (magpies and jackdaws) pecking the milk bottle tops.[132]

Waterborne outbreaks of *Campylobacter* infections have been reported in the United States, Europe, and Israel.[77,82,133–137] In the two largest outbreaks affecting 3000 persons in Vermont[136] and 2000 persons in central Sweden,[133] untreated surface water most likely contaminated drinking water systems. In smaller outbreaks at an English boarding school[134] and in a Florida town,[77] water in open-topped storage tanks became contaminated perhaps by feces from birds or rodents. During heavy rains, an untreated water reservoir in a Norwegian community was contaminated with sheep feces; 680 (66%) of the 1021 community residents who drank the water developed symptomatic *Campylobacter* infection.[82] In a national park in the Rocky Mountains of the western United States, ingestion of untreated surface water was the most important risk factor for *Campylobacter* infection, which was found to be a more common cause of diarrhea than giardiasis.[136] In Colorado, ingestion of raw water is an important risk factor for sporadic cases.[138] *C. lari* was the probable cause of a waterborne outbreak among 162 construction workers in Canada when lake water was cross-connected to the main drinking water supply.[30] This outbreak provided convincing evidence that *C. lari* was a human diarrheal disease pathogen.

With *Campylobacter* excretion among domestic animals so common, it is not surprising that retail meats are frequently contaminated with *C. jejuni*. In surveys in the United States, about 5% of beef or pork and 30% of poultry meats were found to be contaminated.[139,140] Eating sausages was shown to be an important risk factor for sporadic cases of *Campylobacter* infection in Norway.[141] Outbreaks have been associated with undercooked chicken, and in England,[142] Sweden, Washington,[143] and Colorado,[144] eating chicken, particularly undercooked chicken, appears to be a significant risk factor for sporadic *Campylobacter* infections.[101,141] It is possible that increasing reports of *Campylobacter* infection in England may be due partly to the increased consumption of poultry in that country. An outbreak of *Campylobacter* infection occurred among new employees at a poultry abattoir, and serological surveys indicate increased exposure among poultry workers.[102] Other outbreak reports have implicated cross-contamination of foods in kitchens[145,146] and contamination of shellfish with sewage.[95] Nonmeat products such as mushrooms may be contaminated in the soil.[147] Human infection after contact with sick animals, especially puppies and kittens, was one of the first observed modes of transmission, but probably accounts for a relatively small proportion of the total cases.[141,148,149]

As with other enteric infections, infected humans may be a reservoir for further transmission of infection, but *Campylobacter* is microaerophilic and sensitive to desiccation. Person-to-person transmission has been reported[150]; however, the index case has usually been a young child not yet toilet trained. There have been several reports of vertical transmission of *Campylobacter* infection from symptomatic or asymptomatic mothers to their neonates.[151,152] A contaminated bath plug may have caused an outbreak of *C. jejuni* infection among 11 children in the neonatal and pediatric intensive care units of a Dutch hospital.[153] Among 19 reported cases of premature labor, abortion, and perinatal sepsis due to *Campylobacter* species, *C. fetus* subsp. *fetus* was isolated in 9 and *C. jejuni/coli* in 10.[19] Considering that *C. jejuni* infection is many more times (ca. 500) more common than *C. fetus* subsp *fetus* infection, *C. fetus* must be considered to have a propensity for these complications.[27,44] Neonatal infections may be severe. A nosocomial outbreak of meningitis occurred in a neonatal nursery in France.[154] Transmission has not been demonstrated from asymptomatic food handlers or hospital personnel, nor has chronic or convalescent fecal carriage of *Campylobacter* been a source of transmission. There has been a report of laboratory-acquired infection,[155] but transmission to hospital personnel from patients or specimens in the hospital appears to be uncommon.

7. Pathogenesis and Immunity

The minimal dose of *Campylobacter* that produces human infections is not known. A volunteer who ingested 10^6 organisms in milk became ill within 3 days[19]; however, infection has been induced with as few as 500 organisms.[64] In general, attack rates have been dose-dependent in volunteer studies.[65,156] In a large milk-borne outbreak, almost all patients experienced the onset of illness within 2–7 days of drinking the contaminated milk.[157] For most pathogens, the length of the incubation period is inversely related to the dose ingested. The marked sensitivity of *Campylobacter* to gastric pH[39] suggests that it would take a high dose to infect 50–100% of subjects. The ID_{50} when given with sodium bicarbonate was 10^8.[65]

The mechanism(s) by which *C. jejuni* causes disease is not known. All campylobacters have a flagellum at one or both ends; the organisms' motility contributes to their ability to colonize and infect the intestinal mucosa.[158–160] Infection leads to multiplication of organisms in the intestine; patients shed 10^6–10^9 *Campylobacter*/g stool,[39] concentrations similar to those in *Salmonella* and *Shigella* infections. The sites of tissue injury include the jejunum, ileum, and colon,[39] although whether the small or large intestine is more commonly affected is not known. In both organs, acute exudative and hemorrhagic inflammation may occur, and the appendix, mesenteric lymph nodes, and gallbladder may also be affected by the inflammatory process.[15] Patients with severe clinical manifestations frequently have colonic involvement. The pathological lesion may include infiltration of the lamina propria with acute and chronic inflammatory cells and destruction of epithelial glands with crypt abscess formation. This nonspecific colitis may mimic that seen in other types of infectious colitis, acute ulcerative colitis, or Crohn's disease. A pseudomembranous colitis has also been described.

A choleralike enterotoxin has been described by some researchers,[152,161,162] but others have been unable to reproduce these results.[81] More than 10 years after this toxin was first described, considerable evidence suggests that it does not exist. Enterotoxic activity is not found in fecal specimens from *C. jejuni*-infected persons.[163] Furthermore, unlike persons with cholera or those infected with enterotoxigenic *E. coli* persons infected with *C. jejuni* do not possess antibodies to the putative toxin. Even if the presence of an enterotoxin were proven, its biological relevance would be questionable since the biological lesion of *C. jejuni* enteritis is inflammatory enteritis. A Shiga-like cytotoxin is produced *in vitro* by a small number of strains but only at very low titers.[164] The biological significance of this toxin is also uncertain. Increasing evidence suggests that *C. jejuni* is locally invasive,[165–167] although not in high numbers, and that infection with this organism possibly involves novel mechanisms.

Although strains have different pathogenic properties,[152] as yet there is no well-defined association between the clinical illness and any virulence property. In developed countries over 50% of patients with enteritis caused by *C. jejuni* have bloody diarrhea,[20] while in developing countries the proportion varies from 10 to 30%.[93,96] *Campylobacter* serotypes show little geographic variation and there is no other strain difference that can account for the difference in the severity of the illness. Immunity to *Campylobacter* infection, which is higher among persons in developing countries, may prevent illness or modify the illness to a less severe form. Hippurate-negative *Campylobacter* strains may be less virulent than *C. jejuni*, which is hippurate-positive. In most surveys from developed countries, hippurate-negative strains account for a small proportion of the total number of *Campylobacter* isolates; however, *C. coli* accounts for 30 to 40% of strains isolated in Hong Kong[168] and the Central African Republic,[169] a sufficient number to make an impact on the observed spectrum of illness.

Most intestinal isolates of *C. jejuni* are killed by normal human serum (serum-sensitive), while extraintestinal isolates may be either serum-sensitive or serum-resistant.[1] Extraintestinal isolates from normal hosts are usually serum-resistant; those from impaired hosts are serum-sensitive as are the intestinal isolates.[44] Serum resistance in *C. jejuni* strains has been associated with the total amount of lipopolysaccharide (LPS) produced.[44,170] The LPS may serve as a type of capsule that protects the organism from the killing activity of serum.

Studies in Canada,[171] the United States,[172] the United Kingdom,[157] and Sweden[22] have shown the median duration of excretion to be 2–3 weeks from onset of symptoms. Almost all patients were culture-negative by 2 months. In developing countries the duration of excretion is 7 to 10 days.[93,96] A longer excretion period was observed in Thailand among children less than 1 year old (14 days) compared to older children (8 days), suggesting that previous immunity may shorten the convalescent excretion period.[96]

Patients infected with *Campylobacter* develop specific serum antibodies against a variety of *Campylobacter* proteins and its LPS.[29,173,174] The response to LPS is both species and type specific.[175] The IgM antibodies rise and fall earlier than the IgG and do not reach the height of the IgG titer rise. Titers of both classes of antibodies appear to decline within several months of infection.[29] Serum antibodies developed in response to infection with one *Campylobacter* strain are cross-reactive with heterologous strains.[176] In developing countries, infection rates, case-to-infection ratios, as well as the duration and magnitude of convalescent carriage decline with age.[31,177] IgG antibody titers to *Campylobacter* antigens peak in the first few years of life and then decline, while IgA antibody titers continue to increase throughout life[30]; repeated infections may stimulate specific IgA production, but have little effect on systemic IgG production. After acute infection, IgA appears in the serum more rapidly than IgG and is predominantly in polymeric form.[178] Intestinal antibodies have also been detected.[179] Uninfected individuals have low-titer antibody to specific organisms. Volunteers with elevated serum and intestinal antibody levels to *Campylobacter* proteins become infected but are protected from illness. Similarly, habitual raw milk drinkers were protected from illness when exposed to contaminated raw milk that led to illness in other persons.[32] Little is known about the role of the cellular immune response in the control of *C. jejuni* infections. However, the increased severity and duration of these infections among HIV-infected persons suggests that cell-mediated immunity does play some role.

8. Patterns of Host Response

8.1. Clinical Features

The consequences of infection with *C. jejuni* vary from asymptomatic excretion to death. The infection-to-case ratio is not known, but in one large outbreak, 25% of those infected were found to be asymptomatic.[157] Some studies have shown that >50% of infected persons may be asymptomatic.[180] In Sweden, 11% of persons with *Campylobacter* enteritis required hospitalization[181]; in Norway, 13.3% of patients were hospitalized.[70]

In general, the symptoms and signs of *Campylobacter* infection are not so distinctive that the physician would be able to distinguish it from illness caused by other enteric pathogens. At the mild end of the spectrum, symptoms may last for 24 hr and be indistinguishable from those seen with a viral gastroenteritis. Such patients usually do not seek medical attention; the occurrence of those cases has been detected only in outbreaks.[78] In industrialized nations, bloody diarrhea or the presence of fecal leukocytes is often a helpful clinical indication of *Campylobacter* infection.

Most information on the clinical features of *Campylobacter* infection is based on hospital- or laboratory-based studies, and is thus biased toward those who are the most severely ill and who have diarrheal illnesses. In a multicenter study[20] in the United States where diarrhea was the criterion for stool culture, *Campylobacter* infection was associated with abdominal pain (79%), fever ⩾ 37.8°C (74%), and a history of bloody diarrhea (46%). Among those 10 to 29 years old, 31% of persons with a history of fever and ten or more fecal leukocytes had *Campylobacter* enteritis. The abdominal pain has been so severe on occasion as to mimic acute appendicitis.[15,70] Fever has been noted in up to 80% of these patients, although children have been febrile less frequently; convulsions have been reported. A prodrome of constitutional complaints, chiefly fever, may be more prominent than the enteric symptoms.

Illness usually lasts less than 10 days, but up to 20% of the patients studied in the hospital-based series had a more prolonged and severe illness, with persistently high fever and frequently grossly bloody stools.[97] With bloody diarrhea and abdominal pain being common manifestations, many were thought to have an acute bout of inflammatory bowel disease or a surgical abdomen before *Campylobacter* infection was diagnosed.[70] *Campylobacter* colitis may mimic the early presentation of ulcerative colitis. *Campylobacter* infection may be a cause of exacerbation of inflammatory colitis, but there is no evidence that it plays a role in the etiology of these diseases. Endoscopic examination is often helpful in differentiating infectious from idiopathic types of colitis.[182] Cultures obtained by endoscopy at the site of mucosal ulceration may be positive when stool cultures are negative. *Campylobacter* colitis also may present as a surgical abdomen because of severe abdominal pain or bleeding.

C. jejuni bacteremia occurs in approximately 1.5 per 1000 intestinal infections[183]; the rate is highest in the elderly and in immunodeficient persons.[184] In most patients, the bacteremia is associated with diarrhea and other gastroenterological symptoms. In contrast, *C. fetus* bacteremias are infrequently associated with diarrhea. Of all *Campylobacter* bacteremias, 89% are due to *C. jejuni* or *C. coli*; only 8.6% are due to *C. fetus*.[183]

Rarely, *Campylobacter* may infect the biliary tract, giving rise to cholecystitis, pancreatitis, or obstructive hepatitis.[86,185,186] It has been reported to cause splenic rupture.[187] It may cause peritonitis in patients receiving peritoneal dialysis,[188] and occasionally has been isolated from the urinary tract in women. *C. jejuni* infections in pregnant women are likely to be mild and self-limited; however, neonatal sepsis and death can occur if the woman is infected during her third trimester.[189]

A reactive arthritis has been reported after both symptomatic and asymptomatic *Campylobacter* infection. Similar to *Shigella*, *Salmonella*, and *Yersinia* infection, this complication is associated with HLA-B27 in about 60% of the cases.[190] In Scandinavia, 1 to 2% of patients with *Campylobacter* enteritis develop arthritis beginning 4 days to 4 weeks after the onset of diarrhea.[191] Interestingly, in another Scandinavian study, 32 patients in a hospital for rheumatic diseases developed culture-confirmed *C. jejuni* infection during a hospital outbreak; none of these patients developed exacerbations of their existing conditions.[192]

During the past decade, *C. jejuni* infections have been implicated as triggers of the Guillain–Barré syndrome (GBS), an acute demyelinating disease of peripheral nerves. Both serological and cultural studies indicate that 20–40% of GBS patients are infected with *C. jejuni* in the 1–3 weeks before the onset of neurological symptoms.(34,35,193) There is no relation between the severity of gastrointestinal symptoms and the likelihood of developing GBS following infection with *C. jejuni*; in fact, even asymptomatic infections can trigger GBS.

Between 30 and 80% of *C. jejuni* isolates from GBS patients in the United States and Japan belong to Penner serotype O:19.(34,194) This serotype is present in less than 3% of randomly selected *C. jejuni* strains reported to the CDC, and thus is overrepresented in patients with GBS. Antibody cross-reactivity between structures on the cell surface (including *C. jejuni* O:19 LPS) and glycolipids or myelin proteins may explain this association.(195)

In addition to sporadic cases of GBS in the United States, Japan, and other industrialized countries, *C. jejuni* infection has been implicated as a potential cause of acute motor axonal neuropathy (AMAN) in China and other developing nations. AMAN is clinically indistinguishable from GBS but affects the peripheral nerve axon and spares myelin. AMAN occurs in epidemics during the summer and fall and principally affects children living in rural areas of northern China. (196) Case–control studies showed that children with AMAN were more likely than controls to have serological evidence of preceding *C. jejuni* infection.(196) Interestingly, patients in the United Kingdom who developed GBS following *C. jejuni* infection also had axonal degeneration.(193)

Other reported but rare postinfectious complications of *C. jejuni* infections include hemolytic anemia, hemolytic–uremic syndrome, carditis, and encephalopathy.(197–199) Erythema nodosum and migrating urticaria also have been associated with *Campylobacter* infections.(86)

Illness due to *Campylobacter* infection is frequently self-limited and usually ends within 10 days; however, one or more relapses can occur. Those with more severe symptoms may have persistence of illness for 1 month or longer. Rarely, *Campylobacter* infection may cause mild, chronic diarrhea.(34,200,201) Illnesses are more likely to be prolonged and more severe in patients with HIV infection.(23,129,202–204) Among persons with AIDS, *C. jejuni* infections are reported almost 40 times as frequently as in the general population.(24) This excess of *C. jejuni* infections affects only infections in the later stages of HIV disease; patients with early HIV infection and relatively high CD4 counts are not unusually prone to *C. jejuni* infection or relapses of such infections.(205) Hypogammaglobulinemia patients develop severe persistent and relapsing infections due to *C. jejuni*.(206,207) A lack of opsonizing activity also predisposes individuals to bacteremia and other extraintestinal manifestations, including osteomyelitis, cellulitis, and meningitis.(208–210)

Campylobacters are susceptible *in vitro* to a wide variety of antimicrobial agents.(66,72) Because erythromycin is safe, easy to administer, and has less of an inhibitory effect on fecal flora than other antibiotics, it is the recommended therapy. However, most clinical trials performed in adults or children have not found that erythromycin significantly alters the clinical course of *Campylobacter* infection.(211,212) Only one study in Peru demonstrated that children with bloody diarrhea benefitted from erythromycin therapy if treatment was begun early in the course of illness.(63) Treatment of susceptible organisms shortens the duration of convalescent excretion, which in areas of poor sanitation may be useful. Other patients who may benefit from antimicrobial treatment include those with prolonged (>1 week) or worsening symptoms, high fevers, or bloody stools. HIV-infected or other immunocompromised persons also should receive antibodies for *Campylobacter* enteritis. Because infection with *C. jejuni* in pregnant women may have deleterious effects on the fetus, pregnant women also should receive antimicrobial treatment for *C. jejuni* infections.

At one time it appeared that fluoroquinolones such as ciprofloxacin had emerged as the treatment of choice for *Campylobacter* enteritis in particular and for acute bacterial diarrhea in general.(213) Unfortunately, as the use of fluoroquinolones has expanded (especially in food animals), the rate of resistance of campylobacters to these agents has increased.(214,215) Gentamicin and imipenem are active against campylobacters, with resistance in fewer than 1% of strains. Therapy with these agents is indicated in persons with bacteremia and other extraintestinal suppurative infections. Because gentamicin is ineffective against *Campylobacter* in the gut, oral therapy also must be given.

8.2. Diagnosis

The diagnosis of *Campylobacter* infection is based on a positive stool culture or a positive blood culture. The frequency of bacteremia was low (about 1%) in one series of patients hospitalized for acute *Campylobacter* enteritis.(98) Not all commercial blood culture methods support the growth of *Campylobacter*.(47)

Serological diagnosis may be useful in industrialized countries where background asymptomatic infection rates are low. Serodiagnostic techniques may also be useful in determining the role of *Campylobacter* in abortion, postinfectious syndromes, inflammatory bowel disease, and other late manifestations of *Campylobacter* infection.

Serotyping and biotyping of *C. jejuni* and *C. coli* have been useful in epidemiological investigations to determine associated cases and the source of infection. Typing so far has not identified strains of different virulence potential.

9. Control and Prevention

Since poultry, livestock, pets, and wild animals are the major reservoir for these organisms, control is based on interruption of transmission to humans from animals, animal products, or environmental sources contaminated by animals. Because transmission of *Campylobacter* infection to poultry flocks most likely occurs via environmental sources,[216] careful hygienic practices on farms may reduce contamination of flocks. Awareness of the necessity for hand washing after contact with animals or animal products and the importance of proper cooking and storage of foods of animal origin are as important for preventing *Campylobacter* infections as they are for *Salmonella* infections. Similarly, consuming only pasteurized milk and treated water is an important sanitary measure for the prevention of illness by individuals. The majority of *Campylobacter* outbreaks would not have occurred if not for the consumption of raw milk. HIV-infected and other immune-deficient persons should be particularly careful to avoid high-risk foods (such as unpasteurized dairy products or untreated surface water), as the consequences of infection may be more severe. Because many outbreaks and sporadic cases of *Campylobacter* infection are caused by injection of contaminated water, special care should be taken to prevent contamination of community drinking water supplies with animal or bird excrement or with untreated water.

Control of nosocomial transmission from patients hospitalized with *Campylobacter* infection is another important consideration. As such "excretion precautions" are recommended for infected infants, children, and adults with fecal incontinence. In general, the bases for control of enteric infection in the hospital are sanitary disposal of excretions and contaminated linens, and hand washing by the patient and by staff members after contact with the patient, especially following contact with excreta. For *Campylobacter* infection, precautions should be maintained for the duration of the illness.

To date, there have been no reports of transmission of *Campylobacter* infection by asymptomatic excretors. Asymptomatically infected food handlers or hospital employees need not be excluded from work, but the need for hand washing after defecation should be stressed to these individuals. Recommendations are different when persons are infected with *Campylobacter* and continue to have diarrhea. Because of the known risk of transmission of other enteric pathogens from individuals with diarrhea, food handlers and symptomatic hospital employees with patient care responsibilities should not be permitted to work until the diarrheal episode has ended. Because of the diversity of serotypes of *C. jejuni*, the possibility of vaccination for prevention of infection is limited. However, identification of group antigens could make immunization feasible.

10. Unresolved Problems

Epidemiological and clinical research during the last 10 years has done much to define the disease and the sources of infection. The priorities should be directed at public health prevention. First, we must learn how to produce poultry and livestock that are not infected with *Campylobacter*. This strategy would not eliminate *Campylobacter* because of the vast reservoir in wild animals and birds, but it should decrease considerably the number of human infections. Efforts also should be directed at determining how to process meat so that it is not contaminated with animal feces containing campylobacters.

Cheaper and simpler diagnostic methods should be available so that a greater number of patients can be cultured for *Campylobacter*, which in turn might lead to better surveillance and more opportunities to investigate outbreaks to find additional modes of transmission. Efforts should be made to introduce simple and inexpensive isolation methods into all diagnostic microbiology laboratories. This should be combined with training in isolation techniques for technicians. Research on new diagnostic methods such as simple antigen detection kits and nonradioactive DNA probes should be pursued and a simple, standardized serotyping scheme should be widely available and routinely used.

The role of *C. jejuni* infection in triggering GBS was not understood until recent years. The pathogenesis of this association as well as possible prevention and control strategies need to be explored. The pathogenesis of *Campylobacter* infection, the host mechanisms that allow most infections to be self-limited, and the occurrence and mediators of immunity are still not well understood. Research in the area of pathogenesis and immunity should continue and may help provide the basis for effective prophylaxis or intervention.

11. References

1. Blaser, M. J., Smith, P. F., and Kohler, P. A., Susceptibility of *Campylobacter* isolates to the bactericidal activity in human serum, *J. Infect. Dis.* **151:**227–235 (1985).
2. Smibert, R. M., Genus *Campylobacter* Sebald and Vernon 1963, 907[AL], in: *Bergey's Manual of Systematic Bacteriology* (N. R. Krieg and H. G. Holt, eds.), pp. 111–118, Williams & Wilkins, Baltimore, 1984.
3. Romaniuk, P. J., Zoltawska, B., Trust, T. J., *et al.*, *Campylobacter pylori*, the spiral bacterium associated with human gastritis is not a true *Campylobacter* sp., *J. Bacteriol.* **169:**2137–2141 (1987).
4. MacFadyean, F., and Stockman, S., *Report of the Department Committee Appointed by the Board of Agriculture and Fisheries to Inquire into Epizootic Abortion*, Vol. 3, His Majesty's Stationery Office, London, 1909.
5. Smibert, R. M., The genus *Campylobacter*, *Annu. Rev. Microbiol.* **32:**700–773 (1978).
6. Jones, F. S., and Little, R. B., Etiology of infectious diarrhea (winter scours) in cattle, *J. Exp. Med.* **53:**835–843 (1931).
7. Doyle, L. P., A vibrio associated with swine dysentery, *Am. J. Vet. Res.* **5:**3–5 (1944).
8. Vinzent, R., Dumas, J., and Picard, N., Septicemie grave au cours de la grossesse due a un vibrion: Avortment consecutif, *Bull. Acad. Natl. Med.* **131:**90–93 (1947).
9. Bokkenheuser, V., *Vibrio fetus* infection in man I. Ten new cases and some epidemiologic observations, *Am. J. Epidemiol.* **91:**400–409 (1970).
10. Guerrant, R. L., Lahita, R. G., Winn, E. C., Jr., and Roberts, R. B., Campylobacteriosis in man: Pathogenic mechanisms and review of 91 bloodstream infections, *Am. J. Med.* **65:**584–592 (1978).
11. King, E. O., Human infections with *Vibrio fetus* and a closely related vibrio, *J. Infect. Dis.* **101:**119–129 (1957).
12. Cooper, I. A., and Slee, K. J., Human infection by *Vibrio fetus*, *Med. J. Aust.* **1:**1263–1267 (1971).
13. Dekeyser, P., Gossvin-Detrain, M., Butzler, J. P., and Sternon, J., Acute enteritis due to related vibrio: First positive stool cultures, *J. Infect. Dis.* **125:**390–392 (1972).
14. Butzler, J. P., Dekeyser, P., Detrain, M., and Dehaen, F., Related vibrio in stools, *J. Pediatr.* **82:**493–495 (1973).
15. Skirrow, M. B., *Campylobacter* enteritis: A "new" disease, *Br. Med. J.* **2:**9–11 (1977).
16. Vernon, M., and Chatlain, R., Taxonomic study of the genus *Campylobacter* (Sebald and Vernon) and designation of the neotype strain for the type species, *Campylobacter fetus* (Smith and Taylor) Sebald and Vernon, *Int. J. Syst. Bacteriol.* **23:**122–134 (1973).
17. Steele, T. W., Sangster, N., and Lanser, J. A., DNA relatedness and biochemical features of *Campylobacter* spp. isolated in Central and South Australia, *J. Clin. Microbiol.* **22:**71–74 (1985).
18. Smith, G. S., and Blaser, M. J., Fatalities associated with *Campylobacter jejuni* infections, *J. Am. Med. Assoc.* **253:**2873–2875 (1985).
19. Simor, A. E., Karmali, M. A., Jadavji, T., and Roscoe, M., Abortion and perinatal sepsis associated with *Campylobacter* infection, *Rev. Infect. Dis.* **8:**397–402 (1986).
20. Blaser, M. J., Wells, J. G., Feldman, R. A., Pollard, R. A., Allen, J. R., and the Collaborative Diarrheal Disease Study Group, *Campylobacter* enteritis in the United States: A multicenter study, *Ann. Intern. Med.* **98:**360–365 (1983).
21. Kendall, E. J., and Tanner, E. I., *Campylobacter* enteritis in general practice, *J. Hyg.* **88:**155–163 (1982).
22. Svedhem, A., and Kaijser, B., *Campylobacter fetus* subspecies *jejuni*: A common cause of diarrhea in Sweden, *J. Infect. Dis.* **142:** 353–359 (1980).
23. Perlman, D. M., Ampel, N. M., Schifman, R. B., *et al.*, Persistent *Campylobacter jejuni* infections in patients infected with human immunodeficiency virus (HIV), *Ann. Intern. Med.* **108:**540–546 (1988).
24. Sovillo, F. J., Lieb, L. E., and Waterman, S. H., Incidence of Campylobacteriosis among patients with AIDS in Los Angeles County, *AIDS* **4:**598–602 (1991).
25. Stoll, B. J., Glass, R. I., Banu, H., Huq, M. I., Khan, M. U., and Holt, J. E., Surveillance of patients attending a diarrhoeal disease hospital in Bangladesh, *Br. Med. J.* **285:**1185–1188 (1982).
26. Skirrow, M. B., *Campylobacter* enteritis: The first five years, *J. Hyg.* **89:**175–184 (1982).
27. Riley, L. W., and Finch, M. J., Results of the first year of national surveillance of *Campylobacter* infections in the United States, *J. Infect. Dis.* **151:**956–959 (1985).
28. Tauxe, R. V., Hargrett-Bean, N., Patton, C. M., and Wachsmuth, I. K., *Campylobacter* isolates in the United States, 1982–1986. CDC Surveillance Summaries, June 1988, *Morbid. Mortal. Week. Rep.* **37:**1–14 (1988).
29. Blaser, M. J., and Duncan, D., Human serum antibody response to *Campylobacter jejuni* infection as measured in an enzyme-linked immunosorbent assay, *Infect. Immun.* **44:**292–298 (1984).
30. Blaser, M. J., Black, R. E., Duncan, D. J., and Amer, J., *Campylobacter jejuni*-specific serum antibodies are elevated in healthy Bangladeshi children, *J. Infect. Dis.* **151:**227–235 (1985).
31. Taylor, D. N., Perlman, D. M., Echeverria, P. D., Lexemboon, U., and Blaser, M. J., *Campylobacter* immunity and quantitative excretion rates in Thai children, *J. Infect. Dis.* **168:**754–758 (1993).
32. Blaser, M. J., Sazie, E., and Williams, L. P., The influence of immunity on raw milk-associated *Campylobacter* infection, *J. Am. Med. Assoc.* **257:**43–46 (1987).
33. Mancinelli, S., Palombi, L., Riccardi, F., and Marazzi, M. C., Serological study of *Campylobacter jejuni* infection in slaughterhouse workers, *J. Infect. Dis.* **156:**856 (1987).
34. Kuroki, S., Saida, T., Nukina, M., *et al.*, *Campylobacter jejuni* strains from patients with Guillain–Barré syndrome belong mostly to Penner serogroup 19 and contain *B-N*-acetylglucosamine, *Ann. Neurol.* **22:**243–247 (1993).
35. Mishu, B., Amjad, A. A., Koski, C. L., *et al.*, Serologic evidence of previous *Campylobacter jejuni* infection in patients with the Guillain–Barré syndrome, *Ann. Intern. Med.* **118:**947–953 (1993).
36. Wang, W. L., Reller, L. B., Smallwood, B., Leuchtefeld, N. W., and Blaser, M. J., Evaluation of transport media and filtration for the isolation of *Campylobacter* in human fecal specimens, *J. Clin. Microbiol.* **18:**803–807 (1983).
37. Butzler, J. P., and Skirrow, M. B., *Campylobacter* enteritis, *Clin. Gastroenterol.* **8:**737–765 (1979).
38. Blaser, M. J., Berkowitz, I. D., LaForce, M., Cravens, J., Reller, L. B., and Wang, W. L., *Campylobacter* enteritis: Clinical and epidemiologic features, *Ann. Intern. Med.* **91:**179–185 (1979).
39. Blaser, M. J., Hardesty, H. L., Powers, B., and Wang, W. L.

Survival of *Campylobacter fetus* subsp. *jejuni* in biological milieus, *J. Clin. Microbiol.* **11:**309–313 (1980).

40. Merino, F. J., Agulla, A., Villasante, P. A., Diaz, A., Saz, J. V., and Velasco, A. C., Comparative efficacy of seven selective media for isolating *Campylobacter jejuni*, *J. Clin. Microbiol.* **24:**451–452 (1986).
41. Karmali, M. A., Simor, A. E., Roscoe, M., Fleming, P. C., Smith, S. S., and Lane, J., Evaluation of a blood-free charcoal-based selective medium for the isolation of *Campylobacter* organisms from feces, *J. Clin. Microbiol.* **23:**456–459 (1986).
42. Nachamkin, I., *Campylobacter* and *Arcobacter*, in: *Manual of Clinical Microbiology* (P. R. Murray *et al.*, eds.), pp. 483–491, American Society for Microbiology, Washington, DC, 1995.
43. Fennell, C. L., Totten, P. A., Quinn, T. C., Patton, D. L., Holmes, K. K., and Stamm, W. E., Characterization of *Campylobacter*-like organisms isolated from homosexual men, *J. Infect. Dis.* **149:**58–66 (1984).
44. Blaser, M. J., Extraintestinal *Campylobacter* infections, *West. J. Med.* **144:**353–354 (1984).
45. Klein, B. S., Vergeront, J. M., Blaser, M. J., *et al.*, *Campylobacter* infection associated with raw milk: An outbreak of gastroenteritis due to *Campylobacter jejuni* and thermotolerant *Campylobacter fetus* subsp *fetus*, *J. Am. Med. Assoc.* **255:**361–364 (1986).
46. Wang, W. L., Leuchtefeld, N. W., Blaser, M. J., and Reller, L. B., Effect of incubation atmosphere and temperature on isolation of *Campylobacter jejuni* from human stools, *Can. J. Microbiol.* **29:** 468–470 (1983).
47. Wang, W. L., and Blaser, M. J., Detection of pathogenic *Campylobacter* species in blood culture systems, *J. Clin. Microbiol.* **23:**709–714 (1986).
48. Hodge, D. S., Prescott, J. F., and Shewen, P. E., Direct immunofluorescence microscopy for rapid screening of *Campylobacter* enteritis, *J. Clin. Microbiol.* **24:**863–865 (1986).
49. Park, C. H., Hixon, D. L., Polhemus, A. S., Ferguson, C. B., and Hall, S. L., A rapid diagnosis of *Campylobacter* enteritis by direct smear examination, *Am. J. Clin. Pathol.* **80:**388–390 (1983).
50. Thorson, S. M., Lohr, J. A., Dudley, S., and Guerrant, R. L., Value of methylene blue examination, dark-field microscopy, and carbol-fuchsin Gram stain in the detection of *Campylobacter* enteritis, *J. Pediatr.* **106:**941–943 (1985).
51. Tompkins, L. S., and Krajden, M., Approaches to the detection of enteric pathogens, including *Campylobacter*, using nucleic acid hybridization, *Diagn. Microbiol. Infect. Dis.* **4:**71S–78S (1986).
52. Jablonski, E., Moomaw, E. W., Tullis, R. H., and Ruth, J. L., Preparation of oligodeoxynucleotide-alkaline phosphatase conjugates and their use as hybridization probes, *Nucleic Acids Res.* **14:**6115–6128 (1986).
53. Lior, H., New, extended biotyping scheme for *Campylobacter jejuni*, *Campylobacter coli*, and *Campylobacter laridis*, *J. Clin. Microbiol.* **20:**636–640 (1984).
54. Grajewski, B. A., Kusek, J. W., and Gelfand, H. M., Development of a bacteriophage typing system for *Campylobacter jejuni* and *Campylobacter coli*, *J. Clin. Microbiol.* **22:**13–18 (1985).
55. Penner, J. L., and Hennessey, J. N., Serotyping *Campylobacter fetus* subsp *jejuni* on the basis of somatic (O) antigens, *J. Clin. Microbiol.* **12:**732–737 (1980).
56. Lior, H., Woodward, D. L., Edgar, J. A., Laroche, L. J., and Gill, P., Serotyping of *Campylobacter jejuni* by slide agglutination based on heat-labile antigenic factors, *J. Clin. Microbiol.* **15:**761–768 (1982).
57. Jones, D. M., Sutcliffe, E. M., Abbott, J. D., Serotyping of *Campylobacter* species by combined use of two methods, *Eur. J. Clin. Microbiol.* **4:**562–565 (1985).
58. Patton, C. M., Barrett, T. J., and Morris, G. K., Comparison of the Penner and Lior methods for serotyping *Campylobacter* spp., *J. Clin. Microbiol.* **22:**558–565 (1985).
59. Nicholson, M. A., and Patton, C. M., Application of Lior biotyping by use of genetically identified *Campylobacter* strains, *J. Clin. Microbiol.* **31:**3348–3350 (1993).
60. Ruiz-Palacios, G. M., Escamilla, E., and Torres, N., Experimental *Campylobacter* diarrhea in chickens, *Infect. Immun.* **34:**250–255 (1981).
61. Prescott, J. F., and Barker, I. K., *Campylobacter* colitis in gnotobiotic dogs, *Vet. Rec.* **107:**314–315 (1980).
62. Tribe, G. W., and Frank, A., *Campylobacter* in monkeys, *Vet. Rec.* **106:**365–366 (1980).
63. Salazar-Lindo, E., Sack, R. B., Chea-Woo, E., *et al.*, Early treatment with erythromycin of *Campylobacter jejuni*-associated dysentery in children, *J. Pediatr.* **109:**355–360 (1986).
64. Robinson, D. A., Infective dose of *Campylobacter jejuni* in milk, *Br. Med. J.* **282:**1584 (1981).
65. Black, R. E., Levine, M. M., Clements, M. L., Hughes, T. P., and Blaser, M. J., Experimental *Campylobacter jejuni* infection in humans, *J. Infect. Dis.* **157:**472–479 (1988).
66. Karmali, M. A., De Grandis, S., and Fleming, P. C., Antimicrobial susceptibility of *Campylobacter jejuni* with special reference to resistance patterns of Canadian isolates, *Antimicrob. Agents Chemother.* **19:**593–597 (1981).
67. Taylor, D. N., Blaser, M. J., Echeverria, P., Pitarangsi, C., Bodhidatta, L., and Wang, W. L., Erythromycin-resistant *Campylobacter* infections in Thailand, *Antimicrob. Agents Chemother.* **31:**438–442 (1987).
68. Taylor, D. E., De Grandis, S. A., Karmali, M. A., and Fleming, P. C., Transmissible plasmids from *Campylobacter jejuni*, *Antimicrob. Agents Chemother.* **19:**831–835 (1981).
69. Rivera, M. J., Castillo, J., Martin, C., Navvarro, M., and Gomez-Lux, R., Aminoglycoside–phosphotransferases APH (3′)-IV and APH (3′) synthesized by a strain of *Campylobacter coli*, *J. Antimicrob. Chemother.* **18:**153–158 (1986).
70. Kapperud, G., Lassen, J., Ostroff, S. M., and Aasen, S., Clinical features of sporadic *Campylobacter* infections in Norway, *Scand. J. Infect. Dis.* **24:**741–749 (1992).
71. Chau, P. Y., Leung, Y. K., and Ng, W. W., Comparative *in vitro* antibacterial activity of ofloxacin and ciprofloxacin against some selected gram-positive and gram-negative isolates, *Infection* **14:**S237–S239 (1986).
72. Vanhoof, R., Hubrechts, J.M., Roebben, E., *et al.*, The comparative activity of perfloxacin, enoxacin, coprofloxacin and 13 other antimicrobial agents against enteropathogenic microorganisms, *Infection* **14:**294–298 (1986).
73. Finch, M. J., and Riley, L. W., *Campylobacter* infections in the United States: Results of an 11-state surveillance, *Arch. Intern. Med.* **144:**1610–1612 (1984).
74. Rishpon, S., Epstein, L. M., Scmilovitz, M., Kretzer, B., Tamir, A., and Egoz, N., *Campylobacter jejuni* infections in Haifa subdistrict, Israel, summer 1981, *Int. J. Epidemiol.* **13:**216–220 (1984).
75. Tauxe, R. V., Pegues, D. A., and Hargrett-Bean, N., *Campylobacter* infections: The emerging national pattern, *Am. J. Public Health* **77:**1219–1221 (1987).
76. MacDonald, K. L., O'Leary, M. J., Cohen, M. L., *et al.*, *Escherichia coli* O157:H7: An emerging gastrointestinal pathogen, *J. Am. Med. Assoc.* **259:**3567–3570 (1988).

77. Sacks, J. J., Lieb, S., Baldy, L. M., *et al.*, Epidemic campylobacteriosis associated with a community water supply, *Am. J. Public Health* **76:**424–428 (1986).
78. Blaser, M. J., Checko, P., Bopp, C., Bruce, A., and Hughes, J. M., *Campylobacter* enteritis associated with foodborne transmission, *Am. J. Epidemiol.* **116:**886–894 (1982).
79. Tauxe, R. V., Epidemiology of *Campylobacter jejuni* infections in the United States and other industrialized nations, in: *Campylobacter jejuni—Current Strategy and Future Trends* (I. Nachamkin, M. J. Blaser, and L. S. Tompkins, eds.), pp. 9–19, American Society of Microbiology, Washington, DC, 1992.
80. Georges-Courbot, M. C., Beraud-Cassel, A. M., Gouandjik, I., Georges, A. J., Prospective study of enteric *Campylobacter* infections in children from birth to 6 months in the Central African Republic, *J. Clin. Microbiol.* **23:**592–594 (1987).
81. Pérez-Pérez, G. I., Cohn, D. L., Guerrant, R. L., Patton, C. M., Reller, L. B., and Blaser, M. J., Clinical and immunological significance of cholera-like toxin and cytotoxin production by *Campylobacter* species in patients with acute inflammatory diarrhea, *J. Infect. Dis.* **160:**460–468 (1989).
82. Melby, K., Dahl, O. P., Crisp, L., and Penner, J. L., Clinical and serological manifestations in patients during a waterborne epidemic due to *Campylobacter jejuni*, *J. Infect.* **21:**309–316 (1990).
83. Riordan, T., Intestinal infection with *Campylobacter* in children, *Lancet* **1:**992 (1988).
84. Schmilovitz, M., Kretzer, B., and Rotman, N., *Campylobacter jejuni* as an etiological agent of diarrheal diseases in Israel, *Isr. J. Med. Sci.* **18:**935–940 (1982).
85. Lassen, J., and Kapperud, G., Epidemiological aspects of enteritis due to *Campylobacter* spp. in Norway, *J. Clin. Microbiol.* **19:**153–156 (1984).
86. Pitkanen, T., Ponka, A., Pettersson, T., and Kosunen, T. U., *Campylobacter* enteritis in 188 hospitalized patients, *Arch. Intern. Med.* **143:**215–219 (1983).
87. Taylor, D. N., and Echeverria, P., Etiology and epidemiology of travelers' diarrhea in Asia, *Rev. Infect. Dis.* **8:**S136–S141 (1986).
88. Thompson, J. S., Cahoon, F. E., and Hodge, D. S., Rate of *Campylobacter* spp. isolation in three regions of Ontario, Canada, from 1978 to 1985, *J. Clin. Microbiol.* **24:**876–878 (1986).
89. Steingrimsson, O., Thorsteinsson, S. B., Hjalmarsdottir, M., Jonasdottir, E., and Kolbeinsson, A., *Campylobacter* spp. infections in Iceland during a 24-month period in 1980–1982, *Scand. J. Infect. Dis.* **17:**285–290 (1985).
90. De Mol, P., Brasseur, D., Hemelhof, W., Kalala, T., Butzler, J. P., and Vis, H. L., Enteropathogenic agents in children with diarrhoea in rural Zaire, *Lancet* **1:**516–518 (1983).
91. Bokkenheuser, V. D., Richardson, N. J., Bryner, J. H., *et al.*, Detection of enteric campylobacteriosis in children, *J. Clin. Microbiol.* **9:**227–232 (1979).
92. Blaser, M. J., Glass, R. I., Imdadul Hug, M., Stoll, B., Kibriya, G. M., and Alim, A. R. M. A., Isolation of *Campylobacter fetus* subsp *jejuni* from Bangladeshi children, *J. Clin. Microbiol.* **12:**744–747 (1980).
93. Glass, R. I., Stoll, B. J., Huq, M. I., Struelens, M. J., Blaser, M. J., and Kibriya, A. K., Epidemiology and clinical features of endemic *Campylobacter jejuni* infection in Bangladesh, *J. Infect. Dis.* **148:**292–296 (1983).
94. Billingham, J. D., *Campylobacter* enteritis in The Gambia, *Trans. R. Soc. Trop. Med. Hyg.* **75:**641– 644 (1981).
95. Griffin, M. R., Dalley, E., Fitzpatrick, M., and Austin, S. H., *Campylobacter* gastroenteritis associated with raw clams, *J. Med. Soc. N.J.,* **80:**607–609 (1983).
96. Taylor, D. N., Echeverria, P., Pitarangsi, C., Seriwatana, J., Bodhidatta, L., and Blaser, M. J., The influence of strain characteristics and immunity on the epidemiology of *Campylobacter* infections in Thailand, *J. Clin. Microbiol.* **26:**863–868 (1988).
97. Blaser, M. J., Reller, L. B., Leuchtefeld, N. W., and Wang, W. L. L., *Campylobacter* enteritis in Denver, *West J. Med.* **136:**287–290 (1982).
98. Tee, W., Kaldor, J., and Dwyer, B., Epidemiology of *Campylobacter* diarrhoea, *Med. J. Aust.* **145:**499–503 (1986).
99. Hopkins, R. S., and Olmsted, R. N., *Campylobacter jejuni* infection in Colorado: Unexplained excess of cases in males, *Public Health Rep.* **100:**333–336 (1985).
100. Tauxe, R. V., Deming, M. S., and Blake, P. A., *Campylobacter jejuni* infections on college campuses: A national survey, *Am. J. Public Health* **75:**659–660 (1985).
101. Deming, M. S., Tauxe, R. V., Blake, P. A., *et al.*, *Campylobacter* enteritis at a university: Transmission from eating chicken and from cats, *Am. J. Epidemiol.* **126:**526–534 (1987).
102. Christenson, B., Ringer, A., Blucher, C., *et al.*, An outbreak of *Campylobacter* enteritis among the staff of a poultry abattoir in Sweden, *Scand. J. Infect. Dis.* **15:**167–172 (1983).
103. Quinn, T. C., Goodell, S. E., Fennell, C. L., *et al.*, Infections with *Campylobacter jejuni* and *Campylobacter*-like organisms in homosexual men, *Ann. Intern. Med.* **101:**187–192 (1984).
104. Totten, P. A., Fennell, C. L., Tenover, F. C., *et al.*, *Campylobacter cinaedi* (sp. nov.) and *Campylobacter fennelliae* (sp. nov): Two new *Campylobacter* species associated with enteric disease in homosexual men, *J. Infect. Dis.* **151:**131–139 (1985).
105. Devlin, H. R., and McIntyre, L., *Campylobacter fetus* subsp *fetus* in homosexual males, *J. Clin. Microbiol.* **18:**999–1000 (1983).
106. Blaser, M. J., Perez, G. P., Smith, P. F., *et al.*, Extraintestinal *Campylobacter jejuni* and *Campylobacter coli* infections: Host factors and strain characteristics, *J. Infect. Dis.* **153:**552–559 (1986).
107. Dhawan, V. K., Ulmer, D. D., Nachum, R., Rao, B., and See, R. B., *Campylobacter jejuni* septicemia: Epidemiology, clinical features and outcome, *West. J. Med.* **144:**324–328 (1986).
108. Allos, B. M., and Blaser, M. J., *Campylobacter jejuni* and the expanding spectrum of related infections, *Clin. Infect. Dis.* **20:**1092–1101 (1995).
109. Allos, B. M., Lastovica, A., and Blaser, M. J., Atypical campylobacters and related organisms, in: *Infections of the Gastrointestinal Tract* (M. J. Blaser *et al.*, eds.), pp. 849–866, Raven Press, New York, 1995.
110. Lastovica, A. J., and LeRoux, E., Prevalence and distribution of *Campylobacter* spp. in the diarrhoeic stools and blood cultures of pediatric patients, *Acta Gastro-Enterol. Belg.* **56:**34 (1993).
111. Morrison, V. A., Lloyd, B. K., Chia, J. K. S., and Tuazon, C. U., Cardiovascular and bacteremia manifestations of *Campylobacter fetus* infection: Case report and review, *Rev. Infect. Dis.* **12:**387–392 (1990).
112. Rao, G. G., Karim, Q. N., Maddocks, A., Hillman, R. J., Harris, J. R. W., and Pinching, A. J., *Campylobacter fetus* infections in two patients with AIDS, *J. Infect.* **20:**170–172 (1990).
113. Patton, C. M., Shaffer, N., Edmonds, P., *et al.*, Human disease associated with "*Campylobacter upsaliensis*" (catalase-negative or weakly positive *Campylobacter* species) in the United States, *J. Clin. Microbiol.* **27:**66–73 (1989).
114. Goossens, H., Pot, B., Vlaes, L., *et al.*, Characterization and description of *Campylobacter upsaliensis* isolated from human feces, *J. Clin. Microbiol.* **28:**1039–1046 (1990).
115. Edmonds, P., Patton, C. M., Griffin, P. M., *et al.*, *Campylobacter*

hyointestinalis associated with human gastrointestinal disease in the United States, *J. Clin. Microbiol.* **25:**685–691 (1987).

116. Soderstrom, C., Schalen, C., and Walder, M., Septicaemia caused by unusual *Campylobacter* species (*C. laridis* and *C. mucosalis*), *Scand. J. Infect. Dis.* **23:**369–371 (1991).
117. Decker, C. F., Martin, G. J., Barham, W. B., and Paparello, S. F., Bacteremia due to *Campylobacter cinaedi* in a patient infected with human immunodeficiency virus, *Clin. Infect. Dis.* **15:**178–179 (1992).
118. Kemper, C. A., Mickelson, P., Morton, A., Walton, B., and Deresinski, S. C., *Helicobacter* (*Campylobacter*) *fennelliae*-like organisms as an important but occult cause of bacteremia in a patient with AIDS, *J. Infect.* **26:**97–101 (1993).
119. Grayson, M. L., Tee, W., and Dwyer, B., Gastroenteritis associated with *Campylobacter cinaedi*, *Med. J. Aust.* **150:**214–215 (1989).
120. Gebhart, C. J., Fennell, C. L., Murtaugh, M. P., and Stamm, W. E., *Campylobacter cinaidi* is the normal intestinal flora in hamsters, *J. Clin. Microbiol.* **27:**1692–1694 (1989).
121. Keihlbauch, J. A., Brenner, D. J., Nicholson, M. A., *et al.*, *Campylobacter butzleri* sp. nov. isolated from humans and animals with diarrheal illness, *J. Clin. Microbiol.* **29:**376–385 (1991).
122. Taylor, D. N., Diehlbauch, J. A., Tee, W., Pitarangsi, C., and Echeverria, P., Isolation of group 2 aerotolerant *Campylobacter* species from Thai children with diarrhea, *J. Infect. Dis.* **163:** 1062–1067 (1991).
123. Steele, T. W., and Owen, R. J., *Campylobacter jejuni* subspecies doylei (subsp. nov.), a subspecies of nitrate-negative campylobacters isolated from human clinical specimens, *Int. J. Syst. Bacteriol.* **38:**316–318 (1988).
124. Tanner, A. C. R., Dzink, J. L., Ebersole, J. L., and Socransky, S. S., *Wolinella recta*, *Campylobacter concisus*, *Bacteriodes gracilis*, and *Eikenella corrodens* from periodontal lesions, *J. Periodont. Res.* **22:**327–330 (1987).
125. Pitkanen, T., Pettersson, T., Ponka, A., and Kosunen, T. U., Clinical and serological studies in patients with *Campylobacter fetus* spp. *jejuni* infection. I. Clinical findings, *Infection* **9:**274–278 (1981).
126. Blaser, M. J., and Reller, L. B., *Campylobacter* enteritis, *N. Engl. J. Med.* **305:**1444–1452 (1981).
127. Birkhead, G., Vogt, R. L., Heun, E., Evelti, C. M., and Patton, C. M., A multiple-strain outbreak of *Campylobacter* enteritis due to consumption of inadequately pasteurized milk, *J. Infect. Dis.* **157:**1095–1097 (1988).
128. Centers for Disease Control, *Campylobacter* outbreak associated with raw milk provided on a dairy tour—California, *Morbid. Mortal. Week. Rep.* **35:**311–312 (1986).
129. Potter, M. E., Kaufmann, A. F., Blake, P. A., and Feldman, R. A., Unpasteurized milk: The hazards of a health fetish, *J. Am. Med. Assoc.* **252:**2048–2052 (1984).
130. Schmid, G. P., Schafer, R. E., Plikaytis, B. D., *et al.*, A one year study of endemic campylobacteriosis in a midwestern city: Association with consumption of raw milk, *J. Infect. Dis.* **156:**218–222 (1987).
131. Wood, R. C., MacDonald, K. L., and Osterholm, M. T., *Campylobacter* enteritis outbreaks associated with drinking raw milk during youth activities, *J. Am. Med. Assoc.* **268:**3228–3230 (1992).
132. Palmer, S. R., and McGuirk, S. M., Bird attacks on milk bottles and *Campylobacter* infections, *Lancet* **345:**326–327 (1995).
133. Mentzing, L. O., Waterborne outbreaks of *Campylobacter* enteritis in central Sweden, *Lancet* **2:**352–354 (1981).
134. Palmer, S. R., Gully, P. R., White, J. M., *et al.*, Water-borne outbreak of *Campylobacter* gastroenteritis, *Lancet* **1:**287–290 (1983).
135. Rogol, M., Sechter, I., Falk, H., *et al.*, Waterborne outbreak of *Campylobacter* enteritis, *Eur. J. Clin. Microbiol.* **2:**588–590 (1983).
136. Taylor, D. N., McDermott, K. T., Little, J. R., Wells, J. G., and Blaser, M. J., *Campylobacter* enteritis from untreated water in the Rocky Mountains, *Ann. Intern. Med.* **99:**38–40 (1983).
137. Vogt, R. L., Sours, H. E., Barrett, T., Feldman, R. A., Dickinson, R. J., and Witherell, L., *Campylobacter* enteritis associated with contaminated water, *Ann. Intern. Med.* **96:**292–296 (1982).
138. Hopkins, R. S., Olmsted, R., and Istre, G. R., Endemic *Campylobacter jejuni* infection in Colorado: Identified risk factors, *Am. J. Public Health* **74:**249–250 (1984).
139. Harris, N. V., Thomson, D., Martin, D. C., and Nolan, C. M., A survey of *Campylobacter* and other bacterial contaminants of premarket chicken and retail poultry and meats, King County, Washington, *Am. J. Public Health* **76:**401–406 (1986).
140. Stern, N. J., Hernandez, M. P., Blankenship, L., *et al.*, Prevalence and distribution of *Campylobacter jejuni* and *Campylobacter coli* in retail meats, *J. Food Prot.* **47:**595–599 (1985).
141. Kapperud, G., Skjerve, E., Bean, N. H., Ostroff, S. M., and Lassen, J., Risk factors for sporadic *Campylobacter* infections: Results of a case–control study in Southeastern Norway, *J. Clin. Microbiol.* **30:**3117–3121 (1992).
142. Rosenfield, J. A., Arnold, G. J., Davey, G. R., Archer, R. S., and Woods, W. H., Serotyping of *Campylobacter jejuni* from an outbreak of enteritis implicating chicken, *J. Infect.* **2:**159–165 (1985).
143. Harris, N. V., Weiss, N. S., and Nolan, C. M., The role of poultry and meats in the etiology of *Campylobacter jejuni/coli* enteritis, *Am. J. Public Health* **76:**407–410 (1986).
144. Istre, G. R., Blaser, M. J., Shillam, P., and Hopkins, R. S., *Campylobacter* enteritis associated with undercooked barbecued chicken, *Am. J. Public Health* **74:**1265–1267 (1984).
145. Brown, P., Kidd, D., Riordan, T., and Barrell, R. A., An outbreak of food-borne *Campylobacter jejuni* infection and the possible role of cross-contamination, *J. Infect.* **17:**171–176 (1988).
146. Finch, M. J., and Blake, P. A., Foodborne outbreaks of campylobacteriosis: The United States experience, *Am. J. Epidemiol.* **122:**262–268 (1985).
147. Doyle, M. P., and Schoeni, J. L., Isolation of *Campylobacter jejuni* from retail mushrooms, *Appl. Environ. Microbiol.* **51:**449–450 (1986).
148. Elliot, D. L., Tolle, S. W., Goldberg, L., and Miller, J. B., Pet-associated illness, *N. Engl. J. Med.* **313:**985–995 (1985).
149. Salfiedl, N. J., and Pugeh, E. J., *Campylobacter* enteritis in young children living in households with puppies, *Br. Med. J.* **294:**21–22 (1987).
150. Blaser, M. J., Waldman, R. J., Barrett, T., and Erlandson, A. L., Outbreaks of *Campylobacter* enteritis in two extended families: Evidence for person-to-person transmission, *J. Pediatr.* **98:**254–257 (1981).
151. Hershkowici, S., Barak, M., Cohen, A., and Montag, J., An outbreak of *Campylobacter jejuni* infection in a neonatal intensive care unit. *J. Hosp. Infect.* **9:**54–59 (1987).
152. Klipstein, F. A., Engert, R. F., Short, H., and Schenk, E. A., Pathogenic properties of *Campylobacter jejuni*: Assay and correlation with clinical manifestations, *Infect. Immun.* **50:**43–49 (1985).
153. van Dijk, W. C., and van der Straaten, P. J. C., An outbreak of

Campylobacter jejuni infection in a neonatal intensive care unit, *J. Hosp. Infect.* **11:**91–92 (1988).

154. Goossens, H., Henocque, G., Kremp, L., *et al.*, Nosocomial outbreak of *Campylobacter jejuni* meningitis in new born infants, *Lancet* **2:**146–149 (1986).
155. Oates, J. D., and Hodgin, U. G., Laboratory-acquired *Campylobacter* enteritis, *South. Med. J.* **74:**83 (1981).
156. Black, R. E., Perlman, D., Clements, M. L., *et al.* (eds.), *Campylobacter jejuni—Current Strategy and Future Trends*, American Society of Microbiology, Washington, DC, 1992.
157. Porter, I. A., and Reid, T. M. S., A milk-borne outbreak of *Campylobacter* infection, *J. Hyg.* **84:**415–419 (1980).
158. Aguero-Rosenfeld, M. E., Yang, X., and Nachamkin, I., Infection of Syrian hamsters with flagellar variants of *Campylobacter jejuni*, *Infect. Immun.* **58:**2214–2219 (1990).
159. Grant, C. C. R., Konkel, M. E., Cieplack, W., and Tompkins, L. S., Role of flagella in adherence, internalization, and translocation of *Campylobacter jejuni* in a non-polarized and polarized epithelial cell cultures, *Infect. Immun.* **61:**1764–1771 (1993).
160. Wassenaar, T. M., Bleumink-Pluym, N. M., Newell, D. G., Nuijten, P. J., and van der Zeijst, B. A. M., Differential flagellin expression in *flaA* and *flaB*$^+$ mutant of *Campylobacter jejuni*, *Infect. Immun.* **62:**3901–3906 (1994).
161. Baig, B. H., Wachsmuth, I. K., Morris, G. K., and Hill, W. E., Probing of *Campylobacter jejuni* with DNA coding for *Escherichia coli* heat-labile enterotoxin [letter], *J. Infect. Dis.* **154:**542 (1986).
162. Johnson, W. M., and Lior, H., Cytotoxic and cytotonic factors produced by *Campylobacter jejuni*, *Campylobacter coli*, and *Campylobacter laridis*, *J. Clin. Microbiol.* **24:**275–281 (1986).
163. Cover, T. L., Pérez-Pérez, G. I., and Blaser, M. J., Evaluation of cytotoxic activity in fecal filtrates from patients with *Campylobacter jejuni* or *Campylobacter coli* enteritis, *FEMS Microbiol. Lett.* **70:**301–304 (1990).
164. Moore, M. A., and Lior, H., Cytotoxic and cytotonic factor produced by *Campylobacter jejuni*, *Campylobacter coli*, and *Campylobacter laridis*, *J. Clin. Microbiol.* **24:**275–281 (1986).
165. Fauchere, J. L., Rosenau, A., Veron, M., Moyen, E. N., Richard, S., and Pfister, A., Association with HeLa cells of *Campylobacter jejuni* and *Campylobacter coli* isolated from human feces, *Infect. Immun.* **54:**283–287 (1986).
166. Konkel, M. E., Babakhani, F., and Joens, L. A., Invasion-related antigens of *Campylobacter jejuni*, *J. Infect. Dis.* **162:**888–895 (1990).
167. Oelshalger, T. A., Guerry, P., and Kopecko, D. J., Unusual microtubule-dependent endocytosis mechanisms triggered by *Campylobacter jejuni* and *Citrobacter freundii*, *Proc. Natl. Soc. Sci. USA* **90:**6884–6888 (1993).
168. Ho, B. S. W., and Wong, W. T., A one-year survey of *Campylobacter* enteritis and other forms of bacterial diarrhoea in Hong Kong, *J. Hyg.* **94:**55–60 (1985).
169. Georges-Courbot, M. C., Baya, C., Beraud, A. M., Meunier, D. M. Y., and Georges, A. J., Distribution and serotypes of *Campylobacter jejuni* and *Campylobacter coli* in enteric *Campylobacter* strains isolated from children in the Central African Republic, *J. Clin. Microbiol.* **23:**592–594 (1986).
170. Pérez-Pérez, G. I., and Blaser, M. J., Lipopolysaccharide characteristics of pathogenic campylobacters, *Infect. Immun.* **47:**353–359 (1985).
171. Karmali, M. A., and Fleming, P. C., *Campylobacter* enteritis in children, *J. Pediatr.* **94:**527–533 (1979).
172. Blaser, M. J., LaForce, F. M., Wilson, N. A., and Wang, W. L., Reservoirs for human campylobacteriosis, *J. Infect. Dis.* **141:** 665–669 (1980).
173. Kervella, M., Pages, J. M., Pei, Z., Grollier, G., Blaser, M. J., and Fauchere, J. L., Isolation and characterization of two *Campylobacter* glycine-extracted proteins that bind to HeLa cell membranes, *Infect. Immunol.* **61:**3440–3448 (1993).
174. Pei, Z., Ellison, R. T., and Blaser, M. J., Identification, purification, and characterization of major antigenic proteins of *Campylobacter jejuni*, *J. Biolog. Chem.* **266:**16363–16369 (1991).
175. Blaser, M. J., and Pérez-Pérez, G. I., Humoral immune response to lipopolysaccharide antigens of *Campylobacter jejuni* in: *Campylobacter jejuni—Current Strategy and Future Trends* (I. Nachamkin, M. J. Blaser, and L. S. Tompkins, eds.), pp. 230–235, American Society of Microbiology, Washington, DC, 1992.
176. Nachamkin, I., and Hart, A. M., Western blot analysis of the human antibody response to *Campylobacter jejuni* cellular antigens during gastrointestinal infection, *J. Clin. Microbiol.* **21:**33–38 (1985).
177. Taylor, D. N., *Campylobacter* infections in developing countries, in: *Campylobacter jejuni—Current Strategy and Future Trends* (I. Nachamkin, M. J. Blaser, and L. S. Tompkins, eds.), pp. 20–30, American Society of Microbiology, Washington, DC, 1992.
178. Mascart-Lemone, F. O., Duchateau, J. R., Oosterom, J., Butzler, J. P., and Delacroix, D. L., Kinetics of anti-*Campylobacter jejuni* monomeric and polymeric immunoglobulin A1 and A2 responses in serum during acute enteritis, *J. Clin. Microbiol.* **25:**1253–1257 (1987).
179. Winsor, D. K., Jr., Mathewson, J. J., and DuPont, H. L., Western blot analysis of intestinal secretory immunoglobulin a response to *Campylobacter jejuni* antigens in patients with naturally acquired *Campylobacter* enteritis, *Gastroenterology* **90:**1217–1222 (1986).
180. Shulman, S. T., and Moel, D., *Campylobacter* infection, *Pediatrics* **72:**437 (1983).
181. Walder, M., Epidemiology of *Campylobacter* enteritis, *Scand. J. Infect. Dis.* **14:**27–33 (1982).
182. Van Spreeuwel, J. P., Duursma, G. C., Meijer, C. J., Bax, R., Rosekrans, P. C., and Lindeman, J., *Campylobacter* colitis: Histological, immunohistochemical and ultrastructural findings, *Gut* **26:**945–951 (1985).
183. Skirrow, M. B., Jones, D. M., Sutcliffe, E., and Benjamin, J., *Campylobacter* bacteremia in England and Wales, 1981–91, *Epidemiol. Infect.* **110:**567–573 (1993).
184. de Guevara, C. L., Gonzalez, J., and Pena, P., Bactaraemia caused by *Campylobacter* spp., *J. Clin. Pathol.* **47:**174–175 (1994).
185. Ezpeleta, C., de Ursa, P. R., Obregon, F., Goni, F., and Cisterna, R., Acute pancreatitis associated with *Campylobacter jejuni* bacteremia, *Clin. Infect. Dis.* **15:**1050 (1992).
186. van der Hoop, A. G., and Veringa, E. M., Cholecystitis caused by *Campylobacter jejuni*, *Clin. Infect. Dis.* **17:**133 (1993).
187. Frizelle, F. A., and Rietveld, J. A., Spontaneous splenic rupture associated with *Campylobacter jejuni* infection, *Br. J. Surg.* **81:**718 (1994).
188. Wood, C. J., Fleming, V., Turridge, J., Thomson, N., and Atkins, R. C., *Campylobacter* peritonitis in continuous ambulatory peritoneal dialysis: Report of eight cases and a review of the literature, *Am. J. Kidney Dis.* **19:**257–263 (1992).
189. Simor, A. E., and Ferro, S., *Campylobacter jejuni* infection occurring during pregnancy, *Eur. J. Clin. Microbiol. Infect. Dis.* **9:**142–144 (1990).
190. Bremell, T., Bjelle, A., and Svedhem, A., Rheumatic symptoms

following an outbreak of *Campylobacter* enteritis: A five year follow-up, *Ann. Rheum. Dis.* **50:**934–938 (1991).

191. Eastmond, C. J., Rennie, J. A., and Reid, T. M., An outbreak of *Campylobacter* enteritis: A rheumatological follow-up survey, *J. Rheumatol.* **10:**107–108 (1983).
192. Rautelin, H., Koota, K., von Essen, R., Jahkola, M., Sitonen, A., and Kosunen, T. U., Waterborne *Campylobacter jejuni* epidemic in a Finnish hospital for rheumatic diseases, *Scand. J. Infect. Dis.* **22:**321–326 (1990).
193. Rees, J. H., Sovdain, S. E., Gregson, N. A., and Hughes, R. A. C., *Campylobacter jejuni* infection and Guillain–Barré syndrome, *N. Engl. J. Med.* **333:**1374–1379 (1995).
194. Mishu, B., Patton, C. M., and Blaser, M. J., Microbiologic characteristics of *Campylobacter jejuni* strains isolated from patients with Guillain–Barré syndrome (Abstract), *Clin. Infect. Dis.* **17:**538 (1993).
195. Yuki, N., Taki, T., Inagaki, F., *et al.*, A bacterium lipopolysaccharide that elicits Guillain–Barré syndrome has a GM1 ganglioside-like structure, *J. Exp. Med.* **178:**1771–1775 (1993).
196. McKhann, G. M., Cornblath, D. R., Griffin, J. W., *et al.*, Acute motor axonal neuropathy: A frequent cause of acute flaccid paralysis in China, *Ann. Neurol.* **33:**333–342 (1993).
197. Chanovitz, B. N., Harstein, A. I., Alexander, S. R., Terry, A. B., Short, P., and Katon, R., *Campylobacter jejuni*-associated hemolytic–uremic syndrome in a mother and daughter, *Pediatrics* **71:**253–256 (1983).
198. Damani, N. N., Humphrey, C. A., and Bell, B., Haemolytic anaemia in *Campylobacter* enteritis, *J. Infect.* 109–110 (1993).
199. van der Krujik, R. A., Affourtit, M. F., Endtz, H. P., and Arts, W. F. M., *Campylobacter jejuni* gastroenteritis and encephalopathy, *J.Infect.* **28:**99–100 (1994).
200. Berezin, S., and Newman, L. J., Prolonged mild diarrhoea caused by *Campylobacter*, *N.Y. State J. Med.* **29:** 1986.
201. Paulet, P., and Coffernils, M., Very long-term diarrhea due to *Campylobacter jejuni*, *Postgrad. Med. J.* **66:**410–411 (1990).
202. Bernard, E., Roger, P. M., Bonaldi, C. V., Fournier, J. P., and Dellamonica, P., Diarrhea and *Campylobacter* infections in patients infected with human immunodeficiency virus, *J. Infect. Dis.* **159:**143–144 (1989).
203. Peterson, M. C., Farr, R. W., and Castiglia, M., Prosthetic hip infections and bacteremia due to *Campylobacter jejuni* in a patient with AIDS, *Clin. Infect. Dis.* **16:**439–440 (1993).
204. Wheeler, A. P., and Gregg, C. R., *Campylobacter* bacteremia, cholecystitis, and the acquired immunodeficiency syndrome, *Ann. Intern. Med.* **105:**804 (1986).
205. Nelson, M. R., Shanson, D. C., Hawkins, D. A., and Gazzard, B. G., *Salmonella*, *Campylobacter* and *Shigella* on HIV-seropositive patients, *AIDS* **6:**1495–1498 (1992).
206. Melamed, I., Bujanover, Y., Igra, Y. S., Schwartz, D., Zakuth, V., and Spirer, Z., *Campylobacter* enteritis in normal and immunodeficient children, *Am. J. Dis. Child.* **137:**752–753 (1983).
207. Van der Meer, J. W. M., Mouton, R. P., Daha, M. R., and Schuurman, R. K. B., *Campylobacter jejuni* bacteraemia as a cause of recurrent fever in a patient with hypogammaglobulinaemia, *J. Infect.* **12:**235–239 (1986).
208. Hammarstrom, V., Smith, C. I. E., and Hammarstrom, L., Oral immunoglobulin treatment in *Campylobacter jejuni* enteritis, *Lancet* **341:**1036 (1993).
209. Kerstens, P. J. S. M., Endtz, H. P., Meis, J. F. G. M., *et al.*, Erysipelas-like skin lesions associated with *Campylobacter jejuni* septicemia in patients with hypogammaglobulinemia, *Eur. J. Clin. Microbiol. Infect. Dis.* **11:**842–847 (1992).
210. Melamed, A., Zakuth, V., Schwartz, D., and Spirer, Z., The immune system response to *Campylobacter* infection, *Microbiol. Immunol.* **32:**75–82 (1988).
211. Mandal, B. K., Ellis, M. E., Dunbar, E. M., and Whale, K., Double-blind placebo-controlled trial of erythromycin in the treatment of clinical *Campylobacter* infection, *J. Antimicrob. Chemother.* **13:**619–623 (1984).
212. Robins-Browne, R. M., Mackenjee, M. K., Bodasing, M. N., and Coovadia, H. M., Treatment of *Campylobacter*-associated enteritis with erythromycin, *Am. J. Dis. Child.* **137:**282–285 (1983).
213. Ruiz-Palacios, G. M., Norfloxacin in the treatment of bacterial enteric infections, *Scand. J. Infect. Dis.* **48:**S55–S63 (1986).
214. Petrucelli, B. P., Murphy, G. S., Sanchez, J. L., *et al.*, Treatment of travelers diarrhea with ciprofloxacin and loperamide, *J. Infect. Dis.* **165:**557–560 (1992).
215. Kuschner, R., Trofa, A., Thomas, R., *et al.*, Azithromycin for the treatment of *Campylobacter* enteritis in travelers to Thailand: An area where ciprofloxacin resistance is prevalent, *Clin. Infect.* **21:** 536–541 (1995).
216. Jacobs-Reitxma, W. F., van de Giessen, A. W., Bolder, N. M., and Mulder, R. W. A. W., Epidemiology of *Campylobacter* spp. at two Dutch broiler farms, *Epidemiol. Infect.* **114:**413–421 (1995).
217. Brunton, W. A. T., and Heggie, D., *Campylobacter*-associated diarrhoea in Edinburgh, *Br. Med. J.* **2:**956 (1977).
218. Bruce, D., Zochowski, W., and Ferguson, I. R., *Campylobacter* enteritis, *Br. Med. J.* **2:**1219 (1977).
219. Severin, W. P. J., *Campylobacter* enteritis, *Ned. Tijdschr. Geneeskd.* **122:**499–504 (1978).
220. Lopez-Brea, M., Molina, D., and Baquero, M., *Campylobacter* enteritis in Spain, *Trans. R. Soc. Trop. Med. Hyg.* **73:**474 (1979).
221. Delorme, L., Lambert, T., Branger, C., and Acar, J. F., Enteritis due to *Campylobacter jejuni* in the Paris area, *Med. Malad. Infect.* **9:**675–681 (1979).
222. Graf, J., Schar, G., and Heinzer, I., *Campylobacter-jejuni*-enteritis in der Schweiz, *Schweiz Med. Wochenschr.* **110:**590–595 (1980).
223. Velasco, A. C., Mateos, M. L., Mas, G., Pedraza, A., Diez, M., and Gutierrez, A., Three-year prospective study of intestinal pathogens in Madrid, Spain, *J. Clin. Microbiol.* **20:**290–292 (1984).
224. Figura, N., and Rossolini, A., A prospective etiological and clinical study on gastroenteritis in Italian children, *Boll. Ist. Sieroter. Milan* **64:**302–310 (1985).
225. Cevenni, R., Varoli, O., Rumpianesi, F., Mazzaracchio, R., Nanetti, A., and La Placa, M., A two-year longitudinal study on the etiology of acute diarrhea in young children in northern Italy, *Microbiologica* **8:**51–58 (1985).
226. Pien, F. D., Hsu, A. K., Padua, S. A., Isaacson, S., and Naka, S., *Campylobacter jejuni* enteritis in Honolulu, Hawaii, *Trans. Soc. Trop. Med. Hyg.* **4:**492–494 (1983).
227. Pai, C. H., Sorger, S., Lackman, L., Sinai, R. E., and Marks, M. I., *Campylobacter* gastroenteritis in children, *J. Pediatr.* **94:**589–591 (1979).
228. Burke, V., Gracey, M., Robinson, J., Peck, D., Beaman, J., and Bundell, C., The microbiology of childhood gastroenteritis: *Aeromonas* species and other infective agents, *J. Infect. Dis.* **148:**68–74 (1983).
229. Kirubakaran, C., Davison, G. P., Darby, H., *et al.*, *Campylobacter* as a cause of acute enteritis in children in South Australia. I. A 12-month study with controls, *Med. J. Aust.* **2:**333–335 (1981).

230. Skirrow, M. B., A demographic survey of *Campylobacter*, *Salmonella*, and *Shigella* infections in England, *Epidemiol. Infect.* **99**:647–657 (1987).
231. Ringertz, S., Rockhill, R. C., Ringertz, O., and Sutomo, A., *Campylobacter fetus* subsp. *jejuni* as a cause of gastroenteritis in Jakarta, Indonesia, *J. Clin. Microbiol.* **12**:538–540 (1980).
232. Rajan, D. P., and Mathan, V. I., Prevalence of *Campylobacter fetus* subsp. *jejuni* in healthy populations in southern India, *J. Clin. Microbiol.* **15**:749–751 (1982).
233. Nair, G. B., Bhattachary, S. K., and Pal, S. C., Isolation and characterization of *Campylobacter jejuni* from acute diarrhoeal cases in Calcutta, *Trans. R. Soc. Trop. Med. Hyg.* **77**:474–476 (1983).
234. Lim, Y. S., Jegathesan, M., and Wong, Y. H., *Campylobacter jejuni* as a cause of diarrhoea in Kuala Lumpur, Malaysia, *Med. J. Malaysia* **39**:285–288 (1984).
235. Young, D. M., Biao, J., Zheng, Z., Hadler, J., and Edberg, S. C., Isolation of *Campylobacter jejuni* in Hunan, the People's Republic of China: Epidemiology and comparison of Chinese and American methodology, *Diagn. Microbiol. Infect. Dis.* **5**:143–149 (1986).
236. Pazzaglia, G., Bourgeois, A. L., Araby, I., *et al.*, *Campylobacter*-associated diarrhoea in Egyptian infants: Epidemiology and clinical manifestations of disease and high frequency of concomitant infection, *Diarrhoeal. Res.* **11**:6–13 (1993).
237. Nath, G., Shukla, B. N., Reddy, D. C. S., and Sanyal, S. C., A community study on the aetiology of childhood diarrhoea with special reference to *Campylobacter jejuni* in a semiurban slum of Varansi, India, *J. Diarrhoeal Res.* **11**:165–168 (1993).
238. Popovic-Urovic, T., *Campylobacter jejuni* and *Campylobacter coli* diarrhoea in rural and urban populations in Yugoslavia, *Epidemiol. Infect.* **102**:59–67 (1989).
239. Olusanya, O., Adebayo, J. O., and Williams, B., *Campylobacter jejuni* as a bacterial cause of diarrhoea in Ile-Ife, *J. Hyg.* **91**:77–80 (1983).
240. Zaki, A. M., DuPont, H. L., Alamy, M., *et al.*, The detection of enteropathogens in acute diarrhea in a family cohort population in rural Egypt, *Am. J. Trop. Med. Hyg.* **35**:1013–1022 (1986).
241. Mauff, A. C., and Chapman, S. R., *Campylobacter* enteritis in Johannesburg, *S. Afr. Med. J.* **59**:217–218 (1981).
242. Mackenjee, M. K., Coovadia, Y. M., Coovadia, H. M., Hewitt, J., and Robins-Browne, R. M., Aetiology of diarrhoea in adequately nourished young African children in Durban, South Africa, *Ann. Trop. Paediatr.* **4**:183–187 (1984).
243. Lastovica, A. J., Le Roux, E., Congi, R. V., and Penner, J. L., Distribution of sero-biotypes of *Campylobacter jejuni* and *C. coli* isolated from paediatric patients, *J. Med. Microbiol.* **21**:1–5 (1986).
244. Hull, B. P., Spence, L., Bassett, D., Swanston, W. H., and Tikasingh, E. S., The relative importance of rotavirus and other pathogens in the etiology of the gastroenteritis in Trinidadian children, *Am. J. Trop. Med. Hyg.* **31**:142–148 (1982).
245. Mata, L., Simhon, A., Padilla, R., *et al.*, Diarrhea associated with rotaviruses, enterotoxigenic *Escherichia coli*, *Campylobacter*, and other agents in Costa Rican children, 1976–1981, *Am. J. Trop. Med. Hyg.* **32**:146–153 (1983).
246. Guerrant, R. L., Kirchhoff, L. V., Shields, D. S., *et al.*, Prospective study of diarrhea illness in northeastern Brazil: Patterns of disease, nutritional impact etiologies, and risk factors, *J. Infect. Dis.* **148**:986–997 (1983).
247. Olarte, J., and Pérez-Pérez, G. I., *Campylobacter jejuni* in children with diarrhea in Mexico City, *Pediatr. Infect. Dis.* **2**:18–20 (1983).
248. Figueroa, G., Araya, M., Ibanez, S., Clerc, N., and Brunser, O., Enteropathogens associated with acute diarrhea in hospitalized infants, *J. Pediatr. Gastroenterol. Nutr.* **5**:226–231 (1986).
249. Skirrow, M. B., and Benjamin, J., Differentiation of enteropathogenic campylobacter, *J. Clin. Pathol.* **33**:1122 (1980).
250. Georges, M. C., Wachsmuth, I. K., Meunier, D. M., *et al.*, Parasitic, bacterial, and viral enteric pathogens associated with diarrhea in the Central African Republic, *J. Clin. Microbiol.* **19**:571–575 (1984).

12. Suggested Reading

Allos, B. M., and Blaser, M. J., *Campylobacter jejuni* and the expanding spectrum of related infections, *Clin. Infect. Dis.* **20**:1092–1101 (1995).

Blaser, M. J., Wells, J. G., Feldman, R. A., Pollard, R. A., Allen, J. R., and the Collaborative Diarrheal Disease Study Group, *Campylobacter* enteritis in the United States: A multicenter study, *Ann. Intern. Med.* **98**:360–365 (1983).

Butzler, J.-P. (ed.), *Campylobacter Infection in Man and Animals*. CRC Press, Boca Raton, 1985.

Kuroki, S., Saida, T., Nukina, M., Haruta, T., Yoshioka, M., Kobayashi, Y., and Nakanishi, H., *Campylobacter jejuni* strains from patients with Guillain-Barré syndrome belong mostly to Penner serogroup 19 and contain B-N-Acetylglucosamine, *Ann. Neurol.* **22**:243–247 (1993).

Melby, K., Dahl, O. P., Crisp, L., and Penner, J. L., Clinical and serological manifestations in patients during a waterborne epidemic due to *Campylobacter jejuni*, *J. Infect.* **21**:309–316 (1990).

Nachamkin, I., *Campylobacter* and *Arcobacter*. In: Murray, P. R., Baron, E. J., Pfaller, M. A., Tenover, F. C., and Yolken, R. H. (eds), *Manual of Clinical Microbiology*. Washington, DC: American Society for Microbiology, 1995:483–491.

Perlman, D. M., Ampel, N. M., Schifman, R. B., Cohn, D. L., Patton, C. M., Aguirre, M. L., Wang, A. L., and Blaser, M. J., Persistent *Campylobacter jejuni* infections in patients infected with human immunodeficiency virus (HIV), *Ann. Intern. Med.* **108**:540–546 (1988).

Tauxe, R. V., Epidemiology of *Campylobacter jejuni* infections in the United States and other industrialized nations, in: *Campylobacter jejuni—current Strategy and Future Trends* (I. Nachamkin, M. J. Blaser, and L. S. Tompkins, eds.), pp. 9–19, American Society of Microbiology, Washington, DC, 1992.

Taylor, D. N., Perlman, D. M., Echeverria, P. D., Lexemboon, U., and Blaser, M. J., Campylobacter immunity and quantitative excretion rates in Thai children, *J. Infect. Dis.* **168**:754–758 (1993).

Wood, R. C., MacDonald, K. L., and Osterholm, M. T., *Campylobacter* enteritis outbreaks associated with drinking raw milk during youth activities, *JAMA* **268**:3228–3230 (1992).

CHAPTER 9

Chancroid

George P. Schmid

1. Introduction

Chancroid is a sexually transmitted disease characterized by one or more genital ulcers, often accompanied by painful inguinal lymphadenopathy. The etiologic agent is *Haemophilus ducreyi*, a fastidious, small, gram-negative rod.

2. Historical Background

Although chancroid is an ancient disease, it was not clinically differentiated from syphilis until 1852. *H. ducreyi* was identified in 1889 by Ducrey,[1] who found a single organism, compatible with *H. ducreyi*, in smears of exudate from serially passaged ulcers; other workers later isolated the organism. Subsequently, chancroid became recognized as a disease associated with poverty and prostitution, occurring in the wake of traveling carnivals and commonly among troops in World War I.

3. Methodology

3.1. Sources of Mortality Data

H. ducreyi does not spread beyond the genital area and fatalities do not occur.

3.2. Sources of Morbidity Data

In the United States, chancroid is a reportable disease and state health departments and the Centers for Disease Control and Prevention (CDC), to whom the state health departments report their cases, compile statistics on the number of cases reported by physicians. Outside the United States, reporting requirements vary by country.

Unfortunately, chancroid is a difficult disease to confirm by laboratory methods. Culture of *H. ducreyi* is notoriously difficult, and direct detection and serological methods are only now being developed. Thus, the large majority of cases reported worldwide are based on clinical diagnosis, and chancroid can be confused with other diseases. Because of this diagnostic confusion, chancroid is overreported in some areas and underreported in others.[2]

3.3. Surveys

The absence of a widely available serological test, combined with the fact that the large majority of symptomatic individuals seek medical treatment, have precluded meaningful surveys for previous or subclinical disease. The best incidence figures for chancroid come from surveys done in sexually transmitted disease (STD) or medical clinics.

3.4. Laboratory Diagnosis

3.4.1. Isolation and Identification of Organism. Culture is the only definitive means of diagnosis, but the sensitivity of culture depends on the presence of personnel who are experienced in working with *H. ducreyi*, the type and number of media used, and the conditions under which plates are incubated. The sensitivity of culture from patients suspected of having chancroid ranges from 0 to as high as 91%, depending largely on the above factors.[3,4] Many media have been used to culture *H. ducreyi*, and the use of two (or more) media are required for optimal isolation rates. Several standard media exist and use vancomycin (3 μg/ml) to suppress contaminating organisms

George P. Schmid • Division of STD Prevention, National Center for HIV, STD, and TB Prevention, Centers for Disease Control and Prevention, Atlanta, Georgia 30333.

and enrichments of 3–5% fetal calf serum and/or IsoVitaleX to enhance the growth of at least some strains.[3,4]

Material is obtained from the base of the ulcer with either a cotton swab or a wire loop, inoculated onto plates, and the plates are then well streaked to allow the best chance of observing colonies of *H. ducreyi*. Plates should be incubated at 33°C in a candle jar, in the bottom of which should be a moist (but not soaked) paper towel to provide humidity. The highest yield of *H. ducreyi* will be at 48 or 72 hr, although ideally plates should be incubated for up to 5 days. On primary isolation plates, it is common for only a few colonies to be present and outnumbered by larger colonies of commensal bacteria; a dissecting microscope is helpful in identifying colonies of *H. ducreyi*. Colonies of *H. ducreyi* are small (1–2 mm, although occasionally larger variants occur) and gray, and can be differentiated from colonies of other bacteria because they can be pushed intact across the top of the agar. Colonies meeting these criteria, which are oxidase-positive when testing using tetramethyl-*p*-phenylenediamine (the dimethyl reagent will produce a negative result), and which contain small, gram-negative bacilli or coccobacilli, can be presumptively identified as *H. ducreyi*. Further biochemical testing will definitively identify *H. ducreyi*.[5]

3.4.2. Serological and Immunologic Diagnostic Methods. Recently developed serological tests using enzyme immunoassay (EIA) are promising.[6–8] These tests, however, need further testing and are currently only research tools. Direct detection of *H. ducreyi* in ulcer exudate by immunofluorescence or polymerase chain reaction (PCR) are promising diagnostic alternatives,[9–11] and a commercial PCR test is undergoing evaluation.

4. Biological Characteristics of the Organism

H. ducreyi is a short, nonmotile, non-spore-forming, gram-negative rod. Colonies of such organisms that can be pushed intact across the surface of the agar, which are oxidase-positive, catalase-negative, and require X factor for growth can be identified as *H. ducreyi*.[4,5] The virulence factors of *H. ducreyi* are being intensively studied.[12,13] Abraded skin is experimentally needed for ulcer induction, suggesting small abrasions acquired during sexual intercourse may be important for disease acquisition. Subsequently, attachment to cells is important and, intriguingly, fetal foreskin cells seem particularly susceptible to attachment, possibly through pili, but there is conflicting evidence over whether *H. ducreyi* invades cells. Lipo-oligosaccharides (LOS) appear to be important for evasion of ingestion by polymorphonuclear leukocytes and ulcer production, and several toxins have been described but their roles are unclear. Lesions can be produced in rabbits, and rabbits housed at low temperatures are more susceptible, suggesting virulence is increased at "lower" temperatures (and perhaps suggesting one reason why ulcers are uncommon within the vagina, as opposed to surface skin). With serial passage on agar, some strains lose their ability to produce lesions, indicating the loss of one or more virulence factors. A primate model has been reported. *H. ducreyi* has acquired resistance to penicillins, sulfonamides, and tetracyclines by acquiring plasmids encoding resistance to these drugs; resistance to tetracyclines in some cases is chromosomally mediated. Seven plasmids, most of which are known to encode for antimicrobial resistance, have been described in *H. ducreyi* and, as with other bacteria, offer epidemiological tools for distinguishing similarities among strains isolated in varying geographic areas. Restriction fragment length polymorphism (ribotyping) offers a second means of distinguishing epidemiological relationships among strains, as do outer membrane protein profiles, indirect immunofluorescence, enzyme profiles, and lectin typing.[14]

5. Descriptive Epidemiology

5.1. Prevalence and Incidence

Determining the prevalence and incidence of chancroid is difficult because of the problem of accurate diagnosis.[2]

In the United States, a mean of 878 cases were reported annually between 1971 and 1980, an incidence of 0.4/100,000. Since 1980, numerous outbreaks of chancroid occurred and the number of cases reported annually peaked in 1987, when 5047 cases were reported.[15] Since then, for uncertain reasons, the number of cases declined, reaching 606 in 1995 and 386 in 1996.

Outside the United States, chancroid is very common in many developing countries, while in the industrialized countries chancroid occurs only sporadically. In many developing countries, chancroid is the most common cause of genital ulcers, while in the United States this is the case only in exceptional outbreak situations.

5.2. Epidemic Behavior and Contagiousness

The worldwide epidemiology of chancroid is closely linked to prostitution and immigration. Prostitution may occur either out of economic necessity (often in areas where access to medical facilities is limited), or because of the association of prostitution with illegal drug use (where women have many sex partners to earn money to purchase drugs, most frequently cocaine, in the United

States)[16]; in either case, women with this painful disease do not cease having sex, either because medical facilities are unavailable or because they do not use available facilities. Immigration brings infected individuals to areas where chancroid does not occur, thus occasionally beginning epidemics.

Unlike many sexually transmitted diseases, chancroid occurs in only selected communities in the United States[15] and other industrialized countries. In communities where chancroid is first appearing, successful control depends on prompt recognition of the disease and immediate identification and treatment of sexual partners.[15,17] If the individual introducing chancroid has intercourse with a limited number of partners and these partners are not highly sexually active, control efforts may be successful in eliminating disease from the community. Sudden, large outbreaks have occurred among men, however, when female prostitutes have been the source of infection. These outbreaks have proved to be difficult to control because the illegality and anonymity of prostitution makes locating infected individuals difficult. In addition, in the United States, several outbreaks have occurred among illegal entrants, further hampering control efforts. The likelihood of chancroid being transmitted during a single act of unprotected intercourse is unclear, but a figure of 63% for male-to-female transmission was derived in a small study.[18] The lack of circumcision is a risk factor for acquiring chancroid.[19,20] Individuals with human immunodeficiency virus (HIV) infection may have a more severe or prolonged case, thus enhancing transmissibility.

5.3. Geographic Distribution

In the United States, the largest number of cases has occurred in New York City, but numerous cities and towns have had cases.[15]

Specific geographic distribution is generally lacking outside the United States. Chancroid occurs frequently in the large majority of developing countries, with relatively more cases in Africa and Asia. In the industrialized world, scattered cities in Europe and Australia have reported cases.

5.4. Temporal Distribution

Chancroid occurs throughout the year.

5.5. Age

Since national age distribution data are not collected, age-specific data come from information gathered during outbreaks. Cases in males are generally most common in the 20- to 24-year age group, but the mean and median age are higher, indicating that a significant number of men older than 20–24 years acquire the disease. Age distribution data in women are less well defined because of the relative paucity of cases in women, but the onset of disease in females is generally at a younger age than in men.

5.6. Sex

In nine outbreaks in the United States between 1981 and 1987, the male female ratio was 3:1 to 25:1, and was highest in outbreaks involving prostitutes.[15] The preponderance of cases in males is due largely to the role prostitution plays and, less so, to the fact that disease in men is almost always symptomatic and easily visible, while ulcers in women may occasionally occur in the vagina and be less symptomatic, and thus not reported.

5.7. Race

Reported cases of chancroid have occurred preponderantly in non-Caucasians. This occurrence likely reflects worldwide differences among racial groups in socioeconomic status, availability of care, reporting sources (most cases are reported from public clinics), types of outbreaks (outbreaks involving illegal entrants in the United States involve principally Hispanics), frequency of prostitute visitation, and attitudes toward such factors as sexual activity, condom usage, and rates of circumcision.

5.8. Occupation

Occupation per se does not predispose to acquiring chancroid, although individuals involved in certain jobs, e.g., seamen or military personnel on leave, may be more likely to have contact with infected individuals.

5.9. Occurrence in Different Settings

During times of war and social upheaval, chancroid becomes more common (see Section 5.10).

5.10. Socioeconomic Factors

Chancroid increases during times of poverty and war. This increase undoubtedly does not reflect poor nutrition or crowded living conditions, but rather a matrix of availability of medical care, knowledge of and attitudes toward STDs, sexual habits, reporting sources, and prevalence of prostitution (for alcohol, money, or drugs). The latter factor may be related to living standards in that during times of austerity, prostitution becomes more common.

6. Mechanisms and Routes of Transmission

Chancroid is sexually transmitted and lesions outside the genital tract are rare, but may occur from oral or anal intercourse, or autoinoculation.

7. Pathogenesis and Immunity

Lesions arise in the areas of the male genital tract that are most easily traumatized: the prepuce of uncircumcised men and the coronal sulcus area of circumcised men. In women, most lesions are found on the external genitalia and only occasionally on the vaginal walls or cervix; perianal lesions may occur and do not appear to necessarily result from anal sex.[21] The usual incubation period is about 3–7 days, but longer incubation periods occur. Immunity develops but is incomplete, as second infections may occur soon after initial infection; nevertheless, the development of even incomplete immunity in key individuals, e.g., prostitutes, may help explain the termination of epidemics.

8. Patterns of Host Response

8.1. Clinical Features

At the site of inoculation, an inflamed macule or papule appears and rapidly erodes into an ulcer; many patients simply recall a "sore" developing without a distinct macule or papule stage. About one half of patients have more than one ulcer, but it is unusual to have more than four.[21–24] Typically, an ulcer caused by *H. ducreyi* is deep, has a ragged, nonindurated margin with an erythematous edge, and a beefy, necrotic base. Superficial ulcers, however, may occur. A diagnostic feature of chancroid ulcers is that they are exquisitely painful, making examination difficult—retraction of the prepuce due to phimosis may be impossible. Ulcers may coalesce and form large, serpiginous ulcerations that partly encircle the penis.

As the disease progresses, as many as one half of men develop unilateral or bilateral inguinal adenopathy, which is characteristically painful even though nodes may be small. Large, fluctuant lymph nodes (buboes) may occur, a finding not seen in genital herpes or syphilis. In the absence of effective antimicrobial therapy and, occasionally, needle drainage, buboes frequently rupture. Lymphadenopathy in women is unusual, presumably because of differences in lymphatic drainage.

Asymptomatic colonization of *H. ducreyi* of the cervix has been described but appears to be rare.[18] Ulcers of the cervix or vagina occasionally occur, with little or no symptomatology.[21] Without treatment, tissue destruction may be significant, but *H. ducreyi* does not spread outside the genital tract. Patients eventually heal their infection after several (unpleasant) months, but often with scarring.

8.2. Diagnosis

Because few laboratories have diagnostic capability for *H. ducreyi*, Gram's stain diagnosis of chancroid is not specific, and there is no standardized serological test, diagnosis of chancroid is often made on clinical grounds. In cases where ulcers are of "typical appearance" and painful, and accompanied by painful, large inguinal lymph nodes, clinical diagnosis is reasonably accurate. Unfortunately, many cases are not so characteristic and other causes of genital ulceration (syphilis and genital herpes) and painful, large inguinal lymph nodes (lymphogranuloma venereum) must be differentiated from chancroid.[22,23] As a result, clinical diagnosis of all chancroid cases, and not just extremely typical ones, is difficult,[22,23,25] but may be as high as 80%.[22] As a consequence of diagnostic uncertainty and coinfection, all patients with a genital ulcer should have a darkfield examination (ideally) and serological test for syphilis performed to exclude syphilis as best as possible; *Treponema pallidum* coinfects about 10% of chancroid cases.[25,26] Genital herpes may be accompanied by painful, inguinal lymphadenopathy but rarely causes buboes, and is typically accompanied by multiple, shallow ulcerations preceded by vesicles. Lymphogranuloma venereum is often confused with chancroid, but in lymphogranuloma venereum it is unusual for the ulcer to be present at the time inguinal lymphadenopathy is prominent.

Gram-stained smears of ulcer material are sometimes used to diagnose chancroid, but the diagnostic utility of the Gram's stain has not been well studied. Ulcers often contain many species of bacteria, some of which may appear like *H. ducreyi* on smear. Diagnostic specificity is probably enhanced by identifying as presumptive *H. ducreyi* only smears showing strands of bacteria, sometimes appearing like "railroad tracks," along mucus strands. Finding organisms compatible with *H. ducreyi* in a bubo aspirate is more specific, but is uncommon. Specific diagnosis can be made by culture, immunofluorescence, PCR, or serology. A transport medium for ulcer exudate may enhance diagnostic capabilities in areas without local culture capability.(27)

Chancroid is associated with HIV infection, within the United States and in other countries, both at the time of initial evaluation (with seropositivity resulting from previous risky sexual behavior) and later (with seropositivity resulting from infection at the time of chancroid acquisition). The prevalence of HIV infection in individuals seeking medical attention can be striking, with prevalences of >45%(25) in Malawi, but 18% in an American New York City study.(20)

Seroconversion further increases these prevalences. In one study in Africa, 43% of uncircumcised men who acquired chancroid following a single sexual encounter developed HIV infection.(28) Such seroconversion rates are <5% in the United States,(29) where fewer source patients are HIV-seropositive. Thus, patients with chancroid should have an HIV test at their initial visit and 3 months later; a follow-up syphilis test should also be performed at that time.(26)

9. Control and Prevention

9.1. General Concepts

In the United States, cases of chancroid must be reported to local health authorities. Cases should be treated with an appropriate antimicrobial and interviewed to elicit the names of sexual partners. Partners within the 10 days preceding onset should be examined and treated, whether lesions are present or not, because they may be in the incubation stage or may be asymptomatic carriers of *H. ducreyi*.

Outbreaks of disease occurring in an area where chancroid is first appearing must be aggressively managed if chancroid is to be eliminated from the area.(15,17) Identifying and locating prostitutes is crucial in these efforts, but often difficult because of the anonymity of prostitution and evidence that exchange of illegal drugs for sex has been the form of payment in some outbreaks. If initial control efforts fail and chancroid becomes established, elimination becomes very difficult, although experience indicates that outbreaks will subsequently diminish in intensity. Control of chancroid is widely thought to be important in the control of HIV infection, at least in the developing world.(19) Nevertheless, attributable risks of chancroid on HIV infection have not been well characterized. One study attributed 30% of HIV infections in an African cohort of women to genital ulcers, most of which were chancroid.(30)

9.2. Antibiotic and Chemotherapeutic Approaches to Prophylaxis

H. ducreyi has developed resistance to several antimicrobials, primarily via plasmids. Treatment with (1) erythromycin, 500 mg, orally, four times a day for 7 days, (2) ceftriaxone, 250 mg, intramuscularly, once, (3) azithromycin, 1 g, orally, once, are recommended therapies for cases or sex partners in the United States, or (4) ciprofloxacin, 500 mg, orally, two times a day, for 3 days.(26,31) Outside the United States, erythromycin (500 mg, three to four times a day, for 5 to 7 days), azithromycin (1 g, once), and ciprofloxacin (500 mg, twice a day, for 3 or more days, or possibly lower doses)(25) have been successfully used recently, while previously effective single doses of ceftriaxone (due to HIV infection) and multiple doses of trimethoprim–sulfamethoxazole (due to antimicrobial resistance) cannot now be relied on. Patients with HIV infection do not respond as well as patients without HIV infection, particularly to single-dose therapy, and more intensive regimens and follow-up may be needed in such individuals.(25,26,31)

In many clinical situations, it is impossible to diagnose the cause of a genital ulcer adequately; in areas where chancroid and syphilis are common, treatment for both chancroid and syphilis is an acceptable therapeutic strategy.

Patients with fluctuant buboes should have the bubo aspirated through intact, adjacent skin, to prevent rupture and subsequent drainage.

9.3. Immunization

No vaccine is available.

10. Unresolved Problems

The largest scientific impediment in controlling chancroid is the lack of simple, accurate diagnostic tests. The development of rapid diagnostic techniques would greatly enhance the ability to differentiate causes of genital ulcers and lead to immediate efforts to locate sexual partners; currently such efforts are diluted by the uncertainty over whether the patient really has chancroid. Improved culture or direct detection techniques and an accurate serological test would enhance the ability to determine whether asymptomatic carriage is more common than thought, as well as aid in accurately determining the prevalence of chancroid.

Further determining the magnitude of interaction between chancroid and HIV infection would enhance efforts to control chancroid. While it is clear that chancroid increases HIV transmission, determining the attributable risk of chancroid on HIV incidence in an area would assist in assigning the resources that should go into chancroid control. Further quantifying the influence that HIV has on prolonging or increasing the severity of the ulcers of chancroid, and how significantly HIV infection interferes with therapy, are additional important pieces of information.

11. References

1. Ducrey, A., Experimentelle untersuchungen uber den Ansteckungsstoff des weichen Schankers und uber die Bubonen, *Monatsh. Prakt. Dermatol.* **9**:387 (1889).
2. Schulte, J. M., Martich, F. A., and Schmid, G. P., Chancroid in the United States, 1981–1990: Evidence for underreporting of cases, *Morbid. Mortal. Week. Rep.* **41**(SS-3):57–61 (1992).
3. Dangor, Y., Miller, S. D., Koornhof, H. J., *et al.*, A simple medium for the primary isolation of *Haemophilus ducreyi*, *Eur. J. Clin. Microbiol. Infect. Dis.* **11**:930–934 (1991).
4. Morse, S. A., Chancroid and *Haemophilus ducreyi*, *Clin. Microbiol. Rev.* **2**:137–157 (1989).
5. Campos, J. M., *Haemophilus*, in: *Manual of Clinical Microbiology*, 6th ed., pp. 556–565, American Society for Microbiology Press, Washington, DC, 1995.
6. Desjardins, M., Thompson, E. E., Filion, L. G., *et al.*, Standardization of an enzyme immunoassay for human antibody to *Haemophilus ducreyi*, *J. Clin. Microbiol.* **30**:2019–2024 (1992).
7. Museyi, K., Van Dyck, E., Vervoort, T., *et al.*, Use of an enzyme immunoassay to detect serum IgG antibodies to *Haemophilus ducreyi*, *J. Infect. Dis.* **157**:1039–1043 (1988).
8. Roggen, E. L., Hoofd, G., Van Dyck, E., *et al.*, Enzyme immunoassays (EIAs) for the detection of anti-*Haemophilus ducreyi* serum IgA, IgG and IgM antibodies, *Sex Transm. Dis.* **21**:36–42 (1994).
9. Chui, L., Albritton, W., Paster, B., *et al.*, Development of the polymerase chain reaction for diagnosis of chancroid, *J. Clin. Microbiol.* **31**:659–664 (1993).
10. Johnson, S. R., Martin, D. H., Cammarata, C., *et al.*, Development of a polymerase chain reaction assay for the detection of *Haemophilus ducreyi*, *Sex Transm. Dis.* **21**:13–23 (1994).
11. Najima Karim, Q., Finn, G. Y., Easmon, C. S. F., *et al.*, Rapid detection of *Haemophilus ducreyi* in clinical and experimental infections using monoclonal antibody: A preliminary evaluation, *Genitourin. Med.* **65**:361–365 (1989).
12. Abeck, D., and Johnson, A. P., Pathophysiological concept of *Haemophilus ducreyi* infection (chancroid), *Int. J. STD AIDS* **3**:319–323 (1992).
13. Totten, P. A., Lara, J. C., Norm, D. V., *et al.*, *Haemophilus ducreyi* attaches to and invades human epithelial cells *in vitro*, *Infect. Immunol.* **62**:5632–5640 (1994).
14. Sarafian, S. K., Woods, T. C., Knapp, J. S., *et al.*, Molecular characterization of *Haemophilus ducreyi* by ribosomal DNA fingerprinting, *J. Clin. Microbiol.* **29**:1949–1954 (1991).
15. Schmid, G. P., Sanders, L. L., Blount, J. H., *et al.*, Chancroid in the United States: Reestablishment of an old disease, *J. Am. Med. Assoc.* **258**:3265–3268 (1987).
16. Martin, D. H., and DiCarlo, R. P., Recent changes in the epidemiology of genital ulcer disease in the United States. The crack cocaine connection, *Sex. Transm. Dis.* **21**(Suppl. 2):76–80 (1994).
17. Jessamine, P. G., and Brunham, R. C., Rapid control of a chancroid outbreak: Implications for Canada, *Can. Med. Assoc. J.* **142**:1081–1085 (1990).
18. Plummer, F. A., D'Costa, L. J., Nsanze, H., *et al.*, Epidemiology of chancroid and *Haemophilus ducreyi* in Nairobi, Kenya, *Lancet* **2**:1293–1295 (1983).
19. Jessamine, P. G., Plummer, F. A., Ndinya Achola, J. O., *et al.*, Human immunodeficiency virus, genital ulcers and the male foreskin: Synergism in HIV-1 transmission, *Scand. J. Infect. Dis.* **69**(Suppl.):181–186 (1990).
20. McLaughlin, M., Wilkes, M., Blum, S., *et al.*, Risks associated with acquiring chancroid genital ulcerative disease and HIV infection. Abstract A.615, Vth International Conference on AIDS, Montreal, Canada, 1989.
21. Plummer, F. A., D'Costa, L. J., Nsanze, H., *et al.*, Clinical and microbiologic studies of genital ulcers in Kenyan women, *Sex. Transm. Dis.* **12**:193–197 (1985).
22. Dangor, Y., Ballard, R. C., Exposoto, F. D. L., *et al.*, Accuracy of clinical diagnosis of genital ulcer disease, *Sex. Transm. Dis.* **17**: 184–189 (1990).
23. O'Farrell, N., Hoosen, A. A., Coetzee, K. D., *et al.*, Genital ulcer disease: Accuracy of clinical diagnosis and strategies to improve control in Durban, South Africa, *Genitourin. Med.* **70**:7–11 (1994).
24. Taylor, D. N., Duangmani, C., Suvongse, C., *et al.*, The role of *Haemophilus ducreyi* in penile ulcers in Bangkok, Thailand, *Sex. Transm. Dis.* **11**:148–151 (1984).
25. Behets, F. M. T., Liomba, G., Lule, G., *et al.*, Sexually transmitted diseases and human immunodeficiency virus control in Malawi: A field study of genital ulcer disease, *J. Infect. Dis.* **171**:451–456 (1995).
26. Centers for Disease Control and Prevention, 1998 guidelines for treatment of sexually transmitted diseases, *Morbid. Mortal. Week. Rep.* **47** (RR-1):1–116 (1998).
27. Dangor, Y., Radebe, F., Ballard, R. C ., *et al.*, Transport media for *Haemophilus ducreyi*, *Sex. Transm. Dis.* **20**:5–9 (1993).
28. Cameron, D. W., Simonsen, J. N., D'Costa, L. J., *et al.*, Female-to-male transmission of HIV in Nairobi, *Lancet* **2**:403–408 (1989).
29. Telzak, E. E., Chiasson, M. A., Bevier, P. J., *et al.*, HIV-1 seroconversion in patients with and without genital ulcer disease, *Ann. Intern. Med.* **119**:1181–1186 (1993).
30. Plourde, P. J., Plummer, F. A., Pepin, P., *et al.*, Human immunodeficiency virus type 1 infection in women attending a sexually transmitted diseases clinic in Kenya, *J. Infect. Dis.* **166**:86–92 (1992).
31. Schulte, J. M., and Schmid, G. P., The management of chancroid, *Clin. Infect. Dis.* **51**:539–546 (1995).

12. Suggested Reading

Ronald, A. R., and Albritton, W. L., Chancroid and *Haemophilus ducreyi*,in: *Sexually Transmitted Diseases* (M. K. Holmes, P. A. Mardh, P. F. Sparling, *et al.*, eds.), pp. 263–272, New York, McGraw-Hill, 1990.

Schmid, G. P., Approach to the patient with genital ulcer disease, *Med. Clin. North Am.* **74**(6):1559–1572 (1990).

CHAPTER 10

Chlamydial Infections

Julius Schachter and E. Russell Alexander

1. Introduction

There are several quite different disease patterns that result from human infection with chlamydial organisms. Infection with *Chlamydia trachomatis* may result in trachoma, a variety of other syndromes that accompany ocular or genital infection, or lymphogranuloma venereum (LGV). *C. psittaci* has one human disease manifestation—psittacosis. *C. pneumoniae* causes respiratory disease, and infection has been associated with coronary artery disease.

Trachoma causes a cicatrizing keratoconjunctivitis, and its sequelae of keratitis, pannus, entropion, and trichiasis occur in severe form in certain endemic areas, primarily the hot, arid parts of the world. Trachoma is the leading infectious cause of blindness.

From a genital reservoir, *C. trachomatis* is transmitted sexually to cause a variety of diseases (Table 1). In the adult female, disease manifestations include cervicitis, salpingitis, urethral syndrome, Bartholinitis, and postpartum endometritis. In the male, they include urethritis and epididymitis. (Both sexes may contract inclusion conjunctivitis and proctitis.) Infant chlamydial diseases include inclusion conjunctivitis of the newborn, pneumonia, and possibly bronchiolitis and otitis media. In the United States, in other Western countries, and in some developing countries where it has been studied, *C. trachomatis* is the most prevalent sexually transmitted bacterium. In infancy, it is the leading single cause of pneumonia in the first 6 months of life.

LGV is a systemic sexually transmitted disease with worldwide distribution, particularly prevalent in warmer climates. The bubonic form is of declining importance in the United States, although proctitis due to the agent is more often recognized.

Psittacosis is an interstitial pneumonia or generalized toxic disease of children and adults that is transmitted from infected avian species. It has become an infrequent disease, except from occupational exposure or exposure to infected psittacine house pets.

C. pneumoniae causes a range of respiratory disease, from pharyngitis and otitis media to bronchitis and interstitial pneumonia. Clinically and, to a great extent, epidemiologically, the manifestations are very similar to those caused by *Mycoplasma pneumoniae*. From present knowledge, it is exclusively a human disease.

2. Historical Background

The description of trachoma is ancient, trachoma being one of the earliest of human diseases to be recognized as a distinct clinical entity.[1] It was described in the Ebers papyrus (1500 BC.) The name *trachoma* was first used by Dioscorides in 60 AD, and the stages of the disease were described by Galen a century later. From the Middle Eastern reservoir, it spread throughout Europe in many waves from the time of the Crusades to Napoleon, being known as both "Egyptian and military ophthalmia." In the last century, the disease has decreased in incidence in many of the temperate climates of the world. It has disappeared from Europe, for example, and is essentially gone from foci that existed in the central United States. Although sulfonamide treatment was introduced in 1938, and tetracyclines and macrolides in following decades, they cannot be credited with this change. Rather, it has appeared to follow improvements in the standard of living and of hygiene practices. Trachoma has persisted in hot,

Julius Schachter • Department of Laboratory Medicine, University of California, San Francisco, California 94110. **E. Russell Alexander** • Seattle–King County Department of Public Health, Seattle, Washington 98104.

Table 1. Disease Manifestations of *Chlamydia*

Chlamydia trachomatis			
Trachoma			
Oculogenital diseases			
Adult, male or female:	Adult female:	Adult male:	Infant:
Conjunctivitis	Cervicitis	Urethritis	Conjunctivitis
Proctitis	Salpingitis	Epididymitis	Pneumonia
	Urethral syndrome	Arthritis (Reiter's syndrome)	Bronchiolitis
	Postpartum endometritis		Otitis media
Lymphogranuloma venereum			
Chlamydia psittaci			
Psittacosis			
Chlamydia pneumoniae			
Pneumonia			

dry climates and is still a major cause of blindness in many developing countries.

In 1907, Halberstaedter and von Prowazek[2] described cytoplasmic inclusion bodies in epithelial scrapings from trachoma cases. They named them *chlamydozoa* or *mantle bodies*, because reddish elementary particles appeared to be embedded in a blue matrix or mantle. Two years later, the same investigators reported inclusions in infants with nongonococcal ophthalmia neonatorum. Lindner[3] named this disease *inclusion blenorrhea* and reproduced ocular disease in nonhuman primates from a mother's genital secretion. Inclusions were demonstrated in female genital epithelium and in nongonococcal urethritis (NGU) scrapings. Material from each of these sources and from infant conjunctivitis was used to produce follicular conjunctivitis in monkeys. Thus, it was believed as early as 1910 that trachoma and ocular genital diseases were caused by similar agents, and the vertical transmission of these agents was postulated.

In 1911, Nicolle *et al.*[4] in Tunis passed trachoma secretions through Berkefeld V filters and succeeded in producing a conjunctivitis in an ape and a chimpanzee, established to be trachoma by transmission to human conjunctiva. In the 1930s, Julianelle[5] for trachoma and Thygeson[1] for inclusion conjunctivitis expanded these studies with the use of smaller filters. After Bedson had described the unique developmental cycle of the psittacosis agent, Thygeson recognized that the same cycle held true for the agent of inclusion conjunctivitis. Thus, Bedson,[6] in 1953, noting the morphological similarity of the developmental cycles of the agents, termed them members of the psittacosis–LGV group of atypical viruses. This concept was strengthened by the finding by Rake that they all shared a common complement-fixing antigen.[7]

In the period 1930–1950, the clinical and epidemiological features of trachoma and inclusion conjunctivitis were described,[5–8] all on the basis of cytological morphological identification. In 1938, the first effective therapy of trachoma occurred with the introduction of sulfanilamides, although it was recognized early that these drugs did not kill the agents. In the search for *in vitro* isolation techniques for chlamydiae, the chorioallantois of the embryonated hen's egg and a wide variety of tissue culture systems were explored. These attempts failed, and *Chlamydia* was believed to be a virus with propensity for epithelial growth. Machiavello, in 1944, and Stewart, in 1950, claimed organism growth in the yolk sac of embryonated eggs, but their findings could not be confirmed. It remained for Tang *et al.*[9] in China, in 1957, to clearly isolate the agent of trachoma in yolk sac treated with streptomycin to retard bacterial contamination and to demonstrate that this material caused inclusion-positive conjunctivitis in the monkey model. Collier and Sowa[10] confirmed this finding in African studies in The Gambia and, in addition, showed serological response to the agent in human sera. They also showed that the antigen responsible for seroconversion was common to the psittacosis and LGV groups of agents. An explosion of trachoma research followed, including studies in Saudi Arabia, Egypt, Taiwan, and San Francisco. As the trachoma agent was studied, it became clear that it was not a virus but a small bacterium that shared with viruses the property of obligate intracellular parasitism. The agent of inclusion conjunctivitis was isolated by Jones *et al.*,[11] in 1959, using yolk sac techniques. In the period 1960–1980, the development of cell cultures for isolation [12] and microimmunofluorescence methods for antigen identification, immunotyping, and measurement of host response[13,14] permitted clinical and epidemiological characteristics of *C. trachomatis* diseases to be expanded.

Psittacosis and LGV were first described clinically much later than trachoma (1874,[15] and 1786,[16] respectively), but in both cases their real definition took place in the first half of this century. The understanding of the biology of the organisms developed more rapidly than with the trachoma and inclusion-conjunctivitis agents, primarily because of their greater virulence and host range. In particular, their pathogenicity for mice and for the embryonated yolk sac permitted the development of isolation methods and of serological methods (a complement-fixation test was developed as early as 1930).[17] With the advent of tissue culture methods, the exploration of the molecular biology of chlamydiae has expanded considerably.[18]

C. pneumoniae disease was first described by Grayston *et al.*[19] in 1986. The agent had been recovered from the eye of a primary schoolchild in 1965 in a prospective study of trachoma in Taiwan. Two decades later, antibody to this isolate was found in the serum of children and adults with respiratory disease.[19]

3. Methodology

3.1. Sources of Mortality Data

There is no significant mortality for any of the diseases caused by *Chlamydia*, and the rare deaths associated with infant chlamydial pneumonitis or psittacosis are usually in persons with serious accompanying underlying disease. Fatal outcome has no importance in the epidemiology of these conditions.

3.2. Sources of Morbidity Data

Trachoma is not a reportable disease in the United States. For the last 40 years, the World Health Organization (WHO) and many national health agencies have accumulated data on trachoma occurrence by clinical surveys, for planning control efforts, but no continuing statistics on incidence are available. In the United States, the oculogenital chlamydial diseases are not uniformly reportable, but there is some degree of reporting in most of the states. So far, all are underreported, as diagnostic tests are not universally available. Other estimates have been made from sexually transmitted disease (STD) clinics where the ratio of nongonococcal to gonococcal disease has been used, along with other prevalence data, to estimate annual incidence.[20] LGV is a reportable disease, but because of its rarity, data are usually available only in annual summaries published by the US Public Health Service. Psittacosis is reportable, and data on incidence are published weekly in the *Morbidity and Mortality Weekly Report* and are summarized in *Surveillance Reports* by the Centers for Disease Control (CDC). In addition, the same centers accumulate data on the occurrence of psittacosis in pet birds or in fowl flocks when these animals are submitted to state laboratories for inspection. There are no data on the incidence of *C. pneumoniae* infections except for small studies done in selected populations. Seroepidemiological studies show that the infection is a common one in many countries.

3.3. Surveys

Trachoma control programs, often supported by the WHO, have developed on clinical surveys of trachoma prevalence and of trachoma sequelae, including blindness. The WHO has helped to standardize survey methods.[21] Most recently, these have been combined with more general surveys of visual acuity and blindness. Traditionally, such surveys do not utilize laboratory diagnostic methods. This is not necessary for trachoma, since the disease is well defined clinically.

Data on incidence and prevention of genital chlamydial infections are available from research studies. These have included studies in STD clinics, prospective studies in pregnant women, studies of chlamydial genital carriage in normal populations, and surveys in infants.

There are no significant survey data for LGV, psittacosis, or *C. pneumoniae* infections in the United States.

3.4. Laboratory Diagnosis

3.4.1. Cytological Identification. For *C. trachomatis*, the organism can be identified in cytological scrapings or in tissue specimens by recognition of characteristic intracytoplasmic inclusions.[22] Such identification in conjunctival epithelial cells, and less frequently in cervical epithelial cells, constituted the only identification possible from the time when trachoma and oculogenital diseases were first recognized, at the turn of the century, until the organism was isolated in embryonated eggs in 1957.

This diagnostic approach has been supplanted by the use of tissue culture (TC) isolation methods and by the use of modern nonculture diagnostic tests that detect chlamydial antigens or genes. Study of epithelial cell scrapings stained with Giemsa stain (the time-honored method) may still be useful for some studies or when other diagnostic tests are not available.

Cytology is a relatively insensitive way to diagnose chlamydial infection. For many years the most sensitive method for identification of *C. trachomatis* infection of the genital tract was isolation in TC. Antigen detection by direct fluorescent antibody staining or by enzyme immunoassay are somewhat less sensitive and specific, but are widely used.[23]

Direct methods of detection of chlamydial DNA have not been more sensitive than EIA procedures. However, the introduction of amplified DNA probe technology, such as the polymerase chain reaction (PCR) or ligase chain reaction (LCR), in the mid-1990s, promises to revolutionize chlamydial diagnostics. These tests are highly specific and are more sensitive than any other diagnostic tests, including culture. The broad-based use of LCR or PCR should provide wide access to accurate *C. trachomatis* diagnosis.

C. trachomatis can be recognized in tissue sections by Giemsa stain, by immunofluorescence (IF) methods, and by electron microscopy. All these methods have been used in human disease and in experimental models.

C. trachomatis cannot be recognized cytologically with any consistency in bubo aspirates in LGV using any of the staining methods. Inclusions have been seen in biopsy material, but this is a poor method of identification. Similarly, *C. psittaci* is rarely recognized in cytological preparations and rarely in tissue secretions. Fluorescent antibody (FA) methods and Giemsa stains have been used effectively in tissue secretions of experimental animal models of *C. psittaci* infection, but are not useful in routine human diagnosis. *C. pneumoniae* strains are relatively difficult to isolate and have been recovered both from the embryonated egg and from TC.

3.4.2. Isolation

3.4.2a. C. trachomatis. The method of choice for recovery of *C. trachomatis* is by cell culture. Cells used are McCoy cells, the HeLa-229 cell line, BHK-21 cells, or L-929 cells. A necessary step in cell cultivation of *C. trachomatis* strains other than LGV is centrifugation of the inoculum into the cells. In addition, the cells are treated in some manner to enhance infection; Gordon *et al.*,[12] who developed the modern cell culture technique, used irradiation of McCoy cells. Cycloheximide has been substituted for irradiation, and cycloheximide-treated McCoy cells are the most widely used method at present.[24] Specimen material is inoculated into individual vials with cell sheets on coverslips within them or into wells of microtiter plates that have been implanted with cells. They can be examined at 48–96 hr after inoculation. Intracytoplasmic inclusions are recognized by iodine stain, by Giemsa stain, or by FA techniques. The most commonly used stain is iodine, which permits rapid identification. Iodine stain will only identify *C. trachomatis.* Giemsa staining will permit identification of *C. psittaci* strains in cell cultures, but since this is usually not necessary, iodine stains are most widely used. FA stains will be more sensitive and can be species or genus specific. The sensitivity of the culture methods is enhanced by one additional passage through cells. LGV strains may be readily isolated in the same system as for the trachoma and oculogenital strains, although they grow more readily in cell culture and do not require cell pretreatment or centrifugation.

Isolation of *C. trachomatis* from yolk sac was historically the first method of agent recovery. However, it is far less sensitive than TC, and thus is no longer used. Mouse inoculation is another possible method for LGV isolation. Intracranial inoculation is more effective than intranasal instillation, but both are inferior to yolk sac inoculation. Trachoma and inclusion-conjunctivitis strains will not grow in mice.

3.4.2b. C. psittaci. These agents will grow in cell culture, in yolk sac, and in mice, by a variety of routes of inoculation. Cultivation in yolk sac or embryonated chick egg is most commonly used in laboratories that are accustomed to this method, as is true of mouse inoculation. This may be accomplished by intraperitoneal, intracerebral, or intranasal inoculation. Since cell culture methods are now more widely available because of greater interest in *C. trachomatis* infection, they will be more widely used. In experienced laboratories, the methods have equal sensitivities. Care must be taken with any of these methods when attempting to recover *C. psittaci* strains, since they are more likely to result in accidental laboratory infections and in cross-contamination.

3.4.2c. C. pneumoniae Strains. These strains have been isolated from the yolk sac of embryonated eggs and initially from HeLa cell. HL and Hep-2 cells have been found to be preferable.[25,26] *C. pneumoniae* antigen in respiratory tract specimens or isolation systems can be demonstrated with species-specific antibody that is commercially available.

3.4.3. Antigen and Nucleic Acid Probes. In recent years, other nonculture diagnostic methods have been evaluated and widely used. They are direct fluorescent antibody smear (DFA), enzyme immunoassay (EIA), and genetic probe methods.

There are a number of DFA kits commercially available. Although they differ primarily in their specificity and in their ease of laboratory measurement, the general principle is the same. A cytological smear is fixed (at which stage it can be stored), stained with a fluorescein-conjugated monoclonal antibody, and examined under a fluorescence microscope. Elementary bodies are recognized as small apple-green dots. When the test is performed by experienced persons, the sensitivity can be as high as 90% but is more often 70–80%. The specificity is usually 98% or greater. Thus, it is an excellent screening test for high-risk populations, but less useful in low prevalence populations.[23]

The EIA class of tests are designed for immunochemical detection of solubilized antigenic components. They have been designed with the use of plastic to absorb *Chlamydia* lipopolysaccharide or that of antigen capture in a sandwich format. All of them use enzyme-conjugated antibody and a recognition system. They have similar sensitivity and specificity as DFA methods.[22] Confirmatory assays improve the specificity.[27]

Both DFA and EIA are less expensive, technologically easier, and less difficult to transport than cell culture. However, they have decreased sensitivity and specificity. The DFA has the advantage of a verifiable sample quality, a rapid test (as little as 1/2 hour), and no restriction as to specimen site. EIA requires less training and experience, as its indicator is more objective; it is more suitable for batch processing; and it can be automated.

Direct nucleic acid probes are commercially available. They are less sensitive than culture, although they are highly specific.[28] In contrast, the amplified DNA technology, exemplified by LCR and PCR, is far more sensitive than TC and it is extremely specific.[29,30] The chlamydial genes can be detected in epithelial cell specimens and in male and female urines.[31–33] The potential for widespread use of noninvasive screening tests is an important option offered by this technology.

All these tests provide ease of transport, automated batch processing, and the potential of differentiation of chlamydial or gonococcal disease on the same specimen. As with antigen identification methods, there is the drawback that no organism is available for further identification (e.g., serological markers, or testing for antibiotic sensitivity). Also, they may be more expensive than culture.

3.4.4. Serological and Immunologic Diagnostic Methods. Although a variety of serological methods have been used in the past, the FA method, first developed by Bernkopf and then by McComb and Nichols, has been simplified and standardized in an indirect microimmunofluorescence (MIF) test by Wang and Grayston. At present, this is the most commonly used test for evaluation of host response to trachoma or to oculogenital *C. trachomatis* agents.[13] For LGV, the complement-fixation (CF) test can be used, although the MIF test remains more sensitive and specific.

The MIF test employs yolk-sac- or cell-culture-grown *C. trachomatis* of all known immunotypes as antigen. Antigen dots are placed on a slide in a specific pattern. They are attached to the slide in a diluted yolk sac suspension. Serial dilutions of serum, tears, or local secretions are applied, followed by fluorescein-conjugated anti-human globulin. An obvious advantage of the test is that the conjugate may be prepared against any immunoglobulin class, thus permitting titration of IgG-, IgM- or IgA-specific antibody. A counterstain is added to the conjugate to permit clearer identification of specific fluorescence in the dots to which antibody-containing serum has been applied. If differentiation among antibodies to specific immunotypes is sought, the antigens can be evaluated separately. For many purposes, antigen pools can be used.

A CF test is available to measure host response to any chlamydial infection.[34] It is still the most commonly used test for psittacosis and LGV, but it is too insensitive for trachoma or oculogenital infections. Usually, the antigen for the CF is obtained from a yolk-sac-grown LGV strain and is prepared by boiling and treatment with phenol. For *C. pneumoniae* strains, the CF test is intermediate in sensitivity. A CF response can be recognized in approximately one half of cases showing response by MIF.[19] Many other serological tests have been evaluated and rejected.

For many years, skin test hypersensitivity to an LGV antigen (prepared from bubo pus) was used for diagnosis of LGV (Frei test).[35] Before more sensitive and specific antibody measurements were available, it was a useful diagnostic aid. However, because cases of LGV are usually not seen early, conversion from negative to positive is rarely observed. In addition, the possibility that positive skin tests merely reflect earlier infections due to other chlamydiae, along with the relative insensitivity of the test and the difficulty in standardizing antigen, have rendered the test obsolete.

Another immunologic method of importance to epidemiological studies is the immunotyping of *C. trachomatis* organisms. Earlier, using a method that employed the protection from type-specific toxic death resulting from massive intravenous inoculation in mice (a method adopted from analogous methods in rickettsial research), it was learned that there were specific immunotypes of *C. trachomatis*. Type-specific immunity could be demonstrated, and it appeared that there was some relationship of immunotype to broad disease categories.[36] Wang *et al.*[13] subsequently showed that a far simpler method of immunotyping could be developed using an MIF method. By this method, 12 immunotypes that cause trachoma and oculogenital disease have been identified, and another three associated with LGV. More subtypes have continued to be identified. No such immunotyping method has been rigorously applied to *C. psittaci*, where specific immunotypes do exist. For *C. pneumoniae*, only one type has been shown. Immunotyping of *C. trachomatis* strains has no broad diagnostic significance other than the differentiation of LGV and oculogenital strains, but immunotyping can be used as a marker of strains in epidemiological investigations.

4. Biological Characteristics of the Organism

Chlamydiae are unusual in that they are obligate intracellular parasites (characteristic of viruses), but they have other characteristics of bacteria. In fact, they were thought to be viruses for many years and were termed *Bedsonia* or *Miyagawanella*. However, it became clear that they had a complex cell wall (similar to gram-negative bacteria in composition), both DNA and RNA, prokaryotic ribosomes, and metabolic enzymes that would permit independent existence, except that they lack energy production mechanisms. Moulder[37] has thus termed the chlamydiae *energy parasites* and credited their obligate intracellular parasitism to this trait.

The other unusual characteristic of the chlamydiae is their reproductive cycle (Fig. 1). The extracellular form of the organism is the elementary body, and it alone is infectious. Following attachment, the elementary body enters the host cell, apparently by a receptor-mediated endocytosis process. If the particles are live or do not have antibody attached, they prevent lysosomal fusion and permit replication in the phagosome. Within 6–8 hr of ingestion, the elementary body is reorganized into a reticulate body (sometimes called an initial body). This larger, thin-walled body diverts the host cell's synthetic functions for its own metabolic purpose and proceeds to divide by binary fission. In this stage, the reticulate bodies are not infectious. After 18–24 hr, the reticulate bodies become reorganized again into elementary bodies (and thus become infectious again). Subsequently, elementary bodies may disrupt and exit the host cell to infect new cells. The full cycle takes about 40 hr for LGV strains and 72–96 hr for the trachoma biovar. These intracytoplasmic collections of elementary bodies constitute the inclusions that may be seen in cytological smears stained by Giemsa or IF methods.

Although all chlamydiae share a genus-specific antigen, there is little DNA homology between *C. trachomatis*, *C. psittaci*, and *C. pneumoniae* strains.[38] The three species of chlamydiae are distinguished by several features. The elementary body of *C. pneumoniae* is pear-shaped with a large periplasmic space, whereas the elementary bodies of the other two species are round with little or no periplasmic space. The inclusions of *C. trachomatis* accumulate glycogen, and thus stain with iodine, whereas the inclusions of *C. psittaci* and *C. pneumoniae* do not. The inclusions of *C. trachomatis* are more compact than those of *C. psittaci* and *C. pneumoniae*. A fourth difference is their response to sulfonamides: *C. trachomatis* is sensitive and *C. psittaci* and *C. pneumoniae* are not.

C. trachomatis can be further subdivided into strains that cause LGV and strains that cause oculogenital infections. They differ significantly in their biological activity. LGV strains (3 serotypes) are more invasive and can invade many tissues in addition to epithelial cells (e.g.,

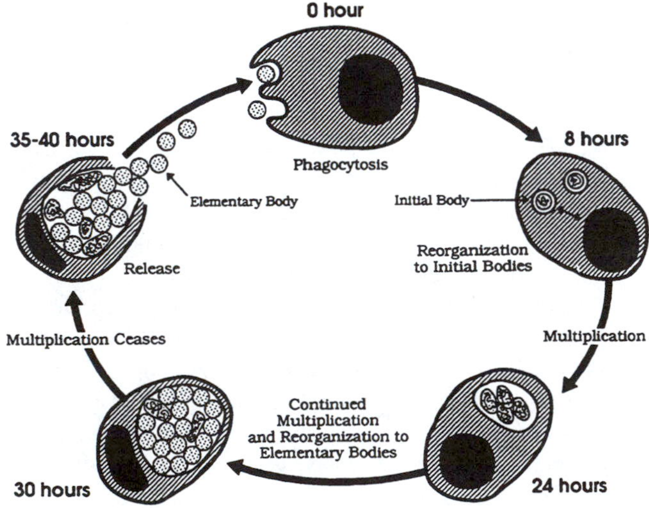

Figure 1. Life cycle of chlamydial organisms. The cycle begins when small elementary bodies infect the host cell by inducing active phagocytosis. During the next 8 hr, they reorganize into the larger reticulated initial bodies, which then divert the cell's synthetic functions to their own metabolic needs, and begin to multiply by binary fission. About 24 hr after infection, the daughter organisms begin reorganizing into infectious elementary bodies. At about 30 hr, multiplication ceases, and by 35–40 hr, the disrupted host cell dies, releasing new elementary bodies that can infect other host cells, and thus continue the cycle. From Alexander.[75]

lymph node invasion, forming the characteristic bubo). This property permits more active cell-to-cell transmission in cell culture and the use of animal inoculation (e.g., mouse) for diagnostic purposes. The oculogenital strains, comprising the trachoma biovar, consist of 12 serotypes. They are not readily invasive in tissue culture and *in vivo* grow only in columnar and squamocolumnar epithelial cells (conjunctivae, respiratory tract, urethra, cervix, rectal mucosa).

C. psittaci will survive for long periods (years) in tissues frozen at −20°C and can persist in dry bird feces for months. Protein (e.g., serum albumin) will aid stability of *Chlamydia. C. trachomatis* strains will lose infectivity within 48 hr at room temperature. They are heat-labile, being inactivated in minutes at 56°C. They are inactivated by common disinfectants (e.g., formalin, phenol).

5. Descriptive Epidemiology

5.1. Trachoma

5.1.1. Prevalence and Incidence. Prevalence surveys of trachoma in endemic countries are repeated frequently for control purposes. In hyperendemic areas, the prevalence of trachoma is essentially 100% by the second or third year of life.[39] Active disease, however, is most common in children, who constitute the reservoir of the disease. By adult life, active infection becomes infrequent, although the sequelae of the disease continue to produce the damaging effects that result in visual defect and blindness. In such areas, trachoma constitutes the major cause of blindness.

In areas of moderate endemicity, infection and disease occur later, often beginning at school entry and going through young adult life.[40] The disease is milder in such settings and sequelae are mild, rarely leading to blindness. Often, within such areas, microfoci of severe disease will persist in certain family groups, where a full range of severity will be found.

The United States represents a nonendemic area where trachoma persists only in isolated population segments. As in the hyperendemic areas, this disease status is constantly changing, as betterment of living standards results in decreasing prevalence. Thus, in southwestern American Indian populations 30 years ago, 10% of Indian schoolchildren were found to have active trachoma at school entrance.[41] Even as active disease is disappearing, sequelae of trachoma can still be seen in the majority of the older population segment.

5.1.2. Epidemic Behavior and Contagiousness. Trachoma is never seen in epidemic form, although perhaps it could return to susceptible populations under disaster conditions if disruption were to result in marked disturbance of hygienic practices. In hyperendemic areas, it persists and is transmitted by a variety of practices that permit eye-to-eye transmission. This may include use of common washing utensils or use of eye drops. The availability of water for washing will greatly affect its transmission. The transmission is potentiated by a variety of ecological factors. In particular, the presence of flies amplifies the transmission of disease. The occurrence of other bacterial eye infections (also transmitted by flies) and the effect of dust on eye irritation also facilitate active infection. When trachoma is reintroduced in nonendemic areas, it is not contagious as long as the hygienic and socioeconomic conditions do not facilitate the transmission.

5.1.3. Geographic Distribution. The trachoma hyperendemic areas of the world are North Africa and sub-Saharan Africa, the Middle East, drier regions of the Indian subcontinent, and Southeast Asia. Foci of trachoma persist in Australia, the South Pacific, and Latin America.

Within the United States, there are no remaining areas of endemicity. At the turn of the century, there was an endemic focus in the south central United States (extending to Texas). A hospital in Missouri devoted to the treatment of trachoma was closed only at midcentury. Similar disappearance of endemic trachoma occurred in Europe, Russia, and the Mediterranean in the same period.

5.1.4. Temporal Distribution. Throughout the world, trachoma vanishes as standards of living improves. Thus, the trends are usually ones of decrease. Within many endemic areas, there are seasonal changes that closely follow the seasonal increase in fly prevalence and the accompanying bacterial conjunctivitis. In some sites (e.g., northern India), two such peaks may occur each year. Such changes will not affect the prevalence of chronic trachoma or the blinding sequelae.

5.1.5. Age. The relationship to age is discussed in Section 5.1.1.

5.1.6. Sex. In hyperendemic areas, there is no sex differential in young children—the reservoir of active trachoma. In adults, reinfection disease occurs more frequently in women taking care of children, and they may also have a higher prevalence of blinding sequelae.

5.1.7. Race. There is no evidence for racial differences.

5.1.8. Occupation. There are no occupational factors that cannot be related to socioeconomic factors.

5.1.9. Socioeconomic Factors. These are predominant epidemiological factors. The important aspects appear to be water availability, fly occurrence, health and hygienic practices, and crowding. Face washing has been identified as a protective behavior.[42] Studies in Saudi Arabia by Nichols *et al.*[43] depicted the decrease of trachoma occurring with the creation of small towns replacing rural foci where trachoma had been hyperendemic. Striking differences could be shown among cities, small towns, and oasis villages. In the United States, as in many other countries, trachoma has vanished with improvement in the standard of living.

5.1.10. Other Factors. Although nutritional factors have been questioned as a possible contributing factor, there is no clear evidence that such is the case, and the factors of water shortage, exposure to bacterial conjunctivitis, fly transmission, and the amplifying factor of dust irritation appear to be most important. Jones[39] summarizes these conditions as those that contribute to "ocular promiscuity" (in contrast to the amplifying factors of "sexual promiscuity" for genital *C. trachomatis* infections) (also see Section 6.1).

5.2. Oculogenital Diseases

5.2.1. Prevalence and Incidence

5.2.1a. Adult Inclusion Conjunctivitis. No incidence or prevalence data in either males or females are available for this illness.

5.2.1b. Cervicitis. Overall population estimates for chlamydial infection are difficult to obtain. However, figures have been obtained for different subgroups. Among pregnant women enrolling for prenatal care, 3–25% have been found to be infected, depending on the group examined. In sexually transmitted disease clinics,[44] up to 30% of symptomatic women have cervical chlamydiae. The prevalence in asymptomatic partners of males with urethritis may be as high as 50%. In asymptomatic nonpregnant college students, chlamydiae were found in the cervices of 5%. In screening women in family planning clinics, infection rates have ranged from about 2–3% in higher socioeconomic settings to 30% in inner-city populations. Up to 70% of the chlamydial infections in these settings have been clinically inapparent.[45]

Etiology in cervicitis is more difficult to define, since multiple organisms may be involved. However, chlamydiae have been isolated from 34 to 63% of women with clinical cervicitis.[44]

5.2.1c. Salpingitis. In the United States, over 200,000 women per year are hospitalized for active pelvic inflammatory disease, and it is estimated that another million are treated as outpatients. If tubal cultures taken at laparoscopy are regarded as identifying the etiological organism, then *C. trachomatis* causes approximately 20–40% of salpingitis in this country and almost 60% in Sweden, although it has become an uncommon disease.[46] Serological data have also implicated *C. trachomatis* as a causal agent in peritonitis or perihepatitis or both (Fitz-Hugh–Curtis syndrome).

5.2.1d. Female Urethral Syndrome The prevalence of acute urethral syndrome is unknown. An estimated 5 million women per year in the United States are seen for symptoms suggestive of urinary tract infection. As many as 30% of these *may* have acute urethral syndrome (acute dysuria, frequent urination, "sterile" urine). Studies in select populations suggest that approximately 30% of the cases of acute urethral syndrome are due to *C. trachomatis*.[44] This has only been shown with young women.

5.2.1e. Postpartum Endometritis. In one study, 7 (22%) of 32 women with *C. trachomatis* cervical infection during pregnancy developed late postpartum endometritis (48 hr to 6 weeks postdelivery).[47] In other studies the association has been less or not found.

5.2.1f. Male Urethritis. In the United States, more than half the estimated 2 million cases of acute urethritis are of nongonococcal etiology. *C. trachomatis* causes 30–50% of these cases.[48] In some populations, e.g., student health clinics, *C. trachomatis* is far more common than gonococcus as a cause of urethritis.

5.2.1g. Epididymitis. This severe complication of acute urethritis occurs in approximately 500,000 men per year in the United States. Roughly half these cases are caused by *C. trachomatis*.[44]

5.2.1h. Arthritis (Reiter's Syndrome). In studies in the United Kingdom, it has been estimated that Reiter's syndrome occurs in about 1% of NGU.[49] An estimate from Finland is 2%.[50] Sexually acquired reactive arthritis (see Section 8.2.1h) as a complication of NGU without the classic triad of Reiter's syndrome occurs four times more frequently.[40]

5.2.1i. Infant Inclusion Conjunctivitis and Pneumonia. Approximately 20–30% of infants exposed to *C. trachomatis* in the birth canal will develop conjunctivitis and 10–15% will develop pneumonia.[44,51] If a conservative figure of 10% maternal carriage rate is used, 3 million babies born each year in the United States would yield 75,000 cases of inclusion conjunctivitis and 30,000 cases of chlamydial pneumonia. *C. trachomatis* has been estimated to cause 20–30% of all pneumonia in infants under 6 months of age ill enough to require hospitalization.

5.2.2. Epidemic Behavior and Contagiousness. The chlamydial oculogenital diseases behave like other STDs. The increasing incidence and prevalence of chlamydial infection probably paralleled that of gonorrhea, but as gonococcal infection rates have declined in recent years, chlamydial infection rates have remained high and may reasonably be termed epidemic at this time.

In the United Kingdom and Sweden, where both gonococcal urethritis and NGU are reportable, the incidence of both diseases rose rapidly from the early 1960s. In fact, the start of the epidemic increase in Sweden preceded the start in the United States by about 4 years. The rest of the curve is very much the same as the United States for gonorrhea. In the mid-1970s, Sweden saw a plateau for the incidence of gonorrhea (the United States experienced the same phenomenon in 1978). In Sweden, the incidence of chlamydial infections has decreased markedly. Chlamydial infections are probably as contagious as gonorrheal infections, but studies to evaluate this have not been done.

Chlamydia and gonorrhea occur together frequently. *C. trachomatis* is recovered from 20–30% of men with gonorrhea, for example; postgonococcal urethritis is now recognized as a chlamydial infection following a gonococcal infection as a result of concomitant infection with *C. trachomatis* not responding to the treatment for gonorrhea. Chlamydial and gonococcal infection may occur together in the cervix (35–45% double infection is not uncommon) and inadequate treatment may result in salpingitis.

Chlamydial conjunctivitis may be transmitted through infected persons by contact. There is no evidence that chlamydial pneumonia of infants can be transmitted in any other way than at birth.

5.2.3. Geographic Distribution. The agent and its various clinical pictures have a worldwide prevalence; it has been identified in all populations in which STDs have been examined.

5.2.4. Temporal Distribution. No seasonal variation is recognized.

5.2.5. Age, Sex, Race, Occupation, Occurrence in Different Settings, Socioeconomic Factors, and Other Factors. *C. trachomatis*, like other genital pathogens, has been found with increased frequency among individuals who are younger, more often nonwhite, unmarried, and of lower socioeconomic status. Both males and females with infection tend to have had more sexual experience in terms of the number of recent sexual partners. Pregnant women with *C. trachomatis* also tend to be of lower gravidity. These factors also characterize the infants who contract conjunctivitis or pneumonia. No distinctive characteristics of diseased versus nondiseased infected infants have been found. Infant conjunctivitis develops at 5–14 days of life (rarely later to 6 weeks, which may be recurrences). Infant pneumonia develops from 2 weeks to 6 months of age. The occurrence of *C. trachomatis* pneumonia in older children and adults is rarely seen.

5.3. Lymphogranuloma Venereum

5.3.1. Prevalence and Incidence. Reported cases of LGV have been decreasing in the last few years from 394 in 1974 to 235 in 1994[52] (the rates have changed from 0.2 to 0.1 in 100,000 population).

5.3.2. Epidemic Behavior and Contagiousness. LGV is transmitted by sexual contact, but the degree of contagiousness has not been measured. Likewise, the epidemic behavior of the disease has not been well documented. The disease was more prevalent in the United States in the first half of this century than it is at present.

5.3.3. Geographic Distribution. In the early part of this century, LGV was more common in the southeastern United States. The present geographic distribution shows a higher prevalence in some of these states (e.g., Virginia, Georgia, and Louisiana). When examined by city, the highest prevalences are in Washington, DC, Atlanta, Houston, and New York. Although some of this concentration can be attributed to better diagnosis in certain centers, it is clear that this also reflects imported disease, particularly in merchant seamen and military personnel. Regarding the source of infection overseas, the disease is more often seen in tropical climates, notably in Africa, Central America, and tropical areas of Asia.

5.3.4. Temporal Distribution. There are no data on temporal distribution.

5.3.5. Age and Sex. This disease is recognized more often in mid-adult life and more often in males than in females.

5.3.6. Race. Although a greater susceptibility of blacks was postulated in years past, such a hypothesis cannot be substantiated, and no difference in racial susceptibility is believed to exist.

5.3.7. Other Factors. The only other population group that appears to be at higher risk are sexually active homosexuals. In recent studies in large cities such as New York, San Francisco, and Seattle, isolates have been found among homosexuals, particularly in men with proctitis.

5.4. Psittacosis

5.4.1. Prevalence and Incidence. Psittacosis is a relatively rare disease in the United States. In 1994, 38 cases were reported (0.2 in 1,000,000 population).[52] Most of these cases are associated with exposure to psittacine birds of domestic or foreign origin. Cases associated with poultry processing decreased in the 1970s and then stabilized. An exception was 1984, when a particular outbreak reversed that trend.[53]

All birds entering the United States (except from Canada) are required by the US Department of Agriculture to undergo a 30-day quarantine, during which time they are treated with chlortetracycline. So far, strains remain susceptible to tetracycline. It has been proposed that the quarantine period be extended to 45 days, particularly for larger psittacine birds. The current importation is about 700,000 birds per year.

5.4.2. Epidemic Behavior and Contagiousness. In 1929, epidemic disease from infected psittacine birds spread from Argentina to England, Germany, and the United States as infected psittacine birds were transported to those countries. Discovery of the cause of this disease and its treatment resulted in control of epidemic disease by the 1950s and cessation of such outbreaks. From the 1950s on, there were sporadic outbreaks in poultry-processing plants. From 1979 to 1984, there were no significant outbreaks in the United States. In 1984, an outbreak occurred in turkey-slaughtering plants.

Human-to-human transmission can occur from a heavily infected pneumonia case, but such occurrence is extremely rare and is of no significance in the epidemiology of the disease. The important epidemiological source remains either psittacine birds or poultry flocks.

5.4.3. Geographic Distribution. Cases are broadly distributed in the United States, but in recent years there have been more cases reported from mountain and Pacific coast states (57% in 1987). Few cases are reported from the northwest, central, and southeastern states. Although this reflects, in part, the distribution of psittacine birds, it also reflects increased disease awareness and better diagnostic facilities in these states.

5.4.4. Temporal Distribution. The distribution of cases has no distinct seasonal pattern.

5.4.5. Age, Sex, Race, and Occupation. Cases occur more often in mid-adult life and more often in males than in females, reflecting the increased exposure in these groups. There is no evidence of racial predilections. Regarding occupation, most cases of psittacosis in recent years have occurred in owners of pet birds, employees of the commercial pet bird trade, bird fanciers, pigeon fanciers, and a variety of miscellaneous avian exposures. Since 1974, few cases have occurred in poultry producers and processors, although the potential for such occurrence still exists. Only about 10% of cases occur in persons without clear-cut exposure. Thus, the majority (93% from 1975 to 1984) of cases occur in persons exposed through vocational or avocational activities.[(53)]

5.4.6. Socioeconomic Factors. Socioeconomic status is not of epidemiological significance.

5.5. *C. pneumoniae* Infections

5.5.1. Prevalence and Incidence. Pneumonia incidence has been measured in a health maintenance organization in Seattle. The incidence of pneumonia averaged 12 per 1000 per year. Fifteen percent had *C. pneumoniae* infection, for an incidence rate of 1 per 1000 per year. This was a little less than half the incidence of *Mucoplasma pneumoniae* infection. It is thought that the *C. pneumoniae* estimate is a little low, as it is based on serology alone.[(54)] Studies in many countries show that 20–80% of adults have antibody, and in most countries that prevalence is 50% or more.[(19)]

5.5.2. Epidemic Behavior and Contagiousness. Epidemics have been studied in military recruits in Finland and in one adjacent civilian community.[(55)] Attack rates varied from 60 to 80 per 1000 men. The case-to-case interval has averaged 30 days and ranged as high as 3 months. Transmission in all instances is slow, with epidemics lasting as long as 6 months in groups such as military and as long as 3 months for households.

5.5.3. Geographic Distribution. The original isolate was from Taiwan. The most extensive studies have been in the United States, but the prevalence of antibody in adults in most countries studied has been 50% or more. Other countries studied heavily have been Finland, Denmark, Sweden, Canada, Taiwan and Japan.[(19)] Serological studies of what appears to be a similar strain from Iran have shown widespread antibody in the United Kingdom.

5.5.4. Temporal Distribution. The disease can occur in any season. There is some evidence of periodicity, with higher incidence rates of infection for 2 or 3 years followed by 4 or 5 years of low incidence.[(54)]

5.5.5. Age and Sex. Antibody is uncommon under the age of 5 years, and then age-specific prevalence increases rapidly from 5 to 20 years. Both of these characteristics are similar to the seroepidemiological findings for *M. pneumoniae*. The prevalence then increases slowly but steadily throughout life. In Seattle, men over 60 have a prevalence of 70%. Rates are higher in men than in women after the age of 20. With current serological methods, there is some loss of antibody with time (3–5 years after the first infection), so that the high rates of antibody after age 70 suggest that virtually everyone is infected at some time in their lives. Reinfections can occur.

5.5.6. Race, Occupation, Occurrence in Different Settings and Socioeconomic Factors. There are no data that suggest significant differences by race or occupation. The significant excess in males in adult life, as well as the experience in epidemics, suggest that infection may occur more often outside the home in settings such as schools, institutions, and the military.

6. Mechanisms and Routes of Transmission

6.1. Trachoma

The conjunctival epithelium of humans constitutes the reservoir of infection for trachoma. It is passed from eye to eye by direct contact. In some instances, this is aided by local practices. For example, in India, it is usual for dye to be applied around the eye, with a small stick or with the finger. This is applied to adult women first and then down to children of both sexes, from the eldest to the youngest. In many Southeast Asian countries, washcloths are applied to the face, again from eldest to youngest and in crowded areas of poverty, usually the same cloth without a change of water. Both are ideal methods for transmission.

Extraocular infections are known to occur in trachoma endemic areas. The organism can be recovered from throat nasopharyngeal and rectal swabs. It is not known what role such infections may play in transmission of the organism. They are likely to be more important in that they provide a rationale for treatment failures to occur following application of topical antibiotics, as they can be a source of reinfection.

Transmission is also potentiated by flies. They will differ as to species, but in each case they are capable of carrying infected secretions from face to face, where they may be self-inoculated into the eye. Jones[39] showed by use of fluorescein dyes that ocular discharges could be transferred from person to person in the household in a matter of minutes. He referred to the sum of these various methods of transfer of infected secretions as "ocular promiscuity" and suggested that this characterizes the epidemiological pattern of endemic trachoma in much the same manner as genital promiscuity characterizes the method of transmission for oculogenital diseases.

Two other factors play some part in the transmission of endemic trachoma in certain areas of the world, perhaps in preparing the eye for more severe infection.One is the occurrence of other bacterial conjunctivitis, often also fly-transmitted. In certain settings, seasonal epidemics of bacterial conjunctivitis precede the peak of trachoma infectivity by a few weeks. A variety of bacterial pathogens have been implicated, particularly certain *Haemophilus* and *Neisseria* species. It is surmised that the bacterial infections increase both conjunctival and corneal inflammation, and thus amplify their subsequent response to trachomatous infection. Anyone who has been in such areas at the height of the fly season can attest to the intensity of fly infestation. Flies cover the faces of children, particularly around the eyes, where there is conjunctival discharge.

A second set of factors, which are less well understood, are the environmental factors that characterize many of the foci of greatest prevalence. These are dust and sunlight—both irritants to conjunctiva and to cornea and both hypothesized to aid *C. trachomatis* in its damaging effects. It is difficult to measure these influences, but trachoma remains most prevalent and most damaging in those locations where these factors predominate.[39]

6.2. Oculogenital Diseases

The columnar cells of the adult male urethra and female endocervix are believed to be the reservoirs of infection. Asymptomatic infection seems to be the rule: depending on the type of clinic, >50% of infected men and women with positive urethral or cervical cultures have no complaints or discharge. The organism is transmitted via sexual contact.

In women, *C. trachomatis* is responsible for a proportion of acute and chronic cervicitis on examination, but how much is difficult to say,since it is often accompanied by other pathogens. Urethral syndrome or acute urethritis may be a result of simultaneous infection, spread from infected cervical secretions. The organism is responsible for at least 20–40% of cases of salpingitis, presumably via direct extension. Postpartum endometritis, thought to be at least partly due to *C. trachomatis*, also occurs via direct extension.

In males, the major illnesses (urethritis and epididymitis) are due to direct extension of infection from the primary urethral focus. Hematogenous dissemination has never been documented in either sex. Adult inclusion conjunctivitis is believed to be transmitted via hand-to-eye contact from infected genital foci.

The only documented mode of transmission of infection to infants is vertically by passage through an infected cervix. No hard evidence for transplacental or postnatal infection exists.

6.3. Lymphogranuloma Venereum

The reservoir of infection is the cervix of the asymptomatic female and, to a lesser extent, for the male homosexual, the rectal mucosa of the asymptomatic male. It is spread exclusively by sexual contact. In the male, primary lesions appear on the penis, usually on the glans (occasionally in the urethra) or the wall of the rectum, and in the female on the labia or on the wall of the vagina. Such lesions are usually painless and may be hidden, adding to the risk of transmission. Extragenital sites for primary lesions include hands (especially fingers) and tongue. Although secondary and tertiary lesions are the ones most easily diagnosed and are the stages of disease that result in damaging sequelae, it is the painless primary lesions that are the source for sexual transmission.

6.4. Psittacosis

The predominant source for human disease are infected avian species, all of which are potential reservoirs. Meyer[(56)] listed 130 species known to be such sources in 1967, and the list could no doubt be lengthened. The risk of exposure is greatly increased in those occupations in which handling birds or their carcasses is common. The most common avian sources are parrots and parakeets, usually resulting in sporadic cases from pet birds. In recent years, about two thirds were from psittacine species. Pigeons are another source, as are poultry, particularly turkeys. Wild birds have infrequently been documented as a source. Domestic and other lower mammals are infected with *C. psittaci* strains, but they rarely cause human disease. An exception may be the chlamydiae associated with ovine abortion. These appear to specially threaten the health of pregnant women. In the overwhelming majority of cases, psittacosis occurs in persons in whom bird processing or handling is a vocation or avocation. Casual exposure is extremely rare.

Transmission between humans can take place, and on rare occasions such transmission has been documented. It has resulted from close exposure to extremely sick or fatal cases. In only one instance, psittacosis has been spread between humans through mildly ill or asymptomatic cases.

The route of infection is airborne and the primary site of infection is the lower respiratory tract. The involvement is in the alveoli, with very little evidence of bronchial or upper respiratory tract infection.

6.5. *C. pneumoniae* Infections

There is no evidence for other than human-to-human transmission of *C. pneumoniae* infection. Clearly, epidemics occur, as described in the pneumonia epidemics in military trainees in Finland.[(55)] Because the organism was originally thought to be a member of the *C. psittaci* species and because it can infect experimental animals, an extensive search for antibody in serum of domestic pets was conducted and yielded no evidence for an animal reservoir. In addition, there is no epidemiological evidence to suggest an unusual frequency of animal contact in cases.[(19)]

7. Pathogenesis and Immunity

7.1. Trachoma

In the early stages of disease, trachoma appears as a follicular conjunctivitis with hyperemia, edema, and distortion of the vascular pattern of the conjunctiva. This is accompanied by papillary hypertrophy of the conjunctiva. The follicles are, in fact, lymphoid germinal centers. In these initial stages, there is involvement of both palpebral and bulbar conjunctivae. Such conjunctival follicles can occur as a response to a number of stimuli, both infectious and toxic. The infant conjunctiva cannot so respond for a number of weeks, and thus chlamydial ocular infection of the newborn (inclusion conjunctivitis) is afollicular, even though the strains are very similar (e.g., as shown by the disease produced in the experimental monkey eye). The chronic follicular conjunctivitis of trachoma heals by scarring. These scars lead to distortion of the lids. This, in turn, results in inability of the lids to close completely, allowing dust particles to damage the cornea. Similarly, the lid distortion results in trichiasis, or inversion of lashes, which adds to the trauma to the cornea. Both these sequelae of trachoma contribute to blindness.[(39)] The incubation period is not known. In volunteer studies and experimental studies in the nonhuman primate it is 5–12 days. It is important to note that in both experimental situations, infection will not occur with simple corneal exposure, but only after vigorous application of concentrated inoculum. Therefore, it might be surmised that the natural incubation period is somewhat longer.

Acute corneal involvement includes follicles, which often ring the limbus and, after rupture, lead to corneal defects termed Herbert's pits. Punctate erosions of the cornea occur (epithelial keratitis). Inflammatory infiltrates of the cornea may be seen. A characteristic feature of trachoma is the vascularization of the cornea, with swelling of the corneal–scleral border, which constitutes pannus. This is an important component of trachoma diagnosis.

Collectively, these features of trachoma constitute the acute and chronic conjunctivitis and their blinding sequelae. The occurrence of these features in all populations increases with age, although the age at which they occur will depend on the intensity of disease in each sample.

All these changes have been reproduced experimentally in the monkey, but never with the initial infection, which produces only acute follicular conjunctivitis, leading to minimal scarring. Pannus is only a result of reinfection (exogenous reinfection or endogenous relapse).[57] Whether this is true for human disease has never been substantiated. If it is, then the disease that is characterized as trachoma (with pannus) is never a primary infection. Nevertheless, it is clear in human disease that the serious sequelae that lead to blindness occur only as a result of many reinfections, abetted by the many other causes of corneal diseases in hyperendemic trachomatous populations, including bacterial infections and various environmental factors (e.g., dust, sunlight). It has been speculated that nutritional factors may also play a role. It has been postulated that hypersensitivity reaction to specific *Chlamydia* heat-shock proteins may be responsible for the inflammation seen on reinfection.[58]

If reinfection is a necessary factor for severe trachoma, what is the role of immunity? In the experimental animal, after infection, for a short period, there is immunity to reinfection with homologous strains (but no immunity to heterologous rechallenge). In the few studies that were made with what are now recognized as relatively crude and antigenically weak vaccines, there was transient immunity to rechallenge. When this immunity waned, not only were the experimental animals susceptible to reinfection, but also the severity of disease produced by such rechallenge was enhanced (a phenomenon similar to that seen in other early and crude experimental vaccines, such as those for *M. pneumoniae* and respiratory syncytial virus). Whether such a period of hyperreactivity exists in natural human infection has not been determined, but immunity in nature is fleeting. Infection in humans and in experimental animals produces both local and circulatory immune responses, but these antibodies do not appear to be protective. One epidemiological fact continues to kindle interest in the prospect of producing an effective vaccine for trachoma: the observation that in all endemic situations studied, active trachoma decreases with age. Although the age at which this occurs will vary with the intensity of disease in the population, eventually the older segment of the population no longer has active disease, suggesting that immunity eventually prevails. This occurs at an early enough age in some populations that one cannot attribute it to decrease in ocular promiscuity alone. It is the aim of proponents of vaccine development to create a vaccine that would mimic the natural occurrence. To date, our knowledge of the immunology of trachoma is relatively primitive (particularly cellular immunity), as is our knowledge of the antigens of *C. trachomatis*.

7.2. Oculogenital Diseases

There are several useful unifying principles in regard to the oculogenital infections caused by *C. trachomatis*: (1) The organism infects superficial columnar epithelial cells in various sites (endocervix, urethra, epididymis, endometrium, salpinx, conjunctiva, nasopharynx, lower respiratory tract) and appears to have little propensity for invasion of or destruction of deeper tissue. (2) The clinical features of chlamydial infection seem to be produced by the host inflammatory response, rather than by the inherent destructiveness of the organism. (3) *C. trachomatis* infections may be present and asymptomatic ("latent" or "silent" infection) for prolonged periods of time. For example, infants have been documented to shed organisms from conjunctivae for up to 2 years postdelivery. Similarly, women with cervical infection have been culture-positive for over 15 months. (4) The stimuli that convert latent infection to chronic disease or that determine symptomatic versus asymptomatic primary infection are unknown. (5) At least in some cases (pregnant women), infection can occur, recur, and persist even in the presence of serum antibody. Cell-mediated immune responses (as measured by lymphocyte blastogenic response) appear to be associated with clearing infection, although the evidence is far from clear.

The incubation periods for oculogenital syndromes vary with the syndrome. Urethritis appears to have an incubation period of 5–14 days. This is longer than the incubation period for gonococcal urethritis, which is 2–7 days. When they occur as a result of concurrent exposure, the chlamydial urethritis usually occurs later, which accounted for the entity known as postgonococcal urethritis that occurred in some cases of gonococcal urethritis treated with penicillin only. The incubation period for cervicitis is probably the same as urethritis, but because of the slow and infrequent development of symptoms, it is harder to define. The incubation period for chlamydial salpingitis is longer, usually following cervical infection by 2–3 weeks. The incubation period for conjunctivitis of infants, children, or adults is 5–12 days. In the case of ophthalmia neonatorum, chlamydial ophthalmia most often has onset in the second week of life, as opposed to gonococcal conjunctivitis which occurs characteristically in the first week. Chlamydial pneumonia of infancy has onset between 3 and 12 weeks of age. From prospective studies, it appears to follow the earliest recognition of posterior nasopharyngeal infection by a week or so. Rectal infection is rarely discovered before the second month of life.

In all illnesses so far studied, the surface chlamydial infection appears to produce an early polymorphonuclear inflammatory response at the surface and a later subepithelial infiltration of lymphocytes, plasma cells, monocytes, and eosinophils. Inclusions have been seen in cervix, conjunctiva, salpinx, and infant airways. Although the antigen load, in terms of inclusions seen, does not appear great, the immune response appears to be profound. In infants with chlamydial pneumonitis, for example, large interstitial and peribronchiolar lymphoid infiltrates and organizing nodules with germinal centers can be seen; these are the "infiltrates" seen on chest radiography.

The preliminary evidence available indicates that chlamydial infections may produce chronic sequelae. The observations are not unexpected, since the intense inflammatory response produced by chlamydial infection can lead to tissue destruction, fibrosis, and scarring. Data from Sweden suggest that chlamydial salpingitis has a higher postinfectious incidence of involuntary infertility and ectopic pregnancy than does gonorrheal disease. Distal tubal obstruction has been reproduced in the nonhuman primate by repeated salpingeal infection.[59] Furthermore, obliterative bronchiolitis has been observed in the lung biopsy specimen taken from an infant recovering from chlamydial pneumonitis.

7.3. Lymphogranuloma Venereum

The primary lesions of LGV is usually painless and may often be missed. The incubation period is variable and has been described as 3–30 days. The primary lesion may be a papule, an ulcer or erosion, a vesicle, or a urethritis. Rarely, the site may be extragenital. Pathologically, there is nothing specific about these lesions. Proctitis commonly accompanies primary anorectal infection.

In most instances, it is the secondary lesions that bring the disease to medical attention. These are involvement of lymph nodes, producing the characteristic bubo. The bubonic form occurs in males more often than females (9:1), in part due to differences in lymphatic drainage patterns. Both inguinal and femoral node chains can be involved (when both are involved, the characteristic groove sign results—a groove between the two chains). Systemic signs (fever, myalgia) may occur at this time, but leukocytosis is rare. Large mononuclear cells proliferate within the nodes, and foci become necrotic. These foci may proceed to suppuration and rupture of the nodes, developing draining fistulas. Alternatively, the nodes may spontaneously harden and then heal. In approximately 5% of cases, a chronic lymphadenopathy may occur, which may persist for many years.

What are sometimes referred to as tertiary lesions of LGV are analogous to the sequelae of trachoma in that they are the result of scarring. They include strictures of the rectum and vagina and fistulas that may be rectovaginal or may involve the urethra. These lesions are characterized by destruction of mucosal epithelium with scarring and plasma cell infiltration. Extragenital involvement may rarely involve the conjunctivae, the skin (e.g., fingers), the oral mucosa, each with respective lymph node involvement. Even less frequent are syndromes of meningitis, salpingitis, arthritis, and pneumonitis.

LGV elicits a marked host response. Nonspecifically, this is reflected in a hypergammaglobulinemia that may result in a reversal of albumin–globulin ratio. Specifically, broad and intense response can be measured with chlamydial antigens. For that reason, CF antibodies are uniformly elevated, and this generally insensitive test is useful in this disease, utilizing *C. psittaci* antigen. Using specific MIF antigens, a brisk response is noted, which is characteristically broad (responding to many *C. trachomatis* antigens). Although the immunological response can be readily measured, less is known concerning immunity in this disease. Reinfection has not been reported, but chronic disease can occur. Cellular immunity is poorly studied in this infection, but skin test reactivity and the prominent tissue damage in lymph nodes suggest that such immunity is operative.

7.4. Psittacosis

The respiratory tract is the organ of entry and initial multiplication. The incubation period is between 6 and 15 days (rarely longer). In the experimental monkey, initial respiratory infection is followed by regional lymphadenopathy (tracheobronchial lymph nodes). Bacteremia occurs, followed by involvement of the reticuloendothelial system, with early hepatic infection and persistent splenic infection. Monocytic and polymorphonuclear infiltration of the tracheal wall marks the initial respiratory lesions, but in human specimens from fatal cases, bronchiolar involvement is not found. The characteristic lesion of psittacosis is a serofibrinous alveolar exudate that results in focal or lobar consolidation. The alveoli contain both fibrinous red cells and polymorphonuclear cells. In later stages, alveolar septal cell hyperplasia with phagocytic infiltration occurs.

The splenomegaly results from lymphoid infiltration with an increase in mononuclear phagocytic cells. Focal necrosis and granulomata may occur in the liver. CNS involvement occurs infrequently and is characterized by congestion and edema of the brain or spinal cord.

Host response to *C. psittaci* infection can be measured in a number of ways, and it is clear that both circulating and cellular immune responses occur. On the other hand, there is no evidence for lasting immunity in either animal or man following this infection. Reinfection is well documented, as is persistent infection under some circumstances.

7.5. *C. pneumoniae* Infections

The pathogenesis of *C. pneumoniae* infections is not understood. There have been no lung biopsies or deaths, and there is no experimental model. Our knowledge is limited to clinical observation and the analogy to *M. pneumoniae* pneumonia. The incubation period for *C. pneumoniae* infection is not known. The case-to-case interval averages 30 days. Reinfection has been documented, even in the same epidemic.(55)

8. Patterns of Host Response

8.1. Trachoma

8.1.1. Clinical Features. The initial response to infection with *C. trachomatis* is a conjunctivitis. This involves both palpebral and bulbar conjunctivae, and in both areas, congestion and edema are the first responses, with papillary hypertrophy prominent in the palpebral conjunctiva. This is followed by follicle formation (except for infants less than 6 weeks of age, in whom follicle formation is not possible). Follicles can also be found on the bulbar conjunctiva. Those that form on the limbal border are most characteristic. After rupture, they leave shallow scars, which are termed Herbert's pits. In hyperendemic trachoma, severe disease is more characteristic of the upper tarsus. The conjunctivitis produces an ocular discharge that is initially serous, but with congestion can become serosanguinous. Since trachomatous conjunctivitis is usually a subacute process, necrosis is minimal, and therefore pure trachomatous disease is not particularly purulent (with the exception of infant conjunctivitis, which has either purulent or mucopurulent discharge). Unfortunately, in hyperendemic areas, bacterial infection often accompanies the initial disease, and thus the discharge is often very purulent. In trachoma, corneal involvement is usually present, producing punctate erosions of the epithelium with cellular infiltrates of the central corneal epithelium and anterior stroma (keratitis). Particularly characteristic of hyperendemic trachoma is a neovascularization (pannus) at the superior limbus. This sign is an important component in the diagnosis of trachoma.

In either classic trachoma or adult inclusion conjunctivitis, the most damaging aspects of the disease are the sequelae of reinfection. Follicles of the palpebral conjunctiva scar, which results in distortion of the lids. This may result in trichiasis (inturning of the lashes to scrape the cornea) and entropion (distortion of the lid margins secondary to scarring, resulting in failure of the lids to close, in turn resulting in disturbance of the protective cleansing action of the lids and therefore further corneal scarring, particularly in dusty environments). These changes, along with the recurrent keratitis, in company with multiple reinfections and bacterial superinfections result in loss of visual acuity and may result in blindness.

All these change are seen, but to a lesser degree, in adult inclusion conjunctivitis. The difference in sequelae between trachoma and inclusion conjunctivitis is probably related more to the greater number of reinfections in hyperendemic trachoma and the adverse physical environment (including the effect of fly-borne bacterial conjunctivitides) than it is to the biological difference between trachomatous and oculogenital chlamydial strains. When reinfection has been studied in nontrachomatous environments (e.g., the studies of Mordhorst(60) in Denmark), each of the sequelae of trachoma has been recognized, but in lesser severity.

8.1.2. Diagnosis. Epidemiologically, trachoma is recognized in restricted areas of the world (see Section 5.1.3) and within those areas can most often be found in populations with poor hygiene and under conditions that favor "ocular promiscuity" (often also favoring fly-borne bacterial conjunctivitis). Other isolated population segments in nonendemic countries may have endemic trachoma.

According to WHO definitions,(21) the clinical diagnosis of trachoma can be made if two of the following signs are present: (1) lymphoid follicles on the upper tarsal conjunctiva; (2) typical conjunctival scarring; (3) vascular pannus; (4) limbal follicles or their sequelae—Herbert's pits. Scales of severity and activity have been used to classify trachoma. The most commonly used staging is the MacCallan classification, which progresses from immature follicles (I) to mature follicular disease (II), active follicles with scarring (III), and scars and other sequelae without activity (IV).

For epidemiological survey purposes , Dawson *et al.*[61] have devised a scale of intensity based on three gradations of follicle activity and papillary hypertrophy. For the potentially disabling irreversible lesions, simple three-grade scores for congenital and corneal scarring and for trichiasis or enteropion or both have also been devised. This method leads to more reproducible and epidemiologically valid results in surveys.

Other syndromes can cause follicular conjunctivitis, including viral and bacterial infections, toxic follicular conjunctivitis, vernal catarrh and atopic conjunctivitis (allergic in origin), and a variety of rarer forms of chronic follicular conjunctivitis of unknown etiology.

The laboratory diagnosis of trachoma depends on the recovery of *C. trachomatis* from conjunctival scrapings or the demonstration of characteristic inclusions in the cytoplasm of conjunctival epithelial cells obtained from such scrapings. These may most easily be recognized with Giemsa stain, but if DFA methodology is available, the sensitivity of this cytological method is greater.

An advantage of the Giemsa stain in cytological diagnosis is the recognition of the characteristic inflammatory response. Whereas viral conjunctivitis usually elicits a lymphocytic response, and vernal catarrh and atopic conjunctivitis can be recognized by the presence of eosinophils or granules, the characteristic picture in trachoma or inclusion conjunctivitis is a mixture of polymorphonuclear leukocytes, immature lymphoid cells, and plasma cells. Also, Leber cells (giant macrophages containing ingested material) are often seen. This inflammatory response, while not in itself diagnostic, may aid in the cytological diagnosis of trachoma.

Although antibodies to *C. trachomatis* may invariably be recognized in the sera of trachomatous patients by MIF methods, it is unusual to detect an antibody rise, since the disease is most often recognized in its chronic state and therefore reflects only past infection with a *C. trachomatis* strain.

8.2. Oculogenital Diseases

8.2.1. Clinical Features (see Table 1)

8.2.1a. Adult Inclusion Conjunctivitis. Adult inclusion conjunctivitis in both the male and the female is an acute follicular conjunctivitis with edema, mucopurulent exudate, and erythema. Inclusions can be found on scrapings of either the tarsal plate or the lower palpebral conjunctiva, and chlamydiae can be cultured from either site. Infection is thought to occur from infected genital tract secretions via hand-to-eye contact. The illness is self-limited, although treatment will shorten the clinical course. Progression to trachoma has not been documented, but pannus and conjunctival scarring may result from reinfection.

8.2.1b. Cervicitis. Chlamydial infection of the endocervix is often associated with a purulent endocervical discharge, congestion, and inflammation. The essential finding is the presence of mucopus (discoloration) on a cervical swab. Initially the criterion of ten or more polymorphonuclear leukocytes per microscopic field was also used, but the difficulties of standardizing the smears made this unreproducible. A more reliable criterion, in addition to mucopurulent exudate, was bleeding induced by swabbing the endocervical mucosa (friability of the mucosa).[62] More than 50% of women with chlamydial cervicitis are asymptomatic, but many may have an abnormal cervical appearance. The difficulty in diagnosing chlamydial cervicitis is that the findings present are often the same as those found with cervicitis of other etiologies. Furthermore, the cervix is often infected with several other organisms simultaneously.

Under the proper stimulus (as yet undefined), chlamydial cervicitis may progress to salpingitis, or to postpartum endometritis in pregnant women, and it may be associated with urethral syndrome. Endometrial infection has been shown to follow cervical infection in more than one third of cases.[63] An inflammation of Bartholin's gland may also be caused by *C. trachomatis*. Without progression to other sites, chlamydial cervical infection may remain active but silent, or it may be cleared by the host either spontaneously or with treatment.

8.2.1c. Salpingitis. Chlamydial pelvic inflammatory disease is similar in presentation to that caused by other organisms, with the exception that it tends to be of more gradual than acute onset, to exhibit low-grade fever, and often has elevation of the erythrocyte sedimentation rate ($>$ 30 min/hr). Like gonorrheal illness, it tends to occur in younger, more sexually active women, and as a first rather than recurrent episode. Major signs and symptoms include fever, lower abdominal pain, and adnexal and uterine tenderness on pelvic examination. The diagnosis of chlamydial infection has proven difficult, however, since the organism may reside solely in the salpinx. Thus, cervical or cul-de-sac cultures may yield gonorrhea or anaerobes, yielding a false diagnosis. The clearest results have been obtained in Sweden using laparoscopy with tubal biopsy,[46] but this is neither a universally available nor an accepted technique for mild illness. The contribution of chlamydial salpingitis to involuntary infertility and to ectopic pregnancy in the United States is not known, although both have increased in parallel with increase in the incidence of salpingitis. Assuming 1 million cases of salpingitis per year in the United States and 15–20% resulting in bilateral tubal occlusion, it has been estimated that 150,000–200,000 women per year become infertile as a result of salpingitis, at least one quarter of which can be attributed to chlamydial infection.[64]

An uncommon complication of salpingitis is perihepatitis (Fitz-Hugh–Curtis syndrome), assumed to be caused by peritoneal spread of the infection. Studies have implicated *C. trachomatis* as an etiologic agent in a proportion of these cases.

8.2.1d. Female Urethral Syndrome. This syndrome is the equivalent in women of NGU in men. It is predominantly manifest as frequency dysuria, with sterile pyuria on microscopic and cultural examination, in young, sexually active women. In this specifically defined group, one study revealed a 62% (10 of 16) prevalence of *C. trachomatis* as the etiologic agent.[65] Other studies show a lesser contribution. Often, there is a history of a new sexual partner in the month prior to symptoms. Untreated, the urethral syndrome will resolve with time. Long-term sequelae are as yet undetermined.

8.2.1e. Postpartum Endometritis. *C. trachomatis* cervical infection in pregnant women has been associated with the development of postpartum endometritis, with onset more than 48 hr after delivery in approximately one third of cases.[47] The disease is not different clinically from that due to other organisms.

8.2.1f. Male Urethritis. Chlamydial infection of the adult male urethra is the most common single cause (30–50%) of nongonococcal urethritis or postgonococcal urethritis. This is a syndrome of dysuria with or without discharge, with pus cells on Gram's smear of an endourethral swab, in which *N. gonorrhoeae* can be neither seen nor cultured. The disease occurs in young, sexually active males and is at least equal in prevalence to gonococcal urethritis in the United States. Untreated, it may lead to epididymitis or resolve spontaneously. Treatment shortens the clinical course.[48]

8.2.1g. Epididymitis. *C. trachomatis* is the most common cause of "idiopathic" acute epididymitis in sexually active man under 35 years of age with no underlying genitourinary pathology.[44] The prevalence of the organism in the urethra, semen, and epididymis of these men far exceeds that of *N. gonorrhoeae*, coliforms, or *Pseudomonas* species. Patients with chlamydial epididymitis tend to have a more chronic course, with more induration of the epididymis, than those with other etiologic diagnoses. The illness will resolve spontaneously, although treatment hastens recovery. The incidence of infertility following chlamydial epididymitis is unknown. However, chlamydial epididymitis is often associated with oligozoospermia.

8.2.1h. Arthritis (Reiter's Syndrome). One of the most serious complications of NGU is Reiter's syndrome. Symptoms appear 1–4 weeks after onset of urethritis. The arthritis is usually asymmetric, involving large joints of the lower extremities or sacroiliac joints. In most patients, arthritis may be the only manifestation. Achilles tendon and plantar fasciae may also be affected. This condition has been termed sexually acquired reactive arthritis (SARA). The full expression (termed Reiter's syndrome) may additionally involve eyes, skin, and mucous membranes. Ocular involvement ranges from a transient mild conjunctivitis to severe uveitis. Skin lesions may involve the penis (balanitis) and a keratoderma of the palms and soles. The mucous membrane lesions are small ulcers of the palate, tongue, and oral mucosa. Symptoms eventually will cease, even without treatment, but recurrences are common.[49] Other infections (not sexually transmitted), such as shigella and salmonella, can also cause Reiter's syndrome.

C. trachomatis has been recovered from the urethra of at least one third of cases of SARA, but serological evidence suggests that one half to two thirds are a result of this infection. Antibody responses are much higher than are usually seen in NGU, suggesting that a brisk immunologic response is a part of the condition. A genetic predisposition to the development of SARA is marked by the presence of histocompatibility determinant HLA-B27 in two thirds of cases. Additional evidence for *Chlamydia* etiology comes from examining synovium or synovial fluid cells with fluorescein-labeled monoclonal antibody to *C. trachomatis* and demonstrating elementary bodies in the joint.[66]

8.2.1i. Infant Inclusion Conjunctivitis. Inclusion conjunctivitis of the newborn is by far the most common cause of neonatal conjunctivitis in the United States and is estimated to be ten times as prevalent as gonococcal ophthalmia neonatorum.[67] Approximately 25% of infants born to cervix-positive mothers will develop some degree of chlamydial conjunctivitis, involving one or both eyes. The illness most commonly has an incubation period of 1–3 weeks. Infants then present with varying degrees of conjunctival erythema, edema, and mucopurulent discharge. Physical examination shows a *nonfollicular* conjunctivitis (as distinct from the conjunctival disease of older children and adults), with diffuse erythema of the conjunctivae. Fever and systemic findings are absent.

Untreated, the disease course is quite variable. Generally, the conjunctivitis remits within 3–4 weeks, although asymptomatic shedding may persist indefinitely. Occasionally, reexacerbations may occur for unknown reasons. Chronic sequelae do occur; in one study, micropannus was observed in a small percentage of infants 1 year following infection.

8.2.1j. Infant Pneumonia. *C. trachomatis* pulmonary infection has been estimated to cause 20–30% of all hospitalized pneumonia in infants less than 6 months old.[(67)] Approximately 10–20% of infants born to cervix-positive mothers will develop pulmonary disease. These infants typically present between 3 and 12 weeks of age, although younger patients have been seen. They have a history of chronic congestion and of a chronic staccato, machine-gun-like cough.[(68)] They are usually afebrile, with minimal malaise, but may have a history of poor growth and weight gain. On examination, they tend to be congested and tachypneic and to have diffuse rales on physical examination. Conjunctivitis is sometimes present. Laboratory examination characteristically reveals eosinophilia (> 300–$400/mm^3$), hyperglobulinemia (especially IgM), and elevated antichlamydial antibody titers. Chest radiographs show hyperexpanded lungs, with variable degrees and patterns of infiltrates. The organism itself may be cultured from nasopharynx, tracheal aspirate material, or lung biopsy, if obtained. Although pneumonia is best studied, other forms of lower respiratory tract disease can occur (e.g., bronchiolitis).

Untreated, the illness tends to be chronic, with multiple exacerbations and remissions, but with gradual recovery over weeks to months. Although placebo-controlled therapy trials have not been performed, appropriate antibiotic therapy does eliminate shedding of the organism and probably shortens the course of the illness.

8.2.2. Diagnosis. The major epidemiological features of chlamydial genital diseases are that they occur in predominantly younger, more sexually active adults who are more often single, of lower socioeconomic status, and more often nonwhite. This is the pattern expected in a sexually transmitted disease. Infant disease may be expected in a proportion of those born to infected women.

In all of the syndromes listed below, antigen detection by DFA or EIA may be substituted for culture as long as one is not dealing with a low-risk group, when predictive power of the test becomes a problem.

8.2.2a. Adult Inclusion Conjunctivitis. The diagnosis is suspect if a follicular conjunctivitis is present. Wright- or Giemsa-stained conjunctival scrapings will reveal inclusion-containing epithelial cells if done carefully and examined in a experienced laboratory. Chlamydial culture is the diagnostic procedure of choice. Similar diseases are caused by bacteria (including *Neisseria meningitidis* and *N. gonorrhoeae*) and viruses (especially adenovirus). Bacterial conjunctivitis is usually purulent, without follicles.

8.2.2b. Cervicitis. Clinical features include mucopurulent discharge and ectopy (redness), with edema, friability, and congestion. Laboratory diagnosis is difficult, at best, since a positive chlamydial endocervical swab or paired serological fourfold titer change is required. Wright- or Giemsa-stained cervical scrapings examined for inclusions are not generally helpful. Other organisms associated with a similar picture include *N. gonorrhoeae*, *M. hominis*, herpes simplex, and possibly *T. vaginalis* and *U. urealyticum*. The presence of mucopurulent exudate is most frequently associated with chlamydial or gonococcal infection.

8.2.2c. Salpingitis. Epidemiological and clinical features are discussed in Section 8.2.1c. Laboratory diagnosis is most definitely made with tubal culture of biopsy under laparoscopy. Endometrial culture has the best correlation with tubal infection. Other sites in which chlamydiae may be cultured with less reliability include cervix and pelvic cul-de-sac. Serologically, a fourfold or greater rise in antichlamydial antibody is usually demonstrable.

Other agents associated with salpingitis include *N. gonorrhoeae*, gram-negative enteric organisms such as *Escherichia coli*, and anaerobic flora.

8.2.2d. Female Urethral Syndrome. Diagnosis of chlamydial etiology is, first, by exclusion of other bacterial etiology on urine and urethral culture and, second, by the culturing of *C. trachomatis* from the urethra or cervix. Other etiologic agents include coliforms, staphylococci, and possibly ureaplasmas.

8.2.2e. Postpartum Endometritis. Information on this syndrome is still limited. However, diagnosis may be established by obtaining *C. trachomatis* from endometrial curetting, aspirates, or swabs. The diagnosis is suspect if *C. trachomatis* is obtained on cervical culture. A serological change also occurs in this infection. Endometritis is also caused by *N. gonorrhoeae*, coliforms, and anaerobes.

8.2.2f. Male Urethritis. Diagnosis is similar to that of urethral syndrome, except that in this case gonococcal infection must be ruled out. The other known cause of NGU is *U. urealyticum*. In 20–30% of cases, no agent is isolated or serological conversion demonstrated.

8.2.2g. Epididymitis. Diagnosis is made by exclusion of bacterial agents in urine, urethra, or epididymis (coliforms, *Pseudomonas*, *N. gonorrhoeae*) and by culture of *C. trachomatis* from urethra or epididymal aspirate, or both, or demonstration of seroconversion.

8.2.2h. Arthritis (Reiter's Syndrome). In either SARA or Reiter's syndrome, the diagnosis is made by recovery of *C. trachomatis* from the urethra of a clinically compatible case or the demonstration of a fourfold rise in specific antibody, or both. Alternatively, the presence of IgM *C. trachomatis* antibody or the presence of high titers of IgG antibody is presumptive evidence of chlamydial involvement.

8.2.2i. Infant Inclusion Conjunctivitis. Conjunctival scraping (stained by Giemsa or FA methods) or culture for *C. trachomatis* are the procedures of choice. Gonococcal ophthalmia neonatorum and other bacterial agents may be excluded by culture and Gram's smear. Chemical conjunctivitis (silver nitrate) rarely presents as late as chlamydial disease.

8.2.2j. Infant Pneumonia. Diagnosis of chlamydial disease is made with a compatible clinical history and physical examination, eosinophilia, hyperinflation, and hyperglobulinemia, coupled with a positive tracheal aspirate, nasopharyngeal, or lung biopsy culture. Serological diagnosis using paired sera may be accomplished retrospectively in patients on antibiotics who are culture-negative. Since this disease occurs early in infancy, active infection may be suspected with a high titer of specific IgG antibody (particularly if it is simultaneously compared with maternal titer) or by a high titer of specific IgM antibody (>1:32 by MIF).

Agents that cause similar pictures are *Bordetella pertussis* and *B. parapertussis*, cytomegalovirus, respiratory syncytial virus, and adenovirus. Recent evidence has also suggested *Pneumocystis carinii* as an etiologic agent.

Another potential diagnostic problem is differentiation from lymphocytic interstitial pneumonia (LIP) associated with human immunodeficiency virus (HIV) and Epstein–Barr virus (EBV) infections. Usually they do not occur at the same age. *C. trachomatis* pneumonia is rare after 4 months of age and LIP is rare before 6 months of age, characteristically occurring in the second year of life. Tachypnea, rather than repetitive cough, is characteristic of LIP, and the radiographic pattern is more diffuse in LIP. Although both may have hyperglobulinemia, eosinophilia is not characteristic of LIP.

8.3. Lymphogranuloma Venereum

8.3.1. Clinical Features. The primary lesion of LGV may develop on the penis, labia, vagina, or cervix, or within the urethra, anus, or rectum, often resulting in proctitis. Rarely, it may be extragenital (e.g., fingers or tongue). Since it is usually painless and may be papular, ulcerative, or bullous, it rarely will cause the patient to seek medical attention and is usually not recognized historically. The secondary lesion of LGV consists of lymphadenopathy, which may follow the primary lesion in 1–6 weeks. With genital involvement, either inguinal or femoral lymph node chains may be involved, starting with a single node, but progressing to involve the whole chain. Abscesses form within the nodes, which expand to necrotic foci that may become fluctuant, spontaneously rupture, and leave chronic draining fistulas. These necrotic abscessed nodes are the buboes that characterize this disease and are most commonly the initial recognition of it. The fact that a far greater number of males than females are recognized to have buboes (up to tenfold in some reports) probably reflects the anatomical differences in lymphatic drainage from the various sites. The vaginal and cervical infections often drain to retroperitoneal chains, as do the anorectal primaries, which may produce manifestations more often confused with appendicitis or inguinal hernia. In the bubo stage, fever, myalgia, and headache may reflect systemic response to the lymphatic infection, and leukocytosis may result. Buboes may spontaneously subside and should not be surgically incised or drained, but may be aspirated. Rarely, chronic lymphadenopathy may result from this disease. The tertiary stage of disease consists of chronic inflammation and scarring, which may result in stricture and fistulas. These changes may follow acute LGV by 5–10 years. Urethral strictures may occur, as may penile fistulas. Anal strictures and rectovaginal fistulas are more often the sequelae in females (perhaps because of the more silent involvement of retroperitoneal lymph nodes). The current increase in the incidence of anorectal LGV in male homosexuals in the United States may be expected to result in increased recognition of resultant anal strictures due to tertiary LGV in the future.

Much rarer clinical manifestations reflect unusual extragenital sites of primary infection, such as axillary buboes with finger sites or submaxillary buboes for oral lesions. Other rare reported manifestations of LGV include meningitis, arthritis, pneumonitis, and conjunctivitis.

8.3.2. Diagnosis. Epidemiologically, LGV is found in sexually active persons, particularly those with past histories of other STDs. At one time, it was prevalent in blacks in the southern United States, but this is probably no longer true. Since the disease is more prevalent in African and Southeast Asian countries, another epidemiological feature of the occurrence in the United States has been overseas contact, such as is found in port cities or in returning military personnel who have served in these areas. In recent years, however, the disease has been found more frequently in the more sexually active male homosexual population in the United States. This segment probably represents the most frequent source of infection in the United States today.

Clinically, the primary lesion rarely comes to medical attention, and the most commonly recognized stage is that of the bubo. They are most often recognized in males, and then by inguinal or femoral node chain involvement. If both chains are involved, the "groove sign" is seen, the groove being formed between enlarged nodes of both chains. Although highly characteristic of this disease, it is seen in only 15–20% of cases.

The differential diagnosis of LGV includes syphilis (although characteristically the nodes are hard and separate in that disease), granuloma inguinale, and chancroid. Other causes of lymphadenopathy, such as various viral infections or cat-scratch disease, can often be differentiated by the discrete and often tender adenopathy they produce and more usually involvement of other chains of nodes. Herpes genitalis may present with lymphadenopathy. Bacterial lymphadenitis may mimic LGV, but sites of invasion should be recognized, and, of course, in these instances, bacteria will be recognized in node aspirates. Lymphoma and leukemia are also a part of the differential diagnosis.

The laboratory diagnosis is most definitely made by tissue culture of bubo aspirate. However, if the node is necrotic enough to rupture spontaneously, it may be too late to recover active organisms. (In the past, yolk sac culture or mouse inoculation was used for diagnosis, but tissue culture methods are more sensitive.)

The Frei antigen—a skin test made of a partially purified elementary body suspension of yolk-sac-grown LGV—was used widely for diagnosis and is still available in the United States today. However, cell culture isolation and serological methods have supplanted the Frei test. The poor sensitivity and specificity and the delay in development of the latter test have made it obsolete.

As with other chlamydial infections, the definitive serological method is the MIF method. However, in the case of LGV, as with psittacosis, CF antibodies usually result from infection within a few weeks of the initial infection and characteristically result in high titers (> 1:64). The CF test is group-specific and may be performed with either LGV or psittacosis yolk-sac- or cell-culture-prepared antigens. Although cross-reactions with the oculogenital trachoma strains would be expected, the general insensitivity of the CF test results in few patients with the oculogenital syndromes who have detectable CF antibody, and then usually at low titer.

8.4. Psittacosis

8.4.1. Clinical Features. The most common human manifestations of infection is an atypical pneumonia. It may be a relatively mild systemic disease (like mycoplasmal pneumonia) or a more severe one (like influenza). An alternative presentation is an acute septiclike illness, with fever and chills and little pneumonitis. Liver and spleen enlargement may occur (particularly in the latter toxic form). Without treatment, fever may extend into the second week, and before chemotherapy, the case-fatality rate averaged 20%, being higher in those 50 years of age and older. With apparent recovery, relapse may later occur, sometimes a matter of years following the original infection. In the 1136 cases reported in the United States in 1975–1984, pneumonia occurred in 54%.[53] Other common symptoms are headache, weakness, and myalgia. Rarely, manifestations such as arthralgia, meningiomas, abdominal pain, photophobia, pleuritis, or pericarditis may result.

8.4.2. Diagnosis. Serological diagnosis is most often employed. The CF test (insensitive for trachoma or oculogenital disease) is sensitive enough for this disease. The usual criterion is a fourfold increase in titer from acute to convalescent sera, but single titers above 1:64 are highly suggestive. *C. psittacii* can be isolated in yolk sac in embryonated eggs, in mice, or in tissue culture systems. The best source for isolation is sputum or bronchial aspirate. Whole blood (heparinized or citrated), serum, or plasma may occasionally yield the agent. Isolation is more common in the second week of disease.

8.5. *C. pneumoniae* Infections

8.5.1. Clinical Features. The limited observations to date suggest that *C. pneumoniae* organisms cause a range of respiratory disease from pharyngitis and otitis media through bronchitis to pneumoniae.[19,54] Illness is more frequent in school-aged children and young adults. It is also apparent that the majority of infections are of low-grade manifestation or are asymptomatic. There appears to be some tendency for more severe manifestations to be seen in the adolescent or young adult. In general, the disease is mild. Onset of illness is gradual and symptoms are often extended over a number of weeks. In all these characteristics, *C. pneumoniae* disease is very similar to *M. pneumoniae* disease.

Pharyngitis (often with laryngitis) appears to precede lower respiratory disease in most cases, often by a week or more, and often gives the impression of a biphasic illness. By the first clinic visit, an average of 13 days has elapsed from the onset of symptoms and the patient is often afebrile. Sinusitis is more often present than in *M. pneumoniae* infections. Chest findings are common on auscultation at this stage. With lower respiratory tract symptoms, the chest radiograph almost always demonstrates pneumonia. There is commonly a single subsegmental lesions, although more extensive involvement is sometimes found. Of pneumonia patients, 84% were outpatients.[(54)] In hospitalized patients, three retrospective serological studies have found 6–10% of community-acquired pneumonia to be due to *C. pneumoniae* infection.[(19)] In this study there were no clinical or radiological features that differentiate this etiology. In this setting the mean age was in the sixth decade and there was often preexisting chronic illness. This reflects the finding that the disease is most common in youth but more severe in the elderly. Bronchospasm and the onset of asthma has recently been associated with *C. pneumoniae* infection, but these findings need to be corroborated.[(69)]

The response to antibiotics is not striking. *In vitro* studies show maximum sensitivity to tetracyclines and erythromycin. Maximum levels of antibiotics are needed for prolonged periods, usually for at least 14 days. New longer-acting macrolides, such as azithromycin, show promise, but there have been no controlled trials reported.

8.5.2. Diagnosis. Isolation of *C. pneumoniae* has been difficult because the organism failed to adapt readily to commonly used cell cultures for other chlamydiae. The use of HL cells has improved this situation.[(24)] The organism can be isolated from respiratory specimens, but the yield from pharyngeal specimens (often all that is available) is not great. Lower respiratory tract specimens yield better results.

The MIF test, developed for *C. trachomatis* is the only sensitive and specific test available, and is useful for serological studies.[(14)] The test is demanding and is available in only a few research and commercial laboratories. Two patterns of response have been described. The first is one of slow development of IgG and IgM antibodies over 1–2 months, with subsequent loss of IgM antibody. This would appear to be a primary type of response. The second pattern is one of rapid IgG response in the absence of any IgM response and is more often noted in older individuals. This is more characteristic of a secondary or reinfection response.

Complement fixing antibodies are not specific among *Chlamydia* species. The test is often used for the diagnosis of psittacosis. In the absence of good epidemiological evidence for *C. psittaci* infection, a positive CF test is more likely to be due to *C. pneumoniae*. CF antibody response is found in two thirds of patients in whom a primary response MIF pattern can be measured. No CF antibody is measured in reinfection pattern sera. Thus, CF antibodies may be useful in screening for primary infection (particularly in younger patients). They are not useful in the diagnosis of reinfections or for seroepidemiological studies.

9. Control and Prevention

9.1. Trachoma

9.1.1. General Concepts. Elimination of trachoma has occurred in large segments of the world, not as a result of specific control programs, but following the changes in lifestyle that accompany a raised standard of living. However, in those areas of the world where trachoma remains hyperendemic, such changes are not likely to occur soon. Therefore, much national and international effort has been expended (with significant contributions from the WHO) on trachoma control programs. In the last few decades, trachoma control programs have been based almost entirely on the mass application of locally applied antibiotics. The results have been far from encouraging. After initial response, trachoma returns to become endemic again. Dawson and Schachter[(70)] have reviewed this subject and suggested that efforts be modified and that programs should be expanded to include the following elements:

1. Assessment of the problem and of the effect of intervention
2. Allocation of resources
3. Chemotherapeutic intervention
4. Surgical intervention to correct lid deformation
5. Training and utilization of local health aides and other non-specialized health workers
6. Health education and community participation

With regard to treatment, satisfactory practical methods have still not been developed.[(71)] Topical tetracylines are effective, but too often, following intensive large-scale chemotherapy, there is failure to follow this by intermittent family-based topical treatment, which depends on easy local availability of inexpensive topical preparations and on vigorous health education by local health workers. Such workers should not only ensure adequate family antibiotic treatment but also actively educate the family regarding the importance of water for hand washing, reduction of crowding, identification and control of breeding sites of eye-seeking flies, and improvement of personal hygiene.

9.1.2. Antibiotic and Chemotherapeutic Aproaches. Community-based antibiotic treatment programs are, in a sense, prophylaxis of reinfection, which is the damaging aspect of trachoma. As stated above, the change in emphasis on use of antibiotics is not one of change of treatment modality but the community application. As is being learned in many public health programs, lasting effects cannot be produced by large, centrally directed mass programs. Success has been achieved in those countries where trachoma control becomes an ongoing part of the broad community-based public health program.[72]

Choice of antibiotic depends on availability, price, and ease of administration. With the exception of rifampin, no significant antibiotic resistance has developed to *C. trachomatis*. Thus, the choices lie with sulfonamides, tetracyclines, erythromycin, and certain other macrolides. Strategies of treatment and control of trachoma have been studied with regard to cost-effectiveness.[71] In areas of high endemicity, mass therapy with ocular antibiotics must be the first resort. When oral antibiotics (tetracycline or doxycycline) are administered as a supplement, the healing rates improve. The use of oral antibiotics can be shown to be a cost-effective strategy, particularly in communities where fewer than 20% of children have active trachoma. Oral administration is theoretically preferable, but topical eye ointments or suspensions have been more practical.

9.1.3. Immunization. Soon after *C. trachomatis* was first recovered in eggs, laboratories in London, Boston, and Taipei (later Seattle) began developing vaccines for trachoma.[40] Even though reinfection can readily occur in humans following prior trachoma, it was found in monkey models that hyperimmunization with vaccine could prevent reinfection, at least under the somewhat artificial environment of an animal trial. In one instance, a similar result was obtained in blind volunteers. However, each of the candidate vaccines was made with relatively crude whole-organism preparations, and all of them gave only fleeting protection. Even more discouraging was the finding that in both animal experiments and human trials, subsequent rechallenge might result in more severe disease than occurred in rechallenge after natural infection (a phenomenon that has also been seen in other experimental vaccines of low antigenic potency). At that point, all vaccine trials were abandoned, pending further study of the molecular biology of the organism, with the hope of discovering antigenic subunits that might result in a more permanent immunity. Such efforts are about to move from the laboratory bench to animal testing.

9.2. Oculogenital Diseases

9.2.1. General Concepts. Since these are STDs, control measures are similar to those for gonorrhea and syphilis. *C. trachomatis* should be sought by culture or antigen detection methods in persons with STD complaints or history. Current recommendations include treatment of all persons with urethritis (gonococcal or nongonococcal), mucopurulent cervicitis, pelvic inflammatory disease, and epididymitis in men under age 35 as if they had both gonococcal and chlamydial infection.[44] They should be treated with a penicillinlike antibiotic (or alternative where penicillin-resistant strains exceed 3%) and a tetracyline antibiotic (or erythromycin in pregnant women). Other individuals recommended for *C. trachomatis* treatment are asymptomatic contacts to patients with the four syndromes mentioned above and others with established gonococcal or chlamydial infections. Similarly, sexual partners of persons with gonococcal infection should be treated. All of these could be treated without a positive laboratory test if diagnostic laboratory sources are limited. Then, diagnostic screening can be saved for highest-risk groups. These would be inner-city women who are sexually active and who are below age 25, particularly adolescents. Of particular concern are those with a history of a prior STD. When possible, contact tracing should be pursued. Both cases and contacts should be treated concurrently and should avoid intercourse (or use condoms) during treatment. In pregnant women, culture and treatment are indicated to protect against postpartum maternal and neonatal consequences.

9.2.2. Prophylaxis. In infected males and nonpregnant females, treatment with azithromycin, tetracyclines, erythromycin, or sulfonamides eliminates infection and therefore provides prophylaxis against the complications of that infection.[44]

Treatment of women during pregnancy or immediately postdelivery will eliminate infection and may protect against postpartum fever and endometritis. Furthermore, for the treatment to be effective during pregnancy, the sexual partner must be treated simultaneously to prevent reinfection. Tetracyclines and sulfonamides are contraindicated during pregnancy; erythromycin remains the only safe and effective drug. If further study elucidates prenatal fetal or maternal complications of infection, or both, routine first-trimester cervical culture and treatment of positive women and partners may be a theoretically useful prophylactic procedure.

For infants, effective prevention of chlamydial disease occurs by treating mothers and partners prior to delivery.[73] Silver nitrate prophylaxis is ineffective against chlamydiae, and topical erythromycin or tetracycline eye prophylaxis at birth for the prevention of inclusion conjunctivitis may reduce it somewhat, but they are not highly effective and will not prevent pneumonia.

Antibiotic resistance of *C. trachomatis* has not been shown and is not currently a clinical problem.

9.2.3. Immunization. No immunization for oculogenital diseases is available.

9.3. Lymphogranuloma Venereum

9.3.1. General Concepts. Prevention of LGV depends on the recognition and treatment of infected persons. Problems exist in both these aims. Although classic cases of LGV are easily recognized, relapse of old disease may occur, particularly in debilitated persons. Furthermore, the occurrence of relatively silent disease in anogenital carriers, particularly in sexually active homosexuals, and the difficulty in availability of simple diagnostic tests result in rather persistent endemic foci. For LGV, unique among other chlamydial diseases, a specific, highly effective method of chemotherapy is also lacking. Sulfonamides were classically used, but more commonly tetracycline therapy is presently preferred. The major difficulty is in assessing the effect of therapy, particularly in treatment of the embryonic or tertiary stage.

9.3.2. Prophylaxis and Immunization. No prophylaxis or immunization for LGV is available.

9.4. Psittacosis

9.4.1. General Concepts. Control of psittacosis depends on control of avian sources of infection. Control of the 1929 pandemic of psittacosis was accomplished by bans on the importation of psittacine birds. This was followed by a method of certification of clean flocks, but many of these efforts were damaged by poor supervision, smuggling, and contamination of susceptible birds from clean flocks during shipment. An effective method for controlling psittacosis in parakeets has been developed: a chlortetracycline-impregnated seed. Current requirements for quarantine of imported birds are for 30 days of treatment. This is probably not enough, and it has been proposed that this be extended to 45 days. It is probable that some birds have suppressed infections that reactivate during shipment following quarantine. The remaining problems are ones of assuring more adequate response to control regulations.

The control of occupational disease in the poultry-processing industry appears to have been successful in recent years, although there is no developed public health program. The epidemics in 1974 served to alert the industry to the problem, and the infection in poultry flocks tends to be rapidly recognized and treated. It is also probable that human disease continues to occur, but is quickly recognized, treated, and not reported in these workers.

9.4.2. Prophylaxis and Immunization. There is no prophylaxis in humans, and although experimental psittacosis vaccines have been developed in birds, they are not cheap enough to replace antibiotic treatment of birds. There is no need to develop human vaccine for such an infrequent disease.

10. Unresolved Problems

10.1. Trachoma

For trachoma, there is no problem of diagnosis, since clinical recognition is relatively simple. The formidable problem is the development of a simple, safe, and easily applied (once daily) chemotherapeutic agent and a public health structure that will assure its application. A vaccine would be far more useful, but development of one depends on a greatly expanded understanding of the immunology and molecular biology of this agent.

10.2. Oculogenital Diseases

10.2.1. Epidemiology and Disease Spectrum. There have been no significant additions to our knowledge of the disease spectrum in the last 5 years. Syndromes such as otitis media, prostatitis, diarrhea, or pharyngitis have not been shown to be caused by *C. trachomatis*. Reports that claimed to find a significant contribution of chlamydia to pharyngitis were based on serological evidence. It is now clear[74] that this phenomenon and the unexplained increment of antibody in early childhood were both a function of cross-reacting antibody to TWAR (Taiwan acute respiratory) organisms.

10.2.2. Diagnostic Tests. Chlamydial cultures and serological techniques are time consuming and expensive; they are not very useful as screening techniques. Amplified DNA technology, such as LCR and PCR, is extremely sensitive and specific, even on urine specimens.[29,30] When these tests are more available and less expensive, they bring the potential of mass screening with noninvasive tests that could revolutionize control approaches. With use of these techniques in high-risk young women and men and with single-dose azithromycin therapy now available, there is the prospect for detection and elimination of asymptomatic infection, and thus an opportunity for major disease control.

10.2.3. Host Response. Data from individuals with asymptomatic infection have shown that infection may persist in the presence of both serum and local antibody. The contribution of other arms of the immune response to clearance of infection is very largely unknown.

10.2.4. Control. Control of oculogenital infections due to *C. trachomatis* constitutes a large-scale public health problem. As has been discussed in other sections, true control of these infections will require definition of all the illnesses caused by *C. trachomatis* and all modes of transmission of infection, coupled with the development of rapid and easily applicable diagnostic techniques.

10.3. Lymphogranuloma Venereum

The outstanding problem in this case, as with the oculogenital syndromes, is the development of a rapid, inexpensive diagnostic method. In this instance, further study of optimal chemotherapy is also needed.

10.4. Psittacosis

In this instance, it would seem that the basic tools are at hand. A vaccine for birds or a more effective antibiotic feed method that would assure elimination of avian infection in less than 30 days would assure better cooperation by the industry.

10.5. *C. pneumoniae* Infections

There are many research needs for this newly discovered agent. Culture and serological methods need to be further adapted for this organism. Basic epidemiological and natural history studies are needed. Although serological studies indicate a ubiquitous agent, there appear to be periods of occurrence and absence in given locations. The transmission of the organism and its infectivity and incubation period need to be defined. Methods of treatment, control, and prevention require extensive research.

11. References

1. Thygeson, P., Trachoma virus: Historical background and review of isolates, *Ann. N.Y. Acad. Sci.* **98**:6–13 (1962).
2. Halberstaedter, L., and von Prowazek, S., Uber Zelleinschliesse parasitarer Natur beim Trachom, *Arb. Kais. Gesund.* **26**: 44–47 (1907).
3. Lindner, K., Zur Trachomforschung, *Z. Augenheilkd.* **22**:547–549 (1909).
4. Nicolle, C., Cuenod, A., and Blaisot, L., Étude experimentalle du trachome, *Arch. Inst. Pasteur Tunis* **3**:185–188 (1911).
5. Julianelle, L. A., *The Etiology of Trachoma*. The Commonwealth Fund, New York, 1938.
6. Bedson, S. P., The psittacosis–lymphogranuloma group of viruses, *Br. Med. Bull.* **9**:226–227 (1953).
7. Rake, G., Shaffer, M. F., and Thygeson, P., Relationship of agents of trachoma and inclusion conjunctivitis to those of lymphogranuloma–psittacosis group, *Proc. Soc. Exp. Biol. Med.* **99**:545–547 (1942).
8. Thygeson, P., and Stone, W., Jr., The epidemiology of inclusion conjunctivitis, *Arch. Ophthalmol.* **27**:91–122 (1942).
9. Tang, F. F., Chang, H. L., Huang, Y. T., *et al.*, Trachoma virus in chick embryo, *Natl. Med. J. China* **43**:81–86 (1957).
10. Collier, L .H., and Sowa, J., Isolation of trachoma virus in embryonated eggs, *Lancet* **1**:993–994 (1958).
11. Jones, B. R., Collier, L. H., and Smith, C. H., Isolation of a virus from inclusion blennorrhea, *Lancet* **1**:902–905 (1959).
12. Gordon, F. B., Harper, I. A., Guan, A. L., *et al.*, Detection of *Chlamydia* (Bedsonia) in certain infections of man. I. Laboratory procedures: Comparison of yolk sac and cell culture for detection and isolation, *J. Infect. Dis.* **120**:451–462 (1969).
13. Wang, S.-P., Kuo, C. C., and Grayston, J. T., A simplified method for immunological typing of trachoma-inclusion conjunctivitis–lymphogranuloma venereum organisms, *Infect. Immun.* **7**:356–360 (1973).
14. Wang, S.-P., Grayston, J. T., Alexander, E. R., *et al.*, A simplified microimmunofluorescence test with trachoma lymphogranuloma venereum (*Chlamydia trachomatis*) antigens for use as a screening test for antibody, *J. Clin. Microbiol.* **1**:250–255 (1975).
15. Jüergensen, T., *Handbuch der Speziellen Pathologie und Therapie. Handbuch der Krankheiten des Respirations-Aparates*, Vogel, Leipzig, 1874.
16. Hunter, J. S., *A Treatise on the Venereal Disease*, J. Webster, Philadelphia, 1818.
17. Bedson, S. P., The use of the complement-fixation reaction in the diagnosis of human psittacosis, *Lancet* **2**:1277–1280 (1935).
18. Moulder, J. W., Comparative biology of intracellular parasitism, *Microbiol. Rev.* **49**:298–337 (1985).
19. Grayston, J. T., Kuo, C. C., Wang, S.-P., *et al.*, A new *Chlamydia psittaci* strain called TWAR from acute respiratory tract infections, *N. Engl. J. Med.* **315**:161–168 (1986).
20. Washington, A. E., Johnson, R. E., Sanders, L. L., *et al.*, Incidence of *Chlamydia trachomatis* infections in the United States using reported *Neisseria gonorrhoeae* as a surrogate, in: *Chlamydia Infections* (D. Oriel, G. Ridgeway, J. Schachter, *et al.*, eds.), pp. 987–990, Cambridge University Press, London, 1962.
21. World Health Organization, *World Health Organization Guide to Trachoma Control*, WHO, Geneva, 1981.
22. Yoneda, C., Dawson, C. R., Daghfous, T., *et al.*, Cytology as a guide to the presence of chlamydial inclusions in Giemsa-stained conjunctival smears in severe endemic trachoma, *Br. J. Ophthalmol.* **59**:116–124 (1975).
23. Stamm, W. E., Diagnosis of *Chlamydia trachomatis* genitourinary infections, *Ann. Intern. Med.* **108**(5):710–717 (1988).
24. Ripa, K. T., and Mårdh, P.-A., Cultivation of *Chlamydia trachomatis* in cycloheximide-treated McCoy cells, *J. Clin. Microbiol.* **6**:328–330 (1977).
25. Cles, L. D., and Stamm, W. E., Use of HL cells for improved isolation and passage of *Chlamydia pneumoniae*, *J. Clin. Microbiol.* **28**(5):938–940 (1990).
26. Hyman, C. L., Roblin, P. M., Gaydos, C. A., *et al.*, The prevalence of asymptomatic nasopharyngeal carriage of *Chlamydia pneu-*

moniae in subjectively healthy adults as assessed by PCR-EIA and culture, *Clin. Infect. Dis.* **20:**1174–1178 (1995).

27. Moncada, J., Schachter, J., Bolan, G. A., *et al.*, Confirmatory assay increases specificity of the chlamydiazyme test for *Chlamydia trachomatis* infection of the cervix, *J. Clin. Microbiol.* **28**(8): 1770–1773 (1990).
28. Clarke, L. M., Sierra, M. F., Daidone, B. J., *et al.*, Comparison of the Syva MicroTrak enzyme immunoassay and Gen-Probe PACE 2 with cell culture for diagnosis of cervical *Chlamydia trachomatis* infection in a high-prevalence female population, *J. Clin. Microbiol.* **31**(4)**:**968–971 (1993).
29. Bobo, L., Coutlee, F., Yolken, R. H., *et al.*, Diagnosis of *Chlamydia trachomatis* cervical infection by amplified DNA with an enzyme immunoassay, *J. Clin. Microbiol.* **28**(9)**:**1968–1973 (1990).
30. Schachter, J., Stamm, W. E., Quinn, T. C., *et al.*, Ligase chain reaction to detect *Chlamydia trachomatis* infection of the cervix, *J. Clin. Microbiol.* **32**(10)**:**2540–2543 (1994).
31. Jaschek, G., Gaydos, C. A., Welsh, L. E., *et al.*, Direct detection of *Chlamydia trachomatis* in urine specimens from symptomatic and asymptomatic men by using a rapid polymerase chain reaction assay, *J. Clin. Microbiol.* **31:**1209–1212 (1993).
32. Chernesky, M. A., Lee, H. H., Schachter, J., *et al.*, Rapid diagnosis of *Chlamydia trachomatis* urethral infection in symptomatic and asymptomatic men by testing first-void urine in a ligase chain reaction assay, *J. Infect. Dis.* **170:**1308–1311 (1994).
33. Lee, H. H., Chernesky, M. A., Schachter, J., *et al.*, Diagnosis of *Chlamydia trachomatis* genitourinary infection in women by ligase chain reaction assay of urine specimens, *Lancet* **345:**213–216 (1995).
34. Schachter, J., Chlamydiae, in: *Manual of Clinical Laboratory Immunology*, 4th ed. (N. R. Rose, E. Conway de Marcario, J. L. Fahey, *et al.*, eds.), pp. 661–666, American Society for Microbiology, Washington, DC, 1992.
35. Schachter, J., Smith, D. E., Dawson, C. R., *et al.*, Lymphogranuloma venereum. I. Comparison of Frei test complement fixation test and isolation of the agent, *J. Infect. Dis.* **120:**372–375 (1969).
36. Alexander, E. R., Wang, S.-P., and Grayston, J. T., Further classification of TRIC agents from ocular trachoma and other sources by the mouse toxicity prevention tests, *Am. J. Ophthmal.* **63:**1469–1478 (1967).
37. Moulder, J. W., The relation of the psittacosis group (chlamydiae) to bacteria and viruses, *Annu. Rev. Microbiol.* **20:**107–130 (1966).
38. Campbell, L. A., Kuo, C. C., and Grayston, J. T., Characterization of the new *Chlamydia* agent TWAR as a unique organism by restriction endonuclease analysis and by DNA–DNA hybridization, *J. Clin. Microbiol.* **25:**1911–1916 (1987).
39. Jones, B. R., Prevention of blindness from trachoma, *Trans. Ophthalmol. Soc. UK* **95:**16–33 (1974).
40. Schachter, J., and Dawson, C. R., *Human Chlamydial Infections*, PSG Publishing, Littleton, MA, 1978.
41. Dawson, C. R., Hanna, L., and Jawetz, E., Controlled treatment trials of trachoma in American Indian children, *Lancet* **2:**961–963 (1967).
42. West, S. K., Congdon, N., Katala, S., *et al.*, Facial cleanliness and risk of trachoma in families, *Arch. Ophthalmol.* **109**(6)**:**885–857 (1991).
43. Nichols, R. I., Bobb, A. A., Haddad, A., *et al.*, Immunofluorescent studies of the microbiologic epidemiology of trachoma in Saudi Arabia, *Am. J. Ophthalmol.* **63:**1372–1408 (1967).
44. Centers for Disease Control and Prevention, *Chlamydia trachomatis* infections. Policy guidelines for prevention and control, *Morbid. Mortal. Week. Rep.* **34**(Suppl)**:**53S–74S (1988).
45. Schachter, J., Stoner, E., and Moncada, J., Screening for chlamydial infections in women attending family planning clinics: Evaluations of presumptive indicators for therapy, *West. J. Med.* **138**(3)**:**375–379 (1983).
46. Mårdh, P.-A., An overview of infectious agents of salpingitis: Their biology and recent advances in methods of detection, *Am. J. Obstet. Gynecol.* **138:**933–951 (1980).
47. Wager, G. P., Martin, D. H., Koutsky, L., *et al.*, Puerperal infectious morbidity: Relationship to route of delivery and to antepartum *Chlamydia trachomatis* infections, *Am. J. Obstet. Gynecol.* **138:** 1028–1033 (1980).
48. Holmes, K. K., Handsfield, H. H., Wang, S.-P., *et al.*, Etiology of nongonococcal urethritis, *N. Engl. J. Med.* **292:**1199–1206 (1975).
49. Keat, A. C., Thomas, B. J., Taylor-Robinson, D., *et al.*, Evidence of *Chlamydia trachomatis* infection in sexually acquired reactive arthritis, *Ann. Rheum. Dis.* **39:**431–437 (1980).
50. Kousa, M., Saikku, P., Richmond, S., *et al.*, Frequent association of chlamydial infection with Reiter's syndrome, *Sex. Transmit. Dis.* **5:**57–61 (1978).
51. Schachter, J., Grossman, M., Sweet, R. L., *et al.*, Prospective study of perinatal transmission of *Chlamydia trachomatis*, *J. Am. Med. Assoc.* **255**(24)**:**3374–3377 (1986).
52. Centers for Disease Control and Prevention, Summary of notifiable diseases: United States, *Morbid. Mortal. Week. Rep.* **42**(53) (1993).
53. Centers for Disease Control and Prevention, *Psittacosis Surveillance Summary (1975–84)*, CDC, Bethesda, MD, 1987.
54. Grayston, J. T., *Chlamydia pneumoniae* strain TWAR pneumonia, *Annu. Rev. Med.* **43:**317–323 (1992).
55. Kleemola, M., Saikku, P., Visakorpi, R., *et al.*, Epidemics of pneumonia caused by TWAR, a new chlamydia organism, in military trainees in Finland, *J. Infect. Dis.* **157:**230–236 (1988).
56. Meyer, K. F., The host spectrum of psittacosis–lymphogranuloma venereum (PL) agents, *Am. J. Ophthalmol.* **63:**1225–1246 (1967).
57. Grayston, J. T., and Wang, S.-P., The potential for vaccine against infection of the genital tract with *Chlamydia trachomatis*, *J. Am. Vener. Dis. Assoc.* **5:**78–79 (1978).
58. Taylor, H. R., Johnson, S. L., Schachter, J., *et al.*, Pathogenesis of trachoma: The stimulus for inflammation, *J. Immunol.* **138**(9)**:** 3023–3027 (1987).
59. Patton, D., Kuo, C. C., Wang, S.-P., *et al.*, Distal tubal obstruction induced by repeated *Chlamydia trachomatis* salpingeal infection in pig-tailed macaques, *J. Infect. Dis.* **155:**1292–1299 (1987).
60. Mordhorst, C. H., Wang, S.-P., and Grayston, J. T., Childhood trachoma in a nonendemic area, *J. Am. Med. Assoc.* **239:**1765–1771 (1978).
61. Dawson, C. R., Jones, B. R., and Darougar, S., Blinding and nonblinding trachoma: Assessment of intensity of upper tarsal inflammatory disease and disabling lesions, *WHO Bull.* **52**(3)**:** 279–282 (1975).
62. Brunham, R. C., Paavonen, J., Stevens, C. E., *et al.*, Mucopurulent cervicitis—the ignored counterpart in women of urethritis in men, *N. Engl. J. Med.* **311**(1)**:**1–6 (1984).
63. Jones, R. B., Mammel, J. B., Shepard, M. K., *et al.*, Recovery of *Chlamydia trachomatis* from the endometrium of women at risk for chlamydial infection, *Am. J. Obstet. Gynecol.* **155**(1)**:**35–39 (1986).
64. Westrom, L., Joesoef, R., Reynolds, G., *et al.*, Pelvic inflammatory

disease and fertility. A cohort study of 1844 women with laparoscopically verified diseases and 657 control women with normal laparoscopic results, *Sex. Transm. Dis.* **19**(4):185–192 (1992).

65. Stamm, W. E., Wager, K. F., Amsel, R., *et al.*, Causes of the acute urethral syndrome in women, *N. Engl. J. Med.* **303**:409–415 (1980).
66. Keat, A., Dixey, J., Sonnex, C., *et al.*, *Chlamydia trachomatis* and reactive arthritis: The missing link, *Lancet* **1**:72–74 (1987).
67. Schachter, J., and Grossman, M., Chlamydial infections, *Annu. Rev. Med.* **32**:45–61 (1981).
68. Beem, M. O., Saxon, E. M., Respiratory tract colonization and a distinctive pneumonia syndrome in infants infected with *Chlamydia trachomatis*, *N. Engl. J. Med.* **296**:306–310 (1977).
69. Hahn, D. L., Dodge, R. W., and Golubjatkinov, R., Association of *Chlamydia pneumoniae* (strain TWAR) infection with wheezing asthmatic bronchitis and adult onset asthma, *J. Am. Med. Assoc.* **266**:225–230 (1991).
70. Dawson, C. R., and Schachter, J., Strategies for treatment and control of blinding trachoma: Cost effectiveness of topical systemic antibiotic, *Rev. Infect. Dis.* **7**:768–773 (1985).
71. Dawson, C. R., and Schachter, J., Proceedings of The Symposium—Human chlamydial infections: Therapeutic considerations in developing and industrialized countries, in: *Economic Implications of Antimicrobial Therapy: Part 2—Genitourinary Tract Infections*, pp. 18–30, Physicians Publications, New York, 1982.
72. Thylefors, B., Development of trachoma control programs and the involvement of natural resources, *Rev. Infect. Dis.* **7**:774–776 (1985).
73. Schachter, J., Sweet, R. L., Grossman, M., *et al.*, Experience with the routine use of erythromycin for chlamydial infections in pregnancy, *N. Engl. J. Med.* **314**(5):276–279 (1986).
74. Schachter, J., Human *Chlamydia psittaci* infection, in: *Chlamydia Infections* (D.Oriel, G. Ridgway, J. S., Schachter, *et al.*, eds.), pp. 311–320, Cambridge University Press, London, 1986.
75. Alexander, E .R., Chlamydia: The organism and neonatal infection, *Hosp. Pract.* **14**:63–69 (1979).

12. Suggested Reading

Grayston, J. T., *Chlamydia pneumoniae*, strain TWAR pneumonia, *Annu. Rev. Med.* **43**:317–323 (1992).

Orfila, J., Byrne, G. I., Chernesky, M. A., *et al.*, *Chlamydial Infections: Proceedings of the Eighth International Symposium on Human Chlamydial Infections*, Societá Editrice Esculapio, Bologna, Italy, 1994.

Schachter, J., Overview of human diseases, in: *Microbiology of Chlamydia* (A. L. Barron, ed.), CRC Press, Boca Raton, 1988.

Schachter, J., and Dawson, C. R., *Human Chlamydial Infections*, Publishing Sciences Group, Littleton, MA, 1978.

CHAPTER 11

Cholera

Robert V. Tauxe

1. Introduction

Cholera is a severe diarrheal illness caused by certain types of *Vibrio cholerae*, which can lead rapidly to dehydration and death. Although other organisms occasionally cause similar illness, the term "cholera" is reserved for illness caused by infection with toxigenic strains of *V. cholerae* O1 or O139, whether the symptoms are mild or severe. Epidemic cholera has appeared relatively recently on the global stage. It spread throughout the world early in the 19th century, causing severe epidemics in the crowded cities of the newly industrializing Europe, and has since recurred in massive multicontinental pandemics. These pandemics had a profound impact on the development of public health itself, stimulating the establishment of standing health departments, ongoing infectious disease surveillance, and swift and effective public health response to epidemics. The discovery that cholera was associated with contaminated municipal water spurred the "sanitary revolution," leading to modern water and sewage treatment systems and the control of many diseases in the developed world. Now as then, epidemic cholera continues to goad countries in the early phases of industrialization to develop adequate infrastructures.

Treatment for cholera is now simple and highly effective. Rapid replacement of the lost fluids and electrolytes with oral and intravenous solutions can reduce the mortality from 25–50% to less than 1%. The organism can be transmitted through contaminated drinking water and through a variety of foods. The specific vehicle of transmission can vary from place to place and during the course of a single epidemic, complicating epidemic control efforts. Efforts to improve drinking water safety and food sanitation can be accelerated by the appearance of epidemic cholera, and prevention can ultimately be achieved by improving the sanitary infrastructure in susceptible areas. Some simple prevention strategies may prove to be sustainable and effective. Natural infection tends to give only limited protection, as do existing and experimental vaccines. Although research has focused recently on the development of effective oral vaccines, as yet, no vaccine is available that has broad public health applicability.

In the 1990s, two events changed the epidemiology of cholera. The appearance of epidemic cholera in Latin America in 1991, after an absence of over 100 years, has stimulated improvements in public health and sanitation throughout the hemisphere, but it is likely to persist as an important public health threat for decades to come. In 1992, a new strain of *V. cholerae*, called O139 Bengal, appeared in India and caused a major epidemic in a population that was already largely immune to cholera caused by *V. cholerae* O1 strains. Although the future of this new epidemic is unknown, it may represent the beginning of a new pandemic. The sudden appearance of this serogroup is a case study in the evolution of bacterial serotypes and in the emergence of new pathogens in general.

2. Historical Background

The history of cholera is linked to the early modern era of industrial civilization. Epidemic cholera is not described in early Mediterranean or Middle Eastern medicine texts, though accounts compatible with cholera exist from medieval India.[1] The disease has a homeland in the Bengal basin, the delta of the Ganges and Brahmaputra Rivers. The vibrio is well-adapted to the estuarine environment and may have been established for many years in this natural reservoir, occasionally infecting those who

Robert V. Tauxe • Foodborne and Diarrheal Diseases Branch, Division of Bacterial and Mycotic Diseases, National Center for Infectious Diseases, Centers for Disease Control and Prevention, Atlanta, Georgia 30333.

drank or consumed raw shellfish from those waters, in an ecological pattern resembling that of many vibrios, including *V. cholerae* other than O1 or O139.

Beginning in 1817, cholera spread from Bengal to other parts of the world in repeated pandemic waves that affected virtually all of the inhabited world. Precisely when each of these waves began and ended is a matter of historical judgment. The most frequently cited account is that of Pollitzer,[1] who divided them into six major pandemics between 1817 and 1923 (Table 1). The global spread of cholera was hastened by the establishment of European empires in Asia, which led to increased international trade. The Hajj, or annual Muslim pilgrimage to Mecca, helped to disseminate cholera in pandemics four through six.[1] Cholera was likely to have been a regular feature of life in Asia in the 19th century. However, the impact was particularly severe in rapidly growing European cities, where huge lethal epidemics occurred. In those cities, immigrants from the countryside crowded into new slums, seeking employment in the new mills and factories of the industrial revolution. Those Dickensian slums bear a striking sociological resemblance to the barrios, favellas, and periurban slums that ring cities in the developing world today. In many respects, Manila in 1995 may be compared to Manchester, England in 1840.[2] Investigations of the 1854 epidemic in London by John Snow[3] showed that the cholera death rate in homes served by the Southwark and Vauxhall Water Company was 31 per 1000 houses, 8.5 times higher than the death rate in homes served by the competing company, which was 3.7 per 1000 houses. Although neither company provided treated water, the former drew water from the Thames below the city sewage outlet, while the latter was supplied from the river above the city. An outbreak of cholera was linked to consuming water drawn from one particular and celebrated pump, located in Broad Street.

Table 1. Cholera Pandemics Since 1817[a]

No.	Years	Origin	Pandemic organism
1	1817–1823	India	?
2	1829–1851	India	?
3	1852–1859	India	?
4	1863–1879	India	?
5	1881–1896	India	*V. cholerae* 01, classical
6	1899–1923	India	*V. cholerae* 01, classical
7	1961–Present	Sulawesi, Indonesia	*V. cholerae* 01, El Tor
8?	1992–Present	Madras, India	*V. cholerae* 0139

[a]Adpated from Pollitzer.[1]

These investigations are classic examples of the application of the epidemiological method even in the absence of a defined microbiological cause. In 1890, similar observations were made in Hamburg, where the incidence of cholera in Hamburg was 34 per 1000 compared with 3.9 per 1000 in surrounding areas that were not supplied by water from the River Elbe.[1] These observations catalyzed efforts to provide safe drinking water and adequate sewer systems in Europe and North America.

The microbiological cause of cholera was described by Robert Koch[4] in 1884, who investigated cholera in Egypt during the fifth pandemic. The strains he described are what we now refer to as the "classical" biotype of *V. cholerae* O1, the cause of pandemics five and six.

Epidemic cholera reached the United States on several occasions.[5] In 1832, the nation responded with prayer and panic, and many believed that the disease was a divine retribution afflicting the wicked. Some cities concealed cholera cases, while others ineffectively banned the transit of goods or passengers from suspected cholera-affected areas. By 1866, a more rational approach prevailed. Temporary boards of health were created in many cities, and began to conduct surveillance, to hospitalize cholera patients, and to take measures to improve the municipal water supply. After 1880, in the fifth and sixth pandemics, resurgent European epidemics again threatened the United States. The value of surveillance was widely appreciated, and many local boards of health became permanent institutions. Laboratory diagnosis was used to identify cases. Many municipal aqueducts and protected watersheds date from that era. Large-scale epidemic spread did not occur, suggesting that the public health infrastructure was sufficiently advanced to protect the population by then.[1]

After the sixth pandemic, cholera entered a curious 50-year lull, and again was largely restricted to the Bengal homeland. This lull broke in 1961, when epidemic cholera appeared in Sulawezi, Indonesia, and then disseminated rapidly[6] This epidemic was caused by the El Tor biotype of *V. cholerae* O1. It spread rapidly across Asia and into Africa by 1970 (Fig. 1). In 1991, a variant El Tor strain appeared in Peru in a new epidemic wave that spread swiftly through Latin America.[7] In the mid-1990s, following the dissolution of the Soviet Union, epidemic cholera appeared in the decaying cities of central Asia.

Thus, in 1993, more countries reported cholera than ever before. Epidemic cholera continues to exert a major influence on the global development of society and public health.

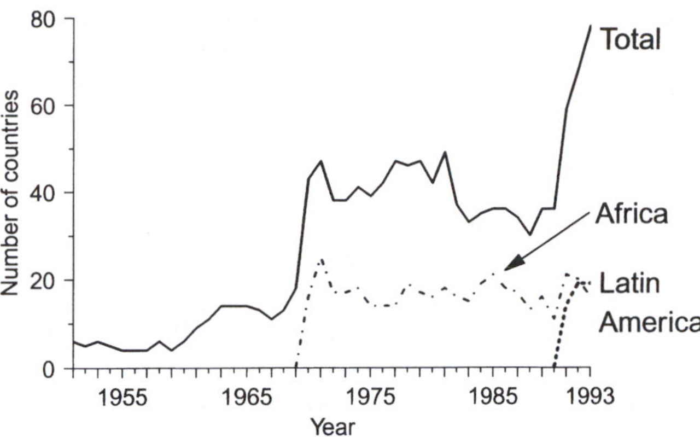

Figure 1. Number of countries reporting cholera to the World Health Organization by year, 1951–1993. Data from the World Health Organization.

3. Methodology

3.1. Sources of Mortality Data

Cholera was the first disease for which modern public health surveillance was organized. Thus, cholera bears the code 001 in the international classification of diseases and, along with plague and yellow fever, cholera is an internationally notifiable disease. Many countries conduct routine surveillance for cholera and report the results to the World Health Organization (WHO). Political concerns, fear of inappropriate trade embargoes or loss of tourism, and other imagined penalties cause some countries to conceal the presence of cholera. In particular, Egypt, China, India, Thailand, and Bangladesh have for years officially denied the presence of cholera, referring instead to "severe diarrheal illness." In many other countries, particularly in Africa, vital statistics are not routinely gathered, disease reporting is limited, and many cases and deaths go unreported. Thus, official global statistics on cholera provide a very incomplete picture.

The definition of a cholera death varies greatly. The definition recommended by the Pan-American Health Organization is "death within 1 week of onset of diarrhea in a person with confirmed or clinically defined cholera."(8)

3.2. Sources of Morbidity Data

Although cholera is a notifiable disease in most countries, the actual number of cases reported is far less than the number that occur. In parts of South Asia, infection with *V. cholerae* is probably nearly universal, yet no cases are reported. The definition of a case used for surveillance purposes varies considerably.(8) In countries where cholera is common, the case is usually defined in clinical terms as watery diarrheal illness associated with severe dehydration. Because there are many other causes of pediatric diarrhea, the precision of this surveillance definition is improved if cases are restricted to those in persons over age 5 years, though this means not counting younger patients.(9) In Peru, the positive predictive value of this simple case definition was better than 80% early in the epidemic.(10)

When cholera is rare, other severe diarrheal illnesses will be more common than cholera, which renders the clinical definition too nonspecific for public health use. Therefore, in most industrialized nations, the surveillance case definition of cholera depends on laboratory isolation of toxigenic *V. cholerae* O1 or O139, or demonstration of diagnostic antibodies.(11) Because many other *V. cholerae* cause occasional illnesses, without the same public health implications, it is important in the setting of a sporadic infection to verify the serogroup of *V. cholerae* as O1 or O139 and the toxigenicity of the organism before calling the illness cholera.

Where cholera is common, case reporting and public health response should not be limited to laboratory-confirmed cases. It is not necessary to expend scarce laboratory resources confirming many thousands of cases during an epidemic; the most useful roles of the laboratory are to define the beginning of the epidemic, to monitor for changes in antimicrobial resistance during the epidemic, and to establish that an epidemic is over.(12)

3.3. Surveys

Serological surveys conducted in the epidemic setting show that the actual number of infections will exceed the reported clinical cases by at least 10-fold.(13) The seroepidemiology of cholera depends on the specific but short-lasting vibriocidal antibody response, so serosurveys like those done for viral pathogens cannot often be meaningfully conducted for cholera. For many years, the International Center for Diarrheal Disease Research in Bangladesh has maintained surveillance over urban and rural populations, defining the epidemiology of cholera in that area.

In the developed world, when a cholera case is detected, it is important to heighten local surveillance to detect other cases, and thereby to establish whether transmission is ongoing. This is done by obtaining cultures from patients with severe diarrhea coming to medical attention and by testing convalescent sera from severe diarrheal cases seen at medical facilities in the preceding weeks.[12,14] If sewage collection is centralized, culturing gauze Moore swabs placed in the main sewer for 24 hr can detect *V. cholerae* in areas drained by the sewer.[15] This is an economical way of maintaining surveillance on a population among whom cholera might be introduced.[12]

3.4. Laboratory Diagnosis

3.4.1. Isolation and Identification of the Organism. *V. cholerae* is excreted in stools of the cholera patient and grows well on several standard bacteriologic media. Efficient isolation depends on the use of a selective medium that suppresses other bacterial species, while permitting *V. cholerae* to grow. Thiosulfate–citrate–bile salts–sucrose (TCBS) agar is the most widely used medium.[12] *V. cholerae* produces large yellow colonies on this medium. The isolates are further characterized biochemically and tested with diagnostic antiserum for the presence of O1 antigen. The O1 strains will agglutinate in the O1 antiserum, producing a coagulated clump on a slide. In the same manner, O139 strains can be identified with O139 antiserum. Strains that agglutinate in neither O1 nor O139 antiserum may be non-O1, non-O139 strains of *V. cholerae* or other closely related vibrios (such as *V. mimicus*). Definitive identification of such strains may require the services of a reference laboratory, but is not necessary if the only concern is cholera. Strains that agglutinate in O1 antiserum can be further characterized as serotype Inaba or Ogawa by using monovalent antisera.

For environmental or food specimens, in which the number of *V. cholerae* organisms may be much lower than in stools, an enrichment step is often necessary. Incubating the specimen in alkaline–peptone broth for 8 hr takes advantage of the affinity *V. cholerae* has for alkaline environments; the broth is subsequently plated on TCBS.[12]

The O1 or O139 strains should be further characterized by whether or not they produce cholera toxin. This was originally measured by the ability of supernatant from a broth culture to induce the outpouring of fluid in the rabbit ileal loop, but is now detected by tissue culture assay, latex bead agglutination, or by enzyme-linked immunosorbent assay.[12]

Strains can be further characterized by biotype. However, because classical biotype is restricted to coastal Bangladesh, the need for biotyping is minimal.

Within biotype El Tor, subtypes can be defined by using traditional and molecular techniques (see Section 4). Subtyping is of value in epidemiological investigations to help determine the source of infecting strains.

Some more rapid presumptive diagnostic methods exist. The characteristic darting "shooting star" motility of vibrios can be observed by microscopy of a wet mount of fresh feces and halts immediately if O1 antiserum is added to the slide.[16] A diagnostic test based on colorimetric immunoassay detection of O1 antigen has been marketed recently and offers rapid presumptive diagnosis in the field without microscopy.[17] The efficiency of this test equals that of traditional microbiological methods; using the test provides greater speed of diagnosis at higher cost. Rapid methods do not yield a living organism for confirmatory or antimicrobial resistance testing. Since a patient with severe diarrhea requires rehydration therapy whether or not cholera is confirmed, using the rapid test should not affect management of the individual patient. Rapid diagnosis may prove most useful when it is linked to public health actions that slow spread of an epidemic.

3.4.2. Serological and Immunologic Diagnostic Methods. The human immune response to infection with toxigenic *V. cholerae* O1 infection has been well characterized.[18] Within 10 days, vibriocidal antibodies appear in the serum, which, like viral neutralizing antibody, rapidly kill target *V. cholerae* O1. This response begins to decline by 1 month and then disappears after a year. There is no difference between antibodies evoked by Ogawa or Inaba strains, though in general, classical strains appear to evoke higher antibody responses than El Tor strains. The somewhat slower antitoxic response peaks by 21–28 days after exposure and remains elevated for several years.

Serodiagnosis of the single case depends on demonstration of a fourfold rise in vibriocidal titers between early and convalescent sera or a fourfold fall between convalescent and late convalescent sera.[12] Detecting antitoxin is suggestive evidence and is helpful when trying to distinguish between vaccine-induced and natural immunity (if the vaccine does not contain toxin subunits). However, similar antibodies appear after infection with *Escherichia coli* producing heat-stable enterotoxin (ETEC-ST). Methods for distinguishing the two responses exist and are applicable in population surveys, but they may not resolve the isolated case.[19]

The immune response to infection with toxigenic *V. cholerae* O139 is incompletely understood.[20] Vibriocidal antibodies are not produced, nor are simple O139 agglutinins. The antitoxin response appears to be similar to that following O1 infection.

4. Biological Characteristics of the Organism

V. cholerae organisms are gram-negative, comma-shaped rods, adapted to life in fresh and brackish water.

They are highly motile, with a long terminal flagellum that propels them through water, and they metabolize a wide variety of nutrients. They grow most rapidly at a pH that is neutral to somewhat basic, in moist environments with traces of salt and organic matter. This includes many foods, such as cooked grains, like rice or lentils, and cooked shellfish.[21] They are exquisitely susceptible to drying, sunlight, and acid, and die rapidly at pH of 4.0 or less. Human beings are the only vertebrate host.

Serogroups of *V. cholerae* have been defined on the basis of their surface antigens. Like other gram-negative organisms, *V. cholerae* produce lipopolysaccharide O-antigen with a variety of terminal sugar groups that can be differentiated serologically. The flagellar antigens (H-antigens) do not vary within the serogroup and are not used for subtyping.[22] The O1 serogroup, until recently, was the only serogroup with recognized ability to cause epidemics. *V. cholerae* of other non-O1 serogroups can sometimes cause human illness, including diarrheal illness and lethal invasive infections, but have not spread in epidemic form. Although they are often isolated from the aquatic environment, most non-O1 *V. cholerae* serogroups are of little importance to public health, and care is needed in the interpretation of reports that do not specify the serogroup under discussion. Within the O1 serogroup, two specific antigenic serotypes, called Ogawa and Inaba, have been defined. Serotype switching has been observed within a given strain, so that these are not stable markers.[10]

A new serogroup, O139, was first detected during outbreaks of choleralike illness in 1992 in India.[23] The O139 strains appear to be derived from O1 strains of biotype El Tor, and they can cause large epidemics. Although the nature of the evolutionary event is not known, it may represent the effects of a phage. A portion of the genome coding for O-antigen synthesis has been deleted from otherwise typical El Tor O1 strains, and genes have been inserted that code for a different antigen expressed as a polysaccharide capsule.[24]

Cholera toxin is an important virulence determinant for *V. cholerae*. Within the O1 or O139 serogroups, nontoxigenic strains occasionally occur but do not cause cholera. Cholera toxin is a protein enterotoxin formed from an active A subunit of 240 amino acids, held within a pentamer ring of five B subunits, each of which has 103 amino acids.[25] The organism varies the amount of toxin produced depending on its immediate environment.[26]

Two other enterotoxins produced by *V. cholerae* O1 have been described, although their role in pathogenesis is uncertain. These are zona occludens toxin (ZOT)[27] and accessory cholera enterotoxin (ACE).[28]

Toxigenic O1 strains can be separated into two biotypes: El Tor and classical. El Tor strains agglutinate chicken red cells and lyse sheep red cells, while classical strains do neither; the two biotypes can be separated by phage susceptibility studies as well.[29] Classical strains caused global pandemics in the late 19th and early 20th centuries, but since then have been restricted to rural Bangladesh.[30] The El Tor biotype of *V. cholerae* O1 is named for a Hajj quarantine station in Egypt, where it was isolated from an asymptomatic pilgrim early in the 20th century. Its epidemic potential was debated until the beginning of the seventh pandemic in 1961. There are important epidemiological differences between the two biotypes. Compared to classical strains, El Tor strains are more likely to produce inapparent infections,[13] persist longer in the environment,[31] multiply more rapidly following inoculation into foods,[21] and evoke less complete immunity.[32]

Molecular subtyping methods have revealed a surprising diversity of subtypes within epidemic strains. Multienzyme electrophoresis identifies four main enzyme types (ET) within El Tor strains, representing the Gulf Coast, Australian, seventh pandemic, and Latin American strains; the same method showed that at least three subgroups could be distinguished in the classical biotype.[33] Ribotyping identified 9 ribotypes (RT) among 176 toxigenic El Tor strains tested.[34] With pulsed field gel electrophoresis (PFGE), 36 patterns were identified among 142 toxigenic El Tor strains tested, offering a fine-grain subtyping that is of use for epidemiological investigations.[35] The Latin American epidemic strain that was introduced in Peru in 1991 remains uniform: ET3, RT5, and PGFE pattern 38, a subtype that has yet to be identified elsewhere.[36] The seventh pandemic in the rest of the world is caused by an overlapping patchwork of strains. Recently, a second strain of *V. cholerae* O1 has spread throughout Central America, so that the Latin American epidemic is now polyclonal. This strain resembles strains found elsewhere in Asia and Romania.[36] Using the same methods, strains associated with the O139 epidemic can be divided into at least two ribotypes and four PGFE types from the beginning, indicating that the epidemic of O139 infections is caused by more than one "epidemic strain."[37]

The genes coding for cholera toxin B subunit also show diversity, and at least three subtypes exist.[38] All toxin types appear to have the same biological activity. Curiously, the Gulf Coast El Tor strains have the same B subunit type as otherwise unrelated classical strains, suggesting that toxin genes have transferred horizontally between unrelated bacteria.

Toxigenic *V. cholerae* O1 El Tor strains can persist in rivers and estuaries for long periods, indicating they have niches in nature that are independent of human fecal contamination. This persistence is best demonstrated for the unique strain found along the US Gulf Coast[39] and for that found in the rivers of northeastern Australia,[40] though other natural foci are likely to exist. The precise nature of the niche is unknown, though several clues point to an association with plankton. *V. cholerae* O1 produces chitinase, an enzyme that dissolves chitin, the structural protein of invertebrate exoskeletons.[41] This suggests they may have a niche in the digestive tracts of marine life that eat crustacea, or even a role in the growth and molting pattern of some crustacea. They can attach directly to crustacea, particularly to zooplanktonic copepods, without harming them.[42] They may persist in association with certain algae.[43] A dormant phase, the so-called "viable but noncultivable state," has been described, though it remains to be shown that bacteria can recover from this state.[44]

5. Descriptive Epidemiology

5.1. Prevalence and Incidence

In 1993, 78 countries reported cholera to the World Health Organization,[45] the greatest number of countries ever to report cholera. This is the result of epidemics in Africa, Latin America, and Asia (Fig. 2). The 376,845 cases and 6,781 deaths reported in 1993 are only a small fraction of the true total and are largely driven by Latin America (from which 209,192 cases and 2,438 deaths were reported in 1993). By June 15, 1995, 1,075,372 cases and 10,098 deaths had been reported since the beginning of the Latin American epidemic in 1991.[46] The case-fatality rate varied by continent in 1993. It was 1.2% in the Americas, 2.0% in Asia, and 3.3% in Africa.[45] These differences reflect differences in reporting (for example, an absurdly low 12 cases and no deaths were reported from Bangladesh) and differences in the delivery of medical care to cholera patients, not an attenuation of the virulence of the organism causing the epidemic in Latin America. In the Amazon, where logistics of health care delivery are daunting, cholera case-fatality rates of 13.5% have been reported.[47]

The incidence of cholera depends on the presence of the causative organism, the opportunities available for transmitting it, and the immunity of the population. Where sanitation is poor and crowded populations are previously uninfected, cholera incidence can be extremely high. However, even then, most infections are asymptomatic. It has been estimated that 2% of infections are severe, 5% are moderate, and 18% have mild symptoms; up to 75% of infections are inapparent.[13] In the first year of the epidemic in Peru, 1.5% of the population was reported to have clinical cholera,[48] and by early 1995, this had risen to 3%.[46] It is likely that most Peruvians have been infected. In remote African villages affected by outbreaks, incidence was 1.5 per 100.[49] In Bangladesh, where infection is likely to be nearly universal and repeated, silent infections maintain a relatively high level of immunity in the population. Nonetheless, the annual incidence of cholera requiring hospitalization ranges from 0.2 to 5 per

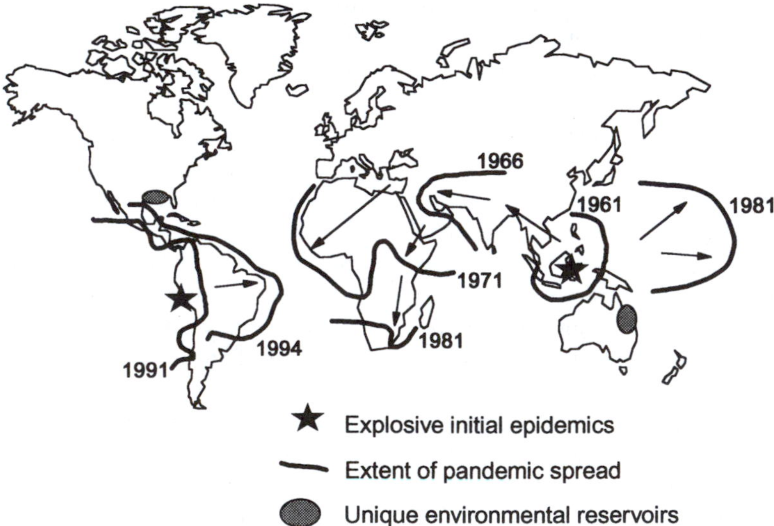

Figure 2. Global spread of the seventh cholera pandemic, 1961–1994, and recently defined areas with environmental reservoirs of toxigenic El Tor *V. cholerae* O1.

1000.[50] In contrast, along the Gulf Coast, although the organism is present in the environment, cases are sporadic and rare, and there is no secondary transmission. Incidence there ranges from 0 to 20 cases per year.[51]

Different strains of *V. cholerae* may compete with each other. In Bangladesh, where El Tor and classical biotypes of *V. cholerae* coexist, the relative prevalence of these strains varies from year to year unpredictably, possibly reflecting shifts in the underlying ecology.[30,50] The impact of O139 strains on the balance of types remains to be seen, and may offer further clues to the ecology of *V. cholerae*.

5.2. Epidemic Behavior and Contagiousness

Cholera can appear as a single isolated case, as focal outbreaks, or in large epidemics. In the developed world, even sporadic cases are rare and are usually the result of travel to the developing world or of consumption of undercooked seafood harvested from a natural reservoir, as with other *Vibrio* infections. When focal outbreaks occur, they are due to a common food source, and secondary transmission is rare.

In the developing world, where sustained transmission is possible, a single case or a focal outbreak can lead to larger epidemics. In small closed groups, such as a village or barracks, transmission halts after several weeks, when there are no more susceptible individuals or when effective control measures are introduced. In larger populations, an epidemic can persist for many months, slowing in the cooler season and then recurring the following year. In some areas, cholera then disappears; in others, it recurs regularly for many years, presumably because the organism finds an environmental niche. A long-term carrier state has been described in humans, but is extremely rare and does not play a defined role in the persistence of the organism.[52]

Throughout the 19th and early 20th century, cholera rarely lasted more than a few years in one location. However, since the beginning of the seventh pandemic, cholera has tended to persist or recur once it was introduced. Cholera remains a public health threat in Africa now, 25 years after it entered that continent in 1970, and it has persisted in many areas of Latin America since 1991. This tendency to persist may be related to the specific properties of El Tor strains. It may also be related to the far greater density and mobility of human populations now compared with 100 years ago. It means that cholera will remain an important global public health threat for years to come.

Because a large inoculum is required to produce disease, cholera is rarely transmitted directly from one person to another without the intervening contamination of food or water. Caregivers themselves are very unlikely to become infected. Episodes of nosocomial transmission are likely to be the result of contaminated water or infant formula, not direct person-to-person spread.[51] Cholera often spreads within households in the developing world. On Truk island, this was particularly likely if the first case in the household occurred in the food preparer.[53] In Calcutta, secondary cases were more likely if the household stored drinking water in a large-mouthed container, where it was easily contaminated.[54] Cholera outbreaks have occurred among persons attending funerals of cholera victims. This is not likely to be due to simple contact with the cadaver, but rather to consuming foods and beverages at a funeral meal that are prepared by bereaved family members after they prepared the corpse for burial.[55]

When an epidemic occurs, it is sometimes possible to determine the original source of the infection. This may be a traveler who arrives while still incubating the infection, or someone bringing contaminated foodstuffs with them, or even the body of a victim being brought back to an ancestral village for burial. It is rare to identify any measure that could have prevented the introduction. *V. cholerae* can also be introduced via ocean freighters, which take on ballast water in one harbor and discharge it in the next, contaminating shellfish beds near harbors in the process.[56] To decrease this risk freighters are now required by the International Maritime Organization to exchange their ballast water while at sea. The source of the unique strain that appeared in Latin America in 1991 remains unknown, though freighters from Asia are a likely possibility.[48] Throughout the world, the tides of humanity that flow from place to place can introduce cholera as long as it persists anywhere.

5.3. Geographic Distribution

The seventh cholera pandemic has affected most of the developing world (Fig. 3). Developing countries with higher levels of sanitation, such as Chile, Argentina, and Costa Rica, tend to have relatively low attack rates, and even in countries affected by epidemics, areas with better sanitation are less likely to be affected. In Mexico, cholera has a north–south incidence gradient, with the highest incidence in the poorest southern states.[48]

Unique strains of *V. cholerae* O1, biotype El Tor, persist in environmental reservoirs along the US Gulf Coast and in rivers of northeastern Australia. Strains of *V. cholerae* O1, classical biotype, are now limited to coastal Bangladesh, while El Tor biotype strains are found farther

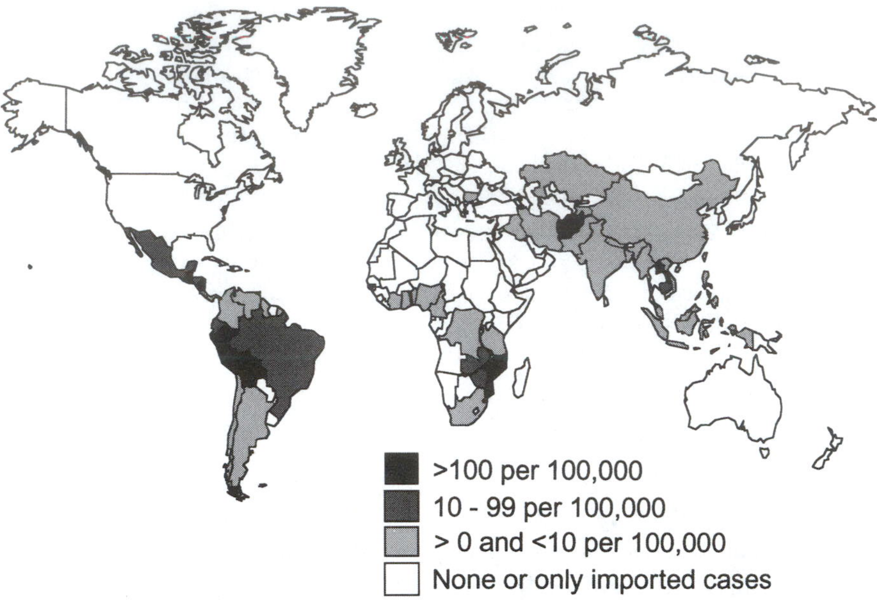

Figure 3. Incidence of cholera reported to World Health Organization, by nation, 1993.[45]

inland in the same country, suggesting that the two differ in their ecological requirements.[30]

The new epidemic strain, *V. cholerae* O139 Bengal, remains restricted to Asia (Fig. 4), but could in the future be introduced into Africa and other parts of the developing world, truly causing the eighth pandemic.

5.4. Temporal Distribution

Cholera is sharply seasonal, becoming rare or undetectable in cooler months. It is not known what determines this seasonality or how the organism survives from one season to the next. In the Latin American epidemic, cholera has increased sharply in the early summer and declines slowly in the fall. The calendar month affected varies with the hemisphere, peaking in July through September in the Northern Hemisphere and from January through March in the Southern Hemisphere.[48] Along the US Gulf Coast, the same seasonal pattern prevails.[57] In Asia, the seasonality tends to be predictable in a given location, but it is not uniform across the continent. Attempts to relate seasonality to rain, monsoon, or water temperature are inconsistent. In the 1950s, the peak season for cholera in Calcutta was May and June, just before the monsoons, while in Madras, farther south on the same coast of India, it was August and September at the end of the monsoons.[1] In rural Bangladesh, the seasonality of El Tor and classical infections differ: the peak for El Tor is October–November, and for classical biotype is in December–January.[50] Seasonal changes in vehicles of transmission or in the biological cycles of an unknown intermediate host could be important but are undocumented.

Year-to-year variation in incidence can be substantial and may also reflect shifts in underlying ecology. No general predictive rule is known. In British Colonial India, it was noted that the year following a year of drought had a higher incidence of cholera.[58] Along the Gulf Coast, the years with highest incidence also happened to be years of drought, when saltwater incursions moved further inland than usual.

5.5. Age

When cholera affects a population that has no preexisting immunity, the age and sex of cholera patients reflect exposure to infection. In Piura, Peru, where the town water and street-vended beverages made with ices were identified sources, nearly all ages were equally exposed. Incidence in the first 3 weeks of the 1991 epidemic was 1.3% among those aged 5–14 years and 1.8% among those over 15 years of age; males and females were equally affected.[59] In Italian outbreaks of 1973, transmission occurred through contaminated raw shellfish that were usually eaten by adults, so the median age of patients was 52 years and 60% were male.[60] Because gastric acidity declines with advancing age, the elderly are often more likely to have severe illness than are younger persons. In Mexico, in 1991, the incidence among those over

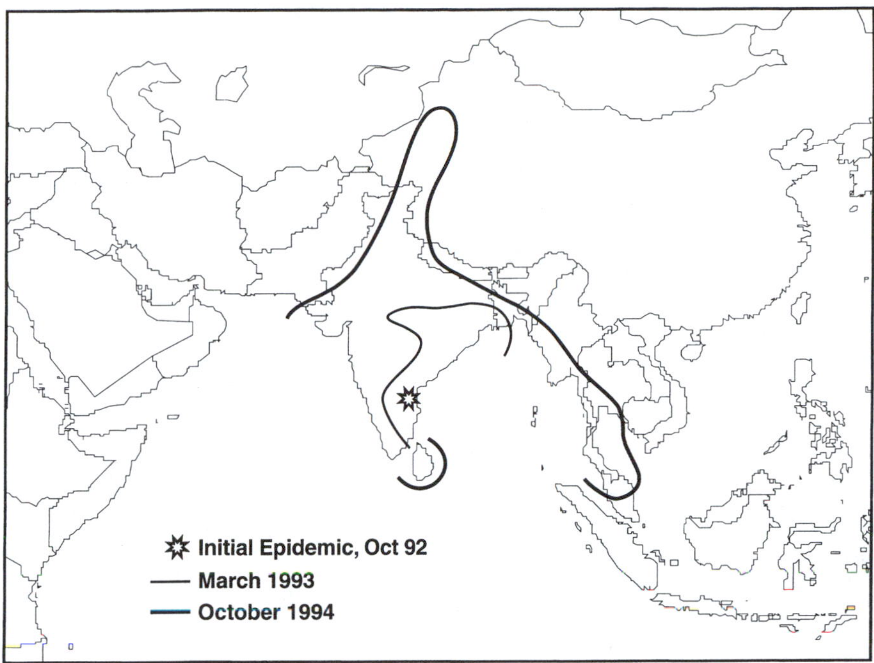

Figure 4. Spread of the epidemic of *V. cholerae* 0139 infections in Asia.

age 65 was 7.1 per 100,000, compared with 2.5 among persons aged 15 to 24.[48] Breast-feeding infants are protected, presumably because they do not consume contaminated water or food.[61]

In Bangladesh, where many adults have natural immunity that may be boosted by repeat exposure, cholera caused by *V. cholerae* O1 is more typically an illness of children, though cases in adults are not rare.[50] Breast-feeding infants are protected because they are not exposed to contaminated water and food and also because of passive protection of antibodies in maternal milk.[62] When epidemic *V. cholerae* O139 infections appeared in the Bengal area, preexisting immunity to O1 strains had little effect, and all ages were affected.[63]

5.6. Sex

The gender of the patient does not affect the outcome of infection or the rate of infection, given equal exposure.

5.7. Race

Cholera and race are not specifically linked. However, severe manifestations of cholera are strongly associated with blood group O, the frequency of which varies among races. Persons of blood group O are more likely to have severe cholera than are persons of other blood groups. In Bangladesh, where blood group O is relatively uncommon, most adults hospitalized with cholera were of blood group O.[64] It has been speculated that the reason that blood group O is so rare in this population is that cholera itself provided a selective pressure over many centuries. In the Americas, most native peoples are blood group O, so this blood group is extremely common throughout Latin America. In Peru, persons with blood group O were no more likely to be infected with *V. cholerae* than others, but if infected they were ninefold more likely to develop life-threatening diarrhea than were persons with other blood groups.[65] The reason for this strong association is unknown.

5.8. Occupation

Few occupational associations are apparent in cholera epidemics or outbreaks. Fisherfolk and harbor workers may be the first to be affected. The first case of cholera in the US Gulf Coast occurred in a shrimp fisherman in 1973.[51]

Notably absent are cases among health staff caring for cholera patients, among microbiologists, and among undertakers preparing the bodies of cholera victims for burial. The extreme rarity of such cases underscores the ease with which simple hygienic precautions prevent cholera transmission.

5.9. Occurrence in Different Settings

Cholera epidemics occur when breaks in sanitation lead to contamination of water and food consumed by many people. The most characteristic setting is the large periurban slum, where people newly arrived from rural areas outstrip the availability of basic urban services (see Section 6). Temporary gatherings have also been recurrent sites of cholera outbreaks, including religious pilgrimages and refugee encampments. Historically, the Islamic Hajj has played an important role in disseminating pandemics, as have the great religious migrations of India.(1) Cholera has not complicated the Hajj in recent years, perhaps because of efforts to provide better sanitation during the pilgrimage; pilgrimages in Bangladesh may have accelerated the spread of *V. cholerae* O139. Concern for the spread of cholera at traditional Andean pilgrimage sites, such as Copacabana on Lake Titicaca, prompted authorities to limit the size of the pilgrim population and to match it with latrine and potable water facilities; to date, pilgrimages have not been a major source of spread of cholera in Latin America.

Refugee camps in Asia and Africa have experienced large epidemics of cholera. These epidemics are most severe when the camps are just being established or are overwhelmed with a new influx of people. The sudden migration of 700,000 Rwandan refugees to fresh lava fields near Goma, Zaire in the summer of 1994, where there were no latrines or wells, led to a catastrophic cholera and dysentery epidemic that killed 5% of the population in the first 3 weeks of the camp.(66) Cholera had recurred in the region for years, suggesting there is an environmental reservoir in Lake Kivu, the water of which was drunk without chlorination. In more organized camps of Mozambican refugees in Malawi, epidemic cholera was recurrent, though with better medical care the mortality was lower. Cases were most common among the most recent arrivals to the camps, who lacked cooking gear, fuel, and water storage pots. However, cholera is not inevitable among refugees.(67) Cholera outbreaks were rare among Vietnamese refugees in Thailand and were easily controlled once the source was determined.(68)

Epidemic cholera has rarely followed natural disasters, except in the Bengal basin. In Bangladesh, epidemics of "severe diarrheal disease" occur after typhoons flood coastal regions, in areas that would have had many cholera cases even without unusual flooding.

5.10. Socioeconomic Factors

In most epidemics, cholera is associated with extreme poverty. In the developing world today, just as in the industrializing cities of Europe 150 years ago, better housing usually implies better water and safer food supplies. Behaviors that protect against cholera cost money: these include boiling water, storing it in special containers, and heating food for each meal rather than eating cold leftovers.

5.11. Other Factors

Because vibrios are exquisitely sensitive to acid, the patient's gastric acid barrier is important. Gastric acid production is decreased by gastric surgery for ulcer disease, by antacid or antiulcer medication, and in the youngest infants and those of advanced age. This risk factor can be an important determinant of who gets ill. For example, in an Italian outbreak in 1973, 27% of patients had had gastric surgery.(60) The positive impact of infection with the gastric bacterium *Helicobacter pylori*, which can induce a state of hypochlorhydria, is less well understood but may be important (see Chapter 17).

6. Mechanism and Routes of Transmission

Cholera follows ingestion of food or water contaminated with an infectious dose of the causative organisms. In epidemics, the source of contamination is usually the feces of infected humans. In sporadic cases associated with natural reservoirs, no fecal contamination need occur.

In the United States, locally acquired cholera is usually associated with eating undercooked seafood harvested on the Gulf Coast.(51) One outbreak on a Texas oil platform in the Gulf of Mexico followed contamination of rice with seawater, which itself was contaminated by the platform's sewage line; it is presumed that fecal contamination played a role.(69) Other cases have been related to foods brought from countries where cholera epidemics were occurring, e.g., two outbreaks were traced to crabs from Ecuador and an outbreak was related to fresh frozen coconut milk imported from Thailand.(51,70)

Travel-associated cases typically occur among persons who are visiting friends or relatives in their own countries of origin in the developing world. These travelers tend to be exposed to the same risks of cholera as the developing country population. Cases among more typical tourists or business travelers are extremely rare. The overall infection rate is remarkably low, approximately 1 per million air travelers to affected countries.[57] Simple precautions should prevent most of these cases (Table 2).

In the developing world, transmission of cholera has been documented through a variety of water- and foodborne mechanisms. During epidemics, infections can be spread by more than one mechanism, and the dominant source of infection may change. In an epidemic on the Gilbert Islands, the initial cases were caused by consumption of partially dried salted fish, but a month later illness was associated with eating a variety of raw clams and shrimp as well as salted fish.[71] In 1974, during a cholera epidemic in Portugal, an initial wave of cases associated with eating raw shellfish was followed by a sudden surge when a popular brand of bottled water became contaminated, thereby infecting those who drank the water precisely to avoid cholera.[72,73] In eight collaborative investigations into the mechanisms of transmission of cholera in Latin America, multiple mechanisms of transmission were identified, including different mechanisms in different cities in the same country (Table 3).

In Latin America, seven of eight collaborative investigations identified waterborne transmission as a major element of risk for epidemic cholera (Table 3). Waterborne transmission occurs when feces from an infected person contaminate a stream, lake, or shallow well used for drinking water; when municipal water supplies draw from a contaminated source; or when water that was initially clean is contaminated during or after distribution. Water pipes are often laid in the same trench as sewer pipes. If water pressure drops, because of an intermittent water or power supply, then the low pressure in the water pipes can draw sewage into the water. In this way, a few cases of cholera that contaminate sewage can multiply rapidly into a citywide epidemic, while authorities who limit their monitoring to the initial quality of water going into the piping system at the wellhead may see no need to chlorinate it.

Table 2. Precautions for Travelers to Areas with Epidemic Cholera[a]

- Drink only water you have boiled or treated with chlorine or iodine. Other safe beverages include tea and coffee made from boiled water and carbonated, bottled beverages with no ice.
- Eat only foods that have been thoroughly cooked and are still hot, or fruit that you have peeled yourself.
- Avoid undercooked or raw fish or shellfish, including ceviche.
- Make sure all vegatables are cooked—avoid salads.
- Avoid foods and beverages from street vendors.
- Do not bring perishable seafood back to the United States.

A simple rule of thumb is: "Boil it, cook it, peel it, or forget it."

[a]From CDC public information brochure, "Cholera Prevention," published May 1992. Available at the Website http://www.cdc.gov/ncidod/diseases/cholera/cholera.htm.

Because water is rarely available 24 hr a day in the developing world, drinking water is usually stored in the home. If the vessel used to store water has a wide mouth and if water is removed by scooping it out by hand, stored water is likely to be further contaminated. Increasing water contamination was measured in Trujillo, Peru in 1991: fecal coliform counts were 1 per 100 ml in water collected at the wellhead, 2 per 100 ml at public taps, and 20 per 100 ml in water stored in the home.[74] Protective practices include using a small-mouthed vessel to store water, pouring water from the vessel rather than scooping it out, treating water in the home with chlorine or by boiling, or adding citrus juice to the water to acidify it.[75]

Foodborne transmission can also occur, particularly through moist grains such as rice or millet. Transmission by foods other than seafood was identified in four of eight collaborative investigations in Latin America (Table 3). When leftover moist grains are held at ambient temperature, a few vibrios can grow to a large dose by the next meal. The risk depends on the sauces that accompany the grain. In Guinea, cholera was associated with the use of a peanut sauce with neutral pH, while an acidic tomato sauce was highly protective.[80] In Mali, cholera was transmitted by millet, a grain that usually would have been made with acidic fermented goats' milk. Because of drought, the goats were dry, and the millet permitted survival of vibrios.[49] Transmission has occurred from fruits and vegetables, which have been documented to have been irrigated with fresh sewage or splashed with sewage on the way to market.[75] *V. cholerae* can be transmitted in street-vended foods and beverages, which are often prepared in unhygienic ways and then held for many hours at ambient temperatures. In Piura, Peru, street beverages made with contaminated ice were an important source of cholera.[59] In Guatemala, frozen fruit drinks were the dominant source.[79]

Seafood can be an important source of cholera in the developing world when shellfish are harvested from heavily contaminated waters and processed with little regard to sanitation. Transmission of cholera through seafood occurred in two of eight collaborative investigations in Latin America (Table 3). Vibrios can easily survive light cooking and then grow to an infectious dose if the seafood is held for several hours at ambient temperature. In Guinea-Bissau, cholera was associated with eating

Table 3. Mechanisms of Transmission of Epidemic Cholera in Latin America Documented in Epidemiological Investigations, 1991–1993

	Peru	Peru	Peru	Ecuador	El Salvador	Bolivia	Brazil	Guatemala
Location	Trujillo	Piura	Iquitos	Guayaquil		Saipina	Fortaleza	Guatemala City
Setting	Urban	Urban	Urban	Urban	Rural	Rural	Rural	Urban
Date	3/91	3/91	7/91	7/91	3/91	2/92	6/93	7/93
Reference	74	59	75	76	77	78	[a]	79
Transmission mechanism								
Waterborne								
Municipal water	+	+		+				
Surface water			+		+	+	+	
Putting hands in water vessel	+	+						
Street vendors								
Foods		+						+
Beverages		+		+				+
Ice/ices		+						+
Other foods								
Uncooked seafood				+				
Cooked seafood				+	+			
Leftover rice		+	+					+
Fruits/vegetables			+					

[a]CDC unpublished data.

small crabs, particularly as leftovers.[55] In Peru, ice used to ship fish was not made from chlorinated water in 1991, because "it was not for human consumption," although the fish were typically eaten without cooking.[59]

In the urban developing world, it is typical to find multiple layers of transmission occurring simultaneously. For example, in a recent investigation in Manila, cholera was associated with municipal water contaminated at the periphery of the distribution system, and with street-vended foods.[81] One common implicated street food was a mussel soup made of shellfish harvested from aquaculture in a contaminated bay.

Cholera has twice affected air travelers on international flights. One outbreak occurred in 1972, on a flight from Great Britain to Australia, and another in 1992, on a flight from Argentina to Los Angeles.[82,83] Following these, the Centers for Disease Control and Prevention (CDC) advised the International Air Transport Association to stock oral rehydration solutions on international flights and to avoid serving cold salads or hors d'oeuvres prepared in cities with cholera epidemics.

Transmission of *V. cholerae* O139 has not been well studied, but is likely to be similar to that of O1. Repeated isolation from water suggest that waterborne transmission is likely. Foodborne transmission to tourists via rice has been documented.[84]

7. Pathogenesis and Immunity

The severity of symptoms varies with the dose of bacteria ingested, the effect of gastric acid, and the patient's blood type (see Section 5.7). In volunteer feeding trials, ingesting 10^6 organism with bicarbonate buffer or mixed in food regularly results in severe diarrheal illness, whereas doses of 10^9 or more are needed if the vibrios are consumed in water without buffering gastric acidity.[85] Even lower doses may result in severe illness if the bacteria are protected by the buffering action of food or if little gastric acid is present for other reasons.

Following ingestion, the bacteria pass through the stomach and reach the small intestine. In that alkaline and bile-rich environment, they attach to mucosal cells and produce cholera toxin. Toxin production is regulated by sensors that react to the surrounding environment. Once toxin is produced, the toxin B-subunits bind to specific ganglioside GM_1 receptors on the surface of intestinal mucosal cells.[86] A portion of the A subunit enters the cell and activates adenylate cyclase, producing high levels of cyclic AMP in the cell and active pumping of chloride ion into the intestinal lumen. As Cl^- is pumped into the intestine, potassium, bicarbonate, and water follow passively. The intestines fill with an alkaline, salty fluid, which is an ideal growth medium for *V. cholerae*. Diarrhea begins when the colon cannot absorb the fluid fast enough, and can reach 1 liter/hr. For the 70-kg adult, this represents a loss of 10% of body weight in 7 hr, unless fluids and electrolytes are replaced. Fluid loss leads to decreased blood pressure, and finally circulation collapses. Loss of bicarbonate leads to profound acidosis, with blood pH below 7.0. Loss of potassium leads to neuromuscular malfunction, painful limb cramps, and ultimately to cardiac arrhythmia, which may be the terminal event

Rapid replacement of lost fluid and electrolytes is the critical lifesaving treatment.[87] For the most severe cases, this is done with intravenous polyelectrolyte fluids such as Ringer's lactate. Oral rehydration solution (ORS), a carefully defined mixture of carbohydrate and electrolytes, can be used to replace losses in patients who are able to drink, saving lives for pennies. This low-cost treatment is widely available throughout the developing world as WHO ORS or UNICEF Salts and represents a major breakthrough in the treatment of cholera and other dehydrating diarrheal diseases. Standard packets of either glucose-based or rice-based solutions are mixed with a standard volume of water and drunk to prevent or correct volume depletion. The presence of the proper amount of carbohydrate drives absorption of the electrolytes by the bowel mucosa. Antibiotic treatment, with, for example, tetracycline or trimethoprim–sulfamethoxazole, is a useful adjunct to fluid therapy, decreasing fluid losses and hastening recovery, but is not sufficient treatment by itself.

The diarrhea decreases after a few days of vigorous fluid therapy, and the patient recovers as soon as the fluid and electrolyte deficits are corrected. The diarrhea stops even though the intestines are still filled with toxigenic *V. cholerae*. Following infection, the patient is resistant to subsequent challenges with *V. cholerae* O1, but this protection is less than perfect and may not last for more than a few years. Infection with classical strains provides nearly complete protection against subsequent infection with any *V. cholerae* O1, while infection with El Tor strains provides only 60–70% protection to subsequent infection with either biotype.[32] This less solid immunity may help explain why the seventh pandemic has lasted so much longer than pandemics five and six. This is also the reason that vaccines are developed from classical strains, even though they are intended to protect against El Tor. Infection with O1 strains appears to provide no subsequent protection to infection with *V. cholerae* O139, although both produce the same toxin. This suggests that antitoxic immunity plays little role in the protective response.

8. Patterns of Host Response

8.1. Clinical Features

The clinical features of cholera are the result of a profound loss of intravascular fluids and electrolytes. The illness begins as a watery diarrhea, accompanied by abdominal cramps, that typically starts 24–72 hr after ingestion of the organisms. The diarrhea becomes voluminous and in severe cases continuous. The feces are like clouded water, with flecks of mucus, and are inoffensive smelling. They have been described since Osler's time as "rice water" stools, but could better be described as looking like thin chicken rice broth. As electrolyte disturbances become more pronounced, acidosis leads to vomiting and hypokalemia produces agonizing leg cramps, particularly in older patients. The signs and symptoms of dehydration are pronounced once fluid losses exceed 5% of body weight: dry mouth, absence of tears, increasing thirst, and loss of skin turgor, leading to the so-called "washerwoman's hands." As fluid losses reach 10% of body weight, the blood pressure drops and the patient becomes obtunded, nearing death from vascular collapse. Fever is rarely pronounced, and the patient's sensorium remains clear until the very end. The disease is reversible to the moment of death, if fluid and electrolyte loses can be vigorously replaced. Transient renal failure may follow rehydration. Cholera can be particularly severe in the pregnant woman, and loss of the fetus is likely if infection occurs in the third trimester.[88] No increase in severity has been described among persons infected with human immunodeficiency virus (HIV).

Clinical manifestations of infection with *V. cholerae* O139 Bengal are similar to those of *V. cholerae* O1. However, several episodes of bacteremia have been documented with *V. cholerae* O139, as well as a case of subsequent reactive arthropathy.[84] It is possible that this organism is more invasive than *V. cholerae* O1, perhaps because of the capsule present in O139 strains.

8.2. Diagnosis

Diagnosis is made by isolation and identification of the causative organism or by demonstrating a diagnostic increase or decrease in the antibody response. In the outbreak setting, persons with similar illnesses may be presumed to have cholera once the etiology of the illness is established for a representative sample.

In the United States, cholera should be suspected and appropriate stool cultures requested from anyone with severe diarrheal illness who recently traveled to the developing world or who has ingested raw shellfish or undercooked crab.

In the developing world, in the setting of a known or threatened epidemic, presumptive diagnosis is made on clinical grounds. The report of two or more adults in the same place with severe watery diarrhea and vomiting or the report of an adult dying of watery diarrhea may be presumed to be cholera until proven otherwise. Immediate action should be taken to bring adequate supplies for treatment, prevention, and diagnosis to that location and to warn surrounding villages of the possibility of cholera. A small number of rectal swabs from persons with fresh diarrheal cases should be collected and transported in Cary-Blair transport medium to a competent laboratory.

9. Control and Prevention

9.1. General Concepts

Toxigenic *V. cholerae* is unlikely to be eradicated, as it is likely to persist indefinitely in environmental reservoirs. Crowded urban populations in the developing world provide the setting for future epidemics of cholera when the organism is introduced, and increasing international mobility makes such introductions likely. As long as the organism persists anywhere, the potential for cholera exists wherever conditions are ripe for sustained transmission.

However, epidemic cholera can be prevented. Avenues of sustained transmission have been closed already in many parts of the world. Between 1961 and 1991, 56 travel-associated cases were reported in the continental United States without subsequent spread.[56] In the United States and other industrialized nations, when a case of cholera occurs, prompt public health action is still warranted to determine the source of infection and to be sure that the feces are properly disposed of. Routine sanitation is adequate to prevent further transmission in most areas, but for some populations, including the homeless, the "colonias" along the Mexican border, and a few Native American reservations, the potential for further transmission still exists. Most populations on the North American and European continents are protected by the engineering triumps of the "Sanitary Revolution," i.e., safe water and sewage treatment systems. Similar efforts now beginning could control cholera by the early 21st century in many rapidly developing countries of Asia and Latin America.

In the rest of the developing world, where industrialization is slower, cholera prevention is an increasing challenge. A targeted health education effort may prevent illness and death by stressing the need for careful water and food handling and the need to seek medical care promptly for diarrheal illness. Emergency control measures such as boiling water are difficult to sustain. large-scale engineering solutions are too costly to build and maintain, and there is a critical need for simpler alternatives. Some promising strategies are being developed and tested. For example, because storage of drinking water in the home is nearly universal in the developing world, modification of the storage vessel to keep stored water from becoming contaminated is a simple and inexpensive strategy.[89] One strategy is to use a narrow-necked water storage container so that the water must be poured out, rather than being scooped out by hand. A simple apparatus can produce a disinfectant chlorine solution by electrolysis of salt water, using solar power. With one such machine, a village of several thousand people can treat their own drinking water and make a net profit selling surplus disinfectant to their neighbors. Larger ventures to produce a water disinfectant product for routine use in the developing world are of potential commercial interest. Closer attention to ice production in the developing world can guarantee that treated water is used to make ice, the cheapest of modern luxury goods.

Simple improvements in food preparation may also greatly reduce the risk of cholera. Acidification of sauces is routine for reasons of taste in many cultures and can be further promoted by public health authorities: tomatoes, tamarind, lemons, and yogurt can all acidify foods sufficiently that *V. cholerae* cannot survive.[90] Foods can be made safer by thorough cooking, by heating or at least acidifying leftovers, and by avoiding raw seafood harvested from dubious waters. Particular attention to the problem of street vendor sanitation can include providing safer carts; promoting the use of clean water, soap, and disinfectants; training street vendors in the elements of food safety; and educating the consumers to look for vendors who are following simple and visible precautions.

In many parts of the world, raw or undercooked seafood is a staple source of protein. Taking precautions to protect harvest waters and using clean water for processing and clean ice for shipping can help prevent seafood-borne cholera. However, as long as raw shellfish from warm waters are consumed, an irreducible minimum number of cases can still be expected because of the natural estuarine reservoirs of toxigenic *V. cholerae*.

When an epidemic of cholera appears, the first priority is to prevent death by assuring adequate treatment and by educating the population to seek treatment rapidly once a diarrheal episode begins. The success of efforts to control the epidemic depends on knowing the actual vehicles of transmission and having the tools available to block them. Because the vehicles may vary, swift epidemiological investigation, including a case–control study, may be critical to guide control efforts. In 1991, in Santiago, Chile, for example, case investigation suggested that cholera was being transmitted through use of fresh sewage to irrigate salad vegetables; halting this practice brought an abrupt end to this specific outbreak as well as decreasing typhoid fever incidence by 90%.[91] In 1974, in Portugal, successful control followed the identification of two sequential vehicles: contaminated raw shellfish and a spring used to make bottled water.[72,73] Throughout Latin America, recommendations to boil water and to avoid street-vended foods and raw seafood followed the identification of these routes early in the epidemic. Such emergency changes are not sustainable, and the persisting epidemic demands more fundamental approaches to prevention.[48]

9.2. Antibiotic and Chemotherapeutic Approaches to Chemoprophylaxis

Antimicrobial prophylaxis plays a limited role in the control of cholera. Prophylactic treatment of family members of cholera patients in the Philippines was shown to decrease the incidence of infection from 13% in the untreated group to 0% in family members taking 20 doses of tetracycline over 5 days.[92] In closed settings, such as prisons, ships, or small and isolated villages, the strategy has potential merit. However, chemoprophylaxis on any scale runs the risk of evoking antimicrobial resistance. Early in the West African epidemic, an extravagant "cordon sanitaire" strategy included forced antimicrobial treatment of all who passed through roadblocks. This had no discernible effect on the progress of the epidemic, but resulted in widespread sulfa resistance in vibrios and avoidance of established roads. In Latin America, where the practice has been to avoid chemoprophylaxis, the organism remained generally susceptible in 1995, after a million cases had been reported. An instructive exception was in Guayaquil, Ecuador, where a vigorous campaign of family chemoprophylaxis in 1991 was associated with rapid emergence of multiple resistance, which forced the strategy to be abandoned.[76] In addition to the risk of causing the emergence of resistant strains and the substantial cost of antibiotics used in this way, mass chemoprophylaxis with sulfa or tetracyclines has been associated with severe adverse reactions to the drugs and with the appearance of folk belief that the antibiotic is a form of vaccine that confers permanent protection.

9.3. Immunization

An inexpensive cholera vaccine that provided long-term protection against cholera would be an important public health tool. Efforts to develop such a vaccine have been ongoing for more than a century. To date, the best vaccines appear to be equivalent to natural infection with El Tor strains, conferring partial and temporary immunity. Three vaccines are now commercially available in some countries (Table 4), of which only the parental killed vaccine tested extensively in the early 1970s is licensed in the United States.[93] Two oral vaccines are marketed in Europe: a whole-cell killed vaccine that includes a B-subunit (WC-BS)[94–97] and a live attenuated vaccine from the Center for Vaccine Development, CVD 103-HgR.[98,99] When WC-BS was tested extensively in a field trial in Bangladesh in a location where both El Tor and classical strains were present, it had a protective efficacy in the first year of the trial of 62%.[94] Efficacy waned after 2 years, and was substantially lower among persons of blood group O,[95] among children, and against infection with El

Table 4. Characteristics of Cholera Vaccines Now in Commercial Production

Characteristic	Type	Route	Number of doses	Time to complete primary series	Efficacy	Duration
Cholera vaccine	Extract of killed organisms	Intramuscular injection	2	1 week	50%	3–6 months
Whole-cell/B subunit	Killed organisms/ B subunit of toxin	Oral	3[a]	12 weeks[a]	62% at 1 year[a,b]	2 years
CVD 103-HgR	Live attenuated organisms	Oral	1	1 day	59%	At least 6 months

[a]In Bangladesh field trials. Recent field trial in Peru used two doses at 1- to 2-week intervals, and obtained efficacy at 1–2 months of 86%.[97]
[b]Against both classical and El Tor strains. Protection against El Tor alone was reported to be lower.

Tor biotype as opposed to classical biotype.[96] In a more recent trial among Peruvian military recruits, short-term efficacy in protecting against El Tor cholera in the first 2 months after vaccination was 86%.[97] The efficacy of the CVD 103-HgR vaccine has been measured in volunteer challenge studies conducted in North America. Efficacy is 62–64% against any diarrhea when challenged with El Tor strains and 100% when challenged with classical strains.[98] Duration of protection has been documented out to 6 months, but has not been tested beyond that. Curiously, the antibody response to CVD 103-HgR is higher in persons with blood group O, though it is unclear whether they are better protected.[99] Although both vaccines are a substantial improvement over the parenteral vaccine, they are too costly and have too brief an effect for use in protecting the public health in the developing world. These vaccines are primarily marketed to international travelers, although the risk of cholera is extremely low in this group and no nation currently requires vaccination for entry.[93] Other live attenuated vaccines are under development, including vaccines against O139 Bengal strains.[100]

Cholera vaccine has not been used successfully in the epidemic setting. The risk of cholera is immediate, whereas protection afforded by vaccines begins a week or two after completion of the primary series. In an extreme example, the cholera epidemic that occurred among refugees at Goma, Zaire, was largely over in 4 weeks, before a two-dose WC-BS vaccine could have provided protection, even had a vaccine campaign commenced the day the camp was created.

The availability of imperfect vaccines leads to pressure to use them, and the issue illustrates what to expect when partially effective vaccines become available for other feared diseases such as acquired immunodeficiency syndrome (AIDS). Humanitarian impulses, coupled with the need for public health departments to "do something," encourage cholera vaccination campaigns. However, long experience has shown that once a campaign is launched, pressure to vaccinate everyone can be irresistible, and scarce public health resources are diverted from other more important activities. It will be difficult to convey the notion of partial protection to a population accustomed to thinking of vaccines as "magic bullets"; vaccinees may falsely believe themselves to be completely protected and may ignore other prevention advice. Vaccination is not the only means of preventing cholera. This means that cholera vaccines need to be shown to be less expensive and more effective than other strategies for preventing cholera before they are adopted as public health tools.

10. Unresolved Problems

Fundamental questions about the nature of the environmental reservoir remain unanswered. We do not know the nature of these niches, nor how *V. cholerae* persists from one season to the next, nor what determines the sharp seasonal increases in disease. Better ecological understanding may lead to improved prevention strategies.

Major questions remain about the bacterial pathogen itself. The mysterious advance and decline of the classical biotype of *V. cholerae* O1 and the potential for competitive interactions among the various strains are of great potential importance. Will *V. cholerae* O139 Bengal persist and continue to spread, becoming the eighth pandemic? The microbial characteristics that permit epidemic spread are undefined. The appearance of *V. cholerae* O139 shows that immunologically important changes can occur in the O-antigen without altering epidemic potential. The appearance of *V. cholerae* O139 offers a case study in the evolution of bacterial serotypes in general. This may be a bacterial example of "antigenic escape" mutation, like the changes that occur regularly in influenza viruses, an evolutionary response by a pathogen to high levels of immunity. Does this change allow this organism to spread more rapidly in a population that was previously immune to cholera because of repeated exposure to O1 strains? Will it continue to spread in less immune populations, where it may have less of an advantage over O1 strains?

Many questions remain unresolved about cholera in relation to the human environment. The development of specific and sustainable control measures is a continuing challenge. Appropriate technologies for water treatment and storage, for sanitation, and for safer food handling are likely to have a direct impact on cholera as well as on a variety of other diseases transmitted through contaminated water and food. In 1854, John Snow demonstrated that water pipes were dangerously efficient at delivering cholera throughout London. Now, throughout the developing world, poorly maintained urban water systems are just as dangerous. Rebuilding such systems depends on the confidence and participation of people in their local government, as well as on the funds for construction and repair. The development of sustainable and locally controlled means of water treatment, such as the combination of better water storage vessels and water disinfection by the consumer at the point of use, may be an interim solution that can help communities gain experience in providing necessary services for themselves.

The search for better cholera vaccines is accelerating. We are soon likely to have a substantially improved understanding of virulence mechanisms and of the nature of the protective immune response. Vaccine research is hampered by the lack of an animal host (so that volunteer trials are inevitable) and is now complicated by the appearance of *V. cholerae* O139. Vaccines may now need to be polyvalent, providing protection against both O1 and O139 serogroups. However, rapid progress in the last decade means that promising vaccine candidates are on the horizon, and the goal of sustained protection may be achievable.

Epidemic cholera is an indicator of severe underdevelopment, a sign that the basic sanitary infrastructure of a society is below a critical threshold that guarantees its citizens safe water and sewage disposal. Communities that make the necessary investments will prevent this and many other diseases that are transmitted through the same routes. Bringing about this investment worldwide, a sustained "Sanitary Revolution," is a central challenge for global public health in the 21st century. The scope of cholera prevention extends beyond public health and clinical medicine to include fisheries, agriculture, shipping, and tourist industries of many nations. Just as cholera spurred the development of sanitary reform and modern public health in Europe and America, so epidemic cholera is likely to be less and less tolerable in the growing democracies of the developing world.

11. References

1. Pollitzer, R., History of the disease, in: *Cholera*, World Health Organization Monograph Series No. 43, pp. 11–50, World Health Organization, Geneva, 1959.
2. Sudjik, D., and Redhead, D., The East is big, *Blueprint* **116:**27–33 (1995).
3. Snow, J., *Snow on Cholera, Being a Reprint of Two Papers*, The Commonwealth Fund, Oxford University Press, London, 1936.
4. Koch, R., An address on cholera and its bacillus, *Br. Med. J.* **2:**403–407 (1884).
5. Rosenberg, C. E., *The Cholera Years: The United States in 1832, 1849, and 1866*, University of Chicago Press, Chicago, 1987.
6. Kamal, A. M., The seventh pandemic of cholera, in: *Cholera* (D. Barua and W. Burrows, eds.), pp. 1–14, Saunders, Philadelphia, 1974.
7. Tauxe, R. V., and Blake, P. A., Epidemic cholera in Latin America, *J. Am. Med. Assoc.* **267:**1388–1390 (1992).
8. Koo, D., Traverso, H., Libel, M., *et al.*, Epidemic cholera in Latin America 1991–1993: Implications of case definitions used for public health surveillance, *Bull. Pan. Am. Health Organ.* **30:**134–143 (1996).
9. Vugia, D. J., Koehler, J. E., and Ries, A. A., Surveillance for epidemic cholera in the Americas: An assessment, CDC Surveillance Summaries, March 1992, *Morbid. Mortal. Week. Rep.* **41**(SS-1)**:**27–34 (1992).
10. Vugia, D. J., Rodriquez, M., Vargas, R., *et al.*, Epidemic cholera in Trujillo, Peru 1992: Utility of a clinical case definition and shift in *Vibrio Cholerae* Ol serotype, *Am. J. Trop. Med. Hyg.* **50:**566–569 (1994).
11. Centers for Disease Control and Prevention, Case definitions for public health surveillance, *Morbid. Mortal. Week. Rep.* **39:** (RR-13) (1990).
12. Bopp, C. A., Kay, B. A., and Wells, J. G., *Laboratory Methods for the Diagnosis of Vibrio cholerae*, Centers for Disease Control and Prevention, Atlanta, GA, 1994.
13. Gangarosa, E. J., and Mosley, W. H., Epidemiology and control of cholera, in: *Cholera* (D. Barua and W. Burrows, eds.), pp. 381–403, Saunders, Philadelphia, 1974.
14. Mintz, E. D., Effler, P., Maslankowski, L., *et al.*, A rapid public health response to a cryptic outbreak of cholera in Hawaii, *Am. J. Public Health* **84:**1988–1991 (1994).
15. Barrett, T. J., Blake, P. A., Morris, G. K., *et al.*, Use of Moore swabs for isolating *Vibrio cholerae* from sewage, *J. Clin. Microbiol.* **11:**385–388 (1980).
16. Benenson, A. S., Islam, M. R., and Greenough, III, W. B., Rapid identification of *Vibrio cholerae* by darkfield microscopy, *Bull. World Health Organ.* **30:**827–831 (1964).
17. Hasan, J. A. K., Huq, A., Tamplin, M. L., Siebeling, R. J., and Colwell, R. R., A novel kit for rapid detection of *Vibrio cholerae* Ol, *J. Clin. Microbiol.* **32:**249–252 (1994).
18. Levine, M. M., Kaper, J. B., Black, R. E., and Clements, M. L., New knowledge on pathogenesis of bacterial infections as applied to vaccine development, *Microbiol. Rev.* **47:**510–550 (1983).
19. Svennerholm, A.-M., Holmgren, J., Black, R., and Levine, M., Serologic differentiation between antitoxin responses to infection with *V. cholerae* and enterotoxin-producing *Escherichia coli*, *J. Infect. Dis.* **147:**514–521 (1983).
20. Morris, J. G., Losonsky, G. E., Johnson, J. A., *et al.*, Clinical and immunological characteristics of *Vibrio cholerae* O139 Bengal infection in North American volunteers, *J. Infect. Dis.* **171:**903–908 (1995).
21. Kolvin, J. L., and Roberts, D., Studies on the growth of *Vibrio cholerae* biotype El Tor and biotype classical in foods, *J. Hygiene* **89:**243–252 (1982).
22. Sakazaki, R., Bacteriology of *Vibrio* and related organisms, in: *Cholera*, 2nd ed. (D Barua and W. B. Greenough III, eds.), pp. 37–55, Plenum Press, New York.
23. Ramamurthy, T., Garg, S., Sharma, R., *et al.*, Emergence of a novel strain of *Vibrio cholerae* with epidemic potential in southern and eastern India, *Lancet* **341:**1347 (1993).
24. Manning, P. A., Stroeher, U. H., and Morona, R., Molecular basis for O-antigen biosynthesis in *Vibrio cholerae* Ol: Ogawa-Inaba switching, in: *Vibrio cholerae and Cholera* (I. K. Wachsmuth, P. A. Blake, and O. Olsvik, eds.), pp. 77–94, American Society for Microbiology, Washington, DC, 1994.
25. Spangler, B. D., Structure and function of cholera toxin and the related *Escherichia coli* heat labile enterotoxin, *Microbiol. Rev.* **56:**622–647 (1992).
26. Ottemann, K. M., and Mekalanos, J. J., Regulation of cholera toxin expression, in: *Vibrio cholerae and Cholera* (I. K. Wachsmuth, P. A. Blake, and O. Olsvik, eds.), pp. 177–185, American Society for Microbiology, Washington, DC, 1994.
27. Fasano, A., Baudry, B., Pumplin, D. W., *et al.*, *Vibrio cholerae* produces a second enterotoxin, which affects intestinal tight junctions, *Proc. Natl. Acad. Sci. USA* **88:**5242–5246 (1991).
28. Trucksis, M., Galen, J. E., Michalski, J., Fasano, A., and Kaper, J. B., Accessory cholera enterotoxin (Ace), the third toxin of a

Vibrio cholerae virulence cassette, *Proc. Natl. Acad. Sci. USA* **90:**5267–5271 (1993).

29. Kay, B. A., Bopp, C. A., and Wells, J. G., Isolation and identification of *Vibrio cholerae* O1 from fecal specimens, in: *Vibrio cholerae and Cholera* (I. K. Wachsmuth, P. A.Blake, and O. Olsvik, eds.), pp. 1–26, American Society for Microbiology, Washington, DC, 1994.
30. Siddique, A. K., Baqui, A. H., Eusof, A., *et al.*, Survival of classic cholera in Bangladesh, *Lancet* **337:**1125–1127 (1991).
31. Benenson, A. S., Ahmad, S. Z., and Oseasohn, R. O., Person-to-person transmission of cholera, in: *Proceedings of the Cholera Research Symposium* (O. A. Bushnell and C. S. Brookhyser, eds.), pp. 332–336, Public Health Service, US Department of Health, Education and Welfare, Bethesda, MD, 1965.
32. Clemens, J. D., Van Loon, F., Sack, D. A., *et al.*, Biotype as determinant of natural immunizing effect of cholera, *Lancet* **337:** 883–884 (1991).
33. Wachsmuth, I. K., Olsvik, O., Evins, G. M., and Popovic, T., The molecular epidemiology of cholera, in: *Vibrio cholerae and Cholera* (I. K. Wachsmuth, P. A. Blake, and O. Olsvik, eds.), pp. 357–370, American Society for Microbiology, Washington, DC, 1994.
34. Popovic, T., Bopp, C., Olsvik, O., and Wachsmuth, K., Epidemiologic application of a standardized ribotype scheme for *Vibrio cholerae* O1, *J. Clin. Microbiol.* **31:**2474–2482 (1993).
35. Cameron, D. N., Khambaty, F. M., Wachsmuth, I. K., Tauxe, R. V., and Barrett, T. J., Molecular characterization of *Vibrio cholerae* O1 strains by pulsed-field electrophoresis, *J. Clin. Microbiol.* **32:**1685–1690 (1994).
36. Evins, G. M., Cameron, D. N., Wells, J. G., *et al.*, The emerging diversity of the electrophoretic types of *Vibrio cholerae* in the Western Hemisphere, *J. Infect. Dis.* **172:**173–179 (1995).
37. Popovic, T., Fields, P. I., Olsvik, O., *et al.*, Molecular subtyping of toxigenic *Vibrio cholerae* O139 causing epidemic cholera in India and Bangladesh, 1992–1993, *J. Infect. Dis.* **171:**122–127 (1995).
38. Olsvik, O., Wahlberg, J., Petterson, B., *et al.*, Use of automated sequencing of polymerase chain reaction generated amplicons to identify three types of cholera toxin subunit B in *Vibrio cholerae* O1 strains, *J. Clin. Microbiol.* **31:**22–25 (1993).
39. Blake, P. A., Endemic cholera in Australia and the United States, in: *Vibrio cholerae and Cholera* (I. K. Wachsmuth, P. A., Blake, and O. Olsvik, eds.), pp. 309–319, American Society for Microbiology, Washington, DC, 1994.
40. Bourke, A. T. C., Cossins, Y. N., Gray, B. R. W., *et al.*, Investigation of cholera acquired from the riverine environment in Queensland, *Med. J. Aust.* **144:**229–234 (1986).
41. Nalin, D. R., Cholera, copepods and chitinase, *Lancet* **2:**958 (1976).
42. Hug, A., West, P. A., Small, B., Huq, M. I., and Colwell, R. R., Influence of water temperature, salinity, and pH on survival and growth of toxigenic *Vibrio cholerae* serovar O1 associated with live copepods in laboratory microcosms, *Appl. Environ. Microbiol.* **48:**420–424 (1984).
43. Islam, M. S., Drasar, B. S., and Bradley, D. J., Attachment of toxigenic *Vibrio cholerae* O1 to various freshwater plants and survival with a filamentous green algae, *Rhizoclonium fontanum*, *J. Trop. Med. Hyg.* **92:**396–401 (1989).
44. Colwell, R. E., and Huq, A., Vibrios in the environment: Viable but nonculturable *Vibrio cholerae*, in: *Vibrio cholerae and Cholera* (I. K. Wachsmuth, P. A. Blake, and O. Olsvik, eds.), pp. 117–133, American Society for Microbiology, Washington, DC, 1994.
45. World Health Organization, Cholera in 1993, *Week. Epidemiol. Rec.* **69:**205–211, 213–216 (1994).
46. Pan-American Health Organization, Cholera in the Americas, *Epidemiol. Bull.* **16**(2)**:**11–13 (1995).
47. Quick, R. E., Vargas, R., Moreno, D., *et al.*, Epidemic cholera in the Amazon: the challenge of preventing death, *Am. J. Trop. Med. Hyg.* **93:**597–602 (1993).
48. Tauxe, R., Seminario, L., Tapia, R., and Libel, M., The Latin American epidemic, in: *Vibrio cholerae and Cholera* (I. K. Wachsmuth, P. A. Blake, and O. Olsvik, eds.), pp. 321–350, American Society for Microbiology, Washington, DC, 1994.
49. Tauxe, R. V., Holmberg, S. D., Dodin, A., Wells, J. G., and Blake, P. A., Epidemic cholera in Mali: High mortality and multiple routes of transmission in a famine area, *Epidemiol. Infect.* **100:** 279–289 (1988).
50. Glass, R. I., Becker, S., Huq, I., *et al.*, Endemic cholera in rural Bangladesh, 1966–1980, *Am. J. Epidemiol.* **116:**959–970 (1982).
51. Blake, P. A., Epidemiology of cholera in the Americas, *Gastroenterol. Clin. North Am.* **22**(3)**:**639–660 (1993).
52. Azurin, J. C., Kobari, K., Barua, D., *et al.*, A long-term carrier of cholera: Cholera Dolores, *Bull. World Health Organ.* **37:**745–749 (1967).
53. Holmberg, S. D., Harris, J. R., Kaye, D. E., *et al.*, Foodborne transmission in Micronesian households, *Lancet* **1:**730–732 (1984).
54. Deb, B. C., Sircar, B. K., Sengupta, P. G., *et al.*, Studies on interventions to prevent eltor cholera transmission in urban slums, *Bull. World Health Organ.* **64:**127–131 (1986).
55. Shaffer, N., Mendes, P., Costa, C. M., *et al.*, Epidemic cholera in Guinea-Bissau: Importance of foodborne transmission, Abstract No. 1459, in: *Program and Abstracts of the 28th Interscience Conference on Antimicrobial Agents and Chemotherapy*, 1988, Los Angeles, p. 370, American Society for Microbiology, Washington, DC, 1988.
56. Centers for Disease Control and Prevention, Isolation of *Vibrio cholerae* O1 from oysters—Mobile Bay, 1991–1992, *Morbid. Mortal. Week. Rep.* **42:**91–93 (1992).
57. Weber, J. T., Levine, W. C., Hopkins, D. P., and Tauxe, R. V., Cholera in the United States, 1965–1991; Risks at home and abroad, *Arch. Intern. Med.* **154:**551–556 (1994).
58. Rogers, L., Thirty years' research on the control of cholera epidemics, *Br. Med. J.* **2:**1193–1197 (1957).
59. Ries, A. A., Vugia, D. J., Beingolea, L., *et al.*, Cholera in Piura, Peru: A modern urban epidemic, *J. Infect. Dis.* **166:**1429–1433 (1992).
60. Baine, W. B., Zampieri, A., Mazzotti, M., *et al.* Epidemiology of cholera in Italy in 1973, *Lancet* **2:**1370–1378 (1974).
61. Gunn, R. A., Kimbal, A. M., Pollard, R. A., *et al.*, Bottle feeding as a risk factor for cholera in infants, *Lancet* **2:**730–732 (1979).
62. Glass, R. I., Svennerholm, A.-M., Stoll, B. J., *et al.*, Protection against cholera in breast-fed children by antibodies in breast milk, *N. Engl. J. Med.* **308:**1389–1392 (1983).
63. Cholera Working Group, Large epidemic of cholera-like disease in Bangladesh caused by *Vibrio cholerae* O139 synonym Bengal, *Lancet* **342:**387–390 (1993).
64. Glass, R. I., Holmgren, J., Haley, C. E., *et al.*, Predispositon for cholera of individuals with O blood group; Possible evolutionary significance, *Am. J. Epidemiol.* **121:**791–796 (1985).
65. Swerdlow, D. L., Mintz, E. D., Rodriguez, M., *et al.*, Severe life-threatening cholera associated with blood group O in Peru: Implications for the Latin American epidemic, *J. Infect. Dis.* **170:**468–472 (1994).
66. Goma Epidemiology Group, Public health impact of the Rwandan refugee crisis: What happened in Goma, Zaire in July, 1994? *Lancet* **345:**359–361 (1995).

67. Hatch, D. L., Waldman, R. J., Lungu, G. W., and Piri, C., Epidemic cholera during refugee resettlement in Malawi, *Int. J. Epidemiol.* **23:**1292–1299 (1994).
68. Morris, J. G., West, G. R., Holck, S. E., *et al.*, Cholera among refugees in Rangsit, Thailand, *J. Infect. Dis.* **145:**131–133 (1982).
69. Johnston, J. M., Martin, D. L., Perdue, J., *et al.*, Cholera on a Gulf Coast oil rig, *N. Engl. J. Med.* **309:**523–526 (1983).
70. Taylor, J. L., Tuttle, J., Pramukul, T., *et al.*, An outbreak of cholera in Maryland associated with imported commercial frozen fresh coconut milk, *J. Infect. Dis.* **167:**1330–1335 (1993).
71. McIntyre, R. C., Tira, T., Flood, T., and Blake, P. A., Modes of transmission of cholera in a newly infected population on an atoll: Implications for control measures, *Lancet* **1:**311–314 (1979).
72. Blake, P. A., Rosenberg, M. L., Costa, J. B., Ferreira, P. S., Guimaraes, C. L., and Gangarosa, E. J., Cholera in Portugal, 1974. I. Modes of transmission, *Am. J. Epidemiol.* **105:**337–343 (1977).
73. Blake, P. A., Rosenberg, M. L., Florencia, J., Costa, J. B., Quintino, L. do P., and Gangarosa, E. J., Cholera in Portugal, 1974. II. Transmission by bottled mineral water, *Am. J. Epidemiol.* **105:** 344–348 (1977).
74. Swerdlow, D. L., Mintz, E. D., Rodriguez, M., *et al.*, Waterborne transmission of epidemic cholera in Trujillo, Peru: Lessons for a continent at risk, *Lancet* **340:**28–32 (1992).
75. Mujica, O. J., Quick, R. E., Palacio, A. M., *et al.*, Epidemic cholera in the Amazon: The role of produce in disease risk and prevention, *J. Infect. Dis.* **169:**1381–1384 (1994).
76. Weber, J. T., Mintz, E. D., Caniazares, R., *et al.*, Epidemic cholera in Ecuador: Multidrug resistance and transmission by water and seafood, *Epidemiol. Infect.* **112:**1–11 (1994).
77. Quick, R. E., Thompson, B. L., Zuniga, A., *et al.*, Epidemic cholera in rural El Salvador: Risk factors in a region covered by a cholera prevention campaign, *Epidemiol. Infect.* **114:**249–255 (1995).
78. Gonzales, O., Aguilar, A., Antunez, D., and Levine, W., An outbreak of cholera in rural Bolivia. Rapid identification of a major vehicle of transmission, Abstract No. 937, in: *Program and Abstracts of the 23nd Interscience Conference on Antimicrobial Agents and Chemotherapy*, Anaheim, 1992, p. 266, American Society of Microbiology, Washington, DC, 1992.
79. Koo, D., Aragon, A., Moscoso, V., *et al.*, Epidemic cholera in Guatemala, 1993: Transmission of a newly introduced epidemic strain by street vendors, *Epidemiol. Infect.* **116:**121–126 (1996).
80. St. Louis, M. E., Porter, J. D., Helal, A., *et al.*, Epidemic cholera in West Africa: The role of food handling and high-risk foods, *Am. J. Epidemiol.* **131:**719–728 (1990).
81. Lim-Quizon, M. C., Benabaye, R. M., White, F. M., Dayrit, M. M., and White, M. E., Cholera in metropolitan Manila: Foodborne transmission via street vendors, *Bull. World Health Organ.* **72:**745–749 (1994).
82. Sutton, R. G. A., An outbreak of cholera in Australia due to food served in flight on an international aircraft, *J. Hyg.* **72:**441–451 (1974).
83. Centers for Disease Control and Prevention, Cholera associated with an international airline flight, 1992, *Morbid. Mortal. Week. Rep.* **41:**134–135 (1992).
84. Boyce, T. G., Mintz, E. D., Greene, K. D., *et al.*, *Vibrio cholerae* O139 Bengal infections among tourists to Southeast Asia: An international foodborne outbreak, *J. Infect. Dis.* **172:**1401–1404 (1995).
85. Levine, M. M., Black, R. E., Clements, M. L., Nalin, D. R., Cisneros, L., and Finkelstein, R. A., Volunteer studies in development of vaccines against cholera and enterotoxigenic *Escherichia coli*: A review, in: *Acute Enteric Infections in Children: New Prospects for Treatment and Prevention* (T. Holme, J. Holmgren, M. Merson, and R. Molby, eds.), pp. 443–459, Elsevier, Amsterdam, 1981.
86. King, C. A., and van Heyningen, W. E., Deactivation of cholera toxin by a sialidase-resistant monosialosylganglioside, *J. Infect. Dis.* **127:**639–647 (1973).
87. Swerdlow, D. L., and Ries, A. A., Cholera in the Americas: Guidelines for the clinician, *J. Am. Med. Assoc.* **267:**1495–1499 (1992).
88. Hirschorn, N., Chowdhury, A. K. M. A., and Lindenbaum, J., Cholera in pregnant women, *Lancet* **1:**1230–1232 (1969).
89. Mintz, E. D., Reiff, F. M., and Tauxe, R. V., Safe water treatment and storage in the home: A practical new strategy to prevent waterborne disease, *J. Am. Med. Assoc.* **273:**948–953 (1995).
90. D'Aquino, M., and Teves, S. A., Lemon juice as a natural biocide for disinfecting drinking water, *Bull. Pan-Am. Health Organ.* **28:**324–330 (1994).
91. Alcayaga, S., Alcagaya, J., and Gassibe, P., Changes in the morbidity profile of certain enteric infections after the cholera epidemic, *Rev. Chile Infect.* **1:**5–10 (1993).
92. McCormack, W. M., Chowdhury, A. M., Jahangir, N., Fariduddin Ahmed, A. B., and Mosley, W. H., Tetracycline prophylaxis in families of cholera patients, *Bull. World Health Organ.* **38:**787–792 (1968).
93. Centers for Disease Control and Prevention, Cholera vaccine: Recommendations of the Immunization Practices Advisory Committee, *Morbid. Mortal. Week. Rep.* **37:**617–624 (1988).
94. Clemens, J. D., Harris, J. R., Sack, D. A., *et al.*, Field trial of oral cholera vaccines in Bangladesh: Results of one year of follow-up, *J. Infect. Dis.* **158:**60–69 (1988).
95. Clemens, J. D., Sack, D. A., Harris, J. R., *et al.*, ABO blood groups and cholera: New observations on specificity of risk, and modification of vaccine efficacy, *J. Infect. Dis.* **159:**770–773 (1989).
96. Clemens, J. D., Sack, D. A., Harris, J. R., *et al.*, Field trial of oral cholera vaccines in Bangladesh: Results from three-year follow-up, *Lancet* **335:**270–273 (1990).
97. Sanchez, J. L., Vasquez, B., Begue, R. E., *et al.*, Protective efficacy of oral whole-cell/recombinant-B-subunit cholera vaccine in Peruvian military recruits, *Lancet* **344:**1273–1276 (1994).
98. Levine, M. M., and Tacket, C. O., Recombinant live oral vaccines, in: *Vibrio cholerae and Cholera* (I. K. Wachsmuth, P. A. Blake, and O. Olsvik, eds.), pp. 395–413, American Society for Microbiology, Washington, DC, 1994.
99. Lagos, R., Avendano, A., Preado, V., *et al.*, Attenuated live cholera vaccine strain CVD 103-HgR elicits significantly higher serum vibriocidal antibody titers in persons of blood group O, *Infect. Immun.* **63:**707–709 (1995).
100. Mekalanos, J. J., and Sadoff, J. C., Cholera vaccines: Fighting an ancient scourge, *Science* **265:**1387–1389 (1994).

12. Suggested Reading

Barua, D., and Greenough, W. B., III (eds.), *Cholera*, Plenum Press, New York, 1992.

Feacham, R. G., Environmental aspects of cholera epidemiology I. A review of selected reports of endemic and epidemic situations during 1961–1980, *Trop. Dis. Bull.* **78:**676–698 (1981).

Feacham, R. G., Environmental aspects of cholera epidemiology III. Transmission and control, *Trop. Dis. Bull.* **79:**2–47 (1982).

Feacham, R. G., Miller, C., and Drasar, B., Environmental aspects of cholera epidemiology II. Occurrence and survival of *Vibrio cholerae* in the environment, *Trop. Dis. Bull.* **78:**866–880 (1981).

Kaper, J. B., Morris, J. G., and Levine, M. M., Cholera, *Clin. Microbiol. Rev.* **8:**48–86 (1995).

Wachsmuth, I. K., Blake, P. A., and Olsvik, O. (eds.), *Vibrio cholerae and Cholera*, American Society for Microbiology, Washington, DC, 1994.

World Health Organization, *Guidelines for Cholera Control*, Geneva, Switzerland, 1993.

CHAPTER 12

Clostridium difficile

Dale N. Gerding and Stuart Johnson

1. Introduction

Clostridium difficile produces gastrointestinal infection in humans and animals, ranging from asymptomatic colonization to diarrhea, pseudomembranous colitis, toxic megacolon, colonic perforation, and death. *C. difficile* has emerged as a major cause of nosocomial diarrhea and is the most frequently identified cause of hospital-acquired infectious diarrhea in patients.[1,2] *C. difficile*-associated disease (CDAD) is a general term used to describe the illness, which is usually diarrheal, that is caused by this organism. Pseudomembranous colitis (PMC) is a descriptive term for the inflammatory colitis with grossly visible colonic exudate composed largely of proteinaceous material and cellular debris. *C. difficile* is the most commonly identified cause of PMC. Not all patients with CDAD have PMC, but PMC is considered a more severe form of diarrheal illness caused by *C. difficile*. *C. difficile* is unprecedented in the bacteriologic world for producing disease almost exclusively in animals or humans who have been exposed to antimicrobial or antineoplastic agents.

2. Historical Background

The historical evolution of the discovery of *Bacillus difficilis* by Hall and O'Toole[3] in 1935 in the feces of asymptomatic newborn infants to the eventual linking of the organism to the new disease, "clindamycin colitis," in the 1970s is a fascinating story of the marriage of an organism without a disease to a disease without an organism. As outlined by Bartlett,[4] three diverse investigative areas, beginning with the first description of PMC by Finney[5] in 1893, the discovery of *C. difficile* by Hall and O'Toole[3] in 1935, and the description of the rodent model of antibiotic-associated colitis by Hambre *et al.*[6] in 1943, were critical to the ultimate discovery of *C. difficile* as the major cause of PMC.

Pseudomembranous colitis was recognized historically before antibiotics were discovered and was noted as a rare complication of gastrointestinal surgery. The increasing use of antibiotics was accompanied by an increase of PMC cases. Chloramphenicol and tetracycline were the most frequently implicated agents, but "staphylococcal enterocolitis" was the usual diagnosis based on the Gram's strain evidence of typical organisms in the stool. It has not been established whether *C. difficile* was the cause of at least some of this illness, but the subsequent publication of the use of oral vancomycin to successfully treat this disease is provocatively suggestive of the possibility.[7] Pathologically, staphylococcal enterocolitis involved both large and small bowel, whereas *C. difficile*-associated PMC is confined to the colon, so they may be separate diseases. In 1974, Tedesco *et al.*,[8] using endoscopy, reported an extraordinary high rate of PMC in patients who had received clindamycin, leading to an intensification of the search for the etiology.

The discovery that antibiotics produced lethal illness in guinea pigs and hamsters was first observed by Hambre *et al.*,[6] using penicillin to treat gas gangrene in guinea pigs. At autopsy these animals demonstrated a consistent finding of a dilated inflamed cecum filled with liquid stool. Although the cause of the illness was vigorously pursued, no etiology was discovered, and the connection of this animal model to human antibiotic-associated enterocolitis was not made. Cytopathic toxicity of animal stool extracts for cell lines used for viral culture led to the mistaken postulate of a viral etiology. When a similar observation was made in human stools from patients with PMC by Larson *et al.*,[9] a similar postulate was made in

Dale N. Gerding and Stuart Johnson • Chicago Health Care System, Lakeside Division, Department of Medicine, University Medical School, Chicago, Illinois 60611.

humans. Protection of animals challenged with clindamycin by giving them oral vancomycin implicated gram-positive bacteria as a cause. This led to the postulate of a toxin as the cause of the cell cytotoxicity[10,11] and eventually implicated a clostridial toxin-producing organism as the cause of both hamster and human disease.[12,13] Subsequent work disclosed that there are two large toxins, A and B, responsible for the production of clinical illness, and that the majority of clinical illness in humans occurs in hospitalized patients, particularly the elderly.[14]

3. Methodology

3.1. Sources of Mortality Data

Mortality data are based on sporadic reports from multiple hospitals and range from 0.6% to 3.5% of patients who acquire CDAD.[15–17]

3.2. Sources of Morbidity Data

CDAD and PMC are not reportable illnesses. Rates of CDAD are reported anecdotally in the medical literature primarily from institutional experiences and range from 0.3 to >22.5 cases per 1000 hospital discharges.[18–22] CDAD rates include cases of PMC, but the proportion of CDAD patients who have PMC is not clear. In one well-studied group of 67 patients with CDAD (diarrhea plus stool culture and toxin assay positive) who underwent flexible sigmoidoscopic examination, PMC was found in 51%.[14]

3.3. Surveys

Population survey data for CDAD are very limited and serological data are not useful. *C. difficile* stool culture surveys are reported sporadically. They reveal less than 5% of stools of asymptomatic adults (range, 1 to 15%) [23,24] contain the organism; however, it is commonly present asymptomatically in infants under 1 year of age (range, 15 to 70%).[25–27]

3.4. Laboratory Diagnosis

3.4.1. Toxin Detection. Detection of cell cytotoxicity in diarrheal stool that is neutralized by the addition of specific *C. difficile* antitoxin prepared from sera of immunized animals (or *C. sordelli* antitoxin, which cross-reacts with *C. difficile* antitoxin) is the most specific diagnostic test for CDAD. Most cell lines used for viral isolation are suitable for detection of the *C. difficile* cytotoxin, toxin B.[28] Proper dilution of the specimen is required for optimal results (dilutions usually range from 1:40 to 1:200); lower dilutions can result in nonspecific cell toxicity and false-positive results. Higher dilutions may result in false-negatives.[28] Sensitivity of the cell cytotoxin test ranges from 67 to 100%, somewhat lower than the sensitivity of organism culture.

Commercial enzyme immunoassays (EIA) for the detection of toxin A and/or B are also available and have undergone evaluation and publication in peer-reviewed journals. The EIA test kits employ monoclonal and/or polyclonal antibodies against the toxin(s) for detection. These tests perform acceptably for the detection of toxin but are slightly less sensitive and specific than cell cytotoxicity; however, they can be performed more rapidly.[28]

3.4.2. Organism Detection. Stool culture for *C. difficile* is the most sensitive laboratory test available, but it is not as specific as toxin testing, primarily because there are often many patients in hospitals who are asymptomatically colonized by toxigenic or nontoxigenic strains of *C. difficile*. Culture of *C. difficile* from such a colonized patient who has diarrhea from another cause could be misinterpreted as CDAD. For this reason, confirmation of the ability of an organism to produce toxin *in vitro* has been suggested as a means to improve the specificity of culture as a diagnostic test in patients who have negative stool toxins or have not had a stool toxin test performed.[28,29] Selective media containing cycloserine, cefoxitin, and fructose (CCFA) is required for the recovery of *C. difficile* from stool specimens; preplacement of CCFA plates in an anaerobic atmosphere for at least 4 hr prior to specimen inoculation enhances organism recovery.[30,31] Stool culture sensitivity is 89–100% and specificity is 84–99%.[28] Stool culture for *C. difficile* is essential for epidemiological investigation of outbreaks so that organism typing can be performed.

Polymerase chain reaction (PCR) employing arbitrary primers is a very sensitive method of organism detection; if the primers are selected from within the toxin gene sequences, it is specific for detection of toxigenic *C. difficile*.[32–35] PCR is not generally available as a diagnostic test and has not undergone rigorous clinical comparative analysis for sensitivity and specificity.

The latex agglutination test for detection of *C. difficile* protein was originally developed to detect toxin A, but subsequently was found to detect another protein: glutamate dehydrogenase.[36,37] Although rapid, inexpensive, and reasonably specific, the sensitivity of this test (58–68%) is not sufficiently high for routine laboratory use.[28]

3.4.3. Detection of Pseudomembranous Colitis. Direct visualization by sigmoidoscopy or colonoscopy is the usual method used to diagnose PMC. Small lesions may require biopsy and histological examination for diagnosis. Visualization of PMC is found in only 51–55% of patients who have diarrhea and have *C. difficile* and its toxin detected in the stool; hence, although endoscopy is essential for the diagnosis of PMC, it is not sufficient to diagnose all cases of CDAD.(14,38)

3.4.3. Pathology. Grossly, PMC appears as a studding of the colonic mucosal surface with white to yellow adherent raised plaques. The distribution of lesions usually includes the whole colon, but it may be variable with occasional rectal sparing. Lesions end abruptly at the ileocecal valve. Microscopically, the membrane is composed of fibrin, mucus, leukocytes, and cellular debris and demonstrates a point of attachment to the mucosal surface. There is a predominantly neutrophilic inflammation of the underlying mucosa, which is typically quite focal and patchy. The superficial epithelium is quite commonly eroded, with necrosis present in the upper half.(39)

4. Biological Characteristics of the Organism

C. difficile is a gram-positive anaerobic spore-forming bacillus. Spores are resistant to drying and persist in the environment for prolonged periods of time. The organism is widespread in distribution worldwide and is found in soil, hay, mud, sand, and the stools of multiple animal species including horses, dogs, cats, camels, donkeys, and cattle. The ability of the organism to produce disease is attributed to two large exotoxins: toxin A, with a molecular weight of 308 kDa, and toxin B, with a molecular weight of 207 kDa.(40) Toxin A is the largest bacterial toxin identified and possesses both enterotoxic and cytotoxic properties. Toxin A binds to carbohydrate receptors on the cell surface. The enterotoxin property of toxin A is not mediated by means of cyclic AMP as it is in cholera, but involves cell destruction as well as fluid accumulation. Cytotoxicity is less for toxin A than for toxin B on most cell lines and appears to be mediated via actin cytoskeletal disruption, probably by action on the Rho protein. Toxin A is also a potent chemoattractant for granulocytes. The toxin B receptor is unknown, but the toxin is a very potent cytotoxin, which has a similar or identical mechanism involving the actin cytoskeleton and Rho protein. Toxins A and B exhibit significant homology (44.8% identity) with the major differences at the C-terminus region of putative receptor binding. Virtually all *C. difficile* organisms either possess the genes to produce both toxin A and toxin B or lack both genes. Strains that lack the ability to produce toxins are not considered to be pathogenic and have not been associated with clinical illness.

5. Descriptive Epidemiology

5.1. Prevalence and Incidence

There are relatively few studies of the incidence of CDAD in the community setting. Most studies have been conducted in hospitals or chronic care facilities. One community-based retrospective cohort study of members of a health maintenance organization identified a CDAD incidence of 7.7 per 100,000 person years.(41) The rate of disease resulting in hospitalization was 0.5–1.0 per 100,000 person years and is comparable to the rate of 1.4 per 100,000 person years published earlier.(42) Two studies from Perth, Australia have determined the proportion of community-acquired diarrhea that is caused by *C. difficile* using stool specimens submitted to a central laboratory by general practitioners in the community as a denominator.(43,44) The incidence of *C. difficile* was 5.5% in the first study, 2.6% in the first phase of the second study, and 10.7% in the second phase following an educational program for the referring physicians.(43,44) *C. difficile* was the most common or second-most common pathogen isolated in the two studies.

The incidence of CDAD in hospitals is considerably higher than in the community and has been studied in two large teaching hospitals over a 10-year period. At the Minneapolis Veterans Affairs Medical Center, the annual CDAD incidence between 1982 and 1991 varied from 3.2 to 9.9 cases per 1000 patient discharges (0.30–0.71 per 1000 patient days).(15,22) A remarkably similar incidence was found at the Sir Charles Gairdner Hospital in Perth from 1983 to 1992, where the annual CDAD rate ranged from 0.22 to 0.55 per 1000 patient days.(45) Both hospitals had active laboratory detection programs utilizing both culture and cytotoxin testing, but the US hospital had a more rigorous CDAD clinical correlation with patient symptoms. Virtually all patients were adult males in the veterans hospital population.

Prevalence data are available for the presence of *C. difficile* in stool specimens of persons without diarrhea. For healthy adults, the prevalence rate of asymptomatic *C. difficile* carriage has been found to be under 3%.(23,27) Prevalence of *C. difficile* in a home for the aged (mean age 86 years) on three surveys was 2.3%, 2.1%, and 8.1%, whereas in an adjoining chronic care hospital it was

14.7%, 7.1%, and 10.2%, rates comparable to other reports of residents of long-term care facilities.[46] A point prevalence rate of 10.8% was found in a survey of 340 asymptomatic adult patients in the acute care Minneapolis Veterans Affairs Medical Center (D. Gerding, unpublished). The prevalence of *C. difficile* in the stool of infants under 1 year of age ranges from 15 to 70%, decreasing to adult levels by the age of 3 years.[25–27]

5.2. Epidemic Behavior and Contagiousness

Epidemics have not been described outside of institutional settings. Only individuals who have received antimicrobial or antineoplastic agents are susceptible to CDAD. Epidemics within acute and chronic care institutions are well described and have been attributed to single predominant strains of *C. difficile* as well as to a variety of strains present simultaneously.[18,19,29,47–49] Outbreaks are characterized by culture of the organism and typing by a variety of methods, which include DNA restriction endonuclease analysis (REA), pulsed field gel electrophoresis, arbitrary-primed PCR, and immunoblot methods.[18,19,33–35,47,48] Contagiousness has been difficult to assess because of the variable susceptibility of exposed persons, the widespread environmental distribution of the spores in epidemic settings, and the possible variable virulence characteristics of the organism. Animal studies indicate that the inoculum required to produce disease is probably <100 colony-forming units (CFU) in susceptible hosts who have received antimicrobials.

5.3. Geographic Distribution

C. difficile and CDAD are considered to be worldwide in distribution.

5.4. Temporal Distribution

No seasonal variation in the incidence of CDAD has been identified.

5.5. Age

The presence of *C. difficile* in stools is highest for children under 1 year of age, but these children are nearly all asymptomatic.[25–27] The rate of CDAD has been found to increase with age, being highest in the eighth and ninth decades.[23,45] The rate of cytotoxin found in stools was also shown to be highest in the ninth decade.[23] McFarland *et al.*[50] identified increased age as a risk factor for CDAD, with a relative risk of 11.77 (2.46–56.39, 95% CI) from ages 61 to 73 years and with a relative risk of 14.30 (3.27–62.51, 95% CI) over the age of 75.

5.6. Sex

Women were found to have significantly higher rates of CDAD between ages 21 and 50 years and over the age of 70 years in one study.[23] In another large hospital study, the ratio of females with CDAD to males was 1.6:1 from ages 40–59 years and 1.7–2.2:1 over the age of 70 years,[45] despite ratios of female to male patients of 0.9:1 in all but the highest decade. Other studies have shown no difference in CDAD rates between the sexes.[20,50] It has been postulated that women may receive more antimicrobial treatment because of the high frequency of urinary tract infections, and thus be at higher risk, but no data are available to support or refute that hypothesis.

5.7. Race

No race-specific attack rate data for CDAD are available. Fecal isolation rates for a Japanese population were higher (15%) than in Sweden (1.9%).[23,24]

5.8. Occupation

No occupational data regarding risk are available. Health care workers have not been noted to be at increased risk of CDAD, although we are aware of sporadic cases in health care employees. Health care workers do not have an increased rate of asymptomatic *C. difficile* colonization.[14,51]

6. Mechanisms and Routes of Transmission

The exact route of transmission is not known, but is assumed to be by way of oral ingestion of *C. difficile* spores, which are found in soil and animal feces. Nosocomial transmission accounts for the majority of CDAD cases reported in the literature. Two potential reservoirs for spread to patients are known: infected patients (symptomatic and asymptomatic) and a contaminated environment including inanimate objects. Infected patients, the environment, and health care workers are likely to be intertwined in the nosocomial transmission process, but the exact mechanism(s) by which transmission occurs still remains somewhat obscure. It is well documented that patients acquire *C. difficile* in the hospital after being admitted free of the organism.[18,19,52] The rate of acquisition over time has been shown to be linear at about 8% per week on one ward of a hospital with an annual CDAD rate that varied from 3.2 to 9.9 cases per 1000 discharges.[52] Most of these acquisitions occur asymptomatically.[18,19,52] Asymptomatic stool carriage of *C. difficile* in hospitals with this rate of CDAD has been found to be approximately 20% of all admitted patients.[14,18,19,52] By using genetic typing techniques, it has been shown that the frequency of CDAD among patients who acquire *C. difficile* in hospital is dependent on the strain acquired, but that even highly virulent strains are asymptomatic in the majority of patients.[19] Admissions of *C. difficile*-colonized patients to a hospital ward were associated temporally with the subsequent acquisition of the identical strain by other patients already on the ward.[52]

The hospital environment is contaminated with *C. difficile* spores in proportion to the status of the patient in the environment: lowest around patients who are free of *C. difficile*, intermediate in rooms of patients asymptomatically colonized, and highest in rooms of patients who have CDAD.[18,53] Persistence in the environment has been documented for 5 months.[53] Inanimate objects in the environment have been implicated as the source of transmission, including contaminated commodes, bathing tubs, and rectal thermometer handles.[54–56]

The hands of hospital personnel have been found to be contaminated with *C. difficile*, and several lines of evidence suggest that personnel transmission on the hands may be an important means of transmission.[18,53] In one outbreak, six of seven new cases of CDAD caused by a specific *C. difficile* strain occurred in patients cared for by the same surgical team caring for a long-term colonized patient with a colostomy.[19] A controlled trial of the use of vinyl gloves by health care personnel handling body substances showed a significant decrease in new CDAD cases.[57] It is not clear how personnel hands become contaminated, as both the patients and their environment could be the source.

7. Pathogenesis and Immunity

We postulate that at least three factors are required for CDAD to occur: (1) antimicrobial exposure, which presumably disrupts the normal protective colonic flora; (2) acquisition of a toxigenic *C. difficile* organism; and (3) unknown host factors that determine if CDAD or asymptomatic colonization will occur. Only two virulence factors have been identified in *C. difficile* organisms—toxin A and toxin B—and virtually all organisms either possess both toxins or neither. Nontoxigenic organisms are not considered capable of producing CDAD, but toxigenic strains appear to differ in their ability to produce CDAD, possibly on the basis of ability to produce toxins.[19,58]

Evidence for host factors in the pathogenesis of CDAD include the observation that asymptomatic colonization, including colonization with toxigenic and epidemic strains, is common and appears to be associated with some protection against subsequent CDAD[19] and the marked variation of clinical CDAD manifestations.[59] The immune response is a potentially important host factor and some indirect evidence supporting a role for immunity has been found in the pediatric population. Among children with chronic diarrhea, *C. difficile* is isolated more often among those with hypogammaglobulinemia than among those with normal immunoglobulin levels.[60] Moreover, children with chronic relapsing *C. difficile* colitis who had low levels of antitoxin A IgG showed both clinical and microbiological responses and increased levels of antitoxin A IgG following treatment with intravenous gamma globulin.[61] Patients with CDAD do develop systemic and mucosal antibody responses to toxin A.[62,63] Data regarding the association of antitoxin A and B antibody and disease manifestations, however, are conflicting. Detection of antibody to toxin B is more frequent if an enzyme-linked immunosorbent assay method is used than if neutralization is the method.[63] Patients who recover from CDAD without specific treatment have a higher rate of antitoxin B antibody than patients who receive antibiotic treatment for CDAD, but it is unclear whether protection is conferred by this antibody.[63] Some investigators have found lower antitoxin A levels in patients with prolonged diarrhea and in those with relapsing CDAD than in patients with diarrhea of shorter duration and in those with CDAD limited to one episode.[64] Other investigators have found higher convalescent levels of serum antitoxin A antibody and toxin A neutralizing activity in patients with relapsing CDAD than those with one episode, suggesting that the serum immune response may reflect the severity of disease rather than influence the clinical course.[62]

8. Patterns of Host Response

8.1. Clinical Features

Most patients with symptomatic *C. difficile* infection present with diarrhea. Fever is present in 28%, abdominal pain in 22%, and leukocytosis ($> 10{,}000/mm^3$) in 50%.[14] Very rarely, patients present with no prior diarrhea and have abdominal pain and tenderness, decreased bowel sounds, and an ileus pattern on abdominal X rays. Severe complications include toxic megacolon and colonic perforation, both of which are very rare but life threatening. Rare cases of extraintestinal infection with *C. difficile* have been reported and include splenic abscess, bacteremia, osteomyelitis, cellulitis, and reactive arthritis.[65,66]

8.2. Diagnosis

The diagnostic definition of CDAD should include (1) diarrhea (variously defined as six watery stools in 36 hr, three unformed stools in 24 hr for 2 days, or eight unformed stools in 48 hr); (2) PMC visualized by endoscopy, or toxin A or B detected in stool, or stool culture positive for toxin-producing *C. difficile*; and (3) no other recognized etiology for diarrhea. In addition, a history of antimicrobial administration within the previous 8 weeks is present in nearly all patients, but is not included in the diagnostic definition, to allow comparison of antimicrobial use as a risk factor. Endoscopy is the only means to diagnose PMC, but the sensitivity of endoscopy in patients with CDAD is only 51–55%, and the procedure is costly and invasive.[14,38] Most diagnoses of CDAD are made by laboratory testing; the cytotoxin test is most specific, but the culture is the most sensitive.

9. Control and Prevention

9.1. General Concepts

Efforts to control and prevent CDAD in institutions have been frustratingly difficult and remain a major area of needed research. Control measures have been of two types: those designed to prevent the patient from acquiring the organism and those designed to minimize risk of clinical illness if the organism is acquired. Barrier precautions are recommended to prevent transmission and include use of gloves by personnel, which has been shown to be effective in one hospital trial,[57] and isolation, cohorting, and hand washing, which are recommended but have not undergone rigorous clinical trials of efficacy. Similarly, efforts to reduce environmental contamination by disinfection and cleaning with sporicidal agents have been recommended but do not have the support of well-controlled clinical trials.[21,67,68] Identification and removal of contaminated inanimate objects such as electronic rectal thermometers has been demonstrated to effectively reduce transmission.[56] Treatment of asymptomatic patients with metronidazole or vancomycin has been proposed as a means to prevent these patients from being a source of contamination of the environment and other patients, but metronidazole has been shown to be ineffective and vancomycin to be only transiently effective in reducing *C. difficile* in the stool.[69] Among the methods directed at reducing the risk of CDAD, the most effective have been control of antimicrobial usage, particularly clindamycin.[20,47]

9.2. Prophylaxis

Prophylactic treatment of patients receiving antimicrobials in order to prevent CDAD has been attempted in a clinical trial using a yeast, *Saccharomyces boulardii*, which significantly reduced antimicrobial-associated diarrhea, but did not reach statistical significance in reducing CDAD.[70] *C. difficile* antibody administered orally has been shown to be effective in the hamster model, but no human data are available.[71] Oral administration of *Lactobacillus* species has been proposed, but no data are available in humans and hamster studies show no benefit from use of yogurt.[72]

9.3. Immunizations

No immunization against CDAD has been developed.

10. Unresolved Problems

10.1. Epidemiology

The major epidemiological question that is unresolved is the mechanism of *C. difficile* transmission in health care institutions. In addition, there is a marked need for simple, rapid, and inexpensive diagnostic tests that will increase the rapidity of patient diagnosis, and thus reduce infection transmission. Much of traditional epidemiology is focused on clinical disease recognition and isolation and cohorting of the clinically ill. It is unclear what role asymptomatic patients play in the transmission process. If it were easier to identify these patients, their role in disease transmission could be better defined. Rapid, inexpensive, and sensitive organism typing methods are needed as a tool to define better the transmission of disease.

10.2. Control and Prevention

Traditional barrier methods other than wearing gloves have not been particularly effective in controlling *C. diffi-*

cile in hospitals. Efforts to more appropriately utilize antimicrobials will help to reduce undue risk to patients, but antimicrobial use in today's high-technology intensive care hospital environment is unavoidable. Vaccines and immunizations do not appear to be likely to prevent CDAD, but efforts to define better the role of immunity should be pursued. Prophylactic measures to prevent disruption of the bowel flora should also be considered.

11. References

1. Siegel, D. L., Edelstein, P. H., and Nachamkin, I., Inappropriate testing for diarrheal diseases in the hospital, *J. Am. Med. Assoc.* **263:**979–982 (1990).
2. Yannelli, B., Gurevich, I., Schoch, P. E., and Cunha, B. A., Yield of stool cultures, ova and parasite tests, and *Clostridium difficile* determinations in nosocomial diarrhea, *Am. J. Infect. Control* **16:**246–249 (1988).
3. Hall, I. C., and O'Toole, E., Intestinal flora in new-born infants, *Am. J. Dis. Child.* **49:**390–402 (1935).
4. Bartlett, J. G., Introduction, in: *Clostridium difficile: Its Role in Intestinal Disease* (R. D. Rolfe and S. M. Finegold, eds.), p. 1, Academic Press, San Diego, CA, 1988.
5. Finney, J. M., Gastro-enterostomy for cicatrizing ulcer of the pylorus, *Johns Hopkins Hosp. Bull.* **11:**53–55 (1893).
6. Hambre, D. M., Raki, G., Mcknee, C. M., and MacPhillamy, H. B., The toxicity of penicillin as prepared for clinical use, *Am. J. Med. Sci.* **206:**642–653 (1943).
7. Khan, M. Y., and Hall, W. H., Staphylococcal enterocolitis treatment with oral vancomycin, *Ann. Intern. Med.* **65:**1–8 (1966).
8. Tedesco, F. J., Barton, R. W., and Alpers, D. H., Clindamycin-associated colitis, *Ann. Intern. Med.* **81:**429–433 (1974).
9. Larson, H. E., Parry, J. V., Price, A. B., *et al.*, Undescribed toxin in pseudomembranous colitis, *Br. Med. J.* **1:**1246–1248 (1977).
10. Bartlett, J. G., Onderdonk, A. B., and Cisneros, R. L., Clindamycin-associated colitis in hamsters: Protection with vancomycin, *Gastroenterology* **73:**772–776 (1977).
11. Browne, R. A., Fekety, R., Silva, J. Jr., *et al.*, The protective effect of vancomycin on clindamycin-induced colitis in hamsters, *Johns Hopkins Med. J.* **141:**183–192 (1977).
12. Bartlett, J. G., Onderdonk, A. B., Cisneros, R. L., and Kasper, D. L., Clindamycin-associated colitis due to a toxin-producing species of *Clostridium* in hamsters, *J. Infect. Dis.* **136:**701–705 (1977).
13. Bartlett, J. G., Chang, T. W., Gurwith, M., Gorbach, S. L., and Onderdonk, A. B., Antibiotic-associated pseudomembranous colitis due to toxin-producing clostridia, *N. Engl. J. Med.* **298:**531–534 (1978).
14. Gerding, D. N., Olson, M. M., Peterson, L. R., *et al.*, *Clostridium difficile*-associated diarrhea and colitis in adults: A prospective case-controlled epidemiologic study, *Arch. Intern. Med.* **146:**95–100 (1986).
15. Olson, M. M., Shanholtzer, M. T., Lee, J. T., Jr., and Gerding, D. N., Ten years of prospective *Clostridium difficile*-associated disease surveillance and treatment at the Minneapolis VA Medical Center, 1982–1991, *Infect. Control Hosp. Epidemiol.* **15:**371–381 (1994).
16. Church, J. M., and Fazio, V. W., A role for colonic stasis in the pathogenesis of disease related to *Clostridium difficile*, *Dis. Colon Rectum.* **29:**804–809 (1986).
17. Jobe, B. A., Grasley, A., Deveney, K. E., *et al.*, *Clostridium difficile* colitis: An increasing hospital-acquired illness, *Am. J. Surg.* **169:**480–483 (1995).
18. McFarland, L. V., Mulligan, M., Kwok, R. Y. Y., and Stamm, W. E., Nosocomial acquisition of *Clostridium difficile* infection, *N. Engl. J. Med.* **320:**204–210 (1989).
19. Johnson, S., Clabots, C. R., Linn, F. V., Olson, M. M., Peterson, L. R., and Gerding, D. N., Nosocomial *Clostridium difficile* colonization and disease, *Lancet* **336:**97–100 (1990).
20. Brown, E., Talbot, G. M., Axelrod, P., Provencher, M., and Hoegg, C., Risk factors for *Clostridium difficile* toxin-associated diarrhea, *Infect. Control Hosp. Epidemiol.* **11:**283–290 (1990).
21. Struelens, M. J., Maas, A., Nonhoff, C., *et al.*, Control of nosocomial transmission of *Clostridium difficile* based on sporadic case surveillance, *Am. J. Med.* **91**(Suppl. 3B)**:**1385–1445 (1991).
22. Olson, M. M., Shanholtzer, M. T., Lee, J. T., Jr., and Gerding, D. N., CDAD rates—reply, *Infect. Cont. Hosp. Epidemiol.* **16:** 64–65 (1995).
23. Aronsson, B., Möllby, R., Nord, C.-E., Antimicrobial agents and *Clostridium difficile* in acute enteric disease: Epidemiologic data from Sweden, 1980–1982, *J. Infect. Dis.* **151:**476–481 (1985).
24. Nakamura, S., Mikawa, M., Takabatake, M., *et al.*, Isolation of *Clostridium difficile* from the feces and antibody in sera of young and elderly adults, *Microbiol. Immunol.* **25:**345–351 (1981).
25. Viscidi, R., Wiley, S., and Bartlett, J. G., Isolation rates and toxigenic potential of *Clostridium difficile* isolates from various patient populations, *Gastroenterology* **81:**5–9 (1981).
26. Tullus, K., Aronsson, B., Marcus, S., and Mollby, R., Intestinal colonization with *Clostridium difficile* in infants up to 18 months of age, *Eur. J. Microbiol. Infect. Dis.* **8:**390–393 (1989).
27. George, R. H., The carrier state: *Clostridium difficile*, *J. Antimicrob. Chemother.* **18**(suppl A)**:**47–58 (1986).
28. Kelly, P. J., and Peterson, L. R., The role of the clinical microbiology laboratory in the management of *Clostridium difficile*-associated diarrhea, *Infect. Dis. Clin. North Am.* **7:**277–293 (1993).
29. Gerding, D. N., and Brazier, J. S., Optimal methods for identifying *Clostridium difficile* infections, *Clin. Infect. Dis.* **16**(Suppl 4)**:** S439–S442 (1993).
30. George, W. L., Sutter, V. L., Citron, D., *et al.*, Selective and differential medium for isolation of *Clostridium difficile*, *J. Clin. Microbiol.* **9:**214–219 (1979).
31. Mundy, L. S., Shanholtzer, C. J., Willard, K. E., Gerding, D. N., and Peterson, L. R., Laboratory detection of *Clostridium difficile*: A comparison of media and incubation systems, *Am. J. Clin. Pathol.* **103:**52–56 (1995).
32. Kato, N., Ou, C.-Y., Kato, H., *et al.*, Identification of toxigenic *Clostridium difficile* by the polymerase chain reaction, *J. Clin. Microbiol.* **29:**33–37 (1991).
33. McMillin, D. E., Muldrow, L. L., Laggette, S. J., *et al.*, Simultaneous detection of toxin A and toxin B genetic determinants of *Clostridium difficile* using the multiplex polymerase chain reaction, *Can. J. Microbiol.* **38:**81–83 (1992).
34. Wren, B., Clayton, C., and Tabaqchali, S., Rapid identification of toxigenic *Clostridium difficile* strains by polymerase chain reaction, *Lancet* **335:**423 (1990).
35. Gumerlock, P. H., Tang, Y. J., Weiss, J. B., and Silva, J. Jr., Specific detection of toxigenic strains of *Clostridium difficile* in stool specimens, *J. Clin. Microbiol.* **31:**507–511 (1993).

36. Lyerly, D. M., and Wilkins, T. D., Commercial latex test for *Clostridium difficile* toxin A does not detect toxin A, *J. Clin. Microbiol.* **23:**622–623 (1986).

37. Lyerly, D. M., Barroso, L. A., and Wilkins, T. D., Identification of the latex test-reactive protein of *Clostridium difficile* as glutamate dehydrogenase, *J. Clin. Microbiol.* **29:**2639–2642 (1991).

38. Bergstein, J. M., Kramer, A., Wittman, D. H., Aprahamian, C., and Quebbeman, E. J., Pseudomembranous colitis: How useful is endoscopy? *Surg. Endosc.* **4:**217–219 (1990).

39. Sumner, H. W., and Tedesco, F. J., Rectal biopsy in clindamycin-associated colitis: An analysis of 23 cases, *Arch Pathol.* **99:**237–241 (1975).

40. Wolfhagen, M. J. H. M., Torensma, R., Fluit, A. C., and Verhoef, J., Toxins A and B of *Clostridium difficile*, *FEMS Microbiol. Rev.* **13:**59–64 (1994).

41. Hirschhorn, L. R., Trnka, Y., Onderdonk, A., Lee, M.-L. T., and Platt, R., Epidemiology of community-acquired *Clostridium difficile*-associated diarrhea, *J. Infect. Dis.* **169:**127–133 (1994).

42. Stergachis, A., Perera, D. R., Schnell, M. M., and Jick, H., Antibiotic-associated colitis, *West. J. Med.* **140:**217–219 (1984).

43. Riley, T. V., Wetherall, F., Bowman, J., Mogyorosy, J., and Golledge, C. L., Diarrheal disease due to *Clostridium difficile* in general practice, *Pathology* **23:**346–349 (1991).

44. Riley, T. V., Cooper, M., Bell, B., and Golledge, C. L., Community-acquired *Clostridium difficile*-associated diarrhea, *Clin. Infect. Dis.* **20**(Suppl. 2)**:**S263–S265 (1995).

45. Riley, T. V., O'Neill, G. L., Bowman, R. A., and Golledge, C. L., *Clostridium difficile*-associated diarrhoea: Epidemiological data from Western Australia, *Epidemiol. Infect.* **113:**13–20 (1994).

46. Simor, A. E., Yake, S. L., and Tsimidis, K., Infection due to *Clostridium difficile* among elderly residents of a long-term-care facility, *Clin. Infect. Dis.* **17:**672–678 (1993).

47. Pear, S., Williamson, T., Bettin, K., Gerding, D. N., and Galgiani, J. N., Decrease in nosocomial *Clostridium difficile*-associated diarrhea by restricting clindamycin use, *Ann. Intern. Med.* **120:**272–277 (1994).

48. Samore, M. H., Bettin, K. M., DeGirolami, P. C., *et al.*, Wide diversity of *Clostridium difficile* types at a tertiary referral hospital, *J. Infect. Dis.* **170:**615–621 (1994).

49. Bender, B. S., Bennett, R., Laughon, B. E., Greenough, W. B. III, *et al.*, Is *Clostridium difficile* endemic in chronic-care facilities? *Lancet* **2:**11–13 (1986).

50. McFarland, L. V., Surawicz, C. M., and Stamm, W. E., Risk factors for *Clostridium difficile* carriage and *Clostridium difficile*-associated diarrhea in a cohort of hospitalized patients, *J. Infect. Dis.* **162:**678–684 (1990).

51. Cohen, R. S., DiMarino, A. J., Jr., and Allen, M. L., Fecal *Clostridium difficile* carriage among medical housestaff, *New Jersey Med.* **91:**327–330 (1994).

52. Clabots, C. R., Johnson, S., Olson, M. M., Peterson, L. R., and Gerding, D. N., Acquisition of *Clostridium difficile* by hospitalized patients: Evidence for colonized new admissions as a source of infection, *J. Infect. Dis.* **166:**561–567 (1992).

53. Kim, K.-H., Fekety, R., Batts, D. H., Brown, D., *et al.*, Isolation of *Clostridium difficile* from the environment and contacts of patients with antibiotic-associated colitis, *J. Infect. Dis.* **143:**42–50 (1981).

54. Larson, H. E., Barclay, F. E., Honour, P., and Hill, I. D., Epidemiology of *Clostridium difficile* in infants, *J. Infect. Dis.* **146:**727–733 (1982).

55. Savage, A. M., and Alford, R. H., Nosocomial spread of *Clostridium difficile*, *Infect. Control* **4:**31–33 (1983).

56. Brooks, S. E., Veal, R. O., Kramer, M., Dore, L., Schupf, N., and Adachi, M., Reduction in the incidence of *Clostridium difficile*-associated diarrhea in an acute care hospital and a skilled nursing facility following replacement of electronic thermometers with single-use disposables, *Infect. Cont. Hosp. Epidemiol.* **13:**98–103 (1992).

57. Johnson, S., Adelmann, A., Clabots, C. R., Peterson, L. R., and Gerding, D. N., Recurrences of *Clostridium difficile* diarrhea not caused by the original infecting organism, *J. Infect. Dis.* **159:**340–343 (1989).

58. Wren, B., Heard, S. R., and Tabaqchali, S., Association between production of toxins A and B and types of *Clostridium difficile*, *J. Clin. Pathol.* **40:**1397–1401 (1987).

59. Bartlett, J. G., *Clostridium difficile*: Clinical considerations, *Rev. Infect. Dis.* **12**(Suppl. 2)**:**S243–251 (1990).

60. Perlmutter, D. H., Leichtner, A. M., Goldman, H., and Winter, H. S., Chronic diarrhea associated with hypogammaglobulinemia and enteropathy in infants and children, *Dig. Dis. Sci.* **30:**1149–1155 (1985).

61. Leung, D. Y. M., Kelly, C. P., Boguniewicz, M., *et al.* Treatment with intravenously administered gamma globulin of chronic relapsing colitis induced by *Clostridium difficilie* toxin, *J. Pediatr.* **118:**633–637 (1991).

62. Johnson, S., Gerding, D. N., and Janoff, E. N., Systemic and mucosal antibody responses to toxin A in patients infected with *Clostridium difficile*, *J. Infect. Dis.* **166:**1287–1294 (1992).

63. Aronsson, B., Granstrom, M., Mollby, R., and Nord, C.-E., Serum antibody response to *Clostridium difficile* toxins A and B in patients with antibiotic-associated diarrhea and colitis, *Infection* **13:**97–101 (1985).

64. Warny, M., Vaerman, J.-P., Avesani, V., and Delmée, M., Human antibody response to *Clostridium difficile* toxin A in relation to clinical course of infection, *Infect. Immun.* **62:**384–389 (1994).

65. Stieglbauer, K. T., Gruber, S. A., and Johnson, S., Elevated serum antibody response to toxin A following splenic abscess due to *Clostridium difficile*, *Clin. Infect. Dis.* **20:**160–162 (1995).

66. Lofgren, R. P., Tadlock, L. M., and Soltis, R. D., Acute oligoarthritis associated with *Clostridium difficile*, *Arch. Intern. Med.* **144:**617–619 (1984).

67. Kaatz, G. W., Gitlin, S. D., Schaberg, D. R., *et al.*, Acquisition of *Clostridium difficile* from the hospital environment, *Am. J. Epidemiol.* **127:**1289–1294 (1988).

68. Delmée, M., Vandercam, B., Avesani, V., and Michaux, J. L., Epidemiology and prevention of *Clostridium difficile* infections in a leukemia unit, *Eur. J. Clin. Microbiol.* **6:**623–627 (1987).

69. Johnson, S., Homann, S. R., Bettin, K. M., *et al.* Treatment of asymptomatic *Clostridium difficile* carriers (fecal excretors) with vancomycin or metronidazole, *Ann. Intern. Med.* **117:**297–302 (1992).

70. Surawicz, C. M., Elmer, G. W., Speelman, P., McFarland, L. V., Chinn, J., and Van Belle, G., Prevention of antibiotic-associated diarrhea by *Saccharomyces boulardii*: A prospective study, *Gastroenterology* **96:**981–988 (1989).

71. Lyerly, D. M., Bostwick, E. F., Binion, S. B., and Wilkins, T. D., Passive immunization of hamsters against disease caused by *Clostridium difficile* by use of bovine immunoglobulin G concentrate, *Infect. Immun.* **59:**2215–2218 (1991).

72. Kotz, C. M., Peterson, L. R., Moody, J. A., Savaiano, D. A., and Levitt, M. D., Effect of yogurt on clindamycin-induced *Clostridium difficile* colitis in hamsters, *Dig. Dis. Sci.* **37:**129–132 (1992).

12. Suggested Reading

Bartlett, J. G., Antibiotic-associated colitis, *Disease-a-Month* **30:**6–55 (1984).

Gerding, D. N., Johnson, S., Peterson, L. R., Mulligan, M. E., and Silva, J. Jr., Society for Healthcare Epidemiology of America position paper on *Clostridium difficile*-associated diarrhea and colitis, *Infect. Control. Hosp. Epidemiol.* **16:**459–477 (1995).

Rambaud, J.-C., and Ducluzeau, R. (Eds.), *Clostridium difficile-Associated Intestinal Diseases*, Springer-Verlag France, Paris, 1990.

Rolfe, R. D., and Finegold, S. M. (Eds.), *Clostridium difficile: Its Role in Intestinal Disease*, Academic Press, San Diego, 1988.

CHAPTER 13

Diphtheria

Iain R. B. Hardy†

1. Introduction

Diphtheria is an acute infectious and communicable disease caused by *Corynebacterium diphtheriae*. The organism infects primarily the respiratory tract, where it causes tonsillopharyngitis and/or laryngitis, classically with a pseudomembrane, and the skin, causing a variety of indolent lesions. If the infecting strain produces exotoxin, organ damage, especially myocarditis and neuritis, may ensue. The incidence of the disease has declined to low levels in most industrialized nations due to mass immunization with diphtheria toxoid. However, a diphtheria epidemic throughout the former Soviet Union, which began in 1990 and by the end of 1994 had resulted in over 75,000 cases, shows that it is not safe to assume that diphtheria will remain a disease of the past.

2. Historical Background

Although possibly recognized as a clinical entity by Hippocrates (4th century BC), Aretaeus of Cappadocia (2nd century AD) gave the first clear description of respiratory diphtheria, which he called Egyptian or Syrian ulcers. Aëtius of Ameda (6th century AD) gave the first description of epidemic diphtheria and mentioned palatal paralysis as a sequel. Repeated epidemics of diphtheria (which was called *garrotillo* in Spain) were reported in Western Europe from the 15th century and in the New England states of the United States from the 16th century. Samuel Bard of New York (1771) described laryngeal diphtheria in a work entitled *Angina Suffocativa*. Bretonneau (1826) gave the disease its present name, using the Greek word for tanned skin or leather, after the tough pseudomembrane, and differentiated it from other diseases of the upper respiratory tract. Klebs (1883) identified the diphtheria bacillus by microscopic examination of diphtheritic membranes and associated it with the disease, and Loeffler (1884) first cultivated the organism on artificial media, established the causal relationship of the diphtheria bacillus by producing the disease in guinea pigs, and identified asymptomatic infections (carriers) among healthy children. Loeffler observed that the organism appeared to remain localized in the membrane without systemic invasion, and hypothesized that damage to cardiac and nervous tissues was due to absorption of toxin elaborated by the organism. This was confirmed by Roux and Yersin (1888), who demonstrated that sterile filtrates of diphtheria cultures would kill guinea pigs and produce lesions identical to those that occurred after injection of the organism. Von Behring (1890–1893) showed that serum obtained from animals immunized against diphtheria toxin could be used for the prevention and treatment of the disease. For this work he received the first Nobel prize for medicine in 1901. Theobald Smith (1907) began the development of active immunization against diphtheria by reporting that durable immunity to the disease could be induced in guinea pigs by the injection of mixtures of diphtheria toxin and antitoxin. Schick (1913) introduced the skin test for susceptibility that bears his name. Ramon (1923) inactivated diphtheria toxin using formalin and heat, producing diphtheria "toxoid," which was nontoxic but able to induce protective antibodies. Vaccination with diphtheria toxoid was gradually introduced after 1930 and became universal in industrialized countries by the late 1940s. Freeman (1951),[1] Groman (1953),[2] and others demonstrated that avirulent *C. diphtheriae* were rendered toxigenic when infected by a specific β-phage. Pappenheimer, Gill, and associates (1952–1973) have

†Deceased.

Iain R. B. Hardy • National Immunization Program, Centers for Disease Control and Prevention, Atlanta, Georgia 30333.

Roland W. Sutter, M.D., assisted in reviewing this chapter.

clarified the molecular mechanisms involved in the pathogenesis of the disease.[3] The evolution of knowledge about diphtheria has been important in the history of medicine, significantly influencing the development of bacteriology, immunology, pathology, epidemiology, and public health.[4,5]

3. Methodology

3.1. Sources of Morbidity and Mortality Data

In the United States, reporting of cases of respiratory diphtheria by health care providers is mandated in all states. In some states, hospitals and other health care facilities are also required to report cases. Cases are reported electronically to the National Notifiable Disease Surveillance System (NNDSS) and published in the weekly *Morbidity and Mortality Weekly Report* (MMWR) and annually in the MMWR Summary of Notifiable Diseases. Because diphtheria is now rare, cases reported to the NNDSS are verified before publication. If the diagnosis of diphtheria is suspected, diphtheria antitoxin for treatment of the patient is usually obtained through the Centers for Disease Control and Prevention (CDC), and less commonly, directly from the manufacturer. A CDC epidemiologist follows the case to collect supplemental data and to determine whether it meets criteria for reporting. It is thus likely that reporting of recognized diphtheria cases and deaths is nearly complete. The CDC maintains a database with supplemental data on diphtheria cases including vaccination status, complications, and outcome, and publishes periodic summaries of the epidemiology of diphtheria in the United States.[6–8]

Since 1980, cutaneous diphtheria has not been reportable in the United States. However, state public health laboratories are requested to send all *C. diphtheriae* isolates from any body site, whether toxigenic or nontoxigenic, to the CDC laboratory for confirmation.

Worldwide, countries report annual numbers of diphtheria cases to their World Health Organization (WHO) regional office, and these data are collated by WHO headquarters in Geneva. The timeliness and completeness of such reporting are variable.

3.2. Surveys

Population immunity to diphtheria is evaluated by measuring serum levels of diphtheria antitoxin in a sample of the population. Assessment of immunity by skin (Schick) testing (Section 3.2.2) has been discontinued in most countries. The National Health and Nutrition Examination Survey (NHANES) is a population-based survey of a representative sample of the US civilian noninstitutionalized population, conducted by the National Center for Health Statistics. Diphtheria antitoxin levels will be determined by *in vitro* neutralization assay of approximately 15,000 sera collected during phase 1 of NHANES III (1988–1991). The testing began in August 1995 and is expected to be completed within 2 years.

Several small studies performed in the last 15 years have examined immunity to diphtheria in convenience samples of children and/or adults. Results from published reports on immunity among adults in the United States are presented in Table 1.

No carrier surveys have been performed in the United States for many years; in the United States, labora-

Table 1. Recent Published Studies of Diphtheria Antitoxic Immunity among Adults in the United States

Site	Assay	Patient group	Age group	Number tested	Percent with titer <0.01 IU/ml[a]
Urban Minnesota[75]	Passive hemagglutination	Outpatients	18–39	74	62
		Outpatients	40–59	51	90
		Residential	>60	58	84
LA County[80]	Passive hemagglutination	Senior citizen center attendees	50–80+	246	51
		Convalescent hospital patients	65–90+	111	44
Boston[79]	Neutralization	Emergency room patients	14–90+	473	20
		General hospital inpatients	14–90+	357	22
		Chronic hospital inpatients	21–90+	153	36
Baltimore[77]	Passive hemagglutination	Mothers of pediatric outpatients	13–19	74	11
			20–30	134	20
			>30	24	33

[a]Lowest level of antitoxin offering protection against diphtheria; levels of >0.1 IU/ml offer more certain protection.

tories do not screen pharyngeal specimens for *C. diphtheriae*, although this is still done in some countries such as the United Kingdom.

3.3. Laboratory Diagnosis

3.3.1. Isolation and Identification of the Organism. *Corynebacterium diphtheriae* is an aerobic, nonmotile, unencapsulated, pleomorphic, gram-positive bacillus. The organism has three biotypes—*mitis*, *gravis*, and *intermedius*—distinguished by colonial morphology and by varying biochemical and hemolytic reactions.

There are several excellent reviews of the recommended procedures for the isolation and identification of *C. diphtheriae*.[9–12] If the diagnosis of diphtheria is suspected, the laboratory should be informed, since on the traditional blood agar used for culture of respiratory specimens the organism may be overgrown or confused with nonpathogenic coryneform bacteria ("diphtheroids"). In respiratory diphtheria, both pharyngeal and posterior nasal swabs should be taken. If possible, specimens should be taken from beneath the margin of the membrane if one is present. If transport to the laboratory will be completed promptly, dry swabs are satisfactory; for periods of up to 24 hr, a general transport medium (e.g., Stuart or Amies) should be used; for longer periods, transport in silica gel sachets is recommended.[13] In stained smears, the organisms are club-shaped (Greek *korynee*, club) and may form characteristic "Chinese letter" patterns. However, diagnosis on the basis of direct smears is not reliable and should instead rely on culture and confirmatory tests.

For primary isolation, swabs should be inoculated onto both blood agar and a tellurite-containing medium, which selectively inhibits the growth of other organisms. On tellurite media, *C. diphtheriae* typically forms brownish-black or grayish-black colonies within 18–48 hr, but other organisms may also produce similar-appearing colonies. Smears of suspicious colonies can be examined under Gram's or methylene blue stain to give a presumptive report. Colonies are taken to set up toxigenicity testing and also inoculated onto Pai or Loeffler's slants for biochemical testing, in which the pattern of metabolism of sugars, nitrate, and urea are used to confirm the species and determine biotype.

Toxigenicity testing may be carried out *in vivo* by cutaneous inoculation of guinea pigs or rabbits,[14] but this is no longer frequently performed. More common is *in vitro* testing using a modified version of the immunodiffusion test originally developed by Elek.[15] In this test, an antitoxin-impregnated strip is laid along the surface of a culture plate containing Elek's medium; test and control cultures are streaked perpendicularly across the strip. Toxigenic organisms are identified by lines of toxin–antitoxin precipitate in the medium. Results are available within 24–48 hr in experienced laboratories. A recently developed polymerase chain reaction (PCR) offers promise as a more rapid toxigenicity test.[16] It appears to be sensitive and specific for screening primary isolates, although occasional false-positive toxigenicity tests have occurred in isolates with nonfunctional *tox* genes. This method has not yet been adequately evaluated for detection of the organism directly from patient specimens.

Cysteinase and pyrazinamidase are useful screening tests to distinguish *C. diphtheriae* and the other two potentially toxin-producing species, *C. ulcerans* (which may cause a diphtherialike illness) and *C. pseudotuberculosis*, from other species of the genus *Corynebacterium*.[12]

A number of molecular techniques, including DNA restriction enzyme analysis with and without use of DNA probes, ribotyping, and pulsed-field gel electrophoresis, have been used in recent years to analyze the molecular epidemiology of diphtheria outbreaks, adding to phage and serological typing further methods for characterizing strains.[17–20]

3.3.2. Serological and Immunologic Diagnostic Methods. Immunity to diphtheria presumably involves both humoral and cell-mediated immunity to multiple antigens of *C. diphtheriae*.[21] In practice, however, only the level of diphtheria antitoxin (antibodies to diphtheria toxin) is measured. Based on the level of antitoxin associated with Schick test conversion and studies of levels of circulating antitoxin in patients at the time of hospitalization with clinical diphtheria,[22–24] it is generally agreed that persons with levels below 0.01 IU/ml have no protection against diphtheria and increasing levels above that correspond to increasing levels of protection. Some authorities differentiate 0.01 IU/ml as the minimum protective level and state that levels from 0.01 to 0.1 IU/ml confer relative or partial protection, levels of ≥0.1 IU/ml provide more reliable protection, and levels ≥1.0 IU/ml confer long-term protection.[12,25] However, no level of antitoxin provides absolute protection against clinical diphtheria.[22]

Formerly, the Schick test was widely used to determine population immunity to diphtheria.[26,27] but this test is now rarely used. The test is performed by subcutaneous injection of a small standardized quantity of diphtheria toxin intradermally in one arm, with a control injection of diphtheria toxoid in the opposite arm. The result is determined after 24 to 48 hr and again 5 to 7 days after inoculation. A positive erythematous skin reaction to toxin but not to toxoid indicates susceptibility. The antitoxin level at which the Schick test conversion occurs is around 0.30 IU/ml.[28]

Several assays for determination of diphtheria antitoxin level in serum have been developed.[29] The "gold standard" tests are neutralization assays: *in vivo* tests performed in animals and the more convenient but equally accurate *in vitro* cell culture methods.[30] Assays that are simpler and/or less costly than neutralization tests include enzyme-linked immunosorbent assay (ELISA) and hemagglutination tests; but while these tests are acceptable for population surveys, they lack sensitivity compared to neutralization tests for antitoxin levels below 0.1 IU/ml, and are therefore not suitable for assessment of the individual patient.[29,31] Use of a radioimmunoassay has been reported.[32,33] This test correlated well with the Schick test and also would be acceptable for population screening; but in the limited number of samples tested in comparison with neutralization assay, there were a number of falsely high results, again limiting its usefulness for the individual patient.

The major role of serological tests is in periodic surveys to determine levels of population immunity to diphtheria. Individual immunity is assessed in two main settings: most commonly in modern practice, to determine antibody response to diphtheria toxoid in vaccine studies or as part of an immunologic assessment; and in the setting of suspected diphtheria, to determine the patient's antitoxin level before therapeutic antitoxin is administered. If this level is later found to be high, the diagnosis of diphtheria is less likely; a low level, while consistent with possible diphtheria, does not prove the diagnosis. Antibody response to diphtheria infection is unreliable for diagnosis, since many patients do not mount a significant antibody response, and available assays in the United States do not distinguish between human antibodies and equine antitoxin used for treatment.

4. Biological Characteristics of the Organism

Humans are apparently the only natural host and reservoir of *C. diphtheriae*. Toxigenic organisms have only been isolated from man and from certain domestic animals closely associated with man, such as horses, cows, sheep, and dogs. It is believed that this represents colonization of such animals due to human contact, rather than representing a source of infection for humans. Experimental infections can be induced in a variety of animals. *C. diphtheriae* is moderately resistant to physical factors such as drying; organisms can be cultured from the environment of patients[34] and may survive in dust for up to several weeks.[35]

The major virulence factor produced by *C. diphtheriae* is diphtheria toxin. Both toxin-producing (toxigenic) and non-toxin-producing (nontoxigenic) strains exist in nature. Expression of toxin depends on infection of the *C. diphtheriae* strain by a number of lysogenic corynephages, which carry the toxin gene (*tox*). Integration of phage DNA into the bacterium allows expression of toxin, which is facilitated by low iron conditions. Nontoxigenic strains can be converted to toxigenic ones *in vitro* by infection with a tox^+ phage. In addition, there have been reports of carriers simultaneously infected with toxigenic and nontoxigenic strains that appear to be identical by phage typing and DNA restriction analysis, differing only in the presence of a tox^+ β-phage.[36] This suggests that conversion of nontoxigenic *C. diphtheriae* strains to toxigenicity may occur *in vivo* in the human pharynx. If so, the *tox* gene could be introduced into a community following the arrival of a toxigenic strain both by direct spread of that strain, but also indirectly by release of the tox^+ phage, which then may spread within the resident population of circulating nontoxigenic strains.[36]

Additional virulence factors that have been described include two cell wall components: K antigens, which appear to be important in the establishment of infection, and a glycolipid named "cord factor," which disrupts mitochondrial function.[37]

Nontoxigenic *C. diphtheriae* may cause pharyngitis without a membrane[34] and a localized diphtherialike membranous tonsillopharyngitis.[24] Although such patients do not suffer toxin-induced complications such as myocarditis and neuritis, their illness may sometimes be severe and occasional deaths are reported.[8,24] Nontoxigenic *C. diphtheriae* may cause invasive disease, including endocarditis and arthritis. Such patients usually, but not invariably, have underlying risk factors.[38–41]

Resistance of *C. diphtheriae* to penicillin has not been demonstrated,[42–45] but organisms resistant to erythromycin, clindamycin, and tetracycline have been described.[46–49] There is one report of erythromycin resistance in four strains isolated from respiratory carriers after a 7-day course of erythromycin.[50] The other reported erythromycin-resistant isolates have been cutaneous isolates, with plasmid-mediated resistance, and associated with previous receipt of erythromycin by the patient or with widespread use of this antibiotic for treatment of pyoderma in the community.[51]

5. Descriptive Epidemiology

5.1. Prevalence and Incidence

In industrialized nations, until the 1920s to 1930s, up to 10% of children in urban areas developed clinical diphtheria. Asymptomatic infection was even more common, and by 15 years of age, 70–80% of children in cities such as New York, Baltimore, and London were immune to diphtheria.(27,52,53) Diphtheria incidence in the United States (but not in England and Wales) declined before the advent of widespread diphtheria vaccination, probably because transmission was reduced as improving social conditions resulted in reduced crowding and improved hygiene. The increasing implementation of diphtheria toxoid vaccination from the late 1920s and its universal use from the late 1940s led to a steady decline in diphtheria incidence.

In the United States, the highest number of diphtheria cases reported since national reporting began in 1920 was 206,939 in 1921, an incidence rate of 191 per 100,000 population. The same year, 15,520 deaths from diphtheria were reported (mortality rate 14.3 per 100,000 population, case fatality ratio 7.5%). Over subsequent decades, diphtheria incidence and mortality rates progressively decreased, while the case fatality rate remained little changed (Fig. 1).(8) Lower case fatality ratios during the 1970s reflected the increased proportion of cutaneous diphtheria cases, which are rarely fatal, reported during that period. The last major outbreak of diphtheria in the United States occurred in King County, Washington, from 1972 to 1982.(51) Of 1100 cases identified during the outbreak, 947 (86%) were cutaneous infections. From 1980 to 1994, a total of 42 cases of diphtheria were reported in the United States, of which 38 were nasopharyngeal cases (average annual incidence 0.001/100,000), two were cutaneous, and two were infections of other sites. Four (10.5%) of the nasopharyngeal cases were fatal. Of the nasopharyngeal cases (Fig. 2), 15 (39%) were confirmed by culture (14 toxigenic and one nontoxigenic strain). The last culture-positive case of diphtheria reported in the United States that was not known to be associated with importation of the organism occurred in 1988.

In less developed nations, diphtheria vaccination was introduced with the Expanded Programme on Immunization (EPI) in the late 1970s. Before this, it was estimated that close to 1 million cases of diphtheria occurred annually in developing countries, with from 50,000 to 60,000 deaths.(54) Until the 1990s, reported diphtheria was decreasing in all regions, and eradication of diphtheria was considered possible.(55) However, since 1990, epidemic diphtheria has returned to the new independent states of the former Soviet Union (Fig. 3).(56) As few as 198 cases (0.08 per 100,000 population) were reported in the entire USSR in 1976; in 1989, 839 cases. The epidemic began in Russia in 1990, and spread to Ukraine in 1991, and in 1993 to 1994, spread to 12 of the 13 remaining new independent states. In 1994, 47,808 cases were reported, of which 1,746 were fatal. This total represents 80% of the diphtheria cases reported worldwide in 1994.

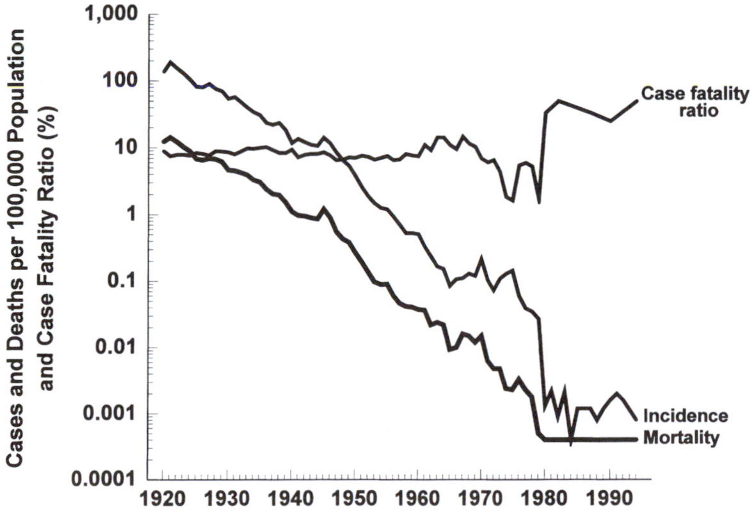

Figure 1. Diphtheria, United States, 1920–1994: Incidence and mortality rate per 100,000 population, and case fatality ratio. The case fatality ratio for the period 1980 to 1994 averaged 9.5% (4 deaths among 42 total cases); but because of the small number of cases, it fluctuated widely from year to year when calculated on an annual basis.

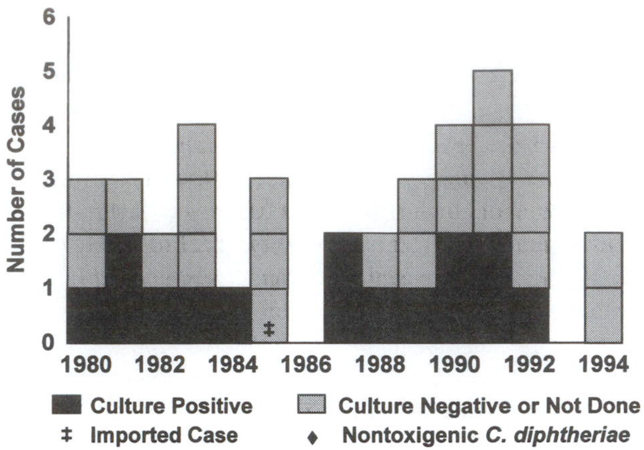

Figure 2. Respiratory diphtheria, United States, 1980–1994. Cases by year and culture status.

A hypothesis to explain why a dramatic drop in the incidence of diphtheria has followed use of a vaccine that induces immunity only to the *tox* gene of *C. diphtheriae* has been advanced by Pappenheimer.(3) The *tox* gene is not essential to the growth of the organism, but likely confers upon it a selective advantage in nonimmune populations. The toxin, by producing tissue necrosis and a site for greater replication of the bacterium in diphtheria cases, facilitates its spread to other susceptible persons. However, in an immune population, infection with toxigenic *C. diphtheriae* does not lead to clinical disease, and this selective advantage is lost, which leads to a reduction in the circulation of toxigenic *C. diphtheriae*. Pappenheimer cites data from Romania in support of this theory. Routine diphtheria immunization began in Romania in 1958, and within several years, the percentage of Schick-negative (immune) individuals in the population had increased from 60% to 97%. The incidence of diphtheria fell rapidly to very low levels. Analysis of *C. diphtheriae* isolates from carriers revealed that, lagging behind the fall in diphtheria incidence, the proportion of strains that were toxigenic fell from 87% in 1958 to only 4% in 1972. Other authors have reported falling carriage rates of toxigenic *C. diphtheriae* in the vaccine era.[21]

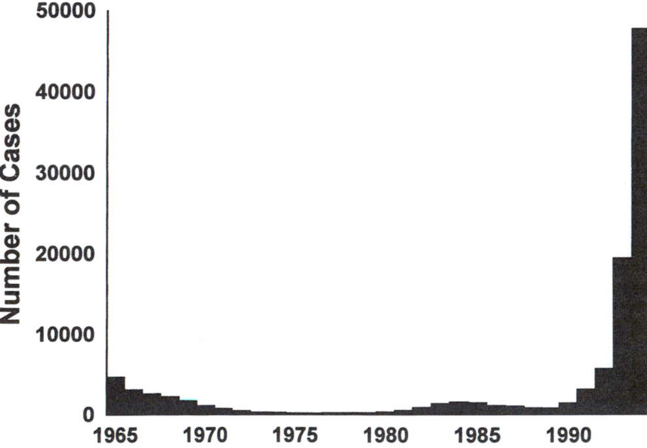

Figure 3. Diphtheria cases in the new independent states of the former Soviet Union, 1965–1995.

There are no current data from the United States, and few worldwide, on the prevalence of carriage with either toxigenic or nontoxigenic *C. diphtheriae*. However, it is believed that toxigenic *C. diphtheriae* has been virtually eliminated from the United States and many other industrialized countries. In King County, Seattle, the site of the last major outbreak of diphtheria in the United States from 1972 to 1982, skin lesions of indigent adults were frequently cultured for several years after the outbreak. From 1984 to 1993, a total of 60 *C. diphtheriae* strains were isolated, of which only two (one each in 1987 and 1988), both from imported cases, were toxigenic (Dr. Marie Coyle, personal communication). There is an impression that the number of nontoxigenic isolates has decreased: from 1984 to 1986, 34 strains were isolated, compared to only five from 1991 to 1993. However, it is not certain that the same intensity of surveillance has been maintained. Two carrier surveys of schoolchildren in Greece in 1970 and in 1980 found no toxigenic *C. diphtheriae* among over 800 children screened. The prevalence of nontoxigenic strains decreased from 3.4% in 1970 to 0.8% in 1980.[57,58] More data are needed to determine whether there has been a general decrease in the prevalence of nontoxigenic strains in industrialized countries.

5.2. Epidemic Behavior and Contagiousness

From at least the 15th century in Europe, diphtheria occurred in epidemics of varying virulence. During some periods there appeared to be a 12- or 15-year periodicity to these outbreaks, but there were also intervals of several decades with little reported diphtheria. Diphtheria incidence increased in the latter part of the 19th century in Europe and the United States, with high case fatality rates.[59] There were significant increases in diphtheria incidence during World War II in many countries, which has been attributed to dissemination of *C. diphtheriae* by military personnel returning from desert or tropical areas.[60,61] In the vaccine era, outbreaks, usually quite limited in geographic extent, have continued to occur in industrialized countries, but with decreasing frequency. However, the current epidemic in the former Soviet Union, which represents the largest epidemic since World War II, represents a significant reversal in this trend.

Both asymptomatic carriers and clinical cases are important in spread of diphtheria. In household settings, up to 27% of close contacts of cases may be found to be infected.[62] Transmission from cases is more efficient than from asymptomatic carriers, presumably because of the greater number of infecting organisms (and perhaps certain features of the infecting organism). Secondary cases are at least 10 times more common after household exposure to cases compared to household exposure to carriers.[63] Although carriers are less infectious than cases, in diphtheria endemic areas, carrier prevalence is many times higher than the prevalence of cases; therefore, carriers have a greater role in transmission. This problem is exemplified by noting that during the first decades of the 20th century, from 2 to 5% of schoolchildren in urban areas were carriers of toxigenic *C. diphtheriae*.[53,63]

5.3. Geographic Distribution

In the prevaccine era, diphtheria had a worldwide distribution. In temperate regions, respiratory diphtheria predominated, with cutaneous diphtheria being relatively uncommon. By contrast, in may (but not all) tropical and desert regions, cutaneous diphtheria was the usual form of the disease, with little or no respiratory diphtheria reported despite moderate rates of pharyngeal carriage of *C. diphtheriae*. In these countries, intense skin transmission appears to occur in the first few years of life, resulting in development of immunity to diphtheria toxin.[64–66]

Since the 1970s, cutaneous diphtheria, which had previously been uncommonly reported, has appeared to play a greater role (generally in association with cases of respiratory diphtheria) in outbreaks in the United States and Canada.[51,67–69] These outbreaks have occurred in three settings: the semitropical South of the United States; among indigent, alcoholic, urban adults; and among Native American populations.

In the 1980s and 1990s, a state of near elimination of toxigenic *C. diphtheriae* has existed in many industrialized countries. However, with the extent and rapidity of travel today, there is a continuing potential for outbreaks in such countries following importation of toxigenic strains from countries where diphtheria is still occurring.[70,71] Such an event was suspected as the reason for a series of outbreaks, with 33 cases of respiratory diphtheria, that occurred in Sweden in the mid-1980s, after the absence of indigenous diphtheria for 20 years.[19,20]

5.4. Temporal Distribution

Diphtheria has a marked seasonal variation in incidence in temperate countries. Incidence peaks in the autumn and early winter, and is at its lowest in late spring and early summer.[56,72]

5.5. Age

Until the 1970s, respiratory diphtheria was a disease of children. The highest attack rates were among preschool children and schoolchildren aged 5 to 9 years. Eighty to ninety percent of cases were among children aged less than 15 years.[53] However, in the vaccine era, there has been a shift in the age distribution toward adults.[73] In the United States from 1980 to 1994, 29 (69%) of the 42 reported diphtheria cases were among persons aged over 14 years. In the outbreak currently occurring in the new independent states of the former Soviet Union, approximately two thirds of cases are among persons aged over 14 years. This change in age distribution is explained by the fact that children are mostly protected by immunization, whereas many adults are now susceptible, because exposure to toxigenic *C. diphtheriae* has become rare and vaccine-induced immunity wanes over time unless periodic booster doses of diphtheria toxoid are given. Reports published during the last two decades indicate that between 11 and 90% of adults in North America (Table 1) and Western Europe are susceptible to diphtheria, if a diphtheria antitoxin level of <0.01 IU/ml is taken as the criterion for susceptibility.[33,74–80]

5.6. Sex

There does not appear to be a particular susceptibility of either gender to clinical diphtheria. If gender-specific differences in incidence occur, they probably reflect differences in levels of exposure of *C. diphtheriae*. In the United States, from 1959 to 1970, 53% of cases reported were among females,[7] whereas from 1971 to 1981, 56% of cases were among males.[6]

5.7. Race

In the United States during the period 1959–1970, the incidence rate among Native Americans was three times higher than persons of black race and 20 times higher than persons of white race.[7] From 1971 to 1981, incidence rates of respiratory diphtheria were approximately equal in whites and blacks, but rates in Native Americans were

100 times higher.[6] A strikingly higher incidence of diphtheria, particularly of the skin and ear, among American Indian populations has also been noted in Canada.[69] A higher incidence of diphtheria, in comparison to whites, has also been reported in Australian aborigines.[81] These racial differences likely represent mostly differences in living conditions (e.g., increased contact rates and reduced hygiene) that promote transmission of diphtheria, particularly in its cutaneous form.

Frost,[52] in his studies in Baltimore during the 1920s, reported that blacks had a lower incidence of clinical diphtheria, while (based on relatively few observations) appearing to have equivalent levels of immunity to whites as determined by Schick testing. He concluded that the ratio of symptomatic to asymptomatic infection with diphtheria was lower in blacks, due to host differences.[52] However, similar findings have not been reported by other workers.

5.8. Occupation

Medical workers exposed to diphtheria in the prevaccine era were reported as having developed higher rates of carriage of the organism compared to the general population.[53] Although cases of clinical diphtheria did occur among medical personnel, frequently the result was asymptomatic infection, since high levels of immunity were maintained by continuing exposure to diphtheria patients. More recent studies of hospital staff contacts of diphtheria cases indicate a low risk of acquisition of the organism.[62]

Diphtheria outbreaks have frequently been reported among military personnel, particularly when deployed in tropical or desert settings, and returning soldiers can import diphtheria into civilian populations.[65,82,83] The Soviet military appears to have played a role in the current epidemic of diphtheria in the former Soviet Union.[56,84] Military personnel are at increased risk of diphtheria because of crowded living conditions and, especially in combat situations, poor hygiene and frequent occurrence of skin lesions, which can become secondarily infected with *C. diphtheriae*.

5.9. Occurrence in Different Settings

The most recent outbreaks in the United States and Western Europe have characteristically involved inner-city, indigent, homeless and/or alcoholic persons (so-called "Skid Road" inhabitants).[19,23,51] Such persons are also said to experience an increased risk of diphtheria in the current outbreak in the former Soviet Union.

Institutional outbreaks have occurred in mental hospitals (where the clinical diagnosis of diphtheria may be delayed), day-care centers, and schools.[62,85–87] Schools and preschool institutions have traditionally been an important setting for transmission among children.[63,85,88,89]

5.10. Socioeconomic Factors

Low socioeconomic status is a risk marker for diphtheria, to the extent that it is associated with crowded living conditions and reduced hygiene and with reduced immunization levels.

6. Mechanism and Routes of Transmission

The organism is carried in the nose and throat[90] and appears to have a particular predilection for tonsillar tissue.[91,92] It also readily infects cutaneous lesions. Transmission occurs in close-contact settings via respiratory droplets or by direct contact with respiratory secretions or skin lesions. The organism survives on clothes and dust in the environment of cases, and fomite transmission via items such as clothes and towels may be important, particularly in settings of crowding and poor hygiene[34,93] Compared to respiratory carriers, persons with skin lesions infected with *C. diphtheriae* (which frequently are unrecognized) apparently both contaminate the environment with the bacterium and transmit it more efficiently to both the skin and respiratory tract of household and school contacts.[34,67,68] However, certain persons with nasopharyngeal infection—both cases and carriers—have been described as "spreaders" because of their apparently efficient dissemination of the organism. *C. diphtheriae* can be readily cultured from the upper lip, hands, and clothes of such individuals.[93] Foodborne transmission, most often by infected milk or milk products, has been occasionally implicated.[25,94,95]

7. Pathogenesis and Immunity

In classical respiratory diphtheria, *C. diphtheriae* colonizes the mucosal surface of the nasopharynx and multiplies locally without bloodstream invasion. The incubation period is from 1 to 7 days (usually, 2 to 5 days). Released toxin causes local tissue necrosis, and a tough, adherent pseudomembrane forms, composed of a mixture of fibrin, dead cells, and bacteria. The membrane usually begins on the tonsils or posterior pharynx. In more severe cases it spreads, extending progressively over the pharyngeal wall, fauces, soft palate, and into the larynx (and on occasions further into the trachea and bronchi), resulting in respiratory obstruction. Toxin entering the bloodstream causes damage at distant sites, particularly the heart (myocarditis), nerves (demyelination), and kidney (tubular necrosis).

Primary infection of the skin may occur, which classically results in a "punched out" ulcer, often with a grayish membrane. However, more frequently *C. diphtheriae* appears to secondarily infect preexisting skin lesions.

Diphtheria toxin, a two subunit protein with a molecular weight of 61,000 kDa, is an extremely potent inhibitor of protein synthesis, with an estimated human lethal dose of 0.1 μg/kg body weight. The B subunit attaches to the cell surface. The A subunit enters the cell and, by ADP-ribosylation, inactivates elongation factor 2, which is an essential factor in the transfer of amino acids to the nascent polypeptide chain.[3,96] The extent of toxin absorption varies with the site of infection, being much less from skin or nose than from the nasopharynx.

Immunity to clinical diphtheria appears largely to depend on the level of diphtheria antitoxin in the serum at the time of onset of illness (Section 3.2.2). Antibodies to fragment B of diphtheria toxin are able to neutralize the effect of toxin and protect against disease. Diphtheria antitoxin is predominantly IgG antibody.[97] It is transmitted transplacentally, providing protection to infants during the first 6 months of life.

Stimulation of antitoxin production occurs with either asymptomatic infection or disease, in addition to immunization with diphtheria toxoid. Following recovery from clinical diphtheria, development of protective immunity is not reliable[98] and vaccination is recommended in convalescence. The possession of protective levels of antibody does not prevent carriage of *C. diphtheriae*, nor does it appear to affect the duration of carriage. On the contrary, identified carriers may have relatively high levels of antitoxin.[23]

Waning of the diphtheria antitoxin level occurs over time, following either natural infection or artificial immunization. Periodic booster doses of diphtheria toxoid are recommended to maintain protective levels of antitoxin. Although a boost in antitoxin levels may occur following the onset of disease in individuals who have been previously immunologically primed but whose antitoxin concentration has fallen below the protective level, in many cases the production of diphtheria toxin by the infecting organism is so overwhelming that the antitoxin response is not swift enough to prevent complications or even death.

8. Patterns of Host Response

8.1. Clinical Features

8.1.1. Carrier State. Asymptomatic nasopharyngeal infection with *C. diphtheriae* occurs more frequently than clinical disease. The duration of carriage was studied by several investigators during the preantibiotic era, by examining the rate of disappearance of *C. diphtheriae* from the nasopharynx of either convalescent cases or identified carriers. Hartley and Martin[91] followed 457 cases and found that 49%, 74%, and 87%, respectively were culture-negative by 15, 30, and 45 days after illness onset. Weaver[99] studied the rate of disappearance of *C. diphtheriae* among 500 cases. After the first week, approximately half of the cases that began the week culture-positive became negative during the following 7 days. By 3 weeks after onset, 71% had become culture-negative, by 4 weeks, 83%, and by 8 weeks, 99%. Weaver also studied the rate of disappearance of *C. diphtheriae* in 52 carriers: by 2 weeks after identification, 55.8% had become culture-negative and by 4 weeks, 80.8%. Two (4%) remained positive after 75 days. Differences between the results of these studies probably largely reflect the greater opportunity for reinfection of Hartley and Martin's patients. Both authors describe the association of chronic carriage with large, irregularly shaped tonsils, and the value of tonsillectomy in eradicating carriage. However, this should not be necessary with the present availability of effective antibiotics.

8.1.2. Respiratory Diphtheria. Infection limited to the anterior nares manifests as chronic serosanguinous or seropurulent discharge, without fever or significant toxicity. A whitish membrane may be observed on the septum. Such patients may readily spread diphtheria. The faucial (pharyngeal) form is the most common. The illness begins insidiously with a sore throat, malaise, and mild to moderate fever. There is an initial mild pharyngeal erythema, usually followed by progressive formation of a whitish tonsilar exudate, which over 24 to 48 hr changes into a gray adherent membrane, which is tightly adherent and bleeds upon attempted removal. In more severe cases, the patient appears toxic and the membrane is more extensive. Gross enlargement of cervical lymph nodes and surrounding tissue edema may occur, resulting in the so-called "bull neck." Laryngeal involvement, which may occur on its own or as a result of membrane extension from the nasopharynx, presents with hoarseness, stridor, and dyspnea. Intubation or tracheostomy may be required.

The likelihood of toxic complications depends on the

severity of disease at presentation and the interval between disease onset and administration of therapeutic antitoxin. Myocarditis typically occurs between 1 and 2 weeks after the onset of respiratory symptoms. Neural impairment occurs in 10 to 20% of patients. In severe cases, palatal and/or pharyngeal paralysis may occur during the acute phase. Cranial nerve involvement may develop after the first week. Peripheral neuritis, symmetrical and predominantly motor, occurs from 2 to 12 weeks after disease onset. Motor deficit may range from minor proximal weakness to complete paralysis. Although slow (several months), recovery of neurological function is usually complete. In fulminant, sometimes called hypertoxic, diphtheria, toxic circulatory collapse with hemorrhagic features occurs. More severe disease occurs in the very young and the elderly and in unimmunized persons.

8.1.3. Cutaneous Diphtheria. Classical cutaneous lesions are indolent deep punched out ulcers, which may have a grayish-white membrane. More commonly, however, *C. diphtheriae* appears as a secondary infecting agent of a variety of dermatoses such as traumatic lesions, pyoderma, or chronic dermatitis, such as stasis dermatitis.[51,67] There is frequently coinfection with *Streptococcus pyogenes* and/or *Staphylococcus aureus*. Recognized toxin-induced diphtheria complications are usually stated to be uncommon, which is said to be because toxin absorption from the skin is much less than from the nasopharynx. However, toxin-induced neuritis and myocarditis were noted following cutaneous diphtheria among soldiers during World War II.[65,82]

8.1.4. Other Sites. The organism may uncommonly infect other sites, including the eye, genitalia, and ear.

8.1.5. Invasive Disease. Uncommonly, *C. diphtheriae*, both toxigenic and nontoxigenic, may cause invasive disease, including endocarditis, osteomyelitis, septic arthritis, and meningitis.[38–41] Frequently, but not always, these patients have predisposing factors such as a prosthetic cardiac valve or underlying immunosuppression.

8.2. Diagnosis

The decision to initiate therapy should be made on clinical grounds, since delay in treatment is associated with worse outcomes, owing to the fact that antitoxin can only neutralize toxin that has not already bound to cells. A high index of suspicion is required. Cultures should be taken from beneath the membrane, from the nasopharynx, and from any suspicious skin lesions. Because special media are required, the microbiology laboratory should be alerted to the concern about diphtheria. Cultures may be negative if the patient received previous antibiotics. The diagnosis of diphtheria is more likely if the patient is unimmunized or has not received recommended booster immunizations; if there is a history of contact with a knowndiphtheriacase;ifthereisahistoryofrecenttravel to a region with endemic diphtheria or of contact with a recent immigrant from such an area; if the patient belongs to a population group that has had a higher risk of diphtheria in the past, such as homeless persons; and if the pretreatment antitoxin titer is <0.01 IU/ml.

The differential diagnosis of respiratory diphtheria includes bacterial (streptococcal, *Arcanobacterium hemolyticum*[100]) and viral tonsillopharyngitis, infectious mononucleosis, peritonsillar abscess, Vincent's angina, candidiasis, and acute epiglottitis. A nasal foreign body produces a unilateral nasal discharge that can mimic nasal diphtheria.

8.3. Treatment

The mainstay of therapy is equine diphtheria antitoxin, which should be administered as the diagnosis is reasonably suspected, without waiting for bacteriologic confirmation, in order to neutralize toxin before it binds to tissues. Antibiotic therapy (penicillin or erythromycin) is necessary to eliminate the organism, thereby halting further toxin production and preventing further transmission. For details about treatment of diphtheria, the reader is referred to textbooks of infectious diseases.[101,102]

9. Control and Prevention

9.1. General Concepts

Recommendations for the prevention and control of diphtheria, including an algorithm to guide investigation and management, were recently published by the CDC and by the WHO Regional Office for Europe.[62,103]

The important first step is recognition of suspected diphtheria by clinicians. Although most practicing clinicians have never seen a case of the disease, it is important that they remain aware of the possibility of diphtheria, particularly in a patient with a nasopharyngeal pseudomembrane. Identification of a suspected case should set in motion a series of activities. The health department should be notified so that the contact investigation can begin as soon as possible. The patient is placed in strict respiratory isolation, the laboratory notified of the suspicion of diphtheria, and the appropriate cultures taken, if possible before antibiotics are commenced. During and after treatment, isolation should be maintained until elimination of the organism is demonstrated by two negative cultures obtained at least 24 hr apart after completion of antimicrobial therapy. The patient should be immunized with diphtheria toxoid during convalescence.

Close contacts (which include household contacts and others spending at least several hours per week in close proximity to the patient, such as preschool and elementary school classmates) irrespective of vaccination status, should be (1) monitored for symptoms and signs of diphtheria for at least 7 days; (2) cultured from the nose and throat for *C. diphtheriae*; and (3) given antibiotic prophylaxis (Section 9.2). The immunization status of all close contacts should be assessed and diphtheria toxoid administered as indicated. Persons who have not previously received at least three doses of diphtheria toxoid should receive a dose of diphtheria toxoid and then further doses as necessary to complete the recommended schedule for age. The schedule can be completed irrespective of the interval between the previous doses. Persons who have received three or more previous doses of diphtheria toxoid should receive a further dose unless their last dose was received within the past 5 years. Contacts found to be carriers of *C. diphtheriae* should receive follow-up cultures a minimum of 2 weeks after completion of antibiotics, to ensure eradication of the organism.

9.2. Antibiotic and Chemotherapeutic Approaches to Prophylaxis

Although the effectiveness of antibiotic prophylaxis in preventing secondary cases among contacts is not proven, it is now recommended by several authorities[62,103,104] that all close contacts should receive antibiotic prophylaxis, after appropriate cultures have been taken. The importance of antibiotic treatment of carriers, in addition to immunization, in the control of diphtheria, has been reinforced by experience during outbreaks in the United States.[85,88] If compliance is assured, a 7- to 10-day course of erythromycin (40 mg/kg per day for children and 1 g/day for adults, in divided doses) is recommended; if compliance is doubtful or there is intolerance to erythromycin, a single intramuscular injection of benzathine penicillin (600,000 units for persons <6 years of age and 1.2 million units for persons $\geqslant 6$ years of age) is preferred. Both clinical and laboratory data indicate that erythromycin may be more effective than penicillin.[105,106]

9.3. Immunization

Both theoretical data and the occurrence of outbreaks in even highly immunized communities[85,88,107,108] suggest that a high level of population immunity, perhaps greater than 85%, is necessary to prevent and to control outbreaks. This contrasts with earlier opinions (offered at a time when levels of natural immunity among adults were high) that diphtheria could be controlled if childhood immunization rates of 70% were achieved.[21] Now that natural exposure to toxigenic *C. diphtheriae* is rare, the necessary levels of immunity can only be realized by achieving childhood vaccination coverage of at least 95% *and* by achieving high coverage of adults with periodic booster doses of diphtheria toxoid. In the United States in 1995, while the level of coverage with three or more doses of diphtheria toxoid among school entrants is at least 95%, 50% or more of adults have not received a diphtheria toxoid booster within the previous 10 years.

Immunization with diphtheria toxoid is the mainstay of diphtheria prevention. Almost always, diphtheria toxoid is administered to children in vaccines in which it is combined with one or more other antigens [tetanus toxoid with or without pertussis vaccine (whole cell or acellular): DT, DTP, and DTaP, respectively]. Quadravalent vaccines in which DTP is additionally combined with inactive polio vaccine or with *Haemophilus influenzae* type B conjugate vaccine are used in some industrialized countries, and similar combinations containing acellular rather than whole cell pertussis vaccine most likely will be soon widely available. Pediatric vaccines usually contain from 10–30 Lf (flocculation units) of diphtheria toxoid. For persons aged 7 years of age or older, adult formulation tetanus and diphtheria toxoids (Td) are used for both primary and booster immunization. The small "d" reflects a reduced amount of diphtheria toxoid (in many countries, approximately 2 Lf) in order to reduce adverse effects, particularly severe local reactions, experienced by some older individuals upon receipt of higher amounts of diphtheria toxoid.[109,110]

Three different vaccination schedules are shown in Table 2. Issues relating to the immunogenicity of different schedules have been reviewed elsewhere.[111] For both adults and children, three doses of diphtheria toxoid are required to raise antitoxin levels above the minimum protective level (0.01 IU/ml) in 100% of recipients.[111,112] In the absence of ongoing natural exposure to toxigenic *C. diphtheriae*, vaccine-induced immunity wanes over time.[113–117] Periodic diphtheria toxoid booster doses are therefore required to maintain immunity: in the United States, decennial boosters are recommended. In some tropical countries, ongoing exposure to cutaneous diphtheria may reduce the need for diphtheria toxoid boosters[111,118]; however, this may change as social and demographic conditions evolve.

Table 2. Schedules for Diphtheria Vaccination Recommended in the United States, in the United Kingdom, and by the World Health Organization Expanded Programme on Immunization

Dose	United States (ACIP, AAP)[121]		United Kingdom (JCVI)[122]		WHO, EPI (GAG)[123]	
Primary						
1	2 months	DTaP or DTP	2 months	DTP	6 weeks	DTP
2	4 months	DTaP or DTP	3 months	DTP	10 weeks	DTP
3	6 months	DTaP or DTP	4 months	DTP	16 weeks	DTP
4	12–18 months	DTaP or DTP	—		—	
Booster						
1	4–6 years	DTaP or DTP	4–5 years	DT		
2	11–16 years	Td	—			
3	Every 10 years	Td				

Abbreviations: ACIP, Advisory Committee on Immunization Practices; AAP, American Academy of Pediatrics; JCVI, Joint Committee on Vaccination and Immunization; WHO, EPI (GAG), World Health Organization Global Advisory Group for the Expanded Programme on Immunization.

The most frequent adverse reactions to diphtheria toxoid are local pain at the site of inoculation, sometimes with associated redness and swelling, and occasionally severe. Systemic reactions (fever and malaise) occur infrequently. Most such reactions are believed to represent hypersensitivity reactions to diphtheria toxoid or to associated impurities.[110] The assessment of adverse reactions is difficult because diphtheria toxoid is now almost always administered in combination with tetanus toxoid and other antigens. Severe generalized anaphylactic reactions rarely have been reported.[119]

The effectiveness of diphtheria toxoid has never been measured in a controlled trial. Its value seemed obvious to early investigators, and the Schick test and serological methods provided measurable correlates of protection. However, studies comparing the incidence of diphtheria in vaccinated and unvaccinated individuals and case–control studies have provided estimates of effectiveness of 71–92%.[120] While immunization with diphtheria toxoid does not provide complete protection against clinical diphtheria, when disease occurs in fully vaccinated persons, it is generally milder and is rarely fatal.

10. Unresolved Problems

In this era of apparent near elimination of toxigenic *C. diphtheriae* from most developed nations, diphtheria is often considered a disease of the past, and therefore interest in research on this disease has waned, with the exception of ongoing molecular studies related to diphtheria toxin. Several issues related to nontoxigenic *C. diphtheriae* strains deserve study. The current epidemiology of nontoxigenic organisms is poorly understood. This information is potentially important, since the introduction, through an imported toxigenic strain, of a *tox*$^+$ phage into the resident pool of nontoxigenic organisms is more likely if they continue to circulate widely. Nontoxigenic organisms may cause local disease, at times severe; in addition, severe local disease due to toxigenic strains may occasionally occur in persons with high levels of diphtheria antitoxin. A better understanding of the pathogenesis of disease caused by nontoxigenic organisms may assist in developing future vaccines that both provide more certain protection against disease and also protect against carriage (asymptomatic infection).

There are surprisingly few published studies from which to establish the current recommendations for prophylaxis of contacts of diphtheria cases and treatment of carriers of *C. diphtheriae*. The current outbreak in the new independent states of the former Soviet Union offers an opportunity to better define the optimal duration of treatment of contacts and the role of alternative antibiotics.

The most important issue, however, is the necessity to maintain vigilance (i.e., surveillance) to ensure that *C. diphtheriae* will not reemerge in those countries where it is now apparently absent. This requires maintaining the clinical and laboratory capacity to recognize and diagnose diphtheria and, crucially, improving levels of immunity among adults by increasing awareness among both the public and medical providers of the importance of regular tetanus–diphtheria boosters.

11. References

1. Freeman, V. J., Studies on the virulence of bacteriophage-infected strains of *Corynebacterium diphtheriae*, *J. Bacteriol.* **61:**675–688 (1951).
2. Groman, N. B., Evidence for the induced nature of the change from nontoxigenicity to toxigenicity in *Corynebacterium diphtheriae* as a result of exposure to a specific bacteriophage, *J. Bacteriol.* **66:**184–191 (1953).
3. Pappenheimer, A. M., Diphtheria: Studies on the biology of an infectious disease, in: *The Harvey Lectures, Series 76*, pp. 45–73, Academic Press, New York, 1982.
4. English, P. C., Diphtheria and theories of infectious disease: Centennial appreciation of the critical role of diphtheria in the history of medicine, *Pediatrics* **76:**1–9 (1985).
5. Holmes, W. H., Diphtheria: History, in: *Bacillary and Rickettsial Infections Acute and Chronic. A Textbook* (W. H. Holmes, ed.), pp. 289–308, MacMillan, New York, 1940.
6. Chen, R. T., Broome, C. V., Weinstein, R. A., Diphtheria in the United States, 1971–81, *Am. J. Public Health* **75:**1393–1397 (1985).
7. Brooks, G. F., Bennett, J. V., and Feldman, R. A., Diphtheria in the United States, 1959–1970, *J. Infect. Dis.* **129:**172–178 (1974).
8. Munford, R. S., Ory, H. W., Brooks, G. F., *et al.*, Diphtheria deaths in the United States, 1959–70, *J. Am. Med. Assoc.* **229:**1890–1893 (1974).
9. Sottnek, F. O., and Miller, J. M., *Isolation and Identification of Corynebacterium diphtheriae*, US Department of Health and Human Services, Atlanta, GA, 1982.
10. Brooks, R., and Joynson, D. H. M., Bacteriological diagnosis of diphtheria: ACP Broadsheet No. 125, *J. Clin. Pathol.* **43:**567–579 (1990).
11. Krech, T., and Hollis, D. G., *Corynebacterium* and related organisms, in: *Manual of Clinical Microbiology*, 5th ed. (A. Balows *et al.*, eds.), pp. 277–286, American Society of Microbiology, Washington, DC, 1991.
12. Efstratiou, A., and Maple, P. A. C., *Manual for the Laboratory Diagnosis of Diphtheria*, Expanded Programme on Immunization, WHO European Region, Copenhagen, 1994.
13. Kim-Farley, R. J., Soewarso, T. I., Rejeki, S., *et al.*, Silica gel as transport medium for *Corynebacterim diphtheriae* under tropical conditions (Indonesia), *J. Clin. Microbiol.* **25:**964–965 (1987).
14. Saragea, A., Maximescu, P., and Meitert, E., *Corynebacterium diphtheriae*: Microbiological methods used in clinical and epidemiological investigations, in: *Methods in Microbiology*, Vol. 3 (T. Bergan and J. R. Norris, eds.), pp. 61–176, Academic Press, New York, 1979.
15. Elek, S. D., The recognition of toxicogenic bacterial strains *in vitro*, *Br. Med. J.* **1:**493–496 (1948).
16. Pallen, M. J., Hay, A. J., Puckey, L. H., *et al.*, Polymerase chain reaction for screening clinical isolates of *Corynebacteria* for the production of diphtheria toxin, *J. Clin. Pathol.* **47:**353–356 (1994).
17. Coyle, M., Groman, N. B., Russell, J. Q., *et al.*, The molecular epidemiology of the three biotypes of *Corynebacterium diphtheriae* in the Seattle outbreak, 1972–1982, *J. Infect. Dis.* **159:** 670–679 (1989).
18. De Zoysa, A., Efstratiou, A., George, R. C., *et al.*, Molecular epidemiology of *Corynebacterium diphtheriae* from northwest Russia and surrounding countries studied by using ribotyping and pulsed-field gel electrophoresis, *J. Clin. Microbiol.* **33:**1080–1083 (1995).
19. Hallander, H. O., Haeggman, S., and Lofdahl, S., Epidemiological typing of *Corynebacterium diphtheriae* isolated in Sweden 1984–86, *Scand. J. Infect. Dis.* **20:**173–176 (1988).
20. Rappuoli, R., Perugnini, M., and Falsen, E., Molecular epidemiology of the 1984–1986 outbreak of diphtheria in Sweden, *N. Engl. J. Med.* **318:**12–14 (1988).
21. Tasman, A., and Lansberg, H. P., Problems concerning the prophylaxis, pathogenesis and therapy of diphtheria, *Bull. World Health Organ.* **16:**939–973 (1957).
22. Ipsen, J., Circulating antitoxin at the onset of diphtheria in 425 patients, *J. Immunol.* **54:**325–347 (1946).
23. Bjorkholm, B., Bottiger, M., Christenson, B., *et al.*, Antitoxin antibody levels and the outcome of illness during an outbreak of diphtheria among alcoholics, *Scand. J. Infect. Dis.* **18:**235–239 (1986).
24. Edward, D. G., and Allison, V. D., Diphtheria in the immunized with observations on a diphtheria-like disease associated with nontoxigenic strains of *Carynebacterium diphtheriae*, *J. Hyg.* **49:**205–219 (1951).
25. Christenson, B., Hellstrom, L., and Aust-Kettis, A., Diphtheria in Stockholm, with a theory concerning transmission, *J. Infect.* **19:**177–183 (1989).
26. Schick, B., Die Diphtherietoxin-Hautreaktion des Menschen als Vorprobe der prophylaktischen Diphtherieheilseruminjektion, *Munch. Med. Wochenschr.* **60:**2608–2610 (1913).
27. Zingher, A., The Schick test performed on more than 150,000 children in public and parochial schools in New York (Manhattan and the Bronx), *Am. J. Dis. Child.* **25:**392–405 (1923).
28. Dudley, S. F., Critical review: Schick's test and its applications, *Q. J. Med.* **22:**321–379 (1929).
29. Craig, J. P., Immune response to *Corynebacterium diphtheriae* and *Clostrium tetani*, in: *Manual of Clinical Laboratory Immunology*, 3rd ed. (N. R. Rose *et al.*, eds.), pp. 408–414, American Society for Microbiology, Washington, DC, 1986.
30. Miyamura, K., Nishio, S., Ito, A., *et al.*, Micro cell culture method for determination of diphtheria toxin and antitoxin titers using VERO cells. I. Studies on factors affecting the toxin and antitoxin titration, *J. Biol. Stand.* **2:**189–201 (1974).
31. Knight, P. A., Tilleray, J., and Queminet, J., Studies on the correlation of a range of immunoassays for diphtheria antitoxin with the guinea-pig neutralization test, *Dev. Biol. Stand.* **64:**25–32 (1986).
32. Menser, M. A., and Hudson, J. R., Population studies of diphtheria immunity using antitoxin radioimmunoassay, *J. Hyg.* **92:** 1–7 (1984).
33. Nelson, L., Peri, B. A., Rieger, C. H. L., *et al.*, Immunity to diphtheria in an urban population, *Pediatrics* **61:**703–710 (1978).
34. Belsey, M. A., Isolation of *Carynebacterium diphtheriae* in the environment of skin carriers, *Am. J. Epidemiol.* **91:**294–299 (1970).
35. Crosbie, W. E., and Wright, H. D., Diphtheria bacilli in floor dust, *Lancet* **1:**656–659 (1941).
36. Pappenheimer, A. M., and Murphy, J. R., Studies on the molecular epidemiology of diphtheria, *Lancet* **2:**923–925 (1983).
37. Willett, H. P., *Corynebacterium diphtheriae*, in: *Zinsser Microbiology*, 18th ed. (W. J. Joklik *et al.*, eds.), pp. 535–543, Appleton-Century-Crofts, Norwalk, CT, 1984.
38. Afghani, B., and Stutman, H. R., Bacterial arthritis caused by *Corynebacterium diphtheriae*, *Pediatr. Infect. Dis. J.* **12:**881–882 (1993).
39. Tiley, S. M., Kociuba, K. R., Heron, I. G., *et al.*, Infective

endocarditis due to nontoxigenic *Corynebacterium diphtheriae*: Report of seven cases and review, *Clin. Infect. Dis.* **16:**271–275 (1993).

40. Efstratiou, A., Tiley, S. M., Sangrador, A., *et al.*, Invasive disease caused by multiple clones of *Corynebacterium diphtheriae* [letter], *Clin. Infect. Dis.* **17:**136 (1993).
41. Trepeta, R. W., and Edberg, S. C., *Corynebacterium diphtheriae* endocarditis: Sustained potential of a classical pathogen, *Am. J. Clin. Pathol.* **81:**679–683 (1984).
42. McLaughlin, J. V., Bickham, S. T., Wiggins, G. L., *et al.*, Antibiotic susceptibility patterns of recent isolates of *Corynebacterium diphtheriae*, *Appl. Microbiol.* **21:**844–851 (1971).
43. Maple, P. A., Efstratiou, A., Tseneva, G., *et al.*, The *in vitro* susceptibilities of toxigenic strains of *Corynebacterium diphtheriae* isolated in northwestern Russia and surrounding areas to ten antibiotics, *Antimicrob. Agents Chemother.* **34:**1037–1040 (1994).
44. Zamiri, I., and McEntegart, M. G., The sensitivity of diphtheria bacilli to eight antibiotics, *J. Clin. Pathol.* **25:**716–717 (1972).
45. Gordon, R. C., Yow, M. D., Clark, D. J., *et al.*, *In vitro* susceptibility of *Corynebacterium diphtheriae* to thirteen antibiotics, *Appl. Microbiol.* **21:**548–549 (1971).
46. Schiller, J., Gorman, N., and Coyle, M., Plasmids in *Corynebacterium diphtheriae* and diphtheroids mediating erythromycin resistance, *Antimicrob. Agents Chemother.* **18:**814–821 (1980).
47. Jellard, C. H., and Lipinski, A. E., *Corynebacterium diphtheriae* resistant to erythromycin and lincomycin [letter], *Lancet* **1:**156 (1973).
48. Rockhill, R. C., Sumaro, Hadiputranto, H., *et al.*, Tetracycline resistance of *Corynebacterium diphtheriae* isolated from diphtheria patients in Jakarta, Indonesia, *Antimicrob. Agents Chemother.* **21:**842–843 (1982).
49. Coyle, M. B., Minshew, B. H., Bland, J. A., *et al.*, Erythromycin and clindamycin resistance in *Corynebacterium diphtheriae* from skin lesions, *Antimicrob. Agents Chemother.* **16:**525–527 (1979).
50. Udgaonkar, U. S., Dharmadhikari, C. A., Kulkarni, R. D., *et al.*, Study of diphtheria carriers in Miraj, *Indian Pediatr.* **26:**435–439 (1989).
51. Harnisch, J. P., Tronca, E., Nolan, C. M., *et al.*, Diphtheria among alcoholic urban adults: A decade of experience in Seattle, *Ann. Intern. Med.* **111:**71–82 (1989).
52. Frost, W. H., Infection, immunity and disease in the epidemiology of diphtheria, with special reference to some studies in Baltimore, *J. Prev. Med.* **2:**325–343 (1928).
53. Russell, W. T., *The Epidemiology of Diphtheria during the Last Forty Years. Medical Research Council Special Report Series*, No. 247, HMSO, London, 1943.
54. Walsh, J. A., and Warren, K. S., Selective primary health care. An interim strategy for disease control in developing countries, *N. Engl. J. Med.* **301:**967–974 (1979).
55. Expanded Programme on Immunization, Feasibility of elimination of vaccine-preventable diseases, *Week. Epidemiol. Rec.* **59:** 143–145 (1984).
56. Hardy, I., Dittmann, S., and Sutter, R. W., Current situation and control strategies for resurgence of diphtheria in newly independent states of the former Soviet Union, *Lancet* **347:**1739–1744 (1995).
57. Kalapothaki, V., Sapounas, T., Xirouchaki, E., *et al.*, Prevalence of diphtheria carriers in a population with disappearing clinical diphtheria, *Infection* **12:**387–389 (1984).
58. Trichopoulos, D., Politou, G., Papoutsakis, G., *et al.*, Diphtheria carriers among schoolchildren in Athens, *Scand. J. Infect. Dis.* **4:**197–201 (1972).
59. Galazka, A. M., Robertson, S. E., and Oblapenko, G. P., Resurgence of diphtheria, *Eur. J. Epidemiol.* **11:**95–105 (1995).
60. Stuart, G., A note on diphtheria incidence in certain European countries, *Br. Med. J.* **2:**613–615 (1945).
61. Liebow, A. A., Diphtheria and the Schick test in the tropics, *Int. Arch. Allergy Appl. Immunol.* **12:**42–58 (1958).
62. Farizo, K. M., Strebel, P. M., Chen, R. T., *et al.*, Fatal respiratory disease due to *Corynebacterium diphtheriae*: Case report and review of guidelines for management, investigation and control, *Clin. Infect. Dis.* **16:**59–68 (1993).
63. Doull, J. A., and Lara, H., The epidemiologic importance of diphtheria carriers, *Am. J. Hyg.* **5:**508–529 (1925).
64. Marples, M. J., and Bacon, D. F., Some observations on the distribution of *Corynebacterium diphtheriae* in Western Samoa, *Tran. R. Soc. Trop. Med. Hyg.* **50:**72–76 (1956).
65. Liebow, A. A., MacLean, P. D., Bumstead, J. H., *et al.*, Tropical ulcers and cutaneous diphtheria, *Arch. Intern. Med.* **78:**255–295 (1946).
66. Bezjak, V., and Farsey, S. J., *Corynebacterium diphtheriae* in skin lesions in Ugandan children, *Bull. World Health Organ.* **43:**643–650 (1970).
67. Belsey, M. A., Sinclair, M., Roder, M. R., *et al.*, *Corynebacterium diphtheriae* skin infections in Alabama and Louisiana, *N. Engl. J. Med.* **280:**135–141 (1969).
68. Koopman, J. S., and Campbell, J., The role of cutaneous diphtheria infections in a diphtheria epidemic, *J. Infect. Dis.* **131:**239–244 (1975).
69. Dixon, J. M. S., Diphtheria in North America, *J. Hyg.* **93:**419–432 (1984).
70. Bowler, I. J., Mandal, B. K., Schlecht, B., *et al.*, Diphtheria—The continuing hazard, *Arch. Dis. Child.* **63:**194–210 (1988).
71. Lumio, J., Jahkola, M., Vuento, R., *et al.*, Diphtheria after a visit to Russia [letter], *Lancet* **342:**53–54 (1993).
72. National Communicable Disease Center, Diphtheria Surveillance, Report No. 8, 1965–1966 Summary, US Public Health Service, Atlanta, GA, 1968.
73. Galazka, A. M., and Robertson, S. E., Diphtheria: Changing patterns in the developing world and the industrialized world, *Eur. J. Epidemiol.* **11:**107–117 (1995).
74. Christenson, B., and Bottiger, M., Serological immunity to diphtheria in Sweden in 1978 and 1984, *Scand. J. Infect. Dis.* **18:**227–233 (1986).
75. Crossley, K., Irvine, P., Warren, J. B., *et al.*, Tetanus and diphtheria immunity in urban Minnesota adults, *J. Am. Med. Assoc.* **242:**2298–3000 (1979).
76. Galazka, A., and Kardymowicz, B., Immunity against diphtheria among adults in Poland, *Epidemiol. Infect.* **103:**587–593 (1989).
77. Koblin, B. A., and Townsend, T. R., Immunity to diphtheria and tetanus in inner-city women of child-bearing age, *Am. J. Public Health* **79:**1297–1298 (1989).
78. Maple, P. A., Efstratiou, A., George, R. C., *et al.*, Diphtheria immunity in UK blood donors, *Lancet* **345:**963–965 (1995).
79. Sargent, R. K., Rossing, T. H., Dowton, S. B., *et al.*, Diphtheria immunity in Massachusetts—A study of three urban patient populations, *Am. J. Med. Sci.* **287:**37–39 (1984).
80. Weiss, B. P., Strassburg, M. A., and Feeley, J. C., Tetanus and diphtheria immunity in an elderly population in Los Angeles County, *Am. J. Public Health* **73:**802–804 (1983).
81. Patel, M., Morey, F., Butcher, A., *et al.*, The frequent isolation of

toxigenic and non-toxigenic *Corynebacterium diphtheriae* at Alice Springs Hospital, *Commun. Dis. Intell.* **18:**310–311 (1994).

82. Livingood, C. S., Perry, D. J., and Forrester, J. S., Cutaneous diphtheria: A report of 140 cases, *J. Invest. Dermatol.* **7:**341–364 (1946).
83. Wheeler, S. M., and Morton, A. R., Epidemiological observations in the Halifax epidemic, *Am. J. Public Health* **32:**947–956 (1942).
84. Liashenko, Y. I., and Velichko, M. A., [The diagnostic and treatment characteristics of diphtheria in troop units and military medical institutions] [Russian]. *Voen. Med. Zh.* **80:**37–40 (1993).
85. Miller, L. W., Older, J. J., Drake, J., *et al.*, Diphtheria immunization. Effect upon carriers and control of outbreaks, *Am. J. Dis. Child.* **123:**197–199 (1972).
86. Gray, R. D., and James, S. M., Occult diphtheria infection in a hospital for the mentally subnormal, *Lancet* **1:**1105–1106 (1973).
87. Anderson, G. S., and Penfold, J. B., An outbreak of diphtheria in a hospital for the mentally subnormal, *J. Clin. Pathol.* **26:**606–615 (1973).
88. Zalma, V. M., Older, J. J., and Brooks, G. F., The Austin, Texas, diphtheria outbreak, *J. Am. Med. Assoc.* **211:**2125–2129 (1970).
89. Gordon, H., and Fleck, D. G., An epidemic of diphtheria carriers, *Public Health* **85:**228–232 (1971).
90. Lyman, E. D., and Youngstrom, J. A., Diphtheria cases and contacts: Is it necessary to take cultures from both nose and throat? *Nebraska State Med. J.* **41:**361–362 (1956).
91. Hartley, P., and Martin, C. J., The apparent rate of disappearance of diphtheria bacilli from the throat after an attack of the disease, *Proc. R. Soc. Med.* **13:**277–289 (1920).
92. Dudley, S. F., May, P. M., and O'Flynn, J. A., *Active Immunization against Diphtheria: Its Effect on the Distribution of Antitoxic Immunity and Case and Carrier Infection*, Medical Research Council Special Report Series No. 195, HMSO, London, 1934.
93. Ouchterlony, O., Air-borne infections. 5. Modes of contagion in diphtheria, *Acta Med. Scand.* **137:**402–410 (1950).
94. Jones, E. E., Kim-Farley, R. J., Algunaid, M., *et al.*, Diphtheria: A possible foodborne outbreak in Hodeida, Yemem Arab Republic, *Bull. World Health Organ.* **63:**287–293 (1985).
95. Goldie, W., and Maddock, E. C. G., A milk-borne outbreak of diphtheria, *Lancet* **1:**285–286 (1943).
96. Gill, D. M., Pappenheimer, A. M., and Uchida, T., Diphtheria toxin, protein synthesis, and the cell, *Fed. Proc.* **32:**1508–1515 (1973).
97. Galazka, A. M., *The Immunological Basis of Immunization. 2. Diphtheria* (WHO/EPI/GEN/93.12), World Health Organization, Geneva, 1993.
98. Madsen, E., Antitoxin production in cases of diphtheria not treated with serum, *Acta Pathol. Microbiol. Scand.* **16:**113–143 (1939).
99. Weaver, G. H., Diphtheria carriers, *J. Am. Med. Assoc.* **76:**831–835 (1921).
100. Kain, K. C., Noble, M. A., Barteluk, R. L., *et al.*, *Arcanobacterium hemolyticum* infection: Confused with scarlet fever and diphtheria, *J. Emerg. Med.* **9:**33–35 (1991).
101. Krugman, S., Katz, S. L., Gershon, A. E., *et al.*, Diphtheria, in: *Infectious Diseases of Children*, 9th ed. (S. Krugman, S. Katz, A. Gerson, and C. Wiltert, eds.), pp. 46–67, Mosby, St. Louis, 1992.
102. MacGregor, R. R., Corynebacterium diphtheriae, in: *Mandell, Douglas and Bennett's Principles and Practice of Infectious Diseases*, 4th ed. (G. L. Mandell, J. E. Bennett, and R. Dolin, eds.), pp. 1865–1872, Churchill Livingstone, New York, 1995.
103. Begg, N., *Manual for the Management and Control of Diphtheria in the European Region*, Expanded Programme on Immunization WHO European Region, Copenhagen, 1994.
104. Committee on Infectious Diseases, American Academy of Pediatrics, Diphtheria, in: *1994 Red Book: Report of the Committee on Infectious Diseases*, 23rd ed., pp. 177–181, American Academy of Pediatrics, Elk Grove, Village, IL, 1994.
105. Beach, M. W., Gamble, W. B., Zemp, C. H., *et al.*, Erythromycin in the treatment of the diphtheria carrier state, *Pediatrics* **16:**335–344 (1955).
106. McCloskey, R. V., Green, M. J., Eller, J., *et al.*, Treatment of diphtheria carriers: Benzathine penicillin, erythromycin, and clindamycin, *Ann. Intern. Med.* **81:**788–791 (1974).
107. Anderson, R. M., and May, R. M., Static aspects of eradication and control, in: *Infectious Diseases of Humans: Dynamics and Control*, pp. 87–121, Oxford University Press, Oxford, 1992.
108. Murphy, W. F., Maley, V. H., and Dick, L., Continued high incidence of diphtheria in a well immunized community, *Public Health Rep.* **71:**481–488 (1956).
109. Edsall, G., Altman, J. A., and Gaspar, A. J., Combined tetanus–diphtheria immunization of adults: Use of small doses of diphtheria toxoid, *Am. J. Public Health* **44:**1537–1545 (1954).
110. Edsall, G., Immunization of adults against diphtheria and tetanus, *Am. J. Public Health* **42:**393–400 (1952).
111. Orenstein, W. A., Weisfeld, J. S., and Halsey, N. A., Diphtheria and tetanus toxoids and pertussis vaccine, combined, in: *Recent Advances in Immunization: A Bibliographic Review*, Scientific Publication No. 451 (N. A. Halsey and C. A. Quadros, eds.), pp. 30–51, Pan American Health Organization, Washington, DC, 1983.
112. Myers, M. G., Beckman, C. W., Vosdingh, R. A., *et al.*, Primary immunization with tetanus and diphtheria toxoids, *J. Am. Med. Assoc.* **248:**2478–2480 (1982).
113. Volk, V. K., Gottshall, R. Y., Anderson, H. D., *et al.*, Antigenic response to booster dose of diphtheria and tetanus toxoids: Seven to thirteen years after primary inoculation of noninstitutionalized children, *Public Health Rep.* **77:**185–194 (1962).
114. Gottlieb, S., Martin, M., McLaughlin, F. X., *et al.*, Long-term immunity to diphtheria and tetanus: A mathematical model. *Am. J. Epidemiol.* **85:**207–219 (1967).
115. Simonsen, O., Vaccination against tetanus and diphtheria, *Dan. Med. Bull.* **36:**24–47 (1989).
116. Kjeldsen, K., Simonsen, O., and Heron, I., Immunity against diphtheria 25–30 years after primary vaccination in childhood, *Lancet* **1:**900–902 (1985).
117. Simonsen, O., Kjeldsen, K., Bentzon, M. W., *et al.*, Susceptibility to diphtheria in populations vaccinated before and after elimination of indigenous diphtheria in Denmark, *Acta Pathol. Microbiol. Immunol. Scand. [C]* **95:**225–231 (1987).
118. Feeley, J. C., Curlin, G. T., Aziz, K. M. A., *et al.*, Response of children in Bangladesh to adult-type tetanus–diphtheria toxoid (Td) administered during a field cholera trial, *J. Biol. Stand.* **7:** 249–252 (1979).
119. Kuhns, W. J., and Pappenheimer, A. M., Immunochemical studies of antitoxin produced in normal and allergic individuals hyperimmunized with diphtheria toxoid, *J. Exp. Med.* **95:**363–374 (1952).
120. Mortimer, E. A., Diphtheria toxoid, in: *Vaccines*, 2nd ed. (S. Plotkin and E. A. Mortimer, eds.), pp. 41–56, W.B. Saunders, Philadelphia, 1994.
121. Centers for Disease Control and Prevention, Recommended

childhood immunization schedule—United States, 1995, *Morbid. Mortal. Week. Rep.* **43:**51–52 (1995).

122. Joint Committee on Vaccination and Immunization, *Immunization against Infectious Disease*, HMSO, London, 1992.

123. World Health Organization, Expanded Programme on Immunization (EPI), *Week. Epidemiol. Rec.* **56:**9–12 (1981).

12. Suggested Reading

Barksdale, L., Immunobiology of diphtheria, in: *Immunology of Human Infection*, Part 1 (A. J. Nahmias and R. J. O'Reilly, eds.), pp. 171–199, Plenum Press, New York, 1981.

Dixon, J. M. S., Noble, W. C., and Smith, G. R., Diphtheria; other corynebacterial and coryneform infections, in: *Topley and Wilson's Principles of Bacteriology*, 8th ed. (W. W. C. Topley, M. T. Park, L. Collier, and G. Wilson, eds.), pp. 56–79, B.C. Decker, Philadelphia, 1990.

Farizo, K. M., Strebel, P. M., Chen, R. T., Kimbler, A., Cleary, T. J., and Cochi, S. L., Fatal respiratory disease due to *Corynebacterium diphtheriae*: Case report and review of guidelines for management, investigation and control, *Clin. Infect. Dis.* **16:**59–68 (1993).

Galazka, A. M., and Robertson, S. E., Diphtheria: Changing patterns in the developing world and the industrialized world, *Eur. J. Epidemiol.* **11:**107–117 (1995).

Harnisch, J. P., Tronca, E., Nolan, C. M., Turck, M., and Holmes, K. K., Diphtheria among alcoholic urban adults: A decade of experience in Seattle, *Ann. Intern. Med.* **111:**71–82 (1989).

Mortimer, E. A., Diphtheria toxoid, in: *Vaccines*, 2nd ed. (S. Plotkin and E. A. Mortimer, eds.), pp. 41–56, W.B. Saunders, Philadelphia, 1994.

Pappenheimer, A. M., Diphtheria: Studies on the biology of an infectious disease, in: *The Harvey lectures*, Series 76, pp. 45–73, Academic Press, New York, 1982.

CHAPTER 14

Escherichia coli Diarrhea

Herbert L. DuPont and John J. Mathewson

1. Introduction

During the 1940s and 1950s, a series of outbreaks of diarrhea in hospital newborn nurseries were reported in which the etiologic agent appeared to be *Escherichia coli* identified by serotype. These strains became known as enteropathogenic *E. coli* (EPEC). Although it is generally recognized that these strains are responsible for diarrhea among children under 2 years of age, only now are we beginning to understand how they produce disease.

In 1969, a strain of *E. coli* was shown to be responsible for diarrhea in a group of British soldiers stationed in the Middle East. The strain was later shown to produce an exotoxin that caused fluid accumulation in a ligated rabbit loop model. Such enterotoxigenic *E. coli* (ETEC) strains have proven to be causes of diarrhea with a worldwide distribution. These strains are responsible for approximately 40% of the diarrhea among United States travelers to developing countries.

Certain nonenterotoxigenic *E. coli* strains are pathogenic by virtue of possessing the ability to penetrate intact epithelial cells. These enteroinvasive *E. coli* (EIEC) strains produce bacillary dysentery clinically indistinguishable from that produced by *Shigella* strains. This form of diarrhea is not common. Enterohemorrhagic *E. coli* (EHEC) strains have been shown to cause hemorrhagic colitis, which is a distinctive clinical syndrome characterized by bloody diarrhea with little or no fever. EHEC belong primarily to serotypes O157:H7 and O26:H11. These strains also have been strongly incriminated in the development of hemolytic uremic syndrome as a sequela.

Herbert L. DuPont • Center for Infectious Diseases, The University of Texas at Houston, and St. Luke's Episcopal Hospital, Houston, Texas 77225. **John J. Mathewson** • Center for Infectious Diseases, The University of Texas at Houston, Houston, Texas 77225.

In this chapter, we will review information available about EPEC, ETEC, EIEC, and EHEC. Since the organisms are biochemically similar (each represents an *E. coli*), they will be discussed in the same sections even though their clinical features and epidemiology are distinctly different.

2. Historical Background

In 1945, Bray[1] identified an organism with similar antigenic properties in stools obtained from 42 of 44 infants who acquired a diarrheal illness during a hospital nursery outbreak. A few years later, Giles *et al.*[2] and Taylor *et al.*[3] described similar outbreaks of diarrhea due to serotype-identified *E. coli*. During the 1950s, serological procedures were outlined that allowed the fingerprinting of *E. coli* strains according to their somatic (O) and flagellar (H) antigens.[4–6] It was reported soon thereafter that EPEC strains had a worldwide distribution. Recently, much has been learned about the pathogenic mechanisms of these strains, although much remains to be resolved.

Taylor *et al.*[7] reported in 1961 that *E. coli* isolated from stools of a number of children with a diarrheal syndrome give a positive rabbit-loop reaction (dilatation from transudation of fluid and electrolytes), while strains recovered from healthy infants, from well water, or from the urine of patients with urinary tract infections produced a negative reaction. In 1970, an O148 strain of *E. coli* was reported to have produced diarrhea in British soldiers stationed in the Middle East.[8] This strain was later shown to be enterotoxigenic. In 1970, two different enterotoxins were shown to be produced by *E. coli* pathogenic for swine.[9] The toxins could be differentiated by a variation in heat susceptibility. In 1971, it was shown that for disease to be produced, ETEC had to colonize the upper gut of the infected host,[10–12] and later, colonization fimbriae were identified with this adherence property.[13] ETEC strains have been shown to be the most important cause of diarrhea among United States travelers to Mexico (see Section 5.1).

EIEC strains were first demonstrated as causative agents of diarrhea in Japan[14] and Brazil.[15] The similarity of these strains to *Shigella* in causing bacillary dysentery was demonstrated in volunteer studies.[10] Except for three widespread outbreaks in the United States associated with contaminated food,[16–18] these strains have been shown to have a low level of endemic occurrence in cases of diarrhea in nearly all parts of the world.

In 1982, two large outbreaks of diarrhea caused by EHEC strains were recognized in the United States.[19] Both outbreaks were associated with the consumption of hamburger served at a "fast-food" restaurant. In 1984, it became clear that O157:H7 was also a cause of sporadic diarrheal illness.[20] It was also recognized at that time that hemolytic–uremic syndrome could be a sequela of infection by EHEC strains.

3. Methodology

3.1. Sources of Mortality Data

Since *E. coli* diarrhea is not a reportable disease in most areas, little is known about the actual incidence and mortality of illness. It is necessary to rely on outbreak data or information obtained from prevalence surveys. The mortality of EPEC diarrhea has varied widely from 0 to as high as 70%. The average mortality rate is 5–6%,[21,22] with an age-specific mortality rate in the neonatal period of 16%.[22] Risk factors that relate directly to increased mortality are age, in that the neonatal period and prematurity are associated with higher death rates, and strain variation, in that EPEC strains appear to differ in virulence. *E. coli* O111 is generally associated with a more striking clinical illness and higher mortality rate.[23] There is a prevailing attitude that mortality of EPEC illness has lessened in recent years. ETEC strains produce mild disease in healthy persons from the United States traveling in Latin America, but severe choleralike illness has been reported in patients studied in cholera-endemic areas.[11,12] Mortality is unusual with ETEC, but it undoubtedly occurs in areas of the world where health standards are low and where fluid and electrolyte replacement is not established in those with dehydrating illness. EIEC is thought to be a fairly uncommon cause of bacillary dysentery. There are no accurate data on mortality rates, but reported studies suggest that deaths would be unusual.[15,17] These reports describe the disease primarily in healthy Western adults and children in developing countries. There is good reason to consider the mortality to approximate that seen in shigellosis due to non-Shiga bacillus strains. Since EHEC infections are newly recognized, little is known about mortality, although infection by *E. coli* O157:H7 has been associated with the development of hemolytic uremic syndrome, which has a mortality rate of about 10% if untreated. In a comprehensive community outbreak of O157:H7 infection, 3 to 501 (0.6%) cases died.[24]

3.2. Sources of Morbidity Data

Since *E. coli* diarrhea is not a reportable disease, data on morbidity must come from survey information.

3.3. Surveys

Sporadic cases and community and hospital nursery outbreaks of EPEC diarrhea have been documented in nearly every country where appropriate studies have been carried out. Three types of studies have been done to determine the importance of EPEC illness: surveys of the relative frequency of recovering EPEC strains in populations with diarrhea, study of newborn nursery outbreaks of EPEC disease, and surveillance of the strains during short periods in communities under study. While it is impossible to state the prevalence and incidence of diarrhea with accuracy, in approximately 10% of diarrhea episodes in infants and young children an EPEC strain can be recovered from stools. Surveillance studies during community epidemics have verified the epidemic potential for EPEC.

Surveys of ETEC, EIEC, and EHEC diarrhea have been restricted to short-term studies of diarrhea cases and outbreaks in several regions around the world.

3.4. Laboratory Diagnosis

3.4.1. Isolation and Identification of Organisms. The methodology for *E. coli* isolation is readily available in microbiology texts, and any diagnostic laboratory that performs bacteriological isolation can isolate *E. coli* with proficiency. Biochemically, diarrheagenic *E. coli* are not distinct from the nonpathogenic *E. coli* always present in the intestine. *E. coli* strains that cause illness can only be differentiated from normal flora strains by the demonstration of a virulence property or specific *E. coli* serotype. This has always presented a problem for the routine clinical bacteriology laboratory because demonstration of *E. coli* virulence properties or serotypes requires sophisticated methodology generally available only in research and reference laboratories. This diagnostic problem has limited what we know about the epidemiology of *E. coli* diarrhea, although recent advancements in molecular techniques have greatly improved our diagnostic capabilities.

E. coli strains can be differentiated by the serological typing system originally developed by Kauffmann.[5] Two different antigens are important in this scheme. Somatic (O) antigens consist mainly of the lipopolysaccharide portion of the cell wall and are heat-stable. Flagellar antigens, also called H antigens, are destroyed by heating to 100°C. Capsular or K antigens also exist but are now rarely used in serotyping. Complete serotyping, a requirement to definitively classify an *E. coli* strain to be EPEC, includes a determination of both the O and H antigen types. There are approximately 164 O groups and 57 H groups. Table 1 lists the 12 O serogroups considered to be EPEC. DNA probes have been constructed to detect EPEC and have largely replaced serotyping for the identification of these strains.[25]

ETEC are diagnosed by the demonstration of the production of one or both of the enterotoxins that they produce. Generally, five to ten *E. coli* strains per patient need to be tested for both toxins. The reference assay for the detection of heat-labile enterotoxin (LT) and heat-stable toxin (ST) is the ligated rabbit ileal-loop assay. Bacteria-free supernatant is injected into ileal loops prepared surgically in a rabbit. Swelling of the loop caused by transudation of fluid and electrolytes within 5–6 hr is indicative of ST and swelling within 12–18 hr is indicative of LT. This assay has been replaced with several other more practical assays that we will discuss.

Table 1. Important *E. coli* Serotypes[a]

EPEC	ETEC	EIEC	EHEC
O44	O6:H16 or H$^-$	O28:H$^-$	O26:H11
O55	O8:H9 or H –	O112:H$^-$	O157:H7
O86	O15:H11 or H$^-$	O115:H$^-$	
O111	O20:H$^-$	O124:H$^-$	
O114	O25:H42 or H$^-$	O136:H$^-$	
O119	O27:H7 or H20	O143:H$^-$	
O125	O63:H12 or H$^-$	O144:H$^-$	
O126	O78:H11, H12, or H20	O147:H$^-$	
O127	O85:H7	O152:H$^-$	
O128	O115:H11 or H40	O164:H$^-$	
O142	O128:H7 or H21	O167:H$^-$	
O158	O148:H28		
	O159:H20		
	O167:H5		

[a]EPEC, enteropathogenic, ETEC, enterotoxigenic, EIEC, enteroinvasive; EHEC, enterohemorrhagic.

LT is often detected using tissue culture techniques. Cell-free supernatants containing LT cause morphological changes and steroidogenesis in Y-1 adrenal cells, which can be neutralized by specific anti-LT sera. ST can be detected in the suckling mouse assay. Cell-free culture supernatants containing ST cause fluid accumulation in the intestines of 2- to 3-day-old mice, which is measured by the gut-to-body-weight ratio. Recently, immunologic methods for detection of LT and ST have become available.[26,27] Most of these methods are enzyme-linked immunosorbent assays (ELISA). Also, DNA probes that hybridize with the genes that encode LT and ST have been developed and now are the most common method for detection of ETEC strains.[28] These probes have proven extremely useful for large-scale field studies because of the ease of testing many hundreds of strains. In the past, ETEC testing had been a limiting factor for the size of many field trials.

Pathogenicity of a *Shigella* or EIEC strain can be verified by testing in the guinea pig eye (Sereny) model.[29] A heavy suspension of bacteria is dropped into the conjunctival sac of a guinea pig, and 1–7 days later, purulent keratoconjunctivitis is seen if the strain possesses the ability to invade epithelial cells. DNA probes are now available to test directly for the presence of genes encoding for invasiveness.[30] One can screen for the presence of EHEC strains by looking for the lack of ability to ferment sorbitol, which is unusual among *E. coli* strains, along with the inhibition of motility in media containing H7 antiserum.[31] Also, strains can be checked for the production of Shiga toxin in a tissue culture assay.[32]

3.4.2. Serological and Immunologic Diagnostic Methods. Although each of the *E. coli* types that produce diarrhea commonly elicits an immunologic response, serology has not been employed routinely as a diagnostic tool. Also, the importance of serum antibody response has been questioned because the intestinal secretory IgA (sIgA) response is more relevant in intestinal infections. Study of the sIgA response has been limited due to technical difficulties, which are just now beginning to be solved and applied to the study of enteric diseases.[33]

During infection with an EPEC strain, seroconversion has been documented,[34,35] but the diverse number of serogroups makes this a poor diagnostic tool. Perhaps serological surveys in populations may play a role in determining the extent of exposure to prevalent strains of EPEC.

In ETEC diarrhea, seroconversion to anti-LT antibody is common[36–38] but not invariable. An ELISA was developed for the detection of IgG and IgM antibody to LT that has allowed the characterization of specific immunoglobulin.[39] Measurement of anti-LT antibody may be useful in determining previous exposure to LT-ETEC, and hence in determining resistance to naturally occurring infection.(37) Also, ELISAs have been recently developed to detect serum antibody to colonization factor antigens.(40) Perhaps these assays will allow the characterization of specific antibody response to these antigens. During infection with EIEC, a serological response can be documented.(10) In view of the similarity to bacillary dysentery, most probably the frequency of seroconversion will correlate with the presence of dysentery (bloody mucous stools), which indicates the extent of mucosal invasion.(41)

An ELISA has been developed to detect serum antibodies against *E. coli* O157:H7.(42) This assay has been used along with culture to increase detection of this EHEC strain.

4. Biological Characteristics of the Organisms

Volunteer experiments have been conducted to establish the virulence of EPEC strains. In 1950, Neter and Shumway(43) produced illness in an infant by feeding an O111 strain of *E. coli*. This strain as well as an O55 strain were fed to additional adult volunteers and the severity of illness was shown to be directly related to dose.(34,35) Adults were found to be relatively resistant to infection. Additional volunteer studies have confirmed the earlier experiments demonstrating the pathogenicity of EPEC strains for adults.(44) EPEC strains have been defined as specific serogroups of *E. coli* that have been epidemiologically incriminated as causes of diarrhea but do not produce conventional enterotoxins and are not invasive.(45) The serogroups recognized as EPEC are listed in Table 1. Biopsies from children infected with O1199 have shown a characteristic lesion consisting of localized adherence of microcolonies, cupping of the enterocyte, and destruction of the microvilli.(46) Cravioto *et al.*(47) developed a tissue culture model of this adherence property using HEp-2 cells. Later, it was discovered that there were at least two patterns of adherence to the HEp-2 cells: localized and diffuse.(48) Localized adherence, which is encoded by genes carried on a plasmid and the bacterial chromosome, is most clearly related to pathogenicity among strains of EPEC.(49) A DNA probe has been isolated and should be useful in studying the epidemiology of these strains.(25) *E. coli* strains exhibiting HEp-2 cell adherence but not belonging to traditional EPEC serogroups have also been associated with diarrhea in US travelers to Mexico and Mexican children.(50,51) Pathogenicity of these isolates has been shown in adult volunteers.(52)

ETEC strains possess a number of virulence properties that relate to their persistence and pathogenicity for men and animals. Both enterotoxins (LT and ST) have been shown to be encoded for by genes carried on plasmids. Plasmids encoding for enterotoxin production tend to be associated with certain *E. coli* serotypes (Table 1) and are easily lost on subculture. Many ETEC strains that occur in nature produce ST alone, LT alone, or both.

LT is a complex protein that resembles cholera toxin in antigenicity and biological activity.(53) There is a single A subunit associated with five identical B subunits. The B subunits appear to be involved in binding to the membrane of the enterocyte. The A subunit enters the cell, causing the production of cyclic AMP, which in turn results in the net secretion of fluids and electrolytes from the cell.

ST is a very small molecule that is poorly antigenic. Two types of ST are recognized: human and porcine ST. Both are important in human disease. The mechanism of action of ST is not as well understood. It is known that this toxin causes fluid accumulation by increasing the intercellular concentrations of cyclic GMP.

ETEC strains show a high degree of host specificity that probably relates to the organism's ability to proliferate in the small bowel of the infected animal and not to differences in any enterotoxin produced. The colonization potential of an ETEC strain generally relates to the presence of fimbrial antigens that serve as ligands in an intestinal binding process. Table 2 lists the known surface antigens that are probably important to intestinal colonization by ETEC strains. K88, K99, and 987-type fimbrial antigens serve as adherence factors for strains of ETEC pathogenic for animals. There is little evidence that strains pathogenic for animals are commonly transmitted to man. This probably relates to the prerequisite of human-adapted colonization factor antigens (CFAs). A K88-positive ETEC strain highly pathogenic for swine was fed to a group of adult volunteers in a dose of 10^{10} viable cells and disease failed to occur, apparently because the strain

Table 2. Adherence Fimbriae of Enterotoxigenic *E. coli*

Surface antigen	Natural host
K88	Piglet
K99	Calf, lamb
987-type	Piglet
CFA/I/II/III/IV	Human
PCFO159	Human
PCFO166	Human

Table 3. Relationship of Colonization Factor Antigen and Serotype in Human Enterotoxigenic *E. coli* Strains

CFA	Serotype
CFA/I	O15:H11, O15:Hw, O25:H42, O25:Hw, O63:H12, O63:Hw, O73:H11, O78:H12
CFA/II	O6:H16, O6:Hw, O8:H9, O8:Hw
CFA/IV	O25:H42, O23:Hw, O115:H40, O167:H5

did not replicate in the upper gut of the men.[10] Human ETEC strains isolated from patients with diarrhea often have one of several colonization fimbriae designated CFA/I, II, III, and IV and putative colonization factors (PCF0159 and PCF0166). The antigens of CFA/I, II, and IV often show a relationship to serotype (Table 3). These adherence properties can be demonstrated by showing colonization in the upper gut of infant rabbits, which can be confirmed by immunofluorescence. There is an unexplained ubiquity of ETEC in the developing but not the industrialized portions of the world. Environmental factors characteristic of these areas must be important prerequisites for persistence of ETEC strains.

EIEC strains possess *Shigella*-like invasive properties that probably represent the important biological activity favoring persistence in nature. This ability to invade epithelial cells is also encoded for by genes carried on a plasmid and are the same as those found in shigellae.[30] The resemblance of these strains to shigellae is further seen in their possession of common antigens.[4] There is a relationship between EIEC and *E.coli* serotype. Table 1 lists the recognized EIEC serotypes. It is unknown why these strains are not more important causes of illness.

EHEC strains are thought to cause disease by production of high levels of Shiga-like toxin.[32] Recently, a fimbrial antigen was described that might enhance the persistence of the organisms in the intestine.[54] There is some evidence that cattle may be an environmental reservoir of EHEC.

5. Descriptive Epidemiology

5.1. Prevalence and Incidence

Studies of diarrhea cases based on hospital data indicate that EPEC strains are responsible for between 10 and 40% of illness presenting to such facilities.[55,56] The frequency of EPEC in stools of diarrhea cases is higher when hospital cases are compared to outpatients.[55] In the reports with the highest frequency of EPEC disease, a single strain usually could be identified in many of the cases, indicating a community wide epidemic. Three geographically distinct areas were involved in one outbreak. In the three epidemic census tracts, attack rates were 73, 118, and 55 per 1000 among nonwhite infants less than 1 year of age. Of index households, 50% had one or more asymptomatic pharyngeal carriers of the epidemic strain, while next-door neighbors and distant community household members harbored the strain in the pharynx in 33 and 0%, respectively. Intestinal carriage in the three household groups was 18, 3, and 0%, respectively. Kessner *et al.*[22] carried out a prospective examination of EPEC in a defined geographic area in Illinois and Indiana. An extensive community epidemic of diarrhea due to *E. coli* O111 during the summer, autumn, and winter of 1960 and 1961 was documented. Age-specific attack rates for the 0- to 6-month age group ranged from 1,800 to 3,700/100,000. Carrier rates of asymptomatic contacts of index cases ranged from 5 to 10%. Pal *et al.*[57] described a community outbreak that occurred in India. The morbidity for the population under study was 0.16%, with age-specific attack rates for the 0- to 2-year-old group of 0.98% and for the 6- to 11-month age group of 2.4%. During another community outbreak in Atlanta, EPEC strains were isolated from 12.7/1000 persons at risk and from 125/1000 infants less than 1 year of age.[21] EPEC strains are responsible for epidemic or sporadic diarrhea as well as community epidemics.[56]

ETEC has variably been reported to cause between 0 and 86% of diarrhea cases in North America.[58–62] The more comprehensive 2-year surveys have indicated that these strains are unusual causes of endemic diarrhea in North America.[60,62] ETEC strains, however, may produce epidemics of diarrhea. Such epidemics have been associated with the consumption of food or water contaminated with ETEC.[10,63–65] Also, outbreaks have been documented in hospital nurseries.[66,67] ETEC infection is more common in developing countries. These organisms were the most frequently isolated pathogen among Mexican children with diarrhea.[52] During the first 3 years of life, Mexican children showed a progressive rise in IgG anti-LT antibody that was statistically greater than that seen for Houston children.[39] Latin Americans possess high serum antibody titers to LT, while North Americans possess relatively low titers.[37] The titer of LT antibody most probably reflects prior exposure to LT-producing *E. coli* and directly relates to resistance to infection.[37] In a cohort study of infants less than 5 years of age, 61% had at least one infection by an ETEC strain.[68] In the study, the annual incidence was 1.2 episodes per child. Seventy-eight percent of the infections were asymptomatic with a decreasing illness-to-infection with increasing age. ETEC strains are the most important cause of diarrhea among US travelers in Latin America,[59,69,70] being responsible for 40–60% of disease. Persons from the United States develop resistance to infection remain in areas where they are at risk to develop diarrhea.

EIEC strains are unusual causes of endemic or epidemic diarrhea. Three outbreaks associated with contaminated food have been documented in the United States.[16–18] EIEC has also been shown to be a cause of endemic diarrhea in Brazil and among travelers to developing nations.[15,71]

EHEC has been incriminated in both endemic and epidemic diarrhea in the United States, Canada, and Europe.[19,20] Outbreaks have occurred in nursing homes, day-care centers, schools, and the community. Investigations have demonstrated that sporadic cases of hemorrhagic colitis occur widely.[20] A community wide investigation of an outbreak of hamburger-associated O157:H7 was carried out in Washington state where it is a notifiable disease.[24] Five hundred and one cases were identified over a 3-month period. The infection resulted from the ingestion of inadequately cooked hamburgers at a fast-food chain.

5.2. Epidemic Behavior and Contagiousness

EPEC strains have a predilection for spread within the hospital, particularly in nursery populations. Although the organism is spread within the community, the hospital probably plays a role in transmission to community members.[22,55] In a community outbreak of EPEC disease, 37% of the cases had been hospitalized within the preceding 30 days, while an additional 17% had direct contact with hospitals.[22] Factors related to contagiousness of EPEC other than exposure to hospitals are age, sex, race, and degree of crowding.

ETEC diarrhea shows epidemic spread to susceptible persons under unusual exposure, which may result from a hospital confinement or travel to a part of the world where ETEC strains are endemic. Epidemic behavior and contagiousness of EIEC strains are unknown.

Very large point source outbreaks of EHEC serotype O157:H7 have been recognized.[19,24] Other EHEC serotypes that have been shown to cause endemic diarrhea have not been recognized in large outbreaks and may not be as contagious. Intrafamilial transmission of O157:H7 has been documented to be 10% during a large community outbreak.[24]

5.3. Geographic Distribution

EPEC diarrhea occurs with a worldwide distribution. The first large outbreaks were recognized in industrialized urban parts of the world. This may have been due to greater reporting and the availability of more sophisticated identification techniques. Recently, EPEC diarrhea has been reported more often in studies of endemic diarrhea in developing countries.[25,48,52]

ETEC diarrhea has been shown to be common only in developing parts of the world. Only two reports suggest that ETEC strains might be common causes of endemic diarrhea in the United States.[72,73] The infection has been reported to occur with frequency in Asia,[11] Brazil,[74] Mexico,[52,69] and Africa.[75] Outbreaks of illness among adults due to ST-only strains have been reported in Japan.[76] EIEC strains have a worldwide distribution, but have been reported to be a frequent cause of diarrhea only in Brazil.[15]

E. coli O157:H7 has only been identified in developed nations. The incidence of the organism in developing countries appears to be lower.

5.4. Temporal Distribution

EPEC diarrhea occurs year-round, and although some investigators have found a peak summertime incidence,[21,56,60] others have shown the disease to have a fall–winter peak.[22] The time of year probably does not greatly influence disease rates.

ETEC diarrhea also occurs year-round. Many of the published studies were conducted during the summer months, and therefore there is a predominance of ETEC isolation during the warmer months. Since most of the areas of the world where ETEC is commonly found to be associated with diarrhea are tropical, it may be that a strong seasonal pattern will not be found.

There is no information about the temporal distribution of EIEC or EHEC infections.

5.5. Age

One study examining the relationship of age to EPEC infection demonstrated that the median age at the time of hospitalization was 8 months and 2 weeks.[22] The distribution by age groups of hospitalized children was: 86% between 0–18 months, 65% under 1 years of age, and 9% in the neonatal period. In the community survey, the age distribution of those with positive stool cultures, and regardless of symptoms, mirrored the age group hospitalized for diarrhea. Most published studies have confirmed that nearly all episodes of culturally confirmed EPEC diarrhea are seen in infants under 2 years of age, with more than half being in the group less than 6 months of age. In Houston, EPEC disease was documented to occur 20 times more frequently in infants below 6 months of age compared to children 1–2 years of age.[77] One study indicated that approximately 25% of infants were infected with an EPEC strain during the first year of life, and the prevalence of EPEC intestinal excretion by a group of infants less than 1 year of age was 1%.[78]

In ETEC diarrhea, most cases of infection occur in children in areas where disease is endemic, as determined by the natural history of antibody to LT during the first 3 years of life plus the observation that adults living in these areas are immune to infection. The highest attack rate of ETEC infection occurs in the age group 6 months to 36 months of age, with decreasing rates with increasing age.[79]

No information is available about the relationship of age to EIEC or EHEC disease. Both are commonly foodborne infections and the age affected usually relates to the group consuming the contaminated food.

5.6. Sex

As with many other infections, males of all ages show a higher infection rate due to EPEC strains. An overall male–female ratio of 4:1 has been reported.[22] Others have documented male predominance.[21,80] Insufficient information is available to determine whether a sex relationship exists for the other diarrheal diseases due to *E. coli*.

5.7. Race

The published studies show a correlation of infection with exposure to hospitals and crowded living conditions, which probably explains the greater occurrence of EPEC in nonwhite children in the United States.[21,22] In rural Guatemala, among a primitive culture wherein hospital exposure was nonexistent and breast-feeding was prevalent, EPEC diarrhea was not encountered during the neonatal period despite shedding of potentially infectious strains by the mothers.[81] EPEC disease occurred later during weaning from breast-feeding in this population. It may be that race is only important in enhancing the probability of exposure and in decreasing the tendency toward breast-feeding.

Insufficient data are available to determine whether there are racial influences on ETEC, EIEC, and EHEC diarrhea.

5.8. Occupation

EPEC is a disease of infants. Those persons taken into tropical climates by their employment might be expected to be at risk for ETEC disease. Occupational factors relating to exposures to EIEC and EHEC are unknown.

5.9. Occurrence in Different Settings

EPEC strains produce diarrhea primarily in hospital populations, particularly in nurseries housing newborn infants. Hospitalized infants and children attending day-care centers represent the major reservoirs for community spread.

ETEC diarrhea is a particular problem among groups traveling from low-risk (United States, northwestern Europe, Canada, and Japan) to high-risk areas (Latin America, Asia, and Africa). It is also a problem among infants and children in these high-risk areas. Hospital outbreaks of ETEC diarrhea have been reported.[66,67] EIEC organisms have been reported as a rare cause of foodborne outbreaks in the United States.[17,18] These organisms have been found rarely in most parts of the world. An exception appears to be Brazil, where there is an unexplained prevalence of EIEIC-associated diarrhea.[15] Hemorrhagic colitis has been shown to occur mainly in developed nations.[19,20]

5.10. Socioeconomic Factors

Socioeconomic factors are important in EPEC diarrhea primarily as they influence crowding, sanitation, breast-feeding, and exposure to hospitals. There is no known relationship between socioeconomic factors and other diarrheal diseases due to *E. coli*, although it can be assumed that the same factors that influence EPEC illness are also important.

6. Mechanisms and Routes of Transmission

Within hospital environments, EPEC organisms are transmitted by direct contact, spread by dust, and from fomites. During one outbreak of diarrhea due to an EPEC strain, nursing personnel and family members were shown to be asymptomatic excretors of the epidemic strain,[82] suggesting a possible role in the transmission of the agent.

In the same study, recovery of an EPEC from stools of mothers just before delivery was documented in 13% (361 mothers), with subsequent isolation of the same serotype of *E. coli* from 40% of the newborn infants of the culture-positive mothers. Asymptomatic adult carriers of EPEC strains undoubtedly play a role in disease transmission to infants and young children.[22,80,83] During one community epidemic, the infecting strain was commonly isolated from pharyngeal cultures, and respiratory symptoms were noted.[82] Others have noted the association of respiratory symptoms and EPEC diarrhea.[22,80] It is possible that a respiratory route of transmission may play a role in disease transmission. As with other enteric diseases, fecal–oral transmission is the most likely mode for spread. Person-to-person contact spread has been suggested by the epidemiological patterns of infection.[22] In a longitudinal study of 40 households, EPEC infection correlated with crowded sleeping arrangements, pork and chicken consumption, and intimate contact with household pets.[84] In one family outbreak, a pet dog was shown to be the index case.

From the available studies, it appears that ETEC strains are spread through ingestion of contaminated food.[85,86] In our studies in Mexico, when students ate at public eating establishments, they were more likely to develop ETEC diarrhea than if they consumed meals prepared by themselves in their own apartments.[86] Food sampled from public eating facilities was commonly found to be contaminated with coliforms. Sack *et al.*[85] found a small percentage of foods in the United States to be contaminated with ETEC. Due to the large inoculum necessary to produce diarrhea in healthy adults ($> 10^8$ viable cells),[10] it is likely that food or water are the most important vehicles of disease transmission. The important transmission kinetics of EIEC are unknown, largely because of the rarity of infection by these strains. All the major documented outbreaks have been associated with consumption of food contaminated with these organisms.[17,18]

Little is known about the transmission of EHEC strains, except that the reported outbreaks have characteristically been associated with eating hamburgers usually at fast-food outlets.[19,24] Lake water also may be a source of infection.[87] Other food and beverages including drinking water may be the source of infection rarely.[88]

7. Pathogenesis and Immunity

Several histopathologic studies have shown that there is a characteristic lesion associated with EPEC infection.[45,46] The EPEC are seen by electron microscopy as microcolonies that adhere to epithelial cells with destruction of the brush border, but with no evidence of invasion. Pedestal formation has also been noted. This lesion can be duplicated in an animal model[89] and there is a tissue culture model (HEp-2 cell assay) available.[47] This adherence property is encoded for by genes carried on a plasmid[49] and has been named the enteroadherence factor (EAF). The product of the EAF gene is unknown and most probably is not fimbrial in nature.[53] Although toxins are suggested by the nature of the lesion in EPEC infection and a few toxins have been reported,[53] it now appears that if enterotoxins are present, they are unrecognized. Although EPEC strains appear to produce illness in adults, the disease is primarily a disease of newborns and young infants. The age distribution suggests that protective immunity develops. The nature and extent of immunity are unknown.

Prior to the development of illness, ETEC strains must colonize the toxin-sensitive upper intestine before elaborating secretory enterotoxins. Specific fimbrial antigens on the surface of ETEC strains have been shown to mediate adherence of the *E. coli* to the mucosa of the small bowel. Table 2 lists the recognized colonization factor antigens of ETEC according to natural hosts. In the small intestine of piglets, the K88 antigen appears to bind to a receptor on the villous epithelial cell.[90–92] Attachments of ETEC to the upper gut depend not only on the fimbriae of the bacteria but also on the presence of specific receptors for the fimbriae.[93] Some strains of pigs genetically lack the receptor for K88, making them immune to disease caused by K88-bearing organisms. Antigenically different fimbriae, K88, K99, 987-type, and type 1 (common) pili, adhere equally to porcine intestinal epithelium.[94] These ligands probably bind to different receptors in view of a lack of competitive inhibition of bacterial adherence.[94] ETEC strains infecting humans usually possess one of several recognized colonization factor antigens known as CFA/I, II, III, and IV and putative colonization factors (PCF0159 and PCF0166). Once an ETEC has adhered to the upper gut of the infected host, enterotoxins produce changes in ion flux across the mucosa of the small intestine. The two classical *E. coli* enterotoxins affect intestinal secretion through two different pathways. ST shows more rapid onset of action and the effect is of shorter duration than LT.

Natural immunity to ETEC infection occurs when persons remain at high risk for infection. In a study of students attending school in Mexico, the attack rate was inversely related to the length of time the student had lived in the endemic area.[69] Newly arrived students from the

United States suffered from diarrhea at a rate of 40% per month, compared to a rate of 20% for the same time period for those students from the United States who had been in Mexico for approximately a year or longer. Newly arrived students from Venezuela did not show an increase in illness, indicating immunity from prior exposure in Venezuela to agents prevalent in Mexico. A decreased frequency and lowered severity of illness among Latin American students correlated with an apparent resistance to ETEC infection. An inverse relationship was found between the geometric mean antibody titer (GMT) to LT and the occurrence of diarrhea associated with LT-producing *E. coli*.(37) Ruiz-Palacios *et al.*(39) examined the titer of IgG and IgM antitoxin antibodies from birth to 3 years of age among children from the United States and Mexico by an ELISA. IgG antitoxin antibodies fell to low levels from birth to 3 months (presumably from natural decay of maternally acquired immunoglobulin) and rose thereafter. The titers were significantly higher among Mexican children than those from the United States. We have found the low GMTs of 3-year-old children from Houston to be essentially the same as those found for adults from various parts of the United States. The lack of exposure to ETEC in the United States appears to explain the remarkable susceptibility to infection among persons from the United States traveling in developing countries. Immunity to ETEC infection does not appear to be strictly antitoxic in origin, since Latin American students exposed to ETEC strains rarely excrete the organism in stools asymptomatically, in contrast to the common finding of asymptomatic fecal shedding of strains in United States students.(69,95) These data suggest that antibacterial immunity is operative because virulent strains are excluded from gut colonization. This could represent intestinal antibody to adhesion fimbriae and/or somatic antigens or other factors.

The pathogenic mechanisms of EIEC are the same as those of shigellae. These organisms invade the colonic mucosa and spread laterally in the epithelium, causing ulcer formation and clinical dysentery. It can be assumed that immunity to EIEC is similar to that seen in shigellosis. Experiments using monkeys have shown that immunity to *Shigella* develops after infection, but the immunity is serotype specific.(96) EHEC apparently causes disease by adherence to the mucosa of the transverse colon mediated by a newly described fimbrial antigen.(54) *E. coli* O157:H7 strains have been shown to elaborate large quantities of Shiga-like toxin that is thought to be responsible for the tissue damage seen in this infection. Since EHEC infection is a relatively newly recognized disease, little information is available concerning immunity to infection. Serum antibodies to Shiga-like toxin and to lipopolysaccharide of the O157 antigen have been demonstrated.(42)

8. Patterns of Host Response

In EPEC infection, inapparent infection and transient colonization are common, especially among older children and adults. In one study, 15–20 per 1000 normal children between birth and 5 years of age harbored an EPEC strain in their stools.(97) Another study found prevalence of EPEC excretion to be 1% for infants less than 1 year of age.(80) In a 1-year longitudinal study of 40 households, transient excretion, infection defined as excretion longer than 4 weeks, and clinical illness were most common in young children.(84) The rate of excretion of EPEC in this study was approximately 11% in children under 1 year of age, while the rate in adults was 5%. Overt illness was seen in 25% of children under 1 year of age who had an EPEC detected in their stools. Illness is uncommon in older children and adults, even though they often carry the organism.

ETEC excretion commonly occurs asymptomatically in persons exposed to these strains.(69,95) It appears that highly susceptible individuals most commonly develop overt disease when exposed to ETEC strains, in contrast to those partially immune, in whom excretion without illness characteristically occurs, and to those with natural immunity through prior exposure, in whom neither disease nor excretion can be documented.

In EIEC infection, as experimentally induced in volunteers, asymptomatic excretion was common and seroconversion occurred without overt illness.(10)

8.1. Clinical Features

While there is marked variation in the duration and severity of EPEC illness, the most common findings are fever (60%), diarrhea (> 90%), respiratory symptoms (50%), abdominal distension suggesting paralytic ileus (10%), and convulsions (< 1%).(22) Dehydration may be seen in one third of cases, especially in infants under 1 year of age, and hypernatremia and metabolic acidosis commonly occur.(80) Dysentery has been reported in EPEC diarrhea. Illness usually lasts about 1 week, yet protracted illness commonly occurs and the illness may result in fatalities.(23,55) In fatal cases and in certain outbreaks of more virulent disease, a picture of septicemia and widespread intestinal inflammation and necrosis is found. A more severe disease with a higher percentage of fatalities has been seen in infection with the O111 serogroup of *E. coli*.[23,84] Mortality is higher for ill infants who are less than 1 month of age.[22] In ETEC diarrhea, the disease resembles mild cholera in most cases, where the most common finding is watery diarrhea. In contradistinction to cholera, abdominal pain and cramps (which may be severe) are common in *E. coli* diarrhea, and low-grade fever may be seen. In our experience in Mexico, the average illness in adults consists of passage of 8 to 12 unformed stools over a 4- to 5-day period. In volunteers with experimentally induced illness, the clinical syndrome in the most severe cases consisted of passage of 5 to 10 watery stools per day, lasting as long as 19 days. We have seen a patient in Houston with ETEC infection present with a choleralike illness requiring more than 30 liters of intravenous fluids to maintain hydration. Of significance was that this person had had a previous gastric resection for peptic ulcer disease. Fatalities are unusual with ETEC disease and probably occur only in the very young, the elderly, and those with marginal cardiovascular reserves. The illness associated with ST-only (strains that produce only ST) *E. coli* appears to be quite similar to that produced by ST/LT strains.[67,76]

EIEC strains produce an illness indistinguishable from shigellosis (bacillary dysentery). Fever, abdominal pain and bloody mucous stools are frequently seen.[10,18] As in shigellosis, the disease is usually self-limiting, and fatalities are probably unusual.

Hemorrhagic colitis is a distinctive clinical syndrome.[19] It normally starts as watery diarrhea and abdominal cramps and progresses to grossly bloody diarrhea with little or no fever. The average duration of symptoms is around 8 days. There does appear, however, to be a spectrum of clinical disease with some patients having only watery diarrhea with no blood in the stool or fever.[20] EHEC has also been associated with hemolytic uremic syndrome as a common sequela to infection with these organisms.[19,20]

8.2. Diagnosis

The features of *E. coli* infections relevant to diagnosis are summarized in Table 4. EPEC diarrhea should be considered in any outbreak that develops in a hospital nursery or on a pediatric hospital ward. In this setting, serotyping is the only way to identify these strains because of the epidemic potential of these strains. Because of the variable clinical syndrome depending on strain variation and host response, any diarrheal illness in a hospitalized pediatric population should be considered as potentially EPEC in origin. Serotyping of *E. coli* from children with sporadic community-acquired diarrhea is of questionable importance and probably does not justify the cost. More studies need to be conducted to determine the importance of the HEp-2 cell adherence assay and the EAF probe in detecting diarrheagenic strains of *E. coli* related to EPEC in endemic diarrhea.

ETEC intestinal infection should be considered in any traveler from the United States, Canada, or northwestern Europe who develops diarrhea without high fever while traveling in Latin America, Asia, or Africa. Unfortunately, the routine diagnostic laboratory is presently unable to assay for LT and ST, which are available only in research and reference laboratories. ELISAs and DNA probes are now being developed for use in the routine diagnostic laboratory.

EIEC infection should be suspected in a patient with bacillary dysentery (bloody mucous stools with prevalent fecal leukocytes on microscopic examination) in whom stool cultures are negative for shigellae. The routine diagnostic laboratory can make a presumptive identification of EIEC by the biochemical reactions of these organisms. EIEC strains, unlike most *E. coli* strains, are lysine decarboxylate-negative and are nonmotile. Presumptively identified strains must then be confirmed in a reference laboratory by DNA probe or the Sereny (guinea pig eye) test.[29]

Table 4. Features of *E. coli* Infections

	EPEC	ETEC	EIEC	EHEC
Laboratory diagnosis	Serotyping, DNA probe	ST and LT detection	Sereny test, DNA probe	Serotyping
Prevalence	10–40% of hospitalized diarrhea	Rare in USA Travelers' diarrhea 40–60%	Rare	Developed countries
Outbreaks	Nurseries	Travelers, infants	Foodborne	Foodborne
Geographic	Worldwide	Developing nations	Worldwide	Developed countries
Temporal	Summer peak	Year-round, summer peak	Unknown	Unknown
Age	< 2 yr	Travelers, infants	Unknown	Unknown

EHEC diarrhea should be suspected in patients with bloody stools and little or no fever. These strains can be definitively identified only by demonstrating Shiga-like toxin productions or possession of genes encoding for Shiga-like toxin. EHEC stains can belong to many *E. coli* serotypes, but O157:H7 and O26:H11 are the most common. The clinical laboratory can screen for these strains by looking for *E. coli* that fail to ferment sorbitol and whose motility can be blocked by antisera to H7 or H11.(31)

9. Control and Prevention

9.1. General Concepts

Since *E. coli* diarrhea is not a reportable condition, we do not have adequate information about the epidemiology and optimal control and intervention procedures. It is clear that during EPEC outbreaks, standard public health and infection control procedures are important in terminating transmission. Isolation of cases, cohorting by area and nursing personnel, institution of strict hand washing, and prevention of common exposure to equipment, bedding, or solutions are all indicated.

In ETEC diarrhea of travelers, careful selection of food by individuals and institutions and enforcement of food hygiene in public eating establishments by departments of public health are the major areas for disease control. For an individual, the selection of a restaurant where a history free of acquisition of diarrheal disease can be elicited from those who frequent the establishment is probably the most important single consideration. Beyond this, ingestion of steaming foods and beverages, carbonated bottled drinks, and citrus fruits, and avoidance of leafy green vegetables, cold meats, desserts, fresh cheese, and milk, are advisable when traveling in parts of the world where food sanitation is substandard. Consumption of tap water of the developing world is never advisable. In EIEC diarrhea, it is not known whether person-to-person spread occurs or whether, due to a large inoculum responsible for disease, food and water represent the important vehicles of transmission. No specific information on the control of EIEC is available.

EHEC infection is best prevented by avoidance of undercooked beef, especially hamburger.

9.2. Antibiotic and Chemotherapeutic Approaches to Prophylaxis

The most important factor in treatment of any diarrheal disease is the maintenance of fluid and electrolyte balance by administering oral rehydration fluids. The value of antimicrobial agents in the control of hospital outbreaks of EPEC diarrhea has not been established. The strains identified in these outbreaks were generally susceptible to the aminoglycosides and polymyxins.(21,34,98–102) Several of these studies demonstrated an apparent effect when neomycin, gentamicin, or colymycin was administered to infants and children during hospital outbreaks. Problems in other reports have related to development of antibiotic resistance by the infecting strain during therapy or failure to affect the spread of the epidemic.(80,100) EPEC strains recently isolated have been very resistant to antimicrobial agents, and these R factors are apparently carried on the same plasmid as the EAF genes.(103)

Antibacterial drugs will significantly shorten the duration of ETEC diarrhea in children and travelers with illness acquired in endemic areas. The antimicrobial drugs of value include trimethoprim–sulfamethoxazole and the fluoroquinolones. In EHEC infection, antibiotics have not been clearly demonstrated to be of value. In fact, there is some evidence to suggest that antimicrobial therapy may predispose infected patients to the development of hemolytic–uremic syndrome.

In studies of ETEC diarrhea, a variety of antimicrobial agents have been used with success in preventing illness among travelers from low-risk to high-risk areas. The drugs include doxycycline, trimethoprim, trimethoprim–sulfamethoxazole, furazolidone, and norfloxicin. A chemical compound, bismuth subsalicylate, has also been found to prevent diarrhea in a group of students from the United States traveling to Mexico.(104) While prophylaxis is not recommended for routine use by travelers, these means of intervention may have value in certain high-risk groups during brief exposures. Groups for which chemoprophylaxis may be useful include businessmen, politicians, the aged, the medically disabled, and those who have had severe diarrhea in the past. Problems to anticipate as groups begin using chemoprophylaxis include adverse reaction to the drugs, selection of more resistant bacterial enteropathogens, and increase in prevalence of resistant pathogens.

Drug prevention of EIEC and EHEC diarrhea is not feasible in view of the facts that populations at high risk are unknown and antibiotic administration is of unknown benefit.

9.3. Immunization

No immunizing agents are available for EPEC, EIEC, or EHEC infections. Efforts are currently underway to develop a vaccine against ETEC and EIEC (*Shigella* vaccines) infection using genetic engineering techniques. An orally administered cholera vaccine made up of killed *Vibrio cholerae* whole cells and the binding subunit of cholera toxin is currently available in some area as a prevention for ETEC diarrhea (see Chapter 11).

10. Unresolved Problems

In EPEC disease, the most important issues to be resolved are the mechanisms of intestinal adherence, the importance of the different adherence patterns, and the pathogenicity and relationship of HEp-2–cell-adherent *E. coli* that do not belong to traditional EPEC serotypes. Further studies using the newer DNA probes should allow the elucidation of the importance of EPEC strains in endemic diarrhea in developing nations.

In ETEC diarrhea, the most pressing problems still center around assays to identify ST and LT in the routine diagnostic laboratory. Progress is being made in this area, and practical serological procedures should be available in the near future. Also, since ETEC disease represents an important childhood illness and immunity occurs naturally, there is great interest in the development of immunoprophylactic agents.

The prevalence and epidemiology of EIEC diarrhea need to be clarified further. This should now be accomplished by using the newly developed DNA probes in field-based studies to determine the prevalence and epidemiology of these organisms.

Hemorrhagic colitis is the most recently recognized of the *E. coli* diarrheas. Much needs to be learned concerning the prevalence, epidemiology, pathogenic mechanisms, detection, and immune response to this O157:H7 strain. Important remaining questions relate to the exact relationship of EHEC infection to the development of hemolytic–uremic syndrome and the role of antimicrobial agents in the pathogenesis of hemolytic–uremic syndrome.

As we continue work with virulent *E. coli* strains, it is essential that we reserve the term enteropathogenic *E. coli* (EPEC) as a designation for those strains that include the specific serotypes that have been epidemiologically incriminated as pathogens. All *E. coli* that cause diarrhea should be referred to as a group as diarrheagenic *E. coli*. Diarrheagenic *E. coli* comprise a diverse group of strains that should be classified by the pathogenic mechanisms they possess.

11. References

1. Bray, J., Isolation of antigenically homogeneous strains of *Bact. coli neapolitanum* from summer diarrhoea of infants, *J. Pathol. Bacteriol.* **57:**239–247 (1945).
2. Giles, C., Sangster, G., and Smith, J., Epidemic gastroenteritis of infants in Aberdeen during 1947, *Arch. Dis. Child.* **24:**45–53 (1949).
3. Taylor, J., Powell, B. W., and Wright, J., Infantile diarrhea and vomiting: A clinical and bacteriological investigation, *Br. Med. J.* **2:**117–125 (1949).
4. Ewing, W. H., (ed.), The genus *Escherichia* in: *Edward's and Ewing's Identification of Enterobacteriaceae*, 4th ed., pp. 93–134, Elsevier, New York, 1986.
5. Kauffman, F., The serology of the *coli* group, *J. Immunol.* **57:**71–100 (1947).
6. Kaufmann, F., and DuPont, A. J., *Escherichia* strains from infantile epidemic gastroenteritis, *Acta Pathol. Microbiol. Scand.* **27:**552–564 (1950).
7. Taylor, J., Wilkins, M. P., and Payne, J. M., Relations of rabbit gut reaction to enteropathogenic *Escherichia coli*, *Br. J. Exp. Pathol.* **42:**43–52 (1961).
8. Rowe, B., Taylor, J., and Bettelheim, K. A., An investigation of travellers' diarrhoea, *Lancet* **1:**1–5 (1970).
9. Smith, H. W., and Gyles, C. L., The relationship between two apparently different enterotoxins produced by enteropathogenic strains of *Escherichia coli* of porcine origin, *J. Med. Microbiol.* **3:**387–401 (1970).
10. DuPont, H. L., Formal, S. B., Hornick, R. B., Snyder, M. J., Libonati, J. P., Sheahan, D. G., LaBrec, E. H., and Kalas, J. P., Pathogenesis of *Escherichia coli* diarrhea, *N. Engl. J. Med.* **285:**1–9 (1971).
11. Gorbach, S. L., Banwell, J. G., Chatterjee, B. D., Jacobs, B., and Sack, R. B., Acute undifferentiated human diarrhea in the tropics. I. Alterations in intestinal microflora, *J. Clin. Invest.* **50:**881–889 (1971).
12. Sack, R. B., Gorbach, S. L., Banwell, J. G., Jacobs, B., Chatterjee, B. D., and Mitra, R., Enterotoxigenic *Escherichia coli* isolated from patients with severe cholera-like disease, *J. Infect. Dis.* **123:**378–385 (1971).
13. Evans, D. J., Jr., Evans, D. G., and DuPont, H. L., Virulence factors of enterotoxigenic *Escherichia coli*, *J. Infect. Dis.* **136:** S118–S123 (1977).
14. Ogawa, H., Nakamura, A., and Sakazaki, R., Pathogenic properties of "enteropathogenic" *Escherichia coli* from diarrheal children and adults, *Jpn. J. Med. Sci. Biol.* **21:**333–349 (1968).
15. Trabulsi, L. R., and de Toledo, M. R. F., *Escherichia coli* serogroup O115 isolated from patients with enteritis: Biochemical characteristics and experimental pathogenicity, *Rev. Inst. Med. Trop. San Palo* **11:**358–362 (1969).
16. Gordillo, M. E., Reeve, G. R., Pappas, J., Mathewson, J. J., DuPont, H. L., and Murray, B. E., Molecular characterization of strains of enteroinvasive *Escherichia coli*, *J. Clin. Microbiol.* **30:**889–893 (1992).
17. Marier, R., Wells, J. G., Swanson, R. C., Callahan, W., and Mehlman, I. J., An outbreak of enteropathogenic *Escherichia coli* foodborne disease traced to imported French cheese, *Lancet* **2:**1376–1378 (1973).
18. Tulloch, E. F., Jr., Ryan, K. J., Formal, S. B., and Franklin, F. A.,

Invasive enteropathogenic *Escherichia coli* dysentery: An outbreak in 28 adults, *Ann. Intern. Med.* **79:**13–17 (1973).

19. Riley, L. W., Remis, R. S., Helgerson, S. D., McGee, H. B., Wells, J. G., Davis, B. R., Herbert, R. J., Olcott, E. S., Johnson, L. M., Hargrett, N. T., Blake, P. A., and Cohen, M. L., Hemorrhagic colitis associated with a rare *Escherichia coli* serotype, *N. Engl. J. Med.* **308:**681–685 (1983).
20. Remis, R. S., MacDonald, K. L., Riley, L. W., Puhr, B. S., Wells, J. G., Davis, B. R., Blake, P. A., and Cohen, M. L., Sporadic cases of hemorrhagic colitis associated with *Escherichia coli* O157:H7, *Ann. Intern. Med.* **101:**624–626 (1984).
21. Boris, M., Thomason, B. M., Hines, V. D., Montague, T. S., and Sellers, T. F., A community epidemic of enteropathogenic *Escherichia coli* O126:B16:NM gastroenteritis associated with asymptomatic respiratory infection, *Pediatrics* **33:**18–29 (1964).
22. Kessner, D. M., Shaughnessy, H. J., Googins, J., Rasmussen, C. M., Rose, M. J., Marshall, A. L., Jr., Andelman, S. L., Hall, J. B., and Rosenblom, P. J., An extensive community outbreak of diarrhea due to enteropathogenic *Escherichia coli* O111:B4. I. Epidemiologic studies, *Am. J. Hyg.* **76:**27–43 (1962).
23. Drucker, M. M., Poliack, A., Yevien, R., and Sacks, T. G., Immunofluorescent demonstration of enteropathogenic *Escherichia coli* in tissue of infants dying with enteritis, *Pediatrics* **46:**855–864 (1970).
24. Bell, B. P., Goldoft, M., Griffin, P. M., Davis, M. A., Gordon, D. C., Tarr, P. I., Bartleson, C. A., Lewis, J. H., Barrett, T. J., Wells, J. G., Baron, R., and Kobayashi, J., A multistate outbreak of *Escherichia coli* O157:H7-associated bloody diarrhea and hemolytic uremic syndrome from hamburgers. The Washington experience, *J. Am. Med. Assoc.* **274:**1349–1353 (1994).
25. Nataro, J. P., Baldini, M. M., Kaper, J. B., Black, R. E., Bravo, N., and Levine, M. M., Detection of an adherence factor of enteropathogenic *Escherichia coli* with a DNA probe, *J. Infect. Dis.* **152:**560–565 (1985).
26. Gustafsson, B., and Mollby, R., GM1 ganglioside enzyme-linked immunosorbent assay for detection of heat-labile enterotoxin produced by human and porcine *Escherichia coli* strains, *J. Clin. Microbiol.* **15:**298–301 (1982).
27. Thompson, M. R., Brandwein, H., LaBine-Racke, M., and Giannela, R. A., Simple and reliable enzyme-linked immunosorbent assay with monoclonal antibodies for the detection of *Escherichia coli* heat-stable enterotoxins, *J. Clin. Microbiol.* **20:**59–64 (1984).
28. Mosely, S. L., Echeverria, P., Seriwatana, J., Tirapat, C., Chaicumpa, W., and Falkow, S., Identification of enterotoxigenic *Escherichia coli* by colony hybridization using three gene probes, *J. Infect. Dis.* **145:**863–869 (1982).
29. Sereny, B., Experimental shigella keratoconjunctivitis: A preliminary report, *Acta Microbiol. Acad. Sci. Hung.* **2:**293–296 (1955).
30. Boileau, C. R., d'Hauteville, H. M., and Sansonetti, P. J., DNA hybridization technique to detect *Shigella* species and enteroinvasive *Escherichia coli*, J. Clin. Microbiol. **20:**959–961 (1984).
31. Farmer, J. J., Jr., and Davis, B. R., H7 antiserum–sorbitol fermentation medium: A single tube screening method for detecting *Escherichia coli* O157:H7 associated with hemorrhagic colitis, *J. Clin. Microbiol.* **22:**620–625 (1985).
32. O'Brien, A. D., Lively, T. A., and Chen, M. S., *Escherichia coli* O157:H7 strains associated with hemorrhagic colitis in the United States produce a *Shigella dysenteriae* 1 (Shiga)-like cytotoxin, *Lancet* **1:**702 (1983).
33. Winsor, D. K., Jr., Mathewson, J. J., and DuPont, H. L., Western blot analysis of intestinal secretory IgA response to *Campylobacter jejuni* antigens in patients with naturally acquired *Campylobacter* enteritis, *Gastroenterology* **90:**1217–1222 (1986).
34. Ferguson, W. W., and June, R. C., Experiments on feeding adult volunteers with *Escherichia coli* 111, B4, a coliform organism associated with infant diarrhea, *Am. J. Hyg.* **55:**155–169 (1952).
35. June, R. C., Ferguson, W. W., and Worfel, M. T., Experiments in feeding adult volunteers with *Escherichia coli* 55, B5 a coliform organism associated with infant diarrhea, *Am. J. Hyg.* **57:**222–236 (1953).
36. Donta, S. T., Sack, D. A., Wallacer, B., DuPont, H-.L., and Sack, R. B., Tissue-culture assay of antibodies to heat-labile *Escherichia coli* enterotoxins, *N. Engl. J. Med.* **291:**117–121 (1974).
37. Evans, D. J., Jr., Ruiz-Palacios, G., Evans, D. C., DuPont, H. L., Pickering, L. K., and Olarte, J., Humoral immune response to heat-labile enterotoxin of *Escherichia coli* in naturally acquired diarrhea and antitoxin determination by passive immune hemolysis, *Infect. Immun.* **16:**781–788 (1977).
38. Sack, R. B., Jacobs, B., and Mitra, R., Antitoxin responses to infections with enterotoxigenic *Escherichia coli*, *J. Infect. Dis.* **129:**330–335 (1974).
39. Ruiz-Palacios, G. M., Evans, D. G., Evans, D. J., Jr., and DuPont, H. L., Enzyme-linked immunosorbent assay (ELISA) for detection of antibody to heat-labile enterotoxin of *Escherichia coli*, *Abstr. Annu. Meet. Am. Soc. Microbiol.* p. 60 (1978).
40. Deetz, T. R., Evans, D. J., Jr., Evans, D .G., and DuPont, H. L., Serologic responses to somatic O and colonization-factor antigens of enterotoxigenic *Escherichia coli* in travelers, *J. Infect. Dis.* **140:**114–118 (1979).
41. DuPont, H. L., Hornick, R. B., Dawkins, A. T., Snyder, M. J., and Formal, S. B., The response of man to virulent *Shigella flexneri* 2a, *J. Infect. Dis.* **119:**296–299 (1969).
42. Greatorex, J. S., and Thorne, G. M., Humoral immune responses to Shiga-like toxins and *Escherichia coli* O157:H7 lipopolysaccharide in hemolytic uremic syndrome patients and healthy subjects, *J. Clin. Microbiol.* **32:**1172–1178 (1994).
43. Neter, E., and Shumway, C. N., *E. coli* serotype D433: Occurrence in intestinal and respiratory tracts, cultural characteristics, sensitivity to antibiotics, *Proc. Soc. Exp. Biol. Med.* **75:**504–507 (1950).
44. Levine, M. M., Bergquist, E. J., Nalin, D. R., Waterman, D. H., Hornick, R. B., Young, C. R., Scotman, S., and Rowe, R., *Escherichia coli* strains that cause diarrhoea but do not produce heat-labile or heat-stable enterotoxins and are noninvasive, *Lancet* **1:**1119–1122 (1978).
45. Edelman, R., and Levine, M. M., Summary of a workshop on enteropathogenic *Escherichia coli*, *J. Infect. Dis.* **147:**1108–1118 (1983).
46. Rothbaum, R., McAdams, A. J., Gianella, R., and Partin, J. C., A clinicopathologic study of enterocyte-adherent *Escherichia coli*: A cause of protracted diarrhea in infants, *Gastroenterology* **83:** 441–454 (1982).
47. Cravioto, A., Gross, R. J., Scotland, S. M., and Rowe, B., An adhesive factor found in strains of *Escherichia coli* belonging to traditional enteropathogenic serotypes, *Curr. Microbiol.* **3:**95–99 (1979).
48. Scaletsky, I. C. A., Silva, M. L. M., and Trabulsi, L. R., Distinctive patterns of adherence of enteropathogenic *Escherichia coli* to HeLa cells, *Infect. Immun.* **45:**534–536 (1984).

49. Baldini, M. M., Kaper, J. B., Levine, M. M., Candy, D. C. A., and Moon, H. W., Plasmid-mediated adhesion in enteropathogenic *Escherichia coli*, *J. Pediatr. Gastroenterol. Nutr.* **2:**534–538 (1983).
50. Mathewson, J. J., Johnson, P. C., DuPont, H. L., Morgan, D. R., Thornton, S. A., Wood, L. V., and Ericsson, C. D., A newly recognized cause of travelers' diarrhea: Enteroadherent *Escherichia coli*, *J. Infect. Dis.* **151:**471–475 (1985).
51. Mathewson, J. J., Johnson, P. C., DuPont, H. L., Satterwhite, T. K., and Winsor, D. K., Pathogenicity of enteroadherent *Escherichia coli* studied in adult volunteers, *J. Infect. Dis.* **154:**524–527 (1986).
52. Mathewson, J. J., Oberhelman, R. A., DuPont, H. L., de la Cabada, F. J., and Garibay, E. V., Enteroadherent *Escherichia coli* as a cause of diarrhea among children in Mexico, *J. Clin. Microbiol.* **25:**1917–1919 (1987).
53. Levine, M. M., Kaper, J. B., Black, R. E., and Clements, M. L., New knowledge of pathogenesis of bacterial enteric infections as applied to vaccine development, *Microbiol. Rev.* **47:**510–550 (1983).
54. Karch, H., Heeseman, J., Laufs, R., O'Brien, A. D., Tacket, C. O., and Levine, M. M., A plasmid of enterohemorrhagic *Escherichia coli* O157:H7 is required for expression of a new fimbrial antigen and adhesion to epithelial cells, *Infect. Immun.* **55:**455–461 (1987).
55. Belnap, W. D., and O'Donnell, J. J., Epidemic gastroenteritis due to *Escherichia coli* O-111: A review of the literature, with epidemiology, bacteriology, and clinical findings of a large outbreak, *J. Pediatr.* **47:**178–193 (1955).
56. Gurwith, M., Hinde, D., Gross, R., and Rowe, B., A prospective study of enteropathogenic *Escherichia coli* in endemic diarrheal disease, *J. Infect. Dis.* **137:**292–297 (1978).
57. Pal, S., Rao, C. K., Kereselidze, T., Krishnaswami, A. K., Murty, D. K., Pandit, C. G., and Shrivastav, J. B., An extensive community outbreak of enteropathogenic *Escherichia coli* O86:B7 gastroenteritis, *Bull. WHO* **41:**851–858 (1969).
58. Echeverria, P., Blacklow, N. R., and Smith, D. H., Role of heat-labile toxigenic *Escherichia coli* and reovirus-like agent in diarrhoea in Boston children, *Lancet* **2:**1113–1116 (1975).
59. Gorbach, S. L., Kean, B. H., Evans, D. G., Evans, D. J., Jr., and Bessudo, D., Travelers' diarrhea and toxigenic *Escherichia coli*, *N. Engl. J. Med.* **292:**933–936 (1975).
60. Gurwith, M. J., and Williams, T. W., Gastroenteritis in children: A two-year review in Manitoba. I. Etiology, *J. Infect. Dis.* **136:**239–247 (1977).
61. Kapikian, A. Z., Kim, H. W., and Wyatt, R. G., Human reovirus-like agent as the major pathogen associated with "winter" gastroenteritis in hospitalized infants and young children, *N. Engl. J. Med.* **294:**965–972 (1976).
62. Pickering, L. K., Evans, D. J., Jr., Munoz, O., DuPont, H. L., Coella-Ramirez, P., Vollet, J. J., Conklin, R. H., Olarte, J., and Kohl, S., Prospective study of enteropathogens in children with diarrhea in Houston and Mexico, *J. Pediatr.* **93:**383–388 (1978).
63. MacDonald, K. L., Eidson, M., Strohmeyer, C., Levy, M. E., Wells, J. G., Puhr, N. D., Wachsmuth, K., Hargrett, N. T., and Cohen, M. L., A multistate outbreak of gastrointestinal illness caused by enterotoxigenic *Escherichia coli* in imported semisoft cheese, *J. Infect. Dis.* **151:**716–720 (1985).
64. Rosenberg, M. I., Koplan, J. P., Wachsmuth, I. K., Wells, J. G., Gangarosa, I. J., Guerrant, R. L., and Sack, D. A., Epidemic diarrhea at Crater Lake from enterotoxigenic *Escherichia coli*: A large waterborne outbreak, *Ann. Intern. Med.* **86:**714–718 (1977).
65. Wood, L. V., Wolfe, W. H., Ruiz-Palacios, G., Foshee, W. S., Corman, L. I., McCleskey, F., Wright, J. A., and DuPont, H. L., An outbreak of gastroenteritis due to heat-labile enterotoxin-producing strain of *Escherichia coli*, *Infect. Immun.* **41:**931–934 (1983).
66. Guerrant, R. L., Dickens, M. D., Wenzel, R. P., and Kapikian, A. Z., Toxigenic bacterial diarrhea: Outbreak involving multiple strains, *J. Pediatr.* **89:**885–891 (1976).
67. Ryder, R. W., Wachsmuth, I. K., Buxton, A. E., Evans, D. G., DuPont, H. L., Mason, E., and Barret, F. F., Infantile diarrhea produced by heat-stable enterotoxigenic *Escherichia coli*, *N. Engl. J. Med.* **295:**849–853 (1976).
68. Lopez-Vidal, Y., Calva, J. J., Trujillo, A., Ponce de Leon, A., Ramos, A., Svennerholm, A.-M., and Ruiz-Palacios, G. M., Enterotoxins and adhesions of enterotoxigenic *Escherichia coli*: Are they risk factors for acute diarrhea in the community? *J. Infect. Dis.* **162:**442–447 (1990).
69. DuPont, H. L., Olarte, J., Evans, D. G., Pickering, L. K., and Evans, D. J., Jr., Comparative susceptibility of Latin American and United States students to enteric pathogens, *N. Engl. J. Med.* **295:**1520–1521 (1976).
70. Merson, M. H., Wells, J. G., Feeley, J. C., Sack, R. B., Cheech, W. B., Kapikan, A. Z., Gangarosa, E. J., Morris, G. K., and Sack, D. A., Travelers' diarrhea in Mexico: A prospective study of physicians and family members attending a congress, *N. Engl. J. Med.* **294:**1299–1305 (1976).
71. Matsushita, S., Yamada, S., Kai, A., and Kudoh, Y., Invasive strains of *Escherichia coli* belonging to serotype O121:NM, *J. Clin. Microbiol.* **31:**3034–3035 (1993).
72. Gorbach, S. L., and Khurana, C. M., Toxigenic *Escherichia coli*: A cause of infantile diarrhea in Chicago, *N. Engl. J. Med.* **287:**933–936 (1972).
73. Sack, R. B., Hirschhorn, N., Brownlee, I., Cash, R. A., Woodward, W. E., and Sack, D. A., Enterotoxigenic *Escherichia coli*-associated diarrheal disease in Apache children, *N. Engl. J. Med.* **292:**1041–1045 (1975).
74. Guerrant, R. L., Moore, R. A., Kirchenfield, P. M., and Sande, M. A., Role of toxigenic and invasive bacteria in acute diarrhea of childhood, *N. Engl. J. Med.* **293:**567–573 (1975).
75. Sack, D. A., Kaminsky, D. C., Sack, R. B., Wamola, I. A., Orskov, F., Orskov, I., Slack, R. C. B., Arthur, R. R., and Kapikian, A. Z., Enterotoxigenic *Escherichia coli* diarrhea of travelers: A prospective study of American Peace Corps volunteers, *Johns Hopkins Med. J.* **141:**64–70 (1977).
76. Kudoh, Y., Zen-yoji, H., Matsushita, S., Sakai, S., and Maruyama, T., Outbreaks of acute enteritis due to heat-stable enterotoxin-producing strains of *Escherichia coli*, *Microbiol. Immun.* **21:**175–178 (1977).
77. Yow, M. D., Melnick, J. L., Blattner, R. J., Stephenson, W. B., Robison, N. W., and Burkhardt, M. A., The association of viruses and bacteria with infantile diarrhea, *Am. J. Epidemiol.* **92:**33–39 (1970).
78. Thomson, S., Watkins, A. G., and Gray, O. P., *Escherichia coli* gastroenteritis, *Arch. Dis. Child.* **31:**340–345 (1956).
79. Black, R. E., Merson, H. H., Huq, I., Alim, A. R. M. A., and Yunus, M., Incidence and severity of rotavirus and *Escherichia coli* diarrhoea in rural Bangladesh, *Lancet* **1:**141–143 (1981).
80. Ironside, A. G., Tuxford, A. F., and Heyworth, B., A survey of infantile gastroenteritis, *Br. Med. J.* **3:**20–24 (1970).
81. Mata, L. J., and Urrutia, J. J., Intestinal colonization of breast-fed children in a rural area of low socioeconomic level, *Ann. NY Acad. Sci.* **176:**93–109 (1971).

82. Cooper, M. L., Keller, H. M., Walters, E. W., Partin, J. C., and Boye, D. E., Isolation of enteropathogenic *Escherichia coli* from mothers and newborn infants, *Am. J. Dis. Child.* **97:**255–266 (1959).
83. Ocklitz, H. W., and Schmidt, E. F., Enteropathogenic *Escherichia coli* serotypes: Infection of the newborn through mother, *Br. Med. J.* **2:**1036–1038 (1957).
84. Smith, M. H. D., Newell, K. W., and Sulianti, J., Epidemiology of enteropathogenic *Escherichia coli* infection in nonhospitalized children, *Antimicrob. Agents Chemother.* **5:**77–83 (1965).
85. Sack, R. B., Sack, D. A., Mehlman, I. J., Orskov, F., and Orskov, I., Enterotoxigenic *Escherichia coli* isolated from food, *J. Infect. Dis.* **235:**313–317 (1977).
86. Tjoa, W., DuPont, H. L., Sullivan, P., Pickering, L. K., Holguin, A. H., Olarte, J., Evans, D. G., and Evans, D. J., Jr., Location of food consumption and travelers' diarrhea, *Am. J. Epidemiol.* **106:**61–66 (1977).
87. Keene, W. E., McAnulty, J. M., Hoesly, F. C., Williams, L. P., Jr., Hedberg, K., Oxman, G. L., Barrett, T. J., Pfaller, M. A., and Fleming, D. W., A swimming-associated outbreak of hemorrhagic colitis caused *Escherichia coli* O157:H7 and *Shigella sonnei*, *N. Engl. J. Med.* **331:**579–584 (1994).
88. Dev, V. J., Main, M., and Gould, I., Waterborne outbreak of *Escherichia coli* O157, *Lancet* **2:**1412 (1991).
89. Moon, H. W., Whip, S. L., Argenzio, R. A., Levine, M. M., and Gianella, R. A., Attaching and effacing activities of rabbit and human enteropathogenic *Escherichia coli* in pig and rabbit intestines, *Infect. Immun.* **41:**1341–1351 (1983).
90. Arbuckle, J. B. R., The location of *Escherichia coli* in the pig intestine, *J. Med. Microbiol.* **3:**333–340 (1970).
91. Jones, G. W., and Rutter, J. M., Role of K88 antigen in the pathogenesis of neonatal diarrhea caused by *Escherichia coli* in piglets, *Infect. Immun.* **6:**918–927 (1972).
92. Smith, H. W., and Linggood, M. A., Observation on the pathogenic properties of the K88 Hly, and Ent plasmids of *Escherichia coli* with particular reference to porcine diarrhoea, *J. Med. Microbiol.* **4:**467–485 (1971).
93. Rutter, J. M., Burrows, M. R., Sellwood, R., and Gibbons, R. A., A genetic basis for resistance to enteric disease caused by *E. coli*, *Nature* **257:**135–136 (1975).
94. Isaacson, R. E., Fusco, P. C., Brinton, C. C., and Moon, H. W., *In vitro* adhesion of *Escherichia coli* to porcine small intestinal epithelial cells: Pili as adhesive factors, *Infect. Immun.* **21:**392–397 (1978).
95. Pickering, L. K., DuPont, H. L., Evans, D. G., Evans, D. J., Jr., and Olarte, J., Isolation of enteric pathogens from asymptomatic students from the United States and Latin America, *J. Infect. Dis.* **135:**1003–1005 (1977).
96. Formal, S. B., Hale, T. L., Kapfer, C., Cogan, J. P., Snoy, P. J., Cung, R., Wingfield, M. E., Elisberg, B. L., and Baron, L. S., Oral vaccination of monkeys with an invasive *Escherichia coli* K-12 hybrid expression *Shigella flexneri* 2a somatic antigen, *Infect. Immun.* **46:**465–469 (1984).
97. Ramsay, A. M., Acute infectious diarrhoea, *Br. Med. J.* **2:**347–350 (1968).
98. Baker, C. J., Barret, F. F., and Clark, D. J., Antibiotic susceptibility patterns of enteropathogenic *Escherichia coli* isolates, *South. Med. J.* **67:**412–414 (1974).
99. Kaslow, R. A., Taylor, A., Jr., Dweck, H. S., Bobo, R. A., Steele, C. D., and Cassady, G., Jr., Enteropathogenic *Escherichia coli* infection in a newborn nursery, *Am. J. Dis. Child.* **128:**797–801 (1974).
100. Neter, E., Enteritis due to enteropathogenic *Escherichia coli*, *J. Pediatr.* **55:**223–239 (1959).
101. Rogers, K. B., Benson, P. R., Foster, W. P., Jones, L. F., Butler, E. B., and Williams, T. C., Phthalylsulphacetamide and neomycin in the treatment of infantile gastroenteritis, *Lancet* **2:**599–604 (1956).
102. Wheeler, W. E., Spread and control of *Escherichia coli* diarrheal disease, *Ann. NY Acad. Sci.* **66:**112–117 (1969).
103. Laporta, M. Z., Silva, M. L. M., Scaletsky, C. A., and Trabulsi, L. R., Plasmids coding for drug resistance and localized adherence to HeLa cells in enteropathogenic *Escherichia coli* O55:H^{-} and O55:H6, *Infect. Immun.* **51:**715–717 (1986).
104. DuPont, H. L., Ericsson, C. D., Johnson, P. C., Bitsura, J. M., DuPont, M. W., and de la Cabada, F. J., Prevention of travelers' diarrhea by the tablet formulation of bismuth subsalicylate, *J. Am. Med. Assoc.* **257:**1347–1350 (1987).

12. Suggested Reading

DuPont, H. L., Formal, S. B., Hornick, R. B., Snyder, M. J., Libonati, J. P., Sheahan, D. B., LaBrec, E. H., and Kalas, J. P., Pathogenesis of *Escherichia coli* diarrhea, *N. Engl. J. Med.* **285:**1–9 (1971).

DuPont, H. L., and Pickering, L. K., *Infections of the Gastrointestinal Tract: Microbiology, Pathophysiology, and Clinical Features*, Plenum Medical, New York, 1980.

Law, D., Adhesion and its role in the virulence of enteropathogenic *Escherichia coli*, *Clin. Microbiol. Rev.* **7:**152–173 (1994).

Riley, L. W., Remis, R. S., Helgerson, S. D., McGee, H. B., Wells, J. G., Davis, B. R., Hebert, R. J., Olcott, E. S., Johnson, L. M., Hargrett, N. T., Blake, P. A., and Cohen, M. L., Hemorrhagic colitis associated with a rare *Escherichia coli* serotype, *N. Engl. J. Med.* **308:**681–685 (1983).

CHAPTER 15

Gonococcal Infections

James DeMaio and Jonathan Zenilman

1. Introduction

Despite currently effective means of diagnosis and treatment, gonorrhea remains a major public health problem throughout the world. In 1993, 439,673 cases of uncomplicated gonococcal infection were reported in the United States,[1] and an additional one to two unreported cases are believed to occur for each reported one. The complications of infection exact the greatest toll in terms of suffering and economic cost. *Neisseria gonorrhoeae* is a major cause of pelvic inflammatory disease, as well as associated infertility and ectopic pregnancies. Furthermore, gonorrhea may facilitate human immunodeficiency virus (HIV) transmission in some settings.

The epidemiology of gonorrhea is determined by the complex interaction of human sexual behavior, social and health-related factors, and the biological characteristics of the organism. Prevention and control of gonococcal infection depends on individual and community education, high standards of diagnosis and treatment, appropriately targeted screening, counseling, and contact tracing.

2. Historical Background

Allusions to gonococcal infection may be found in ancient Assyrian and Chinese writing, as well as in the Book of Leviticus (15:2). Relatively clear clinical descriptions were made by Hippocrates and Galen. Between the 14th and 17th centuries, "gonorrhea" was considered by many to be just another manifestations of syphilis. However, Phillipe Ricord showed that it was a unique, transmissible disease by performing a series of inoculation studies in the 1830s. The organism was identified in secretions by Neisser in 1879, and initially cultured by Bumm in 1885.

Early treatments of gonorrhea consisted of either ineffective oral preparations or potentially dangerous and caustic intraurethral injections. Urethral strictures and secondary infections were apparently common both as complications of the disease and/or therapy. The first major advance in treatment was the use of topical silver nitrate by Karl Crede in the 1880s to prevent gonococcal ophthalmia neonatorum.[2] Topical treatment at birth remains a mainstay in preventing this infection. The second major advance was the discovery of penicillin in the 1940s, which provided the first hope that gonorrhea could be eradicated. Despite some initial success, the 1960s saw a precipitous 12-year rise in gonorrhea incidence. At the same time, relative resistance to penicillin gradually increased. In 1976, the introduction of plasmid-mediated β-lactamase-producing strains foreshadowed an end to penicillin's role as the treatment of choice. Widespread resistance to penicillins and tetracyclines since the 1980s has led to a reliance on newer agents, such as third-generation cephalosporins and quinolones.

The last two decades have witnessed a tremendous expansion in our understanding of the gonococcus and the human response to infection. However, despite our expanded understanding, a successful vaccine appears unlikely in the near future. At the close of the 20th century, the incidence of gonorrhea is more likely to be changed by time-tested public health measures than by advances in molecular biology.

3. Methodology

3.1. Sources of Mortality Data

Fatalities from acute gonococcal infection are rare events, usually resulting from endocarditis or meningitis

James DeMaio and Jonathan Zenilman • Division of Infectious Diseases, Johns Hopkins Hospital, Baltimore, Maryland 21205.

complicating disseminated gonococcal infection (DGI).[3] Data on mortality from the sequelae of gonococcal infection, such as pelvic inflammatory disease (PID) and ectopic pregnancy, are unreliable because the conditions listed on death certificates are rarely specifically linked to the infection. For example, one study estimated the mortality from PID (all causes) to be 0.29 deaths per 100,000 women aged 15 to 44.[4] However, because the underlying microbial etiology is not listed, determining how many of these were related to gonococcal PID is impossible.

3.2. Sources of Morbidity Data

Gonorrhea is a reportable disease in all 50 states. Reporting criteria are based on standardized surveillance definitions that may be clinically or laboratory based.[5] Physicians, laboratories, and institutions have been required to report either positive culture results or the diagnosis, name, address, demographic data, and identity of the reporter to local or state health departments, depending on the jurisdiction. Despite these requirements, there is marked underreporting; an estimated 50–70% of cases are not brought to the attention of local public health authorities.

Data on all reportable infectious diseases, including sexually transmitted diseases (STDs), are reported from the states to the federal Centers for Disease Control and Prevention (CDC). The weekly incidence of gonorrhea is reviewed in the CDC publication *Morbidity and Mortality Weekly Report*. National statistical summaries of STD data are published periodically by the CDC.[6] In addition, antibiotic-resistance surveillance is conducted through a variety of mechanisms. The United States and other countries (e.g., Canada and Australia) monitor antibiotic resistance through periodically collected samples of gonococcal isolates.

In the United States military, gonorrhea and other STD reporting is a function of the Prevention Medicine Units (PMU) for each of the armed services. Military bases located in the United States usually coordinate reporting and disease intervention activities with local county or state health departments. Bases located overseas report STD morbidity to the appropriate Preventive Medicine Command through the PMUs.

Outside the United States, reporting requirements vary, Most countries do not have national-based surveillance for gonorrhea. The areas with the most complete reporting of gonococcal disease are Great Britain and the Scandinavian countries.[7,8] Data from other countries may rely on reports from STD clinics alone, such as in the Netherlands, or on voluntary sentinel networks, such as in France.[9,10]

For a case to be included in the national morbidity statistics, it first must be diagnosed, then reported, and finally correctly tabulated. Misdiagnosis, underdiagnosis, and underreporting probably occur frequently. The extent of these errors, or reporting bias, is partially determined and corrected by special surveys.

Interpretation of disease incidence data must be carefully performed, taking into account possible confounding factors, such as reporting bias, demographic trends, underreporting, and sexual behavior.

3.3. Surveys

Screening programs and surveys have served a multitude of purposes in guiding the emphasis of national and state control programs. For example, the Gonorrhea Screening Program, which provides free cultures for women, has been instrumental in identifying large numbers of asymptomatically infected women. Demographic surveys have indicated that persons infected with gonorrhea are geographically concentrated, and that targeting intervention efforts in these areas may be productive.[11] Microbiological surveys, such as the Gonococcal Isolate Surveillance Project,[12] have been useful in determining the prevalence of gonococcal strains with antimicrobial resistance. These data, in turn, may be useful in developing recommendations for therapy.

However, despite their value in formulating policy, the accuracy of gonorrhea rates determined by surveys is limited by reporting bias. Underreporting is especially common among private physicians serving economically advantaged patients.[13] Although private physicians may underreport cases by as much as 90%,[14] they actually overestimate the incidence of gonorrhea in their practice.[15]

3.4. Laboratory Diagnosis

3.4.1. Isolation of the Organism. Gram's stains of urethral and cervical exudate should be performed when specimens for culture are obtained. In men, demonstration of typical gram-negative diplococci within polymorphonuclear leukocytes in a urethral smear is 95% sensitive and almost 100% specific.[16] In women, sensitivity of cervical smears is only 50%, although specificity is 95%. Gram's stains from rectal and pharyngeal sites are not recommended because of low sensitivity and specificity.

Cultures or other definitive diagnostic tests are preferred in all cases when the diagnosis must be confirmed. In order to prevent overgrowth of contaminating microorganisms, selective media, such as Modified Thayer–Martin or Martin–Lewis media are used. These media contain antibiotics (e.g., vancomycin, colistin, and nystatin) that suppress fungi, gram-negative rods, and gram-positive bacteria. A small proportion of gonococci are hypersusceptible to vancomycin and may fail to grow on selective media.

Presumptive identification may be made on the basis of growth on selected media, characteristic colonial and microbial morphology, and a positive oxidase test. Final identification may be confirmed by either biochemical, immunologic, or molecular biology techniques. Biochemically, the gonococcus will ferment glucose but not maltose, sucrose, or lactose. A variety of immunologic confirmatory tests, such as monoclonal direct fluorescent antibody stains, are commercially available. These include coagglutination tests, as well as both polyclonal and monoclonal direct fluorescent antibody stains.

Specificity of culture without confirmation varies by anatomical site, correlated with the presence of commensal organisms that could produce false-positive results. Specificity of presumptive laboratory diagnosis of urethral cultures (i.e., identification without confirmation by sugar fermentation or monoclonal antibodies) in men is over 95%. For cervical specimens in women, specificity is estimated to be 85%. In pharyngeal, rectal, and ocular infections, the specificity is lower and all isolates from these and other unusual sites should be confirmed. *All* isolates from children and others in whom sexual abuse or assault is a consideration should be confirmed and saved.

In practice, cultures should be obtained from the anatomical sites corresponding to the patient's sexual exposures by history. Pharyngeal and rectal cultures should be performed if indicated. Because up to 30% of women have rectal coinfection with cervical gonorrhea (irrespective of history of rectal intercourse), routine rectal culture is recommended for all women.

Estimates of culture sensitivity are 80 to 90% for a single endocervical culture and greater than 98% for urethral culture in men.[(16)] Rectal cultures probably have a sensitivity similar to cervical cultures. Therefore, either site may be the sole site where infection can be detected. Pharyngeal culture sensitivity is probably somewhat less. In all cases, specificity should approach 100% if confirmatory procedures are used.

Laboratory diagnosis of gonococcal infection from normally sterile sites, such as blood, synovial fluid, cerebrospinal fluid (CSF), and conjunctivae, is often challenging. In these cases, the selective media used for genital cultures should not be used. Blood and synovial fluid should be cultured on enriched broth media. Synovial fluid, conjunctival discharge, and CSF should be plated directly onto supplemented chocolate agar and placed in a Co_2 incubator as soon as possible. Gram's stain of conjunctival discharge, joint fluid, and CSF may be a useful adjunct.

In gonococcal septicemia (DGI), sensitivity of blood culture, under the best conditions, is often less than 50%. However, the presence of positive blood cultures often correlates with the type of DGI syndrome. For example, in cases of dermatitis synovitis (without frank arthritis), half of patients have documented septicemia.

Because resistance to third-generation cephalosporins and fluoroquinolones is rare at present in the United States, antimicrobial susceptibility testing is not necessary for uncomplicated infections. However, direct susceptibility testing using either the disk diffusion method or the agar dilution method should be performed on all isolates where initial treatment failure can result in severe sequelae (e.g., DGI, endocarditis, ophthalmia, and invasive soft tissue infections).

3.4.2. Immunologic and Molecular Diagnostic Methods. Since the late 1980s, there has been a trend toward the use of nonculture methods. These methods offer practical and logistical advantages, such as simple specimen transport, but are generally more expensive.

Leukocyte esterase dipsticks have been suggested as an initial screening test for gonorrhea. The poor sensitivity of the test (40 to 70%) has limited its clinical value.[(17,18)] However, it may be useful in settings, such as adolescent clinics or detention centers, where rapid presumptive diagnosis is necessary.

A variety of antigen detection systems, such as agglutination tests and enzyme-linked immunosorbent assays (ELISA), have been developed to directly detect the presence of *N. gonorrhoeae* in clinical samples. Unfortunately, the efficacy of these tests has been limited by their relatively low sensitivity.

Molecular biology techniques have been applied to the direct detection of gonococcal DNA and RNA with much better results. DNA hybridization assays have been developed with a colorimetric reaction. Although initial studies have shown them to be relatively sensitive and specific,[(19–22)] further studies of nongenital specimens are still necessary.

DNA amplification techniques, such as polymerase chain reaction (PCR) and ligase chain reaction, have been developed utilizing stable DNA sequences from *N. gonor-*

rhoeae.[23] These have been recently approved for clinical use. The sensitivity and specificity (compared to culture) in preliminary studies of genital specimens is 98 to 99%. Because of the high sensitivity of the DNA amplification process, these tests can be used on urine from either men or women. This development may have a positive impact on screening programs and on STD diagnostic capabilities in field settings.

4. Biological Characteristics of the Organism

N. gonorrhoeae is a fastidious aerobic gram-negative diplococcus that grows best at 35–36°C on a rich medium (such as chocolate agar) containing hemoglobin and a variety of other nutrients, in a moist atmosphere containing at least 3% CO_2. Characteristic colonies are small, rounded, and glistening gray after 24 hr of incubation and are nonhemolytic on blood agar.

In the early 1960s, a relationship between gonococcal colonial morphology and virulence was established. Sharply bordered colonies, which contain organisms with pili, were associated with increased virulence, whereas diffuse colonies, consisting of organisms without pili, were associated with lessened virulence. Pili are thin, proteinaceous extensions of cytoplasm that appear to be important for gonococcal adherence to mucosal surfaces and inhibition of phagocytosis.

Besides pilin, the gonococcal cell membrane contains lipopolysaccharide (LPS) and three integral major outer membrane proteins (OMP).[24] Gonococcal LPS has endotoxin activity similar to LPS found in the walls of other gram-negative bacteria. Gonococcal LPS has also been found to have a cytotoxic effect on human Fallopian tube mucosa.[25] Protein I, the major gonococcal OMP, serves as a porin forming a voltage-dependent aqueous channel for the selective passage of solutes through the hydrophobic outer membrane.[26] A variety of serologically distinct forms of protein I exist and are genetically stable over time. This stability has allowed the development of a monoclonal antibody-based serological typing system.[27] Protein II is involved in gonococcal adhesion to mucosal surfaces. The antigenic diversity and rapid antigenic variation of protein II may play a major role in allowing the gonococcus to escape from the immune system.[28] Protein II is closely associated with protein I in the cell membrane. Although the precise function of protein III is unknown, it may play an important role in the pathogenesis of gonorrhea through the induction of blocking antibody. Blocking IgG, which binds to protein III, inhibits complement-mediated phagocytosis and killing of serum-resistant organisms.[29] The presence of antibodies directed against protein III has recently been shown to increase the risk of gonococcal infection.[30]

Most bacteria acquire iron from the environment by excreting siderophores. However, gonococci utilize a unique iron capture system in which gonococcal cell surface proteins remove iron directly from human iron-binding proteins, such as lactoferrin and transferrin.[31,32] This ability to steal iron from the host's iron-sequestering system may be an important factor in gonococcal pathogenesis.

5. Descriptive Epidemiology

Useful data on the trends of reported cases of gonococcal infection are available in countries where most cases are seen in public specialized clinics (United Kingdom), where most laboratory tests are performed in a single central laboratory (Denmark), or where few changes in reporting habits have occurred (United States). Although developed countries have seen a decrease in gonorrhea rates over the last decade, gonorrhea remains a major pubic health threat throughout the world.

5.1. Prevalence and Incidence

The reported cases of uncomplicated gonococcal infection in the United States are depicted in Fig. 1. The total number of reported cases peaked in 1978, with 1,013,436, and has since decreased to 325,883 in 1996. Changes in cases reported among women reflect not only cases presenting for treatment, but also additional case-finding by screening. Trends in acute gonococcal urethritis in men are less influenced by efforts of health workers to find cases.

Despite the decrease in the number of reported cases if gonorrhea, there has been only a minimal change over the last decade in the rate of gonococcal infections among the highest-risk age groups (15 to 44 years old), especially in urban areas. The institution of control programs, greater public awareness, and changes in sexual habits secondary to the risk of HIV infection may have played a minor role in decreasing reported cases of gonorrhea. However, most of the change in total cases simply reflects the fact that baby boomers are aging. As the large cohort of baby boomers leaves the highest-risk age groups, there are fewer individuals at risk.

Reported cases help define trends, but they need to be supplemented by special surveys that count cases in other systems and assess reporting patterns. Published surveys

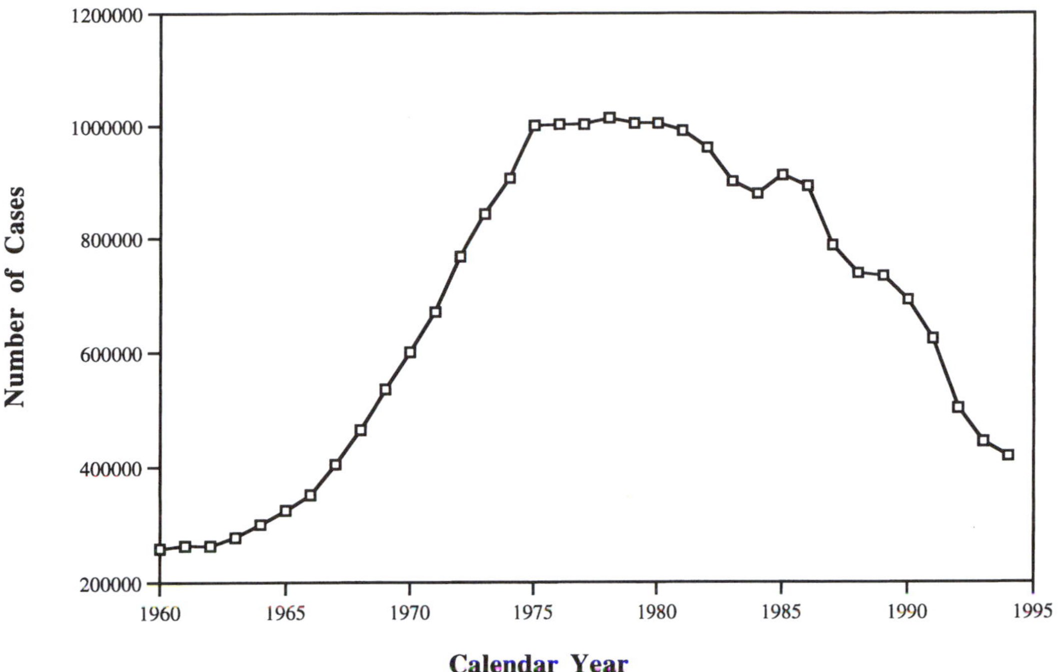

Figure 1. Cases of gonorrhea in the United States, 1960–1994.

of reporting habits have been challenged because of physicians' low response rates and their tendency to overestimate the number of cases they actually see.[14,15] Methods to assess magnitude include surveys of randomly selected physicians who prospectively record all clinical encounters over a specified time and surveys of randomly selected individuals diagnosed by culture. By these approaches, the actual incidence is estimated to be at least twice the reported incidence of disease.

Serious forms of gonococcal infection, such as ophthalmia, acute and recurrent salpingitis, epididymitis, and DGI, have not been systematically recorded even in those countries, such as the United Kingdom and Denmark, that have more complete data on uncomplicated infections. Special studies provide crucial estimates of incidence of these complications and are summarized in the clinical sections.

5.2. Epidemic Behavior and Contagiousness

The spread of gonorrhea in a community is related not only to sexual behavior and the risk of transmission of the disease on exposure, but also to the natural course of the disease, the health behavior of infected individuals, and the behavior of the medical practitioner.

Figure 2 shows the relationship of incubation period, symptoms, and transmission rates to the spread of gonorrhea; it should be useful in correcting several myths about the spread of this disease. It is incorrect to assume that all men with urethral gonorrhea develop typical acute urethritis,[33,34] that the vast majority of women with gonorrhea have no symptoms, or that the cycle of transmission goes from asymptomatic women to symptomatic men and back again. Tracing the course of gonorrhea in Fig. 2 will illustrate these points. Begin with uninfected women being exposed to infected men: the majority of men who infect women have no or atypical urethral symptoms. Although the effectiveness of male-to-female transmission is unknown, it is assumed to be high (50–70%). Once infected, many women will develop either acute salpingitis (20–40%) or a constellation of less specific symptoms (20–30%) (e.g., perineal syndrome, vaginal discharge, abnormal uterine bleeding) within 3 to 45 days of infection. The remaining 30–60% of infected women will have minimal or no symptoms, yet will carry the gonococcus endocervically for 3–12 months.

Next, consider the uninfected men shown in the lower right corner of Fig. 2 who will be exposed mainly to women who are unaware of symptoms; transmission of gonorrhea probably occurs 20 to 30% of the time.[35] Although the majority of men with urethral infection develop frank urethritis (80%), some have atypical signs

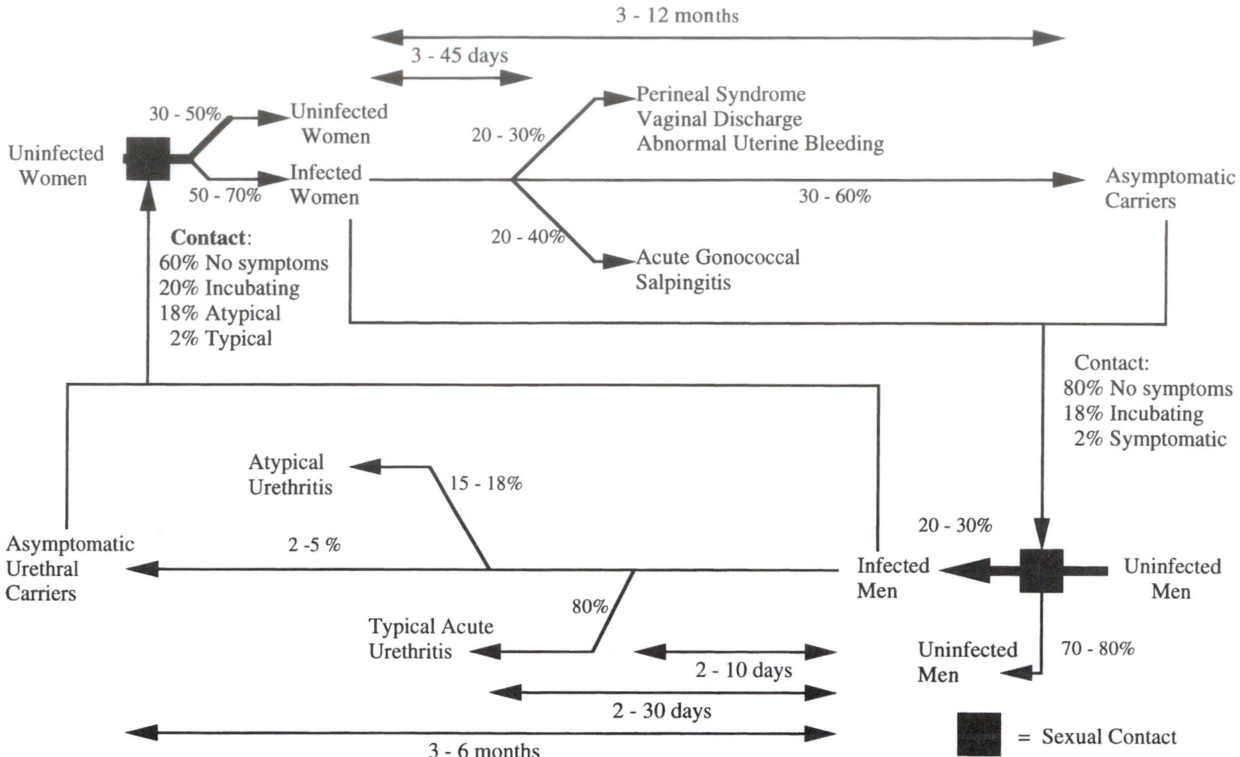

Figure 2. Relationship of incubation period, symptoms, and transmission rates to the spread of gonorrhea.

and symptoms (15–18%). The tendency to seek treatment for either typical or atypical presentations of gonorrhea will vary among different social and psychological groups, so that the perceived incubation period may well vary from 2 to 30 days, if the patient seeks medical advice at all. Some asymptomatic urethral carriers may be of long duration (2–5%) and are very important vectors of gonorrhea; thus, the cycle repeats itself.

Most gonococcal infections are transmitted from asymptomatic individuals or from those who do not recognize atypical signs and symptoms of the disease. This is true for both sexes. Thus, both men and women who seek care for acute symptomatic urethritis or symptomatic pelvic infection will in all but rare cases have acquired their infection from infected sexual partners who have no symptoms. Last, infected women frequently have symptoms, and many men have no symptoms. These asymptomatic men accumulate in high-risk populations and may be major contributors to the spread of disease in the community.

Lesbians rarely transmit the disease to their partners,[36] but the principles of heterosexual transmission of disease in general hold true for homosexual men.[37] Homosexual men can develop symptomatic proctitis with anorectal infection, but the majority are asymptomatic. The course of urethral infection in gay men is similar to that in heterosexual men. Pharyngeal gonococcal infection is usually asymptomatic in both sexes and, although quite common among gay men, is an unlikely but possible source of disease transmission.

5.3. Geographic Distribution

Reported case rates of gonorrhea vary widely among the states. These variations may reflect population factors, such as socioeconomic status, as well as differences in local control programs, such as case-finding activity, reporting practices, and the availability of public clinics. The influence of geographically localized behavioral factors, such as drug abuse (especially "crack" cocaine) and the effect of acquired immunodeficiency syndrome (AIDS) risk-reduction activities have become increasingly appreciated over the last decade.[38]

In 1996, the highest gonorrhea rates in the United States occurred in the Southeast (Fig. 3). The range of disease rates varied between 318 per 100,000 (South Caro-

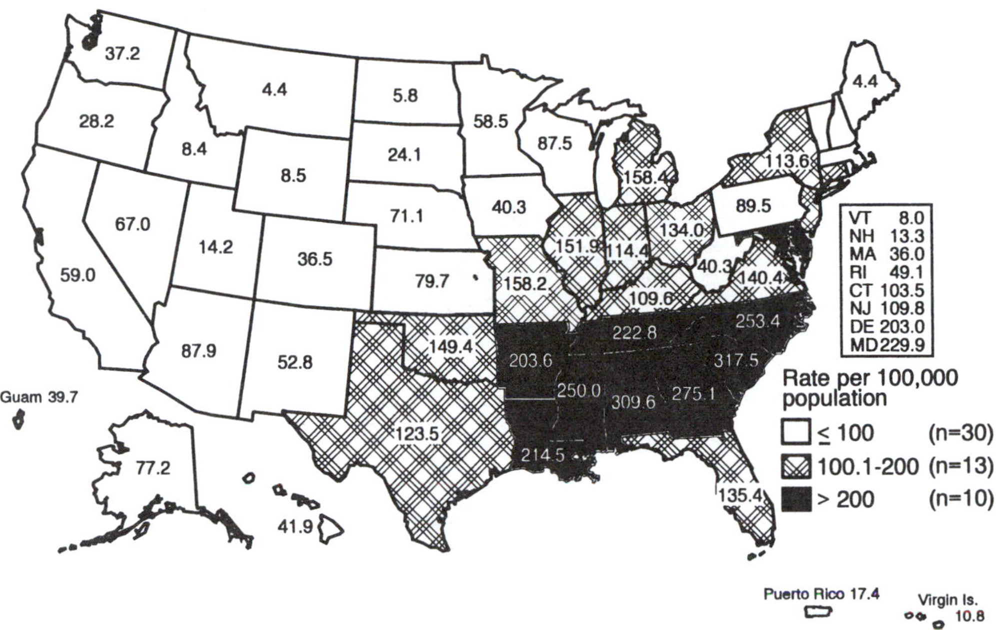

Figure 3. Gonorrhea—rates by state: United States and outlying areas, 1996. Note: The total rate of gonorrhea for the United States and outlying areas (including Guam, Puerto Rico, and Virgin Islands) was 122.4 per 100,000 population. The Healthy People 2000 objective is 100 per 100,000 population.

lina) and 4.4 per 100,000 (Maine). Large cities generally had significantly higher rates than suburban and rural communities: 70% of cities (n = 64) with populations greater than 200,000 had gonorrhea rates exceeding 100 per 100,000.[(4)]

Although the gonorrhea rates determined for large populations are helpful in delineating trends, the "core group" theory may be more valuable for directing control efforts.[(39)] Gonorrhea rates appear to be extremely high in geographically localized, small populations participating in high-risk behavior.[(40,41)] Inner-city areas with low socioeconomic status and poor health care access are most severely affected. For example, out of a total of 202 census tracts in Baltimore, 12 census tracts located in the inner city (core) account for 50% of reported gonorrhea morbidity (Fig. 4). Within these census tracts, the gonorrhea rate is estimated to be five to six times higher than overall citywide rate. Control efforts focused on core groups would potentially have the most cost-effective impact on overall gonorrhea rates.

5.4. Temporal Distribution

A marked seasonality of reported cases has been found ever since data began to be collected in the United States. Consistently, the incidence of reported disease is at least 20% higher in August through October than in February through May. The seasonality of reported gonorrhea cases may reflect combinations of greater mobility, leisure time, and sexual activities in the summer and increased antibiotic use in the winter.[(42)] Different patterns of seasonal prevalence, such as biomodal peaks and no variability over time, have been found in other populations.[(43)] The ability of prevalence rates to change rapidly over a 3- to 6-month period underscores the importance of behavioral factors in the spread of gonorrhea.

5.5. Age and Sex

Young adults and adolescents are at the greatest risk of acquiring gonorrhea. The high rates in these age groups may be secondary to increased risk-taking behavior and to physiological factors, such as increased cervical ectopy in adolescent women. During the last decade, the age group with the highest rate of gonorrhea has become progressively younger. Currently, teenage females (15–19 years of age) have the highest rate of gonorrhea (Fig. 5). Although young adult males (20–24 years of age) have a higher rate than teenage males (15–19 years of age), the difference between these two groups has decreased mark-

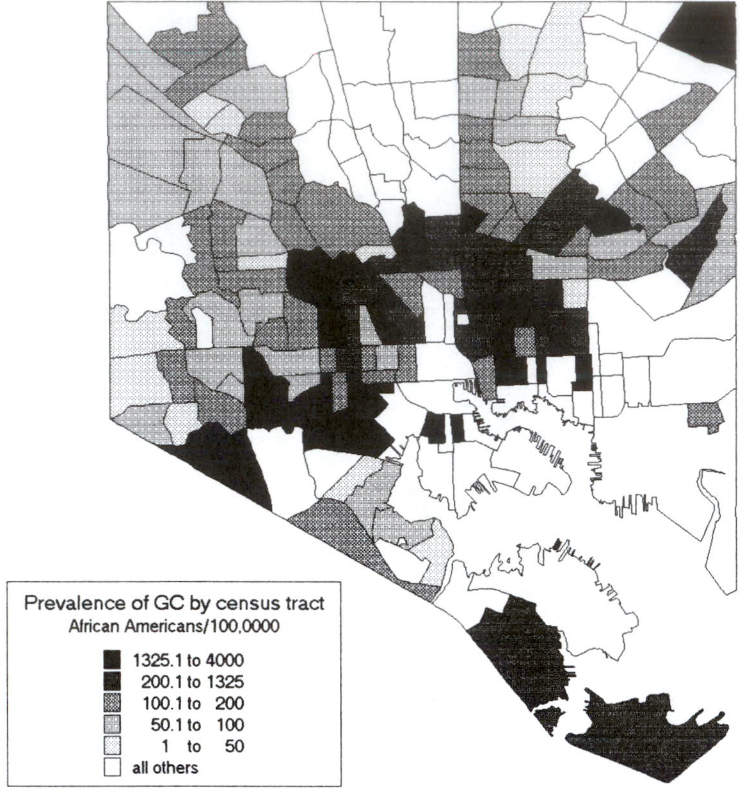

Figure 4. Prevalence of *Neisseria gonorrhoeae* by census tract in Baltimore, Maryland, 1994.

edly since 1987. In light of the long-term sequelae of PID, these trends are highly disturbing.

5.6. Race

Although the reported cases of gonorrhea in all ethnic groups have been decreasing since 1986, the rate of gonorrhea among African Americans is more than 100-fold higher than in other ethnic groups. This difference undoubtedly results in part from the geographic distribution of disease in socioeconomically deprived areas and higher rates of reporting for African-American patients, who are more often seen in public clinics.

5.7. Occupational and Socioeconomic Factors

No reliable data are available on occupation-specific risks for gonorrhea. In general, prostitutes are at higher risk than the general population. Gonorrhea rates of 5 to 10% are seen frequently in incarcerated prostitute populations. However, in areas where prostitutes are routinely screened (e.g., Nevada) gonorrhea rates are low (<1% at screening).

Many factors potentially contribute to the current spread of gonorrhea, including gonococcal antibiotic resistance, differential infectiousness or transmissibility of the organism, the capacity of the gonococcus to cause symptoms or perception of symptoms in various groups, sexual behavior, methods and rates of contraception, homosexuality, illness behavior, other associated high-risk behaviors such as drug abuse, and the quality of clinical and preventive care services available to different groups likely to be infected. The contributions of most of these factors are not easy to document because of insufficient trend data and means of measuring the variable under study.

5.8. Homosexuality

A significant increase in STDs was noted among homosexual males during the late 1970s.[37] However, beginning in the early 1980s, a dramatic fall in gonorrhea rates occurred presumably secondary in behavioral changes in the face of the AIDS epidemic. Unfortunately, investigators from the United States, Europe, and Australia have noted a marked resurgence in both gonorrhea and un-

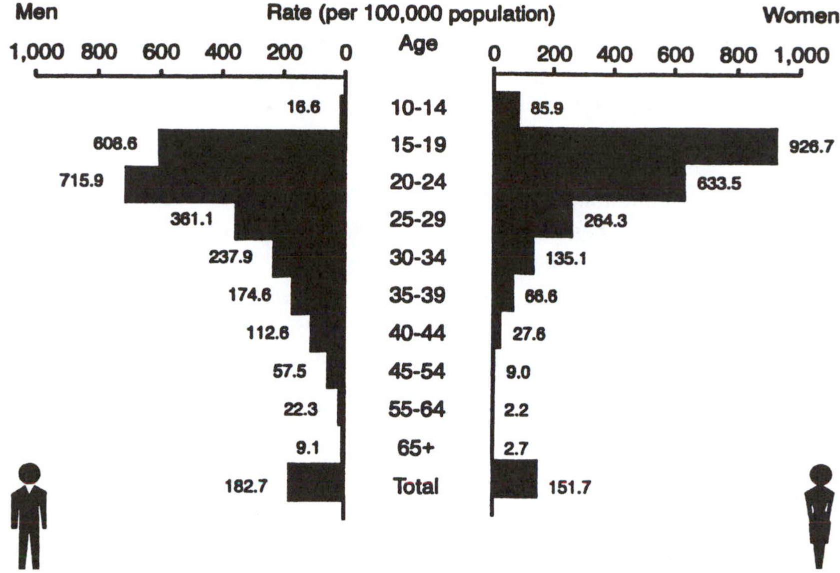

Figure 5. Age-specific case rates of gonorrhea by sex. United States, calendar year 1994.

protected anogenital intercourse in homosexual men since 1988.[44,45] This trend is thought to be secondary to a lower perceived risk in young homosexual males. The increase in gonorrhea and presumably in high-risk behaviors in this population has recently been associated with a rising HIV transmission rate.[46]

5.9. Gonorrhea and HIV

Sexually transmitted diseases that cause genital ulcers, such as syphilis, increase the risk of acquiring HIV.[47] The impact of nonulcerative STDs, such as gonorrhea, is less clear. After controlling for unprotected sexual exposure, Laga and colleagues[48] identified both gonorrhea and chlamydial infections as risk factors for HIV seroconversion. However, the treatment of unprotected sexual exposure as a dichotomous variable, rather than as a continuous variable, may have falsely inflated the calculated odds ratio. When unprotected intercourse was controlled as a continuous variable in a recent study from Cameroon, the impact of gonorrhea on HIV seroconversion decreased to a statistically insignificant level.[49] Because even a small increase in risk from nonulcerative STDs would have major public health implications, further studies are needed.

HIV infection may increase the risk of developing serious complications of gonorrhea, such as salpingitis[30] and keratoconjuctivitis.[50] However, it is unknown whether the immunosuppressed status of HIV-infected patients warrants more aggressive treatment. Anecdotally, HIV-infected patients with uncomplicated gonorrhea appear to respond well to standard treatment regimens.

5.10. Antimicrobial Resistance

The emergence of plasmid-mediated penicillinase-producing *N. gonorrhoeae* (PPNG) in 1976 quickly ended penicillin's role as the treatment of choice for gonorrhea. Currently, third-generation cephalosporins and fluoroquinolones are considered the drugs of choice. However, the ever-increasing development of resistance among all pathogenic organisms in the face of antimicrobial pressure raises serious doubts about the long-term effectiveness of even these newer agents.

5.10.1. Penicillin Resistance. Resistance to penicillin may be either chromosomally (CMRNG) or plasmid (PPNG) mediated. Chromosomally mediated increases in the minimal inhibitory concentration (MIC) of penicillin were noted during the 1950s and 1960s. By 1979, the recommended dose of penicillin was 200-fold higher than that used after World War II. However, these moderately resistant strains still had MICs <1 μg/ml and could be successfully treated with penicillin. CMRNG strains with high-level resistance (MIC >2 μg/ml) were first identified in North Carolina in 1983.[51] Resistance in these strains resulted both from the cumulative effect of multiple genetic mutations leading to altered outer membrane permeability to antibiotics and also from changes in the penicillin-binding proteins. Due to the changes in permeability, CMRNG strains are also frequently resistant to tetracycline and second-generation cephalosporins. Although specific testing to determine the mechanism of resistance is not routinely performed in most laboratories, the proportion of CMRNG strains is approximately 10 to 15% in the United States.

Plasmid-mediated PPNG was introduced into the United States in 1976. The two most commonly identified plasmid types, 3.2 MDa and 4.4 MDa, are thought to have arisen in Africa and Asia, respectively, through acquisition from either *Haemophilus influenzae* or enteric gram-negative rods. Other plasmid types have also been identified. In 1992, 11.6% of isolates submitted in a sentinel survey in the United States were PPNG.[(6)] Similar prevalences (5–13%) have been found recently in other developed countries, such as England and Australia.[(52,53)] However, much higher rates (28–72%) are known to occur in developing areas, such as Africa and Asia.[(54,55)] These high rates are extremely disturbing, given the high cost of nonpenicillin alternatives.

5.10.2. Tetracycline-Resistant Gonorrhea (TRNG). Tetracycline resistance also may be either chromosomally or plasmid mediated. Although many chromosomally mediated TRNG are also resistant to penicillin, chromosomal resistance to these antibiotics may occur independently. Plasmid-mediated TRNG strains carry a 25.2 MDa plasmid, which carries the *tetM* gene. This genetic mechanism is of public health interest for two reasons. First, it represents acquisition of a resistance determinant from other genital flora. Second, *in vitro* studies have been able to transfer *tetM* to other *Neisseria*, including the meningococcus. In 1992, the Gonococcal Isolate Surveillance Project found that 8.1% of gonorrhea isolates possessed plasmid-mediated resistance to tetracycline and a further 13.8% were chromosomally resistant.[(6)]

5.10.3. Spectinomycin Resistance. Spectinomycin resistance occurs via a single step, high-level mutation resulting in an MIC of > 2000 ug/ml. The widespread use of spectinomycin treatment for gonorrhea in Korea led to an 8% failure rate due to resistance.[(56)] Currently, spectinomycin resistant strains are rare in the United States, presumably secondary to minimal selective pressure in the face of infrequent use of the drug. Most strains identified in the United States have been from imported cases.[(57)]

5.10.4. Cephalosporin Resistance. Cephalosporins, such as ceftriaxone, are currently approved for the treatment of gonorrhea. Because these antibiotics are β-lactamase stable, they are active against PPNG strains. Although chromosomally mediated penicillin resistant strains are relatively less sensitive to cephalosporins, this resistance is not clinically significant. At the present time, *N. gonorrhoeae* strains resistant to ceftriaxone have not been identified in the United States. Scattered anecdotal reports suggest that this may be a developing problem in Asia.

5.10.5. Fluoroquinolone Resistance. Fluoroquinolones are widely used for single-dose oral treatment of gonorrhea. However, after less than one decade of clinical use, the value of these agents is already threatened by resistance. Studies from Hong Kong, Australia, and Rwanda have demonstrated the rapid appearance of moderate-level resistance to both ciprofloxacin and ofloxacin.[(58–60)] In the study from Hong Kong, for example, the percentage of strains with an MIC to ofloxacin of >0.1 μg/ml increased from 5.5 to 40% within 3 years. More recently, strains with decreased susceptibility were identified in both Ohio and Hawaii.[(61)] The strains from Hawaii had MICs of 2 μg/ml. Because resistant strains have been associated with treatment failure, close surveillance of fluoroquinolone resistance will be necessary to insure that treatment recommendations remain effective.

6. Mechanisms and Routes of Transmission

The major mode of transmission of gonococcal infection in adults is through sexual intercourse (see Section 5.2). Nonsexual transmission of gonorrhea is extremely rare among adults. Although survival of gonococci can be demonstrated on inanimate objects, such as toilet seats.[(62)] epidemiological data implicating fomites in transmission are lacking. Infants born to infected mothers can acquire conjunctival infection and orogastric colonization before delivery (with premature rupture of fetal membranes) or during delivery. Children up to the age of 5 years rarely acquire the disease from fomites or inoculation with infected adult secretions. However, in all children, family situations must be examined closely because sexual abuse, frequently involving a member of the household, is a significant mode of transmission.[(63)] Most cases of gonorrhea in adolescent children are acquired through sexual intercourse.

7. Pathogenesis and Immunity

7.1. Pathogenesis

The incubation period for gonococcal urethritis in males is 1–7 days with the majority of patients exhibiting symptoms within 72 hr of infection. The incubation period is harder to define in women because cervical infections are often asymptomatic.

Gonococcal infection is initiated by intimate contact of the gonococcus with either epithelial or mucus-secreting cells, usually a nonciliated columnar epithelial surface. Gonococci taken directly from exudate are infectious when inoculated into another human, but serial passage in the laboratory results in reduced virulence. Artificial conditions select against virulence factors, such as the presence of pili and protein II (see Section 4).

The process of mucosal infection is readily observed using an *in vitro* Fallopian tube organ culture system. Four distinct, sequential phases have been delineated[25]:

1. Mucosal attachment to nonciliated cells, mediated by gonococcal pili.
2. Endocytosis of gonococci by epithelial cells.
3. Movement of endocytic vacuoles within the ingesting cell; intracellular replication.
4. Egestion of gonococci by either exocytosis or rupture of the epithelial host cell (usually by day 3).

In most cases, natural infection is accompanied by an intense local polymorphonuclear inflammatory response. Systemic symptoms, such as fever and chills, are unusual.

In about 1% of cases, mucosal infection, often asymptomatic, will progress to septicemia. As discussed in Section 4, serum-resistant organisms may be involved. Patients with defects in terminal complement components are at higher risk for DGI.[64]

7.2. Immunity

When purified antigens, such as pilin, outer membrane protein I, and LPS, are employed in sensitive assays, most patients with gonococcal infection can be shown to produce humoral antibodies. IgG and IgA specific for gonococcal antigens can be found in both serum and mucosal exudates.[65] However, this humoral response is generally short-lived.

Secretory IgA is produced in both men and women in response to mucosal gonococcal infection.[66,67] The gonococcus neutralizes the effectiveness of secretory IgA by two routes. First, gonococci produce IgA proteases, which destroy the host's secretory immunoglobulin. Second, gonococcal pili can shift antigenic determinants through a process called phase variation.[68]

Immunity to *N. gonorrhoeae* is probably only strain specific. Previous infection has little effect on the susceptibility to future infection because of the large antigenic variety of strains, the transient nature of the immune response and the ability of many gonococcal strains to produce IgA protease.

Although effective mucosal immunity is transient and highly strain specific, serum from infected individuals possesses antibodies that are bactericidal for all gonococci except those strains causing disseminated disease. In addition, serum from individuals who presumably have never had a gonococcal infection frequently contains "natural antibodies" that are also bactericidal for gonococci.[69] Natural antibodies are thought to arise from previous infection or colonization with nonpathogenic *Neisseria*. As noted in Section 4, serum-resistant gonococci, which cause the majority of DGI cases, preferentially bind a blocking antibody directed against protein III that successfully competes with bactericidal antibody, thereby protecting the pathogen from complement-mediated destruction.

8. Patterns of Host Response

Gonococcal infection may be limited to mucosal surfaces, such as the urethra, cervix, pharynx, eyes, and rectum. However, more invasive disease, such as ascending infections of the genital tract and gonococcemia, occurs in a significant proportion of these infected.

8.1. Clinical Features

8.1.1. Urethritis in Men.[70] Purulent discharge and dysuria are the most common symptoms. Although most men have one or both symptoms within 1 week of infection, perhaps 5% of cases remain asymptomatic.

The major differential diagnosis is gonococcal urethritis (GCU) and nongonococcal urethritis (NGU). Although GCU is more frequently associated with purulent discharge and dysuria, the diagnosis cannot be confirmed or excluded by history and physical examination alone. Gonorrhea is diagnosed presumptively by urethral smear and Gram's stain and confirmed by culture or DNA-based testing (Section 3.4). Coinfection with *Chlamydia trachomatis* is common and occurs in up to 30% of patients in some areas.

Untreated gonococcal urethritis will usually resolve within 6 months. Because the vast majority of symptomatic men seek early treatment, there are few epidemiological data on the long-term sequelae of untreated gonococcal urethritis. In developing countries, where chronic untreated infections still occur, paraurethral and preputial abscesses, fistula formation, and urethral strictures occur frequently. Epididymitis and prostatitis are also possible sequelae.

8.1.2. Endocervicitis. In most women with gonococcal cervicitis, purulent exudate and cervical friability, erythema, and edema can be detected by a careful visual speculum examination. Infected women may have nonspecific complaints, such as increased vaginal discharge, abnormal menses (increased flow or dysmenorrhea), dyspareunia, or dysuria. Patients often do not associate these symptoms with an STD. Labial tenderness and Bartholin's and Skene's gland abscesses are less frequent signs of infection. Fifty percent of women are asymptomatic at presentation. Bimanual examination of the pelvis is mandatory in evaluating women with gonococcal infection. As many as half of women with endocervical gonorrhea may have upper-tract signs, such as adnexal tenderness, at initial evaluation.[71]

Definitive diagnosis of gonococcal cervicitis is made by culture or DNA-based testing. Gram's stain of cervical secretions may be useful in identifying cases at the bedside, but has a sensitivity of only 50 to 70% (see Section 3.4). Coinfection with other genitourinary pathogens, such as *C. trachomatis* or *Trichomonas vaginalis* is common. Because of the particularly high proportion of coinfection by *C. trachomatis* and the relatively high cost of diagnosis, treatment regimens must be directed against both pathogens.

8.1.3. Upper Genital Tract Infection and PID.[72,73] PID is the most important complication of gonorrhea. Ascending infection from the endocervix through the uterine cavity to the Fallopian tubes usually occurs within one to two menstrual cycles in 10–20% of women with untreated or undertreated gonococcal infection.[74] PID is actually a spectrum of soft-tissue infections, including endometritis and salpingitis. Leakage of infected material can result in tubo-ovarian abscess and/or pelvis peritonitis. Tubal damage impairs the normal host defense mechanisms, such as ciliary motility, setting the stage for superinfection with vaginal flora and secondary abscess formation. Tubal scarring, the major long-term sequelae of PID, leads to increased susceptibility to repeated episodes of PID, as well as to an increased incidence of tubal infertility and ectopic pregnancy.[75,76]

Patients at highest risk for developing PID are under 25 years old, have had previous episodes of PID, have multiple sexual partners, and douche. Use of oral contraceptives as a risk factor for PID is still a subject of considerable debate.

In other 50% of cases, *N. gonorrhoeae* or *C. trachomatis* is isolated.[77,78] Combined infection is common. Other microorganisms implicated in PID are gram-negative enteric bacteria, anaerobes, group B streptococci, and the genital tract mycoplasma.

Clinical diagnosis of PID traditionally has been made by documenting the combination of lower abdominal pain, abnormal cervical or vaginal discharge, and tenderness on bimanual examination. Fever occurs in only half the cases. Women with PID may have crampy, dull, lower abdominal pain occurring with menses or irregular menses over several cycles before the disease becomes overt. On bimanual examination, the signs of PID are uterine traction tenderness, adnexal tenderness, or adnexal enlargement. Although adnexal abscesses are unusual in gonococcal PID, clinical suspicion should lead to further evaluation, such as sonography. The wide spectrum of disease, including mild cases, and the relative nonspecificity of clinical signs make accurate diagnosis difficult. Laparoscopic studies have demonstrated clinicopathological correlation in only two thirds of cases.[79] Therefore, careful clinical observation of the patient is extremely important.

Distinguishing between PID caused by *N. gonorrhoeae*, *C. trachomatis*, and other microorganisms is important but often difficult. Laparoscopic evaluation, although invasive, gives the best diagnostic yield and is being used more widely. Without laparoscopy, properly performed endocervical Gram's stains and culture are the only way to make a microbiological diagnosis. However, diagnostic sensitivity and specificity are both substantially compromised. Culdocentesis without frank pus may not be entirely reliable because specimens may be contaminated with vaginal flora.

Because of the diagnostic problems and the profound sequelae of untreated or undertreated disease, the CDC and other authorities recommend an aggressive approach to PID diagnosis and treatment. Treatment regimens for PID are designed to include adequate antimicrobial coverage for *N. gonorrhoeae*, *C. trachomatis*, gram-negative organisms, and anaerobes.[80,81] Hospitalization may be necessary in severe cases. In addition, if foreign bodies, such as IUDs, are present, they should be removed.

8.1.4. Anorectal Infections. Anorectal gonorrhea occurs in homosexual men with a history of receptive rectal intercourse. Furthermore, 30–50% of women with endocervical gonorrhea have coexistent rectal infection.[82,83] In women, anorectal gonorrhea is not related to rectal intercourse; infected perineal secretions are thought to cause a secondary anorectal mucosal infection.

Most anorectal infections in women are asymptomatic. In homosexual men, symptoms such as tenesmus, mucoid discharge, hematochezia, perianal irritation, and constipation are seen more frequently. Anoscopy in symptomatic cases may show erythema, exudate, and friable mucosa in the anal canal and terminal rectum.[84] In asymptomatic cases, however, anoscopy is often normal.[83]

The differential diagnosis of anorectal gonorrhea,

especially in homosexual men, includes rectal herpes and *C. trachomatis*.[85] Because of the large number of asymptomatic cases and poor specificity of rectal Gram's stain, diagnosis of anorectal gonorrhea is more accurately made by culture.

8.1.5. Pharyngeal Infection. Pharyngeal infection usually results from oral sexual exposure to an infected partner.[86] Among patients with anogenital gonorrhea, pharyngeal infection has been demonstrated in some studies in 3–7% of heterosexual men, 5–20% of women, and 10–25% of homosexual men.[87] Among pregnant women, the proportion may be higher. Although exudative pharyngitis and sore throat are seen in symptomatic cases, pharyngeal gonorrhea is most commonly asymptomatic. Sore throat in some patients may be more related to a postfellatio syndrome rather than an infectious process. Asymptomatic pharyngeal infection resulting in DGI has been well described.

Diagnosis of pharyngeal gonorrhea can only be made by culture. Because of the presence of a large number of commensal *Neisseriaceae*, careful attention must be paid to confirmation of the diagnosis. Pharyngeal gonorrhea is more difficult to cure than gonorrhea at other mucosal sites. Quinolones and third-generation cephalosporins are effective in clearing pharyngeal gonorrhea. However, spectinomycin fails to cure about 50% of the cases.[88] Paradoxically, in studies where patients were followed without antibiotic treatment, spontaneous loss of gonococci from the throat often occurred.[87]

8.1.6. Gonococcal Perihepatitis. This syndrome is probably caused by direct spread of the gonococcus to the capsule of the liver from a pelvic focus via the peritoneal cavity. Again, *Chlamydia* is in the differential diagnosis. Patients, usually women with mucopurulent cervicitis or PID, have right-upper-quadrant pain and mild elevation of liver enzymes. Jaundice is unusual and sonographic studies of the gallbladder and biliary tree are within normal limits. Perihepatitis usually resolves with antibiotic therapy.

8.1.7. Disseminated Gonococcal Infection. Asymptomatic transient gonococcemia probably occurs frequently. Approximately 0.5–1.0% of patients with gonorrhea develop DGI. Patients with DGI have a local infection, either rectal, urogenital, or pharyngeal, that is commonly asymptomatic. Host and organism factors are both important in permitting dissemination. As described earlier, organisms from patients with DGI are more likely to have properties such as serum resistance. Organisms that cause DGI are generally more sensitive to antibiotics than those found in routine anogenital infection.[89] However, DGI due to PPNG or CMRNG does occur.[90] DGI occurs more commonly in women than men; pregnant women are at even higher risk, probably because of suppressed cell-mediated immunity. Persons with terminal complement deficiencies are also at very high risk for dissemination and may experience multiple episodes.

DGI can be separated clinically into two syndromes. The first syndrome is a dermatitis–arthritis.[91–93] Patients present with fevers, chills, polyarthralgias, or tenosynovitis. Joint and tendon symptoms are not migratory, but additive. Three to twenty petechial, papular, pustular, hemorrhagic, or necrotic skin lesions (frequently in combination) may be present on the distal extremities. Fingers, toes, hands, and wrists are commonly involved in an asymmetrical fashion. Painful skin lesions may bring the patient to the physician. Blood cultures are positive for *N. gonorrhoeae* in about half these cases. These clinical findings, together with cultures from mucosal sites, allow a definite or probable diagnosis of DGI in about 85% of cases. Aspiration of small joints is usually not productive. Gram's stain or culture of skin lesions is typically negative; however, gonococci may be demonstrated by fluorescent antibody techniques.

The second common syndrome is a septic arthritis, usually monoarticular, affecting large joints. The knee is involved most commonly. The signs and symptoms are those of any acute joint-space infection. Although the septic arthritis is secondary to a bacteremic process, blood cultures at this stage are rarely positive. Gram's stain and culture of synovial fluid are mandatory diagnostic tests in any suspected septic arthritis and are positive in about half the cases of gonococcal arthritis. Culture-negative cases are thought to result from either immune complex deposition or intra-articular killing of the organisms prior to arthrocentesis. DGI generally responds rapidly to appropriate antibiotic therapy.

In a small proportion of patients with DGI, severe complications such as meningitis, endocarditis, toxic hepatitis, and septic seeding of other organs can develop. Fortunately, these complications are rare.

8.1.8. Gonococcal Ophthalmia. Gonococcal ophthalmia occurs in two groups: neonates born to women with endocervical gonorrhea and adults who are exposed to infected secretions.[94,95]

Neonatal gonococcal ophthalmia is now rare in the United States because of prenatal screening and universal prophylaxis; chlamydial ophthalmia is more common. In developing countries, however, this disease is still a major cause of blindness and is more common than chlamydial disease.[96,97] Infants with gonococcal ophthalmia may also have infection at other sites, such as the throat, anal canal, and respiratory tract. Incubation periods longer than 3 days are not unusual. Clinically, diffuse redness and conjunctival swelling are first seen, followed by a profuse, purulent discharge from which the organism can be easily identified by Gram's stain and culture. Corneal scarring and blindness may occur if the infection is left untreated.

Adult gonococcal ophthalmia is occasionally seen in young adults with anogenital gonorrhea. In one study, infected urine had been used as a folk remedy for acute hemorrhagic viral conjunctivitis.[98] Purulent keratoconjunctivitis is seen clinically. Compared to the neonatal cases, corneal involvement is reported more often.

Diagnosis of gonococcal eye disease is made by Gram's stain and culture. Care must be exercised in confirming the culture result. Cases of pseudogonococcal ophthalmia due to *Moraxella*, other *Neisseria*, and *Acinetobacter* have been reported.[99] Because of the grave sequelae of this disease, all isolates should be tested for antimicrobial susceptibility.

Neonatal gonococcal ophthalmia can be prevented by maternal screening and treatment, where indicated. Additionally, neonatal ocular prophylaxis, first instituted by Crede,[2] is one of the triumphs of preventive medicine. In the United States, routine prophylaxis is given at birth with either erythromycin, silver nitrate, or tetracycline.

8.1.9. Pediatric Gonorrhea. Gonococcal infections in prepubertal children are probably underreported. Clinically, in young girls either a symptomatic or an asymptomatic vulvovaginitis may be seen. Urethritis has been described in boys, and anorectal, rectal, and pharyngeal infection may be seen in both sexes.

Since nonsexual transmission of gonorrhea in children is extremely rare,[100] sexual exposure and child sexual abuse must be seriously considered when the diagnosis is made.[63,101] Because of the forensic implications, specific diagnosis is imperative.[102] The chain of custody must be maintained, cultures from all sites should be confirmed by experienced laboratories, and positive specimens should be archived.

8.2. Diagnosis

Infection with *N. gonorrhoeae* should be included in the differential diagnosis of urethritis, cervicitis, septic arthritis, conjunctivitis, and sepsis in sexually active adults. Most pharyngeal infections with *N. gonorrhoeae* are asymptomatic. However, *N. gonorrhoeae* should be considered as a possible etiology of acute pharyngitis in patients with a history of orogenital sexual exposure. Newborns with conjunctivitis may be infected with *N. gonorrhoeae*.

A specific diagnosis of *N. gonorrhoeae* can usually be made by either Gram's stain or culture. The application of the Gram's stain and culture to specific gonococcal syndromes is detailed in Section 3.4.1. During the last decade, there have been major advances in nonculture diagnostic methods. The application of immunologic and molecular diagnostic tests for *N. gonorrhoeae* is covered in Section 3.4.2.

9. Control and Prevention

9.1. Principles of Control

For control through public health intervention, we emphasize the importance of establishing priorities among gonorrhea cases for the implementation of measures such as intensive case-finding activities and epidemiological treatment. In other words, public health authorities must attempt to identify gonorrhea cases where intervention will have the highest yield in preventing further spread (see Sections 9.1.2, 9.1.3). The mistaken assumption that every case of gonorrhea is equally important for the further spread of the disease must be dispelled. Failure to treat gonorrhea cases and to promote primary prevention among groups with a high rate of disease transmission significantly limits the chances of success. Different degrees of control are possible in different environments. Control programs in many developed countries are currently focused on efforts to decrease the prevalence of the disease. In other areas, attempts may be made to prevent only serious sequelae, i.e., gonococcal ophthalmia neonatorum and gonococcal PID.

9.1.1. Clinical Services. Provision of easily accessible clinical services and proficient laboratory support services are essential to control programs. Clearly, it is futile to engage in widespread screening and elaborate efforts to locate sexual partners, while waiting periods in clinics are long, patients with symptoms are being turned away, and the misdiagnosis and mismanagement of known cases are common. The establishment of practical clinical services should precede attempts at more sophisticated intervention and may in itself have a significant effect on the control of gonorrhea in some communities. To increase accessibility, all services related to the control of gonorrhea should be rendered free of charge or at least not denied because of an inability to pay.

The prevention of gonococcal ophthalmia neonatorum is perhaps the only substantial intervention that is not rooted in STD clinical services. Even ophthalmia prophylaxis requires trained clinical personnel. Community education and promotion of primary prevention (e.g., abstinence, partner selection, personal prophylaxis) should be informed and focused by epidemiological information derived from clinical facilities.

9.1.2. Epidemiological Process. Because of the large reservoir of asymptomatic and minimally symptomatic cases, especially in women, gonorrhea cannot be controlled solely by the application of diagnosis and treatment to cases with apparent symptoms. Public health intervention is targeted both at identifying potentially infected individuals and in preventing the further transmission of disease.

Direct disease control activities are usually a function of local health departments. Ideally, the epidemiological process should focus on five groups: new patients, sexual partners of patients, patients with repeated infections, health care providers, and community sources of health information. The basic information to be obtained from patients is directed toward identifying potentially infected partners and should include age, race, sex, place of residence, mobility, and special sociobehavioral features (e.g., prostitution, employment). Health care providers for the population at highest risk must be determined. Simple measures for doing so include: (1) finding out from patients and their sexual partners where they are seeking health care; (2) making a survey of health care providers located near the places of residence of high risk groups; and (3) seeking "hidden" health care providers (e.g., pharmacists, "street health providers," hotel physicians). In addition, a sample of physicians should be visited to find out the extent of their services to gonorrhea patients, if there is reason to suspect that a significant proportion of cases are not being reported. Health care providers serving high-risk groups must be assisted in the correct diagnosis and treatment of gonorrhea and encouraged to use appropriate intervention techniques. For example, acute detention facilities (e.g., city jails) have been found to have extraordinarily high rates of disease. Therefore, this may be a setting to increase diagnostic and treatment services.

Each community may have unique sources of health information. The quality and influence of these sources (peers, media, social groups, churches, opinion leaders) will vary for subgroups within the community. Liaison with these information sources should be sought by local health authorities.

9.1.3. Transmitters or Nontransmitters. Special emphasis must be placed on finding those infected. Patients who are most likely to be efficient transmitters of the disease deserve special emphasis in case-finding activities. Generally, efficient transmitters are those who are either asymptomatic or tend to ignore symptoms, who have a large number of different sexual partners, and who have limited access to medical care. A good indicator of a group with a high proportion of transmitters is the rate of repeated infection in the group. Efficient transmitters have also been linked epidemiologically to the core group (see Section 5.3).

9.1.4. Diagnostic Screening. Because of cost considerations, culture screening for case detection in gonorrhea control must be targeted to high-risk groups. The cost-effectiveness of screening will depend on the prevalence of the disease in the population and can be increased by concentrating on high-risk groups. However, although this measure will find cases at a lower cost per case, control effectiveness will depend on the proportion of existing cases missed by the screening procedure and other control strategies.

Populations screened should be carefully selected. For example, women presenting with signs or symptoms of other STDs, women distinguished by behavioral or demographic factors characteristic of high-risk groups (e.g., prostitutes), and women from groups in which the prevalence of the disease is high should be those selected for initial screening. The concept of repeated screening may be applied in a retrospective or prospective fashion. Retrospectively, women and men with a history of gonococcal infection should be screened whenever they visit a health facility. Prospectively, most authorities believe that immediate posttreatment evaluation (test of cure) is low yield. However, because of the high reexposure rate, it may be prudent to rescreen in 2–3 months. Available resources will determine the number of screenings and the combinations of initial and repeat screenings that are possible within each locality. In most circumstances, only women are screened for gonorrhea. However, the advent of new urine-based DNA diagnostic assays, which make noninvasive testing in men practical, may change this paradigm. In high-prevalence areas, screening in different clinical settings should also be considered (e.g., in antenatal, gynecological, or family-planning clinics). Endocervical culture is the preferred screening method.

9.1.5. Epidemiological Treatment. Epidemiological treatment consists of providing full therapeutic doses of antibiotics to persons recently exposed to gonorrhea, while awaiting the results of laboratory tests to confirm a diagnosis. This practice is recommended because of the significant chance that the patient has been infected, the serious consequences of the disease, the relative safety and efficacy of treatment, the frequency with which people in high-risk groups default on appointments, and the risk of the spread of the disease in the community.

9.1.5a. Counseling to Obtain the Simultaneous Treatment of Sexual Partners. Since the treatment of patients in isolation would have insufficient effect on disease transmission, every gonorrhea patient should receive counseling with the aim of ensuring that: (1) the patient will return for reexamination; (2) the patient will advise his or her sexual partners to seek examination and treatment; (3) the patient will abstain from sexual contact until the sexual partners have been examined and treated; and (4) should the patient be reinfected in the future, he or she will bring recent sexual partners along to the health care facility.

9.1.5b. More Intensive Case Management. These techniques range from brief motivational educational sessions with individual patients to systems utilizing referral cards and to actual personal interviews with patients that will enable public health workers to visit the patient's sexual partners in the community and offer treatment. Individual personal interviews to learn the names and whereabouts of sexual contacts and, in particular, community visits by health workers to locate these contacts may be possible in some areas. Whatever methods for providing epidemiological treatment to patient's sexual partners are used, they need not be used uniformly for all patients.

9.1.5c. Priorities for Epidemiological Services. The aim of contact tracing is to provide epidemiological treatment for those most likely to have transmitted the disease recently and most likely to continue transmitting it in the future. Contact tracing also requires the accessibility of the index case to the counselor or public health worker. Granting this, priority for epidemiological services should be given to these groups of patients, symptomatic men, and members of high-risk groups (Table 1). When the sexual partners of these groups of patients are examined, the rate of asymptomatic infection is high. If the control organization is still weak, initially it may be the most practical for epidemiological services to concentrate on men with symptomatic gonococcal urethritis.

Table 1. Examples of Priority Criteria for Disease Intervention[a]

Prostitutes
Women with pelvic inflammatory disease
Symptomatic men
Cases of treatment failure (possibility of resistance)
Residence within a defined "core" area
Antimicrobial-resistant infection
Use of "crack" cocaine
Large number of sexual contacts

[a]These are examples of criteria used by different communities. Not all may be applicable to any one community.

9.1.6. Health Education. Health education has been widely accepted as an important tool in the control of STDs because of increased recognition of the behavioral and sociocultural factors involved in their prevention, transmission, diagnosis, and treatment. Medical and organizational measures by themselves have proven to be unsatisfactory. In some countries, sex and health education is neglected, particularly among the young. The consequent ignorance about STDs may hinder their control because infected patients may be slow to take advice. Decisions and action to adopt control and preventive measures in relation to the STD depend on several factors, such as information and misconceptions about these diseases, changes in beliefs about them and in attitudes toward them, prevailing cultural views and social norms, and the way patients are received by the STD health providers.

Health education activities may be aimed at making the public aware of the STD problem in the community, at seeking the active cooperation of groups and individuals in control activities, at informing groups at risk about control and preventive measures and motivating them to adopt these measures, at educating young people to consider the health-related aspects of their sexuality, at preparing personnel for their educational functions in the control program, and at orienting services at the relevant clinics toward the needs of their clients.

9.2. Personal Prophylaxis

Condoms, when used appropriately, are highly effective in preventing transmission of gonorrhea and other STDs.[103] Latex condoms are recommended, since natural membrane condoms contain pores that may allow the transmission of small viral particles, such as HIV. These pores are not present in latex condoms.

A variety of intravaginal capsules, jellies, and creams contain gonococcidal compounds in addition to spermicides.[104] Some have been shown to possess a significant *in vitro* effect against the gonococcus after a 1-minute exposure. Furthermore, the spermicide, nonoxynol-9, may itself reduce the incidence of gonococcal and chlamydial infection.[105] Coordinating the use of these preparations with family-planning programs needs further emphasis.

The overall value of physical and chemical means of personal prophylaxis is limited by factors of motivation, acceptance, and use. The effectiveness of condoms and diaphragms plus spermicide is poor in some populations, both for contraception and for disease prevention, because of poor compliance by users. The effectiveness of the condom must be emphasized to the public to encourage its use by those concerned about disease prevention.

9.3. Antibiotic Prophylaxis against Gonococcal Infection

Systemically administered prophylactic antibiotics, obtained either by prescription or illicitly, have been consistently shown to decrease infection rates.[106] Both sulfa drugs and penicillin were used in mass prophylaxis trials by the military during the 1940s with excellent results.[107,108] Minocycline has also been shown to be effective prophylactically against susceptible strains.[109] Despite the favorable results of early trials, the routine use of prophylactic antibiotics should be discouraged. Widespread prophylactic antibiotic use poses the potential risks of adverse drug reactions, increased antibiotic resistance, and inappropriate use of the antibiotic for serious infections, such as endocarditis in intravenous drug users.

9.4. Possibilities of Immunization

Numerous cell membrane components of *N. gonorrhoeae* have been targeted as potential candidates for vaccine development. Specific antigens have included outer membrane proteins, lipopolysaccharide complexes, and pili.[110] Vaccine development has been complicated by lack of an animal model, antigenic diversity between strains, and antigenic variation within strains over time. Because long-term immunity against gonorrhea does not occur even in the face of natural infection, it is very unlikely that a simple, effective vaccine can be developed using current technology.

10. Unresolved Problems

The gonococcus has historically demonstrated great versatility and adaptability. In the next few years, it would not be unreasonable to expect the continued development of antimicrobial resistance. Quinolone resistance appears to be particularly ominous.

However, we may also expect to see a continued decrease in gonorrhea incidence because of improved diagnosis, which in turn will enhance control. The new DNA-based tests represent a major advance and will facilitate noninvasive screening. From a practical standpoint, these tests will often be combined with *Chlamydia* diagnostics.

Finally, advances in mucosal immunology may yield further insights into local preventive measures for gonorrhea and other STDs.

11. References

1. Centers for Disease Control, Special focus: Surveillance for sexually transmitted diseases, *Morbid. Mortal. Week. Rep.* **42**(SS3): 1–11 (1993).
2. Crede, K., Reports from the obstetrical clinic in Leipzig prevention of eye inflammation in the newborn, *Arch. Gynaek.* **17**:50–53 (1881).
3. Weiss, P. J., Kennedy, C. A., McCann, D. F., Hill, H. E., and Oldfield, E. C., III, Fulminant endocarditis due to infection with penicillinase-producing *Neisseria gonorrhoeae*, *Sex. Transm. Dis.* **19**:288–290 (1992).
4. Grimes, D. A., Deaths due to sexually transmitted diseases, *J. Am. Med. Assoc.* **255**:1727–1729 (1986).
5. Centers for Disease Control, Case definition for public health surveillance, *Morbid. Mortal. Week. Rep.* **39**(RR-13):1–43 (1990).
6. Centers for Disease Control, *Sexually Transmitted Disease Surveillance*, 1996, US Public Health Service, Atlanta, 1997.
7. Cronberg, S., The rise and fall of sexually transmitted diseases in Sweden, *Genitourin. Med.* **69**:184–186 (1993).
8. Danielsson, D., Gonorrhea and syphilis in Sweden—Past and present, *Scand. J. Infect. Dis.* **69**(Suppl.):69–76 (1990).
9. Treurniet, H. F., and Davidse, W., Sexually transmitted diseases reported by STD services in the Netherlands, 1984–1990, *Genitourin. Med.* **69**:434–438 (1993).
10. Meyer, L., Goulet, V., and Massari, V., Surveillance of sexually transmitted diseases in France: Recent trends and incidence, *Genitourin. Med.* **70**:15–21 (1994).
11. Rothenberg, R. B., The geography of gonorrhea, *Am. J. Epidemiol.* **117**:688–694 (1983).
12. Centers for Disease Control, Sentinel surveillance system for antimicrobial resistance in clinical isolates of *Neisseria gonorrhoeae*, *Morbid. Mortal. Week. Rep.* **36**:585–593 (1987).
13. Anderson, J. E., McCormick, L., and Fichtner, R., Factors associated with self-reported STDs: Data from a national survey, *Sex. Transm. Dis.* **21**:303–308 (1994).
14. Gale, J. L., and Hinds, M. W., Male urethritis in King County, Washington 1974–1975: 1. Incidence, *Am. J. Public Health* **68**:20–25 (1978).
15. Eisenberg, M. S., and Wiesner, P. J., Reporting and treating gonorrhea: Results of a statewide survey in Alaska, *J. Am. Venereal Dis. Assoc.* **3**:79–83 (1976).
16. Goodhart, M. E., Ogden, J., Zaidi, A. A., *et al.*, Factors affecting the performance of smear and culture tests for the detection of *Neisseria gonorrhoeae*, *Sex. Transm. Dis.* **9**:63–69 (1982).
17. Knud-Hansen, C. R., Dallabetta, G. A., Reichart, C., Pabst, K. M., Hook, E. W., III, and Wasstheit, J. N., Surrogate methods to diagnose gonococcal and chlamydial cervicitis: Comparison of leukocyte esterase dipstick, endocervical Gram stain, and culture, *Sex. Transm. Dis.* **18**:211–216 (1991).
18. McNagny, S. E., Parker, R. M., Zenilman, J. M., and Lewis, J. S., Urinary leukocyte esterase test: A screening method for the detection of asymptomatic chlamydial and gonococcal infections in men, *J. Infect. Dis.* **165**:573–576 (1992).
19. Hale, Y. M., Melton, M. E., Lewis, J. S., and Willis, D. E., Evaluation of the PACE 2 *Neisseria gonorrhoeae* assay by three public health laboratories, *J. Clin. Microbiol.* **31**:451–453 (1993).
20. Panke, E. S., Yang, L. I., Leist, P. A., Magevney, P., Fry, R. J., and Lee, R. F., Comparison of Gen-probe DNA probe test and culture for the detection of *Neisseria gonorrhoeae* in endocervical specimens, *J. Clin. Microbiol.* **29**:883–888 (1991).

21. Lewis, J. S., Fakile, O., Foss, E., Legarza, G., Lowe, K., and Powning, D., Direct DNA probe assay for *Neisseria gonorrhoeae* in pharyngeal and rectal specimens, *J. Clin. Microbiol.* **31:**2783–2785 (1993).
22. Chapin-Robertson, K., Use of molecular diagnostics in sexually transmitted diseases, *Diagn. Microbiol. Infect. Dis.* **16:**173–184 (1993).
23. Birkenmeyer, L., and Armstrong, A. S., Preliminary evaluation of the ligase chain reaction for specific detection of *Neisseria gonorrhoeae*, *J. Clin. Microbiol.* **30:**3089–3094 (1992).
24. Brooks, G. F., and Lammel, C. J., Humoral immune response to gonococcal infections, *Clin. Microbiol. Rev.* **2**(Suppl.)**:**S5–S10 (1989).
25. McGee, Z. A., Johnson, A. P., and Taylor-Robinson, D., Pathogenic mechanisms of *Neisseria gonorrhoeae*: Observations on damage to human fallopian tubes in organ culture by gonococci of colony type 1 or type 4, *J. Infect. Dis.* **143:**413–422 (1981).
26. Young, J. D. E., Blake, M., Mauro, A., and Cohn, Z. A., Properties of the major outer membrane protein from *Neisseria gonorrhoeae* incorporated into model lipid membranes, *Proc. Natl. Acad. Sci. USA* **80:**3831–3835 (1983).
27. Knapp, J. S., Tam, M. R., Nowinski, R. C., Holme, K. K., and Sandstrom, E. G., Serological classification of *Neisseria gonorrhoeae* with use of monoclonal antibodies to gonococcal outer membrane protein I, *J. Infect. Dis.* **150:**44–48 (1984).
28. Sparling, P. F., Cannon, J. G., and So, M., Phase and antigenic variation of pili and outer membrane protein II of *Neisseria gonorrhoeae*, *J. Infect. Dis.* **153:**196–201 (1986).
29. Joiner, K. A., Scales, R., Warren, K. A., Frank, M. M., and Rice, P. A., Mechanism of action of blocking immunoglobulin G for *Neisseria gonorrhoeae*, *J. Clin. Invest.* **76:**1765–1772 (1985).
30. Plummer, F. A., Chubb, H., Simonsen, J. N., Bosire, M., Slaney, L., MacLean, J., Ndinya-Achola, J. D., Waiyaki, P., and Brunham, R. C., Antibody to Rmp (outer membrane protein 3) increases susceptibility to gonococcal infection, *J. Clin. Invest.* **91:**339–343 (1993).
31. van Putten, J. P. M., Iron acquisition and the pathogenesis of meningococcal and gonococcal disease, *Med. Microbiol. Immunol.* **179:**289–295 (1990).
32. McKenna, W. R., Mickelsen, P. A., Sparling, P. F., and Dyer, D. W., Iron uptake from lactoferrin and transferrin by *Neisseria gonorrhoeae*, *Infect. Immun.* **56:**578–791 (1988).
33. Handsfield, H. H., Lipman, T. O., Harnisch, J. P., Tronca, E., and Holmes, K. K., Asymptomatic gonorrhea in men, *N. Engl. J. Med.* **290:**117–123 (1974).
34. Allard, R., Robert, J., Turgeon, P., and LePage, Y., Predictors of asymptomatic gonorrhea among patients seen by private practitioners, *Can. Med. Assoc. J.* **133:**1135–1146 (1985).
35. Holmes, K. K., Johnson, D. W., and Trostle, H. J., An estimate of the risk of men acquiring gonorrhea by sexual contact with infected females, *Am. J. Epidemiol.* **91:**17–24 (1970).
36. Robertson, P., and Schachter, J., Failure to identify venereal disease in a lesbian population, *Sex. Transm. Dis.* **8:**75–76 (1981).
37. Ostrow, D. G., and Altman, N. L., Sexually transmitted diseases and homosexuality, *Sex. Transm. Dis.* **10:**208–215 (1983).
38. Schwarcz, S. K., Bolan, G. A., Fullilove, M., McCright, J., Fullilove, R., Kohn, R., and Rolfs, R. T., Crack cocaine and the exchange of sex for money or drugs, *Sex. Transm. Dis.* **19:**7–12 (1992).
39. May, R. M., The transmission and control of gonorrhea, *Nature* **291:**376–377 (1981).
40. Garnet, G. P., and Anderson, R. M., Contact tracing and the estimation of sexual mixing patterns: The epidemiology of gonococcal infections, *Sex. Transm. Dis.* **20:**181–191 (1993).
41. Rothenberg, R. B., The geography of gonorrhea, *Am. J. Epidemiol.* **117:**688–694 (1983).
42. Jaffe, H. W., Zaidi, A. A., Thornsberry, C., Reynolds, G. H., and Wiesner, P. J., Trends and seasonality of antibiotic resistance of *Neisseria gonorrhoeae*, *J. Infect. Dis.* **136:**684–688 (1977).
43. Ross, J. D. C., and Scott, G. R., Seasonal variation in gonorrhea, *Eur. J. Epidemiol.* **8:**252–255 (1992).
44. de Wit, J. B. F., Van den Hoek, J. A. R., Sandfort, T. G. M., *et al.* Increase in unprotected anogenital intercourse among homosexual men, *Am. J. Public Health* **83:**1451–1453 (1993).
45. Sherrard, J., and Forsyth, J. R. L., Homosexually acquired gonorrhea in Victoria, 1983–1991, *Med. J. Australia* **158:**450–453 (1993).
46. Evans, B. G., Catchpole, M. A., Heptonstall, J., Mortimer, J. Y., McCarringle, C. A., Nicoll, A. G., Wright, P., Gill, O. N., and Swan, A. V., Sexually transmitted diseases and HIV-1 infection among homosexual men in England and Wales, *Br. Med. J.* **306:**426–428 (1993).
47. Piot, P., and Laga, M., Genital ulcers, other sexually transmitted diseases, and the sexual transmission of HIV, *Br. Med. J.* **298:**623–624 (1989).
48. Laga, M., Manoka, A., Kivuvu, M., Malele, B., Tuliza, M., Nzila, N., Goeman, J., Behets, F., Batter, V., and Alary, M., Non-ulcerative sexually transmitted diseases as risk factors for HIV-1 transmission in women: Results from a cohort study, *AIDS* **7:**95–102 (1993).
49. Weir, S. S., Feldblum, P. J., Roddy, R. E., and Zekeng, L., Gonorrhea as a risk factor for HIV acquisition, *AIDS* **8:**1605–1608 (1994).
50. Lau, R. K., Goh, B. T., Estreich, S., Cox, S. N., and Levy, I., Adult gonococcal keratoconjunctivitis with AIDS, *Br. J. Ophthalmol.* **74:**52 (1990).
51. Faruki, H., Kohmescher, R. N., McKinney, W. P., and Sparling, P. F., A community-based outbreak of infection with penicillin-resistant *Neisseria gonorrhoeae* not producing penicillinase (chromosomally mediated resistance), *N. Engl. J. Med.* **313:**607–611 (1985).
52. Sherrard, J., and Barlow, D., PPNG at St. Thomas' Hospital—A changing provenance, *Int. J. STD AIDS* **4:**330–332 (1993).
53. The Australian Gonococcal Surveillance Program, The incidence of gonorrhea and the antibiotic sensitivity of gonococci in Australia, 1981–1991, *Genitourin. Med.* **69:**364–369 (1993).
54. Otubo, J. A. M., Imade, G. E., Sagay, A. S., and Towobola, O. A., Resistance of recent *Neisseria gonorrhoeae* isolates in Nigeria and outcome of single-dose treatment with ciprofloxacin, *Infection* **20:**339–341 (1992).
55. Clendennen, T. E., Echeverria, P., Saengeur, S., Kees, E. S., Boskeys, J. W., and Wignall, F. S., Antibiotic susceptibility survey of *Neisseria gonorrhoeae* in Thailand, *Antimicrob. Agents Chemother.* **36:**1682–1687 (1992).
56. Boslego, J. W., Tramont, E. C., Takafuji, E. T., Diniega, B. M., Mitchell, B. S., Small, J. W., Khan, W. N., and Stein, D. C., Effect of spectinomycin use on the prevalence of spectinomycin-resistant and of penicillinase-producing *Neisseria gonorrhoeae*, *N. Engl. J. Med.* **317:**272–278 (1987).
57. Zenilman, J. M., Nims, L. J., Menegus, M. A., Nolte, F., and Knapp, J. S., Spectinomycin-resistant gonococcal infections in the United States, 1985–1986, *J. Infect. Dis.* **156:**1002–1004 (1987).

58. Kam, K., Lo, K., Lai, C., Lee, Y. S., and Chen, C. B., Ofloxacin susceptibilities of 5,667 *Neisseria gonorrhoeae* strains isolated in Hong Kong, *Antimicrob. Agents. Chemother.* **37:**2007–2008 (1993).
59. Tapsall, J. W., Shultz, T. R., and Phillips, E. A., Characteristics of *Neisseria gonorrhoeae* isolated in Australia showing decreased sensitivity to quinolone antibiotics, *Pathology* **24:**27–31 (1992).
60. Bogaerts, J., Tello, W. M., Akingeneye, J., Mukantabara, V., Van Dyck, E., and Piot, P., Effectiveness of norfloxacin and ofloxacin for treatment of gonorrhea and decrease of *in vitro* susceptibility to quinolones over time in Rwanda, *Genitourin. Med.* **69:**196–200 (1993).
61. Centers for Disease Control, Decreased susceptibility of *Neisseria gonorrhoeae* to fluoroquinolones—Ohio and Hawaii, 1992–1994, *Morbid. Mortal. Week. Rep.* **43:**325–327 (1994).
62. Gilbaugh, J. H., and Fuchs, P. C., The gonococcus and the toilet seat, *N. Engl. J. Med.* **301:**91–93 (1979).
63. Sgroi, S. M., Pediatric gonorrhea and child sexual abuse: The venereal disease connection, *Sex. Transm. Dis.* **9:**154–156 (1982).
64. Ross, S. C., and Densen, P., Complement deficiency state and infection: Epidemiology, pathogenesis and consequences of neisserial and other infections in an immune deficiency, *Medicine* **63:**243–272 (1984).
65. Tramont, E. C., Inhibition of adherence of *Neisseria gonorrhoeae* by human genital secretions, *J. Clin. Invest.* **59:**117–124 (1977).
66. Kearns, D. H., O'Reilly, R. J., Lee, R. J., and Welch, B. A., Secretory IgA antibodies in the urethral exudate of men with uncomplicated urethritis due to *Neisseria gonorrhoeae*, *J. Infect. Dis.* **127:**99–101 (1973).
67. Ison, C. A., Hadfield, S. G., Bellinger, C. M., Dawson, S. A., and Glynn, A. A., The specificity of serum and local antibodies in female gonorrhea, *Clin. Exp. Immunol.* **65:**198–205 (1986).
68. Meyer, T. F., and van Putten, J. P. M., Genetic mechanisms and biological implications of phase variation in pathogenic *Neisseriae*, *Clin. Microbiol. Rev.* **2**(Suppl.):S139–S145 (1989).
69. Sarafian, S. K., Tam, M. R., and Morse, S. A., Gonococcal protein I-specific opsonic IgG in normal human serum, *J. Infect. Dis.* **148:** 1025–1032 (1983).
70. Hooten, T. M., and Barnes, R. C., Urethritis in men, *Infect. Dis. Clin. North Am.* **1:**165–178 (1987).
71. Platt, R., Rice, P. A., and McCormack, W. M., Risk of acquiring gonorrhea and prevalence of abnormal adnexal findings among women recently exposed to gonorrhea, *J. Am. Med. Assoc.* **250:** 3205–3209 (1983).
72. Centers for Disease Control, Pelvic inflammatory disease: Guidelines for prevention and management, *Morbid. Mortal. Week. Rep.* **40**(RR-5):1–25 (1991).
73. Westrom, L., and Wolner-Hanssen, P., Pathogenesis of pelvic inflammatory disease, *Genitourin. Med.* **69:**9–17 (1993).
74. Westrom, L., Incidence, prevalence, and trends of acute pelvic inflammatory diseases and its consequences in industrialized countries, *Am. J. Obstet. Gynecol.* **138:**880–892 (1980).
75. Westrom, L., Joesoef, R., Reynolds, G., Hagdu, A., and Thompson, S. E., Pelvic inflammatory disease and fertility, *Sex. Transm. Dis.* **19:**185–191 (1992).
76. Hillis, S. D., Joesoef, R., Marchbanks, P. A., Wasserheit, J. N., Cates, W., Jr., and Westrom, L., Delayed care of pelvic inflammatory disease as a risk factor for impaired fertility, *Am. J. Obstet. Gynecol.* **168:**1503–1509 (1993).
77. Sweet, R. L., Pelvic inflammatory disease and infertility in women, *Infect. Dis. Clin. North Am.* **1:**199–215 (1987).
78. Stacey, C. M., Munday, P. E., Taylor-Robinson, D., *et al.*, A longitudinal study of pelvic inflammatory disease, *Br. J. Obstet. Gynaecol.* **99:**994–999 (1992).
79. Jacobson, L., and Westrom, L., Objectivized diagnosis of pelvic inflammatory disease, *Am. J.Obstet. Gynecol.* **105:**1088–1098 (1969).
80. Peterson, H. B., Walker, C. K., Kahn, J. G., Washington, A. E., Eschenbach, D. A., and Faro, S., Pelvic inflammatory disease, *J. Am. Med. Assoc.* **266:**2605–2611, (1991).
81. Walker, C. K., Kahn, J. G., Washington, A. E., Peterson, H. B., and Sweet, R. L., Pelvic inflammatory disease: Meta-analysis of antimicrobial regimen efficacy, *J. Infect. Dis.* **168:**969–978 (1993).
82. Klein, E. J., Fisher, L. S., Chow, A. W., and Guze, L. B., Anorectal gonorrheal infection, *Ann. Intern. Med.* **86:**340–346 (1977).
83. Lebedoff, D. A., Hochman, E. B., Rectal gonorrhea in men: Diagnosis and treatment, *Ann. Intern. Med.* **92:**463–466 (1980).
84. Quinn, T. C., Stamm, W. E., Goodell, S. E., Mkrtichian, E., Benedetti, J., Corey, L., Schuffler, M. D., and Holmes, K. K., The polymicrobial origin of intestinal infection in homosexual men, *N. Engl. J. Med.* **309:**576–582 (1983).
85. Law, C., Sexually transmitted diseases and enteric infections in the male homosexual population, *Semin. Dermatol.* **9:**178–184 (1990).
86. Wiesner, P. J., Tronca, E., Bonin, P., Pedersen, A. H., and Holmes, K. K., Clinical spectrum of pharyngeal gonococcal infection, *N. Engl. J. Med.* **284:**181–185 (1973).
87. Hutt, D. M., and Judson, F. M., Epidemiology and treatment of oropharyngeal gonorrhea, *Ann. Intern. Med.* **104:**655–658 (1986).
88. Judson, F. N., Ehret, J. M., and Handsfield, H. H., Comparative study of certriaxone and spectinomycin for treatment of pharyngeal and anorectal gonorrhea, *J. Am. Med. Assoc.* **253:**1417–1419 (1985).
89. Wiesner, P. J., Handsfield, H. H., and Holmes, K. K., Low antibiotic resistance of gonococci causing disseminated infection, *N. Engl. J. Med.* **288:**1221–1226 (1973).
90. Wise, C. M., Morris, C. R., Wasilauskas, B. L., and Salzer, W. L., Gonococcal arthritis in an era of increasing penicillin resistance, *Arch. Intern. Med.* **154:**2690–2695 (1994).
91. Koss, P. J., Disseminated gonococcal infection—The tenosynovitis–dermatitis and suppurative arthritis syndromes, *Clev. Clin. Q.* **52:**161–173 (1985).
92. Masi, A. T., and Eisenstein, B. I., Disseminated gonococcal infection and gonococcal arthritis: II. Clinical manifestations, diagnosis, complications, treatment, and prevention, *Semin. Arthritis Rheum.* **10:**173–197 (1981).
93. O'Brien, J. P., Goldenberg, D. L., and Rice, P. A., Disseminated gonococcal infection: A prospective analysis of 49 patients and a review of pathophysiology and immune mechanisms, *Medicine* **62:**395–406 (1983).
94. Ullman, S., Roussel, T. J., Culbertson, W. W., Forster, R. K., Alfonso, E., Mendelsohn, A. D., Herdemann, D. A., and Holland, S. P., *Neisseria gonorrhoeae* keratoconjunctivitis, *Ophthalmology* **94:**525–531 (1987).
95. Wan, W. L., Farkas, G. C., May, W. N., and Robin, J. B., The clinical characteristics and course of adult gonococcal conjunctivitis, *Am. J. Ophthalmol.* **102:**575–583 (1986).
96. Fransen, L., Nsanze, H., Klauss, V., Van der Stuyft, P., D'Costa, L., Brunham, R. C., and Piot, P., Ophthalmia neonatorum in Nairobi, Kenya: The roles of *Neisseria gonorrhoeae* and *Chlamydia trachomatis*, *J. Infect. Dis.* **153:**862–869 (1986).

97. Laga, M., Meheus, A., and Piot, P., Epidemiology and control of gonococcal ophthalmia neonatorum, *Bull. WHO* **67:**471–478 (1989).
98. Alfonso, E., Friedland, B., Hupp, S., Olsen, K., Senikowich, K., Sklar, V. E., and Forster, R. K., *Neisseria gonorrhoeae* conjunctivitis. An outbreak during an epidemic of acute hemorrhagic conjunctivitis, *J. Am. Med. Assoc.* **250:**794–795 (1983).
99. Spark, R. P., Dahlberg, P. W., and LaBelle, J. W., Pseudogonococcal ophthalmia neonatorum, *Am. J. Clin. Pathol.* **72:**471–473 (1979).
100. Nenstein, L., Goldenring, J., and Carpenter, S., Nonsexual transmission of sexually transmitted diseases: An infrequent occurrence, *Pediatrics* **74:**67–76 (1984).
101. Potterat, J. J., Markewich, G. S., and Rothenberg, R., Prepubertal infection with *Neisseria gonorrhoeae*: Clinical and epidemiologic significance, *Sex. Transm. Dis.* **5:**1–3 (1978).
102. Whittington, W. L., Rice, R. J., Biddle, J. W., and Knapp, J. S., Incorrect identification of *Neisseria gonorrhoeae* from infants and children, *Pediatr. Infect. Dis. J.* **7:**3–10 (1988).
103. Condoms for prevention of sexually transmitted diseases, *Morbid. Mortal. Week. Rep.* **37:**133–137 (1988).
104. Stone, K. A., Grimes, D. A., and Magder, L. S., Personal protection against sexually transmitted diseases, *Am. J. Obstet. Gynecol.* **155:**180–188 (1986).
105. Niruthisard, S., Roddy, R. E., and Chutivongse, S., Use of nonoxynol-9 and reduction in rate of gonococcal and chlamydial cervical infections, *Lancet* **1:**1371–1375 (1992).
106. Bradbeer, C. S., Thin, R. N., Tan, T., and Thirumoorthy, T., Prophylaxis against infection in Singaporean prostitutes, *Genitourin. Med.* **64:**52–53 (1988).
107. Loveless, J. A., and Denton, W., The oral use of sulfathiazole as a prophylaxis for gonorrhea, *J. Am. Med. Assoc.* **121:**827–828 (1943).
108. Eagle, H., Gude, A. V., Beckman, G. E., *et al.*, Prevention of gonorrhea with penicillin tablets, *J. Am. Med. Assoc.* **140:**940–943 (1949).
109. Harrison, W. O., Hooper, R. R., Wiesner, P. J., Campbell, A. F., Karney, W. W., Reynolds, G. W., Jones, O. A., and Holmes, K. K., A trial of minocycline given after exposure to prevent gonorrhea, *N. Engl. J. Med.* **300:**1074–1078 (1979).
110. Tramont, E. C., Gonococcal vaccines, *Clin. Microbiol. Rev.* **2**(Suppl.):S74–S77 (1989).

12. Suggested Reading

Zenilman, J. M., Gonorrhea: Clinical and public health issues, *Hosp. Pract. (Off. Ed.)* **28**(2A)**:**29–45 (1993).

Moran, J. S., Treating uncomplicated *Neisseria gonorrhoeae* infections: Is the anatomic site of infection important? *Sex. Trans. Dis.* **22:**39–47 (1995).

Cohen, M. S., and Sparling, P. F., Mucosal infection with *Neisseria gonorrhoeae*: Bacterial adaptation and mucosal defenses, *J. Clin. Invest.* **89:**1699–1705 (1992).

Updated sexually transmitted disease incidence data and treatment protocols are available from the CDC via the Internet at http://www.cdc.gov.

CHAPTER 16

Haemophilus influenzae

Joel I. Ward and Constance M. Vadheim

1. Introduction

One of the major public health success stories of the 20th century is the near elimination of invasive *Haemophilus influenzae* type b (Hib) disease in the United States and in most developed countries since 1990, a consequence of the routine immunization of infants with Hib conjugate vaccines. Worldwide, *H. influenzae* has been a leading cause of invasive bacterial infections, which includes bacteremia, epiglottis, pneumonia, and meningitis. Before vaccines were available, Hib was the leading cause of bacterial meningitis, especially for young children. Prior to 1990, an estimated 25,000 persons developed invasive Hib disease (bacteremia and meningitis) each year in the United States. It was estimated that the cumulative incidence of disease during the first 5 years of life was one episode in every 200 children.[1] Despite the availability of effective antimicrobial therapy, invasive Hib infections resulted in substantial mortality and morbidity. The emergence of antibiotic resistance was yet another problem complicating treatment.

In addition to invasive disease, in all age groups *H. influenzae* is a cause of common but less severe mucosal infections, such as otitis media, sinusitis, conjunctivitis, and bronchitis. *H. influenzae* strains are ubiquitous and asymptomatically colonize the upper respiratory tract, and thus can be considered to be part of the normal bacterial flora of man. This wide spectrum of infections and different mechanisms of disease pathogenesis have made it difficult to distinguish pathogenic from nonpathogenic strains and to assess infectivity and incubation period.

There are six serotypes of encapsulated *H. influenzae*, in addition to many nonencapsulated and untypeable strains. However, more than 90% of invasive bacteremic disease is caused by the type b serotype, for which there is now a vaccine. The vaccines developed to date for Hib diseases are derivations of the type b polysaccharide and are very effective against invasive disease. These Hib conjugate vaccines have little or no impact on the incidence of mucosal infections and infections due to nontype b strains (i.e., otitis media or bronchitis). Therefore, in this chapter we will focus on the disease and epidemiology of invasive type b infections, for which there are vaccines.

2. Historical Background

The organism was first described in 1892 by Robert Pfeiffer,[2] who isolated it from the lung and sputum of patients during the 1889–1892 pandemic of influenza. He proposed that the organism was the cause of influenza[3] and it was initially known as the "Pfeiffer influenza bacillus." By the turn of the century the organism had been recovered from the blood and cerebrospinal fluid (CSF) of young children with meningitis. Although there remained doubt about the etiologic role of the Pfeiffer bacillus as the cause of influenza, it was not until the influenza pandemic of 1918 that its etiological role was seriously questioned. In 1920, the Society of American Bacteriologists renamed the organism *H. influenzae* to acknowledge the historic association with influenza and to emphasize its requirement of blood factors for growth (*haemophilus* means "blood loving"). In 1933, Smith *et al.*[4] discovered the influenza virus that finally refuted any remaining confusion about the erroneous association between *H. influenzae* and influenza.

During the 1930s, the classic work by Margaret Pittman[5] demonstrated that *H. infleunzae* existed in encapsu-

Joel I. Ward and Constance M. Vadheim • UCLA Center for Vaccine Research, Harbor–UCLA Medical Center, UCLA School of Medicine, Torrance, California 90509.

lated and unencapsulated forms, and she identified each of the six capsular serotypes (types a–f). Subsequently, it has been shown that each capsular serotype has a chemically distinct polysaccharide capsule. She also observed that virtually all *H. influenza* isolates from CSF and blood were capsular type b, and demonstrated that type b horse antiserum conferred protection against lethal infection in rabbits.(6) This observation led to the use of antiserum as the first treatment for infection, prepared by immunization with formalinized Hib initially in horses and later in rabbits. Prior to this, Hib meningitis and other forms of invasive Hib disease were nearly always fatal.(7) Despite antiserum therapy, the reported case-fatality remained high.(8–10) It was not until the late 1930s that treatment of children with Hib meningitis with rabbit type b antiserum and sulfonamides reduced the case-fatality ratio to about 24%.(10–12)

At about the same time, studies by Fothergill and Wright(13) showed an epidemiological relationship between the age-specific risk for Hib meningitis and the absence of bactericidal antibodies, leading the investigators to propose that the bactericidal activity of serum conferred immunity against Hib meningitis. They hypothesized that disease was uncommon in the first few months of life due to the protective effects of maternally acquired antibody and that it occurred infrequently in later life (older children and adults) due to antibody acquired by natural exposure to the organism.

Antimicrobial agents focused attention away from the need to prevent of Hib disease. Yet even in the early 1990s, with excellent intensive care and many effective antimicrobial therapies, fatality was about 5% and neurological morbidity occurred in about 20% of children with Hib meningitis. And while there was much progress in our understanding of the microbiology, epidemiology, pathogenesis, and immunology of Hib disease, vaccines were late in coming. By the early 1970s, two groups of investigators purified and characterized the type b polysaccharide (polyribosyl–ribitol phosphate) as a potential vaccine candidate. It was shown that serum antibodies to PRP were bactericidal and opsonophagocytic and protected animals against invasive infection.(14,15) The protective efficacy of a PRP vaccine against invasive Hib disease was shown in children 18–71 months of age in a prospective randomized field trial conducted in 1974 in Finland.(16) This and other studies culminated in the licensure of PRP vaccine in the United States in April 1985, the first vaccine available for the prevention of Hib disease. Unfortunately, this vaccine was only licensed for use in children 18 months of age and older, as it induced equivocal immune responses and provided no protection in young infants, those at greatest disease risk. Even in older children the vaccine induced only incomplete protection.

Improved vaccines employed polysaccharide–protein conjugate techniques. The first Hib conjugate vaccine was PRP-D and was licensed in December 1987 for use in older children. In 1988 and 1989, improved Hib conjugate vaccines were licensed: HbOC and PRP-OMP vaccines, respectively.(17,18) In 1990, these Hib conjugate vaccines had been shown to protect young infants.(19–21) With the changes in Hib vaccination practices between 1985 and the present, there have been dramatic decreases in Hib disease incidence in many populations.(22–24)

3. Methodology

3.1. Sources of Mortality Data

The only national data available on deaths caused by invasive *H. influenzae* disease are those compiled by the National Center for Health Statistics (NCHS). To assess the completeness and validity of these data, death certificate data from 1962 to 1968 were compared with population-based retrospective studies of Hib meningitis from four separate areas of the United States.(25) Only 58% of the confirmed cases of fatal *H. influenzae* meningitis in the four study areas were identified in the NCHS registry.

The most reliable mortality data are derived from hospital-based or population-based surveillance studies of invasive Hib disease.(1,26) Such studies identify cases by a variety of overlapping methods, including review of microbiology and hospital records which are considered to be more complete. Passive reporting to the National Bacterial Meningitis Surveillance Study (participation from 27 states that represent 52% of the US population) has also provided estimates of age-specific case-fatality rates.(27)

3.2. Sources of Morbidity Data

Invasive *H. influenzae* disease has not been a nationally reportable disease in the United States, and consequently national incidence and morbidity data are not readily available from a single source. National data are available in Finland and a few other developed countries. Nonetheless, there are active surveillance data from which national incidence and morbidity have been extrapolated. Such data are available from several large populations over considerable periods, including states, large urban counties, health maintenance organizations (HMOs), and the Indian Health Service. Also, several hospital-based studies have been conducted(1) (see Section 5.1). In general, International Classification of Disease-9 hospital discharge diagnoses for meningitis is more sensitive than for other bacteremic *H. influenzae* infections.[28]

3.3. Surveys

There have been survey studies for common diseases like otitis media, but invasive Hib disease is sufficiently uncommon and of too short a duration to make survey data useful. Incidence, morbidity, and mortality data are best derived from prospective population based surveillance studies.

3.4. Laboratory Diagnosis

3.4.1. Isolation and Identification of the Organism. *H. influenzae* is a small gram-negative, nonmotile, nonspore-forming coccobacillus that on Gram's stain of clinical specimens can be pleomorphic, especially in specimens from patients who have received β-lactam antibiotics. The laboratory identification of *H. influenzae* depends on the organism's nutritional need for X and V factors as supplements for growth. The X factor is a heat-stable, iron-containing protoporphyrin essential for activity of the electron transport chain and for aerobic growth. The V factor, a coenzyme, is a heat-labile factor supplied by NAD. Both of these factors are present within erythrocytes and are released in a chocolate agar by heat or enzyme lysis of the red cells. The growth requirements for these factors remain the primary basis for the laboratory differentiation of *H. influenzae* from other *Haemophilus* species. Fermentation and other metabolic activities of the organism are variable between strains, and therefore are not particularly useful for identification. Although not essential for growth, some strains grow better in 5 to 10% CO_2. After overnight incubation on almost any enriched medium that contains X and V factors, colonies appear that are 0.5 to 1.5 mm in diameter and are rough or granular in appearance. Encapsulated strains usually produce slightly larger, mucoid or glistening colonies.

The encapsulated strains (serotypes a–f) can be typed serologically with specific antiserum by agglutination or quellung reaction. The type b capsular polysaccharide consists of a repeating polymer of ribosyl and ribitol phosphate having a 1–1 linkage. This capsular antigen, released both *in vitro* and *in vivo*, can be detected with specific immunologic techniques used for rapid diagnosis.[29–32] Commercially obtained reagent kits using latex agglutination methods are most widely used to detect the type b capsular antigen in body fluids. Although the capsule of Hib and some other encapsulated bacteria may share similar antigenic determinants, cross-reactions causing false-positive antigen tests for Hib rarely occur in clinical practice. Strains without capsules also cause disease, but they rarely cause bacteremia, except in neonates, immunocompromised adults, or compromised children in developing countries (see Sections 7 and 8).

3.4.2. Serological Methods. Serology has not been used to diagnose invasive Hib cases because anticapsular antibodies are not induced in young children and are not reliably induced in older individuals. Further, *Escherichia coli* K100, an enteric nonpathogenic bacteria, can induce cross-reacting type b anticapsular antibody responses. Other immunologic markers, such as immune responses to outer-membrane proteins (OMPs), have the problem that there are different OMPs in different Hib strains and there are shared antigens with cross-reacting bacteria.

4. Biological Characteristics of the Organism

Several surface structures of the organism are important determinants of pathogenicity, and like many invasive bacterial pathogens the outermost structure of Hib is its polysaccharide capsule. The type b capsule is of primary clinical and immunologic importance, inasmuch as type b organisms account for 95% of all strains that cause invasive disease (bacteremia and meningitis).[33] This polysaccharide is known as polyribosyl–ribitol phosphate (PRP) and consists of a repeating polymer of ribosyl and ribitol phosphate. The release of this antigen in body fluids of infected individuals can be detected with specific immunologic techniques used for rapid diagnosis.[30,31,34] The other capsular serotypes have different carbohydrate compositions and only occasionally cause invasive disease. Strains without capsules frequently cause infections of the respiratory tract and adjacent structures, but rarely cause bacteremic infections.[35,36]

Other important components of the *H. influenzae* cell envelope include lipopolysaccharides [(LPS) endotoxin] and a number of proteins and lipids in the outer membrane. Some membrane proteins participate in cell transport (porins) or are adhesions; the functions of other remains undefined. Pili or fimbriae are protein filaments extending from the outer membrane that appear to mediate attachment of the organism to epithelial cells.[37] The electrophoresis of a number of cytoplasmic enzymes has distinguished isoenzyme differences that have been useful in genetic analyses of *H. influenzae* strains.[38]

Methods have been developed for differentiating isolates of Hib by differences in electrophoretic mobility patterns of the major OMPs, and this has been useful for epidemiological studies.[39,40] To date, specific OMP patterns have not been clearly associated with virulence. However, the possibility has been suggested that strains of different OMP subtypes may cause a differing clinical spectrum of illness.[7] LPS or endotoxin of Hib is important in the pathogenicity of the organism and appears to have little antigenic diversity,[41] although there is variability in LPS electrophoretic patterns after passage *in vivo* or *in vitro*.[42] Therefore, electrophoretic characterization of endotoxin has not been useful as an epidemiological tool. Multilocus enzyme electrophoresis is a method used to characterize isoenzymes of the organism. This method has been used to distinguish different genotypes of Hib for epidemiological purposes. This procedure and DNA analysis appear to have the greatest genetic discriminating power.

Another important microbiological feature of *H. influenzae* has been the development of antibiotic resistance. Resistance to a wide variety of antibiotics (e.g., sulfonamides, trimethoprim–sulfamethoxazole, erythromycin, tetracycline, and penicillin) has been described. Of greater importance is resistance to ampicillin,[43] first noted in the mid 1970s, because ampicillin has been the primary antibiotic used for therapy of invasive disease. Since then, ampicillin resistance has become widespread, ranging between 5 and 50% of isolates in various parts of the world.[44,45] The mechanism of resistance usually involves plasmid-mediated β-lactamase enzyme production,[46] and resistant strains can be characterized by their plasmid or β-lactamase enzyme content. Although chloramphenicol-resistant strains are rare in the United States, they are increasingly prevalent in some areas of the world,[39,47] and strains resistant to both ampicillin and chloramphenicol have been reported.[45,48–50] Currently, third-generation cephalosporins, in particular, ceftriaxone and cefotaxime, are the mainstays of antibiotic therapy for invasive disease.[51] Concerns about the potential for the development of resistance to these highly effective agents further emphasizes the need for means to prevent disease.

5. Descriptive Epidemiology

5.1. Disease Incidence

The clinical manifestations of *H. influenzae* infection are discussed in Section 8.1. There are three major categories of manifestations: asymptomatic carriage, noninvasive disease, and invasive disease. The epidemiology of invasive disease is discussed below.

5.1.2. Incidence of Invasive Infections. For epidemiological studies, cases of invasive Hib disease are defined by culturing the organism from normally sterile body fluids such as blood, CSF, joint fluid, or pleural fluid. Laboratory-based studies are useful for determining the incidence of Hib meningitis, because virtually all patients with meningitis are hospitalized and the organism can usually be isolated by routine culture of blood and CSF; or the diagnosis can be confirmed by antigen detection assays. However, the diagnosis of invasive nonmeningitis Hib disease requires recognition by physicians of the need to obtain blood cultures or cultures of other normally sterile body fluids before antibiotics are given. Thus, case definitions that depend on microbiological confirmation underestimate the true incidence of Hib disease, because of the variable use of blood and other cultures by physicians.

Population-based studies with active surveillance provide the most accurate estimates on the incidence of Hib disease and are particularly useful for evaluating risk factors for Hib disease. Data obtained by passive surveillance, such as the National Bacterial Meningitis Surveillance Study, are often affected by substantial underreporting of disease.[27,52] Hospital-based studies, although not providing accurate incidence data, have improved our understanding of the clinical spectrum, complications, and long-term sequelae of Hib disease (see Section 8.1). Inevitably, even the best disease rates underestimate the true incidence of Hib disease, because the cultures necessary for case definition are frequently not obtained prior to antimicrobial treatment.

5.1.2a. Incidence of Endemic (Primary) Disease Prior to Widespread Immunization. Prior to widespread immunization, invasive Hib disease occurred endemically, and communitywide epidemics were not observed. *H. influenzae* caused about 20,000 cases of invasive (bacteremic) disease annually in the United States. More than 95% of all invasive *H. influenzae* clinical isolates were serotype b, and virtually all isolates from infants and young children were serotype b.[53–55] As Hib disease is relatively uncommon in older children (less than 15% of all disease), epidemiological studies of invasive Hib disease have tended to focus on children less than 5 years of age.

The incidence of *H. influenzae* disease in United States and other populations prior to the initiation of infant immunization is summarized in Table 1. Studies conducted just prior to vaccine availability in the United States demonstrate an annual attack rate for all Hib disease of 33 to 129 cases per 100,000.[1,56,57] Incidence rates for meningitis ranged from 45 to 69 cases per 100,000 children less than 5 years of age per year.[10,58–60] Several

Table 1. Comparison of Rates of *Haemophilus influenzae* Meningitis and Other Invasive Disease Among Children Younger than 5 Years of Age

		Annual incidence of *H. influenzae*[a]		
Geographic area	Study period	Meningitis	All invasive disease	Ref.
Fresno Co., CA	1976–1978	60	90	99
Alaska (non-Natives)	1980–1982	69	129	83
Colorado (6 mo)	1981–1982	68	112	56
Jefferson Co., AL	1981–1983	62	NA[b]	10
Monroe Co., NY	1982–1983	55	86	112
Dallas Co., TX	1982–1984	67	109	57
Minnesota	1982–1984	45	67	57
Atlanta, GA	1983–1984	57	82	1
Los Angeles Co., CA	1983–1988	—	33–43	93
Sweden	1971–1983	27–31	NA	66, 342
Finland	1976–1981	27	41	68, 92
Geneva, Switzerland	1976–1989	NA	60	343
France	1980–1989	15	21	65
Israel	1988–1990	18	34	344
Manitoba, Canada	1981–1984	32	NA	345
The Netherlands	1977–1982	22	NA	69
Wales	1988–1990	22	35	346
Bochon, Germany	1971–1992	9	13	347
Scotland	1991	—	25.5	71
Canberra, Australia	1984–1990	—	63.2	348

[a]Rate per 100,000 children per year.
[b]NA, not available.

early studies (1960s and early 1970s) reported rates of meningitis of less than 40/100,000 in some US populations. It is not known whether the higher rates reported since the mid-1970s represent a true increase in disease incidence (due to changes in risk factors such as increased use of day-care facilities) or are due to improvements in diagnosis and surveillance.[24,61,62]

Most studies from other developed countries in the prevaccine era suggest incidence rates substantially lower than in the United States (about 1/3 to 2/3 of the US rates) (see Table 1).[63–65] In Sweden,[63,66] Finland,[67,68] and The Netherlands,[69] *H. influenzae* was until recently the most common cause of bacterial meningitis. Hib also ranked as the leading cause of bacterial meningitis in Canada, with an incidence similar to that in the United States.[70] In other parts of Europe, including the United Kingdom prior to 1980,[71,72] meningococcal meningitis was reported to be more common than Hib meningitis.

Population-based incidence rates for most developing countries are not currently available. However, in areas as geographically diverse as Africa, Oceania, and South America, *H. influenzae* appears to rank first as a cause of bacterial meningitis in some studies of hospitalized patients and second or third behind meningococcal and pneumococcal disease in others.[73–77] Only a few recent studies provide information on the incidence of Hib in young children.[75,77] Reported rates of Hib meningitis in children from The Gambia (60/100,000/year for children <5 years of age) are comparable to those seen in the United States during the prevaccine era. This suggests that invasive Hib disease may become an important child health problem in non-Western countries in the future. In addition, pneumonia caused by *H. influenzae* has been shown to be a significant cause of childhood mortality in Papua New Guinea[77] and The Gambia.[75] Therefore, the next decade may bring increased debate on the use of Hib conjugate vaccines in non-Western countries, with a concurrent increase in studies to document incidence and costs of Hib illness in these countries.[78]

Excessive rates of invasive Hib disease (200 to 1100 cases per 100,000 children < 5 years of age per year) have been reported for selective populations in developed countries, including aboriginal children in central Australia,[64,79,80] Native Alaskans (Indians and Eskimos), and Apache, Yakima, Athabascan, Navajo, and Canadian Indians.[81–84] While these populations reside in developed countries, it should be noted that the living conditions under which these populations reside may more closely approximate those found in developing regions of the world.

5.1.2b. Incidence of Endemic Disease After Universal Immunization. With the licensure and widespread use of Hib conjugate vaccines in infancy, dramatic decreases in Hib disease incidence have occurred. Table 2 summarizes these data for the United States as a whole (National Bacterial Meningitis Reporting System), for six specific US populations, and for several other populations. In each of these populations, Hib incidence decreased by 60–90% between the late 1980s and early 1990s, shortly after the introduction of universal infant immunization. By 1995, there has been greater than a 95% decrease in disease incidence. In all populations, the greatest fall in disease incidence has been in children less than 2 years of age.

5.2. Outbreak Potential

Although the contagious potential of invasive Hib disease has been considered to be limited, certain circumstances in unimmunized populations can lead to outbreaks or direct secondary transmission of disease.[85,86] Secondary disease is usually defined as illness occurring within 60 days following contact with another individual who has Hib disease (family or day-care contact). Secondary cases have never accounted for more than a small proportion of all Hib cases (<5%). As discussed in Section 5.9, the highest risk of secondary Hib disease is in infants, a group currently protected through universal infant immunization. Outbreaks have been described in hospitals, primarily associated with nonencapsulated forms of *H. influenzae* (see Section 5.9).[87,88]

5.3. Age

5.3.1. Prior to Vaccination. In unvaccinated populations, the most important epidemiological feature of invasive Hib disease is its age-related incidence, a feature that has been appreciated for more than half a century.[13] Risk is highest between the ages of 6 and 12 months (see Table 3).[1,57,83] In unvaccinated populations, approximately 85% of all invasive *H. influenzae* disease occurs in children under 5 years of age, and in this age group it is almost exclusively type b disease. Invasive disease is relatively uncommon in infants less than 6 months of age (<15% of cases), presumably because of less exposure, transplacental acquisition of maternal antibodies, and protection conferred by breast-feeding. Although not as well studied, approximately 15% of invasive *H. influenzae* disease occurs in persons 5 years of age or more, most of whom are older adults, often with underlying disease that has increased susceptibility. A substantial proportion of the invasive disease in older individuals is due to non-type b strains.

Table 3 shows the cumulative proportion of disease

Table 2. Rates of *Haemophilus influenzae* type b after Initiation of Universal Infant Immunization in Selected Populations

		Annual incidence of *H. influenzae*[a]		
Geographic area	Study period	Meningitis	All invasive disease	Ref.
Los Angeles Co., CA	1991	—	12.9	93
N CA Kaiser, CA	1991	—	5.7	22
Connecticut	1991	3	4	349
Greater Pittsburgh, PA	1991	2	3	349
Minnesota	1991	—	11 (7–15)	54
Dallas, TX	1991	—	9 (5–14)	23
United States[b]	1991	—	11	350
England and Wales	1991–1994	0.6	—	166
The Netherlands		0.6	—	166
Germany		1.9	—	305
Helsinki, Finland	1990–1991	2.9[a]	NA[c]	165

[a]Rate per 100,000 children per year.
[b]National Bacterial Meningitis Survey.
[c]NA, not available.

Table 3. Age-Specific Incidence of Invasive *H. influenzae* Disease, US Population-Based Studies, 1976–1984

Age (months)	Incidence[a] Meningitis only Median	Range	All invasive disease Median	Range	Cumulative percent of disease[b]
0–5	101	59–141	148	98–197	10–15
6–11	179	143–279	275	218–452	37–43
12–17	146	88–184	223	123–248	60–61
18–23	62	20–64	92	57–107	64–68
24–35	31	18–39	50	37–70	75–78
36–47	17	5–26	31	7–39	80–83
48–59	4	2–16	11	7–41	84–86
>60[b]	0.2	0.1–0.2	1.3	1.2–2.4	100

[a]Cases per 100,000 population/year. Range of point estimates from five studies, including Alaska 1980–1982 (excluding Eskimos, Indians), Atlanta 1983–1984, Fresno County 1976–1978, Dallas 1982–1984, and Minnesota 1982–1984.
[b]Cumulative percent and incidence data for ages ≥60 months are based on studies from Alaska, Atlanta, and Fresno County, where active surveillance for all age groups was conducted.

by age during the first 5 years of life. The age of onset information for a population is important when considering strategies for prevention. For example, the decision to focus US immunization strategies on infants was based on epidemiological data suggesting that at least 85% of all childhood Hib disease could be prevented by vaccinating children by 6 months of age.[(89)]

Each type of invasive disease has a characteristic age occurrence, but as a group the clinical syndromes other than meningitis and cellulitis tend to occur at older ages.[(53,83)] In most unvaccinated US populations, the peak incidence of meningitis occurred in children 6 to 12 months of age and declined markedly after 2 years of age (Table 3).[(59,60,90)] In populations with especially high disease incidence, such as Native Americans, the age-specific incidence is shifted markedly toward younger children[(81–83,91)] and an even younger age spectrum is observed in The Gambia. The social structure of Native American groups (usually with large families living in small dwellings under confined conditions for much of the year) suggests that early or intense exposure to Hib at home or in the community may explain the early age of disease onset and the development of immunity at an earlier age.

The age-specific incidence may be shifted toward older preschool children in populations with a low incidence of Hib disease.[(66,67)] In Finland prior to the late 1980s, the peak incidence of Hib meningitis was reported in children at about 12 months of age,[(67)] and approximately 60% of disease occurred in children older than 18 months of age.[(92)] In contrast, in the United States the figure was only about 30%. Such a shift suggests less intense exposure to Hib in Finland compared to other populations, although other factors cannot be ruled out.

5.3.2. After Vaccination. In all such populations, the greatest fall in disease incidence has been in children less than 2 years of age. As expected, the proportion of cases of Hib meningitis has decreased most dramatically.

5.4. Geographic Distribution

Whether there are true international differences in the incidence of invasive Hib disease is not known with certainty because, outside of North America and Europe, there have been few population-based studies based on active surveillance (see Section 5.1). In Western countries, there is no strong evidence for significant geographic variability. The reported incidence of Hib disease shows some variability in different US populations, but no obvious geographic clustering is evident from these studies. Some of the variability in incidence can be explained by differences in methods of case finding. However, one prospective, laboratory-based incidence study that used similar methodology in two different geographic areas (Dallas County and Minnesota) during the same time period (1982–1984) found substantially different incidences of invasive Hib disease in children under 5 years of age (109 vs. 67 cases per 100,000).[(57)] Differences in the prevalence of risk factors may explain this discrepancy. In some populations, antibiotics are given presumptively before blood or CSF cultures are obtained, and such practices will grossly underestimate disease incidence. Alternatively, there may be true differences in attack rates by geographic area due to differing environmental or host susceptibility factors, or as yet undefined differences in the invasive potential of different strains of Hib.

5.5. Temporal Distribution

Limited data from both the United States and Scandinavian countries suggest that Hib incidence may have increased toward the end of the prevaccine era.[(66)] It is not clear whether this increase was a true increase in disease incidence or merely reflected increased vigilance in case finding.

As discussed in Section 5.1.2b, the incidence of Hib disease decreased dramatically in many developed coun-

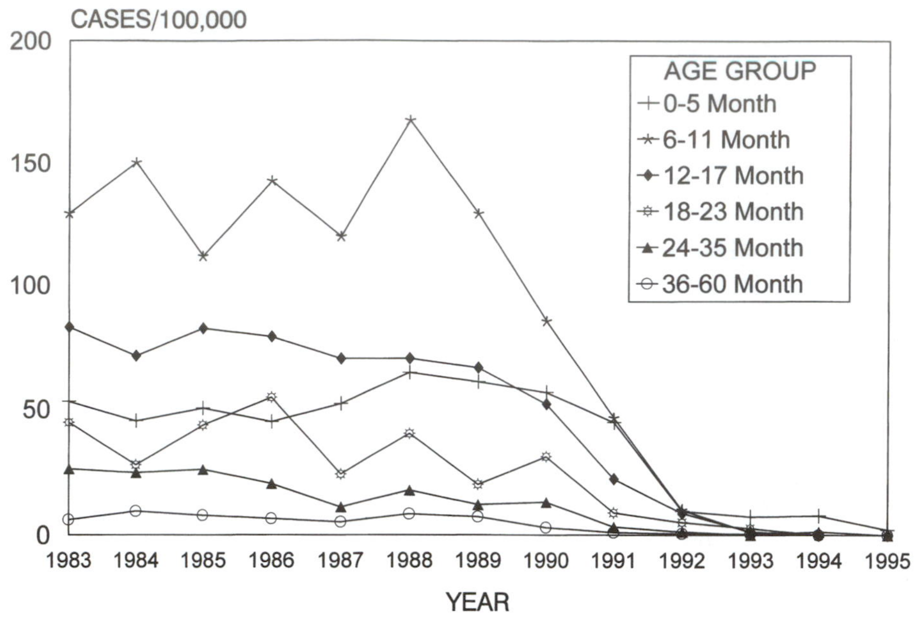

Figure 1. Age-specific incidence rates for *Haemophilus influenzae* type b in Los Angeles County, California, 1983 through 1995. *Haemophilus influenzae* type b polysaccharide vaccine (PRP) was introduced in 1985. PRP-D (*H. influenzae* type b polysaccaride–diphtheria toxoid conjugate) vaccine was licensed for children ≥ 18 months in 1988. Two other Hib conjugate vaccines (HbOC; *H. influenzae* type b polysaccharide CRM_{197} mutant diphtheria toxoid conjugate vaccine and PRP-OMP; *H. influenzae* type b polysaccaride outermembrane protein of group B meningococcus conjugate vaccine) were licensed for children ≥ 15 months of age in 1989 and 1990, respectively. The HbOC and PRP-OMP vaccines were licensed for use in infants in 1991.

tries in the early 1990s, shortly after the introduction of universal infant immunization. Figure 1 shows temporal incidence trends in Los Angeles County.(93) Hib incidence was fairly stable for all age groups until the late 1980s, despite the licensure of PRP and PRP-D vaccines and their use in older children. In 1990, Hib incidence began to decrease in the 0- to 5-month and 6- to 11-month old infants. The decline continued through 1995. Similar trends have been reported for other populations.(22–24)

5.6. Sex

Although most studies show approximately equal rates of disease in males and females, several population-based studies(1,62) and national surveillance data from passively reported cases of meningitis(27) found attack rates to be 1.2- to 1.5-fold higher in boys than in girls.

5.7. Race/Ethnicity

Population-based active surveillance studies have identified African Americans as having increased risk for invasive Hib disease. The incidence of Hib meningitis has consistently been shown to be two to four times higher for black as compared to white children less than 5 years of age in unimmunized US populations.(59,61,94) Also, the incidence of all invasive Hib disease was 1.6- to 4-fold higher in blacks compared with whites.(1,95) An increased incidence of invasive Hib disease has also been observed in Hispanics(95) and Native Americans(81–83,96) (see Section 5.1). Two studies (in Dallas and Los Angeles), however, found no difference in the incidence of Hib disease between white and Hispanic children.(55,57)

Some investigators have suggested that these racial and ethnic differences may be due to genetically determined differences in host susceptibility(97) (see Section 5.10); however, it is equally likely that these differences are explained by confounding socioeconomic variables associated with both race/ethnicity and Hib exposure (see Section 5.8). Factors that increase exposure to Hib carriers (e.g.., household crowding, number of siblings, and day care) are exceedingly difficult to separate from host susceptibility and an increased biological predisposition to Hib disease.

5.8. Socioeconomic Factors

The interplay of many factors influencing exposure to the organism and/or disease susceptibility appears to determine the risk of invasive Hib disease.[55,98] Socioeconomic status may be a marker for increased exposure to Hib, reflecting differences in household size,[99,100] crowding,[55] age, access to antibiotics, or population density. Other surrogate socioeconomic factors, such as low family income[59,60,62,94,101] and low parental education level,[59,100] are also associated with increased risk of disease.[98]

Several studies have analyzed exposure-related risk factors, including socioeconomic factors, using multivariate analysis to assess the independent effects of each potential risk factor. In one case–control study in Atlanta,[1] household crowding (i.e., ≥ 1 person per room) was significantly associated with Hib after controlling for the effects of race, family income, day-care attendance, and breast-feeding. In this study, increased risk was associated with low family income and low maternal education level, although these were not found to be independent risk factors. In a second study from Colorado,[56] the risk of Hib disease was increased in households with at least one member of elementary school age, suggesting that such children may be sources of Hib exposure for younger siblings.

5.9. Occurrence in Different Settings

5.9.1. Secondary Illness in Households In the United States, all studies of secondary Hib disease predate the period of universal immunization of infants. Six such studies have estimated the risk of secondary disease in household contacts in the month (30 days) following onset of disease in an index case.[102–105] Overall, the attack rate for contacts is 0.3%, representing a risk about 600-fold higher than the age-adjusted risk in the general population, but still low compared to other infectious diseases.[106] Attack rates varied significantly by age of the contacts; the attack rate was more than 6% in contacts less than 1 year old, 3.3% in children less than 2 years old, 1.6% in children 24–47 months old, 0.06% in children 4–5 years old, and 0% in children 6 years or older.

Among household contacts, 64% of secondary cases occur within the first week of disease onset in the index patient,[16] and disease risk appears to be related to the prevalence of Hib pharyngeal carriage among household contacts of a case.[107–109] Several studies have documented that Hib colonization can persist for at least 6 months in family members, with up to 40% of culture-negative siblings and mothers of index children subsequently becoming colonized. This may explain the occasional occurrence of late secondary cases.[107,109]

5.9.2. Day-Care Settings

5.9.2a. Primary Disease. Several population-based studies evaluated whether day-care attendance is associated with increased risk of primary (endemic) invasive Hib disease.[1,55,110] Most found that children attending day care were at significantly higher risk for invasive Hib disease than children not in day care. One study estimated that up to 50% of all invasive Hib disease may be attributable to day-care attendance.[1]

While day-care attendance appears to increase risk for Hib disease in infants and young children,[56,110,111] at least three studies have found no day-care-associated risk in children 3 years of age and older.[55,112] Several factors may explain the interstudy differences in day-care results. First, the overall proportion of children in day care varies between populations and may be confounded by differences in day-care utilization between ethnic and socioeconomic groups.[110,111,113,114] Another important factor may be the marked variability in the types of day care available in different populations.[114] Some studies suggest that day-care homes, as opposed to more formal day-care centers, do not increase risk for Hib disease.[55–57,115] A case–control study conducted in Atlanta during 1983–1984 showed that day-care attendance was an independent risk factor after controlling for other known risk factors.[115] The risk was highest in children under 1 year of age and declined with increasing age. In contrast to the Atlanta study, the relative risk was significantly increased only for children ≥ 12 months of age (odds ratio = 3.7, 95% confidence interval 1.6–8.5) in another case–control study.[56] Risk increased with the size of the day-care facility, providing the first clear evidence that specific characteristics of the day-care setting may be associated with risk of Hib disease.

5.9.2b. Risk of Secondary Disease in Day-Care Settings. With universal infant immunization, most US children are now protected against Hib disease prior to day-care enrollment. Five earlier studies estimated the risk for unimmunized day-care classroom contacts during the 30- to 60-day period following onset of disease in the index case.[104,107,113,114,116] Three studies demonstrated a substantial risk, 1.7–3.2%, for contacts younger than 24 months of age,[104,107,113] a risk comparable to that of household contacts of a similar age. However, two other studies failed to demonstrate any increased risk for secondary disease in day-care contacts,[114,116] and even in the studies showing an elevated relative risk, the secondary attack rates were all less than 1%. Because of these divergent results, recommendations for use of rifampin chemoprophylaxis have been vigorously debated (see Section 6). Rates of colonization in day-care contacts appear to be similar to rates seen within households.[107]

5.9.3. Risk of Secondary Disease in Other Institutional Settings. Secondary Hib disease transmission in chronic-care institutions for children has been reported.[117,118] One outbreak affected 5 to 30 young children with chronic illness within a 6-month period, while another affected 4 of 11 young children within 16 days.[119] Nosocomial transmission of invasive Hib disease among elderly adults in a nursing home setting has also been reported,[120] but nosocomial infections appear to be more commonly caused by nonencapsulated *H. influenzae* and serotypes other than type b.[87,118] Only one instance of secondary transmission in children in an acute-care hospital has been reported.[121] However, an outbreak in South Africa of multiply-resistant Hib suggests that there is potential for nosocomial Hib disease transmission when large numbers of susceptible children are kept in close quarters and resistant strains are prevalent.[122]

5.10. Other Factors

5.10.1. Seasonality. A characteristic bimodal seasonal pattern has been observed in several studies, with one peak between September and December, a decrease in cases in January and February, and a second peak between March and May.[27,83] This has been shown in the United States generally and also in Alaska. In contrast, the peak incidence of both pneumococcal and meningococcal meningitis is between January and March.[27] The reason for these differences is not known.

5.10.2. Genetic Factors. Although genetic factors almost certainly play a role in susceptibility to invasive bacterial disease,[123] none of the genetic markers that have been suggested appear to be associated with an unequivocally increased risk for Hib disease.[95,124–126] The suggested genetic associations have included genotypes of the MNS blood system[125–127]; the Aw28, Bw12, Bw14, and Bw17 alleles at the HLA-A and B loci[126]; absence of the immunoglobulin light chain Km(1) allotype in blacks[97]; presence of the immunoglobulin heavy chain G2m(n) allotype[128]; and absence of the G2m(n) allotype.[124] Last, Petersen *et al.*[129] reported an association between a variant of the enzyme uridine monophosphate kinase (UMPK-3) and Hib disease in Alaskan Eskimos.

The reports of genetic marker associations with invasive Hib disease and with response to Hib vaccines support the view that genetic factors may contribute to disease susceptibility. However, studies of genetic susceptibility to infectious diseases are notoriously difficult to conduct and interpret. The choice of control group (controlling for potential confounding variables and correcting for multiple comparisons), relationship between immune response and disease susceptibility, and choice of appropriate genetic markers all are critical.

5.10.3. Occupation. There are no data to suggest any relationship of occupation, including adults who work in hospital or day-care settings, and risk of Hib disease in the small number of adults reported with invasive Hib-disease.

5.10.4. Breast-feeding. Based on the results of three case-control studies, breast-feeding appears to be protective against invasive Hib disease in infants under 6 months of age.[56,130–132] Although the mechanism for protection is not known, it may be due to immune factors or nutritional factors in human milk. These findings are biologically plausible, based on studies demonstrating that human milk contains low levels of secretory antibody to the Hib polysaccharide capsule, which persist for 1 to 6 months after the onset of lactation.[133] Two recent studies of the effect of breast-feeding on infant nasopharyngeal bacterial colonization have produced conflicting results. A study by Kaleida *et al.*[134] found no significant differences in rates of pharyngeal colonization between breast-fed and bottle-fed infants at 1 and 2 months of age. In contrast, Harabuchi *et al.*[135] concluded that levels of secretory IgA in breast milk were inversely related to rates of nasopharyngeal colonization of infants with nontypeable *H. influenzae*.

5.10.5. Underlying Disease. Several hematologic and immunologic disorders are known to be associated with increased risk for Hib disease. These include sickle-cell anemia,[136,137] asplenia or splenectomy,[138] antibody deficiency syndromes,[139,140] complement deficiencies,[141] and malignancies, especially Hodgkin's disease during chemotherapy.[142–144] The precise mechanisms placing such immunocompromised patients at risk have yet to be determined. Reduced reticuloendothelial clearance of bacteria in blood by macrophages in the spleen and liver may be involved. Clearly, complement and antibody are needed to clear bacteremia and to maintain bactericidal activity in blood.

5.10.6. Role of Antecedent Viral Respiratory Infection. Viruses have been implicated in the pathogenesis of bacterial infections for many years, and respiratory viruses have been shown to increase susceptibility to Hib meningitis in experimental animal models.[145,146] A hypothesis has been advanced that antecedent or concurrent viral respiratory infection may alter mucosal immunity or bacterial flora, thereby increasing host susceptibility to invasive Hib disease. Takela *et al.*[147] reported a significant increase in the numbers of Hib cases and family members reporting respiratory symptoms in the month prior to Hib onset compared to controls. Cases from case clusters were most likely to have a clinically diagnostic viral titer [OR = 7.1(1.6;33) compared to isolated cases]. The difficulties and obstacles of conducting prospective studies with appropriate controls continue to hamper the conclusive determination of whether antecedent viral respiratory illness predisposes to invasive Hib disease.

5.11. Summary of Risk Factors for Invasive Hib Disease

The development of invasive Hib disease in a given individual is a consequence of the complex interaction of a variety of factors, including events leading to exposure and characteristics of the organism, the environment, and the host, all acting together in a multifactorial interrelationship.[58] In this discussion, we have enumerated some of those factors. The factors can be divided into those affecting likelihood of exposure to the Hib organism ("exposure factors") and those affecting the host's susceptibility to Hib disease, whether inherently through regulation of the host immune response or because they contribute to a change in the host's ability to defend against the disease ("susceptibility factors"). Some exposure factors such as household crowding and day-care attendance are fairly direct measures of increased exposure to Hib bacteria, while others, such as low family income and low parental education levels, are only indirect measures for increased exposure. Other risk factors cannot be so easily categorized, such as the association of African-American, Alaskan Eskimo, or Native American race with increased risk for Hib disease. Although abundant evidence suggests that more intense and early exposure to Hib may be the primary factors affecting risk in these populations, other lines of evidence suggest that genetic factors may also affect the antibody response to Hib or other susceptibility factors. Factors not reviewed because of a lack of definitive data include antimicrobial use, altered nasopharyngeal flora, the effects of climate, temperature, and humidity, which may affect survival of the bacteria, and the relative efficiency with which Hib carriers versus persons with clinical Hib disease can transmit the organism.

6. Mechanism and Routes of Transmission

Human beings are the only natural hosts for *H. influenzae*, and the vast majority of infections involve asymptomatic colonization of the upper respiratory tract. Although *H. influenzae* are transmitted person-to-person via respiratory droplets or by direct contact with respiratory secretions, the mechanisms and patterns of transmission can be complex. *H. influenzae* are considered part of the normal bacterial flora of the upper airway. Thus, Hib may pass from a patient with disease through many people who remain asymptomatic carriers before the organism again causes illness in a susceptible host. Consequently, the incubation period cannot be accurately assessed. Although some data indicate that transmission is slow, there is also impressive evidence that Hib may be quite contagious for unvaccinated young children exposed in situations of close contact, such as in household or day-care settings.

The role of environmental surfaces and fomites in transmission is unknown. Although Hib is generally regarded as a fastidious organism, Murphy *et al.*[148] demonstrated that Hib in nasal secretions could survive for up to 18 hr on tissue paper, wax paper, and dry gauze. However, they were unable to recover Hib from swab cultures of the cribs and toys of carrier children in day-care settings. This single study raises the possibility that fomites and environmental surfaces could contribute to transmission in circumstances such as the mouthing of toys by young children playing together. It appears unlikely, however, that this is an important mode of transmission.

To prevent the potential for nosocomial transmission of Hib, respiratory isolation of hospitalized patients with invasive Hib disease for 24 hr after initiating antimicrobial therapy is recommended, based on the observation that carriage of the organism is eliminated or suppressed within that period.[149] However, studies show that children with invasive Hib disease can remain Hib colonized for months following the discontinuation of their antimicrobial therapy.[12,150,151] These data suggest that recovery of the Hib organism from the pharynx is suppressed after 24 hr of effective therapy, and the current standard of respiratory isolation for the initial 24 hr of hospitalization is appropriate.

Despite a low overall prevalence of pharyngeal carriage (1–5%), in unvaccinated populations most young children become colonized during the first 2 to 5 years of life.[100,152–154] In some settings the point prevalence of pharyngeal carriage may be higher. Stephenson *et al.*[155] reported a 15% prevalence of Hib colonization among healthy children attending day care. The cumulative rate of pharyngeal acquisition of encapsulated type b strains is such that by 5 years of age most children in unimmunized populations will have acquired Hib and thereby develop specific immunity.[12,155–157] Colonization rates are highest in closed populations exposed to a case, such as household or day-care center classroom contacts of a patient with disease.[105,107,158,159] Type b strains may persist in the nasopharynx for months[12,150,151] and are not eliminated by antimicrobials that do not penetrate into respiratory secretions.[15,160] Culture of throat swabs onto antiserum agar appears to be the most sensitive method for detecting Hib carriage.[161]

With the advent of universal infant immunizations, rates of asymptomatic carriage have decreased. Several studies have shown that rates of Hib carriage are decreased among vaccinated children[162,163] and among household and day-care contacts of vaccinated children.[145,164] In addition, two lines of indirect evidence also support the hypothesis that Hib carriage is decreased generally in populations with high rates of vaccination. The first is the decreased rates of Hib disease seen in infants that occurred in populations even prior to the widespread use of Hib conjugate vaccines in this age group.[21,165,166] Second, rates of Hib disease have decreased both in vaccinated and unvaccinated infants. For example, Hib rates for infants under 2 months of age have been noted to have decreased in several populations after infant immunization beginning at age 2 months was initiated.[93,166]

7. Pathogenesis

Hib is usually transmitted asymptomatically from person to person and there may be many transmission cycles before it causes disease in a susceptible person. The incubation period is unknown. Invasion occurs when there is dissemination of bacteria from the mucosa of the upper respiratory tract to the bloodstream and then elsewhere in the body.[167] Studies in several animal models have shown that the initial stage of invasive disease involves attachment of the organism to the respiratory epithelium, penetration through the mucosa, invasion of the lymphatics, and then to the bloodstream.[167–169] Inflammation of the upper respiratory tissues is not apparent, and the precise mode of entrance of organisms into the vascular space is not well understood. Bacteremia is initially at a low level, but in a susceptible host this increases quantitatively.[168–170] When the bacterial concentration in the blood exceeds 10^4–10^5 organisms/ml, seeding of other body sites frequently occurs, especially to the central nervous system (CNS). In the CNS, invasion appears to occur via the choroid plexus[167]; organisms then circulate through the CSF and infect the arachnoid villi and the leptomeningeal membranes. The resulting increased bacterial density, inflammation, edema, cranial nerve damage, and overall increased CSF pressure cause the morbidity and mortality associated with meningitis. Generally, the magnitude of the bacteremia and the degree of proliferation of organisms in the CNS correlate with the severity of the clinical illness.[171–174] Although meningitis is the most severe form of invasive Hib disease, bacteremic seeding of other body sites may also occur, including to joints, pleural, or pericardial spaces.[167] However, with pneumonia, cellulitis, and epiglottitis, the exact pathogenesis is less well understood, even though these invasive infections are associated with bacteremia. Presumably, pneumonia occurs following the aspiration of a critical number of virulent organisms, epiglottitis involves the focal infection of the epiglottis, and cellulitis occurs by secondary seeding via the bloodstream of deep subcutaneous tissues. With all forms of invasive Hib disease there is an invasion of the bloodstream, either as a primary or as a secondary event.

As discussed elsewhere (Section 8), mucosal infections and infections caused by nontypeable strains have a different pathogenesis. This involves direct extension of organisms through nasal ostia to the sinuses, up the eustachian tubes to cause otitis media and down the bronchi to cause bronchitis and pneumonia. Bacteremia is rarely involved and such infections are generally not life-threatening. Further, such infections appear to be enhanced by antecedent viral infection, eustachian tube malfunction, foreign bodies, or mucosal damage from smoking or other irritants.

7.1. Immunity

The single-most important immunologic factor influencing disease occurrence is the widespread use of Hib conjugate vaccines (see Section 9). The induction of type b anticapsular antibodies has radically changed the patterns of disease, leading to a dramatic decrease in both the number of cases as well as the numbers of asymptomatic carriers.[162,175] Therefore, there is an interplay of vaccine-induced immunity and acquisition of natural immunity. The mechanisms that determine which individuals will be asymptomatically colonized (the vast majority of people in an unimmunized population) and those who will develop invasive disease are related to a multitude of poorly understood factors. Resistance to invasive disease depends on the successful integration of a wide variety of host defenses, including: (1) mucosal factors that prevent attachment or penetration of organisms through the respiratory epithelium; (2) activation of complement-mediated opsonization, killing, and other mediators of inflammation (including the alternative and classical complement pathways); (3) mucosal and humoral antibody; (4) phagocytosis and killing by macrophages and polymorphonuclear cells; and (5) the poorly understood role of cell-mediated immunity.

As discussed above, the severity of disease appears to be related in part to the magnitude of the bacteremia, which, in turn, is determined by several factors that influence bacterial proliferation and bacterial clearance. Although antibody is not the sole defense against bacteremia, it has been the immunologic basis for the development of vaccines that are designed to induce bactericidal, opsonophagocytic, and ultimately protective antibodies. Although antibodies to several surface antigens of Hib probably play a role in conferring protective immunity,[176–178] antibody to the type b capsular polysaccharide appears to be the most important.[179] By 5 years of age most children in unimmunized populations naturally acquire anticapsular antibody. There is considerable evidence that anticapsular antibody protects humans from invasive disease, in that it: (1) activates complement,[180–184] (2) is opsonophagocytic,[185,186] (3) is bactericidal,[186–189] and (4) protects animals from lethal Hib challenge.[190–192] But the most compelling evidence for the protective efficacy of anticapsular antibody is the impressive protective immunity induced by PRP conjugate vaccines.[193]

Different exposures to the organism or to vaccines will induce variable immune responses, and responses to the capsule are markedly influenced by the age of the individual. In children under 2 years of age with invasive Hib disease (i.e., bacteremia) or in those who have been given the plain polysaccharide vaccine, there is rarely an immune response. In contrast, older children and adults will respond with anticapsular antibody following infection or immunization.[194–196] There is also some evidence that anticapsular antibody develops after exposure to other bacteria that have immunologically cross-reacting capsular antigens.[40,160] Therefore, the level of antibody is influenced by the type of exposure, duration of exposure, rate of antigen clearance, and most importantly by the age of the individual. Estimates of the minimum serum concentration of PRP antibody that provides protection range from 0.05 to 0.15 μg/ml, with levels of 1 μg/ml or greater required for long-term protection.[197-199] Unfortunately, these estimates are crude and do not take into account the different functional properties of different immunoglobulins and the contribution of antibodies other than capsular antibody. Several studies show that IgG, IgM, and IgA antibodies to PRP are induced both by disease and by vaccination.[200–203]; however, the idiotype specificity, proportion, and subclass of IgG antibodies vary by age and type of exposure.[204–210]

IgG antibody has been shown to be bactericidal, opsonic in the presence of complement, and protective for animals.[199] IgM is equally as protective; however, it is more bactericidal than IgG in the presence of complement, but it opsonizes organisms in the presence of polymorphonuclear leukocytes poorly. In contrast, IgA antibody is not bactericidal, opsonic, or protective in animals.[199] Some have hypothesized that IgA-specific antibody blocks the activity of other more functional antibodies and that this may depress immunity.[211–213]

The immature antibody response to the plain polysaccharide vaccine appears to result from limited or absent T-helper-cell activation. These cells are normally involved in the maturation, differentiation, and proliferation of specific B-cell populations. T-helper cells also retain immunologic memory, essential to elicit a booster response. Although most of our understanding of the interaction between B cells, T cells, and macrophages derives from extensive research with mice,[205,214,215] it appears that based on the mode of recognition of the antigen, there are T-dependent (thymus-dependent) or T-independent classes of immunogens. Most protein antigens, considered to be T-dependent antigens, induce activation of T-helper cells, which regulate antibody synthesis. Such antigens are recognized and processed by macrophages, T cells, and B cells. The T cells stimulate reactive B-cell subpopulations to proliferate and differentiate specific antibodies and the T cells also retain memory for subsequent booster responses. In contrast, T-independent antigens stimulate little or no T-helper-cell activity. The plain polysaccharide vaccines elicit predominantly T-independent responses, with little or no antibody responses observed in young children, and in older children the antibody produced is predominantly IgM. Furthermore, there is no booster or anamnestic response with repeat exposures. Activation of T cells is necessary: (1) to regulate the magnitude of the immune response, especially in young infants; (2) to regulate the switch in immunoglobulin classes (IgM to IgG); (3) to enhance the functional activity of antibody; and (4) for booster responses.[179]

To create a Hib vaccine that is both immunogenic and protective in young infants, the capsular polysaccharide (PRP) is converted from a T-independent to a T-dependent immunogen, employing hapten-carrier principles first described by Landsteiner[216] early in this century. To achieve this, the polysaccharide is covalently linked to a T-dependent immunogen (a carrier) to form a conjugate vaccine. As a group, Hib conjugate vaccines demonstrate markedly enhanced immunogenicity, as described in Section 9.3.3. Some studies suggest that immune responses are also regulated by genetic factors.[97,124,128,217,218] However, it is not clear whether the degree of variability seen among different populations and among different subjects with different genetic markers (i.e., HLA or immunoglobulin allotypes; see Sections 5.10.2 and 9.3.3) are clinically relevant. No single genetic relationship has been described that appears to regulate susceptibility or the basic immune response to polysaccharide antigens.

The role of mucosal immunity in killing Hib or inhibiting adhesion or penetration of the mucosa is poorly understood, although studies have been reported of secretory IgA antibody to the type capsule.[37,219–221] More importantly, with the more robust immune response of Hib conjugate vaccines, significant amounts of IgG antibodies enter mucosal secretions. This may be the mechanism by which the vaccine interrupts acquisition and transmission. Relatively little is known about direct cell-mediated killing of Hib or other aspects of cellular immunity.[222]

8. Patterns of Host Response

8.1. Clinical Manifestations

Based on the pathogenesis of disease, there are two major categories of *H. influenzae* disease (Table 4). Invasive disease is characterized by the dissemination of bacteria, almost always Hib, from the pharynx to the bloodstream and subsequently to other body sites. Bacteremia is a common characteristic of all invasive forms of Hib disease and it may be the only manifestation of disease in an acutely ill child with high fever and no other recognized focus of infection.

Invasive Hib disease should be distinguished from mucosal infections (Table 4). The latter occurs when *H. influenzae* organisms extend from colonized respiratory passages to contiguous body sites. Although mucosal infections occur frequently, they do not result in bacteremia and therefore are rarely life-threatening. The most common infections of this type include otitis media, sinusitis, conjunctivitis, and bronchitis. The microbiological hallmarks of mucosal infections are: (1) they are produced by the same bacteria that normally colonize the pharynx; (2) they are almost always unencapsulated strains of *H. infleunzaes* (nontypeable)[36]; and (3) extension of these organisms into normally sterile body sites is enhanced by compromise in normal defense mechanisms, such as eustachian tube reflux, foreign bodies, antecedent viral infection, or damage to the bronchopulmonary epithelium due to smoking or selected immune deficiencies.

The clinical separation of invasive and mucosal disease is not absolute, inasmuch as type b strains may cause otitis media or sinusitis.[223] Likewise, other serotypes (nontypeable strains and serotypes other than type b) may occasionally cause bacteremia and meningitis in unimmunized populations, and interestingly they are the predominant cause of invasive *H. influenzae* disease in neonates.[224,225] Many older children experiencing invasive *H. influenzae* non-type b infections have underlying pedisposing medical conditions.[90] In addition, reports from Nigeria, [226] Papua New Guinea,[74,227] and The Gambia[228,229] suggest a higher-than-expected frequency of non-type b pneumonia and meningitis in young children in less-developed countries.[76] Whether these differences relate to poor nutrition or concurrent infections that place such children at risk for invasive disease or whether other unknown factors are involved requires further study. Nonetheless, the clinical categories of disease described above are useful diagnostically and therapeutically and have had important implications regarding strategies for disease prevention.

Hib can produce disease in almost any organ of the body, and the manifestations of invasive infection vary depending on the site involved. The major clinical features of Hib meningitis and the other forms of invasive Hib disease have been thoroughly reviewed elsewhere,[230,231] but are briefly outlined below.

8.1.1. Meningitis. The most commonly recognized and most severe clinical manifestation of invasive Hib disease is meningitis, representing 54–67% of all invasive disease in children in unimmunized populations.[7,53,67] In such populations, most patients with Hib meningitis are less than 3 years of age; however, the disease may occur at any age. The clinical presentation of Hib meningitis is similar to that due to other bacteria. Fever, obtundation, and stiff neck are the hallmarks of illness, although more subtle symptoms may predominate in infancy or early in illness. A fulminating course with rapid neurological deterioration, electrolyte disturbance, and disseminated intravascular coagulation may occur.[52]

Table 4. Spectrum of *H. influenzae* Disease

Invasive disease (predominantly due to type b strains)		
Meningitis	Pneumonia	Empyema
Bacteremia	Arthritis	Osteomyelitis
Epiglottitis	Pericarditis	Cellulitis
	Abscesses	
Mucosal disease (predominantly due to nontypable strains)		
Otitis media	Bronchitis	
Sinusitis	Urinary tract infection	
Conjunctivitis		

8.1.2. Epiglottitis. In both children and adults, Hib is the most common cause of epiglottitis.[232] The disease is characterized by rapid progression of sore throat, fever, toxicity, dysphagia with drooling, and upper airway obstruction. On physical examination, the epiglottis is greatly swollen and cherry red. Rapid diagnosis and prompt institution of therapy are necessary to prevent fatalities. Success of treatment depends on the establishment of an adequate airway, often by nasotracheal intubation.

8.1.3. Pneumonia. Hib is a common cause of the bacteremic form of *H. influenzae* pneumonia in unimmunized persons. The clinical manifestations are indistinguishable from those of other causes of pneumonia; with a lobar or segmental presentation, there may be complications of pleural effusion, empyema, or pericarditis. Less commonly, patients may present with diffuse bronchopneumonia or interstitial disease. Nontypeable *H. influenzae* is a frequent cause of bronchitis and pneumonia in adults and in some children in developing countries.

8.1.4. Cellulitis. Hib cellulitis is associated with high fever and sepsis and usually involves the face, head, or neck (three fourths of all cases). It is characterized by a rapidly developing skin lesion with indistinct margins, induration, tenderness, and purplish discoloration. The most frequently involved sites are the cheeks and periorbital areas, and this manifestation almost invariably occurs only in children under 1 year of age. Hib cellulitis is a bacteremic disease, and diagnosis depends on isolation of the organism from blood or the local lesion.

8.1.5. Septic Arthritis. In unimmunized populations, Hib is the second-most common cause of septic arthritis in children. In general, the large joints, such as hip or knee, are involved and a contiguous osteomyelitis may be present.[233] The clinical manifestations are not different from other bacterial etiologies that cause septic arthritis in children.

8.1.6. Other Infections. Other clinical manifestations of bacteremic invasive Hib disease include osteomyelitis, pericarditis, endocarditis, epididymitis, endophthalmitis, and peritonitis.

8.1.7. Diseases Caused by Other *H. influenzae* Types and Other *Haemophilus* Species. Nontypeable *H. influenzae* strains rarely cause invasive disease in individuals without underlying medical conditions such as prematurity, malignancy, CSF shunts, congenital heart disease, lymphoproliferative disorders, or immunoglobulin deficiencies.[119,142,234–236] However, nonencapsulated and nontype b strains are common causes of a variety of mucosal infections, including otitis media, sinusitis, conjunctivitis, and bronchitis. *H. influenzae* is the second-leading cause of acute otitis media in adults and children.[237]

While *H. influenzae* is a rare cause of endocarditis, two other *Haemophilus* species, *H. parainfluenzae* and *H. aphrophilus*, account for as much as 5% of adult endocarditis.[238] These species are commensal organisms of the oropharynx and due to fastidious growth characteristics are included in the group of pathogens that often cause "culture-negative" endocarditis known as the HACEK group.[239]

H. influenzae biotype *aegyptius* causes Brazilian purpuric fever, a disease characterized by acute onset of high fever, vomiting, abdominal pain, purpura, and vascular collapse. This disease affects Brazilian children under 10 years of age and is associated with a 70% mortality rate.[240]

Chancroid, a sexually transmitted disease caused by *H. dulcreyi* is found worldwide, particularly among populations of lower socioeconomic status and among the HIV infected.[241] This disease causes inguinal and perirectal papules that ulcerate and readily bleed.

8.2. Mortality and Complications

Despite currently available antimicrobial therapy, about 5% of children who acquire invasive Hib disease die.[16] Neurological sequelae of meningitis are relatively common, occurring in 19–45% of such children.[171,242–244] Handicaps include hearing loss, language disorder or delay, mental retardation, motor abnormalities, seizure disorders, and impairment of vision. Deafness is one of the most important and common handicaps associated with Hib meningitis.[245–247] During the 1983–1984 school year, an estimated 8.7% of hearing-impaired children under 18 years of age enrolled in special education programs in the United States had hearing losses attributed to meningitis.[248] Late complications of other forms of invasive Hib disease have generally not been well described, with the exception of functional impairment of joints, including abnormalities in bone growth and limited joint mobility, following septic arthritis.[249,250] Appropriate treatment of empyema caused by Hib has not been associated with functional impairment on long-term follow-up.[33]

9. Control and Prevention

9.1. General Concepts

It is beyond the scope of this chapter to review antimicrobial and other therapies for invasive or other *H.*

influenzae infections. It is nonetheless important to point out that the presumptive treatment of febrile children with antimicrobial agents probably aborts early infections or complicates the likelihood of establishing a definitive microbiological diagnosis. This is important in those developed countries, like Japan, where antibiotics are given to almost all children with febrile illnesses. In such settings, the true incidence and morbidity of Hib disease may not be fully appreciated, and there are problems related to the development of antimicrobial resistance.

Prior to the availability of universal immunization, antimicrobial chemoprophylaxis was used to prevent secondary transmission of Hib disease; it was the only means to prevent disease. The rationale for prophylaxis was to eliminate the carrier state from all contacts of a susceptible child with antimicrobial agents that achieve bactericidal levels in mucosal secretions, saliva, and tears. Interestingly, antibiotics effective in treatment of invasive Hib disease were not necessarily effective in eliminating the carrier state. Universal immunization of infants has nearly eliminated index cases of disease and contacts of the rare cases that do occur usually have been immunized. This modality is not reviewed extensively here because it is now rarely employed. Hyperimmune globulin for passive prophylaxis is high-risk settings was also used transiently and will not be reviewed here. The control of invasive Hib disease depends on widespread use of Hib conjugate vaccines in young infants and the vaccines that are currently available are reviewed.

9.2. Antimicrobial Prophylaxis

Rifampin is the most effective antimicrobial for eradicating Hib from the pharynx, primarily because high concentrations of the antimicrobial are secreted into respiratory secretions, saliva, and tears.[251,252] Several studies involving children and adults indicate rifampin in a dosage of 20 mg/kg per dose once daily (maximum daily dose 600 mg) for 4 days will eradicate Hib carriage in 95% or more of household[107,253] or day-care[107,151,254,255] contacts of a case and significantly decrease secondary disease. Both cohort studies that evaluated the efficacy of rifampin prophylaxis in preventing secondary Hib disease in day-care attendees found a significantly decreased rate of secondary Hib disease in children who received rifampin.[104,113] Rifampin prophylaxis is not 100% effective, as evidenced by the reports of rifampin "failures" in these studies and in anecdotal reports among both household and day-care contacts.[256,257]

Side effects of rifampin include nausea, vomiting, diarrhea, headache, or dizziness, which occurred in 20% of those taking rifampin as compared with 11% of placebo recipients. No serious reactions have been reported.[107] Those taking rifampin, including parents and day-care staff, should be informed that orange discoloration of urine, discoloration of soft contact lenses, and decreased effectiveness of oral contraceptives can occur.[258] Rifampin should not be used in pregnant women, as its effect on the fetus has not been established and it is teratogenic in laboratory animals.[16] Concern over development of Hib resistance to rifampin has arisen from the earlier experience with meningococcal prophylaxis,[259] anecdotal reports of Hib resistance following prophylaxis,[260,261] and *in vitro* studies.[262] However, there is no indication yet that rates of such resistance have become clinically significant.[263] Ampicillin,[255,260] trimethoprim–sulfamethoxazole,[253,264] erythromycin–sulfisoxazole,[265] and cefaclor[262,265] have been shown to be ineffective agents for antimicrobial prophylaxis, eliminating Hib carriage in fewer than 70% of culture-positive contacts. These antimicrobials do not get into secretions in adequate concentrations, and therefore are not recommended for prophylaxis.

9.3. Immunization

9.3.1. Historical Overview. The first type b vaccine available in the early 1970s was the PRP polysaccharide vaccine, which is composed of the purified type b capsular polysaccharide, polyribosyl–ribitol phosphate (PRP).[266,267] In 1985, this became the first vaccine to be licensed for the prevention of Hib disease in U.S. children older than 18 months of age. Beginning in late 1987, this vaccine was supplanted with several improved Hib conjugate vaccines. The polysaccharide vaccine will be briefly reviewed here because it employs the same immunogen contained in the currently licensed vaccines and research studies of this vaccine were important in the evolution of current vaccines and use.

9.3.2. PRP Polysaccharide Vaccine. Antibody to PRP polysaccharide has *in vitro* functional activity and confers *in vivo* protection (in animals and humans) (see Section 7). Responsiveness of children to PRP vaccine is strikingly age-related; infants respond infrequently and even then develop meager antibody levels.[195,196,268] There is a maturation of immune responsiveness by 18 months of age, although children 18–23 months of age do not consistently respond and do not respond as well as those 2 years of age or older.[16,198,201,202,269,270]

PRP vaccine was licensed based on efficacy a large, randomized clinical trial conducted in Finland.[92,268] The data from this trial suggested a protective efficacy of 90%

(95% CI; 56–96%) for children who were immunized between 18 and 71 months of age. Subsequent to the licensure of the polysaccharide vaccine in 1985, it became apparent that routine use of the vaccine resulted in efficacy less than that assessed in the Finnish vaccine trial.[92,270] Some vaccine failures were anecdotally reported both before[271] and after licensure of the vaccine.[92,270] The point estimates from five postlicensure case–control studies ranged from 88% in the multicenter Connecticut/Pittsburgh/Dallas study to −55% in a Minnesota study (a negative efficacy implies greater risk for vaccinees than nonvaccinees). The combined weight of the evidence suggests a variable vaccine efficacy in older children between 40 and 88%. Issues relating to the discrepancy in these studies have been previously reviewed.[272–274]

9.3.3. PRP–Protein Conjugate Vaccines. Currently, there are four PRP conjugate vaccines licensed for routine use in infants and children. As a group, conjugate vaccines offer distinct advantages over the PRP vaccine. These vaccines are novel semisynthetic modifications of the native polysaccharide antigen. The first successful synthesis of a conjugate bacterial vaccine was accomplished by Avery and Goebel[275–277] in 1929, using carrier–hapten principles first defined by Landsteiner in 1924.[216] More recently, Schneerson *et al.*,[278] Gordon,[279] Anderson *et al.*,[280] Tai *et al.*,[281] and Marburg *et al.*[282] developed PRP–protein conjugate vaccines. Basic to all conjugate vaccines is the use of a protein carrier, which is covalently linked or conjugated to PRP; in this context, PRP acts as the hapten. The protein carrier portion of the vaccine is recognized by macrophages and T cells, thereby eliciting a T-dependent immune response. In principle, the immunologic responsiveness of the protein carrier is conferred upon the polysaccharide hapten. This immune response has the following general characteristics: (1) It is quantitatively enhanced, particularly in younger infants. (2) Repeat administration of such vaccines elicit booster responses, thus providing a means of maximizing the level of immunity. This contrasts with the absence of booster responses when repeated doses of the conventional PRP polysaccharide vaccine are administered. (3) There is a maturation of class-specific immunity with a predominance of IgG antibody, indicating T-cell modulation of the immune response. (4) The prior or concurrent administration of the carrier protein alone (e.g., diphtheria or tetanus toxoid) enhances T-cell populations responsive to this antigen, thereby maximizing immune responsiveness to the polysaccharide when the conjugate vaccine is administered (so-called "carrier priming").[283] All four licensed Hib conjugate vaccines employ PRP polysaccharide as the primary immunogen; however, each conjugate vaccine differs in its protein carrier, polysaccharide length, configuration of the linkages, proportions of protein and polysaccharide, and other structural characteristics (Table 5). Therefore, each of the conjugate vaccines is reviewed separately.

9.3.3a. PRP–Diphtheria Toxoid Conjugate Vaccine (PRP-D). PRP-D was the first Hib conjugate vaccine developed by Schneerson and Robbins,[278,284] and later modified and produced commercially by Connaught Laboratories (Swiftwater, PA).[283] It contains medium-sized lengths of polysaccharide (heat-sized) linked to diphtheria toxoid via a size-carbon spacer. Other characteristics of

Table 5. Licensed *Haemophilus influenzae* type b Vaccines

Vaccine	Company	Trade name	Date licensed[b]	Age group (months)
PRP	Praxis	b-CAPSA[a]	April 1985	24–59
	Connaught	Hib-VAX[a]		18–24
	Lederle	HIB-IMUNE[a]		
PRP-D	Connaught	ProHIBiT	December 1987	18–59
			December 1989	15–59
HbOC	Ayerst-Wyeth	HibTITER	December 1988	18–59
			December 1989	15–59
			October 1990	2, 4, 6 and 12–15
HbOC-DTP	Ayerst-Wyeth	TETRAMUNE	March 1993	2, 4, 6 and 15–18
PRP-OMP	Merck Sharp & Dohme	PedvaxHIB	December 1989	15–59
			December 1990	2, 4 and 12–15
PRP-T	PMSV/Connaught	ActHIB	March 1993	2, 4, 6 and 12–15
	SmithKline Beecham	OmniHib	March 1993	2, 4, 6 and 12–15

[a]No longer available.
[b]In United States.

the vaccine are shown in Table 5. This vaccine is less immunogenic than the other conjugate vaccines and is rarely used in the United States.

PRP-D has been extensively evaluated in adults and children of all ages. A single vaccine dose elicits very high levels of antibody (geometric mean titer [GMT] 200 μg/ml) in nearly all adults.[(285)] As with PRP vaccine, the response to PRP-D in children is age-related, though PRP-D induces higher antibody levels than does PRP at all ages. In children 15 months of age and older, high antibody concentrations are achieved with a single dose, and booster doses are not required to provide lasting protection.[(286,287)] In older children and adults, there does not appear to be a detectable difference in immunogenicity between PRP-D and other Hib conjugate vaccines.[(287)]

In children under 15 months of age, PRP-D elicits a weaker immune response than the other Hib conjugate vaccines,[(288)] and in infants younger than 6 months of age, the immune response to PRP-D is very limited and much less than that induced by the other conjugate vaccines (Table 6).[(289,290)] Even after three doses in infants, fewer than half of all infants develop antibody levels greater than 1 μg/ml.[(289,291,292)] In addition, the decline of these meager antibody levels over the ensuing 3 to 12 months may leave many children without protective levels of antibody during the period of greatest disease risk. PRP-D is immunogenic in some high-risk children, including those who do not respond well to invasive Hib disease[(293)]: splenectomized patients with Hodgkin disease,[(294)] children over 18 months of age with sickle-cell disease,[(295)] and children with acute leukemia.[(25,296)]

Before the 1987 licensure of PRP-D in the United States, there was no documentation of its efficacy. Subsequently, a number of case–control studies demonstrated that a single dose of vaccine was at least 80% efficacious in preventing disease in children 18 months of age and older.[(297–301)] There was much controversy about PRP-D's efficacy in young infants, as two clinical efficacy trials in Finland and in Alaskan Natives (Table 7) yielded disparate results.[(193,302)] The discrepancy between the results of the two studies has not been fully explained, but the poor efficacy seen in the Native Alaskan infants paralleled its poor immunogenicity. However, the PRP-D vaccine has been used routinely in European infants, and follow-up studies in Finland,[(303)] Iceland,[(304)] Switzerland, and Germany[(305)] suggest a sustained efficacy.

Between 1988 and 1995, millions of doses of PRP-D have been administered in the United States and Europe without reports of serious adverse consequences. Fewer than 2% of children 18 months of age and older develop fever with PRP-D administration, a rate about threefold lower than with DTP vaccination,[(306)] and local reactions at the injection site are also infrequent.[(286,292,306)] In 1987, the US Food and Drug Administration (FDA) licensed PRP-D for use in children 18–60 months of age, because of its superior immunogenicity to that of PRP vaccine. Currently it is licensed only for use in children 12 months of age and older and it can be given as the booster dose

Table 6. Characteristics of Hib Conjugate Vaccines[a]

Properties	PRP-D	HbOC	PRP-OMP	PRP-T
Polysaccharide (PS):				
Polymer size	Medium (heat sized)	Small (periodate oxidized)	Large (native)	Large (native)
Content	25 μg	10 μg	15 μg	10 μg
Protein carrier	Diphtheria toxoid	CRM_{197}	Mening group B OMP	Tetanus toxoid
Content	18 μg	20 μg	250 μg	20 μg
Linkage				
Activation	Protein	PS	Protein and PS	PS
Reactants	ADH CNBr (protein)	Periodate Cyanoborohydrate	N-ABC (PS) N-AHC (Protein)	ADH CNBr (PS) Carbodiimide HCI
Linkages	Amide/protein Iminocarbamate/PS	2° amino	Amide/protein Carbamate/PS Thioester/spacer	Amide/protein Iminocarbamate/PS
Spacer	6-carbon	None	Bigeneric 1. N-ABC (linked to PS) 2. N-AHC (linked to Protein)	6-carbon

[a]Mening grop B OMP, *Neisseria meningitidis* group B outer membrane protein; CRM_{197}, diphtheria toxin mutant protein; ADH, adipic dihydrazide; the completed reaction cleaves both hydrazide moieties, leaving a 6-carbon linkage; N-ABC, C-NBr, cyanogen bromide; *N*-acetyl butyl carbamate; and N-AHC, *N*-acetyl homocysteine.

Table 7. Efficacy Trial of PRP-D in Native Alaskan Infants

	Episodes of Hib disease/ No. of subjects			
Dose	Vaccinees	Placebo recipients	Protective efficacy	95% Confidence Interval
Post 1	3/1,054	4/1,048	25%	−233 to 83%
Post 2	2/991	3/966	35%	−288 to 89%
Post 3[a]	7/915	12/883	43%	−43 to 78%
Post any[a]	12/1,054	19/1,048	37%	−29 to 69%

[a]One vaccinee had two episodes of Hib infection, the first between the first and second dose and the second after the third dose. In this tabulation, the case is counted once.

after primary immunization with any of the three Hib conjugate vaccines licensed for use in infants. PRP-D is rarely used in the United States because it is not licensed for use in infants.

9.3.3b. PRP Oligosaccharide–CRM$_{197}$ Conjugate Vaccine [HbOC (HibTITER®, Tetraimmune®). HbOC vaccine was developed by Porter Anderson at the University of Rochester, and is now manufactured by Ayerst–Wyeth–Lederle–Praxis Laboratories (Pearl River, NY). It was initially licensed in the United States in 1988 for older children. HbOC differs significantly from the other Hib conjugate vaccines. It consists of a short oligosaccharide of PRP that is covalently linked, without a spacer, to the protein carrier CRM$_{197}$, which is a nontoxic, mutant variant of the diphtheria toxin protein (Table 5).

As with the other Hib conjugate vaccines, a single dose of HbOC is highly immunogenic in children older than 18 months.[22,280,287,307] However, in infants (Table 6), an initial dose at 2 months of age does not induce an antibody response, and a significant number of infants fail to respond to a second dose at 4 months of age.[19] After a third dose at 6 months, high antibody levels are achieved in nearly all infants.[19,308–310] Antibody levels after three doses of HbOC are equivalent to those induced by three doses of PRP-T vaccine and higher than those induced by PRP-D and PRP-OMP vaccines in infants (see below).[310,311] In most infants, antibody persists until at least 1 year of age, when a fourth booster is recommended. An immunization schedule with two doses administered at 2 and 6 months of age yielded similar results, indicating that the age at the time of the booster dose may be the major determinant of the immune response.[312] The HbOC vaccine has been shown to produce good antibody responses in several high-risk groups, including children with immunodeficiency syndromes,[252,313] sickle-cell disease,[314] and prior Hib disease.[315]

Two prospective clinical studies have shown that two or three doses of HbOC administered in the first 6 months of life provide a high degree of protective efficacy,[21,165,316] and several million doses of the vaccine have been given since 1988. The vaccine is safe, with only transient and mild side effects.[19] Fever does not occur significantly more often when HbOC is administered concomitantly with DTP than when DTP is administered alone,[19,317] and a combined HbOC/DTP has similar reaction rates to those reported for coadministration of the two vaccines at different injection sites.[316,318] No serious reactions have been reported with HbOC.

In 1990, HbOC became the first Hib conjugate vaccine to be licensed in the United States for routine use in infants. It is recommended that it be administered at 2, 4, and 6 months of age, with a booster dose at 12–15 months of age.[319] The HbOC vaccine is also available as a combined HbOC/DTP vaccine (licensed in the United States in 1993). This combined vaccine can be used for routine infant immunization or to complete a series begun with the HbOC vaccine.

9.3.3c. PRP–Group B Neisseria meningitidis OMPC Conjugate Vaccine (PRP-OMP). This PRP–protein conjugate vaccine developed by Merck Sharp & Dohme[282] was licensed in 1989 by the US FDA. Structurally and chemically the PRP-OMP vaccine differs markedly from the other Hib conjugate vaccines. It consists of medium lengths of PRP linked via a bigeneric spacer molecule to protein components of outer membrane vesicles of a strain of group B *Neisseria meningitidis* (Table 5).

PRP-OMP induces an immune response that is less age-dependent than is the response to the other Hib conjugate vaccines. Adults and children respond to a single vaccine dose with high antibody levels.[320] Although a booster response is seen in older children, subsequent vaccine doses in infants do not evoke a distinct booster response.[320–323] Unlike the other three vaccines, a single injection of PRP-OMP induces a good antibody response in many infants as young as 6 to 8 weeks of age[310,322,324] (Table 6). A second dose at 4 months of age increases somewhat the proportion of infants with an immune response, but does not elicit a classic booster response.[325] The titers achieved after two doses are, however, higher than those after two doses of any of the other conjugate vaccines.[310,311,321] A third dose at 6 months of age does not boost levels significantly; therefore, a two-dose primary series is used. Surprisingly, infants vaccinated at birth, 2, and 6 months of age showed depressed PRP antibody levels throughout the first year of life, suggesting the potential for tolerance to develop if given at too young an age.[326] There have been concerns about the fall in antibody concentrations during the 3 to 12 months after the two-dose primary immunization series, particularly in those infants with the lowest concentrations of anti-PRP antibodies. About one quarter of vaccine recipients have levels less than 0.15 μg/ml a year after completing their primary immunization series.[327,328] Therefore, a third dose is necessary after 12 months of age to sustain antibody levels that will provide long-term protection.[320,327] PRP-OMP is also immunogenic in high-risk individuals who may not respond to vaccination with PRP.[329] PRP-OMP was evaluated in a randomized, double-blind, placebo-controlled trial in a high-risk Navajo Indian population.[310,330]

In 1990, PRP-OMP vaccine was licensed in the United States for the routine immunization of infants. It is recommended for administration at 2 and 4 months of age, with a booster dose at 12–15 months of age (Table 5). Despite concerns over different recommendations for PRP-OMP as compared to HbOC and PRP-T vaccines, the USFDA decided on the schedules based on available immunogenicity and efficacy data and the concern that vaccine schedules be individually designed so as to maximize efficacy.

9.3.3d. PRP–Tetanus Toxoid Conjugate Vaccine (PRP-T). The PRP–tetanus toxoid conjugate vaccine was developed at the National Institutes of Health,[179,203,278,284] and subsequently produced by Pasteur–Merieux. It is marketed in the United States by Pasteur–Merieux–Connaught and by SmithKline Beecham. PRP-T contains large polysaccharide polymers linked to tetanus toxoid via a six-carbon spacer. Multiple cross-linkages result in a complex three-dimensional structure (Table 5).

PRP-T is highly immunogenic in adults and older children[203,331] In young infants, it requires two or three doses to observe a consistently good immune response.[311,321,322,332] This vaccine also produces good antibody booster responses when given to older children previously given any of the Hib conjugate vaccines.[289] High concentrations of antibody (geometric mean anti-PRP antibody concentrations of 5–10 μg/ml) are achieved in infants with a three dose immunization series at 2, 4, and 6 months of age[20,311,332] (Table 6). The antibody levels wane with time, but most infants sustain protective levels of antibody for at least a year, when a booster dose is recommended.[333] In 1993, the FDA approved the reconstitution of PRP-T with Connaught's DTP.[334] PRP-T is also immunogenic in high-risk individuals with bone marrow transplantation, sickle-cell anemia or malignancies, or prior Hib disease.[117,335]

PRP-T's protective efficacy was evaluated in two large prospective randomized trials that were prematurely terminated due to the licensure of other Hib conjugate vaccines for infants.[20,165,333] In prelicensure studies, PRP-T was administered to over 115,000 children with no serious side effects.[20] Local reactions were more common (up to 32%) after PRP-T than after PRP in children 18–24 months of age,[20,331] possibly due to an Arthur-like reaction in children with preexisting high titers of tetanus antibody. Only 7–15% of infants had local reactions.[20,336] Rates of systemic reactions in infants receiving PRP-T and DTP concurrently were similar to those reported for DTP alone.[20,336] One study suggests that rates of mild reactions may be slightly increased in children receiving PRP-T and DTP in the same syringe.[334]

PRP-T was licensed by the USFDA for use in infants in 1992, based on its immunogenicity profile and the available efficacy data.[319] It is recommended for use in infants at 2, 4, and 6 months of age, with a booster dose at 12–15 months. In 1993, the USFDA approved the reconstitution of PRP-T with Connaught's DTP vaccine to allow simultaneous administration of the two vaccines with a single injection.

9.3.4. Future Vaccine Development. To date, essentially all *H. influenzae* vaccines are based on immunity to the type b capsule. Antibodies to other components of the bacterium also have been shown to be bactericidal, opsonophagocytic, and protective in animal studies. Vaccines containing alternative antigens could provide supplemental protection against Hib, although this does not appear to be necessary based on the efficacy of the available Hib conjugate vaccines. More importantly, these alternative vaccines could provide immunity to non-type b strains, which have substantial phenotypic and genetic variability,[337] but are ubiquitous colonizers of the upper respiratory tract of humans and cause mucosal infections. The basic microbiological problem hindering the development of such vaccines has been the diversity and instability of cell wall antigens between *H. influenzae* strains. Studies have attempted to define OMP, cell wall LPS, and fimbriae surface antigens of the organism.[338] Due to the variability of most of these antigens between heterologous strains and even among homologous strains over time, it has been difficult to find an antigen relevant to all or the majority of strains. Also, not all bacterial antigens elicit protective immunity. The focus of most investigations has been to characterize OMPs.[339] Other efforts have focused on higher-molecular-weight proteins,[340] LPS, or fimbrial antigens.[341] Immunity to these other antigens has not been consistent against heterologous strains.

9.3.5. Comparative Immunogenicity Studies. Comparing immunogenicity data from different studies of different vaccines is difficult. Apparent differences in immunogenicity may be due to differences in study design (e.g., age at immunization or timing of phlebotomy), differences in specific vaccine lots, differences in the laboratory assays used to determine antibody levels, or differences in the statistical methods used to analyze the data. However, several studies have compared the various Hib conjugate vaccines directly in trials using the same vaccine schedules, with the antibody response analyzed in the same laboratory. The studies, however, do reveal consistent patterns of immune response. PRP-OMP is the only vaccine that induces a good immune response with a single dose in young infants. HbOC and PRP-T each require two or three doses in infancy to achieve high antibody levels and these levels are higher than those achieved with PRP-OMP. PRP-D is clearly the least immunogenic of the four vaccines.

While these studies help confirm the pattern of the immune response seen with each of the vaccines, they do not necessarily predict better protection. Because PRP-OMP is the only vaccine that induces an antibody response in 2-month-old infants, it may be the vaccine of choice if there is a high risk of early onset disease (prior to 6 months of age) or if compliance with future doses cannot be assured. HbOC and PRP-T produce higher and more durable antibody levels after completion of the immunization series.Each of the three vaccines licensed for use in infants appears to be highly efficacious, and postlicensure studies suggest that there are not important differences in effectiveness.

10. Unresolved Problems

In the quest to find better ways to prevent invasive Hib disease and other diseases caused by encapsulated respiratory bacteria, investigators have pondered a central enigma: Why some individuals become infected but remain asymptomatically colonized, while others succumb to invasive disease.

In part, the control of invasive Hib disease derived from extensive epidemiological studies over the prior two decades. The lessons from many attempts to prevent Hib disease have direct applicability to the prevention of other encapsulated bacterial respiratory diseases, in particular those caused by *S. pneumoniae* (see Chapter 28) and *N. meningiditis* (see Chapter 23). Indeed, the candidate vaccines for these diseases and the types of vaccine studies that need to be performed will be modeled on the experience with Hib conjugate vaccines.

From a microbial perspective, better understanding of the microbial factors that determine virulence, particularly for disease due to non-type b organisms, would improve our understanding of disease pathogenesis, and it would be useful in the development of new vaccines against all forms of *H. influenzae* disease. The current vaccines are based on the principle that anticapsular antibody alone is sufficient to prevent disease, but it is clear that other antigens of the organism can also elicit antibodies that are protective. Therefore, conjugate vaccines incorporating OMPs or other antigens of the organism might provide significant additional protective benefit. Perhaps most importantly, type b conjugate vaccines do not address the problem of mucosal diseases, especially that caused by non-type b strains. In this regard, the prevention of pneumonia in developing countries may require vaccines with broader specificity than type b conjugate vaccines.

From an immunologic perspective, further understanding of the factors that influence immune response to capsule and to capsule derivatives is of considerable importance. Although epidemiological evidence clearly shows that age is the most important risk factor for disease, the immunologic elements that bring about this unusual susceptibility to disease are not fully understood. Relatively little is known about the determinants of protective immune responses in humans, and there is an inadequate understanding of the role and mechanisms of T-cell responses and mucosal immunity. There is also the issue of providing long-term protection. Markers for these immunologic functions would be useful to optimize the design of newer vaccines. Research in the area of developmental immunology might better explain why young infants and children are so uniquely susceptible to numerous encapsulated bacteria.

Although many questions still remain to be answered, the prevention of Hib disease has been a major achievement of this century. It has implications for the prevention of other encapsulated bacterial diseases. Hib conjugate vaccines now need to be used worldwide to see if there can be benefits in preventing pneumonia and respiratory deaths, the major causes of death in children in developing countries.

11. References

1. Cochi, S. L., Fleming, D. W., Hightower, A. W., Limpakarnjanarat, K., Facklam, R. R., Smith, J. D., Sikes, R. K., and Broome, C. V., Primary invasive *Haemophilus influenzae* type b disease: A population-based assessment of risk factors, *J. Pediatr.* **108:**887–896 (1986).
2. Pfeiffer, R., Vorlaufige mitt Heilungen uber die Erreger der Influenzae, *Dtsch. Med. Wochenschr.* **18:**28–34 (1892).

3. Pfeiffer, R., Die Aetiologie der Influenza, *Z. Hyg. Infektionskr.* **13:**357–386 (1893).
4. Smith, W., Andrewes, C. H., and Laidlaw, P. P., A virus obtained from influenza patients, *Lancet* **2:**66–68 (1933).
5. Pittman, M., Variation and type specificity in the bacterial species *Hemophilus influenzae*, *J. Exp. Med.* **53:**471–495 (1931).
6. Pittman, M., The action of type-specific *Hemophilus influenzae* antiserum, *J. Exp. Med.* **58:**683–706 (1933).
7. Todd, J. K., and Bruhn, F. W., Severe *Haemophilus influenzae* infections: Spectrum of disease, *Am. J. Dis. Child.* **129:**607–611 (1975).
8. Alexander, H. E., Ellis, C., and Leidy, G., Treatment of type-specific *Hemophilus influenzae* infections in infancy and childhood, *J. Pediatr.* **20:**673–698 (1942).
9. Alexander, H. E., Heidelberger, M., and Leidy, G., The protective or curative element in type b *Haemophilus influenzae* rabbit serum, *Yale J. Biol. Med.* **16:**425–440 (1944).
10. Alexander, W. J., and Shaw, J. F. E., Results of a prospective population-based study of the incidence of invasive *Haemophilus influenzae* disease in children, Abstract 7, Symposium on infectious diseases in day care: Management and prevention, Minneapolis, June 1984.
11. Alexander, H. E., Treatment of *Haemophilus influenzae* infections and of meningococcus and pneumococcic meningitis, *Am. J. Dis. Child.* **66:**172–187 (1943).
12. Alpert, G., Campos, J. M., Smith, D. R., Barenkamp, S. J., and Fleisher, G. R., Incidence and persistence of *H. influenzae* type b upper airway colonization in patients with meningitis, *J. Pediatr.* **107:**555–557 (1985).
13. Fothergill, L. D., and Wright, J., Influenzal meningitis: The relation of age incidence to the bactericidal power of blood against the causal organism, *J. Immunol.* **24:**273–284 (1933).
14. Johnston, R. B., Jr., Anderson, P., Rosen, F. S., and Smith, D. H., Characterization of human immunity to polyribophosphate, the capsular antigen of *H. influenzae* type b, *Clin. Immunol. Immunopathol.* **1:**234–240 (1973).
15. Schneerson, R., Rodrigues, L. P., Parke, J. C., Jr., and Robbins, J. B., Immunity to disease caused by *H. influenzae* type b. II. Specificity and some biological characteristics of "natural," infection acquired, and immunization induced antibody to the capsular polysaccharide, *J. Immunol.* **107:**1081–1086 (1971).
16. ACIP, Update: Prevention of *Haemophilus influenzae* type b disease, *Morbid. Mortal. Week. Rep.* **35:**170–174, 179–180 (1986).
17. Committee on Infectious Diseases, *Haemophilus influenzae* type b conjugate vaccine, *Pediatrics* **81:**908–911 (1988).
18. Immunization Practices Advisory Committee (ACIP), Update: Prevention of *Haemophilus influenzae* type b disease, *Morbid. Mortal. Week. Rep.* **37:**13–16 (1988).
19. Black, S. B., Shinefield, H. R., Fireman, B., and Hiatt, R., Safety, immunogenicity, and efficacy in infancy of oligosaccharide conjugate *Haemophilus influenzae* type b vaccine in a United States population: Possible implications for optimal use, *J. Infect. Dis.* **165**(Suppl. 2)**:**S139–43.
20. Fritzell, B., and Plotkin, S., Efficacy and safety of a *Haemophilus influenzae* type b capsular polysaccharide–tetanus protein conjugate vaccine, *J. Pediatr.* **121**(3)**:**355–362 (1992).
21. Vadheim, C. M., Greenberg, D. P., Eriksen, E., Hemenway, L., Christenson, P., Ward, B., Mascola, L., and Ward, J. I., Protection provided by *Haemophilus influenzae* type b conjugate vaccines in Los Angeles county: A case–control study, *Pediatr. Infect. Dis. J.* **13**(4)**:**274–280 (1994).
22. Black, S. B., and Shinefield, H. R., Immunization with oligosaccharide conjugate *Haemophilus influenzae* type b (HbOC) vaccine on a large health maintenance organization population: Extended follow-up and impact on *Haemophilus influenzae* disease epidemiology. The Kaiser Permanente Pediatric Vaccine Study Group, *Pediatr. Infect. Dis. J.* **11**(8)**:**610–613 (1992).
23. Murphy, T. B., White, K. E., Pastor, P., Gabriel, L., Medley, F., Granoff, D. M., and Osterholm, M. T., Declining incidence of *Haemophilus influenzae* type b disease since introduction of vaccination, *J. Am. Med. Assoc.* **269**(2)**:**246–248 (1993).
24. Nicolosi, A., Hauser, W. A., Beghi, E., and Kurland, L. T., Epidemiology of central nervous system infections in Olmsted County, Minnesota, 1950–1982, *J. Infect. Dis.* **154:**399–408 (1986).
25. Feldman, R., Fraser, D., and Koehler, R., Death certificates as a measure of *Haemophilus influenzae* meningitis mortality in the United States 1962–1968, in: *Haemophilus influenzae* (S. Sell and E. Karzon, eds.), pp. 221–230, Vanderbilt University Press, Nashville, 1973.
26. Macleod, C. A., *Haemophilus influenzae*: The efficiency of reporting invasive disease in England and Wales, *Commun. Dis. Rep. CDR Rev.* **4**(2)**:**R13–16 (1994).
27. Schlech, W. F., Band, J. D., Ward, J. I., Hightower, A. W., Fraser, D. W., and Broome, C. V., Bacterial meningitis in the United States, 1978–1982: The national bacterial meningitis surveillance study, *J. Am. Med. Assoc.* **253:**1749–1754 (1985).
28. Wenger, J. D., Hightower, A. W., Harrison, L. H., Broome, C. F., and the *Haemophilus influenzae* Study Group, Use of discharge codes for detection of *Haemophilus influenzae* disease (Abstract), Program and Abstracts of the Twenty-eighth Interscience Conference on Antimicrobial Agents and Chemotherapy, Los Angeles, 1988.
29. Crosson, F. J., Winkelstein, J. A., and Moxon, E. R., Enzyme-linked immunosorbent assay for detection and quantitation of capsular antigen of *Haemophilus influenzae* type b, *Infect. Immun.* **22:**617–619 (1978).
30. Ingram, D. L., Pearson, A. B., and Occhiuti, A. R., Detection of bacterial antigens in body fluids with the Wellcogen *Haemophilus influenzae* b, *Streptococcus pneumoniae* and *Neisseria meningitidis* (ACYW135) latex agglutination tests, *J. Clin. Microbiol.* **18:**1119–1121 (1983).
31. Marcon, M. J., Hamoudi, A. C., and Cannon, H. J., Comparative laboratory evaluation of three antigen detection methods for diagnosis of *Haemophilus influenzae* type b disease, *J. Clin. Microbiol.* **19:**333–337 (1984).
32. Scheifele, D. W., Ward, J. I., and Siber, G., Advantage of latex agglutination over countercurrent immunoelectrophoresis in the detection of *Haemophilus influenzae* type b antigen in serum, *Pediatrics* **68:**888–891 (1981).
33. Mason, E. O., Kaplan, S. L., Lambeth, L. B., Hinds, D. B., Kvernland, S. J., Loiselle, E. M., and Feigin, R. D., Serotype and ampicillin susceptibility of *Haemophilus influenzae* causing systemic infections in children: Three years of experience, *J. Clin. Microbiol.* **15:**543–546 (1982).
34. Daum, R. S., Siber, G. R., Kamon, J. S., and Russell, R. R., Evaluation of a commercial latex particle agglutination test for rapid diagnosis of *Haemophilus influenzae* type b infection, *Pediatrics* **69:**406–471 (1982).
35. McLaughlin, F. J., Goldmann, D. A., Rosenbaum, D. M., Harris,

G. B. C., Schuster, S. R., and Strieder, D. J., Empyema in children: Clinical course and long-term follow-up, *Pediatrics* **73:** 587–593 (1984).

36. Turk, D. C., Clinical importance of *Haemophilus influenzae*—1981, in: *Haemophilus influenzae* (S. H. Sell and P. F. Wright, eds.), pp. 3–9, Elsevier, Amsterdam, 1982.
37. Andersson, B., Porras, O., Hanson, L. A., Lagergard, T., and Svanborg-Eden, C., Inhibition of attachment of *Streptococcus pneumoniae* and *Haemophilus influenzae* by human milk and receptor oligosaccharides, *J. Infect. Dis.* **153:**232–237 (1986).
38. Porras, O., Caugant, D. A., Lagergard, T., and Svanborg-Eden, C. S., Application of multilocus enzyme gel electrophoresis to *Haemophilus influenzae*, *Infect. Immun.* **53:**71–78 (1986).
39. Campos, J., Garcia-Tornel, S., Gairi, J. M., and Fabregues, I., Multiply resistant *Haemophilus influenzae* type b causing meningitis: Comparative clinical and laboratory study, *J. Pediatr.* **108:**897–902 (1986).
40. Robbins, J. B., Schneerson, R., Glode, M. P., Vann, W., Schiffer, M. S., Liv, T. Y., Parke, J. C., and Huntley, C., Cross-reactive antigens and immunity to diseases caused by encapsulated bacteria, *J. Allergy Clin. Immunol.* **56:**141–151 (1975).
41. Gulig, P. A., Patrick, C. C., Hermanstorfer, L., McCracken, G. H., Jr., and Hansen, E. J., Conservation of epitopes in the oligosaccharide portion of the lipooligosaccharide of *Haemophilus influenzae* type b, *Infect. Immun.* **55:**513–520 (1987).
42. Tolan, R. W., Munson, R. S., and Granoff, D. M., Lipopolysaccharide gel profiles of *Haemophilus influenzae* type b are not stable epidemiologic markers, *J. Clin. Microbiol.* **24:**223–227 (1986).
43. Centers for Disease Control, Ampicillin-resistant *Haemophilus influenzae* meningitis—Maryland, Georgia, *Morbid. Mortal. Week. Rep.* **23:**77–78 (1974).
44. Campos, J., Garcia-Tornel, S., and Sanfeliu, I., Susceptibility studies of multiply resistant *Haemophilus influenzae* isolated from pediatric patients and contacts, *Antimicrob. Agents Chemother.* **25:**706–709 (1984).
45. Centers for Disease Control, Ampicillin and chloramphenicol resistance in systemic *Haemophilus influenzae* disease, *Morbid. Mortal. Week. Rep.* **33:**35–37 (1984).
46. Smith, A. L., Antibiotic resistance in *Haemophilus influenzae*, *Pediatr. Infect. Dis. J.* **2:**352–355 (1983).
47. Preston, D. A., Global surveillance of bacterial susceptibility to cefaclor: 1988–1990, *Clin. Ther.* **15**(1):88–96 (1993).
48. Mendelman, P. M., Doroshow, C. A., Gandy, S. L., Syriopoulou, V., Weigen, C. P., and Smith, A. L., Plasmid-mediated resistance in multiply resistant *Haemophilus influenzae* type b causing meningitis: Molecular characterization of one strain and review of the literature, *J. Infect. Dis.* **150:**30–39 (1984).
49. Overturf, G. D., Cable, D., and Ward, J., Ampicillin–chloramphenicol-resistant *Haemophilus influenzae*: Plasmid-mediated resistance in bacterial meningitis, *Pediatr. Res.* **22:**438–441 (1987).
50. Powell, M., Fah, Y. S., Seymour, A., Yuan, M., and Williams, J. D., Antimicrobial resistance in *Haemophilus influenzae* from England and Scotland in 1991, *J. Antimicrob. Chemother.* **29**(5)**:** 547–554 (1992).
51. Daum, R. S., Murphey-Corb, M., Shapir, E., and Dipp, S., Epidemiology of Rob beta-lactamase among ampicillin-resistant *Haemophilus influenzae* isolates in the United States, *J. Infect. Dis.* **157:**450–455 (1988).
52. Jacobs, R. F., Hsi, S., Wilson, C. B., Benjamin, D., Smith, A. L., and Morrow, R., Apparent meningococcemia: Clinical features of disease due to *Haemophilus influenzae* and *Neisseria meningitidis*, *Pediatrics* **72:**469–472 (1983).
53. Dajani, A. S., Asmar, B. I., and Thirumoorthi, M. C., Systemic *Haemophilus influenzae* disease: An overview, *J. Pediatr.* **94:** 355–364 (1979).
54. Murphy, T. V., Granoff, D. M., Pierson, L. M., Pastor, P., White, K. E., Clements, J. F., and Osterholm, M. T., Invasive *Haemophilus influenzae* type b disease in children less than 5 years of age in Minnesota and in Dallas County, Texas, 1983–1984, *J. Infect. Dis.* **165**(Suppl. 1)**:**S7–10 (1992).
55. Vadheim, C. M., Greenberg, D. P., Bordenave, N., Ziontz, L., Christenson, P., Waterman, S. H., and Ward, J. I., Risk factors for invasive *Haemophilus influenzae* type b in Los Angeles County children 18–60 months of age, *Am. J. Epidemiol.* **136**(2)**:**221–235 (1992)
56. Istre, G. R., Conner, J. S., Broome, C. V., Hightower, A., and Hopkins, R. S., Risk factors for primary invasive *Haemophilus infuenzae* disease: Increased risk from day care attendance and school age household members, *J. Pediatr.* **106:**190–195 (1985).
57. Murphy, T. V., Osterholm, M. T., Pierson, L. M., White, K. E., Breedlove, J. A., Seibert, G. B., Kuritsky, J. N., and Granoff, D. M., Prospective surveillance of *Haemophilus influenzae* type b disease in Dallas County, Texas, and in Minnesota, *Pediatrics* **79:**173–180 (1987).
58. Fraser, D. W., *Haemophilus influenzae* in the community and in the home, in: *Haemophilus influenzae* (S. H. Sell and P. F. Wright, eds.), pp. 11–22, Elsevier, Amsterdam, 1982.
59. Fraser, D. W., Hencke, C. E., and Feldman, R. A., Changing patterns of bacterial meningitis in Olmsted County, Minnesota, 1935–1970, *J. Infect. Dis.* **128:**300–307 (1973).
60. Fraser, D. W., Geil, C. C., and Feldman, R. A., Bacterial meningitis in Bernalillo County, New Mexico: A comparison with three other American populations, *Am. J. Epidemiol.* **100:**29–34 (1974).
61. Parke, J. C., Jr., Schneerson, R., and Robbins, J. B., The attack rate, age incidence, racial distribution, and case fatality rate of *Haemophilus influenzae* type b meningitis in Mecklenburg County, North Carolina, *J. Pediatr.* **81:**765–769 (1972).
62. Santosham, M., Kallman, C. H., Neff, J. M., and Moxon, E. R., Absence of increasing incidence of meningitis caused by *Haemophilus influenzae* type b, *J. Infect. Dis.* **140:**1009–1012 (1979).
63. Claesson, B., Trollfors, B., Jodal, U., and Rosenhall, U., Incidence and prognosis of *Haemophilus influenzae* meningitis in children in a Swedish region, *Pediatr. Infect. Dis. J.* **3:**35–39 (1984).
64. Hansman, D., Hanna, J., and Morey, F., High prevalence of invasive *Haemophilus influenzae* disease in central Australia, 1986, *Lancet* **2:**927 (1986).
65. Reinert, P., Liwartowski, A., Dabernat, H., Guyot, C., Boucher, J., and Carrere, C., Epidemiology of *Haemophilus influenzae* type b disease in France, *Vaccine* **11**(Suppl 1)**:**S38–42 (1993).
66. Salwen, K. M., Vikerfors, T., and Olcen, P., Increased incidence of childhood bacterial meningitis: A 25-year study in a defined population in Sweden, *Scand. J. Infect. Dis.* **19:**1–11 (1987).
67. Peltola, H., and Virtanen, M., Systemic *Haemophilus influenzae* infection in Finland, *Clin. Pediatr.* **5:**275–280 (1984).
68. Valmari, P., Kataja, M., and Peltola, H., Invasive *Haemophilus influenzae* and meningococcal infections in Finland, *Scand. J. Infect. Dis.* **19:**19–27 (1987).

69. Spanjaard, L., Bol, P., Ekker, W., and Zanen, H. C., The incidence of bacterial meningitis in The Netherlands—A comparison of three registration systems, 1977–1982, *J. Infect.* **11**:259–268 (1985).
70. Varaghese, P., *Haemophilus influenzae* infection, in Canada, 1969–1985, *Can. Dis. Week. Rep.* **12**:37–43 (1986).
71. Brewster, D., The epidemiology of *Haemophilus influenzae* invasive disease in Scotland prior to immunization, *Health Bull.* **51**(6):385–393 (1993).
72. Dawson, B., and Zinnemann, K., Incidence and type distribution of capsulated *H. influenzae* strains, *Br. Med. J.* **1**:740–742 (1952).
73. Akpede O., Abiodum, P. O., Sykes, M., and Salami, C. E., Childhood bacterial meningitis beyond the neonatal period in southern Nigeria: Changes in organisms/antibiotic susceptibility, *East Afr. Med. J.* **71**(1):14–20 (1994).
74. Gratten, M., and Montgomery, J., The bacteriology of acute pneumonia and meningitis in Papua New Guinea: Assumptions, facts and technical strategies, *Papua New Guinea Med. J.* **34**:185–198 (1991).
75. Greenwood, B., Epidemiology of acute lower respiratory tract infections, especially those due to *Haemophilus influenzae* type b, in The Gambia, West Africa, *J. Infect. Dis.* **165**(Suppl 1):S26–28 (1992).
76. Greenwood, B. M., The epidemiology of acute bacterial meningitis in tropical Africa, in: *Bacterial meningitis*, pp. 61–91, Academic Press, New York, 1987.
77. Lehmann, D., Epidemiology of acute respiratory tract infections, especially those due to *Haemophilus influenzae*, in Papua New Guinean children, *J. Infect. Dis.* **165**(Suppl. 1):S20–25 (1992).
78. Iwarson, S., World-wide strategies for immunization against invasive *Haemophilus influenzae* type b disease, *Vaccine* **11**(Suppl. 1):S28–29 (1993).
79. Hanna, J. N., Wild, B. E., and Sly, P. D., The epidemiology of acute epiglottitis in children in Western Australia, *J. Paediatr. Child Health* **28**(6):459–464 (1992).
80. Hanna, J. N., and Wild, B. E., Bacterial meningitis in children under five years of age in Western Australia, *Med. J. Aust.* **155:** 160–164 (1991).
81. Coulehan, J. L., Michaels, R. H., Hallowell, C., Schults, R., Welty, T. K., and Kuo, J. S. C., Epidemiology of *Haemophilus influenzae* type b disease among Navajo Indians, *Public Health Rep.* **99**:404–409 (1984).
82. Losonsky, G. A., Santosham, M., Sehgal, V. M., Zwahlen, A., and Moxon, E. R., *Haemophilus influenzae* in the White Mountain Apaches: Molecular epidemiology of a high-risk population, *Pediatr. Infect. Dis. J.* **3**:539–547 (1984).
83. Ward, J. I., Lum, M. K. W., Hall, D. B., Silimperi, D. R., and Bender, T. R., Invasive *H. influenzae* type b disease in Alaska: Background epidemiology for a vaccine efficacy trial, *J. Infect. Dis.* **108**:887–896 (1986).
84. Wotton, K. A., Stiver, H. G., and Hildes, J. A., Meningitis in the central Arctic: A 4-year experience, *Can. Med. Assoc. J.* **124:** 887–890 (1981).
85. Granoff, D. M., Gilsdorf, J., Gessert, C., and Basden, M., *Haemophilus influenzae* type b disease in a day care center: Eradication of carrier state by rifampin, *Pediatrics* **63**:397–401 (1979).
86. Centers for Disease Control, Prevention of secondary cases of *Haemophilus influenzae* type b disease, *Morbid. Mortal. Week. Rep.* **31**:672–680 (1982).
87. Anderson, J. R., Smith, M. D., Kibbler, C. C., Holton, J., and Scott, G. M., A nosocomial outbreak due to a non-encapsulated *Haemophilus influenzae*: Analysis of plasmids coding for antibiotic resistance, *J. Hosp. Infect.* **27**:17–27 (1994).
88. Hekker, T. A., van der Schee, A. C., Kempers, J., Namavar, F., and van Alphen, L., A nosocomial outbreak of amoxicillin-resistant non-typeable *Haemophilus influenzae* in a respiratory ward, *J. Hosp. Infect.* **19**:25–31 (1991).
89. Cochi, S. L., Broome, C. V., and Hightower, A. W., Immunization of US children with *Hemophilus influenzae* type b polysaccharide vaccine: A cost-effectiveness model of strategy assessment, *J. Am. Med. Assoc.* **253**:521–529 (1985).
90. Fraser, D. W., Darby, C. P., Koehler, R. E., Jacobs, C. F., and Feldman, R. A., Risk factors in bacterial meningitis: Charleston County, South Carolina, *J. Infect. Dis.* **127**:271–277 (1973).
91. Ward, J. I., Lum, M. K., Margolis, H. S., Fraser, D. W., and Bender, T. R., *Haemophilus influenzae* disease in Alaskan Eskimos: Characteristics of a population with an unusual incidence of invasive disease, *Lancet* **1**:1281–1285 (1982).
92. Peltola, H., Kayhty, H., Virtanen, M., and Makela, P. H., Prevention of *Haemophilus influenzae* bacteremic infections with the capsular polysaccharide vaccine, *N. Engl. J. Med.* **310**:1561–1566 (1984).
93. Vadheim, C. M., Greenberg, D. P., Eriksen, E., Hemenway, L., Bendana, N., Mascola, L., and Ward, J. I., Eradication of *Haemophilus influenzae* type b disease in Southern California. Kaiser-UCLA Vaccine Study Group, *Arch. Pediatr. Adolesc. Med.* **148**(1):51–56 (1994).
94. Floyd, R. F., Federspiel, C. F., and Schaffner, W., Bacterial meningitis in urban and rural Tennessee, *Am. J. Epidemiol.* **99**:395–397 (1974).
95. Granoff, D. M., Boies, E., Squires, J., Pandey, J. P., Suarez, B., Oldfather, J., and Rodey, G. E., Interactive effect of genes associated with immunoglobulin allotypes and HLA specificities on susceptibility to *Haemophilus influenzae* disease, *J. Immunogenet.* **11**:181–188 (1984).
96. Yost, G. C., Kaplan, A. M., Bustamante, R., Ellison, C., Hargrave, A. F., and Randall, D. L., Bacterial meningitis in Arizona American Indian children, *Am. J. Dis. Chil.* **140**:943–946 (1986).
97. Granoff, D. M., Pandey, J. P., Boies, E., Squires, J., Munson, R. S., and Suarez, B., Response to immunization with *Haemophilus influenzae* type polysaccharide–pertussis vaccine and risk of *Haemophilus* meningitis in children with the Km(1) immunoglobulin allotype, *J. Clin. Invest.* **74**:1708–1714 (1984).
98. Takala, A. K., and Clements, D. A., Socioeconomic risk factors for invasive *Haemophilus influenzae* type b disease, *J. Infect. Dis.* **165**(Suppl. 1):S11 (1992).
99. Granoff, D. M., and Basden, M., *Haemophilus influenzae* infections in Fresno County, California: A prospective study of the effects of age, race, and contact with a case on incidence of disease, *J. Infect. Dis.* **140**:40–46 (1980).
100. Michaels, R. H., and Schultz, W. F., The frequency of *Haemophilus influenzae* infections: Analysis of racial and environmental factors, in: *Hemophilus influenzae* (S. H. W. Sell and D. T. Karzon, eds.), pp. 243–250, Vanderbilt University Press, Nashville, 1973.
101. Tarr, P. I., and Peter, G., Demographic factors in the epidemiology of *Haemophilus influenzae* meningitis in young children, *J. Pediatr.* **92**:884–888 (1978).
102. Campbell, L. R., Zedd, A. J., and Michaels, R. H., Household spread of infection due to *Haemophilus influenzae* type b, *Pediatrics* **66**:115–117 (1980).
103. Filice, G. A., Andrews, J. S., Jr., Hudgins, M. P., and Fraser,

D. W., Spread of *Haemophilus influenzae*: Secondary illness in household contacts of patients with *H. influenzae* meningitis, *Am. J. Dis. Child.* **132:**757–759 (1978).

104. Fleming, D. W., Liebenhaut, M. H., Albanes, D., Cochi, S. L., Hightower, A. W., Makintubee, S., Helgerson, S. D., Broome, C. V., and the Contributing Group, Secondary *Haemophilus influenzae* type b in day-care facilities: Risk factors and prevention, *J. Am. Med. Assoc.* **254:**509–514 (1985).
105. Granoff, D. M., Gilsdorf, J., Gessert, C. E., and Lowe, L., *H. influenzae* type b in a day care center: Relationship of nasopharyngeal carriage to development of anticapsular antibody, *Pediatrics* **65:**65–68 (1980).
106. Ward, J. I., Fraser, D. W., Baraff, L. J., and Plikaytis, B. D., *Haemophilus influenzae* meningitis: A national study of secondary spread in household contacts, *N. Engl. J. Med.* **301:**122–126 (1979).
107. Band, J. D., Fraser, D. W., and Ajello, G., *Haemophilus Influenzae* Disease Study Group, Prevention of *Haemophilus influenzae* type b disease, *J. Am. Med. Assoc.* **251:**2381–2386 (1984).
108. Daum, R. S., and Granoff, D. M., A vaccine against *Hemophilus influenzae* type b, *Pediatr. Infect. Dis. J.* **4:**355–357 (1985).
109. Turk, D. C., An investigation of the family background of acute *Haemophilus* infections in children, *J. Hyg.* **75:**315–332 (1975).
110. Harrison, L. H., Broome, C. V., Hightower, A. W., Hoppe, C. C., Makintubee, S., Sitze, S. L., Taylor, J. A., Gaventa, S., Wenger, J. D., Facklam, R. R., and the *Haemophilus* Vaccine Efficacy Study Group, A day care-based study of the efficacy of *Haemophilus* b polysaccharide vaccine, *J. Am. Med. Assoc.* **260:**1413–1418 (1988).
111. Berg, A. T., Shapiro, E. D., and Capobianco, L. A., Group daycare and risk of serious infectious illnesses, *Am. J. Epidemiol.* **133:** 154–163 (1991).
112. Redmond, S. R., and Pichichero, M. E., *Haemophilus influenzae* type b disease: An epidemiologic study with special reference to day care centers, *J. Am. Med. Assoc.* **252:**2581–2584 (1984).
113. Makintubee, S., Istre, G. R., and Ward, J. I., Transmission of invasive *Haemophilus influenzae* type b disease in day care settings, *J. Pediatr.* **111:**180–186 (1987).
114. Murphy, T. V., Clements, J. F., Breedlove, J. A., Hansen, E. J., and Seibert, G. B., Risk of subsequent disease among day-care contacts of patients with systemic *Haemophilus influenzae* type b disease, *N. Engl. J. Med.* **316:**5–10 (1987).
115. Wenger, J. D., Harrison, L. H., Hightower, A., *et al.*, Day care characteristics associated with *Haemophilus influenzae* disease, *Am. J. Public Health* **80:**1455–1458 (1990).
116. Osterholm, M. T., Pierson, L. N., White, K. E., Libby, T. A., Kuritsky, J. N., and McCullough, J. G., Risk of subsequent transmission of *Haemophilus influenzae* type b disease among children in day care, *N. Engl. J. Med.* **316:**1–4 (1987).
117. Bachrach, S., An outbreak of *Haemophilus influenzae* type b bacteraemia in an intermediate care hospital for children, *J. Hosp. Infect.* **11:**121–126 (1988).
118. Goetz, M. B., O'Brien, H., Musser, J. M., and Ward, J. I., Nosocomial transmission of disease caused by nontypeable strains of *Haemophilus influenzae*, *Am. J. Med.* **96**(4)**:**342–347 (1994).
119. Gilsdorf, J. R., *Haemophilus influenzae* non-type b infections in children, *Am. J. Dis. Child.* **141:**1063–1065 (1987).
120. Smith, P. F., Stricof, R. L., Shayegani, M., and Morse, D. L., Cluster of *Haemophilus influenzae* type b infections in adults, *J. Am. Med. Assoc.* **260:**1446–1449 (1988).
121. Barton, L. L., Granoff, D. M., and Barenkamp, S. J., Nosocomial spread of *H. influenzae* type b infection documented by outer membrane protein subtype analysis, *J. Pediatr.* **102:**820–824 (1983).
122. Hussey, G., Hitchcock, J., Schaaf, H., Coetzee, G., Hanslo, D., van Schalkwyk, E., Pitout, J., and van der Horst, W., Epidemiology of invasive *Haemophilus influenzae* infections in Cape Town, South Africa, *Ann. Trop. Paediatr.* **14:**97–103 (1994).
123. Kaslow, R. A., and Shaw, S., The role of histocompatibility antigens (HLA) in infection, *Epidemiol. Rev.* **40:**8–15 (1981).
124. Ambrosino, D. M., Schiffman, G., Gotschlich, E. C., Schur, P. H., Rosenberg, G. A., DeLange, G. G., van Loghem, E., and Siber, G. R., Correlation between G2m(n) immunoglobulin allotype and human antibody response and susceptibility to polysaccharide encapsulated bacteria, *J. Clin. Invest.* **75:**1935–1942 (1985).
125. Granoff, D. M., Boies, E. G., Squires, J. E., Pandey, J. P., Suarez, B. K., Oldfather, J. W., and Rodey, G. E., Histocompatibility leukocyte antigen and erythrocyte MNSs specificities in patients with meningitis or epiglottitis due to *Haemophilus influenzae* type b, *J. Infect. Dis.* **149:**373–377 (1984).
126. Peterson, G. M., Silimperi, D. R., Rotter, J. I., Terasaki, P. I., Schanfield, M. S., Park, M. S., and Ward, J. I., Genetic factors in *Haemophilus influenzae* type b disease susceptibility and antibody acquisition, *J. Pediatr.* **110:**229–233 (1987).
127. Whisnant, J. K., Rogentine, G. N., Gralnick, M. A., Schlesselman, J. J., and Robbins, J. B., Host factors and antibody response in *Haemophilus influenzae* type b meningitis and epiglottitis, *J. Infect. Dis.* **133:**448–455 (1976).
128. Granoff, D. M., Shackelford, P. G., Pandey, J. P., and Boies, E. G., Antibody responses to *Haemophilus influenzae* type b polysaccharide vaccine in relation to Km(1) and G2m(23) immunoglobulin allotypes, *J. Infect. Dis.* **154:**257–264 (1986).
129. Peterson, G. M., Silimperi, D. R., Scott, E. M., Hall, D. B., Rotter, J. I., and Ward, J. I., Uridine monophosphate kinase 3: A genetic marker for susceptibility to *Haemophilus influenzae* type b disease, *Lancet* **2:**417–419 (1985).
130. Cochi, S. L., Fleming, D. W., Hightower, A. W., and Broome, C. V., Does breast-feeding protect infants from *Haemophilus influenzae* infection? [letter], *J. Pediatr.* **110:**162–163 (1987).
131. Lum, M. K., Ward, J. I., and Bender, T. R., Protective influence of breast-feeding on the risk of developing invasive *H. influenzae* type b disease (Abstract), *Pediatr. Res.* **16**(Part 2)**:**151A (1982).
132. Peterson, G. M., Silimperi, Chiu, C. Y., and Ward, J. I., Effects of age, breast-feeding and household structure on *Haemophilus influenzae* type b disease risk and antibody acquisition in Alaskan Eskimos, *Am. J. Epidemiol.* **134:**1212–1221 (1991).
133. Pichichero, M. E., Sommerfelt, A. E., Steinhoff, M. C., and Insel, R. A., Breast milk antibody to the capsular polysaccharide of *Haemophilus influenzae* type b, *J. Infect. Dis.* **142:**694–698 (1980).
134. Kaleida, P. H., Nativio, D. G., Chao, H. P., and Cowden, S. N., Prevalence of bacterial respiratory pathogens in the nasopharynx in breast-fed versus formula-fed infants, *J. Clin. Microbiol.* **31**(10)**:**2674–2678 (1993).
135. Harabuchi, Y., Faden, H., Yamanaka, N., Duffy, L., Wolf, J., and Krystofik, D., Human milk secretory IgA antibody to nontypeable *Haemophilus influenzae*: Possible protective effects against nasopharyngeal colonization, *J. Pediatr.* **124**(2)**:**193–198 (1994).
136. Powars, D., Overturf, G., and Turner, E., Is there an increased risk of *Haemophilus influenzae* septicemia in children with sickle cell anemia? *Pediatrics* **71:**927–931 (1983).

137. Zarkowsky, H. S., Gallagher, D., Gill, F. M., Wang, W. C., Falletta, J. M., Lande, W. M., Levy, P. S., Verter, J. I., Wethers, D., and the Cooperative Study of Sickle Cell Disease, Bacteremia in sickle hemoglobinopathies, *J. Pediatr.* **109:**579–585 (1986).
138. Chilcote, R., Baehner, R., and Hammond, D., Septicemia and meningitis in children splenectomized for Hodgkin's disease, *N. Engl. J. Med.* **275:**709–715 (1966).
139. Farrand, R. J., Recurrent *Haemophilus* septicemia and immunoglobulin deficiency, *Arch. Dis. Child.* **45:**582–584 (1970).
140. Rosen, F. S., and Janeway, C. A., The gamma globulins: III. The antibody deficiency syndromes, *N. Engl. J. Med.* **275:**709–715 (1966).
141. Ross, S. C., and Densen, P., Complement deficiency states and infection: Epidemiology, pathogenesis, and consequences of neisserial and other infections in an immune deficiency, *Medicine* **63:**243–273 (1984).
142. Bartlett, A. V., Zusman, J., and Daum, R. S., Unusual presentations of *Haemophilus influenzae* infections in immunocompromised patients, *J. Pediatr.* **102:**55–58 (1983).
143. Siber, G. R., Bacteremias due to *Haemophilus influenzae* and *Streptococcus pneumoniae*: Their occurrence and course in children with cancer, *Am. J. Dis. Child.* **134:**668–672 (1980).
144. Weitzman, S., and Aisenberg, A. C., Fulminant sepsis after the successful treatment of Hodgkin's disease, *Am. J. Med.* **62:**47–50 (1977).
145. Michaels, R. H., Poziviak, C. S., Stonebraker, F. E., and Norden, C. W., Factors affecting pharyngeal *H. influenzae* type b colonization rates in children, *J. Clin. Microbiol.* **4:**413–417 (1976).
146. Myerowitz, R. L., and Michaels, R. H., Mechanism of potentiation of experimental *Haemophilus influenzae* type B disease in infant rats by influenza A virus, *Lab. Invest.* **44:**434–441 (1981).
147. Takala, A. K., Meurman, O., Kleemola, M., Kela, E., Ronnberg, P. R., Eskola, J., and Makela, P. H., Preceding respiratory infection predisposing for primary and secondary invasive *Haemophilus influenzae* type b disease, *Pediatr. Infect. Dis. J.* **12**(3)**:**189–195 (1993).
148. Murphy, T. V., Clements, J. F., Petroni, M., Coury, S., and Stetler, L., Survival of *Haemophilus influenzae* type b in respiratory secretions, *Pediatr. Infect. Dis. J.* **8:**148–151 (1989).
149. Gardner, J. S., and Simons, B. P., Guideline for isolation precautions in hospitals, *Infect. Control* **4**(Suppl.)**:**245–349 (1983).
150. Shapiro, E. D., Persistent pharyngeal colonization with *H. influenzae* type b after intravenous chloramphenicol therapy, *Pediatrics* **67:**435–437 (1981).
151. Shapiro, E. D., and Wald, E. R., Efficacy of rifampin in eliminating pharyngeal carriage of *Haemophilus influenzae* type b, *Pediatrics* **66:**5–8 (1980).
152. Lerman, S. J., Kucera, J. C., and Brunken, J. M., Nasopharyngeal carriage of antibiotic-resistant *H. influenzae* in healthy children, *Pediatrics* **65:**287–291 (1979).
153. Masters, P. L., Brumfitt, W., Mendez, R. L., and Likar, M., Bacterial flora of the upper respiratory tract in Paddington families, 1952–4, *Br. Med. J.* **1:**1200–1205 (1958).
154. Mpairwe, Y., Observations on the nasopharyngeal carriage of *H. influenzae* type b in children in Kampala, Uganda, *J. Hyg.* **68:**337–341 (1970).
155. Stephenson, W. P., Doern, G., Gantz, N., Lipworth, L., and Chapin, K., Pharyngeal carriage rates of *Haemophilus influenzae*, type b and non-b, and prevalence of ampicillin-resistant *Haemophilus influenzae* among healthy day-care children in central Massachusetts, *Am. J. Epidemiol.* **122:**868–875 (1985).
156. Greenfield, S., Peter, G., Howie, V. M., Ploussard, J. H., and Smith, O. H., Acquisition of type-specific antibodies to *H. influenzae* type b, *J. Pediatr.* **80:**204–208 (1972).
157. Hall, D. B., Lum, M. K. W., Knutson, L. R., Heyward, W. L., and Ward, J. I., Pharyngeal carriage and acquisition of anticapsular antibody to *Haemophilus influenzae* type b in a high-risk population in southwestern Alaska, *Am. J. Epidemiol.* **126:**1190–1197 (1987).
158. Lagos, R., Avendano, A., Horwitz, I., *et al.*, Molecular epidemiology of *Haemophilus influenzae* with families in Santiago, Chile, *J. Infect. Dis.* **164:**1149–1153 (1991).
159. Michaels, R. H., and Norden, C. W., Pharyngeal colonization with *H. influenzae* type b: A longitudinal study of families with a child with meningitis or epiglottitis due to *H. influenzae* type b, *J. Infect. Dis.* **136:**222–228 (1977).
160. Schneerson, R., and Robbins, J. B., Induction of serum *H. influenzae* type b capsular antibodies in adult volunteers fed cross-reacting *Escherichia coli* O75:K100:H5, *N. Engl. J. Med.* **292:** 1093–1096 (1975).
161. Michaels, R. H., Stonebraker, F. E., and Robbins, J. B., Use of antiserum agar for detection of *H. influenzae* type b in the pharynx, *Pediatr. Res.* **9:**513–516 (1975).
162. Takela, A. K., Eskola, J., Leinoene, M., *et al.*, Reduction of oropharyngeal carriage of *Haemophilus influenzae* type b (Hib) in children with a Hib conjugate vaccine, *J. Infect. Dis.* **164:**982–986 (1991).
163. Takela, A. K., Santosham, M., Almeido-Hill, J., *et al.*, Effect of *Haemophilus influenzae* type b (Hib) meningococcal protein conjugate vaccine (Hib-OMP) on oropharyngeal carriage of Hib among American Indian infants and children (Abstract 982), in: *Program and Abstracts of the 32nd Interscience Conference on Antimicrobial Agents and Chemotherapy* (1992).
164. Gilsdorf, J. R., Dynamics of nasopharyngeal colonization with *Haemophilus influenzae* b during antibiotic therapy, *Pediatrics* **77:**242–245 (1986).
165. Peltola, H., Kilpi, T., and Anttila, M., Rapid disappearance of *Haemophilus influenzae* type be meningitis after routine childhood immunization with conjugate vaccines, *Lancet* **340**(8819)**:** 592–594 (1992).
166. Teare, E. L., Fairley, C., K., White, J., and Begg, N. T., Efficacy of Hib vaccine (letter), *Lancet* **344:**828–829 (1994).
167. Smith, A. L., Daum, R. S., Schiefele, D., Syriopoulou, V., Averill, D. R., Roberts, M. C., and Stull, T. L., Pathogenesis of *H. influenzae* meningitis, in: *Haemophilus influenzae* (S. H. Sell and P. F. Wright, eds.), Elsevier, Amsterdam, 1982.
168. Moxon, E. R., Smith, A. L., Averill, D. R., and Smith, D. H., *H. influenzae* meningitis in rats following intranasal inoculation, *J. Infect. Dis.* **129:**154–162 (1974).
169. Ostrow, P. T., Moxon, E. R., Vernon, N., and Kapko, R., Studies on the route of meningeal invasion following *H. influenzae* inoculation of infant rats, *Lab. Invest.* **40:**678–685 (1979).
170. Gregorius, F. K., Johnson, B. J., Stern, W. E., and Brown, W. J., Pathogenesis of hematogenous bacterial meningitis in rabbits, *J. Neurosurg.* **45:**561–567 (1976).
171. Ferry, P. C., Culbertson, J. L., Cooper, J. A., Sitton, A. B., and Sell, S.H., Sequelae of *Haemophilus influenzae* meningitis, in: *Haemophilus influenzae* (S. H. Sell and P. F. Wright, eds.), pp. 111–116, Elsevier, Amsterdam, 1982.
172. Rubin, L. G., and Moxon, E. R., Pathogenesis of bloodstream invasion with *H. influenzae* type b, *Infect. Immun.* **41:**280–284 (1983).

173. Weller, P., Smith, A. L., Anderson, P., and Smith, D. H., The role of encapsulation and host age in the clearance of *H. influenzae* bacteremia, *J. Infect. Dis.* **138:**427–436 (1978).
174. Weller, P., Smith, A. L., Smith, D. H., and Anderson, P., Role of immunity in the clearance of bacteremia due to *H. influenzae*, *J. Infect. Dis.* **135:**34–41 (1977).
175. Murphy, T. B., Pastor, P., Medley, F., Osterholm, M. T., and Granoff, D. M., Decreased *Haemophilus* colonization in children vaccinated with *Haemophilus influenzae* type b conjugate vaccine, *J. Pediatr.* **122**(4):517–523 (1993).
176. Hansen, E. J., Frisch, C. F., and Johnston, K. H., Detection of antibody-accessible proteins on the cell surface of H. influenzae type b, *Infect. Immun.* **32:**950–953 (1981).
177. Inzana, T. J., and Anderson, P., Serum factor-dependent resistance of *H. Influenzae* type b to antibody to lipopolysaccharide, *J. Infect. Dis.* **151:**869–877 (1985).
178. Lagergard, T., Nylen, O., Sandberg, T., and Trollfors, B., Antibody responses to capsular polysaccharide, lipopolysaccharide, and outer membrane in adults infected with *H. influenzae* type b, *J. Clin. Microbiol.* **20:**1154–1158 (1984).
179. Robbins, J. B., Schneerson, R., and Pittman, M., *H. influenzae* type b infections, in: *Bacterial Vaccines* (R. Germanier, ed.), Academic Press, New York, 1984.
180. Crosson, F. J., Jr., Winkelstein, J. A., and Moxon, E. R., Participation of complement in the nonimmune host defense against experimental *H. influenzae* type b septicemia and meningitis, *Infect. Immun.* **14:**882–887 (1976).
181. Quinn, P. H., Crosson, F. J., Jr., Winkelstein, J. A., and Moxon, E. R., Activation of the alternative complement pathway by *H. influenzae* type b, *Infect. Immun.* **16:**400–402 (1977).
182. Steele, N. P., Munson, R. S., Jr., Granoff, D. M., Cummins, J. E., and Levine, R. P., Antibody-dependent alternative pathway killing of *H. influenzae* type b, *Infect. Immun.* **44:**452–458 (1984).
183. Tarr, P. I., Hosea, S. W., Brown, E. J., Schneerson, R., Sutton, A., and Frank, M. M., The requirement of specific anticapsular IgG for killing of *H. influenzae* by the alternative pathway of complement activation, *J. Immunol.* **128:**1772–1775 (1982).
184. Winkelstein, J. A., and Moxon, E. R., Role of complement in the host's defense against *H. influenzae*, in: *Haemophilus influenzae* (S. H. Sell and P. F. Wright, eds.), Elsevier, Amsterdam, 1982.
185. Hayashi, K., Lee, D. A., and Quie, P. G., Chemiluminescent response of polymorphonuclear leukocytes to *Streptococcus pneumoniae* and *H. influenzae* in suspension and adhered to glass, *Infect. Immun.* **52:**397–400 (1986).
186. Newman, S. L., Waldo, B., and Johnston, R. B., Jr., Separation of serum bactericidal and opsonizing activities for *H. influenzae* type b, *Infect. Immun.* **8:**488–490 (1973).
187. Anderson, P., Peter, G., Johnston, R. B., Jr., Wetterlow, L. H., and Smith, O. H., Immunization of humans with polyribophosphate, the capsular antigen of *H. influenzae* type b, *J. Clin. Invest.* **51:**39–44 (1972).
188. Dahlberg-Lagergard, T., Target antigens for bactericidal and opsonizing antibodies to *H. influenzae*, *Acta Pathol. Microbiol. Scand.* **90:**209–216 (1982).
189. Feigin, R. D., Tichmond, D., Hisler, M. W., and Shackelford, P.G., Reassessment of the role of bactericidal antibody in *H. influenzae* infection, *Am. J. Med. Sci.* **262:**338–346 (1971).
190. Lee, C. J., Malik, F. G., and Robbins, J. B., The regulation of the immune response of mice to *H. influenzae* type b capsular polysaccharide, *Immunology* **34:**149–156 (1978).
191. Myerowitz, R. L., and Norden, C. W., Immunology of the infant rat experimental model of *H. influenzae* type b meningitis, *Infect. Immun.* **16:**218–225 (1977).
192. Schneerson, R., and Robbins, J. B., Age-related susceptibility to *H. influenzae* type b disease in rabbits, *Infect. Immun.* **4:**397–401 (1971).
193. Eskola, J., Peltola, H., Takala, A. K., Kayhty, H., Hakulinen, M., Karonko, V., Kela, E., Rekola, P., Ronnberg, P. R., Samuelson, J. S., Gordon, L. K., and Markela, P. H., Efficacy of *Haemophilus influenzae* type b polysaccharide–diphtheria toxoid conjugate vaccine in infancy, *N. Engl. J. Med.* **317:**717–722 (1987).
194. Anderson, P., Smith, D. H., Ingram, D. L., Wilkins, J., Wehrle, P. F., and Howie, V. M., Antibody to polyribophosphate of *H. influenzae* type b in infants and children: Effect of immunization with polyribophosphate, *J. Infect. Dis.* **136**(Suppl.1)**:**S57–S62 (1977).
195. Kayhty, H., Karanko, V., Peltola, H., and Makela, P. H., Serum antibodies after vaccination with *Haemophilus influenzae* type b capsular polysaccharide and responses to reimmunization: No evidence of immunological tolerance or memory, *Pediatrics* **74:**857–865 (1984).
196. Smith, D. H., Peter, G., Ingram, D. L., Harding, A. L., and Anderson, P., Responses of children immunized with the capsular polysaccharide of *Haemophilus influenzae*, type b, *Pediatrics* **52:**637–644 (1973).
197. Anderson P. The protective level of serum antibodies to the capsular polysaccharide of *Haemophilus influenzae* type b, *J. Infect. Dis.* **149:**1034 (1984).
198. Kayhty, H., Peltola, H., Karanko, V., and Makela, P. H., The protective level of serum antibodies to the capsular polysaccharide of *Haemophilus influenzae* type b, *J. Infect. Dis.* **147:**1100 (1983).
199. Schreiber, J. R., Barrus, V., Cates, K. L., and Siber, G. R., Functional characterization of human IgG, IgM, and IgA antibody directed to the capsule of *H. influenzae* type b, *J. Infect. Dis.* **153:**8–16 (1986).
200. Kaplan, S. L., Mason, E. O., Jr., Johnson, G., Broughton, R. A., Hurley, D., and Parke, J. C., Enzyme-linked immunosorbent assay for detection of capsular antibodies against *H. influenzae* type b: Comparison with radioimmunoassay, *J. Clin. Microbiol.* **18:**1201–1204 (1983).
201. Kayhty, H., Jousimies-Somer, H., Peltola, H., and Makela, P. H., Antibody response to capsular polysaccharides of groups A and C *Neisseria meningitidis* and *H. Influenzae* type b during bacteremic disease, *J. Infect. Dis.* **143:**32–41 (1981).
202. Kaythy, H., Schneerson, R., and Sutton, A., Class-specific antibody response to *H. influenzae* type b capsular polysaccharide vaccine, *J. Infect. Dis.* **148:**767 (1983).
203. Schneerson, R., Robbins, J. B., Parke, J. C., Bell, C., Schlesselman, J. J., Sutton, A., Wang, Z., Schiffman, G., Karpas, A., and Shiloach, J., Quantitative and qualitative analyses of serum antibodies elicited in adults by *H. influenzae* type b and pneumococcus type 6A capsular polysaccharide–tetanus toxoid conjugates, *Infect. Immun.* **52:**519–528 (1986).
204. Beuvery, E. C., Van Rossum, F., and Nagel, J., Comparison of the induction of immunoglobulin M and G antibodies in mice with purified pneumococcal type 3 and meningococcal group G polysaccharides and their protein conjugates, *Infect. Immun.* **37:**15–22 (1982).
205. Jennings, H. J., Capsular polysaccharides as human vaccines, *Adv. Carbohydr. Chem. Biochem.* **41:**155–208 (1983).
206. Oxelius, V.-A., Quantitative and qualitative investigations of

serum IgG subclasses in immunodeficiency diseases, *Clin. Exp. Immunol.* **36:**112–116 (1979).

207. Ramadas, K., Peterson, G. M., Heiner, D. C., and Ward, J. I., Class and subclass antibodies to *H. influenzae* type b capsule: Comparison of invasive disease and natural exposure, *Infect. Immun.* **53:**468–490 (1986).
208. Shackelford, P. G., Granoff, D. M., Nahm, M. H., Scott, M. G., Suarez, B., Pandey, J. P., and Nelson, S. J., Relation of age, race, and allotype to immunoglobulin subclass concentrations, *Pediatr. Res.* **19:**846–849 (1985).
209. Shackelford, P. G., Granoff, D. M., Nelson, S. J., Scott, M. G., Smith, D. S., and Nahm, M. H., Subclass distribution of human antibodies to *Haemophilus influenzae* type b capsular polysaccharide, *J. Immunol.* **138:**587–592 (1987).
210. Siber, G. R., Schur, P. H., Aisenberg, A. C., Weitzman, S. A., and Schiffman, G., Correlation between serum IgG-2 concentrations and the antibody response to bacterial polysaccharides, *N. Engl. J. Med.* **303:**178–182 (1980).
211. Griffiss, J. M., and Bertram, M. A., Immunoepidemiology of meningococcal disease in military recruits. II. Blocking of serum bacterial activity by circulating IgA early in the course of invasive disease, *J. Infect. Dis.* **136:**733–739 (1977).
212. Musher, D. M., Goree, A., Baughn, R. E., and Birdsall, H. H., Immunoglobulin A from bronchopulmonary secretions blocks bactericidal and opsonizing, effects of antibody to nontypeable *H. influenzae*, *Infect. Immun.* **45:**36–40 (1984).
213. Rosales, S. V., Lascolea, L. J., Jr., and Ogra, P. L., Development of respiratory mucosal tolerance during *H. Influenzae* type b infection in infancy, *J. Immunol.* **132:**1517–1521 (1984).
214. Davie, J. M., Antipolysaccharide immunity in man and animals, in: *Haemophilus influenzae* (S. H. Sell and P. F. Wright, eds.), pp. 129–134, Elsevier, Amsterdam, 1982.
215. Huber, B. R., B cell differentiation antigens as probes for functional B cell subsets, *Immunol. Rev.* **64:**57–79 (1982)
216. Landsteiner, K., *The Specificity of Serological Reactions*, rev. ed., Harvard University Press, Cambridge, MA, 1945 (reprinted by Dover Publications, New York, 1962).
217. Ambrosino, D. M., Barrus, V. A., DeLange, G. G., and Siber, G. R., Correlation of the Km(1) immunoglobulin allotype with anti-polysaccharide antibodies in Caucasian adults, *J. Clin. Invest.* **78:**361–365 (1986).
218. Pandey, J. P., Fudenberg, H. H., Virella, G., Kyong, C. U., Loadhold, C. B., Galbraith, R. M., Gotschlich, E. C., and Parke, J. C., Jr., Association between immunoglobulin allotypes and immune responses to *Haemophilus influenzae* and meningococcus polysaccharides, *Lancet* **1:**190–192 (1979).
219. Pichichero, M. E., and Insel, R. A., Relationship between naturally occurring human mucosal and serum antibody to the capsular polysaccharide of *Haemophilus influenzae* type b, *J. Infect. Dis.* **146:**243–248 (1982).
220. Pichichero, M. E., and Insel, R. A., Mucosal antibody response to parenteral vaccination with *Haemophilus influenzae* type b capsule, *J. Allergy Clin. Immunol.* **72:**481–486 (1983).
221. Pichichero, M. E., Hall, C. B., and Insel, R. A., A mucosal antibody response following systemic *Haemophilus influenzae* type b infection in children, *J. Clin. Invest.* **67:**1482–1489 (1981).
222. Drexhage, H. A., Van de Plassche, E. M., Kokje, M., and Leezenberg, H. A., Abnormalities in cell-mediated immune functions to *Haemophilus influenzae* in chronic purulent infections of the upper respiratory tract, *Clin. Immunol. Immunopathol.* **28:**218–228 (1983).
223. Harding, A. L., Anderson, P., Howie, V. M., Ploussard, J. H., and Smith, D. H., *Haemophilus influenzae* isolated from otitis media, in: *Haemophilus influenzae* (S. H. W. Sell and D. T. Karzon, eds.), pp. 21–28, Vanderbilt University Press, Nashville, 1973.
224. Campognone, P., and Singer, D. B., Neonatal sepsis due to nontypable *Haemophilus influenzae*, *Am. J. Dis. Child.* **140:**117–121 (1986).
225. Wallace, R. J., Baker, C. J., Quinones, F. J., Hollis, D. G., Weaver, R. C., and Wiss, K., Nontypeable *Haemophilus influenzae* (biotype 4) as a neonatal, maternal, and genital pathogen, *Rev. Infect. Dis.* **5:**123–136 (1983).
226. Silverman, M., Stratton, D., Diallo, A., and Egler, L. J., Diagnosis of acute bacterial pneumonia in Nigerian children, *Arch. Dis. Child.* **52:**925–931 (1977).
227. Shann, F., Gratten, M., Germer, S., Linnemann, V., Hazlett, D., and Payne, R., Aetiology of pneumonia in children in Goroka Hospital, Papua New Guinea, *Lancet* **2:**537–541 (1984).
228. Wall, R. A., Mabey, D. C. W., and Corrah, P. T., *Haemophilus influenzae* non-type b, *Lancet* **2:**845 (1985).
229. Wall, R. A., Corrah, P. T., Mabey, D. C. W., and Greenwood, B. M., The etiology of lobar pneumonia in the Gambia, *Bull. WHO* **64:**553–558 (1986).
230. Klein, J. O., Feigin, R. D., and McCracken, G. H., Jr., Report of the Task Force on Diagnosis and Management of Meningitis, *Pediatrics* **78**(Suppl.)**:**S959–S982 (1986).
231. Mendelman, P. M., and Smith, A. L., *Haemophilus influenzae*, in: *Textbook of Pediatric Infectious Diseases*, 2nd ed. (R. D.Feigin and J. D. Cherry, eds.), pp. 1142–1163, Saunders, Philadelphia, 1987.
232. Mayosmith, M. F., Hirsch, P. J., Wodzinski, S. F., and Schiffman, F. J., Acute epiglottitis in adults: An eight-year experience in the state of Rhode Island, *N. Engl. J. Med.* **314:**1133–1139 (1986).
233. Chusid, M. J., Schneider, J. P., Thometz, J. G., and Dunne, W. M., Osteomyelitis and septic arthritis caused by *Haemophilus influenzae*, type f, in a young girl, *Diagn. Microbiol. Infect. Dis.* **15**(20:157–159 (1992).
234. Clarke, C. W., Hannant, C. A., Scicchitano, R., *et al.*, Antigen of *Haemophilus influenzae* in bronchial tissue, *Thorax* **36:**665–668 (1981).
235. Falla, T. J., Dobson, S. R. M., Crook, D. W. M., *et al.*, Population-based study of non-typeable *Haemophilus influenzae* invasive disease in children and neonates, *Lancet* 851–854 (1993).
236. Pauwels, R., Verschraegen, G., and Van Der Straeten, M., IgE antibodies to bacteria in patients with bronchial asthma, *Allergy* **157:**665–669 (1980).
237. Bluestone, C. D., Stephenson, J. S., and Martin, L. M., Ten-year review of otitis media pathogens, *Pediatr. Infect. Dis. J.* **11:**S7–S11 (1992).
238. Danford, D. A., Kugler, J. D., Cheatham, J. P., *et al.*, *Haemophilus influenzae* endocarditis: Successful treatment with ampicillin and early valve replacement, *Nebr. Med. J.* **69:**88–91 (1984).
239. Wilson, W. R., Karchmer, A. W., Dajani, A. S., *et al.*, Antibiotic treatment of adults with infective endocarditis due to streptococci, enterococci, staphylococci, and HACEK microorganisms, *J. Am. Med. Assoc.* **274:**1706–1713 (1995).
240. Harrison, L. H., da Silva, G. A., Pittman, M., *et al.*, Epidemiology and clinical spectrum of Brazilian purpuric fever. Brazilian Purpuric Fever Study Group, *J. Clin. Microbiol.* **27:**599–604 (1989).
241. Hammond, G. W., Slutchuk, M., Scatiff, J., *et al.*, Epidemiologic, clinical, laboratory and therapeutic features of an urban outbreak of chancroid in North America, *Rev. Infect. Dis.* **2:**867–869 (1980).
242. Dodge, P. R., and Swartz, M. N., Bacterial meningitis—A review

of selected aspects. II. Special neurologic problems, post-meningitis complications and clinicopathological correlations, *N. Engl. J. Med.* **272:**1003–1010 (1965).

243. Sell, S. H. W., Merrill, R. E., Doyne, E. O., and Zinsky, E. P., Jr., Long-term sequelae of *Haemophilus influenzae* meningitis, *Pediatrics* **49:**206–217 (1972).

244. Taylor, H. G., Michaels, R. H., Mazur, P. M., and Liden, C. B., Intellectual neuropsychological and achievement outcomes in children six to eight years after recovery from *Haemophilus influenzae* meningitis, *Pediatrics* **74:**198–205 (1984).

245. Cooper, R. F., Bagwell, C., and Smith, T. B., Hearing loss in pediatric meningitis, *Am. Fam. Physician* **35:**133–138 (1987).

246. Kaplan, S. L., Catlin, F. I., Weaver, T., and Feigin, R. D., Onset of hearing loss in children with bacterial meningitis, *Pediatrics* **73:**575–578 (1984).

247. Vienny, H., Despland, P. A., Lutschg, J., Deonna, T., Dutoit-Marco, M. L., and Gander, C., Early diagnosis and evaluation of deafness in childhood bacterial meningitis: A study using brainstem auditory evoked potentials, *Pediatrics* **73:**579–586 (1984).

248. Wolff, A. B., and Brown, S. C., Demographics of meningitis-induced hearing impairment: Implications for immunization of children against *Hemophilus influenzae* type b, *Am. Ann. Deaf.* **132:**26–30 (1987).

249. Howard, J. B., Highgenboten, C. L., and Nelson, J. D., Residual effects of septic arthritis in infancy and childhood, *J. Am. Med. Assoc.* **236:**932–935 (1976).

250. Welkon, C. J., Long, S. S., Fisher, M. C., and Alburger, P. D., Pyogenic arthritis in infants and children: A review of 95 cases, *Pediatr. Infect. Dis. J.* **5:**669–676 (1986).

251. Devine, L. F., Johnson, L. F., Johnson, D. P., Hagerman, C. R., Pierce, W. E., Rhode, S. L., and Peckinpaugh, R. O., Rifampin: Levels in serum and saliva and effect on the meningococcal carrier state, *J. Am. Med. Assoc.* **214:**1055–1059 (1970).

252. McCracken, G. H., Jr., Ginsburg, C. M., Zweighaft, T. C., and Clahsen, J., Pharmacokinetics of rifampin in infants and children: Relevance to prophylaxis against *Haemophilus influenzae* type b disease, *Pediatrics* **66:**17–21 (1980).

253. Glode, M. P., Daum, R. S., Halsey, N. A., Johansen, T. L., Goldmann, D. A., Ambrosino, D., Boies, E., and Granoff, D. M., Rifampin alone and in combination with trimethoprim in chemoprophylaxis for infections due to *Haemophilus influenzae* type b, *Rev. Infect. Dis.* **5**(Suppl.)**:**S549–S555 (1983).

254. Cox, F., Trincher, R., Rissing, J. P., Patton, M., McCracken, G. H., Jr., and Granoff, D. M., Rifampin prophylaxis for contacts of *Haemophilus influenzae* type b disease, *J. Am. Med. Assoc.* **245:** 1043–1045 (1981).

255. Gilsdorf, J. R., Bacterial meningitis in southwestern Alaska, *Am. J. Epidemiol.* **106:**388–391 (1977).

256. Boies, E. G., Granoff, D. M., Squires, J. E., and Barenkamp, S. J., Development of *Haemophilus influenzae* type b meningitis in a household contact treated with rifampin, *Pediatrics* **70:**141–142 (1982).

257. Murphy, T. V., McCracken, G. H., Jr., Moore, B. S., Gulig, P. A., and Hansen, E. J., *Haemophilus influenzae* type b disease after rifampin prophylaxis in a day-care center: Possible reasons for its failure, *Pediatr. Infect. Dis. J.* **2:**193–198 (1983).

258. Skolnick, J. L., Stoler, B. S., Katz, D. B., and Anderson, W. H., Rifampin, oral contraceptives, and pregnancy, *J. Am. Med. Assoc.* **236:**1382 (1976).

259. Eickhoff, T. C., *In vitro* and *in vivo* studies of resistance to rifampin in meningococci, *J. Infect. Dis.* **123:**414–420 (1971).

260. Glode, M. P., Joffe, L. S., Brogden, R., and Kuo, J., Reimmunization of children immunized at 18 months of age with *Haemophilus influenzae* type b vaccine, *J. Pediatr.* **112:**703–708 (1988).

261. Murphy, T. V., McCracken, G. H., Jr., Zweighaft, T. C., and Hansen, E. J., Emergence of rifampin-resistant *Haemophilus influenzae* after prophylaxis, *J. Pediatr.* **99:**406–409 (1981).

262. Yogev, R., Melick, C., and Glogowski, W., *In vitro* development of rifampin resistance in clinical isolates of *Haemophilus influenzae* type b, *Antimicrob. Agents Chemother.* **21:**387–389 (1982).

263. Doern, G. V., Jorgensen, J., Thornsberry, C., Preston, D. A., Tubert, T., Redding, J. S., and Maher, L. A., National collaborative study of the prevalence of antimicrobial resistance among clinical isolates of *Haemophilus influenzae*, *Antimicrob. Agents. Chemother.* **32:**180–185 (1988).

264. Yogev, R., Lander, H. B., and Davis, A. T., Effect of TMP-SMX on nasopharyngeal carriage of ampicillin-sensitive and ampicillin-resistant *Hemophilus influenzae* type b, *J. Pediatr.* **93:**394–397 (1978).

265. Horner, D. B., McCracken, G. H., Jr., Ginsburg, C. M., and Zweighaft, T. C., A comparison of three antibiotic regimens for eradication of *Haemophilus influenzae* type b from the pharynx of infants and children, *Pediatrics* **66:**136–138 (1980).

266. Anderson, P., and Smith, D. H., Isolation of the capsular polysaccharide from culture supernatant of *Haemophilus influenzae* type b, *Infect. Immun.* **15:**472–477 (1977).

267. Argaman, M., Lin, T. Y., and Robbins, J. B., Polyribitol–phosphate: An antigen of four gram-positive bacteria cross-reactive with the capsular polysaccharide of *Haemophilus influenzae* type b, *J. Immunol.* **112:**649–655 (1974).

268. Makela, P. H., Peltola, H., Kayhty, H., Jousimies, H., Pettay, O., Ruoslathi, E., Sivonen, A., and Renkonen, O. V., Polysaccharide vaccines of group A *Neisseria meningitidis* and *Haemophilus influenzae* type b: A field trial in Finland, *J. Infect. Dis.* **136** (Suppl.)**:**S43–S50 (1977).

269. Berkowitz, C. D., Ward, J. I., Chiu, C. E., Marcy, S. M., Hendley, J. O., Meier, K., Marchant, C. D., McVerry, P., and Gordon, L., Persistence of antibody and responses to reimmunization with *Haemophilus influenzae* type b vaccines polysaccharide and polysaccharide diphtheria toxic conjugate vaccines in children initially immunized at 15 to 24 months, *Pediatrics* **85:**288–293 (1990).

270. Granoff, D. M., Shackelford, P. G., Suarez, B. K., Nahm, M. H., Cates, K. L., Murphy, T. V., Karasic, R., Osterholm, M. T., Pandey, J. P., Daum, R. S., and The Collaborative Group, *Haemophilus influenzae* type b disease in children vaccinated with type b polysaccharide vaccine, *N. Engl. J. Med.* **315:**1584–1590 (1986).

271. Ward, J. I., Is *Haemophilus influenzae* type b disease preventable? *J. Am. Med. Assoc.* **253:**554–556 (1985).

272. Daum, R. S., Marcuse, E. K., Giebink, G. S., Hall, C. B., Lepow, M. L., McCracken, G. H., Peter, G., Phillips, C. F., Wright, H. T., and Plotkin, S. A., *Haemophilus influenzae* type b vaccines: Lessons from the past, *Pediatrics* **81:**893–897 (1988).

273. Murphy, T. V., *Haemophilus* b polysaccharide vaccine: Need for continuing assessment, *Pediatr. Infect. Dis. J.* **6:**701–703 (1987).

274. Ward, J. I., Broome, C. V., Harrison, L. H., Shinefield, H. R., and Black, S. B., *Haemophilus influenzae* type b vaccines: Lessons for the future, *Pediatrics* **81:**886–892 (1988).

275. Avery, O. T., and Goebel, W. F., Chemo-immunological studies on conjugate carbohydrate–proteins. II. Immunological specificity of synthetic sugar–protein antigens, *J. Exp. Med.* **50:**533–550 (1929).

276. Goebel, W. F., Studies on antibacterial immunity induced by artificial antigens. I. Immunity to experimental pneumococcal infection with an antigen containing cellobiuronic acid, *J. Exp. Med.* **69:**353–364 (1939).
277. Goebel, W. F., and Avery, O. T., Chemo-immunological studies on conjugated carbohydrate–proteins. I. The synthesis of *p*-aminophenol β-glucoside, *p*-aminophenol β-galactoside, and their coupling with serum globulin, *J. Exp. Med.* **50:**521–531 (1929).
278. Schneerson, R., Barrera, O., Sutton, A., and Robbins, J. B., Preparation, characterization, and immunogenicity of *Haemophilus influenzae* type b polysaccharide–protein conjugates, *J. Exp. Med.* **152:**361–376 (1980).
279. Gordon, L.K., Characterization of a hapten-carrier conjugate vaccine, *H. influenzae*-diphtheria conjugate vaccine, in: *Modern Approaches to Vaccines* (R. M. Chanock, and R. A. Lerner, eds.), pp. 393–396, Cold Spring Harbor Laboratory, Cold Spring Harbor, NY, 1984.
280. Anderson, P., Antibody responses to *Haemophilus influenzae* type b and diphtheria toxin induced by conjugates of oligosaccharides of the type b capsule with the nontoxic protein CRM_{197}, *Infect. Immun.* **39:**233–238 (1983).
281. Tai, J. Y., Vella, P., and McLean, A. A., *Haemophilus influenzae* type b polysaccharide–protein conjugate vaccine (42460), *Proc. Soc. Exp. Biol. Med.* **184:**154–161 (1987).
282. Marburg, S., Jorn, D., Tolman, R. L., Arison, B., McCauley, J., Kniskern, P. J., Hagopian, A., and Vella, P. P., Biomolecular chemistry of macromolecules: Synthesis of bacterial polysaccharide conjugates with *Neisseria meningitidis* membrane protein, *J. Am. Chem. Soc.* **108:**5282–5287 (1986).
283. Gotoff, S. P., On the surface of *H. influenzae*, *J. Infect. Dis.* **143:**747–748 (1981).
284. Chu, C-Y., Schneerson, R., Robbins, J. B., and Rastogi, S. C., Further studies on the immunogenicity of *Haemophilus influenzae* type b and pneumococcal type 6A polysaccharide–protein conjugates, *Infect. Immun.* **40:**245–256 (1983).
285. Lepow, M. L., Samuelson, J. S., and Gordon, L. K., Safety and immunogenicity of *Haemophilus influenzae* type b polysaccharide–diphtheria toxoid conjugate vaccine in adults, *J. Infect. Dis.* **150:**402–406 (1984).
286. Berkowitz, C. D., Ward, J. I., Meier, K., Hendley, J. O., Brunell, P. A., Barkin, R. A., Zahradnik, J. M., Samuelson, J., and Gordon, L., Safety and immunogenicity of *Haemophilus influenzae* type b polysaccharide and polysaccharide diphtheria toxoid conjugate vaccines in children 15 to 24 months of age, *J. Pediatr.* **110:**509–514 (1987).
287. Holmes, S. J., Murphy, T. V., Anderson, R. S., *et al.*, Immunogenicity of four *Haemophilus influenzae* type b conjugate vaccines in 17- to 19-month old children, *J. Pediatr.* **118:**364–371 (1991).
288. Lepow, M. L., Samuelson, J. S., and Gordon, L. K., Safety and immunogenicity of *Haemophilus influenzae* type b polysaccharide–diphtheria toxoid conjugate vaccine in infants 9 to 15 months of age, *J. Pediatr.* **106:**185–189 (1985).
289. Decker, M. D., Edwards, K. M., Bradley, R., and Palmer, P., Responses of children to booster immunization with their primary conjugate *Haemophilus influenzae* type B vaccine or with polyribosylribitol phosphate conjugated with diphtheria toxoid, *J. Pediatr.* **122**(3)**:**410–413 (1993).
290. Lepow, M., Randolph, M., Cimma, R., Larsen, D., Rogar, M., Schumacher, J., Lent, B., Gainter, S., Samuelson, J., and Gordon, L., Persistence of antibody and responses to booster dose of *H. influenzae* type b polysaccharide diphtheria toxoid conjugate vaccine in infants immunized at 9 to 15 months of age, *J. Pediatr.* **108:**882–886 (1986).
291. Eskola, J., Kayhty, H., Peltola, H., Karanko, V., Makela, P. H., Samuelson, I., and Gordon, L. K., Antibody levels achieved in infants by course of *Haemophilus influenzae* type b polysaccharide/diphtheria toxoid conjugate vaccine, *Lancet* **1:**1184–1186 (1985).
292. Kayhty, H., Eskola, J., Peltola, H., Karanko, V., Makela, P. H., Samuelson, J., and Gordon, L. K., Antibody levels achieved in infants by a course of *H. influenzae* type b polysaccharide/diphtheria toxoid conjugate vaccine, *Lancet* **1:**1184–1186 (1985).
293. Weinberg, G. A., Murphy, T. V., and Granoff, D. M., *Haemophilus influenzae* type b polysaccharide–diphtheria toxoid conjugate vaccine in vaccinated children who developed *Haemophilus disease, Pediatrics* **86:**617–620 (1990).
294. Jakacki, R., Luery, N., McVerry, P., and Lange, B., *Haemophilus influenzae* diphtheria protein conjugate immunization after therapy in splenectomized patients with Hodgkin disease, *Ann. Intern. Med.* **112:**143–144 (1990).
295. Frank, A. L., Labotka, R. J., Rao, S., Frisone, L. R., McVerry, P. H., Samuelson, J. S., Maurer, H., and Yogev, R., *Haemophilus influenzae* type b immunization of children with sickle cell disease, *J. Pediatr.* **82:**571–575 (1988).
296. Lange, B., Jakacki, R., Nasab, A. H., Luery, N., and McVerry, P. H., Immunization of leukemic children with *Haemophilus* conjugate vaccine, *Pediatr. Infect. Dis. J.* **8:**883–884 (1989).
297. Frasch, C. E., Hiner, E. E., and Gross, T. P., *Haemophilus* b disease after vaccination with *Haemophilus* b polysaccharide or conjugate vaccine, *Am. J. Dis. Child.* **145**(12)**:**1379–1382 (1991).
298. Greenberg, D. P., Vadheim, C. M., Bordenave, N., *et al.*, Protective efficacy of *Haemophilus influenzae* type b polysaccharide and conjugate vaccines in children 18 months of age and older, *J. Am. Med. Assoc.* **265:**987–992 (1991).
299. Loughlin, A. M., Marchant, C. D., Lett, S., and Shapiro, E. D., Efficacy of *Haemophilus influenzae* type b vaccines in Massachusetts children 18 to 59 months of age, *Pediatr. Infect. Dis. J.* **11:**374–379 (1992).
300. Shapiro, E. D., and Wald, E. R., Protective efficacy of PRP-D conjugate vaccine against *Haemophilus influenzae* type b (Abstract 604), Program and Abstracts of the 30th ICAAC, Atlanta, GA, 1990.
301. Wenger, J. D., Pierce, R., Deaver, K. A., Plikaytis, B. D., Facklam, R. R., Broome, C. V., and *Haemophilus influenzae* Vaccine Efficacy Study Group, Efficacy of *Haemophilus influenzae* type b polysaccharide–diphtheria toxoid conjugate vaccine in US children aged 18–59 months, *Lancet* **338:**395–398 (1991).
302. Eskola, J., Kayhty, H., Takala, A. K., *et al.*, A randomized, prospective field trial of a conjugate vaccine the protection of infants and young children against invasive *Haemophilus influenzae* type b disease, *N. Engl. J. Med.* **323:**1381–1387 (1990).
303. Eskola, J., Peltola, H., Kayhty, H., Takala, A. K., and Makela, P. H., Finnish efficacy trials with *Haemophilus influenza* type b vaccines, *J. Infect. Dis.* **165**(Suppl. 1)**:**S137 (1992).
304. Jonsdottir, K. E., Steingrimsson, O., and Olafsson, O., Immunization of infants in Iceland against *Haemophilus influenzae* type b, *Lancet* **340:**252–253 (1992).
305. Zielen, S., Ahrens, P., and Hofmann, D., Efficacy of Hib vaccine, *Lancet* **344:**828 (1994).
306. Vadheim, C. M., Greenberg, D. P., Marcy, S. M., Froeschle, J., and Ward, J. I., Safety evaluation of PRP-D *Haemophilus influ-*

enzae type b conjugate vaccine in children immunized at 18 months of age and older: Follow-up study of 30,000 children, *Pediatr. Infect. Dis. J.* **9:**555–561 (1990).

307. Madore, D. V., Johnson, C. L., Phipps, D. C., Myers, M. G., Eby, R., and Smith, D. H., Safety and immunogenicity of *Haemophilus influenzae* type b oligosaccharide–CRM197 conjugate vaccine in infants aged 15 to 23 months, *Pediatrics* **86:**527–534 (1990).
308. Decker, M. D., Edwards, K. M., Bradley, R., and Palmer, P., Responses of children to booster immunization with their primary conjugate *Haemophilus influenzae* type b vaccine or with polyribosylribitol phosphate conjugated with diphtheria toxoid, *J. Pediatr.* **122:**410–413 (1993).
309. Insel, R. A., and Anderson, P. W., Oligosaccharide–protein conjugate vaccines induce and prime for oligoclonal IgG antibody responses to the *Haemophilus influenzae* b capsular polysaccharide in human infants, *J. Exp. Med.* **163:**262–269 (1986).
310. Santosham, M., Rivin, B., Wolff, M., Reid, R., Newcomer, W., Letson, G. W., Almeido-Hill, J., Thompson, C., and Siber, G. R., Prevention of *Haemophilus influenzae* type b infections in Apache and Navajo children, *J. Infect. Dis.* **165**(Suppl. 1):S144–151 (1992).
311. Decker, M. D., Edwards, K. M., Bradley, R., and Palmer, P., Comparative trial in infants of four conjugate *Haemophilus influenzae* type b vaccines, *J. Pediatr.* **120:**184–189 (1992).
312. Makela, P. H., Eskola, J., Peltola, H., Takala, A. K., and Kayhty, H., Clinical experience with *Haemophilus influenzae* type b conjugate vaccines, *Pediatrics* **85:**651–653 (1990).
313. Insel, R. A., and Anderson, P. W., Response to oligosaccharide–protein conjugate vaccine against *Haemophilus influenzae* type b in two patients with IgG2 deficiency unresponse to capsular polysaccharide vaccine, *N. Engl. J. Med.* **315:**499–503 (1986).
314. Rubin, L. B., Voulalas, D., and Carmody, L., Immunogenicity of *Haemophilus influenzae* type b conjugate vaccine in children with sickle cell disease, *Am. J. Dis. Child.* **146:**340–342 (1992).
315. Edwards, K. M., Decker, M. D., Porch, C. R., Palmer, P., and Bradley, R., Immunization after invasive *Haemophilus influenzae* type b disease. Serologic response to a conjugate vaccine, *Am. J. Dis. Child.* **143:**31–33 (1989).
316. Black, S., Shinefield, H., Ray, P., *et al.*, Safety of combined oligosaccharide conjugate *Haemophilus influenzae* type b (HbOC) and whole cell diphtheria–tetanus toxoids–pertussis vaccine in infancy, *Pediatr. Infect. Dis. J.* **12:**981–985 (1993).
317. Madore, D. V., Johnson, C. L., Phipps, D. C., Popejoy, L. A., Eby, R., and Smith, D. H., Safety and immunologic response to *Haemophilus influenzae* type b oligosaccharide–CRM197 conjugate vaccine in 1- to 6-month-old infants, *Pediatrics* **85:**331–337 (1990).
318. Paradiso, P. R., Hogerman, D. A., Madore, D. V., *et al.*, Safety and immunogenicity of a combined diphtheria, tetanus, pertussis and *Haemophilus influenzae* type b vaccine in young infants, *Pediatrics* **92:**827–832 (1993).
319. American Academy of Pediatrics Committee on Infectious Diseases, *Haemophilus influenzae* type b conjugate vaccines: Recommendations for immunization with recently and previously licensed vaccines, *Pediatrics* **92**(3)**:**480–488 (1993).
320. Calandra, G. B., Lukas, L. J., Jonas, L. C., *et al.*, Anti-PRP antibody levels after a primary series of PRP-OMPC and persistence of antibody titres following primary and booster doses, *Vaccine* **11**(Suppl. 1)**:**S58–62 (1993).
321. Bulkow, L. R., Wainwright, R. B., Letson, G. W., Chang, S. J., and Ward, J. I., Comparative immunogenicity of four *Haemophilus influenzae* type b conjugate vaccines in Alaska Native infants, *Pediatr. Infect. Dis. J.* **12:**484–492 (1993).
322. Granoff, D. M., Anderson, E. L., Osterholm, M. T., Holmes, S. J., McHugh, J. E., Belshe, R. B., Medley, F., and Murphy, T. V., Differences in the immunogenicity of three *Haemophilus influenzae* type b conjugate vaccines in infants, *J. Pediatr.* **21:**187–194 (1992)
323. Reid, R., Santosham, M., Croll, J., Thompson, C., Newcomer, W., and Siber, G. R., Antibody response of Navajo children primed with PRP-OMP vaccine to booster doses of PRP-OMP vs. HbOC vaccine, *Pediatr. Infect. Dis. J.* **12**(10)**:**812–815 (1993).
324. Campbell, H., Byass, P., Ahonkhai, V. I., Vella, P. P., and Greenwood, B. M., Serologic responses to a *Haemophilus influenzae* type b polysaccharide–Neisseria meningitidis outer membrane protein conjugate vaccine in very young Gambian infants, *Pediatrics* **86:**102–107 (1990).
325. Yogev, R., Arditi, M., Chadwick, E. G., Amer, M. D., and Sroka, P. A., *Haemophilus influenza* type b conjugate vaccine (meningococcal protein conjugate)**:** Immunogenicity and safety at various doses, *Pediatrics* **85:**690–693 (1990).
326. Ward, J. I., Bulkow, L., Wainwright, R., and Chang, S., Immune tolerance and lack of booster responses to *Haemophilus influenzae* (Hib) conjugate vaccination in infants immunized beginning at birth (Abstract 984), Program and Abstracts of the 32nd ICAAC, Anaheim, CA, 1992.
327. Mulholland, E. K., Todd, J., Rowe, M., Campbell, H., Byass, P., Vella, P. P., Ahonkhai, V. I., and Greenwood, B. M., Persistence of antibody at 18 months following vaccination of young Gambian infants with PRP-OMPC *Haemophilus influenzae* type b conjugate vaccine, *Ann. Trop. Paediatr.* **13**(2)**:**153–158 (1993).
328. Sood, S. K., Ballanco, G. A., and Daum, R. S., Duration of serum anticapsular antibody after a two-dose regimen of a *Haemophilus influenzae* type b polysaccharide–*Neisseria meningitidis* over membrane protein conjugate vaccine and anamnestic response after a third dose, *J. Pediatr.* **119:**652–654 (1991).
329. Granoff, D. M., Chacko, A., Lottenbach, K. R., and Sheetz, K. E., Immunogenicity of *Haemophilus influenzae* type b polysaccharide–outer membrane protein conjugate vaccine in patients who acquired *Haemophilus* disease despite previous vaccination with type b polysaccharide vaccine, *J. Pediatr.* **114:**925–933 (1989).
330. Santhosham, M., Wolff, M., Reid, R., *et al.*, The efficacy in Navajo infants of a conjugate vaccine consisting of *Haemophilus influenzae* type b polysaccharide and *Neisseria meningitidis* outer-membrane protein complex, *N. Engl. J. Med.* **324:**1767–1772 (1991).
331. Claesson, B. A., Trollfors, B., Lagergard, T., Taranger, J., Bryla, D., Otterman, G., Cranton, T., Yang, Y., Reimer, C. B., Robbins, J. B., and Schreerson, R., Clinical and immunologic responses to the capsular polysaccharide of *Haemophilus influenzae* type b alone or conjugated to tetanus toxoid in 18- to 23-month-old children, *J. Pediatr.* **112:**695–702 (1988).
332. Greenberg, D. P., Vadheim, C. M., Partridge, S., Chang, S. J., Chiu, C. Y., and Ward, J. I., Immunogenicity of *Haemophilus influenzae* type b tetanus toxoid conjugate vaccine in young infants. The Kaiser–UCLA Vaccine Study Group, *J. Infect. Dis.* **170**(1)**:**76–81 (1994).
333. Booy, R., Hodgson, S., Carpenter, L., *et al.*, Efficacy of *Haemophilus influenzae* type b conjugate vaccine PRP-T, *Lancet* **344** (8919)**:**362–366 (1984).
334. Kaplan, S. L., Lauer, B. A., Ward, M. A., *et al.*, Immunogenicity and safety of *Haemophilus influenzae* type b–tetanus protein

conjugate vaccine alone or mixed with diphtheria–tetanus–pertussis vaccine in infants, *J. Pediatr.* **124**(2)**:**323–327 (1994).

335. Kaplan, S. L., Duckett, T., Mahoney, D. H., Jr., *et al.*, Immunogenicity of *Haemophilus influenzae* type b polysaccharide–tetanus protein conjugate vaccine in children with sickle hemoglobinopathy or malignancies, and after systemic *Haemophilus influenzae* type b injection, *J. Pediatr.* **120:**367–370 (1992).
336. Vadheim, C. M., Greenberg, D. P., Partridge, S., Jing, J., Ward, J. I., and Kaiser–UCLA Vaccine Study Group, Effectiveness and safety of an *Haemophilus influenzae* type b conjugate vaccine (PRP-T) in young infants, *Pediatrics* **92:**272–279 (1993).
337. Musser, J. M., Kroll, J. S., Moxon, E. R., and Selander, R. K., Evolutionary genetics of the encapsulated strains of *Haemophilus influenzae*, *Proc. Natl. Acad. Sci. USA* **85:**7758–7752 (1988).
338. Barenkamp, S. J., Granoff, D. M., and Munson, R. S., Jr., Outer membrane protein subtypes of *Haemophilus influenzae* type b and spread of disease in day care centers, *J. Infect. Dis.* **144:**210–217 (1981).
339. Nelson, M. D., Murphy, T. F., van Keulen, H., *et al.*, Studies on P6, an important outer-membrane protein antigen of *Haemophilus influenzae*, *Rev. Infect. Dis.* **10:**S331–S336 (1988).
340. van Alphen, L., Eijk, P., Geelen-van den,, B., and Dankert, J., Immunochemical characterization of variable epitopes of outer membrane protein P2 of nontypeable *Haemophilus influenzae*, *Infect. Immun.* **59**(1)**:**247–252 (1991).
341. Karasic, R. B., Beste, D. J., To, S. C., *et al.*, Evaluation of pilus vaccines for prevention of experimental otitis media caused by nontypeable *Haemophilus influenzae*, *Pediatr. Infect. Dis. J.* **8:**S62–S65 (1989).
342. Trollfors, B., Claesson, B. A., Strangert, K., and Taranger, J., *Haemophilus influenzae* meningitis in Sweden, 1981–1983, *Arch. Dis. Child.* **62:**1220–1223 (1987).
343. Gervaix, A., and Suter, S., Need for prevention of invasive *Haemophilus influenzae* type b infections in Geneva, Switzerland, *Vaccine* **11**(Suppl. 1)**:**S34–37 (1993).
344. Dagan, R., Epidemiology of invasive *Haemophilus influenzae* type b (Hib) disease in Israel, *Vaccine* **11**(Suppl. 1)**:**S43–45 (1993).
345. Hammond, G. W., Rutherford, B. E., Mazdrewics, R., *et al.*, *Haemophilus influenzae* meningitis in Manitoba and the Keewatin District, NWT: Potential for mass vaccination, *Can. Med. Assoc. J.* **139:**743–747 (1988).
346. Howard, A. J., Dunkin, K. T., Musser, J. M., and Palmer, S. R., Epidemiology of *Haemophilus influenzae* type b invasive disease in Wales, *Br. Med. J.* **303:**441–445 (1991).
347. Severian, C., and Lehners, T. H., Epidemiology of invasive *Haemophilus influenzae* disease in a German city, *Klin. Padiatr.* **206**(2)**:**108–111 (1994).
348. McGregor, A. R., Bell, J. M., Abdool, I. M., and Collignon, P. J., Invasive *Haemophilus influenzae* infection in the Australian Capital Territory region, *Med. J. Aust.* **156**(8)**:**569–572 (1992).
349. Shapiro, E. D., Wald, E. R., Margolis, A. G., and Ortenzo, M. E., The decreasing incidence of *Haemophilus influenzae* type b disease in both Connecticut and greater Pittsburgh, PA (Abstract 587), *Pediatr. Res.* **31:**100A (1992).
350. Adams, W. G., Deaver, K. A., Cochi, S. L., Plikaytis, B. D., Zell, E. R., Broome, C. V., and Wenger, J. D., Decline of childhood *Haemophilus influenzae* type b (Hib) disease in the Hib vaccine era, *J. Am. Med. Assoc.* **269**(2)**:**221–226 (1993).

12. Suggested Reading

Mendelman, P. M., and Smith, A. L., *Haemophilus influenzae*, in: *Textbook of Pediatric Infectious Diseases*, 2nd ed. (R. D. Feigin and J. D. Cherry, eds.), pp. 1142–1163, Saunders, Philadelphia, 1987.

Proceedings of a roundtable, *Haemophilus influenzae* type b: The disease and its prevention, *Pediatr. Infect. Dis. J.* **6:**773–807 (1987).

Sell, S. H. and Wright, P. F. (eds.), *Haemophilus influenzae: Epidemiology, Immunology, and Prevention of Disease*, Elsevier, Amsterdam, 1982.

Weinberg, G. A., and Granoff, D. M., Polysaccharide–protein conjugate vaccines for the prevention of *Haemophilus influenzae* type b disease, *J. Pediatr.* **113:**621–631 (1988).

CHAPTER 17

Helicobacter pylori

Karen L. Smith and Julie Parsonnet

1. Introduction

Helicobacter pylori is a corkscrew-shaped, gram-negative rod that lives in the mucous layer of the stomach. The organism is extraordinarily common, infecting at least half of the world's population. Once acquired, infection persists chronically, probably continuing in the stomach throughout the host's life. *H. pylori* infection invariably causes acute and chronic gastric inflammation, but in only a minority of cases does it result in overt clinical disease. Yet, the clinical diseases attributed to *H. pylori* infection, peptic ulcer disease, and gastric malignancy are among the world's most important causes of morbidity and mortality in adults. For this reason, the 1980s and 1990s have borne witness to furious activity concerning diagnosis, treatment, and prevention of this newly rediscovered pathogen.

2. Historical Background

Spiral gastric bacteria have been recognized in the human stomach since 1906.[(1)] As early as the 1930s, pathologists linked these organisms with gastric inflammation.[(2,3)] Later, the organisms were deemed postmortem contaminants, however, and work on gastric spiral bacteria largely ceased by the 1950s.[(4)] Some attention continued to be directed to the surprising production of urease within the gastric mucosa, but a specific connection between this enzyme and the previously identified spiral bacterium was not made.[(5,6)]

In the 1970s, interest in gastric spiral organisms was revived by a few, scattered investigators.[(7–9)] In 1979, Robin Warren, a pathologist in Perth, Australia, began to intensively study the organism and connected it with a common form of gastric inflammation: chronic superficial gastritis.[(10)] On the strength of this pathological data, Barry Marshall, a gastroenterologist in Perth, treated an infected, dyspeptic patient with tetracycline; the patient's symptoms and histological gastritis completely resolved. From then, Warren and Marshall's research accelerated. In 1982, their group made two major advances: they cultured the organism for the first time (it was named *Campylobacter pyloridis*, but was later renamed *Helicobacter pylori* when taxonomic studies determined it was not a *Campylobacter*) and linked it with peptic ulcer disease.[(10)] In 1984, after a period of contentious academic debate, Marshall addressed the skeptics by ingesting the organism, thus inducing a self-limited gastritis.[(11)] Soon thereafter, another investigator repeated the experiment and developed sustained gastric inflammation that did not respond to simple antibiotic regimens.[(12)] These final experiments convinced most doubters of a role for *H. pylori* in producing gastric inflammation.

Since 1984, thousands of articles by hundreds of investigators worldwide have been conducted concerning *H. pylori*. The high prevalence of infection in asymptomatic populations has been amply documented. Moreover, infection has been linked to dyspepsia, peptic ulcer disease, hypertrophic gastropathy, gastric cancer, and gastric lymphoma. The links with peptic ulcer disease and gastric adenocarcinoma have been most convincingly demonstrated. Numerous studies have shown that gastric and duodenal ulcers can be cured more effectively with antibiotic therapy than with acid inhibitors alone. As a consequence, the National Institutes of Health declared *H. pylori* to be a major cause of peptic ulcer disease and recommended antibiotic therapy as a mainstay of treatment.[(13)] Others have demonstrated that *H. pylori* increases risk of gastric cancer at least fourfold. In 1994, the

Karen L. Smith • Department of Medicine, Stanford University School of Medicine, Stanford, California 94305-5405. **Julie Parsonnet** • Department of Health Research and Policy, Stanford University School of Medicine, Stanford, California 94305-5405.

International Agency for Research on Cancer declared *H. pylori* a group 1 carcinogen (a definite cause of cancer in humans).[14]

3. Methodology

3.1. Sources of Mortality Data

H. pylori does not invade beyond the gastric mucosa and does not directly cause fatalities. There are, therefore, no mortality statistics available for *H. pylori* infection. Diseases associated with *H. pylori* infection, however, do lead to death. Mortality statistics for peptic ulcer disease have not been systematically collected, although several investigators in the United States and Europe have analyzed data from local areas. These data reveal decreasing mortality rates from peptic ulcer disease over time.[15–17] The highest mortality has been observed in persons born at the time of the Industrial Revolution, with a gradual decline in risk since. Regional cancer registries throughout the United States provide mortality statistics for gastric malignancies.[18]

3.2. Sources of Morbidity Data

H. pylori infection is not a reportable disease. Information on *H. pylori*-related diseases can be obtained from investigator-generated studies and cancer registries.[18–21] Because dyspepsia is often treated empirically without diagnosis of the underlying pathology, morbidity data for gastric and duodenal ulcers are considered unreliable.

3.3. Surveys

Surveys are the most widely used method for studying the population distribution of *H. pylori* infection. Household, institutional, and population surveys have been conducted in numerous populations worldwide (see Section 5.1). Although small surveys have been conducted using endoscopic diagnosis of infection, serological surveys are the most widely employed cross-sectional design. Because a positive serological test is thought to reflect active rather than past infection, seroprevalence studies can determine the burden of ongoing infection in a population. Breath tests are also becoming popular as surveillance tools, particularly in studies of children.[22–24] These tests, which have high sensitivity and specificity, will undoubtedly see wider use when they become commercially available.

3.4. Laboratory Diagnosis

Both endoscopic and nonendoscopic methods exist to diagnose *H. pylori* infection; none is perfect. The sensitivity and specificity of the diagnostic methods and their respective pros and cons are listed in Table 1.

3.4.1. Isolation and Identification. *H. pylori* is a relatively fastidious organism that does not thrive outside of its natural environment. Despite this, the organism can be cultured from gastric mucosa if proper measures are taken. Biopsies obtained from the stomach should be rapidly placed in transport medium (such as Stuart's medium with chocolate or broth with supplemental serum) to prevent desiccation. Ground gastric biopsy specimens should then be plated on a solid medium as soon as possible.[25] Delay in culture mandates freezing of the biopsy specimen at 4°C until the time of plating. *H. pylori* requires an enriched environment for growth. Many agar bases will sustain the organism if supplemented with blood or serum; antibiotic supplementation in the medium may minimally increase culture sensitivity. Plates should be incubated at 37°C under microaerophilic conditions

Table 1. Diagnostic Tests for *Helicobacter pylori* Infection[a]

Test	Sensitivity (%)	Specificity (%)	Comments	Cost
Endoscopic				
Histology	93–99	95–99	Based on at least two antral biopsies	$$$
Culture	77–92	100	Technically demanding; best reserved for research	$$$
Rapid urease test	89–98	93–98	Endoscopic method of choice for diagnosis	$
Nonendoscopic				
13C or 14C breath test	90–100	89–100	Good for children and for patient follow-up; currently not widely available	$$
Serology	88–99	86–95	Nonendoscopic method of choice for initial diagnosis; not good for short-term follow-up	$

[a]Adapted from Brown, K.E., and Peura, D.A. Diagnosis of *Helicobacter pylori* infection. *Gastroenterol. Clin. North Am.* **22**:106 (1993) (with permission).

(10% CO_2 with 98% humidity).[25] *H. pylori* grows slowly and plates may require 7 days incubation to develop recognizable colonies. Presumptive identification can be made if organisms have typical gram-negative, curved morphology on Gram's stain and produce both catalase and urease. In research settings, a more definitive diagnosis can be made with molecular probes and/or electron microscopy. On rare occasion, *H. pylori* has been cultured from stool and saliva[26,27]; this is not routinely effective.

Culture is the least sensitive but most specific method for diagnosis *H. pylori*. It is particularly insensitive in laboratories with little experience. Because other diagnostic tests are widely available, culture is best reserved for research laboratories with an interest in obtaining isolates for research and/or antimicrobial sensitivity testing.

3.4.2. Other Endoscopic Methods of Diagnosis. Histology is still considered by many to be the "gold standard" for diagnosis. Not only does it reliably identify infection, but it also can provide information on underlying gastric pathology. Because *H. pylori* is not evenly distributed throughout the gastric mucosa, however, at least two biopsies need to be performed to sensitively diagnose infection.[28,29] Routine hematoxylin and eosin staining will usually reveal the organism; the more sensitive but more expensive silver stains should be reserved for inconclusive examinations.[30]

Another commonly used endoscopic test is the rapid urease test. This method exploits the organism's rapid hydrolysis of urea to ammonia and carbon dioxide. A biopsy of the stomach is obtained and placed in a urea-containing medium with a pH indicator. Production of ammonia turns the indicator red and confirms the presence of the organism. The rapid urease test can often be interpreted in less than 1 hr and is substantially less expensive than histology. It does require endoscopy none the less. Reported sensitivity and specificity of rapid urease tests vary considerably from study to study.[31–33] Most, however, show approximately 90% sensitivity with even greater specificity.

3.4.3. Nonendoscopic Diagnostic Tests. The primary nonendoscopic method for diagnosing *H. pylori* is serology. The usual assays are quantitative enzyme-linked immunosorbent assays (ELISAs). These measure serum IgG titers (IgA titers have proven less useful) against *H. pylori*-specific antigens. While it is commonly believed that antibody titers cannot distinguish between active and past infection, this is not the case for *H. pylori* infection. In untreated patients, IgG response to *H. pylori* infection is stable over years, reflecting the chronic nature of infection even in the face of routine antibiotic use.[34] Conversely, 6 months following successful eradication therapy against *H. pylori* infection, antibody titers typically decrease at least 50%.[35,36] This drop in titer appears to be quite sensitive and specific for successful treatment. Unfortunately, a single serum obtained following therapy will not necessarily become quantitatively negative. Thus, comparison of pre- and posttreatment titers is necessary for treatment follow-up.

Numerous commercial ELISA methods are available; the antigens used vary from kit to kit as may the simplicity of the assay methods. Consequently, sensitivity and specificity also vary; some kits perform inadequately.[37] At their best, ELISA kits have sensitivity and specificity for active infection exceeding 90% and sometimes exceeding 95%. ELISAs may also have varying performance from population to population, perhaps due to differences among the *H. pylori* strains used for the ELISA and those found in the population.[37,38] Serological tests should be evaluated in a population before being used for epidemiological or clinical purposes.

Carbon-labeled urea breath tests hold much promise for *H. pylori* diagnosis.[30,39,40] In these tests, the subject ingests either ^{13}C- or ^{14}C-labeled urea. If *H. pylori* is present in the stomach, the labeled urea is metabolized by its urease enzyme into ammonia and labeled CO_2. Using either mass spectroscopy (^{13}C) or scintillography (^{14}C), labeled CO_2 will be measured in exhaled air of an infected patient within 1/2 hr. Although widely used in research settings because of their high sensitivity and specificity, breath tests are not yet commercially available in most countries.

Polymerase chain reaction (PCR) can sensitively detects *H. pylori* DNA in the saliva or dental plaque of persons with gastric infection but is currently only a research tool.[41,42]

4. Biological Characteristics of the Organism

H. pylori is a spiral-shaped, gram-negative rod. It has multiple flagella at one end that provide it with corkscrew motility. In humans, *H. pylori* only lives adjacent to gastric epithelium. It colonizes nowhere else in the body. While most organisms on microscopy appear to be free living within the mucous layer, approximately one fifth are adherent to the mucosal surface.[43] This adherence to gastric tissue appears to be highly specific and is related to features of both the host (e.g., blood group type) and the parasite (e.g., production of adhesions such as pili and hemagglutinins).[44–46] Under stress, *H. pylori* loses its spiral morphology and first becomes more simply curved and eventually coccoid. Some believe the coccoid forms to be metabolically active, transmissible, but noncultivable forms of the organism; most recent data, however, suggest that coccoid forms are not viable.[47,48]

One of *H. pylori's* central features is its prodigious production of urease. This enzyme, a 300- to 625-kDa nickel-containing hexamer, hydrolyzes urea to CO_2 and ammonia.[49] It is produced constitutively by *H. pylori*. In animal models, urease is essential for *H. pylori* colonization of the stomach[50]; it does not appear to be essential for survival once colonization occurs.[43] Within the cell, urease is located on the outer membrane, but it is also actively excreted into the gastric lumen.[43]

Hypotheses abound concerning the physiological role of *H. pylori* urease.[51,52] The organism may use the enzyme to produce a surrounding shell of ammonia and protect itself from the stomach's acid environment. Although *H. pylori* prefers to live in a neutral pH environment (such as is found beneath the gastric mucosa), it can survive in artificial media at a pH of 1.5 if given supplemental urea.[53] Damage to the gastric mucosa induced by urease and/or ammonia may also provide the organism with the necessary nutrients and/or an appropriate environment for attachment and growth. Alternatively, urease-induced ammonia may be important for nitrogen assimilation by the organism. Whatever its function, urease must be of critical importance to *H. pylori*, since its production accounts for a considerable portion of the organism's energy expenditure.

Another potentially important protein of *H. pylori* is its vacuolating cytotoxin. This 87-kDa secreted protein has structural homology with the IgA proteases of *Neisseria* and *Haemophilus*.[54] It received its name from the vacuole formation it induces in tissue culture cells.[55] In mouse models, oral administration of purified cytotoxin not only induces vacuolation of gastric mucosal cell, but also results in inflammation and gastric ulceration.[56] All strains of *H. pylori* possess the cytotoxin (*VacA*) gene, although expression of the protein occurs in only 50% of strains.[57] A separate gene, the cytotoxin-associated (*CagA*) gene, has been found to be an excellent marker for cytotoxin expression; generally, only strains that contain the *CagA* gene will produce functional VacA protein. This association is not causal, however, since specific deletion of the *CagA* gene does not reduce cytotoxin expression. Thus, the function of the 128-kDa surface-exposed CagA protein remains unknown.

H. pylori strains exhibit enormous genetic diversity.[58–60] By fingerprinting methods, it is unusual to find identical strains in different subjects. Fortunately, *H. pylori* is reported to be the first free-living organism to have its genome completely sequenced.[61] Although these sequence data have not yet been made publicly available, it is anticipated the information will rapidly transform our understanding of *H. pylori* and related organisms.

5. Descriptive Epidemiology

5.1. Prevalence and Incidence

Many seroprevalence studies of *H. pylori* have been conducted worldwide and the organism has been found wherever it has been sought. The prevalence of infection, however, varies widely between and within population groups. Prevalence in developed countries is considerably lower than in developing countries. Prevalence of infection within populations also varies with age and socioeconomic status.

Figure 1 consolidates prevalence data from many different studies.[62] In developing countries, a majority of the population is infected by age 10 (Fig. 1). Similarly, immigrants from developing countries to developed countries have a high prevalence of infection; these infections are then retained throughout life.[63,64] In developed countries, prevalence of *H. pylori* is lower. Few children are infected.

Because acute *H. pylori* infection virtually always passes undiagnosed, incidence cannot be estimated from clinical data. Some information on incidence can be gleaned from prevalence data, however. In some surveys, an exponential increase in prevalence with age suggests a steady incidence of infection over time.[65] For example, in whites from the United States, prevalence data correspond closely to a 1% per year rate of infection. In contrast, prevalence in one African-American population conformed to an incidence of 3% per year.[23,65] Most prevalence data, however, do not support a constant incidence rate. In some populations, prevalence distributions suggest a higher incidence in children than among adults.[66] In others, particularly populations of developing countries, extrapolations from prevalence data would tend to indicate a lower incidence rate in children than among adults.[67]

Because of the difficulties in determining incidence based on clinical illness or prevalence data, investigators have repetitively tested for *H. pylori* infection in population cohorts followed over several years (Table 2).[65] Despite differences in study design, the data from developed countries are relatively consistent in their estimations of incidence. In adults, a mean of 0.4% of subjects converted from *H. pylori* seronegative to seropositive per year.[65] In the two studies that evaluated children, the incidence rate was higher than in adults: 2.7% per year. Coincidentally, the incidence rate observed in these pro-

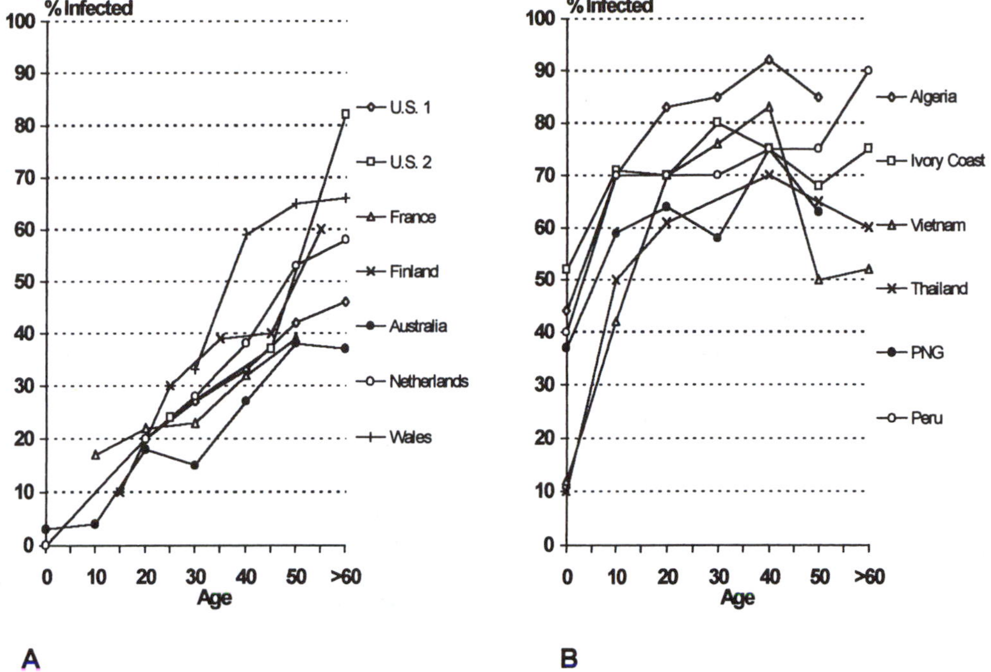

Figure 1. Prevalence of *H. pylori* in healthy persons by age in (A) developed countries and (B) developing countries. From Taylor, D.N., and Blaser, M.J., The epidemiology of *Helicobacter pylori* infection, *Epidemiol. Rev.* **13**:50–51 (1991) (with permission).

spective studies closely matches the incidence of reinfection seen in treated patients. This suggests that prior infection with *H. pylori* neither protects against nor predisposes to reacquisition of the organism.

5.2. Age and Birth Cohort

A disproportionately high prevalence of *H. pylori* infection among older persons may reflect one of two phenomena: an age effect (higher acquisition of infection at older ages) or a cohort effect (older individuals may have been born in times when risk of infection was greater). A birth cohort effect explains better how low incidence rates documented in recent prospective trials can be reconciled with high cross-sectional prevalence. Three of four surveillance studies that examined populations over time demonstrated a decreasing prevalence of *H. pylori* infection with increasing birth year.[34,68–70]

Table 2. Prospective Studies of *H. pylori* Incidence[a]

Population	Follow-up (mean years)	New infections/ total studied	Incidence (%/year)
Dutch endoscopy patients[162]	11.5	2/59	0.3
Australian adults[69]	21	6/89	0.3
American epidemiologists[34]	8.5	11/278	0.5
American heart transplant patients[163]	3.1	1/65	0.5
Canadian cohort[70]	1.5	3/196	1.0
British children[24]	1	4/116[b]	2.7
Okinawa cohort[164]	10	7/64	1.1[c]

[a]Adapted from Parsonnet, J. The incidence of *Helicobacter pylori* infection, *Aliment. Pharamacol. Ther.* **9**(suppl. 2):45–51 (1995).
[b]Used breath test rather than serology to determine infection status.
[c]Incidence = 2.7%/year in children.

Birth cohorts from the United Kingdom ranging from 1900 to 1979 showed a 26% decrease in prevalence per birth decade.[68] Similarly, in a population of US epidemiologists, birth cohort was a stronger predictor of risk than age.[34] Although not all studies confirm a cohort effect,[70] it is generally agreed that *H. pylori* incidence has decreased over time in industrialized countries in parallel with improving hygiene and socioeconomic status.

As mentioned above, prevalence of *H. pylori* infection increases with age in all population groups. An exception to this is seen in the advanced elderly, particularly in developing countries. Serosurveys suggest that the very old may have lower prevalence of *H. pylori* than persons more junior.[62] It has been speculated that this is due to advanced preneoplastic lesions that occur with older age. Since *H. pylori* can only survive adjacent to gastric epithelium, replacement of gastric mucosa by metaplastic intestinal epithelium might result in loss of infection.[71]

5.3. Gender

Men have higher rates of both duodenal ulcer disease and gastric cancer than do women.[72] yet, while *H. pylori* infection is thought to cause both diseases, most studies report no difference between the genders in *H. pylori* prevalence.[73,74] For example, a multinational seroprevalence study found 48.8% prevalence of *H. pylori* in women and 49.1% in men.[75] A recent study of 938 US military recruits did not find gender to be a significant predictor of seropositivity.[76] However, one large study of healthy Californians revealed consistently higher prevalence of antibody to *H. pylori* in men than women (odds ratio = 2.0); this association remained constant across all strata of race/ethnicity, age, education, and income.[72] Meta-analysis of previously published data also showed a modestly elevated risk of infection among men concordant with their elevated risk for *H. pylori*-related diseases.[72] Thus, in some populations, males may have a higher incidence or a higher likelihood of maintaining infection than females. This association may not be uniformly observed worldwide.

5.4. Race–Ethnicity

Serosurveys of *H. pylori* infection have identified pronounced differences in prevalence among racial/ethnic population groups. In the United States, higher prevalence of *H. pylori* has been reported in African-American and Hispanic populations compared to non-Hispanic white populations. The overall seroprevalence in a Maryland population was 57% for African Americans compared with 26% for non-Hispanic whites.[77] This difference was independent of age, gender, dietary practice, and geographic location. Similarly, in Houston, Texas 70% of African Americans were infected compared with 34% of non-Hispanic whites.[23] This remained statistically significant after controlling for age, gender, educational level, current income, and use of tobacco or alcohol. Among male clients of a sexually transmitted diseases (STD) clinic in Denver, 42% of Hispanic and African-American men were infected compared with 12% of white men.[78] Comparable findings have been observed among US Army recruits and healthy young adults from California.[72,76]

Outside of the United States, racial–ethnic variations in *H. pylori* prevalence also have been observed. In Taiwan, the highest seroprevalence (63.4%) was found in a rural indigenous population and the lowest (40.5%) in an urban area inhabited primarily by Hakkas.[79] Indigenous populations in New Zealand also had higher (39–70%) infection rates than white New Zealanders (15%).[80] Somewhat surprisingly, the opposite has been observed in Australia where indigenous populations have less infection (0.5% vs. 15%).[63] Of note, Australian Aborigines have a low incidence of duodenal ulcers. In Belgium, non-Caucasian children were more likely than Caucasian children to be infected.[81]

The reasons for racial–ethnic differences are not entirely understood. Poor socioeconomic conditions during childhood, as measured by household crowding and parental income, are thought to play an important role (see Section 5.5). These cannot, however, completely explain observed differences and a genetic component cannot be entirely excluded.[72] A comparison of *H. pylori* concordance in monozygotic and dizygotic Swedish twins reared apart suggested that a proportion of infection may be attributable to genetic factors.[82]

5.5. Socioeconomic Status

Virtually all studies to date have shown an inverse relationship between *H. pylori* infection and socioeconomic status. A number of markers have been used as indirect measures of socioeconomic status including level of education, crowding, sharing of beds, and availability of indoor plumbing or hot running water in the home. In one large study (the Eurogast serosurvey of 3194 asymptomatic individuals in 17 countries), *H. pylori* seroprevalence showed a significant inverse association with educational level in 11 of the 17 populations[75]; in the remaining six population groups, the inverse relationship remained but did not attain statistical significance. In Wales, age-adjusted prevalence of *H. pylori* was also found to be highest in the lowest social classes (62%), less in the middle class (57%), and lowest in the higher class (49%).(77)

Some studies suggest that socioeconomic status during childhood may serve best as an indicator of *H. pylori* risk. For example, in 150 healthy African Americans and Hispanics between the ages of 19 and 49, a combined index of parental education, occupation, and income was a strong predictor of *H. pylori* infection.(83) Eighty-five percent of adults raised in the lowest socioeconomic stratum had infection compared to 11% in the highest stratum. The association remained after adjustment for age and current social class. Studies of US high-income versus low-income families in Arkansas and in Texas support this finding.(23,84) These data reinforce incidence and prevalence data (Section 5.1) that point to childhood as a critical period for acquiring infection.

6. Mechanisms and Routes of Transmission

6.1. Person-to-Person Transmission

H. pylori has never been isolated from environmental sources or from domesticated animals. Person-to-person spread is therefore considered to be the most likely means of transmission. Whether spread is fecal–oral or oral–oral has yet to be definitively established.

Available data most strongly support a fecal–oral route of transmission, although the evidence is circumstantial. Fecal–oral transmission is most likely to occur in groups where hygiene is suboptimal, such as institutions for the disabled or families with young children, particularly if the children are in diapers. *H. pylori* infection conforms to these expected patterns. Seropositivity rates are higher in individuals in institutionalized populations.(85–87) Clustering also occurs among families, particularly if a child is the index case.(88–90) In Belgium, investigators identified a 2.7-fold increased risk of *H. pylori* among first-degree family members of infected, symptomatic pediatric patients compared to the general population (48.6% compared to 17.8%).(91) Other groups report similar results.(92,93) Strains of *H. pylori* among families are also more likely to be identical in the children. Using the PCR and restriction fragment length polymorphism analysis, children in five families were infected with identical strains of *H. pylori*; in only three of the five families was one parent infected with the identical strain.(93) Seropositivity has also been related to sibship size, birth order, and current number of children in the family, factors that serve as markers for increased risk of fecal–oral transmission within households.(79) Crowding within households particularly engenders greater risk for infection, with sharing of beds during childhood an especially hazardous practice.(67,83,94) Outside of the family setting, crowding and diminished sanitary conditions are also risk factors for development of *H. pylori* infection during adulthood. This is particularly evident in military personnel deployed in close quarters under field conditions.(62,95)

Fecal–oral spread is microbiologically plausible. One investigative team has isolated *H. pylori* from feces of both children and adults, demonstrating that *H. pylori* can pass through the gastrointestinal tract and remain viable.(26,96) These findings, however, still need to be reproduced by other groups.

An oral–oral route is supported by microbiological but not epidemiological studies. *H. pylori* DNA has frequently been recovered by PCR from both saliva and dental plaque.(27,42) Only on a rare occasion, however, has *H. pylori* been actually cultured from the mouth.(27,97) If oral–oral spread is common, however, one would expect rates of infection among dental workers to be elevated compared to age-matched controls. This has not been found to be the case.(98) There is also little concordance of infection among married couples in whom oral–oral transmission might be expected.(64) Moreover, *H. pylori* infection is rare in neonates and young children of infected mothers.(99) Even after 1 year of follow-up in 67 mother–infant pairs, there was no evidence of *H. pylori* transmission from mother to child.(100)

There is currently no evidence to support a role for sexual transmission of *H. pylori* infection. A study of heterosexual couples attending an infertility clinic showed no evidence for partner-to-partner transmission.(64) Similarly, a study of men attending a clinic for STD showed no correlation between *H. pylori* infection and sexual preference, number of sexual partners, history of sexually transmitted diseases, or human immunodeficiency virus (HIV) status.(78)

6.2. Transmission from a Common Environmental Source

Although the preponderance of evidence supports person-to-person spread of infection, there is some evidence to suggest other transmission modalities. A study of children in Lima, Peru revealed an increased risk of *H. pylori* infection in children who drank from the municipal water supply compared with those who drank from private wells.(101) This association was independent of socioeconomic level and presence of indoor plumbing in the household. In Chile, consumption of shellfish and uncooked vegetables was associated with higher rates of *H. pylori* infection, presumably because these vehicles were contaminated by sewage water.[102] Similarities in the epidemiology of *H. pylori* infection and that of the hepatitis A virus have been touted to support of fecal–oral transmission through infected water.[103,104] These correlations may well reflect common socioeconomic conditions, however, rather than common vectors.[105]

No evidence for a food- or waterborne route of transmission has been reported from developed countries. Foods of animal origin also seem an unlikely source since vegetarians and meateaters have similar rates of infection.[77,106]

6.3. Iatrogenic Transmission

Iatrogenic transmission via endoscopy has been well documented through the isolation of identical strains of *H. pylori* from patients undergoing endoscopy in the same suite. Transmission has been estimated to occur in 0.3% of endoscopies when the endoscope is mechanically cleaned with detergent and ethanol alone.[107] More rigorous cleansing methods, however, prevent transmission.[108,109 Endoscopists and endoscopy nurses appear to be at particularly high risk for infection, leading some to call *H. pylori* an occupational hazard.[110,111]

7. Pathogenesis and Immunity

Because acquisition of *H. pylori* infection passes unrecognized, little is known about host and/or bacterial factors required for establishing infection. The only information on incubation period (estimated 3–7 days) derives from a handful of iatrogenic and/or experimental infections of volunteers (see Section 8.1).[11,12] Even when large inocula were given to experimental subjects, however, infection could not be established without altering the natural gastric environment with histamine antagonists. The natural circumstances for acquiring infection are thus unknown. It has been hypothesized that here are "windows of opportunity" (such as periods of hypochlorhydria) when exposed persons are at increased risk for establishing infection. Given the high, but not universal, prevalence of *H. pylori* throughout the world, however, it seems likely that many are exposed who do not develop chronic infection.

H. pylori infection is virtually always accompanied by acute and chronic inflammatory changes in the gastric submucosa. The characteristic, histological lesion has been termed superficial active gastritis, type B gastritis, or, most recently, *H. pylori*-associated chronic gastritis with polymorphonuclear cell activity.[112] In the vast majority of infected patients, lymphoid follicles (mucosal-associated lymphoid tissue) also develop.[113] With rare exception, inflammation is accompanied by elevations in serum IgG against several *H. pylori* antigens including the urease subunits and, when expressed by the bacterium, the vacuolating cytotoxin and the CagA protein. *H. pylori* infection also elicits an IgA response in two thirds of infected persons.[35]

Inflammation is thought to be mediated by several pathogenic factors. *H. pylori* secretes proteins that are absorbed into the lamina propria, causing chemotaxis of both mononuclear and polymorphonuclear and induction of inflammatory cytokines.[114] The vacuolating cytotoxin of *H. pylori* particularly enhances cytokine expression *in vitro*. *In vivo*, persons with cytotoxin-producing strains of *H. pylori* have more severe inflammatory changes.[115] Polymorphonuclear leukocytes undergo an oxidative burst when exposed to *H. pylori* culture supernatant.[116] Secreted proteins of *H. pylori* also appear to directly or indirectly cause epithelial cell damage and death.[56,117) This, too, would tend to augment the inflammatory response as well as precipitate increased epithelial proliferation.

Persons with *H. pylori*-related gastritis can progress to a variety of clinical diseases. The pathogenic mechanisms for the variable outcome of infection, i.e., asymptomatic, ulcer, or cancer, are largely unknown. It is assumed that differences in outcome can be explained by a combination of bacterial, environmental, and host factors. One popular model for peptic ulcer pathogenesis holds that, in some people, *H. pylori* infection increases postprandial gastrin production. This, in turn, increases acid production and predisposes the host to develop gastric metaplasia in the duodenum. Development of gastric metaplasia may be enhanced by environmental factors such as smoking or use of nonsteroidal anti-inflammatory agents. Gastric metaplasia allows *H. pylori* colonization of the duodenal mucosa, where its mucinases and other exoproteins can weaken the mucous barrier in the duodenum, fostering development of peptic ulcer disease.[114,118,119] This process appears to be particularly likely in persons with cytotoxin-producing strains of *H. pylori* and persons with the Lewis(b) blood group phenotype.[44,55]

The pathogenesis of gastric malignancy differs from that of peptic ulcer disease. In some persons with infection, superficial gastritis progresses not to ulcers but to chronic atrophic gastritis, a condition characterized by destruction of the acid-secreting gastric glands.[120] In monkey models, chronic atrophic gastritis can be induced by sustaining *H. pylori* infection in the animal for several years.[121] Persons with atrophic gastritis are predisposed to gastric cancer, but because they have limited acid production, they are largely protected from peptic ulcer disease.[122,123] It is not surprising, however, that this chronic bacterial infection should cause cancer. Chronic inflammation secondary to infection has long been known to predispose to malignancy at the inflamed site. Inflammation typically accelerates cell proliferation, a critical factor in mutation. Inflammation also induces oxidative bursts of free radicals that potentially can damage DNA. Both enhanced cell proliferation and free radical formation have been observed with *H. pylori*-associated gastritis.[124,125] Over a lifetime, one would expect the risk for a carcinogenic mutation to be higher in infected than in uninfected hosts. Undoubtedly, environmental and host factors can augment or minimize cancer risk attributable to *H. pylori* infection. In addition, certain bacterial strains (i.e., those that produce the vacuolating cytotoxin) may be disproportionately associated with malignancy and or cancer precursors than others.[126,127]

Until adequate animal models successfully reproduce human diseases, the above models of *H. pylori* pathogenesis will remain largely hypothetical.

8. Patterns of Host Response

In the absence of specific antimicrobial therapy designed to eradicate the organism, infection with *H. pylori* probably persists throughout life. Restriction fragment length polymorphism analyses demonstrate persistence of specific strains of *Helicobacter* in individuals over several years.[128] Repeated serological testing of infected individuals over time also demonstrates that the serum IgG response does not change in the absences specific eradication therapy.[34,129] Although the majority of infected individuals are asymptomatic, a spectrum of syndromes and diseases, including dyspepsia, peptic ulcer disease, gastric adenocarcinoma, and lymphoma, have been attributed to *H. pylori* infection. While the presence of infection alone may be sufficient in some cases to cause these diseases, it is likely that cofactors such as genetic predisposition, smoking, alcohol, and diet play important roles in determining infection outcome.

8.1. Clinical Spectrum of Disease

Despite histological evidence of inflammation, the majority of individuals infected with *H. pylori* are asymptomatic. In one study, 37% of 113 asymptomatic adult volunteers showed superficial gastritis on gastric biopsy.[130] In another study, 74% of 57 *H. pylori*-positive healthy blood donors were asymptomatic, while 26% reported dyspepsialike symptoms. This was similar to the 24% of *H. pylori*-negative individuals reporting similar symptoms.[131]

8.1.1. Acute Symptomatic Gastritis. While chronic *H. pylori* infection may remain silent, acute infection appears to cause epigastric symptoms. Two investigators experimentally illustrated the clinical features of acute infection by ingesting the organism.[11,12] Each investigator had normal gastric histology prior to the experiment. After neutralization of stomach acid with histamine blockers, 10^9 and 3×10^6 *H. pylori* organisms, respectively, were taken orally. The first investigator developed an acute, self-limited gastritis. He was asymptomatic until day 7 when he developed epigastric discomfort, vomiting, and irritability.[11] Gastroscopy with biopsy on day 10 confirmed infection and revealed antral gastritis. This gastritis had resolved spontaneously by day 14. Neither further symptoms nor an antibody response developed.

The second case of self-induced infection resulted in not only acute but also chronic gastritis.[12] Three days after ingestion, the investigator developed severe epigastric pain, stomach cramping, nausea, vomiting, and insomnia. Mild abdominal discomfort persisted for approximately 11 days after which all symptoms resolved. Biopsies done on day 5 revealed severe inflammation of the antrum with normal fundus. Fasting gastric pH was 1.2 at that time but had increased to 7.6 by day 8. An initial, transient IgM seroconversion was followed by subsequent development of both IgA and IgG antibody against *H. pylori*. Following a 4-week course of bismuth, biopsies revealed no organisms and resolution of inflammatory changes. Biopsy 1 year after ingestion, however, showed persistence of both *H. pylori* and chronic inflammation despite lack of symptoms.[132] The infection and pathological changes remained for over 3 years until combination antimicrobial therapy successfully eradicated the infection.

Acute *H. pylori* infection has also occurred in epidemic form.[133,134] Two endoscopic studies were marred by outbreaks of acute gastritis illness and hypochlorhydria. In the larger of the two studies,[134] an increase in pH was detected in the previously healthy volunteers approximately 1 week after undergoing the gastric secretions studies. This was accompanied by transient epigastric pain, nausea, and vomiting in half of the subjects; the remaining subjects stayed asymptomatic despite increases in gastric pH. Retrospective analysis of biopsy and serum specimens in both series suggested *H. pylori* was the etiologic agent of these outbreaks.

In a serological study of epidemiologists tested for *H. pylori* infection on two occasions spanning a mean of 8 years, chronically infected subjects had similar symptoms to uninfected subjects. Persons who seroconverted in the 8-year interval, however, had significantly higher rates of self-described upper gastrointestinal symptoms. The combined weight of all of these studies suggests that acute infection with *H. pylori* probably causes upper gastrointestinal discomfort in a significant proportion of persons. The clinical illness, however, is not specific and acute infection remains undiagnosed. Once chronic, the majority of infections are silent.

8.1.2. Nonulcer Dyspepsia. The role of *H. pylori* infection in nonulcer dyspepsia (NUD) remains controversial. Exploring the relationship is problematic because of the wide variety of symptoms that fall under this catch-all term. Differences in the selection of patients for studies and the method of diagnosis of *H. pylori* infection makes comparison between them difficult. Some studies have shown a greater prevalence of *H. pylori* infection in patients with NUD, while others have not. Moreover, while some longitudinal studies have shown symptomatic improvement in dyspeptic patients after eradication of *H. pylori*, the results are not uniform.[135] The seeming inconsistencies may reflect the lack of control groups standardized for other known risk factors for *H. pylori* infection.[136] It is likely that some proportion of dyspepsia is due to *H. pylori* infection. It remains impossible, however, to pinpoint *a priori* those that will respond to antimicrobial therapy.

8.1.3. Peptic Ulcer Disease. *H. pylori* is an important cause of both duodenal and gastric ulcers.[13] Although "no acid, no ulcer" is still accepted dogma in duodenal ulcer pathogenesis, *H. pylori* appears to be similarly critical. Over 90% of persons with duodenal ulcer disease will have concomitant *H. pylori* infection. The best evidence for a causal association comes from therapeutic trials. Persons treated with antibiotics in addition to acid inhibitory therapy have much lower rates of ulcer relapse than persons treated with acid inhibitory therapy alone.[137,138] Moreover, if the antimicrobial agents used do not successfully eradicate *H. pylori* infection, there is no benefit over acid inhibition alone. Duodenal ulcers should now be assumed to be related to *H. pylori* infection unless other predisposing conditions such as nonsteroidal anti-inflammatory drug (NSAID) use, Zollinger–Ellison syndrome, or Crohn's disease are present.

Only a minority (approximately 20%) of infected persons will develop duodenal ulcer within a 10-year period.[120] The infected individuals at highest risk are those with duodenitis and gastric metaplasia of the duodenal mucosa.[139] Environmental cofactors may also magnify ulcer risk. These include cigarette and alcohol use, use of NSAIDs, male gender, and blood group O and other hereditary factors.[140]

Clinical trials similar to those conducted for duodenal ulcers support a role for *H. pylori* in gastric ulceration as well.[137] The percent of disease attributable to *H. pylori*, however, is lower for gastric than for duodenal ulcers. In the United States, a substantial proportion of gastric ulcers (about 35%) can be explained not by infection but by NSAID use.[141] Of the remaining 65%, *H. pylori* must be considered the preeminent cause.

8.1.4. Gastric Adenocarcinoma. In 1994, the World Health Organization (WHO) declared *H. pylori* infection to be an important cause of gastric adenocarcinoma.[14] Support for this declaration came from two types of data: studies of the natural history of gastric cancer and epidemiological studies of the association of *H. pylori* infection and cancer. Since gastric cancer usually occurs in the setting of chronic superficial gastritis, a relationship with *H. pylori* can be deduced.[142] The most compelling data linking *H. pylori* infection with cancer, however, come from epidemiological investigations. Several types of studies have been done including studies paralleling the epidemiological features of *H. pylori* infection and gastric cancer, case–control studies of patients with cancer, and nested case–control studies within large cohort populations followed, prospectively, for cancer. These studies show that: (1) gastric cancer occurs at an increased rate in regions with high prevalence of *H. pylori* infection, (2) cancer patients have higher rates of *H. pylori* infection than controls, and (3) *H. pylori* infection precedes cancer by many years.[143–145] The association between *H. pylori* and cancer is restricted to tumors distal to the gastric cardia. Tumors of the gastroesophageal area do not appear to be *H. pylori*-related.

The progression of mucosal changes from superficial gastritis to carcinoma probably requires decades. Therefore, individuals who acquire *H. pylori* infection early in life should have the highest risk of malignancy. Epidemiological studies provide some support for this hypothesis.[146,147] Other factors influencing the development of cancer include dietary exposures (nitrates and salts increase risk, fruits and vegetables decrease risk) and genetic predisposition.[148]

8.1.5. Gastric Lymphoma. Gastric lymphona is the rarest of the diseases associated with *H. pylori* infection, with only seven cases per million population per year.[149] The normal stomach is not a lymphoid organ.

Since *H. pylori* is the preeminent initiator of inflammation and lymphoid follicle formation in the stomach, it seems intuitive that it would be linked to lymphoma. Several cross-sectional and ecological studies have weakly supported this conjecture.(150,151) One somewhat stronger study demonstrated that *H. pylori* infection increased risk of later developing diffuse histiocytic gastric lymphomas sixfold.(152) A particularly strong association of infection has been observed for mucosa-associated lymphoid tissue (MALT) lymphoma, a type of low-grade lymphoma that arises from lymphoid follicles.(153,154) The remarkable feature of these MALT lymphomas is that they may completely regress if *H. pylori* infection is eradicated with antibiotics.(155,156)

Why a scattered few people with *H. pylori* develop these rare lymphomas is unknown. Some believe that infection may precipitate an autoimmune response that predisposes to malignancy.(157,158) Others hypothesize that *H. pylori* antigens themselves may drive lymphoproliferation.(152) It is hoped that understanding the role of *H. pylori* and lymphoma will shed light not only on the pathogenesis of gastric lymphomas but on other extranodal lymphomas as well.

8.2. Diagnosis

The National Institutes of Health recommends that diagnostic tests for *H. pylori* be conducted in: (1) all persons with active gastric or duodenal ulcer, and (2) persons on maintenance histamine antagonists for prevention of recurrent peptic ulcer disease.(13) For patients undergoing endoscopy, a rapid urease test is the diagnostic test of choice. This test is less expensive and more rapid than histological examination and/or culture. For patients in whom endoscopy is not necessary, serology is the best option. A quantitative serological assay is preferable to a qualitative assay since a drop in titer can be used to assess cure.

9. Control and Prevention

9.1. General Concepts

Since the mechanism of transmission of *H. pylori* is still unknown, there are no current recommendations for control and prevention. Based on epidemiological studies indicating person-to-person transmission, it is likely that general improvements in hygiene standards such as hand washing and good household sanitation will decrease transmission.

9.2. Antibiotic and Chemotherapeutic Approaches to Disease Prevention

H. pylori is curable with antimicrobial therapy. The two most widely use regimens are bismuth triple therapy (a combination of metronidazole, tetracycline, and bismuth; 70–90% cure) and proton-pump inhibitor triple therapy (a proton pump inhibitor plus clarithromycon and either amoxicillin or metronidazole; 80–90% cure). Controversy rages, however, over whom to treat. The National Institutes of Health recommend treating only persons with active ulcer disease (gastric or duodenal) or persons on maintenance antihistamine therapy for recurrent ulcer disease.(13) Some investigators, however, have reported that treatment could be a cost-effective approach to preventing ulcer disease, dyspepsia, and/or cancer in populations at high risk.(159) Still others maintain that eradicating infection in all infected persons, regardless of symptoms, is the correct approach.(160) As new information accumulates, it is likely that diagnosis and therapy will be offered to a wider segment of the population in order to prevent adverse outcomes of infection. For now, however, there are no recommendations for diagnostic testing and/or treatment in asymptomatic persons or persons with dyspepsia of unknown etiology.

9.3. Immunization

No vaccine is currently available to prevent or treat *H. pylori* infection. This is an area of considerable interest. Because the brisk, natural immune response neither eliminates infection nor prevents reinfection, one might rightly feel skeptical that a vaccine could be efficacious. Despite this theoretical concern, however, several candidate vaccines are beginning to show promise in animal models.(161) Were such a vaccine available, it is not yet known how it would optimally be used.

10. Unresolved Problems

Since 1982, an enormous amount of research has been conducted on *H. pylori* infection. In the five years from 1990–1994 alone, over 2500 manuscripts were published. Yet many of the critical issues concerning *H. pylori* remain to be understood.

Because acute infection almost always remains undiagnosed, the infectious inoculum has not been established. Moreover, it is unknown whether host factors affect the infectious inoculum or whether all uninfected persons are equally at risk. Because of the absence of acute cases, it is also difficult to discern precisely how *H. pylori* is transmitted. While there is strong, circumstantial evidence for person-to-person transmission, it is debated whether this involves fecal–oral or oral–oral contact. There is also considerable controversy over the role of environmental sources in causing disease.

The interplay of *H. pylori* with other disease cofactors is undoubtedly complex and will take years if not decades to parse out. It is assumed that differences in outcome can be explained by a combination of bacterial factors (e.g., presence of cytotoxin), environmental factors (e.g., diet, cigarettes, etc.), host factors (e.g., blood group type), and temporal factors (e.g., age at acquisition of infection). The interaction of risk factors is undoubtedly complex and will take years if not decades to parse out. Development of suitable animal models will facilitate our understanding of these processes.

From a public health perspective, there remains no good algorithm for disease prevention. Over half of the world's population is infected with *H. pylori*. In developing countries, *H. pylori* infection is almost universal. In developed countries, on the other hand, the incidence of infection has been rapidly decreasing without any specific antibacterial intervention. Adverse outcomes of *H. pylori* infection, such as gastric cancer and ulcer disease, are also on an impressive decline. Improvements in hygiene, diet, and other socioeconomic factors, rather than antibiotic use, probably account for this favorable slope. Should we be focusing on vaccine development for a disease that disappears with improvements in hygiene? Should we be screening and treating persons in order to prevent *H. pylori*-related diseases? Should we be treating the families of infected persons in order to interrupt the cycle of reinfection? Would widespread use of antibiotics to treat *H. pylori* produce more harm in terms of the overall burden of antimicrobial resistance than good? These very fundamental issues remain to be resolved.

Acknowledgment

This work is supported in part by a Clinical Epidemiology Fellowship from Merck and the Society for Epidemiologic Research.

11. References

1. Kreinitz, W., Ueber das Auftreten von Spirochaeten verschiedener Form im Mageninhatl bei Carcinoma ventriculi, *Dtsch. Med. Wochenschr.* **32:**872 (1906).
2. Doenges, J. L., Spirochaetes in gastric glands of macacus rhesus and humans without defined history of related disease, *Proc. Soc. Exp. Biol. Med.* **38:**536–538 (1938).
3. Freedberg, A. S., and Barron, L. E., The presence of spirochaetes in human gastric mucosa, *Am. J. Dig. Dis.* **38:**443–445 (1940).
4. Palmer, E. D., Investigation of the gastric spirochaetes of the human, *Gastroenterology* **27:**218–220 (1954).
5. Fitzgerald, O., and Murphy, P., Studies of the physiological chemistry and clinical significance of urease and urea with special reference to the human stomach, *Ir. J. Med. Sci.* **292:**97–159 (1950).
6. Lieber, C. S., and LeFevre, A., Ammonia as a source of hypoacidity in patients with uraemia, *J. Clin. Invest.* **38:**1271–1277 (1959).
7. Steer, H. W., and Colin-Jones, D. G., Mucosal changes in gastric ulceration and their response to carbenoxolone sodium, *Gut* **16:** 590–597 (1975).
8. Steer, H. W., Ultrastructure of cell migration through the gastric epithelium and its relationship to bacteria, *J. Clin. Pathol.* **28:** 639–646 (1975).
9. Fung, W. P., Papadimitriou, J. M., and Matz, L. R., Endoscopic, histologic and ultrastructural correlations in chronic gastritis, *Am. J. Gastroenterol.* **71:**269–279 (1979).
10. Marshall, B. J., History of the discovery of *C. pylori*, in: *Campylobacter pylori in Gastritis and Peptic Ulcer Disease*, Igaku-Shoin, New York, 1989.
11. Marshall, B. J., Armstrong, J. A., McGeche, D. B., and Glancy, R. J., Attempt to fulfill Koch's postulates for pyloric *Campylobacter*, *Med. J. Aust.* **142:**436–439 (1985).
12. Morris, A., and Nicholson, G., Ingestion of *Campylobacter pyloridis* causes gastritis and raised fasting gastric pH, *Gastroenterology* **82:**192–194 (1987).
13. NIH Consensus Development Panel on *Helicobacter pylori* in Peptic Ulcer Disease, *Helicobacter pylori* in peptic ulcer disease, *J. Am. Med. Assoc.* **272:**65–69 (1994).
14. IARC Working Group on the Evaluation of Carcinogenic Risks to Humans: *Helicobacter pylori*, in: *Schistosomes, Liver Flukes and Helicobacter pylori: Views and Expert Opinions of an IARC Working Group on the Evaluation of Carcinogenic Risks to Humans*, pp. 177–240, IARC, Lyon, 1994.
15. Kurata, J. H., Elashoff, J. D., Haile, B. M., and Honda, G. D., A reappraisal of time trends in ulcer disease and factors related to changes in ulcer hospitalization and mortality rates, *Am. J. Public Health* **73:**1066–1072 (1983).
16. Sonnenberg, A., Occurrence of a cohort phenomenon in peptic ulcer mortality from Switzerland, *Gastroenterology* **86:**398–401 (1984).
17. Sonnenberg, A., and Fritsch, A., Changing mortality of peptic ulcer disease in Germany, *Gastroenterology* **84:**1553–1557 (1983).
18. US Department of Health and Human Services, *Surveillance, Epidemiology and End Results: Incidence and Mortality Data, 1973–1977*, Department of Health and Human Services, Bethesda, 1981.
19. Tilvis, R. S., Vuoristo, M., and Varis, K., Changed profile of peptic ulcer disease in hospital patients during 1969–1984, *Scand. J. Gastroenterol.* **22:**1238–1244 (1987).
20. Jennings, D., Perforated peptic ulcer: Changes in age-incidence and sex-distribution in the last 150 years (Part I), *Lancet* **1:**395–398 (1940).
21. Kurata, J. H., Honda, G. D., and Frankl, H., Hospitalization and mortality rates for peptic ulcers: A comparison of large health maintenance organization and United States data, *Gastroenterology* **83:**1008–1016 (1982).

22. Glupczynski, Y., Bourdeaux, L., Verhas, M., DePrez, C., DeVos, D., and Devreker, T., Use of a urea breath test versus invasive methods to determine the prevalence of *Helicobacter pylori* in Zaire, *Eur. J. Clin. Microbiol. Infect. Dis.* **11:**322–327 (1992).
23. Graham, D. Y., Malaty, H. M., Evans, D. G., Evans, D. J. J., Klein, P. D., and Adam, E., Epidemiology of *Helicobacter pylori* in an asymptomatic population in the United States. Effects of age, race, and socioeconomic status, *Gastroenterology* **100:**1495–1501 (1991).
24. Baker, S., Gummett, P. A., Whittaker, L., *et al.*, A pilot study of the epidemiology of *Helicobacter pylori* in children from London using the ^{13}C-urea breath test (Abstract), *Am. J. Gastroenterol.* **89:**1307 (1994).
25. Hazell, S. L., Cultural techniques for the growth and isolation of *Helicobacter pylori*, in: *Helicobacter pylori: Biology and Clinical Practice* (C. S. Goodwin and B. W. Worsley, eds.), pp. 273–283, CRC Press, Boca Raton, FL, 1993.
26. Thomas, J. E., Gibson, G. R., Darboe, M. K., Dale, A., and Weaver, L. T., Isolation of *Helicobacter pylori* from human faeces, *Lancet* **340:**1194–1195 (1992).
27. Krajden, S., Fuksa, M., Anderson, J., *et al.*, Examination of human stomach biopsies, saliva, and dental plaque for *Campylobacter pylori*, *J. Clin. Microbiol.* **27:**1397–1398 (1989).
28. Nedenskov-Sorensen, P., Aase, S., Bjorneklett, A., Fausa, O., and Bukholm, G., Sampling efficiency in the diagnosis of *Helicobacter pylori* infection and chronic active gastritis, *J. Clin. Microbiol.* **29:**672–675 (1991).
29. Morris, A., Ali, M. R., Brown, P., Lane, M., and Patton, K., *Campylobacter pylori* infection in biopsy specimens of gastric antrum: Laboratory diagnosis and estimation of sampling error, *J. Clin. Pathol.* **42:**727–732 (1989).
30. Brown, K. E., and Peura, D. A., Diagnosis of *Helicobacter pylori* infection, *Gastroenterol. Clin. North Am.* **22:**105–115 (1993).
31. McNulty, C. A., Dent, J. C., Uff, J. S., *et al.*, Detection of *Campylobacter pylori* by the biopsy urease test: An assessment of 1445 patients, *Gut* **30:**1058–1062 (1989).
32. Marshall, B. J., Warren, J. R., Francis, G. J., Langton, S. R., Goodwin, C. S., and Blincow, E. D., Rapid urease test in the management of *Campylobacter pyloridis*-associated gastritis, *Am. J. Gastroenterol.* **82:**200–210 (1987).
33. Lee, N., Lee, T. T., and Fang, K. M., Assessment of four rapid urease test systems for detection of *Helicobacter pylori* in gastric biopsy specimens, *Diagn. Microbiol. Infect. Dis.* **18:**69–74 (1994).
34. Parsonnet, J., Blaser, M. J., Perez-Perez, G. I., Hargrett-Bean, N., and Tauxe, R. V., Symptoms and risk factors of *Helicobacter pylori* infection in a cohort of epidemiologists, *Gastroenterology* **102:**41–46 (1992).
35. Kosunen, T. U., Seppala, K., Sarna, S., and Sipponen, P., Diagnostic value of decreasing IgG, IgA, and IgM antibody titres after eradication of *Helicobacter pylori*, *Lancet* **339:**893–895 (1992).
36. Cutler, A., Schubert, A., and Schubert, T., Role of *Helicobacter pylori* serology in evaluating treatment success, *Dig. Dis. Sci.* **38:**2262–2266 (1993).
37. Andersen, L. P., The antibody response to *Helicobacter pylori* infection, and the value of serologic tests to detect *H. pylori* and for post-treatment monitoring, in: *Helicobacter pylori: Biology and Clinical Practice* (C. S. Goodwin and B. W. Worsley, eds.), pp. 285–305, CRC Press, Boca Raton, FL, 1993.
38. Bodhidatta, L., Hoge, C. W., Churnratanakul, S., *et al.*, Diagnosis of *Helicobacter pylori* infection in a developing country: Comparison of two ELISAs and a seroprevalence study, *J. Infect. Dis.* **168:**1549–1553 (1993).
39. Atherton, J. C., and Spiller, R. C., The urea breath test for *Helicobacter pylori*, *Gut* **35:**723–725 (1994).
40. Dill, S., Payne-James, J. J., Misiewicz, J. J., *et al.*, Evaluation of ^{13}C-urea breath test in the detection of *Helicobacter pylori* and in monitoring the effect of tripotassium dicitratobismuthate, *Gut* **31:** 1237–1241 (1990).
41. Nguyen, A. M., Engstrand, L., Genta, R. M., Graham, D. Y., and el-Zaatari, F. A., Detection of *Helicobacter pylori* in dental plaque by reverse transcription-polymerase chain reaction, *J. Clin. Microbiol.* **31:**783–787 (1993).
42. Mapstone, N. P., Lynch, D. A., Lewis, F. A., *et al.*, Identification of *Helicobacter pylori* DNA in the mouths and stomachs of patients with gastritis using PCR, *J. Clin. Pathol.* **46:**540–543 (1993).
43. Lee, A., Fox, J., and Hazell, S., Pathogenicity of *Helicobacter pylori*: A perspective. *Infect. Immun.* **61:**1601–1610 (1993).
44. Boren, T., Falk, P., Roth, K. A., Larson, G., and Normark, S., Attachment of *Helicobacter pylori* to human gastric epithelium mediated by blood group antigens, *Science* **262:**1892–1895 (1993).
45. Valkonen, K. H., Wadstrom, T., and Moran, A. P., Interaction of lipopolysaccharides of *Helicobacter pylori* with basement membrane protein laminin, *Infect. Immun.* **62:**3640–3648 (1994).
46. Lingwood, C. A., Wasfy, G., Han, H., and Huesca, M., Receptor affinity purification of a lipid-binding adhesion from *Helicobacter pylori*, *Infect. Immun.* **61:**2474–2478 (1993).
47. Eaton, K. A., Catrenich, C. E., Makin, K. M., and Krakowka, S., Virulence of coccoid and bacillary forms of *Helicobacter pylori* in gnotobiotic piglets, *J. Infect. Dis.* **171:**459–462 (1995).
48. Bode, G., Mauch, F., and Malfertheiner, P., The coccoid forms of *Helicobacter pylori*. Criteria for their viability, *Epidemiol. Infect.* **111:**483–490 (1993).
49. Turbett, G. R., Hoj, P. B., Horne, R., and Mee, B. J., Purification and characterization of the urease enzymes of *Helicobacter* species from humans and animals, *Infect. Immun.* **60:**5259–5266 (1992).
50. Eaton, K. A., Brooks, C. L., Morgan, D. R., and Krakowka, S., Essential role of urease in pathogenesis of gastritis induced by *Helicobacter pylori* in gnotobiotic piglets, *Infect. Immun.* **59:** 2470–2475 (1991).
51. Ferrero, R. L., and Labigne, A., The organization and expression of the *Helicobacter pylori* urease gene cluster, in: *Helicobacter pylori: Biology and Clinical Practice* (C. S. Goodwin and B. W. Worsley, eds.), pp. 171–190, CRC Press, Boca Raton, FL, 1993.
52. Hazell, S. L., and Mendz, G. L., The metabolism and enzymes of *Helicobacter pylori*: Function and potential virulence effects, in *Helicobacter pylori: Biology and Clinical Practice* (C. S. Goodwin and B. W. Worsley, eds.), pp. 115–142, CRC Press, Boca Raton, FL, 1993.
53. Marshall, B. J., Barrett, L. J., Prakash, C., McCallum, R. W., Guerrant, R. L., Urea protects *Helicobacter* (*Campylobacter*) pylori from the bactericidal effect of acid, *Gastroenterology* **99:**697–702 (1990).
54. Schmitt, W., and Haas, R., Genetic analysis of the *Helicobacter pylori* vacuolating cytotoxin: Structural similarities with the IgA protease type of exported protein, *Mol. Microbiol.* **12:**307–319 (1994).
55. Cover, T. L., Dooley, C. P., and Blaser, M. J., Characterization of and human serologic response to proteins in *Helicobacter pylori* broth culture supernatants with vacuolizing cytotoxin activity, *Infect. Immun.* **58:**603–610 (1990).

56. Telford, J. L., Ghiara, P., Dell'Orco, M., *et al.*, Gene structure of the *Helicobacter pylori* cytotoxin and evidence of its key role in gastric disease, *J. Exp. Med.* **179:**1653–1658 (1994).
57. Cover, T. L., Cao, P., Murthy, U. K., Sipple, M. S., and Blaser, M. J., Serum neutralizing antibody response to the vacuolating cytotoxin of *Helicobacter pylori*, *J. Clin. Invest.* **90:**913–918 (1992).
58. Akopyanz, N., Bukanov, N. O., Westblom, T. U., and Berg, D. E., PCR-based RFLP analysis of DNA sequence diversity in the gastric pathogen *Helicobacter pylori*, *Nucleic Acids Res.* **20:** 6221–6225 (1992).
59. Hurtado, A., Chahal, B., Owen, R. J., and Smith, A. W., Genetic diversity of the *Helicobacter pylori* haemagglutinin/protease (*hap*) gene, *FEMS Microbiol. Lett.* **123:**173–178 (1994).
60. Taylor, D. E., Eaton, M., Chang, N., and Salama, S. M., Construction of a *Helicobacter pylori* genome map and demonstration of diversity at the genome level, *J. Bacteriol.* **174:**6800–6806 (1992).
61. Nowak, R., Getting the bugs worked out, *Science* **267:**172–174 (1995).
62. Taylor, D. N., and Parsonnet, J., The epidemiology and natural history of *Helicobacter pylori* infection, in: *Infections of the Gastrointestinal Tract* (M. J. Blaser *et al.*, eds.), pp. 553–557, Raven Press, New York, 1995.
63. Dwyer, B., Kaldor, J., Tee, W., Marakowski, E., and Raios, K., Antibody response to *Campylobacter pylori* infection in diverse ethnic groups, *Scand. J. Infect. Dis.* **20:**349–350 (1988).
64. Perez-Perez, G. I., Witkin, S. S., Decker, M. D., and Blaser, M. J., Seroprevalence of *Helicobacter pylori* infection in couples, *J. Clin. Microbiol.* **29:**642–644 (1991).
65. Parsonnet, J., The incidence of *Helicobacter pylori* infection, *Aliment. Pharmacol. Ther.* **9**(Suppl. 2)**:**45–52 (1995).
66. Lin, J. T., Wang, J. T., Wang, T. H., Wu, M. S., Lee, T. K., and Chen, C. J., *Helicobacter pylori* infection in a randomly selected population, healthy volunteers, and patients with gastric ulcer and gastric adenocarcinoma. A seroprevalence study in Taiwan, *Scand. J. Gastroenterol.* **28:**1067–1072 (1993).
67. Mendall, M. A., Goggin, P. M., Molineaux, N., *et al.*, Childhood living conditions and *Helicobacter pylori* seropositivity in adult life, *Lancet* **339:**896–897 (1992).
68. Banatvala, N., Mayo, K., Megraud, F., Jennings, R., Deeks, J. J., and Feldman, R. A., The cohort effect and *Helicobacter pylori*, *J. Infect. Dis.* **168:**219–221 (1993).
69. Cullen, D. J. E., Collins, B. J., Christiansen, K. J., *et al.*, When is *Helicobacter pylori* infection acquired? *Gut* **34:**1681–1682 (1993).
70. Veldhuyzen van Zanten, S. J. O., Pollak, P. T., Best, L. M., Bezanson, G. S., and Marrie, T., Increasing prevalence of *Helicobacter pylori* infection with age: Continuous risk of infection in adults rather than cohort effect, *J. Infect. Dis.* **169:**434–437 (1994).
71. Genta, R. M., and Graham, D. Y., Intestinal metaplasia, not atrophy or achlorhydria, creates a hostile environment for *Helicobacter pylori*, *Scand. J. Gastroenterol.* **28:**924–928 (1993).
72. Replogle, M. L., Glaser, S. L., Hiatt, R. A., and Parsonnet, J., Gender as a risk for *Helicobacter pylori* infection in healthy young adults, *Am. J. Epidemiol.* **142:**856–863 (1995).
73. Taylor, D. N., and Blaser, M. J., The epidemiology of *Helicobacter pylori* infection, *Epidemiol. Rev.* **13:**42–59 (1991).
74. Megraud, F., Brassens,-Rabbe, M. P., Denis, F., Belbari, A., and Hoa, D. Q., Seroepidemiology of *Campylobacter pylori* infection in various populations, *J. Clin. Microbiol.* **17:**1870–1873 (1989).
75. Eurogast Study Group, Epidemiology of, and risk factors for, *Helicobacter pylori* infection among 3194 asymptomatic subjects in 17 populations, *Gut* **34:**1672–1676 (1993).
76. Smoak, B., Kelley, P., and Taylor, D. N., Seroprevalence of *Helicobacter pylori* infections in a cohort of US Army recruits, unpublished manuscript, 1994.
77. Hopkins, R. J., Russell, R. G., O'Donnoghue, J. M., Wasserman, S. S., Lefkowitz, A., and Morris, J. G., Seroprevalence of *Helicobacter pylori* in Seventh-Day Adventists and other groups in Maryland. Lack of association with diet [see comments], *Arch. Intern. Med.* **150:**2347–2348 (1990).
78. Polish, L. B., Doulgas, J. M., Davidson, A. J., Perez-Perez, G. I., and Blaser, M. J., Characterization of risk factors for *Helicobacter pylori* infection among men attending a sexually transmitted disease clinic: Lack of evidence for sexual transmission, *J. Clin. Microbiol.* **29:**2139–2143 (1991).
79. Teh, B. H., Lin, J. T., Pan, W. H., *et al.*, Seroprevalence and associated risk factors of *Helicobacter pylori* infection in Taiwan, *Anticancer Res.* **14:**1389–1392 (1994).
80. Morris, A., Nicholson, G., Lloyd, G., Haines, D., Rogers, A., and Taylor, D., Seroepidemiology of *Campylobacter pyloridis*, *N. Z. Med. J.* **99:**657–659 (1986).
81. Blecker, U., Hauser, B., Lanciers, S., Peeters, S., Suys, B., and Vandenplas, Y., The prevalence of *Helicobacter pylori*-positive serology in asymptomatic children, *J. Pediatr. Gastroenterol. Nutr.* **16:**252–256 (1993).
82. Malaty, H. M., Engstrand, L., Pedersen, N. L., and Graham, D. Y., *Helicobacter pylori* infection: Genetic and environmental influences, *Ann. Intern. Med.* **120:**982–986 (1994).
83. Malaty, H. M., and Graham, D. Y., Importance of childhood socioeconomic status on the current prevalence of *Helicobacter pylori* infection, *Gut* **35:**742–745 (1994).
84. Fiedorek, S. C., Malaty, H. M., Evans, D. L., *et al.*, Factors influencing the epidemiology of *Helicobacter pylori* infection in children, *Pediatrics* **88:**578–582 (1991).
85. Perez-Perez, G. I., Taylor, D. N., Bodhidatta, L., *et al.*, Seroprevalence of *Helicobacter pylori* infections in Thailand, *J. Infect. Dis.* **161:**1237–1241 (1990).
86. Berkowicz, J., and Lee, A., Person-to-person transmission of *Campylobacter pylori* [letter], *Lancet* **2:**680–681 (1987).
87. Reiff, A., Jacobs, E., and Kist, M., Seroepidemiological study of the immune response to *Campylobacter pylori* in potential risk groups, *Eur. J. Clin. Microbiol. Infect. Dis.* **8:**592–596 (1989).
88. Drumm, B., Perez-Perez, G. I., Blaser, M. J., and Sherman, P. M., Intrafamilial clustering of *Helicobacter pylori* infection, *N. Engl. J. Med.* **322:**359–364 (1990).
89. Mitchell, J. D., Mitchell, H. M., and Tobias, V., Acute *Helicobacter pylori* infection in an infant, associated with gastric ulceration and serological evidence of intra familial transmission, *Am. J. Gastroenterol.* **87:**382–386 (1992).
90. Malaty, H. M., Graham, D. Y., Klein, P. D., Evans, D. G., Adam, E., and Evans, D. J., Transmission of *Helicobacter pylori* infection. Studies in families of healthy individuals, *Scand. J. Gastroenterol.* **26:**927–932 (1991).
91. Blecker, U., Lanciers, S., Mehta, D. I., and Vandenplas, Y., Familial clustering of *Helicobacter pylori* infection, *Clin. Pediatr. (Phila)* **33:**307–308 (1994).
92. Mitchell, H. M., Bohane, T., Hawkes, R. A., and Lee, A., *Helicobacter pylori* infection within families, *Int. J. Med. Microbiol. Virol. Parasitol. Infect. Dis.* **280:**128–136 (1993).
93. Wang, J. T., Sheu, J. C., Lin, J. T., Wang, T. H., and Wu, M. S.,

Direct DNA amplification and restriction pattern analysis of *Helicobacter pylori* in patients with duodenal ulcer and their families, *J. Infect. Dis.* **168:**1544–1548 (1993).

94. Webb, P. M., Knight, T., Greaves, S., *et al.*, Relation between infection with *Helicobacter pylori* and living conditions in childhood: Evidence for person-to-person transmission in early life, *Br. Med. J.* **308:**750–753 (1994).
95. Hammermeister, I., Janus, G., Schamorowski, F., Rudolf, M., Jacobs, E., and Kist, M., Elevated risk of *Helicobacter pylori* infection in submarine crews, *Eur. J. Clin. Microbiol. Infect. Dis.* **11:**9–14 (1992).
96. Kelly, S. M., Pitcher, M. C., Farmery, S. M., and Gibson, G. R., Isolation of *Helicobacter pylori* from feces of patients with dyspepsia in the United Kingdom, *Gastroenterology* **107:**1671–1674 (1994).
97. Ferguson, D. A., Li, C., Patel, N. R., Mayberry, W. R., Chi, D. S., and Thomas, E., Isolation of *Helicobacter pylori* from saliva, *J. Clin. Microbiol.* **31:**2802–2804 (1993).
98. Malaty, H. M., Evans, D. J., Abramovitch, K., Evans, D. G., and Graham, D. Y., *Helicobacter pylori* infection in dental workers: A seroepidemiology study, *Am. J. Gastroenterol.* **87:**1728–1731 (1992).
99. Guelrud, M., Mujica, C., Jaen, D., Machuca, J., and Essenfeld, H., Prevalence of *Helicobacter pylori* in neonates and young infants undergoing ERCP for diagnosis of neonatal cholestasis, *J. Pediatr. Gastroenterol. Nutr.* **18:**461–464 (1994).
100. Blecker, U., Lanciers, S., Keppens, E., and Vandenplas, Y., Evolution of *Helicobacter pylori* positivity in infants born from positive mothers, *J. Pediatr. Gastroenterol. Nutr.* **19:**87–90 (1994).
101. Klein, P. D., Graham, D. Y., Gaillour, A., Opekun, A. R., O'Brian Smith, E., and Gastrointestinal Physiology Working Group, Water source as risk factor for *Helicobacter pylori* infection in Peruvian children, *Lancet* **337:**1503–1506 (1991).
102. Hopkins, R. J., Vial, P. A., Ferreccio, C., *et al.*, Seroprevalence of *Helicobacter pylori* in Chile: Vegetables may serve as one route of transmission, *J. Infect. Dis.* **168:**222–226 (1993).
103. Gill, H. H., Desai, H. G., Majmudar, P., Mehta, P. R., and Prabhu, S. R., Epidemiology of *Helicobacter pylori*: The Indian scenario, *Indian J. Gastroenterol.* **12:**9–11 (1993).
104. Gill, H. H., Majmudar, P., Shankaran, K., and Desai, H. G., Age-related prevalence of *Helicobacter pylori* antibodies in Indian subjects, *Indian J. Gastroenterol.* **13:**92–94 (1994).
105. Hazell, S. L., Mitchell, H. M., Hedges, M., *et al.*, Heapatitis A and evidence against the community dissemination of *Helicobacter pylori* via feces, *J. Infect. Dis.* **170:**686–689 (1994).
106. Webberley, M. J., Webberley, J. M., Newell, D. G., Lowe, P., and Melikian, V., Seroepidemiology of *Helicobacter pylori* infection in vegans and meat-eaters, *Epidemiol. Infect.* **108:**457–462 (1992).
107. Langenberg, W., Rauws, E. A., Oudbier, J. H., and Tytgat, G. N., Patient-to-patient transmission of *Campylobacter pylori* infection by fiberoptic gastroduodenoscopy and biopsy, *J. Infect. Dis.* **161:**507–511 (1990).
108. Fantry, G. T., Zheng, Q. X., and James, S. P., Conventional cleaning and disinfection techniques eliminate the risk of endoscopic transmission of *Helicobacter pylori*, *Am. J. Gastroenterol.* **90:**227–232 (1995).
109. Katoh, M., Saito, D., Noda, T., *et al.*, *Helicobacter pylori* may be transmitted through gastrofiberscope even after manual Hyamine washing, *Jpn. J. Cancer Res.* **84:**117–119 (1993).
110. Chong, J., Marshall, B. J., Barkin, J. S., *et al.*, Occupational exposure to *Helicobacter pylori* for the endoscopy professional: A sera epidemiological study, *Am. J. Gastroenterol.* **89:**1987–1992 (1994).
111. Lin, S. K., Lambert, J. R., Schembri, M. A., Nicholson, L., and Korman, M. G., *Helicobacter pylori* prevalence in endoscopy and medical staff, *J. Gastroenterol. Hepatol.* **9:**319–324 (1994).
112. Price, A., The Sydney system: Histological division, *J. Gastroenterol. Hepatol.* **6:**209–222 (1991).
113. Genta, R. M., Hamner, H. W., and Graham, D. Y., Gastric lymphoid follicles in *Helicobacter pylori* infection: Frequency, distribution, and response to triple therapy, *Hum. Pathol.* **24:**577–583 (1993).
114. Blaser, M. J., and Parsonnet, J., Parasitism by the "slow" bacterium *Helicobacter pylori* leads to altered gastric homeostasis and neoplasia (perspectives), *J. Clin. Invest.* **94:**4–8 (1994).
115. Phadnis, S. H., Ilver, D., Janzon, L., Normark, S., and Westblom, T. U., Pathological significance and molecular characterization of the vacuolating toxin gene of *Helicobacter pylori*, *Infect. Immun.* **62:**1557–1565 (1994).
116. Mooney, C., Keenan, J., Munster, D.,*et al.*, Neutrophil activation by *Helicobacter pylori*, *Gut* **32:**853–857 (1991).
117. Tsujii, M., Kawano, S., Tsuji, S., Fusamoto, H., Kamada, T., and Sato, N., Mechanism of gastric mucosal damage induced by ammonia, *Gastroenterology* **102:**1881–1888 (1992).
118. Goodwin, C. S., Duodenal ulcer, *Campylobacter pylori*, and the "leaking roof" concept, *Lancet* **2:**1467–1469 (1988).
119. Tarnasky, P. R., Kovacs, T. O. G., Sytnik, B., and Walsh, J. H., Asymptomatic *H. pylori* infection impairs pH inhibition of gastrin and acid secretion during second hour of peptone meal stimulation, *Dig. Dis. Sci.* **38:**1681–1687 (1993).
120. Sipponen, P., Natural history of gastritis and its relationship to peptic ulcer disease, *Digestion* **5:**70–75 (1992).
121. Shuto, R., Fujioka, T., Kodama, R., and Nasu, M., Experimental study in Japanese monkeys with *Helicobacter pylori* infection, *Nippon Rinsho* **51:**3132–3137 (1993).
122. Sipponen, P., Kekki, M., Haapakoski, J., Ihamaki, T., and Siurala, M., Gastric cancer risk in chronic atrophic gastritis: Statistical calculations on cross-sectional data, *Cancer* **35:**173–177 (1985).
123. Sipponen, P., and Seppala, K., Gastric carcinoma: Failed adaptation to *Helicobacter pylori*, *Scand. J. Gastroenterol.* **27**(Suppl.)**:** 33–38 (1992).
124. Davies, G. R., Simmonds, N. J., Stevens, T. R. J., *et al.*, *Helicobacter pylori* stimulates antral mucosal reactive oxygen metabolite production *in vivo*, *Gut* **35:**179–185 (1994).
125. Lynch, D. A. F., Mapstone, N. P., Clarke, A. M. T., *et al.*, Cell proliferation in *Helicobacter pylori* associated gastritis and the effect of eradication therapy, *Gut* **36:**345–350 (1995).
126. Hirai, M., Azuma, T., Ito, S., Kato, T., Kohli, Y., and Kujiki, N., High prevalence of neutralizing activity to *Helicobacter pylori* cytotoxin in serum of gastric-carcinoma patients, *Int. J. Cancer* **56:**56–60 (1994).
127. Fox, J. G., Correa, P., Taylor, N. S., *et al.*, High prevalence and persistence of cytotoxin-positive *Helicobacter pylori* strains in a population with high prevalence of atrophic gastritis, *Am. J. Gastroenterol.* **887:**1554–1560 (1992).
128. Langenberg, W., Rauws, E. A., Widjojokusumo, A., Tytgat, G. N., and Zanen, H. C., Identification of *Campylobacter pyloridis* isolates by restriction endonuclease DNA analysis, *J. Clin. Microbiol.* **24:**414–417 (1986).
129. Langenberg, W., Rauws, E. A., Houthoff, H. J., *et al.*, Follow-up

study of individuals with untreated *Campylobacter pylori*-associated gastritis and of noninfected persons with non-ulcer dyspepsia, *J. Infect. Dis.* **157**:1245–1249 (1988).
130. Dooley, C. P., Cohen, H., Fitzgibbons, P. L., *et al.*, Prevalence of *Helicobacter pylori* infection and histologic gastritis in asymptomatic persons, *N. Engl. J. Med.* **321**:1562–1566 (1989).
131. Holtmann, G., Goebell, H., Holtmann, M., and Talley, N. J., Dyspepsia in healthy blood donors. Pattern of symptoms and association with *Helicobacter pylori*, *Dig. Dis. Sci.* **39**:1090–1098 (1994).
132. Morris, A. J., Ali, M. R., Nicholson, G. I., Perez-Perez, G. I., and Blaser, M. J., Long-term follow-up of voluntary ingestion of *Helicobacter pylori*, *Ann. Intern. Med.* **114**:662–663 (1991).
133. Gledhill, T., Leicester, R. J., Addis, B.,*et al.*, Epidemic hypochlorhydria, *Br. Med. J.* **290**:1383–1386 (1985).
134. Ramsey, E. J., Carey, K. V., Peterson, W. L., *et al.*, Epidemic gastritis with hypochlorhydria, *Gastroenterology* **76**:1449–1457 (1979).
135. Lambert, J. R., The role of *Helicobacter pylori* in nonulcer dyspepsia. A debate—for, *Gastroenterol. Clin. North Am.* **22:** 141–151 (1993).
136. Talley, N. J., The role of *Helicobacter pylori* in nonulcer dyspepsia. A debate—against, *Gastroenterol. Clin. North Am.* **22**:153–167 (1993).
137. Graham, D. Y., Lew, G. M., Klein, P. D., *et al.*, Effect of treatment of *Helicobacter pylori* infection on the long-term recurrence of gastric or duodenal ulcer. A randomized, controlled study, *Ann. Intern. Med.* **116**:705–708 (1992).
138. Hentschel, E., Brandstatter, G., Dragosics, B., *et al.*, Effect of ranitidine and amoxicillin plus metronidazole on the eradication of *Helicobacter pylori* and the recurrence of duodenal ulcer, *N. Engl. J. Med.* **328**:308–312 (1993).
139. Graham, D. Y., Treatment of peptic ulcers caused by *Helicobacter pylori*, *N. Engl. J. Med.* **328**:349–350 (1993).
140. Sipponen, P., Aarynen, M., Kaariainen, I., Kettunen, P., Helske, T., and Seppala, K., Chronic antral gastritis, Lewis (a+) phenotype, and male sex as factors in predicting coexisting duodenal ulcer, *Scand. J. Gastroenterol.* **24**:581–588 (1989).
141. Marshall, B. J., *Helicobacter pylori*, *Am. J. Gastroenterol.* **89**:S116–128 (1994).
142. Sipponen, P., Kekki, M., and Siurala, M., The Sydney system: Epidemiology and natural history of chronic gastritis, *J. Gastroenterol. Hepatol.* **6**:244–251 (1991).
143. Parsonnet, J., Friedman, G. D., Vandersteen, D. P., *et al.*, *Helicobacter pylori* infection and the risk of gastric carcinoma, *N. Engl. J. Med.* **325**:1127–1131 (1991).
144. Nomura, A. M. Y., Stemmerman, G. N., Chyou, P., Kato, I., Perez-Perez, G. I., and Blaser, M. J., *Helicobacter pylori* infection and gastric carcinoma in a population of Japanese-Americans in Hawaii, *N. Engl. J. Med.* **325**:1132–1136 (1991).
145. Eurogast Study Group, An international association between *Helicobacter pylori* infection and gastric cancer, *Lancet* **341:** 1359–1362 (1993).
146. Forman, D., Webb, P., and Parsonnet, J., *H. pylori* and gastric cancer, *Lancet* **343**:243–244 (1994).
147. Blaser, M. J., Chyou, P. H., and Nomura, A., Age at establishment of *Helicobacter pylori* infection and gastric carcinoma, gastric ulcer, and duodenal ulcer risk, *Cancer Res.* **55**:562–565 (1995).
148. Howson, C., Hiyama, T., and Wynder, E., The decline in gastric cancer: Epidemiology of an unplanned triumph, *Epidemiol. Rev.* **8**:1–27 (1986).
149. Severson, R. K., and Davis, S., Increasing incidence of primary gastric lymphoma, *Cancer* **66**:1283–1287 (1990).
150. Doglioni, C., Wotherspoon, A. C., Moschini, A., de Boni, M., and Isaacson, P. G., High incidence of primary gastric lymphoma in northeastern Italy, *Lancet* **339**:834–835 (1992).
151. Forman, D., Sitas, F., Newell, D. G., *et al.*, Geographic association of *Helicobacter pylori* antibody prevalence and gastric cancer mortality in rural China, *Int. J. Cancer* **46**:608–611 (1990).
152. Parsonnet, J., Hansen, S., Rodriguez, L., *et al.*, *Helicobacter pylori* infection and gastric lymphoma, *N. Engl. J. Med.* **330:** 1267–1271 (1994).
153. Talley, N. J., Zinsmeister, A. R., Weaver, A., *et al.*, Gastric adenocarcinoma and *Helicobacter pylori* infection, *J. Natl. Cancer Inst.* **83**:1734–1739 (1991).
154. Wotherspoon, A. C., Ortiz-Hidalgo, C., Falzon, M. R., and Isaacson, P. G., *Helicobacter pylori*-associated gastritis and primary B-cell gastric lymphoma, *Lancet* **338**:1175–1176 (1991).
155. Hussell, T., Isaacson, P. G., Crabtree, J. E., and Spencer, J., The response of cells from low-grade B-cell gastric lymphomas of mucosa-associated lymphoid tissue to *Helicobacter pylori*, *Lancet* **342**:571–574 (1993).
156. Bayerdorffer, E., Neubauer, A., Rudolf, B., Thiede, C., Lehn, N., Eidt, S., and Stolte, M., Regression of primary gastric lymphoma of mucosa-associated lymphoid tissue type after cure of *Helicobacter pylori* infection. MALT lymphoma study group, *Lancet* **345**:1591–1594 (1995).
157. Isaacson, P. G., Extranodal lymphomas: The MALT concept, *Verh. Dtsch. Ges. Pathol.* **76**:14–23 (1992).
158. Griener, A., Marx, A., Heesemann, J., Leebmann, J., Schmausser, B., and Muller-Hermelink, H. K., Idiotype identity in a MALT-type lymphoma and B cells in *Helicobacter pylori* associated chronic gastritis, *Lab. Invest.* **70**:572–578 (1994).
159. Hack, H. M., Harris, R., Owens, D. K., and Parsonnet, J., Prevention of gastric cancer: A cost-effectiveness analysis of screening for *H. pylori* (Abstract), *Clin. Res.* **42**:23A (1994).
160. Graham, D. Y., Benefits from elimination of *Helicobacter pylori* infection include major reduction in the incidence of peptic ulcer disease, gastric cancer, and primary gastric lymphoma, *Prev. Med.* **23**:712–716 (1994).
161. Marchetti, M., Arico, B., Burroni, D., Figura, N., Rappuoli, R., and Ghiara, P., Development of a mouse model of *Helicobacter pylori* infection that mimics human disease, *Science* **267**:1655–1658 (1995).
162. Kuipers, E. J., Pena, A. S., Van Kamp, G., Uyterlinde, A. M., Pals, G., Pels, N. F., Durz-Pohlmann, E., and Meuwissen, S. G., Seroconversion for *Helicobacter pylori*, *Lancet* **342**:328–331 (1993).
163. Dummer, S., Perez-Perez, G. I., Breining, M. K., Lee, A., and Griffith, B. P., Seroepidemiology of *Helicobacter pylori* infection in heart transplant recipients (Abstract), *Gastroenterology* **104:** A73 (1992).
164. Banatvala, N., Kashiwagi, S., Adbi, Y., Hayoshi, J., Hardie, J. M., and Feldman, R. A., *Helicobacter pylori* seroconversion and seroreversion in an Okinawan cohort followed for 10 years (Abstract), *Am. J. Gastroenterol.* **89**:1300 (1994).

12. Suggested Reading

Blaser, M. J., and Parsonnet, J., Parasitism by the "slow" bacterium *Helicobacter pylori* leads to altered gastric homeostasis and neoplasia, *J. Clin. Invest.* **94**:4–8 (1994).
Goodwin, C. S., and Worsley, B. W. (eds.), *Helicobacter pylori: Biology and Clinical Practice*, CRC Press, Boca Raton, FL, 1993.

IARC Working Group on the Evaluation of Carcinogenic Risks to Humans, *Helicobacter pylori*, in: *Schistosomes, Liver Flukes and Helicobacter pylori: Views and Expert Opinions of an IARC Working Group on the Evaluation of Carcinogenic Risks to Humans*, pp. 177–240, IARC, Lyon, 1994.

NIH Consensus Development Panel on *Helicobacter pylori* in Peptic Ulcer Disease, *Helicobacter pylori* in peptic ulcer disease, *J. Am. Med. Assoc.* **272**:65–69 (1994).

Warren, J. R., and Marshall, B. J., Unidentified curved bacilli in gastric epithelium in active chronic gastritis, *Lancet* **1**:1273–1275 (1983).

CHAPTER 18

Legionellosis

Jay C. Butler and Robert F. Breiman

1. Introduction

Legionellosis is infection with bacteria of the genus *Legionella*. Legionellosis is primarily associated with two clinically and epidemiologically distinct syndromes: Legionnaires' disease, a potentially fatal form of pneumonia, and Pontiac fever, a self-limited, nonpneumonic illness (Table 1.)[1,2] At least 39 *Legionella* species and 61 serogroups have been identified,[3] but one species, *L. pneumophila*, causes over 90% of Legionnaires' disease cases.[4] Most of the other cases are caused by *L. micdadei*, *L. longbeachae*, *L. dumoffii*, and *L. bozemanii*, although a number of other species have been occasionally reported as causing illness.[4,5] The majority of *L. pneumophila* infections are caused by serogroup 1.[4] Legionellosis may occur in outbreaks or as sporadic cases (i.e., not part of a recognized outbreak). Although Legionnaires' diseases outbreaks capture much media attention, the majority of reported cases are sporadic.[4] Pontiac fever is generally recognized only when clusters of illness occur. Legionnaires' disease is an important cause of community-acquired and nosocomial pneumonia; at least 8000–18,000 cases of Legionnaires' disease occur each year in the United States.[6]

2. Historical Background

When the 58th annual convention of the American Legion's Pennsylvania Department was held at the Bellevue-Stratford Hotel in Philadelphia on July 21 though 24, 1976, none of the 4400 attendees could have known that events surrounding the meeting would be chronicled on the front pages of newspapers and in medical journals around the world. Between July 22 and August 3, dozens of conventioneers developed a mysterious febrile illness with pneumonia; no etiology was identified. During the investigation that followed, a total of 182 cases of the illness were identified among persons who had entered the Bellevue-Stratford between July 1 and August 18, 1976.[1] Many of the conventioneers became ill after returning home from the convention, yet illness was not identified among family members who had not attended the convention, indicating that it was not likely transmitted from person to person. Illness was reported for 39 additional persons who had no direct connection to either the convention or the hotel, except all had been within one block of the Bellevue-Stratford at some time after July 1. This finding, together with the higher attack rate among convention delegates who had watched a parade from the sidewalk in front of the hotel,[1] suggested airborne transmission of an agent in the environment. Altogether, 221 people became ill and 34 died of the illness; which initially was dubbed Legionnaires' disease, a name that subsequently by mutual agreement of all involved parties was accepted as the official name. The cause of the outbreak remained unknown for 5 months despite intensive investigation, until early in 1977, when McDade and co-workers[7] recovered a fastidious, weakly gram-negative bacillus (subsequently named *Legionella pneumophila*) from guinea pigs inoculated with lung tissues of patients who had died during the outbreak. Paired acute- and convalescent-phase serum specimens from other ill conventioneers demonstrated rising levels of specific antibody to the organism, and high levels of antibody were present in over 90% of convalescent-phase specimens from ill conventioneers.[7] The source of the organism at the Bellevue-Stratford was not identified.

Serologic tests indicated that the newly identified

Jay C. Butler and Robert F. Breiman • Respiratory Diseases Branch, Division of Bacterial and Mycotic Diseases, National Center for Infectious Diseases, Centers for Disease Control and Prevention, Atlanta, Georgia 30333.

Table 1. Clinical and Epidemiological Characteristics of the Two Major Forms of Legionellosis

Characteristic	Legionnaires' disease	Pontiac fever
Symptoms	Fever, cough, headache, myalgia, dyspnea, chest pain, diarrhea, delirium	Fever, headache, myalgia, cough, sore throat, chest tightness
Chest X ray	Pneumonia	Normal
Primary treatment	Erythromycin	No specific therapy
Attack rate in outbreaks	<5%	>95%
Incubation period	2–10 days	<48 h
Mortality	5–30%	None

organism was also the etiologic agent of earlier, unsolved outbreaks of respiratory illness and cases of sporadic pneumonia.[7] Antibody tests performed on paired serum specimens that had been stored for several years at the Centers for Disease Control and Prevention (CDC) showed that the same organism, or an antigenically similar one, had caused an outbreak of 81 cases of pneumonia with 14 deaths in 1965 at a psychiatric hospital in Washington, DC.[8] Outbreaks of pneumonia occurring as early as 1957 were associated with serological evidence of legionellosis.[9] Also, a "*Rickettsia*-like" organism that had been isolated in 1947, in guinea pigs inoculated with blood of a patient with a febrile illness, was subsequently shown to be *L. pneumophila*.[10] Other organisms that had been isolated before 1976, but only partially characterized, were identified as *Legionella* species. An organism isolated from guinea pigs injected with the blood of a febrile soldier at Fort Bragg, North Carolina, in 1943, was identified as *L. micdadei* (although the role of *L. micdadei* in the soldier's illness is questionable),[11] and the same agent was described by Pasculle *et al.*,[12] in 1979, as the cause of acute pneumonia in renal transplant recipients. Bozeman[13] isolated an organism, later named *L. bozemanii*, from lung tissue of a scuba diver in 1959. *L. pneumophila* was also identified as the etiologic agent of an outbreak with a high attack rate of a self-limited, nonpneumonic illness with fever (Pontiac fever) occurring in 1968 at a health department building in Pontiac, MI.[2] Stored lung tissue from guinea pigs that had been exposed to air in the health department building and had developed pneumonia in 1968 yielded *L. pneumophila* a decade later.[14]

The environmental source and means of transmission of the organism were unknown until 1978, when Morris *et al.*[15] recovered *L. pneumophila* from various environmental specimens in conjunction with investigations of outbreaks that year. Aerosolized water from cooling towers and evaporative condensers (heat rejection devices used in the air-conditioning systems of large buildings) was implicated as the sources of dissemination of *L. pneumophila* in outbreaks of Legionnaires' disease in Memphis and Atlanta during 1978.[16,17] In 1980, Tobin and colleagues[18] isolated the same serogroup of *L. pneumophila* from two people who developed pneumonia after receiving renal transplants in an Oxford, England, hospital and from water taken from the shower in their common hospital room, indicating the role of potable water systems in the dissemination of *Legionella* species. Subsequent investigations conducted in the 1980s and 1990s further documented the role of cooling towers and potable water systems in the transmission of legionellosis, and dissemination of legionellae from other aerosol-producing devices have been reported (Section 6).

3. Methodology

3.1. Sources of Mortality Data

The gross and microscopic pathological findings in material obtained at autopsy from patients who died of Legionnaires' disease do not differ substantially from those found in cases of severe pneumonia caused by other bacteria.[19] Direct immunofluorescent antibody (DFA) staining has been widely used to identify the organisms postmortem in lung tissue.[19,20] Monoclonal DFA reagents are designed to detect only a single species or serogroup. Polyclonal reagents that react with several serogroups and species of *Legionella* are also available, but are more likely to cross-react with bacteria that may colonize the respiratory tract, such as *Pseudomonas* spp.[21] Either method of DFA testing may be performed on formalin-fixed lung scrapings, paraffin-embedded tissue sections, or fresh lung tissue,[19,20] although polyclonal reagents may be preferable for tissues fixed to prolonged periods in formalin.[22] Culture and polymerase chain reaction (PCR) have also been used to identify the organism in lung tissue obtained at autopsy, but care must be taken to avoid false-positive results caused by contamination during specimen processing.[23] The exact role of legionellosis in causing death may be difficult to determine because other serious, life-threatening underlying illnesses are often present. Additionally, bacteria other than *Legionella* spp. occasionally may be isolated from the lungs of persons who have died of Legionnaires' disease.[24]

Comprehensive, systematic, and reliable data on mortality due to Legionnaires' disease are unavailable. Although the National Center for Health Statistics (NCHS) receives copies of death certificates to tabulate national figures on deaths attributed to pneumonia and influenza based on International Classification of Diseases (ICD-9) codes, identification of a specific etiologic agent is lacking in the majority of cases. Data regarding the prevalence of Legionnaires' disease among patients who have died with pneumonia have been systematically sought in one multicity survey of fatal nosocomial pneumonia, in autopsy surveys of one or more hospitals in a city, and in conjunction with investigations of outbreaks.[25,26] Estimates of disease incidence from these studies are limited by small sample sizes and by nonrandom selection of hospitals surveyed. Review of autopsy material during epidemic investigations has been useful for defining the magnitude of the individual outbreaks. The case-fatality rate can be estimated by determining the proportion of fatal cases among those reported through surveillance for Legionnaires' disease; however, these estimates may be inaccurate because of underreporting of cases.[4] Additionally, the diagnosis may be confirmed more often among patients who die than those who survive because of more aggressive diagnostic testing among persons with severe pneumonia.

3.2. Sources of Morbidity Data

Data on the incidence and prevalence of Legionnaires' disease in the general population are based on findings from studies of patients with community-acquired pneumonia.[6,27–34] The most dependable data are from studies that are prospective, because of the difficulty of confirming the diagnosis retrospectively, and population-based, so that incidence of disease may be defined and bias is not introduced because only patients from a particular type of institution are included. The findings of these studies are affected by the criteria used to identify patients for laboratory testing and the type of laboratory tests used for case confirmation. Studies of incidence and prevalence of nosocomial legionellosis.[31,35–39] may be influenced by the same factors that affect studies of patients with community-acquired infection. Additionally, the incidence of nosocomial infection varies greatly from one institution to another because of differences in the potential for transmission and in the susceptibility of the patients.

National surveillance for legionellosis is conducted with varying intensity in many countries. In the United States, Legionnaires' disease is a reportable condition in most states and territories. State health departments are encouraged to submit case reports to CDC for national surveillance; however, data from prospective studies of patients with pneumonia indicate that less than 5% of legionellosis cases are reported to CDC.[4,6] The deficiencies in legionellosis case reporting is likely due in part to the difficulty in confirming the diagnosis. The quality of surveillance data may improve as newer diagnostic tests (e.g., urine antigen detection) become more widely utilized in evaluating patients with illnesses suggestive of Legionnaires' disease.

3.3. Surveys

The indirect immunofluorescent-antibody (IFA) test has been used most widely in serological surveys, although other, less standardized methods, including hemagglutination, indirect hemagglutination, immune adherence, microagglutination test, and enzyme-linked immunosorbent assay (ELISA), have also been used. Differences in methods of preparing test antigens and possible cross-reactions with other organisms, especially at relatively low titers, make the interpretation of serological surveys difficult. Serological tests prepared from heat-killed antigens, the most widely used test in North America, may not be as specific as those using formalinized antigen, which are commonly used in Europe.[40] Rates of elevated IFA titers ($\geqslant$1:128) to *L. pneumophila* in the general population have ranged from 1% to 36%[40–42]; generally, the higher rates are observed when pooled antigens from several *L. pneumophila* serogroups are used for preparation of reagents and the lower rates are seen in studies using tests specific for *L. pneumophila* serogroup 1. The relatively high background rates of elevated titers indicate that the positive predictive value of a single titer for determining recent legionellosis is low. The frequency with which legionellosis can occur as an asymptomatic or subclinical infection has been estimated by testing paired serum specimens from exposed well persons in conjunction with outbreak investigations.[43,44] Serological surveys have also been used to detect outbreaks of mild illness, but because of the low predictive value of serological testing of a single specimen, this approach is valid only if a suitable control group is used for comparison.

3.4. Laboratory Diagnosis

3.4.1. Isolation and Identification. Culture is the "gold standard" diagnostic method for legionellosis and for identifying the organism in the environment. Legionellae are most readily recovered on buffered charcoal–yeast extract agar medium enriched with α-ketoglutarate (BCYE-α) and are not isolated by routine clinical bacteriologic techniques. Three to ten days are generally required for the isolation of legionellae from respiratory secretions on BCYE-α medium.

Although recovery of *Legionella* spp. from clinical specimens is 100% specific for the diagnosis of Legionnaires' disease, a number of factors limit the sensitivity of culture. Laboratories experienced in the isolation of legionellae are more likely to recover the organism. A survey by the College of American Pathologists indicated that as many as two thirds of clinical microbiology labs in the United States are unable to grow a pure and heavy culture of *L. pneumophila*.[45] Moreover, to improve the specificity of the diagnosis of pneumonia caused by pyogenic bacteria, a common practice in hospital laboratories is to reject sputum specimens containing many squamous epithelial cells or few polymorphonuclear leukocytes; however, some patients with Legionnaires' disease produce little or nonpurulent sputum, and sputum specimens that would be routinely discarded may contain culturable legionellae.[46]

3.4.2. Serological Diagnostic Methods. Although serological tests are widely used for the diagnosis of legionellosis, these tests have a number of important and often underrecognized limitations. Even in cases of culture-confirmed Legionnaires' disease, a fourfold rise in antibody by IFA can be documented for only 70–80% of patients, and seroconversion following legionellosis may not occur for up to 2 months following the onset of illness.[40] Reagents that detect all major immunoglobulin classes (IgG, IgM, and IgA) are generally used. Testing for IgM alone has not proved useful for the diagnosis of legionellosis because IgM often increases concomitantly with IgG and may remain elevated for months or years after infection.[47] A single elevated antibody titer does not confirm the diagnosis of legionellosis. In a large study of patients hospitalized with community-acquired pneumonia in Ohio, a single titer of ≥1:256 did not distinguish between Legionnaires' disease and pneumonia due to other agents: only 10% of 68 patients with legionellosis confirmed by culture or fourfold rise in antibody had acute-phase titers of ≥256 compared with 6% of 636 patients with pneumonia caused by other agents.[48]

3.4.3. Antigen Detection and Genetic Probe Methods. Microscopic examination of specimens using DFA staining can be used to detect legionellae in lung tissue (from autopsy or biopsy) and in respiratory secretions. The sensitivity of DFA testing of respiratory secretions for the diagnosis of Legionnaires' disease has ranged from 25 to 75%, and specificity is >95%.[45] While DFA provides a rapid method of identifying *Legionella* spp., immunofluorescent microscopy is technically demanding and should be performed only by laboratory personnel experienced in the procedure. The specificity of polyvalent DFA reagents is probably lower than that of monoclonal reagents, leading some clinical microbiologists to recommend against routine use of polyvalent reagents.[45] Legionellae can be detected in respiratory secretions by DFA for several days after the start of antimicrobial therapy.

L. pneumophila serogroup 1 antigens can be detected in the urine of infected patients by a commercially available radioimmunoassay (RIA) test. The sensitivity of urinary antigen testing by RIA for the diagnosis of *L. pneumophila* serogroup 1 infection is 60–80%, and specificity approaches 100%.[40] Antigens are generally detectable in urine within a few days of illness onset and can remain so for several weeks after initiation of appropriate antimicrobial therapy.[49] A major drawback of urinary antigen testing is the difficulty involved in the handling and disposal of radioisotopes required to perform RIA. Urine tests based on nonradiometric formats, such as ELISA, are not available, and ELISA urinary antigen tests appear to have sensitivity and specificity equivalent to the RIA method.[50] Currently available urinary antigen tests are specific for *L. pneumophila* serogroup 1 and will not detect the 20–30% of Legionnaires' disease cases that are caused by other serogroups and species.[4] Development of a genus-wide urinary antigen test appears feasible and would provide a distinct diagnostic advantage.[51]

A genus-specific DNA probe for detecting legionellae in clinical specimens has been commercially available. The sensitivity and specificity of the DNA probe is similar to that of DFA testing.[40] However, a pseudo-outbreak of legionellosis attributed to false-positive DNA probe tests has been reported.[52] This pseudo-outbreak illustrates the need for clinical microbiology laboratories to confirm test results from new diagnostic modalities by standardized methods (e.g., culture) and for formal evaluation of newly marketed diagnostic tests in clinical settings. A PCR assay for detecting legionellae in water specimens is available, and limited experience using this test on clinical specimens is promising.[53]

4. Biological Characteristics of the Organism

Legionellae are rod-shaped bacteria 0.3–0.9 μm in diameter and ≥2 μm long.[54] Filamentous forms ≥10 μm in length have been seen after growth on artificial media. Ultrastructurally, legionellae resemble typical gram-negative bacilli, with a double membrane envelope and no evident cell wall. Like gram-negative bacteria, legionellae reproduce by cellular "pinching" without formation of septae.[54] Large numbers of organisms can be visualized and recovered from the lungs of patients with Legionnaires' disease; however, the organism does not appear to asymptomatically colonize the respiratory tract.[55] Therefore, any *Legionella* species recovered from respiratory secretions should be viewed as a likely pathogen. Legionellae have not been recovered from patients with Pontiac fever. The association between *Legionella* spp. and Pontiac fever is based on serological findings in patients exposed to confirmed sources of the organism during outbreaks.

Legionellae are readily phagocytized by alveolar macrophages and monocytes and are able to multiply intracellularly within specialized phagosomes.[56–58] Several moieties that may promote cell invasion or intracellular survival and multiplication have been identified.[59,60] The best characterized of these is macrophage infectivity potentiator (Mip), a cell surface protein that is necessary for efficient invasion of phagocytic cells and full expression of virulence.[61,62] When a site-specific mutation was introduced into a gene that encodes Mip in *L. pneumophila*, an 80-fold decrease in infectivity in explanted human macrophages was observed, and the mutant strain produced milder illness in experimentally infected guinea pigs.[61] Full infectivity and virulence was restored when the Mip gene was reintroduced into the attenuated strain.

Legionellae also infect and multiply within at least five genera of free-living amoebae (*Acanthamoeba*, *Naegleria*, *Hartmannella*, *Vahlkampfia*, and *Tetrahymena*) and one genus of ciliated protozoa (*Tetrahymena*) in aquatic environments.[63–65] Although legionellae may be cultivated on special agar media in laboratory settings, growth in nature in the absence of protozoa has not been documented, and intracellular multiplication within protozoa may be the primary means of proliferation.[65] Little is known about the nature of the interaction of these organisms at the cellular level, but the intracellular habitat likely provides the bacterium with a source of nutrients and protection against the biocidal effects of chlorine and heat.[66,67]

Several *Legionella* spp. and serogroups appear to be less virulent than *L. pneumophila* serogroup 1 and cause disease more commonly in immunosuppressed persons.[5] Certain strains of *L. pneumophila* serogroup 1, as determined by monoclonal antibody subtyping, are frequently associated with outbreaks of disease.[68,69] These strains react with a specific monoclonal antibody, MAb2, and are not commonly isolated from the environment.[70] The antigenic determinant reacting with MAb2 is a lipopolysaccharide.[71] The basis for the association of strains bearing this epitope with outbreaks of disease is unknown. In addition to monoclonal antibody testing, a number of other methods have been used for subtyping *L. pneumophila*, including plasmid analysis, electrophoretic alloenzyme typing, ribotyping, restriction length polymorphism analysis, pulsed-field electrophoresis, and arbitrarily primed PCR analysis.[72,73]

Subtyping can provide crucial information in supporting epidemiological evidence of a link between a specific source and human illness; however, these tests alone cannot reliably implicate a source without epidemiological data, because the distribution of isolates of various subtypes in the environment is unknown. The importance of interpreting the results of environmental testing and subtype analysis in the light of epidemiological data is illustrated by an investigation of 33 cases of Legionnaires' disease occurring in Washington Parish, Louisiana in 1989.[74] An industrial plant with several large cooling towers appeared to be the most obvious source of the outbreak, and of 200 water specimens initially collected from the area, only one, a specimen from a cooling tower at the industrial plant, contained the same subtype of *L. pneumophila* serogroup 1 as that isolated from patients. A case–control study systematically assessed the risk of disease associated with activities throughout the area, and infected persons were shown to be much more likely than controls to shop at a specific grocery store. Of those who did, persons with Legionnaires' disease were more likely to have shopped for at least 30 min and to have bought items in one section of the produce display. Adjacent to this display was an ultrasonic mist machine that moistened the vegetables, and the reservoir of this machine contained *L. pneumophila* serogroup 1 matching the epidemic strain by monoclonal antibody testing.[74] The mist machine was removed from the store and the outbreak ended. Had the investigation been limited to collection of water specimens, the cooling tower would have been implicated as the source of the outbreak, while the actual source would have remained undetected and caused additional cases.

5. Descriptive Epidemiology

5.1. Incidence and Prevalence

Few population-based studies have assessed the incidence of legionellosis. In a population-based study of all adults hospitalized during 1991 with pneumonia in two counties of Ohio with a combined population of 1.1 million persons ≥18 years old, the annual incidence of Legionnaires' disease was 7.0 cases per 100,000 adults in the study area.[(6)] In a study of patients participating in a prepaid health plan that covered 10% of the population in Seattle, Washington, 5 (1%) of 500 patients with community-acquired pneumonia (84% treated as outpatients) evaluated between 1963 and 1975 had legionellosis confirmed by a fourfold rise in antibody titer.[(27)] Based on these findings, the annual incidence of legionellosis was estimated to be 12 cases per 100,000 persons (95% confidence interval: 4–28 per 100,000).[(27)] A much lower incidence was observed in a 1-year, community-based study in Nottingham, England (population approximately 70,000): Of 251 patients with pneumonia (78% managed without hospitalization), only one had legionellosis confirmed by serological testing, for an annual incidence of 1.4 cases per 100,000 persons.[(28)]

The majority of studies assessing the prevalence of legionellosis among persons with pneumonia have been hospital-, reference laboratory-, or autopsy-based and have not permitted accurate calculation of incidence. Numerous studies have assessed the prevalence of legionellosis among patients hospitalized with community-acquired pneumonia. In recent studies involving more than 100 patients, the proportion of patients with community-acquired pneumonia who have evidence of legionellosis has ranged from 2 to 15%.[(6,29–34)] Similar proportions have been observed in studies designed to select for patients with severe pneumonia: Among patients prospectively evaluated after admission to intensive care for pneumonia, 3 to 14% had evidence of legionellosis.[(75,76)] In a retrospective examination of formalinized lung tissue from patients who died during hospitalization for pneumonia at either of two hospitals in St. Louis, MO, 1 (1%) of 97 had evidence of legionellosis.[(26)] Fewer data are available on the prevalence of legionellosis among persons with pneumonia not requiring hospitalization. Foy *et al.*[(27)] found evidence of legionellosis in 4 (1%) of 420 pneumonia patients managed as outpatients in a prepaid medical care group, compared with 1 (1%) of 80 patients requiring hospitalization.

The overall proportion of nosocomial pneumonias due to legionellosis is not known, although the percentage at individual hospitals has ranged from 0 to nearly 50%.[(31,35–39)] Of 263 patients who died of nosocomial pneumonia in 40 hospitals participating in the CDC's National Nosocomial Infections Surveillance (NNIS) during the mid-1970s, 3.8% had evidence of legionellosis based on DFA testing of specimens collected at autopsy.[(25)] From the NNIS data, Cohen *et al.*[(25)] estimated that 950 cases of fatal nosocomially acquired legionellosis occurred in the United States annually.

No data are available on the incidence or prevalence of Pontiac fever. Surveillance for Pontiac fever is not possible because the symptoms are mild and nonspecific, and no rapid tests are available to confirm the diagnosis.

5.2. Epidemic Behavior and Contagiousness

Although 80 to 90% of legionellosis cases reported through surveillance in the United States and the United Kingdom are sporadic,[(4,77)] Legionnaires' disease occasionally occurs in explosive, common source outbreaks. Ongoing or recurrent outbreaks occurring over a period of years have been associated with exposure to colonized water systems in buildings such as hotels and hospitals.[(78–80)] During outbreaks of Legionnaires' disease, attack rates among those exposed to the source of the organism are generally less than 5%, while the attack rate for Pontiac fever is much higher, up to 95% of exposed persons become ill.[(81)] In outbreaks of legionellosis, the risk of illness is often associated with the amount of time spent in the area of apparent exposure and, for Legionnaires' disease, the level of host susceptibility.

Although the organism is present in the respiratory secretions of patients with Legionnaires' disease, person-to-person transmission has not been documented. To assess the possibility of person-to-person transmission during the 1976 outbreak in Philadelphia, interviews were conducted with 193 household contacts of persons with Legionnaires' disease; no cases of illness suggestive of secondary spread during the 3 weeks following exposure were identified.[(1)] Similar interviews were conducted with household and hospital contacts of 27 patients during the investigation of an outbreak in Kingsport, Tennessee, in 1977; no evidence of person-to-person transmission was found.[(82)] Yu and colleagues[(83)] found no instances of pneumonia or seroconversion to *L. pneumophila* among 17 household contacts of patients with community-acquired Legionnaires' disease or among 15 hospital roommates of patients with nosocomial infection. There was no evidence of transmission of *L. pneumophila* from symptomatic, experimentally infected guinea pigs to uninfected animals in adjacent cages located <1 inch away.[(84)] One investigation found a higher prevalence of unexplained febrile respiratory illnesses and elevated antibody titers to *L. pneumophila* among hospital personnel in contact with Legionnaires' disease patients compared with health care workers without such exposure,[85] but these findings have not been reproduced. The elevated antibody levels among contacts of persons with legionellosis may reflect common exposure to an environmental source of the organism rather than person-to-person transmission, and the higher prevalence of self-reported respiratory illnesses among persons also reporting exposure to infected patients may be due to recall bias.

5.3. Geographic Distribution

Legionellosis occurs worldwide. Although most surveillance data comes from countries in temperate regions, cases of Legionnaires' disease have been identified in tropical countries when diagnostic testing has been performed.[86,87] In the United States, the incidence of reported Legionnaires' disease cases varies greatly among the states, with the higher rates observed in some northern states.[4] The observed regional variation in incidence may be due to dissimilar diagnostic and reporting practices or may reflect actual differences in incidence resulting from disparate ecological or epidemiological factors.

5.4. Temporal Distribution

Rates of reported Legionnaires' disease cases vary seasonally, with the highest rates occurring during the summer months[4]; outbreaks of Legionnaires' disease associated with cooling towers often have occurred during the summer and fall months.[88] Nonetheless, during a prospective, population-based study of pneumonia in Ohio, where diagnostic tests for legionellosis were systematically obtained, cases of Legionnaires' disease were identified year-round without an excess of cases in the summer.[6] Thus, the reported seasonality of Legionnaires' disease could reflect an ascertainment bias; i.e., clinicians may suspect and order tests for legionellosis more frequently during the summer on the basis of early reports of Legionnaires' disease as a predominantly summer disease.[89]

5.5. Age

In the 1976 outbreak in Philadelphia and in many subsequent Legionnaires' disease outbreaks, attack rates increased progressively with increasing age.[1] The rates of Legionnaires' disease identified through surveillance are highest among persons 60 to 79 years of age.[4] The association between illness and advanced age may be confounded by the high prevalence of medical conditions that predispose to Legionnaires' disease among the elderly (see Section 5.11). Compared with adults, Legionnaires' disease appears to be an uncommon cause of pneumonia among children. Most children with Legionnaires' disease have had underlying immunosuppressive conditions or chronic respiratory diseases.[90] However, seroconversion to *L. pneumophila* without respiratory disease is not uncommon during early childhood.[91] It is not clear whether these asymptomatic seroconversions among young children reflect frequent exposure to the organism or infection with serologically cross-reacting organisms.

Little is known about the role of age in Pontiac fever. In a large outbreak of Pontiac fever associated with a whirlpool spa in Scotland, attack rates were high among both children and adults.[92]

5.6. Sex

Legionnaires' disease occurs more often in men than women.[4] It has not been determined whether this is the result of greater susceptibility, higher prevalence of certain predisposing conditions (e.g., cigarette smoking, chronic lung diseases), more diagnostic testing, or increased risk of exposure. Serosurveys have generally not demonstrated differences in prevalence of elevated titers to *L. pneumophila* among men and women,[41,93] although one study found a greater prevalence of reciprocal titers $\geqslant$ 128 among men age 40 years and older compared with women in the same age range.[42] In outbreaks of Pontiac fever, attack rates among exposed males and females are generally equal.

5.7. Race

No consistent association between race and risk of legionellosis during outbreaks has been observed. One study found that the risk of community-acquired Legionnaires' disease was 14-fold higher among blacks than whites,[94] but among persons with Legionnaires' disease reported through surveillance during the 1980s, the rate of disease was only slightly higher among blacks (rate ratio: 1.1) compared with the general population.[4]

5.8. Occupation

Outbreaks of legionellosis have occurred in a variety of workplace settings, including industrial plants[95] and office buildings.[96,97] Additionally, employees working in hospitals where transmission of nosocomial Legionnaires' disease was occurring have become infected.[98,99] The relative importance of workplace exposure as a setting for transmission of non-outbreak-related legionellosis is unknown.

No particular occupation has been consistently identified as posing an increased risk of legionellosis. Construction workers were found to be at higher risk of contracting sporadic Legionnaires' disease in one case–control study,[94] but a serological survey did not show a higher prevalence of elevated antibody titers to *L. pneumophila* among construction and other outdoor workers compared with white-collar personnel working indoors.[100] A survey comparing air-conditioning maintenance personnel with workers for the same company who had no direct exposure to cooling towers demonstrated no differences in history of pneumonia or elevated titers to *L. pneumophila* serogroup 1.[101] While one study found a higher prevalence of antibody to *L. pneumophila* among workers with greater exposure to colonized power plant cooling towers,[102] another study failed to demonstrate such a difference.[103] Asymptomatic maintenance employees who worked on air-conditioning cooling towers associated with an outbreak of Legionnaires' disease were more likely to have serological evidence of infection compared to co-workers with less exposure.[104]

5.9. Occurrence in Special Settings

5.9.1. Nosocomial Infection. Legionnaires' disease is a common cause of nosocomial pneumonia in some hospitals. Hospitals provide a unique setting where large numbers of persons with underlying medical conditions predisposing to Legionnaires' disease may be exposed to the organism, and numerous outbreaks of nosocomial disease have been reported.[8,16,18,35–37,79,80,99,104–116] Transmission within hospitals with colonized hot water systems can occur intermittently for years.[79,80] Data from surveillance indicate that when one case of nosocomial Legionnaires' disease occurs at a hospital, additional cases are likely to occur.[117] Of 196 cases of nosocomial Legionnaires' disease reported in England and Wales between 1980 and 1992, 69% occurred during 22 nosocomial outbreaks (defined as two or more cases occurring at an institution over a 6-month period).[117] Nine percent occurred as "sporadic" cases (6 or more months before or after additional cases) at hospitals where outbreaks occurred. In five instances, sporadic cases preceded the outbreak, suggesting that a single case of nosocomial Legionnaires' disease may be a sentinel event, indicating the risk of escalating transmission. Another 13% of cases occurred in institutions where other "sporadic" cases, but no outbreaks, were identified. Only 9% of cases occurred at institutions where no outbreaks or additional sporadic cases were identified.[117]

The risk of acquiring Legionnaires' disease during hospitalization is influenced by a number of factors, including the type and intensity of exposure and the exposed person's health status.[118] Specific risk factors for nosocomial Legionnaires' disease identified in case–control studies include immunosuppressive medication (e.g., cytotoxic chemotherapy, corticosteroids), endotracheal intubation, general anesthesia, placement of a nasogastric tube, and occupying a hospital room in the proximity of an aerosol source.[35,99,105–107,109,111] Showering was associated with nosocomial legionellosis in one case control study,[106] while another found showering to be significantly less common among patients with hospital-acquired infection.[107] The lack of consistent association with showering likely reflects different modes of transmission in various hospital settings.

In nosocomial outbreaks of Legionnaires' disease, patients were exposed to contaminated aerosols generated by cooling towers,[110] showers,[106] faucets,[108] and respiratory therapy equipment contaminated with potable water.[105,112] Aspiration of contaminated potable water has also been proposed as a mode of transmission among hospitalized patients.[36,107] In a prospective study of nosocomial pneumonias among patients with head and neck cancer (who may be particularly prone to aspiration of oropharyngeal contents), a large proportion (30%) of 27 cases of nosocomial pneumonia were due to *L. pneumophila*.[36] Among 177 patients who had undergone laryngectomy, making oropharyngeal aspiration into the bronchopulmonary tree impossible, only three cases of pneumonia were identified, and none were due to legionellosis.[36] In a case–control study of patients with nosocomial Legionnaires' disease acquired at a hospital where the potable water system was colonized with *L. pneumophila*, aspiration was proposed as the mode of transmission, in part because of the absence of culturable legionellae from air samples collected in the vicinity of aerosol-producing devices.[107] However, air sampling, particularly with the settling plate method utilized in this study, is an insensitive method of detecting airborne legionellae. While it appears likely that aspiration of contaminated potable water plays some role in the transmission of nosocomial legionellosis, the proportion of infections attributable to aspiration is unknown.

5.9.2. Disease in Travelers. A history of recent travel is associated with many cases of legionellosis. Approximately 25–50% of Legionnaires' disease cases reported through surveillance in the United States and United Kingdom are associated with recent travel (CDC unpublished data).[77] In a case–control study of sporadic community-acquired Legionnaires' disease in the United States, case-patients were more likely to report having traveled during the 2 weeks before illness onset than were their acquaintances.[94] Outbreaks of legionellosis have been identified among guests at hotels and resorts and among passengers on a cruise ship.[1,78,92,119–123] Outbreaks of Legionnaires' disease among travelers are probably underrecognized, because hotel guests and cruise ship passengers exposed during travel often return home before becoming ill; unless several members of the same travel partly become ill, the clustering of cases and the association with travel may not be recognized.

5.10. Socioeconomic Factors

Although socioeconomic status may be linked with risk factors for legionellosis (e.g., smoking, travel, underlying illness), a direct association between socioeconomic status and the risk of legionellosis has not been identified.

5.11. Other Factors

5.11.1. Cigarette Smoking. Cigarette smokers have a two- to fourfold higher risk of developing Legionnaires' disease than do nonsmokers, and the risk is greatest among those who smoke the most cigarettes.[4,94] Alveolar macrophages harvested from healthy smokers have diminished resistance to intracellular replication of *L. pneumophila* compared with those from nonsmokers.[124] Cigarette smoking has not been associated with Pontiac fever.

5.11.2. Alcohol Consumption. Compared with cigarette smoking, alcohol consumption has been less consistently associated with Legionnaires' disease, and the association may be confounded by the higher prevalence of smoking among those who drink alcohol heavily.[125] After controlling for smoking in multivariate analysis, one study of sporadic, community-acquired disease demonstrated an increased risk of infection among persons who consumed three or more alcohol-containing drinks per day.[94]

5.11.3. Underlying Medical Conditions. The risk of acquiring Legionnaires' disease is over 20-fold greater for persons with hematologic malignancies or with end-stage renal disease than for the general population.[4] Risk of disease is also heightened for persons with diabetes mellitus or lung cancer and for patients receiving corticosteroids.[4,94,105,109,111] Legionnaires' disease is increasingly recognized in persons with acquired immunodeficiency syndrome (AIDS).[126] Based on a small number of cases reported through surveillance, the incidence of Legionnaires' disease among person with AIDS is more than 40 times that of the general population.[4] Pontiac fever generally occurs in people who are otherwise healthy.

6. Mechanism and Routes of Transmission

Legionellae are commonly present in natural and manmade aquatic environment.[15,127] The organism is occasionally found in other sources such as potting soil, as shown by an investigation of an outbreak of *L. longbeachae* infection in Australia.[128] However, the overall importance of nonaquatic environmental sources in human disease is not yet known. In natural water sources and municipal water systems, legionellae are generally present in very low concentrations.[129,130] However, under certain circumstances within manmade water systems, the concentration of organisms may increase markedly, a process termed "amplification.[131] Conditions that are favorable for the amplification of legionellae growth include temperatures of approximately 25–42°C, stagnation, scale and sediment, biofilms, and the presence of amoebae.[64,132–136]

Most of what is known regarding the transmission of legionellosis is derived from investigations of disease outbreaks. These data suggest that, in most instances, transmission to humans occurs when water containing the organism is aerosolized in respirable droplet nuclei (1–5 μm in diameter) and inhaled by a susceptible host. A variety of aerosol-producing devices have been associated with outbreaks of legionellosis (Table 2). The role of airborne transmission of Legionnaires' disease has been questioned because of evidence of aspiration in some nosocomial infections, the low attack rate in outbreaks, and implication of potable water rather than cooling towers in many recent nosocomial outbreak investigations.[35,137,138] Aspiration of organisms colonizing the oropharynx is important in the pathogenesis of pneumonia caused by most pyogenic bacteria. However, legionellae can be recovered from the oropharynx for only a very short period (<60 min) after gargling with tap water containing *L. pneumophila*,[137] and colonization of the oropharynx by legionellae occurs rarely, if at all.[55] Low attack rates in Legionnaires' disease outbreaks probably reflect the importance of host susceptibility as a key factor in developing illness following exposure, rather than suggesting a specific mode of transmission. Although most recently published reports of nosocomial outbreaks have implicated hospital potable water as the source of the

Table 2. Aerosol Sources for Transmission of Legionellosis Identified During Outbreak Investigation

Clinical syndrome	Aerosol source	Selected references
Legionnaires' disease	Cooling tower	16, 96, 104, 110, 114, 139–141
	Evaporative condenser	17, 143
	Showers	18, 99, 106
	Faucets	108
	Respiratory therapy equipment	105, 112
	Portable room humidifier	105
	Whirlpool spa	123, 145a, 189
	Decorative fountain	122
	Ultrasonic mist machine	74
Pontiac fever	Cooling tower	97
	Evaporative condenser	14
	Whirlpool spa	92, 121, 190, 191
	Decorative fountain	192
	Water-based lubricant from industrial metal grinder	95
	Cleaning of steam turbine condenser	193

organism, outbreaks associated with exposure to infectious aerosols produced by cooling towers continue to occur.(139) The relative importance of airborne spread via aerosolized water and aspiration of water containing the organism in the transmission of Legionnaires' disease in various settings has not been determined.

Numerous investigations have demonstrated that cooling towers and evaporative condensers have served as the sources *Legionella*-contaminated aerosols causing outbreaks of community-acquired and nosocomial disease.(14,16,97,104,106,110,114,140,141) Cooling towers and evaporative condensers are devices that reject heat from coolant (water) to the atmosphere by maximizing contact of the water with air (Fig. 1). Mechanisms for facilitating heat transfer include spraying the water into droplets and allowing for countercurrent air flow. Some of the water in these systems is broken into airborne particles that are ejected with the airflow. Conditions within cooling towers and evaporative condensers are often ideal for amplification of legionellae,(135) and a substantial proportion of these devices contain water contaminated with *Legionella* spp.(142) The aerosols from these devices may either be directly inhaled(17) or entrained into a building's ventilation system and inhaled by the occupants.(143) Outbreak-associated transmission via cooling towers and evaporative condensers has been most commonly documented when those infected have been in fairly close proximity of the contaminated devices; however, data from one Legionnaires' disease outbreak investigation suggest that legionellae may be carried in cooling tower aerosols for distances of up to 1 to 2 miles (1.6 to 3.2 km).(141) Certain climatic conditions, such as greater relative humidity, prolong the viability of legionellae carried in aerosols and may play a role in disease transmission.(141,144) A number of outbreaks of legionellosis associated with cooling towers and evaporative condensers have occurred after these devices have been started up following a period of inactivity.(2,18,104,139-141) Bentham and Broadbent(88) observed that the concentration of legionellae isolated from water of idle cooling towers increases markedly within 10 min of beginning operation. The increased concentration of organisms, and possibly increased risk of disease transmission, may be caused by disturbance of *Legionella*-containing biofilms and sediments by water flowing through the system after start up. While it has been clearly shown that cooling towers and evaporative condensers are capable of transmitting disease, it is less certain how often they actually do.

Aerosolization of contaminated warm potable water can also transmit legionellosis during outbreaks. Shower heads and tap faucets can produce aerosols containing legionellae in droplets of respirable size.(145) Case–control studies and air sampling conducted during outbreak investigations have established the role of aerosols produced by showers and tap faucets in disease transmission.(106,108) Transmission of disease has occurred via aerosols produced by respiratory therapy equipment that has been filled or rinsed with contaminated potable water in hospitals.(105,112) Some nosocomial outbreaks of Legionnaires' disease have been associated with nearby construction,

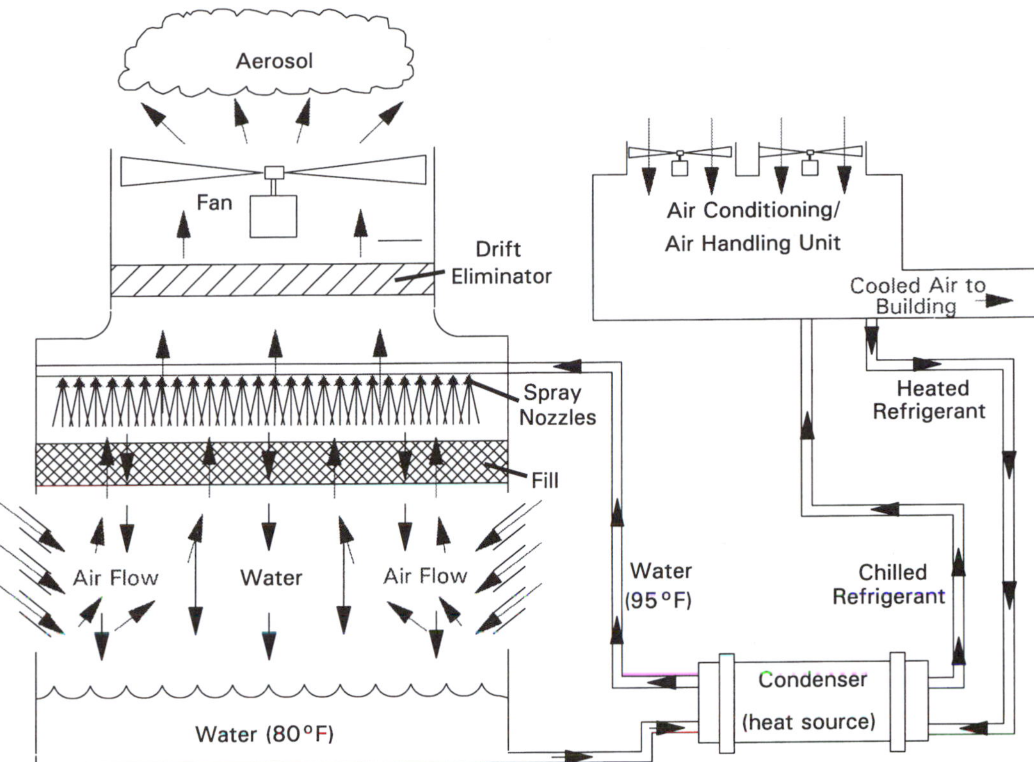

Figure 1. Schematic drawing of a typical air conditioning (induced draft) cooling tower; water temperatures are approximate and may differ substantially according to system use and design. Warm water from the condenser (or chiller) is sprayed downward into a counter- or cross-current air flow. To accelerate heat transfer to the air, the water passes over the fill, a component of the tower designed to increase the surface area of water exposed to air by either breaking the water into small droplets or causing it to spread into a thin film. Some of the water becomes aerosolized during this process, although the volume of aerosol discharged into the atmosphere can be reduced by the placement of a drift eliminator. Water cooled in the tower returns to the heat source to cool refrigerant from the air conditioning unit and to continue the cycle of heat transfer.

most likely due to loosening of sediment and scale containing legionellae within plumbing systems by vibrations or major changes in water pressure that may occur during repairs.[115] In one outbreak, cases of nosocomial infection were identified within a few days after a test of a potable water pump caused a sharp drop in water pressure and left the hospital's water discolored for several weeks.[116] Case-patients did not differ from controls in any measurable exposure to hospital potable water, including number of glasses of water drunk, use of ice, and showers taken; however, *L. pneumophila* was isolated from the potable water, and reproducing the water pressure drop in an isolated segment of the hospital led to a 30-fold increase in *L. pneumophila* concentration and the recurrence of discoloration of the water.[116] Recent outbreaks of Legionnaires' disease among persons in and around whirlpool spas emphasize the potential for transmission from previously unrecognized sources.[123,145a]

Compared with outbreak-associated infection, much less is known about transmission of sporadic legionellosis, although it is likely that transmission occurs by similar mechanisms. Exposure to legionellae in sporadic cases may occur in a variety of settings, including the home, the workplace, and public places visited during routine daily activities or during travel. The proportion of sporadic disease attributable to exposure in each of these settings and to various environmental sources is unknown.

In a retrospective analysis of sporadic cases occurring in Glasgow, Scotland, the homes of persons with Legionnaires' disease were located within close proximity of cooling towers more often than expected in comparison with the distribution of residences in the community.[146] However, the analysis may not have controlled for possible confounders.[81] For example, cooling towers are more likely to be located in inner-city and industrial zones, areas often inhabited by persons of lower socioeconomic status who are at risk of having underlying conditions or behaviors (such as cigarette smoking) that are associated with acquiring Legionnaires' disease.

Exposure to contaminated potable water also plays an important role in transmission of sporadic legionellosis. In an investigation of patients with culture-confirmed, sporadic Legionnaires' disease in Pittsburgh, Pennsylvania, Stout and colleagues[147] recovered identical subtypes of *L. pneumophila* from both the patient and potable water to which patients had been exposed for 8 of 20 cases investigated. Sites from which the identical subtypes were recovered included two nursing homes (accounting for three patients), two patients' homes, two clinics, and an industrial plant.[147] In a study comparing household characteristics of patients with Legionnaires' disease and those of matched controls, recent plumbing work within the home was associated with acquiring Legionnaires' disease.[148] This finding suggests that disruption of biofilm and sediment by changes in water pressure during repairs may result in seeding of the plumbing system with legionellae. Microbiological surveys of residential water systems have shown that detectable levels of legionellae are present in 2 to 32% of residential hot water systems, with the organism more likely to be present in apartment buildings with large hot water distribution systems.[70,149,150] Factors associated with colonization of home water systems have included lower hot water tank temperatures and use of electric rather than gas or oil water heaters.[70,148,151]

7. Pathogenesis and Immunity

The incubation period for Legionnaires' disease is generally 2–10 days from inhalation of the causative agent until onset of pneumonia symptoms.[1,81] Inhaled organisms that reach the terminal alveoli are engulfed by alveolar macrophages and reside within specialized phagosomes that do not fuse with lysosomes, permitting the organism to escape intracellular killing.[58,152] Animal studies indicate that *L. pneumophila* replicates rapidly within the first 24 hr after infection[153]; large numbers of organisms are released from infected macrophages and, in turn, enter other phagocytes. Legionellae also appear to be capable of reproducing within alveolar epithelial cells, but the significance of this observation is not known.[154] An influx of polymorphonuclear leukocytes into the lungs occurs during the initial 3 days of infection, followed by an infiltration of mononuclear phagocytes.[153] Viable organisms are cleared from the lungs of surviving animals within 11 days of infection, and clearance coincides with the appearance of antibodies to *Legionella* in serum and alveolar lavage fluid.[153]

The gross pathological findings in Legionnaires' disease include heavy, congested lungs with consolidation distributed evenly through the lung parenchyma with no predilection for any specific lobe.[24,155,156] Consolidation is usually delineated by the lobular septa.[24] In some cases, consolidation is distinctly nodular and may be mistaken for tumor nodules.[156] Cut surfaces of involved portions of lung appear moist and airless. Although pulmonary cavities are rarely identified radiographically with Legionnaires' disease, multiple small macroscopic lung abscesses are observed in approximately 20% of fatal cases.[156] Overtly hemorrhagic pulmonary parenchyma and empyema are unusual.

Microscopically, there is an acute fibropurulent pneumonia with neutrophils, macrophages, erythrocytes, and fibrin that fill the alveoli and respiratory bronchioles; these findings do not differ substantially from those of bronchopneumonia caused by other bacteria.[19,156] Superimposed features of diffuse alveolar damage, such as hyaline membranes, interstitial inflammation, and pneumocyte regeneration, may be present in severe cases. Although the cellular infiltrate is commonly necrotic and small abscess formation may occur, the underlying pulmonary structure remains intact. Legionellae are difficult to identify by Gram's stain, but will stain nonspecifically with Giemsa, Warthin–Starry, and Dieterle techniques.[19] Bacilli are commonly seen in clusters within macrophages. *L. micdadei* and *L. cincinnatiensis* in clinical specimens may stain with acid-fast techniques (e.g., Kinyoun stain), but will appear morphologically distinct from mycobacteria.[156–158]

Bacteremia may accompany Legionnaires' disease,[159] but whether symptoms referable to the gastrointestinal tract, kidneys, central nervous system, and muscle result from direct bacterial invasion (which has rarely been demonstrated in extrathoracic organs), toxins, or other indirect effects is not known. No consistent histopathologic changes have been demonstrated except in the lungs.

Cell-mediated immunity is important in host defense against legionellae, which multiply in human blood monocytes and alveolar macrophages.[56,57] Three different types of cell-mediated immune mechanisms have been studied.[60] First, human monocytes and alveolar macrophages activated by lymphokines inhibit intracellular multiplication of *L. pneumophila*. Second, activated polymorphonuclear leukocytes have an enhanced capacity to kill the organism, although several days are required for killing, raising some question about the significance of this immune mechanism. Third, cytotoxic lymphocytes may be capable of lysing infected macrophages, although evidence supporting this mechanism has not been reproduced.[60] Moreover, patients receiving medications that impair cell-mediated immunity are at increased risk of Legionnaires' disease. These observations suggest that cell-mediated immunity is the primary host defense against legionellosis, while humoral immunity plays a secondary role. Anti-*L. pneumophila* antibody promotes phagocytosis of the organism by alveolar macrophages but does not promote intracellular killing.[57]

The level of protection against reinfection among humans after legionellosis is poorly understood. Guinea pigs exposed to sublethal doses of *L. pneumophila* in aerosols developed strong humoral and cell-mediated immune responses, and these animals survived subsequent challenge with large doses of aerosolized *L. pneumophila*, which killed control animals that were not previously exposed.[160]

Pontiac fever usually has an incubation period of <48 hr after legionellae are inhaled.[2] The pathogenesis of this syndrome is not understood, in part because the disease is not fatal and no pathological material has been examined. It is also unknown whether proliferation of bacteria is necessary to produce the syndrome and, if it is, where the proliferation occurs. Hypersensitivity to inhaled amoebae that are infected with legionellae has been proposed as a possible cause of Pontiac fever.[161]

8. Patterns of Host Response

8.1. Clinical Features

Legionnaires' disease is a type of pneumonia that may also involve other organ systems. Clinical features may include fever, cough, headache, myalgia, dyspnea, pleuritic chest pain, diarrhea, and delirium. The white blood cell count is normal or elevated, with an increased proportion of immature neutrophils. Chest X rays of patients with Legionnaires' disease typically show alveolar infiltrates, although a variety of radiographic patterns may be seen.[45] Pleural effusions, when present, are typically small. Cavitation of pulmonary infiltrates occasionally occurs, particularly in immunosuppressed patients.

The severity of illness in legionellosis ranges from asymptomatic seroconversion to rapidly fatal pneumonia. Among patients with at least a fourfold rise in antibodies to *Legionella* spp. after admission to hospitals where ongoing nosocomial transmission was occurring, 29 to 69% had no evidence of pneumonia.[43,44] Mortality in Legionnaires' disease outbreaks has ranged from 5 to 30%.[81] Among cases reported through surveillance, 24% were fatal.[4] Death occurs due to progressive pneumonia with hypoxemia and shock. Factors associated with a fatal outcome include advanced age, immunosuppression, nosocomial acquisition of infection, end-stage renal disease, and cancer.[4] The drug of choice for treatment of Legionnaires' disease is erythromycin, and early administration of therapy at the appropriate dosage improves survival.[162] Rifampin is occasionally used in addition to erythromycin in clinically severe infections. Other antibiotics with activity against *Legionella* spp. include trimethoprim–sulfamethoxazole, doxycycline, azithromycin, clarithromycin, and several fluoroquinolone agents.[45] Convalescence following Legionnaires' disease may be prolonged in some cases, with weakness and shortness of breath persisting for months. Residual defects in pulmonary diffusing capacity have been observed.[163] Reinfection with *L. pneumophila* has been reported for severely immunocompromised patients.[164] Manifestations of disease caused by *L. pneumophila* and by other species of *Legionella* appear to be similar.[5]

Extrapulmonary infections during the course of Legionnaires' disease have been recognized, most likely due to bacteremic seeding during the course of pneumonia. Reported extrapulmonary infections with *Legionella* spp. in the absence of clinically apparent pneumonia include involvement of the endocardium, pericardium, peritoneum, bowel, respiratory sinuses, and skin and soft tissues.[45] Extrapulmonary disease generally occurs in immnosuppressed patients. Transmission of extrapulmonary *L. dumoffii* infection by direct inoculation of surgical wounds with colonized tap water during bathing or dressing changes has been reported.[165]

Pontiac fever is characterized by fever, headache, and myalgia. Cough, sore throat, and chest tightness are observed in about 50% of cases.[2] Other symptoms occasionally reported include dizziness, nausea, confusion, and a burning sensation in the eyes. No specific therapy is required for Pontiac fever. Illness may be debilitating for several days, but recovery is complete within 1 week.

8.2. Diagnosis

Clinical studies have not reliably distinguished community-acquired or nosocomial Legionnaires' disease from other causes of pneumonia on the basis of signs, symptoms, routine laboratory tests, or radiographic findings[30,39,166–168]; however, these studies have had limited statistical power because of relatively small numbers of patients. Legionnaires' disease can be diagnosed with certainty only when the diagnosis is considered, appropriate specimens are collected, and specimens are tested using laboratory tests specifically designed to detect legionellosis (Section 3.4). The decision to obtain diagnostic tests for legionellosis from patients with pneumonia must be individualized, but they should be particularly considered for patients who: (1) are immunosuppressed, (2) have pneumonia that is acquired nosocomially in a hospital where transmission of legionellosis is known to occur, (3) are involved in an outbreak of pneumonia, (4) have traveled during the preceding 2 weeks, or (5) have illness not responding to treatment with β-lactam antibiotics. If Legionnaires' disease is suspected, appropriate antibiotic treatment should not be withheld pending the results of specific laboratory tests.

Pontiac fever should be suspected when multiple cases of an acute, influenzalike illness are identified among persons with direct exposure to an aerosol-producing device. Confirmation of the diagnosis is based on serological testing. Detection of *Legionella* spp. in an aerosol source that is epidemiologically linked to cases can help guide selection of antigens for use in serologic testing.[121]

9. Control and Prevention

9.1. General Concepts

Legionellosis can be prevented by interrupting transmission of the bacteria from the environment to humans. This has been accomplished in the context of disease outbreaks (secondary prevention) by disinfecting the water systems of devices that generated contaminated aerosols. Strategies to prevent transmission in settings not associated with recognized cases of legionellosis (primary prevention) should create conditions that are unsuitable for amplification and dissemination to occur. Certain characteristics of legionellae can be exploited to control and eradicate the organism. Legionellae grow poorly at temperatures below 20°C or above 50°C and are readily killed at temperatures above 60°C.[132] Additionally, legionellae are susceptible to a broad range of disinfectants, including chlorine- and bromine-containing compounds, ozone, heavy metal ions, and ultraviolet light.[169–171] However, the results of studies under laboratory conditions may not accurately predict the efficacy of a control measure under operating conditions.[172]

Cooling towers and evaporative condensers associated with legionellosis outbreaks have been decontaminated by hyperchlorination and mechanical cleaning,[118] and further transmission has been prevented. The optimal method for primary prevention of transmission from heat rejection devices has not been identified, but a reasonable strategy might include placement of towers as far from building air intakes and public areas as possible, use of drift eliminators to minimize aerosol dissemination, periodic inspection and cleaning to remove accumulations of sediment and organic matter, and a water treatment program that includes corrosion control and automatic dosing with an effective biocide.[173]

A number of methods have been used to eradicate legionellae from potable water systems.[118,174] In buildings where the heated-water system has been identified as the source of Legionnaires' disease outbreaks, the system has been decontaminated by thermal disinfection (i.e., flushing each distal outlet of the hot water system for at least 5 min with water ⩾65°C) or hyperchlorination (flushing all outlets of the hot water system with water containing ⩾10 mg/liter free residual chlorine), and transmission has been interrupted. Following either of these procedures, the water system is maintained to provide water ⩾50°C at the hot water tap and cold water at <20°C at the cold tap, and/or supplemental chlorine is continuously added to achieve 1–2 mg/liter free residual chlorine at the tap. Disadvantages of thermal eradication include the risk of scalding; supplemental chlorination has caused accelerated corrosion and leaks in plumbing systems and could lead to formation of potentially carcinogenic halogenated organic compounds.[174] Additional measures, such as physical cleaning or replacement of hot water storage tanks, water heaters, faucets, and shower heads, may be required to remove accumulated scale and sediment that protect organisms from the biocidal effects of heat and chlorine. Plumbing system design may need to be altered to remove portions not reached by thermal eradication and chlorination and where amplification may continue to occur (e.g., spur pipes).[175] Experience with alternative methods for control and eradication of legionellae in water systems, such as treatment of water with ozone, ultraviolet light, or heavy metal ions, is more limited. Occasionally, a combination of modalities has been required to prevent transmission from potable water systems.

Additional steps can be taken to prevent transmission of legionellae. Only sterile water should be used to clean and fill nebulizers, other respiratory therapy equipment, and humidifiers.[118] Halogen levels in whirlpool spas should be maintained at 4–10 mg/liter and levels should be monitored frequently. To ensure that free halogen is effective for disinfection, water pH should be maintained at 7.2 to 7.8. The system should be drained and water contact areas should be cleaned regularly—at least daily during periods of heavy use. Whirlpool spa filters should be inspected at least weekly and cleaned or replaced if organic material has accumulated.

An alternative approach to control is based on periodic, routine culturing of water samples from cooling towers, potable water systems, or other aerosol-producing devices, and instituting control measures if legionellae are detected.[176,177] However, this method has not been widely recommended by public health officials because: (1) the results of water culture do not necessarily correlate with the potential for aerosol transmission; (2) the bacterium is frequently present in water systems without being associated with known cases of disease; (3) interpretation of the results of routine culturing of water is confounded by use of different bacteriologic methods in various laboratories, by variable culture results among sites sampled within a water system, and by fluctuations in the concentration of legionellae isolated from a single site,[178,179] and (4) the risk of illness following exposure to a given source is influenced by a number of factors (e.g., strain virulence, host susceptibility) other than the detectability and concentration of organisms in a sample.

9.2. Antibiotic and Chemotherapeutic Approaches to Prophylaxis

Erythromycin chemoprophylaxis of immunosuppressed patients at a hospital with a high incidence of nosocomial Legionnaires' disease due to colonization of the hot water distribution system resulted in protection against Legionnaires' disease.[113] However, in view of the generally low attack rate during outbreaks and the potential of eliminating the source of the organism, chemoprophylaxis is seldom indicated.

9.3. Immunization

Immunization of humans against legionellosis has not been attempted. Given the success of prototypic vaccines in an animal model, a vaccine against Legionnaires' disease in humans seems feasible.[180] From a cost-benefit standpoint, such a vaccine would probably be targeted at patients at highest risk of infection.

10. Unresolved Issues

10.1. Rapid Diagnostic Tests

The clinical presentation of Legionnaires' disease is similar to that of other types of pneumonia; therefore, accurate, rapid diagnostic tests are essential to ensure appropriate clinical management of patients and early recognition of outbreaks so that prevention strategies may be instituted. Continued development and evaluation of new diagnostic modalities, such as antigen detection tests and PCR, are needed. Tests to detect *Legionella* other than *L. pneumophila* serogroup 1 antigens in urine will likely become available in the near future.[51] Additional studies are needed to determine whether PCR is as sensitive and specific as culture for identifying *Legionella* in clinical specimens and whether the effect of substances present in sputum that inhibit PCR can be overcome.[40]

10.2. Risk Assessment

Although environments capable of supporting the growth of legionellae, such as cooling towers and hot water distribution systems, are a part of everyday modern life and the bacterium is frequently present in these systems, transmission resulting in disease occurs relatively infrequently. More information is needed about the specific virulence, host, and environmental factors that increase the risk of transmission. Epidemiological studies in concert with careful environmental investigations can define the risk of Legionnaires' disease attributable to various colonized water systems and aerosol-producing devices. The role of environmental monitoring in risk assessment is yet to be determined, and at present, limited data are available on the association between the concentration of organisms in a water system and the risk of transmission.[181] The utility of nonculture methods (e.g., antigen detection, PCR) for detecting virulent *Legionella* in the environment needs to be further defined.[149,182–184] Additionally, the pathogenic potential of legionellae and related organisms that are not detected by culture methods designed to detect *Legionella* spp. needs to be assessed.[121,185,186]

10.3. Prevention

The most cost-effective methods of primary and secondary prevention of legionellosis in various settings have not been identified. Development of prevention strategies is complicated by the complex ecology of *Legionella* spp. and the limited knowledge of the determinants of disease transmission. Understanding factors in the microbiological milieu that favor amplification of legionellae, such as biofilm formation and the presence of protozoa capable of supporting intracellular growth of the organism, will provide additional insight into methods of prevention. Large field trials of various biocides in operating cooling towers could identify specific compounds and dosing regimens to effectively limit the growth of legionellae.[187] The role of new water quality technologies (e.g., ozone, UV light, heavy metal ions) in the control of legionellae in water systems also needs to be determined. Plumbing system design and materials that deter the growth of legionellae should be identified and utilized.[188]

11. References

1. Fraser, D. W., Tsai, T. R., Orenstein, W., *et al.*, Legionnaires' disease: Description of an epidemic of pneumonia, *N. Engl. J. Med.* **297:**1189–1197 (1977).
2. Glick, T. H., Gregg, M. B., Berman, B., *et al.*, Pontiac fever: An epidemic of unknown etiology in a health department. I. Clinical and epidemiologic aspects, *Am. J. Epidemiol.* **107:**149–160 (1978).
3. Dennis, P. J., Brenner, D. J., Thacker, W. L., *et al.*, Five new *Legionella* species isolated from water, *Int. J. Syst. Bacteriol.* **43:**329–337 (1993).
4. Marston, B. J., Lipman, H. B., and Breiman, R. F., Surveillance for Legionnaires' disease: Risk factors for morbidity and mortality, *Arch. Intern. Med.* **154:**2417–2422 (1994).
5. Fang, G.-D., Yu, V. L., and Vickers, R. M., Disease due to legionellaceae (other than *Legionella pneumophila*): Historical, microbiological, clinical, and epidemiologic review, *Medicine* **68:**116–132 (1989).
6. Marston, B. J., Plouffe, J. F., Breiman, R. F., *et al.*, Incidence of community-acquired pneumonia requiring hospitalization: Results of a population based active surveillance in Ohio. *Arch. Intern. Med.* **157:**1709–1718 (1997).
7. McDade, J. E., Shepard, C. C., Fraser, D. W., *et al.*, Isolation of a bacterium and demonstration of its role in other respiratory disease, *N. Engl. J. Med.* **297:**1197–1203 (1977).
8. Thacker, S. B., Bennett, J. V., Tsai, T. F., *et al.*, An outbreak in 1965 of severe respiratory illness caused by the Legionnaires' disease bacterium, *J. Infect. Dis.* **138:**512–519 (1978).
9. Osterholm, M. T., Chin, T. D. Y., Osborne, D. O., *et al.* . A 1957 outbreak of Legionnaires' disease associated with a meat packing plant, *Am. J. Epidemiol.* **117:**60–67 (1983).
10. McDade, J. E., Brenner, D. J., and Bozeman, F. M., Legionnaires' disease bacterium isolated in 1947, *Ann. Intern. Med.* **90:**659–661 (1979).
11. Tatlock, H., Clarification of the cause of Fort Bragg Fever (pretibial fever)—January 1982, *Rev. Infect. Dis.* **4:**157–158 (1982).
12. Pasculle, A. W., Myerowitz, R. L., and Rinaldo, C. R., Jr., New bacterial agent of pneumonia isolated from renal-transplant recipients, *Lancet* **2:**58–61 (1979).
13. Bozeman, F. M., Humphries, J. W., and Campbell, J. M., A new group of rickettsia-like agents recovered from guinea pigs, *Acta Virol.* **12:**87–93 (1986).
14. Kaufman, A. F., McDade, J. E., Patton, C. M., *et al.*, Pontiac fever: isolation of the etiologic agent (*Legionella pneumophila*) and demonstration of its mode of transmission, *Am. J. Epidemiol.* **114:**337–347 (1981).
15. Morris, G. K., Patton, C. M., Feeley, J. C., *et al.*, Isolation of the Legionnaires' disease bacterium from environmental samples, *Ann. Intern. Med.* **90:**664–666 (1979).
16. Dondero, T. J., Rentdorff, R. C., Mallison, G. F., *et al.*, An outbreak of Legionnaires' disease associated with a contaminated air-conditioning cooling tower, *N. Engl. J. Med.* **302:**365–370 (1980).
17. Cordes, L. G., Fraser, D. W., Skailiy, P., *et al.*, Legionnaires' disease outbreak at an Atlanta, Georgia country club: Evidence for spread from an evaporative condenser, *Am. J. Epidemiol.* **111:**425–431 (1980).
18. Tobin, J. O., Dunnill, M. S., French, M., *et al.*, Legionnaires' disease in a transplant unit: Isolation of the causative agent from shower baths, *Lancet* **2:**118–121 (1980).
19. Pounder, D. J., and Stevens, S., Legionnaires' disease at autopsy, *Am. J. Forensic Med. Pathol.* **2:**139–142 (1981).
20. Cherry, W. B., Pittman, B., Harris, P. P., *et al.*, Detection of Legionnaires' disease bacteria by direct immunofluorescent staining, *J. Clin. Microbiol.* **8:**329–338 (1978).
21. Tenover, F. C., Edelstein, P. H., Goldstein, L. C., *et al.*, Comparison of cross-staining reactions by *Pseudomonas* spp. and fluorescein-labeled polyclonal and monoclonal antibodies directed against *Legionella pneumophila*, *J. Clin. Microbiol.* **23:**647–649 (1986).
22. Edelstein, P. H., Laboratory diagnosis of infections caused by legionellae, *Eur. J. Clin. Microbiol.* **6:**4–10 (1987).
23. Lightfoot, N. F., Richardson, I. R., Shrimanker, J., and Farrell, D. J., Post-mortem isolation of *Legionella* due to contamination, *Lancet* **1:**376 (1991).
24. Winn, W. C., Jr., Glavin, F. L., Perl, D. P., and Craighead, J. E., Macroscopic pathology of the lungs in Legionnaires' disease, *Ann. Intern. Med.* **90:**548–551 (1979).
25. Cohen, M. L., Broome, C. V., Paris, A. L., *et al.*, Fatal nosocomial Legionnaires' disease: Clinical and epidemiologic characteristics, *Ann. Intern. Med.* **90:**611–613 (1979).
26. Sutherland, G. E., Tsai, C. C., Routberg, M., *et al.*, Prevalence of pneumonia caused by *Legionella* species among patients on whom autopsies were performed, *Arch. Pathol. Lab. Med.* **107:**358–360 (1983).
27. Foy, H. M., Hayes, P. S., Cooney, M. K., *et al.*, Legionnaires' disease in a prepaid medical-care group in Seattle 1963–75, *Lancet* **1:**767–770 (1979).
28. Woodhead, M. A., Macfarlane, J. T., McCracken, J. S., *et al.*, Prospective study of the aetiology and outcome of pneumonia in the community, *Lancet* **1:**671–674 (1987).
29. Marrie, T. J., Durant, H., and Yates, L., Community-acquired pneumonia requiring hospitalization: 5-year prospective study, *Rev. Infect. Dis.* **11:**586–599 (1989).
30. Fang, G.-D., Fine, M., Orloff, J., *et al.*, New and emerging etiologies for community-acquired pneumonia with implications for therapy: A prospective multicenter study of 359 cases, *Medicine* **69:**307–316 (1990).
31. Ruf, B., Schürmann, D., Horbach, I., *et al.*, Prevalence and diagnosis of *Legionella* pneumonia: A 3-year prospective study with emphasis on application of urinary antigen detection, *J. Infect. Dis.* **162:**1341–1348 (1990).
32. Blanquer, J., Blanquer, R., Borrás, R., *et al.*, Aetiology of community acquired pneumonia in Valencia, Spain: A multicentre prospective study, *Thorax* **46:**508–511 (1991).
33. Bates, J. H., Campbell, G. D., Barron, A. L., *et al.*, Microbial etiology of acute pneumonia in hospitalized patients, *Chest* **101:**1005–1012 (1992).
34. Ostergaard, L., and Andersen, P. L., Etiology of community-acquired pneumonia: evaluation by transtracheal aspiration, blood culture, or serology, *Chest* **104:**1400–1407 (1993).

35. Muder, R. R., Yu, V. L., McClure, J. K., *et al.*, Nosocomial Legionnaires' disease uncovered in a prospective pneumonia study: Implications for underdiagnosis, *J. Am. Med. Assoc.* **249:**3184–3188 (1983).
36. Johnson, J. T., Yu, V. L., Best, M. G., *et al.*, Nosocomial legionellosis in surgical patients with head and neck cancer: Implications for epidemiological reservoir and mode of transmission, *Lancet* **2:**298–300 (1985).
37. Brennen, C., Vickers, J. P., Yu, V. L., *et al.*, Discovery of occult *Legionella* pneumonia in a long-stay hospital: Results of prospective serologic survey, *Br. Med. J.* **295:**306–307 (1987).
38. Marrie, T. J., MacDonald, S., Clarke, K., and Haldane, D., Nosocomial Legionnaires' disease: Lessons from a four-year prospective study, *Am. J. Infect. Control* **19:**79–85 (1991).
39. Roig, J. D., Aguilar, X., Ruiz, J., *et al.*, Comparative study of *Legionella pneumophila* and other nosocomially acquired pneumonias, *Chest* **99:**344–350 (1991).
40. Edelstein, P. H., Laboratory diagnosis of Legionnaires' disease, in: *Legionella: Current Status and Emerging Perspectives* (J. M. Barbaree, R. F. Breiman, and A. P. DuFour, eds.), pp. 7–11, American Society for Microbiology, Washington, DC, 1993.
41. Storch, G., Hayes, P. S., Hill, D. L., and Baine, W. B., Prevalence of antibody to *Legionella pneumophila* in middle-aged and elderly Americans, *J. Infect. Dis.* **140:**784–787 (1979).
42. Helms, C. M., Renner, E. D., Viner, J. P., *et al.*, Indirect immunofluorescence antibodies to *Legionella pneumophila*: Frequency in a rural community, *J. Clin. Microbiol.* **12:**326–328 (1980).
43. Dowling, J. N., Pasculle, A. W., Frola, F. N., *et al.*, Infections caused by *Legionella micdadei* and *Legionella pneumophila* among renal transplant recipients, *J. Infect. Dis.* **149:**703–713 (1984).
44. Meyer, R. D., Shimizu, G. H., Fuller, R., *et al.*, Prospective survey of acquisition of Legionnaires' disease, in: *Legionella: Proceedings of the 2nd International Symposium* (C. Thornsberry *et al.*, eds.), pp. 218–219, American Society for Microbiology, Washington, DC, 1984.
45. Edelstein, P. H., Legionnaires' disease, *Clin. Infect. Dis.* **16:**741–749 (1993).
46. Ingram, J. G., and Plouffe, J. F., Danger of sputum purulence screens in culture of *Legionella* species, *J. Clin. Microbiol.* **32:**209–210 (1994).
47. Campbell, J. F., and Spika, J. S., The serodiagnosis of non-pneumococcal bacterial pneumonia, *Semin. Respir. Infect.* **3:**123–130 (1988).
48. Plouffe, J. F., File, T. M., Breiman, R. F., *et al.*, Reevaluation of the definition of Legionnaires' disease: Use of the urinary antigen assay, *Clin. Infect. Dis.* **20:**1286–1291 (1995).
49. Kohler, R. B., Winn, W. C., Jr., and Wheat, L. J., Onset and duration of urinary antigen excretion in Legionnaires' disease, *J. Clin. Microbiol.* **20:**605–607 (1984).
50. Sathapatayavongs, B., Kohler, R. B., Wheat, L. J., *et al.*, Rapid diagnosis of Legionnaires' disease by urinary antigen detection: Comparison of ELISA and radioimmunoassay, *Am. J. Med.* **72:** 576–582 (1982).
51. Tang, P., and Krishnan, C., Legionella antigenuria: Six-year study of broad-spectrum enzyme-linked immunosorbent assay as a routine diagnostic test, in: *Legionella: Current Status and Emerging Perspectives* (J. M. Barbaree, R. F. Breiman, and A. P. DuFour, eds.), pp. 12–13, American Society for Microbiology, Washington, DC, 1993.
52. Laussucq, S., Schuster, D., Alexander, W. J., *et al.*, False-positive DNA probe test for *Legionella* species associated with a cluster of respiratory illnesses, *J. Clin. Microbiol.* **26:**1442–1444 (1988).
53. Matsiota-Bernard, P., Pitsouni, E., Legakis, N., and Nauciel, C., Evaluation of commercial amplification kit for detection of *Legionella pneumophila* in clinical specimens, *J. Clin. Microbiol.* **32:**1503–1505 (1994).
54. Chandler, F. W., Cole, R. M., Hicklin, M. D., *et al.*, Ultrastructure of the Legionnaires' disease bacterium: A study using transmission electron microscopy, *Ann. Intern. Med.* **90:**642–647 (1979).
55. Bridge, J. A., and Edelstein, P. H., Oropharyngeal colonization with *Legionella pneumophila*, *J. Clin. Microbiol.* **18:**1108–1112 (1983).
56. Horwitz, M. A., and Silverstein, S. C., The Legionnaires' disease bacterium (*Legionella pneumophila*) multiplies intracellularly in human monocytes, *J. Clin. Invest.* **66:**441–450 (1980).
57. Nash, T. W., Libby, D. M., and Horwitz, M. A., Interaction between the Legionnaires' disease bacterium (*Legionella pneumophila*) and alveolar macrophages. Influence of antibody, lymphokines, and hydrocortisone, *J. Clin. Invest.* **74:**771–782 (1984).
58. Horwitz, M. A., Formation of a novel phagosome by the Legionnaires' disease bacterium (*Legionella pneumophila*) in human monocytes, *J. Exp. Med.* **158:**1319–1331 (1983).
59. Dowling, J. N., Saha, A. K., and Glew, R. H., Virulence factors of the family *Legionellaceae*, *Microbiol. Rev.* **56:**32–60 (1992).
60. Horwitz, M. A., Toward an understanding of host and bacterial molecules mediating *Legionella pneumophila* pathogenesis, in: *Legionella: Current Status and Emerging Perspectives* (J. M. Barbaree, R. F. Breiman, and A. P. DuFour, eds.), pp. 55–62, American Society for Microbiology, Washington, DC, 1993.
61. Cianciotto, N. P., Eisenstein, B. I., Mody, C. H., and Engleberg, N. C., A mutation in the *mip* gene results in an attenuation of *Legionella pneumophila* virulence, *J. Infect. Dis.* **162:**121–126 (1990).
62. Ludwig, B., Rahfeld, J., Schmidt, B., *et al.*, Characterization of *mip* proteins of *Legionella pneumophila*, *FEMS Microbiol. Lett.* **118:**23–30 (1994).
63. Rowbotham, T. J., Preliminary report on the pathogenicity of *Legionella pneumophila* for freshwater and soil amoebae, *J. Clin. Pathol.* **33:**1179–1183 (1980).
64. Fields, B. S., Sanden, G. N., Barbaree, J. M., *et al.*, Intracellular multiplication of *Legionella pneumophila* in amoebae isolated from hospital water tanks, *Curr. Microbiol.* **18:**131–137 (1989).
65. Fields, B. S., *Legionella* and protozoa: Interaction of a pathogen and its natural host, in: *Legionella: Current Status and Emerging Perspectives* (J. M. Barbaree, R. F. Breiman, and A. P. DuFour, eds.), pp. 129–136, American Society for Microbiology, Washington, DC, 1993.
66. Kilvington, S., and Price, J., Survival of *Legionella pneumophila* within cysts of *Acanthamoeba polyphaga* following chlorine exposure, *J. Appl. Bacteriol.* **68:**519–525 (1990).
67. Kuchta, J. M., Navratil, J. S., Shepherd, M. E., *et al.*, Impact of chlorine and heat on the survival of *Hartmannella vermiformis* and subsequent growth of *Legionella pneumophila*, *Appl. Environ. Microbiol.* **59:**4096–4100 (1993).
68. Joly, J. R., McKinney, R. M., Tobin, J. O., *et al.*, Development of a standardized subgrouping scheme for *Legionella pneumophila* serogroup 1 using monoclonal antibodies, *J. Clin. Microbiol.* **23:**768–771 (1986).
69. Breiman, R. F., Modes of transmission in epidemic and nonepidemic *Legionella* infection: Directions for further study, in: *Legionella: Current Status and Emerging Perspectives* (J. M.

Barbaree, R. F. Breiman, and A. P. DuFour, eds.), pp. 30–35, American Society for Microbiology, Washington, DC, 1993.

70. Stout, J. E., Yee, Y. C., Vaccarello, S., *et al.*, *Legionella pneumophila* in residential water supplies: Environmental surveillance with clinical assessment for Legionnaires' disease, *Epidemiol. Infect.* **109:**49–57 (1992).
71. Petitjean, F., Dournon, E., Strosberg, A. D., and Hoebeke, J., Isolation, purification and partial analysis of the lipopolysaccharide antigenic determinant recognized by monoclonal antibody to *Legionella pneumophila* serogroup 1, *Res. Microbiol.* **141:**1077–1094 (1990).
72. Barbaree, J. M., Selecting a subtyping technique for use in investigations of legionellosis epidemics, in: *Legionella: Current Status and Emerging Perspectives* (J. M. Barbaree, R. F. Breiman, and A. P. DuFour, eds.), pp. 169–172, American Society for Microbiology, Washington, DC, 1993.
73. Gomez-Luz, P., Fields, B. S., Benson, R. F., *et al.*, Comparison of arbitrarily primed polymerase chain reaction, robotyping, and monoclonal antibody analysis for subtyping *Legionella pneumophila* serogroup 1, *J. Clin. Microbiol.* **31:**1940–1942 (1993).
74. Mahoney, F. J., Hoge, C. W., Farley, T. A., *et al.*, Communitywide outbreak of Legionnaires' disease associated with a grocery store mist machine, *J. Infect. Dis.* **165:**736–739 (1992).
75. Torres, A., Serra-Batlles, J., Ferrer, A., *et al.*, Severe community-acquired pneumonia: Epidemiology and prognostic factors, *Am. Rev. Respir. Dis.* **144:**312–318 (1991).
76. Moine, P., Vercken, J. B., Chevret, S., *et al.*, Severe community-acquired pneumonia: Etiology, epidemiology, and prognosis factors, *Chest* **105:**1487–1495 (1994).
77. Joseph, C. A., Dedman, D., Birtles, R., *et al.*, Legionnaires' disease surveillance: England and Wales, 1993, *Commun. Dis. Rep.* **4:**R109–R111 (1994).
78. Bartlett, C. L. R., Swann, R. A., Casal, J., *et al.*, Recurrent Legionnaires' disease from a hotel water system, in: *Legionella: Proceedings of the 2nd International Symposium* (C.Thornsberry *et al.*, eds), pp. 237–239, American Society for Microbiology, Washington, DC, 1984.
79. Best, M., Stout, J., Muder, R. R., *et al.*, Legionellaceae in the hospital water supply, *Lancet* **1:**307–310 (1983).
80. Doebbeling, B. N., Ishak, M. A., Wade, B. H., *et al.*, Nosocomial *Legionella micdadei* pneumonia: 10 years experience and a case–control study, *J. Hosp. Infect.* **13:**289–298 (1989).
81. Hoge, C. W., and Breiman, R. F., Advances in the epidemiology and control of *Legionella* infections, *Epidemiol. Rev.* **13:**329–340 (1991).
82. Dondero, T. J., Clegg, H. W., 2nd, and Tsai, T. F., Legionnaires' disease in Kingsport, Tennessee, *Ann. Intern. Med.* **90:**569–573 (1979).
83. Yu, V. L., Zuravleff, J. J., Gavlik, L., and Magnussen, M. H., Lack of evidence for person-to-person transmission of Legionnaires' diseases, *J. Infect. Dis.* **147:**362 (1983).
84. Katz, S. M., Habib, W., Hammel, J. M., and Nash, P., Lack of airborne spread of infection by *Legionella pneumophila* among guinea pigs, *Infect. Immun.* **38:**620–622 (1982).
85. Saravolatz, L., Arking, L., Wentworth, B., and Quinn, E., Prevalence of antibody to Legionnaires' disease bacterium in hospital employees, *Ann. Intern. Med.* **90:**601–603 (1979).
86. Agrawal, L., Dhunjibhoy, K. R., and Nair, K. G., Isolation of *Legionella pneumophila* from patients of respiratory tract disease and environmental samples, *Indian J. Med. Res.* **93:**364–365 (1991).
87. Levin, A. S., Mazieri, N. A., Carvalho, N. B., *et al.*, Five cases of nosocomial and community-acquired Legionnaires' disease in Sao Paulo, Brazil (English abstract), *Rev. Institu. Med. Trop. Sao Paulo* **35:**103–104 (1993).
88. Bentham, R. H., and Broadbent, C. R., A model for autumn outbreaks of Legionnaires' disease associated with cooling towers, linked to operation and size, *Epidemiol. Infect.* **111:**287–295 (1993).
89. England, A. C., Fraser, D. W., Plikaytis, B. D., *et al.*, Sporadic legionellosis in the United States: The first thousand cases, *Ann. Intern. Med.* **94:**164–170 (1981).
90. Carlson, N. C., Kuskie, M. R., Dobyns, E. L., *et al.*, Legionellosis in children: An expanding spectrum, *Pediatr. Infect. Dis. J.* **9:**133–137 (1990).
91. Andersen, R. D., Lauer, B. A., Fraser, D. W., *et al.*, Infections with *Legionella pneumophila* in children, *J. Infect. Dis.* **143:**386–390 (1981).
92. Goldberg, D. J., Wrench, J. G., Collier, P. W., *et al.*, Lochgoilhead fever: Outbreak of non-pneumonic legionellosis due to *Legionella micdadei*, *Lancet* **1:**316–318 (1989).
93. Poshni, I. A., and Millian, S. J., Seroepidemiology of *Legionella pneumophila* serogroup 1 in healthy residents of New York City, *NY State J. Med.* **85:**10–14 (1985).
94. Storch, G., Baine, W. B., Fraser, D. W., *et al.*, Sporadic community-acquired Legionnaires' disease in the United States: A case–control study, *Ann. Intern. Med.* **90:**596–600 (1979).
95. Herwaldt, L. A., Gorman, G. W., McGrath, T., *et al.*, A new *Legionella* species, *Legionella feeleii* species nova, causes Pontiac fever in an automobile plant, *Ann. Intern. Med.* **100:**333–338 (1984).
96. Conwill, D. E., Werner, B. S., Dritz, S. K., *et al.*, Legionellosis: The 1980 San Francisco outbreak, *Am. Rev. Respir. Dis.* **126:**666–669 (1982).
97. Friedman, S., Spitalny, K., Barbaree, J., *et al.*, Pontiac fever outbreak associated with a cooling tower, *Am. J. Public Health* **77:**568–572 (1987).
98. Kirby, B. D., Snyder, K. M., Meyer, R. D., and Finegold, S. M., Legionnaires' disease: Report of sixty-five nosocomially acquired cases and review of the literature, *Medicine* **59:**188–205 (1980).
99. Hanrahan, J. P., Morse, D. L., Scharf, V. B., *et al.*, A community hospital outbreak of legionellosis, *Am. J. Epidemiol.* **125:**639–649 (1987).
100. Snowman, W. R., Holtzhauer, F. J., Halpin, T. J., and Correa-Villasenor, A., The role of indoor and outdoor occupations in the seroepidemiology of *Legionella pneumophila*, *J. Infect. Dis.* **145:**275 (1982).
101. Goldman, W. D., and Marr, J. S., Are air-conditioning maintenance personnel at increased risk of legionellosis? *Appl. Environ. Microbiol.* **40:**114–116 (1980).
102. Buehler, J. W., Sikes, R. K., Kuritsky, J. N., *et al.*, Prevalence of antibodies to *Legionella pneumophila* among workers exposed to a contaminated cooling tower, *Arch. Environ. Health* **40:**207–210 (1985).
103. Deubner, D. C., MacCormick, J. N., Kleeman, K., and Muhibaier, L. H., One-time screening to define the problem: *Legionella* exposure in an electric power company, *J. Occup. Med.* **28:**670–673 (1986).
104. Klaucke, D. N., Vogt, R. L., LaRue, D., *et al.*, Legionnaires' disease: The epidemiology of two outbreaks in Burlington, Vermont, 1980, *Am. J. Epidemiol.* **119:**382–391 (1984).

105. Arnow, P. M., Chou, T., Weil, D., *et al.*, Nosocomial Legionnaires' disease caused by aerosolized tap water from respiratory devices, *J. Infect. Dis.* **146:**460–467 (1982).
106. Breiman, R. F., Fields, B. S., Sanden, G., *et al.*, An outbreak of Legionnaires' disease associated with shower use: Possible role of amoebae, *J. Am. Med. Assoc.* **263:**2924–2926 (1990).
107. Blatt, S. P., Parkinson, M. D., Pace, E., *et al.*, Nosocomial Legionnaires' disease: Aspiration as a primary mode of disease acquisition, *Am. J. Med.* **95:**16–22 (1993).
108. Breiman, R. F., VanLoock, F. L., Sion, J. P., *et al.*, Association of "sink bathing" and Legionnaires' disease, in: Abstracts of the 19st Meeting of the American Society for Microbiology, May 5–9, 1991, Dallas, TX. (Abstract #L18).
109. Carratala, J., Gudiol, F., Pallares, R., *et al.*, Risk factors for nosocomial *Legionella pneumophila* pneumonia, *Am. J. Respir. Crit. Care Med.* **149:**625–629 (1994).
110. Garbe, P. L., Davis, B. J., Weisfeld, J. S., *et al.*, Nosocomial Legionnaires' disease: Epidemiologic demonstration of cooling towers as a source, *J. Am. Med. Assoc.* **254:**521–524 (1985).
111. Guiguet M., Pierre, J., Brun, P., *et al.*, Epidemiological survey of a major outbreak of nosocomial legionellosis, *Int. J. Epidemiol.* **16:** 466–471 (1987).
112. Mastro, T. D., Fields, B. S., Breiman, R. F., *et al.*, Nosocomial Legionnaires' disease and use of medication nebulizers, *J. Infect. Dis.* **163:**667–670 (1991).
113. Vereerstraeten, P., Stolear, J. C., Schoutens-Serruys, E., *et al.*, Erythromycin prophylaxis for Legionnaires' disease in immunosuppressed patients in a contaminated hospital environment, *Transplantation* **41:**52–54 (1986).
114. O'Mahony, M. C., Stanwell-Smith, R. E., Tillett, H. E., *et al.*, The Stafford outbreak of Legionnaires' disease, *Epidemiol. Infect.* **104:**361–380 (1990).
115. Mermel, L. A., Josephson, S. L., Giorgio, C. H., *et al.*, Association of Legionnaires' disease with construction: Contamination of potable water? *Infect. Control Hosp. Epidemiol.* **16:**76–81 (1995).
116. Shands, K. N., Ho, J. L., Meyer, R. D., *et al.*, Potable water as a source of Legionnaires' disease, *J. Am. Med. Assoc.* **253:**1412–1416 (1985).
117. Joseph, C. A., Watson, J. M., Harrison, T. G., and Bartlett, C. L. R., Nosocomial Legionnaires' disease in England and Wales, 1980–92, *Epidemiol. Infect.* **112:**329–345 (1994).
118. Tablan, O. C., Anderson, L. J., Arden, N. H., *et al.*, Guideline for prevention of nosocomial pneumonia, *Respir. Care* **39:**1191–1236 (1994).
119. Schlech, W. F., III, Gorman, G. W., Payne, M. C., and Broome, C. V., Legionnaires' disease in the Caribbean: An outbreak associated with a resort hotel, *Arch. Intern. Med.* **145:**2076–2079 (1985).
120. Mamolen, M., Breiman, R. F., Barbaree, J. M., *et al.*, Use of multiple molecular subtyping techniques to investigate a Legionnaires' disease outbreak due to identical strains at two tourist lodges, *J. Clin. Microbiol.* **31:**2584–2588 (1993).
121. Miller, L. A., Beebe, J. L., Butler, J. C., *et al.*, Use of polymerase chain reaction in an epidemiologic investigation of Pontiac fever, *J. Infect. Dis.* **168:**769–772 (1993).
122. Hlady, W. G., Mullen, R. C., Mintz, C. S., *et al.*, Outbreak of Legionnaires' disease linked to a decorative fountain by molecular epidemiology, *Am. J. Epidemiol.* **138:**555–562 (1993).
123. Jernegan, D. B., Hofmann, J., Cetron, M. S., *et al.*, Outbreak of Legionnaires' disease among cruise ship passengers exposed to a contaminated whirlpool spa, *Lancet* **347:**494–499 (1996).
124. Jensen, W. A., Rose, R. M., Wasserman, A. S., *et al.*, *In vitro* activation of the antibacterial activity of human pulmonary macrophages by recombinant γ interferon, *J. Infect. Dis.* **155:**574–577 (1987).
125. Jensen, G. D., and Bellecci, P., Alcohol and the elderly: Relationships to illness and smoking, *Alcohol Alcohol.* **22:**193–198 (1987).
126. Blatt, S. P., Dolan, M. J., Hendrix, C. W., and Melcher, G. P., Legionnaires' disease in human immunodeficiency virus-infected patients: Eight cases and review, *Clin. Infect. Dis.* **18:**227–232 (1994).
127. Fliermans, C. B., Cherry, W. B., Orrison, L. H., *et al.*, Ecological distribution of *Legionella pneumophila*, *Appl. Environ. Microbiol.* **41:**9–16 (1981).
128. Steele, T. W., Langser, J., and Sangster, N., Isolation of *Legionella longbeachae* serogroup 1 from potting mixes, *Appl. Environ. Microbiol.* **56:**49–53 (1990).
129. Hsu, S. C., Martin, R., and Wentworth, B. B., Isolation of *Legionella* species from drinking water, *Appl. Environ. Microbiol.* **48:**830–832 (1984).
130. Tison, D. L., and Seidler, R. J., *Legionella* incidence and density in potable drinking water, *Appl. Environ. Microbiol.* **45:**337–339 (1983).
131. Fraser, D. W., Sources of legionellosis, in: *Legionella: Proceedings of the 2nd International Symposium* (C. Thornsberry *et al.*, eds.), pp. 277–280, American Society for Microbiology, Washington, DC, 1984.
132. Sanden, G. N., Fields, B. S., Barbaree, J. M., *et al.*, Viability of *Legionella pneumophila* in chlorine-free water at elevated temperature, *Curr. Microbiol.* **18:**61–65 (1989).
133. Stout, J. E., Yu, V. L., and Best, M. G., Ecology of *Legionella pneumophila* within water distribution systems, *Appl. Environ. Microbiol.* **49:**221–228 (1985).
134. Ciesielski, C. A., Blaser, M. J., and Wang, W. L., Role of stagnation and obstruction of water flow in isolation of *Legionella pneumophila* from hospital plumbing, *Appl. Environ. Microbiol.* **48:**984–987 (1984).
135. Yamamoto, H., Sugiura, M., Kusunoki, S., *et al.*, Factors stimulating propagation of legionellae in cooling tower water, *Appl. Environ. Microbiol.* **58:**1394–1397 (1992).
136. Rogers, J., and Keevil, C. W., Immunogold and fluorescein immunolabeling of *Legionella pneumophila* within an aquatic biofilm visualized by using episcopic differential interference contrast microscopy, *Appl. Environ. Microbiol.* **58:**2326–2330 (1992).
137. Yu, V. L., Could aspiration be the major mode of transmission for *Legionella*? *Am. J. Med.* **95:**13–15 (1993).
138. Muder, R. R., Yu, V. L., and Woo, A. H., Mode of transmission of *Legionella pneumophila*: A critical review, *Arch. Intern. Med.* **146:**1607–1612 (1986).
139. Centers for Disease Control and Prevention, Legionnaires' disease associated with cooling towers—Massachusetts, Michigan, and Rhode Island, *Morbid. Mortal. Week. Rep.* **43:**491–499 (1994).
140. Band, J. D., LaVenture, M., Davis, J. P., *et al.*, Epidemic Legionnairees' disease: Airborne transmission down a chimney, *J. Am. Med. Assoc.* **245:**2404–2407 (1981).
141. Addiss, D. G., Davis, J. P., LaVenture, M., *et al.*, Community-acquired Legionnaires disease associated with a cooling tower: Evidence for longer-distance transport of *Legionella pneumophila*, *Am. J. Epidemiol.* **130:**557–568 (1989).

142. Brundrett, G. W., Surveys of legionella in building services not associated with outbreaks, in: *Legionella and Building Services* (G. W. Brundrett, ed.), pp. 167–189, Butterworth-Heinemann, Oxford, 1992.
143. Breiman, R. F., Cozen, W., Fields, B. S., *et al.*, Role of air sampling in investigation of an outbreak of Legionnaires' disease associated with exposure to aerosols from an evaporative condenser, *J. Infect. Dis.* **161:**1257–1261 (1990).
144. Berendt, R. F., Survival of *Legionella pneumophia* in aerosols: Effect of relative humidity, *J. Infect. Dis.* **141:**689 (1980).
145. Bollin, G. E., Plouffe, J. F., Para, M. F., and Hackman, B., Aerosols containing *Legionella pneumophila* generated by shower heads and hot-water faucets, *Appl. Environ. Microbiol.* **50:**1128–1131 (1985).
145a. Centers for Disease Control and Prevention, Legionnaires' disease associated with a whirlpool display—Virginia, September–October, 1996, *Morbid. Mortal. Week. Rep.* **46:**83–86 (1997).
146. Bhopal, R. S., Fallon, R. J., Buist, E. C., *et al.*, Proximity of the home to a cooling tower and risk of non-outbreak Legionnaires' disease, *Br. Med. J.* **302:**378–383 (1991).
147. Stout, J. E., Yu, V. L., Muraca, P., *et al.*, Potable water as a cause of sporadic cases of community-acquired Legionnaires' disease, *N. Engl. J. Med.* **326:**151–155 (1992).
148. Straus, W. L., Plouffe, J. F., File, T. M., *et al.*, Risk factors for domestic acquisition of Legionnaires' disease, *Arch. Intern. Med.* **156:**1685–1692 (1996).
149. Alary, M., and Joly, J. R., Comparison of culture methods and an immunofluorescent assay for the detection of *Legionella pneumophila* in domestic hot water devices, *Curr. Microbiol.* **25:**19–23 (1992).
150. Marrie, T. J., Green, P., Burbridge, S., *et al.*, Legionellaceae in the potable water of Nova Scotia hospitals and Halifax residences, *Epidemiol. Infect.* **112:**143–150 (1994).
151. Alary, M., and Joly, J. R., Risk factors for contamination of domestic hot water systems by legionellae, *Appl. Environ. Microbiol.* **57:**2360–2367 (1991).
152. Horwitz, M. A., The Legionnaires' disease bacterium (*Legionella pneumophila*) inhibits phagosome–lysosome fusion in human monocytes, *J. Exp. Med.* **158:**2108–2126 (1983).
153. Davis, G. S., Winn, W. C., Jr., Gump, D. W., and Beaty, N. H., The kinetics of early inflammatory events during experimental pneumonia due to *Legionella pneumophila* in guinea pigs, *J. Infect. Dis.* **148:**823–835 (1983).
154. Mody, C. H., Paine, R., III, Shahrabadi, M. S., *et al.*, *Legionella pneumophila* replicates within rat alveolar epithelial cells, *J. Infect. Dis.* **167:**1138–1145 (1993).
155. Blackmon, J. A., Hicklin, M. D., Chandler, F. W., and the Special Expert Pathology Panel, Legionnaires' disease: Pathological and historical aspects of a "new" disease, *Arch. Pathol. Lab. Med.* **102:**337–343 (1976).
156. Winn, W. C., Jr., and Myerowitz, R. L., The pathology of the *Legionella* pneumonias: A review of 74 cases and the literature, *Hum. Pathol.* **12:**401–422 (1981).
157. Hilton, E., Freedman, R. A., Cintron, F., *et al.*, Acid-fast bacilli in sputum: A case of *Legionella micdadei* pneumonia, *J. Clin. Microbiol.* **24:**1102–1103 (1986).
158. Jernigan, D. B., Sanders, L. I., Waites, K. B., *et al.*, Pulmonary infection due to *Legionella cincinnatiensis* in renal transplant recipients: Two cases and implications for laboratory diagnosis, *Clin. Infect. Dis.* **18:**385–389 (1994).
159. Babe, K. S., Jr., and Reinhardt, J. F., Diagnosis of *Legionella* sepsis by examination of a peripheral blood smear, *Clin. Infect. Dis.* **19:**1164–1165 (1994).
160. Breiman, R. F., and Horwitz, M. A., Guinea pigs sublethally infected with aerosolized *Legionella pneumophila* develop humoral and cell-mediated immune responses and are protected against lethal aerosol challenge, *J. Exp. Med.* **164:**799–811 (1987).
161. Rowbotham, T. J., Pontiac fever explained? *Lancet* **2:**969 (1980).
162. Roig, J., Carreres, A., and Domingo, C., Treatment of Legionnaires' disease: Current recommendations, *Drugs* **46:**63–79 (1993).
163. Lattimer, G. L., Rhodes, L. V., 3rd, Salventi, J. S., *et al.*, The Philadelphia epidemic of Legionnaires' disease: Clinical, pulmonary, and serologic findings two years later, *Ann. Intern. Med.* **90:**522–526 (1979).
164. Leverstein-van Hall, M. A., Verbon, A., Huisman, M. V., *et al.*, Reinfection with *Legionella pneumophila* documented by pulsed-field gel electrophoresis, *Clin. Infect. Dis.* **19:**1147–1149 (1994).
165. Lowry, P. W., Blankenship, R. J., Gridley, W., *et al.*, A cluster of *Legionella* sternal wound infections due to postoperative topical exposure to contaminated tap water, *N. Engl. J. Med.* **324:**109–113 (1991).
166. Helms, C. M., Viner, J. P., Sturm, R. H., *et al.*, Comparative features of pneumococcal, mycoplasma, and Legionnaires' disease pneumonias, *Ann. Intern. Med.* **90:**543–547 (1979).
167. Yu, V., Kroboth, F. J., Shonnard, J., *et al.*, Legionnaires' disease: New clinical perspectives from a prospective pneumonia study, *Am. J. Med.* **73:**357–361 (1982).
168. Granados, A., Podzamczer, D., Guidol, F., and Manresa, F., Pneumonia due to *Legionella pneumophila* and pneumococcal pneumonia: Similarities and differences on presentation, *Eur. Respir. J.* **2:**130–134 (1989).
169. Skaliy, P., Thompson, T. A., Gorman, G. W., *et al.*, Laboratory studies of disinfectants against *Legionella pneumophila*, *Appl. Environ. Microbiol.* **40:**697–700 (1980).
170. Muraca, P., Stout, J. E., and Yu, V. L., Comparative assessment of chlorine, heat, ozone, and UV light for killing *Legionella pneumophila* within a model plumbing system, *Appl. Environ. Microbiol.* **53:**447–453 (1987).
171. Landeen, L. K., Yahya, M. T., and Gerba, C. P., Efficacy of copper and silver ions and reduced levels of free chlorine in inactivation of *Legionella pneumophila*, *Appl. Environ. Microbiol.* **55:**3045–3050 (1989).
172. Edelstein, P. H., Whittaker, R. E., Kreiling, R. L., and Howell, C. L., Efficacy of ozone in eradication of *Legionella pneumophila* from hospital plumbing fixtures, *Appl. Environ. Microbiol.* **44:**1330–1334 (1982).
173. Broadbent, C. R., *Legionella* in cooling towers: Practical research, design, treatment, and control guidelines, in: *Legionella: Current Status and Emerging Perspectives* (J. M. Barbaree, R. F. Breiman, and A. P. Du Four, eds.), pp. 217–222, American Society for Microbiology, Washington, DC 1993.
174. Muraca, P., Yu, V. L., and Goetz, A., Disinfection of water distribution systems for *Legionella*: A review of application procedures and methodologies, *Infect. Control Host. Epidemiol.* **11:**79–88 (1990).
175. Patterson, W. J., Seal, D. V., Curran, E., *et al.*, Fatal nosocomial Legionnaires' disease: Relevance of contamination of hospital water supply by temperature-dependent buoyancy-driven flow from spur pipes, *Epidemiol. Infect.* **112:**513–525 (1994).
176. Yu, V. L., Beam, T. R., Lumish, R. M., *et al.*, Routine culturing for

Legionella in the hospital environment may be a good idea: A three-hospital prospective study, *Am. J. Med. Sci.* **294:**97–99 (1987).

177. Allegheny County Health Department, *Approaches to Prevention and Control of Legionella Infection in Health Care Facilities*, Allegheny County Health Department, Pittsburgh, PA, 1993.
178. Marrie, T. J., Haldane, D., Bezanson, G., and Peppard, R., Each water outlet is a unique ecologic niche for *Legionella pneumophila*, *Epidemiol. Infect.* **108:**261–270 (1992).
179. Marie, T. J., Berzcason, G., Fox, J., *et al.*, Dynamics of *Legionella pneumophila* in the potable water of one floor of a hospital, in: *Legionella: Current Status and Emerging Perspectives* (J. M. Barbaree, R. F. Breiman, and A. P. DuFour, eds.), pp. 238–240, American Society for Microbiology, Washington, DC, 1993.
180. Horwitz, M. A., Marston, B. J., Broome, C. V., and Breiman, R. F., Prospects for vaccine development, in: *Legionella: Current Status and Emerging Perspectives* (J. M. Barbaree, R. F. Breiman, and A. P. DuFour, eds.), pp. 296–297, American Society for Microbiology, Washington, 1993.
181. Shelton, B. G., Flanders, W. D., and Morris, G. K., Legionnaires' disease outbreaks and cooling towers with amplified *Legionella* concentrations, *Curr. Microbiol.* **28:**359–363 (1994).
182. Vickers, R. M., Stout, J. E., and Yu, V. L., Failure of a diagnostic monoclonal immunofluorescent reagent to detect *Legionella pneumophila* in environment samples, *Appl. Environ. Microbiol.* **56:**2912–2914 (1990).
183. Koide, M., Saito, A., Kusano, N., and Higa, F., Detection of *Legionella* spp. in cooling tower water by the polymerase chain reaction method, *Appl. Environ. Microbiol.* **59:**1943–1946 (1993).
184. Maiwald, M., Kissel, K., Srimuang, S., *et al.*, Comparison of polymerase chain reaction and conventional culture for the detection of legionellas in hospital water samples, *J. Appl. Bacteriol.* **76:**216–225 (1994).
185. Hay, J., Seal, D. V., Billcliffe, B., and Freer, J. H., Non-culturable *Legionella pneumophila* associated with *Acanthamoeba castellanii*: Detection of the bacterium using DNA amplification and hybridization, *J. Appl. Bacteriol.* **78:**61–65 (1995).
186. Rowbotham, T. J., *Legionella*-like amoebal pathogen, in: *Legionella: Current Status and Emerging Perspectives*, (J. M. Barbaree, R. F. Breiman, and A. P. DuFour, eds.), pp. 137–140, American Society for Microbiology, Washington, DC, 1993.
187. Bentham, R. H., and Broadbent, C. R., Field trial of biocides for control of *Legionella* in cooling towers, *Curr. Microbiol.* **30:**167–172 (1995).
188. Rogers, J., Dowsett, A. B., Dennis, P. J., *et al.*, Influence of plumbing materials on biofilm formation and growth of *Legionella pneumophila* in potable water systems, *Appl. Environ. Microbiol.* **60:**1842–1851 (1994).
189. Vogt, R. L., Hudson, P. J., Orciari, L., *et al.*, Legionnaire's disease and a whirlpool spa (letter), *Ann. Intern. Med.* **107:**596 (1987).
190. Magione, E. J., Remis, R. S., Tait, K. A., *et al.*, An outbreak of Pontiac fever related to whirlpool spa use, Michigan, 1982, *J. Am. Med. Assoc.* **253:**535–539 (1985).
191. Spitalny, K. C., Vogt, R. L., Orciari, L. A., Witherell, L. E., Etkind P., and Novick, L. F., Pontiac fever associated with a whirlpool spa, *Am. J. Epidemiol.* **120:**809–817 (1984).
192. Fenstersheib, M. D., Miller, M., Diggins, S., *et al.*, Outbreak of Pontiac fever due to *Legionella anisa*, *Lancet* **2:**35–37 (1990).
193. Fraser, D. W., Deubner, D. C., Hill, D. L., and Gilliam, D. K., Nonpneumonic, short-incubation-period legionellosis (Pontiac fever) in men who cleaned a steam turbine condenser, *Science* **205:**690–691 (1979).

12. Suggested Reading

Barbaree, J. M., Breiman, R. F., and DuFour, A. P. (eds.), *Legionella: Current Status and Emerging Perspectives*, American Society for Microbiology, Washington, DC, 1993.

Fraser, D. W., and McDade, J. W., Legionellosis, *Sci. Am.* **241**(4):82–99 (1979).

Garrett, L., The American Bicentennial: Swine flu and Legionnaires' disease, in: *The Coming Plague: Newly Emerging Diseases in a World Out of Balance*, pp. 153–191, Farrar, Straus, and Giroux, New York, 1994.

Thornsberry, C., Balows, A., Feeley, J. C., and Jakubowski, W. (eds.), *Legionella: Proceedings of the 2nd International Symposium*, American Society for Microbiology, Washington, DC, 1984.

Winn, W. C., Jr., Legionnaires disease: Historical perspective, *Clin. Microbiol. Rev.* **1:**60–81 (1988).

CHAPTER 19

Leprosy

Robert R. Jacobson and Leo J. Yoder

1. Introduction

Leprosy (Hansen's disease) is a chronic infectious disease caused by *Mycobacterium leprae* that primarily affects the skin, peripheral nerves, eyes, and mucous membranes. It has been known for well over 2000 years and afflicts several million people worldwide, mostly in underdeveloped nations. Hansen[1] discovered the etiologic agent over 100 years ago, but it still has not definitely been cultured in artificial media, and there is much about the disease process we do not understand.

As discussed in Section 8, leprosy may present in several different ways, depending on the resistance of the patient to the infection. The earliest form is referred to as indeterminate. The lesion is usually singular and often self-heals. Where self-healing or treatment does not intervene, the disease may remain localized in relatively resistant patients and evolve into tuberculoid disease; but if resistance is poor, generalized (borderline or lepromatous) disease develops. Today, indeterminate and tuberculoid cases are usually referred to merely as paucibacillary (PB) and borderline and lepromatous cases as multibacillary (MB). Where the disease is uncommon, as in the United States, the diagnosis is sometimes made relatively late. It can be a difficult disease to treat. An understanding of the clinical aspects and the problems associated with treatment is probably more vital with this than perhaps with any other infectious disease if one is to understand, for example, why progress in control of the disease has been so slow. Nevertheless, the situation has steadily improved, particularly in the last decade, and today, if the patient cooperates, we are able to manage nearly all cases satisfactorily. Much of this improvement has been due to introduction of short-term therapy and the World Health Organization's (WHO) campaign to eliminate leprosy as a public health problem by the year 2000. Of equal importance is that we now can counteract most of the fears created by the folklore surrounding this disease so that the patient may retain normal position and repute in society.

Robert R. Jacobson and Leo J. Yoder • Gillis W. Long Hansen's Disease Center, Carville, Louisiana 70721.

2. Historical Background

It is uncertain just where and when the disease first appeared and whether biblical "leprosy" was in fact leprosy as we know it today. However, the opinion of most authorities[2] seems to be that it started in the Far East before 600 BC and then spread to the Near East and Africa and later to Europe. The incidence of the disease probably peaked in Europe in the Middle Ages and then gradually declined, ultimately disappearing in most of these countries, though it is still found in those that border the Mediterranean. The reasons for this disappearance are uncertain, but it has been suggested that a general improvement in hygiene and housing played a major role.[2] Leprosy was probably first introduced into the Americas via the early Spanish explorations and later by means of the slave trade. The first definite reference to the disease in the United States, however, was in the Floridas[3] in 1758, and in the 1760s, cases occurring among the French were isolated near the mouth of the Mississippi River. In 1785, a hospital was established in New Orleans for the treatment of leprosy patients, and over 100 years later (1894), this facility was moved to a location near the village of Carville, becoming the Louisiana Leper Home. Because patients from many states began seeking care there, the institution was acquired by the federal government in 1921, becoming the National Leprosarium. As the Gillis W. Long Hansen's Disease Center (GWLHDC) at Carville, it continues in this function today. Nearly all states have some cases, but most are reported from Hawaii,

California, Texas, Louisiana, Florida, and the New York City area. Significant numbers of cases occurred among Scandinavian immigrants residing in and around Minnesota in the 19th century, but this focus has now completely disappeared. A settlement for Hawaiian patients at Kalaupapa on Molokai remains but is gradually being phased out. One formerly existed on Penikese Island, Massachusetts, but this was closed in 1921, and the remaining 13 patients were transferred to Carville.

Significant milestones in the history of leprosy would have to include the discovery by Hansen[(1)] of *M. leprae* as the causative agent of this disease in 1874, the introduction of sulfone therapy in 1941,[(4)] the development of the mouse footpad technique for growing the bacillus in 1960,[(5)] the discovery that the bacillus grows readily in the armadillo in 1971,[(6)] and the development of short-term therapy in 1981.[(7)]

3. Methodology

3.1. Sources of Mortality Data

Leprosy is not, generally speaking, considered a fatal disease. Mortality statistics, therefore, do not reflect incidence.

3.2. Sources of Morbidity Data

Although many countries list leprosy as a reportable disease, existing morbidity data on leprosy are often unreliable. There are still varying degrees of stigma attached to the disease in most countries so that some patients may try to either conceal the diagnosis or seek the care of physicians who will not report it. WHO considers leprosy a communicable disease of major public health importance, and the data collected are usually published annually.[(8)] The data include separate figures for the number of registered cases and estimated cases in member countries, the latter being based on a multiplication factor that was devised for calculating the total number of cases from registered cases. The figure obtained probably represents a somewhat conservative estimate of the size of the world problem. Nonetheless, the number of cases is clearly declining as a result of WHO's effort to eliminate leprosy as a public health problem by the year 2000. In 1985, for example, there were 5.4 million registered cases, but by 1994 this number had dropped to 1.7 million.[(8)]

In the United States, leprosy is a reportable disease in all states except Missouri, Oklahoma, Pennsylvania, South Dakota, and Vermont. National registries are maintained at the GWLHDC at Carville and the Centers for Disease Control and Prevention (CDC) at Atlanta. Cases are reported on a leprosy surveillance form available from either Carville or the CDC. In the United States, as elsewhere, because of attempts to conceal the diagnosis or laxity of physicians, leprosy is undoubtedly somewhat underreported, but to what extent is difficult to ascertain. Cases are reported in the *Morbidity and Mortality Weekly Report* under "Summary—Cases of specified notifiable diseases, United States," and are periodically summarized in statistical reports issued by the GWLHDC. The Texas State Health Department includes leprosy case-reporting data in its *Texas Morbidity This Week*, but only for cases that occur within the state.

3.3. Surveys

Surveys for leprosy to detect new cases and assess prevalence have primarily been done by clinical examination of defined populations. The most common of these have been school surveys, examination of special groups such as military personnel, and household contact examinations; where prevalence is high, whole population surveys have been done. In actual practice most cases are found by voluntary reporting or referral by medical personnel. In countries such as the United States, where the disease is rare, household contact examination is the only kind of survey that has any practical value.

The lepromin skin test has been used for surveys and classification of leprosy for over 60 years and was the only means available to assess the immune status of leprosy patients with regard to *M. leprae*. In recent years, more specific and direct measures of immunity and evidence of infection with *M. leprae* have been developed, such as the lymphocyte transformation test (LTT), antibody assays, and polymerase chain reaction (PCR). The lepromin skin test is an indicator of the capacity of an individual to mount a cell-mediated immune (CMI) response to *M. leprae* if exposed to the bacteria. It is not a diagnostic test, since many individuals who have never had the disease or been exposed to the disease will still have positive lepromin skin tests. Its usefulness is mainly in predicting susceptibility and as an aid in classification of diagnosed cases. The test is invariably positive in tuberculoid leprosy cases and negative in lepromatous cases, and may be positive or negative in borderline and indeterminate cases. A considerable body of epidemiological data has been obtained from surveys of populations and contacts in leprosy endemic areas with lepromin testing. But in general the test is of limited value as an indicator for evidence of infection with *M. leprae*. In the United States, it is considered investigational.

Until armadillo sources of *M. leprae* became available, lepromin was prepared from bacilli obtained from skin nodules from patients with the disease (lepromin H). Standard lepromin H contains 160 million bacilli/ml and for field conditions is further diluted to 40 million bacilli/ml. Virtually all lepromin is now prepared from armadillo tissue and is known as lepromin A. A single 0.1-ml dose of the suspension is injected intracutaneously, and readings are taken at 48 hr (Fernandez reaction) and at 3–4 weeks (Mitsuda reaction). The reaction is read as positive if the induration is 3 mm or more, and doubtful if it is less than 3 mm. The Fernandez reaction is considered to be an indication of actual exposure to *M. leprae*, though its significance is less certain than that of the Mitsuda reaction. The Mitsuda reaction is considered to be a measure of an individual's ability to mount a CMI response to *M. leprae* and is not dependent on previous exposure to the bacteria. Correlation between the Fernandez and the Mitsuda reactions is poor.[9] The Fernandez reaction may be negative even though the Mitsuda is positive. The WHO recommends that only the Mitsuda response be read.

Both human and armadillo lepromin contain variable amounts of tissue. A more purified preparation, Dharmendra lepromin, is occasionally used, especially in India. The Mitsuda reaction is poor with this preparation, and only the 48-hr reaction is generally useful. Since this is a more purified preparation than the standard integral lepromin, the 48-hr reaction is not known as the Fernandez reaction, but its clinical significance is considered equivalent to that of integral lepromin. Other even more highly purified preparations, such as Convit's soluble antigen, have also been used by some investigators.[9,10]

In the 1970s LLTs were developed and showed a higher degree of specificity than the lepromin skin test for detecting previous exposure to *M. leprae*. An 88% response rate was found in a subgroup of health personnel with extensive exposure to leprosy patients and without disease, but complete unresponsiveness was noted in those not exposed.[11] Similar findings have been noted among household contacts.[12] The test has also helped define the immunologic spectrum of leprosy, with responsiveness diminishing as one moves from tuberculoid (high-resistance) toward lepromatous (low-resistance) disease.[13] LTTs are not readily applicable under field conditions and their usefulness in this area is being superseded by other newer tests.[14]

Two of the earliest antibody assays were the fluorescent leprosy antibody absorption (FLA-ABS)[15] and a radioimmunoassay (RIA) for specific and nonspecific *M. leprae* antigens.[16] Both have relatively good sensitivity and specificity in the hands of some investigators; however, they have had only limited use in case-finding activities. More recently a number of species-specific antibody tests have been developed. The one that has generated the most interest is the phenolic glycolipid-I (PGL-1) antibody. The titers of PGL-1 antibodies detected in leprosy patients are proportional to the bacillary load, and elevated titers have also been found in some contacts of multibacillary (MB) patients as well as a portion of noncontacts among inhabitants of endemic areas. Published studies indicate that MB cases can be readily detected, but among paucibacillary cases, only 40–50% will have elevated PGL-1 antibody levels. In a study in Venezuela, high PGL-1 levels were highly predictive for developing leprosy, but most of the 20 cases that occurred during this study were in those who did not have elevated levels. In general, it appears that measuring PGL-1 levels is not a useful strategy for detecting early cases in control programs. It is possible that combining PGL-1 testing with other tests such as lepromin skin testing might be able to assist in defining those at greatest risk for developing overt disease.[17]

The most recent development in this area is the use of the PCR as a direct test for the presence of *M. leprae* DNA. The application of this technique to the epidemiology of leprosy is still being developed, but it appears that this technique may have promise for studying transmission within a population. A study[18] of nasal swabs taken from patients in the Philippines showed that the swabs were PCR-positive for *M. leprae* in 55% of untreated patients, 19% of persons who worked with leprosy patients daily, and in 12% of persons who worked in the same area but had no direct contact with leprosy patients. There were no positives in specimens from persons from outside the country with no exposure to leprosy. It also has been proposed that the combination of PCR and antibody tests might be useful in surveys. A study in an area of high endemicity in Indonesia did not support this theory. The study showed a PGL-1 positivity rate of 33% in both household contacts of patients and in those with no contacts. The positivity rate was 23% in diagnosed patients. *M. leprae* were detected by PCR in 7.7% of nasal swabs in the same population with no correlation between the PCR results and serology.[19] These studies from the Philippines and Indonesia indicate a rate of infection far beyond the rate at which people show any clinical evidence of disease, and indicate that *M. leprae* is transmitted frequently in endemic populations. The study from Indonesia also indicates that nasal carriage of *M. leprae* is common in such areas. Whether these carriers actually transmit *M. leprae* has yet to be determined.

3.4. Laboratory Diagnosis

The only laboratory tests used routinely for diagnosis of leprosy are skin smears and skin biopsies. In a few centers, mouse footpad studies are used for determination of *M. leprae* drug sensitivities.

3.4.1. Isolation and Identification of Organism. Skin smears are obtained by pinching a fold of skin to diminish blood flow, wiping the area with an alcohol sponge, and making a small slit into the dermis with a sterile razor blade or scalpel. The slit is gently scraped and the tissue fluid obtained is smeared on a microscopic slide. Bacilli are more abundant in the skin in cool areas such as the earlobes. In the United States, routine skin smear sites are the ears, elbows, and knees. In new cases additional sites are selected from active or suspected skin lesions. Smears are usually negative in indeterminate, tuberculoid (TT), and borderline tubercoloid (BT) cases, strongly positive in lepromatous (LL) and borderline lepromatous (BL) cases, and mildly positive in midborderline cases. Skin smears should be done in all suspected cases, though negative smears do not exclude the diagnosis. Those with positive sites should have smears repeated at least annually to monitor the clearance of bacilli.

Skin smears are stained for acid-fast bacilli (AFB) with the Fite–Faraco modification of the Ziehl–Neelson stain. The number of AFB found in each smear are quantified using a semilogarithmic scale called the bacterial index (BI), as shown in Table 1. The percentage of intact solid-staining bacilli with respect to size, shape, and uniformity of staining is also determined and is referred to as the morphological index (MI). This is usually 1–5% in a typical newly diagnosed case. The MI correlates to some extent with viability in that when the MI becomes 0, the bacilli can no longer be grown in the mouse footpad system. It usually takes 5–8 years for the BI to become negative.

Biopsies are not always necessary to make the diagnosis, and in areas of the world where the disease is common, most patients are not biopsied. However, in countries such as the United States, where the disease is rare, all patients should have at least an initial biopsy. A biopsy should be taken from entirely within the margin of the chose lesion and fixed in 10% formalin. Some sections are stained with hematoxylin–eosin for routine histopathology and a modified Fite–Faraco stain for AFB is used on other sections.

Table 1. Bacterial Index

0	No bacilli per 100 OIFs[a]
1+	1–10 bacilli per 100 OIFs
2+	1–10 bacilli per 10 OIFs
3+	1–10 bacilli per OIFs
4+	10–100 bacilli per OIFs
5+	100–1000 bacilli per OIFs
6+	>1000 bacilli per OIFs

[a]OIF, oil-immersion field

Shepard first reported that *M. leprae* will grow to a limited extent in mouse footpads in 1960.[(5)] In this system, a skin biopsy is taken from an active site with a BI of at least 4^+. The bacilli are put into a suspension and 5000 bacilli are injected into both hind footpads of each mouse. The number of mice used depends on the number of drugs being evaluated, but normally a group of 10 or more controls will be injected plus groups of 5 or more for each drug concentration to be tested. Typically, treated groups will contain mice fed 0.01%, 0.001%, and 0.0001% dapsone, 0.001% clofazimine, and 0.01% rifampin. Maximal growth is attained in about 6 months, when the original 5000 bacilli will have increased to about 10^6 if viable *M. leprae* were present in the inoculum. Lack of growth in the drug-treated group denotes sensitivity to that dietary level of the drug in question. Six to nine months is required to complete this study.

Although *M. leprae* cannot be cultured *in vitro*, there are now several studies reporting limited metabolism in cell-free *in vitro* radiorespirometric systems. The most promising method at present appears to be a system which measures $^{14}CO_2$ evolution from ^{14}C-labeled palmitic acid such as in the BACTEC or Buddemeyer system utilizing nude-mouse-derived *M. leprae*. These techniques have been used to screen potential antileprosy drugs and are a significant advance from using animal models.[(2)] Several recent studies show that radiorespirometry may also be utilized to assess viability of *M. leprae* in patient biopsies during treatment and could potentially be used to quantify response to antibacterial treatment.[(21)]

3.4.2. Serological and Immunologic Diagnostic Methods. Serological methods of detecting exposure to *M. leprae* are discussed in Section 3.3. Generally, these tests have not proved to be useful for diagnostic purposes. The most widely studied of these, PGL-1 antibody, is always positive in new lepromatous cases, but these cases also are usually easily diagnosed by conventional methods. In tuberculoid cases, more than 50% cannot be detected by this method. Consequently, serology is not generally helpful in difficult cases where it would be most useful. PCR has also been studied as a possible method of diagnosis. In general, most patients who have AFB in routine biopsies can also be detected with PCR; however, in those whose biopsies are negative for AFB, only 50–60% are detected by PCR.[22] It has also been shown to be possible to consistently distinguish *M. leprae* from other mycobacterial species with PCR[23] This would be useful in situations where there may be confusion with other atypical mycobacterial infections. PCR appears to be highly specific and sensitive and offers a new approach to identifying *M. leprae* under clinical conditions.[24] However, the application of PCR to routine patient diagnosis and management will require considerably more study.

Other laboratory studies utilized in the management of leprosy are those required to monitor drug side effects and occasionally measurement of blood sulfone levels. Multiple circulating autoantibodies have been reported, and false-positive serologies are not uncommon.

4. Biological Characteristics of the Organism

Although *M. leprae* organisms can be isolated and positively identified only from patients with high bacterial counts and the Henle–Koch postulates (see Chapter 1, Section 13) have yet to be fulfilled, few would question that *M. leprae* is the causative agent of leprosy. *M. leprae* was first described in 1874 and was one of the first organisms to be identified as a cause of human disease. However, it still has not been grown in artificial media, and the usual methods for studying bacteria have not been applicable. Consequently, less is known about this bacterium than most other bacteria of medical importance.

M. leprae is a gram-positive acid-fast bacillus, 0.3–0.4 mm × 2–7 mm and is an obligate intracellular parasite. It is the only mycobacterial species with a special predilection for peripheral nerves and specifically for Schwann cells. On skin smears or biopsy sections, the bacilli are often clustered in oval formations called globi. Over 90% of the bacilli from a typical new patient stain irregularly and have been shown to be nonviable[25] for the mouse footpad. With effective chemotherapy, all bacilli become granular and disintegrate. Although the disintegrating bacilli appear to slowly clear with treatment, this clearing may be due in part to a loss of acid-fastness by the bacillary remnants rather than actual disappearance of the bacilli. Staining with the Gomori's–methenamine–silver technique has demonstrated bacilli in some biopsy sections that had shown none on a Fite–Faraco stain.[26]

The bacilli will survive in soil and water for up to 3 days[27] and in dried secretions for up to 9 days in a hot, humid climate.[28] At the temperature of wet ice, they may survive 2 weeks or more, and heating at 45°C for 1 hr reportedly kills them.[29] Their antigenic activity persists at temperatures of over 200°C.[30] In the mouse footpad, maximum growth occurs at an average footpad temperature in the 27–30°C range.[31] This corresponds to its growth pattern in humans where the highest bacterial counts occur in the cooler areas of the body such as the skin, extremities, and the anterior portion of the eye. Most authorities regard the ability to oxidize dihydroxyphenylalanine (dopa) a unique characteristic of this bacillus, since it has not been found in any other mycobacteria.[32] Dopa oxidase activity has been included in a list of seven characteristic criteria that must be met to confirm that bacilli are *M. leprae*.[33] The other six requirements are unique drug-sensitivity patterns, identical antigen composition, exclusion of environmental contamination or similarity to other known mycobacteria, similar growth in experimental animals, similar results when used in lepromin testing, and identical chemical composition of the cell wall skeleton. Characteristic growth in the mouse footpad and sensitivity of *M. leprae* to very low levels of dapsone are also unique.[34] In the mouse footpad, there appear to be "fast"- and "slow"-growing strains, but this characteristic seems to have no bearing on human disease. With the development of PCR and related technologies, it is likely that the older criteria for identifying *M. leprae* will eventually be superseded by the newer technology.

The large numbers of relatively tissue-free bacilli obtainable from armadillos has made it possible to begin applying the techniques of molecular biology to the study of this organism. *M. leprae* DNA libraries can be prepared in *Escherichia coli* vectors, which can provide a readily available source of *M. leprae* DNA. Thus, it is now possible to learn a great deal about this organism without the need to culture the organism.[35] The size of the genome in *M. leprae* is about 2.2–4.5 × 10^9 Da, with a guanine plus cytosine (G + C) ratio of 54–58% compared to 65–69% for most other mycobacteria.[36] Advances in molecular biology have led to the construction of genomic libraries of *M. leprae* and the mapping of virtually the entire chromosome. The position of at least 75 genetic loci has been determined.[37] Large numbers of nonspecific *M. leprae* antigens are also known and a number of specific antigens have been identified using monoclonal antibodies. Probably the most thorough investigated from a clinical point of view is PGL-1,[17] which was previously mentioned as serodiagnostic test for leprosy.

5. Descriptive Epidemiology

Statistical data for leprosy has improved significantly in recent years, and since most US cases occur among immigrants, our relatively limited problem in this country is best reviewed in terms of the worldwide leprosy problem.

5.1. Prevalence and Incidence

Worldwide figures are of limited value since significant numbers of cases occur only in a portion of countries and incidence may vary markedly within a given country. The estimated prevalence will also be higher than figures based on the actual number of registered cases and it may not always be clear which figure a given report refers to. Prevalence (1994) and case detection rate (1993) data from the 25 major endemic countries are shown in Table 2. As noted in recent years, the prevalence of leprosy has begun to decline as a result of the widespread application of short-term multidrug therapy, which was first introduced in 1981 and markedly improved control efforts. In 1990, this led the World Health Assembly to recommend an international effort to eliminate leprosy as a public health problem by the year 2000; elimination was defined as a prevalence below 1/10,000 in every country and in the major subunits of highly endemic countries. Since WHO defines a leprosy case as a patient who needs treatment (chemotherapy), the short-term treatment regimens have allowed mild cases (PB) to be removed from registries within 6 to 9 months and severe cases (MB) within 24 to 36 months. Results to date indicate that this effort either will succeed or at least come very close. The total number of registered cases has, as already noted, fallen from 5.4 million in 1985 to 1.7 million in 1994 (prevalence 3.0/10,000) but with an estimated total of 2.4 million cases (prevalence 4.4/10,000). Approximately 93% of these cases reside in 25 countries (Table 2) and 78% within just 6 countries: India, Brazil, Bangladesh, Indonesia, Myanmar, and Nigeria. Prevalence rates per 10,000 are highest in Brazil (14.3), Myanmar (12.6), and India (11.1). About 600,000 new cases are detected annually worldwide, and although this figure had risen through 1992, possibly as a result of increased control efforts, it fell (to 591,000) in 1993. Obviously, for the elimination of leprosy as a public health problem effort to succeed, the incidence must continue to fall.

The United States has only 6000 cases on its national registry; but if one uses the WHO definition of a case, only about 600 of these still require treatment, for a prevalence of approximately 0.26/100,000, with a case detection rate

Table 2. 1994 Prevalence and 1993 Case Detection Rate Data for the 25 Major Leprosy Endemic Countries[a]

Country	Estimated cases	Registered cases	Prevalence (registered cases) 10,000	New cases	Detection rate per 100,000
India	1,167,900	995,285	11.10	456,000	50.86
Brazil	283,800	223,539	14.28	34,235	21.86
Bangladesh	136,000	22,334	1.83	6,943	5.68
Indonesia	130,000	70,961	3.65	12,638	6.49
Myanmar	120,000	56,410	12.64	12,018	26.94
Nigeria	63,000	33,196	3.75	4,381	4.95
Philippines	30,000	15,441	2.32	3,442	5.17
Nepal	29,000	17,756	8.42	6,152	29.18
Sudan	28,000	4,579	1.67	1,489	5.43
Zaire	25,000	8,190	1.99	3,927	9.54
Ethiopia	20,000	15,673	2.87	4,090	7.49
Mozambique	15,100	12,838	8.38	1,930	12.60
Guinea	15,000	4,811	7.63	4,038	64.03
Colombia	15,000	6,628	1.95	645	1.90
Cote D'Ivoire	15,000	3,762	2.81	2,186	16.32
Vietnam	15,000	8,018	1.13	2,620	3.70
Mali	15,000	8,000	7.89	2,000	19.73
Madagascar	12,000	5,369	4.05	740	5.58
Chad	11,000	7,468	12.43	516	8.59
Mexico	10,000	8,938	0.99	335	0.37
Cambodia	10,000	2,038	2.27	945	10.53
Niger	10,000	6,563	7.69	768	9.00
Thailand	10,000	5,917	1.04	543	0.95
Egypt	10,000	3,338	0.60	1,042	1.86
Iran	10,000	2,627	0.42	127	0.20

[a]From World Health Organization.[8]

of only about 0.08/100,000 (200 cases annually). If only endemic areas of the United States are considered, the incidence ranges from approximately 0.2/100,000 in Louisiana and Texas to 0.8/100,000 in Hawaii. Most new cases occur among immigrants, particularly from Southeast Asia, Mexico, and the Philippines, and only 10–15% are native-born.

With all these data, it is important to realize that incidence rates in leprosy will tend to be higher with increasing frequency of examinations.[38] This occurs because more early lesions are detected, and many of these would have regressed spontaneously, and thus would have been missed if examinations had been done very infrequently.

5.2. Epidemic Behavior and Contagiousness

It appears from immunologic, serological, and epidemiological studies on household contacts and others with extensive exposure that, contrary to older beliefs, leprosy has a relatively high infectivity but a low pathogenicity for most individuals.[39] Epidemics in the usual sense of the word do not commonly occur in leprosy. It is true that the spread of leprosy throughout Europe in the Middle Ages is sometimes referred to as an epidemic[2]; however, some of these cases were probably not leprosy, the spread was gradual over a period of many years, and we have relatively little accurate information about it. The Nauru epidemic in the 1920s is probably the best-documented occurrence of a true leprosy epidemic.[40] Leprosy was introduced onto this island by a woman who arrived there about 1912. In 1920, the first case appeared among the native population, and by 1924, there were 284 cases in the population of 1200–1300. By 1929, 438 cases had been found, and apparently the incidence gradually diminished thereafter. Thus, at the peak of the epidemic, 34% of the population had been afflicted. Over 90% of the cases were tuberculoid type, and deformities were uncommon. On the basis of the findings in Nauru, New Guinea, and elsewhere, Leiker[41] noted that where leprosy is newly introduced, what is essentially an "epidemic" of tuberculoid leprosy occurs, the disease spreads rapidly, there are no foci of infection, and adults and children are equally susceptible. In old endemic areas, however, there is more lepromatous disease than in the newly infected population, a higher proportion of the cases are among children and young adults, the disease spreads slowly, and there are foci, i.e., particular villages and families with a higher incidence than others. It is evident that the pattern of leprosy in Nauru (an extreme and unprecedented example) and in other newly infected populations does indeed fit Leiker's postulates. However, it is more difficult to characterize the situation in most countries on the basis of such a hypothesis, particularly since nearly all data are now reported to WHO in terms of PB and MB or unclassified disease. Nonetheless, WHO does report a rise in MB leprosy in Africa, but PB leprosy has become more frequent in the Americas and Asia.[8] The reasons for this are uncertain. In the United States,[42] about 50% of cases are classified lepromatous, 15–20% borderline, and 30–35% tuberculoid and indeterminate.

5.3. Geographic Distribution

Leprosy today is found mostly in developing countries, the majority of which are in tropical and semitropical areas. Since it occurred in much of the north temperate zone in the past, however, climate probably has little to do with its present distribution.

5.4. Temporal Distribution

There is no significant variation in occurrence with the seasons.

5.5. Age

It is difficult to make generalizations about the age of onset of leprosy, but several reviews of the topic are worthy of note. A study of childhood leprosy[43] notes that it is uncommon below 2 years of age, though cases below the age of 6 months have been reported.[44] A significant number of cases below 5 years of age will be found in countries with a high or very high prevalence, and prevalence rates rise up to age 14, reaching values as high as and occasionally higher than those for the general population. Guinto[45] states that "it is a fact that children are much more susceptible than adults," but Newell[46] believes that statistics in this regard could be equally well interpreted as indicating only that children have more opportunity for exposure. More recently, the findings in Goa and from several other series in India and throughout the world have been tabulated.[47] These studies emphasize the great variations seen not only from country to country, but also within the same country. Generally speaking, the median age at onset is somewhere between 20 and 30. The most recent data from the United States[42] show about half the cases being below 35 at the time of diagnosis, with the oldest being in their 80s.

5.6. Sex

Sex ratios are generally 1:1 for children, but for adults the disease is usually more prevalent among males by a ratio of about 1.5 or 1.6:1,[43] except in Africa where females predominate some populations.[48] In the United

States males predominate by a ratio of 1.5:1. The reason for this predominance of adult males is unknown, but it could be due to greater susceptibility or greater exposure outside the household setting in most cultures.

5.7. Race

Although there are wide variations in incidence and prevalence and in the way the disease manifests itself throughout the world, there are no data that indicate any special race-related susceptibility or resistance, all other things being equal.

5.8. Occupation

There is no particular relationship between occupation and the occurrence of leprosy. Some studies[(49)] have found an increased incidence of leprosy among missionaries working with leprosy patients; however, the prevalence was well below that in the population they were serving and was "increased" only over the prevalence in their homelands. In one study,[(50)] native hospital workers actually had less chance of contracting the disease than their counterparts in other occupations, and no cases have occurred among the staff at Carville.

5.9. Occurrence in Different Settings

The incidence of leprosy is generally higher in a family with one or more cases than in families with no cases, but considerable variation exists. Guinto[(45)] notes that in a retrospective study done in the Philippines in 1935, the risk of contracting leprosy was eight times greater in family contacts of lepromatous patients than in the general population. In a follow-up prospective study (1935–1950), however, the risk was about five times, rather than eight times, greater. A study by Kluth[(51)] in Texas found that 2.6% of 1522 household contacts of lepromatous patients developed leprosy. On the other hand, after a review of several other series, mostly foreign ones, Filice and Fraser[(52)] concluded that the long-term risk was such that about 10% of the household contacts of lepromatous patients would ultimately develop the disease. More recent studies have yielded similar data.[(53)] In all these studies, exposure to tuberculoid and probably indeterminate disease had an extremely small effect, i.e., the incidence of leprosy in these families was not significantly higher than in the general population. In US studies, the risks of exposed adults and children have been about the same, but in other countries, the risk for children is considerably higher.[(52)] The chance of one spouse's infecting the other has also been evaluated[(54)] and seems to be about 5%. Institutional exposure can occasionally lead to very high rates. Of 2000 children born in or admitted to Culion Leprosarium in the Philippines in the 1930s without any sign of leprosy, 23% later developed it.[(43)] Over 75% spontaneously healed, however. On the other hand, thus far clinical leprosy is not more common in human immunodeficiency virus (HIV)-positive than in HIV-negative persons in areas where both are endemic.[(55)] Also, among United States military veterans, the incidence of leprosy has been relatively low. A review of the 240 cases known to have occurred among veterans from 1940 through 1968 reported that 46 were considered to have service-connected leprosy from exposure outside the United States.[(56)]

5.10. Socioeconomic Factors

Leprosy today occurs mostly among the poor in underdeveloped countries. Why this is so is uncertain; however, crowded living conditions, poor diet, inadequate medical care, and improper sanitation may all play a role. Good housing conditions and extended schooling, for example, reduced the risk of leprosy in Malawi.[(57)]

5.11. Other Factors

It has long been suspected that a genetic defect determines susceptibility to leprosy and its mode of expression, but definitive proof of this is lacking. Hastings[(58)] points out that familial clusters of leprosy patients, wide variation in prevalence and type of leprosy within a given population, high concordance rates of leprosy in identical twins, the persistence of anergy to *M. leprae* in inactive lepromatous patients, and the study of Dharmendra and Chatterjee[(59)] indicating a preexisting immune defect in patients destined to get lepromatous leprosy all favor the existence of a genetic defect, probably in the immune-response genes. Although the investigations of leprosy in identical twins[(60)] lend support to the theory, they are not conclusive, because the concordance rates, though relatively high, were far from perfect. Multiple studies of histocompatibility antigens in leprosy patients have likewise given variable results,[(61,62)] but an association between HLA-DR3 and predisposition to tuberculoid leprosy, and HLA-DQW1 and lepromatous disease is suggested.

6. Mechanisms and Routes of Transmission

The mechanism by which leprosy is transmitted is unknown, but three possibilities exist. The oldest theory holds that it is the result of prolonged close skin-to-skin-type contact with an active infectious case or through skin via fomites. Since it is unlikely *M. leprae* could penetrate intact skin, a break such as a cut or an abrasion would seem to be necessary for this to occur. Evidence cited[45] to support this theory includes the appearance of the first leprosy lesion in children at the sites most touched by their infected mothers, accidental inoculation by tattooing or at surgery, and inoculation via thorn pricks in animal models.[63] This evidence actually provides relatively little support for transmission via the skin. While the bacillus might occasionally be inoculated via injuries that pierce the skin, a history of such an injury is rare and the literature contains a number of studies showing that the site of the first lesion in children is not related to the extent to which an area is touched.[64] Furthermore, over 50% of cases in low to moderate endemicity areas give no history of contact with a leprosy case.[65] Thus, "prolonged" or "intimate" contact in these instances seems unlikely. The possible role of the nose and upper respiratory tract in the transmission of leprosy has been studied extensively. Pedley[66] demonstrated that although bacilli may easily be found in the nasal discharge, they are difficult to locate on the skin surface. Davey and Rees[67] demonstrated that a high percentage of bacilli passed out in the nasal discharge are viable and can survive up to 7 days. A single nose blow from 31 patients gave a mean discharge of 1.1×10^8 bacilli with a mean morphological index of 16.9%. It has also been shown[68] that mice may be infected with *M. leprae* via the respiratory route followed by dissemination of the infection and many similarities exist between the modes of spread and routes in infection of tuberculosis and leprosy in a population.[38] Of further interest are epidemiological studies[19] in highly endemic areas that show a relatively high incidence of *M. leprae* in nasal swabs from individuals with no evidence of leprosy.

Reports of acid-fast bacilli in the stomachs of insects who had bitten leprosy patients appeared as early as 1912.[45] Proof that transmission by this route is possible was not reported, however, until 1977.[69] After earlier demonstration that mosquitoes and bedbugs took up viable *M. leprae* when biting untreated patients, it was shown that mosquitoes (*Aedes aegypti*) were capable of transmitting the infection to mouse footpads. This important work demonstrated that arthropod transmission of leprosy is possible, but there is no evidence that it is a probable route in humans, and further studies are needed. The question of how leprosy is transmitted, then, remains undecided. On the basis of available data, however, the most likely possibility would seem to be that it is spread by the respiratory route in the majority of instances, though insect vectors or the transcutaneous route may occasionally play a role.

Several other possible sources of infection have been suggested. Beginning in 1975, it was reported that uninoculated armadillos caught in Louisiana were infected with acid-fast bacilli ultimately proven to be *M. leprae*.[70] Numerous other surveys have confirmed that this occurs in 2–6% of armadillos caught in parts of Texas and Louisiana.[71] The significance is uncertain and the problem appears to be confined to the United States and Mexico. Originally it was felt that this was not a likely source of human infection,[72] but some investigators[73,74] have found evidence that transmission of the disease from armadillos to humans may at least occasionally occur. Leprosy has also been found in a chimpanzee from Sierra Leone[75] and a sooty mangabey monkey from Nigeria. These animals might have caught it from handlers, but its apparent transmission to a second mangabey monkey kept with the first indicates that monkey-to-monkey spread could occur.[76] Evidence that *M. leprae* may exist free in nature has also been found,[77] raising the possibility that this may be the source of infection in these various animals and perhaps occasionally in man. Finally, the possibility of a carrier state for leprosy has also been the subject of several studies reviewed by Guinto.[45] No strong evidence supporting such a condition was found, but more recent studies indicate this may occur.[19] It is clear that much more research will be needed to resolve all these issues.

7. Pathogenesis and Immunity

Many newly diagnosed leprosy patients have no known contact, and therefore the specific time of infection and the time of onset of disease are usually difficult to define. Thus, reports regarding incubation periods generally are only estimates. There are reports of incubation periods from less than 1 year to up to 30 years, with reports of average incubation periods ranging from 4 to 8 years.[78] When leprosy bacilli are transmitted from a patient to a contact, the overwhelming majority of individuals (over 95%) appear able to resist the infection and destroy the bacilli without developing any sign of the disease. In contacts who have the specific CMI defect, the macrophages ingest the bacilli, but in effect fail to fully recognize them as pathogens and allow bacilli to multiply and disseminate to varying degrees. Dissemination is probably hematogenous, since it has been demonstrated repeatedly that *M. leprae* bacilli are readily found within neutrophils and mononuclear phagocytes or occasionally free in the buffy coat of centrifuged blood specimens in untreated lepromatous patients,[79] As one might expect, the frequency of this finding diminishes as one moves from disseminated (lepromatous) to localized (tuberculoid) disease.

Although the immune defect in persons who contract leprosy is not clearly defined, our present understanding is that those who are susceptible have a defect in CMI that is specific for *M. leprae*. At least four major mechanisms have been proposed: (1) direct inhibition of T cells and/or macrophages by *M. leprae*; (2) inhibition of T cells by factors released from *M. leprae* stimulated macrophages; (3) T helper and cytolytic T cells may cause suppression of CMI for *M. leprae*; and (4) antigen-specific suppressor T cells are activated in some way.[80] Whatever the nature of the defect, it is not clear whether it is genetic, acquired, or both.

There is also evidence for a moderate general impairment of CMI in untreated lepromatous leprosy patients such as lack of dinitrochlorobenzene sensitization[81] and reduced numbers of T cells.[82] However, these patients are capable of handling other infections, including mycobacterial ones, in a normal fashion. They have no evidence of an increased incidence of cancer,[83] and there appears to be recovery of the generalized CMI impairment with treatment. However, the lack of response of lepromatous patients to lepromin does not recover with elimination of the bacterial load.

Historically, the varied clinical presentations of leprosy have been described as distinct disease entities. While this was satisfactory for clinical purposes, it tended to obscure the fact that these were all merely different manifestations of the same disease. What was needed was a classification that integrated the clinical, immunologic, and histopathologic findings. It was against this background that the Ridley–Jopling classification was introduced in 1962, and with the addition of a classification for reactions has gained widespread acceptance.[84] Figure 1 illustrates our current concept of the disease in terms of the five-part Ridley–Jopling classification.

As shown in Fig. 1, the earliest lesion in all cases is

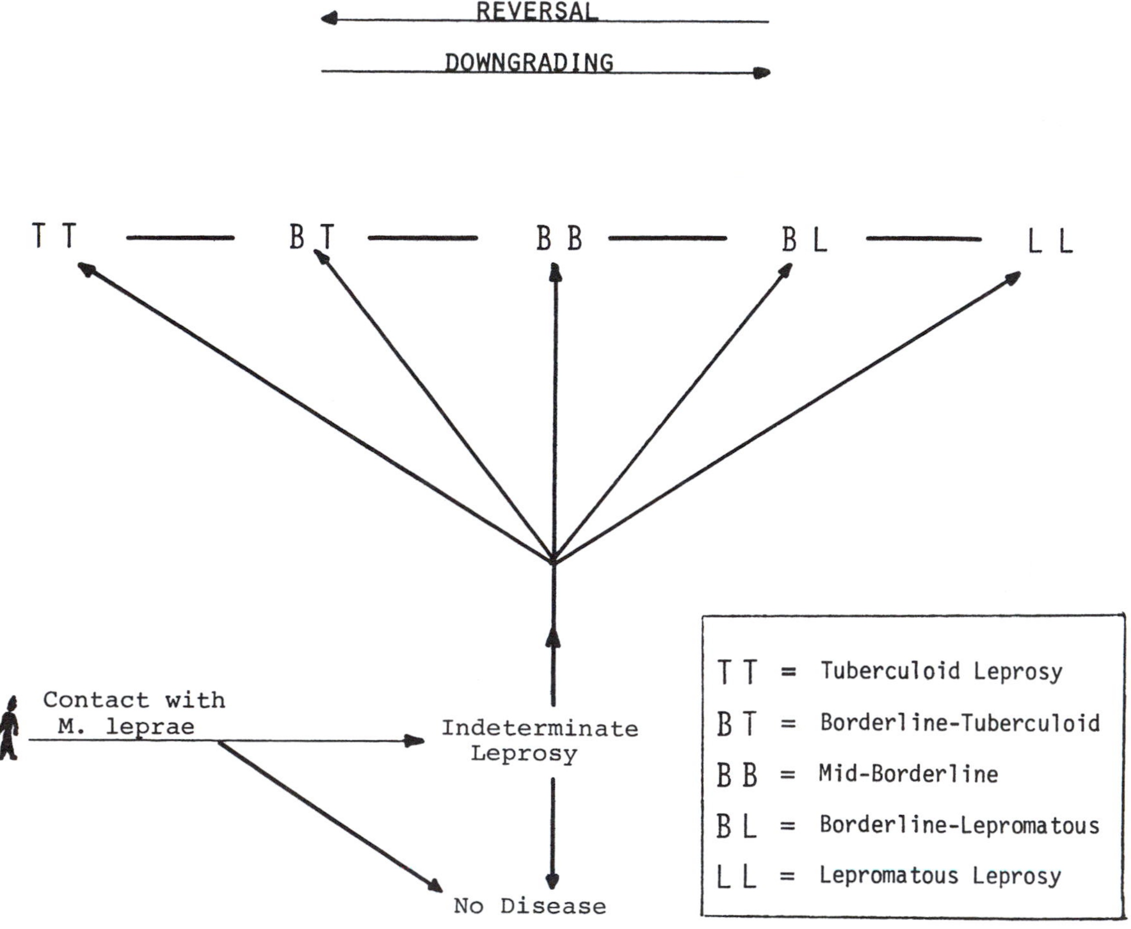

Figure 1. Ridley–Jopling classification of leprosy.

commonly referred to as indeterminate leprosy. It is usually only a single hypopigmented macule, and biopsy sections will show a minimal nonspecific chronic inflammatory infiltrate around nerves, blood vessels, and glands in the upper dermis. Only rare bacilli are likely to be present. Indeterminate leprosy may be self-healing in up to 75% of the cases,[85] but if diagnosed, it is always treated. Those lesions that are not treated or that are self-healing will ultimately progress to one of the three common clinical types: tuberculoid, borderline, or lepromatous. Those with the greatest degree of resistance keep the infection localized and develop tuberculoid disease, referred to as TT in the Ridley–Jopling classification. Biopsy sections in these cases are characterized by epitheloid cell granulomas surrounded by lymphocytes. Nerve bundles are invaded and destroyed, often to the point of being unidentifiable, and the nerve involvement is pathognomonic of leprosy. As with indeterminate disease, there are only rare bacilli.

Those with the least resistance to the infection develop lepromatous disease (LL). Histologically, the infiltrate initially consists of macrophages around dermal appendages, nerves, and blood vessels. The infiltrate gradually increases to the point where in advanced cases it may replace most of the dermis. *M. leprae* increase in macrophages to the point of eventually replacing the cytoplasm, which becomes vacuolated with accumulated lipid, forming foam cells. Bacilli are easily demonstrable (BI = 4–6^+) and lymphocytes are, for practical purposes, absent.

Between the extremes of TT and LL disease, there is a broad zone referred to as borderline leprosy. Histologically, lesions in these cases present a varied picture ranging from a tuberculoid appearance on the borderline tuberculoid (BT) side of the spectrum through the mixed histology of the midborderline (BB) area to a more lepromatous appearance in the borderline lepromatous (BL) region. The infiltrate consists mostly of lymphocytes, epithelioid, and giant cells in BT cases; but as one moves toward BL, the number of lymphocytes steadily diminishes, the infiltrate consists mostly of macrophages, and bacilli increase in numbers (BI = 2–4^+). This change in the number of lymphocytes is consistent with the presumed decrease in immune status as one moves from the tuberculoid end of the spectrum to the lepromatous end.

The Ridley–Jopling classification is important for research purposes, but it is generally too complex to apply under most field conditions. Thus, in 1982, the WHO introduced a simpler two-part classification that is now used almost universally to classify patients for treatment purposes. PB includes indeterminate, tuberculoid, and most borderline tuberculoid disease, and MB includes midborderline, borderline lepromatous, and lepromatous on the Ridley–Jopling scale. Skin smears are used to define PB and MB disease in that MB includes all those who have positive skin smears.[86] The only shortcoming of this definition is that if skin smears are poorly done, a MB case may inadvertently be classified as PB and therefore inadequately treated. In some programs, BT cases with large numbers of lesions are also classified as MB for treatment purposes. This two-group system has greatly simplified classification under field conditions.

While the disease in a patient at either pole (tuberculoid or lepromatous) tends to be stable, in the broad borderline portion of the spectrum some shift in disease type can occur. With treatment, the tendency is for the disease to shift toward tuberculoid with an enhanced immune response. Without treatment, the tendency is for immunity to diminish with a consequent shift of the disease toward lepromatous. If reactions (see Section 8) accompany these immunologic shifts, they are referred to as reversal reaction (type 1) if the shift is toward the tuberculoid pole, or downgrading reaction if the shift is toward lepromatous disease. Thus, a patient's disease may start out as relatively limited BT disease, but if left untreated, it may downgrade and develop more extensive disease and be classified BB or BL when diagnosed. With treatment, immunologic improvement may occur (reversal), moving the patient toward BT again.

8. Patterns of Host Response

As noted in Section 7, leprosy is a spectrum of disease, both clinically and immunologically, ranging from a few hypopigmented skin lesions and rare bacteria in tuberculoid disease to generalized disease with diffuse skin lesions and many bacteria in lepromatous cases. Between these two polar extremes there is a broad range of borderline disease. A large portion of cases fall somewhere in the borderline group.

8.1. Clinical Features

The earliest form of leprosy is usually indeterminate (I) and presents as one or two hypopigmented or occasionally erythematous macules on the face, extremities, or buttocks. Sensation may be slightly diminished or normal, and the diagnosis is confirmed by biopsy. Because of its benign appearance, it is most often diagnosed during contact examinations or case-finding surveys. Tuberculoid (TT) normally presents as one or two hypopigmented or erythematous anesthetic lesions that may be macular, with or without a raised margin, or occasionally plaquelike lesions. The surface is often scaly. Peripheral nerves in the area of the skin lesion may be involved, resulting in anesthesia or motor loss in a hand or foot. The presentation in lepromatous leprosy (LL) is quite variable and is usually a generalized skin eruption of some type. The skin lesions may be disseminated faint erythematous macules, or a generalized papular and nodular eruption, or a diffuse skin infiltration with no distinct lesions. Early in the disease there may be very little evidence of neuropathy, but as the disease progresses there will be diminished sensation in the distal extremities, and in more advanced disease there may be motor loss with claw hands, claw toes, or footdrop. Sensory loss may affect only the distal extremities or may progress to the point of nearly total body anesthesia, sparing only the warmer regions such as the axilla or groin area. In advanced lepromatous cases there may be loss of eyebrows, nasal stuffiness with septal perforation and collapse of the bridge of the nose, epistaxis, hoarseness, and the classic "leonine" facies. Other complications include lagophthalmos and iridocyclitis (which may damage vision if not controlled), testicular atrophy, gynecomastia, and injuries of the extremities as a result of sensory loss.

Borderline disease occupies the broad middle portion of the leprosy spectrum. Skin lesions vary from being tuberculoidlike in the BT region to lepromatouslike in BL disease, with mixed findings for BB cases. Sensory loss is usually present in skin lesions in TT and BT cases, while lesions in BL and LL cases may have minimal loss early in the disease. Nerve involvement leading to extensive sensory and motor loss in the extremities tends to be more severe in borderline cases than in the other types.

Acute immunologic problems commonly known as reactions may develop before diagnosis and treatment, but usually occur afterward and are seen with varying degrees of severity in up to 50% of cases. These reactions are of two main types, erythema nodosum leprosum (ENL, or type 2) and reversal reactions (type 1). ENL occurs in BL and LL cases and is thought to be due to an imbalance of the humoral immune system and to fit into the category of an immune complex disorder. Recently it has also been found that blood tumor necrosis factor levels are increased during ENL and appear to play a role in this reaction.[87] Clinically, ENL can range from mild to a severe generalized illness. It usually presents as fever with erythematous, tender, skin nodules that develop rapidly. The nodules usually subside in 1–2 weeks, but new crops of lesions will tend to occur if patients are not treated. Neuritis, malaise, edema, arthralgia, leukocytosis, iridocyclitis, lymphadenitis, pretibial periostitis, orchitis, and nephritis may also occur. ENL can be controlled with thalidomide, corticosteroids, or clofazimine, or a combination of these.

Reversal reaction, as noted in Section 7, is considered a delayed-type hypersensitivity response to *M. leprae* because an acute change or "reversal" has apparently occurred in the patient's ability to respond to bacterial antigens. Reversal reactions can occur in all borderline cases. Clinically, reversal reactions present as erythema and swelling of previously visible skin lesions and may be associated with peripheral edema and painful neuritis. The neuritis may lead to severe motor or sensory loss, and high doses of corticosteroids often must be used to halt the process and reverse the damage. Patients with BL disease may have either type of reaction and even occasionally appear to have a mixed reaction. A severe ulcerating skin reaction known as Lucio's phenomenon can occur in patients with a rare diffuse nonnodular lepromatous leprosy known as Lucio's leprosy.

8.2. Diagnosis

The skin lesions of leprosy vary considerably and may mimic many skin disorders. However, the combination of skin lesions and sensory loss in skin lesions and/or evidence of neuropathy in an extremity is the hallmark of leprosy. Skin lesions that do not respond to treatment as expected should also raise the suspicion of leprosy. The differential diagnosis for leprosy would be a long list ranging from simple fungus infections to more rare diseases such as leishmaniasis. Occasionally, a rare combination such as necrobiosis lipoidica diabeticorum with a diabetic polyneuropathy may mimic leprosy. However, a careful examination of the skin and peripheral nerves, slit-skin smears, and properly selected and processed biopsies will establish or exclude the diagnosis in the vast majority of cases.

9. Control and Prevention

9.1. General Concepts

Leprosy control today is based mainly on early case detection and treatment. Modern therapy with regimens containing rifampin kills 99.9+% of all viable *M. leprae* within a few days so that bacilli isolated from treated patients cannot be grown in the mouse footpad system. Since treated cases are thereby apparently rapidly rendered noninfectious, isolation is not required nor is hospitalization ever necessary except very occasionally for leprosy-related complications. Success of this approach, of course, depends on having a good overall leprosy control program that can be either vertical or horizontal in type; horizontal programs will generally be integrated to varying degrees into the available primary health care system. Guidelines for all aspects of the control program are contained in a number of the WHO publications,[7,88,89] but obviously all such guidelines must, in various ways, be adapted to the individual country situation.

Case detection is based mainly on the examination of household contacts and an awareness of medical practitioners in general of the early signs and symptoms of the disease. General population surveys, clue surveys, and screening of school children or other special population groups are generally insufficiently productive insofar as detection of new cases to justify their cost. Exceptions would be those areas with a high prevalence rate, particularly where the population has relatively poor access to medical care and/or the control program is just being developed. Another exception would be patients previously "cured" with just dapsone monotherapy, because their relapse rate is known to be high. The Fifth Expert WHO Committee on Leprosy[90] indicated that although all detected cases should be treated, to reduce incidence the program must regularly treat at least 75% of MB patients, ultimately rendering them bacteriologically negative. Most control programs nowadays meet or surpass this goal; recent evidence indicates the incidence worldwide may have started to decline.[8] Another measure of success insofar as early case detection is concerned is a low disability rate in new cases and the extent of disease as measured by clinical and bacteriologic findings.

Treatment is now almost universally with the standard WHO PB and MB short-term regimens developed in 1981.[7] The PB regimen involves giving a supervised dose of 600 mg of rifampin monthly for 6 months, with dapsone 100 mg daily, unsupervised, for 6 months. MB cases receive the same treatment for 24 months with the addition of a supervised dose of 300 mg of clofazimine monthly and 50 mg daily. Relapse rates to date are only about 1% for either regimen, with nearly 10 years follow-up in many instances. A higher relapse rate is found among patients with very advanced disease[91] (average BI on skin scrapings, 5+ or above), but these fortunately represent only a small portion of the total patient population in most countries. Relapse is managed by re-treatment with the same drug regimens, since drug resistance has not yet been noted to develop in relapsed cases treated with multidrug therapy.

While the standard WHO regimens appear to give excellent treatment results, there still is a problem in many areas because access to patients is difficult or because of other problems. Fortunately, several new drugs that are highly bactericidal against *M. leprae* have been found, including ofloxacin, clarithromycin, and minocycline. A trial is now underway using rifampin and ofloxacin daily for only 1 month to treat all types of leprosy, as are trials of combinations of the newer drugs with rifampin just once monthly or whenever the patient is accessible for 3 versus 6 doses for PB cases and 12 versus 24 doses for MB cases. The success of such regimens would make therapy accessible to nearly all patients, even under the most difficult circumstances, and could do much to improve control.

The WHO recommends[88] an evaluation of household contacts only at the time of diagnosis of the index case. Thereafter, contacts are advised to return only if signs or symptoms of the disease occur. Nonetheless, many control programs and the United States' recommendations are for annual follow-up examinations for 5 years. Early detection among contacts or the general population obviously depends on having physicians and other health practitioners who are trained to recognize the early signs and symptoms of the disease. As a result of efforts to eliminate leprosy as a public health problem by the year 2000, there has been significant improvement in this regard in most leprosy-endemic countries in recent years. Nonetheless, the effort must continue even after that goal is reached if we are to avoid a future resurgence of the leprosy problem.

In the United States, our goal should be early detection and appropriate treatment of all patients. Because of the limited extent of the problem in this country, however, only household contacts need be regularly examined. It is doubtful that we can eliminate the disease, since most new cases occur among aliens, but the problem should be easily controllable. The efforts of the Gillis W. Long Hansen's Disease Center and the Regional Hansen's Disease Program have made physicians in this country more aware of and knowledgeable about leprosy, and the multiple clinics of the Regional Hansen's Disease Program operated in 10 cities bring treatment to a majority of patients free of charge.

Health education of patients and their families cannot receive too much emphasis either in the United States or elsewhere. Most patients will require treatment for 6 months to 2 or more years, depending on the occurrence of complications, and they are likely to cooperate with therapy only if they understand it. In this way they are similar to patients with diabetes, epilepsy, or hypertension. They must be aware of why they are being treated, that they may get worse (reactions) before they get better, how long they will need treatment, and what the long-term benefits of treatment are to them and their families.

9.2. Antibiotic and Chemotherapeutic Approaches to Prophylaxis

Chemoprophylaxis as a leprosy control measure has been attempted in a number of studies over the years since the sulfones were first found to be effective for the treatment of leprosy in the 1940s. Many investigators reported a 40 to 80% success rate using dapsone.[92] Unfortunately, most had insufficient follow-up to determine whether the disease was actually prevented or only delayed in those contacts destined to develop MB disease. The best trial in this regard was carried out on two isolated Pacific Islands, with an incidence rate of 7/1,000.[93] A relatively successful attempt was made to treat all of the population with 15 injections of acedapsone over a 3-year period. This drug is the diacetyl derivative of dapsone and, given in a dose of 225 mg every 11 weeks, maintains a low, relatively stable level of dapsone in the blood throughout the interval. As expected, the incidence of new cases fell to zero during the trial, but cases began appearing again shortly after the trial was discontinued and have continued to appear up to the present. Even had dapsone prophylaxis been successful, the prolonged period of time it had to be given would have markedly limited its usefulness under field conditions.

Dapsone is essentially bacteriostatic for *M. leprae*, so that prolonged treatment was required when it was used as monotherapy. Rifampin, on the other hand, is highly bactericidal, and this is the major reason the WHO short-term regimens have thus far been so successful. It is therefore not surprising that trials of a single large dose of rifampin (25 mg/kg in adults) would be tried as a prophylactic measure to prevent leprosy.[94] The trial demonstrated some effectiveness but was too small to clearly define the benefits from this approach. Thus, WHO at this time does not recommend any form of chemoprophylaxis to prevent leprosy.[88] Nonetheless, the availability of several new bactericidal drugs, as noted previously, will probably lead to further trials of these in combination with rifampin for leprosy prevention.

9.3. Immunization

Although no specific antileprosy vaccine is yet available, BCG offers about 50–80% protection against leprosy,[95–97] and is appreciably more effective than against tuberculosis. Giving a vaccine consisting of a mixture of BCG and armadillo-derived heat-killed *M. leprae* did not improve protection,[95] but another trial of BCG versus BCG plus heat-killed *M. leprae* is now underway. Whether these results would justify the use of BCG as a control measure is uncertain. It could conceivably be beneficial in highly endemic areas; but unless a greater protective effect against tuberculosis than is now evident can be demonstrated, its use in areas of low endemnicity for leprosy may not be cost effective. Trials with two other vaccines utilizing *Mycobacterium w*[98] and ICRC,[99] both cultivatable mycobacteria, are also underway. In addition to preventing leprosy, there is evidence that these vaccines may also have an immunotherapeutic effect on this disease.

10. Unresolved Problems

The WHO goal of elimination of leprosy as a public health problem (prevalence less than 1/10,000) by the year 2000 may succeed or at least come close to succeeding. This is, however, not the same as the elimination of leprosy. It will merely indicate that the problem has been brought under relatively good control. Unless there is also a steady decline in the incidence of the disease, the problem could progress again at any time and is likely to do so in some countries where the control effort is not maintained after the WHO goal is achieved. Also, there are large numbers of patients with severe leprosy-related disabilities who will continue to need various services from the control program if they are to be rehabilitated or maintain their ability to work, and so forth. Thus, there are a variety of actions that are necessary if true elimination of leprosy is ever to be achieved or even if our progress to date is to be maintained.

The presently available serological, PCR, and other methods for detecting exposure to *M. leprae*, diagnosis, and follow-up are disappointing because they lack sensitivity and/or specificity and in any event would not be useful under field conditions in most leprosy-endemic countries because of their cost and/or complexity. The most commonly used approach, i.e., skin scrapings, is likewise difficult and often unreliable, and biopsies are impractical particularly because the expertise to evaluate them is often not available. Thus, improved methods for diagnosis and follow-up of patients are important and may become even more so as control programs are more and more integrated into primary health care. The need for shorter-term therapy has already been mentioned and this is the one area where we are likely to see continued progress utilizing the new highly bactericidal antileprosy drugs.

Reaction control continues to be an important aspect of overall patient care since reactive episodes may result in further disabilities. Thalidomide and corticosteroids are the mainstays of therapy at this time, but both are toxic in various ways and somewhat variable in effectiveness and usefulness under field conditions. Thus, safer and more effective drugs are needed.

If leprosy is ever to be completely eliminated, it is unlikely to be accomplished with chemotherapy alone; to the extent that *M. leprae* exist in nature in armadillos, e.g., it may not be possible to completely eliminate it. A highly effective vaccine would perhaps be the most effective approach and would help improve control in some highly endemic areas. It would be costly in areas of lower endeminicity, however, and probably would be impractical unless it were multipurpose as that once proposed by Bloom,[100] using molecular biological techniques to make BCG effective against a variety of pathogens.

Finally, as has been noted, all of these efforts will be of little value unless we find ways to maintain effective control programs without excessive cost. Integration of leprosy control into the general health care scheme as the WHO recommends is almost certainly going to be necessary in most control programs as the prevalence and incidence of the disease decreases, but it is easy for leprosy control to deteriorate under such circumstances. Motivation of health care workers, improving patient compliance, reducing the stigma of leprosy, and obtaining sufficient personnel and funds will still be vital to a good control program. Clearly these problems must be solved lest we succeed in eliminating leprosy as a public health problem by the year 2000, but end up without a satisfactory means of maintaining this control or extending it to the ultimate eradication of leprosy.

11. References

1. Hansen, G. H. A., Undersogelser angaende Spedalskhedens Arsager, *Nor. Mag. Laegevidensk* **4:**76–79 (1874).
2. Browne, S. G., The history of leprosy, in: *Leprosy* (R. C. Hastings, ed.), pp. 1–14, Churchill Livingstone, Edinbrough, 1985.
3. Badger, L. F., Leprosy in the United States, *Public Health Rep.* **70:**525–535 (1955).
4. Faget, G. P., Pogge, R. C., Johansen, F. A., *et al.*, The promin treatment of leprosy: A progress report, *Public Health Rep.* **58:** 1729–1741 (1943).
5. Shepard, C. C., The experimental disease that follows the injection of human leprosy bacilli into footpads of mice, *J. Exp. Med.* **112:**445–454 (1960).
6. Kirchheimer, W. F., and Storrs, E. E., Attempts to establish the armadillo (*Dasypus novencintus* Linn.) as a model for the study of leprosy. I. Report of lepromatoid leprosy in an experimentally infected armadillo, *Int. J. Lepr.* **39:**693–702 (1971).
7. WHO Study Group, Chemotherapy of leprosy for control programmes, *WHO Tech. Rep. Ser.* No. 675, Geneva, WHO, 1982.
8. World Health Organization, Progress towards eliminating leprosy as a public health problem, *Wkly. Epidem. Rec.* **69:**145–151, 153–157 (1994).
9. Sengupta, U., Studies on lepromin and soluble antigens of *M. leprae*, *Ind. J. Lepr.* **63:**457–465 (1991).
10. Meyers, W. M., Kvernes, S., and Binford, C. H., Comparison of human and armadillo lepromins in leprosy, *Int. J. Lepr.* **43:**218–225 (1975).
11. Godal, T., and Negassi, K., Subclinical infection in leprosy, *Br. Med. J.* **3:**557–559 (1973).
12. Menzel, S., Bjune, G., Kronvall, G., *et al.*, Lymphocyte transformation test in healthy leprosy contacts: Influence of household exposure (Abstract), *Int. J. Lepr.* **47:**374 (1979).
13. Job, C. K., Chacko, C. J. G., Taylor, P. M., *et al.*, Evaluation of cell mediated immunity in the histopathologic spectrum of leprosy using lymphocyte transformation test, *Int. J. Lepr.* **44:**256–266 (1976).
14. Ilangumaran, S., Robinson, P., Shankernarayan, N. P., *et al.*, T lymphocyte reactivity of leprosy patients and healthy contacts from a leprosy-endemic population to delipified cell components of *Mycobacterium leprae*, *Lepr. Rev.* **65:**34–44 (1994).
15. Abe, M., Fumishige, M., Yuji, Y., *et al.*, Fluorescent leprosy-antibody absorption (FLA-ABS) test for detecting subclinical infection with *Mycobacterium leprae*, *Int. J. Lepr.* **48:**109–119 (1980).
16. Harboe, M., and Closs, O., A revival of interest in antibody studies in leprosy (Abstract)? *Int. J. Lepr.* **47:**372 (1979).
17. Smith, P. G., The serodiagnosis of leprosy, *Lepr. Rev.* **63:**97–100 (1992).
18. de Wit, M. Y., Douglas, P. T., McFadden, J., *et al.*, Polymerase chain reaction for detection of *Mycobacterium leprae* in nasal swab specimens, *J. Clin. Microbiol.* **31:**502–506 (1993).
19. van Beers, S. M., Izumi, S., Madjid, B., *et al.*, An epidemiological study of leprosy by serology and polymerase chain reaction, *Int. J. Lepr.* **62:**1–9 (1994).
20. Franzblau, S. G., Biswas, A. N., Jenner, P., *et al.*, Double-blind evaluation of BACTEC and Buddeymer-type radiorespirometric assays for *in vitro* screening of antileprosy drugs, *Lepr. Rev.* **63:**125–133 (1992).
21. Chan, G. P., Garcia-Ignacia, B. Y., Chavez, V. E., *et al.*, Clinical trial of sparfloxacin for lepromatous leprosy, *Antimicrob. Agents Chemother.* **38:**61–65 (1994).
22. de Witt, M. Y. L., Faber, W. R., Krieg, S. R., *et al.*, Application of polymerase chain reaction for the detection of *Mycobacterium leprae* in skin tissues, *J. Clin. Microbiol.* **29:**906–910 (1991).
23. Arnoldi, J., Schluter, C., Duchrow, M., *et al.*, Species- specific assessment of *Mycobacterium leprae* in skin biopsies by *in situ* hybridization and polymerase chain reaction, *Lab. Invest.* **66:** 618–623 (1992).
24. Gillis, T. P., and Williams, D. L., Polymerase chain reaction and leprosy, *Int. J. Lepr.* **59:**311–316 (1991).
25. Shepard, C. C., and McRae, D. H., *Mycobacterium leprae* in mice: Minimal infectious dose, relationship between staining quality and infectivity, and effect of cortisone, *J. Bacteriol.* **89:**365–372 (1965).
26. Krieg, R. E., and Meyers, W. M., Demonstration of *Mycobacterium leprae* in tissues from bacteriologically negative treated lepromatous leprosy patients (Abstract), *Int. J. Lepr.* **47:**367 (1979).

27. Harris, E. B., Landry, M. T., Sanchez, R., *et al.*, Viability of *Mycobacterium leprae* in soil, water, and degenerating armadillo tissue and its significance, *Microbios Lett.* **44:**73–76 (1990).
28. Desikan, K. B., Viability of *Mycobacterium leprae* outside the human body, *Lepr. Rev.* **48:**231–235 (1977).
29. Pattyn, S. R., Use of the mouse footpad in studying thermoresistance of *Mycobacterium leprae*, *Int. J. Lepr.* **33:**611–615 (1965).
30. Shepard, C. C., Walker, L. L., and Vanlandingham, R., Heat stability of *Mycobacterium leprae* immunogenicity, *Infect. Immun.* **22:**87–93 (1978).
31. Shepard, C. C., Stability of *Mycobacterium leprae* and temperature optimum for growth, *Int. J. Lepr.* **33:**541–547 (1965).
32. Prabhakaran, K., and Kirchheimer, W. F., Use of 3,4-dihydroxyphenylalanine oxidation in the identification of *Mycobacterium leprae*, *J. Bacteriol.* **92:**1267–1268 (1966).
33. Report of the Workshop on Microbiology of the XI International Leprosy Congress, *Int. J. Lepr.* **47:**291–294 (1979).
34. Shepard, C. C., Experimental chemotherapy in leprosy, then and now, *Int. J. Lepr.* **41:**307–319 (1973).
35. Colston, M. J., The molecular biology of *Mycobacterium leprae*, *Lepr. Rev.* **64:**289–294 (1993).
36. Rees, R. J. W., and Young, D. B., The microbiology of leprosy, in: *Leprosy*, 2nd ed. (R. C. Hastings, ed.), pp. 49–83, Edinburgh, Churchill Livingston, 1994.
37. Colston, M. J., Leprosy 1962–1992. The microbiology of *M. leprae*; Progress in the last 30 years, *Trans. R. Soc. Trop. Med. Hyg.* **87:**504–507 (1993).
38. Rees, R. J. W., and Meade, T. W., Comparison of modes of spread and incidence of tuberculosis and leprosy, *Lancet* **1:**47–49 (1974).
39. Baumgart, K. W., Britton, W. H., Mullins, R. J., *et al.*, Subclinical infection with *Mycobacterium leprae*—A problem for leprosy control strategies, *Trans. R. Soc. Trop. Med. Hyg.* **87:**412–415 (1993).
40. Wade, H. W., and Ledowsky, V., The leprosy epidemic at Nauru: A review with data on status since 1937, *Int. J. Lepr.* **20:**1–29 (1952).
41. Leiker, D. L., Epidemiological and immunological surveys in Netherlands New Guinea, *Lepr. Rev.* **31:**241–259 (1960).
42. Long, Gillis W., Unpublished data of the National Hansen's Disease Registry, Carville, Louisiana.
43. Noussitou, F. M., Sansarricq, H., and Walter, J., *Leprosy in Children*, WHO, Geneva, 1976.
44. Girdhar, A., Mishra, B., Lavania, R. K., *et al.*, Leprosy in infants. Report of two cases, *Int. J. Lepr.* **57:**472–475 (1989).
45. Guinto, R. S., Epidemiology of leprosy: Current views, concepts and problems, in: *A Window on Leprosy* (B. R. Chatterjee, ed.), pp. 36–53, Statesman Commercial Press, Calcutta, 1978.
46. Newell, K. W., An epidemiologist's view of leprosy, *Bull. WHO* **34:**827–857 (1966).
47. Sehgal, V. M., Rege, V. L., and Singh, K. P., The age of onset of leprosy, *Int. J. Lepr.* **45:**52–55 (1977).
48. Ponnighaus, J. M., Fine, P. E. M., Sterne, J. A. C., *et al.*, Incidence rates of leprosy in Karonga District, Northern Malawi; Patterns by age, sex, BCG status and classification, *Int. J. Lepr.* **62:**10–23 (1994).
49. Gray, H. H., and Dreisbach, J. A., Leprosy among foreign missionaries in northern Nigeria, *Int. J. lepr.* **29:**279–290 (1961).
50. Mathai, R., Rao, P. S. S., and Job, C. K., Risks of treating leprosy in a general hospital (Abstract), *Int. J. Lepr.* **47:**322 (1979).
51. Kluth, F. C., Leprosy in Texas: Risk of contracting the disease in the household, *Tex. State J. Med.* **52:**758–789 (1956).
52. Filice, G. A., and Fraser, D. W., Management of household contacts of leprosy patients, *Ann. Intern. Med.* **88:**538–542 (1978).
53. Chaudhury, S., Hazra, S. K., Saha, B., *et al.*, An eight-year field trial on antileprosy vaccines among high-risk household contacts in the Calcutta metropolis, *Int. J. Lepr.* **62:**389–394 (1994).
54. Badger, L. F., Epidemiology, in: *Leprosy in Theory and Practice*, 2nd ed. (R. G. Cochrane and T. F. Davey, eds.), pp. 69–97, John Wright, Bristol, 1964.
55. Lucas, S., Human immunodeficiency virus and leprosy, *Lepr. Rev.* **64:**97–103 (1993).
56. Brubaker, M. L., Binford, C. H., and Trautman, J. R., Occurrence of leprosy in US veterans after service in endemic areas abroad, *Public Health Rep.* **84:**1051–1058 (1969).
57. Ponninghaus, J. M., Fine, P. E. M., Sterne, J. A. C., *et al.*, Extended schooling and good housing conditions are associated with reduced risk of leprosy in rural Malawi, *Int. J. Lepr.* **62:**345–353 (1994).
58. Hastings, R. C., Transfer factor as a probe of the immune deficit in lepromatous leprosy, *Int. J. Lepr.* **45:**281– 291 (1977).
59. Dharmendra, and Chatterjee, B. R., Prognostic value of the lepromin test in contacts of leprosy cases, *Lepr. India* **27:**149–158 (1955).
60. Chakravatti, M. R., and Vogel, F., A twin study on leprosy, Topics in Human Genetics. No. 1, Thieme, Stuttgart, 1973.
61. Kher, S. K., Rao, M. R., Raghunath, D., *et al.*, HLA-linked genetic control of leprosy, *Med. J. Armed Forces India* **48:**116–118 (1992).
62. Rani, R., Zaheer, S. A., Mukherjee, R., Do human leukocyte antigens have a role to play in differential manifestations of multibacillary leprosy—A study on multibacillary leprosy patients from India, *Tissue Antigens* **40:**124–127 (1992).
63. Job, C. K., Chehl, S. K., and Hastings, R. C., Transmission of leprosy in nude mice through thorn pricks, *Int. J. Lepr.* **62:**395–398 (1994).
64. Bechelli, L. M., Garbojosa, P. G., Gyi, M. M., *et al.*, Site of early skin lesions in children with leprosy, *Bull. WHO* **48:**107–111 (1973).
65. Enna, C. D., Jacobson, R. R., Trautman, J. R., *et al.*, Leprosy in the United States, 1967–1976, *Public Health Rep.* **93:**468–473 (1978).
66. Pedley, J. C., The hypothesis of skin to skin transmission, *Lepr. Rev.* **48:**295–297 (1977).
67. Davey, T. F., and Rees, R. J. W., The nasal discharge in leprosy: Clinical and bacteriologic aspects, *Lepr. Rev.* **45:**121–134 (1974).
68. Rees, R. J. W., and McDougall, A. C., Airborne infection with *Mycobacterium leprae* in mice, *J. Med. Microbiol.* **10:**63–68 (1977).
69. Narayanan, E., Sreevatsa, Kirchheimer, W. F., *et al.*, Transfer of leprosy bacilli from patients to mouse footpads by *Aedes aegypti*, *Lepr. India* **49:**181–186 (1977).
70. Walsh, G. P., Storrs, E. E., Burchfield, H. P., *et al.*, Leprosy-like disease occurring naturally in armadillos, *J. Reticuloendothel. Soc.* **18:**347–351 (1975).
71. Job, C. K., Harris, E. B., Allen, J. L., *et al.*, A random survey of leprosy in wild nine-banded armadillos in Louisiana, *Int. J. Lepr.* **54:**453–457 (1986).
72. Centers for Disease Control, Leprosy-like disease in wild-caught armadillos, *Morbid. Mortal. Week. Rep.* **25:**18,23 (1976).
73. Lumpkin, L. R., III, Cox, G. F., and Wolf, J. E., Jr., Leprosy in five armadillo handlers, *J. Am. Acad. Dermatol.* **9:**899–903 (1983).

74. Thomas, D. A., Mines, J .S., Thomas, D. C., *et al.*, Armadillo exposure among Mexican-born patients with lepromatous leprosy, *J. Infect. Dis.* **156:**990–992 (1987).
75. Donham, K. J., and Leininger, J. R., Spontaneous leprosy-like disease in a chimpanzee, *J. Infect. Dis.* **136:**132–136 (1977).
76. Gormus, B. J., Wolf, R. H., Baskin, G. B., *et al.*, A second sooty mangabey monkey with naturally acquired leprosy: First reported possible monkey-to-monkey transmission, *Int. J. Lepr.* **56:**61–65 (1988).
77. Ingrens, L. M., and Kazda, J., The epidemiological significance of the occurrence of *M. leprae*-like microorganisms in the environment, *Int. J. Lepr.* **52:**719 (1984).
78. Noordeen, S. K., The epidemiology of leprosy, in: *Leprosy*, 2nd ed. (R. C. Hastings, ed.), pp. 29–45, Churchhill Livingstone, Edinburgh, 1994.
79. Drutz, D. J., Chen, T. S. N., and Lu, W. H., The continuous bacteremia of lepromatous leprosy, *N. Engl. J. Med.* **287:**159–164 (1972).
80. Kaufmann, S. H. E., Cell mediated immunity, in: *Leprosy*, 2nd ed. (R. C. Hastings, ed.), pp. 157–168, Churchhill Livingstone, Edinburgh, 1994.
81. Waldorf, D. S., Sheagren, J. N., Trautman, J. R., *et al.*, Impaired delayed hypersensitivity in patients with lepromatous leprosy, *Lancet* **2:**773–776 (1966).
82. Lim, S. E., Kiszkiss, E. F., Jacobson, R. R., *et al.*, Thymus dependent lymphocytes of peripheral blood in leprosy patients, *Infect. Immun.* **9:**394–399 (1974).
83. Oleinich, A., Altered immunity and cancer risks: A review of the problem and analysis of the cancer mortality experience of leprosy patients, *J. Natl. Cancer Inst.* **43:**775–781 (1969).
84. Ridley, D. S., and Jopling, W. H., Classification of leprosy according to immunity; a five group system, *Int. J. Lepr.* **34:**255–273 (1966).
85. Nousitu, F. M., Sansarricq, H., and Walter, J., *Leprosy in Children*, WHO, Geneva, 1976.
86. World Health Organization Expert Committee on Leprosy, Sixth Report, *WHO Tech. Rep. Ser.* No. 768, WHO, Geneva, 1988.
87. Sampaio, E. P., Kaplan, G., Miranda, A., *et al.*, The influence of thalidomide on the clinical and immunologic manifestations of erythema nodosum leprosum, *J. Infect. Dis.* **168:**408–414 (1993).
88. WHO Study Group, Chemotherapy of leprosy, *WHO Tech. Resp. Ser.* No. 847, WHO, Geneva, 1994.
89. World Health Organization, *A Guide to Leprosy Control*, 2nd ed. WHO, Geneva, 1988.
90. WHO Expert Committee on Leprosy, Fifth Report, *WHO Tech. Rep. Ser.* No. 607, WHO, Geneva, 1977.
91. Pattyn, S. R., Search for effective short-course regimens for the treatment of leprosy, *Int. J. Lepr.* **61:**76–81 (1993).
92. Noordeen, S. K., Long-term effects of chemoprophylaxis among contacts of lepromatous cases, *Lepr. India* **49:**504–509 (1977).
93. Russell, D. A., Worth, R. M., Scott, G. C., *et al.*, Experience with acedapsone (DADDS) in a therapeutic trial in New Guinea and the chemoprophylactic trial in Micronesia, *Int. J. Lepr.* **44:**170–176 (1976).
94. Cartel, J. L., Chantaeu, S., Moulia-Pelat, J. P., *et al.*, Chemoprophylaxis of leprosy with a single dose of 25 mg per kg rifampin in the Southern Marquesas; Results after four years, *Int. J. Lepr.* **60:**416–420 (1992).
95. Convit, J., Smith, P. G., Zuniga, M., *et al.*, BCG vaccination protects against leprosy in Venezuela: A case-control study, *Int. J. Lepr.* **61:**185–191 (1993).
96. Ponnighaus, J. M., Fine, P. E. M., Sterne, J. A. C., *et al.*, Efficacy of BCG vaccine against leprosy and tuberculosis in Malawi, *Lancet* **1:**636–639 (1992).
97. Orege, P. A., Fine, P. E. M., Lucas, S. B., *et al.*, Case-control study of BCG vaccination as a risk factor for leprosy and tuberculosis in Western Kenya, *Int. J. Lepr.* **61:**542–549 (1993).
98. Reddi, P. P., Amin, A. G., Khandekar, P. S., *et al.*, Molecular definition of unique species status of *Mycobacterium w*; a candidate leprosy vaccine strain, *Int. J. Lepr.* **62:**229–236 (1994).
99. Chiplunkar, S. V., Kudalkar, J. L., Gangal, S. G., *et al.*, Immunoreactivity of mycobacterial strain ICRC and *Mycobacterium leprae* antigens with polyclonal and monoclonal antibodies, *Int. J. Lepr.* **61:**421–427 (1993).
100. Bloom, B. R., New strategies for leprosy and tuberculosis and for development of bacillus Calmette-Guérin into a multivaccine vehicle, *Ann. NY Acad. Sci.* **569:**155–173 (1989).

12. Suggested Reading

Bahong, J., and Noordeen, S. K., Leprosy, in: *Tropical Disease Research: A Global Partnership* (J. Maurice and A. M. Pearce, eds.), pp. 113–124, WHO, Geneva, 1987.

Harboe, M. (ed.), Immunology of leprosy: Proceedings of an international symposium, *Lepr. Rev.* **57**(Suppl. 2)**:**1–308 (1986).

Hastings, R. C. (ed.), *Leprosy*, Churchill Livingstone, Edinburgh, 1994.

World Health Organization Study Group, Chemotherapy of leprosy, *WHO Tech. Rep. Ser.* No. 847, Geneva, WHO, 1994.

World Health Organization, *A Guide to Leprosy Control*, WHO, Geneva, 1988.

CHAPTER 20

Leptospirosis

Solly Faine

1. Introduction

Leptospirosis in humans occurs throughout the world as an acute infection ranging in severity from unnoticed and subclinical to fatal. It is a zoonosis (strictly, an anthropozoonosis) acquired by humans from an animal source. The causal bacterium is a pathogenic member of the genus *Leptospira*, of which there are several species and more than 200 serological varieties (serovars) (see Section 3.4.1a), each of which has some special diagnostic, prognostic, or epidemiological significance.[1–3]

The ultimate reservoir of all leptospirosis is a nonhuman carrier animal that excretes the causal bacteria (leptospires) in its urine. In animals, the leptospires infect primarily young animals, which may become renal carriers and urinary excretors if they survive an acute initial infection. Human-to-human transmission has been recorded extremely rarely, congenital infection has been infrequently reported, and laboratory-acquired infections have been documented.

There are a large number of leptospires identified by serology or by genetic relationships. In general, there is a correlation between animal reservoir, serological type (serovar), and potential severity of the illness. The disease has many local and folk names, frequently originating from historical or clinical features or associated occupations, such as "pretibial fever," "swineherds' disease," "cane-cutters disease," "mud fever."

As it is a zoonosis, leptospirosis is most significant for those whose work or leisure brings them into contact with infected animals or their urine. It is highly related to occupation in societies where animal contact is rare except through work.

In some societies, particularly in tropical areas, it is impossible to avoid direct or indirect contact with feral carrier rodents or with livestock. In others, only those in selected occupations are exposed to significant risks. The public health importance of leptospirosis lies in its occupational, season, and sex- and age-related incidence; the acute and sometimes prolonged incapacity for work; loss of human and livestock productivity; costs for medical care, workers' compensation, or other occupational disease insurance payments; and preventive measures. It can be epidemic, sporadic, or endemic.

The geographic distribution of the literature sources cited (references) reflects the inevitable fact that most research on leptospirosis occurs where there is a high morbidity together with a high level of scientific expertise and funding.

2. Historical Background[2]

The early history of leptospirosis is vague, because it was not possible to differentiate the different forms of "malignant jaundice," which included hepatitis, yellow fever, leptospirosis, and malaria, until scientific clinical and pathological knowledge had progressed into the 1880s. Nevertheless, an account by Wittman, a British military surgeon, in 1803, may well have been of an epidemic of leptospirosis during the Napoleonic wars in Palestine and Egypt. The clinical entity was described by both Mathieu and Weil in 1886, but Weil's description became the classical reference. The syndrome of fever, hemorrhage, jaundice, and enlarged liver and spleen, with renal failure, became known as "Weil's disease." Its etiology was unknown until the discovery of pathogenic leptospires, first seen in stained tissue sections of liver from a "yellow fever" patient, and later cultivated independently from Weil's disease patients among coal miners in Japan in 1914 and troops in trenches in Germany during

Solly Faine • Department of Microbiology, Monash University, Clayton Vic. 3168, Australia.

World War I in 1915. It was named *Spirochaeta icterohaemorrhagiae* by the Japanese; *Spirochaeta icterogenes* by the Germans; and later *Leptospira icterohaemorrhagiae* by Noguchi. Both the Japanese and German workers and their associates quickly published much of the basic knowledge of the microorganisms, as well as the pathogenesis, pathology, clinical features and diagnosis, and rodent source of leptospirosis.

Less severe illnesses were soon recognized as forms of leptospirosis. Dogs were identified as both reservoirs and susceptible animals. Once the wider range of clinical manifestations was recognized, other serovars were isolated from patients and carrier rodents and were identified, so that by the early 1950s, 45 serovars significant for human leptospirosis and their reservoirs had been identified.

A major discovery was that livestock (pigs, cattle) could be carriers and could excrete large numbers of leptospires in urine. Both primary (rodent–rodent) and secondary (rodent–livestock–rodent) cycles were identified. The range of known serovars continued to expand, mainly following research in tropical countries. Although leptospires could be isolated by culturing blood or urine from patients, evidence of leptospirosis was obtained mainly by serological tests on patients' sera. Most culture media required rabbit serum. The use of bovine albumin and oleic acid or polysorbate-linked fatty acids (Tween) to replace rabbit serum was an important advance, facilitating laboratory cultivation and allowing the easier isolation of serovar *hardjo*, a major cause of human leptospirosis wherever there are dairy cattle. The subtype "hardjoprajitno" was originally isolated from an Indonesian patient, and the subtype "hardjobovis" later, from cattle. The serovar is expressed by several genetic species of *Leptospira*. Antibodies to Hebdomadis-group leptospires were already known to be prevalent in both humans and cattle. Genetic typing of leptospires, first done in the 1960s by DNA–DNA hybridization, was a major step that led much later, in 1994, to formal recognition of genospecies of *Leptospira*.

Vaccines for control of leptospirosis in dogs were introduced in 1939 and in pigs and cattle soon after. These vaccines would also indirectly assist in protecting humans by reducing excretion of leptospires by animals. Further developments in knowledge of microbiology of leptospires and of pathology, pathogenesis, immunity, epidemiology, and control of leptospirosis are reflected in improved laboratory and diagnostic methods during the 1980s. Major improvements in control of the disease have not occurred yet as a result of recent rapid progress in the understanding of immunochemistry and molecular biology of leptospires.[2,4,5]

3. Methodology

Except where doctors are experienced with leptospirosis, the diagnosis usually depends on laboratory confirmatory tests. Laboratory tests may be unavailable or delayed, because the diagnosis is not considered at an early state or because the patient is not seen until late in the illness. Failure to use appropriate laboratory tests at the proper time can lead to misdiagnosis in both suspected and unsuspected patients. Because of diagnostic deficiencies, mortality, morbidity, and incidence data based on unconfirmed diagnoses or confirmed diagnoses of a few selected patients are fallacious, almost without exception.

3.1. Sources of Mortality Data

Death notifications and autopsy reports have been used. Accurate postmortem diagnosis is impossible where autopsies are forbidden by custom or belief. Antemortem diagnosis is required for accurate death notification without an autopsy. Mortality rates may be spuriously high if the diagnosis is made only in advanced cases who are nearly moribund when medical or hospital assistance is sought.

3.2. Sources of Morbidity Data

The World Health Organization (WHO) has recommended that leptospirosis be a notifiable disease. Notification may be based on hospital admissions and diagnosis, discharge data, notification by private or community practitioners, or laboratory notification of infections diagnosed by isolation of leptospires, or on seroconversion, or both. Laboratory notification results in the recording of higher morbidity rates than practitioner notification. This is partly because patients are discharged, or recover, or die before all laboratory results are returned to practitioners, who may then see notification as useless. Follow-up of patient contacts has led to detection of cases, not because of the contagiousness of the disease, but because locally epidemic leptospirosis has been detected as a result of inquiries.

Expression of mortality or morbidity statistics in terms of a total population can give a false index of incidence or prevalence if the disease is not homogeneously distributed in that population, or unless a correction is made for risk of exposure. In a large predominantly urban population, an overall low morbidity rate may mask a very high rate in a selected group of that population, such as sewer workers, abattoir workers, or meat packers. Statistics should be refined and expressed in rates relevant to the size of the population at risk.[1,2]

3.3. Surveys

Serological surveys have been used frequently in studies of leptospirosis. They can be used on unselected populations to see whether leptospirosis exists at all. In such studies it is necessary to use a battery of antigens in agglutination tests to ensure that representative serovars of all serogroups are included. Locally prevalent serovars must be included, if they are known. The initial work load can be reduced by testing against pools of antigens, combining up to five serogroups in one suspension. Reactive sera can be tested against individual serogroups. Broadly cross-reactive antigens have been used in enzyme-linked immunosorbent assays (ELISAs) to detect antibodies to any serovar of pathogenic leptospires. At present, polymerase chain reaction (PCR)-based tests are available in some laboratories, usually for specific diagnostic purposes rather than for surveillance.

Survey information can be used to show which serovars are likely to be prevalent, by analyzing results of tests on batteries of antigens, or by retesting broadly reactive sera against individual serovars. Many sera will react with more than one serovar, however, because several serovars have antigens in common, and the highest titer is not necessarily against the infecting serovar, especially following recent infections. The fact that leptospirosis may not be distributed homogeneously in the population should be borne in mind when planning surveys. The survey should be properly planned to request necessary information such as age, sex, occupation, travel, and previous known leptospirosis or similar undiagnosed illness. Adequate statistical planning beforehand is essential to ensure that an appropriate number of samples are taken in each group and that results can be analyzed by statistical techniques.

Once the presence of leptospirosis is known or detected in a survey, the data may be used to determine the population groups exposed to a risk or risks and once those are delineated, to measure the prevalence of antibodies in one or more selected subgroups. Another important function of surveys is to ascertain prevalence for evaluating control measures, both for a baseline level before their introduction and during and after implementation as part of their evaluation.

Either IgM or IgG or both classes of antibody may be measured in surveys using ELISA with specific antigens or cross-reactive antigens. IgM antibodies usually indicate relatively recent infections. Survey information can be important for interpretation of diagnostic serology in acute cases to establish whether the patient is one of a population or subgroup in which there is a known high prevalence of antibodies.

Serological or bacteriological surveys have proved valuable in investigating an epidemic. Information may be obtained retrospectively from serum bank specimens collected from epidemic patients or from patients and their surrounding population in general concurrently with an epidemic. Apart from epidemics, surveys of serum banks have been used to ascertain overall prevalence rates in certain clinical groups, such as patients with jaundice and fever, undiagnosed aseptic meningitis, or pyrexia of unknown origin.

Prospective surveys offer a better chance of understanding incidence of leptospirosis and prevalence of antibodies in selected groups. These may be carried out on selected groups of hospital admissions or patients in primary health care clinics or practices. A suitable protocol is to carry out diagnostic tests for leptospirosis on all clinically suspected patients. If serology is tested, a matched control series, such as nonfebrile patients, must be included.

3.3.1. Ethics of Surveys. The taking of blood or other specimens solely for investigative rather than diagnostic purposes should be done only with the informed consent of the patient or competent relatives. Where surveys are carried out as part of national or international research programs, it is essential that due regard and respect should be paid to the local customs, traditions, and religious practices of the population and with their cooperation.[1,5]

3.4. Laboratory Diagnosis

In the absence of clear characteristic clinical features, especially in mild leptospirosis, laboratory diagnosis is essential. Its importance cannot be overstated, because it is also the basis of epidemiological statistics and preventive policies and programs. Not only must the diagnosis be established as leptospirosis, but the causal leptospire should be identified, at least by serogroup, preferably also by serovar and genospecies, for prognosis, management, and prevention activities.

3.4.1. Isolation and Identification of Leptospires

3.4.1a. Classification and Nomenclature of Leptospires. All leptospires are similar in appearance and culture. Historically, they were classified into serovars and serogroups by serology using cross-agglutination with rabbit antisera and a microscopic endpoint. All pathogens were grouped in a serologically defined species known for years as "*L. interrogans*," and nonpathogens were similarly grouped as "*L. biflexa*." Now the members of the genus *Leptospira* are classified by genetic relationships into distinct species (genospecies). The species *borgpetersenii*, *inadai*, *interrogans*, *kirschneri*, *santa-*

Table 1. Abridged List of Species, Serogroups, and Main Serovars of Pathogenic Members of the Genus *Leptospira*

Species	Serovar	Serogroup	Serovar	Serogroup
L. borgpetersenii	*anhoa*	Celledoni	*javanica*	Javanica
	arborea	Ballum	*jules*	Hebdomadis
	balcanica	Sejroe	*mini*	Mini
	ballum	Ballum	*sejroe*	Sejroe
	guangdong	Ballum	*whitcombi*	Celledoni
	hardjo (hardjobovis)	Sejroe	*tarassovi*	Tarassovi
L. faineii	*hurstbridge*	Hurstbridge	–	–
L. inadai	*icterohaemorrhagiae*	Icterо[a]	*lyme*	Lyme
L. interrogans	*australis*	Australis	*icterohaemorrhagiae*	Ictero.
	autumnalis	Autumnalis	*kennewicki*	Pomona
	bangkok	Australis	*kremastos*	Pomona
	bataviae	Bataviae	*lora*	Australis
	birkini	Ictero.	*medanensis*	Sejroe
	bratislava	Australis	*mwogolo*	Ictero.
	broomi	Canicola	*naam*	Ictero.
	bulgarica	Autumnalis	*paidjan*	Bataviae
	canicola	Canicola	*pomona*	Pomona
	copenhageni	Ictero.	*pyrogenes*	Pyrogenes
	djasiman	Djasiman	*rachmati*	Autumnalis
	grippotyphosa	Grippotyphosa	*robinsoni*	Pyrogenes
	hardjo	Sejroe	*swazijak*	Mini
	(hardjoprajitno)		*saxkoebing*	Sejroe
	hebdomadis	Hebdomadis	*zanoni*	Pyrogenes
L. kirschneri	*bim*	Autumnalis	*grippotyphosa*	Grippotyphosa
	bulgarica	Autumnalis	*mwogolo*	Ictero.
	butembo	Autumnalis	*mozdok*	Pomona
	cynopteri	Cynopteri	*tsaratsova*	Pomona
L. noguchii	*bajan*	Australis	*meunchen*	Australis
	fortbragg	Autumnalis		
L. santarosai	*bataviae*	Bataviae	*pyrogenes*	Pyrogenes
	borincana	Hebdomadis	*tabaquite*	Mini
	kremastos	Hebdomadis	*trinidad*	Sejroe
	maru	Hebdomadis	*weaveri*	Sarmin
	navet	Tarassovi		
L. weilii	*celledoni*	Celledoni	*mengma*	Javanica
	hainan	Celledoni	*sarmin*	Sarmin
Turneria parva	*parva*	Turneria		
Leptonema illini	*illini*	Leptonema		

[a]Serogroup Icterohaemorrhagiae.

rosai, and *weilii* include almost all the pathogenic leptospires (Table 1). A recently described new serovar *hurstbridge* (serogroup Hurstbridge) belongs to a new species for which the name *L. faineii* was proposed.[6] Genera of *Leptonema* and *Turneria* are recognized, comprising morphologically similar spirochetes. Some strains are not yet classified by genotype. Several strains of leptospires classified serologically by their antigens as members of a single serovar are found to belong to different genospecies; that is, more than one species may express the same serovar-specific antigens (see Section 4).[7–9]

3.4.1b. Culture. Culture media containing long-chain fatty acids such as oleic acid or Tween with 1% bovine serum albumin as a detoxicant are used widely. A common formulation is the Ellinghausen–McCullough–Johnson–Harris (EMJH) medium. It is usually used in liquid form in screw-cap containers. In tubes of semisolid media containing 0.1–0.2% agar, growth occurs in one or more zones situated from just below the surface to deep in the medium. In fluid media, growth from inocula of 1–10% of volume can be seen as a birefringent swirl in 3–20 days, depending on the individual strain. Heavier growth, always less than the turbidity seen in cultures of enteric bacteria, may be encouraged by shaking during incubation. Optimum temperature for the cultivation of laboratory strains is 28–30°C. Most strains grow poorly if at all at 37°C.

Cultures of properly collected clinical material cultured shortly after collection are highly sensitive and capable of detecting very small numbers of leptospires in from 2 or 3 days to several weeks. Cultures should be examined at least weekly and incubated for 4 weeks to 2 to 3 months.

3.4.1c. Specimens for Culture (see Section 8.2.2b). Blood cultures taken during the first few days (up to 10 days, especially in the first week) during the fever are frequently positive. Addition of a sulfathiazole–neomycin–cycloheximide mixture has been recommended to reduce risks of overgrowth by bacteria from contaminated specimens; however, subculture after a day or two into medium without antibiotic is advisable. Special culture media are available for isolating fastidious leptospires currently found mainly in veterinary practice.[10,11]

Cultures may also be taken from cerebrospinal fluid (CSF), urine, and tissue samples, including autopsy specimens (see Section 8.2.2b). The antibiotic medium above or a selective medium comprising EMJH with 100 μg/ml of 5-fluorouracil is useful for tissues.

3.4.1d. Microscopy and Examination of Cultures. Microscopy by an experienced person is used to recognize leptospires directly in clinical or pathological specimens and in cultures from them. Leptospires may be seen readily by dark-field microscopy in thin preparations or in direct examination of clinical specimens. Leptospires appear as motile, bright, beaded, rotating, thin rods, usually with one or both ends curved, against a black background. Phase-contrast microscopy is of limited value in diagnostic work because of its strict optical requirements.

3.4.1e. Staining. Leptospires are poorly stained by conventional microscopic stains. They may be visualized by Giemsa or silver deposition methods. Silver deposition by one of several methods can be used for tissue sections, but flawless technique is required to obtain clean interpretable results. Immunologic stains such as immunofluorescence and immunoperoxidase provide a valuable alternative to direct staining methods. Indirect (antiglobulin) labeled antisera are more practical than direct coupled antisera. Good fluorescence technique will allow the detection of small numbers of approximately 10^3–10^4 leptospires/ml specimen. A major disadvantage of all immunostains is the need for specific antiserum. Although the aim of this test is to seek and allow the recognition of leptospires in the specimen, it cannot work if the test antiserum does not match the serovar (or at least serogroup) antigens of the leptospires in the specimen (see Section 3.4.1f). A secondary result is that a positive reaction also serves to identify at least broadly the serovar or serogroup of the fluorescing leptospires. A battery of antisera may be required if the serovar is unknown or unsuspected. In extreme cases, where the infection is due to a new serovar, only convalescent patients' sera can be used as a source of the primary antibody for the test until the new organism has been isolated and immune sera prepared from it. Results of direct microscopy or immunostaining can be obtained in minutes to a few hours.

3.4.1f. Serological Typing. If a leptospire is isolated, it must be identified by agglutination to titer with reference antisera or serogroup- and serovar-specific monoclonal antibodies. These identification procedures are usually performed only in reference laboratories. A list of serogroups recognized currently, with their type serovars and the major serovars in the serogroup, is provided in Table 1. Full lists have been published.[2,12,13]

Monoclonal murine antibodies have been described, with specificities ranging from broad across all pathogenic species, to narrowly reactive with members of particular serogroups, to highly specific to epitopes characteristic of a single serovar. Some of the specific monoclonal antibodies agglutinate leptospires, indicating reaction with a surface epitope. Less serospecific monoclonal antibodies tend to react only with physically, enzymatically, or chemically disrupted leptospires in ELISA. Monoclonal antibodies are obviously useful in allowing rapid presumptive identification of leptospires without the tedium of agglutination and absorption methods. Batteries of selected standardized monoclonal antibodies* can be used for rapid serological identification.

3.4.1g. PCR, Gene Probes, and Other Methods. Gene probes used with PCR are capable of detecting about 10–10^3 leptospires in diagnostic specimens. They are being introduced for primary diagnosis in acute illness and for rapidly identifying leptospires in cultured isolates.[14–17]

Alternative nonserological and molecular methods based on analysis and comparison of restriction fragment length polymorphism (RFLP) and on pulsed field gel electrophoresis of digests also have been used for the characterization and identification of strains of leptospires.[18] Methods for differentiating *L. biflexa* from pathogenic species of leptospires are described in Section 4.

*Availabile from the Leptospirosis Laboratory, Laboratory of Tropical Hygiene, Royal Tropical Institute, Meiberqdreet 39, Amsterdam 20, The Netherlands 1105 AZ.

3.4.2. Serological Methods. Antibodies in sera from patients or survey subjects can be detected and measured directly by agglutination of leptospires or by ELISA (see Section 3.4.2b). Tests used for diagnoses of acutely ill patients need to be specific and performed rapidly if they are to aid in management and prognosis, as well as for detection of sources common to several patients and for prevention. For epidemiological and survey purposes, there is less urgency for obtaining test results, but laboratories should be able to test large numbers of sera rapidly if necessary. Usually, knowledge of the serovar specificity of reacting antibodies is required, especially where several serovars are endemic, each with a different reservoir and pattern of transmission.

Almost all laboratories use the microscopic agglutination test (MAT) as their standard test, although some use ELISA. Agglutination tests are definitive but need specially trained staff and special reagents. Molecular tests are potentially faster, automated, and generally available in laboratories equipped for molecular microbiological diagnosis.

Two milliliters of serum are usually necessary for serological studies. If venous blood is unavailable, capillary blood from an ear, finger, or heel prick may be soaked up on a standard square of absorbent (blotting or filter) paper and allowed to dry. An approximately 1-cm square will hold about 0.1 ml of blood. The paper is eluted in 0.5 ml of saline. The eluate is treated as a nominal dilution of 1:10 of serum for subsequent dilutions, and hemolysis is disregarded. For diagnostic purposes, any blood specimen for serology should be taken as soon as possible in the illness. It should be followed by two further specimens at intervals of 5 days, to look for a rising titer of antibodies, but the first sample should be tested at once without waiting for a paired sample. Occasionally, late seroconversion has been reported. In clinically characteristic cases, where no other diagnosis is confirmed and seroconversion has not occurred in 15 days, another specimen may be taken after 30 days. Serum may be frozen during transport and storage. Only one specimen is required for epidemiological and prevalence surveys.

3.2.4a. Agglutination Tests. The principle of all agglutination tests is that leptospires are agglutinated by serum antibodies. There are two types of agglutination tests: macroscopic and microscopic (MAT). Macroscopic agglutination tests may be performed on a microscope slide, a tile, or in a tube. The test is at best semiquantitative, but it is useful for rapid screening to detect high levels of antibody. It is significantly less sensitive than microscopic or tube agglutination and also less serovar specific because of the greater chance of recording cross-agglutinations. A macroscopic tube agglutination test is sometimes used because its endpoint is read easily by the naked eye. Titers are generally lower than for a corresponding MAT, and the test is less sensitive than MAT but more sensitive than slide agglutination. A positive reaction is taken as agglutination at a dilution of 1:80 or higher.

MAT remains the basic reference test in leptospirosis.[1,2,5] It is extremely sensitive because the endpoint is read microscopically under dark field. The use of live, late-log-phase cultures standardized to 5×10^7 to 10^8 leptospires/ml is recommended, but formalin-killed suspensions may be used where lower sensitivity can be tolerated and in small laboratories or in tropical countries where local production of cultures, transport, and storage free of contamination are problems. They are also safer to handle in the laboratory.

Tests should always be quality controlled by including sera of known high and low specific reactivity as controls. The authenticity of strains used in antigen suspensions should be checked periodically against reference antisera.

Serologically authenticated, local, recently isolated strains should be chosen, but usually standard reference strains obtained from a reference laboratory are used because of their known antigenic composition. Sera generally react specifically with the infecting serovar, but cross-reactions with other serovars are well known, especially early in infection. The highest titer is sometimes recorded against a cross-reacting serovar. Where several serovars from different serogroups are prevalent locally, there is a need to test each patient's serum against each of them or at least against a representative serovar of each serogroup. This means that in many tropical areas or where the likely infecting serovar is unknown, a battery of up to 30 serovars may be used for each serum. The battery may comprise pools of antigens or simply two or three serovars where there is a strong likelihood that no others are present. The same considerations apply in epidemiological prevalence surveys. There is no satisfactory single group antigen with which all patients' sera will react.

Interpretation of MAT depends on the stage of illness, the serovar, and local epidemiology. In an acute infection, a single low titer of under 200 where there is a high prevalence of antibodies to one or more serovars of leptospires may be unrelated to current illness. A rising titer commencing under 400 and either rising fourfold within 1 or 2 weeks, or reaching 400 to 800, is highly suspicious. For diagnostic purposes, an initial low titer of 50 (or 40 depending on the dilution system) in a new patient in a nonendemic area may indicate to clinicians that the patient has leptospirosis. Titers may rise significantly on repeat testing 5 to 7 days later. The early low titer is thus diagnostically useful. Some patients fail to seroconvert for several weeks. In such cases, the positive diagnosis depends solely on culture of the leptospire.

In epidemiological surveys, titers as low as 10 are significant, indicating previous exposure or infection with a leptospire. It is not known for certain how long antibodies persist following clinical or subclinical infection in humans.

MAT is rapid, specific, and sensitive, but it has important disadvantages: subjective endpoint, extreme tedium, and labor-intensive testing leading to observer error and fatigue following prolonged reading of tests; danger due to the use of live cultures; and potential for error if the correct serovars are not chosen. Direct measurement of specific IgM or IgG in MAT is not feasible.

3.4.2b. Enzyme Immunoassay (ELISA). The main advantages of ELISA (including immunoblots) are precision, objectivity, and instrumentation; adaptability for screening large numbers of sera; cost; and ability to measure specific IgM, IgG, or other immunoglobulin classes, which is especially valuable in diagnosing congenital or early infection. Antigens used in diagnosis and epidemiology have been a broadly species-reactive preparation of boiled, formalin-killed leptospiral culture or a sonicated leptospiral suspension.[19,20] Leptospiral polysaccharides and lipopolysaccharide preparations have been used experimentally. ELISA tests do not measure the same antibodies as those in agglutination, so there is little correspondence between the optical densities or titers in ELISA and the agglutinating titer in MAT. In pigs and cattle, blood levels of IgM reacting in ELISA have been correlated with renal excretion of leptospires. A recently developed solid-phase ELISA test for diagnosis gave acceptable results when tested internationally.[21]

4. Biological Characteristics of the Organism

4.1. Morphology

Leptospires are thin, helical, motile, gram-negative bacteria. They are so thin that they can be seen by transmitted light microscopy only with difficulty after staining or by deposition of Giemsa stain or silver to make them thick enough to see. They can be seen unstained by phase-contrast or dark-field illumination. The standard method of observation is by dark-field microscopy of a wet preparation on a thin microscope slide under a thin coverslip. Leptospires seen this way rotate rapidly around their long axis and are translationally motile in either direction. One or both ends are usually hooked, imparting a looped appearance to the end of the leptospire when it rotates rapidly. Straight-ended variants occur and are much less translationally motile. In semisolid agar media, leptospires move like a flexible screw between invisible particles. Within limits of variability for any serovar, all serovars appear the same morphologically.

When seen by electron microscopy, leptospires are made up of a helically wound, protoplasmic cylinder incorporating the cellular contents, surrounded by a cell wall around which a three- or five-layer membrane may be visualized, depending on the methods of preparation and fixation. The whole is enclosed in a trilaminar outer envelope that is easily washed off or damaged in preparation. The cytoplasmic cylinder has a diameter of approximately 0.1 μm and an amplitude of winding of approximately 0.2 μm. Leptospires vary in length from approximately 5 μm after division to more than 20 μm according to age, strain, and culture conditions. The outer envelope is an important source of antigens for immunization and the study of immunity.

A single flagellum, previously called an "axial filament," is attached close to each end of the leptospire by a characteristic gram-negative-type insertion structure. The flagellum has motor functions and runs down the center of the helix applied to the protoplasmic cylinder and surrounded by outer envelope. In purified preparations, flagella appear to be composed of strands of protein surrounded by a sheath for part of their length. They contain characteristic antigens. Microfibrils arising from the cell wall have been described. A variable but relatively high lipid content, including unusual long-chained fatty acids, is a characteristic of the genus *Leptospira*.

4.2. Physiology and Growth

All members of the genus *Leptospira* are obligate aerobes or microaerophiles with the requisite enzymes for aerobic metabolism. Growth may be accelerated and increased substantially in amount by aeration. Anaerobic growth has not been reported. In general, pathogenic serovars are inhibited by 8-azaguanine and cannot grow at temperatures below 13–15°C in EMJH medium, in contrast to nonpathogenic *L. biflexa*. Leptospires are easily killed by drying; heating above 42–45°C for a few minutes; acid conditions below pH 7.0; alkaline conditions above approximately pH 7.8; and disinfectants such as phenolics, quaternary ammonium derivatives, halogens, and aldehydes (formaldehyde, glutaraldehyde). They may be preserved in media containing protein at −70°C or in liquid nitrogen.

The essential requirements for growth of pathogenic leptospires are ammonium ions as a nitrogen source, long-chained fatty acids as a carbon and energy source, and thiamine and cyanocobalamin. There appear to be no major differences in requirements among members of the species. Pyrimidines are not required and carbohydrates are not fermented. A detoxicant, usually 1% bovine serum albumin or whole rabbit serum, is required to bind and detoxify the fatty acids and release them slowly. The optimum pH for growth is in the range 7.2 to 7.8 and the optimum temperature range is 28 to 30°C. Large inocula of up to 10% of culture volume are used routinely to initiate growth.[(2)]

4.3. Biochemical and Genetic Composition

Molecular studies have shown that leptospires have lipopolysaccharide (LPS) similar in structure to but less toxic than that of some other gram-negative bacteria (*Salmonella*, *Shigella*).[(22–26)] They contain a GroE-type heat-shock protein, Ompl porin proteins, and numerous enzymes, including sphingomyelinases, which have been cloned and studied.[(27–31)] The leptospiral genome comprises two genetic elements—one of them 460 kilobase pairs (kbp) and the other 0.35 kbp—and an IS-3-like insertion sequence element.[(32–36)] A bacteriophage specific for nonpathogenic *L. biflexa* was found, but no mechanisms for genetic transfer are known in pathogenic leptospires.[(37)] Several genes have been cloned and characterized. Leptospires have a unique genomic organization, including modification at 5′GTAC and an unusual codon usage.[(38–40)] Isolates of *L. interrogans*, *sensu latu*, have guanosine plus cytosine ratios in the range of 33 to 42 mole% GC.

4.4. Antigens

Surface antigens, probably polysaccharides, allow the separation of leptospires into serum-sensitive and serum-resistant groups correlating with avirulence and virulence for experimental animals, respectively. Antigens on the leptospiral surface are involved in agglutination. Agglutination results from interaction of surface LPS antigens whose determinants and reactive epitopes are polysaccharides or oligosaccharides. Serovar specificity is a property of LPS oligosaccharides and/or glycolipids.[(24–26,41)] Leptospiral LPS has many properties similar to those of other gram-negative bacteria, but it has some significant differences, notably much less pyrogenicity and toxicity, an unknown link sugar that in some serovars only partly resembles ketodeoxyoctonate (KDO), and phosphate-linked sugars and amino sugars. Other characteristic antigens are found in flagella, in a glycolipoprotein highly toxic for tissue-cultured cells and experimental animals, and in a range of protein antigens of undetermined significance.[(22,23,42)] In addition to their toxic and invasive properties, leptospires are able to adhere to cultured tissue cells by an attachment ligand. In experimental studies, virulent leptospires were able to attach to the cellular cytoskeleton while avirulent ones were not. Attachment properties have obvious importance for our understanding of the renal carrier state.[(43–46)]

4.5. Other Properties

A wide range of antibiotics is effective against leptospires in the laboratory, although penicillin, erythromycin, and doxycycline are recommended therapeutic antibiotics, with doxycycline recommended for chemoprophylaxis. It is relatively easy to select streptomycin-resistant leptospires in the laboratory following incubation with high concentrations of streptomycin.[(47)] Strains resistant to antibiotics have not been reported clinically, although antibiotics (especially penicillin) are used widely in treatment.

Leptospires may persist in body tissues following infection (see Section 7.3.7) in the presence of antibodies. Little is known of the properties of the leptospires or the immunologic mechanisms that allow them to live and grow in sequestered sites such as the anterior chamber of the eye, the proximal renal tubules, the genital tracts of carrier animals, and possibly in the brain of rodents.[(48)]

5. Descriptive Epidemiology

5.1. Prevalence and Incidence

Statistics of prevalence and incidence are influenced frequently by the lack of reliability in diagnosis and by failure to recognize the selective risk to population groups. Prevalence figures derived from planned surveys are much more reliable than those based on hospital records or disease notifications (see Section 3.3). Antibody prevalence rates to local serovars in tropical countries with large feral and peridomiciliary rodent populations are higher, often up to 80–90% of the population, than in temperate climates where leptospirosis tends to be more occupationally segregated. In surveys of dairy farming populations in the state of Victoria in southeastern Australia, antibodies to serovar *hardjo* are present in about 25% or 25,000 per 100,000 of the population and almost zero in the rest of the community. It is estimated that dairy farmers and meat workers comprise no more than 20,000 or 1/200th of the 4 million residents of the state, so an overall statistic of 125 per 100,000 would be quite erroneous if extrapolated to the whole population, as would be the almost zero figure for the urban population extrapolated to rural areas. Similarly, notifications of approximately 100 cases per year of leptospires among farmers and meat workers result in an incidence rate of 2.5 per 100,000 in the whole population of 4 million but in a much more significant rate of 500 per 100,000 among the 20,000 in the population at risk. These high rates reflect a high prevalence of antibodies, up to 85% in dairy cattle, a level comparable with that in countries with environments as diverse as Australia, the Netherlands, and the Congo.

Reported statistics are also influenced by technical factors such as the starting dilution for sera, the interpretation of low titers, and the techniques used for serology. These factors are often not clear from reports. When using prevalence statistics for epidemiological and control policy planning, it should be noted that the duration of persistence of antibodies after infection is variable. It ranged from within 1 year, through a median between 3 and 6 years, to indefinite in some patients in a study where the seroconversion rate in the population was about 4% annually. In another study, where the seroconversion rate was 11%, the rate of fall of titer was 10–16%.[49]

Second infections with a different serovar have been reported, indicating that there is little immunity between serogroups. Very rare reports of second infections with the same serovar are poorly documented.

In the United States, fewer than 100 cases of leptospirosis are reported each year, representing an incidence of about 0.05 cases per 100,000 population, with an overall case fatality rate of 5–7%. Cases occur throughout the country, but they are most common in the South Atlantic, Gulf, and Pacific coastal states. Hawaii reported the highest annual incidence (10–12 cases per 100,000 during 1971–1990 in Hawaii and Kauai Islands), reflecting assiduous searching, education of medical personnel, and knowledgeable diagnosis.[50] Leptospirosis is predominantly a disease of males (80% of cases) between the ages of 10 and 59 years (76% of cases). The importance of leptospirosis in children is becoming clearer. The case-fatality rate was age-dependent, averaging 2.9% from 1% under 40 years to 29% over 70 years.

In contrast to other countries, slightly fewer than half of US cases are occupation-associated. Patients usually have a history of exposure to animals, mud, or fresh water. Cases occur with a distinct seasonal predominance from July through October. In descending order of frequency, infections by members of the Icterohaemorrhagiae, Canicola, Autumnalis, Grippotyphosa, Hebdomadis, Australis, Pomona, and Ballum serogroups are most commonly recognized.

5.2. Epidemic Behavior and Contagiousness

Leptospirosis is considered to be of a low order of contagiousness, because spread from human to human is almost unknown and direct inoculation into the body via skin, mucosal, or conjunctival penetration is required for infection. Laboratory infections, a significant occupational problem, have occurred after inoculation into the eye or through the skin. In natural infections an animal source of infection is required, except for transplacental infection. Animal urine is the most important vehicle of infection for man. Direct contact with infected animals also is an important method of transmission.[2]

Epidemics have occurred apart from sporadic endemic zoonotic infections. The precipitating factors in epidemics have been large buildups of carrier animal populations, together with an increase in direct or indirect contact between the animals and humans at risk.[51] Examples of major epidemics include an outbreak of primarily nonicteric leptospirosis characterized by severe pulmonary hemorrhages in Korea in 1984, associated with rice harvesting following a heavy storm. Urine from a large field rodent population, attracted by the crop, contributed to heavy contamination of the rice fields and exposure of harvesters, including many emergency workers who presumably had little if any immunity. Epidemics of leptospirosis following floods and earthquakes are well documented in China, Brazil, and elsewhere. An epidemic of severe-type nonicteric leptospirosis occurred in Nicaragua in October 1995, following extremely heavy rainfall. Clinically, patients presented with fever, headaches, chills, and muscle pains, but the precipitating cause of death was a dramatic massive sudden pulmonary hemorrhage reminiscent of epidemics in Korea and China due to serovar *lai*. More than 2,200 cases, 200 of them hospitalized, were reported in an affected population of about 37,000 (approx. 61 cases per 1,000). The mortality rate was 0.7%. Contrary to the experience with some other epidemics, the highest age-specific incidence (approx. 80 per 1000) occurred in the 1- to 14-year-old age group, while 40 per 1,000 of children under 1 year were affected (see Section 5.5). The serovars isolated were *canicola* and *pyrogenes*. The animal sources were presumed to be dogs, mice, and pigs. Point-source outbreaks have occurred in recent years during military operations and leisure activities such as kayaking, rafting, and hiking, where groups have been exposed simultaneously, and among children or young people bathing in polluted fresh water swimming holes.[52–56] The usual situation in tropical countries and among occupationally exposed risk groups in temperate climates is that sporadic cases occur according to seasonal and other factors. Precipitating factors are wet conditions, buildup of rodent populations, or seasonal occupational conditions. Even where occupation appears to be irrelevant, there is invariably a history of some contact with animals, as in hunting, domestic slaughter of livestock, rat catching, swimming, boating, or cleaning drains or sewers.[57]

Although leptospirosis is solely a zoonosis, human social factors are most important in epidemiology. The way people live, their housing, transport, food, livestock and domestic animals, and social and religious customs will all contribute positively or negatively to their risks of leptospirosis (see Section 5.10).

5.3. Geographical Distribution

Leptospirosis is distributed worldwide. In recent years the most severe clinical forms transmitted via rodent reservoirs have been more commonly diagnosed and reported in tropical rural areas and urban areas lacking good rodent control. The anicteric form is the most prevalent. In temperate climates the pattern tends to be less severe types carried by serovars indigenous to dogs, livestock, or field mice rather than domestic rats, reflecting as much the influence of social factors and efficacy of rodent control as a direct geographic effect. There is a direct relationship with soil and geologic environment, which can affect the ability of leptospires to survive in surface waters and mud and soil through their effects on acidity and porosity. Changes to the environment caused by human activities and subsequent changes in the patterns of human life have potential for profound influence on leptospirosis.[58,59] Draining of swamps and waterway control can obviously create drier conditions. Irrigation and dams can convert desert or dry lands to fertile territories into which animals and birds migrate as the environment changes. The increased food available, moist ground conditions, and ground cover for rodents protecting them from predators create new ecological conditions in which resident fauna can change quite rapidly. With these changes come increased risks to humans whose activities take them into the new wet environments.

5.4. Temporal Distribution

The worldwide experience is that leptospirosis is related to wet periods of the year. The wet seasons, whether monsoon, floods, or spring and summer, are associated with surface conditions favoring leptospirosis in all parts of the world. In temperate climates the risks increase with fresh spring and summer growth of pastures. Risks also increase for harvest workers for many crops but not wheat and corn. Well-documented epidemics have been recorded during rice, sugarcane, and pea harvests. In dairy herds, leptospirosis is seasonal, because young cows are introduced to milking in the spring. It is not clear how the increased incidence of human leptospirosis in milkers in the spring is affected by wet conditions.

5.5. Age

Although leptospiral antibodies can be found in people of all ages, the predominant incidence of acute infection is found in the 20- to 50-year age range, though in developing countries more cases may be seen in younger people. Pediatric and congenital infections have been described. The age distribution reflects the relative amount of environmental exposure to risk factors in the age groups concerned.[54,60]

5.6. Sex

Although some workers have concluded that males and females are equally affected for equivalent risks of exposure, there are contrary facts that the rate in women was considerably lower than in men among women engaged in milking cows in conditions comparable with those for men. The explanation offered is that the women were more careful about personal occupational hygiene. The overall predominance of males in statistics reflects the sex distribution within the occupational or residential populations under review.

5.7. Race

There is no evidence for any risk factors determined by race. Some statistics showing racial tendencies toward or against leptospirosis can be explained by social or occupational factors affecting the chances of exposure to risk. Nothing is known about genetic determinants of susceptibility or resistance to leptospirosis in humans.

5.8. Occupation

There is a strong occupational trend in all areas. Even in tropical climates, those whose jobs bring them into indirect contact with animals via rodent urine contamination in such activities as rice planting and harvesting, fish farming, forestry, mining, boating, and military exercises are at special risk. In addition, those in all climates exposed to urine contamination directly or indirectly from livestock and domestic dogs and rodents have a greater risk and increased incidence of infection. Prevalence rates for antibodies to serovar *hardjo* in dairy farmers may be as high as 25%, or 25,000 per 100,000, matched by comparable rates in slaughtermen. In each case the proved infection rate is also high.[(49)]

Occupational hazards involve special considerations of workers' compensation and preventive measures to protect workers (see Section 9.1). In turn, these create special social needs and expenses for the workers and the industries involved.

5.9. Occurrence in Different Settings

Leptospirosis poses a special problem in military or civilian emergencies. Rodent infestation may increase and with it risks to humans from leptospirosis as well as other zoonoses. Military, paramilitary, police, or civilian emergency workers may be forced into conditions such as floods and destroyed buildings that house rodents. Frequently, troops have been exposed to leptospirosis in rat-infested trench warfare or in jungle warfare or exercises.

Modern leisure activities have attracted city dwellers to rural settings, sometimes in faraway lands, in search of adventures in canoeing, rafting, caving, and climbing. The risks of contracting leptospirosis on these vacations need to be emphasized.[(57,61)]

5.10. Socioeconomic Factors

Social class is no barrier to leptospirosis. The only requirement is contact with infected animal urine or animals. Nevertheless, there are social groups whose occupations are more likely to expose them to these risks than others.

An important socioeconomic consideration, however, is the effect of leptospirosis on productivity of animals used for food or burden. Leptospirosis can cause abortions, stillbirths, failure to thrive, retarded growth, milk failure or spoilage for human consumption, and loss of productivity in meat animals among livestock. These effects can in themselves place an additional burden of malnutrition on people already threatened by the risk of illness.

It is difficult to calculate the costs of the effects of leptospirosis as a cause of community or individual ill health. Some of the factors to be considered are the costs of labor to replace sick workers; the cost to the self-employed or peasant farmer or villager in money to replace his own inability to produce food for his family, and in pain and sometimes chronic illness; costs of medical attention including hospital and medical services; and costs in insurance for lost work, production, and workers' compensation. The first requirement is adequate diagnosis so that the actual impact of the disease can be assessed. However, costs of special diagnostic facilities and surveillance for leptospirosis are hard to justify if there is an impression that the disease is rare or absent, so that the circular logic leads to continued underdiagnosis and underreporting. Existing mild illnesses have frequently and easily been attributed to numerous other causes, including "influenza" or "viral infections," but may well be leptospirosis.

6. Mechanisms and Routes of Transmission

Leptospirosis is transmitted primarily from its animal host reservoirs by urine. Urine from carrier animals, also sometimes called excretors or shedders, may contain undetectably small numbers of leptospires or as many as about 10^9/ml urine intermittently in the same animal. The reasons for the variable output are not known. Urine from carriers frequently contains antibodies to the homologous serovar of leptospires. Carrier animals may shed leptospires constantly or intermittently for short periods or for all of their lives. The intermittent shedding, the difficulties of detecting small numbers of urinary leptospires in livestock, and the potentially enormous load of leptospires excreted into the surface water and soil environment from heavy feral rodent environmental contamination are the main sources of difficulties in control in different situations.[(62,63)]

Pathogenic leptospires can survive free in the environment, depending on soil type and geologic factors in moist conditions such as in soil, mud, swamps, drains, surface waters, streams, and rivers, as long as conditions are not acid. All of these sites are well known as sources of leptospirosis. The leptospires can infect fresh host animals or humans by penetrating sodden or broken skin or mucosal surfaces. It is not clear whether pathogenic leptospires multiply in these inanimate environments, but credible nutritional models have been described.

Food preparation areas can be contaminated by infectious urine from foraging carrier rodents, resulting in infections in food process workers. Urine splash and aerosols can infect milkers (especially in "herringbone"-pattern milking sheds), veterinarians, and animal handlers.

Animal tissues and blood are infrequently causes of leptospirosis, often in workers, inspectors, and transporters of meat. Conception products and autopsy of infected livestock and separated kidneys used for domestic food can transmit leptospirosis to veterinarians, farmers, laboratory workers, and housewives.[64] In a bizarre episode, a medical practitioner farmer who resuscitated newborn anemic piglets by mouth-to-mouth resuscitation developed leptospirosis.[65]

Human-to-human transmission is virtually unknown, apart from *in utero* congenital infection.[66–68]

Laboratory-acquired infections usually have resulted from accidents involving direct skin penetration with cultures or suspensions of infected tissues via syringe and needle, broken glass, or splash into an unprotected eye, and from being bitten by infected animals whose urine contaminated the bite. Rat-bite leptospirosis is rare.[69,70]

Leptospires die rapidly when dry. Drying out of surfaces or environments contaminated by infective material prevents spread, even after rehydration. Heating above about 42°C is lethal to leptospires, but they survive freezing.

Spread of leptospirosis is not known to occur by airborne, respiratory, or gastrointestinal routes. Genital infection and venereal transmission occur in livestock.

7. Pathogenesis and Immunity

7.1. Incubation Period

The incubation period of leptospirosis varies from 2 to 21 days, usually between 3 and 10 days, although longer periods have been reported. It is relatively shorter with larger infective doses or more virulent leptospires. Incubation periods can be calculated from a recognized infection episode, but they are difficult to define when there is continual or repeated exposure.[71,72] The relatively sudden onset makes it easier to detect the first clinical symptoms unless they are very mild or unnoticed. In these cases the incubation period may be erroneously dated to the onset of late presenting symptoms such as hemorrhage, meningitis, or renal failure.

7.2. Virulence and Its Attributes

After they penetrate the integument, leptospires must spread, evade body defenses, grow, and produce pathological changes in tissues. In animals destined to become carriers, leptospires must also take up renal tubular residence. The combination of these attributes contributes to the property of pathogenicity, which is the genetically endowed potential for evading and overcoming the resistance of the host and producing lesions or death. Virulence of a defined strain may be measured by the size of the dose or the time taken to produce a lesion or death in a carefully standardized test system. It is difficult to assess accurately in a clinical or epidemiological environment where one or more of the components of virulence, such as surface antigens or toxins, may operate simultaneously in patients or animal reservoir hosts possessing various degrees of natural or acquired immunity. Some serovars, such as *icterohaemorrhagiae*, *copenhageni*, and *bataviae*, typically produce a more severe clinical picture that resembles classical Weil's disease (jaundice, hemorrhages, renal failure) than do other serovars such as *canicola*, *grippotyphosa*, or *hardjo*.

The ability to produce lesions following experimental inoculation into animals is gradually lost on cultivation of leptospires in the laboratory following isolation from patient or animal tissues. This loss of virulence results from the gradual replacement of the population of leptospires in culture by leptospires better able to grow in laboratory media but less able to damage host tissues. The less virulent organisms in culture presumably arise from spontaneous mutants selected by cultural conditions. Frequently the less virulent forms are straight rather than hooked, less translationally motile, and grow in dense small colonies in agar media. Loss of virulence is accompanied by an increase in susceptibility to killing by naturally occurring innate serum IgM antibody acting on a surface polysaccharide antigen. Nonpathogenic *L. biflexa* are killed by a similar serum leptospiricidal mechanism. Thus, an initial component of virulence—the ability to resist serum killing—is associated with a surface polysaccharide antigen. A virulence-associated protein antigen has been described.[45] Virulence is regained in a single animal passage of a culture, as a result of selection in the host of those members of the inoculated population able to evade leptospiricidal defenses and survive and grow *in vivo*.[73]

There is no information about virulence plasmids or any other mechanism of genetic control of virulence attributes.

7.3. The Course of Events in Infection

7.3.1. Entry. Leptospires gain entry through small abrasions or cuts in the skin or mucosal surfaces. Immersion in water can soften skin to facilitate cutaneous damage. Entry may occur via the conjunctiva or by aerosol into the lungs, as well as by inhalation following immersion in contaminated water. Ingestion into an intact alimentary tract, except for the oral cavity, is not a recognized route of entry. Laboratory infections have occurred through injections, needle-stick injuries and cuts, and eye-splash accidents.

7.3.2. Spread. Leptospires that enter the body spread at once in the lymphatics and bloodstream. There is no initial localizing acute inflammation at the site of entry in natural infection or in models using doses resembling those found in nature, although small abscesses may be produced by local injection of extremely large numbers (e.g., 10^{10} or more) of leptospires intradermally. Leptospires can be found distributed in various tissues within 2 hr of infection. Nonpathogenic leptospires (*L. biflexa*) and avirulent strains of the pathogenic species of *Leptospira* are opsonized by innate serum IgM. All leptospires may be opsonized by specific immune IgM or IgG in hosts previously immunized by infection or vaccination. Phagocytosis occurs rapidly in reticuloendothelial fixed phagocytes in the liver (Kupffer cells) and lung. These phagocytes later migrate to the spleen. The bloodstream is cleared rapidly following opsonization, which may occur with minimal detectable levels of immunoglobulin recognized as agglutinating antibody at titers as low as 2. Polymorphonuclear and mononuclear phagocytes can be observed to take up leptospires from the tissues following the development of antibody.

In the absence of immunity and consequent phagocytosis, leptospires grow in the body in an initial infection as if in culture. Nothing is known of specific nutritional requirements *in vivo*. Both virulent and avirulent leptospires have been shown to adhere to fibroblast-derived cells in the laboratory.[43,44,74]

A threshold level of leptospires is required before lesions occur. The time to reach this level (the incubation period) depends on the number of leptospires in the infecting dose, their rate of growth (possibly related to the fever), the state of the patient's immunity, or the host animal's immunity and genetic makeup. The first and most important lesions to be detected are in small blood vessels throughout the body. Localized endothelial cell degeneration occurs, followed by small localized extravasations that frequently contain leptospires.[73]

Fever occurs at an early stage of infection. It is presumably mediated by pyrogenic toxins released by leptospires following phagocytosis as well as by nonspecific factors associated with all infections. At this stage it is also possible to demonstrate microscopic focal degeneration of skeletal muscle fibers, notably in the calf muscles. The extreme pain in muscles and acute tenderness found clinically are presumably the result of these lesions. Thus, the main presenting symptoms of severe headache, fever, and muscle pains can be attributed to the effects of leptospires growing in the body to threshold levels sufficient to cause characteristic damage to small blood vessels.

The natural history of the further development of leptospirosis in either humans or animals is similar. Exponentially increasing numbers of leptospires lead to severe blood vessel damage, local ischemia, and small hemorrhages in most tissues, and eventually to major organ damage. Depending on the serovar of leptospire, there is greater or lesser hepatocellular degeneration, leading to jaundice; renal tubular degeneration similar to that seen in crush injuries or after renal ischemias, leading to an acute, often hemorrhagic interstitial nephritis; and pulmonary hemorrhages ranging from insignificant to gross and fatal, with hemoptysis. Cholecystitis, symptoms of acute abdominal emergency, meningitis, hemiparesis, myocarditis, adrenal hemorrhage, and placentitis have all been reported. Clearly, there is no single pathognomonic lesion or clinical feature, although typical combinations of lesions with symptoms, associated with particular serovars of leptospires, occur in particular regions and epidemiological circumstances, as in classical severe Weil's disease or the relatively mild serovar *hardjo* infections of dairy farmers.

7.3.3. Lesions. Once the infection is fully developed, the typical lesions described in clinical–pathological and postmortem studies of leptospirosis, usually of the severe and fatal types, appear. Hemorrhage is associated with a sudden drop in platelet numbers, possibly as a result of leptospiral toxin action or of adhesion of leptospires. The role of disseminated intravascular coagulopathy (DIC) syndrome is not clear. Anemia is common, not usually solely as a result of hemorrhage. Evidence of nitrogen retention is found almost universally, albeit transitorily, reflecting the renal ischemia occurring even in mild types of leptospirosis. In these cases, patients whose kidneys are functioning poorly and at the limit of compensation due to other causes of renal insufficiency may be precipitated rapidly into renal failure. In severe cases there is very widespread tubular degeneration, which is the usual main cause of death. Other potentially fatal lesions include hepatocellular degeneration, pulmonary hemorrhages, and myocarditis.[75–78]

7.3.4. Transplacental Spread. Transplacental infection can occur at any stage of leptospirosis. If the fetus or placenta is severely damaged, abortion will occur. Stillbirth or congenital leptospirosis may follow infection late in pregnancy. Abortion is a well-documented cause of loss of productivity of livestock. In human congenital infection, IgM antibodies can be demonstrated in the fetus and cord blood and leptospires in the degenerative lesions in tissues.[2]

7.3.5. Recovery. Recovery from leptospirosis commences as soon as the patient produces opsonizing antibody, which leads to rapid phagocytosis of leptospires in the circulation and in the tissues. Mopping up phagocytosis also follows destruction of leptospires by antibiotics. Opsonizing antibody levels can be correlated with agglutinating antibody levels. Virtually any detectable specific agglutinating antibody in MAT can signify opsonic activity. Bacteriologic clearance of live leptospires from tissues by antibody, however, does not ensure clinical recovery, especially in severe-type leptospirosis, because lesions in organs and tissue damage may have proceeded to stages where vital functions are almost irreversibly impaired. Clinical supportive measures for renal failure (dialysis), hemorrhage (transfusion), myocarditis, and liver failure may be necessary until the patient's tissues regenerate. Complete recovery is the rule in surviving patients, although rare examples of prolonged asymptomatic renal carriage have been recorded in people. Depressive and psychotic symptoms may persist for many weeks.[79]

7.3.6. Carrier State. The carrier state is very rare in humans. In animals it follows recovery from systemic infection, which may be subclinical. Leptospires are attached to the epithelial surface of proximal renal tubule cells, where they grow in the tubular lumen and are excreted in the urine. Homologous antibody may be demonstrated in the urine of carriers. Active excretion may be sporadic or intermittent. The mechanisms of adhesion, immunologic events, and nutritional needs of leptospires in renal tubules need to be elucidated. There is no inflammation around affected tubules, which appear to be morphologically intact in electron microscopic studies. In some animals (especially dogs and pigs) there may be considerable scarring in the kidneys where leptospires occupy renal tubules, apparently related more to the recovery and repair processes following renal damage (acute nephritis) and hemorrhage in the acute state of infection than to the presence of leptospires in the tubules. Leptospires are not found in renal tissue outside renal tubules in carrier animals. Genital carriage of leptospires has been described in livestock.

7.3.7. Autoimmunity and Hypersensitivity. The roles of autoimmunity and hypersensitivity in producing lesions are unclear. The acute nature of infection and absence of chronic infection precludes consideration of these immunopathologic mechanisms in the development of initial lesions. However, leptospires may be sequestered in "privileged sites" during acute infection, leading to later allergic reactions to their presence. A notable example is uveitis that has followed either systemic infection or accidental laboratory inoculation into the conjunctiva. Leptospires may be cultured from the anterior chamber of the eye for long periods after infection. Contact with leptospiral antigen can cause an allergic aggravation of the uveitis. A similar condition known as "moon blindness" occurs in horses.

7.4. Toxins

Numerous toxic properties of leptospirosis have been described. Some have been specific to some serovars, others distributed universally. Hemolysins act on erythrocytes of selected animal species, so that there is a combination of specificity of hemolysin according to serovar and according to animal species. For example, hemolysins produced by serovar *pomona* but not by serovar *icterohaemorrhagiae* are active on bovine but not on human erythrocytes. Most hemolysins act at 37°C. Where they have been characterized, they have been shown to be phospholipases that act on one or more of lecithin, sphingomyelin, phosphatidylcholine, or phosphatidylethanolamine, and accordingly, on the erythrocytes of those animal species whose erythrocyte membranes contain the substrate phospholipid for the phospholipase.[80] Inasmuch as hemolysin activity may be a significant toxin in pathogenesis, this mechanism provides some basis for the range of host specificities seen between leptospiral serovars and animal species. There is electron microscopic evidence for the appearance of holes in erythrocytes of calves infected with serovar *pomona*, but the responsible toxin has not been characterized.[81] In addition, lipase and urease have been identified in some serovars, although their pathogenic role is unclear.

Cytopathic effects on various cultured mammalian cell lines have been demonstrated following incubation with leptospires under a bewildering variety of combinations of cell type, cultural and incubation conditions, and leptospiral serovar and virulence. These studies may be summarized by noting that cytopathology can be observed following incubation with cultures that are either virulent or avirulent for animals and with strains of *L. biflexa*, provided large doses of 10^{10}/ml or more are used. Activity of a toxic leptospiral protein elaborated in hamster blood in leptospirosis was reported but the agent was not characterized. A toxic glycolipoprotein (GLP) is capable of damaging fibroblast cell membranes in culture and is toxic to laboratory animals by virtue of its toxic lipids. These lipids are uniquely leptospiral unsaturated long-chain fatty acids and may act on cell membranes to produce lesions resembling those occurring in the pathogenesis of the essential small blood vessel damage in leptospirosis. The activity of GLP and its fatty acids is neutralized in the presence of serum albumin, which may act as a sponge absorbing the toxic lipid. Presumably the toxin can act in infection once the serum albumin carrying capacity for lipid is saturated. GLP can affect renal sodium transport and can be located in specific renal elements in infection.[82–84] Leptospiral antigens with affinity for cell membranes were identified in infected tissues.[23,82]

LPS may be prepared from leptospires by treatment with hot aqueous phenol and extraction from either the phenol or the aqueous phase. Its chemical and physical properties resemble those of LPS from typical gram-negative enteric bacteria, but it is very poorly pyrogenic. LPS was found not to be toxic, but large amounts may inhibit phagocytosis. Antigenic derivatives of LPS are important in diagnosis and immunity (see Section 7.5.3).

7.5. Immunity[2]

There is no evidence for variability in resistance to leptospirosis in humans on the basis of race, gender, genetics, or immunologic deficiency, although a genetically endowed relative resistance in certain lines of a breed of pigs has been described. Differences in susceptibility in population groups can be explained on social and cultural epidemiological grounds that affect the magnitude of the risk of exposure.

7.5.1. Specific and Nonspecific Immunity. Low levels of innate antileptospiral IgM antibodies, found in the serum of humans and other animals not known to have been exposed to leptospirosis, destroy avirulent leptospires but are inactive against virulent strains. Nothing is known of nonspecific immunity to leptospirosis stimulated by infection with other bacteria or their LPS.

The basic facts about specific immunity to leptospirosis are that it develops rapidly, within a few days of clinical or subclinical infection. Fully effective immunity can be transmitted passively naturally through the placenta and colostrum and artificially with convalescent or hyperimmune serum. Both IgM and IgG antibodies are protective, and presumably colostral IgA antibodies are also, although there is no direct evidence. Immunity is associated with agglutinating antibodies which are also opsonic; moreover, a very low level of agglutinating antibody (titer 1:2) is protective. Immunity to reinfection is specific for the infecting serovar or closely antigenically related serovars, almost exclusively within the same serogroup determined by MAT. Polysaccharide and oligosaccharide antigenic components of LPS are protective and are involved in agglutination and opsonization as shown in studies with monoclonal murine antibodies. Sera from convalescent patients contain antibodies that react with the same antigens as those revealed in immunoblots with monoclonal antibodies.[41,85,86]

Some animal species are relatively resistant to leptospiral infection with certain serovars; the basis of such resistance is unknown. It is not known whether humans are incapable of infection with any serovars. Generally, young animals are much more susceptible than old, provided they have no maternally endowed passive immunity. The development of age-related relative resistance to leptospirosis reflects the rate of maturation of the B-cell immune response.

Cell-mediated responses occur following infection, but there is no evidence for their operation as determinants of immunity. Thus, all the evidence points to antibody-related (humoral) immunity as the sole significant mechanism for protection from leptospirosis. The duration of immunity in humans is not known. Agglutinating antibodies fall in titer after infection, but the rate is very variable in individuals and there are no studies of the relative rates of fall of IgM and IgG antibodies. Some people known to have had leptospirosis are seronegative in 1 or 2 years and others are still seropositive after more than 10 years, although the possibility cannot be excluded that they have had continued exposure to leptospires during this period.[49,87,88] There are no studies of the duration of ELISA-reactive antibodies after infection. Indeed, it is not clear that the loss of detectable agglutinating antibody over time following infection is synonymous with loss of immunity. These deficiencies in knowledge are obviously important for understanding immunity, epidemiology, and planning for vaccines.

7.5.2. Antibodies. Convalescent sera contain specific IgM, IgG, or both. Usually, IgM is elaborated first, within approximately 7–20 days of infection, followed by IgG. In some patients, seroconversion does not occur until 30 days after onset of infection. IgM persists at low levels in certain cases, while in others IgG is sometimes the sole demonstrable immunoglobulin. However, information from this type of retrospective study is necessarily limited in value because one cannot know for certain beforehand the previous history of exposure to leptospirosis. Cross-reactions with related and occasionally with unrelated serovars occur, especially early in infection. These "paradoxical reactions" occur typically, for example, between serovars *icterohaemorrhagiae* and *canicola*, and *icterohaemorrhagiae* and *pomona*. IgG antibodies tend to be more specific. In some patients treated very early with penicillin whose infections were proved with blood cultures, seroconversion did not occur at all or was delayed several weeks.

Immunoglobulins that agglutinate usually also opsonize, react with outer envelope in immunofluorescence, and protect. Murine monoclonal antibodies allow classification based on antigens reacting with the monoclonals in ELISA and in immunoblots of electrophoresed sonicates of leptospires. Batteries of monoclonals are useful for rapid identification of isolates to serogroup and presumptive serovar level. Antibodies to the infecting serovar may be found in the urine of carrier animals.[2,63]

7.5.3. Antigens Related to Pathogenesis and Immunity. Antibodies reacting with antigens in flagellar, subsurface, and outer-envelope locations have been identified in sera from patients who have been proved to have leptospirosis. Some of the antibodies persist for months and years. The only antigens among these for which there is evidence for a role in pathogenesis or immunity are the polysaccharide components of LPS or GLP, found in the outer envelope and on the leptospiral surface. Successful experimental immunization has been achieved with purified LPS or polysaccharides.[26,89]

7.5.4. Vaccines. Vaccines for leptospirosis were introduced soon after leptospires were identified and could be cultivated. Preparations effective in protecting animals and humans have been made by killing the leptospires in cultures with heat or formalin and injecting doses subcutaneously or intramuscularly. Outer-envelope preparations have been used to vaccinate animals, and irradiated live cultures rendered avirulent by irradiation have been used experimentally. Formalin-killed cultures are used widely to vaccinate animals (cattle, pigs, dogs) and are in use in some countries to immunize people. The vaccine is usually given subcutaneously in two doses and repeated annually. There is a high incidence of painful swellings at the injection site, especially on revaccination. The toxicity is considered to be too great to justify widespread use in many countries.[90–92]

In countries where leptospirosis is confined to clearly recognized occupational groups whose source of infection is livestock, the vaccination of livestock is recommended and used widely to decrease shedding by carrier animals with the twofold purpose of reducing and eliminating animal leptospirosis, thus increasing productivity, and protecting humans at risk from unavoidable exposure to these animals. Vaccination of animals requires two doses a month apart and annual revaccination. Serovar-specific vaccines made from leptospires grown in protein-free media are available for use in animals. Pregnant sows are commonly vaccinated to ensure passive protection to growing piglets. Nevertheless, those piglets may acquire asymptomatic leptospirosis after their passive protection has been lost, and they may then become shedders and thus a hazard to handlers, slaughtermen, and other abattoir workers.

8. Patterns of Host Response

Several noteworthy epidemiological features of leptospirosis determine the host responses and clinical features. The disease is almost uniquely acquired from carrier animals, which cannot be identified as carriers or shedders without laboratory tests. Recently developed sensitive PCR tests may indicate very small numbers of leptospires, but the tests, however sensitive, may miss carriers excreting intermittently or shedding only small numbers of leptospires. Inapparent infections and carriers in humans are not relevant to clinical disease or transmission.

The severity and presenting features of clinical leptospirosis result from a complex of climatic, social, and geographic factors influencing the animal host and source, and thus the serovar and the clinical features and in turn the accuracy of diagnosis and notification.[58] Living conditions and social organization, partly dependent on climatic and geographic factors, determine the amount and nature of direct or indirect contact with excretor animals of various types (see Sections 5.2–5.10). In general, different leptospiral serovars are associated with characteristic groups of animal species. The nature and severity of leptospirosis in humans depends on the infecting serovar. Living conditions for most people in tropical countries favor contact with rat or related rodent sources of leptospires rather than other animals. Most of the leptospires that clinically result in the very severe leptospirosis of the classical Weil's disease type, which may be fatal following renal failure, hemorrhages, and jaundice, are borne by rats. Serovars of the Icterohaemorrhagiae, Autumnalis, and Bataviae serogroups are examples. Conversely, in temperate climates, in addition to rats, there are other carriers of leptospires such as field mice, pigs, dogs, and cattle that shed mainly leptospires of those serovars causing a milder form of illness. The disease also tends to be much more occupationally related and confined to people in contact with these animal sources. Serovars *grippotyphosa*, *hardjo*, *pomona*, and *tarassovi* are examples of this group.

Perceptions and statistics of leptospirosis are influenced by whether the disease is seen as the severe or the mild type. Mild infections of either variety have often been overlooked because the symptoms are not pathognomonic. Usually, seriously ill patients with the severe type who needed hospital treatment or died were accurately diagnosed as leptospirosis. Since they were the only ones in whom the diagnosis was made, the clinical features recorded and reported in textbooks have been those of the severe type, emphasizing jaundice, hemorrhages, renal failure, meningitis, and a high case-fatality rate. Overall, these symptoms apply only to a few and late cases of the classical severe Weil's disease type of leptospirosis. Most patients affected with any serovar report initial symptoms as described below. The severe and the mild types differ in their subsequent progress.

8.1. Clinical Features[2,93,94]

Characteristically, leptospirosis commences suddenly with headache, myalgia, fever, and red eyes. Headache develops without warning and may be extremely severe. Myalgia is usually felt in the back and especially in the calf muscles, which may be excruciatingly tender to touch. The fever is generally greater than 39°C and the red eyes are the result of conjunctival suffusion, reflecting a generalized dilation of blood vessels, rather than a conjunctivitis. There is frequently a macular rash on the trunk, lasting only a few hours. Careful examination of the palate may show a similar petechial rash. In untreated patients with the mild type of leptospirosis, the symptoms usually persist for 3 to 10 days, followed by gradual but complete recovery. Occasionally, further acute symptoms may develop. These include oliguria from renal failure; acute abdominal pain, resembling an acute abdominal emergency and sometimes due to acute cholecystitis; meningism, hemiparesis, or other neurological signs; and cough, sometimes with mild hemoptysis. Jaundice is rare in mild-type leptospirosis. Aseptic meningitis may develop as a later complication, but most patients recover fully within 3 to 6 weeks. In patients with severe-type leptospirosis, the symptoms increase in severity, at times following a 1- or 2-day temporary remission. Delirium and confusion may develop, with increasing evidence of renal failure, together with hemorrhages and jaundice. In addition, the spleen may be enlarged. Pulmonary hemorrhages may be diffuse, resembling multiple infarcts or bronchopneumonia, accompanied by coughing of blood, but in some cases the pulmonary hemorrhages and hemoptysis may be gross. Adult respiratory distress syndrome can also occur and cause death. As liver and renal failure progress, jaundice and oliguria increase, confusion and delirium give way to unconsciousness, and death occurs through renal and hepatic failure. Supportive measures such as renal dialysis can tide patients over renal failure until renal structure is regenerated and function restored, but myocarditis causes death. Final recovery is usually complete unless vital organs are irreparably damaged. The earlier severe phase is described as the septicemic stage and the later the tissue phase.

Death from renal failure may occur at any state of the illness. The autopsy appearances will depend on the duration and degree of development of lesions. Usually, there is generalized jaundice and widespread hemorrhage in the skin, muscles, peritoneal surfaces, and lungs. The kidneys are enlarged, bile stained, and have subcapsular hemorrhages. Bleeding into all viscera including the adrenals is common. The liver shows signs of hepatitis and hemorrhages. Death is so rare in mild cases that there is no record of significant and characteristic autopsy appearances.

Uveitis may develop at any time after the second week, and as late as 6 months. It may affect one or both eyes.

8.1.1. Congenital Leptospirosis. Leptospirosis in pregnant women can be transmitted to the developing fetus at any state of pregnancy. The fetus is actively infected. If it is severely damaged, even by serovars causing the mild type of leptospirosis in the mother, it may die. If infection occurs near the time of birth, the child may develop congenital neonatal leptospirosis, whose manifestations are similar to those of adult leptospirosis. Complete recovery follows satisfactory treatment. The diagnosis of intrauterine leptospirosis depends on the correct diagnosis in the mother and evidence that the fetus is infected as shown by fetal distress. Antenatal proof is usually only available if the fetus dies. If the fetus recovers before birth, IgM antibodies will be present in the cord blood. The diagnosis of neonatal congenital leptospirosis involves the same methods as used in adults, except that recognition of specific IgM rather than IgG antibodies proves that the fetus was actively infected and that the antibodies were not passively acquired maternal immunoglobulin.[2]

8.1.2. Clinical Laboratory Findings. Laboratory tests, other than bacteriologic or serological, may help support the clinical diagnosis. In the absence of bleeding, the erythrocyte count and hemoglobin may be normal unless the patient is jaundiced, and then they are both reduced. Leukocytosis of 11–20,000/mm^3 (11–20 $\times$ 10^9/liter) is usual in icteric patients. The platelet count is frequently reduced, especially in severely jaundiced patients. The erythrocyte sedimentation rate is generally raised.

Blood urea and creatinine are always raised at least

transiently, even in mild cases. Liver function tests are useful diagnostically. The serum aminotransferases are normal or high, while the serum bilirubin level is always raised in icteric or preicteric leptospirosis. The combination of raised blood urea, raised direct bilirubin, and normal or slightly elevated aminotransferases serves to differentiate leptospirosis from hepatitis in which the serum aminotransferases are always significantly elevated.

Proteinuria is a constant but sometimes transient finding, even in mild cases. In severe cases, or wherever there is renal failure, granular and hyaline casts will be found in urine, together with bile.

Examination of CSF reveals a leukocytosis and increased protein with normal glucose.

8.1.3. Prognosis. Recovery is usually complete within a few weeks in mild-type patients. However, residual depression, irritability, and psychosis have been reported, lasting up to 6 months and preventing a return to normal life and work. Occasional reports of prolonged headache and backache following mild leptospirosis are hard to evaluate. Patients who survive the severe type of leptospirosis usually show no further signs of illness within a few weeks of full recovery of function in vital organs. Prolonged neurological symptoms and signs have been recorded, but in some of these patients there is room for doubt about the validity of the original diagnosis.

8.1.4. Treatment. Penicillin (or erythromycin in allergic patients) is the recommended treatment of choice as early as possible in the illness.[1] Doxycycline is also used. Given on the first day or two in patients diagnosed in the acute stage of infection, it can abort the symptoms and progress of either the mild or the severe form abruptly, so that the patient is frequently clinically well within 24 hr. Antibiotics given in the late ("tissue") stages may make no difference to the outcome, because the disease process is then a consequence of established lesions, the leptospires usually having been eliminated by the patient's development of antibodies; nevertheless, good results have been reported in late penicillin treatment.[95] A Jarisch–Herxheimer reaction (temporary aggravation of symptoms and fever) may occur when antibiotic treatment is commenced in well-advanced patients.[96–99]

Symptomatic and supportive systemic treatment is required for hemorrhage; shock; renal, hepatic, or cardiac insufficiency; and meningitis and other symptoms, such as headache, fever, and vomiting.

8.2. Diagnosis

8.2.1. Clinical Diagnosis. The clinical features in early leptospirosis of either the mild or the severe type are not pathognomonic and give no indication of the diagnosis to an inexperienced or uneducated clinician. In areas where the disease is common and has been recognized using laboratory confirmation, fresh cases can be diagnosed with a high degree of accuracy. A checklist of symptoms and tests is a valuable aid for primary health workers, especially those not already familiar with clinical leptospirosis. The list provides minimal diagnostic criteria and a point score for likelihood of diagnosis.[1]

Epidemiological factors such as occupational or domestic exposure to risk of infection from carrier animals or recent travel will influence the interpretation of clinical findings, pending results of confirmatory laboratory tests.

8.2.2. Laboratory Bacteriologic Diagnosis.[2,100] The principles of diagnosis are cultivation of leptospires from blood, urine, CSF, or other sites in the acute stages, demonstration of leptospires in tissues and body fluids, and serological tests.

8.2.2a. Diagnosis by Direct Microscopy. Leptospires can be seen in body fluids by dark-field illumination. The most useful specimens in the acute stage are urine and CSF, although examination of anterior chamber fluid from the eye is indicated in uveitis. Inexpert observers looking at body fluids can mistake fibrin threads for leptospires.

Urine to be examined for leptospires, whether by microscopy or by culture, should be alkaline or alkalinized by medication, because leptospires die rapidly in acid.

Leptospires may be found in urine during the first week to 10 days and intermittently thereafter. A negative result for direct microscopy of urine or CSF does not negate the diagnosis.

Leptospires may also be identified directly by immunofluorescence or immunoperoxidase staining or by silver deposition in smears or frozen or wax-embedded histological sections of autopsy or biopsy material. Technical problems inherent in silver staining techniques dictate extremely rigorous cleanliness and care.

Leptospires can be identified in specimens of blood or tissues by direct PCR.[14,17,101]

8.2.2b. Culture. Diagnostic cultures are usually made from specimens, blood, urine, CSF, other body fluids and exudates, and occasionally from tissues obtained at biopsy or autopsy. Tween–albumin fluid culture media such as EMJH are most generally useful, because more exacting strains grow better in it on primary isolation. Protein-free culture media are seldom satisfactory for primary cultivation. Special media are required for primary isolation and growth of fastidious pathogens.

Blood cultures are made by inoculating blood drawn

aseptically by venipuncture directly into culture media. Multiple inoculation of several tubes, each containing 5–10 ml of medium, with one to ten drops of blood, is recommended. Good results can be obtained by adding approximately 0.5 ml of blood to approximately 50 ml of medium, but the volume of medium is not critical. A significant dilution of at least one in ten in culture medium is required to dilute antileptospiral activity in the blood. If blood cannot be inoculated at the bedside, it can be collected in a sterile ammonium oxalate or heparin anticoagulant tube or even as a last resort in a plain tube and transported to a laboratory where the blood or serum can be inoculated into medium. If possible, multiple cultures should be prepared from each specimen. Penicillinase and sodium polyanetholesulfonate (SPS) can be added if required. The inoculated media are incubated at 30°C and examined for growth microscopically daily for the first week and weekly thereafter, up to 2 months, and ideally they should be subcultured weekly. The value of blood culture is positive identification of the etiological agent rather than speed. Isolates may be identified serologically, and relatively rapidly using batteries of monoclonal antibodies (see Section 3.4.1a).

Culture of urine requires an alkalinized fresh midstream or catheter specimen taken with care to minimize contamination. A selective medium containing 100 μg/ml 5-fluorouracil as an inhibitor of contaminant microorganisms is recommended. Media made semisolid with a final 0.1% concentration of agar are preferred by some workers, using at least a tenfold dilution of urine in the medium. Multiple cultures should be prepared from each specimen.

Leptospires may be found in CSF in the first 10 days of illness and can be cultured from it by inoculating 0.1–0.5 ml into 5–10 ml of fluid or semisolid culture medium.

8.2.2c. Serological Diagnosis (see Section 3.4.2). It can take 14 days or even much longer incubation before cultures become positive. Specimens or media for culture are frequently not available. Furthermore, the diagnosis of leptospirosis is often not suspected, or the patient does not seek medical attention until the illness is well advanced, when leptospires may have been eliminated from the body by antibodies. PCR and gene probes are unlikely to help with late retrospective diagnosis. Thus, serological tests may be the most reliable means by which a retrospective, if not concurrent, diagnosis can be made.

The main test used universally is the microscopic agglutination test (MAT) in which a small volume of live leptospiral culture of a standard age and density is mixed with a volume of a known dilution of the patient's serum. Agglutination is recorded following observation by dark-field microscopy. A variant, using formalin-killed cultures, gives slower results and lower titers but has advantages in safety, availability, and longer shelf life of the antigen suspension. A macroscopic slide agglutination test using a heavy suspension of leptospires is available for rapid screening. It is relatively insensitive and prone to false-positive reactions. Negative results cannot be used to rule out the possible diagnosis of leptospirosis. Sera reacting in slide agglutination tests must be titrated by MAT.

Enzyme immunoassays do not supplant MAT for diagnosis, because MAT is extremely sensitive and highly specific for the homologous serovar, provided antigenic overlaps within a serogroup are understood. The highest titer recorded is not necessarily to the infecting serovar, especially early in the illness. Both IgM and IgG antibodies can agglutinate leptospires (see Section 7.5.2). IgM antibodies can be detected by immunoblotting in the sera of patients with concurrently proved leptospirosis, usually within the first week.

Serum specimens for diagnosis by serological tests should be taken immediately at the outset of investigations, preferably on the first day of illness, and tested as soon as possible. A further specimen should be taken on the fifth to seventh days, and further tests if required on the 10th and 12th days (see Section 3.4.2).

In new patients in nonendemic areas, MAT antibodies at titers $\geq$ 400 in a single specimen may be considered diagnostic (see Section 3.4.2a). Titers of between 100 and 400 are suspicious and are indications for retesting where the clinical picture is consistent with leptospirosis. A fourfold or greater rising titer from an initial level of zero, $\geq$ 50, or $\geq$ 100 to $\geq$ 400–800 may be considered diagnostic. In an endemic area or in patients known to have had leptospirosis before, there may be residual background titers of $\geq$ 10 to $\geq$ 1000 from previous infections. A fresh infection in such a patient will be indicated by a rise of titer in paired serum specimens. Cross-reactivity among serovars is not uncommon.

The level of antibody in MAT will be influenced to some extent by the serovar. Characteristically, very low titers follow serovar *hardjo* infections, frequently $\geq$ 800–3200, while typically much higher titers up to $\geq$ 1000–10,000 are seen following serovar *copenhageni* infections. In patients whose sera cross-react with a heterologous serovar, the higher homologous titer prevails eventually, sometimes after several weeks.

It is common practice to commence dilutions at 1:100 or even greater in screening tests used for antibody prevalence surveys in epidemiological studies. The rationale is that people who have had leptospirosis maintain high antibody levels and lower levels of antibodies are nonspecific, meaning that they may be cross-reactive from infection with other serovars than the one used in the test. This rationale is fallacious in diagnosis of clinical cases, where even a very low titer of antibody may indicate the earliest response to current infection. A further MAT within a few days will show a significant rise. Physicians can use the first low titer in clinically characteristic patients to indicate a need to do a further test soon and perhaps treat as leptospirosis in the meantime. The deciding factor is how one interprets low titers in the epidemiological environment. Where leptospirosis is rarely seen, any titer is significant. Where it is common, low MAT titers or even a high MAT titer may be irrelevant to a current illness that is not leptospirosis.

Diagnosis by MAT presupposes that the test antigen used is the appropriate infecting serovar of *L. interrogans* or at least a serovar that shares antigens sufficiently to agglutinate with the patients' sera. A full range of serovars recommended includes representatives of all 23 serogroups. It is also recommended that local isolates be used, where available, for antigen suspensions.

ELISA tests detect antibodies in patients' sera. The serospecificity depends on the type of antigen used, but in general ELISA tests cross-react more widely than MAT. In all ELISA tests, including immunoblots, it is simple to measure reactivity in IgM or IgG separately. The results obtained in ELISA tests using sonicated leptospires correlate with MAT in general qualitatively, but the levels of reaction are often unrelated.

8.2.3. Detection of Leptospires in Urine. Darkfield microscopy is unreliable for small numbers of leptospires. Detection of small numbers of leptospires in carrier animal urine is important. Attempts to improve detection have used radioimmunoassay, DNA hybridization, and gene probes with PCR, immunoperoxidase stains, and chemiluminescence, although unknown substances in urine can reduce the sensitivity of some tests in field conditions (see Section 8.2.2a). Fluorescent antibody testing can also be used and cultures (see Section 8.2.2b) can be prepared.

8.2.4. Differential Diagnosis. At the onset of either mild- or severe-type leptospirosis, there is little to distinguish it from any other acute febrile illness. The very severe headache, fever, and myalgia are characteristic, but at this stage they may be confused with severe influenza, poliomyelitis, dengue, Q fever, and viral meningitis. The main differentiating criteria in leptospirosis are raised blood creatinine and urea, leukocytosis, and in some cases, an early rise in titer of leptospiral antibodies. At a later stage the main differential diagnoses are with viral meningitis and acute abdominal emergencies in mild-type leptospirosis and with malaria, blackwater fever, viral meningitis, hepatitis, yellow fever, and acute glomerulonephritis in severe-type leptospirosis. The main diagnostic criteria are high serum bilirubin with low or normal levels of serum aminotransferases, with significant and rising titers of specific antileptospiral antibodies. The isolation and identification of leptospires from blood, urine, or CSF confirm the diagnosis positively. At autopsy, differential diagnosis depends on characteristic pathological changes of jaundice and widespread hemorrhages with pale, enlarged hemorrhagic kidneys showing histological evidence of renal tubular degeneration and hemorrhage, liver cell degeneration, myocarditis, and pulmonary hemorrhages. Leptospires can be found and stained by immunostaining in tissues up to about 7 to 10 days after onset, but are hard to demonstrate thereafter. Postmortem serum specimens may be tested for antibodies.

In all patients, an epidemiological history of occupational or accidental exposure to risk and animal contact or travel may elucidate the diagnosis.

9. Control and Prevention

9.1. General Concepts

As is the case in all zoonoses, control of leptospirosis in humans is complex, because the primary sources of the disease are in animals, in some of which control is impossible. Regulation if not elimination of leptospirosis may be feasible in livestock and domestic animals, even though carriers are clinically normal and shedders hard to detect, but it cannot be envisaged in wildlife. Control is further complicated by the general and nonspecific clinical picture of mild or early severe leptospirosis, indistinguishable from a variety of other incapacitating fevers common in tropical areas, so that an animal source is often not suspected. The essentials of control and prevention lie in awareness and recognition of the disease and in containment in livestock and domestic sources.

Awareness and recognition require a knowledge of epidemiological facts acquired by selected surveillance, reporting, and notification, which in turn need specialized diagnostic laboratory services and education of physicians, veterinarians, administrators, and the public. Although containment of animal sources may be seen as a veterinary public health and hygiene problem, it is essential to the protection of humans. The main measures are veterinary surveillance, treatment, and prevention; occupational hygiene; rodent control; engineering; laboratory safety; and evaluation of preventive measures. In addition, containment extends to the prevention of human disease by the judicious avoidance of risk, by immunization, and by chemoprophylaxis.

9.1.1. Education, Laboratory Services, and Notification. Ordinary routine microbiological diagnostic laboratories are not usually equipped with skilled staff and specialized techniques for leptospirosis. If specialized diagnosis is not available locally, there should be a central leptospirosis laboratory available for referral of specimens and consultation. Reference laboratories staffed by experts are required only on a regional international basis for stock cultures, standard sera, research, education, and consultation. New methods of molecular diagnosis may make diagnostic facilities more readily available.

Evaluation of diagnostic laboratory results provides a useful form of surveillance. In addition, prevalence surveys for antibodies in selected groups can reveal problems or evaluate control measures. The most effective form of information gathering should be notification by health practitioners. Usually, this is of limited value because of inadequate diagnosis, failure to use appropriate laboratory tests, and failure to notify. Statistics of practitioner notifications frequently indicate an incidence much lower than diagnosed by laboratories.

9.1.2. Control Measures in Animals

9.1.2a. Rodent Control. Removal of rodents from the domestic environment effectively reduces the infection rate of leptospirosis. Standard measures include control of litter and garbage disposal, protecting food sources, trapping, and poisoning. Feral rodents and small marsupials cannot be controlled. When they share the environment with crops, precautions can be taken, such as burning off sugarcane before cutting by hand or mechanization of cutting.[1]

9.1.2b. Environmental Control. Any measure to reduce the load of leptospires in soil, water, or mud will reduce the risk to humans. Simple drainage can prevent seepage of urine into waterlogged soils or yards where livestock are herded. Environmental engineering can also increase the risk by flooding previously dry areas.

9.1.2c. Immunization, Chemotherapy, and Culling of Livestock. Excretor rates in cattle and pig herds frequently reach levels of 65 to 90%. If shedders can be identified and removed from herds, the risks to the herd and to attendant humans can be reduced, provided the remaining animals are immunized, the herd is restocked with immunized animals, fresh excretor animals are not introduced, and the herd is protected from fresh infection from environmental sources. Immunization alone can reduce both animal and indirectly human leptospirosis, but it is hard to evaluate, because most studies have been specially set up under artificial conditions accompanied by education and improvements in occupational hygiene and farming practice. Outer-envelope preparations and leptospiral cultures in protein-free media are available as vaccines. Immunization of livestock or dogs requires two doses of a killed vaccine a month or so apart followed by annual revaccination. Culling or vaccination are both expensive and their use by small holding farmers will depend on the relative values and costs of animals, vaccines, and health (or illness). The associated costs of transport, skilled attention, and equipment may also be relatively high. The control of leptospirosis in stud stock, where leptospires may be found in semen samples used for artificial insemination, requires special methods for testing and transport of semen.

9.1.3. Treatment of the Carrier State. Carrier animals have been cured by streptomycin treatment. The cost is relatively high and the results so difficult to evaluate in field conditions that it is considered impractical for general use.[102,103]

Humans do not become chronic carriers or excretors for any length of time. Elementary domestic, personal, and hospital hygiene ensures little risk from patients and convalescents still excreting leptospires. Urine specimens from convalescent patients are not recognized sources of laboratory infection, but care should be taken nonetheless.

9.1.4. Occupational Hygiene. Preventive measures for people who cannot avoid exposure to risk are centered around methods for physical protection in their work or leisure. Waterproof footwear, watershedding aprons worn outside and over the boots or other clothing, and clear plastic facemasks have all been recommended for milkers and slaughterhouse workers. In hot climates or working conditions, impermeable protective clothing is uncomfortable and poorly accepted. Nevertheless, rubber boots provide obvious protection. Most infections appear to follow penetration of cuts and damaged, abraded, or macerated skin by leptospires. It is therefore important to protect such injuries, but often not practicable to do so in daily working conditions.

Good drainage of floors and herding yards and control of rodent infestation in food preparation areas are important occupational hygienic measures, but no measures will be effective unless the people concerned understand the disease, the means of infection, and the need for precautions so that they are prepared to implement recommended practices. The risk for field workers can be reduced by attempting to control the environmental hazards as outlined in Section 9.1.2.

9.2. Antimicrobial Prophylaxis

Chemoprophylaxis with doxycycline has been used to prevent leptospirosis in soldiers exposed to jungle conditions.[104] It, or prophylactic penicillin, could be used to protect anyone exposed to a significant risk for a brief defined period. People in such categories could include those about to undertake rafting or canoeing trips, cavers, grain farmers and workers at harvest time when risks are serious for a short period only, field ecologists trapping small wild rodents, and people caught in floods. Tetracycline-group antibiotics are leptospirostatic rather than leptospiricidal and in any case contraindicated in pregnant women, in children, and in people with renal insufficiency. Prolonged or permanent chemoprophylaxis is not recommended. It is unlikely that antibiotic treatment of humans before or during leptospirosis will lead to leptospirosis from antibiotic-resistant leptospires, because human-to-human transmission is almost unrecorded, although leptospires develop resistance to some antibiotics readily in the laboratory.

Antibiotic-resistant leptospirosis has not been recorded in animals, despite some decades of use of streptomycin and penicillin in veterinary medicine. Antibiotic susceptibility tests usually are not performed on leptospires isolated from either human or animal sources. Spontaneous resistance to penicillins, aminoglycosides, tetracyclines, or macrolides, all of which have been used in leptospirosis, is not known. On the other hand, it is highly probable that chemoprophylaxis with any antibiotic will aggravate undesirable selection of antibiotic-resistant derivatives of other bacteria including pathogens of the alimentary and respiratory tracts.

9.3. Immunization

Immunization of humans and animals with killed cultures of leptospires has been used almost since leptospires were discovered. Vaccines are serovar specific and currently administered subcutaneously in two or more doses 2 or 4 weeks apart and repeated annually.[5]

Local reactions of pain, redness, and swelling ranging from mild to very severe occur, especially on revaccination. There was always a risk of anaphylaxis or serum sickness from the serum or serum proteins necessarily in the culture media until relatively recently, when protein-free media became available. Some preparations involved washing and resuspending leptospires to reduce the animal protein content, but protein can always be found adherent to the leptospiral surface after washing. Washed or whole culture vaccines have been employed in several countries, mainly in Asia, where the risks to life and health from severe leptospirosis could justify the side effects of the vaccine.[92] There has not been widespread acceptance of an early protein-free vaccine for humans, although more recent studies showed evidence of effective immunization. Increasing worldwide concern about quality control, safety, pyrogenicity, potential teratogenicity, and efficacy of vaccines ensure that rigorous evaluation will be required before a suitable vaccine can be accepted for human use.

10. Unresolved Problems

There is a series of interconnected questions that need answers before great improvements in control of leptospirosis can be achieved. Neither the duration of postinfection immunity nor its specificity is known. Conventional wisdom based mainly on animal experimentation states that immunity is specific for antigens that are serovar specific, or at best shared within a serogroup. Is there any underlying genus- or species-specific immunity in humans mediating a level of resistance to all serovars of pathogenic leptospires?

Leptospiral toxins are able to damage host tissues. Is there antitoxic immunity as well as antileptospiral immunity, and if so, is it significant in recovery or protection?

There are genetic differences in the susceptibility of pigs to primary infection. Are there human genetic differences in susceptibility, and if so, are they reflected in the response to particular serovars or to all serovars, and thus to the pathogenicity of particular serovars for humans?

There are about 200 serovars described among the pathogenic leptospires, based on antigenic surface characteristics mediated by LPS-related polysaccharide epitopes; new serovars are identified every year. Although part of the LPS gene has been characterized, the genetic basis for serovar specificity and variation is still unknown. A plasmid has yet to be described in pathogenic leptospires. What is the basis for genetic exchange in nature? This problem becomes acutely relevant with the recognition that the various species of *Leptospira* each contain serovars also found in other species; that is, serovar specificity overlaps the genetic groupings. The effects of these observations on classification of leptospires have implications for diagnosis, epidemiology, and prognosis. Many more isolates need to be genotyped.

Rapid bedside tests are required that will enable a clinician to identify whether or not a patient has leptospirosis, and if so, which serovar, often at a time in the illness before antibodies have appeared in blood. Methods explored so far are antigen detection and gene probes amplified by PCR. Further development of these or other methods would be invaluable in the early recognition and diagnosis of cases and the institution of appropriate treatment. Direct tests for the leptospira or its antigens would overcome the serious difficulty of evaluating the significance of a positive serological test in a patient in an endemic area where most of the population have antibodies, even residual IgM, to one or more serovars, or where the patient may have residual antibodies from an infection with a serovar unrelated to the present illness. Similar direct diagnostic methods would allow easier and more positive detection of carrier animals than is possible now.

Most people at risk from leptospirosis live in developing countries without ready access to specialized diagnostic or treatment facilities. There is seldom a capacity for new scientific research into the problems identified here. On the other hand, leptospirosis is rarely diagnosed in urban agglomerations in developed countries where most researchers and institutes capable of high technology are found and there are relatively few among them interested in leptospirosis. Knowledge and research in leptospirosis are thus not available in most developed countries, to which developing countries turn for scientific assistance. The situation is aggravated when inadequate statistics in developed countries indicate a spuriously low rate of leptospirosis, leading to an impression that the disease is nonexistent or unimportant and does not justify allocation of funds for the maintenance of existing research and surveillance or for new studies toward solutions to the problems outlined above.

ACKNOWLEDGMENTS

Original research from the author's laboratory was supported by grants to him or Dr. B. Adler from the Australian National Health and Medical Research Council, Canberra, Australia.

11. References

1. Faine, S. (ed.), *Offset Publication*, No. 67: *Guidelines for the control of leptospirosis*, World Health Organization, Geneva, 1982.
2. Faine, S., *Leptospira and leptospirosis*, CRC Press, Boca Raton, FL, 1994.
3. Ellis, W. A., International Committee on Systematic Bacteriology Subcommittee on the Taxonomy of *Leptospira*. Minutes of the meetings, 1 and 2 July 1994, Prague, Czech Republic, *Int. J. Syst. Bacteriol.* **45**:872–874 (1995).
4. Torten, M., Leptospirosis, in: *CRC Handbook Series in Zoonoses. Section A. 1. Bacterial, Rickettsial and Mycotic Diseases* (J. H. Steele, ed.), pp. 363–421, CRC Press, Boca Raton, FL, 1979.
5. Torten, M., and Marshall, R. B., Leptospirosis, in: *Handbook of Zoonoses, Section A: Bacterial, Rickettsial, Chlamydial and Mycotic Diseases* 2nd ed., Vol. 1 (G. W. Beran, ed.), pp. 245–264, CRC Press, Boca Raton, FL, 1994.
6. Perolat, P., Chappel, R., Adler, B., *et al.*, Description, characterization and phylogenetic analysis of *Leptospira faineii* sp. nov., isolated from pigs in Australia. *Int. J. Syst. Bacteriol.*, 1998.
7. Johnson, R. C., and Faine, S., Genus I. Leptospira Noguchi 1917, 755, in: *Bergey's Manual of Systematic Bacteriology*, 1st ed., Vol. 1 (N. R. Krieg and J. C. Holt, eds.), pp. 62–67, Williams and Wilkins, Baltimore, 1984.
8. Johnson, R. C., and Faine, S., Order I. Spirochaetales: Family II. "*Leptospiraceae*" Hovind-Hougen 1979, 245, in: *Bergey's Manual of Systematic Bacteriology*, 1st ed., Vol. 1 (N. R. Krieg and J. G. Holt, eds.), p. 62, Williams and Wilkins, Baltimore, 1984.
9. Faine, S., and Stallman, N. D., Amended descriptions of the genus *Leptospira* Noguchi 1917 and the species *L. interrogans* (Stimson 1907) Wenyon 1926 and *L. biflexa* (Wolbach and Binger 1914) Noguchi 1918, *Int. J. Syst. Bacteriol.* **32**:461–463 (1982).
10. Ellis, W. A., McParland, P. J., and Bryson, D. G., Isolation of leptospires from the genital tract and kidneys of aborted sows, *Vet. Rec.* **118**:294–295 (1986).
11. Wagenaar, J. A., *Leptospirosis*—Diagnosis and Pathogenesis, dissertation, Veterinary Faculty, University of Utrecht, Netherlands, 1994.
12. Dikken, H., and Kmety, E., Serological typing methods of leptospires, in: *Methods in Microbiology*, Vol. 11 (T. Bergan and R. Norris, eds.), pp. 260–295, Academic Press, New York, 1978.
13. Kmety, E., and Dikken, H., *Revised list of "Leptospira" serovars. I Alphabetical Order, II Chronological Order*, Vols. 1 and 2, Groningen, Netherlands: University Press; 1988. [Accepted by the Subcommittee on the Taxonomy of "*Leptospira*" at the Manchester meeting, 6/7 September, 1986 (International Committee on Systematic Bacteriology, International Union of Microbiological Societies).]
14. Gravekamp, C., van de Kemp, H., Franzen, M., *et al.*, Detection of seven species of pathogenic leptospires by PCR using two sets of primers, *J. Gen. Microbiol.* **139**:1691–1700 (1993).
15. Letocart, M., Baranton, G., and Perolat, P., Rapid identification of pathogenic *Leptospira* species (*Leptospira interrogans*, *L. borgpetersenii*, and *L. kirschneri*) with species-specific DNA probes produced by arbitrarily primed PCR, *J. Clin. Microbiol.* **35**:248–253 (1997).
16. Savio, M. L., Rossi, C., Fusi, P., *et al.*, Detection and identification of *Leptospira interrogans* serovars by PCR coupled with restriction endonuclease analysis of amplified DNA, *J. Clin. Microbiol.* **32**:935–941 (1994).
17. Merien, F., Perolat, P., Mancel, E., *et al.*, Detection of *Leptospira* DNA by polymerase chain reaction in aqueous humor of a patient with unilateral uveitis, *J. Infect. Dis.* **168**:1335–1336 (1993).
18. Hookey, J. V., Bryden, J., and Gatehouse, L., The use of 16S rDNA sequence analysis to investigate the phylogeny of Leptospiraceae and related spirochaetes, *J. Gen. Microbiol.* **139**:2585–2590 (1993).
19. Terpstra, W. J., Ligthart, G. S., and Schoone, G. J., Serodiagnosis of human leptospirosis by enzyme-linked immunosorbent-assay (ELISA), *Zentralbl. Bakteriol. Mikrobiol. Hyg. Abt. I Orig. Reihe A* **247**:400–405 (1980).
20. Adler, B., Murphy, A. M., Locarnini, S., *et al.*, Detection of

specific antileptospiral immunoglobulins M and G in human serum by solid-phase enzyme-linked immunosorbent assay, *J. Clin. Microbiol.* **11:**452–457 (1980).

21. Gussenhoven, G. C., van der Hoorn, M. A., Goris, M. G., *et al.*, LEPTO dipstick, a dipstick assay for detection of *Leptospira*-specific immunoglobulin M antibodies in human sera, *J. Clin. Microbiol.* **35:**92–97 (1997).
22. Vinh, T., Adler, B., and Faine, S., Ultrastructure and chemical composition of lipopolysaccharide extracted from *Leptospira interrogans* serovar *copenhageni*, *J. Gen. Microbiol.* **132:**103–109 (1986).
23. Vinh, T., Adler, B., and Faine, S., Glycolipoprotein cytotoxin from *Leptospira interrogans* serovar *copenhageni*, *J. Gen. Microbiol.* **132:**111–123 (1986).
24. Mitchison, M., Bulach, D., Vinh, T., *et al.*, Identification and characterization of the dTDP-rhamnose biosynthesis and transfer genes of the lipopolysaccharide-related *rbf* locus in *Leptospira interrogans* serovar copenhageni, *J. Bacteriol.* **179:**1262–1267 (1997).
25. Vinh, T., Faine, S., Handley, C. J., *et al.*, Immunochemical studies of opsonic epitopes of the lipopolysaccharide of *Leptospira interrogans* serovar *hardjo*, *FEMS Immunol. Med. Microbiol.* **8:**99–108 (1994).
26. Midwinter, A., Vinh, T., Faine, S., *et al.*, Characterization of an antigenic oligosaccharide from *Leptospira interrogans* serovar *pomona* and its role in immunity, *Infect. Immun.* **62:**5477–5482 (1994).
27. Ballard, S. A., Segers, R. P. A. M., Bleumink-Pluym, N., *et al.*, Molecular analysis of the *hsp* (*groE*) operon of *Leptospira interrogans* serovar *copenhageni*, *Mol. Microbiol.* **8:**739–751 (1993).
28. Segers, R. P., van Gestel, J. A., van Eys, G. J., *et al.*, Presence of putative sphingomyelinase genes among members of the family *Leptospiraceae*, *Infect. Immun.* **60:**1707–1710 (1992).
29. Segers, R. P. A. M., *The Molecular Analysis of Sphingomyelinase Genes of Leptospiraceae*, dissertation, Rijksuniversiteit of Utrecht, Netherlands, 1991.
30. Ding, M., and Yelton, D. B., Cloning and analysis of the *leuB* gene of *Leptospira interrogans* serovar *pomona*, *J. Gen. Microbiol.* **139:**1093–1103 (1993).
31. Haake, D. A., Champion, D. I., Martinich, C., *et al.*, Molecular cloning and sequence analysis of the gene encoding OpmL1, a transmembrane outer membrane protein of pathogenic *Leptospira* spp., *J. Bacteriol.* **175:**4225–4234 (1993).
32. Baril, C., and Saint-Girons, I., Sizing of the *Leptospira* genome by pulsed-field agarose gel electrophoresis, *FEMS Microbiol. Lett.* **71:**95–99 (1990).
33. Richaud, C., Margarita, D., Baranton, G., *et al.*, Cloning of genes required for amino acid biosynthesis from *Leptospira interrogans* serovar *icterohaemorrhagiae*, *J. Gen. Micrbiol.* **136:**651–656 (1990).
34. Zuerner, R. L., Nucleotide sequence analysis of IS1533 from *Leptospira borgpetersenii*: Identification and expression of two IS-encoded proteins, *Plasmid* **31:**1–11 (1994).
35. Zuerner, R. L., Herrmann, J. L., and Saint Girons, I., Comparison of genetic maps for two *Leptospira interrogans* serovars provides evidence for two chromosomes and intraspecies heterogeneity, *J. Bacteriol.* **175:**5445–5451 (1993).
36. Ralph, D., and McClelland, M., Phylogenetic evidence for horizontal transfer of an intervening sequence between species in a spirochete genus, *J. Bacteriol.* **176:**5982–5987 (1994).
37. Saint Girons, I., Margarita, D., Amouriaux, P., *et al.*, First isolation of bacteriophages for a spirochaete: Potential genetic tools for *Leptospira*, *Res. Microbiol.* **141:**1131–1138 (1990).
38. Fukunaga, M., and Mifuchi, I., Unique organization of *Leptospira interrogans* rRNA genes, *J. Bacteriol.* **171:**5763–5767 (1989).
39. Penn, C. W., Bassford, P. J., Yelton, D. B., *et al.*, Genetic approaches to cell biology and metabolism of spirochetes, *Res. Microbiol.* **143:**605–613 (1992).
40. Ralph, D., Que, Q., Van Etten, J. L., *et al.*, *Leptospira* genomes are modified at 5′-GTAC, *J. Bacteriol.* **175:**3913–3915 (1993).
41. Vinh, T., Shi, M. H., Adler, B., *et al.*, Characterisation and taxonomic significance of lipopolysaccharides of *Leptospira interogans* serovar *hardjo*, *J. Gen. Microbiol.* **135:**2663–2673 (1989).
42. Chang, A., Faine, S., and Williams, W. T., Cross-reactivity of the axial filament antigen as a criterion for classification of *Leptospira*, *Aust. J. Exp. Biol. Med. Sci.* **52:**549–568 (1974).
43. Vinh, T., Faine, S., and Adler, B., Adhesion of leptospires to mouse fibroblasts (L929) and its enhancement by specific antibody, *J. Med. Microbiol.* **18:**73–85 (1984).
44. Ito, T., and Yanagawa, R., Leptospiral attachment to extracellular matrix of mouse fibroblast (L929) cells, *Vet. Microbiol.* **15:**89–96 (1987).
45. Niikura, M., Ono, E., and Yanagawa, R., Molecular comparison of antigens on proteins of virulent and avirulent clones of *Leptospira interrogans* serovar *copenhageni* strain Shibaura, *Zentralbl. Bakteriol. Mikrobiol. Hyg. Abt. I Orig. Reihe. A* **266:**453–462 (1987).
46. Ono, E., Takase, H., Naiki, M., *et al.*, Purification, characterization and serological properties of a glycolipid antigen reactive with a serovar-specific monoclonal antibody against *Leptospira interrogans* serovar *canicola*, *J. Gen. Microbiol.* **133:**1329–1336 (1987).
47. Takashima, I., and Yanagawa, R., Isolation and chemical characterisation of streptomycin-resistant mutants of leptospiras, *Jpn. J. Microbiol.* **16:**535–537 (1972).
48. Ellis, W. A., Songer, J. G., Montgomery, J., *et al.*, Prevalence of *Leptospira interrogans* serovar *hardjo* in the genital and urinary tracts of nonpregnant cattle, *Vet. Rec.* **118:**11–13 (1986).
49. Palit, A., Hosking, C., Create, L., *et al.*, Leptospirosis in dairy farmers of western Victoria, Australia, in: *Leptospirosis. Proceedings of the Leptospirosis Research Conference, 1990* (Y. Kobayashi, ed.), pp. 126–137, Hokusen-Sha Publishing, Tokyo, 1991.
50. Sasaki, D. M., Pang, L., Minette, H. P., *et al.*, Active surveillance and risk factors for leptospirosis in Hawaii, *Am. J. Trop. Med. Hyg.* **48:**35–43 (1993).
51. Li, Y. [Cluster and multiple regression analysis of leptospirosis epidemic factors]. *Chung Hua Liu Hsing Ping Hsueh Tsa Chih* **13:**151–153 (1992).
52. Philipp, R., King, C., and Hughes, A., Understanding of Weil's disease among canoeists, *Br. J. Sports Med.* **26:**223–227 (1992).
53. Johnston, J. H., Lloyd, J., McDonald, J., *et al.*, Leptospirosis: An occupational disease of soldiers, *J. R. Army Med. Corps.* **129:**111–114 (1983).
54. Jackson, L. A., Kaufmann, A. F., Adams, W. G., *et al.*, Outbreak of leptospirosis associated with swimming, *Pediatr. Infect. Dis. J.* **12:**48–54 (1993).
55. Katz, A. R., Manea, S. J., and Sasaki, D. M., Leptospirosis on Kauai: Investigation of a common source waterborne outbreak, *Am. J. Public Health* **81:**1310–1312 (1991).

56. Gollop, J. H., Pang, G., and Sasaki, D. M., Leptospirosis: A possible cause of "aseptic meningitis," *Hawaii Med. J.* **49:**162, 165 (1990).
57. Ferguson, I. R., Leptospirosis surveillance: 1990–1992, *Commun. Dis. Rep.* **3:**R47–R48 (1993).
58. Shyakov, E. N., Influence de l'activité humaine sur l'épidémiologie des zooanthroponoses, *Med. Mal. Infect.* **13:**784–787 (1983).
59. Galuzo, I. G., Landscape epidemiology (epizootology), *Adv. Vet. Sci.* **19:**73–96 (1975).
60. Giudicelli, J., Lemaitre, D., Fournier, V., *et al.*, [3 pediatric cases of leptospirosis], Trois observations pédiatriques de leptospirose, *Pédiatrie* **48:**455–458 (1993).
61. Self, C. A., Iskrzynska, W. I., and Waitkins, S. A., Leptospirosis among British cavers, *Cave Sci.* **14:**131–134 (1987).
62. Ballard, S. A., Adler, B., Millar, B. D., *et al.*, The immunoglobulin response of swine following experimental infection with *Leptospira interrogans* serovar *pomona*, *Zentralbl. Bakteriol. Mikrobiol. Hyg. Abt. I Orig. Reihe. A* **256:**510–517 (1984).
63. Leonard, F. C., Quinn, P. J., Ellis, W. A., *et al.*, Association between cessation of leptospiruria in cattle and urinary antibody levels, *Res. Vet. Sci.* **55:**195–202 (1993).
64. Peet, R. L., Mercy, A., Hustas, L., *et al.*, The significance of *Leptospira* isolated from the kidneys of slaughtered pigs, *Aust. Vet. J.* **60:**226–227 (1983).
65. Goard, K. E., Infection by *Leptospira pomona* contracted from pigs by mouth-to-mouth resuscitation, *Med. J. Aust.* **1:**897–898 (1961).
66. Spinu, I., Topciu, V., Trinh, T. H. Q., *et al.*, L'homme comme réservoir de virus dans une épidémie de leptospirose survenue dans la jungle, *Arch. Roum. Pathol. Exp. Microbiol.* **22:**1081–1100 (1963).
67. Gsell, H. O., Olafsson, A., Sonnabend, W., *et al.*, Intrauterine *Leptospirosis pomona*, *Dtsch. Med. Wochenschr.* **96:**1263–1268 (1971).
68. Faine, S., Adler, B., Christopher, W., *et al.*, Fatal congenital human leptospirosis, *Zentralbl. Bakteriol. Mikrobiol. Hyg. Abt. I Orig. Reihe. A* **257:**548 (1984).
69. Gollop, J. H., Katz, A. R., Rudoy, R. C., *et al.*, Rat-bite leptospirosis, *West J. Med.* **159:**76–77 (1993).
70. Cerny, A., Ettlin, D., Betschen, K., *et al.*, Weil's disease after a rat bite, *Eur. J. Med.* **1:**315–316 (1992).
71. Korthof, G., Experimentelles Schlammfieber beim Menschen, *Zentralbl. Bakteriol. Parasitenkd. Abt. I* **125:**429–434 (1932).
72. Derrick, E. H., Estimation of the incubation period of canefield leptospirosis from the weekly work pattern, *Pathology* **1:**73–75 (1969).
73. Faine, S., Virulence in *Leptospira*. II. The growth *in vivo* of virulent *Leptospira icterohaemorrhagiae*, *Br. J. Exp. Pathol.* **38:**8–14 (1957).
74. Ballard, S. A., Williams, M., Adler, B., *et al.*, Interactions of virulent and avirulent leptospires with primary cultures of renal epithelial cells, *J. Med. Microbiol.* **21:**59–67 (1986).
75. Edwards, C. N., Nicholson, G. D., and Everard, C. O. R., Thrombocytopenia in leptospirosis, *Am. J. Trop. Med. Hyg.* **31:**827–829 (1982).
76. De Arriaga, A. J. D., Rocha, A. S., Yasuda, P. H., *et al.*, Morphofunctional patterns of kidney injury in the experimental leptospirosis of the guinea-pig (*L. icterohaemorrhagiae*), *J. Pathol.* **138:**145–161 (1982).
77. Sitprija, V., Pipatangul, V., Mertowidjojo, K., *et al.*, Pathogenesis of renal disease in leptospirosis: Clinical and experimental studies, *Kidney Int.* **17:**827–836 (1980).
78. Sitprija, V., Renal involvement in leptospirosis, in: *Nephrology* (R. R. Robinson, ed.), pp. 1041–1052. Springer-Verlag, New York, 1984.
79. Avery, T. L., Leptospirosis and mental illness, *N. Z. Med. J.* **96:**589 (1983).
80. Kasarov, L. B., Degradation of the erythrocyte phospholipids and haemolysis of the erythrocytes of different animal species by Leptospirae, *J. Med. Microbiol.* **3:**29–37 (1970).
81. Thompson, J. C., Morphological changes in red blood cells of calves caused by *Leptospira interrogans* serovar *pomona*, *J. Comp. Pathol.* **96:**512–527 (1986).
82. de Brito, T., Prado, M. J. B. A., Negreiros, V. A. C., *et al.*, Detection of leptospiral antigen (*L. interrogans* serovar *copenhageni* serogroup Icterohaemorrhagiae) by immunoelectron microscopy in the liver and kidney of experimentally infected guinea-pigs, *Int. J. Exp. Pathol.* **73:**633–642 (1992).
83. Younes-Ibrahim, M., Burth, P., Faria, M. V., *et al.*, Inhibition of Na,K-ATPase by an endotoxin extracted from *Leptospira interrogans*: A possible mechanism for the physiopathology of leptospirosis, *C. R. Acad. Sci.* **318:**619–625 (1995).
84. Burth, P., Younes-Ibrahim, M., Goncalez, F. H., *et al.*, Purification and characterization of an Na^+,K^+ ATPase inhibitor found in a endotoxin of *Leptospira interrogans*, *Infect. Immunity* **65:**1557–1560 (1997).
85. Jost, B. H., Adler, B., and Faine, S., Experimental immunisation of hamsters with lipopolysaccharide antigens of *Leptospira interrogans*, *J. Med. Microbiol.* **29:**115–120 (1989).
86. Vinh, T., Faine, S., Handley, C. J., *et al.*, Immunochemical studies of opsonic epitopes of the lipopolysaccharide of *Leptospira interrogans* serovar *hardjo*, *FEMS Immunol. Med. Microbiol.* **8:**99–107 (1994).
87. Everard, C. O. R., and Bennett, S., Persistence of leptospiral agglutinins in Trinidadian survey subjects, *Eur. J. Epidemiol.* **6:**40–44 (1990).
88. Everard, C. O., Baulu, J., Carrington, D. G., *et al.*, Retention of leptospiral agglutinins and long-term response to administration of monoclonal antibodies in vervet monkeys (*Cercopithecus aethiops*) on Barbados, *Eur. J. Epidemiol.* **7:**396–402 (1991).
89. Ruby, K. W., Cardella, M. A., and Knudtson, W. U., Assay for measuring relative potency of leptospiral bacterins containing serovar *pomona*, *Biologicals* **20:**259–266 (1992).
90. Shenberg, E., and Torten, M., A new leptospiral vaccine for use in man. I. Development of a vaccine from "*Leptospira*" grown on a chemically defined medium, *J. Infect. Dis.* **128:**642–646 (1973).
91. Torten, M., Shenberg, E., Gerichter, C. B., *et al.*, A new leptospiral vaccine for use in man. II. Clinical and serologic evaluation of a field trial with volunteers, *J. Infect. Dis.* **128:**647–651 (1973).
92. Chen, T. Z., Development and present status of leptospiral vaccine and technology of production of the vaccine in China, *Ann. Immunol. Hung.* **26:**125–151 (1986).
93. Watt, G., Leptospirosis, *Curr. Opin. Infect. Dis.* **5:**659–663 (1992).
94. Faine, S., Leptospirosis, in: *Infectious Diseases*, 5th ed. (P. D. Hoeprich, M. C. Jordan, and A. R. Roland, eds.), pp. 619–625, Lippincott, Philadelphia (1994).
95. Watt, G., Padre, L. P., Tuazon, M. L., *et al.*, Placebo-controlled trial of intravenous penicillin for severe and late leptospirosis, *Lancet* **1:**433–435 (1988).
96. Watt, G., Padre, L. P., Tuazon, M., *et al.*, Limulus lysate positivity

and Herxheimer-like reactions in leptospirosis: A placebo-controlled study, *J. Infect. Dis.* **162:**564–567 (1990).
97. Friedland, J. S., and Warrell, D. A., The Jarisch–Herxheimer reaction in leptospirosis: Possible pathogenesis and review, *Rev. Infect. Dis.* **13:**207–210 (1991).
98. Emmanouilides, C. E., Kohn, O. F., and Garibaldi, R., Leptospirosis complicated by a Jarisch–Herxheimer reaction and adult respiratory distress syndrome: Case report, *Clin. Infect. Dis.* **18:**1004–1006 (1994).
99. Vaughan, C., Cronin, C. C., Walsh, E. K., *et al.*, The Jarisch–Herxheimer reaction in leptospirosis, *Postgrad. Med. J.* **70:**118–121 (1994).
100. Faine, S., Leptospirosis, in: *Laboratory Diagnosis of Infectious Diseases. Principles and Practice, Bacterial Mycotic and Parasitic Diseases*, Vol. 1 (A. Balows *et al.*, eds.), pp. 344–352, Springer-Verlag, New York, 1988.
101. van Eys, G. J. J. M., Gravenkamp, C., Gerritsen, M. J., *et al.*, Detection of leptospires in urine by polymerase chain reaction, *J. Clin. Microbiol.* **27:**2258–2262 (1989).
102. Ellis, W. A., Montgomery, J., and Cassells, J. A., Dihydrostreptomycin treatment of bovine carriers of *Leptospira interrogans* serovar *hardjo*, *Res. Vet. Sci.* **39:**292–295 (1986).
103. Gerritsen, M. J., Koopmans, M. J., and Olyhoek, T., Effect of streptomycin treatment on the shedding of and the serologic responses to *Leptospira interrogans* serovar *hardjo* subtype hardjobovis in experimentally infected cows, *Vet. Microbiol.* **38:**129–135 (1993).
104. Takafuji, E. T., Kirkpatrick, J. W., Miller, R. N., *et al.*, An efficacy trial of doxycycline chemoprophylaxis against leptospirosis, *N. Engl. J. Med.* **310:**497–500 (1984).

12. Suggested Reading

Faine, S. (ed.), Offset Publication, No. 67: *Guidelines for the Control of Leptospirosis*, World Health Organization, Geneva, 1982.

Faine, S., *Leptospira and Leptospirosis*, CRC Press, Boca Raton, FL, 1994.

Torten, M., and Marshall, R. B., Leptospirosis, in: *Handbook of Zoonoses, Section A: Bacterial, Rickettsial, Chlamydial and Mycotic Diseases* 2nd ed., Vol. 1 (G. W. Beran, ed.), pp. 245–264, CRC Press, Boca Raton, FL, 1994.

Watt, G., Leptospirosis, *Infect. Curr. Opin. Dis.* **5:**659–663 (1992).

Faine, S., Leptospirosis, in: *Infectious Diseases*, 5th ed. (P. D. Hoeprich, M. C. Jordan, and A. R. Roland, eds.), pp. 619–625, Lippincott, Philadelphia, 1994.

Faine, S., *Leptospira*, in: *Topley and Wilson's Microbiology and Microbial Infections*, 9th ed., Vol. 2. *Systematic Bacteriology* (A. Balows and B. I. Duerden, eds.), pp. 1287–1303, Arnold, London, 1998.

Faine, S., Leptospirosis, in: *Topley and Wilson's Microbiology and Microbial Infections*, 9th ed., Vol. 3. *Bacterial Infections* (W. J. Hausler and M. Sussman, eds.), pp. 849–869, Arnold, London, 1998.

Farrar, W. E., *Leptospira* species (Leptospirosis), in: *Principles and Practice of Infectious Diseases*. 4th ed., Vol. 2 (G. L. Mandell, J. E. Bennett, and R. Dolin, eds.), pp. 2137–2141, Churchill Livingstone, New York, 1995.

CHAPTER 21

Listeria monocytogenes Infections

Donald Armstrong and Bruce G. Gellin

1. Introduction

Listeria monocytogenes has been recognized as a human pathogen since the turn of the century. Investigations of listeriosis epidemics in North America and Europe over the past 15 years have confirmed a long-held suspicion that listeriosis is a foodborne disease.[1–6] *Listeria monocytogenes* infections resulting in invasive disease occur most often in the immunocompromised host, specifically those in whom the T-helper cell–mononuclear phagocyte arm of the immune defense system is altered. Severe disease also occurs in the very young and very old as well as in patients with neoplastic disease and in recipients of organ transplants. Alcoholism and diabetes mellitus are also frequently associated risk factors, as are adrenocorticosteroid therapy for underlying disorders such as collagen vascular disease or inflammatory bowel disease. Although not a common opportunistic infection among patients with advanced human immunodeficiency virus (HIV) infections, listeriosis recently has been shown to be at least 100 times as frequent in acquired immunodeficiency syndrome (AIDS) patients than in the general population.[7–10] *L. monocytogenes* has a predilection for pregnant women, with potentially lethal consequences for the fetus *in utero* and the newborn. Normal hosts are not entirely resistant to invasive infections, and the occurrence of listeriosis in such individuals should not warrant an exhaustive search for an underlying but yet undiagnosed immunosuppressive disorder.

In immunocompromised and elderly adults (nonperinatal listeriosis), the clinical presentation is usually sepsis or meningitis, or a more subtle nonmeningitis central nervous system (CNS) infection such as meningoencephalitis, cerebritis, or brain abscess. While these severe forms of listeriosis have been well described, recent investigations of point-source foodborne outbreaks of listeriosis have further confirmed the clinical entity of a milder, noninvasive gastrointestinal illness characterized by fever, nausea, vomiting, diarrhea, and musculoskeletal symptoms, indistinguishable from other common presentations of food poisoning. Such an illness may be a prodrome of a more severe, invasive infection, especially in groups known to be at high risk for invasive disease.[2,11] Table 1 contains a categorization of *L. monocytogenes* infections.

In pregnant women (perinatal listeriosis), infection may present as a flulike illness with fever, headache, and myalgia and progress to amnionitis and premature labor. The corresponding intrauterine infection is usually apparent at birth or within the first few days of life. This congenital infection, granulomatosis infantisepticum, is characterized by a severe, often fatal, disseminated, multiorgan infection. In contrast, newborns who acquire listeriosis at the time of delivery or shortly thereafter are usually full term and the product of an uncomplicated pregnancy. These infants acquire *L. monocytogenes* at delivery when exposed to a contaminated birth canal or via nosocomial transmission in the hospital.[12–16] In this group, the clinical presentation is more likely to be meningitis than overwhelming sepsis.[17]

Sporadic cases are the rule, but outbreaks have been well described due to an expanding variety of contaminated foods including cole slaw, cheese, milk, and processed meats. The number of outbreaks recorded has been small and predominantly in North America and Europe. However, given the nature of the organism, there is no reason to believe that the disease is limited to these regions. Rather, listeriosis may be occurring but not de-

Donald Armstrong • Department of Medicine, Memorial Sloan-Kettering Cancer Center, New York, New York 10021. **Bruce G. Gellin** • Division of Microbiology and Infectious Diseases, National Institute of Allergy and Infectious Diseases, National Institutes of Health, Bethesda, Maryland 20892.

Table 1. *Listeria monocytogenes* **Infection**[a]

Host	Illness	Type of infection
Gravid woman	"Flulike" syndrome	Bacteremia and/or chorioamnionitis
Neonate	Disseminated, lethal septic disease	*In utero*, widely disseminated, multiorgan disease; "granulomatosis infantiseptica"
	Sepsis and/or meningitis	Postpartum bacteremia (may or may not progress to meningitis)
Adult (usually immunocompromised)	Sepsis and/or meningitis	Bacteremia (may or may not progress to meningitis)
	Meningoencephalitis, rhomboencephalitis, cerebritis or brain abscess	Subacute cerebritis (usually does not progress to brain abscess)
Any age	Focal infection[b]	Resulting from bacteremia or direct inoculation
	Gastroenteritis	Mild gastroenteritis following recent exposure to contaminated food product, usually self-limited

[a]Adapted from Armstrong,(131) with permission.
[b]Includes skin, ocular, lymph node, bacterial endocarditis, osteomyelitis, prosthetic joint infection, spinal or brain abscess, peritonitis, cholecystitis, and hepatitis.

tected due to difficulties with bacterial isolation and identification.(18) Nosocomial outbreaks have also been described in newborn nurseries and renal transplant units. Since pregnant women appear to be highly susceptible to this infection, the occurrence of listeriosis in pregnant women should alert public health officials to the possibility of communitywide exposure to *L. monocytogenes*, as it can be assumed that many more people are exposed than develop disease.

A recent Centers for Disease Control and Prevention (CDC) surveillance report documenting the decline in listeriosis incidence in the United States since the mid-1980s suggests that this has resulted from the combination of efforts by food manufacturers to minimize opportunities for *Listeria* to contaminate ready-to-eat products, stringent food regulations, and improved consumer education, and awareness regarding food safety.(19–23)

2. Historical Background

L. monocytogenes was first isolated from necrotic lesions in the liver of rabbits in 1919, and named *Bacillus hepatitis*.(24) This was the same year that French clinicians isolated and preserved a "diphtheroid" from spinal fluid cultures of a patient with meningitis, subsequently identified as *L. monocytogenes*.(25) In 1924, this organism was named *Bacterium monocytogenes* for the monocytosis that is associated with systemic illness in an outbreak among laboratory rabbits in England.(26,27) The etiologic agent of an epizootic among wild gerbils from South Africa was identified as *Listerella hepatolytica* in honor of the father of antisepsis, Joseph Lister.(28) The organism was named *L. monocytogenes* in 1940.(29,30) Despite the name of the organism, monocytosis is an atypical feature of human infections and an unreliable clinical clue.

Initially recognized as an infections of animals, *L. monocytogenes* was considered a veterinary disease, causing epizootics in sheep and cattle, with manifestations of abortions and basilar meningoencephalitis ("circling disease") in mammals. In humans, the association of a *Listeria* infection in pregnancy and severe disease in the fetus was first described in 1936,(31) and the association between *L. monocytogenes* and neoplastic disease was first reported by Louria and colleagues in 1967.(32) Since then, confirmatory reports have further identified a range of underlying conditions that increase the risk of listeriosis. These include: renal and other organ solid transplant patients,(33) alcoholism and cirrhosis,(34) diabetes mellitus, and conditions that are typified by dysfunctional T-helper lymphocytes and an altered mononuclear phagocyte system, including persons on immunosuppressive doses of adrenocorticosteroids,(35–38) and those with HIV infection.(7–10)

Foodborne outbreaks were first described in 1961 and 1962.(39,40) Other well-characterized food outbreaks have been reported more recently,(1–6) including a multihospital outbreak where a hospital food source was implicated but not fully documented.(41) Clusters of cases have also occurred among immunocompromised hosts and in hospital settings. Although the source of nosocomial transmission is rarely identified, a well-documented investigation of an outbreak of listeriosis among newborns at a hospital in Costa Rica linked to aspiration of mineral oil used to bathe infants provided overwhelming evidence that transmission is not limited to the ingestion of contaminated foods.(12,13,15,33,36,42–46)

Gastrointestinal carriage of *L. monocytogenes* without signs or symptoms of systemic listeriosis has been well documented. Prevalence rates in community studies range from 1–2% (patients with diarrhea and hospitalized adult patients) to 5–13% (healthy abattoir workers). Despite these carriage rates, disease has not been described in these populations and secondary cases within a household have not been documented. Recent studies have also documented the increased rate of asymptomatic stool carriage in up to one fifth of the household contacts of patients with listeriosis. This reinforces the importance of the susceptibility of the host that is exposed to this organism, constituting additional evidence that exposure greatly exceeds observed disease.[2,47–52]

3. Methodology

Since *L. monocytogenes* infections have not been reportable in most counties until recently, including the United States, accurate figures on incidence are not generally available. In an effort to improve the accuracy of surveillance data in the United States, in 1986 the Council of State and Territorial Epidemiologists (CSTE) recommended that listeriosis be made a reportable disease and highlighted the importance of clinical microbiology laboratories as an important source of case reports. Prior to this, the most comprehensive US study was based on hospital discharge data from hospitals participating in the Professional Activities Study (PAS) of the Commission on Professional and Hospital Activities (CPHA), a nonprofit, nongovernmental hospital discharge data system.[25] The data set was generated from the data bank of the CPHA-PAS participating hospitals using the discharge diagnosis of listeriosis during 1980, 1981, and 1982. The number of hospitals participating in PAS ranged from 1354 (1980) to 1283 (1982), with a mean of 1309 hospitals per year. These hospitals represented 22–23% of all short-term, nonfederal hospitals in the United States and included 27 to 29% of all US discharges from such hospitals. For each state, total hospitalizations for listeriosis were projected by dividing the number of cases from participating hospitals in a given state by the proportion of all the states' discharges that were from PAS hospitals. A more accurate measure of listeriosis in the United States has been reported by CDC investigators' active surveillance project that began in 1986 and collected data from biweekly communication with infection control coordinators at all acute care hospitals in a several state area (see below).[8,23]

Following four large foodborne outbreaks of listeriosis in North America in the early 1980s, the CDC initiated an active surveillance project with six geographically distinct state and county health departments covering a total population base of approximately 34 million persons, representing over 14% of the US population.[8] In these surveillance areas (Missouri, New Jersey, Oklahoma, Tennessee, Washington, and Los Angeles County), all patients in whom *L. monocytogenes* was isolated from cultures of normally sterile body sites were reported to the state's or county's Listeriosis Study Group coordinator via biweekly telephone reports by hospital-based contacts (usually the infection control nurse) at each of the 666 acute-care hospitals. A single-page case report form with demographic and clinical information was completed for each case. The clinical isolates of *L. monocytogenes* from these case patients were confirmed and serotyping and molecular fingerprinting by multilocus enzyme electrophoresis was performed to further characterize these clinical isolates. This multi-state active surveillance system has been maintained, with some modifications, since 1986, replacing the passive reporting system based on data from hospital discharge diagnoses.[25] This intensive, ongoing assessment of listeriosis in the United States over time has supplied a measure of the impact that educational efforts and the concomitant tightening of regulations of the food industry have had on the health of the public[23]

3.1. Sources of Mortality Data

Sources of mortality data include case reports, descriptions of outbreaks, reviews, and recent epidemiological surveillance and surveys.[8,23,53,54] Mortality rates vary considerably with the age and underlying medical condition of the host. Approximately 20% of pregnancies complicated by listeriosis result in intrauterine fetal death, but only rarely does this infection persist in the mother following delivery. However, the full impact of listeriosis in pregnancy may be underestimated, as suggested by a French study where researchers cultured *L. monocytogenes* from the placentas and/or fetuses of 1.6% of all pregnancies that resulted in preterm labor or spontaneous abortion.[55] In the severest form of congenital infection, granulomatosis infantisepticum, mortality has ranged from 33 to 100%.[47,56,57] In contrast, late-onset neonatal cases (onset between 8 and 28 days of life) are more likely to present with meningitis than sepsis and have a more favorable outcome compared with early-onset neonatal cases.[17] In the largest North American epidemic of listeriosis in Los Angeles in 1985, there was a 63% case fatality rate for early-onset neonatal cases, in contrast with a 37% case fatality rate among late-onset neonatal cases.[5]

The CDC's 1986 *Listeria* surveillance project documented that the case fatality rate in patients with sepsis (40%) was higher than that of patients with meningitis (27%), although the difference was not statistically different and may have been affected by a misclassification bias due to a lack of cerebrospinal fluid (CSF) cultures.[8] In foodborne outbreaks, overall case-fatality rates were approximately 30%.[1,3,5,6,53] Overall mortality rates have been estimated as 19–35%, with the rate increasing with increasing age.[8,23,53]

3.2. Sources of Morbidity Data

Since reported listeriosis cases are usually due to severe invasive disease, patients are usually hospitalized. Therefore, sources of morbidity data are similar to those of mortality data. Among 27 states participating in the National Bacterial Meningitis Surveillance Study, there were 265 cases of *Listeria* meningitis between 1978 and 1981.[58] In some regions, *Listeria* was reported as the second most common cause of neonatal meningitis (after Group B streptococcus) and the second most common cause of meningitis in individuals over 60 years old (after *Streptococcus pneumoniae*). Sources of morbidity data have also been obtained from epidemiological surveillance and from investigations of outbreaks of listeriosis.[2,15,23,47,56,57,59–64] The recent documentation of a mild, self-limited gastrointestinal syndrome associated with the ingestion of *Listeria*-contaminated food products highlights the fact that additional cases of *Listeria* infection in the community may go undetected.[2,11]

3.3. Surveys

The detection and investigation of recent epidemics underscores the need for improved surveillance of listeriosis. Even though the attack rate of epidemic listeriosis may be four- to sixfold higher than the background rate,[65] since the absolute attack rate during an epidemic may be as low as 0.8–2.0 per 10^5 population, an ongoing epidemic may not be observed in a community, especially if patients are being diagnosed and treated at several hospitals in the community. In the epidemic in Los Angeles County in 1985 associated with a contaminated Mexican-type soft cheese, the outbreak was detected by an alert infection control nurse in the county women's hospital that provides care for the largest segment of the Hispanic population. It was only after an unusual number of cases occurred in this hospital that Los Angeles County health official were notified and the full extent of the communitywide outbreak was revealed.[5] Had the 142 cases in Los Angeles County been distributed throughout the hospitals in the county, it is unlikely that the few patients at each hospital would have been other than a clinical curiosity.

3.4. Laboratory Diagnosis

3.4.1. Isolation and Identification of the Organism. Isolation and identification of the organism is not difficult as long as laboratory personnel recognize the importance of scrutinizing gram-positive, diphtheroidlike organisms for the possibility of being *L. monocytogenes*.[32,66] *L. monocytogenes* is motile and hemolytic, unlike other "diphtheroids." The organism's tumbling motility is best seen at room temperature and characteristic hemolysis may be minimal but enhanced with passage. Presumptive identification can be made based on these properties, while final identification requires an additional 24 hr.

In cases of meningitis, the organism is seen on gram stain in only 10% of cases. The absence of organisms on gram stain in the presence of a pleocytosis in the appropriate host should strongly raise the possibility of *L. monocytogenes*. When attempting to isolate the organism from food, stool, or environmental sources, holding specimens at 4°C has resulted in improved yields, but this "cold enrichment" technique has not been demonstrated to be more efficacious with clinical specimens such as CSF, blood, or others.[66] The cold enrichment method has been improved upon by the United States Department of Agriculture's (USDA) culture method.[67,68] Because of concern of *Listeria* contamination in the food industry,[69] a variety of rapid diagnostic techniques have been developed for its detection in food and environmental samples. These have included DNA probes based on the listeriolysin O gene sequence or species-specific rDNA sequences,[46,70,71] monoclonal antibodies to cell surface antigens,[72] and polymerase chain reaction (PCR).[73,74]

Of the seven species of *Listeria*, *L. monocytogenes* is considered to be the principal human pathogen, although there are case reports of invasive listeriosis caused by species other than *L. monocytogenes*.[34,75,76] There are 11 serotypes of *L. monocytogenes*, differentiated on the basis of agglutination of somatic (O) and flagellar (H) antigens.[52,66,77] Serotypes 1/2a, 1/2b, and 4b account for over 90% of all isolates, although the distribution of these serotypes may vary by geographic region.[8,23,61,66,78] Other than the fact that the majority of *Listeria* infections are caused by these three serotypes, no clinical differences in disease presentation or severity have been demonstrated among the various serotypes.[17]

Since just three principal serotypes cause most human disease, this subtyping system has been of limited use in epidemiological investigations, such as attempts to link sporadic cases of listeriosis to an implicated food item or environmental specimen. More discriminatory subtyping techniques include phage typing,[79] multilocus enzyme electrophoresis,[80–83] restriction fragment length polymorphism (RFLP),[84–87] ribosomal DNA fingerprinting (ribotyping),[88–90] and PCR-based randomly amplified polymorphic DNA patterns (RAPD).[91]

3.4.2. Serological and Immunological Diagnostic Methods. *L. monocytogenes* has several antigens that cross-react with other gram-positive organisms; therefore, false-positive serological results may occur. Further, gastrointestinal carriage studies and the recently described mild gastrointestinal manifestations of *L. monocytogenes* infection suggest that exposure may be widespread.[11] Therefore, *Listeria* agglutination titers may be detected in persons without evidence of having experienced invasive listeriosis. Earlier attempts at serological diagnosis were limited by the lack of sensitivity and specificity of the available assays, and false-negative serological tests were observed in patients with culture-proven listeriosis, especially in newborns and immunosuppressed patients,[6,66,77,92–94] however, the use of an improved antilisteriolysin O assay as part of a recent outbreak investigation shows promise for such investigations.[2] Like many serological tests, this one offers little assistance in the clinical management of a patient.

4. Biological Characteristics of the Organism

Its precise ecological niche is unknown, but *L. monocytogenes* has been isolated from a wide variety of environmental sources. Its survival in the environment was best documented from quantitative bacterial counts demonstrating persistence of viable organisms for at least 2 months in various agricultural settings.[95] Carriage studies have repeatedly demonstrated that the organism can survive in the human gastrointestinal track.[47–52] In addition, it has been shown to live in the gastrointestinal and genital tract of a variety of animals ranging from shellfish to birds and most mammals. Its predilection to immunocompromised hosts, including pregnant women, attests to its low pathogenicity in immunologically normal individuals.

5. Descriptive Epidemiology

Initially described as a zoonosis, *L. monocytogenes* is responsible for abortion, mastitis, septicemia, meningitis, and encephalitis in cattle and sheep and is the etiologic agent of circling disease. Zoonotics in sheep and cattle have been attributed to poor-quality silage, a link that has been speculative and only rarely documented.[96,97]

The investigation of a series of outbreaks of human listeriosis since the early 1980s has clearly demonstrated that listeriosis is a foodborne disease. Although the bulk of human listeriosis occurs as individual "sporadic" cases rather than in the setting of an outbreak, investigations of such cases have continued to demonstrate that they often result from an encounter between a susceptible person and a *Listeria*-contaminated food item. Because of concern of *Listeria* contamination in the food industry, a variety of rapid diagnostic methods have been developed to detect *L. monocytogenes* in food and environmental samples, including restriction fragment length polymorphism (RFLP), ribosomal DNA fingerprinting (ribotyping), and PCR-based randomly amplified polymorphic DNA (RAPD) patterns.[21,46,70,72,80] The lessons learned from the investigation of these epidemics regarding foods at high risk of *Listeria* contamination coupled with increased concern of food safety at a microbiological level is likely responsible for the marked decline in human listeriosis in the United States over the past decade.[23] After initially concentrating on dairy products, both FDA and USDA's Food Safety Inspection Service (FSIS) have broadened their surveillance for *Listeria*-contaminated products following a well-documented case of listeriosis that was linked to a contaminated turkey frankfurter.[19–22,98,99] Following the epidemics in the early 1980s, these agencies ultimately developed a "zero tolerance" posture. In 1986, the first full year of the program, over 40 commercial food products were recalled or kept from being distributed due to *L. monocytogenes* contamination.[8] Since then, over 30 food recalls have been initiated each year, including ready-to-eat delicatessen meats and poultry products, prepared salads, and seafoods.[23,54]

5.1. Prevalence and Incidence

5.1.1. Asymptomatic Carriage. Epidemiological evidence that listeriosis is a usually a foodborne infection is further strengthened by studies of asymptomatic gastrointestinal carriage. This has been well documented, although prevalence rates have varied in different studies as a function of the subject selection, sampling frame, and culture technique. However, since the identification of *L. monocytogenes* from cultures of samples contaminated with other bacteria can be difficult and since many of these carriage studies were conducted prior to the development of selective and sensitive culture techniques, it cannot be certain that these rates reflect only pathological strains of *Listeria*. Nevertheless, these rates have ranged from 1–5%

in community-based studies to 5–29% in healthy abattoir workers and poultry workers to 8–26% among household members of listeriosis patients, the latter presumably having similar exposure risks as the case patient, further evidence that exposure may greatly exceed observed disease.[47,50,51,54]

5.1.2. Gastroenteritis. The isolation of *L. monocytogenes* from stool may be problematic. Population-based studies of listeriosis have focused on invasive disease with a case definition that depends on the recovery of *L. monocytogenes* from a normally sterile site. Therefore, the full burden of *L. monocytogenes* morbidity is also likely to have been underestimated. Mild gastrointestinal illness attributed to listeriosis only recently has been documented,[2,11] but it is indistinguishable from a variety of pathogens and conditions that are characterized by similar symptoms.

5.1.3. Invasive Infection. Despite the indirect evidence from food microbiology and gastrointestinal carriage studies that exposure to pathogenic *L. monocytogenes* is common, serious infection is rare. Infection occurs primarily among pregnant women and their neonates, hosts immunocompromised by their underlying illnesses or medications, and the elderly.[18,100] Prior to the CDC's active surveillance studies and the CSTE's recommendation for laboratory reporting of cases of listeriosis in 1986, estimates of the incidence of listeriosis depended on passive reporting systems or hospital discharge data.[53] These methods were acknowledged to underestimate the true burden of disease and made it difficult for direct comparisons of incidence data collected in different ways.[52,53] The CDC's study of hospital discharge data between 1980 and 1982 estimated the annual incidence of listeriosis in the United States to be $0.36/10^5$, accounting for approximately 800 cases and over 150 deaths (case-fatality rate, 19%). In contrast, in the CDC's more intensive 1986 active surveillance study incidence rates were nearly twice that estimated by hospital discharge data.[8] In Europe in 1986–1987, incidence rates ranged from $0.5/10^5$ in the United Kingdom to $1.1/10^5$ in France.[1,101] Whether these differences reflect true difference in incidence or differences in surveillance and reporting have not been assessed.[60–63,102]

The CDC's active surveillance project identified 246 cases of listeriosis that occurred among residents of the surveillance areas in 1986; the overall incidence was $0.7/10^5$: 67 perinatal cases ($12.7/10^5$ live births) and 179 cases in nonpregnant adults (nonperinatal cases, incidence = $0.5/10^5$). From these data it was estimated that in 1986 at least 1700 cases of listeriosis occurred in the United States annually, resulting in approximately 450 deaths. On average, the case-fatality rate among the nonperinatal *Listeria* infections is 35%, with worse clinical outcomes with advancing age. The incidence of listeriosis increases with advancing age; more than 80% of patients with listeriosis are over 50 years of age and over 40% are 70 years of age or more[8] (Fig. 1).

Twenty-one percent of the pregnancies complicated by *L. monocytogenes* infections resulted in intrauterine fetal death, including two multiple gestation pregnancies. Gestational age was not uniformly reported; however, the earliest documented gestational age reported was 11 weeks. Perinatal incidence was four times higher in Los Angeles ($24.3/10^5$) than in other areas ($5.2/10^5$ births, $p = 5 \times 10^{-5}$), and race-specific perinatal rates in Los Angeles were higher among blacks ($51.1/10^5$ births than among whites ($21.7/10^5$ births) or Hispanics ($22/10^5$ births), $p = 0.03$. The perinatal rate for whites and blacks in Los Angeles was higher than comparable race-specific rates in the other areas (whites = $10.7/10^5$ births, blacks $5.6/10^5$ live births, $p = 0.003$). The higher rates could not be attributed to maternal age or serotype distribution. Since this surveillance study occurred during the year following the well-publicized cheese-borne listeriosis epidemic in Los Angeles, it was speculated that clinicians may have had a heightened index of suspicion and increased the number of cultures they performed to rule out a *Listeria* infection.

In the CDC's 1986 surveillance project, 162 clinical isolates were serotyped. Three serotypes (1/2a, 1/2b, and 4b) accounted for nearly 95% of all strains: 30% were

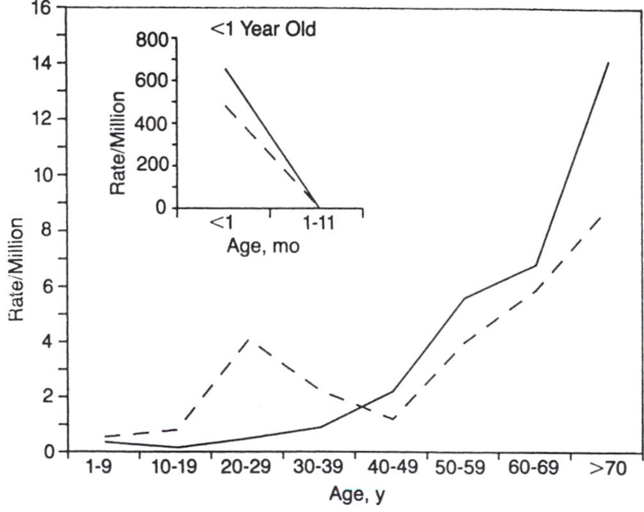

Figure 1. Age-specific incidence of listeriosis, by sex, 1988. Solid line indicates male patients; dashed line, female patients. Reprinted with permission from Ciesielski *et al.*[53]

serotype 1/2a, 32% serotype 1/2b, and 33% serotype 4b. The remaining nine strains were distributed among three additional serotypes: 3a, 3b, and 1/2c. These isolates were further subtyped by multilocus enzyme electrophoresis and found to be distributed among 37 distinct electrophoretic types, a method by which all strains can be typed.[80] This demonstrated both the diversity of the species and the promise of molecular biological techniques to clarify the epidemiology of listeriosis.[8]

The more recent CDC active surveillance system report documents a 44% and 48% reduction in invasive listeriosis infection and death, respectively, compared with 1989 data, and statistically significant decreases in both nonperinatal and perinatal disease to $0.4/10^6$ and $8.6/10^5$ births, respectively. It is likely that multifaceted prevention efforts by industry, food regulatory agencies, and from widely disseminated consumer guidelines have been responsible for this decline[19–23,99] (Fig. 2).

5.2. Epidemic Behavior and Contagiousness

With the marked exception of the well-documented nosocomial outbreak of neonatal listeriosis traced to contaminated mineral oil used to bathe newborns,[15] the majority of listeriosis epidemics have implicated contaminated food items.[103] Foods have included milk,[2,3] soft cheese,[1,5] cole slaw,[6] pate,[104] and processed meats.[4,54,98] Contamination of dairy products may have occurred either from contaminated milk obtained from cows with *Listeria* mastitis or as a result of in-process or postpasteurization contamination of products being prepared and packaged in *Listeria*-contaminated environments. The cole slaw contamination was attributed to the local practice of fertilizing with sheep manure. Unfortunately, in this circumstance the source of manure was from a sheep herd that had apparently suffered a *Listeria* epizootic. Since the cabbage was kept in silos over the winter, enhancement of bacterial growth by an unintentional cold enrichment process was also considered as a contributory factor.

It is apparent that in several of the communitywide outbreaks linked to contaminated food items, many more are exposed than become ill.[2,105] Carriage studies have shown that elevated rates of asymptomatic carriage in household contacts of listeriosis patients and in members of the community at large occur, even among individuals considered to be at high risk of acquiring listeriosis.[37,50,51,106] Other than for vertical transmission from a pregnant woman to her fetus, no cases have been linked to person-to-person transmission although outbreaks among neonates in hospital settings has raised suspicion about cross-contamination.[14,16,107–109] As discussed previously, an outbreak in a neonatal unit in Costa Rica was linked to mineral oil that had been initially contaminated by an infant with listeriosis and was the source of subsequent infections when infants aspirated this contaminated oil while being bathed.

The recent description of a milder, noninvasive form of listeriosis characterized predominantly by gastrointestinal symptoms has demonstrated a broader spectrum of

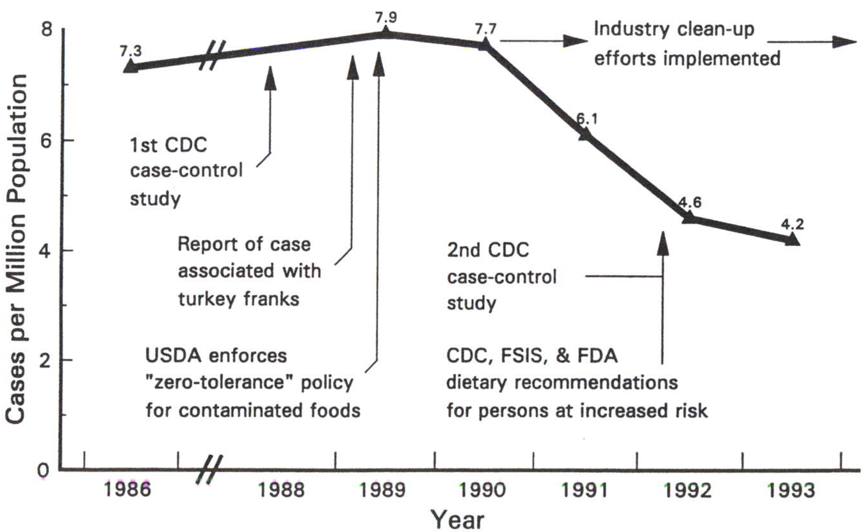

Figure 2. Incidence of listeriosis in the United Staes, 1986–1993. Reprinted with permission from Tappero *et al.*[23]

illness; however, there is no evidence that differences in clinical presentation are linked to strain-specific differences among *L. monocytogenes* isolates. In contrast, although there are case reports of *Listeria* species other than *L. monocytogenes* causing disease, all strains of *L. monocytogenes* are considered to be potential pathogens. The reason why just 3 of the 11 serotypes are responsible for the bulk of disease remains unanswered.[2,11]

The infectious dose of *L. monocytogenes* in humans is not known, although it is likely that there is an interaction between host susceptibility and the size of the inoculum. This is supported by feeding studies of steroid-treated mice,[110] Sprague-Dawley rats with altered gastric acidity,[103] and feeding trials in nonhuman primates.[111,112] Nevertheless, since the bacterial counts of *Listeria*-contaminated food items may increase with prolonged shelf life and since differences in host defense mechanisms influence susceptibility to *L. monocytogenes*, a zero tolerance standard has been adopted by the food industry.[69,112,113]

5.3. Geographic Distribution

Surveillance studies, outbreak investigations, and case reports of listeriosis, coupled with its ubiquity in the environment, suggest that *L. monocytogenes* has a worldwide distribution. Differences in disease rates have been attributed to differences in surveillance and/or the likelihood of exposure to foods that may be contaminated.

5.4. Temporal Distribution

The incidence of listeriosis is generally believed to be higher in humans from the late spring to early fall.[8] In other animals it appears more often in the winter. Presumably this is related to seasonal exposure to contaminated food or environmental sources, but this has not been adequately documented.

5.5. Age

The very young and very old have the highest incidence rates and mortality rates. Beyond the neonatal period, the incidence of listeriosis remains low until the fifth decade of life, when it increases with advancing age. More than 40% of cases occurring in individuals 70 years of age or more.[8,23] In the immunosuppressed patient the age varies with the reason for immunosuppression and the age of onset of the underlying immunosuppressing condition (e.g., pregnancy, organ transplantation, and HIV infection) (Fig. 1).

5.6. Sex

Other than the predilection for pregnant women, there are no significant gender-specific differences in incidence, clinical presentation, or severity of disease.

5.7. Race

Differential rates of disease may be associated with food items to which some groups may be more likely to be exposed; however, there are no data to support differences in disease that are inherent to specific racial or ethnic groups.

5.8. Occupation

Other than a handful of case reports of cutaneous listeriosis among laboratory personnel working with *L. monocytogenes* and veterinarians and ranchers participating in the delivery of infected and aborted calves, there are no defined occupational risks for developing invasive listeriosis.[114–116] Groups with greater exposure to the organism may have higher gastrointestinal carriage rates, however, but there is no evidence that disease is more common.

5.9. Occurrence in Different Settings

In addition to communitywide foodborne epidemics, small outbreaks in organ transplant units and newborn nurseries have been described.[33,52,117]

5.10. Socioeconomic Factors

There are no known socioeconomic factors that affect risk of acquiring listeriosis.

5.11. Other Factors

Several reports have suggested that underlying gastrointestinal conditions such as reduced gastric acidity,[41,103] a concomitant gastrointestinal infection,[118,119] or a recent gastrointestinal procedure[120,121] may facilitate invasion and result in a systemic infection. Whether these represent true risk factors is a hypothesis that has yet to be adequately addressed.

6. Mechanisms and Routes of Transmission

The growing number of reports of sporadic listeriosis traced to a contaminated food product and the evidence of contaminated foods as the source of communitywide outbreaks has confirmed that listeriosis is a principally foodborne infection, although the well-documented epidemic of nosocomial listeriosis traced to contaminated mineral oil aspirated by newborn infants in the nursery demonstrate the epidemic potential in other settings.[15] However, given the ecology of this organism, it is likely that contaminated food products are ultimately linked to an infected animal, with the subsequent direct or indirect contamination of selected food products during preparation, processing, or packaging. The gastrointestinal reservoir offers the potential for person-to-person transmission via fecal–oral spread, but there is no evidence to support this hypothesis.[51] As noted earlier, direct contact with this bacterium has resulted in focal infections in laboratory workers and in those attending the delivery of infected or aborted calves.[114–116]

7. Pathogenesis and Immunity

The investigation of outbreaks and well-documented point-sources of exposure to *Listeria*-contaminated foods has helped to clarify the incubation period of foodborne listeriosis and may range from 2 to 4 weeks.[5,11] Several well-documented sporadic cases linked to ingestion of contaminated food products[80,90,104,122] have also demonstrated that the incubation period may be as short as 2 or 3 days.[2,11,90] In addition, there are also reports that suggest that it may be considerably longer, although documentation of a precise point of exposure limits generalizations of reports of protracted incubation periods.[5] Also, persons with known risk factors for listeriosis may be transient asymptomatic carriers and never develop invasive disease.[123]

Once it invades, the organism appears to reside in the protected environment of nonactivated macrophages where it is shielded from antibiotics, a feature that has important implications for antimicrobial therapy. As *in vitro* human enterocytelike model suggests that *L. monocytogenes* is protected by intracellular vacuoles resulting from phagocytosis and that listerolysin O, a hemolysin with structural and physiological similarities to hemolysins of *Streptococcus pneumoniae* and *Streptococcus pyogenes*, constitutes the virulence factor whereby the intravacuolar bacteria can escape into the cytoplasm proper, an environment conducive to replication.[124–127] Only *L. monocytogenes* and *L. ivanovii*, but not other species of *Listeria*, produce this toxin.[125,128] In the 1960s, the importance of the mononuclear phagocyte in host resistance to *L. monocytogenes* was demonstrated.[129,130] Subsequently, it was shown that antibody, complement, and T-helper lymphocytes were active in this infection.[131] It appears that the nonactivated macrophage may also be important in host defenses in listeriosis and may protect even in the absence of activated macrophages.

8. Patterns of Host Response

8.1. Patterns of Host Response

The response observed in histopathologic studies of both animal models and human disease varies from the production of a neutrophilic exudate to granulomas. This is reflected in the CSF pleocytosis, which varies from a predominantly neutrophilic to a predominantly mononuclear response. The investigation of foodborne epidemics and recent documentation of a mild form of listeriosis with predominantly gastrointestinal manifestations suggests that the gastrointestinal tract is the initial portal of entry; however, no gastrointestinal lesion has been consistently observed. Investigators of an epidemic in Philadelphia caused by several different strains of *L. monocytogenes* hypothesized that a predisposing gastrointestinal infection with another pathogen may have impaired the gastrointestinal barrier, increasing susceptibility for *Listeria* invasion.[118,119]

8.1.1. Nonperinatal Listeriosis. In immunocompromised and elderly adults, the clinical presentation is usually one of sepsis or meningitis, meningoencephalitis, cerebritis, or a brain abscess. A noninvasive gastrointestinal illness characterized by fever, nausea, vomiting, diarrhea, and musculoskeletal symptoms has recently been described; however, this has not consistently been observed as a prodrome of an invasive infection.[11] Focal infections, the result of or a concomitant bacteremia, may occur at virtually any site, most commonly affecting the central nervous system. Similar to patients with *Listeria* sepsis and meningitis, these usually occur in people with T-helper-cell defects.

Relative to other opportunistic infections, there have been relatively few cases of listeriosis reported in patients with AIDS, although recent studies have demonstrated that listeriosis in AIDS patients is at least 100 times more frequent than in the general population.[7,8,10,36] This is particularly ironic since the importance of T-cell immunity and cell-mediated resistance to infection was first demonstrated experimentally with *L. monocytogenes* in the early 1960s.[129,130] That this infection is not more common in HIV infection may reflect that nonactivated macrophages, monocytes, and neutrophils may play an important role in immune protection against *Listeria*.[9,132,133]

8.1.2. Perinatal Listeriosis. Case reports and case series have demonstrated that *L. monocytogenes* infections tend to complicate later stage pregnancies, but perinatal infection can occur as early as the first trimester.[8,134] Perinatal cases of listeriosis may be underdiagnosed, especially when a pregnancy ends in a fetal death. A French study cultured *L. monocytogenes* from the placentas and/or fetuses of 1.6% of all pregnancies that resulted in preterm labor or spontaneous abortion.[55] Listeriosis should be suspected in a pregnant woman with chills and fever with no obvious source, especially if the fever is accompanied by signs of a threatened abortion. A newborn or neonate with evidence of sepsis with or without meningitis should be suspected of *Listeria* infection.

8.2. Diagnosis

The CDC's active surveillance documented a marked difference in perinatal listeriosis in different regions of the United States, with significantly higher rates in Los Angeles Country, the year following the large outbreak among pregnant women and newborns traced to a contaminated locally produced fresh cheese product. However, there was no evidence that the 1985 outbreak was continuing. Rather, it was suspected that a heightened index of suspicion for listeriosis in pregnancy was in large part responsible for the increased detection in this setting.[8] This episode highlights the need for clinicians to suspect listeriosis when confronted with unexplained fever in pregnant women and immunocompromised and elderly hosts. Blood cultures and spinal cultures, when appropriate, should routinely be obtained. Given the difficulty of isolation of *Listeria* from clinical specimens from nonsterile sites and substantial rates of asymptomatic gastrointestinal carriage, stool cultures are not sufficiently sensitive or specific to be a helpful diagnostic aid. Though not of assistance in clinical settings, improved serological tests of antilisteriolysin O may prove useful in clarifying the epidemiology of this infection.

8.3. Differential Diagnosis

The differential diagnosis in a patient with meningitis includes *Streptococcus pneumoniae*, *Neisseria meningitidis*, or *Haemophilus influenzae*. In patients with T-helper-cell defects, *Cryptococcus neoformans* should be included in the differential diagnosis. The absence of organisms on gram stain may suggest tuberculosis or a partially treated bacterial meningitis as well as *Listeria* meningitis; therefore, a patient with meningitis and a CSF pleocytosis without organisms seen on gram stain should be suspected of *Listeria* meningitis.[44] Similarly, a clinical presentation of cerebritis with a normal CSF should also raise suspicion of *Listeria* cerebritis. In the former, the organism can be expected to be isolated from the CSF, even though not seen. In the latter, the bacteria should be isolated from blood, but may not be recovered from the CSF. The picture of clinical sepsis without meningitis or other localizing features in a patient with a T-helper-cell defect may be produced by a number of organisms, including *Salmonella* species, mycobacteria species, *Cryptococcus neoformans*, *Histoplasma capsulatum*, *Coccidioides immitis*, or cytomegalovirus. Rarely, *Pneumocystis carinii* pneumonia may occur without pulmonary symptoms. *Listeria* cerebritis appears to be rather unique in that symptoms and bacteremia may occur over a longer period of time before forming a brain abscess compared with other organisms, a manifestation that has been confused with *Toxoplasma gondii* encephalitis. In the pregnant woman, the illness resembles influenza or a urinary tract infection. In the neonate, the usual causes of neonatal sepsis and meningitis such as *Escherichia coli*, *Klebsiella pneumoniae*, group B streptococci, the enterococci, and *Bacillus* species must be considered.[135]

9. Control and Prevention

9.1. General Concepts

Although two outbreaks have implicated pasteurized milk,[2,3] there is ample evidence that routine pasteurization procedures easily eliminates *Listeria*.[136,137] This stresses the importance of reducing opportunities for post-pasteurization contamination.[30] Immunocompromised hosts, such as those with T-helper-cell defects, and pregnant women should be educated as to the dangers of improperly processed dairy products, poorly washed raw vegetables, and inadequately cooked meat products.

9.2. Antibiotic and Chemotherapeutic Approaches to Prophylaxis and Treatment

As person-to-person transmission is not a feature of listeriosis, isolation of patients with listeriosis is not warranted. Data on treatment for enteric listeriosis or to guide postexposure prophylaxis, especially in pregnant women, are lacking. In high-risk patients with a known exposure, such prophylaxis is not generally recommended. Given its spectrum of activity and its ability to cross the blood–brain barrier, the antibiotic of choice has traditionally been ampicillin with or without gentamicin. Trimethoprim–sulfamethoxazole, generically called cotrimoxazole, has also been used successfully; however, there are too few

Table 2. Differential Diagnosis and Treatment of *Listeria monocytogenes* Infections[a]

Category	Differential diagnosis	Treatment: First choice[b]	Treatment: Second choice[c]
Pregnancy infections	Influenza Pyelonephritis Chorioamnionitis Septic abortion	Ampicillin or penicillin	TMP-SMX, erythromycin; ? vancomycin
Granulomatosis infantiseptica	Neonatal sepsis Neonatal meningitis due to enteric bacilli, group B streptococcus	Ampicillin or penicillin	TMP-SMX, erythromycin; ? vancomycin
Sepsis	Sepsis of unknown source	Ampicillin or penicillin	TMP-SMX, erythromycin; ? vancomycin
Meningoencephalitis	Viral encephalitis, metabolic encephalopathy or psychiatric illness Infection due to *Streptococcus pneumoniae*, *Haemophilus influenzae*, *Neisseria meningitidis*, *Cryptococcus neoformans* or *Mycobacterium tuberculosis* in immunosuppressed patients or group B streptococci or enteric bacilli in neonates	Ampicillin or penicillin, possibly with gentamicin intrathecally	TMP-SMX, erythromycin, and/or chloramphenicol; ? vancomycin
Cerebritis	Brain abscess, tumor, stroke	Ampicillin or penicillin	TMP-SMX, erythromycin; ? vancomycin
Focal infections	Varies with site	Ampicillin or penicillin	TMP-SMX, erythromycin, and/or tetracycline; ? vancomycin
Gastroenteritis	Bacterial gastroenteritis Viral gastroenteritis	No data available	

[a]Adapted from Armstrong, with permission.
[b]Ampicillin, 200 mg/kg/day intravenously in six divided doses; penicillin, 300,000 units/kg/day intravenously in six divided doses; gentamicin, 6 mg/kg/day intravenously in four divided doses.
[c]TMP-SMX, trimethoprim–sulfamethoxazole as 20 mg/kg/day of the trimethoprim component in four divided doses; Erythromycin, 60 mg/kg/day intravenously in four divided doses; tetracycline, 15 mg/kg/day intravenously in four divided doses; chloramphenicol, 60 /mg/kg/day intravenously in four divided doses.

cases nationwide to readily do a comparative trial unless a large multicenter study is organized.[45,138–140] Comparative clinical trials have not been conducted to assess the most efficacious treatment for listeriosis. There are case reports of treatment failures or relapses among patients treated with vancomycin or a cephalosporin[141] (Table 2).

9.3. Immunization

Because of the potential economic consequences of listeriosis outbreaks in farm animals, a variety of *Listeria* vaccines have been developed for agricultural use, but none are routinely used. No vaccine has been developed for use in humans.

10. Unresolved Problems

The CDC's active surveillance system has highlighted the importance of community-based surveillance and prompt reporting of cases. The recent description of a mild form of listeriosis raises the question as to the degree to which *L. monocytogenes* is responsible for self-limited community-acquired gastrointestinal illness. These cases could serve as sentinels for an undetected common-source food item or an outbreak.

A further investigation into the virulence factors that separate pathogenic and nonpathogenic strains of *Listeria* and more specific host factors that determine susceptibility may help to better target preventive strategies for minimizing exposure to these pathogens and further reducing the substantial morbidity and mortality that these ubiquitous organisms have on the health of the public.

11. References

1. Bille, J., Epidemiology of human listeriosis in Europe, with special reference to the Swiss outbreak, in: *Topics in Industrial Microbiology: Foodborne Listeriosis* (A. J. Miller, J. L. Smith, and G. A. Somkuti, eds.), pp. 71–74, Elsevier, Amsterdam, 1990.
2. Dalton, C. B., Austin, C. C., Sobel, J., Hayes, P. S., Bibb, W. F., Graves, L. M., Swaminathat, B., Proctor, M. E., and Griffin, P. M.,

An outbreak of gastroenteritis and fever due to Listeria monocytogenes in milk, *N. Engl. J. Med.* **336:**100–105 (1997).
3. Fleming, D. W., Cochi, S. L., MacDonald, L. K., Brondum, J., Hayes, P. S., Plikaytis, B. O., Holmes, M. B., Audurier, A., Broome, C. V., and Reingold, A. L., Pasteurized milk as a vehicle of infection in an outbreak of listeriosis, *N. Engl. J. Med.* **312:**404–407 (1985).
4. Goulet, V., Lepoutre, A., Roucourt, J., Courtieu, A. L., Dehaumont, P., and Veit, P., Epidemie de listeriose en France: Bilan final et resultats de l'enquete epidemiologique, *Bull. Epidemiol. Hebdomadaire* **39:**13–14 (1993).
5. Linnan, M. J., Mascola, L., Lou, X. D., Goulet, V., May, S., Salminen, C., Hird, D. W., Yonnekura, L., Hayes, P., Weaver, R., Audurier, A., Plikaytis, B. D., Fannin, S. L., Kleks, A., and Broome, C. V., Epidemic listeriosis associated with Mexican-style cheese, *N. Engl. J. Med.* **319:**823–828 (1988).
6. Schlech, W. F., Lavigne, P. M., Bortolussi, R. A., Allen, A. C., Haldane, E. V., Wort, A. J., Hightower, A. W., Johnson, S. E., King, J. H., Nicholls, E. S., and Broome, C. V., Epidemic listeriosis—Evidence for transmission by food, *N. Engl. J. Med.* **308:**203–206 (1983).
7. Ewert, D. P., Lieb, L., Hayes, P. S., Reeves, M. W., and Mascola, L., *Listeria monocytogenes* infection and serotype distribution among HIV-infected persons in Los Angeles County, 1985–1992, *J. Acquir. Immune Defic. Syndr. Hum. Retrovirol.* **8:**461–465 (1995).
8. Gellin, B. G., Broome, C. V., Bibb, W. F., Weaver, R. E., Gaventa, S., Mascola, L., and the Listeriosis Study Group, The epidemiology of listeriosis in the United States—1986, *Am. J. Epidemiol.* **133:**392–401 (1991).
9. Jacobs, J. L., and Murray, H. W., Why is *Listeria monocytogenes* not a pathogen in the acquired immunodeficiency syndrome? [editorial], *Arch. Intern. Med.* **146:**1299 (1986).
10. Jurado, R. L., Farley, M. M., Pereira, E., Harvey, R. C., Schuchat, A., Wenger, J. D., and Stephens, D. S., Increased risk of meningitis and bacteremia due to *Listeria monocytogenes* in patients with human immunodeficiency virus infection, *Clin. Infect. Dis.* **71:**224–227 (1993).
11. Riedo, F. X., Pinner, R. W., Tosca, M. L., Cartter, M. L., Graves, L. M., Reeves, M. W., Weaver, R. E., Plikaytis, B. D., and Broome, C. V., A point-source foodborne listeriosis outbreak: Documented incubation period and possible mild illness, *J. Infect. Dis.* **170:**693–696 (1994).
12. Filice, G. A., Cantrell, H. F., Smith, A. B., Hayes, P. S., Feeley, J. C., and Fraser, D. W., *Listeria monocytogenes* infection in neonates: Investigation of an epidemic, *J. Infect. Dis.* **138:**17–23 (1978).
13. Levy, E., and Nassau, E., Experience with listeriosis in the newborn. An account of a small epidemic in a nursery ward, *Ann. Paediatr.* **194:**321–330 (1960).
14. Pejaver, R. K., Watson, A. H., and Mucklow, E. S., Neonatal cross-infection with *Listeria monocytogenes*, *J. Infect.* **26:**301–303 (1993).
15. Schuchat, A., Lizano, C., Broome, C. V., Swaminathan, B., Kim, C., and Winn, K., Outbreak of neonatal listeriosis associated with mineral oil, *Pediatr. Infect. Dis. J.* **10:**183–189 (1991).
16. Simmons, M. D., Cockroft, P. M., and Okubadejo, O. A., Neonatal listeriosis due to cross-contamination in an obstetric theatre, *J. Infect.* **13:**235–239 (1986).
17. Albritton, W. L., Wiggins, G. L., and Feely, J. C., Neonatal listeriosis: Distribution of serotypes in relation to age at onset of disease, *J. Pediatr.* **88:**481–483 (1976).
18. Gellin, B. G., and Broome, C. V., Listeriosis, *J. Am. Med. Assoc.* **261:**1313–1320 (1989).
19. Food and Drug Administration, Efforts to prevent foodborne listeriosis, *J. Am. Med. Assoc.* **268:**180–181 (1992).
20. Food Safety and Inspection Service, Testing for *Listeria monocytogenes*, *Fed. Reg.* **52:**7464, March 11, 1987.
21. Food Safety and Inspection Service, Revised policy for controlling *Listeria monocytogenes*, *Fed. Reg.* **54:**22345–22346, May 23, 1989.
22. Food Safety and Inspection Service, Microbiological monitoring program: Sampling, testing procedures and actions for *Listeria monocytogenes* and *Salmonella*, FSIS Directive 10.240.1., Washington, DC, August 30, 1990.
23. Tappero, J. W., Schuchat, A., Deaver, K. A., Mascola, L., Wenger, J. D., and the Listeriosis Study Group, Reduction in the incidence of human listeriosis in the United States: Effectiveness of prevention efforts? *J. Am. Med. Assoc.* **273:**1118–1122 (1995).
24. Hulphers, G., Lefvernekros hos kanin orsakad af en ej forut beskrifven bakteria, *Medlemsbl. Sverge Vet. Forb.* **11**(Suppl): 10–16 (1959).
25. Cotoni, L., A proposdes bacteries denommees *Listeria* rappel d'une observation ancienne de meningite chez l'homme, *Ann. Microbiol. Paris* **68:**92–95 (1942).
26. Anton, W., Kritisch-experimenteller Beitrag zur Biologie des *Bakteriium Monocytogenes*, *Zentralbl. Bakteriol. Mikrobiol. Hyg. A* **131:**89–103 (1934).
27. Murray, E. G. D., Webb, R. A., and Swann, M. B. R., A disease of rabbits characterized by a large mononuclear leucocytosis caused by a hitherto undescribed bacillus, *Bacterium monocytogenes*, *J. Pathol. Bacteriol.* **29:**407–439 (1926).
28. Pirie, J. H. H., A new disease of veld rodents "Tiger River Disease," *Publ. S. Afr. Inst. Med. Res.* **3**(13)**:**163–187 (1927).
29. Hoeprich, P. D., Infection due to *Listeria monocytogenes*, *Medicine* **37:**143–160 (1958).
30. Seelinger, H. P. R., and Jones, D., *Listeria*, in: *Bergey's Manual of Systematic Bacteriology*, Vol. 2 (P. H. Sneath, ed.), pp. 1235–1245, Williams and Wilkins, Baltimore, 1986.
31. Burn, C. G., Clinical and pathological features of an infection caused by a new pathogen of the genus *Listerella*, *Am. J. Pathol.* **12:**341–349 (1936).
32. Louria, D. B., Hensle, T., Armstrong, D., Collins, H. S., Blevins, A., Krugman, D., and Buse, M., Listeriosis complicating malignant disease, a new association, *Ann. Intern. Med.* **67:**261–281 (1967).
33. Ascher, N. L., Simmons, R. L., Marker, S., and Najarian, V. S., *Listeria* infection in transplant patients, *Arch. Surg.* **113:**90–94 (1978).
34. Roucourt, J., Hof, H., and Schrettenbrunner, A., Meningite purulente Aigue *Listeria seeligeri* chen un adulte immunocompetent, *Schweiz. Med. Wochenschr.* **116:**248–251 (1986).
35. Cheruik, N. L., Armstrong, D., and Posner, J. B., Central nervous system infections in patients with cancer, changing patterns, *Cancer* **40:**268–274 (1977).
36. Gantz, N. M., Myerowitz, R. L., Medeiros, A. A., Carrera, G. F., Wilson, R. E., and O'Brien, T. F., Listeriosis in immunocompromised patients: A cluster of eight cases, *Am. J. Med.* **58:**637–643 (1975).
37. MacGowan, A. P., Marshall, R. J., MacKay, I. M., and Reeves, D. S., *Listeria* faecal carriage by renal transplant recipients, haemodialysis patients and patients in general practice: its relation to season, drug therapy, foreign travel, animal exposure and diet, *Epidemiol. Infect.* **106:**157–166 (1991).

38. Saad, A. J., Domiati-Saad, R., and Jerrells, T. R., Ethanol ingestion increases susceptibility of mice to *Listeria monocytogenes*, *Alcoholism* **17:**75–85 (1993).
39. Gray, M. L. (ed.), *Second Symposium on Listeric Infections*, Artcraft Printers, Bozeman, MN, 1962.
40. Seeliger, H. P. R., *Listeriosis*, 2nd ed., Hafner, New York, 1961.
41. Ho, J. L., Shands, K. N., Friedland, G., Echkind, P., and Fraser, D. W., An outbreak of type 4b *Listeria monocytogenes* infection involving patients from eight Boston hospitals, *Arch. Intern. Med.* **146:**520–524 (1986).
42. Becroft, D. M. O., Farmer, K., Seddon, R. J., Sowden, R., Stewart, J. H., Vines, A., and Wattle, D. A., Epidemic listeriosis in the newborn, *Br. Med. J.* **3:**747–751 (1971).
43. Green, H. T., and Macaulay, M. B., Hospital outbreak of *Listeria monocytogenes* septicemia: Problems of cross infection, *Lancet* **2:**1039–1040 (1978).
44. Latcha, S., and Cunha, B. A., *Listeria monocytogenes* meningoencephalitis: The diagnostic importance of the CSF lactic acid, *Heart Lung* **23:**177–179 (1994).
45. Nieman, R. E., and Lorber, B., Listeriosis in adults: A changing pattern. Report of eight cases and review of the literature, 1968–1978, *Rev. Infect. Dis.* **2:**207– 227 (1980).
46. Nocera, D., Bannerman, E., Roucourt, J., Jaton-Ogay, K., and Bille, J., Characterization by DNA restriction endonuclease analysis of *Listeria monocytogenes* strains related to the Swiss epidemic of listeriosis, *J. Clin. Microbiol.* **28:**2259–2263 (1990).
47. Bojsen-Moller, J., Human listeriosis, diagnostic, epidemiological and clinical studies, *Acta Pathol. Microbiol. Scand.* (Suppl.) **229:**1–157 (1972).
48. Kampelmacher, E. H., Huysinga, W. T., and van Noorle Jansen, L. M., The presence of *Listeria monocytogenes* in feces of pregnant women and neonates, *Zentralbl. Bakteriol. Mikrobiol. Hyg.* I Abt [A] **222:**258–262 (1972).
49. Kampelmacher, E. H., and van Noorle Jansen, L. M., Isolation of *Listeria monocytogenes* from feces of clinically healthy humans and animals, *Zentralbl. Bakteriol. Mikrobiol. Hyg.* I Abt. **211:** 353–359 (1969).
50. Mascola, L., Sorvillo, F., Goulet, V., Hall, B., Weaver, R. E., and Linnan, M., Fecal carriage of *Listeria monocytogenes*—observations during a community-wide, common-source outbreak, *Clin. Infect. Dis.* **15:**557–558 (1992).
51. Schuchat, A., Deaver, K., Hayes, P. S., Graves, L., Mascola, L., and Wenger, J. D., Gastrointestinal carriage of *Listeria monocytogenes* in household contacts of patients with listeriosis, *J. Infect. Dis.* **167:**1261–1266 (1993).
52. Schuchat, A., Swaminathan, B., and Broome, C. V., Epidemiology of human listeriosis, *Clin. Microbiol. Rev.* **4:**169–183 (1991).
53. Ciesielski, C. A., Hightower, A. W., Parsons, S. K., and Broome, C. V., Listeriosis in the United States: 1980–1982, *Arch. Intern. Med.* **148:**1416–1419 (1988).
54. Schuchat, A., Deaver, K. A., Wenger, J. D., Plikaytis, B. D., Mascola, L., Pinner, R. W., Reingold, A. L., Broome, C. V., and the Listeria Study Group, Role of foods in sporadic listeriosis. I: Case-control study of dietary risk factors, *J. Am. Med. Assoc.* **267:**2014–2045 (1992).
55. Giraud, J. R., Denis, F., and Gargot, F., La listeriose: Incidence dans les interruptions spontanees de la grosse, *Nouvelle Presse Med.* **2:**215–218 (1973).
56. Gray, M. L., and Killinger, A. H., *Listeria monocytogenes* and *Listeria* infections, *Bacteriol. Rev.* **30:**309–382 (1966).
57. Moore, R. M., and Zehmer, R. B., Listeriosis in the United States—1971, *J. Infect. Dis.* **127:**610–611 (1973).
58. Schlech, W. F., Ward, J. I., Band, J. D., Hightower, A., Fraser, D. W., and Broome, C. V., Bacterial meningitis in the United States, 1978–1981: The National Bacterial meningitis Surveillance Study, *J. Am. Med. Assoc.* **253:**1749–1754 (1985).
59. Busch, L. A., Human listeriosis in the United States, 1967–1969, *J. Infect. Dis.* **123:**328–332 (1971).
60. Larsson, S., Epidemiology of listeriosis in Sweden, 1958–1974, *Scand. J. Infect. Dis.* **11:**47–54 (1979).
61. McLauchlin, J., Audurier, A., and Taylor, A. G., Aspects of the epidemiology of human *Listeria monocytogenes* infections in Britain, 1967–1984: Use of serotyping and phage typing, *J. Med. Microbiol.* **22:**367–377 (1986).
62. Newton, L., Hall, S. M., and McLauchlin, J., Listeriosis surveillance: 1992, *Commun. Dis. Rep. CDR Rev.* **3:**R144–R146 (1993)
63. Nolla-Salas, J., Anto, J. M., Almela, M., Coll, P., Gasser, I., and Plasencia, A., Incidence of listeriosis in Barcelona, Spain, in 1990, *Eur. J. Clin. Microbiol. Infect. Dis.* **12:**157–161 (1993).
64. *Proceedings of the Third International Symposium on Listeriosis*, Bilthoven, The Netherlands, 1966.
65. Broome, C. V., Gellin, B. G., and Schwartz, B., Epidemiology of listeriosis in the United States, in: *Topics in Industrial Microbiology: Foodborne Listeriosis* (A. J. Miller, J. L. Smith, and G. A. Somkuti, eds.), pp. 61–65, Elsevier, Amsterdam, 1990.
66. Bortolussi, R., Schlech, W. F., III, and Albritton, W. L., *Listeria: Manual of Clinical Microbiology*, 4th ed., American Society for Microbiology, Washington, DC, 1985.
67. Gellin, B. G., Hayes, P. S., Pine, L., and Weaver, R. E., *Isolation and identification of Listeria monocytogenes*, US Department of Health and Human Services, Washington, 1989.
68. Hayes, P. S., Graves, L. M., Ajello, G. W., Swaminathan, B., Weaver, R. E., Wenger, J. D., Schuchat, A., Broome, C. V., and the Listeriosis Study Group. Comparison of cold enrichment and U.S. Department of Agriculture methods for isolating *Listeria monocytogenes* from naturally contaminated foods, *Appl. Environ. Microbiol.* **57:**2109–2113 (1991).
69. Schlech, W. F., Expanding the horizons of foodborne listeriosis (editorial), *J. Am. Med. Assoc.* **267:**2081–2082 (1992).
70. Chenevert, J., Mengaud, J., Gormley, E., and Cossart, P., A DNA probe specific for *Listeria monocytogenes* in the genus *Listeria*, *Int. J. Food Microbiol.* **8:**317–320 (1989).
71. King, W., Raposa, S., Warshaw, J., Johnson, A., Halbert, D., and Klinger, J. D., A new colorimetric nucleic acid hybridization assay for *Listeria* in foods, *Int. J. Food Microbiol.* **8:**225–232 (1989).
72. Helsel, L., Johnson, S., DeWitt, W., and Bibb, W. F., 1990. Characterization of monoclonal antibodies to the hemolysin of *Listeria monocytogenes* and the use of the antibodies in affinity purification of the protein, Abstracts of the 90th Annual meeting of the American Society of Microbiology (B-168), p. 54, ASM, Washington, DC, 1990.
73. Jatson, K., Sahli, R., and Bille, J., Development of polymerase chain reaction assays for detection of *Listeria monocytogenes* in clinical cerebrospinal fluid samples, *J. Clin. Microbiol. Biol.* **30:**1931–1936 (1992).
74. Kim, C., Swaminathan, B., Holloway, B., Pinner, R., and Varma, V. A., Detection of *Listeria monocytogenes* in formalin-fixed paraffin-embedded tissues using a 2-stage nested polymerase chain reaction, Abstracts of the 90th Annual meeting of the American Society of Microbiology (D-54), p 89, ASM, Washington, DC, 1990.
75. Andre, P., and Genicot, A., First isolation of *Listeria welshimeri* from human beings, *Zentrabl. Bakteriol. Hyg. A.* **263:**605–606 (1987).

76. Cummins, A. J., Fielding, A. K., and McLauchlin, J., *Listeria ivanovii* infection in a patient with AIDS, *J. Infect.* **28:**89–91 (1994).
77. Seeliger, H. P. R., *Listeria monocytogenes*, in *Medical Microbiology and Infectious Diseases* (A. Braude, ed.), p. 205, Saunders, Philadelphia, 1981.
78. McLauchlin, J., Audurier, A., and Taylor, A. G., Aspect of the epidemiology of human *Listeria monocytogenes* infections in Britain 1967–1984: The use of serotyping and phage typing, *J. Med. Microbiol.* **22:**367–377 (1986).
79. McLauchlin, J., Audurier, A., and Taylor, A. G., The evaluation of a phage-typing system for *L. monocytogenes* for use in epidemiological studies, *J. Med. Microbiol.* **22:**357–365 (1986).
80. Bibb, W. F., Gellin, B. G., Schwartz, B., Plikaytis, B. D., and Weaver, R. E., Analysis of clinical and food-borne isolates of *Listeria monocytogenes* by multilocus enzyme electrophoresis and application of the method to epidemiologic investigations, *Appl. Environ. Microbiol.* **56:**2133–2141 (1990).
81. Boerlin, P., and Piffaretti, J. C., Typing of human, animal, food, and environmental isolates of *Listeria monocytogenes* by multilocus enzyme electrophoresis, *Appl. Environ. Microbiol.* **57:** 1624–1629 (1991).
82. Piffaretti, J. C., Kressebuch, H., Aeschbacher, M., Bille, J., Bannerman, E., Musser, J. M., Selander, R. K., and Rocourt, J., Genetic characterization of clones of the bacterium *L. monocytogenes* causing epidemic disease, *Proc. Natl. Acad. Sci. USA* **86:**3818–3822 (1989).
83. Selander, H. P. R., Caugant, D. A., Ochman, H., Musser, J. M., Gilmour, M. N., and Whittman, T. S., Methods of multilocus enzyme electrophoresis for bacterial population genetics and systematics, *Appl. Environ. Microbiol.* **51:**873–884 (1986).
84. Buchrieser, C., Brosch, R., Catimel, B., and Roucourt, J., Pulsed-field gel electrophoresis applied for comparing *Listeria monocytogenes* strains involved in outbreaks, *Can. J. Microbiol.* **39:**395–410 (1993).
85. Harvey, J., and Gilmour, A., Application of multilocus enzyme electrophoresis and restriction fragment length polymorphism analysis to the typing of *Listeria monocytogenes* strains isolated from raw milk, nondairy foods, and clinical and veterinary sources, *Appl. Environ. Microbiol.* **60:**1547–1553 (1994).
86. Lew, A. E., and Desmarchelier, P. M., Restriction fragment length polymorphism analysis of *Listeria monocytogenes* and its application to epidemiological investigations, *Int. J. Food Microbiol.* **15:**347–356 (1992).
87. Saunders, N. A., Ridley, A. M., and Taylor, A. G., Typing of *Listeria monocytogenes* for epidemiological studies using DNA probes, *Acta. Microbiol. Hung.* **36:**205–210 (1989).
88. Graves, L. M., Swaminathan, B., Reeves, M. W., Hunter, S. B., Weaver, R. E., Plikaytis, B. D., and Schuchat, A., Comparison of ribotyping and multilocus enzyme electrophoresis for subtyping of *Listeria monocytogenes* isolates, *J. Clin. Microbiol.* **32:**2936–2943 (1994).
89. Nocera, D., Altwegg, M., Martinetti Lucchini, G., Bannerman, E., Ischer, F., Roucourt, J., and Bille, J., Characterization of *Listeria* strains from a foodborne listeriosis outbreak by rDNA gene restriction patterns compared to four other typing methods, *Eur. J. Clin. Microbiol. Infect. Dis.* **12:**162–169 (1993).
90. Vogt, R. L., Donnelly, C., Gellin, B., Bibb, W., and Swaminathan, B., Linking environmental and human strains of *Listeria monocytogenes* with isoenzyme and ribosomal RNA typing, *Eur. J. Epidemiol.* **6:**229–230 (1990).
91. Czajka, J., and Batt, C. A., Verification of causal relationships between *Listeria monocytogenes* isolates implicated in food-borne outbreaks of listeriosis by randomly applied polymorphic DNA patterns, *J. Clin. Microbiol.* **32:**1280–1287 (1994).
92. Berche, P., Reich, K. A., Bonnichon, M., Beretti, J. L., Geoffroy, C., Raveneau, J., Cossart, P., Gaillard, J. L., Geslin, P., and Kreis, H., Detection of anti-listeriolysin O for serodiagnosis of human listeriosis, *Lancet* **335**(8690)**:**624–627 (1990).
93. Hudak, A. P., Lee, S. H., Issekutz, A. C., and Bortolussi, R., Comparison of three serological methods: Enzyme-linked immunosorbent assay, complement fixation, and microagglutination in the diagnosis of human perinatal *L. monocytogenes* infection, *Clin. Invest. Med.* **7:**349–354 (1984).
94. Rennenberg, J., Persson, K., and Christensen, P., Western blot analysis of the antibody response in patients with *Listeria monocytogenes* meningitis and septicemia, *Eur. J. Clin. Microbiol. Infect. Dis.* **9:**659–663 (1990).
95. Watkins, J., and Sleath, K. P., Isolation of *L. monocytogenes* from sewage, sewage sludge, and river water, *J. Appl. Bacteriol.* **50:** 1–9 (1981).
96. Gitter, M., *Listeria* infections in farm animals, *Vet. Rec.* **112:**314–318 (1983).
97. Vazquez-Boland, J. A., Dominguez, L., Blanco, M., Roocourt, J., Fernandez-Garayzabal, J. F., Gutierrez, C. B, Tascon, R. I., and Rodriguez-Ferri, E. F., Epidemiologic investigation of a silage-associated epizootic of ovine listeric encephalitis, using a new *Listeria*-selective enumeration medium and phage typing, *Am. J. Vet. Res.* **53:**368–371 (1992).
98. Centers for Disease Control, Listeriosis associated with consumption of turkey franks, *Morbid. Mortal. Week. Rep.* **38:**267–268 (1989).
99. Food and Drug Administration, Eating defensively: Food safety advice for persons with AIDS, FDA Publication 92–2232 (1992).
100. Skogberg, K., Syrjanen, J., Jahkola, M., Renkonen, O. V., Paavonen, J., Ahonen, J., Kontiainen, S., Ruutu, P., and Valtonen, V., Clinical presentation and outcome of listeriosis in patients with and without immunosuppressive therapy, *Clin. Infect. Dis.* **14:**815–821 (1992).
101. Campbell, D. M., Human listeriosis in Scotland 1967–1988, *J. Infect.* **20:**241–250 (1990).
102. Anonymous, Listeriosis in France, *Commun. Dis. Resp. CDR Week.* **2**(29)**:**129–130 (1992).
103. Schlech, W. F., Chase, D. P., and Badley, A., A model of food-borne *Listeria monocytogenes* infection in the Sprague-Dawley rat using gastric inoculation: Development and effect of gastric acidity on infective dose, *Int. J. Food Microbiol.* **18:**15–24 (1993).
104. McLauchlin, J., Hall, S. M., Velani, S. K., and Gilbert, R. J., Human listeriosis and pate: A possible association, *Br. Med. J.* **303:**773–775 (1991).
105. Pinner, R. W., Schuchat, A., Swaminathan, B., Hayes, P. S., Deaver, K. A., Weaver, R. E., Plikaytis, B. D., Reeves, M., Broome, C. V., Wenger, J. D., and the Listeriosis Study Group, Role of foods in sporadic listeriosis: II: Microbiologic and epidemiologic investigation, *J. Am. Med. Assoc.* **267:**2046–2050 (1992).
106. MacGowan, A. P., Cartlidge, P. H., MacLeod, F., and McLaughlin, J., Maternal listeriosis in pregnancy without fetal or neonatal infection, *J. Infect.* **22:**53–57 (1991).
107. Campbell, A. N., Sill, P. R., and Wardle, J. K., *Listeria* meningitis acquired by cross-infection in a delivery suite, *Lancet* **2:**752–763 (1981).

108. Isaacs, D., and Libermann, M. N., Babies cross-infected with *L. monocytogenes* (letter), *Lancet* **2:**940 (1981).
109. Larsson, S., *Listeria monocytogenes* causing hospital-acquired enterocolitis and meningitis in newborn infants, *Br. Med. J.* **2:**473–474 (1978).
110. Miller, J. K., and Hedberg, M., Effects of cortisone on susceptibility of mice to *L. monocytogenes*, *Am. J. Clin. Pathol.* **43:**248–250 (1965)
111. Farber, J. M., Daley, E., Coates, F., Beausoleil, N., and Fournier, J., Feeding trials of *Listeria monocytogenes* with a nonhuman primate model, *J. Clin. Microbiol.* **29:**2606–2608 (1991).
112. Schlech, W. F., An animal model of foodborne *Listeria monocytogenes* virulence: Effect of alterations in local and systemic immunity on invasive infection, *Clin. Invest. Med.* **16:**219–225 (1993).
113. Schlech, W. F., *Listeria*, animals and man: Aspects of virulence, in: *Foodborne Listeriosis* (A. J. Miller, J. L. Misth, and G. A. Somkuti, eds.), pp. 51–54, Elsevier, Amsterdam, 1990.
114. Cain, D. B., and McCann, V. L., An unusual case of cutaneous listeriosis, *J. Clin. Microbiol.* **23:**976–977 (1986).
115. Felsenfeld, O., Diseases of poultry transmissible to man, *Iowa State Coll. Vet.* **13:**89–92 (1951).
116. Owen, C. R., Meis, A., Jackson, J. W., and Stonner, H. G., A case of primary cutaneous listeriosis, *N. Engl. J. Med.* **262:**1026–1028 (1960).
117. Stamm, A. M., Dismukes, W. E., and Simmons, B. P., Listeriosis in renal transplant recipients: Report of an outbreak and review of 102 cases, *Rev. Infect. Dis.* **4:**665–682 (1982).
118. Lorber, B., Listeriosis following shigellosis, *Rev. Infect. Dis.* **13:**865–866 (1991).
119. Schwartz, B., Hexter, D., Broome, C. V., Hightower, A. W., Hirschorn, R. B., Porter, J. D., Hayes, P. S., Bibb, W. F., Lorber, B., and Faris, D. G., Investigation of an outbreak of listeriosis: New hypothesis for the etiology of epidemic *Listeria monocytogenes* infections, *J. Infect. Dis.* **159:**680–685 (1989).
120. Shemesh, O., Bornstein, I. P., Weissberg, N., Braverman, D. Z., and Rudensky, B., *Listeria* septicemia after colonoscopy in an ulcerative colitis patient receiving ACTH [letter], *Am. J. Gastroenterol.* **85:**216 (1990).
121. Sheehan, G. J., and Galbraith, J. C. T., Colonoscopy-associated listeriosis: Report of a case, *Clin. Infect. Dis.* **17:**1061–1062 (1993).
122. Farber, J. M., Carter, A. O., Varughese, P. V., Ashton, F. E., and Ewan, E. P., Listeriosis traced to the consumption of alfalfa tablets and soft cheese [letter], *N. Engl. J. Med.* **322:**338 (1990).
123. Gray, J. W., Barrett, J. F., Pedler, S. J., and Lind, T., Faecal carriage of *Listeria* during pregnancy, *Br. J. Ob. Gyn.* **100:**873–874 (1993).
124. Bouwer, H. G. A., Nelson, C. S., Gibbins, B. L., Portnoy, D. A., and Hinrichs, D. A., Listeriolysin O is a target of the immune response to *Listeria monocytogenes*, *J. Exp. Med.* **175:**1467–1471 (1992).
125. Gaillard, J. L., and Alouf, J. E., Purification, characterization and toxicity of the sulfhydryl-activated hemolysin listeriolysin O from *L. monocytogenes*, *Infect. Immun.* **55:**1641–1646 (1987).
126. McKay, D. B., and Lu, C. Y., Listeriolysin as a virulence factor in *Listeria monocytogenes* infection of neonatal mice and urine decidual tissue, *Infect. Immun.* **59:**4286–4290 (1991).
127. Portnoy, D. A., Innate immunity to a facultative intracellular bacterial pathogen, *Curr. Opin. Immunol.* **4:**20–24 (1992).
128. Galworthy, S. B., Monocytosis producing activity from virulent and avirulent strains of *Listeria*, *Acta Microbiol. Hung.* **37:**97–99 (1990).
129. Mackaness, G. B., Cellular resistance to infection, *J. Exp. Med.* **116:**381–406 (1962).
130. Mackaness, G. B., and Hill, W. C., The effect of antilymphocyte globulin on cell-mediated resistance to infection, *J. Exp. Med.* **129:**993–1012 (1969).
131. Armstrong, D., *Listeria monocytogenes*, in: *Principles and Practice of Infectious Diseases*, 4th ed. (G. L. Mandell, J. E. Bennett, and R. Dolin, eds.), pp. 1880–1885, Churchill Livingstone, New York, 1995.
132. Hugin, A. W., Cerny, A., and Morse, H. C., Mice with an acquired immunodeficiency (MAIDS) develop a persistent infection after injection with *Listeria monocytogenes*, *Cell. Immunol.* **155:**246–252 (1994).
133. Real, F. X., Gold, J. W., Krown, S. E., and Armstrong, D., *Listeria monocytogenes* bacteremia in the acquired immunodeficiency syndrome, *Ann. Intern. Med.* **101:**883 (1984).
134. Pezeshkian, R., Fernando, N., and Carne, C. A., Listeriosis in mother and fetus during the first trimester of pregnancy: Case report, *Br. J. Obstet. Gynaecol.* **91:**85–86 (1994).
135. Workowski, K. A., and Flaherty, J. P., Systemic *Bacillus* species infection mimicking listeriosis of pregnancy, *Clin. Infect. Dis.* **14:**694–696 (1992).
136. Donnelly, C. W., Resistance of *Listeria monocytogenes* to heat, in: *Topics in Industrial Microbiology: Foodborne Listeriosis* (A. J. Miller, J. L. Smith, and G. A. Somkuti, eds.), pp. 189–194, Elsevier, Amsterdam, 1990.
137. World Health Organization, *Foodborne Listeriosis*, Report of a WHO Informal Working Group Geneva, WHO/EHE/FOS/88.5, February 1988.
138. Kluge, R. M., Listeriosis: Problems and therapeutic options, *J. Antimicrob. Chemother.* **25:**887–890 (1990).
139. Michelet, C., Avril, J. L., Cartier, F., and Berche, P., Inhibition of intracellular growth of *Listeria monocytogenes* by antibiotics, *Antimicrob. Agents Chemother.* **38:**438–446 (1994).
140. Spitzer, P. G., Hammer, S. M., Karchmer, A. W., Treatment of *Listeria monocytogenes* infection with trimethoprim–sulfamethoxazole: Case report and review of the literature, *Rev. Infect. Dis.* **8:**427–430 (1986).
141. Banerji, C., Wheeler, D. C., and Morgan, J. R., *Listeria monocytogenes* CAPD peritonitis: Failure of vancomycin therapy [letter], *J. Antimicrob. Chemother.* **33:**374–375 (1994).

12. Suggested Reading

Armstrong, D., *Listeria monocytogenes*, in: *Principles and Practice of Infectious Diseases*, 4th ed. (G. L. Mandell, J. E. Bennett, and R. Dolin, eds.), pp. 1880–1885, Churchill Livingstone, New York, 1995.

Dalton, C. B., Austin, C. C., Sobel, J., Hayes, P. S., Bibb, W. F., Graves, L. M., Swaminathat, B., Proctor, M. E., and Griffin, P. M., An outbreak of gastroenteritis and fever due to *Listeria monocytogenes* in milk, *N. Engl. J. Med.* **336:**100–105 (1997).

Gellin, B. G., Broome, C. V., Bibb, W. F., Weaver, R. E., Gaventa, S., Mascola, L., and the Listeriosis Study Group, The epidemiology of listeriosis in the United States—1986, *Am. J. Epidemiol.* **133:**392–401 (1991).

Gellin, B. G., and Broome, C. V., Listeriosis, *J. Am. Med. Assoc.* **261:**1313–1320 (1989).

Goulet, V., Lepoutre, A., Roucourt, J., Courtieu, A. L., Dehaumont, P., and Veit, P., Epidemie de listeriose en France: Bilan final et resultats de l'enquete epidemiologique, *Bull. Epidemiol. Hebdomadaire* **39:** 13–14 (1993).

Jurado, R. L., Farley, M. M., Pereira, E., Harvey, R. C., Schuchat, A., Wenger, J. D., and Stephens, D. S., Increased risk of meningitis and bacteremia due to *Listeria monocytogenes* in patients with human immunodeficiency virus infection, *Clin. Infect. Dis.* **71:**224–227 (1993).

Linnan, M. J., Mascola, L., Lou, X. D., Goulet, V., May, S., Salminen, C., Hird, D. W., Yonnekura, L., Hayes, P., Weaver, R., Audurier, A., Plikaytis, B. D., Fannin, S. L., Kleks, A., and Broome, C. V., Epidemic listeriosis associated with Mexican-style cheese, *N. Engl. J. Med.* **319:** 823–828 (1988).

Pinner, R. W., Schuchat, A., Swaminathan, B., Hayes, P. S., Deaver, K. A., Weaver, R. E., Plikaytis, B. D., Reeves, M., Broome, C. V., Wenger, J. D., and the Listeriosis Study Group, Role of foods in sporadic listeriosis: II: Microbiologic and epidemiologic investigation, *J. Am. Med. Assoc.* **267:**2046–2050 (1992).

Riedo, F. X., Pinner, R. W., Tosca, M. L., Cartter, M. L., Graves, L. M., Reeves, M. W., Weaver, R. E., Plikaytis, B. D., and Broome, C. V., A point-source foodborne listeriosis outbreak: Documented incubation period and possible mild illness, *J. Infect. Dis.* **170:**693–696 (1994).

Schlech, W. F., Listeria gastroenteritis—old syndrome, new pathogen, *N. Engl. J. Med.* **336:**130–132 (1997).

Schlech, W. F., An animal model of foodborne *Listeria monocytogenes* virulence: Effect of alterations in local and systemic immunity on invasive infection, *Clin. Invest. Med.* **16:**219–225 (1993).

Schlech, W. F., Lavigne, P. M., Bortolussi, R. A., Allen, A. C., Haldane, E. V., Wort, A. J., Hightower, A. W., Johnson, S. E., King, J. H., Nicholls, E. S., and Broome, C. V., Epidemic listeriosis—Evidence for transmission by food, *N. Engl. J. Med.* **308:**203–206 (1983).

Schuchat, A., Deaver, K., Hayes, P. S., Graves, L., Mascola, L., and Wenger, J. D., Gastrointestinal carriage of *Listeria monocytogenes* in household contacts of patients with listeriosis, *J. Infect. Dis.* **167:** 1261–1262 (1993).

Schuchat, A., Deaver, K. A., Wenger, J. D., Plikaytis, B. D., Mascola, L., Pinner, R. W., Reingold, A. L., Broome, C. V., and the Listeria Study Group, Role of foods in sporadic listeriosis. I: Case-control study of dietary risk factors, *J. Am. Med. Assoc.* **267:**2014–2045 (1992).

Schuchat, A., Lizano, C., Broome, C. V., Swaminathan, B., Kim, C., and Winn, K., Outbreak of neonatal listeriosis associated with mineral oil, *Pediatr. Infect. Dis. J.* **10:**183–189 (1991).

Schuchat, A., Swaminathan, B., and Broome, C. V., Epidemiology of human listeriosis, *Clin. Microbiol. Rev.* **4:**169–183 (1991).

Seelinger, H. P. R., and Jones, D., *Listeria*, in: *Bergey's Manual of Systematic Bacteriology*, Vol. 2 (P. H. Sneath, ed.), pp. 1235–1245, Baltimore, Williams and Wilkins, 1986.

Tappero, J. W., Schuchat, A., Deaver, K. A., Mascola, L., Wenger, J. D., and the Listeriosis Study Group, Reduction in the incidence of human listeriosis in the United States: Effectiveness of prevention efforts? *J. Am. Med. Assoc.* **273:**1118–1122 (1995).

Wenger, J. D., Hightower, A. W., Facklam, R. R., Gaventa, S., and Broome, C. V., Bacterial meningitis in the United States, 1986: Report of a multistate surveillance study, *J. Infect. Dis.* **162:**1316–1323 (1990).

CHAPTER 22

Lyme Disease

Kristine A. Moore, Craig Hedberg, and Michael T. Osterholm

1. Introduction

Lyme disease is a tick-borne multisystem illness caused by the spirochete *Borrelia burgdorferi*. The clinical manifestations of illness are divided into three stages. Stage 1 is predominantly characterized by erythema migrans (EM), a skin rash that classically begins as a single macule that expands to an annular lesion. The occurrence of EM is often associated with minor constitutional symptoms. Stage 2 is characterized by hematogenous dissemination; neurological involvement (particularly meningoencephalitis) and cardiovascular involvement (endocarditis, endomyocarditis, vasculitis, or fibrinous pericarditis) are classic hallmarks of stage 2 disease. Stage 3 is characterized by persistent infection; recurrent migratory arthritis, primarily of the large joints, occurs in stage 3. Chronic neurological involvement can also be associated with stage 3 disease. Patients may develop EM without further sequelae, or they may present with stage 2 or stage 3 disease without recalling prior EM or a tick bite. Without appropriate antimicrobial therapy, in some instances, Lyme disease can be severely debilitating; therefore, accurate diagnosis and treatment are critical to the clinical management and to the public health control of this illness.

B. burgdorferi is known to be transmitted by at least two tick vectors in the United States: *Ixodes scapularis* (formerly referred to as *I. dammini*) and *I. pacificus*. Other tick vectors in the United States have also been suggested. In addition, *B. burgdorferi* is transmitted by *I. ricinus* in Europe. These three species (*I. ricinus*, *I. scapularis*, and *I. pacificus*) form the *I. ricinus* complex. Lyme disease was first described in 1975; since that time the reported incidence has steadily increased (due to either a true increase in cases or an increased physician awareness and diagnosis of the condition). Currently, Lyme disease is the most commonly reported tick-borne illness in the United States, with endemic areas in the Northeast (particularly from Massachusetts to Maryland); the upper Midwest (Minnesota and Wisconsin); and the Pacific Northwest (particularly southern Oregon, parts of northern California, and Nevada).

Kristine A. Moore, Craig Hedberg, and Michael T. Osterholm • Minnesota Department of Health, Minneapolis, Minnesota 55440-9441.

2. Historical Background

Lyme disease (initially referred to as Lyme arthritis) was first recognized by Steere *et al.*[1] in 1975, following identification of a cluster of children living in Old Lyme, Connecticut, who were diagnosed with juvenile rheumatoid arthritis. Investigation of this cluster demonstrated an exceptionally high prevalence of arthritis in the affected communities. In addition, clustering within families was noted, a majority of affected children had onset of illness in summer or early fall, and a significant proportion of patients recalled the occurrence of an annular skin lesion (originating as a single papule) in the month before onset of arthritis. The skin lesions were typically suggestive of insect bites, and descriptions were compatible with EM. These epidemiological features supported the hypothesis that this particular cluster of arthritis cases represented a vector-borne infection. Steere and colleagues subsequently observed that the clinical spectrum of Lyme disease included not only arthritis and EM, but also neurological and cardiac abnormalities.[2–5] Early descriptions of Lyme disease correctly identified EM as the clinical hallmark of this disorder.[3]

Although Lyme disease with arthritis as a major manifestation was initially described in the United States in the late 1970s, EM following a tick bite had been previously recognized. The lesion was first described by

Afzelius,[6] a Swedish dermatologist, in 1909, and several years later it was designated as EM. Subsequently, the occurrence of neurological abnormalities following EM was noted by investigators in France in 1922, in Sweden in 1930, and in Germany in 1941.[7–9] Additional descriptions confirmed the systemic nature of the disease and suggested an infectious etiology.[10,11] In Europe, this illness became known as erythema migrans disease (EMD). In 1948, Lennhoft[12] described spirochetelike structures in skin specimens in several dermatologic conditions, including erythema migrans. As a result of this report, penicillin was used to treat this disorder in Europe.[11] In 1969, EM was first reported in the United States in a grouse hunter in northwestern Wisconsin, which is an area now recognized as endemic for Lyme disease.[13] In 1975, an additional case of EM was diagnosed in a woman vacationing in northern Minnesota; she reported an arthropod bite 2 days before the development of EM.[14]

Following recognition of Lyme disease as a distinct clinical entity, epidemiological data indicated that *I. scapularis* and *I. pacificus* were the most likely tick vectors for transmission of the etiologic agent in the United States.[15,16] Other potential tick vectors, including *Amblyomma americanum*, have been suggested.[17] In Europe, cases of EM were recognized in the distribution of an additional tick, *I. ricinus*.

Subsequent to evidence implicating *I. scapularis* as the major tick vector for a suspected infectious agent, a spirochete was isolated from *I. scapularis* ticks collected in an endemic area.[18] The spirochetal etiology of Lyme disease was then confirmed clinically in two studies.[19,20] One of these studies clearly demonstrated elevated IgG and IgM antibody titers to the newly recognized spirochete.[20] In the other study, the spirochete was isolated from the blood of 2 of 36 patients with characteristic symptoms.[19]This spirochete was subsequently classified as *B. burgdorferi*.[21]

Additional clinical studies have demonstrated that early Lyme disease can usually be effectively treated with antibiotic therapy (e.g., tetracycline, doxycycline, and penicillin),[22] although treatment failures have been reported.[23] Furthermore, major late manifestations (including myocarditis, meningoencephalitis, and arthritis) can usually be prevented if patients receive appropriate antimicrobial therapy during the early clinical manifestations, when EM and associated constitutional symptoms are present.[24] Late manifestations, particularly arthritis, may be relatively refractory to antimicrobial therapy; high-dose intravenous penicillin or ceftriaxone may be efficacious in treating otherwise refractory arthritis and neurological disease.[25–29]

The term "Lyme borreliosis" was suggested at the Second International *Borrelia* Conference in Vienna, Austria, in 1985, and its worldwide use was recommended for describing all the clinical manifestations of *B. burgdorferi* infection.[30] This was an attempt to find a name that could be accepted globally; however, the term Lyme disease is still often used, especially in the United States.

3. Methodology

3.1. Sources of Mortality Data

Mortality data for Lyme disease are generally lacking. One death due to pancarditis was reported in a patient with concurrent *B. burgdorferi* and *Babesia microti* infections.[31] An additional case, refractory to antimicrobial therapy and associated with fatal adult respiratory distress syndrome, has also been reported.[32] The relative absence of recognized fatal cases of Lyme disease from endemic areas suggests that the case-fatality rate is extremely low.

3.2. Sources of Morbidity Data

In the United States, the Centers for Disease Control and Prevention (CDC) initiated informal national surveillance for Lyme disease in 1980.[33] Cases of Lyme disease reported to the CDC by individual states have been compiled since 1982.[34] Over time, these data have demonstrated the occurrence of Lyme disease in areas of low incidence and in areas where Lyme disease had not previously been recognized. However, the epidemiological importance of these data are limited by the lack of uniform case definition criteria during the 1980s, changes in case definition criteria with the introduction of *B. burgdorferi* antibody serology, and differences in reporting requirements among the states. The current case definition adopted by the Council of State and Territorial Epidemiologists for Public Health Surveillance of Lyme disease includes erythema migrans, or at least one late manifestation, and laboratory confirmation of infection.[35] Case ascertainment in most states is by passive surveillance, and verification of reported information may not be routine. Furthermore, serological tests for antibody to *B. burgdorferi* performed at private laboratories, state health department laboratories, and the CDC have not been standardized. Several studies have demonstrated that wide variation in serology can occur.[36–38] Furthermore, surveillance data that include as cases persons with positive enzyme immunoassay (EIA) serology results not confirmed by immunoblot may lead to significant overreporting of Lyme disease.[39] Recently, consensus has been developed on the need for a two-stage serological testing process with the use of an initial sensitive screening assay such as EIA followed by a confirmatory test such as Western immunoblot.[40] Consistent application of these criteria across states will help standardize the national case definition for Lyme disease and for the first time provide a consistent frame of reference for interpreting surveillance data from state to state.

Due to limitations in interpreting the results of *B. burgdorferi* antibody serology, laboratory-based surveillance for Lyme disease can serve only to identify patients for whom clinical information can be collected and evaluated. Internationally, serological reference laboratories have served as sources for Lyme disease surveillance data through routine collection of clinical information on patients for whom specimens were submitted for testing. Surveillance for Lyme disease will be improved by the use of two-step serological testing. Eventually, polymerase chain reaction (PCR)-based tests may become standardized for use in reference laboratories. In the absence of definitive confirmation of infection, various investigators from public health departments and academic research centers have developed clinical case definitions that are not dependent on serological test results; however, these, too, have not been standardized.

3.3. Surveys

Several incident surveys of Lyme disease have been conducted in defined populations living in endemic areas in the United States.[41–45] Two early studies were conducted of summertime residents of island communities.[41,42] In these studies, investigators excluded short-term residents, sought to include all eligible participants, administered multiple questionnaires over time, included a serosurvey for *B. burgdorferi* antibody, and a medical evaluation of incident cases. Shortly afterward, Lastavica *et al.*[43] conducted a clinical and serological survey of residents of a community adjoining a nature preserve in coastal Massachusetts, and Alpert *et al.*[44] conducted a survey of a residential suburban community just north of New York City.

These studies of 200 or fewer subjects demonstrated cumulative frequencies from 8.8 to 35% and annual incidences from 1.8 to 10%. In each study, clinical Lyme disease was more common than asymptomatic infection as defined by results of immunofluorescent antibody (IFA) or EIA serology without immunoblot confirmation. Feder *et al.*[45] studied the incidence and cumulative frequency of Lyme disease in a school-aged population in Connecticut using only physician-diagnosed clinical histories and immunoblot confirmation of serological test results. Using these more specific and potentially less sensitive methods, they found a cumulative frequency of 7.3% and an annual incidence of 1.4% in 796 patient years of evaluation involving 410 students. As in the other studies, clinical Lyme disease was more common than asymptomatic infection.

In Europe, Gustafson *et al.*[46] found a 3.2 to 4.6% annual rate of clinical illness among 346 residents of an endemic area in Sweden. This was similar to the rate of asymptomatic seroconversion in the same population. Fahrer *et al.*[47] found a 0.8% clinical incidence of Lyme disease among Swiss orienteers who had an 8.1% asymptomatic seroconversion rate over the same 6-month time period. These findings suggest that asymptomatic infection with *B. burgdorferi* appears to be more common in Europe than in North America.

B. burgdorferi infection has been documented in white-tailed deer (*Odocoileus virginianus*), feral mice (*Peromyscus* species), a variety of medium-sized mammals, and ticks in the same geographic areas where Lyme disease occurs in humans.[48–50] A serological survey of dogs in southern Connecticut established the presence of *B. burgdorferi* infection and subsequent lameness in dogs in geographic areas corresponding to the distribution of Lyme disease cases.[51] Serological and clinical evidence of infection in horses and cows have been reported from New England states, New Jersey, and Wisconsin.[52–55] Anderson[56] reviewed 31 mammalian and 49 avian host species for *I. scapularis* and 15 mammalian species that have been infected with *B. burgdorferi*. The presence of infected larval *I. scapularis* on ground-feeding migratory birds has led to suggestions that they may be responsible for the spread of Lyme disease over wide areas.[57] The role of migrating birds in the distribution of infected ticks and *Borrelia* species has been further supported by Scandinavian studies.[58]

3.4. Laboratory Diagnosis

Barbour–Stoenner–Kelly medium is available for isolation of *B. burgdorferi*,[21] and *B. burgdorferi* organisms have been readily isolated from the margins of erythema migrans lesions.[59] However, *B. burgdorferi* organisms have been isolated infrequently from blood, joints, and cerebrospinal fluid (CSF) of patients with Lyme disease.[19,20,60–62] The low yield from clinical specimens has been attributed to the small number of organisms present in affected tissues.[60,62]

Visualization of spirochetes with silver stains and immunofluorescence was used to demonstrate the presence of spirochetes in synovial fluid from a patient with arthritis, in myocardial tissue obtained postmortem from a patient with a fatal case of Lyme disease, and in the remains of a fetus infected *in utero*.[31,63,64] However, direct detection methods are of limited utility because small numbers of organisms are generally present in infected tissues.

During the early 1990s, considerable effort went into developing clinically useful PCR primers and probes for detecting *B. burgdorferi* DNA from patients with Lyme disease. Goodman *et al.*[65] first detected *B. burgdorferi* DNA in urine using a 3.7-kb probe of chromosomal origin. Lebech and Hansen[66] used a 248-bp fragment of the *B. burgdorferi* flagellin gene in both urine and CSF with mixed results. Nine of ten urine samples but only four CSF samples were positive from patients with neuroborreliosis. Keller *et al.*[67] used an outer-surface protein (Osp) A probe on CSF from patients with Lyme neuroborreliosis and showed that clearance of PCR-reactivity following treatment correlated with clinical improvement. Pachner and Delaney[68] evaluated 24 patients with probable or definite Lyme neuroborreliosis and 35 patients with other neurological diseases using a chromosomal DNA probe. In that study, *B. burgdorferi* DNA was detected in CSF of 46% of the neuroborrelosis patients but only 3% of patients with other neurological diseases.

Nocton *et al.*[69] tested a series of primer-probe sets on 88 patients with Lyme arthritis and found the sensitivity of results ranged from 48 to 76% for individual primer-probe sets, with 85% of patients positive by at least one of the PCR assays. Sixty-four patients with other causes of arthritis were negative by all sets.[69] Persing *et al.*[70] subsequently showed that reactivity of genomic DNA targets was weak or absent in synovial fluid of patients with Lyme arthritis, but that plasmid-encoded genes to Osp A and Osp B were easily detected.

PCR testing of skin biopsy specimens has demonstrated sensitivities on the same order as culture.[71,72] Recently, Goodman *et al.*[73] reported the use of PCR to document spirochetemia in patients with clinical evidence of disseminated disease. Ten of 33 patients with systemic symptoms were PCR positive; however, *B. burgdorferi* was isolated from blood from only two of these.[73] Results were confirmed using primers to amplify a 231-bp fragment of the *B. burgdorferi* RNA polymerase C gene and sequences of the plasmid-encoded Osp A gene.

While PCR offers considerable promise as a diagnostic tool, there are major methodological hurdles in its use for the diagnosis of Lyme disease. First, since few *B. burgdorferi* organisms are present in most clinical specimens, the PCR assay needs to be highly sensitive. This sensitivity increases the potential for laboratory contamination and subsequent false-positive test results. Second, because *B. burgdorferi* organisms exhibit significant genetic variability, it will be difficult to identify and standardize suitable primers for target genes. These constraints will likely restrict the use of PCR to a few research or specialized reference laboratories, at least for the near future.

In addition to isolation of *B. burgdorferi* from humans, isolation of spirochetes, or their detection by PCR, from ticks and feral rodents has been proposed as a means of identifying endemic areas.[49,74,75] Marshall *et al.*[76] identified *B. burgdorferi* DNA sequences in two white-footed mouse specimens obtained from a museum collection to show that the agent of Lyme disease had existed in the United States since at least 1894.

In the absence of routine bacterial culture and PCR testing, serology remains the only widely available laboratory procedure to aid in the diagnosis of Lyme disease. *B. burgdorferi* antibody serology tests were developed shortly after the spirochete was identified. Craft *et al.*[77] demonstrated an IgM response in 11 of 12 patients who developed severe disease; the response peaked 3–6 weeks following onset of symptoms and persisted in some patients. An IgG response, which was delayed for several weeks in some individuals, was demonstrated for all 12 patients, and titers remained elevated after months of clinical remission.[77] A prospective study of early Lyme disease using antibody detection by immunoblotting revealed 16 patients (53%) with positive test results in acute-phase sera and 25 patients (83%) with positive test results in convalescent-phase sera.[78] Detectable IgG antibody remains present for years after successful treatment of Lyme disease and limits the usefulness of serological testing to evaluate persistent or recurrent symptoms.[79] In addition to identification of serum antibody, intrathecal production of antibody has also been demonstrated for patients with neurological manifestations of Lyme disease.[80]

Although results of serology are being used in the diagnosis of Lyme disease and have been incorporated into the surveillance case definition of Lyme disease by some state health departments, a number of qualifications must be placed on the interpretation of such results. First, currently available serology has not been standardized, and significant variability of results between laboratories has been reported.[36–38] Significant variability between laboratories has been demonstrated for both IFA and EIA methods, including "standardized" commercial EIA test kits. Second, although EIA tests, regardless of antigenic formulation, may be sensitive screening tests for antibody to *B. burgdorferi*, they are not highly specific. Thus, reliance on EIA results alone may lead to overdiagnosis of Lyme disease and subsequent overreporting of Lyme disease to public health officials. Dressler *et al.*[81] found an IgG EIA to have a specificity of 72% for patients seen in a diagnostic Lyme disease clinic. Cutler and Wright[39] found that only 16% of samples submitted for serological testing and positive by EIA were confirmed as positive by immunoblotting. For these reasons, the Second National Conference on Serologic Diagnosis of Lyme Disease recommended a two-test approach for active disease and previous infection using a sensitive EIA or IFA followed by Western immunoblot confirmation of all specimens positive or equivocal by EIA or IFA.[40] Callister *et al.*[82] developed a test to detect borreliacidal activity of serum from patients with Lyme disease. Although preliminary studies suggested that this may be a highly specific serodiagnostic test for Lyme disease, it has several limitations that make it less useful than Western immunoblots. The borreliacidal assay does not identify which antigens are being targeted by the antibody response and it requires that patients not be on antibiotics at the time the blood sample is collected. In addition, it has not been standardized or prospectively evaluated in a clinical setting. Thus, Western immunoblotting is currently recommended as the confirmatory test for detection of antibodies to *B. burgdorferi*.

Recommendations to use immunoblot confirmation of EIA results should eliminate false-positive results for patients with rheumatoid arthritis, systemic lupus erythematosis,[83] and treponemal infections.[84] However, as noted by Feder *et al.*[79] and documented in several serosurveys, the mere presence of antibody to *B. burgdorferi* in a patient with otherwise nonspecific symptoms and signs may not be diagnostic of Lyme disease. Similarly, one study has shown that immunoblot analysis of sera from dogs in endemic areas failed to distinguish asymptomatic animals from clinically ill animals.[85] In summary, positive results for *B. burgdorferi* antibody serology may be absent during acute disease, preempted by appropriate antimicrobial therapy, found in asymptomatic persons without a history of earlier clinical illness, and need to be distinguished from nonspecific or cross-reacting antibody serology results.

4. Biological Characteristics of the Organism

B. burgdoferi are helically shaped gram-negative bacteria with cell diameters of 0.18 to 0.25 μm, cell lengths of 20 to 30 μm, and possess 7 to 11 flagella. They are not as tightly coiled as other spirochetes.[21,86] Like other borreliae, they are microaerophilic, do not produce catalase,[86] and have their genes encoding outer membrane proteins located on plasmids. A lipopolysaccharide has been isolated from the cell wall of *B. burgdorferi* and endotoxinlike activity has been demonstrated in rabbit pyrogen and *Limulus* assays.[87,88] Three major outer-surface proteins have been identified; these include Osp A (30–32 kDa), Osp B (34–36 (kDa), and Osp C (22–85 kDa).[89,90] *B. burgdorferi* also possess several other outer surface proteins, a 41-kDa flagellar antigen,[91] several heat-shock proteins (66–73 kDa).[92] and a 93-kDa protoplasmic cylinder antigen.[93] Other antigens identified by Western immunoblot remain to be characterized.

Observations on the antigenic differences of *B. burgdorferi* strains in Europe and the United States have led to the recognition of three genomic groups in the *B. burgdorferi sensu lato* complex.[94,95] These include *B. burgdorferi sensu stricto* (which comprises all North American strains), *Borrelia garinii*, and *Borellia afzelii*. All three groups have been isolated in Europe, although most European isolates have belonged to the *B. garinii* or *B. afzelii* groups. Biological characteristics of the groups may account for differences in clinical presentations of Lyme disease between North America and Europe.[96,97]

B. burgdorferi has a distinct affinity for tissue rather than body fluids. The motility of *B. burgdorferi* has been correlated with viscoelasticity,[98] and it appears that the spirochete can only move along its longitudinal axis in a medium with properties that approach fixed tissue.[98] These observations may explain the relative ease of culturing *B. burgdorferi* from skin compared to CSF, synovial fluid, or blood.

The susceptibility *in vitro* and *in vivo* of *B. burgdorferi* to several antimicrobial agents has been studied.[99–102] Using a broth dilution technique to assess *in vitro* susceptibility, Johnson *et al.*[100] measured minimum bactericidal concentrations (MBCs) for the antimicrobials most commonly used to treat Lyme disease. Tests demonstrated the following MBCs: 0.04 μg/ml for ceftriaxone, 0.05 μg/ml for erythromycin, 0.8 μg/ml for tetracycline, and 6.4 μg/ml for penicillin G. In the same report, *in vivo* studies were performed by determining the 50% curative doses of these four antimicrobial agents in Syrian hamsters infected with *B. burgdorferi* by intraperitoneal injection.[100] After a 14-day incubation period, the hamsters were treated with daily subcutaneous injections of the antimicrobials for 5 days. Fourteen days after the last treatment, the hamsters were sacrificed and organs cultured for evidence of *B. burgdorferi* infection. By this method, the 50% curative doses obtained were 240 mg/kg for ceftriax-

Table 1. Lyme Disease in the United States by State Where Reported, 1991–1994

Region	Year 1991	1992	1993	1994	Region	Year 1991	1992	1993	1994
New England	1659	2327	1815	2827	South Atlantic (*cont.*)				
Maine	15	16	18	33	North Carolina	73	67	86	77
New Hampshire	38	44	15	30	South Carolina	10	2	9	7
Vermont	7	9	12	16	Georgia	25	48	44	127
Massachusetts	265	223	148	247	Florida	35	24	30	28
Rhode Island	142	275	272	471	East South Central	100	69	40	43
Connecticut	1192	1760	1350	2030	Kentucky	44	28	16	24
Mid Atlantic	5577	5309	4689	8171	Tennessee	35	31	20	13
New York (excl. NYC)	3807	3345	2758	5105	Alabama	13	10	4	6
New York City	137	103	60	95	Mississippi	8	—	—	—
New Jersey	915	688	786	1533	West South Central	123	167	78	174
Pennsylvania	718	1173	1085	1438	Arkansas	31	20	8	15
East North Central	649	655	505	530	Louisiana	6	7	3	4
Ohio	112	32	30	45	Oklahoma	29	27	19	99
Indiana	16	22	32	19	Texas	57	113	48	56
Illinois	51	41	19	24	Mountain	25	16	20	18
Michigan	46	35	23	33	Montana	—	—	—	—
Wisconsin	424	525	401	409	Idaho	2	2	2	3
West North Central	363	422	319	347	Wyoming	11	5	9	5
Minnesota	84	197	141	208	Colorado	1	—	—	1
Iowa	22	33	8	17	New Mexico	3	2	2	5
Missouri	207	150	108	102	Arizona	1	—	—	—
North Dakota	2	1	2	—	Utah	2	6	2	3
South Dakota	1	1	—	—	Nevada	5	1	5	1
Nebraska	25	22	6	3	Pacific	272	247	152	78
Kansas	22	18	54	17	Washington	7	14	9	4
South Atlantic	697	683	639	855	Oregon	NN[a]	NN[a]	8	6
Delaware	73	219	143	106	California	265	231	134	68
Maryland	282	183	180	341	Alaska	—	—	—	—
District of Columbia	5	3	2	9	Hawaii	—	2	1	—
Virginia	151	123	95	131	Total	9465	9895	8257	13043
West Virginia	43	14	50	29					

[a]NN, not notifiable.

one, 287 mg/kg for tetracycline, > 1975 mg/kg for penicillin G, and 2353 mg/kg for erythromycin. Results of these *in vivo* and *in vitro* studies correlate with available clinical data on treatment of patients with Lyme disease.[24,102] While some cases of Lyme disease are relatively refractory to antimicrobial therapy,[25,27] *in vitro* antimicrobial resistance has not been reported for *B. burgdorferi*. Thus, treatment failures are more likely due to sequestration of organisms in tissues not well penetrated by the antimicrobials used rather than due to specific antimicrobial resistance.

5. Descriptive Epidemiology

5.1. Prevalence and Incidence

The actual incidence of *B. burgdorferi* infection, including clinically apparent disease and asymptomatic infection, is unknown. In part, this is due to the lack of a sensitive and specific serological test for *B. burgdorferi* infection or a method for routine isolation of the organisms from infected tissue or blood.

The CDC has described the distribution of Lyme disease in the United States for 1980 through 1994 as determined by the national surveillance system (Table 1).[103–106] Lyme disease is now the most commonly reported tick-borne illness in the United States. The numbers of cases reported to the CDC for 1991 (9465), 1992 (9895), 1993 (8257), and 1994 (13,043) were 30 times higher than the numbers of cases reported for 1980 (226), 1982 (491), and 1983 (600).[34] The New York State Department of Health, using both tick and communicable disease surveillance systems, found that the range of *I. scapularis* had expanded annually into areas up to 384 km from the original known endemic areas of Long Island, New York, and Connecticut. Cumulative data from human surveillance in New York have documented both temporal and geographic expansion of Lyme disease in that state.[107] However, on a nationwide basis, it remains unclear whether the increased number of reported cases represents improved clinical recognition of the disease and better surveillance or an actual increased incidence of disease. Therefore, the CDC and the Council of State and Territorial Epidemiologists have indicated that national surveillance data should be used to monitor trends, not to represent the true incidence of Lyme disease in the United States.[34,108]

In addition to national surveillance, several states and counties have reported surveillance data. Early studies were conducted in Minnesota, Wisconsin, and Connecticut.[109–111] Officials in Connecticut conducted a laboratory-based program of surveillance for Lyme disease from July 1, 1984, to March 1, 1986.[109] Serological testing was offered without cost to Connecticut physicians for diagnosing Lyme disease. Physicians were requested to include a completed case report form with serum specimens submitted for testing. Patients were considered to have Lyme disease if they had onset of EM and/or neurological, cardiac, or arthritic manifestations characteristic of Lyme disease and a positive *B. burgdorferi* serology. From this study, the incidence of Lyme disease for all Connecticut residents in 1985 was estimated to be 22 per 100,000 person years. Town-specific incidence rates ranged from 0 to 1156 per 100,000 person years. Eighty-three percent of the patients studied had EM, 24% had arthritis, 8% had neurological manifestations, and 2% had cardiac involvement. The authors of this study compared their results with those from a similar study by Steere *et al.*[16] conducted in 1977 in the same communities. They suggested that a 163% increase in the incidence of Lyme disease had occurred from 1977 to 1986 for eight towns studied. In addition, they suggested that the disease had spread inland from the coastal areas. However, it is unclear if this detected increase reflected an actual increase in the incidence of Lyme disease or may have resulted from increased availability of *B. burgdorferi* serology or an increased physician awareness of the disease.

In a second study conducted during 1990–92, by some of these same researchers, the incidence and cumulative frequency of Lyme disease was ascertained in a school-aged population in an area in Connecticut where Lyme disease is endemic.[45] They found at enrollment that 7% of students had a history of Lyme disease and 41% were seropositive for *B. burgdorferi* infection. Seronegative students were followed prospectively over a total of 796 person years. During this period, eight students (10.1 cases/1000 person years) developed clinical Lyme disease and three (3.8 cases/1000 person years) had evidence of asymptomatic infection.

In Ipswich, Massachusetts, 35% of 190 residents of an area next to a nature preserve were affected during a 7-year period.[43] Sixteen percent of 162 residents of Great Island, Massachusetts, developed illness during a 10-year period and 7.5% of 200 people who participated in a study on Fire Island, New York, had the illness during a 5-year period.[41,42] In these studies, most of the individuals with serological evidence of infection also had symptoms of disease. However, in serosurveys done in Europe, the majority of patients with antibody to *B. burgdorferi* have been asymptomatic. Of 346 individuals who were studied in the highly endemic area of Liso, Sweden, 41 (12%) had symptomatic disease and 89 (26%) had evidence of subclinical infection.[46] In a serosurvey of 950 Swiss orienteers, 26% had detectable IgG antibody to *B. burgdorferi*, but only 3% had a past history of definite or probable Lyme borreliosis.[47]

5.2. Epidemic Behavior and Contagiousness

The incidence of Lyme disease in a particular geographic area depends on the population density of the tick and the frequency of contact between the tick and susceptible human and animal populations.[34] In the United States, studies have demonstrated varying rates of *B. burgdorferi* infection in ticks from about 60% in the *I. scapularis* population on Shelter Island, New York, to approximately 1.2% in the *I. pacificus* population in the Western states.[112] An additional study identified *I. scapularis* ticks near the homes of patients with Lyme disease in Westchester County, New York.[113] In that study, 32 ticks from one lawn were examined: 33% of nymphs and 55% of adult ticks contained spirochetes. There is evidence in some areas of temporal increases in *I. scapularis* population density.[103–107] For example, in 1994, in one site in Westchester County, the population density of *I. scapularis* nymphs increased 400% from 0.4 nymphs per square meter in 1993 to 1.6 nymphs per square meter in 1994.[103] *B. burgdorferi* has been demonstrated in other species of ticks and in mosquitoes and deer flies,[114] but only ticks of the *I. ricinus* complex (composed of *I. ricinus*, *I. scapularis*, and *I. pacificus*) seem to be important to the transmission of the spirochete to humans.

The frequency with which transmission of *B. burgdorferi* occurs following a single bite from an infected tick is unclear. Factors associated with transmission included length of the time of tick attachment and prevalence of *B. burgdorferi* infection in the ticks. The pooled estimate of the probability of contracting Lyme disease after a single tick bite in an endemic area found in four studies ranged from 0.012 to 0.05.[115]

5.3. Geographic Distribution

In the United States, the number of states where Lyme disease has been acquired has increased annually, from 18 in 1983 to 44 in 1994 (Table 1). However, the primary endemic area for Lyme disease continues to be the three originally described regions in the United States—coastal areas of the Northeast; the Upper Midwest, including Minnesota and Wisconsin; and the Northwest, including regions in northern California, southern Oregon, and western Nevada. Specifically, 70% of the 40,660 cases reported to the CDC from 1991 through 1994 were acquired in seven states: New York, New Jersey, Massachusetts, Rhode Island, Connecticut, Wisconsin, and Minnesota. Cases of Lyme disease have been documented from at least 21 countries on four continents.[116–120] Cases in Europe have occurred predominantly in the known range of *I. ricinus*, including Scandinavia, the United Kingdom, and many other countries in western Europe.[118,119] Lyme disease has also been described in areas where none of the currently recognized tick vectors are known to exist, including Australia, Japan, and China.[116,120] These reports, and the recent evidence that *A. americanum* and possibly *Ixodes persulcatus* can be infected with *B. burgdorferi*, suggest that cases of Lyme disease in the future may be diagnosed in additional geographic areas throughout the world.[17,118]

5.4. Temporal Distribution

Cases of Lyme disease in the United States have been reported with onsets during all 12 months of the year. However, disease incidence is highest in the summer and early fall months, as would be expected with a tick-borne infection. Seventy percent of patients that have EM are seen by physicians in May through August, a period corresponding with peak human outdoor activity and the presence of nymphal ticks seeking blood meals.[121] A similar pattern for disease onset has been documented for cases of EM in Europe.

5.5. Age

Cases of Lyme disease have occurred in individuals of all ages. However, several studies have demonstrated a higher incidence among children. In Connecticut, the age-specific incidence by 5-year age groups for patients reported in 1993 was 60 per 100,000 person years for children 5 to 10 years of age and 36 per 100,000 person years for those $\geq$15 years of age.[122] In Westchester County, New York, two thirds of all cases of Lyme disease in 1982–1983 occurred in individuals under 40 years of age, with children under 19 comprising almost 43% of the total.[44] In that study, the median age of patients was 27 years. Benach and Coleman[123] documented that 63% of 679 patients reported with Lyme disease to the New York Health Department in 1983 were 19 years of age or younger. A third study by Steere *et al.*[42] demonstrated a different age distribution for patients in Great Island, Massachusetts. The mean age for cases with arthritis alone was 19 years, with EM or "flulike" illness was 42 years, and with asymptomatic infection was 53 years. The age-specific attack rates in that population suggested that the risk of Lyme disease increased with age; however, cases of arthritis alone occurred predominantly in children.

5.6. Sex

To date, all studies have documented a slight predominance of male patients.[33,42,111,124] It has been suggested that this finding reflects a greater exposure for males due to increased likelihood of engaging in activities out-of-doors in areas where tick vectors are found. However, 1994 national surveillance data demonstrated that males and females were nearly equally affected in all age groups except those aged 10–19 years (males: 55%) and those aged 30–39 years (females: 56%).[103]

5.7. Race

The race-specific attack rates for Lyme disease appear to approximate the racial breakdown of the general population in the geographic areas with tick vectors. Further studies are needed to confirm this observation.

5.8. Occupation

Data have been reported by Neubert *et al.*[125] in Bavaria, Smith *et al.*[126] in New York, and Guy *et al.*[127] in the United Kingdom suggesting that outdoor workers in areas with known tick reservoirs of *B. burgdorferi* may have an occupational risk of acquiring Lyme disease. In these studies, employees were surveyed regarding exposure and illness histories, blood specimens were collected for serological determination of antibody to *B. burgdorferi*, and comparisons were made between groups of employees defined as seropositive and seronegative. In addition, Smith *et al.*[126] compared rates of seropositivity in the study group to a group of anonymous blood donors from the same area and to a group of sexually transmitted disease clinic patients who were from a nonendemic area of New York State and whose sera were nonreactive for *B. burgdorferi* when tested by a reagin test. Neubert *et al.*[125] did not use an external control group; however, 3 years after the original survey they reexamined 53 of 71 workers who were initially seropositive.

Neubert *et al.*[125] found that 71 (34%) of 211 forest workers had reciprocal titers of IgM antibody to *B. burgdorferi* $\geqslant 10$ by IFA. Smith *et al.*[126] found that 27 (7%) of 414 outdoor workers had an optical density $\geqslant 0.2$ by EIA and antibody against polypeptides of *B. burgdorferi* by Western immunoblot assay. Apparent differences in rates of seropositivity between the studies may be due to the different serological criteria used to define a positive sample. Despite these and other methodological differences, both studies revealed trends toward associations between the presence of antibody to *B. burgdorferi* and increasing age, history of tick bites, rash compatible with EM, and various cardiac, rheumatological, and neurological disorders.[125,126] However, only age, history of tick bites, and history of EM were significantly associated ($p < 0.05$) with being seropositive. Age was believed to be a surrogate for duration of exposure.[125]

In their reexamination of 53 seropositive forest workers 2½ years following their initial study, Neubert *et al.*[125] found that 14 (26%) had findings compatible with Lyme disease or a history suggestive of earlier Lyme disease. In addition, 33 (62%) had a fourfold or greater decrease in IgG antibody titer between the initial and subsequent examinations.

Smith *et al.*[126] found only 4 (1%) of 362 volunteer blood donors from Suffolk and Westchester counties in New York and none of 100 sexually transmitted disease clinic patients from northwestern New York state (where Lyme disease is not endemic) to be seropositive for antibody to *B. burgdorferi*. Thus, the group of outdoor workers with occupational exposure were 5.9 times as likely to be seropositive than were blood donors from the same area.[126] Taken together, these studies suggest that individuals who work outdoors in areas with a high density of the tick vector and a high prevalence of *B. burgdorferi* infection in ticks are at greater risk of developing Lyme disease than those who do not routinely participate in similar activities.

Guy *et al.*[127] screened 41 forestry workers in the United Kingdom who had a high occupational risk of tick bites. The workers were tested for *B. burgdorferi* antibody by EIA and Western blotting techniques. Workers were also questioned about possible symptoms of Lyme disease. While antibody was detected in 10 (25%) of 40 workers, EM was reported in only 2 workers. They concluded that the clinical implications of finding antibody in such workers is unclear.

6. Mechanisms and Routes of Transmission

B. burgdorferi is transmitted to humans by the bite from one of several related species of tick belonging to the genus *Ixodes*. The principal vectors are *I. scapularis* in the northeastern and northcentral United States, *I. pacificus* in the western United States, and *I. ricinus* in northern and western Europe.[15] *A. americanum* has been identified as a potential tick vector in the United States; however, no human cases are linked to bites by these ticks.[17] Piesman and Sinsky[128] have shown that larval *A. americanum* are inefficient at acquiring *B. burgdorferi* when allowed to feed on spirochete-infected hamsters. In addition, none of the *A. americanum* examined after molting to nymphs contained spirochetes. Thus, the role of *A. americanum* in transmission of *B. burgdorferi* remains unclear. *I. persulcatus* has been associated with the first cases of Lyme disease reported from China and Japan.[116,120]

Steere *et al.*[15,16] first implicated a tick vector for Lyme disease from epidemiological investigations conducted before the causative organism was identified. Ticks had previously been associated with EM in Europe, and the isolation of identical spirochetes from ticks and patients confirmed the etiology and mode of transmission. The nymphal form of the tick is primarily responsible for transmission during the summer months.[129] Adult females have been implicated in transmission during the early spring and late fall.[130]

Ribeiro *et al.*[131] demonstrated that *B. burgdorferi* organisms are generally restricted to the guts of unfed *I. scapularis* nymphs and adults. In their study, infected nymphs produced saliva containing the organisms within 3 days after attachment. For adult female ticks, spirochetes disseminated from the gut to the hemocoel at 4 days after attachment for approximately 50% of the ticks.[131] At that time, approximately one half of those adult female ticks produced saliva containing spirochetes. Thus, a minimum feeding period for infected ticks (which may be longer for adults than for nymphs) appears to be required before transmission of *B. burgdorferi* to the human host will occur. The smaller size and shorter feeding period of nymphal ticks compared to adults make them more effective vectors of *B. burgdorferi*. This is supported by the seasonal abundance of Lyme disease cases corresponding to periods of nymphal tick activity.[33]

The major reservoir for sustaining *B. burgdorferi* in

nature is small rodents, such as the white-footed mouse (*Peromyscus leucopus*). *B. burgdorferi* have also been isolated from raccoons, dogs, and deer.[56] Olsen *et al.*[58] determined the prevalence of *B. burgdorferi*-infected ticks (*I. ricinus*) on migrating birds in Scandinavia. Two percent of birds had such ticks attached. The authors concluded that these data support the notion that birds are partly responsible for the heterogeneous distribution of *B. burgdorferi* in Europe. While spirochetemia has been demonstrated in white-tailed deer, larval ticks that feed on deer do not appear to become infected by *B. burgdorferi*.[48,132] Transmission of *B. burgdorferi* from the rodent reservoir to larval ticks occurs when the ticks feed on rodents that harbor the organisms. Transstadial transmission occurs among *I. scapularis* and related ticks. The ticks, which acquire infection through a blood meal as larvae, remain infected through their development into nymphal and adult stages. Transstadial transmission is important to the vectorial capacity of ticks, which may feed on only one host between molts. Ticks such as *Dermacentor variabilis* and *A. americanum*, which appear able to acquire *B. burgdorferi* but are not able to maintain infection through a molt, do not appear to be competent vectors.[128] Nymphs may subsequently infect other rodents, small and large domestic mammals, and humans. Transovarial transmission from one tick generation to the next has been shown to occur in both naturally and experimentally infected *I. scapularis*. However, relatively few progeny remain infected, perhaps because eggs infected with *B. burgdorferi* fail to mature or incorporated spirochetes gradually die off during oogenesis.[133] Thus, transovarial transmission does not appear to provide an important mechanism for sustaining *B. burgdorferi* in nature.

Spirochetes have been found in deerflies, horseflies, and mosquitoes.[114,134] Individual cases have been reported in which EM has developed at the site of mosquito and deerfly bites.[114,135] However, the importance of these isolated reports is difficult to assess when compared to the strong epidemiological association between the geographic distribution of cases of Lyme disease and vector species of the genus *Ixodes*.[15] Magnarelli and Anderson[136] were not able to transmit *B. burgdorferi* from 11 naturally infected females of two mosquito species to hamsters upon which the mosquitoes were allowed to feed. Thus, the vector potential of these insects for transmission of *B. burgdorferi* remains unproven.

Contact transmission has been demonstrated in the laboratory between mice, and spirocheturic mice that have been collected from the wild.[137,138] These studies housed infected and uninfected mice together and demonstrated transmission to the uninfected mice. Contact transmission between animals may help to maintain the organisms in the small rodent reservoir.[138] Currently, there is no evidence to support person-to-person transmission. Transmission of *B. burgdorferi* through transfusion of blood obtained from an infected donor has not been reported; however, blood-borne transmission is theoretically possible. *B. burgdorferi* inoculated into blood samples collected on citrate phosphate dextrose preservative and held at 4°C remained viable in each of nine samples held for 25 days and for 60 days in a tenth sample.[139]

7. Pathogenesis and Immunity

B. burgdorferi spirochetes enter the susceptible host through the skin following a tick bite. EM, the earliest manifestation of acute infection, occurs at the site where the organisms enter the host. Histologically, EM skin lesions involve perivascular infiltrates predominantly composed of lymphocytes, but plasma cells and mast cells may also be present.[140] Spirochetes can be isolated from EM lesions (particularly the peripheral aspect of such lesions)[59,140–142] and can also be isolated from clinically normal perilesional skin,[141] indicating lateral migration through the skin of *B. burgdorferi* organisms.

In addition to migrating locally from the site of inoculation, the spirochetes also disseminate hematogenously early in the course of infection.[60,61,73,143] During this phase, diffuse visceral involvement can occur and can result in a clinical illness resembling acute mononucleosis. Lymphoid hyperplasia of lymph nodes and spleen can also occur, with prominent germinal centers and numerous perifollicular lymphocytes.[140] A proliferation of plasma cells and plasma cell precursors is also seen.[140] The ability of the spirochetes to disseminate appears to correlate with resistance to elimination by host phagocytic cells.[144]

Following dissemination of the spirochetes, specific organ system involvement occurs weeks (stage 2 disease) to months or years (stage 3 disease) after initial infection. Subsequent involvement predominantly affects the neurological, cardiac, and musculoskeletal systems. Histologically, lesions at each of these sites demonstrate infiltration of lymphocytes and plasma cells, often with vascular damage.[140] Spirochetes have been isolated from the myocardium in patients with active Lyme myocarditis[31,145,146] and from one patient with long-standing cardiomyopathy.[147] Spirochetes have also been isolated from CSF in patients with Lyme neuroborreliosis[60,148] and spirochetal antigens have been identified in CSF by PCR from patients with acute disseminated infection and from patients with symptoms of Lyme neuroborreliosis.[67,149,150] Spirochetes or spirochetal antigens have been identified in patients with acute and chronic Lyme arthritis as well.[64,69,151–153] The organisms have also been identified in other involved sites during the course of illness. These findings indicate that *B. burgdorferi* spirochetes can sequester themselves in selected anatomical sites and persist for years in host tissue. The persistence of spirochetes appears to be the most likely mechanism for pathogenesis of acute and chronic manifestations of Lyme disease.[154] Organisms are identified infrequently on tissue biopsy samples, suggesting that persistent pathology relies on the presence of relatively few organisms. It is also possible that spirochetes may survive in the host at the intracellular level. *B. burgdorferi* have been shown to localize intracellularly in *in vitro* systems[155]; however, the clinical significance of this finding is not yet known.

Small numbers of organisms can apparently maintain host inflammatory responses that may contribute to the pathogenesis of disease. *B. burgdorferi* have been shown to induce immunoregulatory cytokines that mediate inflammation, including tumor necrosis factor-alpha (TNF-α) and interleukin-1β (IL-1β).[154,156,157] *B. burgdorferi* are also capable of adhering to endothelial cells and cells of glial origin.[154,158] Injury to endothelium and endothelial cell activation may contribute to pathogenesis of disease in a variety of organs. In support of this hypothesis, perivasculitis and microvascular lesions have been demonstrated in cardiac, synovial, skin, and neurological tissues from patients with Lyme disease.[140,159–161] Other host factors may also play a role in the pathogenesis of Lyme disease. For example, circulating immune complexes have been demonstrated in several studies.[162–164] A recent study also demonstrated an association between chronic Lyme arthritis refractory to antibiotic therapy and the presence of the HLA-DR4 histocompatibility gene.[165] This susceptibility may be related to an ineffective immune response in such patients or to autoimmune mechanisms stimulated by *B. burgdorferi* infection.

7.2. Immunity

Early in the course of infection, a vigorous specific T-cell response to *B. burgdorferi* occurs.[166] The humoral response begins with appearance of IgM antibody, which generally peaks between the third and sixth week of infection.[77] In some patients, IgM titers may remain elevated throughout the course of illness.[77] Specific IgM antibody to *B. burgdorferi* (generally directed to the 41-kDa flagellar antigen) often is associated with elevated total serum IgM levels.[77] A second delayed IgM response late in the course of illness has also been demonstrated in some patients, suggesting that persistence of spirochetes in the host can trigger a new immune response as the disease process unfolds.[167] The IgG response generally is detectable 4 to 6 weeks after infection and may expand over time. IgG antibody may remain elevated for years after clinical remission,[79] although antibody levels tend to decline slowly over time following treatment. IgG antibodies develop to multiple spirochetal antigens,[167,168] with the response culminating in the development of antibody to the 31-kDa OspA and the 34-kDa OspB spirochetal proteins, from months to years after illness onset.[169] In some patients who receive early antibiotic therapy, the humoral immune response may be aborted due to removal of microbial antigens. Patients with early incomplete therapy and subsequent negative antibody titers may develop late sequelae of Lyme disease.[23] In these cases of seronegative Lyme disease, a vigorous proliferative T-cell response can be detected, supporting a dissociation between T-cell and B-cell immune response in such patients.[23]

Intrathecal production of specific IgG antibody to *B. burgdorferi* has been demonstrated in patients with Lyme neuroborreliosis.[170–172] Identification of local antibody production appears to be greatest (>90%) in patients with early Lyme meningitis,[170] and is less commonly detected in patients with late or chronic neurological manifestations of Lyme disease.[170,173] Antibodies to IgG, IgM, and IgA have been detected in the CSF.[170] In one study, the 41-kDa flagellar antigen was the major antigen leading to a specific intrathecal IgG response.[171] Another study demonstrated a rapid decline in antibody-secreting cells in the CSF following antibiotic therapy and clinical improvement.[172]

Antibody response following natural infection appears to confer immunity to *B. burgdorferi*, since cases of reinfection have not been reported in patients who develop an expanded antibody response. Reinfection may develop, however, in patients who lose IgG antibody or in those who receive early therapy and do not mount an adequate immune response.[174]

8. Patterns of Host Response

8.1. Clinical Features

Lyme disease is a multisystem disorder that generally occurs in stages. Stage 1, early infection, is characterized by localized EM. Stage 2, disseminated infection, occurs several days to weeks after EM is recognized. At the time of hematogenous dissemination, patients often experience a variety of constitutional symptoms including severe migratory arthralgias and myalgias, debilitating malaise and fatigue, generalized lymphadenopathy, splenomegaly, hepatitis, headache, and fever. Secondary annular EM skin lesions often occur at this time, as well as other dermatologic manifestations. A variety of other systems, including neurological and cardiac, are often involved during stage 2 disease. Stage 3, persistent infection, is predominantly characterized by chronic arthritis. Other manifestations of stage 3 disease include chronic neurological involvement, interstitial keratitis, acrodermatitis chronica atrophicans, and persistent fatigue. Stage 3 occurs months to years after initial infection.

8.1.1. Dermatologic Manifestations. Lyme disease typically begins with the characteristic skin lesion, EM, which is the hallmark of stage 1 Lyme disease. EM begins as a red macule or papule at the site of a tick bite, which expands to form an annular lesion, usually with an indurated outer border accompanied by partial central clearing.[175] Initial lesions range in size from a few centimeters to more than 60 cm as expansion occurs. At times, central clearing does not occur; instead, the initial lesion can become intensely erythematous and indurated or the center can become vesicular and necrotic.[175] In one study, 30% of 314 patients evaluated recalled a tick bite in the previous month at the site of the initial lesion.[175] In another study, 14% of patients were aware of having been bitten by a tick.[176] The time interval between tick bite and the appearance of EM in that study was 1 to 36 days, with a median of 9 days. The initial lesion occurs most commonly in the thigh, groin, or axilla. Secondary multiple annular skin lesions develop in approximately 50% of patients within several days after the onset of EM. Secondary lesions tend to be similar to the initial lesion, but are smaller and tend to be less migratory. In one study, EM persisted for a median of 28 days in 55 patients not treated with antimicrobial agents.[175] With antimicrobial therapy, skin lesions typically resolve within several days. Occasionally, patients who are not treated with antimicrobial agents can have a recurrence of EM lesions months after initial onset.

Other dermatologic manifestations that can occur during stage 2 disease include diffuse erythema, urticaria, evanescent lesions, or a malar rash.[175] A spirochetal lymphocytoma can also occur in stage 2 and appears as a solitary skin lesion at the site of a tick bite.[177] The lymphocytoma may present as a small nodule or as a plaque several centimeters in diameter; histopathologic examination demonstrates follicles consisting of small lymphocytes and central larger cells are noted. Both B and T lymphocytes are present; macrophages, plasma cells, and eosinophils may also be noted. If untreated, such lesions may last months to years.

In stage 3 disease, acrodermatitis chronica atrophicans can occur; this condition has been observed primarily in Europe. It is a chronic skin disorder that begins with violaceous discoloration of the skin, associated with inflammation and swelling. In later phases, the skin may become thin and atrophic or sclerotic. *B. burgdorferi* organisms have been cultured from these lesions up to 10 years after onset.[178] Occasionally, involvement of underlying bone or joint tissue can occur.

8.1.2. Neurological Manifestations. Neurological symptoms can occur early in the clinical course when EM lesions are still present. Such symptoms are suggestive of meningeal irritation and include headache and stiff neck; however, examination of CSF from such patients is generally normal.[5] The classic neurological involvement of stage 2 disease generally begins several weeks after onset of EM. The major neurological manifestations of *B. burgdorferi* infection during stage 2 disease include meningitis, cranial neuritis, and peripheral neurological disorders.[26,179–181] Approximately 15% of untreated patients will develop neurological involvement.[179] Patients with Lyme meningitis frequently complain of headache, photophobia, meningismus, and fever. Evaluation of CSF generally reveals a lymphocytic pleocytosis associated with an elevated protein and normal glucose. Patients with meningitis often also have symptoms of mild encephalitis, including confusion, irritability, poor memory, disorientation, and emotional lability. Most patients with stage 2 neurological disease respond well to antibiotic therapy.[26] Cranial neuropathy frequently occurs in the presence of meningitis and may be unilateral or bilateral. In one study of 38 patients, 50% had facial palsies.[179] Isolated Bell's palsy (without recognized prior EM) can be a presenting feature of Lyme disease.[182] Facial nerve palsy is the most common manifestation of cranial neuritis; however, multiple other cranial nerves may be involved and optic neuritis with atrophy can occur.[180,181]

Peripheral neurological disorders associated with stage 2 disease include radiculoneuropathy, diffuse peripheral neuropathy, mononeuropathy multiplex, brachial neuritis, motor neuropathy, lumbosacral plexopathy, Guillain–Barré-like syndrome, and intermittent paresthesias.[179,183,184] Most patients respond to antibiotic therapy.[179,184] Electrophysiological studies suggest axonal degeneration.[160] Biopsies of peripheral nerves demonstrate perivascular lymphocytic infiltrates and distal axonal loss.[140,160]

In stage 3 disease, months to years after initial infection, patients may develop chronic peripheral and/or central neurological manifestations.[173,185–187] Central nervous system involvement during stage 3 disease consists predominantly of subacute encephalopathy, characterized by memory loss, mood changes, or sleep disturbance.[173,185–187] In addition, a variety of neuropsychiatric symptoms have been associated with chronic central nervous system involvement, including paranoia, dementia, major depression, and bipolar disorder.[188] Current evidence indicates that chronic Lyme neuroborreliosis can present with a range of clinical findings and is similar to tertiary syphilis in that regard.[189] In one study of 27 patients with chronic Lyme neuroborreliosis, peripheral neurological symptoms began a median of 16 months after onset of infection and symptoms of the central nervous system began a median of 26 months after disease onset.[173] Sixteen patients (63%) had both peripheral and central nervous system complaints.[173] Of 24 patients with encephalopathy, 18 (75%) had increased CSF protein levels, intrathecal production of antibody to *B. burgdorferi*, or both.[173] Most such patients respond to antibiotic therapy; however, response is not uniform and some patients may relapse.[173,185] Further studies are needed to determine appropriate treatment strategies for such patients.

8.1.3. Cardiac Manifestations. Evidence of cardiac involvement can occur as part of stage 2 disease and symptoms develop several weeks to several months after illness onset.[4] Approximately 5% of patients will develop Lyme carditis (pericarditis and/or myocarditis) in the absence of therapy.[4] Cardiac manifestations of Lyme disease include atrioventricular conduction defects (first degree, second degree, and complete heart block), bundle branch block, atrial and ventricular tachyarrhythmias, and myocardial dysfunction with cardiomegaly.[4,190–192] Ventricular arrhythmias are uncommon and generally occur as escape rhythms, whereas atrial arrhythmias most likely occur as a result of pericarditis.[193] The electrocardiogram may demonstrate evidence of conduction defects or may show nonspecific ST- and T-wave changes.[193] Gallium scan may demonstrate an intense diffuse uptake in the myocardium of some patients.[194,195] Cardiac involvement tends to be of short duration, usually lasting less than 6 weeks. Temporary pacemakers may be needed during the acute phase. Chronic cardiomyopathy apparently caused by *B. burgdorferi* infection has been reported,[4] but this condition appears rare.

8.1.4. Musculoskeletal Manifestations. The classic feature of stage 3 Lyme disease is arthritis. Within several weeks after onset of illness, most untreated patients with Lyme disease will develop migratory myalgias and arthralgias, often without objective joint swelling. True arthritis generally does not begin until months after illness onset.[3] Without treatment, approximately 60% of patients will develop intermittent joint swelling, generally of large joints, particularly the knee. The median duration of arthritis in a single joint was 8 days in one study, with some attacks lasting up to 3 months.[3] In some patients, arthritis may become chronic (defined as a year or more of continuous inflammation), sometimes with erosion of cartilage or bone. Occasionally, permanent joint disability can occur.[196] Lyme disease can mimic rheumatoid arthritis with symmetrical polyarthritis involving smaller joints. Without treatment, attacks of arthritis will often gradually subside in many patients over several years.[196,197] However, joint pain may persist in some patients if not treated. In one study of children, up to one third had sporadic joint pain as long as 10 years after onset of acute arthritis.[196] Lyme arthritis generally responds well to antimicrobial therapy[27]; however, some patients appear to be relatively refractory to treatment. The histocompatibility type HLA-DR4 has been associated with lack of treatment response.[169,198] Some patients who fail to respond have also been shown to have high levels of circulating IgG antibody to the Osp A of *B. burgdorferi*.[169,198] Another study demonstrated that patients with low concentrations of IL-1 receptor antagonist and high concentrations of IL-1β in the synovial fluid recovered slowly from arthritis.[199] This finding suggests that cytokine levels within the joint space may play a role in treatment response.

Joint fluid analysis during episodes of arthritis demonstrates a leukocytosis consisting mostly of granulocytes.[3] Synovial biopsies demonstrate synovial hypertrophy, vascular proliferation, and infiltration of mononuclear cells.[3]

Other musculoskeletal syndromes have been reported with *B. burgdorferi* infection. These include myositis, diffuse fasciitis, osteomyelitis, and panniculitis.[200–204] Myositis tends to be localized and is often demonstrated near an involved joint or localized neuropathy. One case of dermatomyositis associated with periorbital edema, dysphagia, proximal muscle weakness, and elevated creatine phosphokinase has been reported.[201] *B. burgdorferi* organisms have been identified in tissue from two patients with diffuse fasciitis and peripheral eosinophilia.[202] Rarely, in patients with achrodermatitis chronica atrophicans, chronic joint and bone involvement including joint subluxations and periostitis can occur beneath existing skin lesions.

8.1.5. Other Manifestations of Lyme Disease. A variety of ocular findings have been reported in patients with Lyme disease. The optic nerve (i.e., optic neuritis, optic atrophy, papilledema) can be involved in neuroborreliosis. Other ocular findings during stage 2 disease include conjunctivitis early in the clinical course, uveitis, and endophthalmitis.[205] During stage 3 disease, interstitial keratitis, peripheral ulcerative keratitis, and episcleritis may occur.[205]

Adverse outcomes have ben associated with Lyme disease in pregnancy, and maternal–fetal transmission has been documented.[63,206–208] Case reports have included stillbirth or neonatal death, premature birth, rash illness, syndactyly, and cortical blindness. In two cases of neonatal death, cardiac abnormalities were noted on infant autopsies. In some instances, the mothers received antibiotic treatment, and in some, they did not. These case reports suggest that congenital Lyme disease may occur; however, this condition appears to be rare.

8.2. Diagnosis

Direct detection of the organism is of limited utility, since few organisms may be present in infected tissues. The diagnosis of stage 1 disease can usually be made based on the presence of EM, since serological assays may often be negative early in the clinical course. Later stages of disease can generally be diagnosed based on the clinical presentation and an elevated antibody response to *B. burgdorferi*. However, EM as a presenting manifestation may be missed or may be absent; therefore, the diagnosis cannot be ruled out in the absence of a history of EM. Serological antibody assays most commonly used in the diagnosis of Lyme disease include EIA and indirect immunofluorescence assays.[77,209,210] Four to six weeks after infection, most patients will have detectable IgG antibody to *B. burgdorferi*. However, false-positive and false-negative results can occur. False-positive results can occur due to cross-reactivity from other spirochetal infections.[84] In addition, asymptomatic infection with *B. burgdorferi* can occur, leading to a certain proportion of the population having detectable antibody in the absence of symptoms. Thus, if persons with past asymptomatic infection develop suggestive symptoms of Lyme disease from some other etiology, they may be falsely diagnosed with Lyme disease. False-negative results can occur if testing is performed too early in the clinical course, or if the antibody response is aborted due to prior antibiotic therapy.[166] One study has suggested that apparent seronegativity in Lyme disease may be due to sequestration of antibody to *B. burgdorferi* in circulating immune complexes.[211] Western blot testing can improve specificity of serological testing[81] and is recommended for confirming or classifying serological tests that are positive or indeterminant, respectively.[40] *B. burgdorferi* antibody testing on CSF may be useful in the diagnosis of Lyme neuroborreliosis.

8.3. Treatment

Antibiotic treatment of erythema migrans and early febrile symptoms has been shown to prevent late manifestations of Lyme disease.[24,212] Current data indicate that early infection in adults can usually be treated successfully with tetracycline, doxycycline, amoxicillin, or penicillin V, with erythromycin as a second-line drug.[22] The minimum duration of therapy for early disease is 10 days; however, treatment needs to be guided by clinical response, and some patients with early disease need longer therapy. Neurological manifestations, arthritis, and carditis often require parenteral therapy (ceftriaxone, penicillin) for 14–28 days.

9. Control and Prevention

9.1. General Concepts

Prevention of Lyme disease is currently a matter of personal protection. Commonly recommended measures include: avoiding tick-infested areas during the spring, summer, and fall; taking steps to prevent tick attachment such as using repellents and wearing protective clothing; and performing daily body checks for the presence of ticks. The small size of nymphal ticks, their abundance at times when the larger adults may not be active, and their predilection for attachment sites such as the back of the knee, the groin, the axilla, and behind the ear, indicate the need for constant summertime awareness. Since ticks may need to feed for a day or longer before transmission of the organisms is possible, daily removal of attached ticks should help prevent the disease. However, Smith *et al.*[126] found that outdoor workers who took precautions such as wearing long pants or long-sleeve shirts, tucking pants into socks, using insect repellents on skin or clothing, and checking themselves for ticks were as likely to have antibody to *B. burgdorferi* as were workers who did not take similar precautions. If tick avoidance measures fail, early recognition of signs and symptoms and appropriate antimicrobial therapy can generally prevent the later manifestations of Lyme disease.

Several measures to control tick populations also have been evaluated. Wilson *et al.*[213] found acaricidal treatment of deer to be impractical and that removal of 70% of a local deer herd did not markedly reduce the abundance of ticks. However, elimination of the deer herd resulted in reduced abundance of larval ticks the following summer and a more gradual decline in the abundance of nymphs and adults.(214) Duffy *et al.*(215) found that while *I. scapularis* nymphs were less abundant on Shelter Island where there were no white-tailed deer, they were nonetheless present. They conclude that populations of *I. scapularis* can occur and reproduce in the absence of white-tailed deer, so eradication of the deer population would reduce but not eliminate the risk of Lyme disease. Mather *et al.*(216) showed that mice will use permethrin-treated cotton as nesting material. The use of this product in wooded sites resulted in a 90% reduction in the number of ticks carried by mice in the treated sits compared to mice captured in an untreated adjacent area.(216) Schulze *et al.*(217) achieved 97 to 100% reductions of adult *I. scapularis* with ground applications of insecticide following leaf abscission in the fall; however, this strategy is limited by its lack of effect in immature stages. Destruction of mouse habitat by burning and mowing brush may locally reduce the abundance of questing adult ticks; however, displacement of mice by mowing alone resulted in a short-term increase in the abundance of nymphal *I. scapularis* on the freshly mown land.(218) The potential effectiveness of communitywide application of such measures to prevent Lyme disease is unknown.

In the absence of tick control measures, awareness of Lyme disease in endemic areas will remain the primary prevention strategy. Endemic areas can be identified through disease surveillance and through tick surveys or serological surveys of rodents, other mammals, and humans.

9.2. Prophylaxis

Antimicrobial prophylaxis of persons who are bitten by *Ixodes* ticks has not been formally recommended. However, it remains controversial, since some practitioners do recommend such treatment. To date, four studies have been reported that attempt to determine the probability of contracting Lyme disease after a tick bite in an area of endemic disease.(219–222) These results are summarized as a pooled estimate, and a probability has been determined.(115) In these four studies, the probability of contracting Lyme disease after a tick bite ranged from 0.012 to 0.05, with a 95% confidence interval of 0.013 to 0.049. In general, the authors of these studies conclude that even in an area in which Lyme disease is endemic, the risk of infection with *B. burgdorferi* after a recognized bite with *I. scapularis* is so low that prophylactic antimicrobial treatment is not routinely indicated.

9.3. Immunization

Reinfection with *B. burgdorferi* and a subsequent course of Lyme disease has not been observed in patients with a vigorous antibody response following their initial infection. Although reinfection may occur in patients who received inadequate therapy early in the course of Lyme disease, this likely represents an aborted antibody response due to early therapy. Thus, it would appear that protective immunity can be achieved with natural infection. In an experimental animal model of Lyme disease, mice vaccinated with recombinant OspA were protected from infection with *B. burgdorferi* both by antibody-mediated killing of the spirochete within the host and by destruction of the organism within the tick prior to disease transmission.(223,224)

A chemically inactivated whole-cell *B. burgdorferi* vaccine formulated with a proprietary polymer-based adjuvant (Fort Dodge Laboratories, Fort Dodge, IA) was conditionally licensed by the US Department of Agriculture in 1990 for use in dogs. This vaccine was given full licensure in 1992, but published information on its effectiveness and safety is still limited.(225,226) Vaccinated dogs primarily develop antibodies to certain outer-surface proteins (OspA and OspB) of the vaccine strain of *B. burgdorferi*.

In a phase 1 efficacy trial on humans, OspA vaccine was found to be safe and immunogenic.(227) Phases 2 and 3 safety studies and trials are now underway. However, development of a human Lyme disease vaccine may be complicated by several factors. First, antigenic variability of *B. burgdorferi* between strains and during the course of an infection can occur.(228–230) Second, designing a clinical trial of Lyme disease vaccine may be difficult. Incidence rates of 1.5 to 3.3% in endemic areas(41,42) would require enrollment of large numbers of study participants, each of whom would need to be screened to determine prior exposure to *B. burgdorferi*. Also, vaccinating should lead to *B. burgdorferi* antibody production, thereby prohibiting the ability to measure antibody as an endpoint of infection. Thus, vaccine efficacy measurements would need to be based on prevention of certain clinical manifestations, including arthritis, cardiac, and neurological sequelae. Evaluating such endpoints in a large clinical trial poses major diagnostic and logistic difficulties. Third, Lyme disease, like Rocky Mountain Spotted Fever, is a tick-borne illness of regional importance. The potential use for a human vaccine would likely be limited to individuals at high risk of exposure (i.e., those in endemic areas). Vaccine manufacturers may determine that a limited market is insufficient to justify vaccine development costs. Finally, the public health impact of a vaccine may be limited, because Lyme disease can frequently be recognized by clinicians and successfully treated with antimicrobial agents in most instances.

10. Unresolved Problems

10.1. Epidemiology

Much progress has been made in the laboratory diagnosis of infection with *B. burgdorferi*. The use of standardized criteria to interpret Western immunoblot results will allow many chronic and nonspecific illnesses to be ruled out from the diagnosis of Lyme disease. The development of PCR assays will increasingly allow for determination of active versus past infection. These methods need further development and clinical evaluation, but they form the basis for an objective definition of Lyme disease that has been lacking in the past.

A major new problem that needs to be addressed is the role of coinfection with *Babesia microti* and with the agent of human granulocytic ehrlichiosis. These pathogens, along with *B. burgdorferi*, have been shown to infect and to be transmitted by *I. scapularis* and to occur in the same geographic areas. Coinfection could alter both the severity of acute infection and the likelihood of chronic manifestations of illness caused by these agents, including Lyme disease. The extent to which coinfections occur and their relative contributions to morbidity remain to be determined.

10.2. Control and Prevention

Wide-area tick control has not been shown to result in sustained control of tick populations or to reduce the occurrence of Lyme disease in communities. Individual prevention measures have a mixed record of success in reducing reported tick exposures and infection, but remain the primary public health prevention message. Additional studies are needed to evaluate behavioral interventions to allow health officials to better target health education messages.

The continuing development of a human vaccine for Lyme disease offers the potential to reduce Lyme disease in the absence of other personal or area-wide control measures. However, a human vaccine remains on the horizon. In addition, the potential for transmission of *Ehrlichia* and *Babesia* species will continue to require prevention efforts designed to reduce exposures to the tick vectors.

11. References

1. Steere, A. C., Malawista, S. E., Snydman, D. R., *et al.*, Lyme arthritis: An epidemic of oligoarticular arthritis in children and adults in three Connecticut communities, *Arthritis Rheum.* **20:**7–17 (1977).
2. Reik, L., Steere, A. C., Bartenhagen, N. H., *et al.*, Neurologic abnormalities of Lyme disease, *Medicine* **58:**281–294 (1979).
3. Steere, A. C., Malawista, S. E., Hardin, J. A., *et al.*, Erythema chronicum migrans and Lyme arthritis: The enlarging clinical spectrum, *Ann. Intern. Med.* **86:**685–698 (1977).
4. Steere, A. C., Batsford, W. P., Weinberg, M., *et al.*, Lyme carditis: Cardiac abnormalities of Lyme disease, *Ann. Intern. Med.* **93:**8–16 (1980).
5. Steere, A. C., Bartenhagen, N. H., Craft, J. E., *et al.*, The early clinical manifestations of Lyme disease, *Ann. Intern. Med.* **99:** 76–82 (1983).
6. Afzelius, A., Erythema chronicum migrans, *Acta Derm. Venereol.* **2:**120–125 (1921).
7. Bannwarth, A., Chronische lymphocyte meningitis, entzundliche polyneuritis and "Rheumatismus." Ein Beitrag zum problem "Allergie und Nervensystem." *Arch. Psychiatr. Nervenkr.* **113:** 284–376 (1941).
8. Garin Bujadoux, C. H., Paralysie par les tiques, *J. Med. Lyon* **71c:**765–767 (1922).
9. Hellerstrom, S., Erythema chronicum migrans Afzelii, *Acta Derm. Venereol.* **11:**315–321 (1930).
10. Binder, E., Doepfmer, R., and Hornstein, O., Experimentelle Ubertragung des erythema chronicum migrans von Mensch zu Mensch, *Hautarzt* **6:**494–496 (1955).
11. Hollstrom, E., Successful treatment of erythema migrans Afzelius, *Acta Derm. Venereol.* **31:**235–243 (1951).
12. Lennhoff, C., Spirochaetes in aetiologically obscure diseases, *Acta Derm. Venereol.* **28:**295–324 (1948).
13. Scrimenti, R. J., Erythema chronicum migrans, *Arch. Dermatol.* **102:**104–105 (1970).
14. Smith, L., Burgdorfer, W., and Katz, H., Erythema chronicum migrans, *Cutis* **17**(S)**:**962–964 (1976).
15. Steere, A. C., and Malawista, S. E., Cases of Lyme disease in the United States: Locations correlated with distribution of *Ixodes dammini*, *Ann. Intern. Med.* **91:**730–733 (1979).
16. Steere, A. C., Broderick, T. F., and Malawista, S. E., Erythema chronicum migrans and Lyme arthritis: Epidemiologic evidence for a tick vector, *Am. J. Epidemiol.* **108:**312–321 (1978).
17. Schulze, T. L., Bowen, G. S., Bosler, E. M., *et al.*, *Amblyomma americanum*: A potential vector of Lyme disease in New Jersey, *Science* **224:**601–603 (1984).
18. Burgdorfer, W., Barbour, A. G., Hayes, S. F., *et al.*, Lyme disease–A tickborne spirochetosis? *Science* **216:**1319–1320 (1982).
19. Benach, J. L., Bosler, E. M., Hanrahan, J. P., *et al.*, Spirochetes isolated from the blood of two patients with Lyme disease, *N. Engl. J. Med.* **308:**740–742 (1983).
20. Steere, A. C., Grodzicki, R. L., Kornblatt, A. N., *et al.*, The spirochetal etiology of Lyme disease, *N. Engl. J. Med.* **308:**733–740 (1983).
21. Johnson, R. C., Schmid, G. P., Hyde, F. W., *et al.*, *Borrelia burgdorferi* sp. nov.: Etiologic agent of Lyme disease, *Int. J. Syst. Bacteriol.* **34:**496–497 (1984).
22. Steere, A. C., Lyme disease, *N. Engl. J. Med.* **321:**586–596 (1989).

23. Dattwyler, R. J., Volkman, D. J., Luft, B. J., *et al.*, Seronegative Lyme disease: Dissociation of specific T- and B-lymphocyte responses to *Borrelia burgdorferi*, *N. Engl. J. Med.* **319:**1441–1446 (1988).
24. Steere, A. C., Hutchinson, G. J., Rahn, D. W., *et al.*, Treatment of the early manifestations of Lyme disease, *Ann. Intern. Med.* **99:** 22–26 (1983).
25. Dattwyler, R. J., Halperin, J. J., Pass, H., *et al.*, Ceftriaxone as effective therapy in refractory Lyme disease, *J. Infect. Dis.* **155:** 1322–1325 (1987).
26. Steere, A. C., Pachner, A. R., and Malawista, S. E., Neurologic abnormalities of Lyme disease: Successful treatment with high-dose intravenous penicillin, *Ann. Intern. Med.* **99:**767–772 (1983).
27. Steere, A. C., Green, J., Schoen, R., *et al.*, Successful parenteral penicillin therapy of established Lyme arthritis, *N. Engl. J. Med.* **312:**869–874 (1985).
28. Skoldenberg, B., Stiernstedt, G., Karlsson, M., *et al.*, Treatment of Lyme borreliosis with emphasis on neurological disease, *Ann. NY Acad. Sci.* **539:**317–323 (1988).
29. Dattwyler, R. J., Halperin, J. J., Volkman, D. J., *et al.*, Treatment of late Lyme borreliosis—Randomized comparison of cerftriaxone and penicillin, *Lancet* **1:**1191–1194 (1988).
30. Asbrink, E., and Hovmark, A., Classification, geographic variations, and epidemiology of Lyme borreliosis, *Clin. Dermatol.* **11:**353–357 (1993).
31. Marcus, L. C., Steere, A. C., Duray, P. H., *et al.*, Fatal pancarditis in a patient with coexistent Lyme disease and babesiosis. Demonstration of spirochetes in the myocardium, *Ann. Intern. Med.* **103:**374–376 (1985).
32. Kirsch, M., Ruben, F. L., Steere, A. C., *et al.*, Fatal adult respiratory distress syndrome in a patient with Lyme disease, *J. Am. Med. Assoc.* **259:**2737–2739 (1988).
33. Schmid, G. P., Horsley, R., Steere, A. C., *et al.*, Surveillance of Lyme disease in the United States, 1982, *J. Infect. Dis.* **151:**1144–1148 (1985).
34. Ciesielski, C. A., Markowitz, L. E., Horsley, R., *et al.*, The geographic distribution of Lyme disease in the United States, *Ann. NY Acad. Sci.* **539:**283–288 (1988).
35. Centers for Disease Control and Prevention, Case definitions for public health surveillance, *Morbid. Mortal. Week. Rep.* **39**(No. RR-13):19–21 (1990).
36. Hedberg, C. W., Osterholm, M. T., MacDonald, K. L., *et al.*, An interlaboratory study of antibody to *Borrelia burgdorferi*, *J. Infect. Dis.* **154:**1325–1327 (1987).
37. Luger, S. W., and Krauss, E., Serologic tests for Lyme disease: Interlaboratory variability, *Arch. Intern. Med.* **150:**761–763 (1990).
38. Schwartz, B. S., Goldstein, M. D., Ribeiro, J. M., *et al.*, Antibody testing in Lyme disease: A comparison of results in four laboratories, *J. Am. Med. Assoc.* **262:**3431–3434 (1989).
39. Cutler, S. J., and Wright, D. J. M., Predictive value of serology in diagnosing Lyme borreliosis, *J. Clin. Pathol.* **47:**344–349 (1994).
40. Association of State and Territorial Public Health Laboratory Directors, Recommendations for test performance and interpretation from the Second National Conference on Serologic Diagnosis of Lyme Disease, *Morbid. Mortal. Week. Rep.* **44:**590–591 (1995).
41. Hanrahan, J. P., Benach, J. L., Coleman, J. L., *et al.*, Incidence and cumulative frequency of endemic Lyme disease in a community, *J. Infect. Dis.* **150:**489–496 (1984).
42. Steere, A. C., Taylor, E., Wilson, M. L., *et al.*, Longitudinal assessment of the clinical and epidemiological features of Lyme disease in a community, *J. Infect. Dis.* **154:**295–300 (1986).
43. Lastavica, C. C., Wilson, M. L., Berardi, V. P., *et al.*, Rapid emergence of a focal epidemic of Lyme disease in coastal Massachusetts, *N. Engl. J. Med.* **320:**133–137 (1989).
44. Alpert, B., Esin, J., Sivak, S. L., *et al.*, Incidence and prevalence of Lyme disease in a suburban Westchester county community, *NY State J. Med.* **92:**5–8 (1992).
45. Feder, H. M., Gerber, M. A., Cartter, M. L., *et al.*, Prospective assessment of Lyme disease in a school-aged population in Connecticut, *J. Infect. Dis.* **171:**1371–1374 (1995).
46. Gustafson, R., Svenungsson, B., Forsgren, M., *et al.*, Two-year survey of the incidence of Lyme borreliosis and tick-borne encephalitis in a high-risk population in Sweden, *Eur. J. Clin. Microbiol. Infect. Dis.* **11:**894–900 (1992).
47. Fahrer, H., van der Linden, S. M., Sauvain, M. J., *et al.*, The prevalence and incidence of clinical and asymptomatic Lyme borreliosis in a population at risk, *J. Infect. Dis.* **163:**305–310 (1991).
48. Bosler, E. M., Ormiston, B. G., Coleman, J. L., *et al.*, Prevalence of the Lyme disease spirochete in populations of white-tailed deer and white-footed mice, *Yale J. Biol. Med.* **57:**651–659 (1984).
49. Levine, J. F., Wilson, M. L., Spielman, A., Mice as reservoirs of the lyme disease spirochete, *Am. J. Trop. Med. Hyg.* **34:**355–360 (1985).
50. Fish, D., and Daniels, T. J., The role of medium-sized mammals as reservoirs of *Borrelia burgdorferi* in southern New York, *J. Wildlife Dis.* **26:**339–345 (1990).
51. Magnarelli, L. A., Anderson, J. F., Kaufman, A., *et al.*, Borreliosis in dogs from southern Connecticut, *J. Am. Vet. Med. Assoc.* **186:**955–959 (1985).
52. Bosler, E. M., Cohen, D., Schulze, T., *et al.*, Host responses to *Borrelia burgdorferi* in dogs and horses, *Ann. NY Acad. Sci.* **539:**221–234 (1988).
53. Burgess, E. C., *Borrelia burgdorferi* infection in Wisconsin horses and cows, *Ann. NY Acad. Sci.* **539:**235–243 (1988).
54. Cohen, D., Bosler, E. M., Bernard, W., *et al.*, Epidemiologic studies of Lyme disease in horses and their public health significance, *Ann. NY Acad. Sci.* **539:**244–257 (1988).
55. Marcus, L. C., Patterson, M., Gilfillan, R., *et al.*, Antibodies to *Borrelia burgdorferi* in New England horses: Serologic survey, *Am. J. Vet. Res.* **46:**2570–2571 (1985).
56. Anderson, J. F., Mammalian and avian reservoirs for *Borrelia burgdorferi*, *Ann. NY Acad. Sci.* **539:**180–191 (1988).
57. Anderson, J. F., Johnson, R. C., Magnarelli, L. A., *et al.*, Involvement of birds in the epidemiology of the Lyme disease agent *Borrelia burgdorferi*, *Infect. Immun.* **51:**394–396 (1986).
58. Olsen, B., Jaenson, T. G. T., and Bergstrom, S., Prevalence of *Borrelia burgdorferi sensu lato*-infected ticks on migrating birds, *Appl. Environ. Microbiol.* **61:**3082–3087 (1995).
59. Berger, B. W., Kaplan, M. H., Rothenberg, I. R., *et al.*, Isolation and characterization of the Lyme disease spirochete from the skin of patients with erythema chronicum migrans, *J. Am. Acad. Dermatol.* **13:**444–449 (1985).
60. Steere, A. C., Grodzicki, R. L., Craft, J. E., *et al.*, Recovery of Lyme disease spirochetes from patients, *Yale J. Biol. Med.* **57:** 557–560 (1984).
61. Nadelman, R. B., Pavia, C. S., Magnerelli, L. A., *et al.*, Isolation of *Borrelia burgdorferi* from the blood of seven patients with Lyme disease, *Am. J. Med.* **88:**21–26 (1990).

62. Wallach, F. R., Forni, A. L., Hariprashad, J., *et al.*, Circulating *Borrelia burgdorferi* in patients with acute Lyme disease: Results of blood cultures and serum DNA analysis, *J. Infect. Dis.* **168:** 1541–1543 (1993).
63. Schlesinger, P. A., Duray, P. H., Burke, B. A., *et al.*, Maternal–fetal transmission of the Lyme disease spirochete, *Borrelia burgdorferi*, *Ann. Intern. Med.* **103:**67–68 (1985).
64. Snydman, D. R., Schenkein, D. P., Berardi, V. P., *et al.*, *Borrelia burgdorferi* in joint fluid in chronic Lyme arthritis, *Ann. Intern. Med.* **104:**798–800 (1986).
65. Goodman, J. L., Jurkovich, P., Kramber, J. M., *et al.*, Molecular detection of persistent *Borrelia burgdorferi* in the urine of patients with active Lyme disease, *Infect. Immun.* **59:**269–278 (1991).
66. Lebech, A. M., and Hansen, K., Detection of *Borrelia burgdorferi* DNA in urine samples and cerebrospinal fluid samples from patients with early and late Lyme neuroborreliosis by polymerase chain reaction, *J. Clin. Microbiol.* **30:**1646–1653 (1992).
67. Keller, T. L., Halperin, J. J., and Whitman, M., PCR detection of *Borrelia burgdorferi* DNA in cerebrospinal fluid of Lyme neuroborreliosis patients, *Neurology* **42:**32–42 (1992).
68. Pachner, A. R., and Delaney, E., The polymerase chain reaction in the diagnosis of Lyme neuroborreliosis, *Ann. Neurol.* **34:**544–550 (1993).
69. Nocton, J. J., Dressler, F., Rutledge, B. J., *et al.*, Detection of *Borrelia burgdorferi* DNA by polymerase chain reaction in synovial fluid from patients with Lyme arthritis, *N. Engl. J. Med.* **330:**229–234 (1994).
70. Persing, D. H., Rutledge, B. J., Rys, P. N., *et al.*, Target imbalance: Disparity of *Borrelia burgdorferi* genetic material in synovial fluid from Lyme arthritis patients, *J. Infect. Dis.* **169:**668–672 (1994).
71. Schwartz, I., Wormser, G. P., Schwartz, J. J., *et al.*, Diagnosis of early Lyme disease by polymerase chain reaction amplification and culture of skin biopsies from erythema migrans lesions, *J. Clin. Microbiol.* **30:**3082–3088 (1992).
72. Moter, S. E., Hofmann, H., Wallich, R., *et al.*, Detection of *Borrelia burgdorferi sensu lato* in lesional skin of patients with erythema migrans and acrodermatitis chronica atrophicans by Osp A-specific PCR, *J. Clin. Microbiol.* **32:**2980–2988 (1994).
73. Goodman, J. L., Bradley, J. F., Ross, A. E., *et al.*, Bloodstream invasion in early Lyme disease: Results from a prospective, controlled, blinded study using the polymerase chain reaction, *Am. J. Med.* **99:**6–12 (1995).
74. Hofmeister, E. K., Markham, R. B., Childs, J. E., *et al.*, Comparison of polymerase chain reaction and culture for detection of *Borrelia burgdorferi* in naturally infected *Peromyscus leucopus* and experimentally infected C.B-17 scid/scid mice, *J. Clin. Microbiol.* **30:**2625–2631 (1992).
75. Anderson, J. F., Johnson, R. C., Magnarelli, L. A., and Hyde, F. W., Identification of endemic foci of Lyme disease: Isolation of *Borrelia burgdorferi* from feral rodents and ticks (*Dermacentor variabilis*), *J. Clin. Microbiol.* **22:**36–38 (1985).
76. Marshall, W. F., Telford, S. R., Rys, P. N., *et al.*, Detection of *Borrelia burgdorferi* DNA in museum specimens of *Peromyscus leucopus*, *J. Infect. Dis.* **170:**1027–1032 (1994).
77. Craft, J. E., Grodzicki, R. L., and Steere, A. C., Antibody response in Lyme disease: Evaluation of diagnostic tests, *J. Infect. Dis.* **149:**789–795 (1984).
78. Gordzicki, R. L., and Steere, A. C., Comparison of immunoblotting and indirect enzyme-linked immunosorbent assay using different antigen preparations for diagnosing early Lyme disease, *J. Infect. Dis.* **157:**790–797 (1988).
79. Feder, H. M., Gerber, M. A., Luger, S. W., and Ryan, R. W., Persistence of serum antibodies to *Borrelia burgdorferi* in patients treated for Lyme disease, *Clin. Infect. Dis.* **15:**788–793 (1992).
80. Wilske, B., Schierz, G., Preac-Mursic, V., *et al.*, Intrathecal production of specific antibodies against *Borrelia burgdorferi* in patients with lymphocytic meningoradiculitis (Bannworth's syndrome), *J. Infect. Dis.* **153:**304–314 (1986).
81. Dressler, F., Whalen, J. A., Reinhardt, B. N., *et al.*, Western blotting in the serodiagnosis of Lyme disease, *J. Infect. Dis.* **167:**392–400 (1993).
82. Callister, S. M., Schell, R. F., Lim, L. C. L., *et al.*, Detection of borreliacidal antibodies by flow cytometry. An accurate, highly specific serodiagnostic test for Lyme disease, *Arch. Intern. Med.* **154:**1625–1634 (1994).
83. Mertz, L. E., Wobig, G. H., Duffy, J., *et al.*, Ticks, spirochetes and new diagnostic tests for Lyme disease, *Mayo Clin. Proc.* **60:**402–406 (1985).
84. Magnarelli, L. A., Anderson, J. F., and Johnson, R. C., Cross-reactivity in serological tests for Lyme disease and other spirochetal infections, *J. Infect. Dis.* **156:**183–188 (1987).
85. Greene, R. T., Walker, R. L., Nicholson, W. L., *et al.*, Immunoblot analysis of immunoglobulin G response to the Lyme disease agent (*Borrelia burgdorferi*) in experimentally and naturally exposed dogs, *J. Clin. Microbiol.* **26:**648–653 (1988).
86. Hovind-Hougen, K., Asbrink, E., Stiernstedt, G., *et al.*, Ultrastructural differences among spirochetes isolated from patients with Lyme disease and related disorders, and from *Ixodes ricinus*, *Zentrabl. Bakteriol. Mikrobiol. Hyg. A* **263:**103–111 (1986).
87. Fumarola, D., Munno, I., Marcuccio, C., *et al.*, Endotoxin-like activity associated with Lyme disease borrelia, *Zentralbl. Bakteriol. Mikrobiol. Hyg. A* **263:**142–145 (1986).
88. Habicht, G. S., Beck, G., Benach, J. L., *et al.*, *Borrelia burgdorferi* lipopolysaccharide and its role in the pathogenesis of Lyme disease, *Zentralbl. Bakteriol. Mikrobiol. Hyg. A* **263:**137–141 (1986).
89. Bergstrom, S., Bundoc, V. G., and Barbour, A. G., Molecular analysis of linear plasmid-encoded major surface proteins, Osp A and Osp B of the Lyme disease spirochaete *Borrelia burgdorferi*, *Mol. Microbiol.* **3:**479–486 (1989).
90. Fuchs, R., Jauris, S., Lottspeich, F., *et al.*, Molecular analysis and expression of a *Borrelia burgdorferi* gene encoding a 22 kDa protein (pC) in *Escherichia coli*, *Mol. Microbiol.* **6:**503–509 (1992).
91. Coleman, J. L., and Benach, J. L., Identification and characterization of an endoflagellar antigen of *Borrelia burgdorferi*, *J. Clin. Invest.* **84:**322–330 (1989).
92. Luft, B. J., Gorevic, P. D., Jiang, W., *et al.*, Immunologic and structural characterization of the dominant 66- to 73-kDa antigens of *Borrelia burgdorferi*, *J. Immunol.* **146:**2776–2782 (1991).
93. Luft, B. J., Mudri, S., Jiang, W., *et al.*, The 93-kilodalton protein of *Borrelia burgdorferi*: An immunodominant protoplasmic cylinder antigen, *Infect. Immun.* **60:**4309–4321 (1992).
94. Wilske, B., Barbour, A. G., Bergstrom, S., *et al.* Antigenic variation and strain heterogeneity in *Borrelia* spp., *Res. Microbiol.* **143:**583–596 (1992).
95. Baranton, G., Postic, D., Saint-Girons, I., *et al.*, Delineation of

Borrelia burgdorferi sensu stricto, *Borrelia garinii* sp. nov., and group VS 461 associated with Lyme borreliosis, *Int. J. Syst. Bacteriol.* **42:**378–383 (1992).

96. Steere, A. C., *Borrelia burgdorferi* (Lyme disease, Lyme borreliosis), in: *Principles and Practice of Infectious Diseases*, 4th ed. (G. L. Mandell, J. E. Bennett, and R. Dolin, eds.), pp. 2143–2155, Churchill Livingston, New York, 1995.
97. Van Dam, A. P., Kuiper, H., Vos, K., *et al.*, Different genospecies of *Borrelia burgdorferi* are associated with distinct clinical manifestations of Lyme borreliosis, *Clin. Infect. Dis.* **17:**708–717 (1993).
98. Kimsey, R. B., and Spielman, A., Motility of Lyme disease spirochetes in fluids as viscous as the extracellular matrix, *J. Infect. Dis.* **162:**1205–1208 (1990).
99. Agger, W. A., Callister, S. M., and Jobe, D. A., *In vitro* susceptibilities of *Borrelia burgdorferi* to five oral cephalosporins and ceftriaxone, *Antimicrob. Agents Chemother.* **36:**1788–1790 (1992).
100. Johnson, R. C., Kodner, C., and Russell, M., *In vitro* and *in vivo* susceptibility of the Lyme disease spirochete, *Borrelia burgdorferi*, to four antimicrobial agents, *Antimicrob. Agents. Chemother.* **31:**164–167 (1987).
101. Johnson, S. E., Kelin, G. C., Schmid, G. P., *et al.*, Susceptibility of the Lyme disease spirochete to seven antimicrobial agents, *Yale J. Biol. Med.* **57:**99–103 (1984).
102. Luft, B. J., Volkman, D., Halperin, J. J., *et al.*, New chemotherapeutic approaches in the treatment of Lyme borreliosis, *Ann. NY Acad. Sci.* **539:**352–361 (1988).
103. Centers for Disease Control and Prevention, Lyme disease—United States, 1994, *Morbid. Mortal. Week. Rep.* **44:**459–462 (1995).
104. Centers for Disease Control and Prevention, Summary of notifiable diseases, United States, 1991, *Morbid. Mortal. Week. Rep.* **40:**4–9 (1992).
105. Centers for Disease Control and Prevention, Summary of notifiable diseases, United States, 1992, *Morbid. Mortal. Week. Rep.* **41:**4–9 (1993).
106. Centers for Disease Control and Prevention, Summary of notifiable diseases, United States, 1993, *Morbid. Mortal. Week. Rep.* **42:**4–9 (1994).
107. White, D. J., Chang, H. G., Benach, J. L., *et al.*, The geographic spread and temporal increase of the Lyme disease epidemic, *J. Am. Med. Assoc.* **266:**1230–1236 (1991).
108. Vogt, R. L., National survey of state epidemiologists to determine the status of Lyme disease surveillance, *Public Health Rep.* **107:**644–646 (1992).
109. Centers for Disease Control, Lyme disease—Connecticut, *Morbid. Mortal. Week. Rep.* **37:**1–3 (1988).
110. Davis, J. P., Schell, W. L., Amundson, T. E., *et al.*, Lyme disease in Wisconsin: Epidemiologic, clinical, serologic, and entomologic findings, *Yale J. Biol. Med.* **57:**685–696 (1984).
111. Osterholm, M. T., Forfang, J. C., White, K. E., *et al.*, Lyme disease in Minnesota: Epidemiologic and serologic findings, *Yale J. Biol. Med.* **57:**677–683 (1984).
112. Burgdorfer, W., Lane, R. S., Barbour, A. G., *et al.*, The Western black-legged tick, *Ixodes pacificus*: A vector of *Borrelia burgdorferi*, *Am. J. Trop. Med. Hyg.* **34:**925–930 (1985).
113. Falco, R. C., and Fish, D., Prevalence of *Ixodes dammini* near the homes of Lyme disease patients in Westchester County, New York, *Am. J. Epidemiol.* **127:**826–830 (1988).
114. Magnarelli, L. A., Anderson, J. F., and Barbour, A. G., The etiologic agent of Lyme disease in deer flies, horse flies, and mosquitoes, *J. Infect. Dis.* **154:**355–358 (1986).
115. Magid, D., Schwartz, B., Craft, J., *et al.*, Prevention of Lyme disease after tick bites: A cost-effective analysis, *N. Engl. J. Med.* **327:**534–541 (1992).
116. Chengxu, A., Yuxin, W., Yongquo, Z., *et al.*, Clinical manifestations and epidemiological characteristics of Lyme disease in Hailin County, Heilongjaing Province, China, *Ann. NY Acad. Sci.* **539:**302–313 (1988).
117. Dekonenko, E. J., Steere, A. C., Berardi, V. P., *et al.*, Lyme borreliosis in the Soviet Union: A cooperative US–USSR report, *J. Infect. Dis.* **158:**748–753 (1988).
118. Schmid, G. P., The global distribution of Lyme disease, *Rev. Infect. Dis.* **7:**741–750 (1985).
119. Stanek, G., Pletschette, M., Flamm, H., *et al.*, European Lyme borreliosis, *Ann. NY Acad. Sci.* **539:**274–282 (1988).
120. Kawabatha, M., Baba, S., Iguchi, K., *et al.*, Lyme disease in Japan and its possible incriminated tick vector, *Ixodes persulcatus*, *J. Infect. Dis.* **156:**854 (1987).
121. Dennis, D., Epidemiology, in: *Lyme Disease* (P. K. Coyle, ed.), pp. 22–37, Mosby Year Book, St. Louis, 1993.
122. Shapiro, E. D., Lyme disease in children, *Am. J. Med.* **98**(Suppl. 4A):69S–73S (1995).
123. Benach, J. L., and Coleman, J. L., Clinical and geographical characteristics of Lyme disease in New York, *Zentralbl. Bakteriol. Mikrobiol. Hyg. A* **263:**477–482 (1986).
124. Williams, C. L., Curran, A. J., Lee, A. C., *et al.*, Lyme disease: Epidemiologic characteristics of an outbreak in Westchester County, NY, *Am. J. Public Health* **76:**62–65 (1986).
125. Neubert, U., Munchhoff, P., Volker, B., *et al.*, Borrelia burgdorferi infections in Bavarian forest workers: A follow-up study, *Ann. NY Acad. Sci.* **539:**476–479 (1988).
126. Smith, P. F., Benach, J. L., White, D. J., *et al.*, Occupational risk of Lyme disease in endemic areas of New York State, *Ann. NY Acad. Sci.* **539:**289–301 (1988).
127. Guy, E. C., Bateman, D. E., Martyn, C. N., *et al.*, Lyme disease: Prevalence and clinical importance of *Borrelia burgdorferi*: Specific IgG in forestry workers, *Lancet* **1:**484–486 (1989).
128. Piesman, J., and Sinsky, R., Ability of *Ixodes scapularis*, *Dermacentor variabilis*, and *Amblyomma americanum* (Acari: Ixodidae) to acquire, maintain and transmit Lyme disease spirochetes (*Borrelia burgdorferi*), *J. Med. Entomol.* **25:**336–339 (1988).
129. Wilson, M. L., and Spielman, A., Seasonal activity of immature *Ixodes dammini* (Acari: Ixodidae), *J. Med. Entomol.* **22:**408–414 (1985).
130. Schulze, T. L., Bowe, G. S., Lakat, M. F., *et al.*, The role of adult *Ixodes dammini* (Acari: Ixodidae) in the transmission of Lyme disease in New Jersey, USA, *J. Med. Entomol.* **22:**88–93 (1985).
131. Ribeiro, J. M. C., Mather, T. N., Piesman, J., *et al.*, Dissemination and salivary delivery of Lyme disease spirochetes in vector ticks (Acari: Ixodidae), *J. Med. Entomol.* **24:**201–215 (1987).
132. Telsford, S. R. III, Mather, T. W., Moore, S. I., *et al.*, Incompetence of deer as reservoirs of the Lyme disease spirochete, *Am. J. Trop. Med. Hyg.* **39:**105–109 (1988).
133. Burgdorfer, W., Hayes, S. F., and Benach, J. L., Development of *Borrelia burgdorferi* in ixodid tick vectors, *Ann. NY Acad. Sci.* **539:**172–179 (1988).
134. Anderson, J. F., and Magnarelli, L. A., Avian and mammalian hosts for spirochete-infected ticks and insects in a Lyme disease focus in Connecticut, *Yale J. Biol. Med.* **57:**627–641 (1984).

135. Hard, S., Erythema chronicum migrans (Afzelii) associated with a mosquito bite, *Acta Derm. Venereol.* **46:**473–476 (1966).
136. Magnarelli, L. A., and Anderson, J. F., Ticks and biting insects infected with the etiologic agent of Lyme disease, *Borrelia burgdorferi*, *J. Clin. Microbiol.* **26:**1482–1486 (1988).
137. Bosler, E. M., and Schulze, T. L., The prevalence and significance of *Borrelia burgdorferi* in the urine of feral reservoir hosts, *Zentralbl. Bakteriol. Mikrobiol. Hyg. A* **263:**40–44 (1986).
138. Burgess, E. C., Amundson, T. E., Davis, J. P., *et al.*, Experimental inoculation of *Peromyscus* spp. with *Borrelia burgdorferi*: Evidence of contact transmission, *Am. J. Trop. Med. Hyg.* **35:**355–359 (1986).
139. Baranton, G., and Saint-Girons, I., *Borrelia burgdorferi* survival in human blood samples, *Ann. NY Acad. Sci.* **539:**444–445 (1988).
140. Duray, P. H., and Steere, A. C., Clinical pathologic correlations of Lyme disease by stage, *Ann. NY Acad. Sci.* **539:**65–79 (1988).
141. Berger, B. W., Johnson, R. C., Kodner, C., *et al.*, Cultivation of *Borrelia burgdorferi* from erythema migrans lesions and perilesional skin, *J. Clin. Microbiol.* **30:**359–361 (1992).
142. Asbrink, E., and Hovmark, A., Early and late cutaneous manifestations in Ixodes-borne borreliosis, *Ann. NY Acad. Sci.* **539:** 4–16 (1988).
143. Berger, B. W., Johnson, R. C., Kodner, C., *et al.*, Cultivation of *Borrelia burgdorferi* from the blood of two patients with erythema migrans lesions lacking extracutaneous signs and symptoms of Lyme disease, *J. Am. Acad. Dermatol.* **30:**48–51 (1994).
144. Georgilis, K., Steere, A. C., and Klempner, M. S., Infectivity of *Borrelia burgdorferi* correlates with resistance to elimination by phagocytic cells, *J. Infect. Dis.* **163:**150–155 (1991).
145. de Koning, J., Hoogkamp-Korstanje, J. A. A., van der Linde, M. R., *et al.*, Demonstration of spirochetes in cardiac biopsies of patients with Lyme disease, *J. Infect. Dis.* **160:**150–153 (1989).
146. Reznick, J. W., Braunstein, D. B., Walsh, R. L., *et al.*, Lyme carditis: Electrophysiologic and histopathologic study, *Am. J. Med.* **81:**923–927 (1986).
147. Stanek, G., Klein, J., Bittner, R., *et al.*, Isolation of *Borrelia burgdorferi* from the myocardium of a patient with long-standing cardiomyopathy, *N. Engl. J. Med.* **322:**249–252 (1990).
148. Karlsson, M., Hovind-Hougen, K., Svenungsson, B., *et al.*, Cultivation and characterization of spirochetes from cerebrospinal fluid of patients with Lyme borreliosis, *J. Clin. Microbiol.* **28:**473–479 (1990).
149. Luft, B. J., Steinman, C. R., Neimark, H. C., *et al.*, Invasion of the central nervous system by *Borrelia burgdorferi* in acute disseminated infection, *J. Am. Med. Assoc.* **267:**1364–1367 (1992).
150. Coyle, P. K., Deng, Z., Schutzer, S. E., *et al.*, Detection of *Borrelia burgdorferi* antigens in cerebrospinal fluid, *Neurology* **43:**1093–1097 (1993).
151. Bradley, J. F., Johnson, R. C., and Goodman, J. L., The persistence of spirochetal nucleic acids in active Lyme arthritis, *Ann. Intern. Med.* **120:**487–489 (1994).
152. Schmidli, J., Junziker, T., Moesli, P., *et al.*, Cultivation of *Borrelia burgdorferi* from joint fluid three months after treatment of facial palsy due to Lyme borreliosis, *J. Infect. Dis.* **158:**905–906 (1988).
153. Johnson, Y. E., Duray, P. H., Steere, A. C., *et al.*, Lyme arthritis: Spirochetes found in synovial microangiopathic lesions, *Am. J. Pathol.* **118:**26–34 (1985).
154. Garcia-Monco, J. C., and Benach, J. L., The pathogenesis of Lyme disease, *Rheum. Dis. Clin. North Am.* **15:**711–726 (1989).
155. Ma, Y., Sturrock, A., and Weis, J. J., Intracellular localization of *Borrelia burgdorferi* within human endothelial cells, *Infect. Immun.* **59:**671–678 (1991).
156. Habicht, G. S., Beck, G., Benach, J. L., *et al.*, Lyme disease spirochetes induce human and murine interleukin production, *J. Immunol.* **134:**3147–3154 (1985).
157. Defosse, D. L., and Johnson, R. C., *In vitro* and *in vivo* induction of tumor necrosis factor alpha by *Borrelia burgdorferi*, *Infect. Immun.* **60:**1109–1113 (1992).
158. Garcia-Monco, J. C., Fernandex-Villar, B., and Benach, J. L., Adherence of the Lyme disease spirochete to glial cells and cells of glial origin, *J. Infect. Dis.* **160:**497–506 (1989).
159. Miklossy, J., Kuntzer, T., Bogousslavsky, J., *et al.*, Meningovascular form of neuroborreliosis: Similarities between neuropathological findings in a case of Lyme disease and those occurring in tertiary neurosyphilis, *Acta Neuropathol.* **80:**568–572 (1990).
160. Vallat, J. M., Hugon, J., Lubeau, M., *et al.*, Tick-bite meningoradiculoneuritis: Clinical, electrophysiologic, and histologic findings in 10 cases, *Neurology* **37:**749–753 (1987).
161. Steere, A. C., Duray, P. H., and Butcher, E. C., Spirochetal antigens and lymphoid cell surface markers in Lyme synovitis: Comparison with rheumatoid synovium and tonsillar lymphoid tissue, *Arthritis Rheum.* **31:**487–495 (1988).
162. Hardin, J. A., Steere, A. C., and Malawista, S. E., The pathogenesis of arthritis in Lyme disease: Humoral immune responses and the role of intraarticular immune complexes, *Yale J. Biol. Med.* **57:**589–593 (1984).
163. Hardin, J. A., Steere, A. C., and Malawista, S. E., Immune complexes and the evolution of Lyme arthritis: Dissemination and localization of Clq binding activity, *N. Engl. J. Med.* **301:** 1358–1363 (1979).
164. Hardin, J. A., Walker, L. C., and Steere, A. C., Circulating immune complexes in Lyme arthritis: Detection by the ^{125}I-Clq binding, Clq solid phase and Raji cell assays, *J. Clin. Invest.* **63:** 468–477 (1979).
165. Steere, A. C., Dwyer, E., and Winchester, R., Association of chronic Lyme arthritis with HLA-DR4 and HLA-DR2 alleles, *N. Engl. J. Med.* **323:**219–223 (1990).
166. Dattwyler, R. J., Volkman, D. J., Halperin, J. J., *et al.*, Seronegative Lyme disease: Specific immune responses in Lyme borreliosis. Characterization of T cell and B cell responses to *Borrelia burgdorferi*, *Ann. NY Acad. Sci.* **539:**93–102 (1988).
167. Craft, J. E., Fischer, D. K., Shimamoto, G. T., *et al.*, Antigens of *Borrelia burgdorferi* recognized during Lyme disease, *J. Clin. Invest.* **78:**934–939 (1986).
168. Coleman, J. L., and Benach, J. L., Isolation of antigenic components from the Lyme disease spirochete: Their role in early diagnosis, *J. Infect. Dis.* **155:**756–765 (1987).
169. Kalish, R. A., Leong, J. M., and Steere, A. C., Association of treatment resistant chronic Lyme arthritis with HLA-DR4 and antibody reactivity to OspA and OspB of *Borrelia burgdorferi*, *Infect. Immun.* **61:**2774–2779 (1993).
170. Steere, A. C., Berardi, V. P., Weeks, K. E., *et al.*, Evaluation of the intrathecal antibody response to *Borrelia burgdorferi* as a diagnostic test for Lyme neuroborreliosis, *J. Infect. Dis.* **161:**1203–1209 (1990).
171. Hansen, K., Cruz, M., and Link, H., Oligoclonal *Borrelia burgdorferi*-specific IgG antibodies in cerebrospinal fluid in Lyme neuroborreliosis, *J. Infect. Dis.* **161:**1194–1202 (1990).

172. Shahid, B., Olsson, T., Hansen, K., *et al.*, Anti-*Borrelia burgdorferi* antibody response over the course of Lyme neuroborreliosis, *Infect. Immun.* **59:**1050–1056 (1991).
173. Logigian, E. L., Kaplan, R. F., and Steere, A. C., Chronic neurologic manifestations of Lyme disease, *N. Engl. J. Med.***323:**1438–1444 (1990).
174. Pfister, H.-W., Neubert, U., Wilske, B., *et al.*, Reinfection with *Borrelia burgdorferi*, *Lancet* **2:**984–985 (1986).
175. Steere, A. C., Malawista, S. E., Bartenhagen, N. H., *et al.*, The clinical spectrum and treatment of Lyme disease, *Yale J. Biol. Med.* **57:**453–461 (1984).
176. Berger, B. W., Dermatologic manifestations of Lyme disease, *Rev. Infect. Dis.* **11**(Suppl. 6):S1475–S1481 (1989).
177. Weber, K., Schierz, G., Wilske, B., *et al.*, European erythema migrans disease and related disorders, *Yale J. Biol. Med.* **57:**463–471 (1984).
178. Asbrink, E., and Hovmark, A., Successful cultivation of spirochetes from skin lesions of patients with erythema chronicum migrans afzelios and acrodermatitis chronica atrophicans, *Acta Pathol. Microbiol. Immunol. Scand.* **93:**161–163 (1985).
179. Pachner, A. R., and Steere, A. C., The triad of neurologic manifestations of Lyme disease: Meningitis, cranial neuritis, and radiculoneuritis, *Neurology* **35:**47–53 (1985).
180. Reik, L., Burgdorfer, W., and Donaldson, J., Neurologic abnormalities in Lyme disease with erythema chronicum migrans, *Am. J. Med.* **81:**73–78 (1986).
181. Schechter, S., Lyme disease associated with optic neuropathy, *Am. J. Med.* **81:**143–145 (1986).
182. Halperin, J. J., and Golightly, M., Lyme borreliosis in Bell's palsy, *Neurology* **42:**1268–1270 (1992).
183. Halperin, J. J., Neuroborreliosis, *Am. J. Med.* **98**(Suppl. 4A): 52S–59S (1995).
184. Halperin, J. J., Little, B. W., Coyle, P. K., *et al.*, Lyme disease: Cause of a treatable peripheral neuropathy, *Neurology* **37:**1700–1706 (1987).
185. Pachner, A. R., Duray, P. H., and Steere, A. C., Central nervous system manifestations of Lyme disease, *Arch. Neurol.* **46:**790–795 (1989).
186. Kaplan, R. F., Meadows, M.-E., Vincent, L. C., *et al.*, Memory impairment and depression in patients with Lyme encephalopathy: Comparison with fibromyalgia and nonpsychotically depressed patients, *Neurology* **42:**1263–1267 (1992).
187. Halperin, J. J., Luft, B. J., Anand, A. K., *et al.*, Lyme neuroborreliosis: Central nervous system manifestations, *Neurology* **39:** 753–759 (1989).
188. Fallon, B. A., and Nields, J. A., Lyme disease: A neuropsychiatric illness, *Am. J. Psychiatry* **151:**1571–1583 (1994).
189. Pachner, A. R., Neurologic manifestations of Lyme disease, the new "great imitator," *Rev. Infect. Dis.* **11**(Suppl. 6):S1482–S1486 (1989).
190. Cox, J., and Krajden, M., Cardiovascular manifestations of Lyme disease, *Am. Heart J.* **122:**1449–1455 (1991).
191. Van der Linde, M. R., Crijus, H. J., de Koning, J., *et al.*, Range of atrioventricular conduction disturbances in Lyme borreliosis: A report of four cases and review of other published reports, *Br. Heart J.* **63:**162–168 (1990).
192. McAlister, M. F., Klementowicz, P. T., and Andrews, C., Lyme carditis: An important cause of reversible heart block, *Ann. Intern. Med.* **110:**339–345 (1989).
193. Sigal, L. H., Early disseminated Lyme disease: Cardiac manifestations, *Am. J. Med.* **98**(Suppl. 4A):25S–29S (1995).
194. Jacobs, J. C., Rosen, J. M., and Szer, I. S., Lyme myocarditis diagnosed by gallium scan, *J. Pediatr.* **105:**950–952 (1984).
195. Alpert, L. I., Welch, P., and Fisher, N., Gallium-positive Lyme disease myocarditis, *Clin. Nucl. Med.* **10:**617 (1985).
196. Szer, I. S., Taylor, E., and Steere, A. C., The long-term course of Lyme arthritis in children, *N. Engl. J. Med.* **325:**159–163 (1991).
197. Steere, A. C., Schoen, R. T., and Taylor, E., The clinical evolution of Lyme arthritis, *Am. Intern. Med.* **107:**725–731 (1987).
198. Steere, A. C., Levin, R. E., Molloy, P. J., *et al.*, Treatment of Lyme arthritis, *Arthritis Rheum.* **37:**878–888 (1994).
199. Miller, L. C., Lynch, E. A., Isa, S., *et al.*, Balance of synovial fluid IL-1β and IL-1 receptor antagonist and recovery from Lyme arthritis, *Lancet* **341:**146–148 (1993).
200. Granter, S. R., Barnhill, R. L., Hewins, M. E., *et al.*, Identification of *Borrelia burgdorferi* in diffuse fasciitis with peripheral eosinophilia: Borrelial fasciitis, *J. Am. Med. Assoc.* **272:**1283–1285 (1994).
201. Horowitz, H. W., Sanghera, K., Goldberg, N., *et al.*, Dermatomyositis associated with Lyme disease: Case report and review of Lyme myositis, *Clin. Infect. Dis.* **18:**166–171 (1994).
202. Kramer, N., Rickert, R., Brodkin, R., *et al.*, Septal panniculitis as a manifestation of Lyme disease, *Am. J. Med.* **81:**149–157 (1986).
203. Jacobs, J. C., Stevens, M., and Duray, P. H., Lyme disease simulating septic arthritis (Letter), *J. Am. Med. Assoc.* **256:**1138 (1986).
204. Ilowite, N. T., Muscle, reticuloendothelial, and late skin manifestations of Lyme disease, *Am. J. Med.* **98**(Suppl. 4A):63S–68S (1995).
205. Berglöff, J., Gasser, R., and Feigel, B., Opthalmic manifestations in Lyme borreliosis: A review, *J. Neuroophthalmol.* **14:**15–20 (1994).
206. Weber, K., Bratzke, H. J., Neubert, U., *et al.*, *Borrelia burgdorferi* in a newborn despite oral penicillin for Lyme borreliosis during pregnancy, *Pediatr. Infect. Dis. J.* **7:**286 (1988).
207. MacDonald, A. B., Benach, J. L., and Burgdorfer, W., Stillbirth following maternal Lyme disease, *NY State J. Med.* **1:**615–616 (1987).
208. Markowitz, L. E., Steere, A. C., Benach, J. L., *et al.*, Lyme disease during pregnancy, *J. Am. Med. Assoc.* **255:**3394–3396 (1986).
209. Russell, H., Sampson, J. S., Schmid, G. P., *et al.*, Enzyme-linked immunosorbent assay and indirect immunofluorescence assay for Lyme disease, *J. Infect. Dis.* **149:**465–470 (1984).
210. Magnarelli, L. A., Meegan, J. M., Anderson, J. F., *et al.*, Comparison of an indirect fluorescent-antibody test with an enzyme-linked immunosorbent assay for serological studies of Lyme disease, *J. Clin. Microbiol.* **20:**181–184 (1984).
211. Schutzer, S. E., Coyle, P. K., Belman, A. L., *et al.*, Sequestration of antibody to *Borrelia burgdorferi* in immune complexes in seronegative Lyme disease, *Lancet* **335:**312–315 (1990).
212. Steere, A. C., Malawista, S. E., Newman, J. H., *et al.*, Antibiotic therapy in Lyme disease, *Ann. Intern. Med.* **93:**1–8 (1980).
213. Wilson, M. L., Levine, J. F., and Spielman, A., Effect of deer reduction on abundance of the deer tick (*Ixodes dammini*), *Yale J. Biol. Med.* **57:**5697–5705 (1984).
214. Wilson, M., Telford, S. R. III, Presman, J., *et al.*, Reduced abundance of immature *Ixodes dammini* (Acari: Ixodidae) following elimination of deer, *J. Med. Entomol.* **25:**224–228 (1988).
215. Duffy, D. C., Campbell, S. R., Clark, D., *et al.*, *Ixodes scapularis* (Acari: Ixodidae) deer tick mesoscale populations in natural areas: Effects of deer, area, and location, *J. Med. Entomol.* **31:** 152–158 (1994).

216. Mather, T. N., Ribeiro, J. M. C., and Spielman, A., Lyme disease and babesiosis: Acaricide focused on potentially infected ticks, *Am. J. Trop. Med. Hyg.* **36:**609–614 (1987).
217. Schulze, T. L., McDevitt, W. M., Parkin, W. S., *et al.*, Effectiveness of two insecticides in controlling *Ixodes dammini* (Acari: Ixodidae) following an outbreak of Lyme disease in New Jersey, *J. Med. Entomol.* **24:**420–424 (1987).
218. Spielman, A., Prospects for suppressing transmission of Lyme disease, *Ann. NY Acad. Sci.* **539:**212–220 (1988).
219. Falco, R. C., and Fish, D., A survey of tick bites acquired in a Lyme disease endemic area in southern New York State, *Ann. NY Acad. Sci.* **539:**456–457 (1988).
220. Costello, C. M., Steere, A. C., Pinkerton, R. E., *et al.*, A prospective study of tick bites in an endemic area for Lyme disease, *J. Infect. Dis.* **159:**136–139 (1989).
221. Agre, F., and Schwartz, R. M., The value of early treatment for the prevention of Lyme disease (Abstract), *Am. J. Dis. Child.* **145:**391 (1991).
222. Shapiro, E. D., Gerber, M. A., Persing, D., *et al.*, Prevention of Lyme disease: A randomized clinical trial of antimicrobial prophylaxis for people bitten by a deer tick, in: *Proceedings and Abstracts of the Fifth International Conference on Lyme Borreliosis* (Washington, DC, May 30–June 2, 1992), p. A47, Federation of American Societies for Experimental Biology, Bethesda, 1992.
223. Fikrig, E., Barthold, S. W., Kantor, F. S., *et al.*, Protection of mice against the Lyme disease agent by immunizing with recombinant OspA, *Science* **250:**553–556 (1990).
224. Fikrig, E., Berland, R., Chen, M., *et al.*, Serologic response to the *Borrelia burgdorferi* flagellin demonstrated an epitope common to a neuroblastoma cell line, *Proc. Natl. Acad. Sci. USA* **90:**183–187 (1993).
225. *Borrelia burgdorferi* bacterin, Lyme Vax, package insert, Fort Dodge Laboratories, Fort Dodge, IA, 1994.
226. Levy, S. A., Lissman, B. A., and Ficke, C. M., Performance of a *Borrelia burgdorferi* bacterin in borreliosis-endemic areas, *J. Am. Vet. Med. Assoc.* **202:**1834–1838 (1993).
227. Keller, D., Koster, F. T., Marks, D. H., *et al.*, Safety and immunogenicity of a recombinant outer surface protein A Lyme vaccine, *J. Am. Med. Assoc.* **271:**1764–1768 (1994).
228. Barbour, A., and Garon, C. F., The genes encoding major surface proteins of *Borrelia burgdorferi* are located on a plasmid, *Ann. NY Acad. Sci.* **539:**144–153 (1988).
229. Schwan, T. G., and Burgdorfer, W., Antigenic changes of *Borrelia burgdorferi* as a result of *in vitro* cultivation, *J. Infect. Dis.* **156:**852–853 (1987).
230. Wilske, B., Preac-Mursic, V., Schierz, G., *et al.*, Antigenic variability of *Borrelia burgdorferi*, *Ann. NY Acad. Sci.* **539:**126–143 (1988).

12. Suggested Reading

Feder H. M., and Hunt M. S., Pitfalls in the diagnosis and treatment of Lyme disease in children, *J. Am. Med. Assoc.* **274:**66–68 (1995).

Nichol, G., Dennis D. T., Steere A. C., *et al.*, Test-treatment strategies for patients suspected of having Lyme disease: A cost-effective analysis, *Ann. Intern. Med.* **128:**37–48 (1998).

Oliver, J. H. Lyme borelliosis in the southern United States: A review, *J. Parasitol.* **82**(6):926–935 (1996).

Ostrov, B. E., and Athreya, B. H. Lyme disease: Difficulties in diagnosis and management, *Pediatr. Clin. North Am.* **38:**535–553 (1991).

Wormser, G. P., Prospects for a vaccine to prevent Lyme disease in humans, *Clin. Infect. Dis.* **21:**1267–1274 (1995).

Wormser, G. P., Treatment and prevention of Lyme disease, with emphasis on antimicrobial therapy for neuroborreliosis and vaccination, *Semin. Neurol.* **17:**45–52 (1997).

Silver, H. M., Lyme disease during pregnancy, *Infect. Obstet.* **11:**93–97 (1997).

Walker, D. H., Barbour, A. G., Oliver, J. H., *et al.*, Emerging bacterial zoonotic and vectorborne diseases, *J. Am. Med. Assoc.* **275:**463–469 (1996).

CHAPTER 23

Meningococcal Infections

Robert S. Baltimore

1. Introduction

The meningococcal diseases* represent a spectrum of illness caused by *Neisseria meningitidis* (Table 1). Although sporadic endemic cases occur throughout the world, massive, devastating epidemics tend to reflect conditions of crowding, mobilization, and enclosed institutional populations. Such outbreaks tend to be extraordinarily disruptive, especially because of the fear and fright that they induce in the affected populations. Among civilians, children are most often attacked, with mortality rates of 80–90% having been noted in some epidemics that occurred before effective therapeutic agents became available. The disease is also known as "cerebral spinal fever" and "epidemic cerebral spinal meningitis," as well as by other names. Mobilization for war, with the induction of many young men into crowded military camps, has generally been accompanied by outbreaks. This has been in contrast to the absence of such outbreaks among college freshmen, who also represent a mix from many diverse origins, in dormitories and other sometimes crowded living quarters on many campuses. It should also be stated that generalized outbreaks among the military do not arise *de novo*, but may reflect what is occurring in the associated civilian populations. The development of meningococcal capsular polysaccharide vaccines has had a significant effect on prevention of military epidemics of meningococcal epidemics, but its impact on civilian disease is, as yet, unrealized.

*In this chapter, the term *case* or *disease* refers to any instance of meningococcal infection other than asymptomatic pharyngeal (carrier).

Robert S. Baltimore • Departments of Pediatrics and Epidemiology and Public Health, Yale University School of Medicine, New Haven, Connecticut 06520-8064.

In the first edition of this book, this chapter was written by the late Harry Feldman, MD. Substantial historical and epidemiological data come from his original manuscript.

2. Historical Background

Clinical meningococcal disease was first described by Vieusseux[1] in 1805 during an outbreak in the vicinity of Geneva, Switzerland. A year later, Danielson and Mann[2] reported a small, probable epidemic of meningococcal meningitis in Medfield, Massachusetts. This paper appeared in a publication known as the *Medical and Agricultural Register* and was entitled "The history of a singular and very mortal disease, which lately made its appearance in Medfield." The nine fatal cases were so similar that only one was fully described; all occurred during March. Weichselbaum[3] identified meningococci in the spinal fluids of patients in 1887.

During the 19th century, possible epidemics occurred in countries throughout the world in 1805, 1837, 1854, 1876, and 1896. In this century, major outbreaks were noted during World Wars I and II, and subsequent to the latter, there was a massive, lengthy outbreak in sub-Sahara Africa,[4] a more localized one in Morocco,[5] and another affecting more than a quarter of a million people in Brazil,[6] as well as others in Finland[7] and among American military inductees during the Korean and Vietnam mobilizations. Smaller, localized outbreaks have occurred from time to time in various institutions and localities. In the course of the many studies that were conducted during World War I, Gordon[8] identified four serological types of meningococci: I, II, III, and IV. In 1953, Branham,[9] as the result of her careful, meticulous studies, labeled the different serogroups A, B, C, and D. She believed that organisms of group A were those principally responsible for epidemics and that sporadic cases

Table 1. Clinical Spectrum of Symptomatic Meningococcal Infections

Meningitis
With meningococcemia
without meningococcemia
Septicemia
Purpura
Adrenal hemorrhage
Chronic meningococcemia
Occult bacteremia
Pneumonia
Other focal infections
Conjunctivitis
Endophthalmitis
Septic emboli to skin
Pericarditis
Myocarditis
Urethritis
Arthritis
Epididymitis
Recurrent meningococcemia with complement deficiency

tend to be antigenically heterogeneous as the result of infections with groups B and C. Slaterus[10] subsequently demonstrated three additional meningococcal serogroups (X, Y, and Z), and then Evans *et al.*[11] identified serogroups W-135 and 29-E from US Army isolates. Subsequently, groups H, I, K, and L have been described.[12,13]

An enormous step forward was made early in World War II when it was learned not only that sulfadiazine was effective in the treatment of cases, but also that small doses eliminated the organism from the nasopharynx.[14–17] When sulfadiazine was administered on a mass basis to a closed population, cases of disease disappeared almost instantaneously and the carrier rate was reduced to near-zero levels. Thus, an effective, simple, relatively inexpensive control system for preventing meningococcal disease and curtailing epidemics was provided. Unfortunately, this was found to be ineffective in 1963 by Millar *et al.*[18] during several unsuccessful attempts to control the disease among naval recruits in San Diego. It was learned then that many disease-related strains were resistant to large concentrations of sulfadiazine, and thus that the sulfonamides could no longer be used effectively for the prevention or control of epidemics.[19] In a number of subsequent trials conducted under the auspices of the Armed Forces Epidemiological Board, no substitute chemotherapeutic agent was found, although the satisfactory treatment of actual cases could be accomplished with large doses of penicillin. The latter was quickly adopted as routine therapy for both military and civilian use. Eventually, in the 1970s, rifampin was adopted as the recommended chemoprophylactic agent for close contacts of cases.[20]

In the early 1970s, a vaccine for serogroups A and C was developed.[21,22] A tetravalent vaccine (containing vaccines for serogroups A, C, Y, and W135) is available today for the military and individuals considered to be at exceptional risk of contracting meningococcal infection.

3. Methodology

3.1. Sources of Mortality Data

The principal sources of mortality data on meningococcal diseases are local and federal health agencies such as, in the United States, local and state health departments and the Centers for Disease Control and Prevention (CDC) through the *Morbidity and Mortality Weekly Report* (MMWR). In addition, there are publications of the World Health Organization (WHO) and various military sources, but these deal only with the populations that they serve. By and large, mortality data reflect the incidence of the disease, although they can be affected by a number of variables, especially the level of health care available and the rapidity with which treatment can be instituted. The level of completeness of mortality data is reflected to a great extent by how well public health reporting is organized and whether adequate laboratory facilities are available for identifying individual disease-causing agents.

3.2. Sources of Morbidity Data

The disease is generally reportable, and because of the fear that it engenders, reporting is reasonably complete and tends to mirror the availability of proper laboratory facilities to identify etiologic agents in individual cases.

Prevalence and incidence data are regularly supplied in the CDC MMWRs and in the *Annual Summary* of the same publication. Additional sources of information are the *WHO Weekly Epidemiological Record* and the *Canada Diseases Weekly Report*. Other data may be found in the published reports describing individual outbreaks. The latter generally observe geographic limitations, whereas the MMWR considers the United States as a whole. Additional data may be found in the reports of various state and local health departments.

3.3. Surveys

Carrier surveys are often conducted among military populations, whereas among civilians, case contacts are often cultured, especially in schools and families. Carrier surveys are primarily of the posterior nasopharyngeal carrier state. In recent years, carrier surveys have been deemphasized. This is because they generally yield little information about the immune state of the population or the introduction of new, virulent meningococcal strains. These appear to be more predictive of risk for an outbreak. Serological surveys have not been used generally because the available methods do not lend themselves to mass application and, furthermore, because one would have to test for antibodies to all known serogroups.

In the United States, the CDC has sponsored special surveys of meningococcemia and meningitis. These usually target representative states and then are extrapolated to calculate rates for the whole country.[23,24,24a]

3.4. Laboratory Diagnosis

3.4.1. Isolation and Identification of the Organism. *N. meningitidis* is a fastidious, gram-negative diplococcus that grows best on enriched media such as blood or chocolate agar and in the presence of increased CO_2. The latter is especially useful for primary isolation. The organism may be isolated from all body areas and orifices. When *N. meningitidis* is sought in places where competing bacteria are prominent, it is best to use Thayer–Martin medium,[25] which consists of chocolate agar to which several antibiotics inhibitory for gram-negative, gram-positive, and yeast-contaminating organisms have been added. This medium is especially useful for the identification of meningococci in nasopharyngeal secretions and cultures from rectal swabs. Organisms may be cultivated frequently from the male urethra, the cervix, the conjunctivae, and in cases of arthritis, from purulent septic joint fluids. In patients with meningococcal bacteremia or meningitis, cultures of the blood are usually positive, as are those of spinal fluid. Meningococci may be demonstrated in Gram-stained smears from petechiae or the buffy coats of those with severe sepsis. Cultures from normally sterile fluids such as blood, cerebrospinal fluid (CSF), or joint fluid may be cultivated on regular blood or chocolate agar rather than Thayer–Martin medium, as inhibition of normal flora is not necessary. The same is true of subcultures of individual colonies from primary isolation media.

The organism ferments glucose and maltose but not lactose. Sometimes the fermentation of glucose is slow and may require 48 hr or more of incubation. More rarely, glucose may not be fermented at all. Meningococci are oxidase-positive, and this reaction may be helpful in the recognition of colonies on plates with mixed flora. The use of Thayer–Martin medium usually removes the latter requirement. The organism does not grow at room temperature or on simple media such as nutrient agar.[26]

Meningococcal polysaccharide antigens can be detected in body fluids or in the supernatant of growing cultures. Latex beads coated with meningococcal antisera are available commercially. They will agglutinate in the presence of soluble meningococcal antigens.

3.4.2. Serological and Immunologic Diagnostic Methods. While meningococci contain several antigens, the group-specific one is a polysaccharide that is readily detected by slide agglutination.[26] This usually works well with isolates from body fluids of actual cases. Often, throat and sputum isolates are rough and tend to agglutinate spontaneously in saline. They are also agglutinated in normal rabbit serum and all, or nearly all, group-specific antisera. Such organisms are usually identified as "saline agglutinable." Slide agglutination can be performed rapidly, but requires pure cultures and active antisera. These can be done in fairly large numbers on large plates, and thus lend themselves well to population studies and epidemiological investigations. Organisms of serogroups A and C are encapsulated; when freshly isolated or still in original spinal fluids they may be shown to "quell" with potent antisera. This reaction can be used for rapid identification, especially of organisms in spinal fluid. For serogrouping in a reference laboratory, the hemagglutination inhibition test has been reported to be both highly sensitive and specific.[27]

4. Biological Characteristics of the Organism

Under the special conditions that lead to epidemics, encapsulated (virulent) organisms are transmitted rapidly from person to person, probably in respiratory droplets. They tend to localize primarily in the posterior nasopharynx. Thus, attempts to determine the extent, or degree, of infection of a population at any given time requires surveys of the posterior nasopharyngeal prevalence of the organism. This is best achieved with a bent wire swab that is passed up behind the uvula, wiped across the posterior nasopharynx, withdrawn, and immediately plated on Thayer–Martin chocolate agar. The warmed plates should be placed in an incubator as soon as possible thereafter. If the incubator contains CO_2, no other container need be used. If no CO_2 incubator is available, then the newly inoculated plates should be put into candle jars. The spontaneous extinction of the candle flame will indicate that the CO_2 content is elevated; when the jar is put at

37°C, suitable growth for further subinoculation and isolation should appear overnight.

Most of the major epidemics of this century have been caused by group A meningococci, although the massive Brazilian epidemic of the 1970s began as a group C outbreak that was then displaced by group A organisms. Localized outbreaks due to meningococci of groups B, C, or Y have been noted, but more often than not, they are present in sporadic cases.

4.1. Serotypes and Serogroups

Meningococci are grouped according to their polysaccharide capsule antigens into serogroups A, B, C, D, H, I, K, L, X, Y, Z, W135, and 29E. In the United States, serogroups B and C were responsible for 46% and 45% of meningococcal isolates, respectively, in 1989–1991. The next most common serogroups were W135 and Y, accounting for 3% and 2% of isolates, respectively.[(28)] Fewer than 1% are serogroup A. In contrast, in sub-Saharan Africa and Scandinavia serogroups A and C predominate.

Meningococci can also be typed according to protein and lipopolysaccharide (LPS) antigens. A number of systems have been devised for typing meningococci. Three methods were reported in the 1970s. One by Frasch and Chapman[(29)] utilizes the bactericidal-inhibition technique and designated 10 serotypes of group B meningococci. The dominant antigen in this scheme is a protein–LPS complex. Zollinger and Mandrell[(30)] used both outer-membrane protein and LPS to serotype meningococci, but with specific absorptions they could type according to outer-membrane proteins. Subsequently, Apicella[(31)] also used LPS to serotype group B meningococci. Frasch and associates[(32)] subsequently proposed a scheme based on electrophoretic mobility in sodium dodecyl sulfate–polyacrylamide gel electrophoresis (SDS-PAGE) gels of two major proteins and LPS into 21 serotypes, bringing together schema of several laboratories into a unified scheme. Most of these 21 types can be distinguished by monoclonal antibodies.[(32)] Multilocus enzyme electrophoresis is a more recently described method used by a number of laboratories. Achtman[(33)] has utilized mobility of bacterial isoenzyme proteins in an electrophoretic field and typed epidemic strains and has traced clones of serogroup A that have spread from country to country. Ashton *et al.*[(34)] used typing by monoclonal antibodies to differentiate serogroup B isolates from Canada using an enzyme-linked immunosorbent assay (ELISA) technique. These techniques are not generally available for typing strains from individual cases, but when applied by research laboratories can provide additional information for epidemiological studies of transmission, relationships among cases, or the presence of an epidemic strain in a geographically defined area.[(33–36)]

4.2. Antibiotic Susceptibility

The susceptibility and resistance of meningococci to various chemotherapeutic and antibiotic agents have played a significant role in the treatment of individual patients and, perhaps more important, in the management of epidemics. The new era began in 1941 with a publication by Dingle *et al.*[(37)] that demonstrated that sulfadiazine was effective in the treatment of meningococcal meningitis. This finding was subsequently supported by others.[(38)] It was also found during these clinical studies that meningococci were eradicated from the posterior nasopharynx within hours after treatment was initiated. Then came a number of trials in the military in which it was observed that small doses of sulfadiazine given for short periods of time were sufficient to eradicate the carrier state.[(14–16,39)] When 1 g was given twice daily for 2 days to military recruits en masse in a given installation, not only was the carrier rate reduced to negligible levels, but also the effect on disease was almost instantaneous. This simple control measure was instituted as a routine in all military installations as well as in civilian populations with excessive numbers of cases or to prevent secondary cases within households.

All this came to an end in 1963 when such control measures seemed to have no impact on the occurrence of cases at the San Diego Naval Training Center.[(18)] Investigation of this event led to the demonstration by Millar *et al.*[(18)] that resistance to sulfonamides was widespread throughout the United States in both military and civilian populations. Initially, this seemed to be limited to serogroup B and C meningococci, whereas group A infections that were occurring in Africa and in some parts of the Mediterranean Basin continued to be susceptible. However, in a widespread group A epidemic in Morocco,[(5)] the causative organisms were found to be significantly resistant to sulfadiazine. This was soon confirmed in other parts of the world and led to the recommendation that cases be treated with large doses of penicillin. This has proven to be successful. Subsequently, rifampin or minocycline or a combination thereof has been demonstrated to reduce carrier rates,[(40–43)] although proof of efficacy for disease prevention is lacking (see Section 9.2).

For decades, penicillin has been considered to be the antibiotic of choice for treatment of meningococcal disease, although other semisynthetic penicillins and cephalosporins and chloramphenicol are also effective. Recently, there have been reports of meningococcal isolates with reduced susceptibility to penicillin. While susceptible strains have a minimum inhibitory concentration (MIC) of 0.03 μg/ml to penicillin, relative resistant strains with an MIC of 0.1–1.28 μg/ml have been reported from Spain,[44] England,[45] South Africa,[46] Canada,[47] and the United States,[48,49] While an estimated 4% of meningococcal isolates in the United States in 1991 were relatively resistant, the clinical significance of resistance at this level is uncertain if large doses of penicillin are used for treatment.[49] Penicillin-resistant strains are generally susceptible to third-generation cephalosporins and these are frequently employed at the beginning of antibiotic therapy before the organism has been positively identified. Penicillin resistance is not due to production of penicillinase by the organism but by reduced affinity of cell wall penicillin-binding proteins for penicillin. In Spain, where the prevalence of such isolates climbed to 20% in the late 1980s, the types and subtypes of these isolates was quite diverse.[36]

5. Descriptive Epidemiology

5.1. Prevalence and Incidence

Information on prevalence and incidence is complicated by the multiplicity of serogroups of meningococci. Prevalence and incidence are more precisely stated and of greater value when serogroups are identified than when they are categorized under the generic term "meningococci."

Jacobson *et al.*[50] reported that in the United States in 1974, there was 0.60 case/100,000 population per year. As noted in Fig. 1, this was a year of low incidence. Yet, despite this low incidence, the rates were 9.47 in infants less than 1 year old and 2.27 in children 1–4 years old.

In an active surveillance program sponsored by the CDC in 1978, the annual incidence of meningococcal meningitis in the United States was estimated to be 0.72 case/100,000 population. The peak age of meningococcal meningitis was 3–8 months (peak incidence 13/100,000). The peak age of meningococcemia was 6–8 months (peak incidence 5/100,000).[23] A CDC-sponsored laboratory surveillance reported an average annual incidence of 1.1/100,000 in 1989–1991.[28] The highest rate was in infants <4 months of age, 26.4/100,000. In 1990–1994, the rate of meningococcal meningitis averaged 0.96 cases per 100,000.[51] While the rate of meningococcal disease in the United States and other Western countries is 1–3/100,000, in developing countries it is much higher, up to 10–25/100,000.[52]

5.2. Epidemic Behavior and Contagiousness

Glover,[53] in a classic report, concluded that carrier rates were most affected by "overcrowding" of sleeping arrangements. While "standard" accommodations in the British Army had been defined by a Royal Commission in 1861 and 60 square feet of floor space (600 cubic feet of air space and 3 feet spacing between beds) per man, this was reduced to 40 square feet of floor space and 400 cubic feet of air space soon after the outbreak of World War I because of mobilization pressures. At the end of the third year of the war, he found the space between beds in a distinguished unit to be less than 6 inches. Glover concluded that distances between beds were so important that he could predict the meningococcal carrier rate in a barracks by computing the distance between its beds. If the distance was 1 foot 4 inches, the carrier rate would be 10%. A slight decrease sent the carrier rate up to between 10 and 20%. If the beds were closer than 1 foot, 20% was the rate, and if the distance was less than 9 inches, a carrier rate of 28–30% was to be expected. When the recommended distance was maintained, the carrier rate rarely exceeded 5%.

"Overcrowding" (defined as less than 40 square feet per man) was soon followed by a sharp rise in the carrier rate, reaching its maximum in about 2 weeks. The rise was accompanied by an increase in the proportion of epidemic carrier strains. The increase of this rate among noncontact carriers to 20% meant that an outbreak was imminent. The high carrier rates could be reduced, although not as quickly as they had increased, by increasing the space between beds to 2½ feet or more. Thus, he concluded that "to raise the carrier rate by overcrowding was both easier and quicker than to diminish it by spacing out."

In the devastating epidemic of 5885 cases that occurred in Santiago, Chile, during 1941–1942, Pizzi[54] reported that in the area of the city where the epidemic was concentrated, the population density was 7 persons per room and 2.9 per bed. The secondary attack rate overall was 2.5%, but it was 3.9% for those under 15 years of age and 1.5% among those more than 15. This experience tended to support Glover's observations.

Various studies have been reported by other authors in which no cases were seen when carrier rates were high[55] or cases were seen when carrier rates were low. Perhaps a key observation was supplied by Schoenbach,[56] who cultured 200 men in a military unit three times a week for 10 weeks. While the carrier rate averaged 41% during this period, 91% were identified at some time

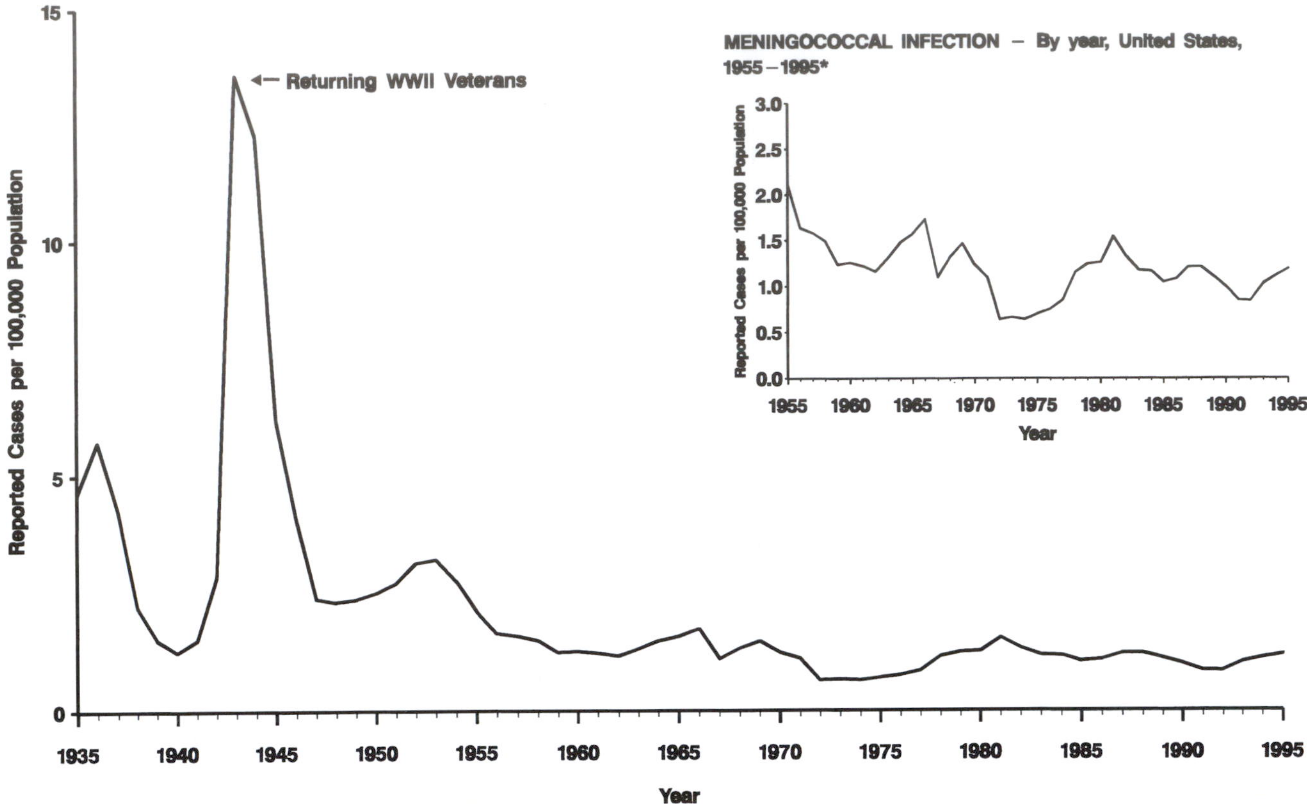

Figure 1. Meningococcal infections: rates by year, United States, 1935–1995. From the CDC (personnal communication).

to be carriers. Similar, but unpublished, observations were made by Dr. Harry A. Feldman in conjunction with colleagues at the Fourth Service Command Medical Laboratory at Fort McPherson, Georgia, during the same period.

A source of great puzzlement for public health workers, epidemiologists, and microbiologists who have studied epidemics of meningococcal disease over the years has been the apparent discontinuous pattern of disease occurrence. Arkwright,[57] in a truly remarkable albeit much neglected report, concluded:

> The large number and widespread distribution of carriers and the small number of cases of meningitis compared to the population forces upon one the view that for a true understanding of an epidemic of meningitis, the total number of persons who harbour the meningococcus should be looked upon as constituting the true epidemic . . . the carriers constitute the mass of the epidemic, and those who subsequently develop meningitis are only a small accidental minority. The cases of meningitis, on account of the severity and fatality of this complication, give to the epidemic its importance, and they necessarily bulk largely in the eyes of the clinician . . . a consideration of all the evidence about carriers leads to the conclusion that the statement that cases of meningitis occur when and where carriers of the meningococcus become numerous, is a more correct way of stating the facts than by saying that many carriers occur in the neighbourhood of cases of meningitis.

The meningococcal situation parallels that of poliomyelitis, in which paralytic cases seemed to occur without rhyme or reason until the presence and importance of the nonparalytic individual was established. It was then determined that only about 1 in 100 infected individuals developed paralytic disease.[58] Maxcy[59] concluded that a similar rate occurred in meningococcal infections.

The key to the occurrence of an epidemic is the carrier or acquisition incidence rate. This has to be rapid for an epidemic to happen, since many individuals must acquire the organism for the relatively few cases to occur. It is the concentration of the latter that defines the presence of an epidemic. The key question remains, namely, what initiates the transmission speedup in a population that results in increased numbers of cases and an epidemic? While the carrier state may persist for months,[60,61] the period of communicability is unknown.

It would seem logical to infer that if there were *no* carriers, there would be no cases. This concept led many to investigate the effectiveness of sulfonamides for the elimination of the carrier state, since it had been observed early in the research on sulfadiazine treatment that organisms disappeared rapidly from the posterior nasopharynx.[14–16,39,56] Typical of reports confirming this effective measure was that of Kuhns *et al.*[16] A simple 2-g dose reduced the carrier rate to near zero, but the effect was prolonged when such treatment was maintained for 2–3 days.[56] Cases disappeared just as promptly.

During World War II, an epidemic in the military was defined as the occurrence of 1 or more cases/10,000 soldiers per week.[62] United States rates for the 65 years from 1930 to 1994 are summarized by 5-year averages per 100,000 population in Table 2. The epidemic that accompanied World War II can be readily seen in Fig. 1, as can the relative increases noted during the Korean and Vietnam conflicts. The latter two reflect recruit outbreaks primarily, while the World War II increase was noted both in the military and in civilians, worldwide.

5.3. Geographic Distribution

Meningococcal infections are limited to humans and have been noted throughout the world in either small circumscribed concentrations[63] of cases or widespread areas[64–68] involving whole countries (Brazil) or geographically large areas such as sub-Sahara Africa.[4] In 1948–1950, there was an epidemic of 92,964 cases with 14,273 deaths in northern Nigeria.[69] The band of countries stretching across sub-Sahara Africa from Gambia to Ethiopia is often referred to as the meningitis belt and epidemics in this area are frequent, with rates of meningococcal disease of up to 1000/100,000 (1%).[52] In recent years, outbreaks of meningococcal disease have occurred in Saudi Arabia at the time of the *Haj*, presumably due both to influx of individuals who carried epidemic strains and to overcrowding. A major outbreak occurred in 1987 with a particular clone of group A that was spread by pilgrims returning from Mecca to many other countries.[33]

Table 2. Average 5-Year US Rates per 100,000 Population of Meningococcal Infections[a]

Years	Rate	Years	Rate
1930–1934	3.596	1965–1969	1.434
1935–1939	3.655	1970–1974	0.8479
1940–1944	6.308	1975–1979	0.9369
1945–1949	3.407	1980–1984	1.274
1950–1954	2.867	1985–1989	1.13
1955–1959[b]	1.602	1990–1994	0.96
1960–1964	1.286		

[a]Compiled from the CDC.[51,134]
[b]Alaska was included beginning in 1958; Hawaii, beginning in 1959.

5.4. Temporal Distribution

Sporadic endemic cases of meningococcal infections are encountered throughout the world at all times. Outbreaks tend to occur in various places for no discernible reason(s). On occasion, epidemics break out almost simultaneously in different places with no apparent connection with each other.

In tropical areas, especially sub-Sahara Africa, cases are most often seen during dry seasons, perhaps because changes in sleeping arrangements accompany the regression of the rainy season. In the dry season the dusty conditions drive workers indoors to sleep in crowded rooms.[64] In the cooler temperate zones, outbreaks tend to be clustered in the winter and spring months.[70] In the United States, the peak incidence of meningococcal disease is in the late winter and early spring (February through May) and the lowest incidence is from July through October.

5.5. Age

Basically, meningitis is a childhood disease most often seen under age 15 years.[50,71] Beeson and Westerman,[72] in a study of 3575 British cases, found that 45.5% occurred in children under 15 years. In the great Detroit epidemic,[73] children under 15 years made up 60% of the patients, while in the German epidemic of 1905–1907, 80% were under 15 years.[72] Recent US data confirm that the age-related predisposition of meningococcal meningitis still exists and that the peak incidence is from age 1 month to 1 year (Table 3).

5.6. Sex

As is true of other severe diseases, males are more often subject to meningitis than are females. In the Beeson and Westerman[72] study, the male–female ratio was 6:4, but fatalities were more frequent in females. The excess of males persisted through age 50 years. This preponderance was also noted in the Detroit civilian outbreak.[73] Since military forces in the past have consisted predominantly of males, an excess prevalence of males is to be expected. Thus, in time of war, one should expect male cases to predominate, especially among recruits.

In a longitudinal study of meningococcal carriage in a population of "normal" families, it was found that males 20 years or older were more likely than adult

Table 3. Annual Age-Specific Incidence of Meningococcal Meningitis, United States, 1978–1981[a]

Age	Rate[b]	Age	Rate
<1 month	2.0	1–2 years	3.8
1–2 months	9.1	3–4 years	1.8
3–5 months	11.5	5–9 years	0.7
6–8 months	10.6	10–19 years	0.6
9–11 months	7.9		

[a]Adapted from Klein *et al.*(71)
[b]Cases of meningococcal meningitis per 100,000 population.

females to become carriers.(60) In recent data (1989–1991) from the CDC, 55% of cases of meningococcal disease occurred in males (annual rate in males = 1.2/100,000 and in females = 1.0/100,000(28)).

5.7. Race

Race seems to be of little significance for either the acquisition or the severity of infections, except that those with sickle-cell disease may be more prone to fatal infections, as they are to those caused by other polysaccharide-encapsulated bacteria. In a review of deaths from bacterial meningitis in the United States from 1962 to 1968,(74) it was concluded that excessive deaths from this cause were noted among African Americans and American Indians. Race per se is not mentioned as a risk factor, but poverty and crowding are. In a population-based study in Charleston County, South Carolina, neither race nor income affected the risk for meningococcal meningitis.(75) In the multistate surveillance study performed by the CDC in 1986, the rate of meningitis in African Americans caused by *N. meningitidis* was twice that of whites (1.5 vs 0.7/100,000), with Hispanics having a rate in-between (1.1/100,000).(24) Recent national data from the CDC continue to show a higher annual incidence of meningococcal disease in African Americans (1.5/100,000) compared with whites (1.1/100,000). The relative risk for African Americans was 1.3 with a confidence interval of 1.0–1.6.(28)

5.8. Occupation

Pike,(76) in an exhaustive review of laboratory-associated infections, records two such fatalities. In 1918, an employee of the State Serum Institute, Copenhagen, Denmark, whose job was concerned with the production of antimeningococcal serum, died of meningococcal meningitis. Another, an employee of the National Institutes of Health, in the United States, while injecting an animal with meningococci, had some of the syringe's contents sprayed into her eyes as the animal struggled. She became ill 4 days later and died after 4 days of illness.

The CDC reported two cases of fatal disease in 1988 in bacteriologists from California and Massachusetts who had handled meningococci in a laboratory, each having the same isoenzyme type as a strain isolated from them at the time of their infection. There was considerable evidence of laboratory-acquired infection.(77)

While these cases indicate a potential occupational hazard, symptomatic infections with this organism are exceedingly rare. Nonetheless, it is prudent that laboratory personnel receive the tetravalent meningococcal polysaccharide vaccine before taking up their work assignments and that laboratory workers who work with large quantities of organisms be protected with gloves and laboratory coats and use a class II biologic safety cabinet in a biosafety level 3 laboratory. Persons exposed to high-concentration aerosols or who have percutaneous exposures should have prophylaxis with treatment doses of penicillin.(7)

There are no other identifiable occupational hazards except for military recruits during periods of mobilization, who seem to have a special susceptibility that becomes manifest in outbreaks among them. Despite great fears and expressed anxieties, physicians and nurses tend not to be excessively susceptible either to sporadic cases or during outbreaks. Arkwright(57) stated:

> It is almost universally accepted that doctors and hospital nurses seldom contract the disease. These and similar facts which have been observed in many epidemics are evidence against the spread of the disease being usually due to direct infection from one patient to another.

This concept has been modified in the present era by two new therapeutic procedures. Several cases of meningococcal disease have occurred among physicians who gave mouth-to-mouth resuscitation to patients severely affected by such infections. Feldman reported a case in which infection was apparently transferred with a kidney transplanted from an undiagnosed fatal case to a susceptible recipient.(78) Other than in the case of direct exposure to respiratory tract secretions of infected patients such as with mouth-to-mouth resuscitation, medical personnel do not require prophylaxis with rifampin following the delivery of medical care to patients with meningococcal disease.

5.9. Occurrence in Different Settings

The most predictable outbreaks have been those that accompanied increased military mobilization and the induction of large numbers of recruits such as were noted in World Wars I and II and the Korean and Vietnamese mobilizations in the United States. The most extensive and largest outbreaks in this century were those in civilians in sub-Saharan Africa and in Brazil. While more than a quarter of a million cases occurred in the latter, even under such conditions, outbreaks are spotty and concentrated in the poor and crowded[42,54]; e.g., during the Vietnamese mobilization, extensive outbreaks occurred among US Army and Navy recruits, while the Air Force and Marines experienced only sporadic cases and were spared the major epidemics that affected the other two services. One would assume that the induction system being what it is, susceptibles would have been distributed more or less equally among all four services. Cases were almost unknown among female recruits, but there were many fewer of them and their housing conditions were relatively uncrowded. Outbreaks of meningococcal disease in the military has not been a problem since the development of the polysaccharide meningococcal vaccine and its widespread use in the military throughout the world in the early 1970s.

Daniels *et al.*[79] reported that whereas a third of the troops at Fort Bragg, North Carolina, had less than 3 months of service, 59% of all patients with meningococcal infections were in this category. In other places, as many as 90% of cases were reported among recruits with less than 90 days of service. In the military, then, meningococcal infections represent a disease of recruits, whereas among seasoned troops or cadres in training, only sporadic cases are likely to be seen.[62] These are probably the result of specific antibody deficiencies.[80] A similar situation has been noted among South African miners, who represent a young population in whom meningococcal infections tend to occur early in their employment in the mines. Those who reenlist for a second tour of service are seldom troubled by this disease. Outbreaks may also be noted on occasion in institutions such as jails, mental asylums, residential schools, and other closed populations.

Outbreaks of meningococcal infection are quite uncommon in day-care centers or other infant-care facilities, but they have been reported, usually as part of a community outbreak. A report from the CDC, published in 1977, described a cluster of three cases of serogroup B disease from a private home day-care center with nine attendees in Georgia. Review of the recent literature at that time revealed a cluster of three group B cases in a crowded church nursery attended by 40 children under 6 years of age in 1966–1967, and two group C cases in a day-care center in Dade County, Florida during an epidemic in 1969–1970.[81]

In 1981, there was a large outbreak of meningococcal disease in an elementary school classroom in Houston. In this outbreak there were five children and two siblings of one child who became ill within a 6-day period with serogroup C *N. meningitidis*. This outbreak was unusual in that the children were 12 years old, older than in other reports of spread among children, and that disease was not noted in other classrooms or the community at large. Other studies of cases in school classrooms have been notable for the absence of secondary cases. Overcrowding may have been the major promoting spread of disease.[82]

5.10. Socioeconomic Factors

Outbreaks among civilians tend to occur among the poor, especially those who are overcrowded, ill-housed, and ill-fed.[54] In the great Brazilian epidemic of the 1970s, cases were concentrated in the barrios and typically were unusual among the middle and upper classes. Thus, even within cities, cases are often localized and confined to small areas rather than spread among the community as a whole. In a surveillance study of bacterial meningitis in Charleston County, South Carolina from 1961–1971, neither race nor income affected the risk of meningococcal meningitis, even though income was inversely correlated with rate of meningitis due to *Haemophilus influenzae* and *Streptococcus pneumoniae*.[75]

5.11. Other Factors

The principal factors that seem to be related to the occurrence of meningococcal infections are climatic conditions. In the sub-Sahara area, the change from the wet to the dry season tends to lead to an increase in cases. The reason for this relationship is unknown, although Belcher *et al.*[64] are of the opinion that considerably more population mixing takes place during the dry season, when farming work is reduced and more time is available for socializing and visiting. Also, there is a shift from sleeping outdoors to sleeping indoors in crowded and poorly ventilated rooms. In northern Ghana, the peak occurrence of cases comes during the dry season, when there is little rainfall, low humidity, and cold nights. Since this is the time when food becomes scarcer, it is popularly known as the "hunger season."

Despite much effort, familial and genetic factors have not been found to play a significant role in the acquisition of meningococcal disease, except among those who lack one of the terminal complement components.[83] (see Section 8.1.1).

6. Mechanisms and Routes of Transmission

Transmission of meningococcal infections is usually assumed to be by way of droplets from the respiratory tract, regardless of the clinical status of the individual. Organisms are present in almost pure culture in the posterior nasopharynx of colonized individuals. Direct transmission may occur during mouth-to-mouth resuscitation, by the transfer of infected blood, such as an accidental needle puncture from a contaminated syringe, or by organ transplant. Nosocomial transmission, while probably very rare, was documented by Cohen *et al.*[84] in New Haven, Connecticut. At a time when two patients on a cancer ward developed group Y meningococcal infections, the prevalence of asymptomatic pharyngeal carriage of group Y strains was 10% among other patients on the ward. The carriage prevalence was significantly lower in ward workers and casual visitors. Spread was presumably due to airborne transmission.

Acute, purulent meningococcal urethritis[85] has been reported increasingly along with more frequent reports of isolations of meningococci from the cervix[86,87] and other unusual areas.[88–96] How often these reflect sexual activity or generalized infection is unclear. It has been suggested that cervical acquisitions may be related to orogenital sex, or perhaps transmitted by a male with meningococcal urethritis, or the result of generalized dissemination during mild meningococcemia. Whether direct cervical implantation leads to clinical systemic disease is unknown.

6.1. Secondary Attack Rate

Considerable confusion has surrounded the calculation and interpretation of secondary attack rates of meningococcal disease. Norton and Gordon,[73] in their study of the meningococcal epidemic of 1929 in Detroit, found among the 724 cases of meningitis 32 (4.4%) additional cases in households. Among these additional cases, they believed that 2 could be eliminated completely, leading to the conclusion that there had been 30 secondary household cases. In the Santiago, Chile epidemic, Pizzi[54] calculated the secondary attack rate to be 3.9% for those less than 15 years of age and 1.5% for those older than 15. For all ages during this epidemic of 5885 cases, the secondary attack rate was 2.5%. During the massive Brazilian epidemic, a study[98] conducted among classmates of children who had meningococcal disease was interpreted as indicating that classroom exposure to cases did not increase the risk of acquiring meningococcal meningitis. The authors concluded that such exposure was an insufficient indication for prophylactic chemotherapy.

The Meningococcal Disease Surveillance Group,[99] organized by the CDC, analyzed 326 cases reported in the United States from November 1973 through March 1974. Three household members manifested meningococcal disease following initial cases in their homes, a secondary attack rate of approximately 3/1000 household members at risk. Among 293 households for whom follow-up data were available, 4 had two cases and none had more than two. In this study, cases in contacts with onset within 24 hr of the case to which they were exposed were labeled "co-primary." In 107 households in which no chemoprophylaxis was administered to any household members, the secondary attack rate was 2.2/1000. The authors concluded that a secondary attack rate of 2–4/1000 is still a thousand times greater than the overall reported rate of 0.23/100,000 of meningococcal disease in the states in the cases studied.

What is not clear here is whether a distinction is drawn between secondary and co-primary cases, as was attempted by Leedom *et al.*[100] in a 3-year study of Los Angeles County cases. There were 290 different families, 3.4% of which had more than one case. From a sample of these cases, it was determined that the average number of people residing in the same household with each patient was 3.71. The risk of multiple cases among household contacts of patients was estimated to be 992/100,000. The 3-year case average (1963–1965) for Los Angeles County was 2.09/100,000. One household had three cases. The onset of disease was basically simultaneous among all family members except for three in which the cases were separated by 5, 7, and 9 days. The remainder, then, would be considered to have been co-primary cases. The high rate of secondary cases during epidemics compared with the rate with endemic disease may be due to multiple factors, but the problem of assigning status as a true secondary case may be more difficult during an epidemic.

What, then, are the implications of using these different designations, or is it solely a matter of semantics? The incubation period for meningococcal disease varies from 2 to 10 days, commonly 3–4 days.[101] Bolduan and Goodwin,[102] in a 1905 study in New York City, identified 88 instances where there was more than one case in a house.

Among 58 of these, the interval between the index and second case was 7 days in 14 and 2 weeks to 3 months in 16. Norton[97] stated that among 6416 household contacts of 1272 cases, there were 36 homes with more than one case. In three, two persons became ill the same day, and in another, there were four simultaneous onsets. The latter had a fifth case sometime later. Norton calculated that while 3.6% of homes had additional cases after their first, there were 46 (0.7%) secondary cases among 6416 contacts. Of these 46, 20 had their onsets within 4 days and 14 within the next 5 days, or 34 (74%) within 9 days of the index patient. Thus, with an incubation period up to 10 days, most of these "secondary" cases are really co-primary. In contrast, Jacobson *et al.*[98] defined a secondary case as "the onset of illness more than 24 hours and less than 31 days after onset of another case in the same classroom." Their definition was more applicable to the issue of prophylaxis where it is unlikely that an oral prophylactic agent would affect an already-invasive infection.

7. Pathogenesis and Immunity

Meningococci are generally transmitted via droplets or through close oral contact. The organisms have a predilection for the posterior nasopharynx and can often be obtained in almost pure culture from that area. It was believed for a long time that the bacteria penetrated to the central nervous system through the cribriform plate, but there is no real evidence for this. Dingle and Finland[70] summarized the evidence for and against this concept and decided, as had most observers, that dissemination from the posterior nasopharynx is via the bloodstream. Once the bloodstream has been entered, a variety of consequences may follow, leading to various clinical expressions.[65] As shown in Table 1, these manifestations may run the gamut from mild, self-limited bacteremia—which may or may not be accompanied by low-grade fever, a pinkish, maculopapular rash, arthralgias with malaise, and muscle pains—to overwhelming sepsis with a coalescing, extensive petechial rash that may lead to large areas of necrosis. Disseminated intravascular coagulation, meningitis, septic arthritis, epididymitis, myocarditis, conjunctivitis, adrenal collapse (Waterhouse–Friderichsen syndrome), and death within an hour or two may follow. Fortunately, it is only the rare individual who falls into this latter category. What there is about such individuals that makes them especially susceptible to such severe disease manifestations is unknown, but they arouse the greatest interest and serve to direct attention to the disease. Probably as many as 90% of those who acquire meningococci have infections that are limited to the posterior nasopharynx with, occasionally perhaps, self-limited bacteremia. Whether infection limited to the posterior nasopharynx leads to clinical signs has been debated for decades and remains unresolved. Unfortunately, most such studies have been performed among military recruits, who are notorious for the amount of bacterial, mycoplasmal, and viral upper-respiratory infections that they support. Each of these agents would have to be excluded before one could conclude that meningococci are producing the reference symptoms. It is the prevalence of posterior nasopharyngeal infections and the paucity of clinical disease that complicate our understanding of the epidemiology of these diseases. That relationship led Arkwright[57] to conclude that epidemics basically affect the nasopharynx and that cases of meningitis and other complications are incidental. This also explains the apparent indiscriminate occurrence of clinical disease and the lack of evidence for direct connections between cases.

Immunity has been studied extensively during the past three decades. Serum antibodies have been demonstrated by a variety of techniques, including radioimmunoassay,[103] bactericidal,[80,104] hemagglutination,[105] agglutination,[104,106] and others. The solid-phase radioimmunoassay is particularly suited to determination of antibody to noncapsular antigens.[107] Immunity is acquired as the result of infection even when this seems to have been limited to the posterior nasopharynx.[104,108] Thus, the carrier state can induce immunity to the serogroup of the organism carried. The presence of bactericidal antibodies correlates well with protection from disease.[80,108] The presence of bactericidal antibody to serogroups not in circulation in specific populations suggests the importance of antibody to protein and LPS type-specific antigens. Since antibodies are free in the circulation, their protective value supports well the concept that the serum antibodies play an important role in the dissemination of meningococci.

An alternative hypothesis for the role of antibody, in military recruits, has been proposed by Griffiss.[109] He has found antimeningococcal IgA in the acute sera of military recruits who had meningococcal disease. This IgA was able to inhibit the lytic function IgM in sera. Removal of IgA made sera that appeared to lack bactericidal antibody functionally lytic. Thus, it is Griffiss' contention that susceptibility, in addition to being defined by the *absence* of functional antibody, may be due, in some cases, to the presence of blocking IgA.[109] Thus, as it is the acquisition of new strains of meningococci that represents the major risk factor for invasive disease, true susceptibility may also be related to exposure to successive waves of meningococci. The role of this mechanism, if any, in civilian endemic disease is unknown.

Another factor influencing susceptibility of individuals to meningococcal infections is deficiency of terminal complement components. It is known that in antibody-mediated bacteriolysis the late components of complement (C5–C9) are required. Individuals who lack one or more of these components are susceptible to invasive meningococcal infections and even recurrent infections (see Section 8.1).

8. Patterns of Host Response

Inapparent infections play an important role in meningococcal disease because they constitute the majority and account for the bulk of carriers. As has been expressed previously, the acquisition of the carrier state leads to immunity,[80,104] and thus protection against the disease itself. We have no information as to why, among children, an occasional individual is unable to restrict the acquired meningococci to the posterior nasopharynx and becomes the victim of a life-threatening disease episode. Among adults, deficiency of lytic antibody appears to be the major predisposing factor accounting for biological susceptibility to meningococcal disease. The reason why a small number of adults lack antibody is unknown. Either they were never colonized or colonization did not result in the production of a long-lasting antibody response.

8.1. Clinical Features

Meningococcal infections may manifest themselves clinically by several different syndromes (see Table 1). These may overlap or be noted sequentially in the same patient. The most common occurrence is represented by the asymptomatic acquisition of meningococci in the posterior nasopharynx or the carrier state. While there are some who believe that an acute pharyngitis may be clinically manifest in this stage, this has never really been proven and, while only a possibility, may account for as much as 90% or more of all acquisitions. Thus, disease as such is limited to less than 10% of those who acquire meningococci. The next stage may be that of a mild, self-limited bacteremia that may be accompanied by an evanescent rubellalike rash, arthralgias, fever, malaise, and myalgias. A blood culture taken at this time is often positive for meningococci. This may regress completely or for several days, only to be followed by an explosive onset of severe illness. This is generally heralded or accompanied by a severe petechial rash that may be very extensive and coalescent, with large areas of necrotic skin and muscle. Similar lesions probably occur in the deeper viscera.

Prostration and shock may follow in short order, with death close behind. Smears made from petechial lesions or from the buffy coat of peripheral blood may contain gram-negative diplococci within or without cells. This is the most devastating form of the infection, in which septicemia is so severe and overwhelming that it often kills before there is localization in the CNS, joints, or other organs.

A less virulent form of septicemia is more common, and while this too is identifiable with a petechial rash, progression is slower and permits other complications to become evident. These patients often are the cases with meningitis, septic arthritis, epididymitis, pneumonitis with pneumonia, conjunctivitis, and myocarditis. All these may occur in a single patient, or in any combination thereof.

In infants, "mild" meningococcemia may present with fever as the only symptom. This presentation of meningococcemia is very similar to that of occult pneumonococcemia, which occurs more frequently than meningococcemia in ambulatory pediatric patients.[110,111]

Discrete meningococcal pneumonia has also been reported, especially from the military. Group Y meningococcus has often been implicated in this form of infection.[112] Koppes *et al.*[112] reported on 88 cases of group Y meningococcal disease in Air Force recruits, 68 of whom had primary bacterial pneumonia. All but one did well with penicillin therapy. It is possible that the predominance of group Y in these cases reflected immunization with group C polysaccharide vaccine, which had been instituted as a routine procedure in the Air Force. In this study, 52 of 64 individuals sampled had pure cultures of group Y meningococci in transtracheal aspirates. In the remainder, growth was due primarily to group Y meningococci, with relatively small amounts of contaminants such as α-streptococci, *Haemophilus influenzae* type b, and others. Primary meningococcal pneumonia, either alone or in concert with other evidence of septic meningococcal infections, has been reported often enough to constitute a disease entity, establishment of the identity of which should be sought in cases of otherwise undefined pneumonia.

Group Y meningococcal infections have also occurred in children.[110,113,114] Pneumonia was reported in one case.[114] Group W-135, which has increased in incidence in the past two decades, has also been reported to have a varied presentation in children, similar to other serogroups.[115,116]

There is an unusual and infrequently seen form of the disease that is identified as chronic meningococcemia. This may be a manifestation of subacute bacterial endocarditis or the result of continuous seeding into the bloodstream from an unknown nidus. Such patients may go for weeks or months with recurring fever and evanescent rashes, as either pink macules or small petechiae. They respond rapidly to treatment and are often cured by penicillin administered for other reasons, such as a suspected infectious cause of the fever, malaise, and rash.

8.1.1. Complement Deficiency and Meningococcal Infections. Petersen *et al.*[83] summarized information from various reports of 24 patients who had had recurrent episodes of meningococcal or (generalized) gonorrheal infections. Their distinguishing characteristic is that they lack one or more of the late components of the complement system: C6, C7, or C8. Of the 24 patients, 6 were deficient in either C6 or C7 and 8 in C8. In all, 13 of the 24 had had either *N. meningitidis* or *N. gonorrhoeae* bacteremia, and all recovered. The patient with C7 deficiency apparently recovered from four episodes of meningococcal meningitis. The frequency of this abnormality is unknown, but it would seem that while the propensity to have recurrent neisserial infections is present in such individuals, the disease does not appear to be overwhelming or fatal, since so many seem to have recovered. From subsequent reports it appears that deficiency of C5 and C9 are also risk factors for neisserial infections.

Ellison *et al.*[117] studied 20 adults with a first episode of meningococcal infection. Six of them had a complement deficiency. Of these six, three had a specific terminal component deficiency and three had multiple component deficiencies due to an underlying illness. In children, the prevalence of underlying complement deficiency in those with one meningococcal infection was 18% in one study.[118] In a larger study, of 544 patients with meningitis or bacteremia due to encapsulated organisms, seven had complement deficiencies; of those seven, six experienced meningococcal infection and one had pneumococcal bacteremia.[119] While the rate of complement deficiencies varies between ethnic groups, the estimate of prevalence is 0.03%. The prevalence of patients with complement deficiencies among those with meningococcal infections is higher when the case is sporadic, in an area of low incidence, than when it is part of a meningococcal outbreak. In a study comparing complement-sufficient patients who had meningococcal disease with patients with complement defects, those with complement defects were older (mean age of 17 years vs. 3 years), more likely to have recurrence and relapse, and had a much lower mortality rate (1.5 vs. 19%).[119] Immunization with meningococcal polysaccharide vaccine appears to offer some individuals with complement deficiencies protection from meningococcal disease.[120]

Corfield[121] may have recorded the first such case in 1945 and suggests another, seen by Boudin, in whom three episodes occurred in 1849, 1850, and 1851. These cases are to be separated from the recurrent disease that was encountered before modern therapy prevented the frequent bacterial relapses common to that era. Patients who have recurrent disseminated neisserial disease should be screened with CH_{50} assays, and if they are positive, specific deficiencies should be sought.

8.2. Diagnosis

As is true of many diseases, the frequency of the diagnosis of meningitis often reflects the observer's index of suspicion. The carrier state is not diagnosable except by culture and is of little importance except under some very special circumstances. In the case of expressed disease, diagnosis generally requires laboratory confirmation. With this in mind, blood cultures should be obtained as quickly as possible. If there are clinical signs of meningitis, an immediate lumbar puncture is mandatory, followed by prompt examination of the fluid. Its cellular content should be ascertained as to type and number. Sugar and protein should be measured. (It is well to determine the comparative blood sugar at the same time.) A Gram's stain should be performed on a smear made from the fluid if the fluid is cloudy; but if it is clear, it should be spun and a thick, stained smear made from the residual drop after the supernate is decanted. Fluid should be cultured on chocolate agar in an atmosphere of increased CO_2. If organisms are visible in the direct smear, it is well to mix a small volume with specific grouping antiserum. Organisms of groups A and C usually have good capsules in spinal fluid, and mixing with specific antiserum may lead to a "quellung" reaction, or capsular swelling. This is a specific reaction that can provide definitive identification. A sensitive modification of this procedure was described by Thomas *et al.*[104]

Additionally, Gram's stains of smears of fluid from petechial lesions or buffy coats of peripheral blood may also yield gram-negative diplococci. If these are present, then they are most likely meningococci. The peripheral white blood count is usually elevated, but in severely ill patients, it may be less than 4000/mm^3. A culture of the posterior nasopharynx on Thayer–Martin chocolate agar

Table 4. Chemoprophylaxis for Contacts of Patients with Infection due to *Neisseria meningitidis*

Drug	Age of contact	Dose/regimen/duration
Rifampin (orally)	Adult	600 mg every 12 hr for 2 days
	1 month to 12 years	10 mg/kg every 12 hr for 2 days
	Less than 1 month	5 mg/kg every 12 hr for 2 days
Sulfadiazine (orally)	Adult	1 gram every 12 hr for 2 days
	1 to 12 years	500 mg every 12 hr for 2 days
	Less than 1 year	500 mg every 24 hr for 2 days
Ceftriaxone (inramuscularly)[a]	15 years or older	250 mg as a single injection
	Less than 15 years	125 mg as a single injection

[a]Ceftriaxone has shown to be very effective for elimination of meningococcal carriage in contacts of casees with group A meningococcal strains but there is a lack of data on reduction of the rate of secondary cases.[123,124]

is indicated on admission for all patients with a suspected diagnosis of meningococcal disease. If a patient has been treated with antibiotics prior to obtaining samples for culture detection of antigens in blood, urine or spinal fluid using the latex agglutination test may be helpful in making a diagnosis even if the cultures are sterile.

Because of the nature of the rash and the clinically severe illness, the diagnosis may be confused with Rocky Mountain spotted fever. Less severe cases may be confused with endemic typhus and, when very mild, even with rubella.

9. Control and Prevention

9.1. General Concepts

Because cases of meningococcal disease tend to be distributed indiscriminately in a population and because death may be sudden, the appearance of a case frequently leads to generalized hysteria in the associated population, whether it be open or closed. Outbreaks tend to occur in closed groups such as institutions, recruit military camps, and crowded, impoverished districts of major cities.[6,54] As with poliomyelitis, cases do not seem to lead to other cases, an observation that understandably tends to increase fear and hysteria among the populace in which the cases occur.

Sporadic cases of meningococcal disease occur throughout the year in all places. They often appear as isolated instances for reasons that are not understood. More incomprehensibly, cases may begin to occur in rapid succession in a given population. These are usually closed, institutionalized settings, but numerous cases may be noted in the community at large and constitute an epidemic.

9.2. Antibiotic and Chemotherapeutic Approaches to Prophylaxis: Suggestions for the Management of Outbreaks

Before rational intervention can be instituted or attempted when it is suspected that excessive cases of meningococcal disease are occurring, two important questions must be answered. First, can the affected population be defined; and second, what are the characteristics of the causative agent? In respect to the latter, is it of a single serogroup, and most important, is the predominant organism sulfonamide-sensitive or -resistant?

If the affected population can be reasonably well defined, and if only one meningococcal serogroup accounts for most of the cases, and is sulfonamide-sensitive (i.e., susceptible to $\leqslant$ 0.1 mg/100 ml of sulfadiazine), then the quickest, simplest, and most effective way to institute control is to provide each member of the population at risk with sulfadiazine for 2 consecutive days (see Table 4). In these dosages and with the further precaution that the drug not be administered to individuals with histories of previous sulfonamide reactions, the drug is safe and exceedingly effective. The carrier rate may be expected to drop to near zero almost immediately, slowly rebuilding itself over a period of weeks. Cases also stop occurring as the carrier rate diminishes. It is required, for maximum benefit, that treatment be simultaneous for the total target population.

If the causative organism is sulfonamide-resistant, then there are still two options. One is to attempt chemoprophylaxis with drugs other than sulfonamides; the other is to attempt to immunize the population with a polysaccharide vaccine. The latter is feasible only if the causative organisms are of serogroups A, C, Y, or W-135. The licensed vaccine contains the polysaccharides of groups A, C, Y, and W-135, and only a single dose is required. When the vaccine is used, it must be anticipated that maximum beneficial effects will be noted after 10–14 days, although diminution in the severity of the disease in some cases may be observed by the 7th day.

The other drugs that have been used for meningococcal prophylaxis, and that were alluded to in Section 4, are rifampin and minocycline.[43] The dose of rifampin is listed in Table 4. Minocycline is rarely used for this indication because of gastrointestinal and vestibular toxicity,[41,42] but the recommended dose is 100 mg every 12 hr for 5 days.[43] Resistance to rifampin has been noted in as many as one fourth of strains. This proportion increased with repeated courses of the drug in the same population. It should be borne in mind that there are no data on the therapeutic effectiveness of either minocycline or rifampin, and thus neither should be used for treatment.[122] In the case of sulfadiazine, part of its effectiveness may be related to its efficiency as a therapeutic agent, so that even small doses may effect cures of mild bacteremias. It cannot be emphasized too much that knowledge of the sulfonamide-resistance pattern of the offending organism(s) and the predominant serogroup presented in the target population is an essential requirement for the intelligent management of suspected outbreaks. A single intramuscular dose of ceftriaxone is effective in eradicating meningococci from the pharynx,[123,124] and it can be used for meningococcal prophylaxis. Its high cost and difficulty of administration limit the usefulness of this option to special circumstances where repeated oral dosing is not practical.

9.3. Immunization

Gotschlich, Artenstein, and their colleagues,[80,105,108] in the search for an effective alternative to sulfonamide prevention of meningococcal disease, successfully reopened the investigation of vaccines, an approach that had lain dormant for a quarter of a century. A series of publications beginning with the demonstration of the importance of serum antibodies in protection against the disease,[80] the effectiveness of pure carbohydrate antigens[105,108] in stimulating specific immunity against infection with organisms of the various serogroups, and finally the value of such antigenic stimulation in providing protection against the disease during epidemic periods[22] was probably the most important contribution to the meningococcal problem in this century. Subsequently, group A meningococcal vaccine was used in the management of large epidemics of disease in Finland,[7] Brazil,[6] and Egypt.[125] Effective polysaccharide immunogens for groups Y and W135 appeared later.[126]

Greenwood *et al.*[127] evaluated the effectiveness of group A vaccine in preventing secondary cases when administered to household contacts of group A cases and found the secondary attack rate to be 18/1000 among control household contacts who received tetanus toxoid. Among the 520 case contacts who had received group A meningococcal vaccine, there was only one instance of meningococcal disease. The efficacy of the group A meningococcal vaccine was clearly demonstrated in the trial of Peltola *et al.*[21] in Finland in 1974–1975. In two trials conducted during an epidemic of group A meningococcal disease, 49,295 and 21,007 children, aged 3 months to 5 years, received the vaccine. None developed group A meningococcal disease. In the first trial there were two control groups that had significantly more cases than the vaccine group.

Despite the Finnish experience, there is good evidence that in children the degree of antibody response to the groups A and C vaccine, measured as the concentration of anticapsular antibody in the serum, is proportional to age. Children under 1 year of age have a poor response and no immunologic memory.[128,129] As is seen for other polysaccharide vaccines that are non-T-cell-dependent immunogens, it is not until 2 years of age that there is sufficient maturation of the immune system for there to be a protective antibody response to group C polysaccharide, although the response to the group A polysaccharide appears to occur earlier.[128,129]

Initially, meningococcal vaccine was marketed for civilian use as 50 μg of group A polysaccharide, 50 μg of group C polysaccharide, or a combination of both. Later, a tetravalent vaccine consisting of 50 μg each of groups A, C, Y, and W-135 capsular polysaccharides has been shown to be safe and immunogenic and has been licensed (Menomune, manufactured by Connaught Laboratories, Swiftwater, PA).[130] After group B, the commonest, these four are the most common groups causing meningococcal disease in the United States. No vaccine for group B has been produced because the B polysaccharide is not immunogenic. Despite extensive research into production of a nonpolysaccharide vaccine or a polysaccharide conjugated with another immunogen, there is no candidate group B vaccine at this time.

A single 0.5-ml dose of vaccine is sufficient to immunize a child over 2 years of age or an adult. Adverse reactions have not presented a problem, generally being limited to local erythema or soreness or both, usually persisting for no more than 24 hr.[131] Reactions are more likely to increase with repeated doses of polysaccharide, which are not required and should be discouraged. While there was some problem originally with stability and persistence of antigenicity, these problems have largely been solved with manufacturing modifications currently in use. One of the difficulties in the production of this vaccine was that it is essentially not immunogenic in animals other than man and therefore must be standardized in humans.

Protection conveyed by vaccines requires about 7 days before noticeable benefits are observed. The initial effect is that of modification of the illness so as to reduce mortality; total protection from disease requires approximately 14 days after inoculation. In various trials, the effectiveness level has been calculated to be in the vicinity of 90%.[125,132] Antibody responses have been found to persist for at least 5 years,[132] and may be expected to last much longer in further studies. The American Academy of Pediatrics recommends revaccination in 1 year for those children at continued high risk who were vaccinated before 4 years of age and after 5 years for those first immunized at 4 years of age or older.[133]

9.3.1. Application. Except during World War II, the incidence of meningococcal disease in the US general population has been too low to warrant wide-scale immunization with the available meningococcal vaccines. In the United States, demonstrated group A infections have been very rare since the end of World War II, while groups B and C have provided most of the interim cases. Over the past decade, groups Y and W-135 have emerged as common where previously they had been rare.

On the other hand, the 4-year Brazilian epidemic[6] of the 1970s resulted in more than a quarter of a million cases. In the first 2 years, this was essentially a group C epidemic that then became a group A outbreak. A massive countrywide immunization campaign was undertaken, which eventually meant that more than 80 million persons received bivalent A and C, or monovalent A or C, vaccines. This brought the epidemic to a close and it has not recurred. In Finland, a large outbreak in the military, accompanied by many civilian cases, was also treated with vaccine and was soon brought under control.[7]

When, then, should vaccine be expected to be effective? Meningococcal diseases represent a serious health hazard for military recruits, especially during periods of increased mobilization. Thus, since the early 1970s all recruits entering the United States military have received a single dose of group C, A/C, or more recently A/C/Y/W-135 vaccine with evident benefit. In the light of extensive past experience, it would seem prudent to continue this policy for recruits entering the military in all its branches.

Usage in civilians is more limited. Since current vaccines are only protective when given at over 2 years of age, and the great majority of civilian cases occur in younger children, routine vaccination is not recommended. Vaccination would seem to be indicated where localized or institutional outbreaks can be defined and the causative strain identified as either group A, C, Y, or W-135. A possible guideline being considered by the Advisory Committee on Immunization Practices, is that if there are three or more cases with the same serogroup and the serogroup-specific rate of meningococcal infection in a defined population exceeds 10 times the baseline or expected rate for that serogroup over a 3-month period, vaccination may be considered. Usage to prevent secondary cases among close contacts is recommended by the Immunization Practices Advisory Committee of the CDC,[130] but the overall risk is low and most such cases occur within less than 6 or at most 9–10 days of the index case. Thus, chemotherapeutic measures should be more effective.

In addition, patients with functional or anatomic asplenia, such as in sickle-cell disease or traumatic rupture of the spleen, are prone to severe or fatal infections with polysaccharide-encapsulated bacteria. Individuals with deficiencies of the terminal complement components may also have recurrent meningococcal infections. Patients over 2 years of age who fit any of these categories should receive the current meningococcal vaccine as part of their preventive care. While younger patients might have benefit from the serogroup A component, the risk of group A disease is too low to warrant vaccine in most Western countries.

Meningococcal vaccine is also recommended for travelers to countries known to have an epidemic of meningococcal disease or where the endemic rate is very high such as sub-Saharan Africa or in certain regions of Saudi Arabia at the time of the *Haj*.

10. Unresolved Problems

The greatest unresolved problems are the elucidation of the factors that lead to the occurrence of a case; i.e., of the many individuals who acquire meningococci carriage, why do only so few (probably less than 10%) develop meningococcal disease? In parallel with this is the question of which factor or factors lead to the occurrence of an epidemic in a given locality or institution. Such epidemics arise suddenly and for no apparent reason persist for varying periods of time—days, weeks, months, or years—and then either disappear completely or are replaced by meningococci of another serogroup. Are the factors responsible for these fluxes changes in the pathogen, the host or a combination of the two?

Questions remain concerning the use of the current meningococcal capsular polysaccharide vaccine. This involves questions of optimal timing and the definition of the population that would benefit most from their use, as well as the definition of the conditions under which they achieve maximum effectiveness. There are few data that address the question of revaccination. Finally, we still need new vaccines. Despite immunogenic preparations for adults, we lack vaccines for children under 2 years of age that will protect against the major serogroups, and we still lack an effective vaccine for group B *N. meningitidis*.

11. References

1. Vieusseux, M., Mémoire sur le maladie qui a regné à Génève au printemps de 1805, *J. Med. Chir. Pharmacol.* **11:**163 (1805).
2. Danielson, L., and Mann, E., The history of a singular and very mortal disease, which lately made its appearance in Medfield, *Med. Agric. Register.* **1:**65–69 (1806).
3. Weichselbaum, A., Ueber die Aetiologie der akuten Meningitis cerebrospinalis, *Fortschr. Med.* **5:**573 (1887).
4. Lapeyssonnie, L., La méningite cérébro-spinale en Afrique, *Bull.WHO* **28**(Suppl.) (1963).
5. Alexander, C. E., Sanborn, W. R., Cherriere, G., Crocker, W. H., Jr., Ewald, P. E., and Kay, C. R., Sulfadiazine-resistant group A *Neisseria meningitidis, Science* **161:**1019 (1968).
6. Pan American Health Organization, Report of the first hemispheric meeting on meningococcal disease, *Pan. Am. Health Organ. Bull.* **10:**163–174 (1976).
7. Mäkelä, P. H., Peltola, H., Käyhty, H., Jousimies, H., Pettay, O., Ruoslahti, E., Sivonen, A., and Renkonen, O.-V., Polysaccharide vaccines of group A *Neisseria meningitidis* and *Haemophilus influenzae* type b: A field trial in Finland, *J. Infect. Dis.* **136:**S43–S50 (1977).
8. Gordon, M. H., Identification of the meningococcus, *J. R. Army Med. Corps* **24:**455–458 (1915).
9. Branham, S. E., Serological relationships among meningococci, *Bacteriol. Rev.* **17:**175–188 (1953).
10. Slaterus, K. W., Serological typing of meningococci by means of microprecipitation, *Antonie van Leeuwenhoek J. Microbiol. Serol.* **27:**304–315 (1961).
11. Evans, J. R., Artenstein, M. S., and Hunter, D. H., Prevalence of meningococcal serogroups and description of three new groups, *Am. J. Epidemiol.* **87:**643–646 (1968).
12. Diong, S., Ye, R., and Zhang, H., Three new serogroups of *Neisseria menigitidis*, *J. Biol. Stand.* **9:**305–315 (1981).
13. Ashton, F. E., Ryan, A., Diena, B., and Jennings, H. J., A new serogroup (L) of *Neisseria meningitidis*, *J. Clin. Microbiol.* **17:**722–727 (1983).
14. Cheever, F. S., The control of meningococcal meningitis by mass chemoprophylaxis with sulfadiazine, *Am. J. Med. Sci.* **209:** 74–75 (1945).
15. Gray, F. C., and Gear, J., Sulphapyridine, M and B 693, as a prophylactic against cerebrospinal meningitis, *S. Afr. Med. J.* **15:**139–140 (1941).
16. Kuhns, D. M., Nelson, C. T., Feldman, H. A., and Kuhn, L. R., The prophylactic value of sulfadiazine in the control of meningococcic meningitis, *J. Am. Med. Assoc.* **123:**335–339 (1943).
17. Phair, J. J., Schoenbach, E. B., and Root, C. M., Meningococcal carrier studies, *Am. J. Public Health* **34:**148–154 (1944).
18. Millar, J. W., Siess, E. E., Feldman, H. A., Silverman, C., and Frank, P., *In vivo* and *in vitro* resistance to sulfadiazine in strains of *Neisseria meningitidis*, *J. Am. Med. Assoc.* **186:**139–141 (1963).
19. Feldman, H. A., Sulfonamide-resistant meningococci, *Annu. Rev. Med.* **18:**495–506 (1967).
20. The Medical Letter, Inc., Preventing the spread of meningococcal disease, *Med. Lett.* **23:**37–38 (1981).
21. Peltola, H., Mäkelä, H., Käyhty, H., Jousimies, H., Herva, E., Hällström, K., Sivonen, H., Renkonen, O.-V., Péttay, O., Karanko, V., Ahvonen, P., and Sarna, S., Clinical efficacy of meningococcal group A polysaccharide vaccine in children three months to five years of age, *N. Engl. J. Med.* **297:**686–691 (1977).
22. Artenstein, M. S., Gold, R., Zimmerly, J. G., Wyle, F. A., Schneider, H., and Harkins, C., Prevention of meningococcal disease by group C polysaccharide vaccine, *N. Engl. J. Med.* **282:**417–420 (1970).
23. Centers for Disease Control, Bacterial meningitis and meningococcemia—United States, 1978, *Morbid. Mortal. Week. Rep.* **28:**277–279 (1979).
24. Wenger, J. D., Hightower, A. W., Facklam, R. R., Gaventa, S., Broome, C. V., and the Bacterial Meningitis Study Group, Bacterial meningitis in the United States, 1986: Report of a multistate surveillance study, *J. Infect. Dis.* **162:**1316–1323 (1990).

24a. Schuchat, A., Robinson, K., Wenger, J. D., Harrison, L. H., Farley, M., Reingold, A. L., Lefkowitz, L., and Perkins, B. A., For the active surveillance team, Bacterial meningitis in the United States in 1995. *N. Engl. J. Med.* **337:**970–976 (1997).

25. Thayer, J. D., and Martin, J. E., Jr., A selective medium for the cultivation of *N. gonorrhoeae* and *N. meningitidis*, *Public Health Rep.* **79:**49–57 (1964).
26. Feldman, H. A., *Neisseria* infections other than gonococcal, in: *Diagnostic Procedures for Bacterial, Mycotic and Parasitic Infections* (H. L. Bodily, E. L. Updyke, and J. O. Mason, eds.), pp. 135–152, American Public Health Association, New York, 1970.
27. Cohen, R. L., and Artenstein, M. S., Hemagglutination inhibition for serogrouping *Neisseria meningitidis*, *Appl. Microbiol.* **23:** 289–292 (1972).
28. Jackson, L. A., and Wenger, J. D., Laboratory-based surveillance for meningococcal disease in selected areas, United States, 1989–1991, *Morbid. Mortal. Week. Rep.* **42:**21–30 (1993).
29. Frasch, C. E., and Chapman, S. S., Classification of *Neisseria meningitidis* group B into distinct serotypes. III. Application of a new bactericidal-inhibition technique to distribution of serotypes among cases and carriers, *J. Infect. Dis.* **127:**149–154 (1973).
30. Zollinger, W. D., and Mandrell, R. E., Outer-membrane protein and lipopolysaccharide serotyping of *Neisseria meningitidis* by inhibition of a solid-phase radioimmunoassay, *Infect. Immun.* **18:**424–433 (1977).
31. Apicella, M. A., Lipopolysaccharide-derived serotype polysac-

charides from *Neisseria meningitidis* group B, *J. Infect. Dis.* **140:**62–72 (1979).

32. Frasch, C. E., Zollinger, W. D., and Poolman, J. T., Serotype antigens of *Neisseria meningitidis* and a proposed scheme for designation of serotypes, *Rev. Infect. Dis.* **7:**504–510 (1985).
33. Achtman, M., Clonal properties of meningococci from epidemic meningitis, *Trans. R. Soc. Trop. Med. Hyg.* **85**(Suppl. 1)**:**24–31 (1991).
34. Ashton, F. E., Mancino, L., Ryan, A. J., Poolman, J. T., Abdillahi, H., and Zollinger, W. D., Serotypes and subtypes of *Neisseria meningitidis* serogroup B strains associated with meningococcal disease in Canada 1977, 1989, *Can. J. Microbiol.* **37:**613–617 (1991).
35. Block, C., Raz, R., Frasch, C. E., Ephros, M., Areif, Z., Talmon, Y., Rosin, D., and Bogokowsky, B., Re-emergence of meningococcal carriage on three-year follow-up of a kibbutz population after whole-community chemoprophylaxis, *Eur. J. Microbiol. Infect. Dis.* **12:**505–511 (1993).
36. Sáez-Nieto, J. A., Lujan, R., Berrón, S., Campos, J. A., Viñas, M., Fusté, C., Vazquez, J. A., Zhang, Q-Y., Bowler, L. D., Martinez-Suarez, V., and Spratt, B. G., Epidemiology and molecular basis of penicillin-resistant *Neisseria meningitidis* in Spain: A 5-year history (1985–1989), *Clin. Infect. Dis.* **14:**394–402 (1992).
37. Dingle, J. H., Thomas, L., and Morton, A. R., Treatment of meningococcic meningitis and meningococcemia with sulfadiazine, *J. Am. Med. Assoc.* **116:**2666–2668 (1941).
38. Feldman, H. A., Sweet, L. K., and Dowling, H. F., Sulfadiazine therapy of purluent meningitis including its use in 24 consecutive patients with meningococcic meningitis, *War Med.* **2:**995–1007 (1942).
39. Cheever, F. S., Breese, B. B., and Upham, H. C., The treatment of meningococcus carriers with sulfadiazine, *Ann. Intern. Med.* **19:**602–608 (1943).
40. Devine, L. F., Johnson, D. P., Hagerman, C. R., Pierce, W. E., Rhode, S. L., III, and Peckinpaugh, R. O., The effect of minocycline on meningococcal nasopharyngeal carrier state in naval personnel, *Am. J. Epidemiol.* **93:**337–345 (1971).
41. Drew, T. M., Altman, R., Black, K., and Goldfield, M., Minocycline for prophylaxis of infection with *Neisseria meningitidis*: High rate of side effects in recipients, *J. Infect. Dis.* **133:**194–198 (1976).
42. Munford, R. S., Sussuarana de Vasconcelos, Z. J., Phillips, C. J., Gelli, D. S., Gorman, G. W., Risi, J. B., and Feldman, R. A., Eradication of carriage of *Neisseria meningitidis* in families: A study in Brazil, *J. Infect. Dis.* **129:**644–659 (1974).
43. Sivonen, A., Renkonen, O.-V., Weckstrom, P., Koskenvuo, K., Raunio, V., and Mäkelä, P. H., The effect of chemoprophylactic use of rifampin and minocycline on rates of carriage of *Neisseria meningitidis* in Army recruits in Finland, *J. Infect. Dis.* **137:**238–244 (1978).
44. Campos, J., Mendelman, P. M., Sako, M. U., Chaffin, D. O., Smith, A. L., and Sáez-Nieto, J. A., Detection of a relatively penicillin G-resistant *Neisseria meningitidis* by disk susceptibility testing, *Antimicrobiol. Agents. Chemother.* **31:**1478–1482 (1987).
45. Sutcliffe, E. M., Jones, D. M., El-Sheikh, S., and Percival, A., Penicillin-insensitive meningococci in the UK, *Lancet* **1:**657–658 (1988).
46. Botha, P., Penicillin-resistant *Neisseria meningitidis* in Southern Africa (letter), *Lancet* **1:**54 (1988).
47. Riley, G., Brown, S., and Krishnan, C., Penicillin resistance in *Neisseria meningitidis* (letter), *N. Engl. J. Med.* **324:**997 (1991).
48. Woods, C. R., Smith, A. L., Wasilauskas, B. L., Campos, J., and Givner, L. B., Invasive disease caused by *Neisseria meningitidis* relatively resistant to penicillin in North Carolina, *J. Infect. Dis.* **170:**453–456 (1994).
49. Jackson, L. A., Tenover, F. C., Baker, C., Plikaytis, B. D., and Reeves, M. W., Prevalence of *Neisseria meningitidis* relatively resistant to penicillin in the United States, 1991, *J. Infect. Dis.* **169:**438–441 (1994).
50. Jacobson, J. A., Weaver, R. E., and Thornsberry, C., Trends in meningococcal disease, 1974, *J. Infect. Dis.* **132:**480–484 (1975).
51. Centers for Disease Control and Prevention, Summary of notifiable diseases, United States, 1994, *Morbid. Mortal. Week. Rep.* **43:**69–80 (1994).
52. Riedo, F. X., Plikaytis, B. D., and Broome, C. V., Epidemiology and prevention of meningococcal disease, *Pediatr. Infect. Dis. J.* **14:**643–657 (1995).
53. Glover, J. A., Observations of the meningococcus carrier rate, and their application to the prevention of cerebrospinal fever, Medical Research Council of the Privy Council, Special Report Series, No. 50, pp. 133–165, H.M. Stationery Offices, London, 1920.
54. Pizzi, M., A severe epidemic of meningococcus meningitis in Chile, 1941–1942, *Am. J. Public Health* **34:**231–238 (1944).
55. Dudley, S. F., and Brennan, J. R., High and persistent carrier rates of *Neisseria meningitidis*, unaccompanied by cases of meningitis, *J. Hyg.* **34:**525–541 (1934).
56. Schoenbach, E. B., The meningococcal carrier state, *Med. Ann. DC* **12:**417–420 (1943).
57. Arkwright, J. A., Cerebro-spinal meningitis: The interpretation of epidemiological observations by the light of bacteriological knowledge, *Br. Med. J.* **1:**494–496 (1915).
58. Paul, J. R., *Clinical Epidemiology*, University of Chicago Press, Chicago, 1966.
59. Maxcy, K. F., The relationship of meningococcus carriers to the incidence of cerebrospinal fever, *Am. J. Med. Sci.* **193:**438–445 (1937).
60. Greenfield, S., Sheehe, P. R., and Feldman, H. A., Meningococcal carriage in a population of "normal" families, *J. Infect. Dis.* **123:**67–73 (1971).
61. Rake, G., Studies on meningococcus infection. VI. The carrier problem, *J. Exp. Med.* **59:**553–576 (1934).
62. Gauld, J. R., Nitz, R. E., Hunter, D. H., Rust, J. H., and Gauld, R. L., Epidemiology of meningococcal meningitis at Fort Ord, *Am. J. Epidemiol.* **82:**56–72 (1965).
63. Olcén, P., Barr, J., and Kjellander, J., Meningitis and bacteremia due to *Neisseria meningitidis*: Clinical and laboratory findings in 69 cases from Orebro County, 1965 to 1977, *Scand. J. Infect. Dis.* **11:**111–119 (1979).
64. Belcher, D. W., Sherriff, A. C., Nimo, K. P., Chew, G. L. N., Voros, A., Richardson, W. D., and Feldman, H. A., Meningococcal meningitis in northern Ghana: Epidemiology and control measures, *Am. J. Trop. Med. Hyg.* **26:**748–755 (1977).
65. Feldman, H. A., Meningococcal infections, *Adv. Intern. Med.* **18:**117–140 (1972).
66. Greenwood, B. M., Bradley, A. K., Cleland, P. G., Haggie, M. H. K., Hassan-King, M., Lewis, L. S., MacFarlane, J. T., Taqi, A., and Whittle, H. C., An epidemic of meningococcal infection at Zaria, northern Nigeria. 1. General epidemiological features, *Trans. R. Soc. Trop. Med. Hyg.* **73:**557–562 (1979).

67. Greenwood, B. M., Cleland, P. G., Haggie, M. H. K., Lewis, L. S., MacFarlane, J. T., Taqi, A., and Whittle, H. C., An epidemic of meningococcal infection at Zaria, northern Nigeria. 2. The changing clinical pattern, *Trans. R. Soc. Trop. Med. Hyg.* **73:**563–566 (1979).
68. Hassan-King, M., Greenwood, B. M., and Whittle, H. C., An epidemic of meningococcal infection at Zaria, northern Nigeria. 3. Meningococcal carriage, *Trans. R. Soc. Trop. Med. Hyg.* **73:**567–573 (1979).
69. Horn, D. W., The epidemic of cerebrospinal fever in the northern provinces of Nigeria, 1949–1950, *J. R. Sanit. Inst.* **71:**573–588 (1951).
70. Dingle, J. H., and Finland, M., Diagnosis, treatment and prevention of meningococcic meningitis, with a resume of the practical aspects of treatment of other acute bacterial meningitides, *War Med.* **2:**1–58 (1942).
71. Klein, J. O., Feigin, R. D., and McCracken, G. H., Jr., Report of the task force on diagnosis and management of meningitis, *Pediatrics* **78**(S)**:**959–982 (1986).
72. Beeson, P. B., and Westerman, E., Cerebrospinal fever: Analysis of 3,575 case reports with special reference to sulphonamide therapy, *Br. Med. J.* **1:**497–500 (1943).
73. Norton, J. F., and Gordon, J. E., Meningococcus meningitis in Detroit in 1928–1929. I. Epidemiology, *J. Prev. Med.* **4:**207–214 (1930).
74. Feldman, R. A., Koehler, R. E., and Fraser, D. W., Race-specific differences in bacterial meningitis deaths in the United States, 1962–1968, *Am. J. Public Health* **66:**392–396 (1976).
75. Fraser, D. W., Darby, C. P., Koehler, R. E., Jacobs, C. F., and Feldman, R. A., Risk factors in bacterial meningitis: Charleston County, South Carolina, *J. Infect. Dis.* **127:**271–277 (1973).
76. Pike, R. M., Laboratory-associated infections: Incidence, fatalities, causes, and prevention, *Annu. Rev. Microbiol.* **33:**41–66 (1979).
77. Centers for Disease Control and Prevention, Epidemiologic notes and reports. Laboratory-acquired meningococcemia—California and Massachusetts, *Morbid. Mortal. Week. Rep.* **40:**46–55 (1991).
78. Feldman, H. A., Meningococcal Infections, in: *Bacterial Infections of Humans. Epidemiology and Control* (A. S. Evans and H. A. Feldman, eds.), pp. 327–344, Plenum Press, New York, 1982.
79. Daniels, W. B., Solomon, S., and Jaquette, W. A., Jr., Meningococcic infections in soldiers, *J. Am. Med. Assoc.* **123:**1–9 (1943).
80. Goldschneider, I., Gotschlich, E. C., and Artenstein, M. S., Human immunity to the meningococcus. I. The role of humoral antibodies, *J. Exp. Med.* **129:**1307–1326 (1969).
81. Jacobson, J. A., Filice, G. A., and Holloway, J. T., Meningococcal disease in day-care centers, *Pediatrics* **59:**299–300 (1977).
82. Feigin, R. D., Baker, C. J., Herwaldt, L. A., Lampe, R. M., Mason, E. O., and Whitney, S. E., Epidemic meningococcal disease in an elementary-school classroom, *N. Engl. J. Med.* **307:**1255–1257 (1982).
83. Petersen, B. H., Lee, T. J., Snyderman, R., and Brooks, G. F., *Neisseria meningitidis* and *Neisseria gonorrhoeae* bacteremia associated with C6, C7, or C8 deficiency, *Ann. Intern. Med.* **90:**917–920 (1979).
84. Cohen, M. S., Steere, A. C., Baltimore, R. S., von Graevenitz, A., Pantelick, E., Camp, B., and Root, R. K., Possible nosocomial transmission of Group Y *Neisseria meningitidis* among oncology patients, *Ann. Intern. Med.* **91:**7–12 (1979).
85. Carpenter, C. M., and Charles, R., Isolation of meningococcus from the genitourinary tract of seven patients, *Am. J. Public Health* **32:**640–643 (1942).
86. Blackwell, C., Young, H., and Bain, S. S. R., Isolation of *Neisseria meningitidis* and *Neisseria catarrhalis* from the genitourinary tract and anal canal, *Br. J. Vener. Dis.* **54:**41–44 (1978).
87. Reiss-Levy, E., and Stephenson, J., Vaginal isolation of *Neisseria meningitidis* in association with meningococcaemia, *Aust. N.Z. J. Med.* **6:**487–489 (1976).
88. Eschenbach, D. A., Buchanan, T. M., Polock, H. M., Forsyth, P. S., Alexander, E. R., Lin, J.-S., Wang, S.-P., Wentworth, B. B., McCormack, W. M., and Holmes, K. K., Polymicrobial etiology of acute pelvic inflammatory disease, *N. Engl. J. Med.* **293:**166–171 (1975).
89. Fallon, R. J., and Robinson, E. T., Meningococcal vulvovaginitis, *Scand. J. Infect. Dis.* **6:**295–296 (1974).
90. Faur, Y. C., Weisburd, M. H., and Wilson, M. E., Isolation of *Neisseria meningitidis* from the genito-urinary tract and canal, *J. Clin. Microbiol.* **2:**178–182 (1975).
91. Givan, K. F., Thomas, B. W., and Johnston, A. G., Isolation of *Neisseria meningitidis* from the urethra, cervix, and anal canal: Further observations, *Br. J. Vener. Dis.* **53:**109–112 (1977).
92. Gregory, J. E., and Abramson, E., Meningococci in vaginitis, *Am. J. Dis. Child.* **121:**423 (1971).
93. Hammerschlag, M. R., and Baker, C. J., Meningococcal osteomyelitis: A report of two cases associated with septic arthritis, *J. Pediatr.* **88:**519–520 (1976).
94. Laird, S. M., Meningococcal epididymitis, *Lancet* **1:**469–470 (1944).
95. Miller, M. A., Millikin, P., Griffin, P. S., Sexton, R. A., and Yousuf, M., *Neisseria meningitidus* urethritis: A case report, *J. Am. Med. Assoc.* **242:**1656–1657 (1979).
96. Murray, E. G. D., Meningococcus infections of the male urogenital tract and the liability to confusion with gonococcus infection, *Urol. Cutaneous Rev.* **43:**739–741 (1939).
97. Norton, J. F., Meningococcus meningitis in Detroit: 1928–1929. V. Secondary cases, *J. Prev. Med.* **5:**365–367 (1931).
98. Jacobson, J. A., Camargos, P. A. M., Ferreira, J. T., and McCormick, J. B., The risk of meningitis among classroom contacts during an epidemic of meningococcal disease, *Am. J. Epidemiol.* **104:**552–555 (1976).
99. Meningococcal Disease Surveillance Group, Meningococcal disease: Secondary attack rate and chemoprophylaxis in the United States, 1974, *J. Am. Med. Assoc.* **235:**261–265 (1976).
100. Leedom, J. M., Ivler, D., Mathies, A. W., Jr., Thrupp, L. D., Fremont, J. C., Wehrle, P. F., and Portnoy, B., The problem of sulfadiazine-resistant meningococci, in: *Antimicrobial Agents and Chemotherapy 1966* (Hobby, G. L., ed.), pp. 281–292, American Society for Microbiology, Ann Arbor, Michigan, 1967.
101. Benenson, A. S., *Control of Communicable Diseases in Man*, 12th ed., American Public Health Association, Washington, DC, 1975.
102. Bolduan, C., and Goodwin, M. E., A clinical and bacteriological study of the communicability of cerebrospinal meningitis and the probable source of contagion: Part I of an investigation of cerebrospinal meningitis carried out under the auspices of the special commission of the Department of Health of New York City, *Med. News* **87:**1222–1228, 1250–1257 (1905).
103. Gruss, A. D., Spier-Michl, I. B., and Gotschlich, E. C., A method for a radioimmunoassay using microtiter plates allowing simultaneous determination of antibodies to two non cross-reactive antigens, *Immunochemistry* **15:**777–780 (1978).

104. Thomas, L., Smith, H. W., and Dingle, J. H., Investigation of meningococcal infection. II. Immunological aspects, *J. Clin. Invest.* **22:**361–373 (1943).
105. Gotschlich, E. C., Liu, T. Y., and Artenstein, M. S., Human immunity to the meningococcus. III. Preparation and immunochemical properties of the group A, group B, and group C meningococcal polysaccharides, *J. Exp. Med.* **129:**1349–1365 (1969).
106. Mayer, R. L., and Dowling, H. F., The determination of meningococcic antibodies by a centrifuge-agglutination test, *J. Immunol.* **51:**349–354 (1945).
107. Zollinger, W. D., Brandt, B. L., and Tramont, E. C., Immune response to *Neisseria meningitidis*, in: *Manual of Clinical Laboratory Immunology*, 3rd ed. (N. R. Rose, H. Friedman, and J. L. Fahey, eds.), pp. 346–352, American Society for Microbiology, Washington, DC, 1986.
108. Gotschlich, E. C., Goldschneider, I., and Artenstein, M. S., Human immunity to the meningococcus. V. The effect of immunization with meningococcal group C polysaccharide on the carrier state, *J. Exp. Med.* **129:**1385–1395 (1969).
109. Griffiss, J. M., Epidemic meningococcal disease: Synthesis of a hypothetical immunoepidemiologic model, *Rev. Infect. Dis.* **4:**159–172 (1982).
110. Baltimore, R. S., and Hammerschlag, M., Meningococcal bacteremia: Clinical and serologic studies of infants with mild illness, *Am. J. Dis. Child.* **131:**1001–1004 (1977).
111. Dashefsky, B., Teele, D. W., and Klein, J. O., Unsuspected meningococcemia, *J. Pediatr.* **102:**69–72 (1983).
112. Koppes, G. M., Ellenbogen, C., and Gebhart, R. J., Group Y meningococcal disease in United States Air Force recruits, *Am. J. Med.* **62:**661–714 (1977).
113. Hersh, J. H., Gold, R., and Lepow, M. L., Meningococcal group Y pneumonia in an adolescent female, *Pediatrics* **64:**222–224 (1979).
114. Stephens, D. S., Edwards, K. M., and McKee, K. T., Meningococcal group Y disease in children, *Pediatr. Infect. Dis.* **3:**523–525 (1984).
115. Griffiss, J. M., and Brandt, M. S., Disease due to W135 *Neisseria meningitidis*, *Pediatrics* **64:**218–221 (1979).
116. Hammerschlag, M. R., and Baltimore, R. S., Infections in children due to *Neisseria meningitidis* serogroup 135, *J. Pediatr.* **92:**503–504 (1978).
117. Ellison, R. T., III, Kohler, P. F., Curd, J. G., Judson, F. N., and Reller, L. B., Prevalence of congenital or acquired complement deficiency in patients with sporadic meningococcal disease, *N. Engl. J. Med.* **308:**914–916 (1983).
118. Laggiado, R. J., and Winkelstein, J. A., Prevalence of complement deficiencies in children with systemic meningococcal infections, *Pediatr. Infect. Dis.* **6:**75–76 (1987).
119. Densen, P., Complement deficiencies and meningococcal disease, *Clin. Exp. Immunol.* **86**(Suppl.)**:**57–62 (1991).
120. Densen, P., Weiler, J. M., Griffiss, J. M., and Hoffman, L. G., Familial properidin deficiency and fatal meningococcemia. Correction of the bactericidal defect by vaccination, *N. Engl. J. Med.* **316:**922–926 (1987).
121. Corfield, W. F., Multiple attacks of cerebrospinal fever, *Lancet* **1:**402–403 (1945).
122. Feldman, H. A., Editorial comment, in: *Year Book of Pediatrics* (S. S. Gellis, ed.), pp. 81–82, Year Book Medical, Chicago, 1975.
123. Schwartz, B., Chemoprophylaxis for bacterial infections: Principles of and application to meningococcal infections, *Rev. Infect. Dis.* **13**(Suppl. 2)**:**S170–S173 (1991).
124. Schwartz, B., Al-Tobaiqi, A., Al-Ruwais, A., Fontaine, R. E., A'ashi, J., Hightower, A. W., Broome, C. V., and Music, S. I., Comparative efficacy of ceftriaxone and rifampicin in eradicating pharyngeal carriage of group A *Neisseria meningitidis*, *Lancet* **1:**1239–1242 (1988).
125. Wahdan, M. H., Rizk, F., El-Akkad, A. M., El Ghoroury, A. E., Hablas, R., Girgis, N. I., Amer, A., Boctar, W., Sippel, J. E., Gotschlich, E. C., Triau, R., Sanborn, W. R., and Cvjetanovic, B., A controlled field trial of a serogroup A meningococcal polysaccharide vaccine, *Bull. WHO* **48:**667–673 (1973).
126. Griffiss, J. M., Brandt, B. L., Altieri, P. L., Pier, G. B., and Berman, S. L., Safety and immunogenicity of group Y and group W135 meningococcal capsular polysaccharide vaccines in adults, *Infect. Immun.* **34:**725–732 (1981).
127. Greenwood, B. M., Hassan-King, M., and Whittle, H. C., Prevention of secondary cases of meningococcal disease in household contacts by vaccination, *Br. Med. J.* **1:**1317–1319 (1978).
128. Gold, R., Polysaccharide meningococcal vaccines—Current status, *Hosp. Pract.* **14:**41–48 (1979).
129. Gold, R., Lepow, M. L., Goldschneider, I., Draper, T. L., and Gotschlich, E. C., Clinical evaluation of group A and group C meningococcal polysaccharide vaccines in infants, *J. Clin. Invest.* **56:**1536–1547 (1975).
130. Centers for Disease Control, Recommendation of the Immunization Practices Advisory Committee (ACIP): Meningococcal vaccines, *Morbid. Mortal. Week. Rep.* **34:**255–259 (1985).
131. Lepow, M. L., Beeler, J., Randolph, M., Samuelson, J. S., and Hankins, W. A., Reactogenicity and immunogenicity of a quadrivalent combined meningococcal polysaccharide vaccine in children, *J. Infect. Dis.* **154:**1033–1036 (1986).
132. Artenstein, M. S., Control of meningococcal meningitis with meningococcal vaccines, *Yale J. Biol. Med.* **48:**197–200 (1975).
133. American Academy of Pediatrics, Meningococcal infections, in: *1997 Red Book Report of the Committee on Infectious Diseases, 24th Edition* (G. Peter, ed.), pp. 357–362, American Academy of Pediatrics, Elk Grove Village, IL, 1997.
134. Centers for Disease Control, Reported morbidity and mortality in the United States, annual summary 1979, *Morbid. Mortal. Week. Rep.* **28:**53–56 (1980).

12. Suggested Reading

Arkwright, J. A., Cerebro-spinal meningitis: The interpretation of epidemiological observations by the light of bacteriological knowledge, *Br. Med. J.* **1:**494–496 (1915).

Dingle, J. H., and Finland, M., Diagnosis, treatment and prevention of meningococcic meningitis, with a resume of the practical aspects of treatment of other acute bacterial meningitides, *War Med.* **2:**1–58 (1942).

Goldschneider, I., Gotschlich, E. C., and Artenstein, M. S., Human immunity to the meningococcus. I. The role of humoral antibodies, *J. Exp. Med.* **129:**1307–1326 (1969).

Gotschlich, E. C., Liu, T. Y., and Artenstein, M. S., Human immunity to the meningococcus. III. Preparation and immunochemical properties of the group A, group B, and group C meningococcal polysaccharides, *J. Exp. Med.* **129:**1349–1365 (1969).

Greenfield, S., Sheehe, P. R., and Feldman, H. A., Meningococcal carriage in a population of "normal" families, *J. Infect. Dis.* **123:**67–73 (1971).

Jackson, L. A., and Wenger, J. D., Laboratory-based surveillance for meningococcal disease in selected areas, United States, 1989–1991, *Morbid. Mortal. Week. Rep.* **42:**21–30 (1993).

Riedo, F. X., Plikaytis, B. D., and Broome, C. V., Epidemiology and prevention of meningococcal disease, *Pediatr. Infect. Dis. J.* **14:**643–657 (1995).

Wenger, J. D., Hightower, A. W., Facklam, R. R., Gaventa, S., Broome, C. V., and The Bacterial Meningitis Study Group, Bacterial meningitis in the United States, 1986: Report of a multistate surveillance study, *J. Infect. Dis.* **162:**1316–1323 (1990).

CHAPTER 24

Mycoplasma pneumoniae and Other Human Mycoplasmas

Hjordis M. Foy

1. Introduction

Mycoplasmas are small pliable pleomorph bacteria lacking cell walls. They were first called pleuropneumonia-like organisms (PPLOs) for the disease they caused in cattle. The first human isolation of a mycoplasma, probably *Mycoplasma hominis*, was made from a Bartilin's gland in 1937. However, their role as human parasites did not become recognized until the 1950s. They belong to the order Mycoplasmatales, family Mycoplasmataceae, and class Mollicutes.(1)

Mycoplasma pneumoniae is well established as a human pathogen, a cause of pneumonitis and of a wide spectrum of milder respiratory symptoms, such as bronchitis, bronchiolitis and pharyngitis.(2) Because the pneumonia is usually mild and leads to recovery even without antibiotic treatment, it is frequently called "walking pneumonia" or mistaken for virus pneumonia. However, the organism may also cause a wide array of hematologic, neurological, and visceral complications.(3–7)

Other mycoplasmas—*M. orale*, *M. salivarium*, *M. buccale*, and *M. faucium*—are commensals in the oral cavity.(1) *M. genitalium* has recently been recognized as a cause of male urethritis.(8,9) *M. hominis* and *Ureaplasma urealyticum*, a minor cause of male urethritis, also inhabit primarily the genital tract and often act as opportunistic invaders.(9–11) They may colonize infants at birth.(12) *M. fermentans*, *M. penetrans*, and *M. pirum* may have a role as cofactors in acquired immunodeficiency syndrome (AIDS).(13) *M. incognitus*, first seen in AIDS patients, is a substrain of *M. hominis*.

Specific methods for diagnosis of *M. pneumoniae* became available in the 1960s.(14) They are still not widely available in routine laboratories, and methods to isolate the other mycoplasmas are usually only available in research laboratories. PCR technology offers rapid diagnosis for the future.

2. Historical Background

The microscopic features of lung specimens obtained as far back as the Civil War suggest that *M. pneumoniae* has been circulating for a long time. *M. pneumoniae* pneumonia has flourished in wartime; cold-agglutinin-positive pneumonia was a frequent diagnosis during World War II.(2,14) In the 1930s, almost any bacterial pneumonia responded to the newly introduced sulfapyridine derivatives. However, one type of pneumonia was an exception because it failed to respond to the new drugs or to penicillin, and for this reason was named "primary atypical pneumonia" (PAP). This category was probably made up of pneumonia of several etiologies, including pneumonia caused by viruses. In 1943, cold agglutinins were discovered in the serum of patients with PAP, particularly in the type of PAP occurring in epidemics in the military.(15) The Commission on Acute Respiratory Diseases conducted experiments that showed that the disease agent could be passed to human volunteers by means of bacteria-free filtrates of secretions from ill persons.(16) Thus, this disease-causing organism was first thought to be a virus. However, unlike true viruses, the agent re-

Hjordis M. Foy • Department of Epidemiology, School of Public Health and Community Medicine, University of Washington, Seattle, Washington 98195-7236.

sponded to the tetracycline type of antibiotics. As far back as 1944, Eaton *et al.*[17] reported that the organism caused pneumonia in cotton rats and hamsters and could be passed in egg yolk. It was after this discovery that the organism was named "Eaton agent."[17] Doubt was first cast on this achievement because of the possibility that the agent was indigenous in rats. Liu,[18] using the fluorescent-antibody technique, established that the agent was present in human lung tissue from fatal cases and also succeeded in isolation, cultivation, and serial passage of the agent in chick embryos. Liu *et al.*[19] applied immunofluorescent-antibody testing for the serological diagnosis of pneumonia. Retrospective testing of sera from volunteers participating in the earlier transmission studies confirmed an infection with Eaton agent. Also, milder respiratory symptoms and asymptomatic infections following challenge of volunteers came to light with the new methods.[20] Microscopic examinations of tissues led to the speculation that they were PPLOs (mycoplasmas). The true character of the organism was confirmed when Chanock *et al.*[21] grew it on artificial media enriched with serum and yeast extract in 1962. Chanock and co-workers[21] conducted the first field studies of the agent with the newly developed diagnostic tools. Challenge studies among human volunteers were repeated using agar-grown organisms, confirming that the organism was a human pathogen.

A mycoplasma, in retrospect thought to be *M. hominis*, was first isolated from an abscessed Bartolin's gland in 1937. Shepard[11] drew attention to the ureaplasmas, a minor cause of urethtitis, in the 1950s. Interest in the genital mycoplasmas has risen since the 1960s.[1,9] Since some of them, especially *U. urealyticum*, occur with high frequency in the genital tract of asymptomatic persons, their role in disease has been controversial.[12] *M. hominis* is also a frequent genital isolate that has also been found in purulent infections at peripheric sites.[9] *M. fermentans*, *M. penetrans*, and *M. pirum* have drawn attention as possible cofactors in AIDS in the 1990s.[13] *M. fermentans* has previously been considered a contaminant; *M. penetrans* and *M. pirum* have similarities with *M. pneumoniae*.[13]

3. Methodology

3.1. Sources of Mortality Data

Although national data are available on deaths due to pneumonia and influenza, these statistics do not reflect mortality due to *M. pneumoniae* pneumonia, since the latter disease is rarely fatal. Furthermore, the diagnosis cannot be made by autopsy without appropriate microbiological testing. Deaths due to this disease have not been reported in the many studies of epidemics among military personnel since the 1950s[21–24] or in the long-term studies of a civilian population in Seattle.[25] However, such studies often rely on antibody-titer rises between acute and convalescent sera and would not easily detect fatal cases if death occurred early. Back in the 1940s, when the United States appears to have experienced a major wave of *M. pneumoniae* infections, several deaths due to PAP, diagnosed by the cold-agglutinin test, were described.[15] Since the 1960s, when specific laboratory methods for diagnosis gained general use, many reports of fatalities have appeared in the literature,[5,6,26–28] Although the incidence of the disease is highest in children and adults, most fatal cases have been reported in middle-aged or older persons. All evidence suggests that death is a rare occurrence.

Data on oral, genital, and other mycoplasmas are generally available only from surveys and research projects, and death due to these mycoplasma would be rare.

3.2. Sources of Morbidity Data

M. pneumoniae infections are not reportable and the Centers for Disease Control (CDC) do not usually monitor the disease. However, in 1993, the CDC reported on three outbreaks occurring in various settings in New York, Ohio, and Texas.[29] The World Health Organization (WHO) has reported on *M. pneumoniae* infections in its surveillance of neurological disease.[30] Public health laboratories that carry out serological testing of persons with respiratory disease are able to monitor the fluctuations in incidence. So far, this avenue of surveillance has been utilized primarily in Denmark and England.[31,32] In Japan, surveillance of school children has elucidated the epidemiology of the disease.[33] Morbidity data in the United States derive from research funded to carry out in-depth studies in selected representative population samples.

Population-based studies have been conducted in pediatric practices in North Carolina,[34–36] among families in Tecumseh, Michigan,[37] and in a prepaid-medical-care group in Seattle, Washington.[25,38–40] Studies of incidence of the infection and disease have been carried out in military recruit populations,[16,21–24] children's homes,[36,41–43] day-care facilities,[35,44] and schools,[45,46] and among college students[40] and family units[47–49] (see Section 5.9). Studies of families with an index case of pneumonia have provided information on the secondary attack rates, the spectrum of clinical manifestations, the duration of shedding, and the incubation period.[47–49] On the other hand, families under continuous observation during both health and illness have provided community infection rates and epidemiological patterns.[25,37,50] Studies of *M. pneumoniae* pneumonia in hospitalized patients in the United States reflect incidence poorly, since only severe cases of pneumonia or its complications are generally hospitalized. In Scandinavia, where the policy for hospitalization is more liberal than in the United States, statistics of hospitalized pneumonia patients reflect seasonal and annual variations of incidence.[51] High proportions (up to 37%) of outpatient pneumonia due to *M. pneumoniae* have been reported in Sweden.[52]

Studies of volunteers inoculated with *M. pneumoniae* have yielded data on immunity and the spectrum of disease manifestations.[20] Ear involvement occurred frequently after artificial inoculation in the nasopharynx by nebulizer.[20]

The oral mycoplasmas have primarily been of interest in dentistry. Studies of genital mycoplasmas have been carried out in sexually transmitted disease (STD) clinics[1,8,9] and women's clinics,[12] and colonization with these agents have been studied in newborn, older children, and adults.[1]

3.3. Serological Surveys

Serum samples have been collected to compare the prevalence of *M. pneumoniae* antibodies in different populations and age groups.[53,54] Caution must be exercised in interpreting these data, unless the serological testing is carried out in the same laboratory, because of inherent variability in the tests. Furthermore, knowledge regarding the correlation of immunity and various antibodies and the persistence of antibodies is incomplete. Nevertheless, such studies indicate that the organism is ubiquitous in most parts of the world, and the age distribution of antibody acquisition appears similar in tropical and temperate climates. Prospective serological studies measure the incidence of infection (seroconversion) and reinfection.[22,24,34,53,55]

3.4. Laboratory Diagnosis

3.4.1. Isolation. Culture of mycoplasma is still the gold standard, but may be insensitive and impractical. The polymerase chain reaction (PCR) is likely to become a more practical method, especially for *M. pneumoniae*, but the method has yet to be tested further in clinical and epidemiological settings to determine sensitivity and specificity.

Because it may take several weeks to grow *M. pneumoniae* in the laboratory, isolation of the organism has more use in epidemiological studies than in clinical decision making. Isolation of the agent from respiratory specimens usually indicates current or recent infection, since prolonged asymptomatic carrier states are rare.[36,40,46] *M. pneumoniae* pneumonia patients rarely have a productive cough at onset of illness, and throat swabs and nasopharyngeal aspirates but not nasal swabs are a good substitute for sputum in isolation attempts. A single culture is positive in 65% of cases in the acute stage (Fig. 1).[49] Especially in children, the organism is often shed for several weeks, although in decreasing amount.[49] Antibiotic therapy does not eliminate the carriage state. The collection medium commonly used contains bovine albumin in trypticase soy broth with penicillin.[55] The SP-4 medium, utilized since 1979, may be superior to some of the previously used media.[56] Specimens can be stored refrigerated for several days and withstand transportation and freezing.[55] Penicillin is added to suppress bacterial growth; thallium acetate may be used for the same purpose. Both agar plates and broth cultures are utilized. It may taken 1–4 weeks for *M. pneumoniae* colonies to become visible under the microscope; most other human mycoplasma species can be detected with magnification within a couple of days. Colonies have a fried-egg appearance, measure 10–150 μm and are embedded in the agar. Isolates can be presumptively identified by hemolysis of guinea pig red blood cells and fermentation of glucose. In the broth, the organisms cause faint turbidity, but their presence is best demonstrated by pH changes of indicators. Diphasic media, which have an agar base overlaid with a fluid medium and incorporate a pH indicator for

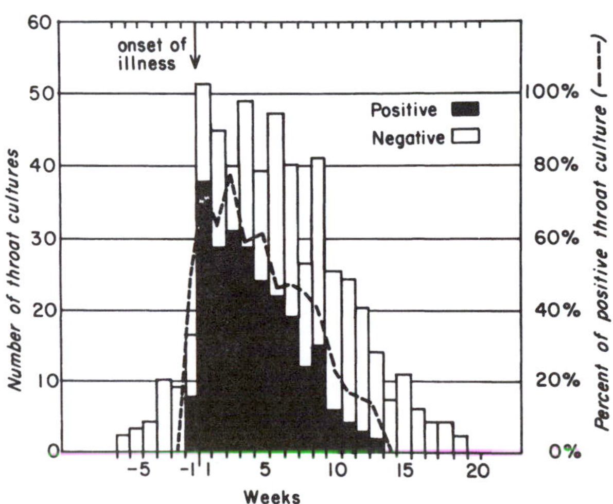

Figure 1. Isolation of *M. pneumoniae* from throat-swab cultures in ill persons by time in relation to onset of illness. Reproduced from Foy *et al.*,[49] with permission.

glucose fermentation, are especially suited to *M. pneumoniae* isolation, since even small inocula will grow. Subculture is necessary for definite identification, which is best carried out by inhibition with species-specific antisera.

Rapid identification for clinical use by use of fluorescent-tagged antisera of throat and sputum specimens or DNA probes has not proven successful, whereas antigen capture enzyme immunoassays (Ag-EIA) and PCR have yielded better results.[57,58] PCR is highly sensitive, but specificity may vary in different laboratories. Finding of mycoplasma DNA does not necessarily indicate living organisms. Several PCR tests have been developed using different primers, and which PCR is most effective is not known.

3.4.2. Serological Tests. The first epidemiological studies of PAP were carried out with cold agglutinins as the diagnostic test.[14,16] Cold agglutinins appear 1 week after onset of illness in approximately two thirds of *M. pneumoniae* pneumonia patients, usually those with more severe disease. Cold agglutination can be used as a rapid presumptive test, since it can sometimes be visualized at the bedside as the blood cools off, but the test is properly carried out at +4°C.

The original complement-fixing (CF) antibody test for *M. pneumoniae* utilized whole organisms, and the test appears to measure antibody to cytoplasm.[59] The major antigen in *M. pneumoniae* is found in the lipid fraction of the organism, located in the triple-layer membrane. Most antibody tests measure antibody to the membrane. The CF test using lipid antigen, obtained through chloroform–methanol extraction, correlates better with infection than does the original CF test; also, fewer anticomplementary reactions are encountered. This test is widely used to diagnose acute infection. In evaluating the literature regarding serological data, it is worthwhile to note which antigen has been used in the CF test. The CF test measures primarily IgM antibodies,[60] and may thus not detect all repeated infections.

Enzyme-linked immunosorbent assays (ELISA) measure primarily antibody to protein. IgM response has been observed in about 80% of sera collected 9 days or later after onset. Older persons may respond with only IgG. An ELISA test for IgA promises to be a rapid and specific serological test; IgA antibody rises can be seen 1 week after onset of illness.[61] *M. pneumoniae* cross-reacts serologically with *M. genitalium*, and false-positive reactions in both CF and ELISA tests occur in patients with bacterial meningitis, and at least in the CF test in those with acute pancreatitis. Concurrent rises to *Legionella pneumophila* and *Chlamydia trachomatis* may also cause confusion as to which is the causative agent. In such cases, polyclonal B-cell activation by *M. pneumoniae* may be the cause of an aberrant antibody response.[62]

Whereas the CF and ELISA antibody test may be the most practical method to diagnose acute infections serologically, its value in serological surveys to determine immunity is compromised by the relatively fast disappearance of antibodies, although a few pneumonia patients have measurable CF antibody for up to 5 years after infection.[40] Western blots are somewhat cumbersome, but more specific.[59]

The clinical and epidemiological experience with all these tests is insufficient to make strong recommendations as to which ones best reflect naturally acquired immunity to *M. pneumoniae*. Most antibodies appear to decay with time. Also, the great variability in the outcome of tests run in different laboratories jeopardizes comparisons of the prevalence of antibodies among communities.

4. Biological Characteristics of the Organism

Mycoplasmas are the smallest free-living organisms known; individual organisms measure 300–500 nm.[1,63] Unlike regular bacteria, they lack a cell wall. This renders them insensitive to antibiotics that interfere with cell wall synthesis (penicillins and cycloserine). They are sensitive to tetracyclines, macrolides, and quinolones, but antibiotic treatment has not eradicated the organisms from the host; however, this has not been studied for the newer antibiotics. Lack of a cell wall also allows for pleomorphism and pliability. Morphologically, they resemble cell-wall-defective bacteria (L forms), but the latter revert to normal morphology when cultured on appropriate media. They contain both RNA and DNA and carry out their own reproductive processes. *M. pneumoniae* ferments glucose, produces a hemolysin and grows under atmospheric conditions. The other human mycoplasmas have their own growth requirements and laboratory characteristics.

M. pneumoniae adheres to respiratory epithelium with an elongated terminal structure, often called a tip.[63] Protein P1 (approximately 170 kDa) is thought to be the major adhesion. No plasmids or phages have been recognized. *M. pneumoniae* have been shown to move on glass surfaces and to react with neuraminic acid receptors. The ability of *M. pneumoniae* to agglutinate cells, including erythrocytes and spermatozoa, is possibly a virulence factor.[63] They survive drying relatively well, but may be sensitive to small fluctuations in humidity.[64,65] Specimens can be frozen and thawed repeatedly without significant loss of viability. They are vulnerable to treatment with lipid solvents, formalin solutions, and other antiseptics.

The outer triple-layer cell membrane of *M. pneumoniae* contains glycolipids as major determinants. Antigenically related compounds are found in many animal cells, possibly the cause of cross-reacting antibodies and infection-induced autoimmunity. Information regarding antigenic variability is sparse, but antigenic changes occur after repeated passages in the laboratory, and temperature-sensitive mutants have been developed.[66] Two variants have been found by fingerprinting. Antibiotic-resistant strains have been produced in the laboratory and are also found in nature.[33]

M. hominis adheres to eukaryotic cells, but not to erythrocytes.[1] Toxicity appears mild. *U. urealyticum*, of which there are 14 serovars, metabolize urea by the enzyme urease and can lyse erythrocytes.[1] *M. genitalium* has many properties in common with *M. pneumoniae*, and these two organisms can easily be confused in the laboratory.[1,8]

5. Descriptive Epidemiology

5.1. Prevalence

Data on the prevalence of *M. pneumoniae* based on throat culture varies with the epidemic cycles of the organism in the community. During low endemic period, the organism is rare in the population, but can increase substantially during epidemics, which commonly occur in 4-year intervals. Since *M. pneumoniae* infections can be very mild and the carriage state may last for several months, the finding of *M. pneumoniae* in a throat culture may be difficult to interpret. PCR tests tend to show higher prevalence rates than culture, which could be due to higher sensitivity or the detection of inactive DNA. In military populations, the carriage rate can be high: among US Marine recruits, the carriage rate was estimated as 0 on induction, 1% after 5 weeks, and 9–10% after 9 weeks.[67]

Seroepidemiological studies show similar antibody patterns among military recruits in Argentina, Colombia, and the United States and among Peace Corps volunteers, with prevalence rates ranging from 49 to 66%.[53]

Using a macrohemagglutination-inhibition test that may measure different antibodies than the more commonly used tests, Suhs and Feldman[54] found increasing antibody levels with increasing age. The prevalence of antibody at Point Barrow, Alaska, was higher than in New York. Prevalence estimates with the highly sensitive radioimmunoprecipitating antibody test suggested that 97% of Americans may have been exposed to the organism by the age of 18.[68] However, the specificity of this test has been questioned, since plant antigens may induce similar antibody.[59]

M. orale and *M. salivarium* are ubiquitous organisms in the oral cavity, and *M. salivarium* is found in dental pockets and is absent from edentous persons. *M. faucium* and *M. buccale* are less frequently isolated. More than half of sexually active women and a high proportion of men carry *U. urealyticum* in the genital tract. *M. hominis* is less common, but follows the same general pattern. *M. fermentans* was first recognized in genital specimens, then in bone marrow specimens, and often was found as a contaminant; the role of this organism in disease other than AIDS is virtually unknown.[66]

5.2. Epidemic Behavior and Contagiousness

M. pneumoniae infections are endemic in larger urban areas, and epidemic increases are observed at 4- to 7-year intervals.[32,33,37,38,51] The spread is slow because of the limited communicability and long case-to-case interval, approximately 3 weeks. Epidemics may last 1–2 years in larger communities. A high incidence is observed among schoolchildren, who often transmit the infection to playmates,[37,38,45,46] but the schoolroom itself appears not to be the focus of spread.[45,46] Neighborhood spread has been observed and microepidemics occur within the larger community.[46,69] In military recruits, the attack rates vary among platoons,[24] and in institutional settings the spread can be traced between buildings.[41]

Although most epidemics appear to be propagated person to person, a few common-source outbreaks have been reported. A party at a fraternity house resulted in nearly half the students becoming infected; 7 of 23 required hospitalization for pneumonia.[70] An outbreak in a prosthodontic laboratory may have been transmitted by aerosolization from abrasive drilling of false teeth.[71] In an outbreak on a nuclear submarine, the closeness of the onset dates suggests a common source, and recirculated air could possibly have been the vehicle.[72] An explosive outbreak peaking 1 month after opening was reported from a boys' summer camp.[73] These outbreaks are further discussed in Section 6.

The transmission and the spectrum of symptoms have been studied in detail in family units with index cases of *M. pneumoniae* pneumonia (see further discussion in Section 5.9.1). The incidence among military-recruit populations can be exceedingly high. Thus, the rate of *M. pneumoniae* pneumonia was 1.5% at Parris Island in 1955, and infection rates regardless of diagnosis were about 30 times higher[21] (see Section 5.9.3). Military outbreaks are probably due to the herding together of susceptibles and to behavior patterns that favor transmission.

M. pneumoniae pneumonia was monitored among the 150,000 members of a prepaid medical care group in Seattle in 1963–1975.[25,38,40] This 10% population sample was considered representative of the total urban–suburban community. The disease was diagnosed by isolation and significant antilipid CF-antibody titer rises. The rate of total pneumonia averaged 1200/100,000. *M. pneumoniae* was recognized as the etiologic agent in 15%, for an average rate of 180/100,000 per year. It varied between a low endemic rate of 60/100,000 in 1966 and an epidemic rate of 300/100,000 in 1974. However, the rate of recognized *M. pneumoniae* pneumonia constituted only the tip of the iceberg of all infections with this organism. In Seattle schoolchildren who were bled annually, the infection rate was estimated to have been at least 35% during the 1974 epidemic. Since CF antibodies sometimes decay quickly after infection, the rates may have been even higher. Studied with the same CF-antibody test, families who were bled annually in Seattle in 1972–1977 had infection rates averaging 8% for 5- to 9-year-old children and 2% for adults.[39] In Tecumseh, Michigan, where families were bled every 6 months, the annual infection rates were 9 and 4%, respectively, in similar age groups.[37]

5.3. Geographic Distribution

Infection with mycoplasmas are worldwide. *M. pneumoniae* has been demonstrated in all continents except Antarctica. It is present in tropical countries as well as in the Arctic.[54] However, the epidemiology of the infection has been studied primarily in the United States, Europe, and Japan. The epidemiology in different climatic entities has not been extensively studied. So far, the evidence suggests that no geographic differences occur except those due to crowding and other socioeconomic variables.

5.4. Temporal Distribution

Although *M. pneumoniae* infections have been endemic in most civilian communities where the infection has been thoroughly sought, epidemic cyclicity is evident from most long-term population studies (Table 1). In Denmark, centrally located public health laboratories have monitored infections since 1958 by serological diagnosis of paired sera forwarded from physicians.[31] A cyclicity of approximately 4½ years was observed, until the 1980s when the infection became endemic. Similar studies in Great Britain and Japan also showed that cycles took about 4½ years. Epidemic periods lasted for up to 2 years.[32,33] Epidemic periods coincided between these two countries. Epidemic patterns in the Scandinavian countries have been similar, but not identical.[74]

Epidemic cycles appear not to be synchronized throughout the United States, although epidemics were reported in several areas around 1965 (Table 1). In Seattle, where rates were closely monitored, *M. pneumoniae* pneumonia rates started to rise in early 1966, but not until January 1967 did the epidemic reach a peak. Rates were low the subsequent year. Slightly increased rates were

Table 1. Recorded *Mycoplasma pneumoniae* Epidemics by Location, Season, Year, and Population Sampled

Location	Season	Years	Study origins	Ref.
Europe				
Denmark	Winter	1958–1959, 1963, 1967–1968, 1972, 1978, 1987	Public health laboratories	31
United Kingdom	Winter	1967–1968, 1971–1972, 1975, 1978–1979, 1983, 1986	Public health laboratories	32
Finland	Winter	1962–1963, 1967–1968, 1973, 1977	Infectious disease hospital	51, 74
United States				
New Orleans, Louisiana	Late summer–fall	1960, 1961, 1965	Military	23
Madison, Wisconsin	Fall–winter	1954–1955, 1960, 1965	College students	75
Chapel Hill, North Carolina	Fall–winter	1964–1965, 1969, 1972–1973	Pediatric practices	34, 35
Omaha, Nebraska	Fall	1964	Boy's school	43
West Virginia	Winter	1964–1965	Hospital	78
La Crosse, Wisconsin	Fall	1965–1966	In- and outpatients	45
Tecumseh, Michigan	Fall	1968–1969	Community surveillance	37
Seattle, Washington	Winter, summer	1966–1967, 1974, 1981	Prepaid medical care group	25
New York, Ohio, Texas	—	1993	Special settings	29
Asia				
Sendai, Japan	—	1968, 1972, 1976, 1980	School children	33

noticed again in the spring of 1972, but a clear-cut epidemic did not recur until 1974, and that epidemic peaked in the summer. The subsequent epidemic occurred in 1981. Epidemic increase was noticed in Tecumseh in 1968–1969.(37) Outbreaks were reported from New York, Ohio, and Texas in 1993.(29) Many studies report epidemics in the fall, and this appears to be characteristic of college populations, where epidemics also have recurred at 4- to 5-year intervals.(40,75) In the military, the highest rates have been observed in late summer, regardless of the influx of new soldiers.(22,23)

Because community rates of pneumonia of other etiologies are at their highest by far in the winter and spring, and *M. pneumoniae* infections are endemic, the proportion of pneumonia due to *M. pneumoniae* is highest in the summer.

5.5. Age

The incidence of all pneumonia regardless of etiology is highest by far in children under the age of 2 and in the elderly.(39,40) The rates are low among teenagers (Fig. 2). The incidence of *M. pneumoniae* pneumonia follows a reverse pattern and is highest among school-age children. The Seattle studies of *M. pneumoniae* pneumonia suggested that the incidence in children under the age of 5 was half that in school-age children, and adolescents 15–19 years old had a lower incidence than all younger age groups (Fig. 2). On the other hand, infection rates, regardless of symptoms, are about equal for children of all age groups in family epidemics.(48,49) The Seattle studies were carried out before it became common practice to care for preschool children in day care.

It has often been stated that the incidence of *M. pneumoniae* pneumonia is highest among young adults. Such statements probably originate from military studies, where the incidence of *M. pneumoniae* infection can be extraordinarily high.(21,23) But in civilian populations the incidence declines with age after puberty. The over-40 age group has the lowest incidence, suggesting that immunity builds up over time. Yet, pneumonia in older persons may lead to more severe complications,(26–28,30) and most

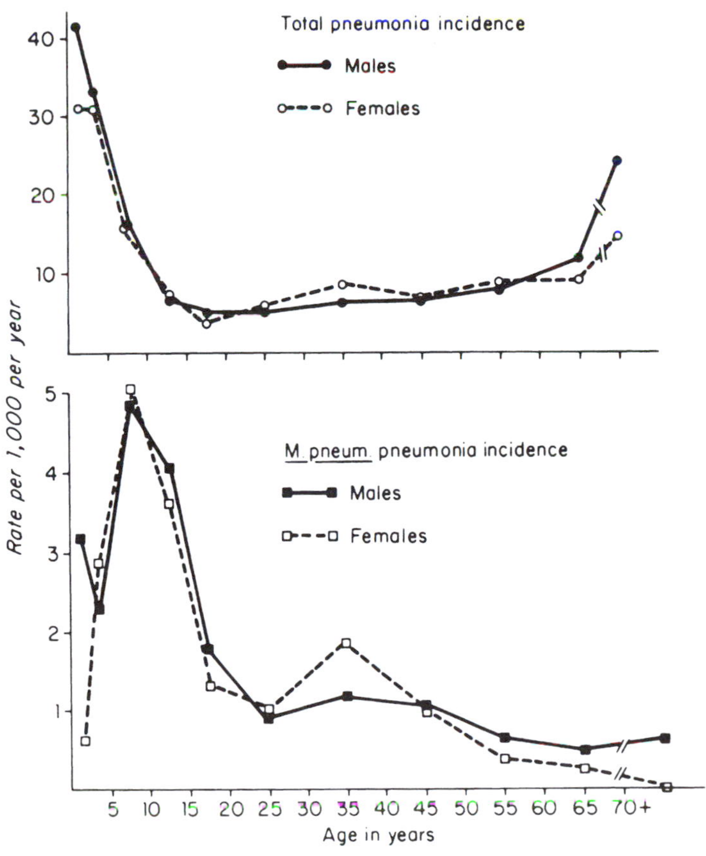

Figure 2. Incidence of *M. pneumoniae* pneumonia by age and sex, Group Health Cooperative, December 1, 1963–Feburary 28, 1975. Infection was determined by isolation or fourfold or greater antilipid CF-antibody rise or both. Reprinted from Foy *et al.*,(25) with permission of the University of Chicago Press. © 1979 by the University of Chicago.

deaths due to *M. pneumoniae* infections have been reported in persons over 40 years of age.

Higher *M. pneumoniae* pneumonia rates were observed in Seattle in those 30–39 years old than in slightly younger and older adults.[38] Similar observations were made regarding infection rates in Tecumseh.[37] This age group includes the parents of school-age children, and the high rate is probably a consequence of intensive exposure.

Infection rates, regardless of illness, have been studied through semiannual bleedings of families under continuous surveillance in Seattle and Tecumseh. Infection rates in Seattle in 1965–1968 were estimated at 12% per year for all age groups, based on fourfold antibody-titer rises or on a rise from no antibody to the lowest detectable titer (1:8) as indicators of infection.[50] In Tecumseh, the infection rate was highest, 9%, in the 5- to 9-year age group, being about 2.5% in children under 5 years of age and declining to 4% after the age of 20. Only fourfold antibody-titer rises were accepted as evidence of infection.[37] In a subsequent study in Seattle (1972–1975), infection rates paralleled those in the Tecumseh studies, possibly because now only fourfold rises were accepted for diagnosis or because the age composition of the families was now different.[38]

The estimates of proportion of infections expressed in pneumonia vary according to study methods. They have been highest by far (60–70%) in studies of families under intensive surveillance because of an index case with pneumonia.[47–49] On the other hand, among families followed continuously with serological testing as the primary means, pneumonia in those infected has only rarely been recorded.[37,50]

The proportion of infections that leads to pneumonia varies with age and appears highest in the 5- to 14-year age group.[39] Studies among children under the age of 5 have led to diverse findings. Thus, in surveillance in a day-care facility in North Carolina, five of seven children carrying the organisms were totally asymptomatic.[35] The same held true for children with serological rises. In a day-care center in Sweden, three of four children under the age of 2 with positive throat cultures responded with febrile respiratory disease and cough.[44] Family studies with an index case of *M. pneumoniae* have indicated milder symptoms in children under the age of 5 than in older age groups[47,49] (see further discussion in Section 5.9.1). The low rate of verified pneumonia in children under 5 has led to the theory that the primary infection leads to sensitization and the succeeding infection to pneumonia. The hypothesis has been challenged in studies from Europe and Japan, which reported high *M. pneumoniae* pneumonia rates in children under the age of 5,[40] and by a family study in Israel.[76] In surveillance studies in children's homes, the proportion of *M. pneumoniae* infections leading to pneumonia has been 13–18% in the 5- to 9-year age group.[41–43] But in older age groups, this proportion has been lower in most studies: about 2–7% of older teenagers and recruits.[21,24,41]

Figure 3 shows the outcome of isolation from throat swabs and CF-antibody tests in all pneumonia patients in the Seattle studies. Isolation was more efficient than serological methods in the age group 2–30 years, but in young children and older adults about half the infections were diagnosed by CF-antilipid tests. A proportion of pneumonia patients with only high antibody titers probably represented *M. pneumoniae* pneumonia where the initial serum was taken too late for an antibody-titer rise to be demonstrated.

5.6. Sex

The infection rate for *M. pneumoniae* is similar for both sexes, but the rate of *M. pneumoniae* pneumonia is slightly higher in males, except in the age group 30–39, where rates for women were higher (see Fig. 2). Also, infection rates regardless of clinical manifestations were higher in women in the Tecumseh studies.[37] Women may contract the infection by close contact with children. The rate of complications in the form of otitis is higher in males,[49] and most cases of Stevens–Johnson syndrome

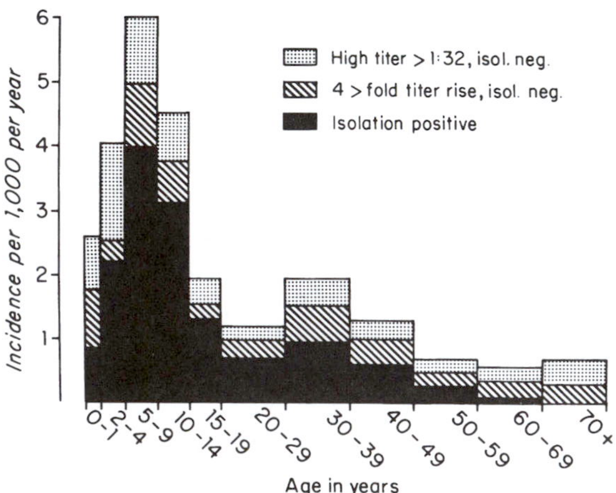

Figure 3. Incidence of pneumonia with evidence of *M. pneumoniae* infection by age measured by different laboratory tests, Goup Health Cooperative, December 1, 1963–February 28, 1975. Those who were isolation-positive also had fourfold or higher antibody titers. Reprinted from Foy *et al.*,[25] with permission of the University of Chicago Press. © 1979 by the University of Chicago.

attributed to *M. pneumoniae* infection have occurred in males.

Colonization of the genital tract with especially *U. urealyticum*, but also *M. hominis*, is higher in the genital tract of women than that of men.[9]

5.7. Race

M. pneumoniae infection probably affects all races equally and with similar symptoms. Sickle-cell anemia, SS or SC hemoglobulinopathy, a congenital disorder of the red blood cells seen among blacks, predisposes to a more severe form of *M. pneumoniae* pneumonia.[77] Surveillance for genital mycoplasmas show higher rates for blacks than whites.[9]

5.8. Occupation

The high rates of *M. pneumoniae* infection observed among military recruits are probably due to crowding and herding during basic training. The disease is frequently observed among physicians and other hospital personnel,[58] although no "hard data" on comparative incidence by occupation are available. The risk associated with being a mother of a school-age child has already been noted.

5.9. Occurrence in Different Settings

5.9.1. Family. Studies of the transmission and symptomatology of *M. pneumoniae* infections in families have contributed substantially to our understanding of the epidemiology of this infection.[47–49,76] In Seattle, 114 families were under observation after an index case of suspect pneumonia had been identified.[49] Throat cultures were collected weekly and paired sera when feasible. In 36 of these families, the laboratory results subsequently showed the etiologic agent to have been *M. pneumoniae*. Transmission to other family members was demonstrated by isolation in 23 of these 36 families, of whom 84% of the children and 41% of the adults became infected. The case-to-case interval centered around 3 weeks, much longer than for most other acute respiratory diseases. In some families, several cycles of 3- to 4-week intervals passed before all family members were infected.

A typical family episode is illustrated in Fig. 4. The 7-year-old boy became ill with *M. pneumoniae* pneumonia, complicated with otitis, on June 12. He made an uneventful recovery. Despite treatment with tetracycline, his throat cultures remained positive. His 8- and 10-year-old sisters became ill with sore throat, slight fever, and cough at the beginning of July. The mother did not consider their symptoms, which did not interfere with daily activities, severe enough to warrant a visit to the clinic. Only because of our urging were they brought to the clinic, and chest films revealed pneumonitis in one of them. On July 18, the father developed malaise and fever, and was first diagnosed by his physician as having influenza. A subsequent chest film revealed an extensive infiltrate, although physical examination of the chest was almost normal. Figure 4 illustrates negative throat cultures prior to illness and then intermittent positive throat cultures for several weeks. The mother and oldest child escaped infection despite low CF-antibody titers. Although in this particular family those who were not treated with antibiotics showed a higher antibody response than those who were, no such relationship between treatment and antibody response has been found when a large number of treated and untreated cases have been compared.

In the Seattle study of families with a suspected index case of pneumonia, asymptomatic infection was seen in 27% of children under the age of 5, in 19% of the age group 5–14, and in 8% of the group 15 years and older.[49] Pharyngitis without cough was the only manifestation in 10% of family cases. The duration of pneumonia illness generally increased with advancing age. Boys had pneumonitis and ear complications more frequently than did girls.

Balassanian and Robbins[47] studied nine families in Cleveland. They observed high infection rates regardless of age, but the rate of pneumonia was lower in those under age 10 than in older persons. Similar family studies were conducted by Biberfeld and Sterner[48] in Sweden. They were able to obtain serological specimens and refer patients for radiological examination to a greater degree than were the American investigators. Transmission was observed in 24 of 25 families. *M. pneumoniae* was isolated from 71% of 45 children and 53% of 62 adults. Chest film demonstrated pneumonia in 13 of 18 infected children and in 27 of 32 adults; only 1 infected person was classified as asymptomatic. A high rate (73%) of pneumonia in children was also reported from a family study in Israel.[76]

Whereas the family studies described above started with index cases of *M. pneumoniae* infection, other investigators have observed *M. pneumoniae* infection in families kept under continuous prospective observation.[37,50] In such studies, sera collected at 6-month intervals have yielded information on infection rates (see Section 5.5), but the information on illness becomes sketchy, because of the multitude of intercurrent viral infections.

5.9.2. Hospital. Epidemics of *M. pneumoniae* pneumonia have been encountered in hospital settings.[51,58,78]

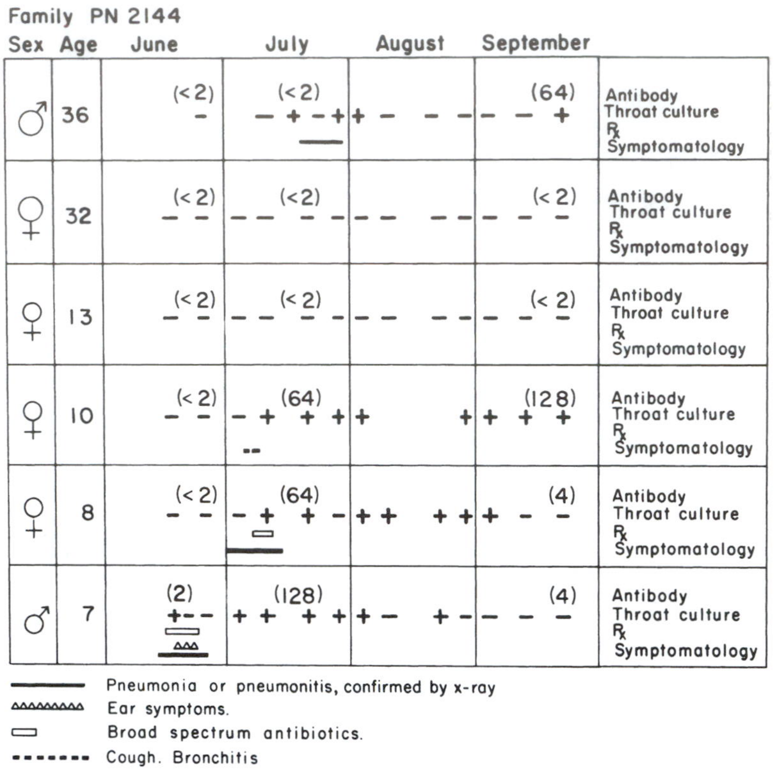

Family PN 2144

Sex	Age	June	July	August	September	
♂	36	(< 2) -	(< 2) — + — +	+ — — —	(64) — — +	Antibody Throat culture ℞ Symptomatology
♀	32	(< 2) — —	(<2) — — — —	— — — —	(< 2) — — —	Antibody Throat culture ℞ Symptomatology
♀	13	(< 2) — —	(< 2) — — — —	— — — —	(< 2) — — —	Antibody Throat culture ℞ Symptomatology
♀	10	(< 2) — —	(64) — + + +	+ +	(128) + + +	Antibody Throat culture ℞ Symptomatology
♀	8	(< 2) — —	(64) — + + —	+ + + +	(4) + — —	Antibody Throat culture ℞ Symptomatology
♂	7	(2) + — —	(128) + + + +	+ — + —	(4) — — —	Antibody Throat culture ℞ Symptomatology

——— Pneumonia or pneumonitis, confirmed by x-ray
ΔΔΔΔΔΔΔ Ear symptoms.
▭ Broad spectrum antibiotics.
------- Cough. Bronchitis

Figure 4. Example of a family epidemic with *M. pneumoniae.* Reproduced from Foy *et al.*,[49] with permission.

Serologically diagnosed *M. pneumoniae* infections also occurred in 20% of patients undergoing open-heart surgery in one hospital, but no cases of pneumonia were reported and the mode of transmission was not determined. Serological cross-reaction with myocardial antigen could not be ruled out.[79] Nosocomial *M. pneumoniae* pneumonia has been described. Because the incubation period for *M. pneumoniae* infection is so long, most hospital-acquired *M. pneumoniae* infection may not be manifest until the patient is discharged.

5.9.3. Military. *M. pneumoniae* infections have posed special problems in the military. Probably the most intensive epidemic reported was among Marine recruits at Parris Island, with rates of *M. pneumoniae* pneumonia of 1,500/100,000 per training period[21,24] (Fig. 5). The rate of infection was 41% over a 14-week period. The infection spread slowly through the population, and infection rates varied among battalions.[24] Navy recruits were studied prospectively for 4 years at Great Lakes, Illinois, and in Florida.[22] Rates of seroconversion were as high as 45–57%, especially during late summer, but usually rates were lower. They were remarkably similar in the two installations over a 4-year period despite climatic differences; a slight epidemic peak was seen in spring and a major one in late summer. Similarly, among airmen studied in Mississippi, *M. pneumoniae* rates were highest in late summer, and 44% of all pneumonia could be attributed to *M. pneumoniae*.[23] In all these studies, it is clear that a clinical diagnosis of pneumonia was made in only a small fraction of recruits who seroconverted. This fraction has been estimated to be 3–5%.[21,24] Pneumonia occurred primarily in those without any or with low antibody titer to the organism.[24]

M. pneumoniae infection is also a problem in recruit training in Europe. In South America, seroconversion rates among Argentinean and Colombian recruits, 17–30% over 1–2 years, are similar to those observed in the United States, suggesting that *M. pneumoniae* infections spread readily during military training in most countries and climates. In susceptible recruits, the infection rate approximated 50%. *M. pneumoniae* is also a leading cause of pneumonia among seasoned troops. Thus, during the Vietnam conflict, 43% of hospitalized pneumonia patients had evidence of *M. pneumoniae* infection.[80] However, the total incidence of pneumonia may have been low.

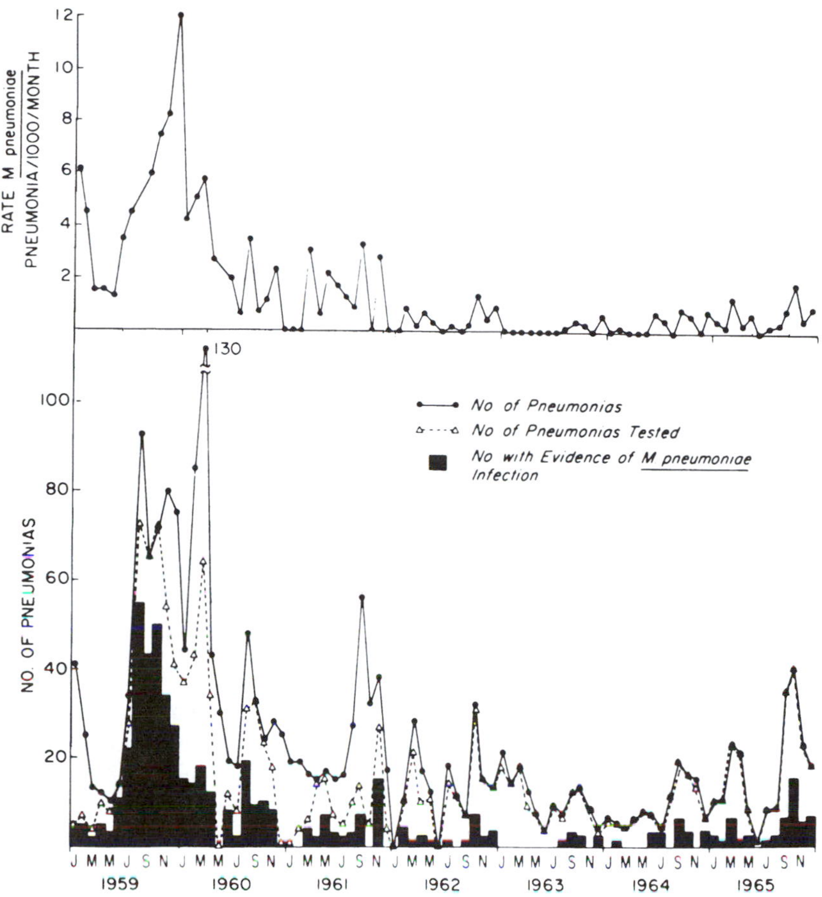

Figure 5. Seven-year surveillance of *M. pneumoniae* pneumonia at Marine Corps Recruit Depot, Parris Island, South Carolina. Reproduced from Chanock *et al.*,[21] with permission.

5.10. Socioeconomic Factors

The disease of *M. pneumoniae* pneumonia has been described primarily from economically advanced societies, which suggests that this relatively mild disease is cause for concern primarily among those who can afford to seek medical attention for relatively minor respiratory disease. An alternate explanation is that in a society with high hygienic standards, exposure to the organism is postponed until later childhood, when the disease takes on more severe symptoms. This is in analogy with the relationship of poliovirus infection to age.

5.11. Other Factors

Little is known of the role, if any, of nutritional and genetic factors in *M. pneumoniae* infections. Any relationship to histocompatibility complexes, such as HLA antigens, is not known, but should be explored in severe complications such as hemolytic anemia and Stevens–Johnson syndrome. No difference in antibody prevalence or in the incidence of infection has been found among persons with different blood groups.[53]

Persons with deficiencies of the humoral antibody system are at greater risk of severe *M. pneumoniae* infection,[40,81] including joint symptoms. Similarly, *M. hominis* and *U. urealyticum* may invade distant sites in immunodeficiency.[1,9,10] Children with Down's syndrome also suffer more severe symptoms,[41] as do persons with sickle-cell disease[77] (Section 5.7). *M. pneumoniae* infection has also been reported as a severe complication in immunosuppressed patients.[40] Persons with asthma are at risk of more severe manifestations of *M. pneumoniae* infection.[82,83]

Neither smoking nor chronic pulmonary disease has been found to predispose to *M. pneumoniae* pneumonia. However, *M. pneumoniae* infection in persons with impaired pulmonary function may do further damage to the ventilatory capacity, and some exacerbation of chronic pulmonary disease has been associated with rise in *M. pneumoniae* antibody titer.[84]

6. Mechanisms and Routes of Transmission

Transmission of *M. pneumoniae* requires close contact such as in the family setting. Several cycles with 3-week case-to-case intervals are sometimes required before the family epidemic is over.[49] The propagation of epidemics in the community is also exceedingly slow, and epidemics may last 1–2 years.[38] Microepidemics in neighborhoods were identified in studies in Seattle,[40,46] LaCrosse, Wisconsin,[45] and Japan.[69] The school-age child seemed to be the most important vector in both intra- and interfamilial spread, yet, as noted in Section 5.2, the school itself appears not to be the focus of spread.[45,46] Introduction of an index case in a school rarely results in classroom epidemics, but the infection spreads among close playmates. Transmission has been described in an amateur wrestling team.[46] Children carry *M. pneumoniae* longer than do adults, but the potential for an asymptomatic carrier to transmit the infection is not known and is probably low.

It is not known whether spread is primarily by droplet or direct or indirect contact, or by all these means. The slow community spread makes airborne spread seem unlikely. Nevertheless, airborne transmission was suggested in a prosthodontal laboratory, where dental drilling of false teeth may have aerosolized the organisms.[71] Similarly, the outbreak on a nuclear-powered submarine may have been airborne.[72] In the common-source outbreak that occurred at a fraternity celebration, the exact mode of transmission was not identified.[70]

In the hamster model, exposure to small particles (2–3 μm) of *M. pneumoniae* resulted in both upper- and lower-respiratory-tract infection, whereas infection remained limited to the upper respiratory tract when hamsters were given inocula of large-particle aerosol (8 μm).[34] Larger doses of the small-particle (2–3 μm) aerosol resulted in more extensive pneumonia than lower doses,[85] suggesting that type and dose of aerosol may affect clinical manifestations of exposure.

Oral and genital mycoplasmas are endemic and do not occur in epidemics. The mode of spread is presumed to be by droplets for oral mycoplasmas and vertical and sexual contact for genital mycoplasmas.

Colonization with *U. urealyticum* to various orifices occurs in a high proportion of newborn infants and seems not to cause disease, at least not in full-term infants.[12] *M. hominis* occurs less frequently than *U. urealyticum*, but is spread by the same routes. The organisms seem to disappear from infants with time. Colonization with these mycoplasmas increases again after puberty and increases with the number of sexual partners.[1] *M. genitalis* is fastidious and only a few laboratories have succeeded in isolating it, and then primarily from the male urethra in patients with urethritis but also from oropharynx.[1,8]

7. Pathogenesis and Immunity

7.1. Incubation Period

The incubation period observed in volunteers inoculated with *M. pneumoniae* in the pharynx has been short (6–12 days), probably due to the large infecting dose.[20] In the common-source outbreak related to one single-day exposure, the median incubation period was 13 days.[73] However, the case-to-case interval observed in families and similar settings is considerably longer; the mode was 20 days in one study and 23 in the other.[48,49] This suggests that a person is not infective until after a week of illness, probably when the cough becomes productive.

The incubation period for *U. urealyticum* is only 1 to 2 days, based on inoculation of volunteers and colonization of newborns. Colonization of infants with *M. hominis* is evident within a week of birth. Inoculation studies of chimpanzees suggest that the incubation period for *M. genitalium* is about a week.

7.2. Pathogenesis

M. pneumoniae is a surface parasite[1] and has primarily been isolated from sites other than the respiratory tract. The organisms can be isolated from the pharynx 1 week prior to onset of illness; recovery rates are highest during the first week of illness, and the shedding from the pharynx subsequently decreases, so that few persons have positive cultures after 6 weeks[49] (see Fig. 1).

The organism has been recovered as late as 4 months after the onset of illness[46] and for a much longer period in hypogammaglobulinemic patients.[40] Healthy controls rarely carry *M. pneumoniae* (see Section 5.1). On the other hand, carriage has not been extensively studied among children under the age of 5, and in surveillance in a daycare center in North Carolina, 11 of 15 infected children (identified by isolation or serological rise) were thought to be asymptomatic.[35]

Many attempts have been made to isolate the organism from sites other than the nasopharynx in *M. pneumoniae* disease. Isolates have been reported from the ear, cerebrospinal fluid (CSF), synovial fluid, pleural and pericardial fluid, and from skin lesions including blisters from a case of Stevens–Johnson syndrome.[3–7,26,27,34,38,86] Of special interest is the detection of *M. pneumoniae* using PCR in the acute sera of 10 of 17 patients with encephalitis.[87] In postmortem, *M. pneumoniae* has been recovered from the blood in the heart,[28] and from the pericardial sac,[6] spleen, brain, and kidney.[27]

By electron microscopy, the organisms are found embedded between the cilia of the bronchial tree and attached to the respiratory epithelium with a terminal organelle.[1] This attachment is formed by a 165- to 190-kDa protein called P1. Antibody to the P1 protein inhibits adherence. At least five additional protein antigens may be important and may be detected by immunoblotting.[1] Some of the proteins may be shared by other organisms. The attachment has been studied in detail in the hamster model and in tracheal culture. Ciliary movements ceased after a couple of days; the latter effect is not observed in the case of nonpathogenic mycoplasmas. An infiltrate formed adjacent to the bronchial regions consisted primarily of mononuclear cells and some cells defined as plasma cells.[1,63] A proportion of the cells were rosette-forming, probably leukocytes and T cells. Polymorphonuclear cells increased with time. *M. pneumoniae* rarely invades the alveoli or the interstitial tissues. Tissue damage may be produced by catalase inhibition, allowing the toxicity of hydrogen peroxide to damage the cells.[1,63] Nonpathogenic strains, recovered through repeated passage in the laboratory, often fail to cause hemolysis and have lost some protein bands as seen by immunoblotting.[1,59] Cold agglutinins probably constitute cross-reacting autoantibodies to the I antigen on human erythrocytes and the membrane of *M. pneumoniae*.[1,63] Erythrocyte receptors are sialylated oligosaccharides of the I type.

Although the number of fatalities due to *M. pneumoniae* infection coming to autopsy is small, the postmortem findings are similar to those seen in the hamster model: interstitial infiltrates surround bronchi and bronchioles.[5–7,27] The infiltrates consist primarily of mononuclear cells, especially macrophages, lymphocytes, and plasma cells. The alveolar lining cells are swollen. Exudate, consisting of fibrin and leukocytes, has been observed primarily in the bronchial spaces. The mechanism of death from this disease is often thromboembolism, including disseminated intravascular coagulation.[5,77] Some patients appear to have died from pulmonary insufficiency.

Interferon is produced during *M. pneumoniae* infection, lasts for a prolonged period, and may be related to prolonged symptomatology.[33]

7.3. Immunity

The mechanism of immunity to *M. pneumoniae* is incompletely understood. When previously infected hamsters were rechallenged with *M. pneumoniae* organisms, the immunologic response and the development of exudates were accelerated and exaggerated.[88] It was shown that leukocytes played a role in the response.[88] Chimpanzees who had been infected previously and shown symptoms similar to human disease were protected on rechallenge.[89] Similarly, chimpanzees who had been given a formalin-inactivated vaccine were protected.[89] In humans, the presence of most humoral antibodies correlates with immunity. Infection rates and pneumonia rates are low in persons with antibodies.[24,25,66] However, serum antibodies, most of which are directed toward the lipid membrane, may constitute only an indirect measure of immunity. Repeated episodes of *M. pneumoniae* pneumonia, 2–7 years after the initial episode, have been documented in children and in young adults by isolation and fourfold titer rises.[40] Recurrences were seen only in children under the age of 10 during a 9-month epidemic in two kibbutzim.[90] Yet, the immunity to repeated infection is much better in persons who have had *M. pneumoniae* pneumonia than in those who had no infection or only mild infection.[40] Persons with immunodeficiency in the humoral antibody system suffered prolonged and severe disease,[40,81] but paradoxically, no infiltrates were observed on the chest film.[40] This may indicate that the pulmonary infiltrate, consisting primarily of various immune cells, serves a useful purpose in normal persons.

Children under the age of 5 sometimes appear to suffer mild or no symptoms when infected with *M. pneumoniae*.[40] This may support the hypothesis that the first infection primarily sensitizes the individual, and at subsequent exposure disease develops. However, in some studies, where children were under close clinical observation, a high rate of pneumonia was observed.[40,48,76] This relationship deserves further study.

M. pneumoniae elicits a variety of immunologic responses. The CF antibodies are of both the IgM and the IgG type.[60] Antibodies of the IgA class are induced in nasal and bronchial secretions after infection with live *M. pneumoniae*; these may be more related to protection than are humoral antibodies.[60,61,66] An increase in IgG relative to IgM antibodies has been noticed with time after onset of illness. Adults respond with a higher IgG antibody ratio than do children[60] and may respond with only IgG antibodies. Family studies suggest that persons may be immune without detectable CF antibody, and the adults, who appear to be immune to a high degree, usually lack CF antibody.[49] *M. pneumoniae*-specific IgE antibodies develop in asthmatic children, suggesting that *M. pneumoniae* can act as an allergen.[91]

The individual variability in response is considerable. In some cases, antilipid CF antibodies appear to decay rapidly, particularly in children; in others, especially those with pneumonia, they may decay slowly over 5 years.[40]

Cold agglutinins are of the IgM type and not identical with any of the *M. pneumoniae*-specific antibodies.[63] Genetic variability in response is suggested in experiments with different strains of mice, some of which developed cold agglutinins and some of which did not. Since the I antigens are not completely developed until the age of 18 months, immunologic immaturity may partially explain the milder *M. pneumoniae* infection in infants.

M. pneumoniae patients may also develop antibodies that cross-react with various other human tissues, e.g., brain, liver, heart, and lung.[63] Such antibodies may explain some of the complications of *M. pneumoniae* infections, although these antibodies are found in patients both with and without complications. Also, circulating antigen–antibody complexes have been demonstrated in patients both with and without complications. *M. pneumoniae* is a polyclonic B-cell activator[62] and induces tuberculin anergy after infection, suggesting temporary suppression of cell-mediated immunity. Cross-reacting antibodies to streptococcus MG (*Streptococcus anginosus*) were observed as early as the 1940s.[14] Rheumatoid factor may develop. This is also a nonspecific reaction. *M. pneumoniae* patients have been observed to have positive skin tests for *Micropolyspora faeni* (cause of farmer's lung).[92] Patients with sarcoidosis have a high prevalence of antibodies to *M. pneumoniae*, possibly reflecting a generalized increase in antibody formation.[93]

Cell-mediated immunity to *M. pneumoniae* following infection has been shown by lymphocyte stimulation, inhibition of migration of leukocytes, and skin testing. Lymphocytes responded to sonicated *M. pneumoniae* antigen up to 10 years after infection. Sensitivity to *M. pneumoniae* skin tests, which is induced by internal (nonlipid) antigens, increases with advancing age.

In the hamster model, circulating antibody, acquired by parenteral immunization, did not correlate with protection.[34,66,88] IgG activity, also IgA, was demonstrated in bronchial washings. Local immune response, whether cell-mediated or secretory, appears important in immunity.

Compared with the body of knowledge of immune response of *M. pneumoniae*, the knowledge of immune response of the genital mycoplasmas in sparse.[1,63] The mechanism for immune response to *M. genitalis* has similarities with *M. pneumoniae*.[8]

8. Patterns of Host Response

8.1. Clinical Features

8.1.1. *M. pneumoniae* Infection. The pattern of host response to *M. pneumoniae* infection ranges from asymptomatic infection to pharyngitis, bronchitis, bronchiolitis, croup, tracheobronchitis, pneumonitis, and pneumonia[2,21,34,36,39,69] (Table 2). The onset of *M. pneumoniae* pneumonia is usually insidious, in contrast to the abrupt onset of classic pneumococcal pneumonia. The symptoms include chills (55%), headache (66%), sore throat (54%), malaise (89%), and cough (99%).[39] The disease may mimic any viral respiratory disease such as influenza or adenovirus infection and even the common cold. In contrast to most viral respiratory diseases, frank coryza is infrequent. Cough is characteristically nonproductive and irritating at onset and may be paroxysmal. In young children, it may have a staccato character and be exaggerated at night. Although the disease resolves spontaneously even without treatment, relapses occur, convalescence may be prolonged, and patients may keep on coughing for months. Wheezing is common.[9]

Asthmatic children may be at higher risk of *M. pneumoniae* pneumonia and even normal children may develop wheezing that may persist.[83,91] Follow-up studies of *M. pneumoniae* patients have shown a decrease in tracheobronchial clearance that may last for a year or more.[94]

A great variety of complications have been described (Table 2). Otitis,[49] bullous hemorrhagic myringitis,[20,49] pleuritis, abscess of the lung, and adult respiratory distress syndrome[78] can be considered extensions of the respiratory tract infections. Complications related to the action of cold agglutinins consist of hemolytic anemia, thrombocytopenia, clot formation (thrombosis), and disseminated intravascular coagulation.[5,14] It may be speculated that myocarditis,[4] temporary arthritis,[81] and encephalitis and meningitis[3] have been due to cross-reacting antibodies or circulating immune complexes. However, the recovery of the organism from CSF[3] and synovial fluid[81] suggests direct invasion. Skin rashes, usually described as maculopapular or urticarial, occur in about 10–20% of cases.[49,86] Since these manifestations often appear rather late in the disease when the patient has started to improve, they may also be an effect of immune response. Stevens–Johnson syndrome (erythema multiforme

Table 2. Manifestation of *Mycoplasma pneumoniae* Infections

Pneumonitis/pneumonia	**Rare complications**
Bronchitis, tracheobronchitis	Hemolytic anemia
Bronchiolitis	Disseminated intravascular coagulation
Tracheobronchitis	Thromboembolism
Pharyngitis	Lung abscess
Croup	Hyperlucent lung syndrome
Otitis	Pneumothorax
Common complications	Respiratory distress syndrome
Otitis, including bullous hemorrhagic myringitis	Pericarditis, myocarditis
Skin rashes, maculopapular or urticarial	Glomerulitis
Pleuritis	Arthritis
Thrombocytopenia	Erythema nodosum
Meningitis–encephalitis	Stevens–Johnson syndrome
Mild anemia	**Neurological complications**
Asthmatic bronchitis	Meningitis
	Encephalitis
	Psychosis
	Gullain–Barré syndrome
	Cerebellar ataxia
	Brain-stem syndrome
	Poliomyelitislike syndrome
	Transverse myelitis
	Focal encephalopathy

major of pluriorificialis) is a rare and sometimes life-threatening complication that mostly affects boys.

Secondary invasion with bacterial pathogens has not been a major problem in *M. pneumoniae* pnuemonia, although superimposed or concurrent *Haemophilus influenzae*, *Streptococcus pneumoniae*, and *Staphylococcus aureus* infections have been described. Evidence of concurrent viral infection is common, but appears not to aggravate the disease,[39]

8.1.2. Genital Mycoplasma Infections. Carriage of *U. urealyticum* and *M. hominis* is so common, especially in women, that it may be considered normal flora.[9,12,95]

M. hominis has been recovered from the tubes of women with salpingitis and thought to be a cause of pelvic inflammatory disease, especially since antibody titer rises have also been observed.[1,9] It has been found in higher proportion of men with prostatitis than in those without. *M. hominis*[9] has also been isolated from various abscesses and from joints, especially in immunosuppressed patients.

U. urealyticum plays a minor role as a cause of nongonococcal urethritis. A role in infertility spontaneous abortion, low birth weight, and prematurity has been proposed, but the evidence for this is controversial and not convincing.[9,12,81,95] It is frequently isolated from the amniotic fluid and other products of conception.[12,95] It may have a role in chronic lung disease following prematurity.[96] It has been isolated from joints in immunosuppressed patients.[81]

Both *M. hominis* and *U. urealyticum* have been isolated from blood postpartum and after abortion, and such isolation may be associated with slight fever.[9] Both organisms have been found in CSF in premature infants with meningitis.[95]

8.2. Diagnosis

A diagnosis of *M. pneumoniae* pneumonia should be suspected in persons with gradual onset of sore throat, headache, chills, cough, fever, and pneumonitis. The white blood cell count is usually normal or slightly elevated; eosinophilia has been reported. The sedimentation rate is high. Many mild cases escape proper diagnosis even if seen by a physician. Dullness is rarely present on examination of the chest, since consolidation is seldom complete. Only a few rales may be heard despite an extensive infiltrate on the chest film. The radiological infiltrate is more often unilateral (84%) than bilateral.[39] It is often described as segmental and patchy and with punctate mottling.[2,39] Hilar infiltrates are common and characteristically fan out in a wedge-shaped manner, but any configuration and location of the infiltrate is possible, including upper lobar infiltrates. Attempts are being made to diagnose *M. pneumoniae* infection rapidly with immunofluorescence and with electron microscopy of throat specimens, but these techniques have not found general use. In patients with pneumonia, a high titer of cold agglutinins (1:32) is highly suggestive of *M. pneumoniae* infection. As noted in Section 3.4.2, the test can sometimes be conducted at the bedside, when agglutination occurs as the blood cools off; placing the tubes in an ice bath will accentuate the effect. The Coombs test, which measures antibody against erythrocytes, is also positive in cold agglutinin-positive pneumonia. The reticulocyte count may be low. Epidemiological clues may be helpful: since pneumonia of other etiologies is infrequent among persons 15–29 years of age, a high proportion of pneumonia is due to *M. pneumoniae* in this age group.

Likewise, a high proportion of pneumonia encountered in the summer is due to *M. pneumoniae*, because then other respiratory agents are at a low ebb. A history of other family members or contacts having had similar disease about 3 weeks previously is also suggestive.

Isolation of the organism from respiratory secretions is almost diagnostic, since the organism is rarely isolated from healthy individuals.[40] However, it may take 1–4 weeks for the laboratory to grow the organism. Thus, PCR test and Ag-EIA, which are rapid and sensitive, offer a better alternative, although it has not yet been tried out in epidemiological studies.[57,58] Probes may give a rapid result, but they are not always reliable. In lieu of isolation, which is offered in only a few specialized laboratories, a significant rise in *M. pneumoniae* antibody titer (see Section 3.4.2) between acute and convalescent specimens taken 2–3 weeks apart can be considered diagnostic, as well as presence of specific IgM and IgA antibody.[55,60]

9. Control and Prevention

9.1. Treatment

9.1.1. *M. pneumoniae* Infections. Controlled studies of *M. pneumoniae* pneumonia have shown that treatment with tetracycline, its derivatives, and erythromycin shortens the duration of illness in *M. pneumoniae* pneumonia. Clindamycin, another macrolide antibiotic similar to erythromycin, is not effective. New macrolides such as azithromycin and clarithromycin promise to be superior, as well as new quinolones such as sparftloxacin.[98–100] However, controlled studies have not been done. The response to antibiotic treatment is far less dramatic than that to treatment of other bacterial pneumonias. Occasionally, relapses are seen after a short duration (5 days) of treatment. Despite the patient's clinical improvement, shedding of the organisms continues unabated at least for the older antibiotics. Since tetracycline may stain developing teeth, erythromycin is the preferred drug for children. Although antibiotic treatment does not eradicate the organism, it is possible that the number of excreted organisms decreases. Strains resistant to tetracycline and erythromycin have been isolated. Patients with hemolytic anemia may require transfusion of blood, preferably i-erythrocytes, and the blood should be warmed to prevent hemolysis due to cold agglutinins in the host.

9.1.2. Genital Mycoplasma Infection. *M. hominis* is treated with doxycycline or other tetracyclines, but quickly develops resistance.[9,101] It responds to clindamycin, but is resistant to erythromycin. *U. ureaplasma* can be treated with erythromycin. However, the consensus appears to be that carriage of *U. urealyticum* in the vagina does not warrant treatment.[9,101] Quinolones may work on these organisms, but there are as yet no clinical trials of this and other new drugs.

9.2. Antibiotic Prophylaxis

This has been studied in elegant experiments in the hamster model: Early prophylaxis soon after inoculation only postponed the development of *M. pneumoniae* pneumonia, which appeared as the antibiotics were stopped.[34] Prophylactic treatment with antibiotics of persons incubating the infection has given mixed results, but may be more successful with newer antibiotics.

9.3. Vaccines

As early as 1964, challenge studies with organisms that had been passed a varying number of times on agar were conducted.[20,66] Challenge with the agar-grown mycoplasmas was followed by less severe illness than was challenge with tissue-grown organisms; furthermore, high-passage-number strains appeared to be less virulent. A small-scale trial of egg-grown vaccine, in which vaccinated and control subjects were challenged with aerosolized *M. pneumoniae* organisms, showed protection among those who had responded serologically to the vaccine.[20] Those who failed to respond, however, suffered relatively severe disease compared with the total control group. This raised the question of whether low-dose vaccine may sensitize rather than protect. These symptoms may also have been caused by sensitization to egg protein that may have been present in their vaccine. It has been suggested that in this challenge study, only those who had previously undergone natural infection responded serologically to the vaccine and that the nonresponders were a subset of persons without previous natural infection. Comparing this subset with controls composed of persons both with and without natural immunity may have yielded falsely alarming results. Subsequently, two large vaccine trials have been carried out among military personnel using two inactivated vaccines made from organisms grown on glass surfaces.[66,67] The trials showed moderate protection against pneumonia, at most 66–67% in the first year following inoculation. The data on protection from bronchitis are conflicting. Carriage rates were not affected by vaccine, but, as in other military studies, increased from 0 to 10% after 9 weeks of training.[67] In neither trial did vaccinees who contracted pneumonia have more severe disease than controls, although such a phemonemon was diligently sought. Challenge studies of chimpanzees vaccinated with a killed vaccine have also yielded promising results.[89] Concern remains about the feasibility of giving vaccines to children, since the response in *M. pneumoniae* pneumonia appears to be immunologic in character.[35] New approaches to vaccine development are being tested out, including acellular and recombined vaccines, and incorporating the PI antigen.[66]

10. Unresolved Problems

Clinical trials of promising new antibiotics, such as the new macrolides and quinolones, have not been carried out. Thus, the optimal antibiotic treatment of *M. pneumoniae* pneumonia is not known. PCR and the antigen capture methods of identification offer promise for a more rapid diagnosis; methods need to be standardized and compared with established methods of diagnosis. Improvement in laboratory diagnosis could result in availability of rapid clinical diagnosis, which may shed further light on complications of *M. pneumoniae* infections. The multitude of acute neurological syndromes attributed to *M. pneumoniae* infections and listed in Table 2 need further investigation. What proportion of such syndromes can be attributed to *M. pneumoniae* infection? What is the mechanism of such complications? What is the role in heart disease?

The impact of present-day child care, utilizing day-care facilities even for infants, is unknown. Prospective studies in day-care facilities are desirable.

The hypothesis that primary infections with *M. pneumoniae* are asymptomatic but sensitize to more severe disease on second exposure needs to be confirmed or refuted, or studies of vaccine efficacy in children cannot be carried out. Considering not only the respiratory disease caused by *M. pneumoniae* but also the many complications, a vaccine seems desirable. Vaccine development should be encouraged.

The role of *M. fermentans*, as well as *M. genitalis*, *M. pirum*, and *M. penetrans* in human populations, is practically unknown and needs to be pursued. The role of *U. urealyticum* as a commensal and disease agent needs to be clarified.

11. References

1. Krause, D. C., and Taylor-Robinson, D., Mycoplasmas which infect humans, in: *Mycoplasmas: Molecular Biology and Pathogenesis* (J. Maniloff, R. N. McElhaney, L. R. Finch, and J. B. Baseman, eds.), pp. 417–444, American Society for Microbiology, Washington, DC, 1992.
2. Clyde, W. A., Jr., Clinical overview of typical *Mycoplasma pneumoniae* infections, *Clin. Infect. Dis.* **17**(Suppl. 1)**:**S32–S36 (1993).
3. Koskiniemi, M., CNS manifestations associated with *Mycoplasma pneumoniae* infections: Summary of cases at the University of Helsinki and review, *Clin. Infect. Dis.* **17**(Suppl. 1)**:**S52–S57 (1993).
4. Kenney, R. T., Li, J. S., Clyde, Jr. W. A., *et al.*, Mycoplasma pericarditis: Evidence of invasive disease, *Clin. Infect. Dis.* **17**(Suppl. 1)**:**S58–S62 (1993).
5. Maisel, J. C., Babbit, L. H., and John T. J., Fatal *Mycoplasma pneumoniae* infection with isolation of organisms from lung, *J. Am. Med. Assoc.* **202:**287–290 (1967).
6. Naftalin, J. M., Wellisch, G., Kahana, Z., *et al.*, *Mycoplasma pneumoniae* septicemia, *J. Am. Med. Assoc.* **228:**565 (1974).
7. Meyers, B. R., and Hirschman, S. Z., Fatal infections associated with *Mycoplasma pneumoniae*: Discussion of three cases with necropsy findings, *Mt. Sinai J. Med.* **39:**258–264 (1972).
8. Taylor-Robinson, D., Gilroy, C. B., and Hay, P. E., Occurrence of *Mycoplasma genitalium* in different populations and its clinical significance, *Clin. Infect. Dis.* **17**(Suppl. 1)**:**S66–S68 (1993).
9. Glatt, A. E., McCormack, W. M., and Taylor-Robinson, D., Genital mycoplasmas, in: *Sexually Transmitted Diseases* (K. K. Holmes, P. A. Mårdh, P. F. Sparling, *et al.*, eds.), pp. 279–293, McGraw-Hill, New York, 1990.
10. Meyer, R. D., and Clough, W., Extragenital *Mycoplasma hominis* infections in adults: Emphasis on immunosuppression, *Clin. Infect. Dis.* **17**(Suppl. 1)**:**S243–S249 (1993).
11. Shepard, M. C., The recovery of pleuropneumonia-like organisms from Negro men with and without nongonococcal urethritis, *Am. J. Syph. Gonorrhea Vener. Dis.* **38:**113–124 (1954).
12. Eschenbach, D. A., *Ureaplasma urealyticum* respiratory disease in newborns, *Clin. Infect. Dis.* **17**(Suppl. 1)**:**S100–S106 (1993).
13. Blanchard, A., and Montagnier, L., AIDS-associated mycoplasmas, *Annu. Rev. Microbiol.* **48:**687–712 (1994).
14. Marmion, B. P., Eaton agent—science and scientific acceptance: A historical commentary, *Rev. Infect. Dis.* **12:**338–353 (1990).
15. Parker, F., Jr., Jolliffe, L. S., and Finland, M., Primary atypical pneumonia: Report of eight cases with autopsies, *Arch. Pathol.* **44:**581–608 (1947).
16. Commission on Acute Respiratory Diseases, Transmission of

primary atypical pneumonia to human volunteers, *J. Am. Med. Assoc.* **127:**146–149 (1945).

17. Eaton, M. D., Meikeljohn, G., and Van Herick, W., Studies on the etiology of primary atypical pneumonia: A filterable agent transmissible to cotton rats, hamsters, and chick embryos, *J. Exp. Med.* **79:**649–668 (1944).
18. Liu, C., Studies on primary atypical pneumonia. I. Localization, isolation, and cultivation of virus in chick embryos, *J. Exp. Med.* **106:**455–456 (1957).
19. Liu, C., Eaton, M. D., and Heyl, J. T., Studies on primary atypical pneumonia. II. Observations concerning the development and immunological characteristics of antibody in patients, *J. Exp. Med.* **109:**545–556 (1959).
20. Couch, R. B., Cate, T. R., and Chanock, R. M., Infection with artificially propagated Eaton agent, *J. Am. Med. Assoc.* **187:**442–447 (1964).
21. Chanock, R. M., Fox, H. H., James, W. D., *et al.*, Epidemiology of *M. pneumoniae* infection in military recruits, *Ann. NY Acad. Sci.* **143:**484–496 (1967).
22. Edwards, E. A., Crawford, Y. E., Pierce, W. E., *et al.*, A longitudinal study of *Mycoplasma pneumoniae* infections in Navy recruits by isolation and seroepidemiology, *Am. J. Epidemiol.* **104:**556–562 (1976).
23. Mogabgab, W. J., *Mycoplasma pneumoniae* and adenovirus respiratory illnesses in military and university personnel, 1959–1966, *Am. Rev. Respir. Dis.* **97:**345–358 (1968).
24. Steinberg, P., White, R. J., Fuld, S. L., *et al.*, Ecology of *Mycoplasma pneumoniae* infections in Marine recruits at Parris Island, South Carolina, *Am. J. Epidemiol.* **89:**62–73 (1969).
25. Foy, H. M., Kenny, G. E., Conney, M. K., *et al.*, Long-term epidemiology of infections with *Mycoplasma pneumoniae*, *J. Infect. Dis.* **139:**681–687 (1979).
26. Abramovitz, P., Schvartzman, P., Harel, D., *et al.*, Direct invasion of the central nervous system by *Mycoplasma pneumoniae*: A report of two cases, *J. Infect. Dis.* **155:**482–487 (1987).
27. Koletsky, R. J., and Weinstein, A. J., Fulminant *Mycoplasma pneumoniae* infection. Report of a fatal case, and a review of the literature, *Am. Rev. Respir. Dis.* **122:**491–496 (1980).
28. Naftalin, J. M., Wellisch, G. K., Kahana, Z., *et al.*, *Mycoplasma pneumoniae* septicemia, *J. Am. Med. Assoc.* **228:**565 (1974).
29. Centers for Disease Control, Outbreaks of *Mycoplasma pneumoniae* respiratory infection—Ohio, Texas, and New York, 1993, *Morbid. Mortal. Week. Rep.* **42:**931–1039 (1993).
30. Assaad, F., Gispen, R., Kleemola, M., *et al.*, Neurological diseases associated with viral and *Mycoplasma pneumoniae* infections, *Bull. WHO* **58:**297–311 (1980).
31. Lind, K., and Bentzen, M. W., Changes in the epidemiological pattern of *M. pneumoniae* infections in Denmark, *Epidemiol. Infect.* **101:**377–386 (1988).
32. Noah, N. D., and Urquhart, A. M., Epidemiology of *Mycoplasma pneumoniae* infection in the British Isles, 1974–9, *J. Infect.* **2:**191–194 (1980).
33. Niitu, Y., *Mycoplasma pneumoniae* infections, *Acta Paediatr. Jpn.* **27:**73–90 (1984).
34. Denny, F. W., Clyde, W. A., Jr., and Glezen, W. P., *Mycoplasma pneumoniae* disease: Clinical spectrum, pathophysiology, epidemiology, and control, *J. Infect. Dis.* **123:**74–92 (1971).
35. Fernald, G. W., Collier, A. M., and Clyde, W. A., Jr., Respiratory infections due to *Mycoplasma pneumoniae* in infants and children, *Pediatrics* **55:**327–334 (1975).
36. Glezen, W. P., Thornburg, G., Chin, T. D. Y., *et al.*, Significance of *Mycoplasma* infections in children with respiratory disease, *Pediatrics* **39:**516–525 (1967).
37. Monto, A. S., Bryan, E. R., and Rhodes, L. M., The Tecumseh study of respiratory illness. VII. Further observations on the occurrence of respiratory syncytial virus and *Mycoplasma pneumoniae* infections, *Am. J. Epidemiol.* **100:**458–468 (1974).
38. Foy, H. M., Kenny, G. E., McMahan, R., *et al.*, *Mycoplasma pneumoniae* pneumonia in an urban area, *J. Am. Med. Assoc.* **30:**1666–1672 (1970).
39. Foy, H. M., Cooney, M. K., McMahan, R., *et al.*, Viral and mycoplasmal pneumonia in a prepaid medical care group during an eight-year period, *Am. J. Epidemiol.* **97:**93–102 (1973).
40. Foy, H. M., Infections caused by *Mycoplasma pneumoniae* and possible carrier state in different populations of patients, *Clin. Infect. Dis.* **17**(Suppl. 1)**:**S37–S46 (1993).
41. Cordero, L., Cuadrado, R., Hall, C. B., *et al.*, Primary atypical pneumonia: An epidemic caused by *Mycoplasma pneumoniae*, *J. Pediatr.* **71:**1–12 (1967).
42. Dowdle, W. R., Stewart, J. A., Heyward, J. T., *et al.*, *Mycoplasma pneumoniae* infections in a children's population: A five-year study, *Am. J. Epidemiol.* **85:**137–146 (1967).
43. Saliba, G. S., Glezen, W. P., and Chin, T. D. Y., *Mycoplasma pneumoniae* infection in a resident boys' home, *Am. J. Epidemiol.* **86:**409–418 (1967).
44. Sterner, G., De Hevesy, G., Tunevall, G., *et al.*, Acute respiratory illness with *Mycoplasma pneumoniae*: An outbreak in a home for children, *Acta Paediatr. Scand.* **55:**280–286 (1966).
45. Copps, M. K., Allen, V. D., Sueltmann, S., *et al.*, A community outbreak of *Mycoplasma pneumoniae*, *J. Am. Med. Assoc.* **204:** 123–128 (1968).
46. Foy, H. M., Kenny, G. E., McMahan, R., *et al.*, *Mycoplasma pneumoniae* in the community, *Am. J. Epidemiol.* **93:**55–67 (1971).
47. Balassanian, N., and Robbins, F. C., *Mycoplasma pneumoniae* infection in families, *N. Engl. J. Med.* **277:**719–725 (1967).
48. Biberfeld, G., and Sterner, G., A study of *Mycoplasma pneumoniae* infections in families, *Scand. J. Infect. Dis.* **1:**39–46 (1969).
49. Foy, H. M., Grayston, J. T., Kenny, G. E., *et al.*, Epidemiology of *Mycoplasma pneumoniae* infection in families, *J. Am. Med. Assoc.* **197:**859–866 (1966).
50. Cooney, M. K., Fox, J. P., and Hall, C. E., The Seattle virus watch. VI. Observations of infections with and illness due to parainfluenza, mumps and respiratory syncytial viruses and *Mycoplasma pneumoniae*, *Am. J. Epidemiol.* **101:**532–551 (1975).
51. Jansson, E., von Essen, R., and Tuuri, S., *Mycoplasma pneumoniae* pneumonia in Helsinki 1962–1970, *Scand. J. Infect. Dis.* **3:**51–54 (1971).
52. Berntsson, E., Lagergård, T., Strannegård Ö., *et al.*, Etiology of community-acquired pneumonia in out-patients, *Eur. J. Clin. Microbiol.* **5:**446–447 (1986).
53. Evans, A. S., Serologic studies of acute respiratory infections in military personnel, *Yale J. Biol. Med.* **48:**201–209 (1975).
54. Suhs, R. H., and Feldman, H. A., Serologic epidemiologic studies with *M. pneumoniae*. II. Prevalence of antibodies in several populations, *Am. J. Epidemiol.* **83:**357–365 (1966).
55. Kenny, G. E., Mycoplasmas, in: *Manual of Clinical Microbiology*, 5th ed. (A. Balows, W. J. Hausler, Jr., K. L. Herrmann, H. D. Isenberg, and H. Y. Shadomy, eds.), pp. 478–482, American Society for Microbiology, Washington, DC, 1991.
56. Tully, J. G., Rose, D. L., Whitcomb, R. F., *et al.*, Enhanced

isolation of *Mycoplasma pneumoniae* from throat washings with a newly modified culture medium, *J. Infect. Dis.* **139:**478–482 (1979).

57. Marmion, B. P., Williamson, J., Worswick, D. A., *et al.*, Experience with newer techniques for the laboratory detection of *Mycoplasma pneumoniae* infection: Adelaide, 1978–1992, *Clin. Infect. Dis.* **17**(Suppl. 1)**:**S90–S99 (1993).
58. Kleemola, M., Jokinen, C., *et al.*, Outbreak of *Mycoplasma pneumoniae* infection among hospital personnel studied by a nucleic acid hybridization test, *J. Hosp. Infect.* **21:**213–221 (1992).
59. Kenny, G. E., Serodiagnosis, in: *Mycoplasma, Molecular Biology and Pathogenesis* (J. Maniloff, R. N. McElhaney, L. R. Finch, and J. B. Baseman, eds.), pp. 505–512, American Society for Microbiology, Washington, DC, 1992.
60. Jacobs, E., Serological diagnosis of Mycoplasma pneumoniae infections: A critical review of current procedures, *Clin. Infect. Dis.* **17**(Suppl. 1)**:**S79–S82 (1993).
61. Granström, M., Holme, T., Sjögren, A. M., *et al.*, The role of IgA determination by ELISA in the early serodiagnosis of *Mycoplasma pneumoniae* infection, in relation to IgG and μ-capture IgM methods, *J. Med. Microbiol.* **40:**288–292 (1994).
62. Biberfeld, G., and Gronowicz, E., *Mycoplasma pneumoniae* is a polyclonal B-cell activator, *Nature* **261:**238–239 (1976).
63. Tryon, W., and Baseman, J. B., Pathogenic determinants and mechanisms, in: *Mycoplasmas, Molecular Biology and Pathogenesis* (J. Maniloff, R. N. McElhaney, L. R. Finch, and J. B. Baseman, eds.), pp. 457–471, American Society for Microbiology, Washington, D.C. 1992.
64. Hatch, M. T., Wright, D. N., and Bailey, G. D., Response of airborne *Mycoplasma pneumoniae* to abrupt changes in relative humidity, *Appl. Microbiol.* **19:**232–238 (1970).
65. Wright, D. N., and Bailey, G. D., Effect of relative humidity on the stability of *Mycoplasma pneumoniae* exposed to simulated solar ultraviolet and to visible radiation, *Can. J. Microbiol.* **15:**1449–1452 (1969).
66. Ellison, J. S., Olson, L. D., and Barile, M. F., Immunity and vaccine development, in: *Mycoplasmas, Molecular Biology and Pathogenesis* (J. Maniloff, R. N. McElhaney, L. R. Finch, and J. B. Baseman, eds.), pp. 491–504, American Society for Microbiology, Washington, DC, 1992.
67. Wenzel, R. P., Craven, R. B., Davies, J. A., *et al.*, Field trial of an inactivated *Mycoplasma pneumoniae* vaccine. I. Vaccine efficacy, *J. Infect. Dis.* **143:**571–576 (1976).
68. Brunner, Z. H., and Chanock, R. M., A radioimmunoprecipitation test for detection of *Mycoplasma pneumoniae* antibody (37261), *Proc. Soc. Exp. Biol. Med.* **143:**97–105 (1973).
69. Nakao, T., and Umetsu, M., An outbreak of *Mycoplasma pneumoniae* infection in a community, *Tohoku J. Exp. Med.* **102:**23–31 (1970).
70. Evatt, B. L., Dowdle, W. R., Johnson, M., Jr., *et al.*, Epidemic *Mycoplasma* pneumonia, *N. Engl. J. Med.* **285:**374–378 (1971).
71. Sande, M. A., Gadot, F., and Wenzel, R. P., Point source epidemic of *Mycoplasma pneumoniae* infection in a prosthodontics laboratory, *Am. Rev. Respir. Dis.* **112:**213–217 (1975).
72. Sawyer, R., and Sommerville, R. G., An outbreak of *Mycoplasma pneumoniae* infection in a nuclear submarine, *J. Am. Med. Assoc.* **195:**958–959 (1966).
73. Broome, C. V., La Venture, M., Kaye, H. S., *et al.*, An explosive outbreak of *Mycoplasma pneumoniae* infection in a summer camp, *Pediatrics* **66:**884–888 (1980).
74. Pönkä, A., Occurrence of serologically verified *Mycoplasma pneumoniae* infections in Finland and in Scandinavia in 1970–1977, *Scand. J. Infect. Dis.* **12:**27–31 (1980).
75. Evans, A. S., Allen, V., Sueltmann, S., Mycoplasma pneumoniae infections in University of Wisconsin students, *Am. Rev. Respir. Dis.* **96:**237–244 (1967).
76. Hanukoglu, A., Hebroni, S., and Fried, D., Pulmonary involvement in *Mycoplasma pneumoniae* infection in families, *Infection* **14:**1–6 (1986).
77. Shulman, S. T., Bartlett, J., Clyde, W. A., Jr., *et al.*, The unusual severity of mycoplasmal pneumonia in children with sickle-cell disease, *N. Engl. J. Med.* **287:**164–167 (1972).
78. Andrews, C. E., Hopewill, P., Burrell, R. E., *et al.*, An epidemic of respiratory infection due to *Mycoplasma pneumoniae* in a civilian population, *Am. Rev. Respir. Dis.* **95:**972–979 (1967).
79. Freeman, R., King, B., and Hambling, M. H., Infection with *Mycoplasma pneumoniae* after open-heart surgery, *J. Thorac. Cardiovas. Surg.* **66:**642–644 (1973).
80. Arnold, K., Kilbridge, T. M., Miller, W. C., Jr., *et al.*, Mycoplasma pneumonia: A study on hospitalized American patients with pneumonia in Vietnam, *Am. J. Trop. Med. Hyg.* **26:**743–747 (1977).
81. Gelfand, E. W., Unique susceptibility of patients with antibody deficiency to *Mycoplasma* infection, *Clin. Infect. Dis.* **17**(Suppl. 1)**:**S250–S253 (1993).
82. Seggev, J. S., Lis, I., Siman-Tov, R., *et al.*, *Mycoplasma pneumoniae* is a frequent cause of exacerbation of bronchial asthma in adults, *Ann. Allergy* **57:**263–265 (1986).
83. Mertsola, J., Ziegler, T., Ruuskanen, O., *et al.*, Recurrent wheezy bronchitis and viral respiratory infections, *Arch. Dis. Child.* **66:**124–129 (1991).
84. Westerberg, S. C., Smith, C. B., and Renzetti, A. D., *Mycoplasma* infections in patients with chronic obstructive pulmonary disease, *J. Infect. Dis.* **127:**491–497 (1973).
85. Jemski, J. V., Hetsko, C. M., Helms, C. M., *et al.*, Immunoprophylaxis of experimental *Mycoplasma pneumoniae* disease: Effect of aerosol particle size and site of deposition of *M. pneumoniae* on the pattern of respiratory infection, disease, and immunity in hamsters, *Infect. Immun.* **16:**93–98 (1977).
86. Cherry, J. D., Anemia and mucocutaneous lesions due to *Mycoplasma* pneumoniae infections, *Clin. Infect. Dis.* **17**(Suppl. 1)**:** S47–S51 (1993).
87. Narita, M., Matsuzono, Y., Itakura, O., *et al.*, Survey of mycoplasmal bacteremia detected in children by polymerase chain reaction, *Clin. Infect. Dis.* **23:**522–525 (1996).
88. Clyde, W. A., Jr., Immunopathology of experimental *Mycoplasma pneumoniae* disease, *Infect. Immun.* **4:**757–763 (1971).
89. Franzoso, G., Hu, P-C., Meloni, G. A., *et al.*, Immunoblot analyses of chimpanzee sera after infection and after immunization and challenge with *Mycoplasma pneumoniae*, *Infect. Immun.* **61:** 1008–1014 (1994).
90. Leibowitz, Z., Schvartzman, P., Epstein, L., *et al.*, An outbreak of *Mycoplasma pneumoniae* pneumonia in two kibbutzim: A clinical and epidemiologic study, *Isr. J. Med. Sci.* **24:**88–92 (1988).
91. Tipirneni, P., Moore, B. S., Hyde, J. S., *et al.*, IgE antibodies to *Mycoplasma pneumoniae* in asthma and other atopic diseases, *Ann. Allergy* **45:**1–7 (1980).
92. Davies, B. H., Edwards, J. H., and Seaton, A., Cross-reacting antibodies to *Micropolyspora faeni* in *Mycoplasma pneumoniae* infection, *Clin. Allergy* **5:**217–224 (1975).
93. Putman, C. E., Baumgarten, A., and Gee, J. B. L., The prevalence of mycoplasmal complement-fixing antibodies in sarcoidosis, *Am. Rev. Respir. Dis.* **3:**364–365 (1975).

94. Sabato, A. R., Martin, A. J., Marmion, B. P., *et al.*, *Mycoplasma pneumoniae*: Acute illness, antibiotics, and subsequent pulmonary function, *Arch. Dis. Child.* **59:**1034–1037 (1984).
95. Sánchez, P. J., Perinatal transmission of *Ureaplasma urealyticum*: Current concepts based on review of the literature, *Clin. Infect. Dis.* **17**(Suppl. 1)**:**S107–S111 (1993).
96. Wang, E. E. L., Cassell, G. H., Sanchez, P. J., *et al.*, *Ureaplasma urealyticum* and chronic lung disease of prematurity: Critical appraisal of the literature on causation, *Clin. Infect. Dis.* **17**(Suppl. 1)**:**S112–S116 (1993).
97. Shames, J. M., George, R. B., Holliday, W. B., *et al.*, Comparison of antibiotics in the treatment of mycoplasmal pneumonia, *Arch. Intern. Med.* **125:**680–684 (1970).
98. Ishida, K., Kaku, M., Irifune, K., *et al.*, *In vitro* and *in vivo* activities of macrolides against *Mycoplasma pneumoniae*, *Antimicrob. Agents Chemother.* **38:**790–798 (1994).
99. Kaku, M., Ishida, I., Irifune, K., *et al.*, *In vitro* and *in vivo* of sparfloxacin against *Mycoplasma pneumoniae*, *Antimicrob. Agents Chemother.* **38:**738–741 (1994).
100. Bébéar, C., Dupon, M., Renaudin, H., *et al.*, Potential improvements in therapeutic options for mycoplasmal respiratory infections, *Clin. Infect. Dis.* **17**(Suppl. 1)**:**S202–S207 (1993).
101. McCormack, W. M., Susceptibility of mycoplasmas to antimicrobial agents: Clinical implications, *Clin. Infect. Dis.* **17** (Suppl. 1)**:**S200–S201 (1993).

12. Suggested Reading

Blanchard, A., and Montagnier, L., AIDS-associated mycoplasmas, *Annu. Rev. Microbiol.* **48:**687–712 (1994).

Casalta, J. P., Piquet, P., Alazia, M., *et al.*, *Mycoplasma pneumoniae* pneumonia following assisted ventilation, *Am. J. Med.* **101:**165–169 (1996).

Cassell, G. H., and Cole, B. C., Mycoplasmas as agents of human disease, *N. Engl. J. Med.* **304:**80–89 (1981).

Changing role of mycoplasmas in respiratory disease and age (a symposium) *Clin. Infect. Dis.*, **17**(Suppl. 1)**:**S2–S315 (1993).

Maniloff, J., McElhaney, R. N., Finch, L. R., and Baseman, J. B. (eds.), *Mycoplasmas: Molecular Biology and Pathogenesis*, American Society for Microbiology, Washington, DC, 1992.

Narita, M., Matsuzono, Y., Itakura, O., *et al.*, Survey of mycoplasmal bacteremia detected in children by polymerase chain reaction, *Clin. Infect. Dis.* **23:**522–525 (1996).

Pönkä, A., The occurrence and clinical picture of serologically verified *Mycoplasma pneumoniae* infections with emphasis on central system, cardiac and joint manifestations, *Ann. Clin. Res.* **22**(Suppl. 24)**:**1–60 (1979).

CHAPTER 25

Nosocomial Bacterial Infections

Louise M. Dembry, Marcus J. Zervos, and Walter J. Hierholzer, Jr.

1. Introduction

From the combination of Greek *nosos* (disease) with *komein* (to take care of) as *nosokomeion* (hospital) and through Latin *nosocomium* (hospital) comes the English *nosocomial* (pertaining to a hospital). Nosocomial infections, then, are infections that develop and are recognized in patients and personnel in health care institutions. These infections are not present or incubating on admission, with the exception that a nosocomial infection may be present on admission if it is directly related to or is the residual of a previous admission. Certain nosocomial infections may not be clinically evident until after discharge. It is common to classify all other infections that fail to meet these criteria as "community-acquired" infections. It is estimated that over 5% of all hospitalized patients fall victim to these infections each year in the United States.(1) Prevalence studies conducted in other countries with collaboration by the World Health Organization (WHO) have found rates from 3 to 20%, with a mean of 8.7 infections per 100 patients surveyed.(2) One third to one half of all nosocomial infections may be preventable.(3) Approximately 90% of reported nosocomial infections are of bacterial etiology, with viral, fungal, protozoal, and other classes of microorganisms associated with a lesser but significant number of cases.(1)

2. Historical Background

Since the use of temples by the Egyptians, there have been documented attempts to provide special care, protection, and segregation for the sick. This collection of the sick has frequently resulted in rapid transmission of infectious agents among patients and personnel and from unrecognized reservoirs within the institution with resultant high morbidity and mortality. Public recognition of hospitals as "pesthouses" was common up to modern times. The role of improved environmental sanitation and the importance of hygienic practices in reducing transmission and infection rates were recognized in the earliest medical traditions and were periodically rediscovered in the following centuries. The medical workers of the middle 1800s were especially productive. Florence Nightingale introduced broad hospital hygiene, transmission of puerperal fever was recognized by Semmelweis and controlled by hand washing with an antiseptic, and Lister introduced antisepsis to surgery. After Pasteur, the putrefaction associated with trauma and surgery was understood as related to transmissible microorganisms, and the importance of aseptic technique became well understood and practiced.(4,5)

The stunning early success of penicillin in controlling gram-positive coccal infections led to the misconception that antibiotics could control and eventually eradicate all infectious disease. The carefully learned lessons of the past concerning aseptic technique were no longer given priority and support. The appearance of penicillin-resistant staphylococci in this milieu led to devastating hospital epidemics with these agents.(6) The current resurgent interest in nosocomial infection grew out of the need to control these epidemics.

With the discovery of penicillinase-resistant penicillins, infections by resistant staphylococci became treatable, and associated epidemics decreased in importance. At the same time, the marketing of antibiotics with effectiveness against a broad spectrum of other microorganisms again led the unwary to discount the need for other control methods. However, the control of nosoco-

Louise M. Dembry and Walter J. Hierholzer, Jr. • Department of Hospital Epidemiology and Infection Control, Yale University School of Medicine, Yale–New Haven Hospital, New Haven, Connecticut 06504. **Marcus J. Zervos** • Division of Infectious Diseases, William Beaumont Hospital, Royal Oak, Michigan 48072.

mial infection was not forthcoming. During the years 1960 to 1980, a new spectrum of agents, in which the gram-negative organisms played a major role, assumed a place of importance in nosocomial infection.[7] More recently, new gram-positive agents, especially resistant staphylococci and enterococci, have assumed increasing significance.[1,8–10]

3. Methodology

3.1. Criteria for Infection

Widely accepted criteria for the identification and classification of nosocomial infection have been suggested by the Centers for Disease Control and Prevention (CDC).[11,12] These criteria satisfy both the need for scientific validity and the practical requirement for easy and uniform recognition necessary to discovery and enumeration. Examples are listed in Table 1. It is common practice to designate most bacterial infections that appear within the first 48 hr of hospital stay as community and not nosocomially acquired. In these criteria both infections from endogenous flora and infections transmitted from exogenous sources are included. Since microbiological sampling in clinical situations is neither routine nor uniform, the criteria are not dependent on the laboratory for data for fulfillment. Such clinical definition is mandated by studies indicating that from 16 to 59% of otherwise well-documented nosocomial infections are not supported by microbiological data in that no tests were submitted or tests were invalidated because of poor sampling, inadequate handling, or laboratory error.[2,9,13] Since both preventable and unavoidable infections are included in these criteria, care in assignment of causation and liability must be taken in the individual case (Table 1).

3.2. Sources of Mortality Data

The usual hospital discharge and death certificate data rarely include comments on complications of nosocomial infection. Some individual studies[14,15] and an autopsy study[16] have been reported. Autopsy data may provide confirmation or documentation of unsuspected nosocomial infection through gross, microscopic, or microbiological cultural evidence. However, autopsy data are biased for patients dying in the hospital with the most severe, interesting, or puzzling illnesses. These factors are associated with prolongation of hospital stay and other comorbid events predisposing to increased nosocomial infection. Since 1970, the National Nosocomial Infections Surveillance (NNIS) has reported selected mortality and morbidity data from a volunteer group of hospitals in the United States, currently numbering over 200 hospitals.[1,17–20] These hospitals range in size from 100 beds to over 1000 beds and are geographically an inadequate representation of US hospitals. While the system does not represent a probability sample of US hospitals, by stratifying hospitals by size and teaching characteristics, it has provided useful data. The NNIS data have tended to be confirmed by Study of Efficacy of Nosocomial Infection Control (SENIC) and other published reports.[3,21] Recent changes in the requirements for participation in the NNIS system and improvements in definitions and methods, including computer-assisted reporting, should improve the quality in the value of this database as a potential source of national estimates of nosocomial infections in the United States.[22–24] Prospective data on the role of nosocomial infection in institutional mortality controlled for conditions that predispose to nosocomial infection are lacking.

3.3. Sources of Morbidity Data

Nosocomial bacterial infections are generally not reportable through any routine public health system. The uniform hospital discharge summary rarely indicates the complication of a nosocomial infection. In a study of risk factors important in nosocomial infection, Freeman and McGowan[25] found only 59% of nosocomial infections labeled with any diagnosis of infection as a primary or secondary discharge diagnosis and only 2% labeled as clearly indicating infection of a nosocomial origin. In a study conducted after the beginning of the new prospective payment systems in the United States, Massanari *et al.*[26] found that only 57% of nosocomial infections were properly recorded in the discharge abstracts of their university hospital. The retrospective audit of medical records to determine the frequency of nosocomial infection has been complicated by difficulties in completeness, illegibility, and inaccessibility. However, the results of a large, statistically complex, and well-controlled evaluation of the efficacy of nosocomial infection practice and control, using a measured and highly reliable retrospective medical record review methodology, have been reported by the CDC. The methodology and analysis of the SENIC project have been published in detail.[3,27,28]

The focal point of hospital infection control must be the patient. The most successful acquisition of data on nosocomial infection has been accomplished through nosocomial infection surveillance. Of critical importance is a specifically trained individual, the infection control practitioner or nurse epidemiologist.[29,30] This sur-

Table 1. Sample Criteria for Determination of Nosocomial Infection[a]

Site	Clinical data	Laboratory data
Urinary tract	Suprapubic tenderness, dysuria, frequency, pyuria	Standard quantitative urine culture[b]
Wound	Purulent drainage	Wound culture[b]
Respiratory tract	Physical signs, sputum change	X ray
	Purulent sputum	Sputum culture[b]
Intravenous	Purulent drainage, pain, erythema	Semiquantitative culture[b]
Gastrointestinal tract	Diarrhea	Stool culture[b]
Skin	Purulent drainage, physical signs	Culture[b]

[a]Modified from Garner *et al.*(11)
[b]Combinations of clinical data may be used to document infection in thr absence of laboratory microbiological isolation (see the text).

veillance method actively acquires data from multiple laboratory(31,32) and clinical sources and uses it to fulfill criteria set to definitions to confirm the presence of a nosocomial infection at a particular site. These data sources have included concurrent review of the patient's clinical record, review of the medical nursing Kardex and other data sheets for evidence of infection, and coordinated supplement of these clinical sources with radiology reports, pharmacy data, and microbiological laboratory reports.(17,29,31–33)

3.4. Surveillance

In addition to the NNIS and SENIC projects of the CDC, some statewide incidence and prevalence studies have been reported in the United States,(34) and the WHO and others have sponsored surveys in other regions of the world.(2,35–37)

3.4.1. Microbiological Surveys. Data routinely generated in the hospital microbiology laboratory have been widely used as a source of information of infections in hospitalized patients, and the increased use of diagnostic tests has been documented to increase the recognition of infectious diseases in acute care institutions.(38,39) The site of infection (e.g., urinary tract, blood, pulmonary, wound), patient location, causative organism(s), and antimicrobial susceptibility data can be determined and evaluated. Computerized data-processing methods have eased the collation and review of these data for recognition of clusters of infections at specific sites, in geographic locations, or of specific species or strains of bacteria.(31,32,40) Patterns of antibiotic resistance and changes in resistance that may be related to antibiotic use are also conveniently followed by this method.(41) Although laboratory reports are a good source for initial case finding, the specificity of the survey of laboratory isolations is low. Isolation of an organism does not separate community-acquired from nosocomial infection and does not specify causation in differentiating commensal from infecting bacteria without additional clinical information. Furthermore, the sensitivity of this system is dependent on the uniformity of the collection of specimens and of culturing practices, features of laboratory practice that are known to vary widely. However, when laboratory data are combined with information from other databases in a highly computerized hospital information system, sensitivities for the identification of nosocomial infection were reported that were equal to or exceeded other methods and at an efficiency that required approximately one third of personnel devoted to routine surveillance.(41)

Routine microbiological surveys of hospitalized patients or the hospital environment are unnecessary and economically unjustifiable. In the absence of epidemic situations, there is no evidence that this type of routine sampling has contributed significantly to detection or prevention of nosocomial infections. In epidemic situations, environmental cultures should be considered only if epidemiological evidence indicates an environmental source for the organism. The incidence of nosocomial infection has not been related to levels of microbial contamination of air, surfaces, or fomites, and meaningful standards for permissible levels of such contamination do not exist.(42–45)

The spread of nosocomial organisms in endemic and most epidemic situations is associated with contact transmission via personnel hands or due to contamination of an item that should be sterile. Therefore, the role of environmental microbiological sampling is currently reduced to: (1) assisting in epidemic investigation in selected circumstances, (2) evaluation of new techniques, (3) serving as an important adjunct to educational programs in the support of nosocomial infection control, and (4) quality control routine monitoring of sterilization, dialysis fluids, infant formula prepared in the hospital, and samples of certain disinfected equipment.

An exception to these limitations has been suggested to determine the presence of certain *Legionella* species in the potable water of hospitals with populations of highly immunocompromised patients known to be at high risk of morbidity and mortality when infected by these agents.[46,47] The CDC recommends culturing of hospital water supplies for *Legionella* when a definite laboratory-confirmed case of nosocomial Legionnaires' disease is identified, particularly if it occurs in a severely immunocompromised patient or severely immunocompromised patients are cared for in the hospital. The CDC has made no recommendation regarding routine culturing of hospital water supply systems in the absence of nosocomial Legionnaires' at this time.[48]

3.4.2. Prevalence Surveys. A prevalence survey based on application of uniform criteria to all patients in an institution during a single day or time period has provided a rapid, inexpensive, and corroborative means of assessing nosocomial infection risk within an institution. Periodic prevalence data have been used as an evaluative tool in infection control programs,[25] as an estimator of risk across a wide variety of institutions,[13,49] including programs of the WHO,[2] and as an important quality control feature of other data collection methods.[30] As with all prevalence studies, bias inherent in sampling of a single day's experience as an indicator of typical risk must be recognized.

3.4.3. Surveillance Studies. Currently the most widely propagated surveillance method for the collection of nosocomial infection data employs a trained individual, a nurse epidemiologist, or infection control practitioner.[33,50] This individual concurrently provides a coordinated review of each patient's clinical and laboratory data, recording those instances that satisfy the standard criteria for identification of a nosocomial infection. These data are summarized on a periodic (monthly, quarterly, yearly) basis, collated, analyzed, and reported to a specific multidisciplinary committee within the hospital and to certain key hospital personnel.[29,30] The importance of the unbiased collection of these data by a trained professional has been repeatedly documented by studies indicating reduced efficiency and accuracy of reporting by other methods[51,52] and by the results of the SENIC project.[28]

The institutional infection control committee recommends appropriate control measures, based on the priorities of risk indicated by the data previously collected and evaluated. The continuous collection of nosocomial infection data allows concurrent evaluation of these control efforts. This form of nosocomial infection data collection, evaluation, and recommendation has been termed "a nosocomial infection surveillance and control program."[53] This format has been widely promoted and supported by the Hospital Infections Program of the CDC since the first reports of its successful use in 1969.[30]

Three demonstration projects by the CDC have investigated this format as the prime method to investigate and control nosocomial infections in US hospitals. The Comprehensive Hospital Infection Project (CHIP) collected intensive surveillance data in nine community hospitals between January 1970 and June 1973, using definitions and methods suggested by the CDC.[30,53] At 4-month intervals, CDC medical epidemiologists conducted onsite prevalence surveys to evaluate surveillance efficiency.

The NNIS system, while not statistically representative of all US hospitals, does contain community, community teaching, state, local, and university hospitals. Large hospitals with more than 500 beds are overrepresented and small hospitals with fewer than 200 beds are underrepresented in the system.[20] Each hospital is required to have an active infection control program, but until recently there was little attempt to evaluate or control the quality of the submitted data. Recently the requirements for membership in the system have been increased, criteria for infection have been improved and standardized, and reliable submission of data has been required in an attempt to improve both the scope and the quality of the information submitted. On the basis of selected prevalence surveys comparing NNIS and CHIP methods, an earlier recommendation was that NNIS data should be inflated by a factor of 1.5 to compensate for their lower efficiency. The relevance of that suggestion for current data is unknown. Data reported by the NNIS system are reviewed in Section 5.

In 1974, the CDC initiated the SENIC project, which thereafter collected data in 338 randomly selected US hospitals. The objectives of this study were to estimate the magnitude of the nosocomial infection problem in US hospitals, to describe the extent of hospitals' infection surveillance and control programs, and to evaluate the efficacy and effectiveness of these programs in reducing nosocomial infection risks. The extensive and complex methodology of the study was reported in 1980 and the results and evaluation were reported in 1985.[27,37,54] The results indicate that in the one third of hospitals supporting the lowest levels of surveillance and control programs, nosocomial infections had increased in the period between 1970 and 1976 by 18%. In the same time period in the 0.5% of hospitals with the highest levels of surveillance and control, nosocomial infections had decreased by approximately one third.

Of the approximately one third of infections estimated to be reduced by the most intensive surveillance and control programs, surgical wound infections were found to be the risk most amenable to control and the problem that demonstrated the greatest risk of both increased cost and length of stay. Bacteremias and urinary tract infections were intermediate in reduction by CDC methods; pneumonias proved to be the most refractory and nosocomial medical pneumonias were not being significantly reduced.

The most effective programs conducted high-level balanced surveillance and control activities, had a trained hospital epidemiologist, supported an infection control practitioner for each 250 beds, and had a system of reporting wound infection rates to individual surgeons. Unfortunately, it was estimated that only 6% of nosocomial infections were being prevented at the end of the study. A follow-up study in 1983 indicated that this figure had risen to 9%, or approximately 28% of the potential estimated to be possible by current methods.[55]

3.5. Laboratory Diagnosis

Standard, reliable laboratory identification of bacteria in clinical samples from suspected nosocomial infection is important epidemiologically to link sources of transmitted microorganisms. The most important steps in assuring the validity of this process begin at the bedside with the collection of body fluids for testing. Inappropriate collection of specimens magnifies the usual difficulties in differentiation of normal flora of the body from truly infecting microbes.

3.5.1. Isolation and Identification of Organisms. The use of expectorated sputum in identification of the causal agents of pneumonia typifies this problem.[56] Pulmonary secretions collected through the oropharynx may be heavily contaminated by commensal oropharyngeal bacteria. Similarly, urine specimens may become contaminated when not obtained by "clean catch, midstream voiding" or by direct bladder catheterization. Cultures from other normally sterile sites must be obtained only after proper preparation of the location to be sampled for results of cultures to be meaningful.

A delay in transport to the laboratory or transport under inappropriate environmental conditions or in a hostile medium may hinder identification of important infecting bacteria. Urine cultures held at room temperature may allow bacteria therein to multiply beyond the usual criteria for identification of a nosocomial urinary tract infection. A collection of anaerobic organisms in cold medium and carriage at ambient oxygen levels may inhibit subsequent growth to an extent that thwarts laboratory rescue and identification.

Many laboratory findings suggest improper collection or transport of specimens. Isolations of skin flora, such as diphtheroids or coagulase-negative staphylococci from normally sterile sites, suggest contamination at the time of collection. The recovery of three or more species of bacteria from urine specimens suggests unsatisfactory technique in collection or handling. The inability to recover anaerobes seen on Gram's stain suggests inappropriate transport of specimens or culturing technique. Negative cultures for *Mycobacterium tuberculosis* in patients at high risk may suggest inappropriate sputum collection. Delayed receipt of sputum specimens diminishes the laboratory's ability to isolate pneumococci from specimens due to overgrowth of the organism by normal oropharyngeal flora. If such inappropriate sampling, mishandling, and delay are not recognized by the laboratory, they may result in the unintentional misreporting of no organisms or of microbes of no clinical significance.

3.5.2. Evaluation of Specimens: Initial Screening. The laboratory specialist is guided by the description of the site of sampling and other clinical information forwarded by the requesting physician. The absence of such information accompanying the specimen may lead to serious mishandling or delay in identification in the laboratory. Recording the time of arrival of the specimen in the laboratory as compared to time of collection may be used to determine delays in transport that will result in an inability to culture fastidious organisms. Specimens received in improper collection containers can also be noted at the time of initial evaluation. In these instances, repeat cultures should be requested.

Assessment of specimens at the time they are received in the laboratory by direct microscopic examination is important in evaluating the acceptability of a specimen for further diagnostic testing. The laboratory use of differential cellular characteristics of sputum and saliva has been helpful in clarifying the source of specimens and their acceptability for diagnostic testings.[57] Specimens containing more than ten squamous epithelial cells per low-power (×10) field suggest contamination with oropharyngeal flora. Material from wounds that do not show polymorphonuclear leukocytes is also unlikely to yield a causative organism when cultured. Smears and other recently developed rapid diagnostic tests that evaluate antigen or antibody detection are of enormous importance in patient management. Smears are also important for detecting organisms of epidemiological significance, such as *Haemophilus*, *Legionella*, or *M. tuberculosis*, that may not be reflected by culture or that may take long periods of time to grow.

Sufficient sophistication in the laboratory is necessary to assure speciation of the common bacteria endemic to the institution. Standard methods are available in many manuals and texts.[58] Reference bacteriology should be conveniently available to assist in the identification of more unusual microbes. The degree to which organisms are speciated can also have epidemiological importance. For example, a report of *Pseudomonas* species fails to distinguish between a variety of related organisms, such as *P. aeruginosa* and *P. cepacia*, which have different reservoirs and modes of transmission. Identifying organisms as *P. cepacia* has etiologic significance, since *P. cepacia* are associated with outbreaks or pseudoepidemics caused by contaminated water or solutions.[59]

3.5.3. *In Vitro* Susceptibility Testing. Testing of the sensitivity of isolates to a spectrum of antibiotics is a commonly used clinical and epidemiological tool. Standardized Kirby–Bauer disk diffusion testing or the more exacting microdilution minimum inhibitory concentration (MIC) tests provide useful information regarding the susceptibility of the bacterial isolate.[58] Disk diffusion testing is performed by measuring the zone of inhibition around an antibiotic-impregnated disk. Zone diameter are interpreted in signifying susceptible, intermediate, or resistant organisms. Microdilution testing provides a quantitative measurement of the MIC, which is defined as the lowest concentration of antibiotic that results in inhibition of growth of the organism. Automated antimicrobial susceptibility testing methods may fail to detect some antibiotic-resistant organisms, particularly antibiotic-resistant enterococci. Recently, it was shown that some of the automated systems could not reliably detect low and intermediate level vancomycin-resistant enterococci.[60,61]

The results of susceptibility studies provide guidance both to the clinician for appropriate therapy and to the epidemiologist as an inexpensive screen for possible common identity of speciated organisms.[39] However, antibiotic sensitivity does not ensure similarity of speciated organisms; organisms may have similar antibiotic resistances and yet be epidemiologically unrelated.[62–64] Also, modification of susceptibility under pressure of antibiotic use may take place without other recognized biological changes.[65]

3.5.4. Quality Control in the Laboratory. Quality control is essential to effective microbiology laboratory and infection control programs. Pseudoepidemics due to contamination of specimens in the laboratory by automated laboratory equipment or other routes have occurred.[66,67] New procedures in the laboratory related to susceptibility testing, new culture techniques, or new ways of reporting results or of naming organisms can also lead to confusion, pseudoepidemics, or lack of recognition of related organisms.

3.5.5. Special Studies for Examining the Relatedness of Isolates. A variety of tests of biological characteristics not generally available in the routine laboratory have proved of value in epidemiological investigations of nosocomial infections. Traditional methods as well as newer molecular methods have been used to differentiate bacterial strains. Phage typing, serotyping, and biotyping are examples of traditional typing methods. The traditional methods can be difficult to perform, often lack the ability to differentiate unrelated strains, and cannot type all isolates. The following are some of the molecular methods that have been evaluated for strain typing purposes.

3.5.5a. Plasmid Typing. Molecular methods that analyze bacterial plasmid DNA increasingly have been used to determine relatedness of isolates. Diverse species of gram-negative and gram-positive bacteria have been studied using this approach.[63,68,69] The relatedness of strains is evaluated by comparison of the plasmid DNA. Bacteria cannot always be typed successfully using this method, as plasmids can undergo molecular rearrangement, recombination, or deletion, and not all bacteria contain plasmids.

3.5.5b. Chromosomal DNA Typing. The chromosome is a stable marker of strain identity. This method allows a larger amount of genetic material to be compared than with plasmid typing. The technique has been particularly useful for bacteria that lacks plasmids. The extracted chromosomal DNA is cleaved with a restriction enzyme and the resulting linear fragments of DNA are separated by agarose gel electrophoresis. The banding patterns generated may be complex and difficult to interpret.

3.5.5c. DNA–DNA Hybridization. The complex banding patterns generated with chromosomal DNA restriction enzyme analysis are more easily interpreted when a few discrete DNA fragments are highlighted by hybridizing the chromosomal DNA with a DNA probe that recognizes a specific gene or region of a gene that is present on a few fragments. Several bacteria have been typed with this technique, including *M. tuberculosis*. Ribotyping is another chromosomal typing technique that uses ribosomal RNA as the probe. This technique is based on the finding that the genes that encode subunits of ribosomal RNA are conserved between species and scattered throughout the chromosome of most bacteria. Ribotyping has been useful for typing gram-negative organisms. It is not as successful with gram-positive organisms, particularly enterococci.

3.5.5d. Pulsed-Field Gel Electrophoresis. Pulsed-field gel electrophoresis allows for the separation of large genomic DNA molecules generated by rare cutting restriction enzymes. The large DNA fragments are separated on agarose gels that are subjected to alternating electric fields. Relatively clear patterns that can be compared are generated in this manner. Although special equipment is required to perform this technique, it is becoming the method of choice for typing many bacteria.[70]

3.5.5e. Polymerase Chain Reaction (PCR). With this technique it is possible to detect very small amounts or sequences of DNA by amplifying specific nucleotide sequences and increasing the number of DNA copies. The technique is much more sensitive than DNA–DNA hybridization with a specific DNA probe. PCR is rapid and technically easy to do, although its extreme sensitivity and problems with cross-contamination may hamper its development as a method for typing bacteria as compared to other currently available methods.

Much of this reference bacteriological testing is available in state and regional public health laboratories. For many of the research techniques, samples may be referred to regional university research centers or to the CDC in Atlanta.

4. Biological Characteristics of Nosocomial Organisms

The relative frequency of the species of bacteria causing nosocomial infection has changed remarkably over the past 30 years.[1,19,71] Changes in sensitivity to antimicrobial agents have also been observed. These changes in the development and persistence of resistant strains have been related to the selective pressure of the widespread use and misuse of antimicrobial agents. These patterns appear to be an extremely important phenomenon in local institutions and geographical areas,[72] as well as on a national level.[19] The biological characteristics important in these resistance changes may be generalized to: (1) the ability of bacteria to survive in the normal flora of the host, (2) the ability of bacteria to survive in the animate and inanimate environments of the health care facility, and (3) the ability of the bacteria to survive antimicrobial stress through acquired resistance.

4.1. Infecting Normal Flora

Bacteria that normally reside as commensals on the internal and external surfaces of the host have been increasingly recognized as causal in nosocomial infections.[10,73–75] In hospitalized patients, the normal pharyngeal and intestinal flora may be displaced by antibiotic-resistant strains. The changes brought about by modification in the host by disease and by treatment factors occur within a few days of hospitalization. These bacteria then can serve as sources for infection in the colonized patient or are transmitted between patients nosocomially. The ability of bacteria to infect is determined by the product of their number and virulence and inversely related to the quality and quantity of host defenses. In this context the term *normal flora* has become suspect in the recognition that virtually any microorganism that appears in the host may be invasive and disease-causing, given a sufficiently impaired patient.[76]

4.2. Antimicrobial Resistance

The emergence of antibiotic resistance plays a critical role in bacterial nosocomial infections. Epidemic penicillin-resistant staphylococci were controlled by a return to antiseptic techniques and the development of successful penicillinase-resistant antistaphylococcal drugs. Concurrent with these events there began to appear, with increasing frequency, infections with gram-negative bacilli, many of which had been considered nonpathogens heretofore.[7,71] Many of these bacteria are naturally resistant to antibiotics successful in the treatment of gram-positive bacteria. Thereafter, epidemic staphylococci resistant to methicillin appeared and spread throughout hospitals worldwide.[8,77–79] More recently, multi-drug-resistant enterococci have emerged as important pathogens, posing therapeutic challenges because of their intrinsic resistance to many antimicrobial agents.[10,80] Concurrent with the rise in tuberculosis has been a rise in multi-drug-resistant tuberculosis, which has been implicated in several nosocomial outbreaks of tuberculosis.[81] Over time, new antibiotics of broader spectrum or of specific usefulness have been developed. In virtually every situation, bacteria in resistant forms equal to the pressure of antibiotic use have emerged.

5. Descriptive Epidemiology

5.1. Prevalence and Incidence

A large number of studies from the United States and other countries have estimated the magnitude of nosocomial infection by a variety of methods. Examples of data from those that have used criteria for infection compatible with those developed and used by the CDC are presented in Table 2. Based on these criteria, these studies routinely include in their totals infections for which no cultures were done or for which no pathogens were isolated. These infections identified by clinical criteria alone make up from 16 to 59% of the data.[2,13,27]

The nosocomial infection "rate," more precisely a ratio, has commonly been determined by citing the num-

Table 2. Prevalence and Incidence Rates of Nosocomial Infection[a]

Location	Years	Type of hospitals	Type of study	Rate (%)
United States				
Virginia	1972–1975[21]	University	Incidence	6.7
Utah	1972–1973[13]	Community < 75 beds	Prevalence	7.2
	1977[49]	Community < 75 beds	Incidence	2.0
West Germany	1976[16]	University	Incidence	6.6
United Kingdom	1980[211]	Community	Autopsy	13.7
			Prevalence	9.2
Israel	1975–1976[212]	University	Incidence	12.2
United States	1984[1]	Mixed NNIS-CDC[b]	Incidence	3.4
		Community NNIS-CDC[b]	Incidence	2.2
		University NNIS-CDC[b]	Incidence	4.1
WHO	1983–1985[2]	Mixed	Prevalence	9.9

[a]Infections per 100 hospital discharges.
[b]NNIS, National Nosocomial Infections Study.

ber of nosocomial infections per 100, 1,000, or 10,000 patient discharges.[30,53] A preferred ratio expressed in infection per 1,000 or 10,000 patient days of risk[25,82–85] has been used in reports of incidence data. This latter ratio is especially valuable in considering nosocomial risk in institutions or services with widely varying length of stay and in extended-care facilities. Although this ratio adjusts for length of stay, it does not take into account the use of invasive devices, which are a major risk factor for specific nosocomial infections, e.g., intravascular catheters for bloodstream infections, urinary catheters for urinary tract infections, and ventilators for pneumonias.[86] Risk-factor-specific infection rates have been developed to account for exposure to these extrinsic risk factors. The rate is expressed as the number of device-associated infections for a site per 1000 device days of risk. These rates are considered more appropriate for inter- as well as intrahospital comparison than the overall nosocomial infection rate, as they partially control for length of stay and device use.

5.1.1. Mortality Data. Estimates of the role of nosocomial infection in mortality have varied widely. CDC–NNIS data estimated that 0.7% of nosocomial infections directly caused death and 3.1% of infections contributed to death.[1] In a retrospective study of 1000 autopsies from a university hospital, in which 75% of patients who died were examined, Daschner *et al.*[16] found an overall nosocomial infection rate of 13.7%. In those individuals with nosocomial infection, 54% of the deaths resulted directly from infection. In a retrospective study of 100 consecutive deaths at each of two hospitals, Gross *et al.*[15] found death causally related to nosocomial infections in 2.5% and contributing in 3.4% of patients without underlying terminal illness. In those with terminal illness on admission, the rates increase to 9.2 and 10.9%, respectively.

5.1.2. Prevalence Studies. Prevalence studies conducted in US acute-care hospitals, using CDC–NNIS-compatible criteria, have reported rates ranging from 7.2% in small, predominantly rural hospitals[13] to as high as 15.5% in a large, metropolitan teaching hospital.[71]

A WHO cooperative hospital infection prevalence survey was carried out between 1983 and 1985 in 55 hospitals in 14 countries in the four regions Europe, Mediterranean, Southeast Asia, and western Pacific.[2] Results reported from 47 hospitals and 28,861 patients showed a mean prevalence rate of 8.7% with regional means from 7.7 to 11.8% and individual institutional rates from 3.0 to 20.7%. Since multiple infections were not recorded, an adjusted mean of 9.9% for the total was estimated, suggesting that approximately one patient in ten in these hospitals was infected while under care.

Prevalence data reported from extended-care facilities have ranged from 3 to 18%.[87–89] These studies have used varying criteria and methodology, making comparisons difficult. Studies in these institutions will require special criteria and methods different from those commonly used in acute-care institutions, since the availability of laboratory data, the extent of daily medical record documentation, and the resources available for data collection and analysis are less in this setting. Standard definitions for nosocomial infections for use in extended-care facilities have been proposed and are currently being tested.[90] These proposed definitions for nosocomial infections in extended-care facilities have been applied in a prevalence study for nosocomial infections in home health care.[91] Over 20% of patients were found to have an infection on the day of the survey; 5% of those infections had occurred during the course of home health care.

5.1.3. Incidence Studies. Using definitions and methodologies outlined by the CDC for NNIS, a large number of incidence studies have been reported. The most recently reported CDC–NNIS data indicate a mean crude annual nosocomial infection rate of 3.4 for the 51 hospitals contributing data for 1984.[1] The 20 nonteaching hospitals reported a mean rate of 2.2, the 18 small teaching hospitals a mean rate of 3.4, and the 13 large teaching hospitals a rate of 4.4. If the CDC–NNIS data are inflated by a factor of 1.5, as suggested (see Section 3.4.3), a mean crude nosocomial infection rate of approximately 5 infections per 100 discharges is observed.[30] Other programs and authors report rates from less than 3 to over 13% (Table 2).

5.1.4. Site–Pathogen Analysis. The site of nosocomial infection and the pathogen(s) reported as responsible for them vary in incidence, relative frequency, morbidity, and mortality. The distribution of nosocomial infections by site varies by hospital service. This variation probably reflects differences in exposure to devices and procedures. Recent CDC–NNIS data[92] reports the site distribution of nosocomial infection based on the hospital-wide surveillance component as follows: urinary tract infection (27.2%), surgical site infection (18.7%), pneumonia (17.3%), primary bloodstream infection (15.8%), and other (21%). Site–pathogen data from the NNIS for the period 1990–1992 are given in Table 3. During the period 1990 to 1995, there has been a trend toward fewer urinary tract infections and increased bloodstream infections. Pediatric services and extended-care facilities report higher comparative rates of cutaneous infections than those reported for other services in acute care. Bacterial infections account for over 85% of those for which an etiology is recognized.

5.1.4a. Urinary Tract Infections. Infections of the urinary tract are consistently reported in Europe and the United States as comprising 30–45% of the total infections identified and are the most common cause of nosocomial infections.[2,19,21] Over 60% of these infections are caused by gram-negative bacilli, with *Escherichia coli* causing approximately one quarter. Enterococci and *P. aeruginosa* appear next in frequency in hospitals in the United States, while *Proteus* species are more frequently reported in the WHO data and in extended-care facilities in the United States. Secondary bacteremia appears in approximately 1% of individuals with nosocomial urinary tract infections, and 30 to 40% of hospital-associated gram-negative bacteremias originate at this site. Platt *et al.*,[93] in a carefully controlled study for other risk factors, have reported a threefold increase in risk of death in patients with nosocomial bacteriuria.

5.1.4b. Surgical Site Infections. Postoperative surgical site infections make up from approximately 15 to 25% of reported nosocomial infections. In some developing areas, up to one third of reported infections have

Table 3. Relative Frequency of Nosocomial Infection by Site and Selected Pathogens[a]

	Site (% of isolates)					
Pathogen	UTI	SSI	Pneumonia	BSI	Other	Percent
E. coli	25	8	4	8	4	12
S. aureus	2	19	20	16	17	12
Coagulase-negative staphylococci	4	14	2	31	14	11
Enterococci	16	12	2	9	5	10
P. aeruginosa	11	8	16	3	6	9
Candida spp.	10	4	6	8	6	7
Enterobacter spp.	5	7	11	4	4	6
Klebsiella spp.	8	4	10	5	4	6
Gram-positive anaerobes	0	1	0	1	19	4
Proteus mirabilis	5	3	2	1	2	3
Other *Streptococcus* spp.	1	3	1	4	2	2
Other fungi	3	0	1	1	1	2
Acinetobacter spp.	1	1	4	2	1	1
Serratia marcescens	1	1	3	1	1	1
Citrobacter spp.	2	1	1	1	1	1
Group B *Streptococcus*	1	1	1	2	1	1
Haemophilus influenzae	0	0	5	0	2	1
Other non-*Enterobacteriaceae* aerobes	0	1	4	1	2	1
Number of isolates	25,371	11,724	8,891	9,444	14,981	70,411

[a]Adapted from Emori and Gaynes[91]; NNIS 1990–1992.
[b]No other pathogens accounted for more than 2% of isolates at any site.

involved surgical sites.[2] Following a classification system for wounds (clean, clean contaminated, contaminated, or dirty) used in The National Research Council Study reported in 1964,[94] recent studies usually have reported risk of infection in postoperative surgical sites based on the probability of wound contamination during surgery. While risk classification and reduction have been thought to be most effective in treating "clean wounds," a simplified multivariate risk index successfully differentiating low, medium, and high risk across all contamination groups has been reported by the CDC, using data gathered during the SENIC project.[54] Surgical site infections usually arise as a result of intraoperative seeding of exogenous bacteria or as a result of dissemination of endogenous bacteria to the operative site. A number of factors determine the risk of surgical site infection, including the degree of microbiological contamination during the procedure, the duration of the procedure, and the patient's intrinsic risk. In order to use surgical site infection rates for comparative purposes, the rates should be adjusted for these risks. The NNIS has developed a surgical site infection risk index, which takes into account the patient's wound class, the American Society of Anesthesiology score, and the duration of the procedure; the NNIS index has a value of 0 to 3.[86] It is simple to use, and the required data are generally readily accessible. In order to make comparisons between institutions or surgeons, surgical site infection rates should be stratified by risk categories.[95]

Staphylococcus aureus remains the most common isolate from wound infections in the WHO studies[2] and in the CDC–NNIS data.[19] *E. coli* had been second in frequency in the 1980s in many reports but has now been exceeded by coagulase-negative staphylococci and enterococci in the most recent CDC–NNIS report.[19] Other gram-negative bacilli remain important etiologic agents. *Bacteriodes* and other anaerobes are probably underreported in these data, since many laboratories outside the university setting in the developed world lack sufficient resources and sophistication to collect and process isolates appropriately to identify these agents with sensitivity.

5.1.4c. Respiratory Infections. Respiratory infections in the form of pneumonias make up a portion equal in importance to surgical site infections in most reports (approximately 15–25%). *P. aeruginosa* is the most frequently reported pathogen in WHO reports and the second most common pathogen, first being *S. aureus*, in the United States.[19] Other gram-negative agents are also causal agents reported with significant frequency in most studies.[2,19,96] Nosocomial pneumonias are the leading cause of death from nosocomial infection. Secondary bacteremias are higher in nosocomial pneumonia than for either urinary or wound infections, and case-fatality rates for nosocomial pneumonias are only exceeded by those for bacteremia.

5.1.4d. Nosocomial Bloodstream Infection. Nosocomial bloodstream infections are reported as secondary to another site if there is documented infection at the primary site (in which case they are not included as an additional infection in determining rates) or primary if there is a culture-confirmed bacteremia without evidence for an underlying site of infection. Secondary bacteremias are documented in over 5% of infections at all sites and are most commonly associated with cardiovascular, intra-abdominal, and intravascular sites of primary infection. Infections with gram-negative organisms, including *Acinetobacter*, *Bacteroides*, and *Serratia*, have the highest rates of secondary bacteremias but are far exceeded in relative frequency by *S. aureus* and coagulase-negative *Staphyloccus* infections. Primary bacteremia rates are highest in teaching hospitals in the CDC–NNIS system, making up over 16% of infections in the larger teaching hospitals. The gram-positive organisms of coagulase-negative staphylococci and *S. aureus* have increased to become the most common agents of primary bacteremia in all but gynecology services where *E. coli* and *Bacteroides* species remain the most frequent. This marks a major change from the past 20 years' experience where gram-negative bacteria held preeminence at this site. Bacteremias remain the site with the highest case-fatality rate, exceeding 25% in most reports and 50% or more in many.[97–99]

5.1.4e. Cutaneous Infection. Cutaneous infections make up approximately 6% of the infections reported from the NNIS system, with high rates in the larger university hospitals and on the newborn units. A larger portion of infections in the developing countries and in extended-care facilities in the United States are reported at the cutaneous site.[85,87] *S. aureus* is the most frequently reported isolate at this site, with aerobic and anaerobic gram-negative rod organisms of increasing importance at this site in pressure ulcers common to the elderly in extended care.

An important subgroup of infections reported at this site are related to intravascular devices and intravenous therapy. Infections secondary to intravenous fluids,[100] intravenous fluid additives,[101] administration apparatus,[102] infusion devices, and a series of different types of implements have been documented.[103–105] These infections are attended by a high rate of continuing secondary bacteremia if the devices are not removed, and case-fatality rates are reported in the 20 to 40% range. In the United States, coagulase-negative staphylococci are an important and increasing cause of these infections.[74,97]

5.1.4f. Other Types of Nosocomial Infections. It is common to identify several other sites of nosocomial infection (gynecological, upper respiratory, eye, gastrointestinal),[53] and events, including epidemics, have been recorded for each. Gastrointestinal infections were especially prominent in data reported from the Southeast Asia and western Pacific areas in the WHO prevalence surveys, apparently indicating important intrahospital endemic transmission of this illness in these predominantly developing countries.[2]

5.2. Epidemic Behavior and Contagiousness

The epidemic form of nosocomial infections represents only 5% of all nosocomial infections, yet it has been the most extensively reported. Epidemic behavior is determined by the causal bacteria, the route of transmission, and the characteristics of the host population at risk. These epidemics have mirrored advances in medicine just as the most common causal agents have moved from gram-positive streptococcal wound and puerperal infections, through resistant staphylococcal epidemics, to gram-negative bacilli of increasing antibiotic resistance infecting hosts with decreasing ability to resist.[106,107] In contrast, endemic nosocomial infections with gram-positive organisms have been increasing over the last decade compared to endemic gram-negative infections. Nosocomial epidemics investigated by the CDC have doubled each 5-year period since 1960.[103] During the period 1970–1975, 42% of the epidemics investigated were associated with some medical device, and 70% were due to gram-negative bacilli.[103] From 1980 to 1985, 46.6% of the outbreaks investigated were related to products, procedures, or devices, and this proportion rose to 67.3% of investigations for the period 1986–1990.[107] Gram-negative bacteria accounted for 66% of the investigated outbreaks. Outbreaks of infection due to vancomycin-resistant enterococci have been increasingly reported in intensive-care units and oncology units, especially from large teaching hospitals.[108] While this experience may represent unusually interesting or difficult outbreaks, it is not unusual for larger medical centers to experience several epidemics per year. The role of the human carrier as either biological or mechanical transmitter has been commented on repeatedly in reports of outbreaks with methicillin-resistant *S. aureus*.[1,8,78]

Several pseudoepidemics have been reported.[109,110] A pseudoepidemic is the occurrence of an increased number of isolates of a microorganism misinterpreted as a true epidemic of infection. The main factors in the psuedo-epidemics have been improper specimen processing, surveillance artifact, and clinical misdiagnosis.[66]

5.3. Geographic Distribution

Nosocomial infections are not limited by geography (Table 2.)[2] Lack of reported nosocomial infection has indicated inadequate study more frequently than an absence of risk. Service, organism, and extent of morbidity and mortality vary within and among different institutions. This variation frequently reflects differing case mix (severity of disease, comorbid factors) in the samples admitted from the population served. As a result, it is common for tertiary-care centers to exhibit higher rates than primary-care hospitals.[1] A direct relationship between rates of specific community-acquired infections and nosocomial risk has not been documented. However, the appearance of nosocomial epidemics as extensions of community-acquired and propagated epidemics has been recognized, as has the converse.[78]

5.4. Temporal Distribution

An unexplained seasonal variation in certain gram-negative rods, including *Acinetobacter* with summer peaks, has been reported.[111,112] Other common bacteria have not been reported to show a seasonal trend in nosocomial infections.

A direct correlation has been suggested between length of stay in a hospital and the incidence of nosocomial infection, but the confounding variables of disease severity, age, and comorbidity have not been sufficiently separated to confirm this observation.

In the one third of the hospitals in the SENIC project that had established no infection control programs or ineffective programs between 1970 and 1976, an increase in nosocomial infection rates of 18% was reported. In the 5% of hospitals in the same study with the highest efficacy programs, an overall decrease of 36% was estimated. These increases would seem to be supported by what is known about changes in length of stay, case mix, and severity in patient populations in acute care institutions in the United States during the same time period.

5.5. Age

Extremes of age have been reported as directly associated with increasing nosocomial infection rates,[113] and the special problems in children[114] and in surgical site infection[115] have been recorded. Since extremes of age are known to be correlated with host defects resulting in increased susceptibility to infection, this hypothesis seems reasonable and attractive. Unfortunately, most studies have reported only relative frequency of infection by age group and have not been well controlled for length of exposure, disease severity, treatment, or other patient-related conditions that predispose to infection. Daschner *et al.*,[16] in a retrospective autopsy study, found an excess of nosocomial deaths in the 20- to 60-year-old age range. In a controlled study of risk factors for nosocomial infection in a university medical setting, age of 65 years or more increased the risk of nosocomial infection three times.[25]

Morbidity and mortality from nosocomial infection increase directly with age in the elderly, as for most infections, and the special problems of the neonate are similar to other infections in that age group.

5.6. Sex

Incidence of nosocomial infection has been reported to be greater in males than in females, but as with most other variables, these studies have not been well controlled.[99] Sex-related morbidity and mortality for nosocomial infection seem to parallel the site–pathogen experience for individual diseases.

5.7. Race

No race difference has been suggested or reported for nosocomial infections independent of other disease processes.

5.8. Occupation

Clinical health care professionals, medical laboratory workers, and other support personnel who come into contact with patients or patient specimens have potential increased risk of bacterial infection related to their employment.[116] While individual cases and outbreaks of a variety of bacterial infectious diseases have been reported,[117–119] the only well-documented increased risk for clinical workers appears to be tuberculosis.[120,121] Medical laboratory personnel share this increased risk of tuberculosis and may have increased rates of brucellosis, shigellosis, and other enteric bacterial diseases.[122]

5.9. Occurrence in Different Settings

Nosocomial infections have been reported in both acute- and extended-care settings. Within acute-care hospitals several high-risk units for nosocomial infection have been recognized. These include burn units,[120] high-risk nurseries,[114] intensive-care units,[106,123] dialysis units,[124,125] transplantation units,[126,127] and oncology units.[83] The common denominator in these units appears to be the use of specific hospital procedures and the presence of more severely compromised patients. The high nosocomial infection rates reported for university teaching hospitals may be directly related to the presence of these high-risk units. In one study of 38 US hospitals, 25% of all nosocomial infections reported occurred in intensive-care unit patients.[106]

Information on nosocomial bacterial infections in extended-care facilities is limited.[87,89,128] No data are available on the risk of nosocomial infection related to ambulatory care. With the increased use of ambulatory care facilities as sites of health care delivery, including surgical procedures, there is a need for increased understanding of the epidemiology of nosocomial infections in this setting.[129]

5.10 Socioeconomic Factors

While the importance of socioeconomic factors in infectious disease epidemiology is well recognized, no differential has been reported for nosocomial infections independent of other disease processes.

5.11. Other Host Factors

In addition to age, the genetic and acquired modifications of host defenses usually important in increased susceptibility to infection contribute to nosocomial risk (Table 4). They include metabolic disease, cardiovascular disease, respiratory disease, cutaneous disease, and a spectrum of hematologic and immunologic abnormalities. Among the host defenses altered by these diseases are modifications in normal flora, changes in anatomical barriers to microorganisms, suppression of inflammatory response, and modifications in the reticuloendothelial system. Among the hematologic and immunologic factors important in nosocomial infection are those that decrease the number of neutrophils, cause defective function of neutrophils, reduce or cause defective immunoglobulin production, or interfere with cellular immunity. A single underlying condition may contribute to several defects in host defenses. A solid tumor may cause obstruction, erode a mucosal surface, and metastatically replace bone marrow. The resultant malnutrition, easy portal of entry, and loss of leukocyte function all contribute to infection by opportunistic microorganisms.

Table 4. Examples of Factors that Modify Host Defenses

Host defenses	Disease modifiers	Treatment modifiers	Frequent sites of infection	Common organism of infection
Normal flora	Thermal burn	Antibiotic therapy	Soft tissue	*Pseudomonas*
		Gastric surgery	Intestine	*Salmonella*
Anatomical barriers	Trauma	Medical devices	Intravenous site	Coagulase-negative staphylococci
		Surgery	Wound	*S. aureus*
Mucociliary clearance	Cystic fibrosis	Irradiation	Pulmonary	*S. aureus*
		Tracheostomy	Pulmonary	*Pseudomonas*
Reticuloendothelial system	Sickle-cell disease, asplenia	Hemodialysis	Bloodstream	*S. pneumoniae* *H. influenzae* *Salmonella*
Leukocyte function	Chronic granulomatous disease, Job's syndrome, diabetic ketoacidosis	Corticosteroids Drug-induced neutropenia	Soft tissue Pneumonia	*S. aureus*
Humoral immunity	Agammaglobulinemia, chronic lymphocytic leukemia, multiple myeloma	Immunosuppression Cancer chemotherapy	Soft tissue Pulmonary	*H. influenzae* *S. pneumoniae* Gram-negative aerobes
Cell-mediated immunity	Thymic aplasia, malnutrition, Hodgkin's disease, HIV/AIDS	Immunosuppression Corticosteroids	Soft tissue	Gram-negative aerobes *Mycobacterium tuberculosis*

The conditions that predispose to such opportunistic infections and the types of organisms involved have been well reviewed elsewhere.[130,131] The epidemic of infections with the human immunodeficiency virus (HIV) and the resultant acquired immunodeficiency syndrome (AIDS) have resulted in a major increase in individuals subject to such infections.[132]

5.12. Treatment Factors

5.12.1. Antibiotics. Between 25 and 35% of hospitalized patients receive systemic antibiotics. Antibiotic treatment, including prophylactic antibiotic use, contributes to the risk of nosocomial infection by several means. In addition to modifying the endogenous microflora of the host, several antibiotics interfere with immune function (chloramphenicol, rifampin) or contribute to renal (aminoglycosides), hepatic (erythromycin, isoniazid), or cutaneous (β-lactams) side effects that increase susceptibility to infection.

Under pressure of antibiotic use or abuse, the environmental microbial flora of medical care institutions increases in antibiotic resistance.[19,133,134] Patient acquisition of these resistant microbial flora begins shortly after admission and is accelerated by antibiotic treatment or prophylaxis, reaching as much as 60% of the patient population by the third week in some studies.[74] This acquisition is paralleled by an increase in the appearance of these bacteria in the causation of nosocomial infection.

5.12.2. Other Drugs. Those drugs with side effects that decrease normal host defenses have the most profound role in increasing risk of nosocomial infection. Corticosteroids modify inflammatory response, interfere with leukocyte function, and depress cellular and humoral immune responses. Antimetabolites and a variety of other cancer chemotherapy drugs have profound effects on all rapidly proliferating tissue, resulting in hemopoietic side effects that decrease immune function and gastrointestinal side effects that interfere with secretory protection and cause loss of anatomical barriers through ulceration. The patient treated with a combination of intensive chemotherapy, immunosuppressive agents, and antibiotic prophylaxis in an attempt to induce remission of leukemia or in preparation for bone marrow or organ transplantation epitomizes the host at special high risk of nosocomial infection secondary to drug effects.

5.12.3. Device- and Procedure-Related Infections. Medical implements and devices and the procedures associated with them have assumed a common necessary part of modern medical practice. These devices include intravenous catheters, drains, urinary catheters, indwelling tubes into normally closed body cavities of the peritoneum or the cardiothoracic spaces, prosthesis in the cardiovascular system, the central nervous system, or the skeletal system, as well as a variety of implements in the respiratory system, including nasotracheal, endotracheal, and tracheostomy tubes. Each of these devices provides a route of entry for microorganisms by penetrating host

Table 5. Common Device-Related Nosocomial Infections[a]

Device[b]	Hospitalized patients with the device (%)	Most common related infection	Patients developing infection (%)	Case-fatality rate (%)
Urinary catheter	10	Bacteruria	20	<1
Intravascular infusion	12	Suppurative phlebitis	<0.01	20–40
Scalp vein needle	12	Suppurative phlebitis	<0.01	20–40
Plastic catheter	12	Suppurative phlebitis	0–8	20–40
TPN	0.1	Suppurative phlebitis	0–27	20–40
Arterial catheter	0.2	Suppurative phlebitis	0.2	20–40
Respiratory therapy				
Continuous ventilator	2	Pneumonia	—	40
IPPB	7	Pneumonia	—	40
Hemodialysis		Shunt infection	15–20	5

[a]Modified from Stamm.(213)
[b]TPN, total parenteral nutrition; IPPB, intermittent positive-pressure breathing.

defense mechanisms and acts as inanimate foci for the proliferation of microorganisms. One or another of the devices is used in the care of approximately 10% of patients hospitalized in acute-care facilities. It has been estimated that 45% of all nosocomial infections, over 850,000 per year in the United States, are device-related (Table 5). Coagulase-negative staphylococci have become important causes of infections, complicating use of central vascular lines, grafts, and other devices.(75)

6. Mechanisms and Routes of Transmission

Patients may be infected with bacteria acquired from either endogenous or exogenous sources. Microorganisms from endogenous sources may appear by reactivation of some previous infection, as in tuberculosis, or by invasion of commensal flora, which infect because of some reduction in host defenses. Transmission from exogenous sources may take place by hands, by the airborne route, through fomites, by insects, or by ingestion of contaminated food or water. While each of these routes, with the exception of insects, has been described in individual outbreaks, transmission by direct and indirect contact remains the common and most significant route in acquiring nosocomial infection. Exogenous sources are found in three specific reservoirs: (1) within the fixed structures of the facility itself; (2) in devices or equipment used within the institution; and (3) in medical personnel, other patients, or visitors.

6.1. Inanimate Reservoirs

The microenvironment of the hospital, rich in water and nutrient sources, has provided a continuing niche for gram-negative bacilli that have evolved as important agents in nosocomial infection. *Enterobacter*, *Serratia*, *Acinetobacter*, *Citrobacter*, *Flavobacteria*, *Legionella*, and *Pseudomonas* species have been repeatedly identified as important nosocomial pathogens because of their ability to survive in the aqueous and other fluid reservoirs of our institutions.(135–138) Clean environmental surfaces are generally not important sources of bacteria-causing nosocomial infections.(43) However, environmental surfaces contaminated with *Clostridium difficile* or vancomycin-resistant enterococci have been implicated in the nosocomial transmission of these organisims.(61) Extensive reviews of reported inanimate reservoirs are available.(138,139)

6.1.1. Structural or Engineering Reservoirs. The medical care field is one of rapid change, and this is evident in frequent requirements for modification of structures used for medical care. With limited funding, compromises in terms of structure, space, and function that are less than ideal may be accepted. The result may be crowding, which encourages cross-contamination, or the inconvenient placement of certain fixed equipment (e.g., hand-washing sinks), which makes the use of the equipment problematical. Reconstruction may disguise an inadequate air-conditioning system, resulting in the recirculation of unfiltered air from an "isolated" tuberculosis patient(116) or of air exhausted from microbiological laboratories or other areas of high biohazard.

Legionella pneumophila is ubiquitous in water and may be present in potable water. Nosocomial Legionnaires' disease has been described as resulting from contaminated cooling towers of air-conditioning systems and potable water as well as from construction activity in the vicinity of the hospital.(60,140,141) Reservoirs of nosocomial bacteria within water supplies or plumbing have been a recurrent problem in hospitals caring for high-risk patients.[135,136,142]

6.1.2. Equipment Reservoirs. In addition to the common medical devices, a wealth of new and increasingly complex equipment attends patient care. Respiratory assistance equipment, cardiovascular assistance pumps, microelectronic monitoring devices, dialysis machinery, and numerous other "black boxes" have reached the bedside. Appropriate use of these instruments is understood by fewer and fewer individuals, and the safe techniques for appropriate disinfection between patients may be overlooked or misunderstood. Portions of this equipment may be expensive, fragile, nondisposable, and unable to withstand the usual harsh but sure techniques of heat sterilization. Alternate methods are often less well understood than classic heat sterilization, and inadequate attention is paid to the detail necessary to assure their full implementation. As a result, residual microorganisms may be transmitted to subsequent patients as has occurred with a variety of devices, including bronchoscopy and endoscopy equipment.[134,143–145] Other problems have arisen when bacterial endotoxins have remained on equipment, causing severe reactions, or residual chemical sterilants themselves have caused toxic effects.[146]

6.2. Animate Reservoirs

Bacteria causing nosocomial infection reside in the animate reservoirs[10,79,147–151] of the health care worker or of the chronically institutionalized patient. Patients colonized with nosocomial organisms at clinical sites, such as wounds or urine, or colonized in their gastrointestinal or genitourinary tract, or their oropharyngeal flora serve as reservoirs for these organisms. Hospital personnel are occasionally personal carriers of nosocomial organisms such as *Salmonella*, staphylococci, or enterococci that are transmitted to hospitalized patients. Of these characteristics, the ability to survive at the time of transmission in mechanical carriage remains the most significant factor in nosocomial infection.

Hospital professionals, medical support workers, and patients provide the animate reservoirs for microorganisms. Biological transmission through symptomatic or asymptomatic carriage of bacteria has led to serious and extensive epidemics.[147,150] While visitors are a potential for microorganisms, they have rarely been implicated in such transmission.

Even more commonly, healthy but careless individuals mechanically transmit large numbers of bacteria from reservoirs within the facility, from equipment, and from patient to patient during their daily rounds.[152] Hand carriage of microorganisms is recognized as the most important factor in endemic and most epidemic spread of nosocomial infection. In one study in a university neurosurgical unit, 44% of randomly sampled personnel carried gram-negative bacilli and 11% had *S. aureus* on their hands.[153] More important, serial culturing demonstrated that all persons at various times carried gram-negative bacilli and two thirds carried staphylococci. Indirect contact spread via transient hand carriage has been implicated in other nosocomial transmission of staphylococci, enterococci, and gram-negatives.[10,79,148,151,154] Such carriage is instrumental in the nosocomial colonization that precedes infection in the compromised host.[10,73,74,149,155]

7. Pathogenesis and Immunity

The pathogenesis of nosocomial infection is determined by host and environmental factors that are uniquely combined in health care institutions.

The susceptible patient is prey to all the conventional pathogens. The compromised host is infected by a much smaller dose of bacteria and by species that are usually considered commensal and "nonpathogenic."[130] Thus, the host with underlying severe disease and impaired host defenses has higher rates of infection, secondary bacteremia, refractory infection, and case fatality.[15,156] As in the example of hematologic cancers, disease and treatment have so devastated the immune system that response is lethargic or nonexistent, infection is poorly controlled, even by appropriate antibiotic therapy, and case mortality is high.[157] Following infection with agents that persist in endogenous sites (e.g., *M. tuberculosis*), significant immune depression may result in reactivation and uncontrolled dissemination. Pathogenicity by nosocomial agents has not been related to the presence of resistant bacteria, but resistance does contribute to difficulty in treatment with conventional drugs. The ecological press of antibiotic use assures the presence of resistant forms available for transmission in the health care setting. At each site, colonization precedes local multiplication and tissue infection.[73,158] Colonization with nosocomial organisms results from alterations in "normal flora" by broad-spectrum therapy, hospitalization, and instrumentation. Colonization is directly related to the organisms' survival ability, ability to adhere to mucosal surfaces and catheters, and organism virulence. Special procedures and devices allow bacteria to be delivered past the superficial barriers and to sustain a milieu important to implantation and multiplication.

8. Patterns of Host Response: Clinical Features and Diagnosis

Patterns of host response to nosocomial infection are those classically described with bacterial disease of the sites involved. As with pathogenesis, clinical features and morbidity are determined by the virulence of the agent, the dose and route of transmission, and the character of the host defense mechanisms.

Signs and symptoms in the compromised host may be altered or reduced. Fever may be low or absent. The site of infection may be unusual, as in the predilection to perirectal abscess in cancer patients.[159]

8.1. Urinary Tract Infection

Infections of the urinary tract account for one third of all nosocomial infections. *E. coli*, *E. faecalis*, and *P. aeruginosa* are the most common causal organisms.[19] Almost all nosocomial urinary tract infections are associated with indwelling bladder catheters or instrumentation, and females, the elderly, and persons with severe underlying illness are at increased risk.[145] The overall risk of bacteriuria in hospitalized patients with indwelling catheters is about 25%. Bacteria gain access to the catheterized bladder by either of two routes. They may migrate from the collection bag or the catheter drainage tube junction, or in the majority of cases, bacteria ascend extraluminally within the periurethral space.[158] Bacteria can adhere to and grow on the inner surface of the catheter, leading to a biofilm that also includes urinary proteins and salts. Bacteria embedded in this biofilm are then less susceptible to antibiotics.[160] Fever in a catherized patient or in a patient with recent urinary tract instrumentation should lead one to suspect urinary tract infection. Greater than 10^5 colony-forming units per milliliter of urine represent significant bacteriuria from a clean-catch midstream urine specimen. In catheterized patients, however, a concentration of microorganisms considerably less than 10^5 can be shown to be progressive in the absence of antimicrobial therapy and can be associated with symptomatic infection.[161] The significance of asymptomatic bacteriuria in patients with indwelling bladder catheters remains under discussion.[93,162]

8.2. Nosocomial Pneumonia

Pneumonia appears frequently in those patients in whom aspiration has taken place or in whom the upper airway is bypassed by endotracheal intubation. The diagnosis of nosocomial pneumonia is difficult to make and often relies on the combination of clinical criteria and microbiological data. Purulent sputum, pulmonary infiltration on X ray, fever, and hypoxia may indicate the presence of this complication. In individuals with community-acquired pneumonia, a change in microbial flora in the sputum accompanied by a worsening in clinical course usually indicates a pulmonary superinfection. Culture and Gram's or other staining of the sputum, transtracheal aspirate, endotracheal aspirate, or percutaneous lung aspirate are essential to the establishment of etiologic diagnosis.[48,56,96] Organisms simultaneously isolated from the blood and pleural fluid are strong evidence of pulmonary infection with that agent.

8.3. Surgical Site Infection

Infection of the surgical site is suspected in any febrile postoperative patient. Drainage of purulent material or disruption of the wound are considered prima facie evidence of wound infection with or without bacterial isolates. Unfortunately, up to 60% of surgical site infections are not evident until after the patient is discharged from the hospital.[95] Following certain procedures involving implantation of a prosthesis or other foreign material, infection may not be evident for months.

8.4. Bacteremia

Bacteremia is usually accompanied by fever and a decline in clinical condition. In the absence of evidence of infection at other sites, an intravenous source of infection should be suspected. Intravascular catheters in place for more than 48 hr should be investigated, even in the absence of inflammation. Blood cultures, cultures of infusates, and semiquantitative cultures of the catheter itself may establish the diagnosis.[163]

8.5. Infection at Other Sites

Nosocomial infection of the skin, soft tissue, gastrointestinal tract, urogenital tract, and other sites is frequently found. A detailed discussion of the appearances, diagnosis, and treatment of the more common and the less common infections has been published.[164]

9. Control and Prevention

9.1. General Concepts

The methods for conducting a successful nosocomial infection control program are outlined in Table 6 and paraphrase the classic scientific method. Identification of nosocomial infections through application of standard

Table 6. Elements of Nosocomial Infection Control

1. Elaborate criteria for infection
2. Establish surveillance
3. Determine endemic rates
4. Evaluate endemic problems
5. Recognize and control epidemic
6. Effect control program
   a. Orientation
   b. In-service education
   c. Behavior modification
7. Evaluate control programs
8. Evaluate cost benefit

criteria is widely accepted. Routine, continuous collection, collation, evaluation, and reporting of these data by a trained nursing specialist using "surveillance" tools are recommended and have been tested for efficacy by the CDC during the SENIC Project.[28] The presence of the nurse practitioner on the clinical unit is also of value in: (1) reinforcing the importance of infection control measures; (2) providing early identification of epidemics; (3) providing informal, concurrent, in-service education; and (4) assisting in providing new information for research efforts in the area of nosocomial risk control. The presence of one of these infection control practitioners (ICP) for approximately every 250 inpatient beds was important to efficacy, as measured by the evaluation models in this study, as was the presence of a trained hospital epidemiologist. The expense of this methodology has been of concern, but the SENIC evaluation estimated an approximate 6-to-1 benefit-to-cost ratio in its application, and alternative reporting methods have been of low efficiency, poor specificity, and slow to recognize outbreaks.[21,29,51,52] Evaluation of institutional nosocomial data through these techniques has allowed identification of priority infection problems and planning, implementation, and evaluation of interventions to control them. Control programs usually fall into three areas: preventive engineering, equipment control, and personnel programs.

9.1.1. Preventive Engineering. A careful review of engineering plans for nosocomial risk should be undertaken before construction or reconstruction is begun. Guidelines have been published by some state and national agencies,[165,166] including guidelines on engineering controls for preventing airborne spread of bacteria.[167] Efficient function follows appropriate form in the hospital as in other industries. If hand-washing sinks are present and conveniently placed in patient care areas, it is more likely that they will be used. Traffic flow will be determined by design and will be difficult to alter by placing signs thereafter. Control of environmental bacterial contamination will be affected by surface features, air-conditioning, and the convenient presence of housekeeping and other service modules.

9.1.2. Equipment Control. As with structure, the design of equipment is important to its correct use, maintenance, and disinfection. Initially inexpensive devices may multiply future costs by requiring complicated disassembly, cleaning, and time-consuming disinfection in order to render them safe for multiple patient use. Component parts may not tolerate heat sterilization and may require gas or chemical sterilization. Gas and chemical sterilization are more demanding in detail and may leave residuals that present toxic problems.[146] The use of disposable equipment has exploded in the hospital industry, contributing to major increases in cost and in problems of waste disposal. Reuse of disposable equipment on individual patients, under strict protocols, has been found acceptable in a few limited situations (e.g., hemodialyzer reuse).[42,48,168] However, attempts to modify this expense by reuse of disposable equipment on multiple patients have been responsible for several outbreaks of nosocomial infection and are to be decried.[105] Intrinsic contamination of industrially prepared medical devices and supplies has been a rare cause of epidemic nosocomial outbreaks and has usually been associated with and identified by the unique bacteria involved.[100,153] Routine sterility testing of commercially prepared products is tedious, difficult to control, and usually of insufficient benefit-to-cost to be justified.

9.1.3. Personnel Programs. Health care personnel are the common final factor in the transmission of most nosocomial infections. Orientation and in-service education programs are important in gaining staff appreciation of infection control programs and techniques. The direct availability of the ICP during on-the-ward surveillance activities provides important one-on-one education and consultation in support of bedside infection control. Behavior modification through management techniques of observation, retraining, and the use of incentives and penalties is recommended and under expanding use as effective infection control efforts.[169] Occupational health programs, which assure that health care workers are screened for transmissible diseases on employment and have the opportunity to have subsequent illnesses evaluated for potential transmission, are also an important feature of control of animate reservoirs.[170]

9.2. Special Control Programs

9.2.1. Hand Washing. Routine hand washing before, between, and after contact with patients is recognized as the most important feature of successful infection control. The use of an antiseptic soap is recommended in high-risk areas and when vancomycin-resistant enterococcus is isolated,[61] but otherwise is of little documented improvement over the routine use of a vigorous scrub with soap and running water. The use of gloves does not replace the need for hand washing. Extensive reviews of hand-washing procedures and guidelines have been published.[42,152,17,172]

9.2.2. Standard Precautions and Isolation Control. Techniques for the recognition and appropriate care of patients with potentially communicable disease have been recommended in a guideline published by the CDC.[173] The recognized inability to identify accurately all such individuals on admission and the potential for health care worker exposure to HIV and other blood-borne disease(s) have led to the recommendation that a modified method of care be used for all patients with whom there is expected to be contact with blood or body fluids. This system of "universal precautions" or "universal blood and body fluid precautions" recommends the use of gloves in any patient care situation where such contact is expected and the additional use of gown, mask, and eye protection where splashing, aerosolization, or more extensive exposure is common.[174]

When appropriately used and expanded to all potentially infectious body fluids, universal, precautions are reported both to increase patient protection from all nosocomial infection except those transmitted by the airborne route and at the same time to protect the health care worker from occupational exposure. The misuse of gloves—not changing between patients and not hand washing—has been implicated in the transmission of infection between patients.[175] Major concerns in changing to this new "isolation" system included issues of risk, retraining, efficacy, availability of materials (gloves), and cost. The appropriate and concurrent use of these two barrier systems, in order to optimize both patient care and worker protection, has been intensely debated and has led to a new set of isolation guidelines.

The new isolation system proposed by the CDC is expected to both simplify and improve the efficacy of isolation precautions.[173] There are two tiers to the new isolation system. The first tier is referred to as *standard* precautions and is to be used for the care of all patients, regardless of diagnosis. Standard precautions incorporate the major features of both universal precautions and body substance isolation and are designed to reduce the risk of transmission of organisms, including blood-borne pathogens, to patients and health care workers. The second tier, referred to as *transmission-based* precautions, includes airborne precautions, droplet precautions, and contact precautions. These precautions are designed for the care of specific patients infected or colonized with epidemiologically significant organisms that are spread by the airborne or droplet route or by contact with dry skin or contaminated environmental surfaces. These precautions are to be used in addition the standard precautions.

An important feature of all barrier isolation programs has been the recognition that isolation is frequently over-restrictive, so that it interferes with patient care, and that a significant portion of isolation needs are satisfied by hand washing and very modest geographic groupings. It has been estimated that over 90% of the isolation used in hospitals is inappropriately restrictive, adding significantly to patient hospital costs.[176]

Protective isolation, a form of isolation designed to protect noninfected patients with seriously impaired resistance to infection from exposure to potentially infective microorganisms, remains a disputed entity in the control of nosocomial infection. Limited protective isolation of the hospitalized immunocompromised patient has not been demonstrated to reduce nosocomial infections significantly. It is estimated that 80–90% of the infections in these patients are from endogenous sources. However, approximately half the bacteria involved in these infections have come from nosocomial colonization. Total protective environments using sterilized food, filtered laminar-flow units, and prophylactic intestinal and systemic antibiotics have been unable to decontaminate the human being effectively.[177] These environments have achieved some reduction of infection in patients, but their contribution to increased longevity has been minimal. These procedures are complicated by high levels of side effects and prohibitive cost.

9.2.3. Epidemic Investigation and Control. The routine collection of surveillance data on nosocomial infections allows one to establish endemic rates by type of nosocomial infection, by organism, and by area and service within the medical facility. This allows rapid recognition of unusual or epidemic events, whether through the appearance of a new or highly resistant microorganism or through a grouping of similar infections. An outline of an epidemic investigation is given in Table 7. The careful documentation and reporting of epidemic investigations are important features in every infection control program.[178]

9.2.4. Nosocomial Urinary Tract Infection. About 80% of documented nosocomial urinary tract infections are associated with catheter use. The use of a closed sterile drainage system with indwelling catheters provides a significant (50%) short-term reduction in infection related to

Table 7. Outline of Epidemic Investigation[a]

1. Establish the existence of an epidemic
2. Complete case count
3. Make analysis of pertinent characteristics
4. Form hypothesis
5. Test hypothesis
6. Institute control measures
7. Evaluate control measures
8. Document and report

[a]Adapted from a CDC training pamphlet.[178]

this device.[179] Appropriate care in the placement and maintenance of these devices is essential to their success in preventing nosocomial infection.[158] Breaks in aseptic technique in placement and disruption and entry into the closed system are the most significant factors in the development of catheter-related urinary tract infection.[180] Guidelines for the control of nosocomial urinary tract infection have been developed and published by the CDC.[181] An outline for catheter use and care is seen in Table 8.[182] In the SENIC project analysis, the combination of high levels of surveillance activity, a modest level of control activity, and the presence of a full-time ICP yielded an estimated 31% reduction of infection in patients at high risk for this event.[28]

9.2.5. Nosocomial Surgical Site Infection. Nosocomial surgical site infections are usually initiated at the time of surgery.[183–185] The responsible microorganisms originate either from the patient's endogenous flora, from operating room personnel, or from the operating room environment. Guidelines featuring the etiology and control of surgical site infections have been reviewed and published by the CDC.[186] Debate over the importance of airborne bacterial contamination of surgical sites continues,[187,188] and most modern operating rooms use air-filtration systems. However, a large cooperative study failed to correlate reduction in airborne levels of bacteria with reduced infection rates in most operations.[94] In a more recent cooperative study of certain high-risk operations (e.g., placement of artificial hip joint), improvement in bacterial air quality appeared to be associated with a reduction in surgical site infections.[189] This has led some investigators to advocate even stricter air-quality standards, including the use of special exhaust headgear and laminar-flow air systems.[190]

Cruse and Foord,[115] in a large study of nosocomial surgical site infections, reduced their clean wound rates to 1% or less. They report the most important factors in the control of surgical site infection as being: (1) the length of preoperative stay, (2) the type of preoperative skin care, including avoidance of shaving, (3) meticulous surgical technique, and (4) the dissemination of surgeon-specific nosocomial surgical site infection data to all surgeons. Analyses of the SENIC project by the CDC support these findings, especially the success of reporting surgical site infection rates to individual surgeons.[28]

The routine use of prophylactic antibiotics just prior to selected surgical procedures has been well studied and supported by a growing number of investigations. Prophylactic antibiotics are meant to decrease microbial proliferation at the incision site. The timing of prophylactic antibiotics is crucial in determining efficacy in preventing surgical site infections. The optimum time for administration has been shown to be in the 2-hr period before the incision.[191] Antibiotic prophylaxis is recommended for clean-contaminated procedures and clean procedures involving the implantation of a foreign body. Several reviews of these recommendations have been published.[192–194] General guidelines for the approach to surgical prophylaxis are reviewed in Table 9.

9.2.6. Nosocomial Respiratory Infections. Attention to the details of disinfection of various respiratory assistance devices and the use of careful technique and sterile equipment in the suctioning of the endotracheal

Table 8. Guidelines for Urinary Catheter Use[a]

1. Do not use unless necessary
2. Use aseptic techniques
3. Use sterile closed drainage system
4. Maintain system closed
5. Keep bag below level of bladder, but not on floor
6. Culture aseptically
7. Discontinue early
8. Sanitize measuring devices after each use

[a]Modified from Hustinx and Verbrugh.[182]

Table 9. Guidelines for Perioperative Antibiotic Prophylaxis[a]

1. Clean-contaminated procedure or clean procedure with foreign body
2. Antibiotic spectrum effective
3. Effective concentrations of antibiotic present at incision time
4. Use single dose regimen—additional intraoperative dose for lengthy procedure
5. Use low-toxicity regimen
6. Avoid antibiotic critical to therapy
7. Benefits should outweigh risk

[a]Modified from Page *et al.*[193]

tree are emphasized as important in the reduction of nosocomial respiratory infection.(96,143,195) Prevention of contamination of humidification devices by routine and frequent disinfection and the use of sterile water have contributed to this control.(137,144) Specific details and background for these methods are outlined in another of the CDC guidelines.(48) Data from the SENIC project suggest that a high level of surveillance and the presence of an ICP were a necessary feature for the 27% reduction in postoperative pneumonia reported. Reductions in medical pneumonia appeared much less successful. Some studies have suggested that specific methods or therapies that maintain or reduce microorganisms to a low level in the stomach are associated with lower risk of nosocomial aspiration and pneumonia.(196) Other studies have failed to show similar benefits, and thus there are no current recommendations to routinely use selective decontamination of the digestive tract as a method for preventing nosocomial pneumonia in intensive-care unit patients.(48)

9.2.7. Nosocomial Intravascular Infection. Proper choice of device, correct placement, and careful maintenance of intravenous systems are important in the control of infections at this site.(197) Teflon and polyurethane catheters are associated with lower inflammation and infection rates than are other catheters.(198) While no improvement in infection rate has been associated with the use of antiseptic or antibiotic creams at the skin site in short-term intravenous use, the effectiveness of a detailed maintenance routine with antibiotic creams has been reported for long-term catheterization for central venous nutrition.(199) Care in prevention of contamination of the delivery system is important as is the documentation of the appropriate use of additives through dating and labeling. New guidelines for the prevention of nosocomial intravascular infections have been prepared by the CDC.(200) Important features for intravenous care are outlined in Table 10.

Table 10. Guidelines for Intravenous Device Use[a]

1. Do not use unnecessarily
2. Choose a low-risk site
3. Use good technique
   a. Wash hands
   b. Use aseptic prep and fixation
   c. Date site
   d. Label appropriately
4. Maintain appropriately:
   a. Discontinure emergent site early
   b. Observe daily
   c. Change set no more frequently than every 72 hr
5. Remove early
6. With sepsis, suspect iv site

[a]Modified from CDC guidelines.(200)

9.2.8. Antimicrobial Prophylaxis. The routine prophylactic use of antibiotics has not been demonstrated to control nosocomial infections in most sites and situations. The use of prophylactic antibiotics for surgical procedures is discussed in Section 9.2.5.

Prophylactic antibiotics, in the form of selective digestive decontamination, have been studied in the prevention of nosocomial pneumonia. Selective digestive decontamination regimens usually include systemic antibiotics combined with topical, nonabsorbable antibiotics in the oropharynx and stomach. Decreased rates of carriage of gram-negative bacilli in the upper and lower airways have been demonstrated, along with decreased rates of nosocomial pneumonia. However, mortality was not affected in most studies.(48,201)

Routine bathing of the newborn with hexachlorophene-containing soaps for control of staphylococcal colonization and nursery infection is no longer recommended. Cutaneous absorption of hexachlorophene has been demonstrated, especially in the premature infant. Such absorption has been associated with pathological changes in the brain, and in cases of high dosage, permanent neurological damage and death have ensued.(202)

Triple dye and a number of other compounds successfully inhibit the colonization of the umbilical stump with staphylococci.(203)

Antibiotic prophylaxis in oncology and burn patients, whose severely compromised host defenses allow repeated endogenous infections, is also in limited use and under continued investigation. Prophylaxis is not recommended in most clinical situations for cancer and burn patients. Prophylactic fluoroquinolone administration appears to delay the time to fever and decreases gram-negative infections in neutropenic patients; however, breakthrough infections with gram-positive organisms may occur and the emergence of fluoroquinolone-resistant organisms is of concern. Early treatment following diagnostic microbiological studies remains the suggested therapeutic program. The recognition of a recurrent infection in a compromised patient with a specific organism may justify the use of continued antibiotic prophylaxis specific to that bacterium.

9.2.9. Immunization. Immunization for the prevention of bacterial nosocomial infection has not been exploited, largely due to the lack of effective vaccines.

However, in other institutional situations pneumococcal and meningococcal vaccines have been tested and found successful. Both passive and active immunization for control of nosocomial *Pseudomonas* infections in oncology and burn units have been investigated.[204,205] Passive immunization has been reported to provide limited protection. Active immunization has been reported to reduce infection in some high-risk units.[206,207] Side effects, however, have been significant.

9.2.10. Cellular and Transplantation Methods. Granulocyte transfusions have improved the response to infection in some leukemia patients with increased survival. This technique is limited by lack of sources for sufficient cells and recurrent concern about the ability to ensure their safe use in excluding occult microbial agents. Bone marrow transplantation is an increasingly successful technique, but one that requires great sophistication and resources. It remains apparent that further advances in basic immunology and transplantation will be required before wider success with these procedures is achieved.

Hematopoietic growth factors, such as granulocyte and granulocyte–macrophage colony-stimulating factors, are increasingly being used in neutropenic patients. These growth factors stimulate the bone marrow to produce neutrophils, thereby shortening the duration of neutropenia following chemotherapy. These growth factors are costly and should only be considered for patients with prolonged neutropenia at high risk of infection.

10. Unresolved Problems

10.1. Efficacy and Cost-Benefit Evaluation: Acute Care

The program of surveillance and infection control recommended by the CDC and mandated by governmental and accreditation agencies has benefited in the support offered in the publication of the results of the SENIC project,[28] indicating a 32% overall reduction in nosocomial infection through application of the program. Since the data on which he study was based were gathered in 1970 and 1975–1976, the applicability to hospital practice two decades later remains open to some question. Medical care continues to change at a rapid pace with new technologies and shifts in practice, which have markedly altered the case mix and intensity of services offered in acute hospital care in the United States. As a result, an even higher portion of nosocomial infections may not be preventable by classic CDC methods, especially those from endogenous sources in highly immunocompromised patients.[159] Continued studies on the characteristics of patients in acute care who are at high risk for preventable nosocomial infection are needed.

The analysis of the SENIC data suggested a 6:1 benefit-to-cost ratio for effective CDC-type programs. Changing costs and efficacy in the past decade may have altered this finding, and continued monitoring is important to affirm these data.

The above problems notwithstanding, these programs appear well justified in the competition for resources in acute medical care. These findings must continue to find their way into the medical and administrative discussions that determine program priorities in hospitals.

10.2. Routine Application of Standard Methods

For many infection control procedures (e.g., catheter care programs), no new information is needed. Uniform, correct implementation of such procedures by all individuals involved in patient care would significantly reduce nosocomial infections at these sites. Responsibility here falls most heavily on the senior professional staff. Whether demonstrating careful surgical technique or simple hand washing, leadership through role-modeling and monitoring through acceptance of authority are the key to success. Hospital leadership and administration is being called on to be more involved in the prevention of nosocomial infections, particularly with regards to the emergence and control of antibiotic resistant organisms.[208] Employee health programs are another underused risk-control program in most hospitals.[170] Absence of physician leadership as providers and participants in these programs is frequently responsible for their lack of success.

Where demonstration and persuasion fail to gain compliance, behavior modification through rewards and penalties may be indicated.

10.3. Coordinated Programs

The many common features in nosocomial infection control and other quality improvement programs should be recognized. In US hospitals the quality assessment and improvement programs are commonly thought to include nosocomial infection control, risk management, monitoring of clinical outcomes, and care coordination. These programs are notable in using common data sources, applying common epidemiological methods, implementing similar analysis, sharing similar committee structures, and sharing similar goals of improved quality of patient care largely by avoiding increased nosocomial risk.[209] Many institutions are now attempting to coordinate these programs through shared personnel and mutually derived and exploited computerized databases. The sharing should have a potential for markedly increasing both the efficiencies and effectiveness of these programs.

10.4. Need and Efficacy in Developing Countries

With the exception of the WHO prevalence studies[2] and a few individual reports,[35] data on nosocomial infection risk in the developing countries are not available. Opinions are repeatedly expressed and assumptions made that medical needs in these areas are such that infection control programs are not a potential priority for consideration.

However, the major potential requirement for resources lost to the community in morbidity and mortality from nosocomial illness and in the cost to treat the infectious complications of medical care caused by the relatively inexpensive but often absent tools for sterilization, materials for disinfection, and training in basic aseptic technique would make the basics of infection control appear even more mandatory in these developing countries.

10.5. Efficacy in Nonacute Care

Most studies of nosocomial infections, including the CDC-NNIS, WHO, and CDC-SENIC projects, have taken place in acute-care hospitals. A small but growing number of investigations are being reported in extended care, but these must be separated by type (e.g., rehabilitation, domiciliary, skilled nursing), Nosocomial infection risk in other care settings, including ambulatory care, physician's office, and home care, is in the early stages of being studied and further characterized.[91,129]

10.6. Education

Several professional groups, including the Association for Professionals in Infection Control and Epidemiology, the Hospital Infections Society, and the Society for Healthcare Epidemiology of America, have been organized and are supporting communication and educational efforts in infection control as has the CDC for several decades. Despite this interest, few medical schools, microbiology training programs, infectious disease training programs, or nursing curricula provide material pertinent to nosocomial infection risk and control. Organizational acceptance of responsibility for these areas of education is important to further program success.[210]

Standards for training ICPs, nurse epidemiologists, infection control committee chairpersons, and hospital epidemiologists remain undefined. They continue to be an intense topic of discussion within these professional organizations.

10.7. Technological Standards

Information on standards of construction important to infection control is neither readily available nor widely implemented in hospital architectural planning. Modern facilities are frequently built with no infection control review, resulting in high-risk units that defy or discourage appropriate application of procedures important to the control of nosocomial infection thereafter. Construction standards important to infection control should be formed at a national level and incorporated into planning, much like current fire-control standards. Special programs for hospital architects may assist in achieving this goal.

Medical equipment design and function frequently provide a reservoir for nosocomial bacteria. Design and manufacturing techniques that allow assembly and disassembly for easy disinfection of critical parts between patients or protection of such parts from contamination should be a part of the engineering of all medical devices. Close cooperation between infectious disease consultants and design engineers will be important to this effort.

10.8. Managed Care Programs

Managed care programs are becoming increasingly common in the United States and have grown out of the demand for quality health care at less cost. These programs attempt to optimize the use of health care resources, particularly in the acute-care setting, by balancing cost and care outcomes, such as surgical site infection rates. Noninfectious and infectious outcomes, including nosocomial infection rates, are generally measured and compared between institutions and providers. However, only nosocomial infection data consistently collected using standard definitions and adjusted for intrinsic risk factors can be compared.[24] As managed care programs grow, data collection will need to be standardized and analysis precise in order to make valid judgments regarding cost and outcome of care for individual providers and institutions. Optimizing the quality of health care, as measured in outcomes, while controlling the cost of care continues to be a challenge.

11. References

1. Centers for Disease Control, Nosocomial infection surveillance, 1984, *Morbid. Mortal. Week. Rep.* **35:**17SS–29SS (1986).
2. Tikhomirov, E., WHO programme for the control of nosocomial infections, *Chemoterapia* **6:**148–151 (1987).
3. Haley, R. W., Culver, D. H., White, J. W., *et al.*, The nationwide nosocomial infection rate: A new need for vital statistics, *Am. J. Epidemiol.* **121:**159–167 (1985).
4. Brieger, G. H., Hospital infection: A brief historical appraisal, in: *Handbook on Hospital Associated Infections, I: Occurrence, Diagnosis, and Source of Hospital Associated Infections* (W. J. Fahlberg and D. Groschel, eds.), pp. 1–12, Marcel Dekker, New York, 1978.
5. Toledo-Pereyra, L. H., and Toledo, M. M., A critical study of Lister's work on antiseptic surgery, *Am. J. Surg.* **131:**736–744 (1976).
6. Ravenholt, R. T., History, epidemiology and control of staphylococcal disease in Seattle, *Am. J. Public Health* **11:**1796–1808 (1962).
7. Williams, R. E. O., Changing perspectives in hospital infection, in: *Proceedings of the International Conference on Nosocomial Infections*, pp. 1–10, Centers for Disease Control, Atlanta, 1970.
8. Haley, R. W., Hightower, A. W., Khabbaz, R. F., *et al.*, The emergence of methicillin-resistant *Staphylococcus aureus* infections in United States hospitals: Possible role of the house staff-patient transfer circuit, *Ann. Intern. Med.* **97:**297–308 (1982).
9. Marples, R. R., Mackintosh, C. A., and Meers, P. D., Microbiological aspects of the 1980 national prevalence survey of infections in hospitals, *J. Hosp. Infect.* **5:**172–180 (1984).
10. Zervos, M. J., Kauffman, C. Z., Therasse, P. M., *et al.*, Nosocomial infection by gentamicin-resistant *Streptococcus faecalis*: An epidemiologic study, *Ann. Intern. Med.* **106:**687–691 (1987).
11. Garner, J. S., Jarvis, W. R., Emori, T. G., *et al.*, CDC definitions for nosocomial infections, 1988, *Am. J. Infect. Control* **16:**128–140 (1988).
12. Horan, T. C., Gaynes, R. P., Martone, W. J., *et al.*, CDC definitions of nosocomial surgical site infections, 1992: A modification of CDC definitions of surgical wound infections, *Am. J. Infect. Control* **20:**271–274 (1992).
13. Britt, M. R., Burke, J. P., Nordquist, A. G., *et al.*, Infection control in small hospitals: Prevalence surveys in 18 institutions, *J. Am. Med. Assoc.* **236:**1700–1703 (1976).
14. Gross, P. A., and Van Antwerpen, C., Nosocomial infections and hospital deaths, a case–control study, *Am. J. Med.* **75:**658–662 (1983).
15. Gross, P. A., Neu, H. C., Aswapokee, P., *et al.*, Deaths from nosocomial infection: Experience in a university and a community hospital, *Am. J. Med.* **68:**219–223 (1980).
16. Daschner, F., Nadjem, H., Langmaack, H., *et al.*, Surveillance, prevention, and control of hospital acquired infections. III. Nosocomial infection as cause of death; retrospective analysis of 1000 autopsy reports, *Infection* **6:**261–265 (1978).
17. Hughes, J. M., Nosocomial infection surveillance in the Untied States: Historical perspective, *Infect. Control* **8:**450–453 (1987).
18. Hughes, J. M., Culver, D. H., White, J. W., *et al.*, Nosocomial infection surveillance, 1980–1982, *Morbid. Mortal. Week. Rep.* **32:**(4SS)**:**1SS–15SS (1983).
19. Emori, T. G., and Gaynes, R. P., An overview of nosocomial infections, including the role of the microbiology laboratory, *Clin. Microbiol. Rev.* **6:**428–442 (1993).
20. Sartor, C., Edwards, J. R., Gaynes, R. P., *et al.*, Evolution of hospital participation in the national nosocomial infections surveillance system, 1986–1993, *Am. J. Infect. Control* **23:**364–368 (1995).
21. Wenzel, R. P., Osterman, C. A., and Hunting, K. J., Hospital-acquired infections. III. Infection rates by site, service, and common procedures in a university hospital, *Am. J. Epidemiol.* **104:**645–651 (1976).
22. Hughes, J. M., Setting priorities: Nationwide nosocomial infection prevention and control programs in the USA, *Eur. J. Clin. Microbiol.* **6:**348–351 (1987).
23. Emori, G. T., Culver, D. H., Horan, T. C., *et al.*, National nosocomial infections surveillance system (NNIS): Description of surveillance methods, *Am. J. Infect. Control* **19:**19–35 (1991).
24. Martone, W. J., Gaynes, R. P., Horan, T. C., *et al.*, Nosocomial infection rates for interhospital comparison: Limitations and possible solutions, *Infect. Control Hosp. Epidemiol.* **12:**609–621 (1991).
25. Freeman, J., and McGowan, J. E., Jr., Risk factors for nosocomial infection, *J. Infect. Dis.* **138:**811–819 (1978).
26. Massanari, R. M., Wilkerson, K., Streed, S. A., *et al.*, Reliability of reporting nosocomial infections in the discharge abstract and implications for receipt of revenues under prospective reimbursement, *Am. J. Public Health* **77:**561–564 (1987).
27. Centers for Disease Control, Special issue: The SENIC project, *Am. J. Epidemiol.* **111:**465–653 (1980).
28. Haley, R. W., Culver, D. H., White, J. W., *et al.*, The efficacy of infection surveillance and control programs in preventing nosocomial infections in US hospitals, *Am. J. Epidemiol.* **121:**182–205 (1985).
29. Wenzel, R. P., Osterman, C. A., Hunting, K. J., *et al.*, Hospital acquired infections. I. Surveillance in a university hospital, *Am. J. Epidemiol.* **103:**251–260 (1976).
30. Eickhoff, T. C., Brachman, P. S., Bennett, J. V., *et al.*, Surveillance of nosocomial infections in community hospitals. I. Surveillance methods, effectiveness, and initial results, *J. Infect. Dis.* **120:**306–316 (1969).
31. Laxson, L. B., Blaser, M. J., and Parkhurst, S. M., Surveillance for the detection of nosocomial infections and the potential for nosocomial outbreaks. I. Microbiology culture surveillance is an effective method of detecting nosocomial infection, *Am. J. Infect. Control* **12**(6)**:**318–324 (1984).
32. Parkhurst, S. M., Blaser, M. J., Laxson, L. B., *et al.*, Surveillance for the detection of nosocomial infections and the potential for nosocomial outbreaks. II. Development of a laboratory-based system, *Am. J. Infect. Control* **13**(1)**:**7–15 (1985).
33. Garner, J. S., Bennett, J. V., Scheckler, W. E., *et al.*, Surveillance of nosocomial infections, in: *Proceedings of the International Conference on Nosocomial Infections*, pp. 277–281, Centers for Disease Control, Atlanta, 1970.
34. Wenzel, R. P., Osterman, C. A., Townsend, T. R., *et al.*, Development of a statewide program for surveillance and reporting of hospital acquired infections, *J. Infect. Dis.* **140:**741–746 (1979).
35. Sociedad Española de Hygiene y Medicina Preventiva Hospitalarias, *Proyecto EPINE 1992*, Barcelona, Spain, 1992.
36. Nystrom, B., Hospital infection control in Sweden, *Infect. Control.* **8**(8)**:**337–338 (1987).

37. Mertens, R., Jones, B., and Kurz, X., A computerized nationwide network for nosocomial infection surveillance in Belgium, *Infect. Control Hosp. Epidemiol.* **15:**171–179 (1994).
38. Haley, R. W., Culver, D. H., Morgan, W. M., *et al.*, Increased recognition of infectious diseases in US hospitals through increased use of diagnostic tests, 1970–1976, *Am. J. Epidemiol.* **121:**168–181 (1985).
39. Weinstein, R. A., and Mallison, G. F., The role of the laboratory in surveillance and control of nosocomial infections, *Am. J. Clin. Pathol.* **69:**130–136 (1978).
40. Hansen, L., Kolmos, H. J. J., and Siboni, K., Detection of cumulations of infections in hospitals over a three year period using electronic data processing, *Dan. Med. Bull.* **25:**253–257 (1978).
41. Evans, R. S., Larsen, R. A., Burke, J. P., *et al.*, Computer surveillance of hospital-acquired infections and antibiotic use, *J. Am. Med. Assoc.* **256:**1007–1011 (1986).
42. Garner, J. S., and Favero, M. S., *Guidelines for Handwashing and Hospital Environmental Control, 1985*, Centers for Disease Control, Atlanta, 1985.
43. Maki, D. G., Alvarado, C. J., Hassemer, C. A., *et al.*, Relation of the inanimate hospital environment to endemic nosocomial infection, *N. Engl. J. Med.* **307:**1562–1566 (1982).
44. Mallison, G. F., and Haley, R. W., Microbiologic sampling of the inanimate environment in US hospitals, 1976–1977, *Am. J. Med.* **70:**941–946 (1981).
45. Statement on microbiological sampling in the hospital, Committee on Infections within Hospitals, American Hospital Association, *Hospitals* **48:**125–126 (1974).
46. Vickers, R. M., Lu, V. L., Hanna, S. S., *et al.*, Determinants of *Legionella pneumophila* contamination of water distribution systems: 15-hospital prospective study, *Infect. Control* **8**(9)**:**357–363 (1987).
47. Yu, B. L., Beam, T. R., Lumish, R. M., *et al.*, Routine culturing for *Legionella* in the hospital environment may be a good idea: A three-hospital study, *Am. J. Med. Sci.* **30:**97–99 (1987).
48. Tablan, O. C., Anderson, L. J., Arden, N. H., *et al.*, Guideline for prevention of nosocomial pneumonia, *Am. J. Infect. Control.* **22:** 247–292 (1994).
49. Britt, M. R., Infectious diseases in small hospitals, prevalence of infections and adequacy of microbiology services, *Ann. Intern. Med.* (Part 2) **89:**757–760 (1978).
50. Emori, T. G., Haley, R. W., and Stanley, R. C., The infection control nurse in US hospitals, 1976–1977, *Am. J. Epidemiol.* **111:**592–607 (1980).
51. Bartlett, C. L. R., Efficacy of different surveillance systems in detecting hospital acquired infection, *Chemioterapia* **6:**152–155 (1987).
52. Freedman, J., and McGowan, J. E., Jr., Methodological issues in hospital epidemiology, *Rev. Infect. Dis.* **3:**658–667 (1981).
53. *Outline for Surveillance and Control of Nosocomial Infections*, Centers for Disease Control, Bureau of Epidemiology, Bacterial Diseases Division, Hospital Infections Branch, Atlanta, November 1976.
54. Haley, R. W., Culver, D. H., Morgan, W. M., *et al.*, Identifying patients at high risk of surgical wound infection: A simple multivariate index of patient susceptibility and wound contamination, *Am. J. Epidemiol.* **121:**206–215 (1985).
55. Haley, R. W., Morgan, W. M., Culver, D. H., *et al.*, Update from the SENIC project. Hospital infection control: Recent progress and opportunities under prospective payment, *Am. J. Infect. Control* **13:**97–108 (1985).
56. Meduri, G. U., Ventilator-associated pneumonia in patients with respiratory failure: A diagnostic approach, *Chest* **97:**1208–1219 (1990).
57. Murray, P. R., and Washington, J. A., II, Microscopic and bacteriologic analysis of expectorated sputum, *Mayo Clin. Proc.* **50:**339–344 (1975).
58. Murray, P. R., Baron, E. J., Pfaller, M. A., *et al.* (eds.), *Manual of Clinical Microbiology*, 6th ed., American Society for Microbiology, Washington, DC, 1995.
59. Martone, W. J., Tablan, O. C., and Jarvis, W. R., The epidemiology of nosocomial epidemic *Pseudomonas cepacia* infections, *Eur. J. Epidemiol.* **3:**222–232 (1987).
60. Tenover, F. C., Tokars, J., Swenson, J., *et al.*, Ability of clinical laboratories to detect antimicrobial agent-resistant enterococci, *J. Clin. Microbiol.* **31:**1695–1699 (1993).
61. Hospital Infection Control Practices Advisory Committee, Recommendations for preventing the spread of vancomycin resistance, *Infect. Control Hosp. Epidemiol.* **16:**105–113 (1995).
62. Archer, G. L., and Mayhall, C. G., Comparison of epidemiological markers used in the investigation of an outbreak of methicillin-resistant *Staphylococcus aureus* infection, *J. Clin. Microbiol.* **18:**395–399 (1983).
63. Schaberg, D. R., and Zervos, M. J., Plasmid analysis in the study of the epidemiology of gram-positive cocci, *Rev. Infect. Dis.* **8:** 705–712 (1986).
64. Wachsmuth, K., Molecular epidemiology of bacterial infections: Examples of methodology and investigation of outbreaks, *Rev. Infect. Dis.* **8:**682–692 (1986).
65. Darland, G., Discriminant analysis of antibiotic susceptibility as a means of bacterial identification, *J. Clin. Microbiol.* **2:**391–396 (1975).
66. Maki, D. G., Through a glass darkly: Nosocomial pseudoepidemics and pseudobacteremias (Editorial), *Arch. Intern. Med.* **140:**26–28 (1980).
67. Weinstein, R. A., and Stamm, W. E., Pseudoepidemics in hospitals, *Lancet* **2:**862–864 (1977).
68. Tompkins, L. S., The use of molecular methods in infectious diseases, *N. Engl. J. Med.* **327:**1290–1297 (1992).
69. Patterson, T. F., Patterson, J. E., Masecar, B. L., *et al.*, A nosocomial outbreak of *Branhamella catarrhalis* confirmed by restriction endonuclease analysis, *J. Infect. Dis.* **157**(5)**:**996–1001 (1988).
70. Bannerman, T. L., Hancock, G. A., Tenover, F. C., *et al.*, Pulsed-field gel electrophoresis as a replacement for bacteriophage typing of *Staphylococcus aureus*, *J. Clin. Microbiol.* **33:**551–555 (1995).
71. Barrett, F. F., Casey, J. I., and Finland, M., Infections and antibiotic use among patients at Boston City Hospital, *N. Engl. J. Med.* **278:**5–9 (1968).
72. Ellner, P. D., Fink, D. J., Neu, H. C., and Parry, M. F., Epidemiologic factors affecting antimicrobial resistance of common bacterial isolates, *J. Clin. Microbiol.* **25:**1668–1674 (1987).
73. Johanson, W. G., Jr., Pierce, A. K., Sanford, J. P., *et al.*, Nosocomial respiratory infections with gram-negative bacilli: The significance of colonization of the respiratory tract, *Ann. Intern. Med.* **77:**701–706 (1972).
74. Selden, R., Lee, S., and Wang, W. L. L., Nosocomial *Klebsiella* infections: Intestinal colonization as a reservoir, *Ann. Intern. Med.* **74:**657–664 (1971).
75. Rupp, M. E., and Archer, G. L., Coagulase-negative staphylococci: Pathogens associated with medical progress, *Clin. Infect. Dis.* **19:**231–245 (1994).

76. Mackowiak, P. A., The normal microbial flora, *N. Engl. J. Med.* **307:**83–93 (1982).
77. Crossley, K., Loesch, D., Landesman, B., *et al.*, An outbreak of infections caused by strain of *Staphyloccus aureus* resistant to methicillin and aminoglycosides, *J. Infect. Dis.* **139:**273–279 (1979).
78. Saravolatz, L. D., Pohlod, D. J., and Arking, L. M., Community-acquired methicillin-resistant *Staphylococcus aureus* infections: A new source for nosocomial outbreaks, *Ann. Intern. Med.* **97:**325–329 (1982).
79. Thompson, R. L., Cabezudo, I., and Wenzel, R. P., Epidemiology of nosocomial infections caused by methicillin-resistant *Staphylococcus aureus*, *Ann. Intern. Med.* **97:**309–317 (1982).
80. Centers for Disease Control and Prevention, Nosocomial enterococci resistant to vancomycin, United States, 1989–1993, *Morbid. Mortal. Week. Rep.* **42:**597–599 (1993).
81. Pearson, M. L., Jereb, J. A., Frieden, T. R., *et al.*, Nosocomial transmission of multidrug-resistant *Mycobacterium tuberculosis*, *Ann. Intern. Med.* **117:**191–196 (1992).
82. Hierholzer, W. J., Jr., Streed, S. A., and Rasley, D. A., Comparison of nosocomial infection risk with varying denominators at a university medical center [Abstract], 2nd International Conference on Nosocomial Infections, Centers for Disease Control, Atlanta, 1980.
83. Madison, R., and Afifi, A. A., Definition and comparability of nosocomial infection rates, *Am. J. Infect. Control* **10**(2)**:**49–52 (1982).
84. Rotstein, C., Cummings, K. M., Nicolaou, A. L., *et al.*, Nosocomial infection rates at an oncology center, *Infect. Control* **9**(1)**:**13–19 (1988).
85. Vlahov, D., Tenney, J. H., Cervino, K. W., *et al.*, Routine surveillance for infections in nursing homes: Experience at two facilities, *Am. J. Infect. Control* **15**(2)**:**47–53 (1987).
86. Culver, D. H., Horan, T. C., Gaynes, R. P., *et al.*, Surgical wound infection rates by wound class, operation, and risk index in US hospitals, 1986–90, *Am. J. Med.* **91**(Suppl. 3B)**:**152–157 (1991).
87. Garibaldi, R. A., Biodine, S., and Matsumuya, S., Infections among patients in nursing homes, *N. Engl. J. Med.* **305:**731–735 (1981).
88. Smith, P. W., Infections in long-term care facilities, *Infect. Control* **6**(11)**:**435–441 (1985).
89. Jackson, M. M., and Fierer, J., Infections and infection risk in residents of long-term care facilities: A review of the literature, 1970–1984, *Am. J. Infect. Control* **13**(2)**:**63–77 (1985).
90. McGeer, A., Campbell, B., Emori, T. G., *et al.*, Definitions of infection surveillance in long-term care facilities, *Am. J. Infect. Control* **19:**1–7 (1991).
91. White, M. C., Infections and infection risks in home care settings, *Infect. Control Hosp. Epidemiol.* **13:**535–539 (1992).
92. Hospital Infections Program, National Nosocomial Infections Surveillance (NNIS) Semiannual Report, May 1995, *Am. J. Infect. Control* **23:**377–385 (1996).
93. Platt, R., Polk, B. F., Murdock, B., *et al.*, Mortality associated with nosocomial urinary tract infection, *N. Engl. J. Med.* **307:** 637–642 (1982).
94. Howard, J. M., Chairman Ad Hoc Committee, Postoperative wound infections: The influence of ultraviolet irradiation of the operating room and of various other factors. A report of an ad hoc committee of the Committee on Trauma, Division of Medical Sciences, National Academy of Sciences—National Research Council, *Ann. Surg.* **160**(2)**:**Suppl. (1964).
95. Sherertz, R. J., Chairperson Surgical Wound Infection Task Force, Consensus paper on the surveillance of surgical wound infections, *Am. J. Infect. Control* **20:**263–270 (1992).
96. Pugliese, G., and Lichtenberg, D. A., Nosocomial bacterial pneumonia: An overview, *Am. J. Infect. Control* **15**(6)**:**249–265 (1987).
97. Miller, P. J., and Wenzel, R. P., Etiologic organisms as independent predictors of death and morbidity associated with bloodstream infections, *J. Infect. Dis.* **156:**471–476 (1987).
98. Setia, U., and Gross, P. A., Bacteremia in a community hospital, *Arch. Intern. Med.* **137:**1698–1701 (1977).
99. Stamm, W.E., Martins, S. M., and Bennett, J. V., Epidemiology of nosocomial infections due to gram-negative bacilli: Aspects relevant to development and use of vaccine, *J. Infect. Dis.* **136** (Suppl.)**:**S151–S160 (1977).
100. Maki, D. G., and Martin, W. T., Nationwide epidemic of septicemia caused by contaminated infusion products. IV. Growth of microbial pathogens in fluids for intravenous infusion, *J. Infect. Dis.* **131:**267–272 (1975).
101. Maki, D. G., Goldmann, D. A., and Rhame, F. S., Infection control in intravenous therapy, *Ann. Intern. Med.* **79:**867–887 (1973).
102. Maki, D. G., Control of colonization and transmission of pathogenic bacteria in the hospital, *Ann. Intern. Med.* **89**(Part 2)**:**777–780 (1978).
103. Stamm, W. E., Infection related to medical devices, *Ann. Intern. Med.* **89**(Part 2)**:**764–769 (1978).
104. Stamm, W. E., Colella, J. J., Anderson, M. S., *et al.*, Indwelling arterial catheters as a source of nosocomial bacteremia, *N. Engl. J. Med.* **292:**1099 (1977).
105. Weinstein, R. A., Stamm, W. E., Kramer, L., *et al.*, Pressure monitoring devices, overlooked source of nosocomial infection, *J. Am. Med. Assoc.* **236:**936 (1976).
106. Wenzel, R. P., Thompson, R. L., Landry, S. M., *et al.*, Hospital-acquired infections in intensive care unit patients: An overview with emphasis on epidemics, *Infect. Control* **4**(5)**:**371–375 (1983).
107. Jarvis, W. R., and the Epidemiology Branch, Hospital Infections Program, Nosocomial outbreaks: The Centers for Disease Control's Hospital Infections Program experience, 1980–1990, *Am. J. Med.* **91**(Suppl. 3B)**:**101–106 (1991).
108. Montecalvo, M. A., Horowitz, H., Gedris, C., *et al.*, Outbreak of vancomycin-, ampicillin-, and aminoglycoside-resistant *Enterococcus faecium* bacteremia in an adult oncology unit, *Antimicrob. Agents Chemother.* **38:**1363–1367 (1994).
109. Centers for Disease Control, False-positive blood cultures related to use of evacuated nonsterile blood collection tubes, *Morbid. Mortal. Week. Rep.* **24:**387–388 (1978).
110. Kaslow, R. A., Mackel, D. C., and Mallinson, G. F., Nosocomial pseudobacteremia: Positive blood cultures due to contaminate benzalkonium antiseptic, *J. Am. Med. Assoc.* **236:**2407–2409 (1976).
111. Allen, J. R., Hightower, A. W., Martin, S. M., *et al.*, Secular trends in nosocomial infections: 1970–1979, *Am. J. Med.* **70:**389–392 (1981).
112. Retailliau, H. F., Hightower, A. W., Dixon, R .E., *et al.*, *Acinetobacter calcoaceticus*: A nosocomial pathogen with an unusual seasonal pattern, *J. Infect. Dis.* **139:**371–375 (1979).
113. Gross, P. A., Rapuano, C., Adrignolo, A., *et al.*, Nosocomial infections: Decade-specific risk, *Infect. Control* **4:**145–147 (1983).

114. Welliver, R. C., and McLaughlin, S., Unique epidemiology of nosocomial infections in a children's hospital, *Am. J. Dis. Child.* **138:**131–135 (1984).
115. Cruse, P. J. E., and Foord, R., The epidemiology of wound infection: A 10-year prospective study of 62,939 wounds, *Surg. Clin. North Am.* **60:**27–40 (1980).
116. Patterson, W. B., Craven, D. E., Schwartz, D. A., *et al.*, Occupational hazards to hospital personnel, *Ann. Intern. Med.* **102:**658–680 (1985).
117. Ehrenkrans, J. J., and Kicklighter, J. L., Tuberculosis outbreak in a general hospital: Evidence for airborne spread of infection, *Ann. Intern. Med.* **77:**377–382 (1972).
118. Fisher, B., Yu, B., Armstrong, D., *et al.*, Outbreak of *Mycoplasma pneumoniae* infection among hospital personnel, *Am. J. Med. Sci.* **271:**205–209 (1978).
119. Smith, R. T., The role of a chronic carrier in an epidemic of staphylococcal disease in a newborn nursery, *Arch. Dis. Child.* **95:**461–468 (1958).
120. Ayliffe, G. A. J., and Lilly, H. A., Cross-infection and its prevention, *J. Hosp. Infect.* **6**(Suppl. B)**:**47–57 (1985).
121. Douglas, B. E., Health problems of hospital employee, *J. Occup. Med.* **13:**555–560 (1971).
122. Harrington, J. M., and Shannon, H. S., Incidence of tuberculosis, hepatitis, brucellosis, and shigellosis in British medical laboratory workers, *Br. Med. J.* **1:**759–762 (1976).
123. Daschner, F. D., Frey, P., Wolff, G., *et al.*, Nosocomial infections in intensive care wards: A multicenter prospective study, *Int. Care Med.* **8:**5–9 (1982).
124. Cheesbrough, J. S., Finch, R. G., and Burden, R. P., A prospective study of the mechanisms of infection associated with hemodialysis catheters, *J. Infect. Dis.* **154:**579–589 (1986).
125. Copley, J. B., Prevention of peritoneal dialysis catheter-related infections, *Am. J. Kidney Dis.* **10:**401–407 (1987).
126. Lobo, P. I., Rudolf, L. E., and Krieger, J. N., Wound infections in renal transplant recipients—A complication of urinary tract infections during allograft malfunction, *Surgery 5* **92:**491–496 (1982).
127. Rogers, T. R., Infection complicating bone marrow transplantation: What are the risks and can they be reduced? *J. Hosp. Infect.* **3:**105–109 (1982).
128. Lester, M. R., Looking inside 101 nursing homes, *Am. J. Nurs.* **64:** 111–116 (1964).
129. Goodman, R. A., and Solomon, S. L., Transmission of infectious diseases in outpatient health care settings, *J. Am. Med. Assoc.* **265:**2377–2381 (1991).
130. Burke, J. P., and Hildeck-Smith, G. Y., *The Infection Prone Hospital Patient*, Little Brown, Boston, 1978.
131. van Gravenitz, A., The role of opportunistic bacteria in human disease, *Annu. Rev. Microbiol.* **31:**447–471 (1977).
132. Human immunodeficiency virus infection in the United States: A review of current knowledge, *Morbid. Mortal. Week. Rep.* **36:** (S-6) (1987).
133. McGowan, J. E., Jr., Antimicrobial resistance in hospital organisms and its relation to antibiotic use, *Rev. Infect. Dis.* **5:**1033–1048 (1983).
134. Spach, D. H., Silverstein, F. E., and Stamm, W. E., Transmission of infection by gastrointestinal endoscopy and bronchoscopy, *Ann. Intern. Med.* **118:**117–128 (1993).
135. Chadwick, P., The epidemiological significance of *Psuedomonas aeruginosa* in hospital sinks, *Can. J. Public Health* **67:**323–328 (1976).
136. Favero, M. W., Petersen, N. J., Carson, L. A., *et al.*, Gram-negative water bacteria in hemodialysis systems, *Health Lab. Sci.* **12:**321–334 (1975).
137. Spaepen, M. S., Berryman, J. R., Bodman, H. A., *et al.*, Prevalence and survival of microbial contaminants in heated nebulizers, *Anesth. Analg.* **57:**191–196 (1978).
138. Wenzel, R. P., Veazey, J. M., Jr., and Townsend, T. R., Role of the inanimate environment in hospital acquired infection, in: *Infection Control in Health Care Facilities* (K. R. Cundy and W. Ball, eds.), pp. 71–146, University Park Press, Baltimore, 1977.
139. Newman, K. A., and Schimpff, S. C., Hospital and hotel services as risk factors for infection among immunocompromised patients, *J. Infect. Dis.* **9**(1)**:**206–213 (1987).
140. Helms, C. M., Massanari, R. M., Zietler, R., *et al.*, Legionnaires' disease associated with a hospital water system: A cluster of 24 nosocomial cases, *Ann. Intern. Med.* **99:**172–178 (1983).
141. Marks, J. S., Tsai, T. F., Martone, W. J., *et al.*, Nosocomial Legionnaires' disease in Columbus, Ohio, *Ann. Intern. Med.* **90:**65–659 (1979).
142. Favero, M. S., Carson, L. A., Bond, W. W., *et al.*, *Pseudomonas aeruginosa*: Growth in distilled water from hospitals, *Science* **173:**836–838 (1971).
143. Phillips, J., Spencer, G., *Pseudomonas aeruginosa* cross-infection due to contaminated respiratory apparatus, *Lancet* **2:**1325–1327 (1965).
144. Smith, P. W., and Massanari, R. M., Room humidifiers as the source of *Acinetobacter* infections, *J. Am. Med. Assoc.* **237:**795–797 (1980).
145. Martin, M. A., and Reicheiderfer, M., APIC guideline for infection prevention and control in flexible endoscopy, *Am. J. Infect. Control.* **22:**19–38 (1994).
146. Bruch, C. W., Sterilization of plastics: Toxicity of ethylene oxide residues, in: *Industrial Sterilization* (G. B. Phillips and W. S. Miller, eds.), pp. 49–77, Duke University Press, Durham, NC, 1972.
147. Burke, J. P., Ingall, D., Klein, J. O., *et al.*, *Proteus mirabilis* infections in a hospital nursery traced to a human carrier, *N. Engl. J. Med.* **284:**115–121 (1971).
148. Craven, D. E., Reed, C., Kollisch, N., *et al.*, A large outbreak of infections caused by a strain of *Staphylococcus aureus* resistant to oxacillin and aminoglycosides, *Am. J. Med.* **71:**53–58 (1981).
149. Schaffner, W., Humans, the animate reservoir of nosocomial pathogens, in: *Infection Control in Health Care Facilities* (K. R. Cundy and W. Ball, eds.), pp. 55–70, University Park Press, Baltimore, 1976.
150. Stamm, W. E., Taley, J. C., and Facklam, R. R., Wound infections due to group A *Streptococcus* traced to a vaginal carrier, *J. Infect. Dis.* **138:**287–292 (1978).
151. Korten, V., and Murray, B. E., The nosocomial transmission of enterococci, *Curr. Opin. Infect. Dis.* **6:**498–505 (1993).
152. Doebbeling, B. N., Stanley, G. L., Sheetz, C. T., *et al.*, Comparative efficacy of alternative hand-washing agents in reducing nosocomial infections in intensive care units, *N. Engl. J. Med.* **327:**88–93 (1992).
153. Maki, D. G., Control of colonization and transmission of pathogenic bacteria in the hospital, *Ann. Intern. Med.* **89**(Part 2)**:**777–780 (1978).
154. Graham, D. R., Anderson, R. L., Ariel, F. E., *et al.*, Epidemic nosocomial meningitis due to *Citrobacter diversus* in neonates, *J. Infect. Dis.* **144:**203–209 (1981).
155. Speck, W. T., Driscoll, J. M., Polin, R. A., *et al.*, Staphylococcal

and streptococcal colonization of the newborn infant, *Am. J. Dis. Child.* **131:**1005–1008 (1977).

156. Britt, M. R., Schluepner, C. J., and Matsumiyu, S., Severity of underlying diseases as a predictor of nosocomial infections: Utility in the control of nosocomial infection, *J. Am. Med. Assoc.* **239:**1047–1051 (1978).
157. Schimpff, S. C., Therapy of infection in patients with granulocytopenia, *Med. Clin. North Am.* **61:**1101–1118 (1977).
158. Garibaldi, R. A., Burke, J. P., Dickman, M. L., *et al.*, Factors redisposing to bacteriuria during indwelling urethral catheterization, *N. Engl. J. Med.* **291:**215–219 (1974).
159. Schimpff, S. C., Young, V. M., Greene, W. H., *et al.*, Origin of infection in acute nonlymphocytic leukemia, *Ann. Intern. Med.* **77:**707–714 (1972).
160. Nickel, J. C., Ruseska, I., Wright, J. B., *et al.*, Tobramycin resistance of *Pseudomonas aeruginosa* cells growing as a biofilm on urinary catheter material, *Anitmicrob. Agents Chemother.* **27:**619–624 (1985).
161. Stark, R. P., and Maki, D. G., Bacteriuria in the catheterized patient: What quantitative level of bacteriuria is relevant? *N. Engl. J. Med.* **311:**560–564 (1984).
162. Boscia, J. A., Abrutyn, E., and Kaye, D., Asymptomatic bacteriuria in elderly persons: Treat or do not treat? *Ann. Intern. Med.* **106:**764–766 (1987).
163. Maki, D. G., Weise, C. E., and Sarafin, H. W., A semi-quantitative method for identifying intravenous catheter-related infection, *N. Engl. J. Med.* **296:**1305–1309 (1977).
164. Bennett, J. V., and Brachman, P. S. (eds), *Hospital Infections*, 3rd ed., Little Brown, Boston, 1992.
165. Connecticut Public Health State Code and Other Department Regulations, Chapter 4, Infection Control, pp. 205–206 (Sect. 19-13-D3), January 1983.
166. The American Institute of Architects Committee on Architecture for Health with assistance from the US Department of Health and Human Resources, *Guidelines for Construction and Equipment of Hospital and Medical Facilities*, The American Institute of Architects Press, Washington, DC, 1993.
167. US Department of Health and Human Services, *Proceedings of the Workshop on Engineering Controls for Preventing Airborne Infections in Workers in Health Care and Related Facilities*, National Institute for Occupational Safety and Health, Cincinnati, July 1993.
168. Alter, M. J., Reuse of hemodialyzers. Results of nationwide surveillance for adverse effects, *J. Am. Med. Assoc.* **260:**2073–2076 (1988).
169. Axnick, K. J., and Yarbrough, M. (eds.), *Infection Control: An Integrated Approach*, Mosby, St. Louis, 1984.
170. American Occupational Medical Association Committee on Medical Center Employee Occupational Health, Robert Lewy, Chairman, Committee report, Guidelines for employee health services in health care institutions, *J. Occup. Med.* **28:**518–523 (1986).
171. Larson, E., Guideline for use of topical antimicrobial agents, *Am. J. Infect. Control* **16**(6)**:**253–266 (1988).
172. Sproat, L. J., and Inglis, T. J. J., A multicentre survey of hand hygiene practice in intensive care units, *J. Hosp. Infect.* **26:**137–148 (1994).
173. Garner, J. S., Guideline for isolation precautions in hospitals, *Infect. Control Hosp. Epidemiol.* **17:**53–80 (1996).
174. Centers for Disease Control, Recommendations for prevention of HIV transmission in health-care settings, *Morbid. Mortal. Week. Rep.* **36:**3S–18S (1987).
175. Patterson, J. E., Vecchio, J., Pantelick, E. L., *et al.*, Association of contaminated gloves with transmission of *Acinetobacter calcoaceticus* var. *anitratus* in an intensive care unit, *Am. J. Med.* **91:**479–483 (1991).
176. Hyams, P. J., and Ehrenkranz, N. J., The overuse of single patient isolation in hospitals, *Am. J. Epidemiol.* **196:**325–329 (1977).
177. Pizzo, P. A., and Levine, A. S., The utility of protected environment regimens for the compromised host: A critical assessment, *Prog. Hematol.* **10:**311–332 (1977).
178. Centers for Disease Control, Training Pamphlet 00-023, *Outline of Procedure in Investigation and Analysis of an Epidemic*, Centers for Disease Control, Atlanta, January 1974.
179. Kunin, C. M., and McCormick, R. C., Prevention of catheter-induced urinary tract infections by sterile closed drainage, *N. Engl. J. Med.* **274:**1155–1161 (1966).
180. Warren, J. W., Platt, R., Thomas, R. J., *et al.*, Antibiotic irrigation and catheter associated urinary tract infection, *N. Engl. J. Med.* **299:**570–573 (1978).
181. Wong, E. S., and Hooton, T. M., *Guidelines for Prevention of Catheter-associated Urinary Tract Infections*, Centers for Disease Control, Atlanta, October 1982.
182. Hustinx, W. N. M., and Verbrugh, H. A., Catheter-associated urinary tract infections: Epidemiological, preventive and therapeutic considerations, *Int. J. Antimicrob. Agents* **4:**117–123 (1994).
183. Kluge, R. M., Calia, F. M., McLaughlin, J. S., *et al.*, Sources of contamination in open heart surgery, *J. Am. Med. Assoc.* **230:**1415–1418 (1974).
184. Nichols, R. L., Techniques known to prevent postoperative wound infection, *Infect. Control* **3**(1)**:**34–37 (1982).
185. Polk, H. C., Prevention of surgical wound infection, *Ann. Intern. Med.* **89**(Part 2)**:**770–773 (1978).
186. Garner, J. S., *Guidelines for Prevention of Surgical Wound Infections*, Centers for Disease Control, Atlanta, 1985.
187. Howorth, F. H., Prevention of airborne infection during surgery, *Lancet* **1:**386–388 (1985).
188. Ravitch, M. M., and McAuley, C. E., Airborne contamination of the operative wound, *Surg. Gynecol. Obstet.* **159:**177–178 (1984).
189. Lidwell, O. M., Lowbury, E. J. L., Whyte, W., *et al.*, Effects of ultraclean air in an operating room on deep sepsis in the joint after total hip or knee replacement: A randomised study, *Br. Med. J.* **285:**10–14 (1982).
190. Franco, J. A., Baer, J., and Enneking, W. F., Airborne contamination in orthopedic surgery: Evaluation of laminar air flow system and aspiration suit, *Clin. Orthop.* **122:**231–234 (1977).
191. Classen, D. C., Evans, R. S., Pestotnik, S. L., *et al.*, The timing of prophylactic administration of antibiotics and the risk of surgical-wound infection, *N. Engl. J. Med.* **326:**281–286 (1992).
192. Waldvogel, F. A., Vaudeaux, P. E., Pittet, D., *et al.*, Perioperative antibiotic prophylaxis of wound and foreign body infections: Microbial factors affecting efficacy, *Rev. Infect. Dis.* **13**(Suppl. 10)**:**S782–S798 (1991).
193. Dellinger, E. P., Gross, P. A., Barrett, T. L., *et al.*, Quality standard for antimicrobial prophylaxis in surgical procedures, *Clin. Infect. Dis.* **18:**422–427 (1994).
194. Platt, R., Methodologic aspects of clinical studies of perioperative antibiotic prophylaxis, *Rev. Infect. Dis.* **13**(Suppl. 10)**:**S810–814 (1991).
195. Favero, M. S., Chairman Committee on Microbial Contamination of Surfaces, Proposed microbiologic guidelines for respiratory therapy equipment and materials. A report of the Committee on

Microbial Contamination of Surfaces, Laboratory Science, American Public Health Association, *Health Lab. Sci.* **15**:177–179 (1978).

196. Tryba, M., Risk of acute stress bleeding and nosocomial pneumonia in ventilated intensive care unit patients: Sucralfate versus antacids, *Am. J. Med.* **83**(3B):117–124 (1987).
197. Mermel, L. A., Prevention of intravascular catheter-related infections, *Infect. Dis. Clin. Pract.* **3**:391–398 (1993).
198. Maki, D. G., and Ringer, M., Risk factors for infusion-related phlebitis with small peripheral venous catheters, *Ann. Intern. Med.* **114**:845–854 (1991).
199. Goldman, D. A., and Maki, D. G., Infection control in total parenteral nutrition, *J. Am. Med. Assoc.* **233**:1360–1364 (1973).
200. Pearson, M. L., and Hospital Infection Control Practices Advisory Committee, Guideline for prevention of intravascular device-related infections, *Infect. Control Hosp. Epidemiol.* **17**(7):438–473 (1996).
201. Craven, D. E., Steger, K. A., and Barber, T. W., Preventing nosocomial pneumonia: State of the art and perspectives for the 1990s, *Am. J. Med.* **91**(Suppl. 3B):44S–53S (1991).
202. Kimbrough, R. D., Review of recent evidence of toxic effects of hexachlorophene, *Pediatrics* **51**(Suppl.):391–394 (1973).
203. Johnson, J. D., Malachowski, N. C., Vosti, K. L., *et al.*, Sequential study of various modes of skin and umbilical care and the incidence of staphylococcal colonization and infection in the neonate, *Pediatrics* **58**:354–361 (1976).
204. Morrison, A. J., Jr., and Wenzel, R. P., Epidemiology of infections due to *Pseudomonas aeruginosa*, *Rev. Infect. Dis.* **6**(Suppl. 3):S627–S642 (1984).
205. Pollack, M., Antibody activity against *Pseudomonas aeruginosa* in immune globulins prepared for intravenous use in humans, *J. Infect. Dis.* **147**:1090–1098 (1983).
206. Fisher, M. W., Development of immunotherapy for infections due to *Pseudomonas aeruginosa*, *J. Infect. Dis.* **130**(Suppl.):S149–S151 (1974).
207. Young, L. S., Meyer, R. D., and Armstrong, D., *Pseudomonas aeruginosa* vaccine in cancer patients, *Ann. Intern. Med.* **79**:518–527 (1973).
208. Goldmann, D. A., Weinstein, R. A., Wenzel, R. P., *et al.*, Strategies to prevent and control the emergence and spread of antimicrobial-resistant microorganisms in hospitals, *J. Am. Med. Assoc.* **275**:234–240 (1996).
209. Hierholzer, W. J., Jr., The practice of hospital epidemiology, *Yale J. Biol. Med.* **55**:225–230 (1982).
210. Eickhoff, T. C., Standards for hospital infection control, *Ann. Intern. Med.* **89**(Part 2):829–831 (1978).
211. Ayliffe, G. A. J., Brightwell, K. M., Collins, B. J., *et al.*, Surveys of hospital infection in the Birmingham region, *J. Hyg.* **79**:299–314 (1977).
212. Egoz, N., and Michaeli, D., A program for surveillance of hospital-acquired infections in a general hospital: A two-year experience, *Rev. Infect. Dis.* **3**:649–657 (1981).
213. Stamm, W. E., Guidelines for prevention of catheter-associated urinary tract infections, *Ann. Intern. Med.* **83**:386–390 (1975).

12. Suggested Reading

Bennett, J. V., and Brachman, P. S. (eds.), *Hospital Infections*, 4rd ed., Little Brown, Boston, 1998.

Wenzel, R. P. (ed.), *Prevention and Control of Nosocomial Infections*, 2nd ed., Williams & Wilkins, Baltimore, 1993.

Mayhall, C. G. (ed.), *Hospital Epidemiology and Infection Control*, Williams & Wilkins, Baltimore, 1996.

CHAPTER 26

Pertussis

Edward A. Mortimer, Jr.

1. Introduction

Bordetella pertussis produces a single disease syndrome in man known as pertussis or whooping cough. Affecting children primarily, it characteristically displays a protracted course measured in weeks, with the development of vigorous paroxysmal coughing often associated with vomiting that sometimes results in inanition and occasionally with brain damage. At the turn of the century, it was a major cause of infant mortality worldwide. Largely due to immunization, it is presently of less consequence in developed countries such as the United States, but continues to be a major child health problem in developing nations.

2. Historical Background

The first recorded description of the disease dates from the 16th century.(1) Its absence from prior literature is curiously unexplained for a disease syndrome with such characteristic symptoms. Perhaps it attracted less attention than more devastating epidemic diseases such as plague and smallpox(1) or it may have been a disease of lower animals that became adapted to man.(2) It also has been suggested that the smaller, isolated populations of the past and little contact among them could not maintain an organism with no carrier state or animal vector but productive of clinical immunity.(3) Identification and isolation of culture of the responsible organism did not occur until the first part of this century.(4) Because of poor understanding of the organism's biological anatomy as well as difficulties in propagation, attempts to develop effective vaccines were unsuccessful until the late 1930s. In the United States, whole, killed bacterial vaccines appeared to be of sufficient efficacy to warrant licensure and general use in young infants in the 1940s. Current federal regulations for vaccine production were established in 1953.(5)

Mortality from pertussis in the United States and other developed nations has declined throughout this century, even before the development and widespread use of pertussis vaccine and antimicrobial drugs.(6–8) Further decreases in death rates have occurred subsequently; the decline prior to the vaccine is not satisfactorily explained (see Section 5.1). But the fact that a decrease in mortality rates antedated widespread use of pertussis vaccine caused some authorities to question the necessity for the vaccine as a routine preventive measure for children,(9) particularly since the vaccine displays undesirable reactivity.

Edward A. Mortimer, Jr. • Department of Epidemiology and Biostatistics, Case Western Reserve University School of Medicine, Cleveland, Ohio 44106-4945.

3. Methodology

3.1. Sources of Mortality Data

In the United States and other developed nations, the only sources of mortality information are published vital statistics. Case-fatality rates are inaccurate because the disease is underreported.(10,11) In addition, it is likely that an uncertain proportion of fatal cases are incorrectly diagnosed as other types of bronchopulmonary infections. Nonetheless, mortality rates reflect the occurrence of pertussis more accurately than do other measures currently available.

3.2. Sources of Morbidity Data

Determination of the precise incidence of pertussis in the United States and elsewhere is not presently possible for four reasons. First, the disease is often not reported.

Second, the diagnosis may often be missed. Third, it is clear that there are mild unrecognized forms of the disease, especially in older children and adults with waning immunity. Fourth, a syndrome that is clinically indistinguishable from true pertussis may be produced occasionally by two other *Bordetella* species: *B. parapertussis* and *B. bronchiseptica*. Additionally, certain adenoviruses or other viruses may produce the syndrome,[12–14] although it is possible that in some way pertussis causes reactivation of these infections. Therefore, except during clear-cut, laboratory-confirmed outbreaks in defined populations, estimates of the incidence of pertussis are unreliable, because nearly 90% or more cases are not reported.[10] Recently Sutter and Cochi[11] employed a unique method to estimate the true incidence of hospitalizations for pertussis in the United States. The technique utilized two independent reporting systems, and, in brief, estimated the number of cases that actually occurred by determining the number of cases reported to both systems and those reported only to one or the other. In this way it was possible to estimate the number of cases missed by both methods and to develop an overall estimate by summating the data. Using this approach, it was concluded that the number of hospitalizations for pertussis in the United States, during 1985–1988, was more than 13,000, three or four times the numbers identified by either of the two reporting systems alone. Because this approach considered only hospitalized cases, which are likely to be reported because of their severity, undoubtedly many more cases, usually milder, occurred. Using a similar approach, these authors also estimated that approximately one third of all deaths due to pertussis, during 1985–1988, were unreported. Nonetheless, mortality rates, although of less-than-optimum precision, are the best indicators of changes in incidence. It should be recognized, however, that mortality rates may not reflect the true incidence of pertussis in all age groups because of the inverse relationship of case-fatality rates to age.[14]

3.3. Surveys

Surveys to determine proportions of the population immune to pertussis are of limited value for the reasons noted above and, in addition, because of failure to recall the disease or prior immunization and the lack of a serological test that has been shown to correlate with clinical protection.[15] In the past, household surveys were used to determine the incidence during outbreaks.

3.4. Laboratory Diagnosis

Most clinicians consider absolute lymphocytosis of 10,000 or more lymphocytes/mm^3 to be strong circumstantial evidence of pertussis in a child with appropriate symptoms. The magnitude of lymphocytosis roughly parallels the severity of the cough. However, in very young infants lymphocytosis may be absent. Additionally, disease-induced lymphocytosis may be reduced in previously immunized persons because of the presence of antibodies to pertussis toxin (PT), which is responsible for the lymphocytic response.

The single, time-tested, unequivocal diagnostic test for pertussis is isolation of the organism on culture from a nasopharyngeal swab[10] or, perhaps preferably, nasopharyngeal wash.[16] The usual medium for isolation of this fastidious, slow-growing organism is either modified Bordet–Gengou agar enriched with 15% defibrinated sheep blood or Regan–Lowe medium containing horse blood. Swabs should be inoculated immediately; delay of as little as 1 hr reduces the likelihood of recovery of the organisms. When inoculation must be delayed, Stuart's transport medium may be employed, although this is less satisfactory than direct inoculation. The addition of methicillin or cephalexin to the culture medium appears to enhance the likelihood of recovery of *B. pertussis* by suppressing the growth of other organisms. Cultures should be incubated at 35°C in moist air and examined daily for 5 days, preferably by a bacteriologist skilled in the recognition of *B.pertussis*. Colonies are small and pearly and display a small zone of hemolysis on blood-containing media. Further identification of colonies may be achieved by agglutination with commercially available sera or by direct immunofluorescence.

In experienced hands, identification by culture is nearly 100% specific; unfortunately, the sensitivity of culture methods is far less even in experienced hands. Fresh media are required, and after the fourth week of illness, recovery of the organism is much less likely. Other factors that reduce the likelihood of recovering the organism on culture include prior administration of erythromycin, past pertussis immunization, delays in transport to the laboratory, and increasing age.[17] Additionally, currently most clinical bacteriology laboratories lack experience in the identification of *B. pertussis* on culture due to the relative infrequency of the disease.

Examination of direct smears from nasopharyngeal swabs by direct immunofluorescence (DFA) appears in some but not all studies to be approximately as sensitive as culture, but unfortunately in most laboratories lacks optimum specificity. Observers may disagree on the interpretation of the same slide,[18] and overdiagnosis by the inexperienced may lead to needless, expensive treatment and prophylaxis and unwarranted concern. However, in very experienced hands, with careful quality control, DFA testing appears to be not only as sensitive but also as specific as culture.[17] DFA testing may be of maximum use during outbreaks, when false-positives are less frequent. The DFA method also has the advantage of rapidity of results compared to culture.

In recent years, considerable efforts have been made to develop more sensitive and specific means for the identification of *B. pertussis* in respiratory secretions. These efforts were in part stimulated by the need to differentiate pertussis from other respiratory infections during clinical field trials of new pertussis vaccines. A promising approach is the polymerase chain reaction (PCR), which has been employed in the diagnosis of other infections due to hard-to-recover organisms.[19–21] In brief, this technique identifies gene sequences unique to the organism in question. For detection, the method requires very few organisms in the specimen and therefore is highly sensitive. To date it appears that PCR is more sensitive than culture and more specific than DFA for the diagnosis of pertussis. To date, however, it is available only as a research tool.

Better, though as yet incomplete, identification of the antigens of *B. pertussis* and their relation to disease in man offer promise not only of means for assessment of immunity but also for recognition of infection by serological methods.[22–25] For the present, these serological methods are of utility for pertussis vaccine research but are impractical and too costly for routine use (see Section 4).

4. Biological Characteristics of the Organism

Bordetella pertussis is a small, poorly staining, gram-negative organism that appears in coccobacillary form on fresh isolation. Older cultures display pleomorphism, ranging from filamentous forms to larger bacilli. It can be distinguished from *B. parapertussis* and *B. bronchiseptica* by various biochemical characteristics and immunofluorescence.

Colonies of freshly isolated strains of *B. pertussis* comprise morphologically homogeneous coccobacilli ("smooth" colonies), and the organisms display full virulence in experimental animals such as the mouse or in the hamster tracheal tissue culture model. Such virulent strains are designated phase I organisms; on repeated passage in culture, certain biological characteristics associated with virulence are lost. The so-called "rough" strains are designated as phases II, III, and IV, in order of decreasing virulence. For vaccine production, phase I strains are preferred.

A major problem in understanding the disease and its epidemiology and in developing an optimum vaccine has been that the biological anatomy of the organism in relation to man has been difficult to determine precisely. Although a multiplicity of cellular antigens of *B. pertussis* has been identified, those responsible for the various manifestations of the disease, for clinical immunity, and for the apparent reactivity of the current relatively crude whole-cell vaccine are only now being defined. Indeed, it is not clear whether the immunologically protective and toxic antigens are the same or different. Table 1 lists some of the identified somatic antigens and biological activities of *B. pertussis*.

From what is known of the biological activities of several of these antigens, it is possible to hypothesize about their roles in disease pathogenesis.[3,26,27] Of prime interest is what has now been variously called pertussis toxin (PT), pertussigen, or lymphocytosis-promoting factor (LPF). This component of the organism has been shown to be a complex protein that contains LPF, the histamine-sensitizing factor, and the insulin-stimulating factor and others. PT appears to participate in the pathogenesis of pertussis at several stages by enhancing attachment of the organism to respiratory cilia, interfering with host defenses, and causing cell toxicity. Antibodies to PT can be measured serologically following immunization or natural disease, including mild or inapparent infections.[22]

Filamentous hemagglutinin (FHA) appears to partic-

Table 1. Major Components of *B. pertussis*, Their Actions, and Their Putative Roles in Pertussis

Component	Physiologic actions	Pathogenetic role	Role in immunity
Pertussis toxin (pertussigen, LPF)	Lymphocytosis promotion Histamine sensitization Insulin stimulation Mitogenicity	Attachment to cilia Cell toxicity	Major antigen
Filamentous hemagglutinin	None known	Probably facilitates attachment to cilia	Probably contributes
Agglutinogens	None known	None known	Possible
Adenylate cyclase	Compromises cell metabolism	Compromises bacterial killing	Possible
Endotoxin	Many	Probably none in pertussis	Probably none
Tracheal cytotoxin	Toxic to respiratory epithelium	Possible cell toxicity	Probably none
Heat-labile toxin	Dermonecrotic and lethal in animals	Unknown	Probably none
69K protein	None known	Unknown	Possible

ipate with PT in facilitating attachment of the organism to respiratory cilia; whether it has other activities in relation to humans is unclear. Measurable antibodies to FHA develop following immunization and the disease, including mild or asymptomatic infection, as with PT.[3,22]

Strains of *B. pertussis* can be serotyped and studied epidemiologically by heat-labile K agglutinogens, antibodies to which can be measured serologically in humans. Among the three species of the genus *Bordetella*, 14 such agglutinogens have been identified; those designated 1 through 6 are unique to *B. pertussis*. Agglutinogens 1, 2, and 3 are those most commonly identified.[27] Whether these agglutinogens play a role in disease pathogenesis is uncertain. A question of major importance is whether clinical efficacy of pertussis vaccine may depend, at least in part, on correspondence between the agglutinogens of other characteristics of vaccine strains and those of the strain(s) of *B. pertussis* circulating in the community.[28,29]

Adenylate cyclase is a component of the organism, largely somatic, that contributes to overcoming host defenses and, perhaps more importantly, facilitates cellular damage by inducing wasteful cell hypermetabolism.[26] Whether antibodies to adenylate cyclase, which is antigenic, contribute to clinical immunity is unknown. There are several other components of *B. pertussis* that may well play roles in disease pathogenesis.[3,26,27] Among these are tracheal cytotoxin, which probably damages tracheal and bronchial epithelium, and a heat-labile toxin that is dermonecrotic or lethal and cytotoxic for bronchial epithelium in animal models. Antibodies to an outer-membrane protein, originally designated 69K from its molecular weight and now called pertactin, may play a role in clinical immunity.[30,31] Antibodies to this antigen appear following natural disease and pertussis immunization. Whether these and other cellular components of the organism participate in disease pathogenesis in humans as well as in the development of immunity is unknown at present. It should be noted that IgG, IgM, and IgA antibodies to these antigens arise from pertussis disease; immunization induces IgG and IgM but not IgA responses.[32] This phenomenon may compromise the efficacy of pertussis vaccines because of the presumed importance of secretory IgA in preventing respiratory colonization.

5. Descriptive Epidemiology

The epidemiology of pertussis has been strikingly modified by immunization. However, even prior to widespread immunization in highly developed countries such as the United States and currently in less developed countries, pertussis has displayed distinctive epidemilogical characteristics.

5.1. Prevalence and Incidence

Pertussis is a reportable disease. Because it is very contagious and is associated with high mortality in infants and young children, it is important to make every effort to establish the diagnosis and report probable and proven cases to local health authorities. As noted above (Section 3.2), pertussis is vastly underreported, for the reasons that the diagnosis is often missed, medical care may not be sought, and some physicians may not be convinced of the importance of reporting. Since the disease is underreported, case-fatality rates have been difficult to determine. In 1992, 1993, and 1994, respectively, 4,083, 6,586, and 4,617 cases of pertussis were reported in the United States.[33] There has been an increase in reported cases in the past decade. Indeed, for the 10 years, 1985–1994, 40,789 cases were reported in the United States compared to 18,223 for the 10 years, 1975–1984. This more than two fold increase is too great to be accounted for by population growth. Figure 1 shows the morbidity and mortality rates for pertussis, 1922–1990, and Fig. 2 portrays the increase in cases and incidence rates 1980–1991 as reported to two different surveillance systems.[34] How much this increase is an artifact attributable to augmented reporting because

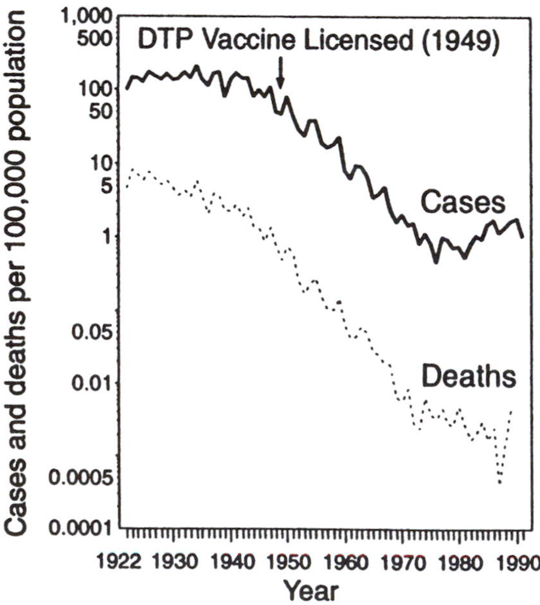

Figure 1. Reported incidence of pertussis and deaths attributed to pertussis, United States, 1922–1991.[34]

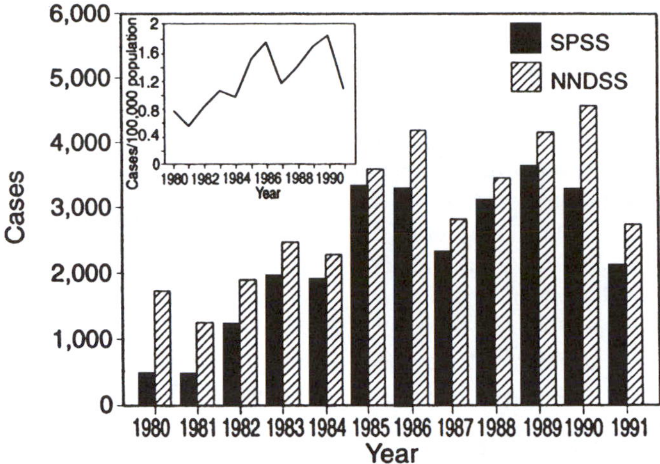

Figure 2. Cases and incidence of pertussis, United States, 1980–1991, as reported to two different but overlapping surveillance systems, the National Notifiable Diseases Surveillance System (NNDSS) and the National Supplementary Pertussis Surveillance System (SPSS).[34]

of better diagnostic procedures, enhanced awareness due to the alleged risks of pertussis vaccine being dramatically portrayed in public media, or other factors is unclear. It does not appear that parental refusal to accept pertussis vaccine for their children because of fears of reactions has played a measurable role. This change in reported cases is remarkable in that the incidence in persons 15 years and older has increased proportionately more than in young children (Fig. 3).[34] However, reported mortality from pertussis in the United States has been low in recent years; during the 10 years, 1983–1992, 56 deaths (none in 1991) from pertussis were recorded in the United States.[33,35]

Although it is clear that case-fatality rates from pertussis are inversely related to age, precise rates are difficult to determine, largely because of underreporting of the disease. Moreover, mortality rates in the developed world decreased in this century independent of immunization or any other form of specific intervention.[6,8,36,37] Direct evidence of the decline in mortality is limited to areas with optimum reporting of cases as well as deaths, such as Providence, Rhode Island,[38] where case-fatality rates steadily declined from 1.36% in 1930–1934 to 0.24% in 1945–1949. Unfortunately, most information related to age-specific case-fatality rates is derived from children

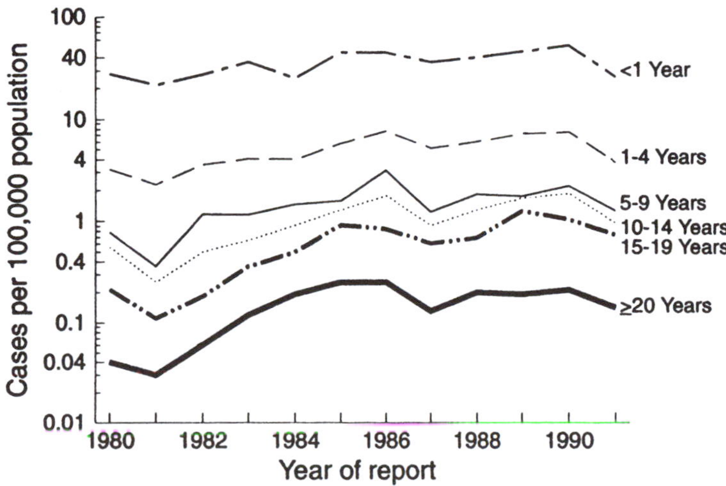

Figure 3. Age-specific incidence rates of reported cases of pertussis, United States, 1980–1991.[34]

hospitalized with pertussis and thus is subject to the biases of such data. However, because almost everyone born in the first half of this century experienced the disease during childhood, the decline in pertussis mortality in the developed world must be attributed to a decrease in case-fatality rates. For example, in the United States, annual deaths attributed to pertussis in children less than 1 years of age were 4.34/1000 for the years 1900–1904; for 1935–1939, before specific measures such as immunization and antimicrobial therapy were developed, the annual death rate in this age group had declined 70% to 1.30/1000.[8] The reasons for this decline are unclear, but may be a consequence of a number of factors. These include better nutrition, the decline of debilitating conditions such as diarrheal diseases that compromised survival, quarantine of recognized cases, better supportive care, and decreasing birth rates that resulted in proportionately fewer infants being exposed to affected older siblings. There is little doubt that in the last decade the remarkable technology available in intensive care units has resulted in the survival of the majority of infants critically ill with pertussis, many or most of whom would have otherwise succumbed. However, in less developed parts of the world, pertussis persists as a major cause of infant mortality. In 1994, the World Health Organization (WHO) estimated that 400,000 of the 104 million children born annually in developing countries die of this preventable disease prior to their fifth birthdays.[39]

5.2. Epidemic Behavior and Contagiousness

In the absence of immunization, essentially no child escapes pertussis.[15] Indeed, during both World War I and World War II, pertussis, in contrast to other childhood contagious diseases, was rarely seen in military personnel, suggesting high prevalence of naturally acquired immunity.[38] Secondary attack rates in susceptible family members may reach 90% or more,[15,40] and have been recorded as 100% in some studies.[14] There is, however, some suggestion that mild atypical cases occur in fully susceptible children.[38] Few data from the pre-vaccine era exist regarding transmission in school settings. However, one study examined an outbreak in an elementary school in Rochester, New York.[41] Excluding children with a past history of pertussis and those with exposure to a sibling with the disease at home, 40 (42%) of 95 school-exposed children developed the disease. Among presumably susceptible children, rates of whooping cough were higher in the lower grades, indicating that some of the older children had experienced forgotten or unrecognized infections in the past. In the United States, pertussis has been both an endemic and an epidemic disease. Since the widespread use of vaccine, large-scale outbreaks are unusual, but local or regional outbreaks continue to occur as in Cincinnati,[42] Chicago,[43] Canada,[21,28] and elsewhere.[44,45] Additionally, institutional outbreaks occur.[46–48]

5.3. Geographic Distribution

The distribution of pertussis is worldwide, though clearly modified by immunization and other poorly defined social, economic, and nutritional factors. The number of cases of pertussis occurring worldwide cannot be estimated with accuracy. Reported incidence rates vary among different nations; the low incidence in some countries may represent poor case reporting, herd immunity from preceding outbreaks, or high levels of immunization. The highest rates occur in those developing countries where immunization programs are inadequate. However, as measured by death rates from pertussis, the incidence must be declining as a consequence of the Expanded Programme on Immunization (EPI).[49]

5.4. Temporal Distribution

Pertussis is both endemic and epidemic. Outbreaks occur at any time, but are perhaps more frequent in the summer. At present in the United States there is a tendency for endemic and epidemic pertussis to be reported more often in summer and early fall months.[44] In the past this was believed to be due to increased contacts between young children during warmer months. However, different seasonal patterns have been reported from various countries.[50] In the past, year-to-year variations occurred, with outbreaks every 2 or 3 years; in isolated areas, intervals of relative freedom from pertussis sometimes extended for 5 or 6 years.[38] This cycle of changes in rates approximately every 3 years continues, even in areas with high vaccine coverage, although rates are much lower.[44]

5.5. Age

In recent years there has been a noticeable shift in the age distribution of reported cases of pertussis, probably largely due to widespread use of pertussis vaccine and the advent of mandatory immunization before school entry. For the years 1935–1939, prior to the availability of pertussis vaccine, data from ten states indicated that for whites about half of all cases of pertussis were reported in 5- to 14-year-old children[6]; for blacks this proportion was lower (20 to 40%), with the preponderance of cases occurring before 5 years. Less than 15% of cases in whites occurred before 1 year of age, but the proportion of cases in infancy among blacks was nearly twice that in whites, probably for socioeconomic reasons.[6] The proportion of reported cases in persons 15 years and older was less than 2% in the late 1930s.[6]

Widespread use of pertussis vaccine during the past four decades has been associated with a marked decline in reported cases and with a striking shift in the proportions of cases in various age groups. For the years 1992–1993, 42% of cases were reported in infants, 20% in children 1 to 4 years old, and about 20% in children 5 to 14 years old.[33,51] In contrast, 17% of cases were reported in persons 15 years and older. Undoubtedly, the paucity of cases in school-age children reflects the impact of school immunization laws, which do not affect younger children. The increased proportion of cases in persons 15 years and older may be an artifact of better diagnosis and enhanced reporting or waning immunity (see Section 7.2).

5.6. Sex

Although both sexes are presumably equally affected, pertussis is unusual in that, inexplicably, the disease is more often reported in females, who also exhibit higher mortality rates. It may be that the smaller larynx of female infants places them in greater jeopardy of severe disease.

5.7. Race

Death rates are higher in blacks[6]; it is likely that these higher rates are attributable to socioeconomic and other factors, rather than to race.

5.8. Other Factors

Mortality rates are higher in lower socioeconomic groups, probably because of exposure earlier in life due to crowding and close contact. But case-fatality rates are also inversely related to socioeconomic status for reasons that are unclear,[13] and access to health care though nutrition may play a role. In contrast to many infectious diseases, mortality from pertussis has been higher in rural than in urban areas.[38]

6. Mechanisms and Routes of Transmission

Pertussis is transmitted via close contact by droplets. It is highly contagious; indeed, up to 90% of susceptible family contacts will develop clinical disease from an index case in the household.[40,52–56] There is no evidence of spread by other routes, such as airborne droplet nuclei, fomites, or dust. The disease appears to be most contagious during the catarrhal stage (the first week of symptoms) and declines so that, as the paroxysmal cough begins to wane, infectivity disappears. An important unanswered question is whether pertussis can be transmitted by individuals without overt disease, because it is likely that individuals immunized in young childhood ultimately experience a mild, clinically unrecognizable disease in adolescence or young adulthood, and thus may serve as a source of exposure. There is, however, no evidence of a carrier state.

7. Pathogenesis and Immunity

7.1. Pathogenesis

The pathogenesis of the disease, better defined in recent years, comprises attachment of the organism to tracheal and bronchial cilia with loss of function and ultimate destruction. Tissue invasion does not occur. The cough appears to be due to interference with normal mechanisms of bronchial toilet; mucoid secretions accumulate and are responsible for ineffective, repetitive, paroxysmal coughing and, ultimately, for varying degrees of bronchial obstruction, atelectasis, and bronchopneumonia.[56] Bronchopneumonia is the most frequent serious complication of pertussis. It most often results from invasion by nonspecific respiratory flora; uncommonly, pneumococcal lobar pneumonia or invasion by *B. pertussis* itself may occur. Among 3826 persons in the United States requiring hospitalization for pertussis and its complications during the years 1989–1991, 1096 (29%) had radiologically diagnosed pneumonia.[34]

A major complication of pertussis is encephalopathy, varying in manifestations from short-lived convulsions to intractable seizures, coma, and permanent cerebral damage.[8,14] The mechanism of pertussis encephalopathy is unclear. The assumption that encephalopathy results from the direct effects of one or more of the toxins of *B. pertussis* no longer appears tenable, and instead it is likely that anoxia and, in some instances, cerebral hemorrhages are responsible.

The experience of contagious disease hospitals and institutions for the handicapped in the past indicate that pertussis encephalopathy is far from rare,[14,57,58] but few data are available. One estimate may be derived from cases reported from the contagious disease hospital that served residents of Brooklyn, New York, in the 1930s.[59]

The childhood population of Brooklyn can be approximated from birth records and, assuming that every child in Brooklyn experienced pertussis, the incidence of severe encephalopathy was approximately 1 in 22,000 cases. A more precise estimate was made by the British National Childhood Encephalopathy Study (NCES),[(60)] from which the frequency was about 1 in 11,000 cases. During 1989–1991 in the United States, among 3826 individuals (mostly children) reported as hospitalized with pertussis, 153 exhibited seizures and 12 were diagnosed as having encephalopathy.[(34)] However, because of considerable underreporting of the disease, the rates of these complications in the general population cannot be determined at present in the United States.

7.2. Immunity

Clinical pertussis is followed by long-lasting immunity. Although occasional anecdotal reports of second attacks in adults have appeared, because of lack of laboratory confirmation, it is not clear whether these episodes represented true second attacks.[(38)] In recent years, however, several well-documented series of pertussis in adults have been reported.[(23–25,61–64)] In many instances these illnesses are mild and atypical. It appears, however, that pertussis in adults is more common than formerly appreciated and may occur in persons who experienced the disease in the past as well as in those who were actively immunized as children.[(48)] Whether the disease is more frequently recognized in adults at present or whether there is an actual increase in rates in older persons is uncertain. If there is a true increase, it is tempting to hypothesize that immunity, whether induced by pertussis or by the vaccine, has been more apt to wane in recent decades due to the present infrequency of exposure to the disease and the consequent lack of repeated, casual "streetcar" boosters.[(64)] Whatever the reason, it is apparent that pertussis in adolescents and young adults is a problem of some importance, particularly because such persons may constitute a reservoir of infection and a source of transmission to others, including young infants.[(23,61,63,64)]

The mechanisms of clinical immunity to pertussis have escaped definition for many years, and only in the last decade has much progress been made. This progress has resulted from laboratory studies that have defined much better the components of the organism and from new methods of measuring antibodies serologically. Several antigens have been identified that appear to be important in the pathogenesis of pertussis and in addition induce antibodies, one or more of which may provide clinical protection against the illness (see Section 4). One of these is PT, which appears to be the major antigen that produces immunity in the mouse protection test, long used for laboratory evaluation and standardization of pertussis vaccine. FHA also may be important not only in disease pathogenesis but also for induction of clinical immunity. FHA is thought to facilitate attachment of *B. pertussis* to respiratory cilia. The agglutinogens may relate to the induction of clinical immunity as well; three of them appear to be of consequence. Their relation to disease pathogenesis is uncertain, but general studies in the past have suggested correlation between clinical immunity and levels of antibody against agglutinogens.[(40)] Further, there is some indication that a mismatch between the specific agglutinogens in pertussis vaccine and those of circulating *B. pertussis* strains is associated with diminished vaccine efficacy.[(28)]

There is a probable role for secretory IgA-mediated immunity, which is expected following natural disease but not immunization.[(32)] The role of cellular immunity in man is uncertain.[(65)]

8. Patterns of Host Response

8.1. Clinical Features

The incubation period of clinical pertussis is usually 7–10 days, and rarely longer than 2 weeks. The first week or two of the illness is called the catarrhal stage, because initial symptoms of the disease are nonspecific, including mild but gradually increasing cough, nasal symptoms suggestive of a cold, slight fever, and some anorexia.

As the catarrhal stage progresses, the cough increases so that severe spells of coughing with the characteristic whoop appear about 2 weeks after onset, marking the beginning of the paroxysmal stage. The paroxysmal cough results from inability to expel tenacious mucus; the whoop is created by vigorous inspiration through the glottis at the end of the paroxysm. Paroxysms may occur repeatedly and may be initiated by eating, drinking, talking, crying, examination of the throat, or even by hearing another individual cough (such as occurs on a hospital division where there are other children with pertussis). During paroxysms, cyanosis may occur. Repetitive post-paroxysmal vomiting may be sufficiently prolonged in young infants to result in inanition, and tetany in infancy has been attributed to alkalosis from repeated emesis. Fever is usually low and may be throughout the course of pertussis in the absence of secondary infection. Subconjunctival and cerebral hemorrhages and epistaxis may be seen. Convulsions, with or without encephalopathy, and pulmonary complications occur during the paroxysmal stage.

In classic pertussis, the duration of the paroxysmal whooping stage is 4 or more weeks, with increasingly frequent paroxysms for 1 to 2 weeks and gradual subsidence and ultimate disappearance of the whoop thereafter. However, cough may persist for some weeks beyond the paroxysmal stage, and exacerbations may occur if an intercurrent respiratory infection occurs. Mortality from pertussis is inversely related to age. The case-fatality rate in very young infants (less than 3 months) may be as high as 50%; after 5 years of age, it is negligible.

The major causes of mortality appear to be pulmonary complications and encephalopathy, but the relative contributions of each are unsatisfactorily defined. In the past in the United States, secondary or intercurrent affections, such as otitis media, mastoiditis, inanition, and diarrhea, undoubtedly contributed to mortality and continue to do so in developing countries.

Permanent neurological sequelae from pertussis, especially from pertussis in infancy, undoubtedly occur.[57,59,60] More subtle intellectual or behavioral abnormalities also may result in some instances.[58,66] Long-term pulmonary damage has not been described,[67,68] although such might be expected in the future, given the success of modern technology in maintaining infants through the course of severe acute pulmonary disease.

8.2. Diagnosis

The diagnosis of the full-blown pertussis syndrome is readily made on clinical grounds by most clinicians who have had experience with the disease. The protracted course, paroxysmal coughing, and whoop are unmistakable. A history of exposure or knowledge of other cases in the area is of help.

Immediate support for the diagnosis of pertussis may frequently be obtained from the leukocyte count. Absolute lymphocytosis, often striking, parallels the severity of the cough, but is said to be less characteristic in young infants.[13]

A definitive diagnosis may be established in two ways. First, recovery and identification of *B. pertussis* by culture of respiratory secretions is definitive (see Section 3.4). However, isolation on culture is not easily accomplished. Identification of the organism in respiratory secretions by fluorescent-antibody techniques is compromised by frequent false-positive tests[10,18] and may be less sensitive. As noted above (Section 3.4), the PCR method is more sensitive and specific but is not readily available. Second, a rise in agglutinating or complement-fixing antibodies by testing acute and convalescent sera is of use retrospectively; unfortunately, such serological testing is not available for routine use. In recent years the efficacy of serological testing for the diagnosis of pertussis has been considerably improved by testing paired acute and convalescent sera by enzyme-linked immunosorbent assays (ELISA).[10,23] Using this technique, antibody responses to PT, FHA, pertactin, and agglutinogens of *B. pertussis* can be measured, and the method appears to be highly sensitive and specific.[10,23,32,47,69] Although IgM responses to infection (and immunization) occur, the rise and fall of these responses is usually too rapid to be of diagnostic utility. Potential limitations of the ELISA method include failure to recognize an IgG response in a previously immunized individual, because the rapidity of anamnestic responses may result in a rise in IgG antibodies before the acute serum is obtained. In such instances, infection may be recognized by a primary IgA response, because IgA antibodies are not induced by immunization.[32] It also has been shown that single convalescent ELISA serum antibody levels that exceed the mean of a control population by three standard deviations are of diagnostic value when timely acute serum samples were not obtained.[22–24,47] Treatment of pertussis with erythromycin appears to have little or no effect on antibody responses.[70] The fact that there is no serological test or other surrogate measure that has been shown to reflect clinical immunity to pertussis with precision has necessitated controlled field trials of new pertussis vaccines in which the outcome variable is clinical pertussis. Because the manifestations of pertussis vary in severity and occur in other respiratory infections, because microbiological diagnostic precision is not optimum, and because what are significant disease-related antibody rises is subject to disagreement and further may be obscured by high titers from prior immunization, it is desirable to establish case definitions for the diagnosis that permit comparisons among studies. This laudable goal has not yet been met. Additionally, two or more sets of definitions that range from indicating maximum probability of pertussis to less probability have seemed desirable. The strictest criteria obviously reflect high specificity but less sensitivity, thus undoubtedly excluding some cases of pertussis.[71,72] More liberal definitions provide high sensitivity but less specificity and would include more cases of pertussis but also more cases of pertussislike syndromes of other causation.

As examples of case definitions for field trials that differ among authorities, the WHO has recommended 21 or more days of paroxysmal cough plus one or more of the following: a positive culture; a significant rise in IgA or IgG antibodies to FHA, PT, or agglutinogens 2 and 3; or household exposure to a culture-positive case within 20 days before or after disease onset in the subject in question. In contrast, for purposes of surveillance, the Centers for Disease Control and Prevention (CDC) has defined pertussis clinically as increasingly severe cough for 2 or more weeks plus one or more of the following: Paroxysms followed by apnea or cyanosis, posttussive emesis or whoop, subconjunctival hemorrhage, or a lymphocyte count of 15,000 or more.

An approach that used four different categories of diagnostic precision was employed in a controlled field trial of two acellular pertussis vaccines in Sweden.[73] The strictest definition (category 1) required a positive culture and cough of any duration. The second category included cough of any duration with serological but not bacteriologic confirmation. Category 3 included cases with cough of more than 7 days that was spasmodic or associated with whoop or emesis without laboratory confirmation but with direct epidemiological linkage to a culture-proven case. Category 4 included cases with more than 21 days of cough with whoop but without positive laboratory or epidemiological evidence. The analysis included vaccine efficacy in these categories individually and in combination. The more recent clinical field trials of pertussis vaccines of varying composition have employed diagnostic criteria used in these studies that, in general, will have been sufficiently similar to permit comparisons.

9. Control and Prevention

In the absence of widespread immunization, outbreaks of pertussis cannot be prevented and control is difficult. Rates of transmission to susceptible households may be 90% or higher; in classroom situations, up to 50% of susceptible students in the same room may acquire the disease following exposure to an infected child (see Section 5.2).

9.1. Isolation

Isolation or quarantine of children with clinical whooping cough is of limited value in controlling spread of the disease, for the reason that children in the catarrhal stage, before the characteristic whoop appears, are quite infectious.

To prevent transmission, recognized cases should be excluded from school and contact with other children for approximately 4 weeks after the onset of the paroxysmal stage. Transmission after that time is very unlikely. The carrier state in pertussis has not been demonstrated; if such exists, it is doubtful that it plays an important role in transmission. Milder forms of the disease, which occur in partially immune individuals, probably play a role in transmission (see Section 6).

9.2. Antibiotics

Pertussis is relatively insusceptible to antimicrobial therapy clinically. Although the organism is susceptible *in vitro* to various antimicrobial drugs effective against gram-negative organisms, such as ampicillin, streptomycin, chloramphenicol, the tetracyclines, and erythromycin, these therapeutic agents do not modify the full-blown disease. Most of them will reduce the length of time to 4 or 5 days during which the organism can be recovered from patients with clinical pertussis. Erythromycin appears to be the most efficacious of these agents.[70,74,75]

Erythromycin may prevent or ameliorate the disease in nonimmune, exposed individuals prior to the onset of symptoms and perhaps has some effect early in the catarrhal stage. The earlier the drug is administered to such individuals, the more likely is success. By the time the patient is well into the catarrhal stage or has begun to whoop, benefit is not expected. Because exposure is often unrecognized and because the disease is rarely suspected during the catarrhal stage, antibiotics do not comprise a satisfactory approach to disease control.

9.3. Passive Immunization

Passive protection of exposed, susceptible individuals was attempted in the past with varying results. In the late 1930s, convalescent and hyperimmune sera were administered to susceptible children exposed within the same household. In one small controlled study, protection appeared to be as high as 70%.[76] Subsequently, pertussis IgG, prepared from human or rabbit sera, was employed with negative results.[77] Whether passive immunization is useless or whether there is protective serum antibody in fractions other than IgG is unknown. Cellular immunity may play a role in protection. More recently, reports from Sweden and Japan have indicated that human hyperimmune globulin containing anti-FHA and anti-PT effectively ameliorated the course of pertussis.[78,79] Studies of the use of this preparation in prophylaxis are not yet available. No preparation for passive immunization is currently available in the United States.

9.4. Active Immunization

Prior to World War I, ill-controlled, hit-or-miss attempts were made to develop an effective pertussis vaccine with inconclusive or uninterpretable results. Studies of the forerunner of the present whole-cell vaccine against pertussis were initiated in the 1930s. By the mid-1940s, in the United States, whole-cell killed pertussis vaccine was widely used, and current criteria for standardization of the vaccine in the United States were established in 1953 by federal regulation. At present in the United States, it is recommended that children receive three injections of pertussis vaccine combined with diphtheria and tetanus toxoids (DTP) adsorbed onto an aluminum salt at 2, 4, and 6 months of age, followed by booster doses of this triple combination at 12 to 18 months and prior to school entry.[80–82]

There is little question that most properly immunized children are protected against pertussis on exposure.[27,82] However, the proportion of children actually protected when intimately exposed, such as in the home, is less than 100%,[83] although the severity of the disease is previously immunized children is usually mild. Estimates of vaccine efficacy in studies of exposed immunized and unimmunized children vary remarkably because of differences in study methods and in ascertainment, particularly in relation to recognition of infection versus clinical disease.[84] Nonetheless, it appears that pertussis vaccine is between 80 to 95% efficacious in preventing clinical disease following intimate exposure.[82] In spite of less than *perfect* efficacy, only 4617 cases of pertussis were reported in the United States in 1994.[33] Even assuming such gross underreporting that the actual number of cases of clinical pertussis is fivefold greater (about 23,000 in 1994), less than 1% of each birth cohort ultimately experiences the disease. Therefore, on a population basis the vaccine is about 99% efficacious in preventing clinical pertussis. Accordingly, the near disappearance of clinical pertussis in such countries as the United States must be attributed in part to herd immunity as a result of widespread vaccine use.

However, in the past decade concerns have been expressed about universal childhood immunization for two reasons: first, it is well established that mortality from pertussis in the developed world was declining long before development and widespread use of the vaccine (see Section 5.1). Whatever the cause of this decline, some have argued that the low rates of mortality from pertussis observed in recent years in developed countries would have occurred even in the absence of the vaccine, and therefore the vaccine may be superfluous.[9] In contradistinction, several studies have indicated that, although mortality from the disease clearly declined remarkably before the vaccine was extensively used, the decline accelerated significantly in association with its widespread use.[8,83] Further, in countries in which use of pertussis vaccine declined or was abandoned, widespread pertussis recurred.[83–85]

Second, concerns have been expressed about the safety of the vaccine itself. Three general types of reactions have been attributed to DTP. The first of these comprises mild local reactions at the site of injection and slight systemic reactions, such as fever and malaise, as observed following receipt of most vaccines. These are usually of no concern. A second group of reactions includes two that are quite disturbing but appear to be without permanent sequelae. These include incessant, inconsolable crying and a strange, shocklike syndrome following injection in young infants. The crying is very likely due to pain at the site of injection. The cause of the shocklike hypotonic hyporesponsive episodes has not been identified. Though these episodes are frightening, death in association with them has not been described. The third group of events includes those related to the central nervous system. These events range from what appear clearly to be simple febrile convulsions without sequelae[86] to severe encephalopathy with permanent brain damage or death. Although it is clear that pertussis vaccine is the antigen in DTP that contributes most to fever and local reactions, it has not been shown that it is the component primarily responsible for the other phenomena.

A 1981 study provided somewhat more precise information about the frequency of the first two groups of side effects.[87] In this study, infants and children who received a total of 15,752 inoculations of DTP and 784 of DT (diphtheria and tetanus toxoids absorbed) were followed for 48 hr. Local and systemic reactions, including fever, were considerably more frequent following DTP than DT. Nine children experienced short seizures following DTP; all but one episode were associated with fever. Nine other children had hypotonic–hyporesponsive episodes. Thus, each of these reactions occurred at a rate of 1 per 1750 injections (95% confidence interval: 1 per 925 to 1 per 3850). However, attribution of these two more worrisome types of reactions solely to the pertussis component of DTP was not feasible because too few immunizations (784) with DT were monitored to permit comparison.

Estimates of rates of post-pertussis-vaccine encephalopathy have ranged from 1/50,0000 to 1/300,000 or more[88]; subsequently, a well-designed study that controlled for background rates of encephalopathy suggested that serious neurological reactions occur following 1/110,000 injections, and that about one third of children so affected incur sequelae that may be evident 10 years later.[89,90] However, there are doubts about the precision of this rate, and indeed it has been concluded by the investigators that the results show that pertussis vaccine produces permanent brain damage very rarely or not at all.[90] Instead, it may be that the majority, if not all, of the instances of alleged pertussis vaccine encephalopathy represent either coincidence or the precipitation of inevitable manifestations of preexisting disorders by the well-known systemic effects of DTP. Most authorities have concluded that permanent brain damage as a result of DTP is either a myth or is so rare that it cannot be differentiated from coincidence. Although occasional reports have suggested that DTP may precipitate the sudden infant death syndrome on rare occasions, several have indicated that these events represent simple coincidence.(91) A full review of all reports and studies has absolved the vaccine of most, if not all, of the alleged high incidence of serious or fatal reactions.(91) This and other assessments have resulted in lessening of public concerns about risks attributable to the vaccine.(92)

Doubts about the continuing need for pertussis vaccine plus anxiety about its safety, widely publicized in the media, resulted in striking diminutions in pertussis vaccine use in the late 1970s in Britain and Japan because of the concerns not only of parents but also of physicians. In both countries, widespread outbreaks of pertussis with its attendant mortality, particularly in unimmunized infants, ensued.(83,84) In Sweden, pertussis immunization was discontinued in 1979, because of doubts about vaccine efficacy, and similarly a recrudescence of the disease occurred.(85) These natural or inadvertent experiments provide strong evidence of the public health merit of widespread immunization against pertussis. Any risk of serious disability or death from pertussis vaccine is negligible or nonexistent, and therefore the benefits far outweigh this possibility.

In spite of this, it was clear that it would be advantageous to have an improved pertussis vaccine. First, the whole-cell vaccine undoubtedly contains antigens and other substances that not only are reactive (though not truly dangerous) but also are irrelevant to immunity and contribute to DTP being of concern to physicians and parents, under criticism from the media, and the subject of hundreds of lawsuits that have no merit. Second, from the standpoint of children, a less unpleasantly reactive vaccine is desirable and would result in its being more acceptable in both developed and developing countries. Third, the possibility that booster doses for adults may be needed to control pertussis makes a less reactive vaccine highly desirable. Fourth, the prospect of genetically engineered vaccines demands definition of the protective components. For these reasons plus the fact that much better understanding of the biological anatomy of *B. pertussis* has steadily evolved over the past decade, efforts were made to develop, evaluate, and market a cellular pertussis vaccines. Indeed, acellular vaccines have been licensed and used exclusively in Japan since 1981.(93) Two adsorbed DTP preparations containing acellular pertussis components were licensed in the United States for use as the fourth and fifth doses by 1992.

It is clear that these acellular vaccines are at least as immunogenic and far less reactive than whole-cell DTP, including in infants.(27,94,95) In addition, studies in Japan and Sweden demonstrated protection against clinical pertussis.(54,73,96) However, because the compositions of these vaccines varied and the components of the organism responsible for immunity to infection and/or disease have not been identified with precision, controlled fields trials to assess clinical protection, particularly for infants, have been required (see Section 4).

Accordingly, starting in 1991, a number of randomized, controlled clinical trials of various acellular DTP products (DTaP) were conducted in infants. Efficacy was compared with whole-cell DTP. The results of these studies showed clinical protection comparable to the whole cell product.(80,81,97) As a result, three DTaP products were licensed for use in the United States in 1996, and are preferred over the whole-cell product.

From these studies it may be concluded that acellular pertussis vaccines appear to be as protective as whole-cell DTP in infancy. Further, there is no evidence that these less reactive acellular vaccines are less apt to produce pertussis vaccine-induced encephalopathy, although the question is now probably moot because of the rarity or absence of permanent brain damage from whole-cell DTP. Data from Japan's public recompense system for vaccine injuries show a striking decline in claims for pertussis vaccine injury following the 1975 recommendation that the age of initiation of whole-cell DTP be shifted from infancy to 2 years of age. No change of consequence occurred subsequent to 1981, when the acellular preparations replaced the whole-cell vaccine in DTP in Japan.(93) It stands to reason that temporally associated reactions not caused by DTP will continue to occur with DTP containing an acellular pertussis component. However, it is also logical to believe that the precipitation of inevitable manifestations of underlying CNS disease, such as seizures, will be observed less frequently following administration of the less pyrogenic pertussis vaccine. Thus, less confusion about causation of such events in the minds of the public, physicians, courts, and the media should ensue.

10. Unresolved Problems

Several important unresolved problems regarding pertussis and its control remain. First, although remarkable progress has been made in understanding the biological anatomy of *B. pertussis* and its relation to man, the relation of that anatomy to immunity to the disease is not precisely defined. In short, which antigen (or antigens) is (or are) necessary for the production of clinical immunity remains to be determined before an optimum vaccine can be produced. This is a task that is not easily subject to study for several reasons. There is no satisfactory animal model for pertussis. Because the time-tested whole-cell vaccine has nearly eliminated pertussis in the developed world, the number of subjects, the costs, and the logistics of such a study in the United States and similar countries present nearly insurmountable problems. Studies in developing countries where pertussis is rife present both ethical dilemmas and enormous difficulties in follow-up. If a vaccine containing two or more components is only fractionally more efficacious than a single-component vaccine, assessment of the relative merits of differently constituted acellular vaccines would require numbers of subjects that stagger the imagination. Thus, the question of the antigenic composition of an optimum acellular pertussis vaccine may not be answered by field trials in which clinical pertussis is the outcome measure. As a corollary, a serological surrogate for clinical protection is sorely needed.

Second, although remarkable progress is being made in controlling pertussis in developing nations, achievement of universal, worldwide immunization against pertussis is some years away. Third, better definition is needed of the role of asymptomatic or atypical pertussis, particularly in partially immune adolescents and young adults. The increasing evidence that such persons comprise a hitherto unrecognized or ignored reservoir for pertussis suggests the need for special attention. It is not unreasonable to predict that, with the anticipated development of a less reactive acellular pertussis vaccine, reinforcing doses will be needed into adolescence and adulthood.[64]

11. References

1. Holmes, W. H., *Bacillary and Rickettsial Infections*, Macmillan, New York, 1940.
2. Kloos, W. E., Mohapatra, N., Dobrogosz, W. J., *et al.*, Deoxyribonucleotide sequence relationships among *Bordetella* species, *Int. J. Syst. Bacteriol.* **31:**173–176 (1981).
3. Wardlaw, A. C., and Parton, R., The host–parasite relationship in pertussis, in: *Pathogenesis and Immunity in Pertussis* (A. C. Wardlaw and R. Parton, eds.), pp.327– 352, John Wiley, London, 1988.
4. Bordet, J., and Gengou, O., Le microbe de la coqueluche, *Ann. Inst. Pasteur* **20:**731–741 (1906).
5. Pittman, M., The concept of pertussis as a toxin-mediated disease, *Pediatr. Infect. Dis. J.* **3:**467–486 (1984).
6. Dauer, C. C., Reported whooping cough morbidity and mortality in the United States, *Public Health Rep.* **58:**661–676 (1943).
7. Miller, D. L., Alderslade, R., and Ross, E. M., Whooping cough and whooping cough vaccine: The risks and benefits debate, *Epidemiol. Rev.* **4:**1–24 (1982).
8. Mortimer, E. A., Jr., and Jones, P. K., An evaluation of pertussis vaccine, *Rev. Infect. Dis.* **1:**927–932 (1979).
9. Stewart, G. T., Pertussis vaccine: The United Kingdom's experience, in: *International Symposium on Pertussis* (C. R. Manclark and J. C. Hill, eds.), pp. 262–278, Government Printing Office, Washington, DC, 1979.
10. Onorato, I. M., and Wassilak, S. G. F., Laboratory diagnosis of pertussis: The state of the art, *Pediatr. Infect. Dis. J.* **6:**145–151 (1987).
11. Sutter, R. W., and Cochi, S. L., Pertussis hospitalizations and mortality, 1985–1988. Evaluation of the completeness of national reporting, *J. Am. Med. Assoc.* **267:**386–391 (1992).
12. Baraff, L. J., Wilkins, J., and Wehrle, P. F., The role of antibiotics, immunizations, and adenoviruses in pertussis, *Pediatrics* **61:**224–230 (1978).
13. Linneman, C. C., Host–parasite interactions in pertussis, in: *International Symposium on Pertussis* (C. R. Manclark and J. C. Hill, eds.), pp. 3–18, US Government Printing Office, Washington, DC, 1979.
14. Olson, L. C., Pertussis, *Medicine* **54:**427–469 (1975).
15. Fine, P. E. M., and Clarkson, J. A., Distribution of immunity to pertussis in the population of England and Wales, *J. Hyg.* **92:**21–26 (1984).
16. Hallander, H. O., Reizenstein, E., Renemar, B., *et al.*, Comparison of nasopharyngeal aspirates with swabs for culture of *Bordetella pertussis*, *J. Clin. Microbiol.* **31:**50–52 (1993).
17. Strebel, P. M., Cochi, S. L., Farizo, K. M., *et al.*, Pertussis in Missouri: Evaluation of nasopharyngeal culture, direct fluorescent antibody testing, and clinical case definitions in the diagnosis of pertussis, *Clin. Infect. Dis.* **16:**276–285 (1993).
18. Broome, C. V., Fraser, D. W., and English, W. J., II, Pertussis—Diagnostic methods and surveillance, in: *International Symposium on Pertussis* (C. R. Manclark and J. C. Hill, eds.), pp. 19–22, US Government Printing Office, Washington, DC, 1979.
19. He, Q., Mertsola, J., Soini, H., and Vijanen, M. K., Sensitive and specific polymerase chain reaction assays for detection of *Bordetella pertussis* in nasopharyngeal specimens, *J. Pediatr.* **124:** 421–426 (1994).
20. Schlapfer, G., Cherry, J. D., Heininger, V., *et al.*, Polymerase chain reaction identification of *Bordetella pertussis* infections in vaccinees and family members in a pertussis vaccine efficacy trial in Germany, *Pediatr. Infect. Dis. J.* **14:**209–214 (1995).
21. Ewanowich, C. A., Chui, L. W.-L., Paranchych, M. G., *et al.*, Major outbreak of pertussis in northern Alberta, Canada: Analysis of discrepant direct fluorescent-antibody and culture results by using polymerase chain reaction methodology, *J. Clin. Microbiol.* **31:**1715–1725 (1993).
22. Steketee, R. W., Burstyn, D. G., Wassilak, S. G. F., *et al.*, A comparison of laboratory and clinical methods for diagnosing pertussis in an outbreak in a facility for the developmentally disabled, *J. Infect. Dis.* **157:**441–449 (1988).
23. Long, S. S., Welkon, C., and Clark, J. L., Widespread silent transmission of pertussis in families: Antibody correlates of infection and symptomatology, *J. Infect. Dis.* **161:**480–486 (1990).
24. Mink, C. A. M., Cherry, J. D., Christenson, P., *et al.*, A search for *Bordetella pertussis* infection in university students, *Clin. Infect. Dis.* **14:**464–471 (1992).

25. Cromer, B. A., Goydos, J., Hackell, J., *et al.*, Unrecognized pertussis infection in adolescents, *Am. J. Dis. Child.* **147:**575–577 (1993).
26. Weiss, A., Hewlett, E. L., Virulence factors of *Bordetella pertussis*, *Annu. Rev. Microbiol.* **40:**661–686 (1986).
27. Mortimer, E. A., Jr., Pertussis vaccine, in: *Vaccines*, 2nd ed. (S. A. Plotkin and E. A. Mortimer, Jr., eds.), pp. 91–135, W.B. Saunders, Philadelphia, 1994.
28. Knowles, K., Lorange, M., Matthews, R. C., and Preston, N. W., Characterization of outbreak and vaccine strains of *Bordetella pertussis*—Quebec, *Can. Comm. Dis. Rep.* **91–21:**182–183, 186–187 (1993).
29. Preston, N. W., Effectiveness of pertussis vaccines, *Br. Med. J.* **2:**11–13 (1965).
30. Thomas, M. G., Redhead, K., and Lambert, H. P., Human serum antibody responses to *Bordetella pertussis* infection and pertussis vaccination, *J. Infect. Dis.* **159:**211–218 (1989).
31. Shahin, R. D., Brennan, M. J., Li, Z. M., *et al.*, Characterization of the protective capacity and immunogenicity of the 69-kD outer membrane protein of *Bordetella pertussis*, *J. Exp. Med.* **171:**63–73 (1990).
32. Winsnes, R., Serological responses to pertussis, in: *Pathogenesis and Immunity in Pertussis* (A. C. Wardlaw and R. Parton, eds.), pp. 283–307, John Wiley, New York, 1988.
33. Centers for Disease Control and Prevention, Summary of notifiable diseases, United States, 1994, *Morbid. Mortal. Week. Resp.* **43** (53):3–80 (1994).
34. Centers for Disease Control and Prevention, Pertussis surveillance—United States, 1989–1991, *Morbid. Mortal. Week. Rep.* **41**(No. SS)**:**11–19 (1992).
35. Kochanek, K. D., and Hudson, B. L., *Advance Report of Final Mortality Statistics*, 1992. *Monthly Vital Statistics Report*; Vol. 43 (No. 6, Suppl)., Hyattsville, MD, National Center for Health Statistics, 1994.
36. Bassili, W. R., and Stewart, G. T., Epidemiological evaluation of immunization and other factors in the control of whooping cough, *Lancet* **1:**471–474 (1976).
37. Ehrengut, W., Whooping cough vaccination: Comment on report from the Joint Committee on Vaccination and Immunisation, *Lancet* **1:**370–371 (1978).
38. Gordon, J. E., and Hood, R. I., Whooping cough and its epidemiological anomalies, *Am. J. Med. Sci.* **222:**333–361 (1951).
39. Grant, J. P., *UNICEF: State of the World's Children, 1994,* Oxford University Press, London, 1994.
40. Sako, W., Studies on pertussis immunization, *J. Pediatr.* **30:**29–40 (1947).
41. Clark, A. C., Bradford, W. L., and Berry, G. P., An epidemiological study of an outbreak of pertussis in a public school, *Am. J. Public Health* **36:**1156–1162 (1946).
42. Christie, C. D. C., Marx, M. L., Marchant, C. D., and Reising, S. F., The 1993 epidemic of pertussis in Cincinnati. Resurgence of disease in a highly immunized population of children, *N. Engl. J. Med.* **331:**16–21 (1994).
43. Centers for Disease Control and Prevention, Resurgence of pertussis—United States, 1993, *Morbid. Mortal. Week. Rep.* **42:**952–953, 959–960 (1993).
44. Farizo, K. M., Cochi, S. L., Zell, E. R., *et al.*, Epidemiological features of pertussis in the United States, 1980–1989, *Clin. Infect. Dis.* **14:**708–719 (1992).
45. Centers for Disease Control and Prevention, Pertussis outbreaks—Massachusetts and Maryland, 1992, *Morbid. Mortal. Week. Rep.* **42:**197–200 (1993).
46. Addiss, D. G., Davis, J. P., Meade, B. D., *et al.*, A pertussis outbreak in a Wisconsin nursing home, *J. Infect. Dis.* **164:**704–710 (1991).
47. Marchant, C. D., Loughlin, A. M., Lett, S. M., *et al.*, Pertussis in Massachusetts, 1981–1991: Incidence, serological diagnosis, and vaccine effectiveness, *J. Infect. Dis.* **169:**1297–1305 (1994).
48. Steketee, R. W., Wassilak, S. G. F., Adkins, W. N., Jr., *et al.*, Evidence for a high attack rate and efficacy of erythromycin prophylaxis in a pertussis outbreak in a facility for the developmentally disabled, *J. Infect. Dis.* **157:**434–440 (1988).
49. Expanded Programme on Immunization, *EPI for the 1990s*, World Health Organization, Geneva, 1992.
50. Fine, P. E. M., and Clarkson, J. A., Seasonal influences on pertussis, *Int. J. Epidemiol.* **15:**237–247 (1986).
51. Centers for Disease Control and Prevention, Summary of notifiable diseases, United States, 1992, *Morbid. Mortal. Week. Rep.* **41**(55)**:** 2–73 (1992).
52. Bradford, W. L., Use of convalescent blood in whooping cough, *Am. J. Dis. Child.* **50:**918–928 (1935).
53. Church, M. A., Evidence of whooping-cough-vaccine efficacy from the 1978 whooping-cough epidemic in Hertfordshire, *Lancet* **2:**188–190 (1979).
54. Noble, G. R., Bernier, R. H., Esber, E. C., *et al.*, Acellular and whole-cell pertussis vaccines in Japan. Report of a visit by US scientists, *J. Am. Med. Assoc.* **257:**1351–1356 (1987).
55. Kendrick, P. L., Secondary attack rates from pertussis in vaccinated and unvaccinated children, *Am. J. Hyg.* **32:**89–91 (1940).
56. Lapin, J. H., *Whooping Cough*, Charles C. Thomas, Springfield, IL, 1943.
57. Byers, R. K., and Rizzo, N. D., A follow-up study of pertussis in infancy, *N. Engl. J. Med.* **242:**887–891 (1950).
58. Rosenfeld, G. B., and Bradley, C., Childhood behavior sequelae of asphyxia in infancy with special reference to pertussis and asphyxia neonatorum, *Pediatrics* **2:**74–83 (1948).
59. Litvak, A. M., Gibel, H., Rosenthal, S. E., and Rosenblatt, P., Cerebral complications in pertussis, *J. Pediatr.* **32:**357–379 (1948).
60. Miller, D., Wadsworth, J., Diamond, J., and Ross, E., Pertussis vaccine and whooping cough as risk factors for acute neurological illness and death in young children, *Dev. Biol. Stand.* **61:**385–394 (1985).
61. Aoyama, T., Takeuchi, Y., Goto, A., *et al.*, Pertussis in adults, *Am. J. Dis. Child.* **146:**163–166 (1992).
62. Trollfors, B., and Rabo, E., Whooping cough in adults, *Br. Med. J.* **283:**696–697 (1981).
63. Nelson, J. D., The changing epidemiology of pertussis in young infants. The role of adults as reservoirs of infection, *Am. J. Dis. Child.* **132:**371–373 (1978).
64. Mortimer, E. A., Jr., Perspectives. Pertussis and its prevention: A family affair, *J. Infect. Dis.* **161:**473–479 (1990).
65. Mills, K. H. G., and Redhead, K., Editorial. Cellular immunity in pertussis, *J. Med. Microbiol.* **39:**163–164 (1993).
66. Butler, N. R., Haslum, M., Golding, J., and Stewart-Brown, S., Recent findings from the 1970 child health and education study: Preliminary communication, *J. Roy. Soc. Med.* **75:**781–784 (1982).
67. Britten, N., and Wadsworth, J., Long-term respiratory sequelae of whooping cough in a nationally representative sample, *Br. Med. J.* **292:**441–444 (1986).
68. Johnston, I. D. A., Bland, J. M., and Ingram, D., Effect of whooping cough in infancy on subsequent lung function and bronchial reactivity, *Am. Rev. Respir. Dis.* **134:**270–275 (1986).
69. Steketee, R. W., Burstyn, D. G., Wassilak, S. G. F., *et al.*, A comparison of laboratory and clinical methods for diagnosing

pertussis in an outbreak in a facility for the developmentally disabled, *J. Infect. Dis.* **157:**441–449 (1988).

70. Granstrom, G., and Granstrom, M., Effect of erythromycin treatment on antibody responses in pertussis, *J. Infect. Dis.* **26:**453–457 (1994).
71. Patriarca, P. A., Biellik, R. J., Sanden, G., *et al.*, Sensitivity and specificity of clinical case definitions for pertussis, *Am. J. Public Health* **78:**833–836 (1988).
72. Blackwelder, W. C., Storsaeter, J., Olin, P., *et al.*, Acellular pertussis vaccines. Efficacy and evaluation of case definitions, *Am. J. Dis. Child.* **145:**1285–1289 (1991).
73. Ad Hoc Group for the Study of pertussis Vaccines, Placebo-controlled trial of two acellular pertussis vaccines in Sweden—Protective efficacy and adverse events, *Lancet* **1:**956–960 (1988). [Erratum, *Lancet* **1:**1238 (1988).]
74. Altemeier, W. A., III, and Ayoub, E. M., Erythromycin prophylaxis for pertussis, *Pediatrics* **59:**623–625 (1977).
75. Sprauer, M. A., Cochi, S. L., Zell, E. R., *et al.*, Prevention of secondary transmission of pertussis in households with the early use of erythromycin, *Am. J. Dis. Child.* **146:**177–181 (1992).
76. Bradford, W. L., Use of convalescent blood in whooping cough, *Am. J. Dis. Child.* **50:**918–928 (1935).
77. Morris, D., and McDonald, J. C., Failure of hyperimmune gamma globulin to prevent whooping cough, *Arch. Dis. Child.* **32:**236–239 (1957).
78. Granstrom, M., Olinder-Nielsen, A. M., Holmblad, P., *et al.*, Specific immunoglobulin for treatment of whooping cough, *Lancet* **338:**1230–1233 (1992).
79. Ichimaru, T., Ohara, Y., Hojo, M., *et al.*, Case report. Treatment of severe pertussis by administration of specific gamma globulin with high titer anti-toxin antibody, *Acta Paediatr.* **82:**1076–1078 (1993).
80. Centers for Disease Control, Pertussis vaccination: Use of acellular pertussis vaccines among infants and young children. Recommendations of the Immunization Practices Advisory Committee (ACIP), *Morbid. Mortal. Week. Rep.* **46**(No. RR-7):1–25 (1997).
81. Halsey, N. A., Chesney, P. J., Gerber, M. A., *et al.*, Acellular pertussis vaccine: Recommendations for use as the initial series in infants and children. Committee on Infectious Diseases, American Academy of Pediatrics, *Pediatrics* **99:**282–288 (1997).
82. Onorato, I. M., Wassilak, S. G., and Meade, B., Efficacy of whole-cell pertussis vaccine in preschool children in the United States, *J. Am. Med. Assoc.* **267:**2745–2749 (1992).
83. Cherry, J. D., The epidemiology of pertussis and pertussis vaccine in the United Kingdom and the United States: A comparative study, in: *Current Problems in Pediatrics*, Vol. 14, No. 2 (J. D. Lockhart, ed.), pp. 7–77, Year Book Medical Publishers, Chicago, 1984.
84. Kanai, K., Japan's experience in pertussis epidemiology and vaccination in the past thirty years, *Jpn. J. Sci. Biol.* **33:**107–143 (1980).
85. Romanus, V., Jonsell, R., and Bergquist, S. E., Pertussis in Sweden after the cessation of general immunization in 1979, *Pediatr. Infect. Dis. J.* **6:**364–371 (1987).
86. Hirtz, D. G., Nelson, K. B., and Ellenberg, J. H., Seizures following childhood immunizations, *J. Pediatr.* **102:**14–18 (1983).
87. Cody, C. L., Baraff, L. J., Cherry, J. D., *et al.*, Nature and rates of adverse reactions associated with DTP and DT immunizations in infants and children, *Pediatrics* **68:**650–660 (1981).
88. Department of Health and Social Security, Committee on Safety of Medicines and Joint Committee on Vaccination and Immunization, *Whooping Cough*, Her Majesty's Stationery Office, London, 1981.
89. Miller, D., Wadsworth, J., Diamond, J., and Ross, E., Pertussis vaccine and whooping cough as risk factors for acute neurological illness and death in young children, *Dev. Biol. Stand.* **61:**389–394 (1985).
90. Miller, D., Madge, N., Diamond, J., *et al.*, Pertussis immunization and serious acute neurological illness in children, *Br. Med. J.* **307:**1171–1176 (1993).
91. Howson, C. P., and Fineberg, H. V., Adverse events following pertussis and rubella vaccines: Summary of a report of the Institute of Medicine, *J. Am. Med. Assoc.* **267:**392–396 (1992).
92. Halsey, N. A., Chesney, P. J., Gerber, M. A., *et al.*, The relationship between pertussis vaccine and central nervous system sequelae: Continuing assessment. Committee on Infectious Diseases, American Academy of Pediatrics, *Pediatrics* **97:**279–281 (1996).
93. Kimura, M., and Kuno-Sakai, H., Developments in pertussis immunisation in Japan, *Lancet* **336:**30–32 (1990).
94. Edwards, K. M., Meade, B. D., Decker, M. D., *et al.*, Comparison of 13 acellular pertussis vaccines: Overview and serologic response, *Pediatrics* **96**(Suppl.)**:**548–557 (1995).
95. Decker, M. D., Edwards, K. M., Steinhoff, M. C., *et al.*, Comparison of thirteen acellular pertussis vaccines: Adverse reactions, *Pediatrics* **96**(Suppl.):557–566 (1995).
96. Mortimer, E. A., Jr., Kimura, M., Cherry, J. D., *et al.*, Protective efficacy of the Takeda acellular pertussis vaccine combined with diphtheria and tetanus toxoids following household exposure of Japanese children, *Am. J. Dis. Child.* **144:**899–904 (1990).
97. Cherry, J. D., Comparative efficacy of acellular pertussis vaccines: An analysis of recent trials, *Pediatr. Infect. Dis. J.* **16:**S90–96 (1997).

12. Suggested Reading

Institute of Medicine, Howson, C. P., Howe, C. J., and Fineberg, H. V. (eds.), *Adverse Effects of Pertussis and Rubella Vaccine*, National Academy Press, Washington, DC, 1991.

Mortimer, E. A., Jr., Pertussis vaccine, in: *Vaccines*, 2nd ed. (S. A. Plotkin and E. A. Mortimer, eds.), pp. 91–135, W.B. Saunders, Philadelphia, 1994.

Wardlaw, A. C., and Parton, R. (eds.), *Pathogenesis and Immunity in Pertussis*, John Wiley, London, 1988.

CHAPTER 27

Plague

Jack D. Poland and David T. Dennis

1. Introduction

Plague is a flea-transmitted infection of rodents caused by *Yersinia pestis*. Fleas incidentally transmit the infection to humans and other susceptible mammalian hosts. Percutaneous inoculation of the plague bacillus in humans typically initiates inflammation of lymph nodes draining the inoculation site, resulting in *bubonic plague*. Bloodstream invasion may lead to *septicemic plague* or to established infection of other organ systems such as the lung or the meninges. Spread of infection to the lungs may result in *secondary pneumonic plague*, which can then be transmitted from person to person via the respiratory route. Respiratory transmission may result in one or a few cases or, rarely, an epidemic of *primary pneumonic plague*.

Historical epidemics of plague spread rapidly through populations. The cause, sources, and modes of transmission of the disease were unknown, and the death rate for bubonic plague was 50–60%. Essentially all pneumonic and septicemic plague patients rapidly died of a terrifying fulminant illness, and prevention measures seemed futile. Consequently, epidemics of plague caused panic and chaos. Even today, despite the availability of antibiotics to treat the infection in humans and proven methods to control both epidemics and epizootics, plague provokes alarm and sometimes irrational responses.

2. Historical Background

The earliest description of plague as we know it today is that of the Great Plague of Justinian in the 6th century AD, which was first recognized in Egypt and then extended through Syria, North Africa, and much of Europe. According to some accounts, half the population of the Roman Empire died in this epidemic. However, reports of clinical illness and mortality in this and other historical epidemics are not reliable because of the intense social disruptions and concomitant outbreaks of other diseases that confound efforts to establish a clear clinical picture arising from a single causative agent. There were political reasons for misrepresenting the real effects of catastrophic events and a lack of organized attempts to record the vital statistics and demographics that we now take for granted.[1,2]

In the 14th century, pandemic plague again appeared. This pandemic is thought to have begun in central Asia, first striking China and northern India and then moving along trade routes to the Crimea and the Levant. From these points, it spread by ship to Sicily and Sardinia, to Italy in 1347, and onward to England in 1348. The records claim fatality rates of 40 to 80% in concentrated European population centers, and the epithet "The Great Mortality" was applied with good reason.[3] The often-used term "Black Death" was coined later, specifically in relation to epidemics that had great numbers of pneumonic plague.[4]

Plague reappeared in Europe during each of the four succeeding centuries. The "Great Plague" of London peaked in 1665 when deaths during August and September of that year were reported to be 7,000 per week in a population of 500,000. Plague gradually disappeared from Europe in the 18th century, and the entire continent was apparently free of plague by 1840.[3] Zinsser[5] considered that this disappearance ". . . presents one of the unsolved mysteries of epidemiology . . ." and Pollitzer[6] notes that ". . . this has been the subject of much debate and few conclusions." Others[3] attribute this freedom from plague to the displacement of the black rat in European homes by the less dangerous plague host, the Nor-

Jack D. Poland and David T. Dennis • Division of Vector-Borne Diseases, National Center for Infectious Diseases, Centers for Disease Control and Prevention, Public Health Service, US Department of Health and Human Services, Fort Collins, Colorado 80522.

way rat. Whatever may have been the true number of deaths, the great epidemics of plague produced extensive political, religious, demographic, and social changes, residua of which persist today. The practice of quarantine, a waiting period before docking of ships arriving from plague affected areas, was initiated by Italian authorities during this pandemic.

Plague reappeared in the last years of the 19th century as the Third (Modern) Pandemic, apparently originating in southwestern China and reaching Hong Kong in 1894.[6] From this seaport, it spread by cargo vessels to all inhabited continents, newly affecting North and South America. India experienced especially severe epidemics that recurred for more than 20 years and resulted in more than 10 million deaths. It was in Hong Kong in 1894 that Alexandre Yersin first isolated the causative organism,[7] and it was in India that the association of rat deaths (ratfalls) and subsequent human illness was described. Studies in India also proved the role of fleas in the transmission of the plague bacillus.[3] To combat epidemics of bubonic plague, various types of vaccines, live attenuated and inactivated whole cell, were made and tested,[8] and antisera received extensive study. Effective antibiotic therapy was first demonstrated in the late 1940s and early 1950s using streptomycin, chloramphenicol, and tetracycline.[9,10]

Although plague is a widespread zoonosis, in the past 40 years the world has experienced mostly sporadic cases and clusters of human plague, punctuated by occasional epidemics of the disease. A notable exception is the prolonged epidemic plague activity that occurred in war-disrupted Vietnam during 1962–1975.[11–14]

3. Methodology

3.1. Sources of Morbidity and Mortality Data

International agreements require telegraphic notification to the World Health Organization (WHO) of the first case of plague in any area previously free of the disease, as well as regular reporting of all confirmed cases. Additionally, individual countries have regulations governing reporting in their jurisdictions. Plague surveillance information is published in the WHO *Weekly Epidemiological Record*, in the *Weekly Epidemiological Report* of the Pan American Health Organization, and in the United States in the *Morbidity and Mortality Weekly Report*. Current WHO-published worldwide figures are thought to be approximately correct, although significant lapses occur; e.g., plague deaths are not routinely reported by some countries, and plague epidemics are sometimes not officially reported to WHO. Frequently, there is underreporting at the onset of an epidemic and overreporting during its course. Sporadic cases may be misdiagnosed, especially those that are treated effectively with antibiotics in early illness and fail to develop a typical clinical picture.

Variations in reporting criteria also contribute to unreliable statistics. For instance, the United States reports only confirmed and presumptive cases, whereas in some countries, once there is reason to believe an outbreak is in progress, suspect cases are reported with or without laboratory evidence of infection. Not infrequently, political and personal interests confound efforts to either confirm or to report cases. Governments are sometimes slow to admit the existence of a new case or cases of plague in an effort to prevent public alarm and to avoid political and economic repercussions. Information on recently reported epidemics of plague in India (1994) was confused by the use of various and nonspecific case definitions and unreliable laboratory confirmation of cases.[15,16] Consequently, there was overreporting of cases and conflicting statistics, and important epidemiological and etiologic features of the outbreaks are not yet fully elucidated.[16–18]

3.2. Surveys

Routine microbiological methods are available for the isolation of *Y. pestis* and for serodiagnosis in humans, rodents, and carnivores. Environmental surveys are based on evaluating ecosystems of affected rodents, collection and identification of rodents and rodent fleas and determination of *Y. pestis* infection in them, and collecting and testing of carnivore serum.[19–23] These surveys are helpful in assessing the public health risk, in determining the need for control and prevention measures (such as issuing warnings to the public, insecticiding burrows, and restricting access), and in evaluating such interventions. Serological surveys to detect unrecognized infections in humans have largely been unrewarding. In 1966–1980, the Centers for Disease Control (CDC) (unpublished) surveyed 784 community or household contacts of US plague cases without finding any evidence of subclinical infection (see Section 5.4).

4. Biological Characteristics of the Organism

4.1. Etiologic Agent, *Yersinia pestis*

Y. pestis is a gram-negative, nonmotile, nonsporulating, coccobacillus in the family Enterobacteriaceae. It is microaerophilic, oxidase- and urease-negative, and biochemically unreactive. *Y. pestis* is nonfastidious and grows slowly but well on simple bacteriologic media.[24] It grows best at 28°C and a pH of 7.4. When incubated on agar plates, it produces pinpoint colonies at 24 hr and 1- to 2-mm diameter colonies at 48 hr. Colonies are gray-white with irregular surfaces that have a hammered-metal appearance when viewed under magnification. In broth, the organism grows in clumps that cling to the sides of the culture tube and the broth itself remains clear. *Y. pestis* readily infects laboratory rodents, which are routinely used in specialized laboratories for virulence testing and for isolating the organism from contaminated materials.

4.2. Virulence Factors

Virulence factors are important in the organism's ability to replicate in mammals and produce disease.[25] Genes for most of these virulence factors are carried on plasmids, but some are associated with chromosomes. At least six determinants of *Y. pestis* virulence in guinea pigs and in mice have been identified, and it is thought that most of these are important in human infection. Fraction 1 antigen (F1) is contained in the diffusible envelope of the organism and is associated with protection against neutrophilic phagocytosis. Expression of this antigen is temperature dependent; maximum F1 production occurs between 32 and 37°C and does not occur below 28°C. Because of the temperature dependence, *Y. pestis* in the flea gut lacks F1, and organisms inoculated into a mammalian host by the bite of a flea are initially vulnerable to neutrophilic phagocytosis. The bacilli that survive and replicate do produce F1 and develop *in vivo* resistance to neutrophilic phagocytosis.[26] F1 antigen produced by organisms transmitted to humans from animal tissues or blood, or in expelled droplets from a person or animal with plague pneumonia is thought to enhance their virulence.

Yops, V, and W virulence proteins are known as low calcium response proteins and are thought to inhibit phagocytosis and to mediate the inflammatory and cell-mediated immune response to infection.[25] Pesticin (Pst) and plasminogen activator protease (Psa) are products of virulent *Y. pestis* that are associated with the production of a fibrinolytic factor and a coagulase. The interplay between Pst and chromosomal iron regulatory genes influences hemin storage and iron transport. Strains that are able to utilize exogenous hemin bind congo red in culture and produce pigment. Murine toxin is specific and highly lethal to mice and less so to rats.[27]

In routine culture of *Y. pestis*, some colonies may be found that lack certain virulence factors. Pigment-negative colonies are the most common finding. Several plague strains from humans have been described that lack other virulence factors, including a strain deficient in F1 recovered from a fatal case of plague in the United States, a pesticin-negative strain from another US case, and a pigment-negative strain from a plague patient in South Africa.[28] Laboratory procedures for isolating *Y. pestis* by inoculating laboratory animals may select against isolates that lack certain virulence factors. Testing for virulence factors should be done on fresh isolates, because laboratory manipulation, particularly prolonged incubation at 37°C, may result in loss of virulence.[29]

4.3. Geographic Biotypes

Biotypes of *Y. pestis* have been described by Devignat[30] based on nitrate reduction and ability to ferment glycerol. These biotypes are not related to virulence, but are of epidemiological interest. The *Y. pestis* biotype that was spread over much of the globe in the Third Pandemic, including the Western Hemisphere, is the variety *orientalis*, characterized by its ability to reduce nitrate and an inability to ferment glycerol. Variety *mediaevalis*, which occurs around the Caspian Sea and is thought to have been associated with the Great Plague epidemic of medieval Europe, does not reduce nitrate but ferments glycerol. Variety *antigua*, present in southeastern Russia, Central Asia, and parts of Africa, both reduces nitrate and ferments glycerol. Recent ribotyping studies of various plague strains generally support the biotyping distinctions.[31]

5. Descriptive Epidemiology

5.1. Fleas

Fleas are small, wingless, bloodsucking ectoparasites of warm-blooded animals that will leave a dead host as its body temperature drops and seek another host, usually of the same species as the one abandoned. Many flea species are strongly host specific; others, such as *Xenopsylla cheopis* (the oriental rat flea), which is the principal vector of urban epidemic plague, are quite promiscuous in their host selection. Other important vectors of plague to humans are *X. astia*, *X. braziliensis*, *X. vexabilis*, *Nosopsyllus fasciatus*, and *Oropsylla montana*.[6,19]

When *X. cheopis* and some other species ingest blood containing *Y. pestis*, bacilli multiply and form an alimentary canal blockage at the level of the proventriculus. As blocked fleas make repeated attempts to feed, blood is sucked into the esophagus where, at the proventricular blockage, it mixes with the clotted mass of plague bacilli and is regurgitated into the bite wound, thus enhancing transmission of infection. The observation that epidemic plague stops when ambient temperatures exceed 28°C led to studies that demonstrated that *X. cheopis* enzymatically lyse their intestinal blockage when held at temperatures above 28°C. As a result, the cleared fleas could feed without regurgitation and no longer served as efficient vectors of the organism.[32] *Y. pestis* strains that are unable to bind congo red in culture do not block fleas; and, recent studies show that blocking can be restored to non-pigment-forming mutants by complementing them with a recombinant plasmid containing genes for hemin storage.[33] The vector competency of fleas is evaluated by comparing them to the "classic," highly efficient vector, *X. cheopis*.[20,34,35]

5.2. Rodents

Of the more than 200 species of rodents found to be naturally infected by *Y. pestis*, many are unimportant in maintaining zoonotic cycles of infection and only a few pose significant risks to humans. *Rattus rattus*, the domestic black rat (house rat, roof rat), is the most dangerous rodent in regard to human plague. The black rat has a cosmopolitan distribution, lives in close association with humans (nesting in attics, wall-spaces, etc.), is a vigorous breeder, is a host favorable to *X. cheopis*, and develops fulminating, fatal plague. In epizootics involving black rats, both the rat and the flea serve as amplifying hosts of *Y. pestis*. "Rat-fall" refers to the extensive die-off of the black rat associated with epizootic plague and serves as a prognosticator of epidemic plague. However, rats that have experienced extended periods of plague may become relatively resistant to infection, and rat-falls may cease even though transmission of *Y. pestis* continues. *R. norvegicus* (Norway rat, sewer rat) is an aggressive territorial competitor of the black rat. It is generally a burrowing rodent that lives peridomestically and frequents cellars, drains, crawl spaces, and foundation areas of buildings. Because of its propensity to live in peridomestic habitats, in rural areas the Norway rat provides an efficient vectorial link between wild rodents and the more domestic black rat. When wild rodent plague is contiguous with abundant black rat and oriental rat flea populations, the potential for epidemic plague is great.[6] When stored grains and other foods serve as an enticement in and around houses, normally wild rodent species may establish peridomestic and domestic lifestyles. Under these circumstances, relatively plague-resistant rodents may introduce plague into residential sites. Without large commensal rat populations, however, such introductions result in sporadic human cases rather than epidemics.

In rural plague foci, several rodent species may intermingle and provide opportunity for interspecies spread of plague; however, because of relative host specificity of most wild rodent fleas, epizootics in an area are often confined to a single species. The likelihood of interspecies spread is enhanced when a susceptible rodent population is severely reduced by an epizootic, forcing fleas of the dead rodents to seek alternate hosts. The risk of spread to humans is also greatly increased by epizootic activity, and control efforts may be required to prevent human cases (see Section 6.1).

Important noncommensal sources of plague throughout the world include marmots, gerbils, and ground squirrels in northern Asia; gerbils and ground squirrels (susliks, sisels) in Central Asia and the Near East; gerbils and bandicoot rats in India; the Polynesian rat (*Rattus exulans*) and shrews in Vietnam; *R. exulans* in Indonesia; gerbils, grass rats, and some species of multimammate mice in Africa; ground squirrels (*Spermophilus* spp.), prairie dogs (*Cynomys* spp.), and chipmunks (*Tamias* spp.) in the United States; and, cavies (*Cavia* spp), rice rats (*Oryzomys* spp.), and cotton rats (*Sigmodon* spp.) in South America.[6,19,36] Although many flea species feed only reluctantly on humans, any plague-infected animal and its associated flea species is a potential source of infection to humans.

5.3. Occurrence of Human Plague

During 1980–1994, a total of 18,739 human cases of plague was reported to the WHO from 24 countries (mean of 1,087 cases per year) (Table 1).[37] The reported fatality rate was about 10%. More than half (10,155) of the total number of cases was reported from countries in eastern and southern Africa; about a third (5,661) from Asia; and the rest from the Americas (2,923). Countries reporting the most numbers of cases were Tanzania, Zaire, and Madagascar in the African region; Vietnam and Myanmar in Asia; and Peru and Brazil in the Americas. Recent outbreak activity has been reported from India, Tanzania, Zaire, Madagascar, Mozambique, Vietnam, and Peru. India, in 1994, reported a total of 876 bubonic and pneumonic plague cases with 54 deaths, but the number of confirmed cases was much less.[15–18]

In the United States, 341 cases of plague in humans were reported during 1970–1995 (average 13 cases per year). Of these cases, 80% occurred in the southwestern states of New Mexico, Arizona, and Colorado; 9% were reported from California; and nine other western states

Table 1. Reported Cases of Plague in Humans by Country, 1980–1994[a]

Continent	Country	No. of cases	No. of deaths
Africa	Angola	27	4
	Botswana	173	12
	Kenya	49	10
	Libya	8	0
	Madagascar	1390	302
	Malawi	9	0
	Mozambique	216	3
	South Africa	19	1
	Tanzania	4964	419
	Uganda	660	48
	Zaire	2242	513
	Zambia	1	1
	Zimbabwe	397	31
	Total	10,155	1344
America	Bolivia	189	27
	Brazil	700	9
	Ecuador	83	3
	Peru	1722	112
	United States	229	33
	Total	2923	184
Asia	China	252	76
	India	876	54
	Kazakhystan	10	4
	Mongolia	59	19
	Myanmar	1160	14
	Vietnam	3304	158
	Total	5661	325
World Total		18,739	1853

[a]From World Health Organization.[37]

reported small numbers of cases.[38] Most likely modes of transmission were determined for 286 of these cases and included flea bite (n = 223; 78%); direct contact with infected animals (n = 56; 20%); and inhalation of respiratory droplets from infected animals (n = 7; 2%). Five of the seven persons infected by inhalation were known to be exposed to infected domestic cats. The overall mortality rate was 15%. In the United States, most cases of plague occur in the summer months when rodent and rodent flea activity is greatest. The majority of cases, especially those in the southwestern states, are acquired in or near the patient's home[39,40]; less often, plague in the United States is acquired while working or during recreational activities, the latter occurring most often in California.

5.4. Contagiousness

Uncomplicated bubonic plague is not contagious and patients do not place their family, other social contacts, or attendants at risk. Household members, however, may be at risk of exposure to the same zoonotic source as the index case. In the United States and other developed countries, most plague exposures occur in rural foci, and plague cases are more likely to be sporadic than epidemic. When a bubonic or septicemic plague patient develops secondary plague pneumonia, person-to-person transmission becomes possible but rarely occurs; no person-to-person plague cases have occurred in the United States since 1924, even though 37 pneumonic plague cases have been recorded since then, including five with primary pneumonic plague acquired from domestic pets with respiratory plague.[39,40] The presence of *Y. pestis* in the throats of presumably healthy individuals has been described,[41,42] but there are no data to suggest that such "carriers" play any role in the transmission of the infection. Any draining buboes or other cutaneous lesions of plague patients should be considered infectious, but experience indicates that risk of secondary spread is minimal.

The plague bacillus does not survive well saprophytically. Temperatures above 40°C and desiccation are rapidly lethal to the organism and aerosolized organisms have a short survival period. Pneumonic plague is transmitted by respiratory droplet, and *Y. pestis* does not become truly airborne or disseminate via ventilation systems. Person-to-person transmission of plague can occur from either a primary or secondary plague pneumonia source when there is close direct contact with the infected patient (usually within 2 m).

5.5. Geographic Distribution

Countries reporting human plague cases are noted in Table 1. The probable distribution of active enzootic plague foci throughout the world is shown in Fig. 1.

5.6. Environmental Factors

Ambient temperature and humidity regulate rodent host populations as well as the survival and continued infectiousness of their fleas. Bubonic plague epidemics have occurred most notably in temperature ranges of 10 to 26°C associated with a high relative humidity.[6,32,36] These conditions are most favorable for plague epizootics in rats. On the other hand, enzootic plague foci are most often associated with semi-arid regions.[19,36,43] Where enzootic plague foci are entrenched in zones adjacent to desert areas of Eurasia, Africa, and North and South America, human plague cases occur primarily in the warmer months, when rodent and flea activity is greatest. In tropical environments, outbreaks tend to occur at the

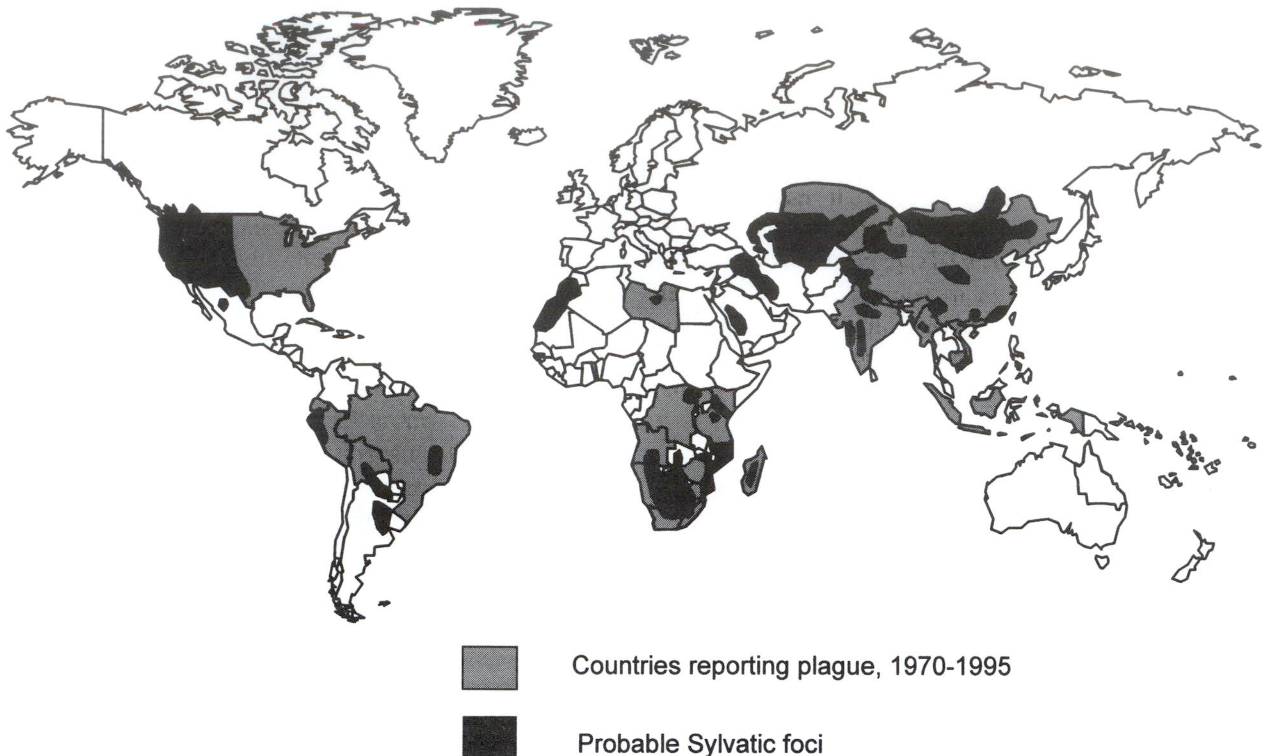

Figure 1. Distribution of natural foci of plague. Compiled from WHO, CDC, and other sources.

end of the dry season, when the temperature falls and humidity rises. In India the rainy season differs between the northern and southcentral plague foci, so that no generalization as to time of year for greatest plague activity can be given for the country as a whole.(6) In Vietnam, human plague incidence was found to be sensitive to slight variations in temperature, relative humidity, and vapor pressure.(32,35,44)

Pneumonic plague epidemics have occurred in winter in circumstances of high relative humidity and overcrowding; this was most dramatically demonstrated in Manchuria during two major epidemics in the early 20th century, when tens of thousands of persons died in epidemics of pneumonic plague.(4) The California urban plague outbreaks in 1919 and 1924 are examples of limited transmission of pneumonic plague in moderate climates.(45)

5.7. Demographic Factors

Plague affects persons of all ages and races. There does not seem to be an age-associated difference in susceptibility to plague. Demographic differences in rates of disease can be explained by exposures associated with place of residence, cultural and sociological factors, and occupational and recreational activities.(46) These factors explain the relatively large numbers of cases that occur among Native Americans in the southwestern United States.(47,48)

5.8. Occupation and Recreation

Certain occupational and recreational activities are associated with an increased risk of exposure to infected fleas. In the United States, persons who live or work on or adjacent to enzootic or epizootic foci, and hunters, trappers, naturalists, pet owners, and campers, are at highest risk of infection.(43,49)

5.9. Occurrence in Different Settings

When family or household clusters of bubonic cases occur, the dates of disease onset usually occur within days of each other. Where multiple cases have occurred within a larger community from a single epizootic source in the United States, dates of onset are usually separated by weeks and involve multiple and geographically separated households.(43) Pneumonic plague patients pose a threat to immediate contacts including family members, friends, and medical personnel. Travel during the incubation period of plague, especially long distance air travel, has been described in the United States as peripatetic plague.[50,51] Some of these traveling patients developed secondary pneumonic plague and were not properly diagnosed prior to death. Fortunately, the risk of pneumonic transmission is high only when there is a productive cough and close face-to-face exposure.[17,52] Disruptions of war have often been associated with plague epidemics. Invading or retreating troops have introduced the disease by transporting infected rodent hosts or their fleas in shipments of grain, other food stuffs, and materiel.[6,36] Movement and crowding of refugees provides the opportunity for preexisting plague to become epidemic.[53] Under conditions of war and other disasters, basic hygiene and sanitation and routine infectious disease prevention and control measures are disrupted.

5.10. Socioeconomic Factors

In rat-borne epidemics, persons with low incomes are generally the most affected. Factors include poor-quality housing that allows ready access to and harborage for rats; housing located near docks, warehouses, or granaries; crowding; and poor environmental hygiene and sanitation. In the United States, cases arise primarily from wild rodent epizootic sources and all socioeconomic groups are affected. The affluent build expensive homes in rural areas with the intention of retaining as much of the natural habitat as possible, sometimes in the midst of an enzootic plague focus. Decorative rock walls form ideal "rocky outcroppings," the principal habitat of *S. variegatus* (rock squirrel), an important plague host in the Rocky Mountain region. On the other hand, some persons who live in close proximity to enzootic plague foci encourage rodent encroachment by providing peridomestic food and harborage in the form of garbage, junk piles, old cars, tires, and wood piles.[49] Prairie dogs may invade overgrazed pastures surrounding or adjacent to human dwellings, which has been especially problematic on Native American lands in the southwestern United States.

6. Mechanisms and Routes of Transmission

The sources of *Y. pestis* infection of humans in order of decreasing frequency are bites by infected fleas; direct contact with the blood or tissues of infected animals captured, hunted, or found dead; persons or pets with plague pneumonia; ingestion of raw or undercooked meat from an infected animal; and rarely the mishandling of plague cultures in the laboratory. Infection can take place through the skin, the respiratory tract, the conjunctiva, the oropharyngeal mucosa, and the digestive tract. Infection by direct conjunctival or mucous membrane exposure is of concern to persons caring for patients with plague pneumonia, laboratorians, and persons who dissect or butcher infected animals.

Entry of the plague bacillus through the respiratory tract may result in two clinical patterns, depending on the size of aerosolized particles introduced. Experiments in guinea pigs showed that bacilli contained in large-particle (10–12μm) sprays were most likely to lodge in the oropharynx resulting in pharyngeal plague and secondary septicemic plague, while smaller particles (< 1μm) initiated bronchopneumonia; in experiments with monkeys, inhalation either of single organism clouds or infectious particles 12 μm in diameter produced lobar pneumonia.[52,54] Domestic cats develop submandibular and/or cervical lymphadenopathy, ulceration, and abscesses, pharyngeal, or pneumonic plague as a result of ingesting infected rodents.[55,56] Humans can acquire plague from cats by inhaling infective respiratory particles, by skin or mucous membrane contact with infectious exudates secretions, or by being bitten or scratched. Ingestion of undercooked infected wild rodents (especially marmots and prairie dogs) and of infected camel and goat meat has resulted both in sporadic cases and limited outbreaks of human plague, which manifest as plague pharyngitis, septicemia, and meningitis.[23,57]

7. Pathogenesis and Immunity

7.1. Pathogenesis

Following the bite of an infected flea or other cutaneous introduction, local *Y. pestis* proliferation ensues but is often not apparent; a small papule or vesicle containing a clear or hemorrhagic fluid (a phlyctenule) sometimes occurs at the site of inoculation and rarely a craterlike tularemic ulcer develops at the site.

From the site of inoculation, organisms travel by way of the lymphatics to regional lymph nodes. The disease may be contained at this level as in simple bubonic plague, or localized infection may be followed by bloodstream invasion with intermittent bacteremia or septicemia. Septicemic plague may develop with no apparent local lymphatic involvement (primary septicemic plague). Bloodstream dissemination may lead to secondary plague pneumonia, plague meningitis, multiple lymphadenopathy, and involvement of other organs, such as the liver, spleen, and rarely the eye.

Pulmonary infection is an urgent public health concern, since respiratory plague is transmissible from person to person. Secondary plague pneumonia occurs more frequently than primary plague pneumonia. Fortunately, patients with secondary plague pneumonia are less likely to transmit the disease than patients with primary pneumonia. The secondary pneumonia patient usually has been severely ill for 2 or more days with sepsis, is less capable of mustering a vigorous cough, and most often produces sputum that tends to be thick, mucopurulent, and tenacious. In comparison, the primary pneumonic plague patient is likely to produce a thin, watery, serosanguinous sputum and to cough with more vigor.

7.2. Incubation Period

The incubation period of bubonic plague is generally 2–6 days,(6) and of pneumonic plague is usually 1–3 days, but longer intervals have been reported.(11,12,58)

7.3. Immunity

Susceptibility of rodents to *Y. pestis* varies from one species to another. Species that are moderately resistant and have a low mortality are important in maintaining plague in a focus and are termed *enzootic* or *maintenance hosts*. They usually coexist with susceptible rodent species that experience a high mortality from infection (epizootic, amplifying hosts). In the United States, inherent species susceptibilities range from highly resistant (kangaroo rats) to highly susceptible (prairie dogs).(21,43) Studies of the natural resistance in rats from a plague-free area showed that some survivors of a small challenge inoculum that developed antibody responses survived a rechallenge with a similar or larger inoculum, while most of those that did not develop antibodies died.(59)

Most humans develop antibody responses to infection with *Y. pestis*.(24,60) In a recent CDC review (unpublished) of 89 confirmed plague cases in the United States, only 4 (4.5%) cases did not develop antibodies to F1 of *Y. pestis*. Asymptomatic infection in humans appears to be rare, but some evidence for this was found in Madagascar by detecting plague antibodies in persons from whom no history of illness could be elicited.(61) On the other hand, serosurveys of 716 community and household contacts of cases living in plague enzootic areas of the United States and 167 residents of two villages in Indonesia during a rat-borne plague epidemic there revealed only four seropositive samples. One, with a titer of 1:128, was a missed bubonic plague case who had onset of illness 3 weeks prior to the survey; one was a Vietnam veteran with a titer of 1:32 who had been previously immunized; two were residents of an Indonesian village with titers of 1:16 and 1:32, respectively, and who had no history of recent illness or of vaccination.(43) This suggests that subclinical infection was rare to nonexistent in those cases.

Persons immunized with formalin-inactivated plague vaccine USP may develop titers against *Y. pestis* that persist for decades. Prior plague vaccination may confound results of serological testing if a history of vaccination is not considered.

The degree of protection provided by plague antibodies in humans is not fully known. Experience in Vietnam suggests that natural infection may not produce complete immunity.(60) And, although the inactivated plague vaccine currently available in the United States has been shown to be an efficient immunogen, its protective efficacy has never been tested in controlled clinical trials. Comparisons of immunologic responses to vaccination by humans and animals and field experiences with vaccinated military personnel, however, do provide indirect evidence that the vaccine is protective in humans.(62)

8. Patterns of Host Response

The clinical response of humans to *Y. pestis* infection is diverse, ranging from mild, ambulatory bubonic plague to rapidly progressing septicemia with bleeding, shock, multiple organ failure, and death.(63–67)

8.1. Clinical Features

The clinical forms of plague that arise from primary exposure include bubonic, septicemic, pneumonic, and pharyngeal plague; secondary manifestations that result from hematogenous spread to other organ systems include plague pneumonitis, meningitis, multiple lymphadenitis (sometimes involving intra-abdominal and thoracic lymph nodes), abscess formation in the liver or spleen, and endophthalmitis.(14,29,63,68)

Two to six days after exposure, bubonic plague patients typically experience sudden onset of illness characterized by severe malaise, headache, shaking chills, fever, and pain in the area of affected regional lymph nodes, which may not be palpably enlarged at this stage. Progression of symptoms is usually rapid with the affected nodes (buboes) often becoming excruciatingly tender and painful. Palpable definition of small to moderately enlarged buboes may be obscured by extensive perinodal edema, erythema, and induration. During the course of the first 3–5 days of illness, the patient may, if not treated, develop gram-negative sepsis, endotoxin-induced systemic inflammatory response syndrome, consumptive coagulopathy, subcutaneous and widely disseminated hemorrhages, septic shock, multiple organ failure and adult respiratory distress syndrome (ARDS), mental confusion, and death.[63–67] Buboes may or may not suppurate.

In primary pneumonic plague, usually within 1–3 days after exposure, the patient experiences a chill followed by fever, splinting of the chest, and cough with production of a thin, serosanguinous sputum. Segmental pulmonary consolidation may occur, manifested by dullness to percussion and decreased breath sounds. A more diffuse interstitial pneumonitis may develop and spread rapidly. Not infrequently, auscultatory findings are surprisingly minimal compared to what is seen by roentgenography. Lobar pneumonia, abscess formation, and cavitation are unusual complications of pulmonary infection. Without administering appropriate antibiotics and providing aggressive supportive care within 18 h or so of onset, primary pneumonic plague almost always follows a fulminating course and death within 2–3 days.

8.2. Differential Diagnosis

When bubonic plague occurs in epidemic form, it is readily diagnosed. Conversely, the diagnosis of an isolated case is often missed. Plague should be considered in any patient presenting with acute lymphadenitis and a history of residence or travel in a known plague area. Other causes of the lymphadenopathy, however, must be investigated: gram-positive bacteria are probably the most common cause, and a Gram's stain of a bubo aspirate should quickly differentiate between gram-positive cocci or gram-negative bacilli. The list of differential causes of lymphadenopathy is long, and plague cases have been misdiagnosed as cat scratch fever, lymphoma, and incarcerated inguinal hernia, to name a few. Bubonic plague and tularemia may be confused in areas where both diseases occur.[69] A skin lesion at the site of inoculation may be seen in both diseases. From a clinical standpoint this may not be a critical distinction, since both respond to the same antibiotic therapy; however, for public health and epidemiological reasons, a missed case of plague is potentially quite serious. Clinically, the severe tenderness and pain of affected lymph nodes of bubonic plague patients present a sharp contrast to the relatively milder discomfort that occurs with most other infectious causes of lymphadenitis.

Pneumonic plague may be confused with ARDS or with any pneumonitis of sudden onset. A history of recent exposure to a person with severe or fatal pneumonia, or to a pet cat with an acute febrile illness, cervical or submandibular lymphadenopathy or abscess, or bloody respiratory discharge[39,56,70,71] should prompt the clinician to consider plague. It is critically important to obtain a careful and thorough history of animal exposures from every suspect plague patient.

When plague is suspected, an examination of bubo aspirate or sputum by Gram's stain and by a polychrome stain should guide the clinician in choosing an appropriate antibiotic. When plague is suspected and other causes of illness cannot be implicated, specific plague therapy should be started pending the outcome of definitive testing. It may also be prudent to initially include therapy for gram-positive causes of lymphadenopathy; gram-positive bacteria grow rapidly on culture so that a microbiological diagnosis can usually be made within 12 to 24 hr. Based on clinical and laboratory findings, cases of plague can be categorized as suspect, presumptive, or confirmed. A *suspect case* is one in which the patient has disease manifestations suggestive of plague as well as nonspecific supportive laboratory findings such as gram-negative, bipolar bacilli seen in stained smears of a lymph node aspirate, sputum, tracheal wash, or other appropriate clinical materials. A *presumptive case* is one in which the patient has compatible clinical manifestations and the laboratory findings are more specific, such as a single seropositive test result for *Y. pestis* infection, or positive fluorescent antibody (FA) testing for the plague bacillus in clinical materials or cultural isolates. A *confirmed case* is one in which there is a fourfold or greater change in *Y. pestis* antibody titer between acute- and convalescent-phase serum samples, or in which a bacterial culture of suspected *Y. pestis* is lysed by the uniquely specific bacteriophage used for this purpose.

8.3. Laboratory Diagnosis

8.3.1. Specimen Collection and Processing. When plague is suspected, laboratory diagnostic specimens should be collected immediately, chest radiographs obtained, and the patient begun on appropriate antibiotic therapy pending microbiological confirmation. Specimens routinely collected include blood on all patients, lymph node aspirates from those with suspected buboes, sputum samples or tracheal washes from those with suspected respiratory plague, and cerebrospinal fluid from patients with suspected meningitis.

Blood is aseptically collected for culture, for preparation of blood smears on glass slides, and for leucocyte counts. For bubo aspiration, a small, sterile syringe containing a few milliliters of sterile saline is inserted into the central part of the suspect lymph node and an attempt is made to aspirate fluid. If this is not successful, the saline is injected and aspirated. A portion of the aspirate is used to make films on two or more glass slides for routine staining, and at least two slides for direct FA testing. Slides for staining are prepared by placing drops of the aspirate on glass slides, which are then air-dried and lightly heat-fixed. For routine staining, one slide should be stained by Giemsa or Wayson's method and one by a Gram's stain. To identify *Y. pestis*, specimens of blood, sputum, tracheal washes, and cerebrospinal fluid should be similarly stained. Under light microscopy, *Y. pestis* is a plump gram-negative bacillus that, with polychrome stains, typically shows a bipolar, closed safety-pin configuration. Fluorescence-stained organisms are identified using dark-field microscopy.[24]

8.3.2. Cultural Isolation of *Y. pestis*. Cultural isolation of *Y. pestis* is critical for early confirmation of infection. If the patient's condition allows, at least three blood cultures should be taken over a 45-min period immediately after the diagnosis of plague is suspected and before antibiotic treatment is begun. Blood and other materials, such as bubo aspirates and sputum, should be inoculated onto media such as sheep blood agar, brain–heart infusion (BHI) broth, or MacConkey or deoxycolate agar; when immediate culture is not possible, specimens may be placed in Cary–Blair transport medium. Confirmation of isolates as *Y. pestis* is made by specific bacteriophage lysis.[24]

8.3.3. Serological Diagnostic Methods. The standard serodiagnostic method is the passive hemagglutination (PHA) test utilizing *Y. pestis* Fl antigen (see Section 3.1.1). The specificity of a positive antibody–antigen reaction should be validated by hemagglutination inhibition testing. An acute serum should be taken for testing and a second serum taken 3–4 weeks after onset. Serum samples taken 3–4 weeks after onset of symptoms will confirm more than 95% of cases. PHA antibodies tend to remain at high titer (⩾64) for months and may persist at low titer for years or for life. Prior vaccination may confuse the interpretation of results (see Sections 5.4 and 6.3). An enzyme-linked immunosorbent assay to detect the Fl antigen in serum or blood clot is quite sensitive, especially for detecting IgM antibodies in early disease; however, this procedure does not recognize all blood culture-positive patients.[72] A complement-fixation test with Fl antigen is comparatively insensitive, especially in early infection. Latex particles coated with Fl antigen have been used successfully as nonbiological carriers in direct and passive agglutination tests, although some reports of its use have described problems with sensitivity and with specificity.[20,24]

8.3.4. Reference Diagnostic Testing. Whenever the diagnosis of plague is considered in the United States, materials should be sent to clinical laboratories experienced in testing for plague and to the CDC, Fort Collins, Colorado 80522, for microbiological confirmation. The CDC should be contacted by telephone (970-221-6400) or fax (970-221-6476) for reporting of a suspected case, for assistance in diagnostic testing (including the confirmation of an isolate as *Y. pestis*), and for other consultation.

9. Control and Prevention

9.1. General Concepts

The major objective of control is reduction of bites by infected fleas. Education of the general public and health professionals in areas where plague occurs is the first line of defense in plague prevention. Risk factors in those areas must be publicized, especially at the outset of known plague seasons.[49] Physicians, veterinarians, and the public must be alerted to the possibility of plague and know its signs and symptoms. Persons in endemic areas need to know the potential danger from rodent die-offs and report changes in rodent activity to public authorities. They should also be educated on the need to control fleas on pet dogs and cats; to properly store grains and other foodstuffs that may attract rodents to home, work, or play areas; to rodent-proof homes; and to take appropriate action when there is severe illness, death, or disappearance of a pet cat. Hikers, campers, and others who take part in outdoor recreational activities in areas where plague occurs should (1) avoid handling sick or dead animals, (2) avoid rodent nests and burrows, (3) use insect repellents containing *N,N*-diethyl-m-toluamide (DEET) on skin and repellents or appropriate insectidical sprays on clothing, and (4) treat accompanying pets with insecticides. Hunters should use gloves when handling dead animals.

During epidemics of bubonic plague, flea control must precede or effectively coincide with rodenticiding. Death of rodent hosts without prior flea control will deprive fleas of their normal hosts, forcing them to seek alternate hosts including humans, and greatly increasing the risk of human exposure. Appropriate insecticides should be applied to rodent burrows, nests, rat runs, and other sites where rodents are active. This should be done under the supervision of persons qualified in pest control.

Tests should be set up to determine whether the target fleas are susceptible to the insecticides considered for use and to evaluate the effectiveness of flea control efforts.[19,20] After reduction of the flea population, trapping or poisoning of rodents may be appropriate in certain situations.[19,20] Killing of commensal rodents will provide no benefit unless rodent-proofing of houses and elimination of food and harborage is also aggressively undertaken. Rodents will quickly move into the vacated spaces and may aggravate an epidemic situation, since in-migrating rodents are apt to be young and more susceptible to *Y. pestis* than the removed population. During rat-borne epidemics, bubonic plague patients, their clothing, and other effects may still be carrying infected fleas, and decontamination measures may be needed.

Plague is a quarantinable disease covered under international regulations.[73] Prior to departure from an area where pneumonic plague is occurring, exposed persons may be placed in isolation for 6 days. On arrival at their destination, travelers from pneumonic plague areas may be held for observation for 6 days after the day of arrival.[73,74] Following reports of outbreaks of plague in India in 1994, international and national health authorities became involved for the first time in many decades in reviewing, interpreting, and implementing regulations concerning the threat of international spread of plague.[17,74] Travel and trade with India was severely disrupted, and the outbreaks were estimated to have cost India more than a billion dollars in lost tourism, commerce, and investment values, disruption of services, and prevention and control efforts. This experience will hopefully lead to improved understanding by public health authorities of the true risks for international spread of plague and the use of more appropriate control measures in future similar occurrences.

Pneumonic plague patients may incubate very large numbers of organisms, but appropriate therapy almost always results in a marked decrease in a matter of hours.

9.2. Antibiotic Prophylaxis

Unless there is a suppurative discharge, bubonic plague patients do not pose a risk to their contacts. However, in circumstances where infection results from rat and flea infestation of houses, drug prophylaxis may be advisable for other members of the household and possibly adjacent households, depending on the environmental circumstances. Persons in close contact with infectious pneumonic plague patients in a previous 6-day period should be given postexposure treatment for 7 days. This is both to protect the individual and to prevent spread. Those who decline drug treatment should be placed under surveillance for 7 days since last exposure. Short-term antibiotic prophylaxis may be recommended in unusual situations for travelers who cannot avoid plague epidemic areas and for health care workers caring for suspected plague cases in an epidemic situation.

Recommended prophylactic drugs include the tetracyclines for adults and older children and sulfonamides in children younger than 9 years of age; chloramphenicol is also effective.[75]

9.3. Immunization

Since 1895, various plague vaccines have been used. The protective value of any of these is still a matter of debate. In some countries, living "avirulent" *Y. pestis* organisms have been used as immunogens. Studies in the United States have confirmed that such preparations are effective in experimental animals, but none of these is commercially available and their safety and efficacy in humans has not been adequately tested.[8,38,76] Since 1942, the vaccine licensed for use in the United States has been a formalin-killed suspension of whole virulent plague bacilli with phenol added as a preservative.[38] Different strains of *Y. pestis* have been tried, the quantity of organisms per dose has been varied, and the dose schedule has been altered repeatedly.[38,77] After vaccination and after recovery from plague, antibodies to many *Y. pestis* antigens are present; it is not known which antigens are most responsible for protection, although recombinant F1 and V antigens are protective in experimental animals.[78,79] In Vietnam during 1961–1971, there were eight plague cases in vaccinated Americans, while thousands of cases occurred in the indigenous peoples. US military personnel were undoubtedly exposed to the fleas that transmit plague, since they experienced a relatively high incidence of murine typhus, which is also transmitted by *X. cheopis*.[13,62] Acute and convalescent serum specimens were collected from 59 Americans who had received killed plague vaccine and who experienced clinical and serologically proved murine typhus. F1 antibody was found in the initial serum samples of 39 individuals, and this was attributed to prior vaccination. Serological tests showed a greater than fourfold rise in F1 titer in four patients and seroconversion in three patients. This was interpreted as evidence of subclinical *Y. pestis* infection in persons previously immunized.[62] There were, however, reports also of inapparent infections in unvaccinated persons in Vietnam.[53] A 1973 report describes the serological response in US military personnel initially immunized with 2×10^9 killed organisms followed by 4×10^8 bacilli on days 90 and 270. Of 29 subjects, two did not develop antibodies at a level considered to be protective.[80] Experts have concluded that the vaccine protected military personnel against bubonic plague during both World War II and the Vietnam conflict.[62] There was some evidence in Vietnam that vaccination modified but did not fully protect against pneumonic plague.

With the exception of the military, persons should be vaccinated only if they are at high risk for exposure.[38] Thus, vaccine is recommended for persons in the following high-risk groups: (1) laboratory personnel who routinely perform procedures that involve viable *Y. pestis*; and (2) persons who have regular contact with wild rodents or their fleas in areas in which there is zootic plague (e.g., mammologists, ecologists, and other field workers). The vaccine is given intramuscularly in a series of three injections, and booster doses can be administered three times at approximately 6-month intervals for vacinees who have a continuing high risk of exposure. Adverse reactions following injection of the first dose of vaccine generally are mild, but the frequency and severity of reactions can increase with repeated doses. Common adverse reactions include pain, erythema, and induration at the site of injection, malaise, fever, headache, and lymphadenopathy.[77] These reactions usually do not persist beyond 48 hr. The formalin-inactivated plague vaccine, USP, in use today is available from Greer Laboratories, Inc., P.O. Box 800, Lenoir, NC 28645-0800.

10. Unresolved Problems

The dynamics of enzootic plague and factors responsible for its introduction, maintenance, spread, or disappearance are not well known. Enzootic foci are widespread and readily available for study, but funding of field research is inconstant. Enzootic plague seems to be dependent on a complex interplay between moderately susceptible and resistant rodents, their fleas, modifications in the landscape, and climate. In the early part of this century, plague was introduced repeatedly into some areas without becoming established in wild rodents; in some areas, enzootic foci have advanced (western United States) and in other areas they have apparently regressed (India, Indonesia). There are currently no feasible means of eliminating enzootic foci for purposes of plague control.

Little is known about *Y. pestis* virulence in humans, the mechanism of action of *Y. pestis* endotoxin, and the means to protect against it. It is not well understood why plague endotoxin sometimes causes an irreversible immunologic cascade and death in spite of effective antibiotic therapy. Studies will hopefully identify the means for preventing these immunopathogenic events; however, the relative rarity of plague in the world today makes it difficult to investigate the pathogenesis and treatment response in humans.

Finally, a significant problem that has defied resolution is the politicization of plague throughout the world. Outbreaks go unreported, some countries impose unrealistic quarantine measures against countries that report cases, and plague continues to be treated as a highly charged economic and political issue, which can be both costly and counterproductive to plague prevention and control.

11. References

1. Eli, S. R., Three days in October of 1630: Detailed examination of mortality during an early modern plague epidemic in Venice, *Rev. Infect. Dis.* **11:**,128–141 (1989).
2. Tuchman, B. W., *A Distant Mirror*, Alfred A. Knopf, New York, 1978.
3. Hirst, L. F., *The Conquest of Plague*, Oxford University Press, London, 1953.
4. Wu Lien-The, *A Treatise on Pneumonic Plague*, League of Nations Health Organization, Geneva, 1926.
5. Zinsser, H., *Rats, Lice and History*, Little, Brown, Boston, 1934.
6. Pollitzer, R., *Plague*, World Health Organization, Geneva, 1954.
7. Butler, T., Yersinia infections: Centennial of the discovery of the plague bacillus, *Clin. Infect. Dis.* **19:**655–663 (1994).
8. Meyer, K. F., Cavanaugh, D. C., Bartelloni, P. J., and Marshall, J. D., Jr., Plague immunization. I. Past and present trends, *J. Infect. Dis.* **129:**S13–S18 (1974).
9. McCrumb, F. R., Jr., Mercier, S., Robic, J., *et al.*, Chloramphenicol and terramycin in the treatment of pneumonic plague, *Am. J. Med.* **14:**284–293 (1953).
10. Lewin, W., Becker, B. J. P., Horwitz, B., Two cases of pneumonic plague: Recovery of one case treated with streptomycin, *S. Afr. Med. J.* **22:**699–703 (1948).
11. Marshall, J. D., Jr., Joy, R. J. T., Ai, N. V., *et al.*, Plague in Vietnam 1965–1966, *Am. J. Epidemiol.* **86:**603–616 (1967).
12. Trong, R., Nhu, T. Q., and Marshall, J. D., Jr., A mixed pneumonic-bubonic plague outbreak in Vietnam, *Mil. Med.* **132:**93–97 (1967).
13. Cavanaugh, D. C., Dangerfield, H. G., Hunter, D. H., *et al.*, Some observations on the current plague outbreak in the Republic of Vietnam, *Am. J. Public Health* **58:**742–752 (1968).
14. Butler, T., *Plague and Other Yersinia Infections*, Plenum Press, New York, 1983.
15. Anonymous, *Plague in India: World Health Organization International Plague Investigative Team Report, December 9, 1994*, World Health Organization, Geneva, 1994.
16. Ramalingaswami, V., An overview of the work carried out by the Technical Advisory Committee on Plague, *Curr. Sci.* **71:**783–786 (1996).
17. Campbell, G. L., and Hughes, J. M., Plague in India: A new warning from an old nemesis, *Ann. Intern. Med.* **122:**151–153 (1995).

18. Mavalankar, D. V., India "plague" epidemic: Unanswered questions and key lessons, *J. R. Soc. Med.* **88:**547–551 (1995).
19. Gage, K. L., and Quan, T. J., Plague and other yersinioses, in: *Topley and Wilson's Microbiology and Microbial Infections, Vol. 3–Bacterial Infections, 9th ed.* (L. Collier *et al.*, eds.), pp. 885–904, Edward Arnold, London, 1998.
20. Bahmanyar, M., and Cavanaugh, D. C., *Plague Manual*, World Health Organization, Geneva, 1976.
21. Barnes, A. M., Surveillance and control of bubonic plague in the United States, *Symp. Zool. Soc. Lond.* **50:**237–270 (1982).
22. World Health Organization, Technical guide for a system of plague surveillance, *Week. Epidemiol. Rec.* **14:**149–160 (1973).
23. Poland, J. D., Quan, T. J., and Barnes, A. M., Plague, in: *Handbook of Zoonoses*, Section A: *Bacterial, Rickettsial, Chlamydial, and Mycotic Diseases* (B. W. Beran and J. H. Steele, eds.), pp. 93–112, CRC Press, Boca Raton, FL, 1993.
24. Quan, T. J., Barnes, A. M., and Poland, J. D., Yersinioses, in: *Diagnostic Procedures for Bacterial Mycotic and Parasitic Infections*, 6th ed. (A. Balows and W. Hausler, eds.), pp. 723–745, APHA, Washington DC, 1981.
25. Brubaker, R. R., Factors promoting acute and chronic diseases caused by yersiniae, *Clin. Microbiol. Rev.* **4:**309–324 (1991).
26. Cavanaugh, D. C., and Randall, R., The role of multiplication of *Pasteurella pestis* in mononuclear phagocytes in the pathogenesis of flea-borne plague, *J. Immunol.* **89:**348–363 (1959).
27. Montie, T. C., Properties and pharmacological action of plague murine toxin, *Pharmacol. Ther.* **12:**491–499 (1981).
28. Williams, J. E., Harrison, D. N., Quan, T. J., *et al.*, Atypical plague bacilli isolated from rodents, fleas, and man, *Am. J. Public Health* **68:**262–264 (1978).
29. Barnes, A. M., and Quan, T. J., Plague, in: *Infectious Diseases* (S. L. Gorbach, J. G. Bartlett, and N. R. Blacklow, eds.), pp. 1285–1291, W.B. Saunders, Philadelphia, 1992.
30. Devignat, R., Varieties de l'espece *Pastuerella pestis*. Nouvelle hypothese, *Bull. WHO* **4:**247–263 (1951).
31. Guiyoule, A., Grimont, F., *et al.*, Plague pandemics investigated by ribotyping of *Yersinia pestis* strains, *J. Clin. Microbiol.* **32:**634–641 (1994).
32. Cavanaugh, D. C., The specific effect of temperature upon the transmission of the plague bacillus by the oriental rat flea (*Xenopsylla cheopis*), *Am. J. Trop. Med. Hyg.* **20:**264–273 (1971).
33. Hinnebusch, B. J., Perry, R.. D., and Schwann, T. G., Role of the *Yersinia pestis* hemin storage (*hms*) locus in the transmission of plague in fleas, *Science* **273:**367–370 (1996).
34. Eskey, C. R., and Haas, V. H., Plague in the western part of the United States, *Public Health Bull.* **254:**1–82 (1940).
35. Kartman, L., and Prince, F. M., Studies on *Pasteurella pestis* in fleas. V. The experimental plague-vector efficiency of wild rodent fleas compared with *Xenopsylla cheopis* together with observations on the influence of temperature, *Am. J. Trop. Med. Hyg.* **5:**1058–1070 (1956).
36. Pollitzer, R., and Meyer, K. F., The ecology of plague, in: *Studies in Disease Ecology* (J. H. May, ed.), pp. 433–501, Hefner, New York, 1961.
37. World Health Organization, Human plague in 1994, *Week. Epidemiol. Rec.* **22:**165–172 (1996).
38. Centers Disease Control and Prevention, Prevention of plague. Recommendations of the Advisory Committee on Immunization Practices (ACIP), *Morbid. Mortal. Week. Rep.* **45:**(RR-14)**:**1–15 (1996).
39. Centers Disease Control and Prevention, Human plague—United States, 1993–1994, *Morbid. Mortal. Week. Rep.* **43:**242–246 (1994).
40. Gage, K. L., Lance, S. E., Dennis, D. T., and Montenieri, J., Human plague in the United States: A review of cases from 1988–1992 with comments on the likelihood of increased plague activity, *Border Epidemiol. Bull.* **19:**1–10 (1992).
41. Marshall, J. D., Jr., Quy, D. V., and Gibson, F. L., Asymptomatic pharyngeal plague infection in Vietnam, *Am. J. Trop. Med. Hyg.* **16:**175–177 (1967).
42. Craven, R. B., and Poland, J. D., Plague, in: *Public Health and Preventive Medicine*, 13th ed. (J. M. Last and R. B. Wallace, eds.), pp. 237–240, Appleton & Lange, Norwalk, CT, 1992.
43. Poland, J. D., and Barnes, A. M., Plague, in: *CRC Handbook Series in Zoonoses, Section A: Bacterial, Rickettsial, and Mycotic Diseases*, Vol. 2 (J. H. Steele, ed.), pp. 523–540, CRC Press, Boca Raton, FL, 1979.
44. Cavanaugh, D. C., and Marshall, J. D., Jr., The influence of climate on the seasonal prevalence of plague in the Republic of Vietnam, *J. Wildl. Dis.* **8:**85–94 (1972).
45. Link, V. B., *A History of Plague in the United States of America*, Public Health Monograph No. 26, Government Printing Office, Washington, DC, 1955.
46. Craven, R. B., Maupin, G. O., Beard, M. L., *et al.*, Reported cases of human plague infections in the United States, 1979–1991, *J. Med. Entomol.* **30:**758–761 (1993).
47. Barnes, A. M., Quan, T. J., Beard, M., and Maupin, G. O., Plague in American Indians, 1956–1987, *Morbid. Mortal. Week. Rep. CDC Surv. Summary* **37:**11–16 (1988).
48. Centers for Disease Control, Plague—United States, 1992, *Morbid. Mortal. Week. Rep.* **41:**787–790 (1992).
49. Mann, J. M., Martone, W. J., Boyce, J. M., *et al.*, Endemic human plague in New Mexico: Risk factors associated with infection, *J. Infect. Dis.* **140:**397–401 (1979).
50. Mann, J. M., Schmid, G. P., Stoetz, P. A., Skinner, M. D., and Kaufmann, A. F., Peripatetic plague, *J. Am. Med. Assoc.* **247:**46–47 (1982).
51. Centers for Disease Control, Plague—South Carolina, *Morbid. Mortal. Week. Rep.* **32:**417–419 (1983).
52. Meyer, K. F., Pneumonic plague, *Bacteriol. Rev.* **25:**249–261 (1961).
53. Legters, L. J., Cottingham, A. J., and Hunter, D. H., Clinical and epidemiological notes on a defined outbreak of plague in Vietnam, *Am. J. Trop. Med. Hyg.* **19:**639–652 (1970).
54. Druett, H. A., Robinson, J. M., Henderson, D. W., *et al.*, Studies on respiratory infection. II. The influence of aerosol particle size on infection of guinea pigs with *Pasteurella pestis*, *J. Hyg.* **54:**37–48 (1956).
55. Gasper, P. W., Barnes, A. M., Quan, T. J., *et al.*, Plague (*Yersinia pestis*) in cats: Description of experimentally induced disease, *J. Med. Entomol.* **30:**20–26 (1993).
56. Eidson, M., Thilsted, J. P., and Rollag, O. J., Clinical, clinicopathologic, and pathologic features of plague in cats: 119 cases (1977–1988), *J. Am. Vet. Med. Assoc.* **199:**1191–1197 (1991).
57. Christie, A. B., Chen, T. C., and Elberg, S. S., Plague in camels and goats: Their role in human epidemics, *J. Infect. Dis.* **141:**724–726 (1980).
58. Burmeister, R. W., Tigertt, W. D., and Overholt, E. L., Laboratory-acquired pneumonic plague, *Ann. Intern. Med.* **56:**789–800 (1962).
59. Chen, T. H., and Meyer, K. F., Susceptibility and antibody response

of *Rattus* species to experimental plague, *J. Infect. Dis.* **129:**S62–S71 (1974).
60. Butler, T., and Hudson, B. W., The serologic response to *Yersinia pestis* infection, *Bull. WHO* **55:**39–42 (1977).
61. Payne, F. E., Smadel, J. E., and Courdurier, J., Immunologic studies on persons residing in a plague endemic area, *J. Immunol.* **77:**24–33 (1956).
62. Cavanaugh, D. C., Elisberg, B. L., Llewellyn, C. H., *et al.*, Plague immunization. V. Indirect evidence for the efficacy of plague vaccination, *J. Infect. Dis.* **129:**S37–S49 (1974).
63. Butler, T., A clinical study of bubonic plague: Observations of the 1970 Vietnam epidemic with emphasis on coagulation studies, skin histology, and electrocardiograms, *Am. J. Med.* **53:**268–276 (1972).
64. Hull, H. F., Montes, J. M., and Mann, J. M., Septicemic plague in New Mexico, *J. Infect. Dis.* **155:**113–118 (1987).
65. Welty, T. K., Grabman, J., Kompare, E., *et al.*, Nineteen cases of plague in Arizona. A spectrum including ecthyma gangrenosum due to plague and plague in pregnancy, *West. J. Med.* **142:**641–646 (1985).
66. Crook, L. D., and Tempest, B., Plague—A clinical review of 27 cases, *Arch. Intern. Med.* **152:**1253–1256 (1992).
67. Finegold, M. J., Pathogenesis of plague. A review of plague deaths in the United States during the last decade, *Am. J. Med.* **45:**549–554 (1968).
68. Sites, V. R., and Poland, J. D., Mediastinal lymphadenopathy in bubonic plague, *Am. J. Roentgenol. Radium Ther. Nucl. Med.* **66:** 567–570 (1972).
69. Sites, V. R., Poland, J. D., and Hudson, B. W., Bubonic plague misdiagnosed as tularemia: Retrospective serologic diagnosis, *J. Am. Med. Assoc.* **222:**1642–1643 (1972).
70. Doll, J. M., Zeitz, P. S., Ettestad, P., *et al.*, Cat-transmitted fatal pneumonic plague in a person who traveled from Colorado to Arizona, *Am. J. Trop. Med. Hyg.* **51:**109–114 (1994).
71. Werner, S. B., Weidmer, C. E., Nelson, B. C., *et al.*, Primary plague pneumonia contracted from a domestic cat at South Lake Tahoe, Calif. *J. Am. Med. Assoc.* **251:**929–931 (1984).
72. Williams, J. E., Arntzen, L., Tyndal, G. L., and Isaacson, M., Application of enzyme immunoassays for the confirmation of clinically suspect plague in Namibia, *Bull. WHO* **64:**745–752 (1982).
73. World Health Organization, *International Health Regulations (1969)*, World Health Organization, Geneva, 1983.
74. World Health Organization, Plague, India, *WHO Week. Epidemiol. Rec.* **40:**295–299 (1994).
75. Campbell, G. L., and Dennis, D. T., Plague and other *Yersinia* infections, in: *Harrison's Principles of Internal Medicine, 14th ed.* (A. S. Fauci *et al.*, eds.), pp. 975–983, McGraw-Hill, New York, 1997.
76. Meyer, K. F., Smith, G., Foster, L., *et al.*, Live, attenuated *Yersinia pestis* vaccine: Virulent in nonhuman primates, harmless to guinea pigs, *J. Infect. Dis.* **129:**S85–S120 (1974).
77. Marshall, J. D., Jr., Bartelloni, P. J., Cavanaugh, D. C., *et al.*, Plague immunization. II. Relation of adverse clinical reactions to multiple immunizations with killed vaccine, *J. Infect. Dis.* **129:** S19–S25 (1974).
78. Leary, S. E., Williamson, D. E., Griffin, K. F., *et al.*, Active immunization with recombinant V antigen from *Yersinia pestis* protects mice against plague, *Infect. Immun.* **63:**2854–2858 (1995).
79. Simpson, W. J., Thomas, R. E., and Schwann, T. G., Recombinant capsular antigen (fraction 1) from *Yersinia pestis* induces a protective antibody response in BALB/C mice, *Am. J. Trop. Med. Hyg.* **43:**389–396 (1990).
80. Bartelloni, P. J., Marshall, J. D., Jr., and Cavanaugh, D. C., Clinical and serological responses to plague vaccine U.S.P., *Mil. Med.* **138:**720–722 (1973).

12. Suggested Reading

Bahmanyar, M., and Cavanaugh, D. C., *Plague Manual*, World Health Organization, Geneva, 1976. (The last edition of the World Health Organization standard reference manual of the control and prevention of plague. A new edition, with new authors, is scheduled for publication.)

Butler, T., *Plague and Other Yersinia Infections*, Plenum Press, New York, 1983. (A review of human plague by an author who has had considerable firsthand experience in the diagnosis and treatment of plague and study of the pathophysiological mechanisms of infection with *Yersinia pestis*. The book includes fascinating material on the history of Alexandre Yersin and his discovery of the plague bacillus. Other yersinioses are also reviewed.)

Centers Disease Control and Prevention, Prevention of plague. Recommendations of the Advisory Committees on Immunization Practices (ACIP), *Morbid. Mortal. Week. Rep.* **45**(RR-14)**:**1–15 (1996). (Reviews information on plague control, with general background information on plague, and a focus on the formalin killed plague vaccine, USP.)

Eskey, C. R., Haas, V. H., Plague in the western part of the United States, *Public Health Bull.* **254:**1–82 (1940). (The classic description of the ecology of plague in the United States.)

Gage, K. L., and Quan, T. J., Plague and other yersinioses, in: *Topley and Wilson's Microbiology and Microbial Infections, Vol. 3–Bacterial Infections, 9th ed.* (L. Collier *et al.*, eds.), pp. 885–904, Edward Arnold, London, 1998. (A current review of the biology and ecology of plague worldwide.)

Gregg, C. T., *Plague, an Ancient Disease in the Twentieth Century*, rev. ed., University of New Mexico Press, Albuquerque, 1985. (Interesting overview of some epidemiological aspects of plague in the United States, with selected case histories.)

Link, V. B., *A History of Plague in the United States of America*, Public Health Monograph No. 26, Government Printing Office, Washington, DC, 1955. (Excellent history of the introduction and spread of plague in the United States in the early part of the 20th century, with fascinating descriptions of human plague outbreaks in California.)

Pollitzer, R., Plague, *WHO Monogr. Ser.* 22 (1954). (Still the most comprehensive plague "text.")

World Health Organization, *International Health Regulations (1969)*, World Health Organization, Geneva, 1983. (Regulations governing the reporting and control of the three remaining class 1 quarantinable diseases: plague, cholera, yellow fever.)

Wu Lien-The, *A Treatise on Pneumonic Plague*, League of Nations Health Organization, Geneva, 1926. (A compendium of all information known on pneumonic plague at the time of writing, with descriptions of occurrences throughout the world, and especially the extraordinary Manchurian epidemics of 1910 and 1920.)

CHAPTER 28

Pneumococcal Infections

Robert S. Baltimore and Eugene D. Shapiro

1. Introduction

The pneumococcus (*Streptococcus pneumoniae*) is a major cause of pneumonia and meningitis worldwide. In his classic book entitled *The Biology of the Pneumococcus*, published in 1938, Benjamin White[1] listed 19 different names applied to the pneumococcus between 1897 and 1930, the year the designation *Diplococcus pneumoniae Weichselbaum* was approved in 4th edition of *Bergey's Manual*.[2] In a more recent (8th) edition of Bergey's *Manual*,[3] it is listed as *Streptococcus pneumoniae*, the designation that is now generally accepted.

Although any of a large number of microorganisms may cause acute inflammation of the lungs (pneumonia),[4] typical (primary) lobar pneumonia is nearly always caused by the pneumococcus, which is also the most frequent cause of bronchopneumonia. Pneumococcal pneumonia of either variety is generally preceded by a simple acute infection of the upper respiratory tract such as the common cold and may also occur as a complication of influenza. It has been called the "captain of the men of death" and "the friend of the aged," because it had long been the principal immediate cause and most frequent contributing cause of death in the aged and infirm and in those with otherwise fatal diseases. Since public health statistics of morbidity and mortality are usually reported by diseases and not by etiologic agents, most of the references are to data on "pneumonia," of which the majority are presumed to be due to the pneumococcus, except during unusual epidemics due to other organisms.

The pneumococcus is also the most frequent cause of acute bacterial meningitis in those over age 3 months, being exceeded in frequency only by the meningococcus during periods of epidemic prevalence.[5,5a] The pneumococcus is also the most frequent cause of purulent empyema of the pleura[6] (usually as a complication of primary pneumonia) and of otitis media at all ages.[7,7a] Less frequently, it may cause focal infections at other sites in the body. It is also the most common organism cultured from the blood of patients with acute febrile illness, usually pneumonia or meningitis, but not infrequently also from infants and young children with no demonstrable localized site of infection.[8,9]

2. Historical Background

The early history of the discovery of the pneumococcus and its pathogenic potentials for animals and humans was presented chronologically and in some detail by White,[1] subsequently by Finland,[10] and recently and more concisely by Austrian[11] in 1981. According to the latter, the pneumococcus was probably first visualized in pulmonary tissues by Klebs in 1875, later by Eberth in 1880, and then by Koch in 1881. However, the organism was first isolated in the laboratory independently by Pasteur in France and Sternberg in the United States and reported by both in 1881; both these workers had injected saliva subcutaneously in rabbits, who died and were shown to have the organisms in large numbers in their blood. Pasteur used saliva of an infant that died of rabies; Sternberg injected his own saliva. Both thus demonstrated the occurrence of pneumococcus in the pharynges in carriers without relation to disease.

During the next few years, a considerable controversy resulted from the descriptions and characterizations of the bacteria seen in pneumonic lungs by Friedlander,

Robert S. Baltimore and Eugene D. Shapiro • Departments of Pediatrics and Epidemiology and Public Health, Yale University School of Medicine, New Haven, Connecticut 06520-8064.

The first edition of this chapter was written by the late Maxwell Finland. In this chapter, significant parts of the background and epidemiological data come from Dr. Finland's manuscript.

Weichselbaum, and Freinkel (quoted by Austrian[11]); this was eventually resolved by the application of the Gram's stain described in 1884. The stain permitted the differentiation of Friedlander's bacillus, now known as *Klebsiella pneumoniae*, which was decolorized by the Gram's method (gram-negative), from the pneumococcus, which was not decolorized (gram-positive).

During the late 1880s, reports were published of the presence of pneumococci in focal infections other than those of the lung, including valvular lesions of cases of endocarditis, purulent meningitis, otitis, arthritis, sinusitis, and conjunctivitis, and from other organs and sites.

At the turn of the century, Neufeld[12] reported on the solubility of pneumococci in bile, which became a useful tool in the differentiation of pneumococci from other streptococci, especially the viridans variety. Most important were the demonstrations of the development of antibodies against the homologous pneumococcus following infection or vaccination, which protected animals against subsequent infection with that organism, and the description of the specific agglutination and quellung reactions in homologous antisera by Neufeld[13] in 1902. The agglutination reaction led to the more definite segregation of pneumococci into specific types in 1913 by Lister[14] in South Africa and by Dochez and Gillespie[15] at the Rockefeller Institute in New York. Some partially successful attempts were made to protect the highly susceptible workers in the gold and diamond mines in South Africa by vaccination with mixtures of these pneumococcal types.[16,17] This also led to the development of specific antisera for therapy and the use of the agglutination reaction to identify the causative type before administering the therapeutic antisera. It was not until 1931, however, that Armstrong[18] in England first reported the clinical use of the quellung reaction for the rapid typing of pneumococci. By 1932, Cooper *et al.*[19] in New York City had segregated more than 30 specific types; subsequently, workers in the United States and in Denmark increased that number to the 90 types known at present.[20,21] The typing of pneumococci and the type-specific antibody response to infection or to immunization, first with whole organisms[22] and later with type-specific capsular polysaccharides,[23] proved to be potent tools that enhanced the capabilities for epidemiological studies of pneumococcal infections[24] and offered the possibility of control of infections in individuals and in susceptible population groups.

Meanwhile, progress was being made, notably at the Rockefeller Institute, in delineating the biology of the pneumococcus and its biochemical constituents and immunogenic properties. Most important was the demonstration that the type specificity, pathogenicity (virulence), and eventually also its immunogenicity resided in the specific chemical composition of its capsular polysaccharide. When purified, this component proved to be essentially nontoxic when injected in humans and capable of inducing type-specific antibodies in varying quantities. When it was also shown that 80% of all serious and life-threatening pneumococcal infections, bacteremia, meningitis, endocarditis, and infections of normally sterile body cavities were caused by only 14 of the known 80 or more types, a vaccine incorporating these 14 types was made available,[23] and early trials showed it to be effective in many circumstances. Its effects on the control of pneumococcal infections are a major subject of contemporary investigation of pneumococcal disease. A separate section of this chapter is devoted to the development of pneumococcal vaccine and the benefits of its use. Since the late 1970s, there has been concern about the existence of pneumococci resistant to penicillin and other antibiotics. In the 1980s and 1990s, the rising rates of antibiotic resistance have been alarming.

3. Methodology

3.1. Sources of Epidemiological Data

In introducing his chapter on the epidemiology of pneumonia, Heffron[25] indicated that the absolute frequency of its occurrence is unknown. Statistics from various health organizations throughout the world provide information on the total number of deaths from all causes, including pneumonia, but in many instances, especially in Africa, where the disease is widely prevalent, deaths are frequently unreported and inaccurate. In the United States, pneumonia and influenza deaths from 121 cities are reported in the Centers for Disease Control (CDC) *Morbidity and Mortality Weekly Report* (MMWR), but they are generally regarded as an index of influenza mortality. In 1934, Collins and Gover[26] reported that acute infections of the respiratory tract caused more deaths and a higher morbidity in the United States than did any other group of diseases. However, it is impossible in the United States or elsewhere to obtain exact figures on morbidity or mortality because pneumonia has not been a reportable disease in most states; it is estimated that even in those states wherein it is reportable, only about half the cases are actually reported. Also, there is no uniform method of reporting cases (as lobar pneumonia, bronchopneumonia, or both). In temperate zones, lobar pneumonia, but not bronchopneumonia, has a definite seasonal incidence, but their differentiation is often impossible. In the United

States, the best estimate of the incidence of pneumococcal pneumonia has come from special surveys (see Section 3.2). Pneumococcal meningitis, while also not a reportable disease, has been included in special meningitis surveys.[5a,27,28]

3.2. Surveys

A number of surveys have been carried out to estimate the incidence of pneumonia. These include a population study of 2,602,000 people conducted by the federal government for 1935–1963, data from the Cleveland family study reported in 1936, health records from the Kaiser-Permanente Health Center, and reports from hospitals such as the large retrospective regional study performed in Sweden, 1964–1980.[29] These have been summarized by Mufson,[30] Austrian,[11] and the CDC.[31] In the past decade there have been a number of studies that have focused on specific populations of interest. Children were the subject of nationwide prospective studies from Finland[32] and Israel.[33] In the United States, specific populations at exceptional risk for pneumococcal infections have been surveyed, including inmates of a correctional facility,[34] Alaskan natives,[35] and Native Americans.[36] Data on these populations are presented in Table 1 and discussed in Section 5.1. Antibody surveys have not been reported except when associated with vaccine trials. The assays are not sufficiently specific to use in establishing estimates of incidence.

3.3. Laboratory Diagnosis

3.3.1. Isolation and Identification of the Organism. Growth of pneumococci requires suitable media such as nutrient broth to which serum or defibrinated blood, preferably rabbit's or sheep's, is added. For epidemiological purposes, however, reliance has been placed on three methods: (1) direct culture on solid media (blood agar); (2) in the past by mouse inoculation, particularly of materials that may contain mixed cultures, such as sputum or broth-moistened swabs of environmental materials; mouse peritoneal exudate may be withdrawn by capillary pipette after 3 or 4 hr, mixed with specific sera, stained, and examined for type-specific agglutination[37]; (3) application of the Neufeld quellung method to cultures or to fresh materials (sputum, exudate, blood cultures) for specific typing of pneumococci. Use of the quellung test has the advantage of being type-specific for the pneumococcus; it can rapidly diagnose the type and also detect multiple types of pneumococci in the same specimen (e.g., in sputum, mouse peritoneal exudate, environmental swab, or any purulent materials). Currently, agglutination of antibody-coated latex beads has replaced the quellung test in many laboratories and can be used for rapid identi-

Table 1. Focused Studies of the Incidence of Pneumococcal Disease[a]

Years of study	Population surveyed	Size of population surveyed[b]	Incidence (per 100,000), unadjusted	Case fatality rate (per 100)	Reference
1986–1990	Native Alaskans	81,368	74	13–14	35
1986–1990	Non-native Alaskans	438,763	16	13–14	35
1986–1990	Native Alaskans, less than 2 years of age	4,068	624	1–2	35
1983–1991	Native Americans, White River Indian Health Service Hospital, total unadjusted	9,814	207	5%	36
1983–1991	Native Americans, White River Indian Health Service Hospital, Children less than 2 years old	654	1,820 (2,396, 1–2 yrs old)	0%	36
1989 (4 weeks)	Correctional facility, USA	6,700	687		34
1988–1990	Israeli, children 0–12 years old	2,400,000 est	19.9	2.2	33
1988–1990	Israeli, children, less than 1 year old	NA	104	30 (first month of life); 2.1 (one month to 12 months of life)	33
1985–1989	Finland, children, 0–15 years old	5,000,000 est	8.9	1.3	32
1985–1989	Finland, children, less than 1 year old	NA	37	NA	32

[a]Standard of diagnosis, isolation of *Streptococcus pneumoniae* from usually sterile sites.
[b]NA, data not available.

fication in the laboratory by testing culture supernates. For cultures of materials from air, dust, skin, or fomites, broth-moistened swabs of the material or surfaces may be streaked directly on blood agar, and characteristic colonies of pneumococci are easily recognized after incubation for 12–24 hr (as are those of hemolytic or viridans streptococci and staphylococci). The swab may then be placed in blood broth and pneumococci identified from subcultures on blood agar or by mouse inoculation or both. Initiation of growth of pneumococci may be enhanced by incubation in 5% carbon dioxide or in a candle jar. Additional cultures in broth and mouse inoculation enhance the yield. Nasal or pharyngeal swabs may be plated directly on blood agar or cultivated in broth and some of the latter inoculated into mice after incubation for 3–4 hr. Prior exposure to antibiotics (during prophylaxis or therapy) markedly reduces or may eliminate the chance of growing pneumococci from the nose and throat.

3.3.2. Serological Methods. Serological tests for demonstrating type-specific antibodies include opsonic or pneumococcidal tests in fresh defibrinated or heparinized whole blood, the mouse protection test on serum, macroscopic or microscopic agglutination of heat- or formalin-killed suspensions of organisms, or precipitin and diffusion tests with supernatant fluids of cultures or exudates or with type-specific polysaccharides. These tests differ in sensitivity and also somewhat in specificity. Specific antibody has been quantitated with specific polysaccharides and used in surveys for susceptibility in relation to immunization and to measure the response to polysaccharide vaccines and enzyme-linked immunoassay (ELISA).[24] A highly type-specific radioimmunoassay (RIA) can also be used to derive similar data,[38,39] and most recent information on responses to pneumococcal vaccine is based on this method.

4. Biological Characteristics of the Organism

Morphologically, the pneumococcus typically appears as an ovoid or spherical, coccoidlike form of 0.5–1.25 μm, in pairs, the distal ends of which tend to be pointed or lancet-shaped, and surrounded by a distinguishable capsule that contains a polysaccharide [soluble specific substance (SSS)]. The diplococci may occur in chains, particularly in liquid medium, hence the designation streptococcus. The chemical composition of the SSS determines its specific serological type, of which there are now at least 90,[21] including several that are closely related serologically. The diplococci usually stain gram-positive, but may decolorize and appear gram-negative in old cultures or after exposure to antibacterial agents. When grown on blood agar, pneumococci form clear, round, mucoid, colorless, umbilicated colonies surrounded by an area of green hemolysis. Heavily capsulated organisms, such as those of type 3, grow in dome-shaped, clear, mucoid colonies.

Resistance of pneumococci to chemotherapeutic agents was recognized as emerging during therapy with ethylhydrocupreine (optochin) in 1918, the first chemical to receive extensive clinical trials in pneumonia.[40] Resistance to sulfapyridine was also recognized as a possible cause of failure of that drug in the treatment of pneumococcal pneumonia in 1938.[41,42] Although significant resistance of pneumococci to penicillin had been infrequent and limited in geographic distribution in the 1970s and early 1980s, in the past decade this has become a serious and increasing worldwide problem (see Section 5.1.1). Resistance to other antibacterial agents has been reported from many areas and has accounted for therapeutic failures. Reports have included resistance to sulfonamides, tetracycline, erythromycin, lincomycin, and chloramphenicol, in addition to β-lactam antibiotics.[43] Pneumococci are also relatively resistant to aminoglycosides and some are highly resistant to streptomycin. Multiantibiotic-resistant pneumococci have been reported from South Africa and in occasional strains isolated in the United States (see Section 5.1.1).

5. Descriptive Epidemiology

5.1. Prevalence and Incidence

In the United States, a federal government survey over a 12-month period in 1935 that involved over 2.6 million people in 83 widely scattered cities and 24 rural counties suggested an incidence rate of 558 cases of pneumonia per 100,000.[44] Data from several centers reported for 1920–1928 indicated that deaths from pneumonia generally accounted for 7.4–8.3% of deaths from all causes. On the basis of data from various sources, Austrian[44] estimated ("with limited confidence") that the attack rate of pneumococcal pneumonia in the United States lay somewhere in the range of 1.5–10 (more likely between 2 and 5)/1000 man years of exposure.

The Cleveland study of illness in middle-class families comprising 292 adults and their school-aged children, reported in 1953, has been summarized by Austrian.[44] There were three illnesses diagnosed as pneumococcal over a 3-year period, 1974–1976, an attack rate of 10.3/1000 man years. At the Kaiser-Permanente Health Center, the estimated attack rate of pneumococcal pneumonia of all types was 1.4/1000 among Californians 45 years of age or older. However, among institutionalized patients, the attack rate was calculated to be 12.5/1000 for pneumonia due to all pneumococcal types.[44]

Data on the incidence of pneumococcal infections has come from the CDC[31] and from a detailed review of morbidity and mortality by Mufson.[30] In the early 1980s, the CDC estimated rates per 100,000 of pneumococcal pneumonia of 68–260, of pneumococcal meningitis of 1.2–2.8, and of pneumococcal bacteremia of 7–25; the case-fatality rates of these syndromes have been 5–7%, 32%, and 20%, respectively.[31] Mufson's estimates of incidence, converted to rates per 100,000, were 100–200 for pneumonia and 0.3–4.9 for pneumococcal meningitis based on published studies from the mid-1970s. Higher rates of pneumococcal infection were observed in patients with sickle-cell anemia, congenital asplenia, renal transplants, Hodgkin's disease, and multiple myeloma than in subjects without these preexisting conditions.[30]

The importance of *S. pneumoniae* in different clinical syndromes and at different ages has been reviewed by Klein[7] in infants and children and by Mufson[30] in the general population. On the basis of recent cooperative studies, the pneumococcus was shown to be the most common pathogen cultured from the respiratory tract in infants (other than neonates) and children, and it is also the most frequent cause of serious infections, including pneumonia and bacteremia.[7]

In the general population of nine cities, *S. pneumoniae* was the most common cause of community-acquired pneumonia requiring hospitalization: pneumococcal pneumonia accounted for 26–78% of all pneumonia cases in the nine areas and in most studies exceeded 50%.[30] Mortality rate varied from 6 to 19%, but was 2–5 times higher in the 20% of adults who developed bacteremia. Indeed, this organism is the most common cause of bacteremia in adults, as well as in children over 1 month old.[30] This may be changing, however. In a recent study from the Johns Hopkins Hospital in Baltimore, Maryland, which was a 1-year prospective study, 385 patients with pneumonia were divided by preadmission status according to whether they were infected with human immunodeficiency virus (HIV) or not. Of the 205 HIV-uninfected patients, 15% had their pneumonia caused by *S. pneumoniae* and of 180 HIV-infected patients 21.1% had their pneumonia caused by *S. pneumoniae*. Of patients who had community-acquired pneumonia the rate of isolation of pneumococcus was about 15% irrespective of HIV status.[45] This suggests that in hospitalized patients *S. pneumoniae* may be less important than it had been in the past. In the late 1980s to early 1990s, there have been a number of focused studies of populations at high risk for pneumococcal infections. The impetus for performing these studies to some extent was the development of conjugate pneumococcal vaccines, which would potentially need to be tested on populations with a high risk of disease. As shown in Table 1, children and residents of closed communities, such as prisoners and infants, all have a risk of invasive pneumococcal infection far above the estimates for normal populations. While populations can be found with an annual rate of 20 or less per 100,000, children in the first 2 years of life and certain populations such as Native Americans have a much higher rate of illness. In the Israeli study by Dagon *et al.*,[33] it was shown that within Israel the rate of pneumococcal illness was much higher among the Arab population than among Jews, and the case fatality rate was 5.7% among non-Jews and 0.3% among Jews.

Pneumococcal meningitis occurs at a rate of about 0.3–4.9 persons/100,000, with children under age 5 at higher risk.[30] In a summary from the CDC reviewing reports of meningitis from 38 states in 1978, the incidence per 100,000 of *S. pneumoniae* meningitis was 0.30.[27] It was exceeded by *Haemophilus influenzae* meningitis and *Neisseria menigitidis* meningitis, with rates per 100,000 of 1.24 and 0.72, respectively (see Chapters 16 and 23). The incidence of pneumococcal meningitis was highest in the first year of life (age-specific rate of 8.0/100,000). While the absolute incidence is much less in older age groups (0.1–0.4/100,000), its *relative* importance increases, and this organism is the most common cause of meningitis for elderly individuals in the United States. In a CDC-sponsored study of six states surveying 34 million people in 1986, the incidence of pneumococcal meningitis was 1.1 per 100,000 compared with rates of 2.9 and 0.9 per 100,000 for *H. influenzae* and *N. meningitidis*, respectively.[28] With the dramatic decline of *H. influenzae* meningitis in the early 1990s due to the success of the conjugate vaccines, *S. pneumoniae* is currently the most common cause of bacterial meningitis.[5a] In a study of children from Israel, 1988–1990, the rate of pneumococcal meningitis was 5.4/100,000 for children less than 5 years of age, but in infants less than 1 year of age it was 16.7/100,000.[33] In Finland, 1985–1989, the rate of pneumococcal meningitis was 2.1 per 100,000 of those under 5 years of age and 6.8/100,000 for those under 1 year of age.[32] *S. pneumoniae* is also the most common aerobic organism grown from blood of febrile infants and children in whom no focus of infection is determined. The highest rate of pneumococcal carriage in the United States is also among preschool children; it is somewhat lower in older children and is about the same in adolescents as in adults, but in the last two groups, carriers are more frequent in households with preschool children.

About one third of all pneumococcal disease affects the respiratory tract, another one third is associated with focal infections (mostly otitis media), and one third is associated with fever and bacteremia without a discernible focus.[8,9] The pneumococcus is the most frequent organism grown from middle-ear fluid; the most common types in such fluid are 3, 9, 19, and 23, the same as in healthy carriers. The most frequent types in bacteremia and meningitis are 6, 15, 18, 19, and 23. Healthy carriers may harbor the same serotypes as are encountered in invasive infections, but carrier strains are often the higher-numeral types rarely associated with disease.

5.1.1. Occurrence of Penicillin-Resistant Pneumococci. Penicillin has historically been the antibiotic of choice for most cases of pneumococcal infection. There has been monitoring of pneumococci worldwide for susceptibility to this agent, and in the past growth of pneumococci has generally been inhibited by a concentration of less than 0.05 μg/ml of penicillin. Relatively resistant strains (now referred to as intermediately resistant) have been reported with low-frequency prevalence worldwide since 1967 when a well-documented case of respiratory infection due to a pneumococcal strain with an MIC of 0.6 μg/ml of penicillin G was reported from Sydney, Australia.[46] The patient involved was a 25-year-old with hypogammaglobulinemia and bronchiectasis who had received many courses of antibiotic treatment in the past. Since then there have been many reports of such isolates. Until the 1980s, there were only sporadic reports of strains intermediately resistant, with MICs of 0.1 to 1.0 μg/ml of penicillin. Strains resistant to 1.0 μg/ml of penicillin have been termed high-level resistant strains.

Beginning in South Africa in 1977,[47,48] there have been reports of pneumococcal isolates resistant to penicillin, with MICs at 2–10 μg/ml. These strains generally had resistance to multiple antibiotics including tetracyclines, streptomycin, chloramphenicol, erythromycin, clindamycin, and sulfonamides. Only a small number of pneumococcal serotypes have been associated with high-level resistance. Generally, the level of resistance to penicillin correlates with resistance to all semisynthetic penicillins and cephalosporins.[43] Resistance of pneumococci has not been associated with the production of β-lactamases but with the alteration in the cell-membrane-associated enzymes that are responsible for cell wall assembly and that bind penicillin. Alteration of these penicillin-binding proteins has been associated with high resistance[49] as well as low-level resistance,[50] and penicillin tolerance.[51,52] (Penicillin tolerance refers to strains requiring a substantially higher concentration of penicillin to kill them than to inhibit their growth.) Strains of pneumococci can develop increasing resistance in a stepwise fashion,[52] and the genes for altered penicillin-binding proteins may come from heterologous organisms as well as pneumococci.[51] It appears that resistant clones have spread throughout the world, although the rates of resistance vary considerably in different countries.[43]

The outbreak of multiply-resistant pneumococci that began in Johannesburg, South Africa, in 1977, deserves special mention. The first isolate was a Danish type 19A from the sputum of a hospitalized 3-year-old with pneumonia. Additional isolates were recovered by screening patients and hospital personnel from the same hospital using an agar–disk diffusion method for screening pneumococcal respiratory isolates. It was clear that these were virulent strains as there was considerable morbidity and some deaths attributable to invasive infection due to these pneumococci. These isolates were resistant to penicillin concentrations of 0.12 to 4 μg/ml and were found in 29% of 543 pediatric patients and 2% of 436 hospital staff members.[48] The year 1977 appeared to be a watershed year as resistant pneumococcal strains were reported from Durban, South Africa; Minneapolis, Minnesota; and London, England.[48] The report from Durban involved five cases of meningitis or sepsis in children from 3 months to 2 years of age. Each had severe malnutrition, with recent courses of antibiotic treatment. Three cases occurred while the children were hospitalized and receiving antibiotics. The isolates were serotype 19A and had MICs of 4–8 μg/ml of penicillin and exhibited resistance to other β-lactams, aminoglycosides, and chloramphenicol. The three children with meningitis died and the two with septicemia responded to treatment with alternative antibiotics.[47]

Intermediately susceptible strains are clearly less susceptible than are usual strains, but in the absence of meningitis, infections due to these strains are often successfully treated with high doses of penicillin.[52,53] In an older case-control study of 18 patients from whom relatively resistant strains of pneumococci were isolated, there was no difference in prior antibiotic treatment or other infectious disease in the household, compared with matched patients from whom susceptible strains were isolated.[54] Response to antibiotic therapy was less prompt, but the number of patients was too small for this to be statistically evaluated. A recent prospective study of 504 patients in Spain demonstrated a similar outcome in patients treated with penicillin or cephalosporins whether their pneumococcal isolate was fully susceptible to penicillin or less susceptible.[53] In a study of patients with pneumococcal pneumonia from whom resistant strains were isolated, it appeared that only strains with an MIC of penicillin of >2 μg/ml were resistant to treatment with high-dose penicillin *in vivo*.[55]

In the past few years the incidence of infections due to resistant strains and prevalence of resistance in colonization has increased considerably and alarmingly. In a recent study from Atlanta, Georgia, isolates from 431 patients with invasive pneumococcal infections were studied. Isolates from 25% of patients were resistant to penicillin (7% were high-level: ⩾2 μg/ml) and the incidence of such infections was 30 cases per 100,000 population. Within the population, blacks had a higher incidence of pneumococcal infections but the incidence of resistant pneumococci was higher in the white population.[56] Many recent studies have demonstrated a high incidence of infections due to relatively resistant strains in children. In a study of 205 hospitalized children with bacteremia or meningitis from Johannesburg, South Africa, 40% of community-acquired isolates and 95% of nosocomially acquired isolates were resistant to penicillin and often other antibiotics as well. While the rate of penicillin resistance in South Africa had been 6.9% from 1983 to 1986, in the 2 years of the study, 1989 to 1991, the rate of resistance of community-acquired strains rose from 32 to 45%.[57] Serotypes 6, 14, 19, and 23 accounted for 70% of all isolates and 99% of resistant isolates, but these are common pediatric serotypes in many populations. In the Johannesburg study, children with resistant isolates tended to be more likely to have an underlying disease, to have previously visited the clinics, and to have recently been treated with antibiotics. There was no particular age predisposition. Mortality was similar for patients with sensitive and resistant strains in non-central nervous system infections but higher for patients with resistant strains in the central nervous system.[57]

In the United States, similar reports have appeared. In a study from Texas Children's Hospital in Houston,[58] the rate of resistance was 12.1% of all isolates. Fifteen of 19 highly resistant isolates were recovered from middle ear fluid. Fifteen of these 19 isolates were serotype 6. In a study of 108 isolates from children in Washington, DC,[59] 12.9% were resistant (8.3% intermediate, 4.6% high level) and many were resistant to multiple antibiotics. In a study from Kentucky,[60] 246 ambulatory children with otitis media were studied. Of the 157 patients with *S. pneumoniae* isolated from middle ear fluid, 25 (16%) were relatively resistant to penicillin and 23 (15%) had high-level resistance. Of the highly resistant strains most were resistant to other antibiotics, and serotypes 6B, 19F, and 23F accounted for 95% of isolates. The same group performed a prevalence study in 240 children attending a day-care center, using nasopharyngeal swabs.[61] *S. pneumoniae* was isolated from 126 (53%). Of the 123 strains tested, 65 (53%) were resistant, and of these 41 (33%) were highly resistant.

While early reports were of infections that were acquired nosocomially, more recent reports indicate that in patients who had previously received penicillin there can be community acquisition of resistant strains in previously healthy individuals.[62] A cluster of serotype 19A isolates was reported from Brooklyn, New York. Of nine isolates with penicillin MICs of 1.0 to 2.0 μg/ml, six came from asymptomatically colonized adults and three from patients with lower-respiratory-tract infections. These isolations were made in 1983–1984 as part of a vaccine-related pneumococcal surveillance program. These strains were also resistant to other penicillins, cephalosporins, tetracycline, chloramphenicol, and trimethoprim/sulfamethoxazole. No common source for the strains was discovered.[63]

The cause of the increase of antibiotic resistance is unclear but probably is multifactorial. There is some evidence that prior exposure to antibiotics is a risk factor for infection due to resistant strains and may play an important role in rising rates of resistance.[51,64] The exceptional risk of children and the high prevalence of "pediatric" serotypes among resistant strains (serotypes 6, 14, 19, 23) provides evidence that indiscriminate use of antibiotics for minor pediatric infections may be a major factor driving this epidemic.

5.1.2. Distribution of Pneumococcal Types. The importance of pneumococcal types and their distribution in various populations need to be stressed. In the past, when immunotherapy with type-specific serum was used, typing of organisms and provision of the proper sera required knowledge of the prevalent serotypes. Since the introduction of the pneumococcal polysaccharide vaccine, which induces type-specific immunity, it is now necessary to know the prevalence of pneumococcal serotypes in order to prepare an appropriate multivalent vaccine. Because the frequency of the different serotypes varies with time and with different clinical syndromes,[65] constant monitoring continues to be a necessity for inclusion of the appropriate types in vaccine formulations.[66]

Pneumococci are serotyped according to the presence of specific carbohydrate antigens that make up the capsule of the bacterium. Rabbit antisera specific for each serotype are used. There are two serotype designation schemes in use. The Danish system is more widely used and classifies strains with a number designation and sometimes a letter following the number. A serogroup number represents a group of antigenically related strains. Each type within the group is indicated by a suffix letter (e.g., serogroup 6 contains serotypes 6A and 6B). In the American system each serotype is given a separate letter. The occurrence of specific types of pneumococci in pneumonia, bacteremia, focal infections, and carriers has been reported from various locations, including South Africa,[67,68] Boston City Hospital,[5,65,69] Denmark,[20] Germany,[70] Britain,[71] Mexico,[72] and worldwide.[25] Essentially all known types have been identified in infections but in different orders of frequency, with lobar pneumonia, bronchopneumonia, otitis media, and other focal infections, as well as in healthy carriers. However, the type distribution in bronchopneumonia and in focal infections is similar to that in carriers, but in roughly inverse relationship to that in lobar pneumonia. The distribution of types in infected individuals and healthy carriers among infants and children[30,73,74] is different than in adults. Multiple types of pneumococci can be isolated from infected patients and carriers at the same time or at different times and may persist for varying lengths of time, continuously or intermittently in carriers as well as after recovery from pneumonia. The role of these types of infections in the individual patient may be surmised from the clinical findings of the demonstration of antibodies to the homologous types during the infection or convalescence. They may also account for recrudescences, recurrences, and reinfections by those types.[69,75,76] The serotypes present in the current vaccine and those most commonly encountered in bacteremic pneumococcal diseases of adults and children are summarized in Tables 2 and 4 from several sources. These change with time and place, so that individual reports may vary from the data shown. In the United States and most western countries the most common serotypes encountered in adults are 3, 4, 7, 8, and 14[44] while in children the most common serotypes are 6, 14, 18, 19, and 23. Types 1 and 5 continue to be reported frequently in developing countries.[44,66,74] Tables 2 and 4 demonstrate that: (1) the vaccine includes the types most commonly responsible for bacteremic disease in children and adults; (2) there is broad overlap in the serotypes seen in children and adults but some differences exist; and (3) bacteremic diseases are largely due to serotypes with lower numbers; the higher-numbered serotypes are more commonly found in the pharynges of healthy carriers.

Table 2. Serotypes Most Commonly Associated with Bacteremic Pneumococcal Infections in Children and Adults

American serotype designation		Danish serotype designation
Adults	Children	
1	1	1
	2	2
3	3	3
4	4	4
6	6	6A
8	8	8
9	9	9N
12	12	12F
14	14	14
19	19	19F
23	23	23F
	25	25
	51	7F
	56	18C

5.1.3. Occurrence in Carriers. Pneumococci are present in the nose or throat or both of about one fourth of all healthy persons at any given time; they are more prevalent in the winter months, and nearly all individuals carry them transiently or intermittently in the course of a year. In young infants, they are usually found only if they occur in the mother, but in older infants, they are more frequent. The presence of upper-respiratory infections is not ordinarily a determinant in the individual, but epidemics of respiratory infections tend to increase the spread of disease-producing types of pneumococci, particularly in families of cases.

The epidemiology of pneumococcal infections was discussed in some detail at a symposium on the *Pneumococcus*[77] in 1980 in which Riley and Douglas from Papua New Guinea, likened the situation in their country to that in the New World at the turn of the century.[78] Acquisition of pneumococci in the nasopharynx begins there in infancy, reaches the highest rates in preschool children, and then declines in advancing age groups. The rates in New Guinea, as elsewhere, are generally related to the amount, degree, and duration of contact with cases or other carriers. There is an inverse ratio of case rates and carrier rates of the common invasive types. The findings in Papua New Guinea confirm the general well-known epidemiological principles developed and established in South Africa in 1914,[22] among recruits in military camps in 1918[79,80] and 1921.[81]

5.2. Epidemic Behavior and Contagiousness

As early as 1888, Netter[82] presented evidence, mostly on clinical grounds, for the contagiousness of pneumonia and for the part played by the pneumococcus. He described family outbreaks of pneumonia and other pneumococcal infections even in the same household. He and others[83,84] traced cases to direct or close contact with other cases or convalescents. He found that pneumococci survived in dried sputum for many months and he recovered the organisms from the dust of hospital rooms.

Epidemics involving multiple cases in families[85,86] or in institutions[87,88] were described in which direct contagion was traced either separately or during outbreaks in small communities. In some of them, the pneumococcus was identified by culture or mouse inoculation.[89] Outbreaks of focal pneumococcal infections have been recorded both in association with pneumonia and independently. Pneumonia acquired in foundling homes was early recognized as an important cause of high death rates in infant asylums and as a frequent cause of deaths in babies who were healthy on arrival. Direct contagion was also recognized as the case of the spread of pneumonia among workers in mining camps in South Africa,[17,67,68] as well as during the construction of the Panama Canal[25,90] in which overcrowding, especially in sleeping quarters, and high attack rates soon after arrival were the two most important features.

Although pneumonia was the leading cause of death in army camps during World War I,[79,80,89,91] it occurred mostly in relation to epidemics of measles and influenza associated with hemolytic streptococci, but the majority of cases and deaths after and even during such epidemics were typical pneumococcal lobar pneumonia. In 1919, epidemics of type I pneumococcal pneumonia were reported from Camp Jackson[91] and Camp Upton[92] and of type II from Camp Grant.[93] New draftees and southern blacks were the most susceptible. Direct contagion was later demonstrated when typing was used. In 1940, spread of pneumococcal pneumonia could also be traced in some hospitals from bed to bed.[94] In 1937, Harris and Ingraham[95] described an epidemic of type II pneumonia in the Civilian Conservation Corps confirmed in many cases by serological studies; these involved primarily members of the corps in the same barracks and only two officers who had the most contact with the men. Recent reports have stressed smaller epidemics and nosocomial spread of resistant strains,[47,48,63] the association of pneumococcal disease with influenza,[30] and conditions responsible for greater susceptibility to pneumococcal infection (see Section 7.1). A recently reported outbreak of pneumococcal pneumonia in a jail reinforced the importance of overcrowding and poor ventilation as contributing factors.[34] Epidemics of meningitis separate from pneumonia have not been described.

5.3. Geographic Distribution

As already noted, reliable information on the geographic distribution, prevalence, and incidence of pneumonia and particularly of other pneumococcal infections is unknown because of lack of adequate reporting in most parts of the world and the unreliability of those reports that are available. It may be said, however, that such infections are ubiquitous, worldwide, and endemic and, under some conditions, may occur in well-circumscribed epidemics. Although usually thought to be particularly prevalent in temperate zones, they also occur in warmer regions and in the tropics.[25] Temperature and humidity appear to influence the prevalence of pneumonia, and in countries where the most abrupt and severe changes occur in winter, the incidence of the disease is correspondingly high during such times.[96,97]

Among admissions to the Boston City Hospital, the incidence of pneumococcal bacteremia[98] and meningitis[5] decreased after 1935 and again after 1941 with the general use of sulfonamides and penicillin, but it has fluctuated within a moderate range after that. The case-fatality rate after 1941, however, still remained high in cases of meningitis and varied with age in other bacteremic cases, being highest in infants and in persons 70 or older.

5.4. Age

Pneumococcal infections occur at all ages. They are most frequent in the first year of life, decrease rapidly to a low between 10 and 15 years, and then increase in incidence steadily in advancing age groups. Deaths from such infections are also most frequent in the first year of life, least frequent between 15 and 20 years, and rise with advancing age groups more steeply than do the case rates.[25] The estimates of incidence for invasive pneumococcal infection in Goteborg, Sweden, which are typical, are 25.8/100,000 in the first year of life, falling to 2/100,000 in the second decade, then rising by decade and peaking in the eighth decade at 16.4/100,000[29] (see Fig. 1). The case-fatality rate from pneumonia and meningitis increases with each decade, from under 10% in the young to over 50% in the eighth decade. The age distribution of cases of pneumococcal meningitis followed the same trend among patients at Boston City Hospital during 12 selected years between 1935 and 1972, but the case-fatality rates were higher, about 60%, for those in the first decade of life, 50% in the second decade, and increased with each decade thereafter to 81% in patients 70 years old or older.[5] In addition to age, another major risk factor for

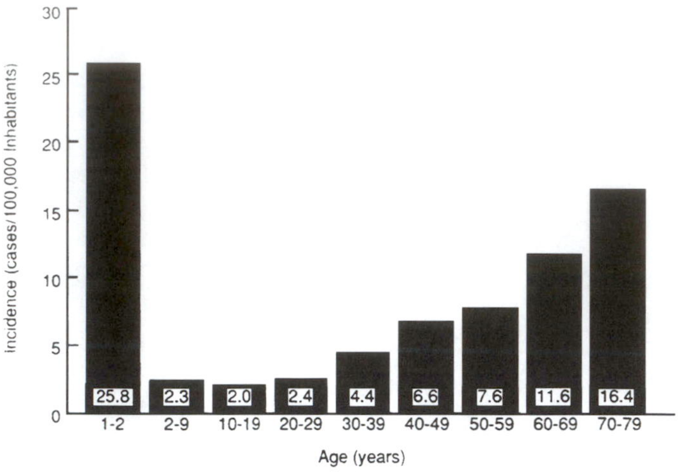

Figure 1. Age-specific incidence (cases/100,000 inhabitants per year) of invasive pneumococcal disease in Goteborg, Sweden, 1970–1980. From Ref. 29.

increased mortality rate from pneumococcal pneumonia is the development of a nonpneumococcal superinfection. The use of high doses of antibiotics and prolonged administration of broad-spectrum antibiotics predisposes to superinfection.(99)

5.5. Sex

Among cases of lobar pneumonia occurring in Massachusetts between 1921 and 1930, males predominated over females (58/42) in all age groups, but male predominance was less among infants and young children.(25) Among bacteremic patients at Boston City Hospital in 1972, the ratio was 51.7% males and 48.3% females for all patients.(98) The ratio of males to females among cases of pneumococcal meningitis for the 12 selected years between 1935 and 1972(5) was much higher and averaged 65% male for all ages, but varied in different age groups: 67% males among infants (<1 year old), 78% males in those 1 to 9 years old, 100% males among the small number of 10 to 19 years, and dropping steadily with each decade to 50% males among patients 70 or older.

5.6. Race

It has long been recognized that blacks are peculiarly susceptible to pneumonia when they reside in cold climates, especially when moved from warm tropical regions. Under certain conditions, there is also a pronounced susceptibility in blacks to pneumonia and pneumococcal infections in general even in warm climates. For example, high rates were encountered among the construction workers, who were predominantly blacks, during the building of the Panama Canal and among pneumonia patients elsewhere in Central America and tropical Africa.(25) Death rates from lobar pneumonia in various widely scattered states in this country are also considerably higher in blacks, sometimes twice as high as among whites. Thus, while true genetic susceptibility has not been separated from socioeconomic factors, blacks are most likely to be subject to crowding in occupational as well as residential life (which is related to risk of infections), and may have a higher incidence of certain lifestyle risks(30,44) and reduced availability of medical care.

5.7. Occupation

Pneumonia has been known to be unusually prevalent in certain mining and milling industries.(100) In some mills, this has been associated with a high carrier rate that has been followed by an outbreak of pneumonia in the community.(101) In certain mining regions, the living conditions of the workers themselves, rather than the circumstances surrounding the work, may be the determining factor in spread of the disease. This was true in a group of steel workers who were crowded into small shanties in 1917,(102) among workers and their families during the construction of the Panama Canal in 1913,(90) among miners in South Africa,(17,103–105) and among plantation workers.(106)

5.8. Occurrence in Families

Today little attention is paid to the spread of pneumococcus within families, and the occurrence of a single case of invasive disease in a family does not merit the attention and use of prophylactic antibiotics that cases of meningococal or *H. influenzae* disease do. Nevertheless, since prolonged intimate contact is required for spread of the pneumococcus, it is not surprising that spread in families does occur. Heffron[25] mentions a number of reports of multiple family members being infected with the same serotype of pneumococcus. In some cases affected family members were carriers, but in many there was an outbreack of invasive infections. The occurrence and spread of pneumococcal infections among members of the households of patients admitted to Boston City Hospital with lobar pneumonia were reported by Finland and Tilghman[86] and by Brown and Finland.[85] They included multiple cases of infections with the same type as the index case; some had lobar pneumonia and others had empyema, primary pneumococcal meningitis, otitis media, simple upper-respiratory infections, or bronchopneumonia, or were carriers without evidence of infection. Some cases admitted with lobar pneumonia were traced to contacts with other cases already in the hospital, but not from the same household. Serological studies demonstrated the presence or development of antibodies to the same types. The appearance and spread of additional new types among members of the household were also noted; these were also associated with pneumonia or focal infections or mild upper-respiratory infection and with the development of specific antibodies to the homologous types in a large percentage of members of these households.

5.9. Occurrence in Animals

The occurrence of pneumococcal carriers and of widespread epidemics of pneumococcal infections among animals was reviewed by Finland.[10] They probably play very little or no part in infections and outbreaks in humans beyond causing occasional cases among animal handlers and will not be considered here.

5.10. Laboratory Infections

Cases of pneumonia acquired in the laboratory are not frequent. They have been associated with exposure to aerosols[107] or droplets or with handling of sputum.[108] They are of interest in delineating the incubation periods of pneumonia in man, since the clinical evidence of infection was manifest from 36 hr to 3 days after a single exposure. Various types, including 1, 2, 7, and 18, were involved, and the same individual has been subject to more than one attack, but with different types and at different times.

5.11. Nutrition

The effect of specific nutritional deficiencies in predisposing to pneumonia is not known. Undernutrition, particularly of calories and proteins, is recognized as predisposing to infectious diseases in general (see Chapter 1). Deficiencies and abnormality in cellular (phagocytes) and circulating immune factors (e.g., complement) may play a role.[109] Alcoholism has been regarded as a major predisposing factor for invasive pneumococcal infections. In a Swedish study it was the most important risk factor in adults.[29] In a US study, alcoholics also had a higher fatality rate from pneumococcal sepsis than did nonalcoholics, but only when accompanied by leukopenia.[110]

6. Mechanisms and Routes of Transmission

The most common route of transmission of pneumococci is by droplets from cases and carriers. In hospitals, the most frequent spread is from one patient to the patient in the adjacent bed, the disease rarely skipping a distance of more than two beds. Physicians, nurses, attendants, and others with frequent and close contact with patients are subject to colonization or infection from the patients unless they take special precautions to avoid or reduce exposure to the patients' droplets (coughing and sneezing), such as by masking the patient or themselves or both. Although pneumococci may be cultured from the air or from the dust on the floors or in the rooms of patients with pneumonia and remain viable in dried secretions for long periods, probably as long as many days if not in direct sunlight,[1,25] documented infections from such sources are rare.

In cases of pneumococcal meningitis following fractured skulls, the infecting organism comes from the patient's own nasopharynx or accessory sinuses, and these foci are probably the sources of "primary" pneumococcal meningitis. The route by which the organism reaches the meninges in "primary" cases can often be traced to previous head trauma involving small fractures in the cribriform plate, difficult to recognize even by X-ray. Such fractures may be associated with recurrent pneumococcal (and other bacterial) meningitis that no longer recurs after the defect in the cribriform plate has been repaired.

Otitis media in the acute form, and probably also acute sinusitis, usually occurs during or after simple upper-respiratory-tract infections and is caused by the same type of pneumococcus found in the nose and/or pharynx or both. Experimentally, inflammation associated with occlusion of the eustachian tube (produced by influenza virus) is required to produce otitis media in the chinchilla after colonization of the nasopharynx with pneumococcus.[111,112]

7. Pathogenesis and Immunity

7.1. Pathogenesis

The incubation period for pneumococcal pneumonia is not known. Most sources state that it is 1–3 days. Heffron[25] suggests that it is "in the neighborhood of a few hours to about 48 hours." This would be for an infection from an exogenous source. Endogenous infection in a person who was previously an asymptomatic carrier and then developed invasive disease can occur with an "incubation period" of weeks.

While significant details of human immunity to the pneumococcus are known, the exact mechanisms by which it can multiply in tissues and produce local inflammation or invasive disease remain to be fully elucidated. Pneumococci attach to respiratory epithelial cells by interaction with cell surface receptors. The mouse, rabbit, rat, and dog, and probably also humans, can remove large numbers of inhaled virulent pneumococci. This is done in part by the ciliary epithelium of the trachea and bronchi but in greater measure by the phagocytic cells, predominantly the pulmonary macrophage system, and is effected with or without the mediation of humoral antibodies.[113] It is known that damage to the ciliary system, particularly to the macrophages, by alcohol or other inhaled toxic substances or by minor viral respiratory infections is necessary to establish pulmonary infection by pneumococci. In experimental animals, intrabronchial inoculation of pneumococci in a gelatin or starch plug is necessary to establish the pneumonia, which extends out from the local alveoli to other parts of the lung.[114] In the dog, infection occurs in the local alveoli, and the pneumococci appear very rapidly in the local lymphatics, then in the hilar lymph nodes, then in the thoracic duct and subclavian vein, and finally in the peripheral blood.[115,116] The healthy mouse, in which a single virulent (e.g., type I) pneumococcus injected intraperitoneally produces a lethal infection, can inhale a large number of the same organism from an aerosolized culture without ill effect; but the same aerosol will produce bronchopneumonia, bacteremia, and death if inhaled after the mouse has been anesthetized or alcoholized to unconsciousness. Intranasal instillation of the broth culture will also produce pneumonia and death in the mouse[117] and in the rabbit.[118] A dermal pneumococcal infection has been produced by intradermal inoculation in rabbits; this lesion can be prevented by previous immunization and terminated by specific antiserum.[119] The same is true of experimental infections in the mouse and the dog. The importance of inflammation and obstruction of the eustachian tube for the establishment of pneumococcal otitis media was mentioned in Section 6. A counterpart to this in human pneumococcal pneumonia is the increased susceptibility of acutely alcoholic patients and the higher mortality among those who develop bacteremic pneumococcal infections.[120]

The pneumococcal specific capsular substances (referred to as SSS in the past) are complex polysaccharides, and the chemical structures of many have been elucidated in detail. These polysaccharides are responsible for the type specificity of protective antibodies that are elicited during infection[121] and the serological classification of which can be determined by the quellung reaction. The presence of the capsule is required for a strain to be pathogenic, and a larger amount of capsule production is associated with increased pathogenic potential. As with other encapsulated organisms, the primary pathogenetic role of the capsule is to allow the organism to avoid phagocytosis by leukocytes. By itself the capsule does not elicit inflammation.[122] There is some clinical and laboratory evidence that when the concentration of free polysaccharide antigen in the blood is very high, there is spontaneous activation of complement that could result in disseminated intravascular coagulation and shock.[123,124] The cell wall component of the bacterium appears to play an important role in pathogenesis. Components of the cell wall stimulate the recruitment of leukocytes, enhance endothelial permeability, which leads to local edema formation, and induce the production of cytokines. Thus, cell wall components may be responsible for the pathological picture characteristic of pneumococcal pneumonia and meningitis. Consistent with this model is the belief that treatment with antibiotics that cause cell lysis is the release of cell wall components that may temporarily augment the inflammatory response.[122]

In humans, host defenses against the pneumococcus can be divided into natural and acquired. Some of the natural host defenses have been deduced from experimental studies, but to a large extent they have been inferred from high rates of disease in people with underlying (predisposing) abnormalities.

The natural defenses in individuals with normal lungs include the production of an inflammatory response and the transport of bacteria out of the lungs by coordinated motion of the cilia. Damage to the lungs by previous infections, smoking, occupational exposure to lung toxins, or chronic obstructive pulmonary disease is associated with defective clearance by these mechanisms and therefore susceptibility to infection by *S. pneumoniae*.

Humoral immunity is of considerable importance in acquired resistance to infection with the pneumococcus.

Individuals whose B-cell function is abnormal are predisposed to infection on this basis. This includes infants, children, and adults who have congenital B-cell deficiency and hypogammaglobulinemia. This predisposition can be ameliorated by treatment with intramuscular or intravenous gamma globulin every 3 to 4 weeks. Acquired dysgammaglobulinemias including multiple myeloma and acquired immunodeficiency syndrome (AIDS) are associated with unusual susceptibility to infection by the pneumococcus. Children and adults with AIDS are highly susceptible to pneumococcal infections.[125–129] Children with AIDS treated prophylactically with intravenous immune globulin have significantly fewer bacterial infections, especially pneumococcal infections.[130]

The presence of a normal spleen is important in containing pneumococcemia. In persons with anatomical or functional asplenia, there is a high risk of overwhelming sepsis. Congenital asplenia is often part of a complex of midline defects and is termed Ivemark's syndrome.[131] Individuals with this syndrome frequently die from severe cardiac disease in infancy. Of those who survive past 6 months of age, sepsis is a frequent occurrence and *S. pneumoniae* is most frequently the cause of sepsis.[132] Of those who have a splenectomy in later life, overwhelming pneumococcal sepsis is a significant threat. Posttraumatic splenectomy may be associated with a lower risk than is elective surgical splenectomy because splenic rupture is often associated with splenosis (implantation of functioning spleen cells in the abdominal cavity). In the absence of splenosis, susceptibility to overwhelming pneumococcal sepsis is lifelong. The characteristic syndrome of overwhelming postsplenectomy infection is associated with *S. pneumoniae* in 50–90% of cases with a mortality rate of 50 to 70% despite treatment with appropriate antibiotics.[133]

The condition most clearly associated with acquired hypofunction of the spleen and hypersusceptibility to pneumococcal infection is sickle-cell anemia. In this disease the spleen is normal in the early months of life and then develops progressive autoinfarction due to stasis of sickled red cells. Finally, there is loss of splenic function even though the spleen may be anatomically present. This is the time of maximum susceptibility to life-threatening pneumococcal infection. The threat of pneumococcal sepsis and meningitis may be decreased by the use of prophylactic penicillin, or in those over 2 years of age, pneumococcal vaccine.[134,135]

The complement system has an important role in the pathogenesis of pneumococcal infections. Using animal models, it has been possible to demonstrate that opsonization of pneumococci, which is necessary for eradication of bacteremia, requires participation of the complement system.[136] Pneumococci can activate the terminal complement components via the classical or alternative complement pathways. The alternative complement pathway can be activated by pneumococci and immunoglobulin that does not have to be specific for pneumococcal antigens. This pathway is responsible for "natural immunity" in nonimmune individuals and activates opsonic C3b. Activation of the classical complement pathway is more efficient and occurs in immune individuals who have specific antipneumococcal antibody in the serum. It also involves activation of C3b. Hypersusceptibility to pneumococcal infection may be a consequence of dysfunction of either system. With congenital absence of any of the early components of the complement cascade, there is frequently recurrent infection, especially with pneumococci. In sickle-cell disease there is abnormally low function of the alternative complement system and this appears to be part of the susceptibility to overwhelming pneumococcal infections.[137]

7.2. Immunity

Type-specific anticapsular antibody appears about the fifth or sixth day of illness in untreated patients and promotes the ingestion of bacteria by leukocytes. The antibody appears to be protective and long-lasting and is specific for the pneumococcal capsular type. Recurrent systemic infection due to the same serotype is rare except in patients with impaired defenses or persistent foci of infection. However, the pneumococcus may persist in the upper respiratory tract for days or weeks in the presence of humoral antibody.

Type-specific capsular antibodies also appear about 11 days after immunization, peak in 3–4 weeks, and persist at protective levels for at least 5 years.[39] Numerous studies have demonstrated that antibody production in response to pneumococcal vaccine is poor below the age of 2 years and is probably not effective in preventing infection in children of that age.[138,139]

8. Patterns of Host Response

8.1. Clinical Features

Pneumococcal infections in humans are manifested in various ways (Table 3). These range from the healthy carrier state or minor respiratory infection to pneumonia and meningitis, otitis media, conjunctivitis, and other focal purulent infections. Bacteremia may occur in asso-

Table 3. Clinical Spectrum of Pneumococcal Infections

Minor respiratory infections	Meningitis
Conjunctivitis	Focal infections
Otitis media	Bacteremia with:
Sinusitis	Pharyngitis
Lobar pneumonia	Fever
Bronchopneumonia	Septicemia with:
Empyema of pleura	Purpura
Endocarditis	Adrenal hemorrhage

ciation with manifestations ranging from simple pharyngitis and fever without a demonstrably localized lesion[8,9] to fulminating septicemia with purpura and adrenal hemorrhage (Waterhouse–Friderichsen syndrome), which may be rapidly lethal in the immunocompromised or asplenic patient.[140] Pneumococcal meningitis is most commonly a complication of skull fracture, sinusitis, mastoiditis, or pneumonia. Pneumococcal empyema of the pleura is the most frequent complication of lobar pneumonia, with vegetative endocarditis generally a late complication.

Clinically, "primary" pneumococcal lobar pneumonia begins characteristically, most often after a few days of mild upper-respiratory symptoms and bronchitis, with a sudden severe chill or pleuritic pain or both. This is accompanied by a hacking cough, with production of small amounts of orange-, rust-, or prune-juice-colored sputum, and followed by fever and the appearance of physical and X-ray signs of moisture and consolidation of the lung(s). If the condition is untreated, the organism invades the bloodstream (bacteremia), and the consolidation spreads to involve an entire lobe. It may spread to other parts of the lung, with a stormy course that ends in death or in recovery by rapid drop in fever and cessation of symptoms (crisis) or by slow resolution of fever, symptoms, and signs over several days (lysis).

8.2. Diagnosis

The diagnosis may be made by demonstrating the specific type of pneumococcus (by the quellung reaction) in the sputum or in the blood culture if obtained before effective chemotherapy is instituted. Meningitis, otitis media, and other focal pneumococcal infections are diagnosed by characteristic physical signs and by demonstrating the organism in a similar manner in the purulent spinal fluid or local exudate. Serological tests have not been used routinely for the diagnosis of pneumococcal infections. Counterimmunoelectrophoresis and latex agglutination using latex beads coated with pneumococcal antisera both detect free antigen in body fluids. They can be used in clinical situations for rapid diagnosis of sepsis, meningitis, and other focal infections. Agglutination of antibody-coated latex beads can be used for rapid identification of *S. pneumoniae* from colonies picked off of primary isolation plates in the diagnostic laboratory.

9. Control and Prevention

9.1. Prevention

Although controversy about the efficacy of active immunization with a polyvalent vaccine persists, it has been the mainstay for the prevention of invasive pneumococcal infections. More recently, investigators have used passive immunization with specific immune intravenous immunoglobulin preparations to attempt to prevent invasive infections in selected patients.

9.2. Pneumococcal Vaccine

Because of the extremely high incidence of serious pneumococcal infections among South African goldminers,[141] Wright and his co-workers, in 1911,[22] immunized miners with a crude whole-cell pneumococcal vaccine. Subsequently, a number of other investigators conducted clinical trials of the safety and efficacy of polysaccharide vaccines against pneumococci of various serotypes.[142–144] However, the validity of the results of many of these trials was questionable because of such methodological flaws as nonrandomization, inadequacies in the clinical follow-up of subjects, and inadequacies in the bacteriological confirmation of the outcomes. However, controlled trials of bivalent, trivalent, and quadrivalent polysaccharide vaccines that were conducted in the 1940s provided stronger evidence that vaccines were efficacious.[145,146] Two different hexavalent vaccines subsequently were commercially produced and marketed. At about the same time, antimicrobials that were effective against pneumococci became available and the outcomes of patients with pneumococcal infections improved substantially. Interest in the vaccines rapidly diminished and they were eventually withdrawn from the market.

However, in 1964, Austrian and Gold[147] reported a mortality rate of 25% in adults with bacteremic pneumococcal pneumonia. Many of these patients died despite early treatment with appropriate antibiotics. Furthermore, most of the patients were either elderly or had a chronic illness which represented a population at increased risk of serious pneumococcal disease. This population could be targeted for immunization if an effective vaccine could be developed. Accordingly, Austrian and others worked together to develop a polyvalent vaccine.[148] The vaccine was tested with prospective double-blind randomized controlled trials in young South African goldminers. This group of subjects was chosen because of the extraordinarily high incidence of pneumococcal disease they experienced, which enabled these trials to be conducted expeditiously and at a relatively low cost.[149] These well-designed trials produced conclusive evidence of the efficacy of these vaccines in this population (the estimates of protective efficacy ranged from 76 to 92%).[149,150]

Two large clinical trials were conducted to try to assess the vaccine's efficacy in the populations at high risk of serious pneumococcal disease in the United States.[151] These trials were conducted among 13,600 ambulatory patients over 45 years of age at the Kaiser-Permanente Health Plan in San Francisco and among 1300 subjects at a chronic-care facility in North Carolina. Despite the relatively large number of subjects, these studies were inconclusive because of the low incidence of invasive pneumococcal infections and the consequent poor statistical power of these trials.[151,152] A small clinical trial conducted among patients with sickle-cell disease found excellent efficacy for these patients, but the study was flawed because the trial was neither randomized nor blinded.[153]

Despite these equivocal results, a quadradecavalent vaccine that contained 50 μg each of the polysaccharide antigen of 14 serotypes of pneumococci was licensed by the FDA in 1977 (Table 4). This vaccine was replaced in 1983 by one containing polysaccharide antigens of 23 capsular types. The vaccine was recommended for use in persons over 2 years of age with a variety of chronic conditions that placed them at increased risk of serious pneumococcal infection.[154] These conditions included anatomical or functional asplenia and chronic pulmonary, cardiac, or renal diseases. The recommendations for the exact target population were rather vague, in part because of a lack of firm data on the magnitude of the increased risk of serious pneumococcal infections associated with various chronic conditions. These original recommendations about whom to vaccinate have been updated several times.[31,155–157] The most recent recommendations from the Immunization Practices Advisory Committee (ACIP) of the CDC are as follows:[31,156]

Adults

1. Immunocompetent adults who are at increased risk of pneumococcal disease or its complications because of chronic illnesses (e.g., cardiovascular disease, pulmonary disease, diabetes mellitus, alcoholism, cirrhosis, or cerebrospinal fluid leaks) or who are ⩾ 65 years old.

Table 4. Antigenic Serotypes of Pneumococcal Polysaccharides Contained in Pneumococcal Vaccine

14-valent vaccine		23-valent vaccine	
Danish system	American system	Danish system	American system
1			
1	1	1	1
2	2	2	2
3	3	3	3
4	4	4	4
6A	6	5	5
7F	51	6B	26
8	8	7F	51
9N	9	8	8
12F	12	9N	9
14	14	9V	68
18C	56	10A	34
19F	19	11A	43
23F	23	12F	12
25	25	14	14
		15B	54
		17F	17
		18C	56
		19A	57
		19F	19
		20	20
		22F	22
		23F	23
		33F	70

2. Immunocompromised adults at increased risk of pneumococcal disease or its complications (e.g., persons with splenic dysfunction or anatomic asplenia, Hodgkin's disease, lymphoma, multiple myeloma, chronic renal failure, nephrotic syndrome, or conditions such as organ transplantation associated with immunosuppression).
3. Adults with asymptomatic or symptomatic HIV infection.

Children

1. Children ⩾2 years old with chronic illnesses sporadically associated with increased risk of pneumococcal disease or its complications [e.g., anatomic or functional asplenia (including sickle cell disease), nephrotic syndrome, cerebrospinal fluid leaks, and conditions associated with immunosuppression].
2. Children ⩾2 years old with asymptomatic or symptomatic HIV infection.
3. The currently available 23-valent vaccine is *not* indicated for patients having only recurrent upper-respiratory-tract disease, including otitis media and sinusitis.

Special Groups

1. Persons living in special environments or social settings with an identified increased risk of pneumococcal disease or its complications (e.g., certain Native American populations).

Adverse Reactions

1. Approximately 50% of persons given pneumococcal vaccine

develop mild side effects, such as erythema and pain at the injection site. Fever, myalgia, and severe local reactions have been reported in <1% of those vaccinated. Severe systemic reactions, such as anaphylaxis, rarely have been reported.

Precautions

1. The safety of pneumococcal vaccine for pregnant women has not been evaluated. Ideally, women at high risk of pneumococcal disease should be vaccinated before pregnancy.

Timing of Vaccination

1. When elective splenectomy is being considered, pneumococcal vaccine should be given at least 2 weeks before the operation, if possible. Similarly, for planning cancer chemotherapy or immunosuppressive therapy, as in patients who undergo organ transplantation, the interval between vaccination and initiation of chemotherapy or immunosuppression should also be at least 2 weeks.

Revaccination

1. In one study, local reactions after revaccination in adults were more severe than after initial vaccination when the interval between vaccinations was 13 months. Reports of revaccination after longer intervals in children and adults, including a large group of elderly persons revaccinated at least 4 years after primary vaccination, suggest a similar incidence of such reactions after primary vaccination and revaccination.
2. Without more information, persons who received the 14-valent pneumococcal vaccine should not be routinely vaccinated with the 23-valent vaccine, as increased coverage is modest and duration of protection is not well defined. However, revaccination with the 23-valent vaccine should be strongly considered for persons who received the 14-valent vaccine if they are at highest risk of fatal pneumococcal infection (e.g., asplenic patients).
3. Revaccination should also be considered for adults at highest risk who received the 23-valent vaccine ≥6 years before and for those shown to have rapid decline in pneumococcal antibody levels (e.g., patients with nephrotic syndrome, asplenia, or sickle-cell anemia who would be ≤10 years old at revaccination). New recommendations from the Advisory Committee on Immunization Practices for the prevention of pneumococcal disease were issued in April, 1997. The major change is that revaccination with polyvalent pneumococcal polysaccharide vaccine is recommended for patients 65 years of age or older who received the vaccine five or more years earlier and were <65 years of age when they last received the vaccine. Reimmunization also is recommended both for persons with either functional or anatomic asplenia and for immunocompromised persons if 5 or more years have elapsed since the last dose (for persons <11 years of age, if 3 or more years have elapsed since the last dose).[156]

Strategies for Vaccine Delivery

1. Recommendations for pneumococcal vaccination have been made by the ACIP, the American Academy of Pediatrics, the American College of Physicians, and the American Academy of Family Physicians. Recent analysis indicates that pneumococcal vaccination of elderly persons is cost-effective. The vaccine is targeted for approximately 27 million persons aged ≥65 years and 21 million persons ages <65 years with high-risk conditions. Despite Medicare reimbursement for costs of the vaccine and its administration, which began in 1981, annual use of pneumococcal vaccine has not increased above levels observed in earlier years. In 1985, <10% of the 48 million persons considered to be at increased risk of serious pneumococcal infection were estimated to have ever received pneumococcal vaccine.
2. Opportunities to vaccinate high-risk persons are missed both at time of hospital discharge and during visits to clinicians' offices. Two thirds or more of patients with serious pneumococcal disease had been hospitalized at least once within 5 years before their pneumococcal illness, yet few had received pneumococcal vaccine. More effective programs for vaccine delivery are needed, including offering pneumococcal vaccine in hospitals (at the time of discharge), clinicians' offices, nursing homes, and other chronic-care facilities. Many patients who receive pneumococcal vaccine should also be immunized with influenza vaccine.

Based on systematic surveillance of the serotypes of pneumococci that caused serious invasive disease, the vaccine was formulated to include serotypes that were responsible for approximately 80% of the cases of systemic pneumococcal infections in the United States.[158,159] However, soon after the vaccine was licensed and distributed, reports of clinical failures of the vaccine began to appear.[160,161] Furthermore, studies suggested that some high-risk patients had poor antibody responses to the vaccine.[162–164] In addition, surveillance data from the CDC suggested that the vaccine's efficacy was poor for many high-risk patients.[165,166] Thus, there was considerable uncertainty about the vaccine because it was shown to be effective in a very select population (young goldminers), but there were serious questions about its efficacy for the population in the United States that was at increased risk of serious pneumococcal infections. However, because of the low incidence of bacteremic pneumococcal infections in developed countries, even in high-risk patients, there are formidable logistical and financial obstacles to conducting a randomized clinical trial in the United States.[167] Furthermore, because the vaccine is licensed (and presumably is efficacious), it may be unethical to allocate high-risk patients randomly to receive placebo, as would be necessary in a randomized trial.

Alternatives to randomized clinical trials to assess the vaccine's efficacy were necessary.[167] Shapiro and Clemens[168] conducted a case–control study that found the vaccine's efficacy to be 67% (95% confidence interval: 13–87%) in high-risk patients. Although there were too few subjects to assess the vaccine's efficacy accurately in immunocompromised patients, its efficacy in high-risk patients with chronic conditions such as diabetes mellitus or chronic pulmonary, cardiac, or renal disease was 77% (95% confidence interval: 27–93%). Bolan and colleagues[169] from the CDC extended their estimates of the vaccine's efficacy based on their surveillance data of reports of serotypes of pneumococci that caused bacteremic disease from 1978 to 1984. They found the vaccine's efficacy against bacteremic disease to be 64% (95% confidence interval: 47–76%). Based on these results, experts have concluded that the vaccine is cost-effective and that it is underutilized.[31,170–173]

Despite the serious obstacles to such a study, Simberkoff and colleagues[174] conducted a randomized clinical trial of the protective efficacy of the 14-valent vaccine at several different Veterans Administration medical centers. Although they were unable to demonstrate that the vaccine was efficacious, there were a number of serious flaws in their methodology that compromise the validity of their conclusions.[175] Many of the events that the investigators counted as episodes of pneumococcal infection were really of uncertain cause since their definition of pneumococcal infection included patients with a cough and isolation of pneumococci from their sputa (even in the absence of an abnormal chest X ray). Because it is known that immunization with pneumococcal vaccine will not affect colonization of the respiratory tract with pneumococci, the definitions of pneumococcal infection used in this study limit its usefulness. By the investigators' own criteria, there were only two subjects with proven (bacteremic) pneumococcal infection. As a result, the statistical power of the study to assess the vaccine's efficacy against proved pneumococcal infections was extraordinarily poor (only 6%).

In July 1983, the 14-valent vaccine was replaced by a new vaccine that contains 25 μg each of the polysaccharides of 23 different serotypes of pneumococci (Table 4). These serotypes were included in the vaccine after extensive examination of data on the serotypes that had been isolated from the blood of cerebrospinal fluid of infected individuals, as well as data on the cross-reactivity of antibodies against the different serotypes.[176] As was true of the 14-valent vaccine, serious adverse reactions to the 23-valent vaccine are extremely rare.[157]

Despite the recommendations of official bodies such as the ACIP[31] and the American College of Physicians[157] that pneumococcal vaccine be administered to high-risk patients, physicians have been slow to implement these recommendations. Studies have indicated that fewer than a quarter of the eligible patients have received the vaccine.[168,177] Consequently, one of the major issues in maximizing the full potential benefit of this vaccine is to find a strategy to increase its utilization among high-risk patients. Fedson[177] and others have found that a large majority of the patients who develop pneumococcal bacteremia had been hospitalized in the preceding several years. Consequently, he suggests a strategy of immunizing with pneumococcal vaccine hospitalized patients who have indications for the vaccine.[177] This strategy would specifically target the group at highest risk of serious invasive pneumococcal disease, and thus enhance the efficiency of an immunization program.

The most definitive postlicensure study of the vaccine's protective efficacy is a case–control study by Shapiro *et al.*,[178] conducted from 1984–1990, of 1054 adults with systemic (usually bacteremic) pneumococcal infection who had one or more indications for pneumococcal vaccine and 1054 matched controls. The case subjects were stratified into a very-high risk, immunocompromised group (18% of the cases) and an immunocompetent group (82% of the cases). The estimate of the vaccine's aggregate protective efficacy (against serotypes in the vaccine) was 61% (95% confidence interval: 47–72%; $p < 0.00001$) among the immunocompetent patients but was only 21% (95% confidence interval: 55–60%; $p = 0.48$) for the immunocompromised group. Although this was an observational study, the findings were robust and did not change after statistical adjustment for potential confounders. In addition, using the same methods, the investigators found that the vaccine was not efficacious in preventing infections caused by serotypes not included in the vaccine and that there was no statistically significant difference in the proportion of cases and controls who had received influenza vaccine. These observations help assure that the findings are not substantially affected by bias and that the conclusions of the investigators are valid.

A report from the CDC in which the vaccine's protective efficacy was assessed based on an indirect cohort method had results similar to those of Shapiro *et al.* In that study (based on isolates of pneumococci from normally sterile sites that were submitted to the CDC from 1978–1992) the investigators found that the vaccine was efficacious in immunocompetent persons with indications for the vaccine (estimates of efficacy ranged from 65–75%, depending on the underlying disease), but that it was not efficacious (although the confidence intervals around the estimates were wide) for severely immunocompromised patients such as those with sickle-cell disease, lymphoma, or multiple myeloma.[179]

An area of particular controversy that has not been resolved is whether there is a significant decline in the efficacy of the vaccine over time. Although there does seem to be some decline, the magnitude of the decline (at least over 5–8 years) is relatively modest and some of this decline may be attributable to increased cumulative risk over time of exposure to serotypes of pneumococci in the vaccine. It is not clear that revaccination will reverse this effect. Nevertheless, the risk of adverse side effects from revaccination is small and is related to how soon after the first vaccination it occurs (if >1 year after the first vaccination, the risk of severe adverse reactions is extremely small). Consequently, revaccination is recommended for those at particularly high risk of serious pneumococcal infections.

The type-specific pneumococcal polysaccharide appears to be a T-cell-independent antigen. Booster (anamnestic) responses to repeated exposure to the polysaccharide antigen are not observed.[180] Although the attack rate of invasive pneumococcal infection is very high in young children, most of the serious infections occur in children under 2 years of age. Unfortunately, children under 2 years of age have a poor immunologic response to T-cell-independent antigens such as those in pneumococcal vaccine. Consequently, universal immunization of children with pneumococcal vaccine has not been recommended, since most cases of serious disease occur among young children who are unlikely to respond to the vaccine.[181] The vaccine also has not been effective in preventing otitis media in young children.[181] Pneumococcal vaccine is indicated for children 2 years of age or older with chronic conditions that place them at increased risk of serious pneumococcal infections.[181,182]

Although there continues to be some controversy about the protective efficacy of polyvalent pneumococcal polysaccharide vaccine for adults, there is no doubt that it is not efficacious in children <2 years of age—the group at highest risk of serious pneumococcal infections. However, polysaccharide–protein conjugate pneumococcal vaccines, which contain from five to eight different serotypes of pneumococci, are being developed. The 7-valent vaccine contains serotypes 4, 6B, 9V, 14, 18C, 19F, and 23F (an 8-valent version also contains serotype 3, which is a relatively common cause of otitis media). The serotypes in these vaccines are responsible for 80–85% of the invasive pneumococcal infections (and for about 75% of the cases of pneumococcal otitis media) in the United States. Addition of other serotypes, such as serotypes 1 and 5, will be important to increase the proportion of serious infections that might be prevented by the vaccine in developing countries.[66] These vaccines have been shown to be immunogenic in infants and primes them for anamnestic antibody responses to a booster dose of either the conjugate or the plain polysaccharide vaccine.[183] If these vaccines prove to be as efficacious as the conjugate vaccines against *H. influenzae* type b, they will become important to prevent serious pneumococcal infections in children at risk.

9.3. Passive Immunization

Commercial preparations of immunoglobulins contain substantial concentrations of antibodies against specific serotypes of pneumococci.[184] These preparations, administered on a regular basis, may prove to be useful in preventing pneumococcal infections in certain very high-risk patients.[184,185] An experimental preparation of a hyperimmune globulin against pneumococci, prepared from the serum of adult volunteers who were immunized with pneumococcal vaccine, may also be useful for certain patients.[186] Infusion of hyperimmune serum is not practical for widespread prophylaxis and it is unlikely to be used when conjugate pneumococcal vaccines become available.

10. Unresolved Problems

The detailed studies of the pneumococcus have been the basis of modern molecular biology and immunochemistry. Probably more is known about the biology of the pneumococcus than about that of any other bacterium. However, the exact mechanism(s) whereby this organism is able to multiply in animal and human tissue and produce its more or less unique type of inflammation in the lung is not fully known. Some progress has been made in the elucidation of the function of various chemical and morphological constituents of the pneumococcus other than the capsular polysaccharide.[121,187] Although many of the defects in cellular and humoral immunity that predispose to pneumococcal infections have been revealed, there are still others that need to be elucidated. Also, the exact mechanism whereby viral infection and chemical irritants predispose local pulmonary tissues to pneumococcal disease needs further elucidation. The reasons for the predominance of infection in males need to be clarified, as does the peculiar increased susceptibility of blacks, apart from environmental factors. The chemical basis for the cross-reactions between some types has been clarified,[188] but for others it is not known. The basis for virulence of pneumococci needs further study. Transformation of types has been shown to be mediated by DNA,[189] but whether transformation occurs under natural conditions is not known. The significance of skin reaction to various fractions of pneumococcus other than SSS[190] also remains unknown. Finally, while a pneumococcal vaccine is currently in use, the extent of its use in target populations is too low, and a protein–polysaccharide conjugate vaccine for use in infants and children under 2 years of age is only now being developed.

11. References

1. White, B. (with the collaboration of Robinson, E. S., and Barnes, L. A.), *The Biology of Pneumococcus: The Bacteriological, Biochemical and Immunological Characters and Activities of Diplococcus pneumoniae*, Commonwealth Fund, New York, 1938; reprinted by Harvard University Press, 1979.

2. Bergey, D. H., A key to the identification of organisms of the class Schizomycetes, in: *Bergey's Manual of Determinative Bacteriology*, 4th ed., p. 48, Williams & Wilkins, Baltimore, 1934.
3. Buchanan, R. E., and Gibbons, W. E., (eds.) *Bergey's Manual of Determinative Bacteriology*, 8th ed., Williams & Wilkins, Baltimore, 1974.
4. Finland, M., Pneumonia and pneumococcal infections, with special reference to pneumococcal pneumonia: The 1979 J. Burns Amberson Lecture, *Am. Rev. Respir. Dis.* **120:**481–502 (1979).
5. Finland, M., and Barnes, M. W., Acute bacterial meningitis at Boston City Hospital during 12 selected years, 1935–1972, *J. Infect. Dis.* **136:**400–415 (1977).
5a. Schuchat, A., Robinson, K., Wenger, J. D., Harrison, L. E., Farley, M., Reingold, A. L., Lefkowitz, L., Perkins, B. A., For the active surveillance team, Bacterial meningitis in the United States in 1995, *N. Engl. J. Med.* **337:**970–976 (1997).
6. Finland, M., and Barnes, M. W., Changing ecology of acute bacterial empyema: Occurrence and mortality at Boston City Hospital during twelve selected years from 1935 to 1972, *J. Infect. Dis.* **157:**274–291 (1978).
7. Klein, J. O., The epidemiology of pneumococcal disease in infants and children, *Rev. Infect. Dis.* **3:**246–253 (1981).
7a. Block, S. L., Causative pathogens, antibiotic resistance and therapeutic considerations in acute otitis media. *Pediatr. Infect. Dis. J.* **16:**449–456 (1997).
8. McGowan, J. E., Jr., Bratton, L., Klein, J. O., and Finland, M., Bacteremia in febrile children in a "walk-in" pediatric clinic, *N. Engl. J. Med.* **288:**1309–1312 (1973).
9. Teele, D. W., Pelton, S. I., Grant, M. J. A., Herskowitz, J., Rosen, D. J., Allen, C. E., Wimer, R. S., and Klein, J. O., Bacteremia in febrile children under 2 years of age: Results of cultures of blood in 600 consecutive febrile children in a "walk-in" clinic, *J. Pediatr.* **87:**227–230 (1975).
10. Finland, M., Recent advances in the epidemiology of pneumococcal infections, *Medicine* **21:**307–344 (1942).
11. Austrian, R., Pneumococcus, the first hundred years, *Rev. Infect. Dis.* **3:**183–189 (1981).
12. Neufeld, F., Ueber eine specifische bakteriolytische Wirkung der Galle, *Z. Hyg. Infektionskr.* **34:**454–464 (1900).
13. Neufeld, F., Ueber die Agglutination der Pneumokokken und Ueber die Theorien der Agglutination, *Z. Hyg. Infektionskr.* **40:**54–72 (1902).
14. Lister, F. S., Specific serological reactions with pneumococci from different sources, *Publ. S. Afr. Inst. Med. Res.* **1:**1–14 (1913).
15. Dochez, A. R., and Gillespie, L. J., A biological classification of pneumococci by means of immunity reactions, *J. Am. Med. Assoc.* **61:**727–730 (1913).
16. Lister, F. S., An experimental study of prophylactic inoculation against pneumococcal infection in the rabbit and in man, *Publ. S. Afr. Inst. Med. Res.* **1:**231–287 (1916).
17. Orenstein, A. J., Vaccine prophylaxis in pneumonia: A review of fourteen years' experience with inoculation of native mine workers on the Witwatersrand against pneumonia, *J. Med. Assoc. S. Afr.* **5:**339–346 (1931).
18. Armstrong, R. R., A swift and simple method for deciding pneumococcal "type," *Br. Med. J.* **1:**214–215 (1931).
19. Cooper, G., Rosenstein, C., Walter, A., and Peizer, L., The further separation of types among the pneumococci hitherto included in group IV and the development of therapeutic antisera for these types, *J. Exp. Med.* **55:**531–554 (1932).
20. Lund, E., Types of pneumococci found in blood, spinal fluid and pleural exudate during 15 years (1954–1969), *Acta Pathol. Microbiol. Scand. Sect. B* **78:**333–336 (1970).
21. Henrichsen, J., Six newly recognized types of *Streptococcus pneumoniae*, *J. Clin. Microbiol.* **33:**2759–2762 (1995).
22. Wright, A. E., Morgan, W., Colbrook, L., and Dodgson, R. W., Observations on prophylactic inoculations against pneumococcus infection, and on the results which have been achieved by it, *Lancet* **1:**1–10, 87–95 (1914).
23. Kass, E. H. (ed.), Assessment of the pneumococcal polysaccharide vaccine: A workshop held at the Harvard Club of Boston, Boston, Massachusetts, October 6, 1980, *Rev. Infect. Dis.* **3:** (Suppl.)**:**S1–S197 (1981).
24. Schiffman, G., Immune response to pneumococcal polysaccharide antigens: A comparison of the murine model and the response in humans, *Rev. Infect. Dis.* **3:**224–231 (1981).
25. Heffron, R., *Pneumonia with Special Reference to Pneumococcus Lobar Pneumonia*, Commonwealth Fund, New York, 1939; reprinted by Harvard University Press, 1979.
26. Collins, S. D., and Gover, M., Age and seasonal incidence of minor respiratory attacks classified according to clinical symptoms, *Am. J. Hyg.* **20:**533–554 (1934).
27. Centers for Disease Control, Surveillance summary: Bacterial meningitis and meningococcemia, *Morbid. Mortal. Week. Rep.* **28:**277–279 (1979).
28. Wenger, J. D., Hightower, A. W., Facklam, R. R., Gaventa, S., Broome, C. V., and the Bacterial Meningitis Study Group, Bacterial meningitis in the United States, 1986: Report of a multistate surveillance study, *J. Infect. Dis.* **162:**1316–1323 (1990).
29. Burman, A., Norrby, R., and Trollfors, B., Invasive pneumococcal infections: Incidence, predisposing factors and prognosis, *Rev. Infect. Dis.* **7:**133–142 (1985).
30. Mufson, M. A., Pneumococcal infections, *J. Am. Med. Assoc.* **246:**1942–1948 (1981).
31. Centers for Disease Control, Recommendations of the Immunization Practices Advisory Committee (ACIP): Pneumococcal polysaccharide vaccine, *Morbid. Mortal. Week. Rep.* **30:**410–419 (1981).
32. Eskola, J., Takala, A., Kela, E., Pekkanen, E., Kalliokosk, R., and Leinonen, M., Epidemiology of invasive pneumococcal infections in children in Finland, *J. Am. Med. Assoc.* **268:**3323–3327 (1992).
33. Dagon, R., Englehard, D., Piccard, E., and the Israeli Pediatric Bacteremia and Meningitis Group, Epidemiology of invasive childhood pneumococcal infections in Israel, *J. Am. Med. Assoc.* **268:**3328–3332 (1992).
34. Hoge, C. W., Reichler, M. R., Dominguez, E. A., Bremer, J. C., Mastro, T. D., Hendrick, K. A., Musher, D. M., Elliott, J. A., Facklam, R. R., and Breiman, R. F., An epidemic of pneumococcal disease in an overcrowded, inadequately ventilated jail, *N. Engl. J. Med.* **331:**643–648 (1994).
35. Davidson, M., Parkinson, A. J., Bulkow, L. R., Fitzgerald, M. A., Peters, H. V., and Parks, D. J., The epidemiology of invasive pneumococcal disease in Alaska, 1986–1990—Ethnic differences and opportunities for prevention, *J. Infect. Dis.* **170:**368–376 (1994).
36. Cortese, M. M., Wolff, M., Almeido-Hill, J., Reed, R., Ketcham, J., and Santosham, M., High incidence rates of pneumococcal disease in the White Mountain Apache population, *Arch. Intern. Med.* **152:**2277–2282 (1992).
37. Sabin, A. B., "Stained slide" microscopic agglutination test:

Application to (1) rapid typing of pneumococci, (2) determination of antibody, *Am. J. Public Health* **19:**1148–1150 (1929).

38. Rytel, M. W., Pneumococcal pneumonia, in: *Rapid Diagnosis in Infectious Disease* (M. W. Rytel, ed.), pp. 91–103, CRC Press, Boca Raton, FL, 1979.
39. Schiffman, G., Douglas, R. M., Bonner, M. J., Robbins, M., and Austrian, R., A radioimmunoassay for immunologic phenomena in pneumococcal disease and for the antibody response to pneumococcal vaccines. 1. Methods for the radioimmunoassay of anticapsular antibodies and comparison of other techniques, *J. Immunol. Methods* **33:**133–144 (1980).
40. Moore, H. F., and Chesney, A. M., A further study of ethylhydrocupreine (optochin) in the treatment of acute lobar pneumonia, *Arch. Intern. Med.* **21:**659–681 (1918).
41. Lowell, F. C., Strauss, E., and Finland, M., Observations on the susceptibility of pneumococci to sulfapyridine, sulfathiazole and sulfamethoxazole, *Ann. Intern. Med.* **14:**1001–1023 (1940).
42. Whitby, L., Chemotherapy of bacterial infections (Bradshaw Lecture), *Lancet* **2:**1095–1103 (1938).
43. Applebaum, P. C., Antimicrobial resistance in *Streptococcus pneumoniae*: An overview, *Clin. Infect. Dis.* **15:**77–83 (1992).
44. Austrian, R., Some observations on the pneumococcus and on the current status of pneumococcal disease and its prevention, *Rev. Infect. Dis.* **3:**(Suppl.):S1–S17 (1981).
45. Mundy, L. M., Auwaerter, P. G., Oldach, D., Warner, M. L., Burton, A., Vance, E., Gaydos, C. A., Joseph, J. M., Gopalan, R., Moore, R. D., Quinn, T. C., Charache, P., and Bartlett, J. G., Community-acquired pneumonia: Impact of immune status, *Am. J. Respir. Crit. Care Med.* **152:**1309–1315 (1995).
46. Hansman, D., and Bullen, M. M., A resistant pneumococcus, *Lancet* **2:**264–265 (1967).
47. Applebaum, P. C., Bhamjee, A., Scragg, J. N., Hallett, A. F., Bowen, A. J., and Cooper, R. C., *Streptococcus pneumoniae* resistant to penicillin and chloramphenicol, *Lancet* **2:**995–997 (1977).
48. Jacobs, M. R., Koornhof, H. J., Robins-Brown, R. M., Stevenson, C. M., Vermaak, Z. A., Freiman, I., Miller, G. B., Witcomb, M. A., Isaäcson, M., Ward, J. I., and Austrian, R., Emergence of multiply resistant pneumococci, *N. Engl. J. Med.* **299:**735–740 (1978).
49. Zighelboim, S., and Tomasz, A., Multiple antibiotic resistance in South African strains of *Streptococcus pneumoniae*: Mechanism of resistance to β-lactam antibiotics, *Rev. Infect. Dis.* **3:**267–276 (1981).
50. Handwerger, S., and Tomasz, A., Alterations in penicillin-binding proteins of clinical and laboratory isolates of pathogenic *Streptococcus pneumoniae* with low levels of penicillin resistance, *J. Infect. Dis.* **153:**83–89 (1986).
51. Tomasz, A., The pneumococcus at the gates, *N. Engl. J. Med.* **333:**514–515 (1995).
52. Caputo, G. M., Applebaum, P. C., and Liu, H. H., Infections due to penicillin-resistant pneumococci. Clinical, epidemiologic, and microbiologic features, *Arch. Intern. Med.* **153:**1301–1310 (1993).
53. Pallares, R., Liñares, J., Vadillo, M., Cabellos, C., Manresa, F., Viladrich, P. F., Martin, R., and Gudiol, F., Resistance to penicillin and cephalosporin and mortality from severe pneumococcal pneumonia in Barcelona, Spain, *N. Engl. J. Med.* **333:**474–480 (1995).
54. Saah, A. J., Mallonee, J. R., Tarpay, M., Thornsberry, C. T., Roberts, M. A., and Rhoades, E. R., Relative resistance to penicillin in the pneumococcus, *J. Am. Med. Assoc.* **243:**1824–1827 (1980).
55. Pallares, R., Gudiol, F., Liñares, J., Ariza, J., Rufi, G., Murgui, L., Dorca, J., and Viladrich, P. F., Risk factors and response to antibiotic therapy in adults with bacteremic pneumonia caused by penicillin-resistant pneumococci, *N. Engl. J. Med.* **317:**18–22 (1987).
56. Hofmann, J., Cetron, M. S., Farley, M. M., Baughman, W. S., Facklam, R. R., Elliott, J. A., Deaver, K. A., and Breiman, R. F., The prevalence of drug-resistant *Streptococcus pneumoniae* in Atlanta, *N. Engl. J. Med.* **333:**481–486 (1995).
57. Friedland, I. R., and Klugman, K. P., Antibiotic-resistant pneumococcal disease in South African children, *Am. J. Dis. Child.* **146:**920–923 (1992).
58. Mason, E. O., Kaplan, S. L., Lamberth, L. B., and Tillman, J., Increased rate of isolation of penicillin-resistant *Streptococcus pneumoniae* in a children's hospital and *in vitro* susceptibilities to antibiotics of potential therapeutic use, *Antimicrob. Agents Chemother.* **36:**1703–1707 (1992).
59. Pikis, A., Akram, S., Donkersloot, J., Campos, J. M., and Rodriguez, W. J., Penicillin-resistant pneumococci from pediatric patients in the Washington, DC area, *Arch. Pediatr. Adolesc. Med.* **149:**30–35 (1995).
60. Block, S., Harrison, C. J., Hedrick, J. A., Tyler, R. D., Smith, R. A., Keegan, E., and Chartrand, S. A., Penicillin-resistant *Streptococcus pneumoniae* in acute otitis media: Risk factors, susceptibility patterns and antimicrobial management, *Pediatr. Infect. Dis. J.* **14:**751–759 (1995).
61. Duchin, J. S., Breiman, R. F., Diamond, A., Lipman, H. B., Block, S. L., Hedrick, J. A., Finger, R., and Elliott, J. A., High prevalence of multidrug-resistant *Streptococcus pneumoniae* among children in a rural Kuntucky community, *Pediatr. Infect. Dis. J.* **14:**745–750 (1995).
62. Feldman, C., Kallenbach, J. M., Miller, S. D., Thorburn, J. R., and Koornhof, H., Community-acquired pneumonia due to penicillin-resistant pneumococci, *N. Engl. J. Med.* **313:**615–617 (1985).
63. Simberkoff, M. S., Lukaszewski, M., Cross, A., Al-Ibrahim, M., Baltch, A. L., Smith, R. P., Geisler, P. J., Nadler, J., and Richmond, A. S., Antibiotic isolates of *Streptococcus pneumoniae* from clinical specimens: A cluster of serotype 19A organisms in Brooklyn, New York, *J. Infect. Dis.* **153:**78–82 (1986).
64. Koornhof, H. J., Wasas, A., and Klugman, K., Antimicrobial resistance in *Streptococcus pneumoniae*: A South African perspective, *Clin. Infect. Dis.* **15:**84–94 (1992).
65. Finland, M., and Barnes, M. W., Changes ion occurrence of capsular serotypes of *Streptococcus pneumoniae* at Boston City Hospital during selected years between 1935 and 1974, *J. Clin. Microbiol.* **5:**154–166 (1977).
66. Baltimore, R. S., New challenges in the development of a conjugate pneumococcal vaccine, *J. Am. Med. Assoc.* **268:**3366–3367 (1992).
67. Ordman, D., Pneumococcus typing: Its value in pneumonia, *S. Afr. Med. J.* **11:**569–573 (1937).
68. Ordman, D., Pneumococcus types in South Africa: A study of their occurrence and the effect thereon of prophylactic inoculation, *Publ. S. Afr. Inst. Med. Res.* **9:**1–27 (1938).
69. Finland, M., The present status of the higher types of antipneumococcus serums, *J. Am. Med. Assoc.* **120:**1294–1307 (1942).
70. Lund, E., Pulverer, G., and Jeljaszewicz, J., Serological types of *Diplococcus pneumoniae* strains isolated in Germany, *Med. Microbiol. Immunol.* **159:**171–178 (1974).
71. Parker, M. T., Type distribution of pneumococci isolated from serious diseases in Britain, in: *Pathogenic Streptococci* (M. T. Parker, ed.), pp. 191–192, Redbooks, Chertsey, England, 1979.

72. Echániz-Aviles, G., Carnalla-Barajas, N., Velázquez-Meza, M. E., Soto-Noguerón, A., Espiñosa-de los Monteros, L. E., and Solórozano-Santos, F., Capsular types of *Streptococcus pneumoniae* causing disease in children from Mexico City, *Pediatr. Infect. Dis. J.* **14:**907–909 (1995).
73. Nemir, R. L., Andrews, E. T., and Vinograd, J., Pneumonia in infants and children: Bacteriologic study with special reference to clinical significance, *Am. J. Dis. Child.* **51:**1277–1295 (1936).
74. Shapiro, E. D., and Austrian, R., Serotypes responsible for invasive *Streptococcus pneumoniae* infections among children in Connecticut, *J. Infect. Dis.* **169:**212–214 (1994).
75. Finland, M., and Winkler, A. W., Recurrences in pneumococcus pneumonia, *Am. J. Med. Sci.* **188:**309–320 (1934).
76. Strauss, E., and Finland, M., Further studies on recurrences in pneumococcic pneumonia with special reference to the effect of specific treatment, *Ann. Intern. Med.* **16:**17–32 (1942).
77. Quie, P. G., Giebink, G. S., and Winkelstein, J. A. (guest eds.), The *Pneumoncoccus*: A symposium held at the Kroc Foundation Headquarters, Santa Ynez Valley, California, February 25–29, 1980, *Rev. Infect. Dis.* **3:**183–371 (1981).
78. Riley, I. D., and Douglas, R. M., An epidemiologic approach to pneumococcal disease, *Rev. Infect. Dis.* **3:**233–245 (1981).
79. Cole, R., and MacCallum, W. G., Pneumonia at a base hospital, *J. Am. Med. Assoc.* **70:**1146–1156 (1918).
80. Small, A. A., Pneumonia at a base hospital: Observations in one thousand and one hundred cases at Camp Pike, Ark., *J. Am. Med. Assoc.* **71:**700–702 (1918).
81. Opie, E. L., Blake, F. G., Small, J. C., and Rivers, T. M., *Epidemic Respiratory Disease: The Pneumonias and Other Infections of the Respiratory Tract Accompanying Influenza and Measles*, Mosby, St. Louis, 1921.
82. Netter, Contagion de la pneumonie, *Arch. Gen. Med. (Paris)* **21:** 530–544, 699–718; **22:**42–59 (1888).
83. Cruickshank, R., Pneumococcal infections (Milroy Lectures), *Lancet* **1:**563–568, 621–626, 680–685 (1933).
84. Johnston, H., Pneumonia as contagious disease, *Can. Med. Assoc. J.* **38:**270–271 (1938).
85. Brown, J. W., and Finland, M., A family outbreak of type V pneumococcus infections: Clinical, bacteriological and immunological studies, *Ann. Intern. Med.* **13:**394–401 (1939).
86. Finland, M., and Tilghman, R. C., Bacteriological and immunological studies in families with pneumococcic infections: The development of type-specific antibodies in healthy contact carriers, *J. Clin. Invest.* **15:**501–508 (1936).
87. Smillie, W. E., Study of an outbreak of type II pneumococcus pneumonia in Veterans' Administration Hospital at Bedford, Massachusetts, *Am. J. Hyg.* **24:**522–535 (1936).
88. Smillie, W. E., Warnock, G. H., and White, H. J., Study of a type I pneumococcus epidemic at the State Hospital at Worcester, Mass., *Am. J. Public Health* **28:**293–302 (1938).
89. Tomforde, Eine Endemie von croupöser Pneumonie im Dorfe Laumuhlen, Kreis Neuhaus an der Oste, Januar 1902, *Dtsch. Med. Wochenschr.* **28:**577–579 (1902).
90. Gorgas, W. C., Sanitation on the Panama Canal, *J. Am. Med. Assoc.* **40:**953–955 (1913).
91. Park, J. H., Jr., and Chickering, H. T., Type I pneumococcal lobar pneumonia among Puerto Rican laborers of Camp Jackson, South Carolina, *J. Am. Med. Assoc.* **73:**183–186 (1919).
92. Tenny, C. F., and Rivenburgh, W. T., A group of 68 cases of type I pneumonia occurring in 30 days at Camp Upton, *Arch. Intern. Med.* **24:**545–552 (1919).
93. Hirsch, E. F., and McKinney, M., An epidemic of pneumococcus bronchopneumonia, *J. Infect. Dis.* **24:**594–617 (1919).
94. Holle, H. A., and Bullowa, J. G. M., Pneumococcal cross-infections in home and hospital, *N. Engl. J. Med.* **223:**887–890 (1940).
95. Harris, A. H., and Ingraham, H. S., Study of carrier condition associated with type II pneumonia in camp of Civilian Conservation Corps, *J. Clin. Invest.* **16:**41–48 (1937).
96. Greenberg, D., Relation of meteorological conditions to the prevalence of pneumonia, *J. Am. Med. Assoc.* **72:**252–257 (1919).
97. Rogers, L., Relationship between pneumonia incidence and climate in India, *Lancet* **1:**1173–1177 (1925).
98. McGowan, J. E., Jr., Barnes, M. W., and Finland, M., Bacteremia at Boston City Hospital: Occurrence and mortality during 12 selected years 1935–1972, with special reference to hospital-acquired cases, *J. Infect. Dis.* **132:**316–335 (1975).
99. Tillotson, J. R., and Finland, M., Bacterial colonization and clinical superinfection of the respiratory tract complicating antibiotic treatment of pneumonia, *J. Infect. Dis.* **119:**597–624 (1969).
100. Brundage, D. K., Russell, A. E., Jones, R. R., Bloomfield, J. J., and Thompson, R., Frequency of pneumonia among iron and steel workers, *Public Health Bulletin*, No. 202, US Government Printing Office, Washington, DC, 1932.
101. Gilman, B. B., and Anderson, G. W., Community outbreak of type I pneumococcus infection, *Am. J. Hyg.* **28:**345–358 (1938).
102. Sydenstricker, V. P. W., and Sutton, A. C., An epidemiological study of lobar pneumonia, *Bull. Johns Hopkins Hosp.* **38:**312–315 (1918).
103. Lister, S., and Ordman, D., Epidemiology of pneumonia on the Witwatersrand goldfields and prevention of pneumonia and other acute respiratory diseases in native laborers in South Africa by means of vaccine, *Publ. S. Afr. Inst. Med. Res.* **7:**1–124 (1935).
104. Ordman, D., Pneumonia in the native mine workers of the Witwatersrand goldfields: A bacteriological and epidemiological study, *J. Med. Assoc. S. Afr.* **5:**108–116 (1931).
105. Ordman, D., Pneumonia in the native mine labourers of northern Rhodesia copperfields with an account of an experiment in pneumonia prophylaxis by means of a vaccine at the Roan Antelope Mine, *Publ. S. Afr. Inst. Med. Res.* **7:**1–124 (1935).
106. Ebgert, J. H., Epidemic pneumonia in the tropics, *NY Med. J.* **103:**1125 (1916).
107. Robertson, O. H., Instance of lobar pneumonia acquired in the laboratory, *J. Prev. Med.* **5:**221–224 (1931).
108. Benjamin, J. E., Ruegsegger, J. M., and Senior, F. A., Cross-infection in pneumococcic pneumonia, *J. Am. Med. Assoc.* **112:** 1127–1130 (1939).
109. Verhoef, J., Effects of nutrition on antibiotic action, in: *Action of Antibiotics in Patients* (L. D. Sabath and G. G. Grassi, eds.), Huber, Bern, 1982.
110. Perlino, C. A., and Rimland, D., Alcoholism leukopenia and pneumococcal sepsis, *Am. Rev. Respir. Dis.* **132:**757–760 (1985).
111. Giebink, G. S., The pathogenesis of otitis media in chinchillas and the efficacy of vaccination on prophylaxis, *Rev. Infect. Dis.* **3:** 342–352 (1981).
112. Giebink, G. S., Berzins, J. K., Marker, S. C., and Schiffman, G., Experimental otitis media after nasal inoculation of *Streptococcus pneumoniae* and influenza A in chinchillas, *Infect. Immun.* **30:**445–450 (1980).
113. Kass, E. H., Green, G. M., and Goldstein, E., Mechanism of antibacterial action in the respiratory tract, *Bacteriol. Rev.* **30:**488–496 (1966).

114. Coonrod, J. D., and Yoneda, K., Complement and opsonins in alveolar secretions and serum of rats with pneumonia due to *Streptococcus pneumoniae*, *Rev. Infect. Dis.* **3**:310–322 (1981).
115. Drinker, C. K., and Field, M. E., *Lymphatics, Lymph and Tissue Fluid*, Williams & Wilkins, Baltimore, 1933.
116. Terrell, E. E., Robertson, O. H., and Coggeshall, L. T., Experimental pneumococcus lobar pneumonia in the dog. I. Method of production and course of disease, *J. Clin. Invest.* **12**:393–432 (1933).
117. Stillman, E. G., and Branch, A., Experimental production of pneumococcus pneumonia in mice by inhalation method, *J. Exp. Med.* **40**:733–742 (1924).
118. Stillman, E. G., Susceptibility of rabbits to infection by the inhalation of type II pneumococcus, *J. Exp. Med.* **52**:215–224 (1930).
119. Goodner, K., Development and localization of dermal pneumococcic infection in the rabbit, *J. Exp. Med.* **54**:847–858 (1931).
120. Tilghman, R. C., and Finland, M., Clinical significance of bacteremia in pneumococcal pneumonia, *Arch. Intern. Med.* **59**:602–619 (1937).
121. Finland, M., and Sutliff, W. D., Specific cutaneous reactions and circulating antibodies in the course of lobar pneumonia. I. Cases receiving no serum therapy, *J. Exp. Med.* **54**:637–652 (1931).
122. Tuomanen, E. I., Austrian, R., and Masure, H. R., Pathogenesis of pneumococcal infection, *N. Engl. J. Med.* **332**:1280–1284 (1995).
123. Giebink, G. S., Grebner, J. V., Kim, Y., and Quie, P. G., Severe opsonic deficiency produced by *Streptococcus pneumoniae* and by capsular polysaccharide antigens, *Yale J. Biol. Med.* **51**:527–538 (1978).
124. Rytel, M. W., Dee, T. H., Ferstenfeld, J. E., and Hensley, G. T., Possible pathogenic role of capsular antigens in fulminant pneumococcal disease with disseminated intravascular coagulation, *Am. J. Med.* **57**:889–896 (1974).
125. Bernstein, L. J., Krieger, B. Z., Novick, B., Sicklick, M. J., and Rubinstein, A., Bacterial infection in the acquired immunodeficiency syndrome of children, *Pediatr. Infect. Dis.* **4**:472–475 (1985).
126. Andiman, W. A., Mezger, J., and Shapiro, E., Invasive bacterial infections in children born to women infected with human immunodefiency virus type 1, *J. Pediatr.* **124**:846–852 (1994).
127. Farley, J. J., King, J. C., Jr., Nair, P., Hines, S. E., Tressler, R. L., and Vink, P. E., Invasive pneumococcal disease among infected and uninfected children of mothers with human immunodeficiency virus infection, *J. Pediatr.* **124**:853–858 (1994).
128. Hirschtick, R. E., Glassroth, J., Jordan, M. C., Bacterial pneumonia in persons infected with the human immunodeficiency virus, *N. Engl. J. Med.* **333**:845–851 (1995).
129. Janoff, E., Breiman, R. F., Daley, C. L., Pneumococcal disease during HIV infection, *Ann. Intern. Med.* **117**:314–324 (1992).
130. The National Institutes of Child Health and Human Development Intravenous Immunoglobulin Study Group, Intravenous immune globulin for the prevention of bacterial infections in children with symptomatic human immunodeficiency virus infection, *N. Engl. J. Med.* **325**:73–80 (1991).
131. Ivemark, B., Implications of agenesis of the spleen on the pathogenesis of conotruncus anomalies in children, *Acta Pediatr. Scand.* (Suppl. 104) **44**:590–592 (1955).
132. Waldman, J. D., Rosenthal, A., Smith, A. L., Shurin, S., and Nadas, A. S., Sepsis and congenital asplenia, *J. Pediatr.* **90**:555–559 (1977).
133. Styrt, B., Infection associated with asplenia: Risks, mechanisms, and prevention, *Am. J. Med.* **88**:33N–44N (1990).
134. Pearson, H. A., Splenectomy: Its risks and its roles, *Hosp. Pract.* **15**(August):85–94 (1980).
135. Gaston, M. H., Verter, J. I., Woods, G., Prophylaxis with oral penicillin in children with sickle cell anemia. A randomized trial, *N. Engl. J. Med.* **314**:1593–1599 (1986).
136. Brown, E. J., Hosea, S. W., and Frank, M. M., The role of antibody and complement in the reticuloendothelial clearance of pneumococci from the blood stream, *Rev. Infect. Dis.* **5**:S797–S805 (1983).
137. Winkelstein, J. A., The role of complement in the hosts' defense against *Streptococcus pneumoniae*, *Rev. Infect. Dis.* **3**:289–298 (1981).
138. Davies, J. A. V., The response of infants to inoculation with type 1 pneumococcus carbohydrate, *J. Immunol.* **33**:1–7 (1937).
139. Sell, S. H., Wright, P. F., Vaughan, W. K., Thompson, J., and Schiffman, G., Clinical studies of pneumococcal vaccine in infants. 1. Reactogenicity and immunogenicity of two polyvalent polysaccharide vaccines, *Rev. Infect. Dis.* **3**:S97–S107 (1981).
140. Wara, D. W., Host defense against *Streptococcus pneumoniae*: The role of the spleen, *Rev. Infect. Dis.* **3**:299–309 (1981).
141. Maynard, G. D., An enquiry into the etiology, manifestations and prevention of pneumonia amongst natives on the Rand from tropical areas, *Publ. S. Afr. Inst. Med. Res.* **1**:1–101 (1913).
142. Ekwurzel, G. M., Simmons, J. S., Dublin, H., and Felton, L. D., Studies of immunizing substances in pneumococci. VIII. Report on field test to determine the prophylactic value of a pneumococcus antigen, *Public Health Rep.* **53**:1877–1893 (1938).
143. Felton, L. D., Studies on immunizing substances in pneumococci. VII. Response in human beings to antigenic pneumococcus polysaccharides, type I and II, *Public Health Rep.* **53**:2855–2877 (1938).
144. Lister, F. S., Prophylactic inoculation of man against pneumococcal infections, and more particularly against lobar pneumonia, *Publ. S. Afr. Inst. Med. Res.* **10**:304–322 (1917).
145. Kaufman, P., Pneumonia in old age. Active immunization against pneumonia with pneumococcus polysaccharides: Results of a six year study, *Arch. Intern. Med.* **79**:518–531 (1947).
146. MacLeod, C. M., Hodges, R. G., Heidelberger, M., and Bernhard, W. G., Prevention of pneumococcal pneumonia by immunization with specific capsular polysaccharides, *J. Exp. Med.* **82**:445–465 (1945).
147. Austrian, R., and Gold, J., Pneumococcal bacteremia with especial reference to bacteremic pneumococcal pneumonia, *Ann. Intern. Med.* **60**:759–776 (1964).
148. US Congress, Office of Technology Assessment, *A Review of Selected Federal Vaccine and Immunization Policies*, US Government Printing Office, Washington, DC, 1979.
149. Austrian, R., Douglas, R. M., Schiffman, G., Coetzee, A. M., Koornhof, H. J., Hayden-Smith, S., and Reid, R. D. W., Prevention of pneumococcal pneumonia by vaccination, *Trans. Assoc. Am. Physicians* **89**:184–194 (1976).
150. Smit, P., Oberholzer, D., Hayden-Smith, S., Koornhof, H. J., and Hilleman, M. R., Protective efficacy of pneumococcal polysaccharide vaccines, *J. Am. Med. Assoc.* **238**:2613–2616 (1977).
151. Austrian, R., *Surveillance of Pneumococcal Infection for Field Trials of Polyvalent Pneumococcal Vaccine*, Report DAB-VDP-12-84, National Institutes of Health, Bethesda, 1980.
152. Schwartz, J. S., Pneumococcal vaccine: Clinical efficacy and effectiveness, *Ann. Intern. Med.* **96**:208–220 (1982).
153. Ammann, A. J., Addiego, J., Wara, D. W., Lubin, B., Smith, W. B., and Mentzer, W. C., Polyvalent pneumococcal–polysaccharide immunization of patients with sickle-cell anemia and patients with splenectomy, *N. Engl. J. Med.* **297**:897–900 (1977).

154. Centers for Disease Control, Recommendation of the Public Health Service Advisory Committee on Immunization Practices: Pneumococcal polysaccharide vaccine, *Morbid. Mortal. Week. Rep.* **27:**25–31 (1978).
155. Centers for Disease Control, Recommendations of the Immunization Practices Advisory Committee (ACIP) update: Pneumococcal vaccine usage—United States, *Morbid. Mortal. Week. Rep.* **33:**273–281 (1984).
156. Centers for Disease Control, Recommendations of the Immunization Practices Advisory Committee (ACIP): Prevention of Pneumococcal Disease, *Morbid. Mortal. Week. Rep.* **46**(suppl. RR-8)**:** 1–24 (1997).
157. Health and Public Policy Committee, American College of Physicians, Pneumococcal vaccine, *Ann. Intern. Med.* **104:**118–120 (1986).
158. Broome, C. V., and Facklam, R. R., Epidemiology of clinically significant isolates of *Streptococcus pneumoniae* in the United States, *Rev. Infect. Dis.* **3:**277–281 (1981).
159. Broome, C. V., Facklam, R. R., Allen, J. R., Fraser, D. W., and Austrian, R., Epidemiology of pneumococcal serotypes in the United States, 1978–1979, *J. Infect. Dis.* **141:**119–123 (1980).
160. Ahonkhai, V. I., Landesman, S. H., Fikrig, S. M., Schmalzer, E. A., Brown, A. K., Cherubin, C. E., and Schiffman, G., Failure of pneumococcal vaccine in children with sickle-cell disease, *N. Engl. J. Med.* **301:**26–27 (1979).
161. Giebink, G. S., Schiffman, G., Krivit, W., and Quie, P. G., Vaccine-type pneumococcal pneumonia after vaccination in an asplenic patient, *J. Am. Med. Assoc.* **241:**2736–2737 (1979).
162. Ammann, A. J., Schiffman, G., Addiego, J. E., Wara, W. M., and Wara, D. W., Immunization of immunosuppressed patients with pneumococcal polysaccharide vaccine, *Rev. Infect. Dis.* **3** (Suppl.)**:**S160–S167 (1981).
163. Giebink, G. S., Le, C. T., Cosio, F. G., Spika, J. S., and Schiffman, G., Serum antibody responses of high-risk children and adults to vaccination with capsular polysaccharides of *Streptococcus pneumoniae*, *Rev. Infect. Dis.* **3**(Suppl.)**:**S168–S178 (1981).
164. Lazarus, H. M., Lederman, M., Lubin, A., Herzig, R. H., Schiffman, G., Jones, P., Wine, A., and Rodman, H. M., Pneumococcal vaccination: The response of patients with multiple myeloma, *Am. J. Med.* **69:**419–423 (1980).
165. Broome, C. V., Efficacy of pneumococcal polysaccharide vaccines, *Rev. Infect. Dis.* **3**(Suppl.)**:**S82–S83 (1981).
166. Broome, C. V., Facklam, R. R., and Fraser, D. W., Pneumococcal disease after pneumococcal vaccination: An alternative method to estimate the efficacy of pneumococcal vaccine, *N. Engl. J. Med.* **303:**549–552 (1980).
167. Clemens, J. D., and Shapiro, E. D., Resolving the pneumococcal vaccine controversy: Are there alternatives to randomized clinical trials? *Rev. Infect. Dis.* **6:**589–600 (1984).
168. Shapiro, E. D., and Clemens, J. D., A controlled evaluation of the protective efficacy of pneumococcal vaccine for patients at high risk for serious pneumococcal infections, *Ann. Intern. Med.* **101:** 325–330 (1984).
169. Bolan, G., Broome, C. V., Facklam, R. R., Pilkaytis, B. D., Fraser, D. W., and Schlech, W. F., III, Pneumococcal vaccine efficacy in selected populations in the United States, *Ann. Intern. Med.* **104:** 1–6 (1986).
170. Austrian, R., A reassessment of pneumococcal vaccine [editorial], *N. Engl. J. Med.* **310:**651–653 (1984).
171. LaForce, F. M., and Eickhoff, T. C., Pneumococcal vaccine: The evidence mounts, *Ann. Intern. Med.* **104:**110–112 (1986).
172. Patrick, K. M., and Woolley, F. R., A cost-benefit analysis of immunization of pneumococcal pneumonia, *J. Am. Med. Assoc.* **245:**473–477 (1981).
173. Sisk, J. E., and Riegelman, R. K., Cost effectiveness of vaccination against pneumococcal pneumonia: An update, *Ann. Intern. Med.* **104:**79–86 (1986).
174. Simberkoff, M. S., Cross, A. P., Al-Ibrahim, M., Baltch, A. L., Geisler, P. J., Nadler, J., Richmond, A. S., Smith, R. P., and Van Eeckhout, J. P., Efficacy of pneumococcal vaccine in high-risk patients: Results of a Veterans Administration cooperative study, *N. Engl. J. Med.* **315:**1318–1327 (1986).
175. Shapiro, E. D., Pneumococcal vaccine failure [letter], *N. Engl. J. Med.* **316:**1272–1273 (1987).
176. Robbins, J. B., Austrian, R., Lee, C.-J., Rastogi, S. C., Schiffman, G., Henrichsen, J., Makela, P. H., Broome, C. V., Facklam, R. R., Tiesjema, R. H., and Parke, J. C., Jr., Considerations for formulating the second-generation pneumococcal capsular lysaccharide vaccine with emphases on the cross-reactive types within groups, *J. Infect. Dis.* **148:**1136–1159 (1983).
177. Fedson, D. S., Improving the use of pneumococcal vaccine through a strategy of hospital-based immunization: A review of its rationale and implications, *J. Am. Geriatr. Soc.* **33:**142–150 (1985).
178. Shapiro, E. D., Berg, A. T., Austrian, R., *et al.*, The protective efficacy of polyvalent pneumococcal polysaccharide vaccine, *N. Engl. J. Med.* **325:**1453–1460 (1991).
179. Butler, J. C., Breiman, R. F., Campbell, J. F., Lipman, H. B., Broome, C. V., and Facklam, R. R., Pneumococcal polysaccharide vaccine efficacy: An evaluation of current recommendations, *J. Am. Med. Assoc.* **270:**1826–1831 (1993).
180. Borgono, J. M., McLean, A. A., Vella, P. P., Woodhour, A. F., Canepa, I., Davidson, W. L., and Hilleman, M. R., Vaccination and revaccination with polyvalent pneumococcal polysaccharide vaccines in adults and infants, *Proc. Soc. Exp. Biol. Med.* **157:**148–154 (1978).
181. Giebink, G. S., Preventing pneumococcal disease in children: Recommendations for using pneumococcal vaccine, *Pediatr. Infect. Dis.* **4:**343–348 (1985).
182. Committee on Infectious Diseases, American Academy of Pediatrics, Recommendations for using pneumococcal vaccine in children, *Pediatrics* **75:**1153–1158 (1985).
183. Käyhty, H., Åhman, H., Rönnberg, P.-R., Tillikainen, R., and Eskola, J., Pneumococcal polysaccharide–meningococcal outer membrane protein complex conjugate vaccine is immunogenic in infants and children, *J. Infect. Dis.* **172:**1273–1278 (1995).
184. Wood, C. C., McNamara, J. G., Schwarz, D. F., Merrill, W. W., and Shapiro, E. D., Prevention of pneumococcal bacteremia in a child with AIDS-related complex, *Pediatr. Infect. Dis. J.* **6:**564–566 (1987).
185. Calvelli, T. A., and Rubinstein, A., Intravenous gammaglobulin in infant acquired immunodeficiency syndrome, *Pediatr. Infect. Dis.* **5:**S207–S210 (1986).
186. Siber, G. R., Thompson, C., Reid, G. R., Almeido-Hill, J., Zachet, B., Wolff, M., and Santosham, M., Evaluation of bacterial polysaccharide immune globulin for the treatment or prevention of *Haemophilus influenzae* type b and pneumococcal disease, *J. Infect. Dis.* **165**(Suppl.)**:**S129–S133 (1992).
187. Tomasz, A., Surface components of *Streptococcus pneumoniae*, *Rev. Infect. Dis.* **3:**190–211 (1981).
188. Lee, C.-J., Fraser, B. A., Szu, S., and Lin, K.-T., Chemical structure of and immune response to polysaccharides of *Streptococcus pneumoniae*, *Rev. Infect. Dis.* **3:**323–331 (1981).
189. Avery, O. T., MacLeod, C. M., and McCarty, M., Studies on the

chemical nature of the substance inducing transformation of pneumococcal types: Induction of transformation by a desoxyribonucleic acid fraction isolated from pneumococcus type III, *J. Exp. Med.* **79:**137–158 (1944).

190. Finland, M., and Sutliff, W. D., Specific antibody response of human subjects to intracutaneous injection of pneumococcus products, *J. Exp. Med.* **55:**853–865 (1932).

12. Suggested Reading

Applebaum, P. C., Antimicrobial resistance in *Streptococcus pneumoniae*: An overview, *Clin. Infect. Dis.* **15:**77–83 (1992).

Austrian, R., and Gold, J., Pneumococcal bacteremia with especial reference to bacteremic pneumococcal pneumonia, *Ann. Intern. Med.* **60:**759–776 (1964).

Heffron, R., *Pneumonia with Special Reference to Pneumococcal Lobar Pneumonia*, Commonwealth Fund, New York, 1939; reprinted by Harvard University Press, 1979.

Mufson, M. A., Pneumococcal infections, *J. Am. Med. Assoc.* **246:**1942–1948 (1981).

Tuomanen, E. I., Austrian, R., and Masure, H. R., Pathogenesis of pneumococcal infection, *N. Engl. J. Med.* **332:**1280–1284 (1995).

White, B. (with the collaboration of Robinson, E. S., and Barnes, L. A.), *The Biology of Pneumococcus: The Bacteriological, Biochemical and Immunological Characters and Activities of Diplococcus pneumoniae*, Commonwealth Fund, New York, 1938; reprinted by Harvard University Press, 1979.

CHAPTER 29

Q Fever

Paul Fiset and Theodore E. Woodward

1. Introduction

Q fever is an acute infectious disease caused by *Coxiella burnetii*. The infection has been reported from all continents and occurs in sporadic and epidemic forms. Human infection is usually acquired by inhalation of the organisms from the tissues of infected domestic animals or their contaminated environment. In its classic form, Q fever has a sudden onset with fever, chills, malaise, weakness, and a severe headache. There is frequently a pneumonitis and, in some cases, signs of hepatic involvement. Infection with *C. burnetii*, however, is usually mild and clinically unrecognized. In contrast to the other rickettsioses, there is no rash and *Proteus* agglutinins do not develop. Chloramphenicol and the tetracyclines are highly effective except in the severe cases of Q fever endocarditis.

2. Historical Background

In 1935, Derrick[1] investigated an outbreak of a febrile illness that occurred in abattoir workers in Brisbane, Australia. The disease was characterized by a sudden onset with fever, chills, and an intractable headache. His first report included nine cases. Respiratory signs and symptoms were not prominent; one patient had signs of hepatic involvement. All attempts to isolate bacterial pathogens failed. Lacking a better name, Derrick called the disease Q (for query) fever. Although the etiology is now well known, the term Q fever has been retained.

Burnet and Freeman[2] isolated an organism from specimens received from Derrick that were passaged in mice. It was characterized as a rickettsia unrelated to any other rickettsia known at that time. Derrick[3] suggested that the organism be called *Rickettsia burnetii*. Working on the principle that rickettsiae had natural vertebrate hosts and were transmitted by specific arthropod vectors, Derrick and Smith[4] conclusively demonstrated that bandicoots and their ticks were involved in the natural life cycle of *R. burnetii*. This observation did not help in popularizing Q fever abroad. It was considered merely as another Australian oddity.

Meanwhile, halfway across the world, Davis and Cox,[5] during their studies on the ecology of Rocky Mountain spotted fever in western Montana, isolated an agent from *Dermacentor andersoni* that they characterized as a rickettsia. It was unrelated to any other known rickettsiae and, because of its filterability through Berkfeld candles, they named it *R. diaporica*.[6] Its potential as a human pathogen was unknown until several laboratory infections occurred. The clinical picture was similar to that of Q fever, and the organism isolated from these patients was identical to *R. diaporica* and *R. burnetii*.[7,8].

Emulsions of rickettsiae extracted from infected mouse spleens were specifically agglutinated by sera of patients convalescent from Q fever.[8] Parker and Davis[9] demonstrated that *R. diaporica* could be transmitted to laboratory animals by *D. andersoni*. However, neither the role of ticks in natural transmission nor the broad prevalence of infection in animals and man was known at the time. Although Q fever had been shown to exist outside Australia in the late 1930s, its importance as a cause of human disease outside the abattoirs of Brisbane or the laboratories of the National Institutes of Health was not fully appreciated. These observations were overshadowed by the onset of World War II.

Until 1944, Q fever was generally considered an

Paul Fiset • Department of Microbiology and Immunology, University of Maryland School of Medicine, Baltimore, Maryland 21201. **Theodore E. Woodward** • Department of Medicine, University of Maryland School of Medicine, Baltimore, Maryland 21201.

Australian disease. By this time, Derrick[10] had reported 176 cases occurring among abattoir and farm workers in Queensland. During the winter of 1944–1945, however, Q fever emerged as a serious infectious disease of military significance. There were several outbreaks of severe respiratory infections with systemic manifestations among American and British troops in Italy. The disease was recognized as Q fever, and approximately 1000 cases were identified.

One outbreak merits a brief description since its study led to a better understanding of the epidemiology of Q fever. The 3rd Battalion of the 362nd Infantry, US Army, was withdrawn from the front and billeted in the Apennine Mountains north of Florence, for rest and recuperation. Headquarters were established in a farmhouse; troops were settled in tents, and a barn was used as a makeshift cinema where training and recreational films were shown. Much dust was created by the movement of men in the barn. Between April 7 and 29, 1945, of 900 men stationed in the base, 269 came down with Q fever. At the 15th Medical General Laboratory in Naples, where specimens from the outbreaks were processed, 20 cases occurred among the personnel.[11]

Study of the 1944–1945 outbreak led to the following important epidemiological conclusions: (1) arthropod vectors were not involved in transmission; (2) infection seemed to be associated with the respiratory route through contaminated dust; (3) although there was a high morbidity rate, Q fever was not a lethal illness; (4) Q fever, as it occurred among the troops, was unknown in the local population; and (5) the local population showed a high incidence of *C. burnetii* antibodies.

It was learned that German troops, during 1943–1944, in Bulgaria, Greece, Italy, and the Crimea had experienced an illness called "Balkan grippe." During an outbreak of Balkan grippe, Caminopetros in Athens isolated an organism that was maintained through passages in guinea pigs. Blood samples obtained from Caminopetros by Zarafonetis were transported to Washington, unrefrigerated for several weeks. *R. burnetii* was isolated from the specimens, which established it as the etiologic agent of Balkan grippe.[12] The observation demonstrated the amazing stability of the agent. Q fever was then recognized as a disease with considerable epidemic potential.

Because the agent of Q fever differed markedly from other rickettsiae (no rash, no Weil–Felix reaction, relatively more resistant to chemical and physical agents, no requirement for arthropod vectors), Philip[13] proposed a new genus, *Coxiella*. *C. burnetii* is the only member of the genus.

3. Methodology

The intensive study of the outbreaks of Q fever among Allied troops in Europe in 1944–1945 resulted in a greater awareness on the part of the medical profession to recognize outbreaks of the disease in other areas of the world.

Investigation of the wartime outbreaks among allied troops was greatly facilitated by the observation of Cox[14] that rickettsiae of Rocky Mountain spotted fever, typhus, and Q fever groups grew profusely in the yolk sac of chick embryos. This simple methodology, unavailable to German scientists at the time, resulted in the production of excellent antigens for agglutination and complement-fixation (CF) reactions. This methodology also led to the production of an effective typhus vaccine.

Experience acquired from the investigation of the outbreaks of Q fever among Allied troops in Europe undoubtedly was instrumental in the recognition of several outbreaks that occurred in the United States shortly after World War II.

3.1. Source of Mortality Data

Q fever is rarely fatal and has a mortality of under 1%, even untreated. Furthermore, the diagnosis requires laboratory confirmation. Thus, mortality data are not useful for assessing the importance of the disease.

3.2. Source of Morbidity Data

Q fever is not a reportable disease in the United States, so incidence rates are not available. Infection is often mild or subclinical. The data on recognized cases come from investigation of epidemics, studies of high-risk exposure groups, and public health and veterinary hospital laboratories where the diagnosis is made. The laboratory information is probably the most reliable source of morbidity data and is periodically reported in national health reports and the *WHO Weekly Epidemiological Record*.

3.3. Surveys

With the use of isolation procedures and the CF reaction for serosurveys, it became quite obvious that infection of man and domestic animals with *C. burnetii* occurred frequently without recognizable clinical manifestations. It was also evident that death following Q fever was rare.

The CF test with phase II antigen (see Section 4) has

been most commonly used in serological surveys; however, since phase II antibody disappears in 2–3 years, it reflects only more recent infection (see Section 8). A skin test for detecting hypersensitivity to *C. burnetii* has been very useful in epidemiological surveys because skin positivity persists longer than detectable CF antibody.

3.4. Laboratory Diagnosis

3.4.1. Isolation Procedures. *C. burnetii* is readily isolated from the blood of patients during the febrile period; it has been recovered also from urine. Milk, birth fluids, urine, and tissues of infected domestic animals yield *C. burnetii*. The guinea pig is exquisitely sensitive to experimental infection, although large inocula are usually required to cause death. Infection can be recognized by serological conversion 21–28 days after inoculation. *C. burnetii* will also grow profusely in the yolk sac of chick embryos. With strains adapted to chick embryos, yields are of the order of 10^{11} rickettsiae/g yolk sac,[(15)] which is considerably more than that achieved with other rickettsiae.

Because of the high risk of infection, attempts at isolation of *C. burnetii* from human or animal specimens should be made only in laboratories with proper skills and facilities.

3.4.2. Serological Procedures. In the past the most commonly used serological procedure for diagnosis and epidemiological surveys was the CF test carried out with yolk-sac-grown *C. burnetii* in phase II (see Section 4). The antigen is available commercially, and the procedure was carried out by most state health department laboratories.

Phase I CF antibodies (see Section 4) rarely develop following acute Q fever; however, they reach high titers and are considered pathognomonic of chronic infections, i.e., hepatitis and endocarditis.[(16)]

Phase II CF antibodies usually become detectable by about 7 days after onset of illness, reach a peak at 21–28 days, and slowly decline thereafter. By 24–36 months after onset, CF antibody titers have usually dropped to levels that, on random serological surveys, would be considered insignificant (<1:8).[(17)]

Over the years, many agglutination tests have been devised. Burnet and Freeman[(8)] used suspensions of infected mouse spleens. Lennette *et al.*[(18)] and Ormsbee[(16)] used rickettsiae extracted from yolk sacs. These procedures require large amounts of antigen. Microscopic techniques have been developed to overcome this problem.[(19)] Although these latter procedures have been quite useful, they are time-consuming and do not lend themselves to the processing of large numbers of sera. A capillary agglutination test (CAT) was developed by Luoto[(20)] and was shown to be useful for detecting antibodies in milk. An agglutination reaction was adapted to the microtiter technique[(21)] for the detection and measurement of rickettsial antibodies. It is simple to perform, rapid, and economical of reagents, and seems to be as sensitive and specific as the CF reaction. Although it is gaining general acceptance by laboratories around the world involved in rickettsial diagnosis and research, it has certain limitations. The antigens must be highly purified and are not at present commercially available. It should be noted that phase II agglutinins appear at about the same time as phase II CF antibodies. Although phase I CF antibodies are rarely detected after acute Q fever in man, phase I agglutinins usually are detectable after the appearance of phase II antibodies.[(22)]

An indirect fluorescent-antibody (IFA) technique is available.[(23)] It has the distinct advantages that highly purified antigen is not required and that immunoglobulin classes of specific antibody can be identified. The procedure is sensitive and can detect specific antibodies many years after the acute illness (see Table 1). This procedure is now considered the method of choice and is carried out in most state health laboratories.

Although enzyme-linked immunosorbent assay (ELISA) technology has been developed, its application has been limited mainly to research and has not yet been extensively adapted to Q fever diagnosis or serosurvey.

3.4.3. Skin-Testing Procedure. The need to identify hypersensitive individuals became obvious as a consequence of field trials of experimental Q fever vaccines. Q fever vaccines developed for military use proved to be highly effective in protecting against experimental Q fever.[(24)] However, there was a high incidence of local and systemic reactions that were more likely to occur in individuals receiving repeated injections of vaccine[(25)] or in individuals previously sensitized by infection.

Lachman *et al.*[(26)] developed a skin test antigen that was initially standardized in CF units but subsequently standardized in term of dry weight of highly purified phase I antigen. It contains 0.02 μg of organisms per dose (R. A. Ormsbee, personal communication). At the Rocky Mountain Laboratory of the National Institutes of Health, Hamilton, Montana, this skin test antigen has been used on all incoming personnel since the early 1960s. Only skin-test-negative individuals receive Q fever vaccine. After the introduction of this practice, no reactions to the vaccine occurred, and only a few laboratory-acquired infections have been reported (R. A. Ormsbee, personal communication).

Table 1. Q Fever Serology[a]

Sera (FITC)	Rabbit antihuman IgG Fc specific		Goat antihuman IgM μ chain specific		Goat antihuman IgA α chain specific	
Antigen[b]	PhI	PhII	PhI	PhII	PhI	PhII
PF 7/12/71[c]	256	512	16	<16	32	<16
PF 11/11/91	256	512	16	<16	16	<16
Controls						
SI (Q fever hepatitis) 4/30/81	128	32,960	512	256	<16	16
CR (Q fever endocarditis) 3/28/88	16,384	65,936	2048	512	1024	16
SC (Q fever endocarditis) 9/25/81	32,960	32,960	256	512	512	<16
EV (Normal human serum)	<16	<16	<16	<16	<16	<16

[a]Microimmunofluorescence tests courtesy of M. G. Peacock.[15]
[b]Phase I and Phase II antigens from plaque purified *C. burnetii*.
[c]This patient had laboratory-acquired Q fever in 1954. He had his aortic valve replaced with a porcine valve in 1989. In 1991 he developed a sudden febrile illnesss with shaking chills. A diagnosis of endocarditis was established. The possibility of recurrent Q fever was considered but was not confirmed serologically.

4. Biological Characteristics of the Organism

C. burnetii possesses the general properties of the other rickettsiae; i.e., it is an obligate intracellular parasite with a cell wall similar to that of gram-negative bacteria. It is pleomorphic, ranging from coccobacillary forms measuring 0.2 μm by 0.5 μm to forms measuring 0.25 μm by 1.5 μm. Tiny spheres about 0.2 μm in diameter also exist, hence its early name, *R. diaporica*. It is considerably more resistant to hostile environmental conditions than other rickettsiae. For instance, *C. burnetii* will survive a temperature of 60°C (140°F) for 30–60 min, while other rickettsiae are inactivated following exposure to 50°C (122°F) for 15 min. *C. burnetii* will survive exposure to 0.5% formalin for 4 days, whereas the other rickettsiae are inactivated following exposure to 0.1% formalin for less than 24 hr.[27] Babudieri and Moscovici[28] demonstrated that *C. burnetii* is much more resistant to UV inactivation than the other rickettsiae. These resistant characteristics allow *C. burnetii* to survive for weeks or even months in dust, which contributes markedly to its epidemiological potential. It can be stored at freezer temperatures for years without any loss of infectivity.[29] McCaul and Williams[30] have shown the presence of sporelike structures inside *C. burnetii*. Whether these structures are similar to the small spheres that led to the early designation of *R. diaporica*[6] is not clear nor is it clear whether these structures have anything to do with the unusual resistance of *C. burnetii* to hostile environmental conditions.

C. burnetii undergoes an antigenic phase variation very similar to that of the rough–smooth variation of bacteria.[31] In nature, *C. burnetii* is found only in phase I, the smooth phase, whereas phase II is a laboratory artifact obtained after adaptation to growth in chick embryos or tissue cultures. Phase I organisms possess a cell-wall-associated surface antigen[32] that behaves as a capsule masking the phase II antigenic component.[31,33–35] The phase I antigen is antiphagocytic[36,37] and appears related to virulence.[10]

Phase II organisms lack the surface phase I antigen, are of lesser virulence than the parent strains,[38] and are readily phagocytized inn the absence of specific antisera. The phenomenon is reversible. Phase II organisms revert to phase I by passage in animals (guinea pigs, mice, hamsters).[31] Ormsbee *et al.*,[39] have demonstrated that repeatedly plaque-purified phase II organisms are completely avirulent for guinea pigs, in which they do not seem to replicate and therefore do not revert to phase I. Repeatedly plaque-purified phase I organisms, on the other hand, are fully virulent for guinea pigs and, when serially passed in developing chick embryos, revert to phase II.

Experimental infection of guinea pigs with either phase I or phase II or vaccination with killed phase I leads to a similar antibody response. Phase II CF antibodies and agglutinins appear early, within 7–10 days after inoculation, reach a peak by about 20 days, and decline thereafter. Phase I agglutinins appear about a week after phase II antibodies. Phase I CF antibodies are not detectable until 40–60 days after inoculation. Vaccination of guinea pigs or rabbits with thoroughly egg-adapted killed phase II organisms leads to a phase II antibody response only.[33,35] The significance of the phase variation in relation to the epidemiology of Q fever is not clear, except that in nature, *C. burnetii* is found only in phase I.

High titers of CF phase I antibodies rarely develop in

man following acute Q fever.[31] High phase I titers are considered pathognomonic of chronic disease, i.e., hepatitis and endocarditis.[40] Peacock *et al.*[15] have refined this observation by demonstrating that elevated levels of IgA phase I antibodies, as measured by the IFA technique, are indicative of Q fever endocarditis (see Table 1).

There seems to be only one serotype of *C. burnetii*.[22] The antigenic differences observed by early investigators can be explained, for the most part, on the basis of the phase-variation phenomenon.[34] However, Hackstadt,[41] in his studies of the lipopolysaccharide (LPS) of several strains of *C. burnetii* phase I by polyacrylamide gel electrophoresis (PAGE) and immunoblotting techniques, has demonstrated that strains isolated from cases of endocarditis have an LPS that is different from that of other strains isolated from cases of acute Q fever or Q fever hepatitis. The important implication of this observation is that only certain strains of *C. burnetii* are likely to cause endocarditis. Also, there is some suggestive evidence that a plasmid is associated with certain strains involved in endocarditis.[42]

5. Descriptive Epidemiology

Q fever is a zoonosis. There is probably no other organism pathogenic for man with a host range as broad as that of *C. burnetii*. It has been isolated from over 40 species of ticks and about a dozen species of chiggers.[43,44] It has been isolated from a large variety of animals including wild and domestic mammals and birds.[43,44]

5.1. Prevalence and Incidence

Since Q fever is not on the list of nationally notifiable diseases in the United States and in many other countries, the information concerning its epidemiology has been acquired either from investigations of defined outbreaks, from serosurveys in human and animal populations conducted in various countries, or from public health laboratory data.

In the United States, Q fever is not a disease reportable to the Centers for Disease Control (CDC). It is, however, reportable in some states.[45] Between 1948 and 1977, 1169 cases have been optionally reported to the CDC from 26 states. Of these cases, 67% (785) were reported from California. Between 1948 and 1977, there has been an average of 39 cases per year reported to the CDC, with peaks of 105 in 1953 and 106 in 1954.[45] Between 1978 and 1986, there were 228 cases reported to CDC.

In the United Kingdom, the public health laboratories reported between 48 and 78 cases annually between 1967 and 1974, averaging about 59 cases a year. In 1976 and 1977, there were 215 reported cases.[46] Although we do not have more recent data for the incidence in the United Kingdom, there is no reason to believe that the situation has changed significantly in recent years.

The prevalence of infection has been determined by serological surveys. A serological survey carried out on 12,000 human sera collected in Los Angeles and vicinity[47] yielded the following information: (1) A first group (5,000 individuals) were selected as representatives of the general population of Los Angeles without any particular association with livestock. In this population, 1.4% had phase II CFG antibodies at significant titers. Considering the fairly rapid decay of CF antibodies after Q fever, 2–3 years,[17] these results would imply that within the past few years there had been 50,000 cases of Q fever in the Los Angeles area. (2) In groups selected because of their association with livestock, the incidence varied depending on the closeness of the association. In packing plants where few or no dairy cows were slaughtered, the incidence was 4.0%. In plants where dairy cows or young calves were slaughtered, it was 11%. Among dairy workers, it was 23%. (3) Of raw-milk drinkers, 12% were seropositive, as opposed to 1.2% of non-raw-milk drinkers.

The incidence and prevalence of infection in animals are also relevant to human exposure. Important observations that led to a better understanding of the epidemiology of Q fever were that dairy cows frequently have a recrudescent infection during pregnancy, that *C. burnetii* can be recovered from the placentas and birth fluids in extremely large numbers [10^8 guinea pig infective doses ($GPID_{50}$)/g], and that the organism is excreted in the milk over a long period.[48] Such massive infections seemed to have no deleterious effect on gestation, parturition, or the newborn. The excretion of such massive numbers of organisms into the environment and the unusual resistance of *C. burnetii* to desiccation indicated that effective transmission to man and domestic animals could occur by inhalation. A serosurvey of the dairy cattle in Los Angeles and vicinity revealed that 10% were constantly infected. When uninfected cows were introduced into the enzootic area, 40% became infected within 6 months.[49] Several serosurveys were carried out on dairy cattle in Los Angeles County over the subsequent 25 years. By 1960, 62% were seropositive,[50] and by 1967, 98% were positive.[51] By 1973, 92% were positive and 62% were shedding *C. burnetii* in their milk.[52] Gross *et al.*[51] suggest that the insignificant increase of prevalence of evidence of Q fever infection in the human population from 1.3% in 1949 to 2.3% in 1967, despite an increase of prevalence in cattle from 10 to 90%, is probably due to (1) a requirement for a higher temperature for pasteurization of milk; (2) a drop in the consumption of raw milk from 20,196 gallons per day to 4,400 while the population doubled in the same time; and (3) a 55% decrease in the number of dairy farms in the area (from 595 to 268).

The involvement of domestic animals as a source of infection for man has been confirmed by numerous other serosurveys carried out in various parts of the world in the last four decades. There are, however, some different epidemiological patterns conditioned by different cultural factors and lifestyles. For example, in a serosurvey carried out in Egypt in the 1950s, Taylor *et al.*[53] demonstrated that 18.3% of the sera were positive. However, there was great variation from one area to another. For instance, in the rural Sinbis Sanitary District, about 30 km north of Cairo, the incidence was 37.4%, with the highest incidence (47%) and highest titers found in children under the age of 2 years. Thereafter, there was a decline to about 25% in the age group of 5–9 years, with a leveling off at this figure in the adult population. The evidence of infection was slightly higher in females than in males. Approximately 60% of sheep and goats had serological evidence of infection. The high incidence of infection in this rural population, particularly in the young, could be explained by the intimate and constant contact of people with their livestock. It was customary for a family and its domestic animals to be housed under the same roof. Despite evidence for widespread infection with *C. burnetii*, Q fever, in its classic form, had never been recognized in the native Egyptian population. However, of 55 Americans residing in Egypt and observed for approximately 2 years, 11 had a serological conversion, of whom 7 had clinically recognized Q fever.

There have been several other epidemiological surveys carried out in other parts of the world. They all have provided strong evidence for incriminating domestic animals as a source of human infection, directly (by contact with infected animal tissues or excretions) or indirectly (by contaminated dust). They also clearly indicate that human infection is usually mild and clinically unrecognized.

5.2. Epidemic Behavior and Contagiousness

The first major outbreak recognized in the United States occurred in Amarillo, Texas, in 1946. There were 55 cases with 2 deaths among 136 employees of three packing houses.[54] In the same year, another outbreak occurred in a Chicago packing house, where 33 of 81 employees acquired Q fever.[55]

In 1947, several cases of Q fever were identified among patients in Artesia, a dairy community located in Los Angeles County.[56] The clinical diagnosis was "viral pneumonia." The observation that Q fever seemed to be endemic in California led to extensive investigations conducted by Huebner and his co-workers[49] in southern California and by Lenette and his co-workers[57] in northern California. Most of the current knowledge of the epidemiology of Q fever and the ecology of *C. burnetii* stems from these studies.

In northern California in 1947–1948, there were 350 confirmed cases of Q fever.[58] The epidemiological investigation that followed these observations demonstrated that sheep and goats were the main source of infection.[59] Serosurveys of sheep, goats, and cattle indicated that in areas where Q fever occurred, a high percentage of animals were seropositive.[48] It was also shown that sheep, whether naturally or experimentally infected, undergo a recrudescence during pregnancy and shed enormous amounts of *C. burnetii* in their birth fluids, placentas (10^8 guinea pig infective doses/g), milk, feces, and urine.[60,61] Although most animals shed *C. burnetii* only following their first lambing, about one third shed the organisms twice, and a few shed them during three consecutive parturitions.[47]

DeLay *et al.*[62] and Lennette and Welsh[63] demonstrated that *C. burnetii* could be isolated from the air of premises harboring infected animals.

The California studies clearly showed that *C. burnetii* infection of domestic animals is not a veterinary problem. Infection does not lead to loss of weight, does not effect gestation or parturition, and has no deleterious effect on the young. Infection is clinically inapparent. The studies also showed that most human infections are either completely asymptomatic or so mild that the diagnosis of Q fever is seldom considered. Classic Q fever, as described by Derrick, seems to be a rare event, whereas silent, inapparent infection seems to be common.

Over the years there have been several outbreaks of Q fever in different parts of the world. All of them have been associated with direct or indirect contact with domestic animals. Suffice it to consider, as an example, an outbreak that occurred in Switzerland in 1983. In the Valais (at val de Bagnes, population 4,642), between mid-October and the first week of December, there were 191 symptomatic and 224 asyptomatic cases of serologically confirmed Q fever. The outbreak began suddenly, 3 weeks after herds of sheep, returning from alpine pasture, were led through the village.[55] Several similar outbreaks have occurred in Slovakia over the years as herds of sheep or cattle are led through small villages.[64]

5.3. Geographic Distribution

Q fever has a worldwide distribution and has been reported from all continents.[17,65,66]

5.4. Temporal Distribution

Most of the infections in California occurred in adult males (ratio of 10:1), suggesting occupational exposure.[56] In northern California, most of the cases occurred in March, April, and May, coinciding with the lambing season, when contamination of the environment was at its maximum.[67] In southern California, where dairy cattle produce milk the year around and where calving is not seasonal, cases occurred through the year.[47] In the United Kingdom, they tended to occur in the summer months.[54]

5.5. Age

The age of infection and disease is related to the opportunity for exposure to infected animals and their products. In Egypt, serosurveys have shown infection without classic disease to occur in some districts in persons under the age of 2.[53] Clinical cases are most common in adults. In the United Kingdom, the age distribution of 215 clinical cases was as follows: 0–10 years, 4.1%; 11–20 years, 14.0%; 21–40 years, 44.6%; and above 40 years it was 37.3%.[46]

5.6. Sex

Males are more commonly involved than females. In the United Kingdom, 72% of 215 cases were males and 28% females. The higher rate in males is related to greater exposure.

5.7. Race

There is no known difference by race except as related to exposure in different geographic areas or by occupation.

5.8. Occupation

Persons whose occupations directly or indirectly involve them in exposure to infected sheep, goats, cattle, and other animals, to the contaminated products of conception, or to airborne particles from such contaminated sources are at highest risk. This includes sheep and goat herders, dairy farmers, dairy and slaughterhouse workers, and workers in plants that process wool and hair. Laboratory personnel working with the agent are also at risk, especially via the airborne route.[69–72] Sheep, particularly pregnant ewes, used for medical research have been responsible for several outbreaks of Q fever in recent years.[71–74]

5.9. Occurrence in Different Settings

Enclosed environments containing infected animals or their products of parturition have been the source of many outbreaks. This includes packing houses,[55] wool and hair processing plants,[75] and soldiers' billets in many different areas. Any time susceptible individuals are exposed to infected animals, outbreaks of Q fever are likely to occur.

In recent years there have been several outbreaks of Q fever associated with sheep used for perinatal research. The scenarios of these outbreaks were remarkably similar. Pregnant ewes were held on a farm or some similar facility at some reasonable distance from the research laboratory to which they were transported at an appropriate time for experimental manipulations. The animals were carted to their destination, in a hospital environment, through elevators and corridors, passing by various secretarial and laboratory personnel not involved with sheep. A major outbreak occurred in 1979 at the University of California at San Franscisco where 600 sheep were used annually for perinatal research. Between March and June 1979, 88 cases of clinical and subclinical Q fever were identified[71,72] Another outbreak occurred at the University of Colorado School of Medicine, where 65 clinical and 72 subclinical cases were identified between April and October 1980.[69] An outbreak occurred at The Hospital for Sick Children in Toronto where, between July and October 1982, 12 clinical and 47 subclinical cases of Q fever were diagnosed.[71] Another laboratory outbreak of Q fever acquired from sheep occurred at the University of Bristol, England, where, in April and May 1981, there were 28 clinical and subclinical cases.[74]

5.10. Socioeconomic Factors

No relationship other than through occupation has been noted.

5.11. Other Factors

The presence of infected cattle, goats, sheep, and other animals and that of the appropriate vector for spread among the animals is the most important determinant as to whether human infection will occur. This is discussed in detail in Section 6.

6. Mechanisms and Routes of Transmission

Human infection with *C. burnetii* is usually acquired by inhalation. Whether milk-associated infection is acquired by ingestion or by aerosolization in the process of drinking is still not known. Although there is a possibility that infection may be acquired from ticks or tick feces, this is unlikely to be a frequent occurrence. The overwhelming evidence incriminates domestic animals as a primary source of human infection. The massive contamination of the environment at time of parturition and the unusual resistance of *C. burnetii* to desiccation are important factors in transmission to other domestic animals and to man. Derrick[(10)] has calculated that an infected bovine placenta weighing 4 kg, powdered and dispersed on the ground, would provide enough coxiellae to dust each square millimeter of a 100-acre field with one organism, which is sufficient to infect one guinea pig. It is easy to understand that during dry periods wind can blow contaminated dust, thus exposing to infection individuals living in proximity to infected animals. Outbreaks can also occur at a considerable distance from the original focus through contaminated straw used as packing material, wool, hides, clothing, and other materials.[(43)]

It should be stated that the infective dose of *C. burnetii* for man is less than ten organisms.[(75)]

Person-to-person transmission, if it occurs, seems to be a rare event. There have been outbreaks associated with the performance of autopsies.[(76)]

The role of arthropods in the overall maintenance of *C. burnetii* in nature is not fully understood; their role may be significant. In some species of ticks, transovarial and transstadial transmission have been demonstrated. In some species of ticks, *C. burnetii* has been shown to persist for as long as 1000 days[(77)] and propagate in tick tissues to extraordinary numbers. One gram of feces from infected *Rhipicephalus sanguineus* (brown dog tick), for example, may contain as many as 10^8 $GPID_{50}$.[(43)] Although several ecological systems have been described in various parts of the world whereby *C. burnetii* seems to be efficiently maintained in wild animals and their ectoparasites, they seem to have no significant bearing on human infection.

Domestic animals are far more important as a source of human infection. Derrick *et al.*[(78)] suspected cattle as a source of human infection, but assumed that ticks were the vectors of transmission. Caminopetros[(79)] demonstrated that sheep and goats in Greece were infected and concluded that they were the probable source of human infection. Huebner *et al.*[(49)] demonstrated a close association between infected cattle and human cases in southern California. Lennette *et al.*[(59)] demonstrated a similar association with infected sheep and goats in northern California. Several studies carried out in other parts of the world since World War II have confirmed the California findings.[(52,54,80–82)]

It became evident from the California studies and others that infection of domestic animals was benign, clinically unrecognizable, did not lead to unthriftiness, and did not interfere with good husbandry.

A study of 300 cases of Q fever in Los Angeles and vicinity investigated in 1947–1948[(83)] indicated that human infections were related to association with cattle. More than half the patients either worked in the dairy or livestock industries, resided close to dairies or livestock yards, or consumed raw milk. Huebner *et al.*[(84)] recovered *C. burnetii* from 40 of 50 milk samples from serologically positive cows obtained from five dairies in the Los Angeles area. Infected milk may contain as many as 10^5 $GPID_{50}/g$.[(85)]

7. Pathogenesis and Immunity

The mechanisms by which *C. burnetii* cause infection and illness are not known. It is assumed that the surface phase I antigen is a virulence factor.[(35)] It is antiphagocytic,[(36,37)] and organisms that lack this component (phase II organisms) are considerably less virulent than the parent phase I.[(38,86)] Ormsbee *et al.*[(39)] demonstrated that a pure phase II strain obtained by repeated plaque purification was unable to infect guinea pigs.

Immunity following infection, whether overt or inapparent, seems to be solid and long-lasting. However, it seems to be a nonsterile immunity maintained by persistence of the organism in the host. This immunity seems to be able to prevent disease but not recrudescence of infection. Luoto and Huebner[(48)] have demonstrated such recrudescence in cattle, and Abinanti *et al.*[(60,61)] reported recrudescence during successive gestations in sheep. Recrudescence also occurs in women. Babudieri[(28,87)] reported that a woman who had contracted Q fever in the laboratory gave birth, 6 months later, to a healthy child. *C. burnetii* was isolated from her placenta and, 1 month after delivery, from her milk. Syrucek *et al.*[(88)] isolated *C. burnetii* from the placentas of three women and from the curettage material of another in whom pregnancy was interrupted in the 3rd month. All four women had had Q fever 2–3 years previously. None of these women, at time of recrudescence, had any clinical manifestation of Q fever. The mechanisms, probably immune, that allow massive infections of the host and yet protect the host from disease are unknown.

8. Patterns of Host Response

As noted several times previously, most infections of man with *C. burnetii* are probably mild and not recognized as Q fever. The situation encountered in Egypt by Taylor *et al.*[53] indicated that there was widespread infection in children without evidence of Q fever. It is likely that in this setting, *C. burnetii* was responsible for a mild febrile illness clinically indistinguishable from that caused by a multitude of other microbial agents.

The patterns of host response may thus be grouped into (1) inapparent infection, (2) acute febrile illness, (3) pneumonic forms, and (4) forms with extrapulmonary localization (hepatitis and endocarditis).[43]

8.1. Clinical Features

Q fever in its classic form as first described by Derrick[1] and subsequently by others[89–91] does not pose a difficult diagnostic problem, particularly if the appropriate epidemiological background is present.

The most accurate data on the incubation period were obtained by Tigertt and his colleagues[75] from experimental aerosol infection of young, healthy adult volunteers. The duration of the incubation period was clearly dose-dependent and varied from 18 days to 9 days with aerosol challenges ranging from 10 $GPID_{50}$ to 1.5×10^5. Onset of disease is usually sudden, with headache, chilly sensations, fever, and malaise, followed by myalgia and anorexia. For several days, the temperature ranges from 101 to 104°F; the entire course rarely exceeds 2 weeks and usually lasts from 3 to 6 days. There may be wide fluctuations in the fever. During the early stages, respiratory symptoms are not conspicuous. A dry cough and chest pain occur after about 5 days, when rales are usually audible. The cough usually produces a small amount of mucoid sputum that is occasionally streaked with blood. *C. burnetii* has been recovered from the sputum, but not visualized directly. Although pneumonitis may be prominent in some cases, it must be emphasized that Q fever is a systemic disease, and serious illness may occur in the absence of pneumonitis.

Respiratory symptoms and physical findings produced by the lung lesion of Q fever are often minimal. During the peak of illness, fine crepitant rales may be heard after deep inspiration. Dullness to percussion is occasionally elicited and may indicate consolidation or the presence of pleural effusion. *C. burnetii* has been isolated from pleural fluid. Other clinical signs are relative bradycardia, hepatomegaly, and splenomegaly.

The roentgen lung findings are often indistinguishable from those of viral atypical pneumonia and may at times closely resemble those of pneumococcal pneumonia. Infiltration is usually present by the 3rd to 4th day of disease, first as patchy areas of consolidation involving a portion of one lobe, giving a homogeneous ground-glass appearance. The lesions tend to occur in the peribronchial and alveolar areas, rather than the hilar regions, and often in the lower lobes. These manifestations persist beyond the febrile period and may appear in patients who are unaware of pulmonary involvement. Segmental or lobar infiltrations occur more commonly in Q fever than in many atypical pneumonias. The sputum of patients with pneumococcal lobar pneumonia differs significantly from that of Q fever. In Q fever, there are small amounts of mucoid sputum occasionally streaked with blood and a few mononuclear cells; frequently in pneumococcal pneumonia, there is rusty mucoid sputum with leukocytes, erythrocytes, and identifiable *Streptococcus pneumoniae*.

The incidence of pneumonia in Q fever varies considerably from one series of reports to another, Powell[91] recognized only 3 in a series of 72 cases of Q fever reported from Brisbane. Clark *et al.*[89] observed it in about one third of 180 cases; Marmion *et al.*,[92] in 25 of 30 cases (83%); and in a recent report from Britain,[46] it was observed in 111 of 215 cases (52%).

Complications are rare, and coincident with defervescence, the appetite begins to return. Convalescence progresses slowly for several weeks, during which time the principal disability is weakness. It is not uncommon for patients to lose 15–20 pounds during the active stages of disease. The disease may be protracted in approximately 29% of cases, with fever persisting for longer than 4 weeks, particularly in elderly patients. Occasionally, relapse occurs, especially in patients treated with antibiotics during the first days of disease.

Hepatitis, with the development of clinically detectable icterus, occurs in approximately one third of patients with the protracted form. This form of Q fever is characterized by fever, malaise, absence of headache or respiratory signs, and hepatomegaly with right upper quadrant pain. Liver biopsy specimens show diffuse granulomatous changes with multinucleated giants cells and scattered infiltrations of polymorphonuclear leukocytes, lymphocytes, and macrophages. *C. burnetii* may be demonstrated in such specimens with the fluorescent antibody technique. Therefore, Q fever must be in the differential diagnosis of liver granulomas such as tuberculosis, sarcoidosis, histoplasmosis, brucellosis, tularemia, syphilis, and others.[93]

Endocarditis has also been reported, and *C. burnetii* has been identified by smear and isolation from vegetations on the heart valves obtained at operation or autopsy. The aortic valve is most commonly involved, often with large vegetations. It is important, therefore, to suspect the possibility of Q fever in cases of apparent subacute bacterial endocarditis with persistently negative blood cultures. Because antibiotics seem unable to penetrate the valvular vegetations, they are ineffective in treating Q fever endocarditis. Surgical valve replacement is required.

As mentioned earlier, high phase I titers are indicative of chronic Q fever, hepatitis, or endocarditis. High IgA phase I titers, however, are characteristic of endocarditis (see Table 1).[15,16,94,95]

8.2. Diagnosis

The clinical diagnosis of Q fever, in its classic form, is easy. The sudden onset of chills, severe headache, fever, and signs of pneumonitis are fairly characteristic. Q fever should be considered in the differential diagnosis of atypical pneumonias. If, along with signs and symptoms suggestive of the disease, there is a history of association with domestic animals, a tentative diagnosis can be made. The diagnosis should be confirmed by demonstrating a rise in specific antibodies by CF, microagglutination, or indirect immunofluorescence tests. However, since most infections with *C. burnetii* do not manifest themselves as Q fever, the diagnosis is rarely made. To get an estimate of the incidence of *C. burnetii* infection, it might be necessary to carry out specific serological tests on all cases of unidentified febrile illnesses.

C. burnetii infection should be considered in the differential diagnosis of granulomatous hepatitis and in the differential diagnosis of subacute endocarditis when repeated blood cultures are negative. In these instances, there is usually a high phase I titer (see Section 8.1). Attempts at isolation of the organism should be made only in laboratories that have the facilities and expertise to do so.

9. Control and Prevention

Livestock are the main source of human infection. In some parts of the world, most of the livestock is infected and shedding *C. burnetii* in massive quantities in milk, birth fluids, urine, and feces. These infections, however, are of little importance to the livestock industry, since they do not result in significant economic loss. Dairy cattle do not have reduced milk production. Abortion does not seem to be a serious problem, although abortions have been reported in goats and cattle. In the case of meat animals, there is no unthriftiness or food wastage.[96] There certainly is no economic justification for massive slaughtering to control infection. There is good evidence that vaccination of cattle with phase I vaccine will prevent infection.[97–99] Whether the livestock industry can be convinced that this should be done is another question.

Prevention of human infection can be achieved, to a certain degree, by pasteurization of milk. Standard pasteurization at 143°F for 30 min is not adequate, whereas, remarkably, pasteurization at 145°F for 30 min or flash pasteurization at 161°F for 15 seconds is sufficient.[100]

Effective vaccines for human use have been developed over the years.[12,101] Ormsbee *et al.*[102] demonstrated that a phase I vaccine was approximately 300 times more effective than the corresponding phase II vaccine. Such a vaccine has been used routinely at the Rocky Mountain Laboratory since the early 1960s with excellent results. To avoid side effects, it is important that the vaccine be administered only to individuals who are skin-test-negative.[103] Such a vaccine would be of benefit to laboratory workers, slaughterhouse and dairy workers, and others at risk, though one is not yet commercially available in the United States. A phase I vaccine (Q-Vax-CSL) has been used with great success by Marmion and co-workers among slaughterhouse workers in Australia since 1985.[103]

Laboratory personnel working with *C. burnetii* are aware of the risks and usually take appropriate precautions to avoid infection. The situation is different, however, with researchers who unknowingly carry out experimental surgery on *C. burnetii*-infected sheep. There is a potential for serious problems if one considers that, in the United States alone, in fiscal year 1987–1988, the National Institutes of Health funded 328 projects in which sheep are used for research. Investigators working with sheep should abide by the recommendations set forth by the CDC.[104]

10. Unresolved Problems

As noted in Section 6, Q fever can be induced in man by aerosol administration of 1–10 organisms,[75] and the infective dose for guinea pigs is about one organism.[87]

Given the efficacy with which experimental disease can be induced, how can one explain the high incidence of inapparent, subclinical infection in endemic areas? It was suggested that milk-borne, opsonized *C. burnetii* might lead to a passive–active immunization without overt disease. There is no experimental proof to support this concept, and even if there were, it would account for only a small number of infections.

Phase I organisms are the only forms found in nature, their phase II counterparts having little survival value outside chick embryos and tissue cultures. The phase I surface antigen seems to endow *C. burnetii* with antiphagocytic activity and is therefore assumed to be a virulence factor. However, Ormsbee *et al.*[102] have demonstrated that a pure phase II immune response can protect guinea pigs from a phase I challenge. The biological significance of phase variation and its involvement in pathogenesis and immunity are unknown. It was suggested that the phase I surface antigen may behave as an adjuvant for the phase II antigenic component.[35]

The most baffling problem is the recrudescence of infection during gestation. What are the mechanisms that allow such massive infections to occur without any evidence of pathological changes? What modulates the immune response in such a way that immunopathologic changes do not develop? How can the mammary gland excrete 10^5 $GPID_{50}$/g milk in the presence of high levels of antibody for long periods without the stimulation of an inflammatory reaction? What inhibits the host from reacting violently to the presence of 10^8 infective organisms/g of placenta?

Although there is evidence that human fetal infections occur,[105] there is, at present, no evidence that such infections lead to neonatal or early childhood pathology. By what mechanism is the fetus protected from damage?

11. References

1. Derrick, E. H., Q fever: A new fever entity. Clinical features, diagnosis and laboratory investigation, *Med. J. Aust.* **2:**281–299 (1937).
2. Burnet, F. M., and Freeman, M., Experimental studies on the virus of Q fever, *Med. J. Aust.* **2:**299–305 (1937).
3. Derrick, E. H., *Rickettsia burneti*. The cause of Q fever, *Med. J. Aust.* **1:**14 (1939).
4. Derrick, E. H., and Smith, D. J. W., Studies on the epidemiology of Q fever, 2. The isolation of three strains of *Rickettsia burneti* from the bandicoot, *Isoodon torosus*, *Aust. J. Exp. Biol. Med. Sci.* **18:**99–102 (1940).
5. Davis, G. E., and Cox, H. R., A filter passing infectious agent isolated from ticks. I. Isolation from *Dermacentor andersoni*. Reactions in animals and filtration experiments, *Public Health Rep.* **53:**2259–2267 (1938).
6. Cox, H. R., Studies of a filter passing infectious agent isolated from ticks. V. Further attempts to cultivate it in cell-free media: Suggested classification, *Public Health Rep.* **54:**1822–1827 (1939).
7. Bengtson, I. A., Immunological relationship between the rickettsiae of Australian and American Q fever, *Public Health Rep.* **56:**272–281 (1941).
8. Burnet, F. M., and Freeman, M., A comparative study of rickettsial strains from an infection of ticks in Montana (USA) and from Q fever, *Med. J. Aust.* **1:**887–891 (1939).
9. Parker, P. R., and Davis, G. E., A filter passing agent isolated from ticks. II. Tranmission by *Dermacentor andersoni*, *Public Health Rep.* **53:**2267–2270 (1938).
10. Derrick, E. H., The epidemiology of Q fever. A review, *Med. J. Aust.* **1:**245–253 (1953).
11. Robbins, F. C., Gauld, R. L., and Warner, F. B., Q fever in the Mediterranean area: Report of its occurrence in Allied troops. II. Epidemiology, *Am. J. Hyg.* **44:**23–50 (1946).
12. Commission on Acute Respiratory Diseases, Identification and characteristics of the Balkan grippe strain of *Rickettsia burneti*, *Am. J. Hyg.* **44:**110–122 (1946).
13. Philip, C. B., Comments on the name of the Q fever organism, *Public Health Rep.* **63:**58 (1948).
14. Cox, H. R., Cultivation of rickettsiae of the Rocky Mountain spotted fever, typhus and Q fever groups in embryonic tissues of developing chicks, *Science* **94:**399–403 (1941).
15. Peacock, M. G., Williams, J. C., and Faulkner, R. S., Serological evaluation of Q fever in humans: Enhanced phase I titers of immunoglobulins G and A are diagnostic for Q fever endocarditis, *Infect. Immun.* **41:**1089–1098 (1983).
16. Ormsbee, R. A., An agglutination resuspension test for Q fever antibodies, *J. Immunol.* **92:**159–166 (1964).
17. Murphy, A. M., and Field, P. R., The persistence of complement fixing antibodies to Q fever (*Coxiella burnetii*) after infection, *Med. J. Aust.* **1:**1148–1150 (1970).
18. Lennette, E. H., Clark, W. H., Jensen, F. W., *et al.*, Q fever studies. XV. Development and persistence in man of complement fixing and agglutinating antibodies to *Coxiella burnetii*, *J. Immunol.* **68:**591–598 (1952).
19. Babudieri, B., and Secchi, P., La reazione di agglutinazione nella serodiagnosi dell'infezione da *Coxiella burneti*, *Rend. Ist. Super. Sanita.* **15:**584–608 (1952).
20. Luoto, L., A capillary agglutination test for bovine Q fever, *J. Immunol.* **71:**226–231 (1953).
21. Fiset, P., Ormsbee, R. A., Silberman, R., *et al.*, A microagglutination technique for detection and measurement of rickettsial antibodies, *Acta Virol.* **13:**60–66 (1969).
22. Fiset, P., Wike, D. A., Pickens, E. G., *et al.*, An antigenic comparison of strains of *Coxiella burnetii*, *Acta Virol.* **15:**161–166 (1971).
23. Philip, R. M., Casper, E. A., Ormsbee, R. A., *et al.*, Microimmunofluorescence test for the serological study of Rocky Mountain spotted fever and typhus, *J. Clin. Microbiol.* **3:**51–61 (1976).
24. Benenson, A. S., Q fever vaccine: Efficacy and present status, Symposium on Q fever, *Med. Sci. Publ. Walter Reed Army Inst. Res.* **6:**47–60 (1959).
25. Bell, J. F., Lackman, D. B., Meis, A., *et al.*, Recurrent reaction at site of Q fever vaccination in a sensitized person, *Mil. Med.* **129:**591–595 (1964).

26. Lackman, D. B., Bell, E. J., Bell, J. F., *et al.*, Intradermal sensitivity testing in man with a purified vaccine for Q fever, *Am. J. Public Health* **52:**87–93 (1962).
27. Ramsom, S. E., and Huebner, R. J., Studies on the resistance of *Coxiella burnetii* to physical and chemical agents, *Am. J. Hyg.* **53:** 110–119 (1951).
28. Babudieri, B., and Moscovici, C., Ricerchi sul corportamento di *Coxiella burneti* di fronte ad alguni agenti fisici e chimici, *Rend. Ist. Super. Sanita.* **13:**739–748 (1950).
29. Ormsbee, R. A., Q Fever Rickettsia, in: *Viral and Rickettsial Diseases of Man* (F. L. Horsfall and T. Tamm, eds.), pp. 1144–1160, Lippincott, Philadelphia, 1965.
30. McCaul, T. F., and Williams, J. C., Developmental cycle of *Coxiella burnetii*: Structure and morphogenesis of vegetative and sporogenic differentiations, *J. Bacteriol.* **147:**1063–1076 (1981).
31. Stoker, M. G. P., and Fiset, P., Phase variation of the Nine Mile and other strains of *Rickettsia burneti*, *Can. J. Microbiol.* **2:**310–321 (1956).
32. Jerrells, T. R., Hinrichs, D. J., and Mallavia, L. P., Cell envelope analysis of *Coxiella burnetii*, phase I and phase II, *Can. J. Microbiol.* **20:**1465–1470 (1974).
33. Fiset, P., Phase variation of *Rickettsia* (*Coxiella*) *burneti*: Study of the antibody response in guinea pigs and rabbits, *Can. J. Microbiol.* **3:**435–445 (1957).
34. Fiset, P., Serological diagnosis, strain identification and antigenic variation. Symposium on Q fever, *Med. Sci. Publ. Walter Reed Army Inst. Res.* **6:**28–37 (1959).
35. Fiset, P., and Ormsbee, R. A., The antibody response to antigens of *Coxiella burnetii*, *Zentralbl. Bakteriol. Parasitenkd. Infektionskr. Hyg. Abt. 1 Orig.* **206:**321–328 (1968).
36. Brezina, R., and Kazar, J., Phagocytosis of *Coxiella burnetii* and the phase phenomenon, *Acta Virol.* **7:**476 (1963).
37. Wisseman, C. L., Jr., Fiset, P., and Ormsbee, R. A., Interaction of rickettsiae and phagocytic host cells. V. Phagocytic and opsonic interactions of phase I and phase II *Coxiella burnetii* with normal and immune human leukocytes and antibodies, *J. Immunol.* **99:** 669–674 (1968).
38. Pinto, M. R., Alguns aspects da biologia da *Coxiella burnetii*, Proceeding of the Seventh International Congresses of Tropical medicine and Malaria, Vol. III, pp. 261–262, Rio de Janeiro, September 1–11, 1963.
39. Ormsbee, R. A., Peacock, M. G., and Tallent, G., Dynamics of phase I to phase II antigenic shift in populations of *Coxiella burnetii*, in: *Proceedings of IIIrd International Symposium on Rickettsiae and Rickettsial Diseases* (J. Kazar, ed.), pp. 146–149, Publishing House of the Slovak Academy of Sciences, 1985.
40. Marmion, B. P., Higgins, F. E., Bridges, J. B., *et al.*, A case of acute rickettsial endocarditis with a survey of cardiac patients with this infection, *Br. Med. J.* **11:**1264–1268 (1960).
41. Hackstadt, T., Antigenic variation in the phase I lipopolysaccharide of *Coxiella burnetii* isolates, *Infect. Immun.* **52:**337–340 (1986).
42. Samuel, J. E., Frazier, M. E., and Mallavia, L. P., Correlation of plasmid type and disease caused by *Coxiella burnetii*, *Infect. Immun.* **49:**775–779 (1985).
43. Babudieri, B., Q fever: A zoonosis, *Adv. Vet. Sci.* **5:**81–181 (1959).
44. Cracea, E., and Popovici, V., *Fevra Q la Om si Animale*, Editura Ceres, Bucharest, 1975.
45. D'Angelo, J. L., Baker, E. F., and Schlosser, W., Q fever in the United States, 1948–1977, *J. Infect. Dis.* **139:**613–615 (1979).
46. World Health Organization, Q fever, *Week. Epidemiol. Rec.* **54:**45–46 (1979).
47. Bell, J. A., Beck, M. D., and Huebner, E. J., Epidemiologic studies of Q fever in southern California, *J. Am. Med. Assoc.* **142:**868–872 (1950).
48. Luoto, L., and Huebner, R. J., Q fever studies in southern California. IX. Isolation of Q fever organisms from parturient placentas of naturally infected dairy cows, *Public Health Rep.* **65:**541–544 (1950).
49. Huebner, R. J., and Bell, J. A., Q fever studies in southern California: Summary of current results and a discussion of possible control measures, *J. Am. Med. Assoc.* **145:**301–305 (1951).
50. Luoto, L., Report on the nationwide occurrence of Q fever infections in cattle, *Public Health Rep.* **75:**135–140 (1960).
51. Gross, P. A., Portnoy, B., Salvatore, M. A., *et al.*, Q fever in Los Angeles County: Serological survey of human and bovine populations, *Calif. Med.* **114:**12–15 (1971).
52. Biberstein, E. L., Bushnell, R., Crenshaw, G., *et al.*, Survey of Q fever (*Coxiella burnetii*) in California dairy cows, *Am. J. Vet. Res.* **35:**1577–1582 (1974).
53. Taylor, R. M., Kingston, J. R., and Rizk, F., Serological (complement-fixation) surveys for Q fever in Egypt and the Sudan, with special reference to its epidemiology in areas of high endemicity, *Arch. Inst. Pasteur Tunis* **36:**529–556 (1959).
54. World Health Organization, Q fever, *Week. Epidemiol. Rec.* **60:** 121–122 (1985).
55. Shepard, C. C., An outbreak of Q fever in a Chicago packing house, *Am. J. Hyg.* **46:**185–192 (1947).
56. Young, F. W., Q fever in Artesia, California, *Calif. Med.* **6:**10–16 (1948).
57. Lennette, E. H., and Clark, W. H., Observations on the epidemiology of Q fever in northern California, *J. Am. Med. Assoc.* **145:** 306–309 (1951).
58. Clark, W. H., Lennette, E. H., and Romer, M. S., Q fever studies in California. XI. An epidemiologic summary of 350 cases occurring in northern California in 1948–1949, *Am. J. Hyg.* **54:**319–330 (1951).
59. Lennette, E. H., Clark, W. H., and Dean, B. H., Sheep and goats in the epidemiology of Q fever in northern California, *Am. J. Trop. Med.* **29:**527–541 (1949).
60. Abinanti, F. R., Lennette, E. H., Winn, J. F., *et al.*, Q fever studies. XVIII. Presence of *Coxiella burnetii* in the birth fluids of naturally infected sheep, *Am. J. Hyg.* **58:**385–388 (1953).
61. Abinanti, F. R., Welsh, H. H., Lennette, E. H., *et al.*, Q fever studies. XVI. Some aspects of the experimental infection induced in sheep by the intratracheal route of inoculation, *Am. J. Hyg.* **57:** 170–184 (1953).
62. DeLay, P. D., Lennette, E. H., and DeOme, K. B., Q fever in Calfornia. II. Recovery of *Coxiella burnetii* from naturally infected airborne dust, *J. Immunol.* **65:**211–220 (1950).
63. Lennette, E. H., and Welsh, H. H., Q fever in California. X. Recovery of *Coxiella burnetii* from the air of premises harboring infected goats, *Am. J. Hyg.* **54:**44–49 (1951).
64. Palanova, A., Rehacek, J., and Brezina, R., Epidemiology of Q fever in Slovakia, in: *Rickettsiae and Rickettsial diseases*, pp. 435–441, Veda, Bratislava, 1978.
65. Kaplan, M. M., and Bertagna, P., The geographical distribution of Q fever, *Bull. WHO* **13:**829–860 (1955).
66. Thiel, N., *Das Q-Fieber und Seine Geographische Verbreitung*, Dunker and Humbolt, Berlin, 1974.

67. Abinanti, F. R., The varied epidemiology of Q fever infections. Symposium on Q fever, *Med. Sci. Publ. Walter Reed Army Inst. Res.* **6:**8–14 (1959).
68. Johnson, J. E., and Kadull, P. J., Laboratory acquired Q fever: A report of fifty cases, *Am. J. Med.* **41:**391–403 (1966).
69. Meiklejohn, G., Reimer, L. G., Graves, P. S., *et al.*, Cryptic epidemic of Q fever in a medical school, *J. Infect. Dis.* **144:**107–113 (1981).
70. Simor, A. E., Brunton, J. L., Salit, I. E., *et al.*, Q fever; hazard from sheep used in research, *Can. Med. Assoc. J.* **130:**1013–1016 (1984).
71. Spinelli, J. S., Managing the Q fever crisis: How UCSF made bureaucracy work fast, *Lab. Anim.* **10:**29–38 (1981).
72. Spinelli, J. S., Ascher, M. S., Brooks, D. L., *et al.*, Q fever crisis in San Fransisco: Controlling a sheep zoonosis in a lab animal facility, *Lab. Anim.* **10:**24–27 (1981).
73. Sigel, M. M., Scott, T. F. McN., Henle, W., *et al.*, Q fever in a wool and hair processing plant, *Am. J. Public Health* **40:**524–532 (1950).
74. Hall, C. J., Richmond, S. J., Caul, E. O., *et al.*, Laboratory outbreak of Q fever acquired from sheep, *Lancet* **1:**1004–1006 (1982).
75. Tigertt, W. D., Benenson, A. S., and Gochenour, W. S., Airborne Q fever, *Bacteriol. Rev.* **25:**285–293 (1961).
76. Marmion, B. P., and Stoker, M. G. P., Q fever in Great Britain: Epidemiology of an outbreak, *Lancet* **2:**611–616 (1950).
77. Davis, G. E., American Q fever: Experimental transmission by the argasid ticks *Ornithodorus moubata* and *O. hermsi*, *Public Health Rep.* **58:**984–987 (1943).
78. Derrick, E. H., Smith, D. J. W., and Brown, H. E., Studies on the epidemiology of Q fever. 9. The role of the cow in the transmission of human infection, *Aust. J. Exp. Biol. Med. Sci.* **20:**105–110 (1942).
79. Caminopetros, J., La "Q fever" en Grece: Le lait source de l'infection pour l'homme et les animaux, *Ann. Parasitol. Hum. Comp.* **23:**107–108 (1948).
80. Marmion, B. P., Stoker, M. G. P., Walker, C. B. B., *et al.*, Q fever in Great Britain: Epidemiological information from a serological survey of healthy adults in Kent and East Anglia, *J. Hyg.* **54:**118–140 (1956).
81. Stoker, M. G. P., and Marmion, B. P., The spread of Q fever from animals to man: The natural history of a rickettsial disease, *Bull. WHO* **13:**781–806 (1955).
82. Wagstaff, D. J., Janney, J. H., Crawford, K. L., *et al.*, Q fever studies in Maryland, *Public Health Rep.* **80:**1095–1099 (1965).
83. Beck, M. D., Bell, J. A., Shaw, E. W., *et al.*, Q fever studies in southern California. II. An epidemiological study of 300 cases, *Public Health Rep.* **64:**41–56 (1949).
84. Huebner, R. J., Jellison, W. L., Beck, M. D., *et al.*, Q fever studies in southern California. I. Recovery of *Rickettsia burneti* from raw milk, *Public Health Rep.* **63:**214–222 (1948).
85. Bell, E. J., Parker, R. R., and Stoenner, H. G., Q fever: Experimental Q fever in cattle, *Am. J. Public Health* **39:**478–484 (1949).
86. Ormsbee, R. A., Peacock, M. G., Gerloff, R., *et al.*, Limits of rickettsial infectivity, *Infect. Immun.* **19:**239–245 (1978).
87. Babudieri, B., La febbre Q o *rickettsiosi burnetii*, *G. Mal. Infett. Parassit.* **6:**449–476 (1954).
88. Syrucek, L., Sobeslavsky, O., and Gutvirth, I., Isolation of *Coxiella burnetii* from human placentas, *J. Hyg. Epidemiol.* **2:**29–35 (1958).
89. Clark, W. H., Lennette, E. H., Railsback, O. C., *et al.*, Q fever in California. VII. Clinical features in 180 cases, *Arch. Intern. Med.* **88:**155–167 (1951).
90. Derrick, E. H., The epidemiology of Q fever, *J. Hyg.* **43:**357–361 (1944).
91. Powell, O., Q fever: Clinical features in 72 cases, *Aust. Ann. Med.* **9:**214 (1960).
92. Marmion, B. P., Stoker, M. G. P., McCoy, J. H., *et al.*, Q fever in Great Britain, *Lancet* **1:**503–510 (1953).
93. Dupont, H. L., Hornick, R. B., Levin, H. S., *et al.*, Q fever hepatitis, *Ann. Intern. Med.* **74:**198–206 (1971).
94. Turck, W. P., Howitt, G., Turnberg, L. A., *et al.*, Chronic Q fever, *Q. J. Med.* **178:**193–221 (1976).
95. Wilson, H. G., Neilson, G. H., Galea, E. G., *et al.*, Q fever endocarditis in Queensland, *Circulation* **53:**680–684 (1976).
96. Gochenour, W. S., Veternary importance of Q fever. Symposium on Q fever, *Med. Sci. Publ. Walter Reed Army Inst. Res.* **6:**20–22 (1959).
97. Biberstein, E. L., Riemann, H. P., Franti, C. E., *et al.*, Vaccination of dairy cattle against Q fever (*Coxiella burnetii*): Results of field trials, *Am. J. Vet. Res.* **38:**189–193 (1977).
98. Luoto, L., Winn, J. F., and Huebner, R. J., Q fever studies in southern California. XIII. Vaccination of dairy cattle against Q fever, *Am. J. Hyg.* **55:**190–202 (1952).
99. Sadecky, E., Brezina, R., Kazar, J., *et al.*, Immunization against Q fever of naturally infected dairy cows, *Acta Virol.* **19:**486–488 (1975).
100. Enright, J. B., Sadler, W. W., and Thomas, R. C., Thermal inactivation of *Coxiella burnetii* and its relation to pasteurization of milk, *Public Health Rep.* **72:**947–948 (1957).
101. Fiset, P., Vaccination against Q fever. 1st International Conference on Vaccines against Viral and Rickettsial Diseases of Man, Scientific Publ. No. 147, PAHO/WHO, pp. 528–531, 1967.
102. Ormsbee, R. A., Bell, E. J., Lackman, D. B., *et al.*, The influence of phase on the protective potency of Q fever vaccine, *J. Immunol.* **92:**404–412 (1964).
103. Ackland, J. R., Worswick, D. A., and Marmion, B. P., Vaccine prophylaxis of Q fever. A follow-up study of the efficacy of Q-Vax (CSL) 1985–1990, *Med. J. Aust.* **160**(11)**:**704–708 (1994).
104. Bernard, K. W., Parham, G. L., Winkler, W. G., *et al.*, Q fever control measures: Recommendations for research facilities using sheep, *Infect. Control* **3:**461–465 (1982).
105. Fiset, P., Wisseman, C. L., Jr., and El Batawi, Y., Immunologic evidence of human fetal infection with *Coxiella burnetii*, *Am. J. Epidemiol.* **101:**65–69 (1975).

12. Suggested Reading

Annals of the New York Academy of Sciences, Vol. 590, 1990, contains several papers on Q fever and on the biology and molecular biology of *Coxiella burnetii.*

Baca, O. G., and Paretsky, D., Q fever and *Coxiella burnetii*: A model for host–parasite interactions, *Microbiol. Rev.* **47:**127–149 (1983).

Leedom, J. M., Q fever: An update, in: *Current clinical topics in infectious diseases*, Vol 1 (J. S. Remington and M. N. Swartz, eds.), pp. 304–331, McGraw-Hill, New York, 1980.

Marrie, T. J. (ed.), *Q Fever, Vol. 1. The Disease*, CRC Press, Boca Raton, FL, 1990.

Sawyer, L. A., Fishbein, D. B., and McDade, J. E., Q fever: Current concepts, *Rev. Infect. Dis.* **9:**935–946 (1987).

CHAPTER 30

Rocky Mountain Spotted Fever

Theodore E. Woodward and J. Stephen Dumler

1. Introduction

Rocky Mountain spotted fever is an acute febrile illness transmitted to man by ticks infected with *Rickettsia rickettsii*. Usually sudden in onset, it is characterized by chills, headache, and fever lasting 2 or more weeks. A characteristic rash appears on the extremities on about the 4th febrile day and, later, on the trunk. The exanthem and other anatomical manifestations result from focal areas of vasculitis and perivascular inflammation scattered throughout the body. Central nervous system (CNS) manifestations of delirium and coma as well as shock and renal failure occur in the severely ill. Serum antibodies to specific rickettsial antigens appear during the 2nd and 3rd weeks of illness. Chloramphenicol and the tetracyclines are highly specific therapeutically.

2. Historical Background

Idaho physicians described a form of "black measles" in the Snake River Valley as early as 1873. In 1899, Maxcy described a febrile illness with delirium and a blotchy-skin, red–purple–black rash that appeared first on the ankles, wrists, and forehead, with rapid general body spread. This was the "spotted fever of Idaho." It was noted to be sporadic and more common in the spring, and local opinion attributed it to the drinking of water from melted snow or inhalation of sawdust.[1] Dr. Earl Strain, a practicing physician in Great Falls, Montana, first suspected the role of ticks, having noted a relationship between death and a history of a tick bite. Wilson and Chowning[2] concurred with this relationship and concluded that the disease was transmitted by a local wood tick and the ground squirrel (gopher) as a possible reservoir.

They proposed *Piroplasma hominis*, an erythrocyte parasite, as the causative agent. In a series of brilliant studies carried out from 1906 to 1909, usually during the spring and summer months, Howard Taylor Ricketts successfully transmitted the disease to guinea pigs and monkeys by inoculation of blood from patients with spotted fever, incriminated the wood tick, *Dermacentor andersoni*, as vector by feeding experiments on animals and demonstrated the occurrence of naturally infected ticks. He observed bacterialike bodies in smears prepared from tick tissues and showed the transovarial transmission of infection to offspring of infected female ticks. Ticks were shown to be infected throughout their life span. Studies of immunity showed that blood from animals that survived the infection protected other animals if blood was administered several days before infection.[3,4] Wilder and Ricketts showed through cross-immunity studies that spotted fever and typhus were distinct entities. Ironically, the Montana legislature in 1909 allocated the sum of $6000 for Rickett's research studies, which the board of examiners failed to appropriate.[1] In July 1909, Ricketts proceeded to Mexico to study typhus fever; there, his life was cut short by this disease, which is closely related to Rocky Mountain spotted fever. In 1916, Dr. da Rocha Lima, another pioneer in this field, gave the name *Rickettsia* to those agents that cause the typhus and spotted fever disorders. An independent study conducted by McCalla and Brereton of Boise, Idaho, in 1905, unknown to Ricketts, showed that the bite of a tick removed from one of their patients transmitted spotted fever to two human subjects—a healthy prisoner and a woman—in whom a moderate and a mild attack, respectively, of Rocky Mountain spotted fever occurred. This work was not published until 1908.[5]

Theodore E. Woodward • Department of Medicine, University of Maryland School of Medicine, Baltimore, Maryland 21201. **J. Stephen Dumler** • Department of Pathology, Johns Hopkins Medical Institution, Baltimore, Maryland 21287.

Wolbach[6] was the first to detail the microscopic lesions of Rocky Mountain spotted fever with descriptions of the classic focal lesions of blood vessels. He distinguished between pathogenic and nonpathogenic organisms in ticks and demonstrated the intranuclear multiplication of rickettsiae in tick tissues.

Much knowledge was added by Spencer and Parker,[7] who showed that guinea pigs could be infected readily by intraperitoneal injection of macerated tick tissue. Ticks obtained in the Bitter Root Valley during early spring failed to cause illness in guinea pigs. Ticks fed on infected goats killed inoculated animals. These workers demonstrated "reactivation" by showing that unfed ticks immunized animals despite their inability to cause demonstrable infection and that virulence could be revived by providing ticks a blood meal (see Section 4). Also, phenolyzed tick juice effectively afforded protection in guinea pigs. Vaccinated humans developed antibodies, and their sera protected guinea pigs from experimental infection. Inactivated infected tick-tissue vaccine for man became a reality.[7]

Cox[8] provided an additional milestone by showing that rickettsiae propagated well in chick-embryo yolk sacs, particularly after death of the embryo. The yolk sac vaccine was simpler to produce and gave fewer reactions.

Therapeutically, immune serum did not prove to be really effective in patients with Rocky Mountain spotted fever. This is principally because rickettsiae are localized intracellularly at the time when the clinical diagnosis becomes apparent, on about the 5th or 6th day. The first effective and specific treatment was para-aminobenzoic acid, which did reduce mortality and morbidity, but it proved awkward to use.[9]

In 1948, first with chloramphenicol and later with the tetracyclines, specific treatment was placed on a firmer basis, and therapy for Rocky Mountain spotted fever became readily available.[10]

It is quite likely that Rocky Mountain spotted fever was prevalent in the eastern Atlantic states before its reported recognition in 1930. Most of the cases in the East probably masqueraded as endemic typhus or were called Brill's disease. Pinkerton and Maxcy[11] reported a case in Charlottesville, VA, that was undoubtedly Rocky Mountain spotted fever. Dyer *et al.*[12] noted, in 1930, that patients whose illness occurred in the spring and summer along the Eastern Seaboard states closely resembled Rocky Mountain spotted fever. One of these patients was recognized in Maryland by Maurice C. Pincoffs[13]; Dr. Pincoffs's case was published by Dyer *et al.*[12] In 1901, Sir William Osler diagnosed a patient with typhus at the Johns Hopkins Hospital in Baltimore, MD. The patient died and the autopsy performed by William Henry Welch revealed findings consistent with the emerging pathological characteristics of typhus fever. Ninety years later, the autopsy materials were retested using an immunohistological technique and were clearly demonstrated to contain *R. rickettsi*, proof that Rocky Mountain spotted fever existed in the eastern United States concurrent with its discovery in the West.[14]

3. Methodology

3.1. Sources of Mortality Data

The mortality from Rocky Mountain spotted fever has been variable, especially after the introduction of antibiotics, so that mortality data are not a reliable indicator of incidence. Prior to specific antibiotic usage, the overall mortality rate annually averaged about 20% for all ages. In the mountain and eastern states, where occupational pursuits exposed adults to infected feces, fatality exceeded 50% in those persons aged 40 or older. It was appreciably lower in children and young adults. Two developments have drastically improved treatment, reduced fatality, and shortened the clinical course of infection. The broad-spectrum antibiotics, first chloramphenicol and later the tetracyclines, were introduced in 1948. When they were given early during the course of Rocky Mountain spotted fever, when the rash was noted, usually on the 3rd–6th day of illness, recovery ensued rapidly. Of equal importance was the elucidation of the pathophysiological abnormalities responsible for the severe manifestations and complications that occur during the 2nd febrile week. Properly applied supportive measures and antibiotic treatment led to recovery in patients who did not come under medical care until late in the illness. Despite these advances in supportive care in managing the late sequelae of late-stage Rocky Mountain spotted fever, a fatal outcome is strongly associated with a delay in diagnosis and therapy.[15]

3.2. Sources of Morbidity Data

Rocky Mountain spotted fever is a reportable disease. In patients whose illness is not detected early and treated properly, serious sequelae and a long hospitalization often follow. The Centers for Disease Control and Prevention (CDC) publish the number of cases that occur weekly in various states under the category of typhus fever ("Tick-borne RMSF"). The data are published in an annual supplement. Criteria for diagnosis are reliable, since confirmatory serological tests, including the indirect fluorescent antibody (IFA) test or the complement-fixation (CF) reaction, and identification of the *Rickettsia* in skin biopsy by immunohistology are generally available.

3.3. Laboratory Diagnosis

Several types of confirmatory laboratory tests are useful for diagnosis of Rocky Mountain spotted fever: (1) serological tests to detect the presence and increase of specific antibodies in the patient's blood during convalescence[16]; (2) isolation and identification of *R. rickettsii* from blood or tissues; (3) identification of the agent in skin, tissues, or blood by the use of labeled antibodies; and (4) identification of rickettsial nucleic acids in the blood or tissues of infected patients by polymerase chain reaction (PCR) amplification.[17] It is important to remember that all of these techniques have a threshold of sensitivity, and a negative result must be carefully judged during the time when initiation of therapy is most important for a favorable outcome. Since no test is 100% sensitive, a negative laboratory result should not dissuade from institution or continuation of effective therapy. In particular, reliance on serological results during the acute illness is hazardous, and these tests are most useful for confirmation of infection in convalescence.

3.3.1. Serological Tests. To be useful, serological tests require at minimum two and preferably three serum samples: during the 1st, 2nd, and 4th–6th weeks of illness.[18] Some serological tests such as the latex agglutination and complement-fixation tests are most useful for detection of IgM and for confirmation early after infection; however, the IFA test, enzyme-linked immunosorbent assay (ELISA), and solid-phase enzyme immunoassay tests (dipsticks)[19] may be useful for detection of IgG, IgM, or both.[20] Antibodies of the IgG type persist for months to years after the acute infection, and thus tests that detect these immunoglobulins are also useful for seroepidemiological investigations. Typically, a serological diagnosis is rendered when a patient with a consistent illness develops a fourfold rise in antibody titer in convalescence or has a minimum titer that is technique dependent. No serological test has been shown to be sensitive during the first 2 weeks of illness, and thus these tests must be considered as confirmatory in convalescence only. No therapeutic decision should be made based on the results of a negative test for antibodies during infection.

3.3.1a. Weil–Felix Reaction. Strains of *Proteus* OX-19 and OX-2 are agglutinated by sera of patients with Rocky Mountain spotted fever. These agglutination tests are now considered to be of historic importance only. The poor sensitivity and very low specificity make these reactions poor predictors of the diagnosis, given the relatively low prevalence of the disease in some geographic regions.

3.3.1b. Complement-Fixation Reaction. The CF reaction was previously useful as a specific diagnostic tool, since it employed specific rickettsial antigens. However, the test detects predominantly IgM antibodies and often later in the course of convalescence than other more recently developed tests. CF antibodies usually appear during the 2nd and 3rd weeks of Rocky Mountain spotted fever and later in those treated with antibiotics within the first 3–5 days of illness. Under these circumstances, a late convalescent specimen should be taken at 4–6 weeks.

3.3.1c. Indirect Fluorescent Antibody and Microimmunofluorescent Tests (MIF). The standard for rickettsial serological diagnosis is the IFA or MIF test. This test utilizes whole, tissue-culture-propagated rickettsiae, and thus is approximately 99% sensitive.[21,22] In addition, the test has a high degree of specificity for antibodies reactive with spotted fever group rickettsiae; it is rapid and highly sensitive. Some cross-reactivity with typhus group rickettsiae is occasionally seen. Moreover, the test can be used to determine IgG or IgM responses to differentiate recent infection from remote disease. The high sensitivity and ability to distinguish among immunoglobulin classes also makes this test useful for seroepidemiological investigation.

3.3.1d. Other Serological Tests. Because of the lack of a rapid, specific, and sensitive test to replace the outdated Weil–Felix reaction, the latex agglutination test was developed.[23] This serological test uses highly purified rickettsial antigens coated on latex beads, may be rapidly performed within minutes, and is simple to perform and interpret. The test is very sensitive and specific and detects predominantly IgM antibodies useful for early serological confirmation in local hospital and public health laboratories. Another recent addition combines the exquisite sensitivity of enzyme immunoassay methods with the ease of rapid dipstick testing.[19] Although not complete, the results of evaluations are encouraging because of a high degree of both sensitivity and specificity and commercial availability. A recurring problem with the serological diagnosis of species in the genus *Rickettsia* is the lack of specificity to the species level. Thus, with a reactive serological test by any of the above methods, it is impossible to distinguish among agents of the spotted fever group rickettsiae and occasionally it is impossible to exclude typhus group rickettsiae as the causative agent of the disease. The development of a highly sensitive and specific ELISA for Rocky Mountain spotted fever for serological testing, coupled with the use of species-specific monoclonal antibodies that are blocked from attachment by the human antibodies in the test sera, provides a serological tool capable of rendering a diagnosis at the species level.[24] The other serological tests, including the microagglutination test (MA), the indirect hemagglutination test (IHA), and other serological tests, are no longer used in clinical circumstances.

3.3.2. Isolation and Identification of *R. rickettsii*. If isolation is attempted, blood should be obtained from the febrile patient prior to antibiotic treatment. Usually, the mononuclear cells are harvested from peripheral blood and used as an inoculum in a centrifugation-assisted shell vial method.[25] Many cell types are susceptible to rickettsial infection, including cells often used in standard virological laboratories, such as Vero cells (African green monkey kidney), L929 mouse fibroblasts, and human embryonal lung (HEL) fibroblast cells, among others. Coupled with the early detection of rickettsial antigen in shell vials by immunofluorescence with species-specific monoclonal antibodies, the diagnosis may be established within as early as 48 hr. Isolation in guinea pigs by intraperitoneal inoculation or in chicken embryo yolk sacs is a cumbersome, expensive method rarely used for clinical diagnosis.

3.3.3. Identification of *R. rickettsii* in Tissues. Immunohistologic techniques, including immunofluorescence and immunoenzymatic methods, are useful for detection of *R. rickettsii* in tissues of patients.[26–28] The most useful specimen is a punch biopsy of a petechial skin lesion. However, the rickettsial infection may be extremely focal, and thus multiple sections must be examined to maximize sensitivity, which averages approximately 70%. The specificity is excellent. Although rickettsia have been observed late after institution of antibiotic therapy, the best opportunity to visualize the organisms by these methods is before initiating treatment, as detection diminishes rapidly thereafter. It must be remembered that a negative result does not exclude Rocky Mountain spotted fever, and thus in suspected cases, therapy should be continued to assure a favorable outcome. The method is useful on both frozen sections and formalin-fixed, paraffin-embedded tissues.[29]

A recently described method, which has been useful for the diagnosis of Mediterranean spotted fever and holds promise for Rocky Mountain spotted fever, harvests circulating endothelial cells by using antiendothelial cell monoclonal antibodies, which are then tested for the presence of rickettsiae by immunofluorescence.[30]

3.3.4. Identification of Rickettsial Nucleic Acids in Clinical Samples. Given the low titer of rickettsiae that are present in peripheral blood of infected patients even at peak rickettsemia, the highly sensitive PCR technique for amplification of rickettsial nucleic acids has been proposed as a specific diagnostic method. Several target genes have been described, including a 16S ribosomal DNA, 190-kDa and 120-kDA *R. rickettsii* outer-membrane protein (rOMP) genes, a gene encoding the genus-common 17-kDa lipoprotein, and the citrate synthase (CS) gene. The best described is amplification of the 17-kDa antigen gene, and several cases where PCR has allowed a rapid, early diagnosis have been reported.[17] The specificity is dependent on the design of the oligonucleotide primers, but is usually very high. However, even the PCR method is no more sensitive than immunohistologic demonstration in skin biopsies,[17] because of the relative lack of rickettsiae in blood at any time. It is likely that application of this PCR method to skin biopsies will prove very useful, since the *Rickettsia* are plentiful in sites of vasculitis.

4. Biological Characteristics of the Organism

R. rickettsii, which possesses the general properties of other rickettsiae, is an obligate intracellular, coccobacillary bacterium. They are minute, averaging 0.6–1.2 μm, and stain purple with Giemsa, light blue with Castenada, red with Machiavello, and bright red with Giménez techniques.[16] These rickettsiae grow in the nucleus and cytoplasm of infected cells of ticks, mammals, and embryonated eggs. Electron micrographs reveal a gram-negative-like cell envelope containing chromosomal material and ribosomes. In some preparations, a microcapsular "slime" layer may be detected. They appear to divide by binary fission.[10,31]

Biochemically, *R. rickettsii* simulate other rickettsiae in chemical composition, metabolic consistency, and nutritional requirements. They contain both RNA and DNA and oxidize certain intermediates of the Krebs cycle.[31,32]

The agent is relatively labile and readily inactivated by heat and chemical agents. Suspensions of infected tissues are inactivated within 24 hr by 0.1% formaldehyde or 0.5% phenol. They remain viable for long periods of time when stored at −70°C. When carefully lyophilized from buffered sucrose–glutamate media and stored at 5°C, they remain viable for years.[10]

The antigenic and molecular constituents are becoming increasingly described and form the basis for understanding the mechanisms of rickettsial attachment, invasion, and intracellular multiplication. Although *R. rickettsii* has abundant lipopolysaccharide (LPS) demonstrable by chemical and immunoblotting methods, this component contributes little to pathogenesis.[33] In fact, it is likely that the LPS accounts for a large proportion of genus- and group-common antigenicity. By immunoblot analysis, two major immunodominant proteins are evident: a 190-kDa outer-membrane protein (rOMP-A) and a 120-kDa outer-membrane protein (rOMP-B).[34] The genes encoding these proteins have been cloned and considerable study has revealed likely functions for both. rOMP-A is the putative rickettsial adherence ligand[35] and rOMP-B is most likely to function as a structural protein.[34] Recombinant rOMP-A has been successfully employed as a protective vaccine in challenged guinea pigs and mice. Mutants lacking normal processing of rOMP-B lack *in vitro* correlates of virulence.[34] A previously described "mouse toxin" is a by-product of an artificial analytical system not associated with endothelial infection, and is now known to occur as a result of massive release of tumor necrosis factor when rickettsiae are inoculated directly into mice intravenously.

After rickettsiae attach to an unknown cellular ligand, they gain access to a transiently formed vacuole, presumably a phagosome, from which they rapidly escape. Once in the cytoplasm, *R. rickettsii* influences the polymerization of intracellular F-actin in a manner similar to that described for *Shigella*.[36] This polymerization rapidly mobilizes the organisms and enables cell escape and cell–cell transfer.

R. rickettsii exists in ticks in a nonvirulent form that con be reactivated to a virulent infection-producing phase with a fresh blood meal or when incubated at 37°C for 24 hr. This phenomenon probably accounts for the failure of infected ticks, after overwintering, to transmit illness to humans in the early spring until they have attached and fed for at least several hours. Later, during spring and summer, when natural reactivation has presumably occurred, ticks may infect humans after shorter exposure. Virulence of *R. rickettsii* is altered by the metabolic state.[10,31]

5. Descriptive Epidemiology

5.1. Prevalence and Incidence

The annual number of patients with Rocky Mountain spotted fever in the United States during the years 1950 to 1993 is shown in Fig. 1. In 1981, there were 1176 cases, which exceeded the number of cases reported in any other of these years. For many years, approximately 500 cases occurred annually in the United States; then, after the introduction of specific therapy in 1948, the number of infected cases decreased to a low of about 200 in 1959, 1960, and 1961. This decrease, however, was primarily an artifact of the widespread use of broad-spectrum antibiotics early in the illness, which led to underreporting and the use of pesticides.

Beginning in 1969, there was a gradual increase in annual incidence in the United States. There were approximately 900 cases reported in 1975 and 1976, and cumulative totals of 1115 in 1977, 1011 in 1978 (see Fig. 1), and 1067 in 1979.[16,37] Transformation of farms into housing developments and recreation of children and adults in wooded areas probably account for the added exposure to infected ticks, particularly in the southeastern Atlantic states, where the largest number of cases occur. The cumulative totals for 1980, 1981, 1982, 1983, 1984, 1985, and 1986 were 1163, 1176, 976, 1126, 836, 700, and 755, respectively. From 1987 to 1991, over 600 cases were reported annually. During 1992 and 1993, there were 502 and 456 cases, respectively. The lowered incidence during the past several years is unexplained but could relate to a cyclic reaction involving vector and parasite (see Fig. 1).

Rocky Mountain spotted fever in the United States and Sao Paulo typhus in Brazil are the most significant and clinically severe types of the tick-borne group. In the Eastern Hemisphere and elsewhere, the tick-borne rickettsioses are milder and are known variably as fièvre boutonneuse, South African, North Asian, Indian, Siberian, Queensland tick typhus, and others. Mite-borne rickettsialpox with its rodent reservoir is meddlesome rather than important.

5.2. Epidemic Behavior and Contagiousness

The epidemiology of spotted fever is associated with the biology of the ticks that transmit this disease. Man is entirely an accidental victim and is in no way responsible for the maintenance of the infection in nature, which is due largely to ticks and the animals on which they feed. A number of species of ticks are found infected with *R. rickettsii* in nature. Four species of ixodid ticks have been recognized as natural carriers of *R. rickettsii*: the Rocky Mountain wood tick, *Dermacentor andersoni*; the American dog tick, *D. variabilis*; the Lone Star tick, *Amblyomma americanum*; and the rabbit tick, *Haemaphysalis leporis-palustris*.[38,39] *D. andersoni* is the principal vector in the West and *D. variabilis* in the East. Infected adult female ticks transmit the agent transovarially to many of their offspring. Ticks that become infected, either through the egg or by feeding on an infected mammal at one of the stages during their developmental cycle, harbor the rickettsiae throughout their life span, which may be as long as

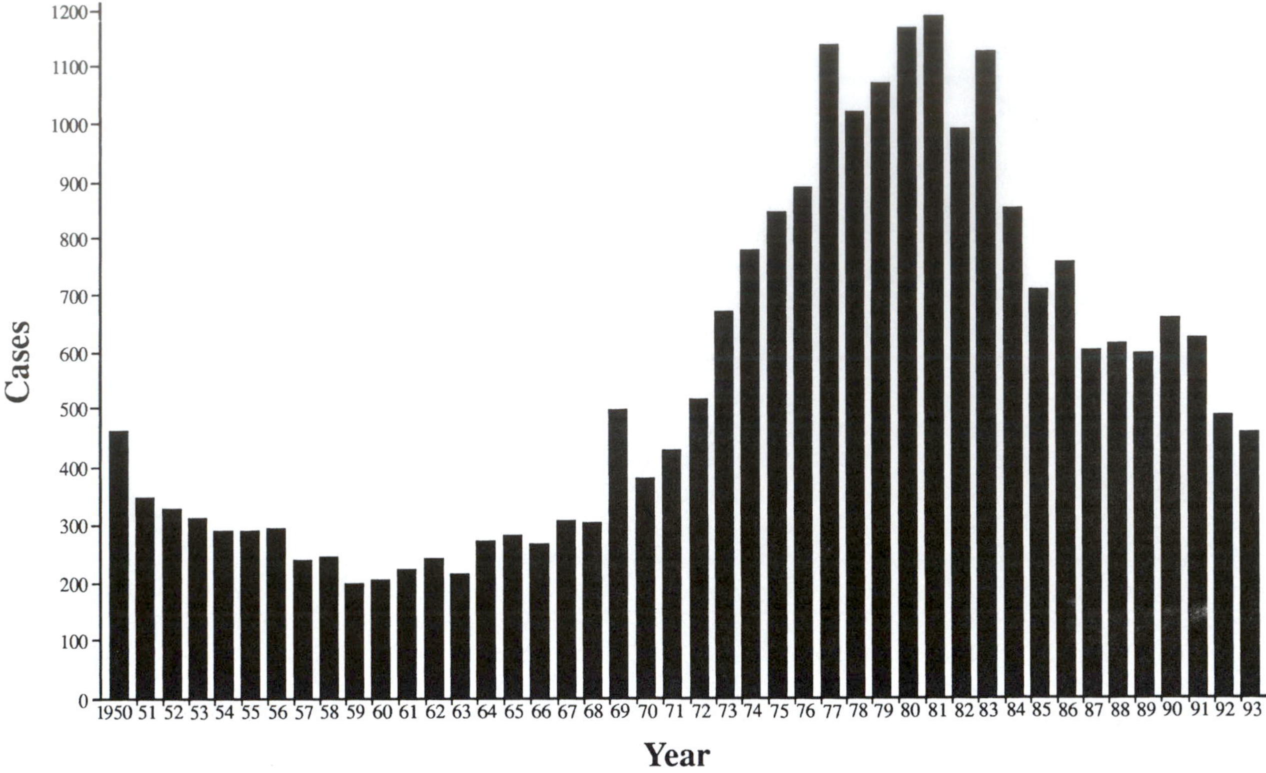

Figure 1. Rocky Mountain spotted fever cases reported in the United States, 1950–1994. Courtesy of the CDC.

several years. Usually, cases occur sporadically within an endemic area, although there appears to be an increasing clustering of patients within families, which have numbered up to four. Person-to-person infection does not occur. Thus, the tick probably serves as a reservoir in addition to being a vector. Small wild animals and puppies may play an important role in spreading rickettsiae in nature by infecting those new ticks that feed on them during the period of disease when rickettsemia is occurring. Most of the natural hosts show only inapparent infections with no diagnostic gross lesions.[10]

5.3. Geographic Distribution

Spotted fever caused by *R. rickettsii* is limited to the Western Hemisphere. During the latter 19th century, the first reports were in Idaho and Montana, which led to the name Rocky Mountain spotted fever. The disease has been recognized throughout the United States except in Vermont. It occurs in Canada, Mexico, Panama, Colombia, and Brazil (see Fig. 2). Now, many more cases occur in the East rather than in the West.

5.4. Temporal Distribution

There are seasonal variations in the incidence of cases of spotted fever. Most cases occur during the period of maximal tick activity, usually during the late spring and summer; however, confirmed cases are reported in every month of the year, particularly from the southeastern and south-central states.[10,37]

5.5. Age, Sex, and Occupational Factors

Differences in age and sex distribution of cases relate to exposure to ticks. In the western United States, a relatively higher proportion of adult males contract the disease because of occupational pursuits, whereas in the East, children and women are infected. This distribution is undoubtedly influenced by occupational propinquity to wood and dog ticks and is not due to variations in susceptibility of various ages or sexes.[10,37]

The age and sex distributions are virtually the same for confirmed and unconfirmed cases. Nearly two thirds of the cases are in persons less than 15 years of age, and 61% were in males. The case-fatality rates are significantly

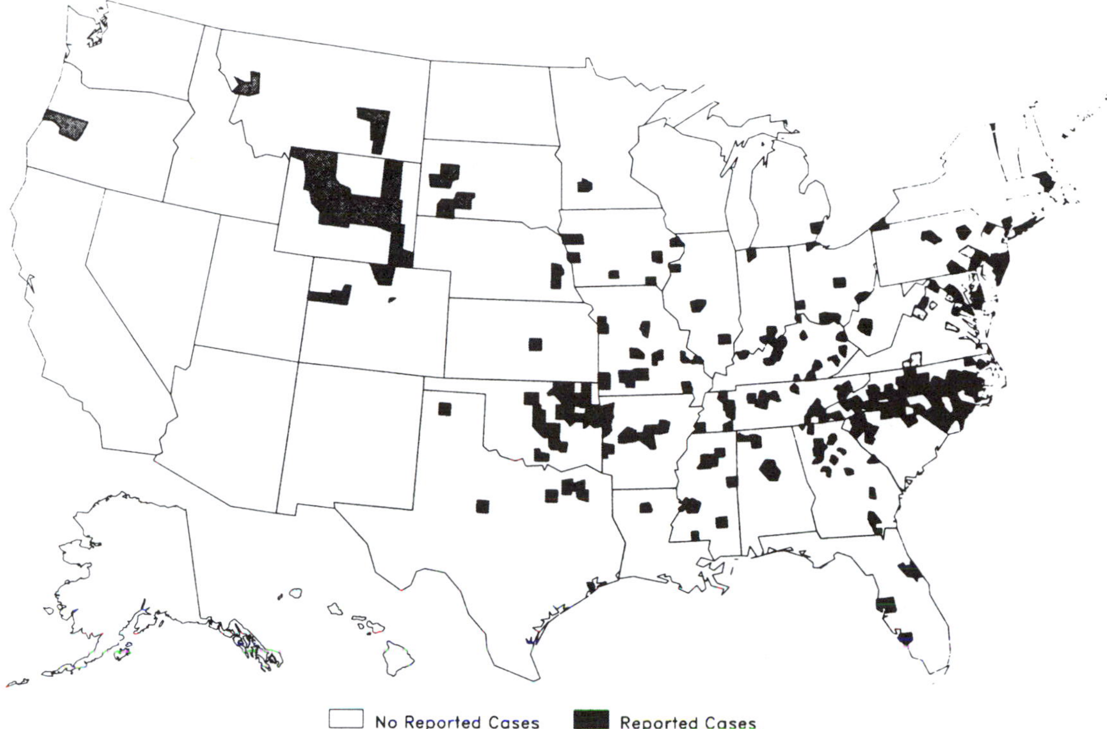

Figure 2. Geographic distribution of Rocky Mountain spotted fever in the United States for 1994, by county. Note the heavy localization in the south eastern Atlantic States. Courtesy of the CDC.

higher for nonwhites (13.9%) than for whites (5.8%), higher for male patients (8.2%) than for female patients (4.5%), and higher for persons older than 30 (13.9%) than for persons younger than 30 (5.4%).[37] Delay in diagnosis with absence of an identifiable rash in the dark-skinned patient probably accounts for the variable mortality data.

6. Mechanisms and Routes of Transmission

Man is generally infected by the bite of an infected tick. The need for ticks to "reactivate" their infection from a nonvirulent immunizing phase in unfed adult ticks to a virulent infection-producing phase brought about by the ingestion of fresh blood probably explains why ticks do not cause illness unless they have attached and have fed for several hours. Infection may also be acquired through abrasions in the skin or through mucous membranes that become contaminated with infected tick feces or tissue juices. Hence, there is a hazard associated with crushing ticks between the fingers when removing them from persons or animals.[10] Quantitative studies conducted to test the efficacy of vaccines in volunteers showed that a very small number of viable rickettsiae given intradermally cause illness in man, i.e., 0.1 $GPIPID_{50}$ (50% guinea pig intraperitoneal infectious dose), which is about one rickettsial organism.[40]

7. Pathogenesis and Immunity

7.1. Pathogenesis

Rocky Mountain spotted fever in man follows infection through the skin or respiratory tract. The bite of a tick usually transmits *R. rickettsii* after the tick has been attached for several hours. Infection may be acquired through an abrasion in the skin contaminated with infected tick feces or juices. Local lesions (eschars) develop with considerable rapidity at sites of arthropod attachment and initial multiplication of rickettsiae in scrub typhus, the tick-borne rickettsioses of the Eastern Hemisphere, and rickettsialpox. A primary lesion occurs occasionally at the site of tick attachment in Rocky Mountain spotted fever (Fig. 3). An eschar also occurs as an initial lesion in tick-borne tularemia, which may confuse the diagnostic picture.[10,41]

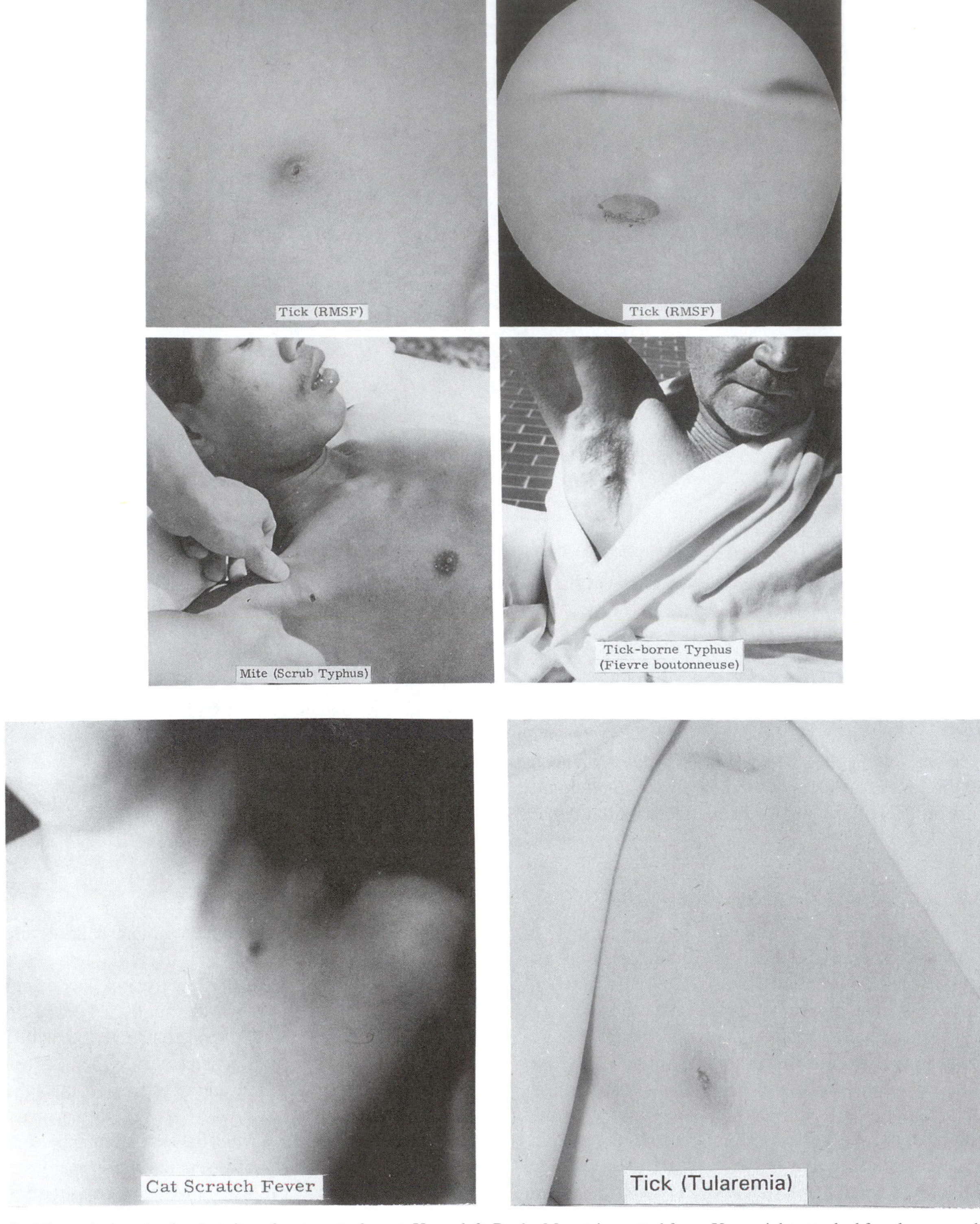

Figure 3. Primary lesions (eschars) at sites of vector attachment. Upper left, Rocky Mountain spotted fever. Upper right, attached female engorged tick, Rocky Mountain spotted fever. Middle left, scrub typhus (mite). Middle right, fiévre boutonneuse (*R. conorii*) tick. Lower left, cat scratch fever; note small primary lesion and adenitis. Lower right, tularemia, tick transmitted.

After infection, illness occurs within a period varying from 3 to 12 days, the mean being about 7 days. A short incubation period usually indicates a more serious infection. Studies in volunteers have shown that patients with scrub typhus and Q fever have rickettsemia late in the incubation period prior to onset of fever.[42,43]

Similar events probably occur in all rickettsial diseases; circulating rickettsiae can be detected during the early febrile period in practically all patients. Little is known about the pathogenesis of infection during the midportion of the incubation period. Presumably, during this time in patients with Rocky Mountain spotted fever, a transient low-grade rickettsemia results from release of organisms multiplying at the initial site of infection, which then seeds infection within endothelial cells of the vascular tree. The presence of rickettsial antigens and tissue damage elicits an inflammatory response rich in lymphocytes and macrophages, both important components of ensuing cell-mediated immunity. The accumulation of these inflammatory cells at the site of infection leads to the characteristic histopathologic finding of vasculitis. Widespread vascular lesions that develop account for the physical findings such as rash and explain the pathophysiology of the infection as intravascular volume, plasma proteins, and electrolytes are lost into the interstitial spaces.

The exact mechanism by which rickettsiae enter and damage the endothelial cell is not known. *R. rickettsii* binds to an unknown cellular ligand by the rOMP-A.[35] This binding triggers or is followed by an unknown mechanism that leads to endothelial cell invasion. Initially this process is mediated by phagocytosis associated with changes in intracellular calcium and the presence of phospholipase A (PLA) activity,[44,45] presumably of rickettsial origin. It is likely that this putative rickettsial PLA damages host cell membranes and may serve a role in (1) induced phagocytosis as a host-mediated reparative process, and (2) escape from the phagosome into the cytoplasmic compartment before phagosome-lysosome fusion occurs. Once within the endothelial cell, the rickettsiae mediate F-actin polymerization and become actively mobile. The rickettsiae multiply by binary fission, and via actin polymerization the rickettsiae escape the cell, often prior to any evident cell injury. In most cases, endothelial cell damage is irreversible, and ultrastructural and biochemical evidence point to free radical and oxidative membrane injury.[46]

Later in the course of illness, the cascade of immune events is activated and matures. The macrophages attracted to the focus of infection undoubtedly process and present rickettsial antigens to T lymphocytes and secrete important cytokine mediators of inflammation including tumor necrosis factor-α and interferon-γ.[47] Recent data from animal models and *in vitro* studies suggest that cytokines such as tumor necrosis factor may act on infected cells to result in cell destruction and death of the rickettsiae contained within. Cytokine-mediated alteration or damage coupled with rickettsial-mediated injury to critical endothelial cells compromises not only vascular flow but also enhances procoagulant activities, clinically resulting in thromboses or abnormalities in coagulation.[48] The activation of T lymphocytes leads to local secretion of interferon-γ, perhaps the most important cytokine factor elaborated by immune cells for enhancing intracellular rickettsial killing and protective immunity.[49] The balance of the degree of host injury (mediated by both the rickettsiae and host cytokines) and the degree to which rickettsiae are eliminated (via specific immune and nonimmune mechanisms) determines the overall amount of endothelial cell and vascular injury and is likely to be directly related to the clinicopathological findings and course in any given patient. This cellular and molecular pathogenetic sequence is consistent with *in vitro* experiments, animal models, and the experiences gleaned from human disease. In patients, infection is associated with induction of cutaneous delayed-type hypersensitivity reactions,[50] lymphocyte transformation, and the development of serum antibody. However, antibody clearly lacks a protective effect and is unable to reverse an established infection.[50] The use of corticosteroids has some beneficial effect in human disease, probably by diminishing local inflammation and suppressing additional cytokine-mediated effects. When used in animal models, corticosteroids do not prevent death. Overall, it appears that induction of inflammation and immunity is beneficial to the infected human host, since the major goal is the elimination of the spread of intracellular infection by sacrificing the large numbers of infected endothelial cells and perhaps some critical vascular beds.

The current concept of how pathophysiological changes caused by rickettsiae, particularly severe types of Rocky Mountain spotted fever, epidemic typhus, and scrub typhus, affect the patient is shown in Fig. 4. When severe vasculitis is present, later in the illness, there is increased capillary permeability and vascular leakage that expands the extravascular space. This can lead to leakage of fluid into the lungs, brain, and peripheral tissues, particularly when excess fluids are administered intravenously.

7.2. Immunity

Second attacks of Rocky Mountain spotted fever have not been reported, although recurrent infection has developed in patients treated with antibiotics very early in

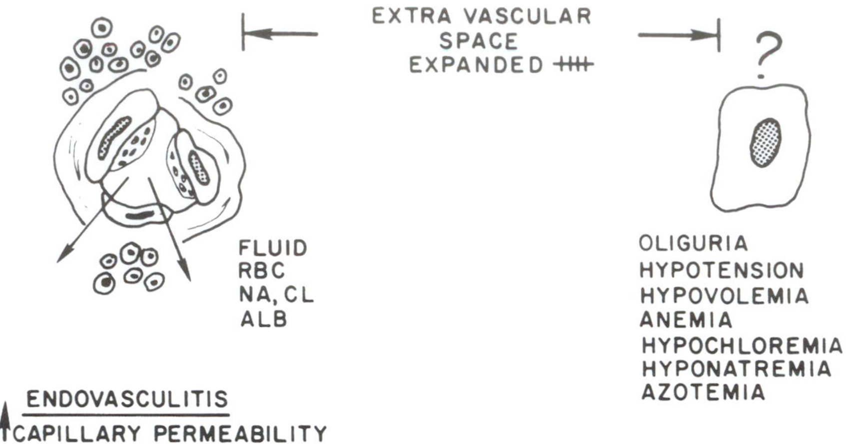

Figure 4. The current concept of how pathophysiological changes caused by rickettsiae, particularly in severe types of Rocky Mountain spotted fever, epidemic typhus, and scrub typhus, affect the patient are shown. When severe vasulitis is present, later in the illness, there is increased capillary permeability and vascular leakage that expands the extravascular space. This can lead to leakage of fluid into the lungs, brain, and peripheral tissues, particularly when excess fluids are administered intravenously.

illness. These are really continuing infections and not true recurrences.[40]

A recurrent type of Rocky Mountain spotted fever such as Brill–Zinnser epidemic louse-borne type has not been reported. Clinicians should be alert to this possibility. Studies of cross-immunity in susceptible animals show protection among the various rickettsiae of the tick-borne group and rickettsialpox. Always, the protection derived from homologous antigens is more significant.

The underlying protective effectors after recovery from natural infection are not precisely identified; however, it is clear from *in vitro* and in *in vivo* experiments, that interferon-γ is a critical factor. Infection and illness has been elicited in patients with high levels of preexisting antibody and preexisting *in vitro* correlates (lymphocyte transformation) of cell-mediated immunity.[50] The specific host and rickettsial factors that influence the development of an acquired protective immune state are actively being sought.

8. Patterns of Host Response

A history of tick bite is elicited in approximately 80% of patients. In a recent report, this was said to be 58%.[10,37,41]

8.1. Common Clinical Features

The onset is usually abrupt in nonvaccinated persons, with severe headache, a shaking chill, prostration, generalized myalgia, especially in the back and leg muscles,[10] nausea with occasional vomiting, and fever that reaches 102–104°F within the first several days. Onset in children and adults may be mild, accompanied by lethargy, anorexia, headache, and low-grade fever. These symptoms are similar to those of many infectious diseases and make specific diagnosis difficult during the first several days. It is doubtful whether many human inapparent infections occur.

Fever: In severe cases, fever continues for approximately 15–20 days; the febrile course in children may be shorter. Usually, the fever maintains a high continuous course with morning remissions that do not reach normal. Hyperpyrexia of 105°F or greater is usually an unfavorable sign, although death may occur when the patient is hypopyrexic with associated vasomotor collapse. Defervescence usually occurs by lysis over several days; rarely, there is a crisis. Recurrent fever is unusual except in the presence of pyogenic complications.

Headache: Headache is usually general and severe, with frontal intensity. It persists during the 1st and 2nd weeks of illness in untreated cases; occasionally, it is mild. Malaise and muscle pain continue during the 1st week. Irritability is common, and the patient shows distraction in such circumstances as during questioning and examination.

Rash: One of the most characteristic and helpful diagnostic signs is the rash, which usually appears on the 4th febrile day; the range is 2 to 6 days. Initial lesions are on the wrists, ankles, soles, palms, and forearms. They are macular, pink, nonfixed, and irregularly defined, and measure 2–6 mm. A warm compress on the extremities may accentuate a faint rash, and the rash is more prominent with elevated temperature. After about 12–24 hr, the rash extends centrally to the legs, buttocks, arms, axillae, trunk, neck, and face. In epidemic typhus fever, the rash spreads from the trunk to the extremities. In about 2–3 days, the rash becomes maculopapular and assumes a deeper red hue. After 4 days or so, the rash is petechial and fails to fade on pressure. Often, the hemorrhagic lesions coalesce to form large ecchymoses. These lesions often form over bony prominences and may slough to form indolent, slow-healing ulcers. In convalescence, the petechiae fade to form brown-pigmented discolorations for several weeks. In mild cases, the rash does not become petechial or purpuric and may disappear within several days. Antibiotic treatment may abort the early exanthem; the late fixed lesions fade slowly with specific therapy. In some patients, particularly dark-skinned patients, a rash does not occur or is unnoticed. When tourniquets are applied to the extremities for several minutes or when the blood pressure is taken, additional petechiae may appear (Rumpel–Leade phenomenon); this is further evidence of capillary abnormalities. Photophobia and redness of the peripheral conjunctivae are often present.

Cardiovascular and Respiratory Signs: In severe cases, the pulse is rapid and the blood pressure is lower. Circulatory failure with shock is an ominous sign and is an indication of the peripheral vascular atonicity and collapse. Ecchymotic skin lesions, cyanosis, and gangrene of the fingers, toes, genitalia, and buttocks are all unfavorable signs. The electrocardiogram shows changes indicative of myocardial involvement, and arrhythmias of various types indicate myocarditis, which may lead to cardiac arrest and death. In severely ill patients, edema of the arms, legs, and face indicates vascular decompensation and capillary abnormalities.

Respiration is usually rapid, and a nonproductive cough with pulmonary rales is indicative of a form of rickettsial pneumonitis. Lung consolidation is rare.

Unwarranted use of intravenous fluids may provoke pulmonary edema.

Hepatic and Renal Signs: Hepatomegaly occurs; usually, there is no jaundice. Hypoalbuminemia results from leakage of albumin into subcutaneous tissues and abnormal hepatic function. Oliguria, anuria, and azotemia are indicators of vascular decompensation and renal involvement.

Gastrointestinal Signs: Abdominal distension is frequent and occasionally some degree of intestinal ileus is observed. Constipation is usual. More acute manifestations with abdominal pain may suggest the presence of either appendicitis or cholecystitis.

Neurological Signs: Headache, restlessness, insomnia, and back stiffness are common neurological manifestations. Coma, muscular rigidity, athetoid movements, convulsive seizures, and hemiplegia (rare) are grave signs and indicate the presence of encephalitis. Deafness during the acute illness and in convalescence is common. Most of the CNS signs abate with time.

8.2. Clinical Course and Complications

In mild and moderately severe cases, the illness abates in about 2 weeks. Convalescence is rapid. If death occurs, it is usually during the latter part of the 2nd week as a result of toxemia, vasomotor weakness, and shock or renal failure with azotemia. In a few patients, the course is rapidly fulminant with death outdistancing treatment, occurring as early as the 6th day of illness.[10,37]

In vaccinated persons who contract the disease, the illness is usually milder, with a short febrile course and a sparse pink rash.

8.3. Diagnosis

During the early stages of infection before the rash has appeared, differentiation from other acute infections is difficult. History of tick bite while living or traveling in a high endemic area is helpful. The rash of meningococcemia resembles that of Rocky Mountain spotted fever in certain aspects, since it is macular, maculopapular, or petechial in the chronic form, and petechial, confluent, or ecchymotic in the fulminant type. The meningococcic skin lesion is tender and develops with extreme rapidity in the fulminant form, whereas the rickettsial rash occurs on about the 4th day of disease and gradually becomes petechial. High blood leukocyte counts are common in meningococcal infections. The exanthem of rubella rapidly becomes confluent, while that of rubeola almost never becomes petechial. The exanthem of varicella or variola is first erythematous and later becomes vesicular. The rose spots of typhoid fever are usually on the lower chest or abdomen and remain delicate, without hemorrhagic character. Rocky Mountain spotted fever skin lesions, in con trast to those of typhoid, begin on the periphery of the skin and later become petechial. The rash of infectious mononucleosis is usually morbilliform on the trunk and rarely becomes petechial. Angina, lymphadenopathy, and atypical lymphocytes in the blood are differentiating features. Murine typhus is a milder disease than Rocky Mountain spotted fever; the rash is less extensive and is nonpurpuric and nonconfluent; renal and vascular complications are uncommon. Not infrequently, differentiation of these two rickettsial infections must await the results of specific serological tests. Epidemic typhus fever is capable of causing all the pronounced clinical, physiological, and anatomical alterations seen in cases of Rocky Mountain spotted fever, i.e., hypotension, peripheral vascular failure, cyanosis and gangrene of digits, renal failure with azotemia, and neurological manifestations. However, the rash of classic typhus is noted initially in the axillary folds and on the trunk and later extends peripherally, rarely involving the palms, soles, or face. The serological patterns in these two diseases are distinctive when specific rickettsial antigens are employed in tests. Moreover, louse-borne typhus is not recognized in the United States except in the form of Brill–Zinsser disease (recurrent typhus fever). Recently, the agent has been isolated from flying squirrels and human cases have occurred. Rickettsialpox, although caused by a member of the spotted-fever group of organisms, is usually readily differentiated from Rocky Mountain spotted fever by the initial lesion, the relative mildness of the illness, and the early vesiculation of the maculopapular rash.

The laboratory findings in Rocky Mountain spotted fever are nonspecific. However, several laboratory findings may aid in establishing the differential diagnosis. Rocky Mountain spotted fever is often associated with normal or low leukocyte counts and significant left-shifts in patients who are quite obviously ill and would be expected to have leukocytosis. Platelet counts are frequently diminished. Careful evaluation of coagulation tests may reveal mild abnormalities, and despite the occasional clinical appearance of a state suggestive of disseminated intravascular coagulation, fibrinogen levels in serum are usually within normal ranges. Electrolyte abnormalities occur often, particularly hyponatremia, and these are best explained on the basis of appropriate antidiuretic hormone release in response to the loss of intravascular volume into interstitial spaces and by the actual loss of electrolytes into third space tissue compartments. Elevations in serum hepatic transaminases, creatine phosphokinase, lactate dehydrogenase, and other enzymes are likely to result from bystander inflammatory injury to hepatocytes or injury secondary to ischemia and hypoperfusion. The development of hyperbilirubinemia and hepatic failure is an ominous sign indicative of severe, probably impending fatal infection. Abnormalities in urea nitrogen and creatinine levels usually indicate renal injury secondary to hypovolemia; however, rickettsial interstitial nephritis is well recognized and may be a contributor in some circumstances. Careful intrepretation of laboratory findings and correlation with the clinical examination is imperative. Most often, the clinical findings and laboratory examination will reveal evidence of a systemic disease, findings that will discourage unwarranted surgical interventions.

Scrub typhus and boutonneuse fever patients are being increasingly reported in the United States among travelers from the Far East[51] and from Africa.[52] The clinical features simulate Rocky Mountain spotted fever. The vector of scrub typhus is a mite and the vector of boutonneuse fever is a tick. The illness may be severe or fatal; however, when detected early, antibiotic treatment is very effective.

9. Control and Prevention

9.1. Vector Control

Avoiding or reducing the chance of contact in tick-infested areas of known endemicity is the principal preventive measure. When this is impractical, area control of spotted fever ticks may include the following prophylactic measures:

1. Spraying the ground with dieldrin or chlordane for tick control. Although there are environmental objections to the use of residual insecticides, such procedures may be warranted under special conditions.
2. Application of repellents such as diethyltoluamide or dimethylphthalate to clothing and exposed parts of the body, or in very heavily infected areas, the wearing of clothing that interferes with the attachment of ticks, i.e., boots and a one-piece outer garment preferably impregnated with repellent.[10]
3. Daily inspection of the entire body, particularly of children, including the hairy parts, to detect and remove attached ticks. Care should be taken in removing attached ticks to avoid crushing the arthropod, which will contaminate the bite wound. Touching the tick with gasoline or whiskey encourages detachment, but gentle traction with small forceps applied close to the mouth parts allows ready extraction. The skin area should be disinfected with soap and water or other antiseptics such as alcohol. These precautions should be employed in removing engorged ticks from dogs and other animals because infection through minor abrasions in the hands is possible.

9.2. Immunization

Spencer and Parker[7] were aware that infected ticks, when they first come out of hibernation, produce either no or low-grade infections in guinea pigs. They found that one infected egg from an infected female tick produced spotted fever in a guinea pig and that suspensions of infected ticks treated with phenol protected guinea pigs against virulent challenge. Spencer and Parker[7,53,54] tested the new vaccine on themselves and showed that a sample of their blood. taken after vaccination, mixed with virulent rickettsiae protected guinea pigs against infection. They developed a tick-derived vaccine, inactivated and preserved with 1.6% phenol and 0.4% formalin. The vaccine was difficult to produce and expensive, originally costing $20.00 per injection. Studies of efficacy were carried out over a number of years. Although no carefully controlled experimental trials were conducted, it appeared, on the basis of differences of attack rates in small groups of vaccinees and control volunteers, that the vaccine prevented the mild type of spotted fever and sharply reduced the mortality in the highly fatal type.[55]

The vaccine was moderately reactive, producing malaise, nausea, slight fever, arthralgia, myalgia, and serum sickness in about 1% of recipients.

Cox developed an inactivated vaccine prepared from rickettsiae grown in yolk sacs of fertile hens' eggs. This was the standard preparation for a number of years.[56] Immunization consisted of a course of three injections of 1.0 ml each given subcutaneously at weekly intervals. Vaccination was preferably performed in the spring before the advent of the spotted fever season, and a 1.0-ml stimulating dose was recommended each year for those at risk. There was little reaction from the vaccine. This chick-tissue vaccine produced commercially (Lederle) was not conclusively tested in the field, and furthermore, the relationship between the immunity demonstrated in guinea pigs and that induced in man following administration of vaccine was inconclusive.

A quantitative trial of inactivated vaccines made from infected tissue and embryonated hens' eggs was conducted in volunteers followed by a challenge with virulent (viable) *R. rickettsii*.[40] Humoral antibodies appeared in a low percentage of vaccinees after use of either available vaccine. It was noted in the vaccinated group that when they were injected with a few virulent rickettsiae 3–6 months after a full course of vaccination, the incubation period was prolonged and the frequency of early clinical relapse was lessened. Vaccinated volunteers were not protected (when compared with controls) against development of clinical illness. In vaccinees, the clinical illness appeared to be shortened,[40] which coincided with the earlier findings of Parker.

There was great hope that a cell-culture-derived, inactivated *R. rickettsii* vaccine would provide greater protective effect than the previously approved vaccines. Initial studies in nonhuman primates suggested efficacy; however, when administered to humans as a challenge trial, the results were disappointing.[50] No vaccinated volunteer was protected from illness, despite induction of serum antibody and *in vitro* correlates of cell-mediated immunity. The interpretation of all the studies suggests that the vaccine might be useful if the regimen were modified to include more rickettsial mass and more booster immunizations. To date no proven or approved vaccine for Rocky Mountain spotted fever exists. Research designed to investigate the important rickettsial factors toward which protective immune responses may be directed is in progress. The successful elucidation of rOMPs as targets for human vaccine development using recombinant proteins has revealed promising results in animal models.[57] A clearer understanding of the mechanisms by which intracellular infections are resolved and protective immunity is established are mandatory before another human vaccine can be proposed. Until then, the need will not diminish, but other methods for control will be required.

9.3. Treatment

Tetracycline (doxycycline) and chloramphenicol are specifically effective for treatment of Rocky Mountain spotted fever. They are rickettsiostatic, not rickettsicidal. Clinical manifestations subside promptly, if initiated early when the rash first appears. Any seriously ill child or adult who lives in a wooded area with unexplained fever, headache, and prostration, with or without a history of tick contact should be suspected of having Rocky Mountain spotted fever. Specific treatment should be initiated after blood is taken for diagnostic tests. Optimal antibiotic regimens include an initial dose of 25 mg/kg (tetracycline), 250 mg (doxycycline, adult dose), or 50 mg/kg (chloramphenicol). Subsequent daily doses of the same amounts are divided equally and given at 6- to 8-hr intervals until the patient has improved and has been afebrile for about 48 hr. Intravenous preparations are used in patients too ill to take oral medications.

Critically ill patients, first observed late in the course of illness, may be given large doses of corticosteroids (for treatment of the vasculitis) in combination with specific antibiotics for about 3 days. Such patients often show circulatory collapse, oliguria, anuria, azotemia, hyponatremia, hypochloremia, edema, and coma. In such patients who manifest increased capillary permeability, intravenous fluids should be given cautiously to avoid increasing pulmonary and cerebral edema. In mildly or moderately ill patients, these pathophysiological abnormalities are not present.

9.4. Antibiotic Prophylaxis

The question is often raised whether antibiotics should be given prophylactically after human exposure to virulent *R. rickettsii*. In guinea pigs, a single dose of oxytetracycline prevented the disease when the antibiotic was given shortly before expected onset. However, relapses occurred when treatment preceded expected onset by 48 hr or more.[58] This regimen is not recommended. After a tick bite in a known endemic area, an exposed person should be observed for signs of fever, headache, prostration, and rash; therapy is very effective at the early stage of illness.

10. Unresolved Problems

Specific chemotherapy of the rickettsial diseases was achieved in 1948. This event inadvertently diverted attention from pursuit of studies aimed at elucidating pathogenesis, pathophysiological abnormalities, and control by vaccines. Some unanswered puzzles awaiting solution are:

1. What is the nature of the increased capillary permeability and the cause of the characteristic vascular lesion? The specific molecular events leading to *Rickettsia*-mediated host membrane damage and the relative contributions of host derived "pathological" cytokine responses and their reversal needs clarification. There are favorable advances in understanding control of illness mediated by the untoward effects of cytokines. Are the changes a result of direct effects by rickettsiae within endothelial cells, an action of their toxins, a combination of both, or an immunopathologic reaction? Evidence does not permit the exclusion of any one mechanism.
2. Hematologic findings in severely ill patients with spotted fever and typhus show a disseminated intravascular coagulation defect late in illness. Its mechanism and the relationships of complement abnormalities merit study. Whether heparin treatment is indicated is not clear.
3. Therapy for early cases is simple and effective. For seriously ill patients during later stages, there is a need for better antitoxemic measures, which will evolve only when the nature of the pathological lesions and the toxic manifestations is understood. Short-term high-dose steroid treatment for several days combined with antibiotics is helpful and is unassociated with sequelae.
4. Spotted and typhus fever rickettsiae persist indefinitely within human cells, presumably within macrophages; Brill–Zinsser disease is a recurrence of epidemic typhus years after the initial infection. This is a remarkable example of microbial persistence. Conceivably, there is a Brill–Zinsser pattern for other rickettsial diseases such as spotted fever, murine and scrub typhus, and Q fever. An understanding of the intracellular growth requirements might provide leads to the complete inactivation of rickettsiae. An important lead will be the cultivation of rickettsiae on artificial media.
5. There is a need for better biological vaccines for prevention of typhus, spotted, and *Q* fevers. Inactivated Q fever vaccine is effective but causes reaction on repeated inoculation. A tissue-culture-derived inactivated vaccine for spotted fever is under development and appears promising. This system may be useful for production of better epidemic typhus vaccines. Live strain E vaccine for typhus is effective but reactive. There are no effective vaccines for scrub typhus. Whether the threat of certain of the rickettsial diseases for humans warrants research directed toward developing attenuated viable vaccines is a major concern.
6. The interrelationships of rickettsiae in animal hosts, vectors, and other environmental factors for epidemic and murine typhus, Rocky Mountain spotted fever, and Q fever are really underdeveloped. For example, there may be a significant reservoir of *R. prowazekii* other than man, such as flying squirrels. Fleas or lice may serve as vectors.

Current work by several investigators is directed to these questions.

11. References

1. Aikawa, J. K., *Rocky Mountain Spotted Fever*, Thomas, Springfield, IL, 1966.
2. Wilson, L. B., and Chowning, W. M., Studies in pyroplasmosis hominis ("spotted fever" or "tick fever" of the Rocky Mountains), *J. Infect. Dis.* **1:**31 (1904).
3. Ricketts, H. T., The study of "Rocky Mountain spotted fever" (tick fever) by means of animal inoculations, *J. Am. Med. Assoc.* **47:**1–10 (1906).
4. Ricketts, H. T., The role of the wood-tick (*Dermacentor occidentalis*) in Rocky Mountain spotted fever, and the susceptibility of local animals to this disease, *J. Am. Med. Assoc.* **49:**24 (1907).
5. McCalla, L. P., Direct transmission from man to man of the Rocky Mountain spotted (tick) fever, *Med. Sentinel* **16:**87 (1908).
6. Wolbach, S. B., Studies on Rocky Mountain spotted fever, *J. Med. Res.* **41:**1–97 (1919).
7. Spencer, R. R., and Parker, R. R., *Studies in Rocky Mountain Spotted Fever*, National Health Service, Hygienic Library Bull. No. 154, US Government Printing Office, Washington, DC, 1930.
8. Cox, H. R., Use of yolk sac of developing chick embryo as medium for growing rickettsiae of Rocky Mountain spotted fever and typhus groups, *Public Health Rep.* **53:**2241–2247 (1938).
9. Rose, H. M., Duane, R. B., and Fischell, E. E., The treatment of spotted fever with para-aminobenzoic acid, *J. Am. Med. Assoc.* **129:**1160–1163 (1945).
10. Woodward, T. E., and Jackson, E. B., Spotted fever rickettsiae, in: *Viral and Rickettsial Infection of Man*, 4th ed. (F. L. Horsfall, Jr., and T. Tamm, eds.), pp. 1095–1129, Lippincott, Philadelphia, 1965.
11. Pinkerton, H., and Maxcy, K. F., Pathological study of a case of endemic typhus in Virginia with demonstration of *Rickettsia*, *Am. J. Pathol.* **7:**95–103 (1931).
12. Dyer, R. E., Rumreich, A. S., and Badger, L. F., The typhus Rocky Mountain spotted fever group in the United States, *J. Am. Med. Assoc.* **97:**589 (1931).
13. Pincoffs, M. C., and Shaw, C. C., The eastern type of Rocky Mountain spotted fever. Report of a case with demonstration of *Rickettsia*, *Med. Clin. North Am.* **16:**1097–1113 (1933).
14. Dumler, J. S., Fatal Rocky Mountain spotted fever in Maryland—1901, *J. Am. Med. Assoc.* **265:**718 (1991).

15. Helmick, C. G., Bernard, K. W., and D'Angelo, L. J., Rocky Mountain spotted fever: Clinical, laboratory, and epidemiological features of 262 cases, *J. Infect. Dis.* **150:**480–486 (1984).
16. Pederson, C. E., Jr., Rocky Mountain spotted fever: A disease that must be recognized, *J. Am. Med. Technol.* **39:**190–198 (1977).
17. Sexton, D. J., Kanj, S. S., Wilson, K., *et al.*, The use of a polymerase chain reaction as a diagnostic test for Rocky Mountain spotted fever, *Am. J. Trop. Med. Hyg.* **50:**59–63 (1994).
18. Smadel, J. E., and Jackson, E. B., Rickettsial infections, in: *Diagnostic Procedures for Viral and Rickettsial Disease*, 3rd ed., pp. 743–771, American Public Health Association, New York, 1964.
19. Kelly, D. J., Serologic diagnosis of rickettsial diseases, *Clin. Immunol. Newslett.* **14:**57–61 (1994).
20. Dumler, J. S., and Walker, D. H., Diagnostic tests for Rocky Mountain spotted fever and other rickettsial diseases, *Dermatol. Clinics* **12:**25–36 (1994).
21. Clements, M. L., Dumler, J. S., Fiset, P., *et al.*, Serodiagnosis of Rocky Mountain spotted fever: Comparison of IgM and IgG enzyme-linked immunosorbent assays and indirect fluorescent antibody test, *J. Infect. Dis.* **148:**876–880 (1983).
22. Philip, R. N., Casper, E. A., Ormsbee, R. A., *et al.*, Microimmunofluorescence test for the serological study of Rocky Mountain spotted fever and typhus, *J. Clin. Microbiol.* **3:**51–61 (1976).
23. Hechemy, K. E., Michaelson, E. E., Anacker, R. L., *et al.*, Evaluation of latex–*Rickettsia rickettsii* test for Rocky Mountain spotted fever in 11 laboratories, *J. Clin. Microbiol.* **18:**938–946 (1983).
24. Radulovic, S., Speed, R., Feng, H.-M., *et al.*, EIA with species-specific monoclonal antibodies: A novel seroepidemiologic tool for determination of the etiologic agent of spotted fever rickettsiosis, *J. Infect. Dis.* **168:**1292–1295 (1993).
25. Marrero, M., and Raoult, D., Centrifugation-assisted shell vial technique for rapid detection of Mediterranean spotted fever rickettsiae in blood culture, *Am. J. Trop. Med. Hyg.* **40:**197–199 (1989).
26. Dumler, J. S., Gage, W. R., Pettis, G. L., *et al.*, Rapid immunoperoxidase demonstration of *Rickettsia rickettsii* in fixed cutaneous specimens from patients with Rocky Mountain spotted fever, *Am. J. Clin. Pathol.* **93:**410–414 (1990).
27. Walker, D. H., Cain, B. G., and Olmstead, P. M. Laboratory diagnosis of Rocky Mountain spotted fever by immunofluorescent demonstration of *Rickettsia rickettsii* in cutaneous lesions, *Am. J. Clin. Pathol.* **69:**619–623 (1978).
28. Woodward, T. E., Pedersen, C. E., Jr., Oster, C. N., *et al.*, Prompt confirmation of Rocky Mountain spotted fever: Identification of rickettsiae in skin tissues, *J. Infect. Dis.* **134:**293–301 (1976).
29. Walker, D. H., and Cain, B. G., A method for specific diagnosis of Rocky Mountain spotted fever on fixed, paraffin-embedded tissues by immunofluorescence, *J. Infect. Dis.* **137:**206–209 (1978).
30. Drancourt, M., George, F., Brouqui, P., *et al.*, Diagnosis of Mediterranean spotted fever by indirect immunofluorescence of *Rickettsia conorii* in circulating endothelial cells isolated with monoclonal antibody-coated immunomagnetic beads, *J. Infect. Dis.* **166:**660–663 (1992).
31. Fuller, H. S., Biologic properties of pathogenic rickettsiae, *Arch. Inst. Pasteur Tunis* **36:**311–338 (1959).
32. Price, W. H., The epidemiology of Rocky Mountain spotted fever: The characterization of strain virulence of *Rickettsia rickettsii*, *Am. J. Hyg.* **58:**248–268 (1953).
33. Kaplowitz, L. G., Lange, J. V., Fischer, J. J., and Walker, D. H., Correlation of rickettsial titers, circulating endotoxin and clinical features in Rocky Mountain spotted fever, *Arch. Intern. Med.* **143:**1149–1151 (1983).
34. Hackstadt, T., Messer, R., Cieplak, W., and Peacock, M. G., Evidence for proteolytic cleavage of the 120-kilodalton outer memebrane protein of rickettsiae: Identification of an avirulent mutant deficient in processing, *Infect. Immun.* **60:**159–165 (1992).
35. Li, H., and Walker, D. H., Characterization of rickettsial attachment to host cells by flow cytometry, *Infect. Immun.* **69:**2030–2035 (1992).
36. Heinzen, R. A., Hayes, S. F., Peacock, M. G., and Hackstadt, T., Directional actin polymerization associated with spotted fever group *Rickettsia* infection of Vero cells, *Infect. Immun.* **61:**1926–1935 (1993).
37. Hattwick, M. A., O'Brien, R. J., and Hanson, B. F., Rocky Mountain spotted fever: Epidemiology of an increasing problem, *Ann. Intern. Med.* **84:**732–739 (1976).
38. Cox, H. R., The spotted fever group, in: *Viral and Rickettsial Diseases of Man*, 3rd ed. (T. M. Rivers and F. L. Horsfall, Jr., eds.), pp. 828–868, Lippincott, Philadelphia, 1959.
39. Kohls, G. M., Vectors of rickettsial diseases, in: *Rickettsial Diseases of Man* (F. R. Moulton, ed.), pp. 83–96, American Association for the Advancement of Science, Washington, DC, 1948.
40. DuPont, H. L., Hornick, R. B., Dawkins, A. T., *et al.*, Rocky Mountain spotted fever: A comparative study of the active immunity induced by inactivated and viable pathogenic *Rickettsia rickettsii*, *J. Infect. Dis.* **128:**340–344 (1973).
41. Woodward, T. E., Rickettsial diseases in the United States, *Med. Clin. North Am.* **43:**1507–1535 (1959).
42. Ley, H. L., Jr., Diercks, F. H., Paterson, P. Y., *et al.*, Immunization against scrub typhus. IV. Living Karp vaccine and chemoprophylaxis in volunteers, *Am. J. Hyg.* **56:**303–312 (1952).
43. Tigertt, W. D., Studies on Q fever in man, in: *Symposium of Q Fever*, Med. Sci. Publ. Walter Reed Army Inst. Res., No. 6, pp. 39–46, US Government Printing Office, Washington, DC 1959.
44. Walker, D. H., Firth, W. T., Ballard, J. F., and Hegarty, B. C., Role of the phospholipase-associated penetration mechanism in cell injury by *Rickettsia rickettsii*, *Infect. Immun.* **40:**840–842 (1983).
45. Walker, T. S., Rickettsial interactions with human endothelial cells *in vitro*: Adherance and entry, *Infect. Immun.* **44:**205–210 (1984).
46. Silverman, D. J., and Santucci, L. A., Potential for free radical-induced lipid peroxidation as a cause of endothelial cell injury in Rocky Mountain spotted fever, *Infect. Immun.* **56:**3110–3115 (1988).
47. Feng, H.-M., and Walker, D. H., Interferon-γ and tumor necrosis factor-α exert their antirickettsial effect via induction of synthesis of nitric oxide, *Am. J. Pathol.* **143:**1016–1023 (1993).
48. Sporn, L. A., Lawrence, S. O., Silverman, D. J., Marder, V. J., E-selectin-dependent neutrophil adhesion to *Rickettsia rickettsii*-infected endothelial cells, *Blood* **81:**2406–2412 (1993).
49. Feng, H.-M., Wen, J., and Walker, D. H., *Rickettsia australis* infection: A murine model of a highly invasive vasculopathic rickettsiosis, *Am. J. Pathol.* **142:**1471–1482 (1993).
50. Clements, M. L., Wisseman, C. L., Woodward, T. E., *et al.*, Reactogenicity, immunogenicity, and efficacy of a chick embryo cell-derived vaccine for Rocky Mountain spotted fever, *J. Infect. Dis.* **148:**922–930 (1983).
51. Watt, G., and Strickman, D., Life-threatening scrub typhus in a traveller returning from Tahiland, *Clin. Infect. Dis.* **186:**624–626 (1994).

52. McDonald, J. C., MacLean, J. D., and McDade, J. E., Imported rickettsial disease: Clinical and epidemiologic features, *Am. J. Med.* **85:**799–805 (1988).
53. Spencer, R. R., and Parker, R. R., Rocky Mountain spotted fever: Infectivity of fasting and recently fed ticks, *Public Health Rep.* **38:**33 (1923).
54. Spencer, R. R., and Parker, R. R., Studies on Rocky Mountain spotted fever: Vaccination of monkeys and man, *Public Health Rep.* **40:**2159 (1925).
55. Parker, R. R., Rocky Mountain spotted fever: Results of fifteen years of prophylactic vaccination, *Am. J. Trop. Med.* **21:**369 (1941).
56. Smadel, J. E., Rocky Mountain spotted fever vaccine, in: *Symposium on the Spotted Fever Group*, Med. Sci. Publ. No. 7 WRAIR 55-61, US Government Printing Office, Washington, DC, 1960.
57. McDonald, G. A., Anacker, R. L., Mann, R. E., and Milch, L. J., Protection of guinea pigs from experimental Rocky Mountain spotted fever with a cloned antigen of *Rickettsia rickettsii*, *J. Infect. Dis.* **158:**228–231 (1988).
58. Kenyon, R. H., Williams, R. G., Oster, C. N., and Pedersen, C. E., Jr., Prophylactic treatment of Rocky Mountain spotted fever, *J. Clin. Microbiol.* **8:**102–104 (1978).

12. Suggested Reading

Harrell, G. T., Rocky Mountain spotted fever, *Medicine* **28:**333–370 (1949).

Hattwick, M. A. W., O'Brien, R. J., and Hanson, B. F., Rocky Mountain spotted fever: Epidemiology of an increasing problem, *Ann. Intern. Med.* **84:**732–739 (1976).

Hechemy, K. E., Laboratory diagnosis of Rocky Mountain spotted fever, *N. Engl. J. Med.* **300:**859–860 (1979).

Philip, R. N., Casperie, A., MacCormack, J. N., *et al.*, A comparison of serologic methods for diagnosis of Rocky Mountain spotted fever, *Am. J. Epidemiol.* **105:**56–67 (1977).

Soneshine, D. E., Bozeman, M. F., Williams, M. S., *et al.*, Epizootiology of epidemic typhus (*Rickettsia prowazeki*) in flying squirrels, *Am. J. Trop. Med. Hyg.* **27:**339–349 (1978).

Woodward, T. E., Section 10, The Rickettsioses, *Harrison's Principles of Internal Medicine*, 9th ed., pp. 746–759, McGraw-Hill, New York, 1980.

Woodward, T. E., and Jackson, E. B., Spotted fever rickettsiae, in: *Viral and Rickettsial Infections of Man*, 4th ed. (F. L. Horsfall, Jr., and T. Tamm, eds.), pp. 1095–1129, Lippincott, Philadelphia, 1965.

CHAPTER 31

Salmonellosis: Nontyphoidal

Robert V. Tauxe and Andrew T. Pavia

1. Introduction

Nontyphoidal salmonellosis refers to disease caused by any serotype of organisms in the genus *Salmonella*, other than *Salmonella* Typhi, the causative agent of typhoid fever (see Chapter 42). The most common manifestation of nontyphoidal salmonellosis is acute enterocolitis, but the organism can cause focal infection, bacteremia, meningitis, as well as "enteric fever" that may be clinically indistinguishable from that caused by *S.* Typhi. Nontyphoidal salmonellosis is a disease of considerable clinical and public health importance. An estimated 2 to 4 million cases of salmonellosis occur each year in the United States, of which a small fraction are cultured and reported. The direct patient care costs alone have been estimated to exceed $2 billion annually, but when one considers the added costs of plant closings, product recalls, and losses of food production, the true economic impact of salmonellosis is likely to be substantially greater.[1]

Over 2000 serotypes of *Salmonella* have been described.[2] The nomenclature of *Salmonella* has undergone considerable evolution over recent years, which has led to some confusion. By DNA hybridization, six subgroups have been identified within what is now referred to as the species *Salmonella enterica*. Most *Salmonella* serotypes associated with human diseases belong to subgroup 1, but strains in subgroup 3, referred to as the Arizona group, are occasionally isolated. Previously, the genus *Salmonella* was classified into three primary species: *S.* Typhi, *S.* Cholerae-suis, and *S.* Enteritidis; Arizona organisms were in a separate genus. The species *Salmonella* Typhi and *Salmonella* Cholerae-suis consisted of a single serotype each; the remaining 2000 serotypes were in the species *Salmonella* Enteritidis. Now, all *Salmonella* and Arizona are subsumed under the single species *Salmonella enterica*.[2] The formal designation of a serotype might be *S. enterica* serotype Typhimurium or *S. enterica* serotype Enteritidis. To avoid the awkwardness present in this and previous nomenclatures, we will designate each serotype directly, without reference to the full species name. Thus, *Salmonella enterica* serotype Typhimurium is written *Salmonella* Typhimurium and *Salmonella enterica* serotype Enteritidis is written *Salmonella* Enteritidis.

Salmonellae probably evolved with the reptiles and birds and are well adapted to a variety of host animals. The diversity of serotypes reflects this diversity of hosts, as many serotypes have a narrow host range. For example, clinically important infections due to *S.* Typhi occur only in humans, and humans are the only known reservoir for this organism. The primary reservoir of *S.* Pullorum, *S.* Gallinarum, and *S.* Heidelberg is chickens; the reservoir of *S.* Cholerae-suis is pigs; for *S.* Bovis-morbificans it is cows; *S.* Marinum is the marine iguana; and *S.* Java, *S.* Urbana, and *S.* Litchfield are predominantly turtle-associated. Nonetheless, all serotypes should be considered potentially pathogenic for humans and animals. In addition to distinctive host ranges, many serotypes exhibit unique patterns of virulence, antibiotic resistance, and geographic distribution that make the epidemiology of *Salmonella* particularly fascinating and complex.[3]

2. Historical Background

Salmon and Smith[4] reported the isolation of "hog cholera bacillus," later named *S.* Cholerae-suis, from

Robert V. Tauxe • Foodborne and Diarrheal Diseases Branch, Division of Bacterial and Mycotic Diseases, National Center for Infectious Diseases, Centers for Disease Control and Prevention, Atlanta, Georgia 30333. **Andrew T. Pavia** • Department of Medicine, Division of Pediatric Infectious Diseases, University of Utah Medical Center, Salt Lake City, Utah 84132.

diarrheic swine in 1885. Three years later, Gaertner[5] reported the first foodborne outbreak of nontyphoidal salmonellosis, in which 58 persons fell ill after eating raw meat from an ill cow; "Gaertner's bacillus," later named *S.* Enteritidis, was isolated from the meat, and from the spleen of a man who died in the outbreak. In 1889, Loeffler isolated *S.* Typhimurium during an outbreak of diarrheal illness in a laboratory mouse colony; the same organism was demonstrated among victims of a meat-associated outbreak in Aertrycke, Belgium, in 1899.[6,7] By the turn of the century, the pathogenic potential of *Salmonella* for humans was widely appreciated in Europe, and following World War I, salmonellosis emerged as a common public health problem on that continent. Between 1923 and 1938, 374 outbreaks due to 11 different serotypes of nontyphoidal salmonellae were reported in the United Kingdom.[6] *S.* Enteritidis infections associated with duck eggs became common in Europe and led to the decline of this once popular food before World War II.[8] In 1941, Kauffmann[6] presented an expanded version of White's approach to the great antigenic diversity of *Salmonella*. The Kauffmann–White schema defined the antigenic formula of each serotype, and provided the widely used nomenclature that we have followed here.

In the United States, nontyphoidal salmonellosis did not emerge as a public health problem until after World War II. The number of reported clinical cases increased from 502 in 1942, the first year that the condition was made nationally reportable, to 65,347 in 1985 (the year of a large milk-associated outbreak) and declining to 41,641 in 1993 (Fig. 1). Over the same time, typhoid fever, caused by *S.* Typhi, became rare. In 1962, following a

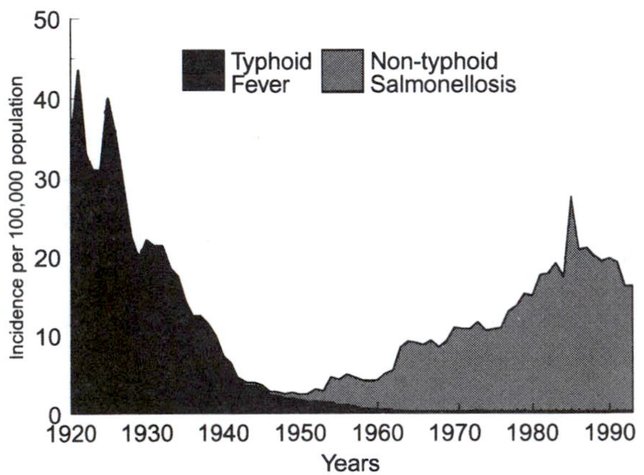

Figure 1. Reported incidence of clinical typhoid fever and nontyphoidal salmonellosis in the United States, 1920–1993. Data from the CDC.[12]

large multistate outbreak of egg-associated *S.* Derby infections, a second national surveillance system for *Salmonella* was instituted, based on reports of laboratory isolates, which thus includes serotype. This surveillance system, coupled with intensive epidemiological investigations, has helped to clarify our understanding of the complex routes of *Salmonella* transmission. As a result of this improved understanding, specific control measures have been implemented. The reported incidence of salmonellosis increased rapidly from the late 1970s until 1988, and has declined slightly since then, indicating the need for further improvements in our efforts to control this pathogen of the modern era.

3. Methodology

3.1. Sources of Mortality Data

Data are limited on the mortality resulting from salmonellosis in the United States. Deaths due to salmonellosis are not routinely reported to the Centers for Disease Control and Prevention (CDC) surveillance systems. Mortality can be estimated from periodic nationwide surveys of sentinel counties (see Section 3.3), from death certificates, and from epidemiological investigations. The surveys of sentinel counties probably give the most reliable overall estimate of mortality, since all reported cases are actively investigated. These studies yielded a mortality rate of between 0.5 and 1.4%, which is similar to that found in 16 years of surveillance in Massachusetts,[9] but lower than the 4.1% mortality rate observed in New York between 1939 and 1955.[10] Applied to the approximately 40,000 infections that are reported annually, this yields an estimate of 200–560 deaths per year. A similar number of deaths may occur related to the much larger number of unreported infections that occur. In outbreaks, the typical case-fatality rate is 0.1% of affected persons.[11] This is lower than the mortality for reported cases because outbreak investigations identify many milder cases that would not be cultured, diagnosed, or reported had they occurred as sporadic cases. Sixty to one hundred deaths per year due to salmonellosis are identified from death certificate data.[12] Death certificates may not reflect the bacteriologic diagnosis in patients dying of gastroenteritis, dehydration, sepsis, or meningitis if appropriate cultures are not obtained or culture results are not available at the time of death. Deaths due to *Salmonella* may be hidden in those attributed to septicemia, meningitis, or cardiopulmonary arrest.

3.2. Sources of Morbidity Data

Since 1962, the laboratory-based National *Salmonella* Surveillance Program has been conducted by the CDC working jointly with the Council of State and Territorial Epidemiologists, the Association of State and Territorial Public Health Laboratory Directors, the US Department of Agriculture, and the US Food and Drug Administration. This program is based on weekly reports of *Salmonella* isolations from the states and from the District of Columbia, and regular summaries of nonhuman isolates from the Food and Drug Administration and the US Department of Agriculture. All laboratories are requested to forward clinical isolates of *Salmonella* to the state or regional laboratory for serotyping, and the results are reported along with information on sex, age, county of residence, and site of isolation. Since 1993, these data are transmitted, collected and analyzed electronically via the Public Health Laboratory Information System (PHLIS).[13] The purpose of this laboratory-based surveillance program is to define patterns of endemic salmonellosis in the United States, to identify trends in disease transmission, and to monitor control efforts. The predecessor to this system, based on physicians' reports of cases, began in 1942 when nontyphoidal salmonellosis became a notifiable disease, and continues to function in parallel. The clinical case-reporting system yields comparable numbers of cases, but because case definitions vary from state to state and the reports do not include serotype, it is of limited epidemiological use.

Limitations and biases exist in the laboratory-based data as well. The reports do not discriminate between symptomatic and asymptomatic cases, and cases of salmonellosis without laboratory confirmation are not included. Several factors influence whether a case of salmonellosis will be reported to the *Salmonella* surveillance system, including the following: the severity of illness, access to medical care, and the association with a recognized outbreak. Physicians may be more likely to obtain stool cultures from infants and elderly persons with gastroenteritis than from young adults, and illness in these age groups may be oversampled. By comparing the number of cases detected in outbreak investigations with the number of outbreak-related cases that are reported to the *Salmonella* surveillance system, it is possible to estimate the sensitivity of the system. Reviewing a series of outbreaks in the 1960s, Aserkoff[14] estimated that 1% symptomatic infections were reported to the laboratory-based surveillance system. Using a variety of methods, including extrapolation from the carrier rate, estimating sequential error in the reporting system, and reviewing recent outbreaks, Chalker and Blaser[15] estimated that between 1 and 5% of infections are reported. Laboratory-based incidence rates can also be obtained from limited defined populations such as health maintenance organizations.

3.3. Surveys and Investigations

Because of the inherent limitations of nationwide surveillance, other studies have been performed to obtain a more detailed picture of the epidemiology of salmonellosis. In 1979– 1980, the CDC performed a survey of all persons from whom *Salmonella* was isolated in a randomly selected, stratified sample of counties.[16] Patients were administered a detailed epidemiological questionnaire concerning exposures, symptoms, and complications, and the isolates were examined for antimicrobial resistance. A similar survey was repeated in the same sentinel counties at 5-year intervals since: 1984–1985,[17] 1989–1990,[18] and 1994–1995 (in progress).

The most detailed information on the epidemiology of salmonellosis has come from outbreak investigations. These investigations provide the opportunity to determine vehicles of transmission, the spectrum of illness, and risk factors for infection and for poor clinical outcomes. Case–control methods and molecular biological techniques for precisely defining the strains involved have made the outbreak investigation an occasion for extraordinarily fruitful research,[19] and outbreak investigations have in turn spawned systematic studies. Examples include studies of the decline of turtle-associated serotype[20] and studies of the dissemination of chloramphenicol-resistant *S.* Newport following an outbreak in California.[21]

3.4. Laboratory Diagnosis

3.4.1. Isolation and Identification. Members of the *Salmonella–Arizona* group are gram-negative, flagellated, nonsporulating, aerobic bacilli. *Salmonella* can usually be directly isolated from primary plates inoculated with stool or rectal swabs from persons with *Salmonella* enterocolitis. The diagnostic yield may be slightly higher if one uses an aliquot of 5–10 g of feces rather than a rectal swab, particularly when attempting to identify *Salmonella* carriers, who may be shedding only small numbers of organisms. As carriers may shed *Salmonella* intermittently, culturing specimens on two or more occasions may increase the likelihood of detection. In clinical laboratories, an enrichment broth is also recommended to increase the isolation of Salmonella from stool specimens.[22] Three selective enrichment media are in widespread use to isolate *Salmonella*: tetrathionate broth, tetrathionate broth with brilliant green, and selenite F broth. Many microbiologists prefer to use either selenite or tetrathionate without the brilliant green dye because neither inhibits *S.* Typhi, in contrast to tetrathionate brilliant green broth. Numerous selective plating media, varying from low to high selectivity, have been used to isolate *Salmonella* from fecal specimens. The purpose of these selective media is to suppress the growth of other Enterobacteriaceae. MacConkey, eosin–methylene blue (EMB), and deoxycholate agar are media of low selectivity. *Salmonella–Shigella* (SS), Hektoen enteric (HE), and xylose–lysine–desoxycholate–citrate (XLD) agars are widely used to screen for *Salmonella* and *Shigella* because they support the growth of both organisms and are considered moderately selective media. When laboratory resources permit the use of an additional plate, highly selective media such as brilliant green or bismuth sulfite agar may be superior to the less selective media. Bismuth sulfite agar is the preferred medium for isolating *S.* Typhi. For specimens obtained from a normally sterile source such as blood or cerebrospinal fluid (CSF), using selective media has no advantage.

Colonies that are suspicious for *Salmonella* should be further identified by a chemical test. At least two representatives of each type of suspicious colony should be selected and transferred to either triple sugar iron (TSI) or Kliger's iron (KI agar). Lysine iron agar (LIA) indicates the decarboxylation or deamination of lysine and the production of hydrogen sulfide, and is particularly helpful when used in conjunction with TSI agar for the presumptive identification of *Salmonella*. The usual reaction of *Salmonella* on TSI or KI will be an alkaline slant and acid butt, and they will produce gas and H_2S. Lactose-positive strains may occasionally occur that will produce an acid slant and do not produce H_2S or gas. On LIA, the usual reaction is an alkaline slant and alkaline butt with production of H_2S. Isolates can be screened for *Salmonella* antigens using a polyvalent O or H antiserum. Colonies with typical TSI and LIA reactions that react to polyvalent O and H antisera are presumptively considered to be *Salmonella*.

If stool specimens must be transported, as is often necessary in epidemiological investigations, a swab coated with feces should be placed in a transport medium and held refrigerated until it can be examined. Commonly used transport media include Stewart's, Amies, Cary Blair, and buffered glycerol saline. Of these, Cary Blair is the most suitable general transport medium.[22]

Rapid diagnostic tests using enzyme immunoassay, latex agglutination, or other immunologic methods to detect *Salmonella* in feces and in foods are under development.

3.4.2. Serological Diagnostic Methods. Salmonellae, as do other Enterobacteriaceae, possess somatic (O) and flagellar (H) antigens. The O antigenic determinants define the serogroup, and the H antigens further break these down into more than 2000 serotypes, according to the Kauffmann–White schema. This great variety is achieved because most *Salmonella* have a unique ability to express at least two separate sets of flagellar antigens. When they encounter antibodies to their usual flagella, they produce a second set, with unrelated antigens. Variations in each set of antigens and in the order in which they appear define the large number of serotypes present in each serogroup. Each serogroup has a major determinant and one or more minor somatic antigens. Serogroups A through I have been identified; most serotypes that cause human disease fall into serogroups A through E. Many clinical laboratories can readily identify serogroup using commercial polyvalent group antisera. Further identification of specific serotype is usually performed by a public health laboratory or other reference laboratory. Serotype determination is extremely useful in epidemiological investigations since many serotypes have specific reservoirs, host ranges, virulence, and age specificity.

Since the ten most common serotypes account for 70% of human isolates in the United States, laboratory techniques for further subtyping a common serotype are often useful for epidemiological purposes.[19] Antimicrobial resistance patterns are the simplest method of further characterizing an epidemic strain. Plasmid profiles have proved useful in defining outbreak strains.[23–26] Phagetyping schemes for *S.* Typhimurium and other serotypes have been used extensively for epidemiological purposes in England and Canada and are the most practical means available for subtyping *S.* Enteritidis.[27] Pulsed-field gel electrophoresis of chromosomal digests is also under investigation as a tool for answering specific epidemiologic questions.

The antibody response to human *Salmonella* infection has not been useful for serodiagnosis. *Salmonella* enterocolitis does not always provoke a measurable serological response. The Widal reaction, used historically to diagnose *S.* Typhi infection, measures agglutinating antibodies to O and H antigens of *S.* Typhi. The usefulness of this test has been severely hampered by nonspecific cross-reactivity with other *Salmonella* antigens, elevated titers due to nonspecific inflammatory disease, antibodies due to typhoid vaccination, and the suppression of O and H agglutinins by early treatment.[28]

4. Biological Characteristics of the Organism

Salmonellae are a hardy and resourceful group of organisms. They successfully parasitize a broad variety of hosts including insects, reptiles, amphibians, birds, and mammals. Although not true spore-formers, they are resistant to drying and freezing and may survive for long periods in a nutrient-poor environment. The organism can survive for over 200 days in contaminated soil, 10 months in dust, more than 5 months in roach and rodent feces, and more than 4 years in dried whole egg. They multiply in food at temperatures ranging from 44 to 114°F (7 to 46°C) and can survive at a pH as low as 4.5.[29]

Many salmonellae have life cycles in nature that guarantee long-term survival. Some have the ability to colonize specific loci in the gastrointestinal tract, tolerating the mild acidity of the animal's rumen or crop, or the bile in the gallbladder. Others have the ability to colonize the reproductive tracts of reptiles and birds, which means that the bacteria can infect the contents of eggs as they are formed, passing vertically to the next generation before it emerges from the shell; the evolution of this capacity well insulates such salmonellae from the environment.

Antimicrobial Resistance

The resistance of *Salmonella* to antimicrobial agents has been a matter of increasing concern. Antimicrobial resistance is important for clinical and public health reasons. Although antimicrobial treatment is not necessary in uncomplicated *Salmonella* enterocolitis and appears to prolong carriage,[30] antimicrobial treatment is essential in extraintestinal infections. The emergence of multiply resistant strains can lead to treatment failures in this setting and may require the use of new and more expensive antibiotics. Antimicrobial resistance in *Salmonella* also has several important public health ramifications because simultaneous exposure to antimicrobials is associated with an increased risk of infection with resistant *Salmonella*. In one outbreak, 12 of 18 persons infected with the outbreak strain of multiply resistant *S.* Newport had taken a penicillin derivative in the week before the onset of their illness, compared to 0 of 11 persons infected with sensitive strains of *S.* Newport.[23] In most cases, illness began within 3 days after taking the antibiotic, suggesting that the antibiotic provided a selective advantage for the resistant organism and converted asymptomatic colonization to overt infection. Exposure to antimicrobials can also lower the infectious dose for a resistant strain. This was demonstrated in a massive outbreak of multiply resistant *S.* Typhimurium infections in 1985.[31] In that outbreak, two brands of milk were contaminated, and the amount of implicated milk that persons reported drinking was an index of the dose of *Salmonella* they had received. Some persons affected by the outbreak had taken an antimicrobial to which the outbreak strain of *S.* Typhimurium was resistant just before becoming ill with salmonellosis. These persons reported drinking smaller volumes of implicated milk than ill persons not taking such antimicrobials, suggesting that a smaller dose of *Salmonella* caused illness in the former group.

At any given moment, some fraction of the population is taking antimicrobials for a variety of reasons. Because those persons appear to have heightened susceptibility to resistant strains of *Salmonella*, an outbreak due to a resistant strain may produce a somewhat larger number of cases than would an outbreak due to a sensitive strain. From 16 to 64% of cases in outbreaks of resistant *Salmonella* infections can be called "excess cases," occurring as a result of this interaction between resistance and prior or concurrent use of antimicrobials.[32]

The overall level of antimicrobial resistance of *Salmonella* isolates appears to be increasing. In the sentinel county survey of *Salmonella* isolates conducted by the CDC in 1989–1990, 31% of isolates were resistant to at least one antimicrobial,[18] a significant increase over the 16% resistance demonstrated in a similar survey in 1979–1980. The number of multiply resistant strains rose from 12% to 25%. The most frequent resistance was to streptomycin, an antibiotic seldom used to treat humans (Table 1). Resistance is increasing to tetracycline, sulfamethoxazole, ampicillin, and, most worrisomely, to gentamicin, which was recently introduced into common use for the treatment of poultry. The level of resistance and specific resistance patterns closely resemble those found in *Salmonella* isolated from slaughtered chickens.[33]

Considerable evidence has accumulated that points to the major role of antimicrobial use in food animals that become a source of human infections with antimicrobial-resistant *Salmonella* in the United States. In the 1984 sentinel county survey, the drugs to which *Salmonella* were likely to be resistant were frequently ones that are seldom used in treating human infections, including streptomycin, nitrofurantoin, and kanamycin, yet these drugs are frequently used in animal husbandry.[32] This increase in tetracycline resistance noted above occurred despite the fact that the number of prescriptions dispensed for human use of tetracycline decreased 61% between 1973 and 1984. During that period, tetracyclines continued to be used extensively as growth enhancers, particularly among cattle. More compelling evidence comes from outbreak investigations in which resistant strains have been traced

Table 1. Rates of Resistance to Specific Antimicrobials for Salmonellosis, Sentinel County Surveys, 1979–1980, 1984–1985, and 1989–1990[a]

	Percent of isolates resistant		
Antimicrobial	1979–1980 (*n* = 511)	1984–1985 (*n* = 485)	1989–1990 (*n* = 484)
Ampicillin	8	9	14
Cephalexin	1.4	0.8	0.2
Chloramphenicol	0.8	2	3
Colistin	0	0.4	0
Gentamicin	0	0.6	4
Kanamycin	3.5	3.5	8
Nalidixic acid	0	1.2	0.2
Nitrofurantoin	1	3.7	1
Streptomycin	12	12.2	23
Sulfisoxazole	8	7	14
Tetracycline	8.6	13	24
Trimethoprim–sulfamethoxazole	0.2	0.6	0.4
Any agent	17	26	31
Two or more agents	12	17	25

[a]Adapted from MacDonald,[17] 1978–1980 and 1984–1985, and Lee,[18] 1989–1990.

from ill persons back through the food distribution chain to the farm. In one outbreak a multiply resistant strain of *S.* Newport was traced from ill persons in one state back through supermarket distribution and the meat processing plant to a farm where the beef cattle had been fed nontherapeutic doses of chlortetracycline.[23] In another outbreak, almost 1000 persons in California became infected with a strain of chloramphenicol-resistant *S.* Newport with a unique plasmid profile. The chain of transmission was followed from ill persons, to hamburger, to beef from meat packers, to slaughterhouses, and, finally, to cows and calves on farms where chloramphenicol had been used.[25] At each stage, the unique epidemic strain of *S.* Newport was isolated. Experience in other countries suggest that decreased use of antimicrobials in animal feed may result in a decrease in antimicrobial-resistant strains of *Salmonella* causing human infection.

5. Descriptive Epidemiology

5.1. Prevalence and Incidence

Between the inception of national laboratory-based *Salmonella* surveillance in 1962 and 1976, the incidence of reported *Salmonella* isolations in humans increased slightly. Between 1976 and 1986, the incidence rose by more than 60%, from 10.6/100,000 in 1976 to 17.4/100,000 in 1986, and then declined to 15 per 100,000 in 1994. This overall trend includes a sharp peak in *S.* Typhimurium infections related to a massive milk-associated outbreak in 1985, a dramatic increase in the isolation rate of *S.* Enteritidis more recently, and an increase and then decrease in *S.* Heidelberg (Fig. 2). This increase in reported isolates was paralleled by an increase in clinical cases reported to the *Morbidity and Mortality Weekly Report* during the same period (Fig. 1). The actual number of infections occurring is likely to be 2 million, the vast majority of which are mild and undiagnosed (see Section 3.2). The isolation rate in a Washington health maintenance organization (HMO) in 1985 was 21/100,000, close to the national surveillance figure.[34]

The epidemiology of *Salmonella* infection varies considerably by serotype. *S.* Typhimurium accounts for 15–25% of human isolates and comes from a variety of different sources, including meat, poultry, and eggs. *S.* Enteritidis has emerged as a dominant serotype in the United States and many other industrialized nations.[35,36] This serotype is strongly egg-associated: between 1985 and 1991, 82% of *S.* Enteritidis outbreaks with known vehicle were egg-associated and the same is true for sporadic infections.[37,38]

The 10 most common serotypes account for 67% of infections. Six of these are also among the top ten reported from nonhuman sources (Table 2).[39] *S.* Newport has an important bovine reservoir. *S.* Heidelberg, *S.* Thompson, and *S.* Montevideo appear to have poultry reservoirs. *S.* Hadar, first isolated in the United States in 1976, has become a common serotype, with a reservoir first in turkeys and more recently in chickens.

The general increase in the incidence of salmonellosis in the United States parallels similar increases seen in many industrialized countries. Several factors contributed to the increase, including changes in methods of producing food animals and shipping them to slaughter and the increased mechanization of animal slaughter. Changes in the cooking practices of the population are also of concern, including a greater reliance on precooked convenience foods, on foods eaten outside of the home, and a decline in what children learn about cooking at home and in school. The more recent decrease in salmonellosis, particularly in serotypes other than *S.* Enteritidis, may reflect greater attention to contamination control in animal husbandry and slaughter, as well as efforts to improve food-handling practices.

The prevalence of *Salmonella* carriage among the general population is not known with accuracy in the

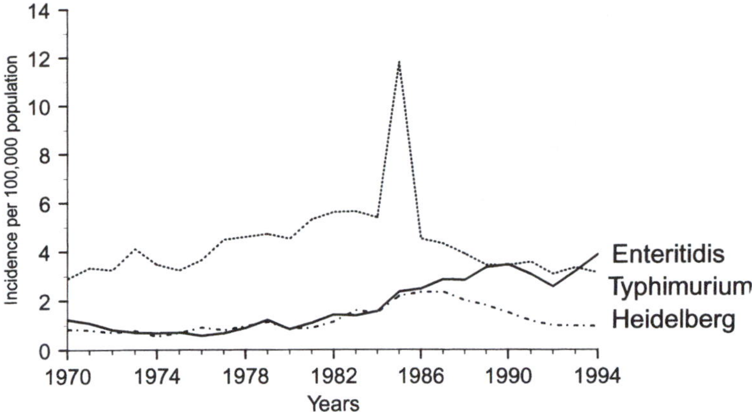

Figure 2. Isolation rates for selected serotypes of *Salmonella* in the United States by year, 1970–1994. From the CDC (unpublished data).

United States, but it is estimated to be between 0.15 and 0.2%.[15,40]

5.2. Epidemic Behavior and Contagiousness

Most cases of human salmonellosis result from contaminated food, although infection has been transmitted by an enormous variety of other vehicles (see Section 6). Cases may occur as part of recognized outbreaks but the majority occur as sporadic cases.

Recognized outbreaks of salmonellosis that are reported to the CDC account for less than 10% of reported isolates in most years. In 1973–1987, the median size of reported outbreaks of *Salmonella* infections was 20 persons, suggesting that only relatively large outbreaks were identified and reported.[12] In the 1979–1980 sentinel county survey, only 21% of reported isolates were associated with outbreaks or linked to other cases reported to local health departments. The remaining cases were not associated with other cases or recognized outbreaks and are considered "sporadic."[16] Case–control studies of sporadic cases relate illness to the same exposures as outbreaks, and in some cases it has been possible to link many "sporadic" cases to a common source.[24,38]

Salmonella outbreaks often have distinctive patterns. Most distinctive is the explosive outbreak from a common source of exposure, dramatically exemplified by the massive milk-borne outbreak in Illinois in 1985 involving more than 16,000 reported cases.[31] A pattern more difficult to recognize is the prolonged epidemic curve associated with continued exposure to a widely distributed contaminated food source or product, such as the outbreaks due to *S.* Newport-contaminated roast beef in several northeastern states,[24] *S.* Eastborne in contaminated chocolate,[41] *S.* Newbrunswick in powdered milk,[42] or marijuana contaminated with *S.* Muenchen.[26] These outbreaks are most easily recognized when they involve an unusual serotype. It is likely, though, that many small foodborne outbreaks occur in families, and this has led to difficulty determining the relative importance of foodborne versus intrafamilial spread. In one study, 39% of cases of salmonellosis in infants were preceded by gastroenteritis in an adult family member, suggesting that intrafamilial spread to infants may follow salmonellosis in other family members.[43] In general, sustained person-to-person transmission of salmonellosis is unlikely (see Section 5.8).

Table 2. The Ten Most Common Serotypes Identified Among Human *Salmonella* Infections and Nonhuman Sources in 1992[a]

Human			Nonhuman		
Serotype	No. of isolates	%	Serotype	No. of isolates	%
Typhimurium	7894	22.9	Enteritidis	4734	19.4
Enteritidis	6547	19.0	Typhimurium	3270	13.4
Heidelberg	2519	7.3	Heidelberg	2409	9.9
Hadar	1526	4.4	Choleraesuis	1307	5.4
Newport	1478	4.3	Hadar	1207	5.4
Agona	748	2.2	Montevideo	904	3.7
Thompson	689	2.0	Agona	828	3.4
Javiana	646	1.9	Kentucky	755	3.1
Oranienberg	595	1.7	Reading	619	2.5
Montevideo	558	1.6	Senftenberg	571	2.3
Other	11320	32.8	Other	7798	32
Total	34520		Total	24402	

[a]From the CDC.[39]

5.3. Geographic Distribution

Nontyphoidal salmonellosis appears to be predominantly a disease of industrialized nations and industrialized agriculture. Worldwide, the proportion of *Salmonella* infections due to nontyphoid serotypes of *Salmonella* appears to increase with the degree of economic development, while the proportion due to *S.* Typhi declines (Fig. 3).

Isolation rates vary considerably across the United States. Differences in reported isolation rates between states must be interpreted with caution since it has been shown that isolation rates correlate with per capita state laboratory expenditure and with the number of stool cultures submitted to the state laboratory.[46] Consistent regional differences exist, however, with the highest rates observed in the New England, Middle Atlantic, and Pacific states and the lowest rates in the West and West–North Central states, suggesting that real variations may exist in *Salmonella* exposure.

Within the United States, considerable geographic variation exists among serotypes. For example, *S.* Enteritidis has been particularly common in the Northeastern part of the United States, often greatly exceeding the number of *S.* Typhimurium isolates there, and is now increasing rapidly in the West, where *S.* Newport and *S.* Dublin have long been concentrated (Fig. 4). *S.* Javiana is associated with the South.

5.4. Temporal Distribution

Salmonella isolation shows a consistent seasonal pattern, with a summer and fall peak. This seasonal pattern is the result of seasonal variation in levels of infection of animals and in the resulting contamination of foods, as well as from the more rapid growth of *Salmonella* at warmer temperatures. The seasonal distribution varies among the different serotypes.

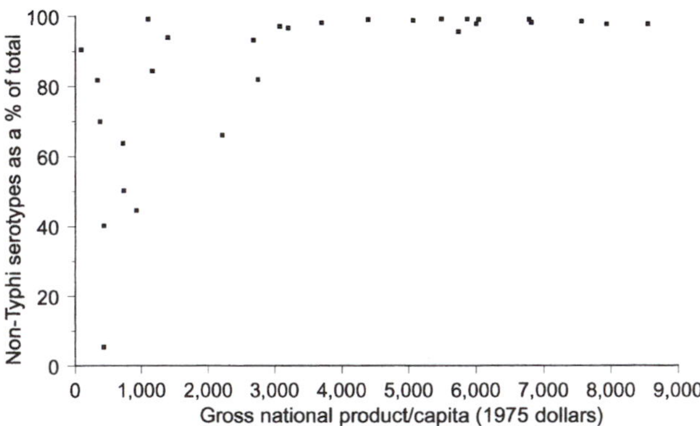

Figure 3. Nontyphoid serotypes as a percentage of all *Salmonella* isolates (including *S.* Typhi) as a function of per capita gross national product, showing the increasing importance of nontyphoidal salmonellosis with increased economic development. Data from Rowe[44] and United Nations.[45]

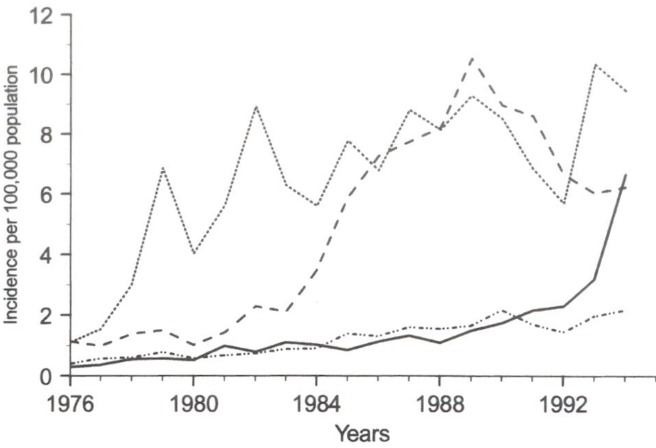

Figure 4. Annual isolation rate of *Salmonella* Enteritidis, United States 1976–1994, by region. From the CDC (unpublished data).

5.5. Age and Sex

The age- and sex-specific isolation rates for *Salmonella* is shown in Fig. 5. The isolation rate is highest in the first year of life, peaking at more than 180 cases per 100,000 population per year in the second month of life. The rate of infection declines rapidly among individuals 10 to 19 years old and then begins to rise among those older than 60. Some degree of detection bias probably exists, since infants and the elderly may be more likely to have stool cultures performed when they are diagnosed with gastrointestinal infection. Nonetheless, this pattern

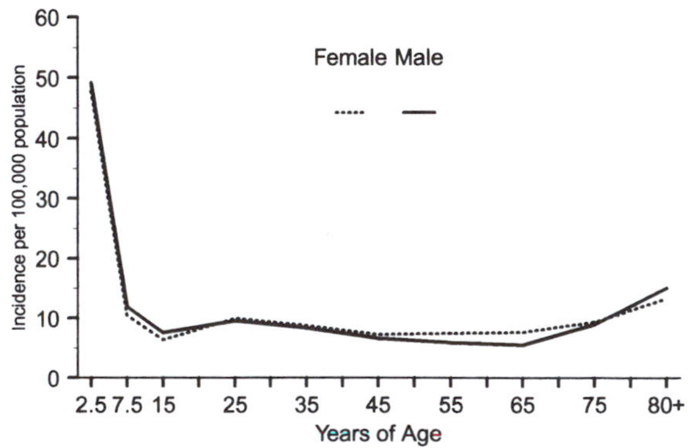

Figure 5. *Salmonella* isolation rates by age and sex, per 100,000 population, United States, 1992. From the CDC (unpublished data).

probably reflects real age-specific differences in host susceptibility and in exposure rates. Substantial differences exist in the age specificity among the various serotypes, which are poorly understood but which presumably reflect differences in vehicle of transmission or of underlying serotype-specific immunity.

5.6. Race

Data on race are not routinely collected in national laboratory-based surveillance and no national data on the relative isolation rates by race have been reported. For unknown reasons, the risk that a *Salmonella* infection will be caused by a resistant strain is higher among black than white infants.[18]

5.7. Occupation

Few data are available to demonstrate that high-risk occupations for salmonellosis exist. Some studies have found higher rates of *Salmonella* carriage among food handlers, which may reflect their high level of contact with raw food and the frequency with which they are cultured.[47] In the past, sewage workers were considered to be at high risk of *Salmonella* infections, particularly typhoid fever, but existing evidence does not suggest that they are currently at increased risk.[48]

5.8. Occurrence in Different Settings

Salmonella outbreaks may create particular problems at institutions, including schools, prisons, nursing homes, hospitals, mental hospitals, and institutions for the retarded. Between 1963 and 1972, 28% of all *Salmonella* outbreaks reported to the CDC occurred in institutions; two thirds of these occurred in acute-care hospitals, pediatric wards, and newborn nurseries.[49] Institutional outbreaks tend to be more serious than those in other settings; the case-fatality rate for all institutional outbreaks between 1963 and 1972 was 2.3% and for those occurring in nursing homes, 8.7%. In the past, nosocomial outbreaks have occurred due to the use of contaminated medical and pharmaceutical products including carmine dye, pancreatic enzymes, platelets, and extracts of thyroid, adrenal cortex, pancreas, and pituitary.[49] Other important hospital outbreaks have been caused by contaminated foods, including powdered eggs, dried milk, and human breast milk.[50] The number of nosocomial *Salmonella* outbreaks reported to the CDC has decreased in recent years, but several outbreaks due to *S.* Enteritidis in shell eggs have occurred in nursing homes and hospitals in the northeastern United States, reflecting an increase in the role of eggs as the vehicle of *S.* Enteritidis.[35] Among 52 foodborne outbreaks of known etiology in nursing homes reported to the CDC between 1975 and 1987, 27 (52%) were caused by *Salmonella*, particularly *S.* Enteritidis.[51] *Salmonella* accounted for 81% of deaths associated with these outbreaks.

Although person-to-person spread is frequently suspected in institutional outbreaks of *Salmonella*, it has been rigorously demonstrated in relatively few. Most recent institutional outbreaks are caused by food products of animal origin. The risk of secondary transmission within hospitals probably varies according to the patient population and setting. Transmission is particularly likely to occur in neonatal nurseries, where peripartum transmission may result in an infected infant and the high level of nursing intervention and the susceptibility of neonates to *Salmonella* predispose to secondary transmission. On regular hospital wards the risk may be considerably less. No secondary transmission was documented in a recent hospital outbreak involving more than 200 nurses who developed salmonellosis after a "nurse appreciation day" meal.[52] Infection control measures included emphasis on hand-washing and exclusion of nurses with enterocolitis until symptoms resolved; negative stool cultures before returning to duty were only required for those working in the neonatal or adult intensive care unit, nursery, or renal dialysis unit.

5.9. *Salmonella* Infections in the Compromised Host

A variety of conditions have been associated with increased risk of *Salmonella* infections, including gastric surgery, decreased gastric acidity, sickle-cell anemia, lymphoma, Hodgkin's disease, metastatic cancer, and infection with human immunodeficiency virus (HIV).[40,53,54] These are related to different mechanisms of defense against *Salmonella* infections (see Section 7). Patients with sickle-cell anemia and other diseases that compromise the reticuloendothelial system have an increased rate of *Salmonella* bacteremia and *Salmonella* osteomyelitis. The decreased ability to clear opsonized bacteria of these patients and perhaps the increased availability of iron may play a major role.[55] Patients with neoplastic disease are also at increased risk of salmonellosis, and lymphoproliferative disorders appear to be more strongly associated with salmonellosis than are solid tumors[54] (see Section 8).

5.10 *Salmonella* Infections and AIDS

Salmonella has emerged as an important pathogen among patients with acquired immunodeficiency syndrome (AIDS). In a San Francisco study, the annual incidence of salmonellosis among patients with AIDS was almost 20 times higher than that in men in a similar age group who did not have AIDS.[53] The proportion of bacteremic *Salmonella* infections is also increased in patients with AIDS; *S.* Typhimurium and *S.* Dublin were more likely to cause bacteremia among these patients than among patients without HIV infection. *Salmonella* bacteremia in patients with AIDS often occurs in the absence of an identifiable episode of enterocolitis and frequently recurs after appropriate antimicrobial treatment.[56] Recurrent *Salmonella* bacteremia was made an indicator disease in the AIDS case definition in 1987. *Salmonella* bacteremia in HIV-infected individuals may precede and foreshadow the development of AIDS; in one third of the patients in the San Francisco study, salmonellosis occurred shortly before they were diagnosed to have AIDS.[53] Increases in *Salmonella* bacteremia, particularly caused by *S.* Enteritidis and *S.* Typhimurium, mirror the demography of the AIDS epidemic.[57,58] *Salmonella* infections represent a large and potentially preventable source of mortality in this group. Patient education and the avoidance of high-risk foods have an important role in prevention.

6. Mechanisms and Routes of Transmission

Human infections are often related directly or indirectly to infection in animals. Transmission can occur via a variety of specific routes, including foodborne, waterborne, animal-to-person contact, person-to-person contact (either direct or indirect), and transfusion. However, up to 90% of infections with *Salmonella* in the United States are foodborne in origin.[32] Data on the sources of foodborne salmonellosis outbreaks indicate that foods of animal origin are the most common source (Table 3). The typical foodborne outbreak is the result of at least two food-handling errors: one that permits the contamination to occur or persist and another that permits sufficient bacterial growth to reach the infectious dose.

The epidemiological complexity of tracing the sources of specific contaminated foods can be challenging. A few serotypes are associated with a specific vehicle. For instance, *S.* Dublin infection is strongly associated with the consumption of raw milk and *S.* Enteritidis with undercooked eggs.[35,59] When a convenient bacteriologic strain marker is available, however, it has been possible to retrace the chain of transmission to farms of origin.[23,25] If the serotype is rare, it may be possible to trace it considerably further. For instance, the international epidemic of *S.* Agona infections was traced to Peruvian fish meal, used in poultry feed, that introduced this formerly rare serotype to several continents simultaneously, where it has since persisted in poultry.[60] *Salmonella* can be introduced and perpetuated on a farm through contaminated feeds, the introduction of infected stock, or by wild animals. Foods may be contaminated in different ways: meat by contents of the gastrointestinal tract during the slaughter process or *in vivo* if the animal was bacteremic at the time of slaughter; milk by feces during the milking process or by mastitis in the milked cow; prepared foods during processing by the use of contaminated ingredients or by cross-contamination within the processing plant itself. In the kitchen, food may be cross-contaminated from raw foods or other sources. Although food handlers are often found to be infected in the course of investigating a foodborne outbreak investigation, they are most often infected because of their exposure to contaminated foods and are rarely shown to be the source of the contamination themselves.[46] Fruits and vegetables have also been increasingly recognized as sources of *Salmonella* outbreaks, including domestic tomatoes and imported cantaloupes.[61] *Salmonella* can multiply within tomatoes and on the cut surfaces of melons.

Table 3. Foodborne Outbreaks of Salmonellosis Reported 1973–1987, by Implicated Vehicle[a]

Food vehicle	No. of outbreaks	Percent of outbreaks of known vehicle
Beef	77	16
Poultry	66	14
Eggs, ice cream	44	9
Pork/ham	25	5
Dairy products	22	5
Bakery products	12	3
Fruits and vegetables	9	2
Fish and shellfish	8	2
Other foods/multiple vehicles	207	44
Unknown	320	
Total	790	

[a]Adapted from Bean and Griffith.[11]

In addition to foodborne transmission, large waterborne outbreaks of salmonellosis have occurred, when drinking water supplies have been contaminated in the absence of proper chlorination.[62]

Salmonella can reach an individual from animal reservoirs via a variety of other routes. Persons in direct contact with ill animals may become infected themselves. Pet turtles, which were almost universally colonized with *Salmonella*, emerged as an important source of the disease in the United States in the early 1970s.[63] Pet iguanas and other reptiles are now a growing source of salmonellosis.[64] Chameleons, aquarium fish, chicks, snakes, and other potential pets may also be colonized with *Salmonella* and may occasionally be sources of infection.[65,66] Marijuana contaminated with *S.* Muenchen was the source of an interstate outbreak probably due to the presence of animal feces.[26] A series of outbreaks of *S.* Cubana infections was traced to carmine dye made from powdered insects and used as a marker of gastrointestinal motility.[67] An outbreak of *S.* Arizona was traced to powdered rattlesnake capsules sold as a folk remedy.[68]

Salmonellosis can also be transmitted from one infected person to another, particularly among a group of unusually susceptible individuals (see Section 5.2). Nosocomial outbreaks of salmonellosis that are not foodborne typically occur in the nursery, and transmission from one child to the next occurs on the unwashed hands of the health care worker. Many other routes of nosocomial transmission are possible. Infection can follow transfer of the organism via endoscope from one patient to the next.[23] *S.* Kottbus has been transmitted through unpasteurized human milk, collected for infants at a human milk bank, from a woman with asymptomatic mammary carriage.[69] *S.* Cholerae-suis was transmitted through platelet transfusions after the platelets were collected from a bacteremic donor.[70] Infection has been transmitted from soiled patient bedclothes to hospital laundry workers.[71]

Although epidemiological data from developing countries are limited, transmission of salmonellosis in those countries may include all of the above routes. Nosocomial reservoirs may be of greater importance than in industrialized countries, particularly for multiply resistant and invasive strains, such as those described in Brazil, Rwanda, and the Ivory Coast.[72–74]

7. Pathogenesis and Immunity

The incubation period after ingestion of *Salmonella* usually ranges from 6 to 48 hr. The pathogenesis of *Salmonella* infections is incompletely understood. The multiplicity of serotypes and animal hosts involved introduces much complexity; a serotype that is nonpathogenic in one animal species may produce severe illness in another. Laboratory models need to be interpreted with caution. For instance, *S.* Typhimurium infections in the mouse may be more analogous to *S.* Typhi than to *S.* Typhimurium infections in humans. The clinical expression of infection is affected by serotype and strain of the bacteria; the status of the underlying health and gut flora of the host; and the dose, vehicle, and route of transmission. Following ingestion, the organisms traverse the gastric acid barrier and multiply in the small intestine. The bacteria penetrate and damage the intestinal mucosa, are ingested by macrophages, and may multiply in a limited fashion in mesenteric lymphoid tissues. In severe invasive infection, bacteremia and focal infections in distant tissues occur.

After more than a century of study, the virulence properties of these organisms remain incompletely understood. Many potential factors and mechanisms have been described, which may be variably present in different serotypes and strains. Some have been well-characterized and undoubtedly more remain to be discovered. The O-specific side-chain portion of lipopolysaccharide (LPS) is associated with invasiveness, and rough mutants with incomplete O-side-chains have markedly diminished virulence.[75] The lipid A portion of LPS is responsible for the endotoxin-mediated effects of the *Salmonella* infection.[76]

The process includes several distinct steps, no single one of which explains the entire pathogenic spectrum: (1) Attachment and penetration. Adhesins facilitate the attachment of salmonellae to intestinal mucosal cells and may be necessary for mucosal invasion.[77] *Salmonella* can induce ordinarily nonphagocytic mucosal cells to engulf them, an unusual ability that gives them rapid access to protected intracellular sites.[78] (2) Inflammation and tissue destruction. The fever, diarrhea, and evidence of colitis that often accompany salmonellosis may be the result of local inflammation, effects of bacterial endotoxin, or of specific cytotoxins that cause mucosal cell death.[79] (3) Intracellular multiplication in macrophages. Lethality in the mouse model is associated with the ability to multiply in macrophages, which may be a function of the presence of flagella, plasmid-associated factors, and an ability to slow acidification within the macrophage.[80–82]

The outcome of infections is partly dependent on the number of ingested bacteria that reach the intestine. Small numbers of ingested *Salmonella* may cause transient asymptomatic intestinal colonization, while larger doses of the same strain may produce overwhelming or even fatal illness. The minimum dose necessary to cause illness varies with the serotype, the vehicle, and a variety of host factors. Although early volunteer studies indicated the infectious dose ranged from 10^5 to 10^{10} organisms, the minimal dose that causes illness in some circumstances may be substantially lower, even as low as 10 organisms.[83]

There are several major barriers in the host's defense against *Salmonella* infection. The first is gastric acidity, which can reduce the number of viable organisms by several logs within minutes. The degree of protection provided by gastric acid depends on the vehicle of infection; *Salmonella* may traverse the stomach more rapidly when consumed in liquids than in solid foods, and contaminated foods that buffer gastric acid well, such as chocolate, cheese, or milk, may transmit infection more efficiently than foods that do not. Persons with high gastric pH, such as the elderly, those taking antacids or other antiulcer medications, and those who have had gastric surgery, are at increased risk for infection.[16,40]

The normal intestinal flora are a second major barrier to infection with salmonellosis. Disruption of the flora, particularly with antimicrobials that are active against the anaerobic flora such as penicillin or tetracycline, decreases the infectious dose needed to produce illness.[31,84] If the infecting strain is resistant to the antimicrobial used, therapy for an unrelated condition may convert a silent transient colonization to overt clinical infection, when the normal flora are suppressed.[16,23] Cellular immunity is the third major defense against bacteremia and invasive illness. This can be overcome in the normal host by certain highly invasive serotypes, such as *S.* Cholerae-suis, or *S.* Paratyphi, or by very large doses of other serotypes.[86] Hemolytic conditions, such as sickle-cell disease, bartonellosis, or malaria, predispose to invasive infection.[87] Persons with defective cellular immunity, such as those receiving immunosuppressive therapy, with advanced malignancies, or infected with HIV, are also at increased risk for invasive illness (see Sections 5.9 and 5.10).

Immunity to *Salmonella* infection is partial at best. In volunteer experiments, patients rechallenged with the homologous strain became ill a second time, although with somewhat milder symptoms than on initial exposure.[88] In animal models, experimental vaccines can prevent death, but not infection. A vaccine against *S.* Cholerae-suis, an economically important pathogen in swine, has now been licensed for use in swine.[89]

The humoral response of humans to experimental infection has been defined. Agglutinating antibodies develop against the somatic (O) and flagellar (H) antigens, even following asymptomatic infections.[90] These antibodies do not always appear, they wane after several months, and sufficient cross-reactions occur with other enteric bacteria that they have been of little diagnostic or epidemiological utility. The nature of the cellular immune response to salmonellosis in humans has not been clearly defined.

8. Patterns of Host Response

The host response to *Salmonella* infection includes asymptomatic colonization, gastroenteritis, focal soft tissue infection, meningitis, bacteremia, sepsis, and death. The pattern of host response may be dictated by the virulence of the specific strain, the size of the inoculum, and specific host factors including age, gastric acidity, immunologic competence, prior antimicrobial exposure, and specific illnesses. Disorders of the gastrointestinal tract (gastrectomy, achlorhydria, esophageal, gastric, or intestinal malignancies) may predispose to enterocolitis, and defects of cellular immunity (leukemia, lymphoma, HIV infection) or reticuloendothelial cell function (sickle-cell anemia, bartonellosis, malaria) may predispose to bacteremia and invasive disease.[40,54] Age is also an important determinant of host response. The incidence of salmonellosis is higher among infants and the elderly and the frequency of bacteremia is higher in both of these age groups.[91] The mortality of *Salmonella* infection is also considerably higher at the extremes of age, as demonstrated by outbreaks in nurseries and nursing homes.[49]

After infection occurs, the organism persists in the gut for a median of 5 weeks, even after all symptoms have ceased. This convalescent carriage can be prolonged in young children.[92] Paradoxically, treatment with antimicrobials does not shorten the duration of carriage, but typically prolongs it, suggesting that the final resolution of infection may depend on the competitive effects of other gut bacteria as well as on the immune response of the host.[30,93] In persons of the HLA-B27 genotype, acute salmonellosis can trigger the reactive arthropathy, Reiter's syndrome, leading to prolonged and recurrent episodes of joint pain, urethritis and uveitis.[94]

The most important determinant of host response may be the organism itself. Certain serotypes appear to be unusually virulent and are isolated more often from the blood and CSF relative to their overall isolation rate. *S.* Cholerae-suis, *S.* Dublin, *S.* Paratyphi A, and *S.* Schottmuelleri (formerly *S.* Paratyphi B) are more commonly isolated from blood, and *S.* Panama, *S.* Heidelberg, and *S.* Saint-Paul are disproportionately common isolates from CSF.[95,96]

8.1. Clinical Features

The clinical manifestations of infection with non-typhoidal *Salmonella* can be grouped into several clinical syndromes with some overlap.

Acute enterocolitis, or gastroenteritis, is the most common syndrome of *Salmonella* infection. Initial symptoms often include nausea, vomiting, and headache, followed by abdominal cramps and diarrhea, which are the predominant manifestations. The stools are normally loose and of moderate volume; blood is occasionally seen. Voluminous, choleralike diarrhea has been reported, as have small-volume, dysenteric stools associated with tenesmus, but these are unusual manifestations. Fever, often accompanied by chills, is present in about 50% of patients. Diarrhea usually lasts 3 to 7 days, but may be prolonged.[(11,40)] The larger the dose of organisms ingested, the shorter the incubation period and the more likely the patient is to have fever, vomiting, and a more severe illness in general.[(97)]

The enteric fever syndrome is classically associated with *S.* Typhi, but may at times occur with other serotypes. This syndrome is characterized by a prolonged course with prominent fever, anorexia, abdominal pain, splenomegaly, and headache. Respiratory symptoms may be prominent and hepatomegaly, neurological manifestations, and relative bradycardia may occur in nontyphoidal enteric fever. Complications include intestinal hemorrhage and perforation, myocarditis, seizures, and localized infections, but are less common than in enteric fever due to *S.* Typhi.

Bacteremia without enteric fever may also occur due to nontyphoidal *Salmonella*. In children, "silent" bacteremia during enterocolitis may occur in 5–10% of patients,[(98)] but *Salmonella* bacteremia with high fever may occur without other signs of enterocolitis or enteric fever, particularly among persons with AIDS. Localized extraintestinal infections may result. Endarteritis, particularly infection of atherosclerotic aortic aneurysms, may occur in patients with preexisting atherosclerotic disease. Endocarditis is rare, and usually occurs on abnormal valves; infection of prosthetic heart valves has also been reported. *S.* Cholerae-suis is responsible for a disproportionate number of endothelial infections. These infections can rarely be cured by antibiotics alone and surgical intervention is often necessary.[(40)] *Salmonella* meningitis occurs primarily in infants, and even with adequate antibiotic therapy, the mortality is high. Osteomyelitis and arthritis due to *Salmonella* may occur in normal hosts but are more common in immunocompromised persons, particularly those with hemolytic disorders. *Salmonella* is the most common cause of osteomyelitis in patients with sickle-cell anemia. Other complications of *Salmonella* bacteremia include pneumonia, empyema, endocarditis, intracranial abscess, urinary tract infections, and abscesses of the spleen, liver, and other soft tissue.[(87)]

8.2. Diagnosis

The diagnosis of *Salmonella* enterocolitis is made by stool culture. The diagnosis should be considered in any patient with moderate to severe gastroenteritis; the presence of headache or fever makes the possibility of this disease more likely. Fecal leukocytes may be present, but are not diagnostic. The differential diagnosis of *Salmonella* enterocolitis includes viral gastroenteritis and other bacterial enteric infections, including those caused by *Shigella*, enterotoxigenic, enterohemorrhagic, and enteropathogenic *E. coli*, *Campylobacter* species, *Vibrio* species, and *Yersinia enterocolitica*. The disorder must also be differentiated from toxin-mediated foodborne illnesses including those caused by *Staphylococcus aureus*, *Bacillus cereus*, and *Clostridium perfringens*. Compared to patients with these toxin-mediated disorders, persons with salmonellosis usually have less prominent vomiting and are more likely to have prolonged diarrhea and fever. The shorter incubation periods of toxin-mediated foodborne illness can be an important clue to distinguish them from salmonellosis. The presence of frequent, small-volume, bloody or mucus-streaked stools, tenesmus, and large numbers of fecal leukocytes makes campylobacterosis or shigellosis more likely than salmonellosis. A recent history of ingestion of raw milk, undercooked eggs or meat, or exposure to lizards or farm animals within the 48 hr before onset of illness may suggest the diagnosis of salmonellosis. Ultimately, however, the diagnosis depends on cultures of stool, or in the case of high fever or invasive disease, blood, CSF, or other body fluids.

9. Control and Prevention

The control of salmonellosis depends on understanding the routes and cycles of transmission well enough to interrupt them. Control of foodborne salmonellosis can occur at many levels, at the farm, during truck transport, the slaughter plant, or food production facility, to the cook and consumer. Once the transmission is understood and the critical control points are understood, intervention can be highly successful.

Interventions at the level of the farm can succeed. In Scandinavia, the prevalence of salmonellae in chicken flocks has been greatly reduced by exposing the chicks to normal fecal flora shortly after they hatch, thus increasing their resistance to subsequent colonization with *Salmonella*.[99] In many countries, including the United States, two serotypes that are highly pathogenic to poultry—*S.* Pullorum and *S.* Gallinarum—have been virtually eradicated by a vigorous program of serological testing and destruction of infected birds.[100]

Animals entering the slaughter plant may be free of *Salmonella*, may have silent colonization, or may be ill or even moribund with systemic salmonellosis. Existing visual inspection methods will detect some of the last group; the proportion of slaughtered cattle that are moribund correlates with the level of carcass contamination.[25] However, visual inspection cannot detect silent colonization, which is far more common. Reassessment of current practices of slaughter and inspection is necessary.[101] Condemned carcasses are sold for pet food or are sent to rendering plants to be converted to meal used to make animal feed. Unfortunately, the rendered product is routinely recontaminated with *Salmonella* before it leaves the rendering plant, so that animal feed in the United States is often contaminated with *Salmonella*. Many countries, but not the United States, require the routine pasteurization of animal feeds to interrupt this cycle.

Salmonellosis related to fresh fruits and vegetables can be controlled if the level of contamination occurring in the field and during processing can be reduced. Strategies include providing adequate sanitary facilities for field workers, washing fruits and vegetables after harvest in carefully disinfected water, shipping them on ice made from disinfected water, and not cutting or slicing them until immediately before consumption.

Changes in food production practices can increase or decrease the likelihood of contamination of the finished product. For example, the pasteurization of milk protects the consumer against many raw-milk-associated pathogens, including *Salmonella*. Because of documented risk of salmonellosis and campylobacteriosis, the interstate sale of raw milk was banned in 1987. In a series of *S.* Newport outbreaks traced to precooked roast beef in the late 1970s, the cooking process was found to be inadequate to kill *Salmonella* present on raw beef. These outbreaks ended after the required time and temperature of cooking were changed in 1980 and 1981.[102] New technologies may reduce contamination of poultry during slaughter and processing, including trisodium phosphate dips that rinse *Salmonella* off carcasses, air-cooling devices to replace the cold water chill tanks, better eviscerators that decrease the likelihood of rupture of the crop or gut, and better decontamination procedures for the machinery used. Irradiating raw meat and poultry would be an effective step in controlling salmonellosis, but one which thus far is unacceptable to some segments of society.[103]

Licensing and inspection of food-service establishments, particularly when coupled with food-handler education and certification, is an integral part of the public health effort to prevent foodborne illnesses of all sorts, including salmonellosis. Educating consumers themselves is a constant effort, requiring the cooperation of the food production and retailing industries, the education establishment, and public health officials.

S. Enteritidis has been shown to contaminate the contents of the intact egg, as a result of ovarian infection in the hen. The hens themselves may be infected *in ovo* or by contact with infected mice or a contaminated environment. A series of control measures are now being implemented throughout the US egg industry, including screening flocks for infection, pasteurizing the eggs from infected flocks, better rodent control in henhouses, and a requirement for refrigeration of eggs during transport and distribution, so that a small number of contaminating *Salmonella* do not have the opportunity to multiply. These measures may explain the recent decline in *S.* Enteritidis infections in the mid-Atlantic region, where they were first pilot tested. At the same time, hospitals, nursing homes, and restaurants are switching from shell eggs to pasteurized eggs and traditional recipes that use raw egg, such as homemade ice cream, eggnog, and Caesar salad, are being rewritten.

Many control measures are implemented to prevent person-to-person transmission. The potential for this transmission makes it prudent to exclude from work food handlers or health care workers with acute *Salmonella* enterocolitis, and convalescent persons in sensitive occupations who continue to shed the organism are often excluded until stool cultures no longer yield *Salmonella*. The risk posed by the entirely asymptomatic shedder is low and does not justify routine periodic stool cultures of food handlers or health care providers. Nosocomial salmonellosis can be controlled by taking routine precautions to prevent transmission of enteric organisms from patients with acute salmonellosis, including strict hand washing and other basic tenets of hospital infection control.[50]

Reptile-associated salmonellosis also has required specific control measures. The ban on the sale of small pet turtles in 1975, following unsuccessful efforts to educate the turtle-owning public in methods to reduce risk, led to a dramatic decrease in the isolation rate of turtle-associated serotypes.[20] Efforts to educate the public about the new risk of iguana-associated salmonellosis are just beginning.[64]

10. Unresolved Problems

There are many control points in the chain of transmission of *Salmonella*. However, it is difficult to achieve coordinated control efforts among the many industrial, professional, and regulatory groups involved. Therefore, salmonellosis will continue to be an important public health problem in the industrialized world and an increasing problem in developing countries. Although the pathogen has been well known for more than 100 years, fundamental questions remain unanswered. Microbiological issues in need of further study include clarifying the mechanisms of virulence, which may ultimately permit the successful development of vaccines. More rapid and sensitive means of detecting the organism in foods are needed if programs of food safety that depend on bacteriologic monitoring are to be widely implemented. A reliable and simple method of subtyping based on molecular methodologies will be needed to replace the time- and labor-intensive serotyping system.

Several important clinical issues are unresolved. The risk factors for invasive infection in infants, particularly meningitis, are poorly defined and the use of antimicrobials to treat *Salmonella* enterocolitis in infants to prevent invasive infections is presently unproven. The paradoxic and important ability of the organism to persist in the individual who is treated with antimicrobials, even when the organism is sensitive to those antimicrobials *in vitro*, needs to be explained. Developing a treatment that would eliminate long-term carriage would be of benefit. The increasing antimicrobial resistance of strains isolated from humans in the United States poses clinical challenges for the treatment of invasive infections and increases the risk that resistant salmonellosis will complicate the therapy of other infections. The problem of increasing antimicrobial resistance would benefit greatly from a rational approach to defining the choice and indications for use of antimicrobials in animal husbandry. Invasive infections are likely to be an increasing clinical problem, as the population ages and the prevalence of AIDS increases.

Unresolved public health issues include the need for active population-based surveillance to estimate the burden and sources of infection, including the relative contributions of fruits and vegetables and of reptile pets to the overall problem. Careful case–control studies of sporadic cases are needed to define precise behaviors and exposures that transmit salmonellosis, such as handling raw chicken viscera or preparing a baby bottle in the area of the kitchen used for meat preparation. Such data would lead to targeted prevention education. Cluster detection methods are needed to identify widely distributed outbreaks related to low-level contamination of a commercial food item and expanded international collaboration can help identify and control foodborne sources of infection. Effective prevention strategies need to be demonstrated for salmonellosis in infants and HIV-infected individuals. Reducing the contamination of our food supply will require a continuing effort to identify specific critical control points at the farm, the rendering plant, the slaughterhouse, and the food-processing factory and to implement cost-effective control measures.

11. References

1. Cohen, M. L., Fontaine, R. E., Pollard, R. A., *et al.*, An assessment of patient-related economic costs in an outbreak of salmonellosis, *N. Engl. J. Med.* **299:**459–460 (1978).
2. McWhorter-Murlin, A. C., and Hickman-Brenner, F. W., *Identification and Serotyping of* Salmonella *and an Update of the Kauffmann–White Scheme*, Centers for Disease Control and Prevention, Atlanta, GA, 1994.
3. Martin, S. M., Hargrett-Bean, N., and Tauxe, R. V., *An Atlas of* Salmonella *in the United States: Serotype-Specific Surveillance 1968–1986*, Centers for Disease Control, Atlanta, GA, 1989. National Technical Information Service, catalogue number PB89-213441-AS.
4. Salmon, D. E., and Smith, T., *Report on Swine Plague*, US Bureau of Animal Industry, 2nd Annual Report, 1885.
5. Karlinski, J., Zur kenntnis des *Bacillus enteritidis* gaertner, *Zentralbl. Bakteriol. Parasitenkd.* **6:**289–292 (1889).
6. Kauffmann, F., *Die Bakteriologie der Salmonella gruppe*, Munksgaard, Copenhagen, 1941.
7. Loeffler, F., Ueber Epidemieen unter den im hygienischen Institute zu Greifswald gehaltenen maeusen und ueber die Bekaempfung der Feldmausplage, *Zentralbl. Bakteriol. Parasitenkd.* **12:** 1–17 (1892).
8. Anonymous, Eggs and *Salmonella* infections, *Br. Med. J.* **2:**760–761 (1944).
9. MacCready, R. A., Reardon, J. P., and Saphra, I., Salmonellosis in Massachusetts. A sixteen-year experience, *N. Engl. J. Med.* **256:** 1121–1127 (1957).
10. Saphra, I., and Winter, J. W., Clinical manifestations of salmonellosis in man: An evaluation of 7779 human infections identified at the New York *Salmonella* Center, *N. Engl. J. Med.* **256:** 1128–1134 (1957).
11. Bean, N. H., and Griffin, P. M., Foodborne disease outbreaks in the United States, 1973–1987: Pathogens, vehicles and trends, *J. Food Protection* **53:**804–817 (1990).
12. Centers for Disease Control and Prevention, Summary of notifiable diseases, United States, 1993, *Morbid. Mortal. Week. Rep.* **42**(53) (1993).
13. Bean, N. H., Morris, S. M., and Bradford, H., PHLIS: An electronic system for reporting public health data from remote sites, *Am. J. Public Health* **82:**1273–1276 (1992).
14. Aserkoff, B., Schroeder, S. A., and Brachman, P. S., Salmonellosis in the United States—A five-year review, *Am. J. Epidemiol.* **92:**13–24 (1970).
15. Chalker, R. B., and Blaser, M. J., A review of human salmo-

nellosis: III. Magnitude of *Salmonella* infection in the United States, *Rev. Infect. Dis.* **9:**111–124 (1988).
16. Riley, L. W., Cohen, M. L., Seals, J. E., *et al.*, Importance of host factors in human salmonellosis caused by multiresistant strains of *Salmonella, J. Infect. Dis.* **149:**878–883 (1984).
17. MacDonald, K. L., Cohen, M. L., Hargrett-Bean, N. T., *et al.*, Changes in antimicrobial resistance of *Salmonella* isolated from humans in the United States, *J. Am. Med. Assoc.* **258:**1496–1499 (1987).
18. Lee, L. A., Puhr, N. D., Maloney, K., *et al.*, Increase in antimicrobial-resistant *Salmonella* infections in the United States, 1989–1990, *J. Infect. Dis.* **170:**128–134 (1994).
19. Wachsmuth, K., Molecular epidemiology of bacterial infections: Examples of methodology and investigations of outbreaks, *Rev. Infect. Dis.* **8:**682–692 (1986).
20. Cohen, M. L., Potter, M. E., Pollard, R., and Feldman, R. A., Turtle-associated salmonellosis in the United States: Effect of public health action, 1970–1976, *J. Am. Med. Assoc.* **243:**1247–1249 (1980).
21. Pacer, R. E., Spika, J. S., Thurmond, M. C., *et al.*, Prevalence of *Salmonella* and multiple antimicrobial-resistant *Salmonella* in California dairies, *J. Am. Vet. Med. Assoc.* **195:**59–63 (1989).
22. Farmer, J. J., Wells, J. G., Griffin, P. M., and Wachsmuth, I. K., *Enterobacteriaceae* infections, in: *Diagnostic Procedures for Bacterial, Mycotic and Parasitic Infections*, 7th ed. (B. Wentworth, ed.), pp. 233–296, American Public Health Association, Baltimore, 1987.
23. Holmberg, S. D., Osterholm, M. T., Senger, K. A., and Cohen, M. L., Drug-resistant *Salmonella* from animals fed antimicrobials, *N. Engl. J. Med.* **311:**617–622.
24. Riley, L. W., DiFerdinando, G. T., DeMelfi, T. M., and Cohen, M. L., Evaluation of isolated cases of salmonellosis by plasmid profile analysis: Introduction and transmission of a bacterial clone by precooked roast beef, *J. Infect. Dis.* **148:**12–14 (1983).
25. Spika, J. S., Waterman, S. H., Soo Hoo, G. W., *et al.*, Chloramphenicol-resistant *Salmonella newport* traced through hamburger to dairy farms, *N. Engl. J. Med.* **316:**565–570 (1987).
26. Taylor, D. N., Wachsmuth, I. K., Schangkuan, Y.-H., *et al.*, Salmonellosis associated with marijuana: A multistate outbreak traced by plasmid finger-printing, *N. Engl. J. Med.* **306:**1249–1253 (1982).
27. Rodrigue, D. C., Cameron, D. N., Puhr, N. D., *et al.*, Comparison of plasmid profiles, phage types, and antimicrobial resistance patterns of *Salmonella enteritidis* isolates in the United States, *J. Clin. Microbiol.* **30:**854–857 (1992).
28. Sack, R. B., Serologic tests for the diagnosis of enterobacterial infections, in: *Manual of Clinical Laboratory Immunology* (N. Rose, ed.), pp. 359–362, American Society for Microbiology, Washington, DC, 1986.
29. Mitscherlich, E., and Martin, E. H., *Microbial Survival in the Environment*, Springer-Verlag, Berlin, 1984.
30. Aserkoff, B., and Bennett, J. V., Effect of therapy in acute salmonellosis on *Salmonellae* in feces, *N. Engl. J. Med.* **281:**3–7 (1969).
31. Ryan, C. A., Nickels, M. K., Hargrett-Bean, N. T., *et al.*, Massive outbreak of antimicrobial-resistant salmonellosis traced to pasteurized milk, *J. Am. Med. Assoc.* **258:**3269–3274 (1987).
32. Cohen, M. L., and Tauxe, R. V., Drug-resistant *Salmonella* in the United States: An epidemiologic perspective, *Science* **234:**964–969 (1986).
33. Lee, L. A., Threatt, V. L., Puhr, N. D., *et al.*, Antimicrobial-resistant *Salmonella* spp isolated from healthy broiler chickens after slaughter, *J. Am. Vet. Med. Assoc.* **202:**752–755 (1993).
34. MacDonald, K. L., O'Leary, M. J., Norris, P., *et al.*, *Escherichia coli* O157:H7, an emerging population-based study, *J. Am. Med. Assoc.* **259:**3567–3570 (1988).
35. St. Louis, M. E., Morse, D. L., Potter, M. E., *et al.*, The emergence of grade A eggs as a major source of *Salmonella enteritidis* infections. New implications for the control of salmonellosis, *J. Am. Med. Assoc.* **259:**2103–2107 (1988).
36. Rodrigue, D. C., Tauxe, R. V., and Rowe, B., International increase in *Salmonella enteritidis*: A new pandemic? *Epidemiol. Infect.* **105:**21–27 (1990).
37. Mishu, B., Koehler, J. E., Lee, L. A., *et al.*, Outbreaks of *Salmonella enteritidis* infections in the United States, 1985–1991, *J. Infect. Dis.* **169:**547–552 (1994).
38. Hedberg, C. W., David, M. J., White, K. E., *et al.*, Role of egg consumption in sporadic *Salmonella enteritidis* and *Salmonella typhimurium* infections in Minnesota, *J. Infect. Dis.* **167:**107–111 (1993).
39. Centers for Disease Control and Prevention, Salmonella *surveillance—Annual Summary—1992*, Atlanta, GA, 1994.
40. Black, P. H., Kunz, L. J., and Swartz, M. N., Salmonellosis—A review of some unusual aspects, *N. Engl. J. Med.* **262:**811–816, 846–870, 921–927 (1960).
41. Craven, P. C., Mackel, D. C., Baine, W. B., *et al.*, International outbreak of *Salmonella eastbourne* infection traced to contaminated chocolate, *Lancet* **1:**788–793 (1975).
42. Collins, R. N., Treger, M. D., Goldsby, J. B., *et al.*, Interstate outbreak of *Salmonella new-brunswick* infection traced to powdered milk, *J. Am. Med. Assoc.* **203:**838–844 (1968).
43. Wilson, R., Feldman, R. A., Davis, J., and LaVenture, M., Salmonellosis in infants: The importance of intrafamilial transmission, *Pediatrics* **69:**436–438 (1982).
44. Rowe, B., *Salmonella* surveillance: Reports received from centers participating with WHO Programme, 1981, Central Public Health Laboratory, London, 1984.
45. United Nations, *Demographic Yearbook*, United Nations, New York, 1983.
46. Ryder, R. W., Merson, M. H., Pollard, R. A., Jr., and Gangarosa, E. J., Salmonellosis in the United States, 1968–1974, *J. Infect. Dis.* **133:**483–486 (1976).
47. Cruickshank, J. G., and Humphrey, T. J., The carrier food-handler and non-typhoid salmonellosis, *Epidemiol. Infect.* **98:**223–230 (1987).
48. Ryan, C. A., Hargrett-Bean, N. T., and Blake, P. A., *Salmonella typhi* infections in the United States, 1975–1984: Increasing role of foreign travel, *Rev. Infect. Dis.* **11:**1–8 (1989).
49. Baine, W. B., Gangarosa, E. J., Bennett, J. V., and Barker, W. H., Jr., Institutional salmonellosis, *J. Infect. Dis.* **128:**357–360 (1973).
50. Weickel, C. S., and Guerrant, R. L., Nosocomial salmonellosis, *Infect. Control* **6:**218–220 (1985).
51. Levine, W. C., Smart, J. F., Archer, D. L., *et al.*, Foodborne disease outbreaks in nursing homes, 1975–1987, *J. Am. Med. Assoc.* **266:**2105–2109 (1991).
52. Tauxe, R. V., Hassan, L. F., Findeisen, K.O., *et al.*, Salmonellosis in nurses: Lack of transmission to patients, *J. Infect. Dis.* **157:**370–373 (1988).
53. Celum, C. L., Chaisson, R. E., Rutherford, G. W., *et al.*, Incidence of salmonellosis in patients with AIDS, *J. Infect. Dis.* **156:**998–1002 (1987).
54. Wolfe, M. S., Armstrong, D., Louria, D. B., and Blevins, A., Salmonellosis in patients with neoplastic disease. A review of 100 episodes at Memorial Cancer Center over a 13-year period, *Arch. Intern. Med.* **128:**546–554 (1971).

55. Barrett-Connor, E., Bacterial infection and sickle cell anemia: An analysis of 250 infections in 166 patients and a review of the literature, *Medicine* **50:**97–112 (1971).
56. Jacobs, J. L., Gold, M. W., Murray, H. W., *et al.*, *Salmonella* infections in patients with the acquired immunodeficiency syndrome, *Ann. Intern. Med.* **103:**186–188 (1985).
57. Levine, W. C., Buehler, J. W., Bean, N. H., and Tauxe, R. V., Epidemiology of nontyphoidal *Salmonella* bacteremia during the human immunodeficiency virus epidemic, *J. Infect. Dis.* **164:** 81–87 (1991).
58. Gruenewald, R., Blum, S., and Chan, J., Relationship between human immunodeficiency virus infection and salmonellosis in 20- to 59-year-old residents of New York City, *Clin. Infect. Dis.* **18:**358–363 (1994).
59. Taylor, D. N., Bied, J. M., Munro, J. S., and Feldman, R. A., *Salmonella dublin* infections in the United States, 1979–1980, *J. Infect. Dis.* **146:**322–327 (1982).
60. Clark, G. M., Kaufmann, A. F., Gangarosa, E. J., and Thompson, M. A., Epidemiology of an international outbreak of *Salmonella agona*, *Lancet* **2:**1–10 (1973).
61. Centers for Disease Control and Prevention, Multistate outbreak of *Salmonella poona* infections—United States and Canada, 1991, *Morbid. Mortal. Week. Rep.* **40:**550–552 (1991).
62. Anonymous, A waterborne epidemic of salmonellosis in Riverside, California, 1965: Epidemiologic aspects, *Am. J. Epidemiol.* **93:**33–48 (1971).
63. Lamm, S. H., Taylor, A., Gangarosa, E. J., *et al.*, Turtle-associated salmonellosis. 1. An estimation of the magnitude of the problem in the United States, 1970–1971, *Am. J. Epidemiol.* **95:**511–517 (1972).
64. Centers for Disease Control and Prevention, Iguana-associated salmonellosis—Selected States, 1994–1995, *Morbid. Mortal. Week. Rep.* **44:**347–350 (1995).
65. Chiodini, R. J., and Sundberg, J. P., Salmonellosis in reptiles: A review, *Am. J. Epidemiol.* **113:**494–499 (1981).
66. Trust, T. J., and Bartlett, K. H., Aquarium pets as a source of antibiotic-resistant salmonellae, *Can. J. Microbiol.* **25:**535–541 (1979).
67. Lang, D. J., Kunz, L. J., Martin, A. R., *et al.*, Carmine as a source of nosocomial salmonellosis, *N. Engl. J. Med.* **276:**829–832 (1967).
68. Riley, K. B., Antoniskis, D., Maris, R., and Leedom, J. M., Rattlesnake capsule-associated *Salmonella arizona* infections, *Arch. Intern. Med.* **148:**1207–1210 (1988).
69. Ryder, R. W., Crosbie-Ritchie, A., McDonough, B., and Hall, W. J., Human milk contaminated with *Salmonella kottbus*: A cause of nosocomial illness in infants, *J. Am. Med. Assoc.* **238:**1533–1534 (1977).
70. Rhame, F. S., Raat, R. K., MacLowry, J. D., *et al.*, *Salmonella* septicemia from platelet transfusions: Study of an outbreak traced to a hematogenous carrier of *Salmonella cholerae-suis*, *Ann. Intern. Med.* **78:**633–641 (1973).
71. Standaert, S. M., Hutcheson, R. H., and Schaffner, W., Nosocomial Transmission of *Salmonella* gastroenteritis to laundry workers in a nursing home, *Infect. Control Hosp. Epidemiol.* **15:**22–26 (1994).
72. Lepage, P., Bogaerts, J., Nsengumuremyi, F., *et al.*, Severe multiresistant *Salmonella typhimurium* systemic infections in central Africa—Clinical features and treatment in a pediatric department, *J. Antimicrob. Chemother.* **14**(Suppl. B):153–159 (1984).
73. Riley, L. W., Ceballos, B. S., Trabulsi, L. R., *et al.*, The significance of hospitals as reservoirs for endemic multiresistant *Salmonella typhimurium* causing infection in urban Brazilian children, *J. Infect. Dis.* **150:**236–241 (1984).
74. Vugia, D. J., Kiehlbauch, J. A., Yeboue, K., *et al.*, Pathogens and predictors of fatal septicemia associated with human immunodeficiency virus infection in Ivory Coast, West Africa, *J. Infect. Dis.* **168:**564–570 (1993).
75. Roantree, R. J., *Salmonella* O antigens and virulence, *Annu. Rev. Microbiol.* **21:**443–466 (1967).
76. Murray, M. J., *Salmonella*: Virulence factors and enteric salmonellosis, *J. Am. Med. Assoc.* **189:**145–147 (1986).
77. Jones, G. W., and Richardson, L. A., The attachment to, and invasion of HeLa cells by *Salmonella typhimurium*: The contribution of mannose-sensitive and mannose-resistant haemagglutinating activities, *J. Gen. Microbiol.* **127:**361–370 (1981).
78. Finlay, B. B., Gumbiner, B., and Falkow, S., Penetration of *Salmonella* through a polarized MDCK epithelial cell monolayer, *J. Cell. Biol.* **107:**221–230 (1988).
79. Giannella, R. A., Importance of intestinal inflammatory reaction in *Salmonella*-mediated intestinal secretion, *Infect. Immun.* **23:** 140–145 (1979).
80. Alpuche-Aranda, C. M., Swanson, J. A., Loomis, W. P., *et al.*, *Salmonella typhimurium* activates virulence gene transcription within acidified macrophage phagosomes, *Proc. Natl. Acad. Sci. USA* **89:**10079–10083 (1992).
81. Gulig, P. A., and Curtiss, R., Plasmid-associated virulence of *Salmonella typhimurium*, *Infect. Immun.* **55:**2891–2901 (1987).
82. Weinstein, D. L., Carsiotis, M., Lissner, C. R., and O'Brien, A. D., Flagella help *Salmonella typhimurium* survive within murine macrophages, *Infect. Immun.* **46:**819–825 (1984).
83. Blaser, M. J., and Newman, L. S., A review of human salmonellosis: I. Infective dose, *Rev. Infect. Dis.* **34:**1096–1106 (1982).
84. Bohnhoff, M., Miller, C. P., and Martin, W. R., Resistance of the mouse's intestinal tract to experimental *Salmonella* infection. II. Factors responsible for its loss following streptomycin treatment, *J. Exp. Med.* **120:**817–828 (1964).
85. Pavia, A. T., Shipman, L. D., Wells, J. G., *et al.*, Epidemiologic evidence that prior antimicrobial exposure decreases resistance to infection by antimicrobial-sensitive *Salmonella*, *J. Infect. Dis.* **161:**255–260 (1990).
86. Taylor, D. N., Bopp, C., Birkness, K., and Cohen, M. L., An outbreak of salmonellosis associated with a fatality in a healthy child: A large dose and severe illness, *Am. J. Epidemiol.* **119:**907–912 (1984).
87. Cohen, J. I., Bartlett, J. A., and Corey, G. F., Extra-intestinal manifestations of *Salmonella* infections, *Medicine* **66:**349–388 (1987).
88. McCullough, N. B., and Eisele, C. W., Experimental human salmonellosis. II. Immunity studies following experimental illness with *Salmonella meleagridis* and *Salmonella anatum*, *J. Immunol.* **66:**595–608 (1951).
89. Kramer, T. T., Roof, M. B., and Matheson, R. R., Safety and efficacy of attenuated strain of *Salmonella choleraeusis* for vaccination of swine, *Am. J. Vet. Res.* **53:**444–448 (1992).
90. Gotoff, S. P., Lepper, M. K., and Fiedler, M. A., Immunologic studies in an epidemic of *Salmonella* infections, *Am. J. Med. Sci.* **251:**61–66 (1966).
91. Hook, E. W., Salmonellosis: Certain factors influencing the interaction of *Salmonella* and the human host, *Bull. NY Acad. Med.* **37:** 499–512 (1961).
92. Buchwald, D. S., and Blaser, M. J., A review of human salmonellosis: II. Duration of excretion following infection with nontyphi *Salmonella*, *Rev. Infect. Dis.* **16:**345–356 (1984).
93. Neill, M. A., Opal, S. M., Heelan, J., *et al.*, Failure of ciprofloxacin to eradicate convalescent fecal excretion after acute salmo-

nellosis: Experience during an outbreak in health care workers, *Ann. Intern. Med.* **114:**195–199 (1991).

94. Swerdlow, D. L., Lee, L. A., Tauxe, R. V., *et al.*, Reactive arthropathy following a multistate outbreak of *Salmonella typhimurium* infections (Abstract 916), 30th Interscience Conference on Antimicrobial Agents and Chemotherapy, Atlanta, October 21–24, 1990.
95. Blaser, M. J., and Feldman, R. A., *Salmonella* bacteremia: Reports to the Centers for Disease Control, 1968–1979, *J. Infect. Dis.* **143:**743–746 (1981).
96. Wilson, R., and Feldman, R. A., Reported isolates of *Salmonella* from cerebrospinal fluid in the United States, 1968–1979, *J. Infect. Dis.* **143:**504–506 (1981).
97. Mintz, E. D., Cartter, M. L., Hadler, J. L., *et al.*, Dose-response effects in an outbreak of *Salmonella enteritidis*, *Epidemiol. Infect.* **112:**13–23 (1994).
98. Torrey, S., Fleisher, G., and Jaffe, D., Incidence of *Salmonella* bacteremia in infants with *Salmonella* gastroenteritis, *J. Pediatr.* **108:**718–721 (1986).
99. Nurmi, E., Use of competitive exclusion in prevention of salmonellae and other enteropathogenic bacteria infections in poultry, in: *Proceedings of the International Symposium on Salmonella*, New Orleans, July 1984 (G. H. Snoeyenbos, ed.), pp. 64–73, University of Pennsylvania, Kennett Square, 1984.
100. Anonymous, The national poultry improvement plan and auxiliary provisions, Animal Science Research Division, Agriculture Research Service, US Department of Agriculture, Beltsville, MD, 1982.
101. National Research Council, *Poultry Inspection: The Basis for a Risk-Assessment Approach*, National Academy Press, Washington, DC, 1987.
102. Parham, G. L., Salmonellae in cooked beef products, in: *Proceedings of the International Symposium on Salmonella*, New University of Pennsylvania, Kennett Square, 1984.
103. Roberts, T., Microbial pathogens in raw pork, chicken and beef: Benefit estimates for control using irradiation, *Am. J. Agric. Econ.* **67:**957–965 (1985).

12. Suggested Reading

Hargrett-Bean, N., Pavia, A. T., and Tauxe, R. V., *Salmonella* isolates from humans in the United States, 1984–1986, in CDC Surveillance Summaries, June 1988, *Morbid. Mortal. Week. Rep.* **37**(No. 55-2)**:** 25–31 (1988).

Hook, E. W., *Salmonella* species (including typhoid fever), in: *Principles and Practice of Infectious Diseases*, 3rd ed. (G. L. Mandell, R. G Douglas, and J. E. Bennett, eds.), pp. 1700–1716, New York: Wiley, 1989.

Kelterborn, E., *Salmonella Species: First Isolations, Names, and Occurrence*, The Hague, Junk, 1967.

National Research Council, *Poultry Inspection: The Basis for a Risk-Management Approach*, National Academy Press, Washington, DC, 1987.

Martin, S. M., Hargrett-Bean, N., and Tauxe, R. V., An atlas of *Salmonella* in the United States: Serotype-specific surveillance 1968–1986. Centers for Disease Control, Atlanta, Georgia, 1989. National Technical Information Service, catelogue number PB89-213441-AS.

McCapes, R. H., Osburn, B. I., and Riemann, H., Safety of foods of animal origin: Model for elimination of *Salmonella* contamination of turkey meat, *J. Am. Vet. Med. Assoc.* **199:**875–880 (1991).

Tauxe, R. V., *Salmonella*: A post-modern pathogen, *J. Food Protection* **54:**563–568 (1991).

CHAPTER 32

Shigellosis

Gerald T. Keusch and Michael L. Bennish

1. Introduction

Shigellosis is an acute, infectious, inflammatory enteritis of humans and, on occasion, subhuman primates. Because it is often clinically manifested by the dysentery syndrome (a triad of frequent, small-volume, bloody-mucoid stools, abdominal cramps, and tenesmus) it is often referred to as bacillary dysentery to distinguish this infection from amebic dysentery. However, watery diarrhea without blood or mucus is common in infection due to all *Shigella* species, and may be the only intestinal sign of infection. In addition to these clinical presentations, there are a myriad of manifestations described in shigellosis, some common and some rare, that without doubt qualify the organism as a protean pathogen. The objective of this chapter is to present the salient features of shigellosis in sufficient detail to understand the spectrum of the disease and its distinctive epidemiology.

2. Historical Background

Dysentery has long been clinically recognized. The classic syndrome is depicted in the Old Testament, and it is mentioned in the descriptions of war, so common in our history, from Thucydides in the Levant to Montgomery at the battle of El Alamein.

There are two principal causes of this syndrome–*Shigella* species and *Entamoeba histolytica*—and a number of minor causes, including *Salmonella* and *Campylobacter*. Under circumstances of epidemic dysentery, *Shigella* is more likely to be the agent involved, while sporadic disease in adults associated with liver involvement is probably due to *E. histolytica*. However, in individual patients, the specific etiology of the syndrome can be determined only by laboratory investigation. This first became possible after Losch described *E. histolytica* and demonstrated its virulence in dogs in 1875, and Councilman and Lafleur reported the anatomic criteria for the diagnosis in humans in 1891. The problem of assigning etiology to cases of dysentery in which neither the organism nor characteristic histology was present, however, remained. The loop was closed in 1898 by Dr. Kioshi Shiga,[1] who isolated the organism now known as *Shigella dysenteriae* 1 (Shiga's bacillus). The bacterium was found in the stools of patients with epidemic dysentery in Japan during a particularly widespread (almost 90,000 cases) and severe (25% mortality) outbreak. Shiga was able to demonstrate the presence of specific serum agglutinins in individuals convalescent from the disease but not in the healthy or in patients with other diseases. In fact, the identical organism had been reported a decade earlier by Chantemesse and Widal as the cause of nonamoebic dysentery, but the description was less complete and lacked the epidemiological proof of Shiga's study, and it is the Japanese microbiologist who is honored in the genus name. Two years later, Shiga's results were confirmed by Flexner in the Philippines and by Kruse in Germany.

Soon thereafter, Kruse isolated a similar but serologically distinct organism during an outbreak of "asylum dysentery," an epidemic disease common in institutions for the mentally ill, which he called *Bacillus pseudodysentery*. Identical organisms were soon described by Flexner, Strong, and Musgrave, and Castellani, who suggested the name *B. paradysenteriae* instead. Todd referred to this same strain as *B. dysenteriae* Flexner, and to clear the confusion the name *Shigella flexneri* was ultimately adopted. A third species was defined by Duval, Castellani,

Gerald T. Keusch • Department of Medicine, Tupper Research Institute, Division of Geographic Medicine and Infections Diseases, New England Medical Center, Boston, Massachusetts 02111. **Michael L. Bennish** • Departments of Pediatrics and Medicine, Tupper Research Institute, Division of Geographic Medicine and Infections Diseases, New England Medical Center, Boston, Massachusetts 02111.

and Kruse, who found a serologically distinct, late lactose-fermenting *Shigella*, which Kruse originally called *B. pseudodysenteriae* type E. To honor the subsequent extensive work of Sonne on Kruse's type E organism, the name was first modified to *B. dysenteriae* Sonne and then shortened to *Shigella sonnei*.

The final stage in classification of shigellae began in 1929 with Boyd's studies in Bangalore, India, of non-lactose-fermenting, mannitol-positive organisms resembling *S. flexneri* that were not agglutinated by *flexneri* antisera. Boyd showed the presence of well-defined distinctive serological reactions with homologous antisera to the inagglutinable Flexner group, and on this bases such strains were classified together as *S. boydii*. By 1938, then, fully 40 years after the first complete description of the prototypic organism, *S. dysenteriae* 1, the four species of *Shigella* were defined [*dysenteriae* (10 serotypes), *flexneri* (6 serotypes), boydii (15 serotypes), and *sonnei* (1 serotype but multiple colicin types)].

At the beginning of the 20th century, when it was commonly believed that pathogenic bacteria exerted their effects via toxins, investigators looked for and found that cell-free culture supernates of Shiga's bacillus, but not of the other related species, were toxic to animals.[2] This toxic activity was known as Shiga neurotoxin, because when injected into certain animals, it caused a characteristic limb paralysis, terminating in death. Over the next 50 years, the neurotoxic material was clearly shown to be distinct from lipopolysaccharide and, when the protein toxin was partially purified, to be one of the most potent known poisons. From the time of its discovery, however, neurotoxin remained a biological activity in search of pathogenetic relevance until 1972 when neurotoxin-containing cell-free preparations from recent epidemic isolates of Shiga's bacillus were shown to be enterotoxic as well, capable of inducing both fluid secretion by rabbit small intestine and an inflammatory enteritis resembling the colitis of human dysentery.[3] Although this finding suggested the importance of the toxin in pathogenesis of the intestinal phase of shigellosis, the gene for Shiga toxin is now known to be restricted to *S. dysenteriae* 1 alone, and it is considered to be a salient accessory factor in causing the particularly severe disease associated with this species.

3. Methodology

3.1. Sources of Mortality and Morbidity Data

It is difficult to accurately determine morbidity or mortality rates due to shigellosis, except during epidemics or in microbiologically proven hospital series. There is first of all a "numerator problem"; that is, unless there is bloody diarrhea or frank dysentery, the clinical manifestations of shigellosis can be indistinguishable from other bacterial or viral enteritides, and without laboratory studies the etiology of the illness cannot be ascertained. A clinical diagnosis can be made with greater confidence if the case occurs among a cluster of related cases, as in a common source or a day-care center outbreak, at least one of which is laboratory confirmed. The "laboratory" diagnosis of an individual case depends on good microbiological technique. Certain media used for isolation of enteric pathogens are inhibitory to the growth of shigellae and multiple cultures may be needed to establish the diagnosis. In addition, shigellae do not survive well in certain transport media, such as Cary–Blair, that are commonly used to transport fecal specimens in community studies from the field to the laboratory for investigation. Second, there is a "denominator problem," because not all groups are equally at risk and because prior assumptions that asymptomatic infections were uncommon may not be true.[4] *Shigella* infection is most often identified in patients, usually children, who either have the dysenteric or bloody diarrhea forms of the illness or have specific complications, such as seizures. More mildly affected patients, particularly those without clinical dysentery, are usually treated symptomatically and specific etiology is not determined. The problem of underdiagnosis is even more pronounced in many less-developed countries, where access to health care facilities is limited and laboratory services are, as a general rule, not available.

Available data generally come from three sources: (1) hospital-based reports, (2) etiologic investigations of diarrhea in the community setting, and (3) national surveillance. The first source will miss most of the disease in the community. The third, such as the national surveillance system maintained by the United States Centers for Disease Control and Prevention (CDC), depends on multiple reporting sources based on cultures submitted to local and state health departments. Only community studies of the second sort can provide reliable estimates of morbidity or mortality. As these data are usually time and place specific, they are not necessarily universally applicable.

3.2. Surveys

Both bacteriologic and serological methods have been used in prospective community-based surveys of the incidence and prevalence of *Shigella* infection. However, bacteriologic surveys can underestimate the true infection prevalence because the stool sample may be inadequate or poorly handled, which allows organisms to die before they can be cultured on appropriate media, or because patients are sampled either too late in the course of their illness or after antibiotic therapy has been initiated.

A variety of serological methods have been employed for detecting both acute infection as well as evidence of past infection, but their usefulness is limited because there can be serological cross-reactivity between *Shigella* and other genera of bacteria as well as between different serotypes of *Shigella*, they may have limited sensitivity, and titers may wane rather quickly after infection. Serotype-specific enzyme-linked immunosorbent assays (ELISAs) have been developed for the somatic antigens of *S. dysenteriae* 1, *S. flexneri* 1–5, *S. flexneri* 6, and *S. sonnei*.[5] ELISAs for shared *Shigella* virulence traits, such as invasion plasmid antigens or other outer-membrane proteins or toxins have been developed, but their utility for diagnostic or epidemiological purposes has not been fully explored.[6]

3.3. Laboratory Diagnosis, Isolation, and Identification of the Organism

Shigellae are slender, gram-negative, nonmotile rods. They are members of the family Enterobacteriaceae and tribe Escherichia, and are closed related to *Escherichia coli*. Routine isolation and identification of *Shigella* species involves the use of selective bacteriologic media that spotlight certain biochemical properties of the genus and allow a presumptive microbiological diagnosis. Identity can be quickly confirmed by the use of serological agglutination reactions, employing group-specific anti-O (somatic) antigen sera. Unfortunately, many of the commercially available typing sera are of poor quality, being too dilute or too cross-reactive to identify group- or type-specific antigens.[7] Even so, the grouping sera are reasonably good for *S. dysenteriae* 1, *S. flexneri* (except *flexneri* 6), and *S. sonnei* bearing form I antigen, which are the most important isolates to identify in the United States.

Because feces is the most frequently submitted specimen for isolation of *Shigella*, representing a complex ecosystem of many different organisms, differential bacteriologic media are used with two purposes in mind: (1) to suppress the growth of the usual nonpathogenic normal flora that might numerically overwhelm and obscure the growth of *Shigella* and (2) to dramatically contrast the colonial appearance of the possible pathogen with that of the common commensal so that suspect colonies may be picked for further study. This is accomplished by inclusion in the media of either substances inhibitory to the growth of nonpathogens or a dye indicator system to detect rapid fermentation of lactose, since all shigellae are unable to perform this reaction, while commensals can. A variety of media have been developed for this purpose; the most successful and currently used are MacConkey's bile salt, xylose–lysine–deoxycholate (XLD), Hektoen enteric (HE), and tergitol-7-triphenyl tetrazolium chloride agars. These media permit the growth of all *Shigella* species reasonably well, are inhibitory to normal flora, and clearly distinguish the lactose-negative organisms by color reactions. *Salmonella–Shigella* (SS) agar is far too inhibitory to shigellae, especially to *S. dysenteriae* 1, to be recommended for general use, particularly if only one differential medium is to be used.[8] Indeed, it is microbiologically sound to employ more than one screening medium to maximize the yield of positives. When the number of organisms in the sample is small, isolation may be facilitated by brief enrichment in broth inhibitory to nonpathogens, such as Hajna's gram-negative broth. After 6–8 hr of incubation of the sample in broth, the resulting growth is streaked onto the same differential media used in direct isolation as above.

Three technical details should be followed to minimize the number of false-negative cultures: (1) whenever possible, inoculate from a stool sample, rather than a swab, selecting blood-tinged mucus plugs as the source of culture; (2) if a swab is to be used, be certain that it passes beyond the anal sphincter; and (3) if there is to be any appreciable delay in processing the sample, place it in buffered glycerol–saline holding medium.[9]

Lactose-negative colonies are picked to a medium such as triple sugar iron (TSI) agar, which allows confirmation of the lactose-negative phenotype and detects glucose fermentation and lack of motility, which are additional properties of shigellae. Both the agar surface (slant) and the butt are inoculated with the colony to be tested, to achieve aerobic and anaerobic conditions, respectively. In the butt, fermentation of glucose results in a pH change and a change in the color of the phenol red indicator to yellow (acid) but without gas bubbles, while on the slant, the failure of the organism to use lactose (or sucrose, which is also contained in TSI) precludes sufficient drop in pH to change the pink (alkaline) color. In contrast to the non-lactose-fermenting enteric pathogens in the genus *Salmonella*, no black reaction product is deposited due to H_2S formation. The presumptive diagnosis is then confirmed by serological agglutinations using group-specific antisera. More thorough biochemical studies can be done, but this is rarely necessary, and the criteria enumerated above, included in standard schemata for the identification of Enterobacteriaceae, are sufficient for diagnostic purposes.

4. Biological Characteristics of the Organism

The ability to invade epithelial cells has been considered the single most important characteristic of *Shigella* mediating its characteristic pathogenesis. Studies over the past decade have shown that invasiveness per se is just one characteristic of a set of traits that allows the organism to enter the host cell, then multiply, spread within the infected cell and, most importantly for virulence, from cell to cell, and ultimately kill the contiguously infected cells.[10] These properties are enlisted in a sequential manner during infection and are dependent on multiple virulence genes encoded on both the chromosome and a large 120- to 140-MDa plasmid present in all virulent *Shigella* and the phenotypically similar enteroinvasive *E. coli* (EIEC).[11] These virulence genes are, in turn, under the control of multiple regulator genes.[12] Once invasion of a single host cell has occurred, the entire process from invasion, escape from the phagocytic vesicle, intracellular multiplication, cell-to-cell spread, and death of the newly infected cell can occur without exposure of the internalized organism to the external milieu. In this manner, *Shigella* secures a secure ecological niche for itself, sequestered away from host antibacterial factors including antibody, complement, and phagocytic cells. It is presumably this sequestration from host defenses that permits establishment of infection in a significant number of adults challenged with as few as 100–200 viable *Shigella* in 30 ml of milk without bicarbonate ingested by mouth[13] (Table 1). The tiny infective dose, in turn, permits effective contact spread from host to host without the need for enrichment growth in some vehicle such as food or water.

Table 1. Infectious Inoculum in Experimental Shigellosis in Normal Adult Volunteers[a]

Species (strain)	Dose[b]	Number of volunteers	Number (%) ill
S. dysenteriae 1			
(A1)	200	8	3 (38)
	10^4	6	2 (33)
(M131)	10	10	1 (10)
	200	4	2 (50)
	2×10^3	10	7 (70)
	10^4	6	5 (83)
S. flexneri 2a			
(2457-T)	100	36	14 (39)
	180	36	9 (25)
	5×10^3	49	28 (57)
	10^4	103	58 (56)
	$\geqslant 10^5$	59	38 (64)
S. sonnei			
(53 G)	500	58	26 (45)

[a]Data from DuPont *et al.*[13]
[b]Estimated number of bacteria given in oral inoculum, suspended in 30 ml of milk.

4.1. Invasiveness and Intercellular Spread

It is now clear that invasion of host cells by virulent *Shigella* within a host cell membrane-bounded vesicle must be followed by escape from the vesicle to the cytoplasm, growth and division of the organism, spread within cells and to adjacent cells, and host cell death, since interruption of any of these stages renders the organism avirulent. The process has been arbitrarily divided into four stages, including (1) entry into the host cell, (2) vesicle lysis and bacterial growth, (3) intra- and intercellular spread, and (4) death of the host cell.[14] This model for virulence has been developed largely on the basis of studies of *S. flexneri* strains, and it is largely assumed that other *Shigella* serotypes and the biologically similar EIEC act in the same manner.

4.1.1. Invasion. Penetration of the host cell proceeds by a process analogous to leukocyte phagocytosis.[15] There is some controversy about the specific cell type initially invaded. The earlier concept was based on tissue culture models and suggested that *Shigella* invade directly across the apical membrane of intestinal epithelial cells. More recent studies indicate that the initial site of invasion from the intestinal lumen might be the antigen-sampling M cell. The use of new model systems raises the possibility that bacteria may also cross the apical mucosa at intercellular junctions after initial inflammatory damage to the brush border and secondary opening of tight junctions. Thus, invasion of villuslike human colonic-cancer-derived $CaCo_2$ cells occurs over the domes formed during cellular differentiation, specifically at intercellular junctions.[16] If these junctions are disrupted by addition of the Ca^{2+} chelator EGTA, the rate of cell invasion is greatly enhanced. Furthermore, when *S. flexneri* are placed on the apical surface of the cryptlike human colon-cancer-derived T-84 cells growing on semipermeable filters in the upper chamber, in the presence of human neutrophils in the basal chamber, the leukocytes migrate across the monolayer, reaching a maximum by 1 hr, after which bacteria invade the monolayer at the intercellular junctions.[17] Limited *in vivo* experimental animal data support these conclusions.[18] In rabbit ligated intestinal loops, for example, early invading organisms are primarily associated with lymphoid follicles; however, subsequent neutrophil infiltration interrupts the cohesion of the epithelial layer and leads to a markedly increased invasion of bacteria. This invasion was significantly inhibited in the presence of anti-CD18 antibody, which also reduced the migration of neutrophils into the mucosa.

Organisms enter the cell, as in phagocytosis, within a vesicle formed from host cell membrane, initiated by at least three surface proteins of the microbe.[19] These are called invasion plasmid antigens (Ipa) B, C, and D, because they are encoded by a plasmid operon common to all invasive and virulent shigellae and EIEC. These essential virulence factors are transported to and inserted in the outer membrane of the organism under the control of two regulatory gene sets, *mxi* (membrane export of Ipa)[20] and *spa* (surface presentation of invasion plasmid antigens).[21] Ipa proteins lead to complex changes in the cytoskeleton of the host cell that underlie vesicle formation and bacterial entry.[15] Growth of the organism on cultured epithelial cells results in the enhanced release of Ipa molecules into the surrounding medium where they can act on the host cell.[22]

4.1.2. Vesicle Lysis and Intracellular Multiplication. To be virulent, *Shigella* must also rapidly escape the vesicle to reach the cytoplasm of the host cell. Lysis of the vesicle has been associated with a temperature-dependent contact hemolytic activity.[23] When virulent strains are grown at 30°C, however, expression of hemolysin is inhibited and bacteria do not reach the host cell cytoplasm. Hemolytic activity of organisms grown at 37°C also increases 100- to 1000-fold when the pH is lowered from neutral to 5.5,[24] as occurs within the phagocytic vesicle, supporting a physiological role for this phenomenon. The molecular basis for vesicle lysis appears to reside in the Ipa proteins involved in bacterial invasion. Nonpolar inactivation mutants of Ipa B, C, or D are inhibited in both entry and lysis of the vesicle,[25] indicating the role of Ipa proteins in both processes.

Intracytoplasmic multiplication of *Shigella* begins soon after vesicle lysis. The organism is avirulent if this too is blocked, for example, by inhibiting folic acid synthesis via the aromatic pathway, or secondary to mutations of the porins, OmpC and OmpF, or their regulatory gene, *ompB*.[26,27]

4.1.3. Intra- and Intercellular Spread. Although they are without flagellae and therefore nonmotile, virulent *Shigella* must move within the host cell cytoplasm to reach the plasma membrane if they are to invade adjacent cell from the intracellular niche. An elaborate mechanism allows the organisms to use the host cell cytoskeleton to accomplish this, via the plasmid-encoded protein IcsA.[28] IcsA is expressed during bacterial division at the back pole of the organism (defined in terms of its subsequent direction of movement),[29] and is associated with localized actin polymerization, leading to the formation of an actin tail just behind the organism. The actin-binding host protein, plastin, which has two actin-binding sites per monomer, colocalizes with the polymerized actin, resulting in actin cross-linking and a sphincterlike contraction, which provides a forward propulsive force. This so-called "actin motor" is energized by ATP generated by IcsA, an ATPase[30] that is regulated by cyclic nucleotide-dependent host cell protein kinases that phosphorylate IcsA.[31] Thus, phosphorylation mutations enhance microbial spread, whereas protein kinase inhibitors block the invasion of HeLa cell monolayers by *S. flexneri*.[32] These data suggest that host protein kinases modulate virulence through phosphorylation of IcsA and, in a sense, act as a molecular host defense mechanism.

To spread from cell to cell, *Shigella* are first propelled to the plasma membrane where they cause long fingerlike protrusions, still membrane bounded, into the adjacent cell.[33] When these subsequently fuse with the plasma membrane of the second cell, the organism is located within a vesicle in the newly invaded cell. One host target for this process is the cadherin, L-CAM,[34] which appears to proceed by homotypic binding of the extracellular domain of cadherin and anchoring of the actin tail via molecular interactions with intermediate junction proteins. Defects in L-CAM result in the formation of abortive protrusions that do not lead to the intercellular transfer of organisms. *IcsB*, the second gene of the Ics operon, is essential for this final stage in cell to cell invasion.[33] Mutational inactivation of *icsB* blocks the ability of the organism to lyse the double membrane vesicle formed by the protrusions from one host cell to the next, and such mutants are avirulent.

A second mechanism for intracellular spread has been noted, wherein *Shigella* move in an organized manner by binding to actin stress fibers. This movement follows the cytoskeletal architecture and has therefore been termed organellelike movement (OLM).[35] In cultured intestinal $CaCo_2$ cells, bacteria move to the perijunctional actin filament ring by means of OLM movement in a manner distinct from the Ics-mediated cell-to-cell spread of infection.[36] Since OLM movement could enhance the likelihood of successful intracellular spread and subsequent intercellular spread, the two mechanisms may be interactive and complementary.

4.1.4. Cell Death. The end result of invasion and cell-to-cell spread is host cell death. Although the mechanism by which this occurs remains uncertain, at least when the target cell is a macrophage, uptake of *S. flexneri* induces apoptosis.[37] IpaB plays a critical role in this process, since strains with mutational inactivation of IpaC or D but still expressing low levels of an inserted *E. coli* hemolysin to allow escape from the phagocytic vesicle still induce apoptosis but and IpaB mutant does not.[38]

4.2. Acid Resistance

Because gastric acid secretion acts as an effective barrier for enteric pathogens to reach their preferred locale in the gut, resistance to acid can serve as an accessory virulence trait. This property could explain one of the unique characteristics of *Shigella* pathogenesis, the very small inoculum required to cause disease. Indeed, *S. flexneri*, and probably other species as well, are significantly more acid resistant *in vitro* than are *Salmonella* or *E. coli*.[39] This phenotype is growth phase dependent and is acquired as bacteria reach late log and stationary phase. Genetic recombination experiments have identified some of the involved genes, including a global regulatory system in which a stationary growth phase sigma factor encoded by *rpoS* plays a key role.[40] Acid resistance is especially marked when cells are grown anaerobically at low pH, conditions encountered in the colon during infection. This suggests that as *Shigella* pass through the colon and enter stationary phase prior to being excreted in feces, they acquire acid resistance. Since this would occur before or as they enter the environment, the excreted organisms would be better equipped to face the gastric acid barrier when ingested by a new susceptible host. There is an apparent trade-off, at least *in vitro*, as acid-exposed bacteria have a reduced capacity to invade tissue culture cells. However, once past the stomach, the bacteria would begin to grow, rapidly lose acid resistance properties, and acquire the invasive phenotype.

4.3. Soluble Virulence Proteins

Shigella siderophores (aerobactin-type in most *Shigella*, except some *S. sonnei*, which express enterobactins), iron chelator proteins essential for bacterial growth, also have an impact on virulence. Although tissue culture models show no differences between invasion or growth of siderophore-positive or -negative organisms *in vivo*, where free iron is virtually completely protein bound, the kinetics of infection with *iuc* aerobactin mutants is delayed,[41] suggesting that functional siderophores facilitate the initial multiplication of the organism.

The specific structure of the O side chain of the somatic antigen may also affect virulence. Conjugal transfer of *E. coli* somatic antigens 8 or 25 into *S. flexneri* 2a renders the former but not the latter avirulent.[42] Interestingly, the O-25 antigen resembles *S. flexneri* 2a somatic antigen in its high mannose content. Rough *Shigella* lacking O side chains invade and multiply intracellularly but do not spread from cell to cell, and they too are avirulent *in vivo*.[43] Moreover, they do not cause disease in humans accidently infected in the laboratory, in contrast to smooth (O-antigen complete) strains.[44] Lack of virulence of rough mutants appears to be, in part, the failure to transport and correctly localize IcsA in the bacterial cell outer membrane.[45] A Tn5 insertion mutant in the *rfa* locus involved in the synthesis of the lipopolysaccharide (LPS) basal core region delays cell-to-cell spread *in vitro* as well as the extent of the inflammatory mucosal reaction *in vivo*.[46]

Superoxide dismutase (SodB) is another protein in *Shigella* that may enhance virulence by blocking the bactericidal effects of host-derived reactive oxygen radicals.[47] Thus, an inactivated *sodB S. flexneri* mutant obtained by allelic exchange is extremely sensitive to oxidative stress and is readily killed by mouse macrophages or human neutrophils and is avirulent in the ligated rabbit ileal loop model.

4.4. Toxins

Shiga toxin, a lethal protein toxin made by *S. dysenteriae* 1, is of the same order of potency as botulinum and tetanus toxins. It is not required for virulence of *Shigella* since the non-Shiga toxin-producing *S. flexneri*, *boydii*, and *sonnei* cause disease; however, its presence increases the severity of illness when isogenic toxin-positive and -negative *S. dysenteriae* 1 mutants are compared in primate infection models.[48] Shiga toxin may play a role in pathogenesis of systemic manifestations of infection with the latter organism, such as hemolytic–uremic syndrome and thrombotic thrombocytopenic purpura, since *E. coli* producing structurally and functionally homologous toxins can cause the same problems.[49]

Shiga toxin (and its homologues in *E. coli* commonly referred to as Shiga-like toxins or Verotoxins, but now renamed Shiga toxin 1 and Shiga toxin 2) are heterodimeric proteins composed of a single enzymatically active A subunit and a cluster of five identical B subunit monomers that mediate binding of toxin to target cell receptors. All share the same enzymatic specificity, an RNA glycohydrolase activity that specifically inactivates the 28S rRNA of the mammalian ribosome and blocks protein synthesis, as well as the same binding specificity for globoseries glycolipids terminating in a galactose-$\alpha 1 \rightarrow 4$-galactose disaccharide.[50]

Using a monoclonal antibody capture ELISA test, Shiga toxin has been found in stool of approximately 80% of patients in Bangladesh with *S. dysenteriae* 1 infection but in fewer than 20% of those with *S. flexneri* infection.[51] Clinical evidence also indicates that the highly toxigenic *S. dysenteriae* 1 strain produces a more severe form of illness than does either *S. flexneri* or *S. sonnei*.[52,53] In volunteers with induced experimental shigellosis, the mean incubation period is shorter and the severity of clinical disease is greater in individuals infected with a fully toxigenic *S. dysenteriae* 1 strain compared to a derived hypotoxigenic mutant.[54]

Recent data have demonstrated two distinctive new *Shigella* enterotoxins: ShET-1 and -2.[55–57] These toxins alter electrolyte transport by rabbit small bowel tissue *in vitro* and cause net fluid secretion *in vivo* in ligated rabbit ileal loops, although they are much less active on a weight basis compared to Shiga toxin. Humans appear to develop neutralizing antibody, which suggests that they are produced *in vivo*; however, their role, if any, in pathogenesis of the watery diarrhea phase of shigellosis remains uncertain. ShET-1 appears to be encoded by a chromosomal gene, whereas ShET-2 is controlled by an iron-regulated plasmid gene and is highly homologous with a previously described EIEC enterotoxin.[55,56] The potential importance of ShET-1 is limited by the observation that the ShET-1 gene appears to be present almost exclusively in *S. flexneri* 2a and not in other species or serotypes.[58]

4.5. Antimicrobial Resistance

Resistance to antimicrobial agents commonly used in the treatment of shigellosis is a continuing major problem, both in developed and in developing countries.[59,60] Increasing resistance to ampicillin and trimethoprim–sulfamethoxazole (T-SMX), the least-cost drugs of choice for the treatment of drug-susceptible shigellosis, has in many situations forced practitioners to use alternative drugs, which are generally more expensive and/or unavailable in the Third World, such as new β-lactams or third-generation cephalosporins, less effective drugs (oral nonabsorbable drugs) or drugs that have not yet been approved by the US Food and Drug Administration for use in shigellosis (naladixic acid) or in children (ciprofloxacin or ofloxacin) (Fig. 1).[61] Resistance to these antimicrobials can also be expected to become more common as well as they are increasingly used (Table 2).[60,61]

5. Descriptive Epidemiology

5.1. Prevalence and Incidence

In 1986, it was estimated that 140 million cases and 576,000 deaths occur annually due to *Shigella* infection in children under 5 years of age, even excluding data from China.[62] Because of the problems described in Section 3, such an estimate of worldwide prevalence is only a gross approximation of the actual number. In the United States, endemic isolation rates for all *Shigella* spp. derived from the CDC's national laboratory-based surveillance system approximated 6 per 100,000 between 1967 through 1988, punctuated by periods of increased endemicity, when rates increased to around 9–10 per 100,000.[63] The periodic increases were primarily due to outbreaks of *S. sonnei*. Rates in children 1 to 4 years of age were tenfold higher than among 20 year and older adults (27 vs. 2.6 per 100,000) and were highest in counties with relatively high

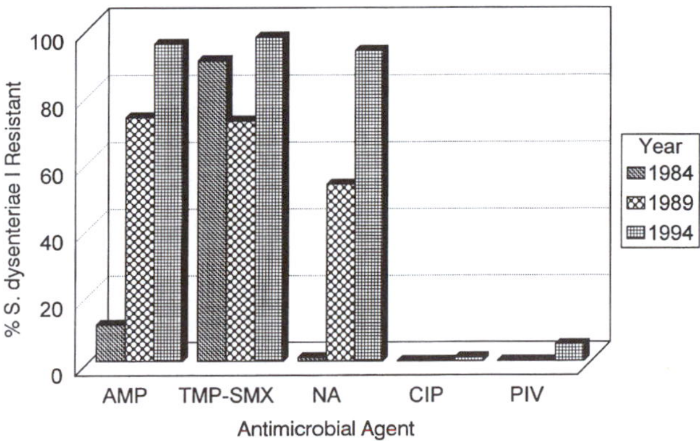

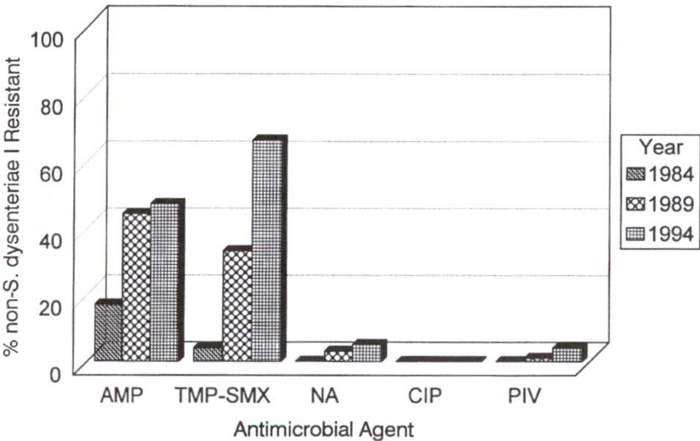

Figure 1. Antimicrobial resistance patterns of *S. dysenteriae* type 1 (upper panel) and other *Shigella* species, predominantly *S. flexneri* (lower panel), to the most commonly used drugs in Dhaka, Bangladesh, in 19984, 1989, and 1994. Following the development of resistance by *S. dysenteriae* type 1 to ampicillin (AMP) and trimethoprim–sulfamethoxazole (TMP-SMX), there was a marked increase in the use of naladixic acid (NAL), with a marked increase in the prevalence of NAL resistance. At this time, nearly all isolates are susceptible to ciprofloxacin (CIP) and pivamdinocillin (PIV). Resistance to AMP and TMP-SMX also has increased among other *Shigella* spp., but not as dramatically, and most isolates remained susceptible to NAL, CIP, and PIV in 1994.

Table 2. Selected Recent Surveys of Antimicrobial Resistance of *Shigella* Species

				Percent (%) susceptible to the listed antimicrobial agent[a]					
Year	Location	*Shigella* spp.	Number	Amp	TMP-SMX	Nal	Pivam	Cipro	Ceph
1994	Bangladesh	*dysenteriae* 1	229	2	0.5	2	95	100	100
		flexneri	461	44	33	95	95	100	100
		boydii	175	74	51	99	99	100	100
		sonnei	72	86	32	77	97	100	100
1991–1992	Israel	*flexneri*	39	49	60	100	NT	100	80
		sonnei	557	16	14	100	NT	100	99
1993	Spain	*flexneri*[b]	14	36	50	NT	NT	100	NT
		flexneri[c]	35	40	63	NT	NT	100	NT
		sonnei[b]	26	69	92	NT	NT	100	NT
		sonnei[c]	22	68	46	NT	NT	100	NT
1989–1992	Brazil	*flexneri*	21	6	19	10	NT	100	93
1991	Guatemala	*flexneri*	36	NT	25	NT	83	NT	NT
		sonnei	15	NT	13	NT	93	NT	NT
1990	Burundi	*dysenteriae* 1	50	0	0	0	100	100	100
		flexneri	23	87	87	100	100	100	100
1990	Canada	*dysenteriae* 1	24	54	71	NT	NT	NT	NT
		flexneri	254	33	79	NT	NT	NT	NT
		boydii	30	43	73	NT	NT	NT	NT
		sonnei	290	61	62	NT	NT	NT	NT

[a]Antibiotics: Amp, ampicillin; TMP-SMX, trimethoprim–sulfamethoxazole; Nal, naladixic acid; Cipro, ciprofloxacin; Ceph, third-generation cephalosporin.
[b]Local isolates.
[c]Traveler's diarrhea isolates, primarily from developing countries.

proportions of low-income minority group residents, including African Americans, Hispanics, and Native Americans, especially in urban communities. Over the same period of time, a prospective surveillance study among 321 children living in a rural Guatemalan village followed for 24 months or until their third birthday showed a striking isolation rate for *Shigella* of 9,800 per 100,000 with diarrheal illness.[(64)] Half of the *Shigella*-infected children had more than one documented episode during the study period, and the incidence rate approximated 125,000 per 100,000. These are similar to the rates observed in prospective studies from similar rural villages in Guatemala two decades earlier. That this is not atypical for developing countries is indicated by analysis of carefully collected prospective surveillance data from rural Bangladesh, where the *Shigella* isolation rate was 9,700 per 100,000 among individuals with diarrhea.[(65)] In both settings, a substantial but significantly lower prevalence of asymptomatic infections was identified.

In an earlier study, nearly one-third of a group of 110 young children recovering from acute *Shigella* infections in a convalescent home in Guatemala were initially positive for *Shigella*.[(66)] Twenty of these children, including 6 documented *Shigella*-infected subjects, were then followed with daily examinations and cultures. Of these 20, 8 remained negative for *Shigella*, while 12 subsequently harbored the agent at one time or another during the study. Of the latter, eight were asymptomatic carriers, one was an acute case, and three had chronic recurrent diarrheal disease. In two patients, there was transition from carrier to acute case after 12 and 15 days of symptomless documented carriage. These two patients highlight the problem of differentiating the healthy carrier state from carriers who subsequently develop disease. It is generally believed that clinical illness occurs within a period of 5–6 days or not at all, but this may not be correct. The chronic relapsing form of illness was characterized by continuous presence of organisms and periods of acute active diarrhea, with intervals of low-grade or indefinite symptomatology. The organism was excreted during 75 of 154 person weeks of observation (in 27 weeks of acute illness and 48 weeks of asymptomatic carriage). Following shigellosis, 17% of the children excreted organisms for at least 1 month and 11% for more than 2 months.

However, there are groups in the United States that have incidence and prevalence rates that begin to resemble those seen in developing countries. One such group are Native Americans, with an incidence rate 3.6 times that of the general population, typically *S. flexneri* rather than *S. sonnei* that infects the rest of the American population. Another group with high incidence are developmentally disabled and mentally retarded persons, because of the difficulty in controlling their fecal contamination of the environment. This has historically been referred to as "asylum dysentery." In studies 25 years ago, as many as 10% of long-time residents of residential schools had *Shigella* infections during a prospective observation study, with incidence rates for new admissions approximating 37,000 per 100,000. Long-term, intermittent excretion of the organism was present in 7%, due either to prolonged carriage or frequent reinfection. In a more recent study in New York state during 1982 to 1987, the relative risk (RR) for diarrhea outbreaks at summer camps for the developmentally disabled compared to summer camps for normal children was 8.6, and all the *Shigella* infections occurred in the former (RR = infinity).[67]

Children in day-care centers are a third group with a high incidence of shigellosis.[68] With the increase in the number of children in day-care facilities in recent years, these centers are playing an increasingly important role in transmission of the disease in the United States. In prospective studies in some centers, the incidence of culture-confirmed shigellosis has approached 7,000 per 100,000, with secondary cases in as many as one quarter of families when a child in day care developed shigellosis. In other settings, infection was first introduced into the household by a child attending day care in 25% of affected families investigated.

The prototypic *Shigella* species, *S. dysenteriae* 1, was the cause of numerous outbreaks of shigellosis throughout the world in the first two decades of the 20th century, with high morbidity and mortality.[69] Inexplicably, this organism became less prevalent after 1920, and various serotypes of *S. flexneri* became dominant. After World War II, *S. sonnei* gradually replaced *S. flexneri* in industrialized nations,[70] while *S. flexneri* persisted in developing countries.[65] In the first decade of surveillance by the CDC in the United States from the mid-1960s to the mid-1970s, the proportion of *S. flexneri* went from 60.6% in 1964 to 15.5% in 1973, while the percent isolation of *S. sonnei* rose from 38.1 to 83.6%.[71] The absolute number of *S. flexneri* decreased and that of *S. sonnei* increased, so that over the course of the decade approximately two thirds of the isolates were *S. sonnei* and one third were *S. flexneri*, a complete reversal in the relative frequency of the two organisms. From 1970 through 1994, 269,890 confirmed isolates of *Shigella* were reported to the CDC through the national surveillance system. Species information was available in nearly 98% (Table 3). Isolation of *S. sonnei* exceeded that of *S. flexneri* by 3:1, and the two species accounted for over 97% of all isolates.

Table 3. Prevalence of *Shigella* Species in the United States, 1970–1994[a]

	Percent (%) of identified isolates during reporting period		
	1970–1979	1980–1989	1990–1994
S. dysenteriae	0.6	0.8	0.5
S. flexneri	22.6	23.7	15.6
S. boydii	1.0	1.9	1.1
S. sonnei	75.8	73.6	82.8

[a]Adapted from the Laboratory Confirmed *Shigella* Surveillance Annual Summary, 1991–1992, Foodborne and Diarrheal Diseases Branch, Centers for Disease Control and Prevention, Atlanta, GA.

A similar change in prevalence has been observed in Israel, where *S. sonnei* overtook *S. flexneri* as the main isolate in the 1960s.[72] Between 1986 and 1991, the proportion of *S. sonnei* increased further from 60 to 91%, while *S. flexneri* decreased from 29 to 8% over the same period.[73] In regions of Israel where both westernized and nonwesternized populations live in the same geographic area, *S. sonnei* was the dominant organism among the former (73.2%), whereas *S. flexneri* continued to predominate in the latter group (66.7%).[74]

5.2. Epidemic Behavior

Engrafted on this unexplained, changing world picture in prevalence of *Shigella* species has been the reappearance of epidemic *S. dysenteriae* 1 dysentery since 1969. After many years of playing a minor role in the etiology of shigellosis in Central America, *S. dysenteriae* 1 suddenly and dramatically became the dominant enteric pathogen in 1969–1970.[75] It resulted in epidemic spread of infection, affecting adults as well as children, with the index case often an adult, and it caused a degree of severity in the disease much beyond the accustomed level. For example, in 18 Guatemalan communities surveyed, the dysentery mortality increased from 39 per 100,000 in 1968 to 170 per 100,000 in 1969 when the outbreak occurred.[75] All age groups were affected, the youngest and the oldest most significantly. The death rate for the entire country was estimated to be 250 per 100,000, varying from 334 per 100,000 in the lowlands to 190 per 100,000 in the highlands. The case fatality rate was also quite high in untreated patients, ranging from 8.4% of community cases to 10–15% of those hospitalized because of acute illness. This rate decreased later in the epidemic when the cause was appreciated and appropriate therapy was employed. These features are in contrast to endemic shigellosis, principally due to *S. flexneri* and *S. sonnei*, primarily affecting young children in the under 5-year-old group, with the index case in families generally a preschool or school-age child and with mortality in adults an unusual event.

Epidemic *S. dysenteriae* 1 dysentery subsequently appeared in South Asia in the mid-1970s and in Africa in the early 1980s. After the initial large-scale outbreaks, it has become a part of endemic dysentery, with periodic surges in incidence. For example, prospective bacteriological data from 1978 to 1987 obtained in rural Bangladesh show a dominance of *S. flexneri* between 1978 and 1982 (56–67%), a rise in *S. dysenteriae* 1 prevalence between 1983 and 1985 (45–50%), and a return of *S. flexneri* in 1986 and 1987 (55–61%).(75) Wherever this organism lurks in the background, the potential for epidemic spread remains a threat. When a sudden influx of nearly three quarters of a million refugees fleeing Rwanda entered into Zaire in 1994, explosive outbreaks of cholera and then *S. dysenteriae* 1 occurred sequentially, with a crude mortality rate of 200–350/100,000 per day and around 50,000 cumulative deaths.(76) This was followed by widespread acute malnutrition, especially in those with a recent history of dysentery and in families without a male adult. Epidemic disease remains a possibility in many parts of the world, often in association with civil disruption and migration of large numbers of people, as occurred in Central Africa in the mid-1990s.(77)

5.3. Geographic Distribution

Shigella is worldwide in distribution. The incidence of infection in different regions will vary, of course, with the level of sanitation and exposure. *S. sonnei* has become the main isolate in industrialized countries, whereas *S. flexneri* remains the most common isolate in developing countries. *S. dysenteriae* 1 is now endemic, and occasionally epidemic, in the poor countries of Asia, Africa, and Latin America. *S. boydii* remains relatively uncommon everywhere (<1–2%) except in the Indian subcontinent. In the United States, the highest *Shigella* isolation rates are from the southwestern states, where the relative proportion of *S. flexneri* is higher than elsewhere in the country. This may be related to the proximity to Mexico and the cross-border flow of legal and illegal immigrants and migrant workers. Infection with *S. dysenteriae* 1, and to a lesser extent *S. flexneri*, is related to travel to developing countries.(78)

5.4. Temporal Distribution

Different temporal patterns of shigellosis have been found in different regions of the world. In the United States, peak incidence of both *S. sonnei* and *S. flexneri* infection occurs in summer and early fall. In both urban and rural Bangladesh, *Shigella* isolation peaks in the post-monsoon season of December and January, and again in the hot, dry premonsoon period of April and May. In Calcutta, India, the incidence of shigellosis is highest during the monsoon season itself, while in Calabar, Nigeria, the peak occurs during the dry season. In Egypt and among Bedouins in southern Israel peak incidence is during the early summer months of June and July. In contrast to the Bedouins, Jews with a Western lifestyle living in southern Israel experience summer and winter peaks, while in nearby Saudi Arabia a winter peak for *S. flexneri* has been reported. In Guatemala, the illness tends to peak just before and in the early weeks of the rainy season. In other locales, there is no clear seasonal peak, and cases occur all year round.

A variety of explanations, none entirely satisfactory, have been offered for the different temporal patterns observed, which must relate to specific epidemiological features in the various environments that lead to seasonal transmission. Explanations for summertime peaks in temperate climates include increased social activity of children during this time, promoting person-to-person transmission, and perhaps longer survival of organisms in the environment. Summertime peaks during the hot, dry season in tropical climates have been explained by decreased availability of water and the attendant decrease of water use for personal hygiene. Last, peaks before or during the rainy season have been explained by increased contamination of water supplies due to water washing feces from ground sources, or seasonal worsening of nutritional status and increased susceptibility to infection.

5.5. Age

Endemic shigellosis is a childhood disease in both developed and developing nation settings, whereas epidemic shigellosis can be expected to affect all age groups. But, even where shigellosis is highly endemic, neonatal shigellosis, generally originating from an infection in the mother, is rare. This is probably attributable to the high prevalence of antibody in breast milk among mothers in this setting.(79) Breast-feeding has been shown to be protective against disease among infected infants,(80) and perhaps this is why neonatal infection has been considered to be transient and usually asymptomatic in developing countries but systemic and severe in bottle-fed neonates in the United States.(81) In countries with a high endemicity of disease, shigellosis rates increase dramatically in the 3 months following cessation of breast-feeding, with an adjusted odds ratio of 6.6 (95% confidence interval, CI =

2.19–14.6, $p < .001$).[82] Although weanling diarrhea has traditionally been attributed to the risks associated with ingestion of contaminated weaning food, the addition of food supplements while breast-feeding is maintained does not increase shigella infection rates over the first 3 months of supplementary feeding if breast-feeding continues, with an odds ratio of just 1.2 for addition of food supplements (95% CI = 0.4–3.0).

However, even in developing countries, neonatal shigellosis may not be as benign as first believed. In a retrospective 5-year review of admissions from 1984 to 1989 to an international diarrhea treatment center in Bangladesh, 4741 patients with culture-proven shigellosis were identified.[83] Of these, 169 (3.1%) were 3 months of age or younger, of whom 19% were neonates under 1 month of age. Records were available on 159 subjects ≤3 months of age, including 30 (18.9%) neonates, and were compared with findings in 156 children 1 to 10 years old, with a mean age of 27 months. Infants were much less likely to have bloody diarrhea (17.2 vs. 57.3%), fever (32.7 vs. 58.6%), pedal edema (3.8 vs. 27.2%), or rectal prolapse (0 vs. 8.3%) on admission; however, they were significantly more likely to be moderately to severely dehydrated (59.9 vs. 31.1%) or to have abdominal distension (19.5 vs. 10.1%) or bacteremia (12 vs. 5%), and were twice as likely to die (16.4 vs. 8.2%). Multivariate analysis showed that concomitant gram-negative bacteremia, ileus, decreased bowel sounds, or severe hyponatremia or hypoproteinemia were significantly associated with fatal outcome. Interestingly, although three fifths of the cases in each age group were due to *S. flexneri*, neonates had a significantly greater prevalence of *S. boydii* (21.4 vs. 6.3%) and *S. sonnei* (7.6 vs. 1.3%), while a smaller proportion had *S. dysenteriae* 1 (9.4 vs. 31.5%).

Shigella infection rates increase after weaning, when poor diets and frequent infections combine to adversely affect host nutritional status. This postweaning increase in infection can also be demonstrated by seroepidemiological methods.[84] In Bangladesh, the highest incidence of Shigella bacteremia and death is in infants under the age of 1, and the associated risk factors are weaning and malnutrition.[85] During the recent epidemics of dysentery due to *S. dysenteriae* 1, the very young and elderly have experienced the most severe illness, with clustering of mortality at the extreme ages of life as well.

Beyond the first few years of life, increasing age is associated with lowered prevalence, diminished severity of illness, and a relative increase in the proportion of mild and subclinical infections. With decreasing prevalence of infection in the community, there is an apparent shift in the age-specific peak to a somewhat older age group. Thus, in contrast to Bangladesh, where the vast majority of cases are in the under 10-year-old children, primarily in those under 4 years old, in the United States, the proportion of isolates in the under 5-year-olds decreased from around 47 to 37% from 1967 to 1988, while the proportion occurring in those over 20 years of age increased from 17.3 to 37.1%, especially after 1974.[63] The proportional rise in the adults is sevenfold greater than the proportional increase in the US population over 20 years of age during the same period of time. Approximately three quarters of these adult patients were 20–39 years old.

5.6. Sex

Age-specific attack rates for *Shigella* infection in children show no sex differences. However, in the United States, the ratio of females to males among young adults with *Shigella* varies from 1.5 to 1.8, presumably reflecting the greater exposure of mothers to young children from whom they acquire the infection.[63] Another relative increase in the ratio of female-to-male cases occurs in 60- to 79-year-olds, suggesting possible transmission from young children to their grandmothers. In 1994, the female-to-male ratio in subjects with proven shigellosis in these two age groups was 2.0 and 1.6, respectively. In contrast, in areas with a large male homosexual population, there has been a discernible increase of infection in young and middle-aged males due to venereal transmission, especially during the period from 1976 to 1985 and primarily involving *S. flexneri*.[86] As a result, the median age of patients with *S. flexneri* infection has risen over time (Table 4). Surveillance data compiled by the CDC from 1977–1991 show an increase in the median age for *S.*

Table 4. Median Age of Persons Infected with *S. flexneri* or *S. sonnei*, United States, 1977–1991[a]

	Surveillance year, median age in years														
Serogroup	1977	1978	1979	1980	1981	1982	1983	1984	1985	1986	1987	1988	1989	1990	1991
S. flexneri	9	6	10	11	11	19	20	23	21	21	22	22	18	18	18
S. sonnei	6	7	6	6	7	7	7	7	8	7	7	7	7	8	7

[a]Adapted from the Laboratory Confirmed *Shigella* Surveillance Annual Summary, 1991–1992, Foodborne and Diarrheal Diseases Branch, Centers for Disease Control and Prevention, Atlanta, GA.

flexneri infection from 9 to over 20 years, peaking in 1984, and perhaps somewhat lower in more recent years, without a change in the median age (around 7 years) for *S. sonnei* infections. This may indicate a return to the pre-1975 trend toward diminishing *S. flexneri* prevalence, perhaps reflecting changing sexual practices among this group of young men.

5.7. Race

There is no evidence that race per se affects susceptibility to the disease. Genetic factors, such as HLA-B27 antigen, clearly predispose to joint involvement and post-dysenteric Reiter's syndrome; this may explain the frequency of these complications in Scandinavia, where the prevalence of histocompatibility antigen B27 in the population is relatively high.

5.8. Occupation

Certain occupations may increase exposure to shigellae. Notable examples are the increased incidence of shigellosis in women caring for young children at home. Teachers in day-care centers are also at greater risk than the general population,[87] and theoretically, so are attendants in custodial institutions for the mentally retarded, clinical microbiology laboratory technicians, and health care workers.[44] The lack of a striking incidence of shigellosis among laboratory technicians and health care workers may point to the protective value of good personal hygiene and ready access to clean water for washing.

5.9. Occurrence in Different Settings

Shigellosis can readily spread among individuals living in close quarters where personal hygiene and environmental sanitation are inadequate. The 1994 epidemic among refugees fleeing Rwanda is evidence of this.[76] Bacillary dysentery has been a classic problem of the army at war. When US military personnel were sent to Somalia in 1992–1993 to safeguard emergency feeding programs, the diarrheal disease rates were unexpectedly low; however, *Shigella* were isolated from 33% of those affected.[88] Other settings in which close contact among people is assured and common meals are taken, such as aboard ship or in airplanes, also lead to outbreaks of shigellosis.

Introduction of illness into the household often results in intrafamilial spread, and the family should therefore be considered an epidemiological entity in this instance. The secondary attack rate is greater in children than in adults (Table 5) and infection is more likely to be symptomatic in the young as well. Nosocomial spread of shigellosis in a newborn nursery can result in serious clinical manifestations, frequently systemic illness and shock, which often terminates fatally.[81]

Table 5. Secondary Attack Rates among Household Contacts of Shigellosis Patients

Age of exposed	Secondary attack rates	
	S. flexneri	*S. sonnei*
Child	42	42
Adult	14	20

5.10. Socioeconomic Factors

Endemic shigellosis is associated with poverty, crowding, poor sanitation, water sources inadequate in quantity and quality, and malnutrition.[64–66,75–77] Using specific ELISAs for serum antibody to *Shigella* lipopolysaccharides and invasion plasmid antigens, recent studies have documented that prevalence of specific antibody is inversely related to socioeconomic status.[5,89] Thus, water availability, water quality, sanitary disposal of feces, and control of flies each affect the infection rate individually. Recent data on fly control using a simple baited trap reveal an 85% reduction in the prevalence of shigellosis (Table 6).[90] However, these factors usually occur together in impoverished populations, which may exacerbate the problem and limit the results of any single intervention.[62] Preexisting malnutrition exerts additional adverse effects and is associated with more severe illness and sequelae. Bottle-feeding young infants in such environments will considerably worsen the situation, whereas

Table 6. Efficacy of a Simple Baited Fly Trap on Shigellosis Rates in Military Camps[a]

Parameter	Intervention camps	Control camps	"P" value	% Efficacy
Fly count	4.20	11.7	0.024	64
% diarrhea	14.60	25.2	0.146	42
% *Shigella* isolated	0.06	4.0	0.015	85
% *Shigella* seroconversions	11.90	49.5	0.024	76

[a]Data from Cohen *et al.*[89]

breast-feeding appears to be protective until full weaning occurs.[82]

6. Mechanisms and Routes of Transmission

The shigellae are, like the typhoid bacillus, highly host-adapted; the only natural hosts for *Shigella* are humans and a few nonhuman primates. For this reason, more than 99% of all *Shigella* isolates in the United States are from human sources. Thus, the route of transmission is inevitably traceable to an infected human (or, on rare occasion, to a simian contact). The route can be further described as a circle from the stool to the mouth and back to the stool again. While intervening vehicles can be involved, shigellosis is most frequently spread by person-to-person contact. Large numbers of shigellae (10^5–10^8) are present in stools of clinical cases, whereas healthy carriers have less than 10^3 organisms/g feces. Even under epidemic conditions, epidemiological evidence may favor contact spread.[76] This is encouraged by conditions of poverty, crowding, and poor sanitation, as in refugee camps, which facilitate the transfer of the small inoculum needed to initiate the infection. Contact with a recent case of dysentery is one of the prominent risk factors in developing countries[64,77]; the index case within households is most often a young child under the age of 10. Interestingly, the use of pit or other protected latrines may not be associated with a reduction in *Shigella* transmission (odds ratio = 0.96, CI 0.43–2.15), but use of a hanging latrine in which feces are discharged directly onto the ground or into a body of water can be associated with a significantly increased risk for infection (odds ratio = 1.42, 95% CI: 1.02–1.98, $p < 0.05$).[91]

Organisms, of course, can find their way to food or water sources and thereby initiate common-source epidemics.[92,93] The list of documented vehicles and settings for such common-source outbreaks has been increasing over time. Foodborne infection is commonly traceable to an infected food handler, with raw vegetables being the most common vehicle.,[94] Large outbreaks have also been traced to commercially prepared shredded lettuce, and imported iceberg lettuce was the source of an outbreak in Norway, with 110 proven cases of *S. sonnei* spread via salad bars.[95,96] Thousands of individuals in Norway and other countries were undoubtedly exposed to the tainted lettuce as well, with an unknown number of additional cases. Newly reported and different vehicles include interesting items such as moose soup in Alaska and raw oysters along the Texas Gulf coast.[97,98] In the latter outbreak, an infected crew member of an oystering boat may have contaminated the oyster beds, since the toilet facilities aboard ship consisted only of 5-gallon pails that were dumped overboard directly into the harvesting area.

Any mass gathering at which centrally prepared food is served can be associated with outbreaks of *Shigella* infection, especially when toilet and hand-washing facilities are primitive or limited. For example, a large *S. sonnei* outbreak occurred in 1988 at an outdoor 5-day summer music festival, affecting over 3000 persons.[99] Major factors in this outbreak were the large number (>2000) of volunteer food handlers preparing communal meals, limited access to soap and running water for hand washing, and a documented small outbreak of shigellosis among the staff before the festival participants arrived. Transmission from staff to attendees likely occurred early but was amplified by a large common-source outbreak due to contamination of an uncooked tofu salad served on the last day. Onset of illness peaked 2 days later, after the festival ended.

Another large outbreak happened in 1987 at a mass gathering in a national forest, where over 50% of almost 13,000 attendees were infected with *S. sonnei* transmitted via multiple routes, including food, water, and person-to-person spread.[100] Further national dissemination of the outbreak strain followed when the participants returned home, with at least three additional confirmed outbreaks linked to the first by the unique antibiotic-resistance pattern, phage type, and plasmid profile of the outbreak strain. Similarly, high attack rates were documented in a foodborne outbreak at summer camps for mentally retarded and developmentally disabled persons.[67] During the same period of time, nearby camps for normal youngsters recorded no shigella outbreaks.

Surveillance for waterborne disease outbreaks during 1986 to 1988 uncovered 50 outbreaks associated with drinking water.[93] Although *Giardia lamblia* was the most frequently identified pathogen, *S. sonnei* was the most common bacterial agent. Infection due to water sources also varies from year to year. Subsequent surveillance by the CDC from 1990 to 1991 identified 34 water-associated diarrhea outbreaks, only one of which was due to *Shigella* spp., in this case due to contaminated well water. Recreational water use has increasingly been implicated in shigella outbreaks.[93] In 1991, a particularly interesting outbreak of bloody diarrhea and hemolytic–uremic syndrome due to *E. coli* O157:H7 and *S. sonnei* occurred at a lakeside park near Portland, Oregon.[101] No association with food or beverage consumption was detected; however, case–control studies strongly associated illness with swimming, especially in persons reporting prolonged time in the water and swallowing of lake water.

Although neither outbreak organism was recovered from the lake, enterococci counts indicated significant fecal contamination. A similar outbreak involving 65 persons occurred at a park pond in Michigan in 1989.[102] Increased risk was associated with swimming with the head submerged. There were no detectable defects in the park's toilets or sewage disposal system, implicating bather contamination of the waters. Waterborne transmission is not restricted to swimming in contaminated water; even wind surfing on contaminated waters can lead to infection.[103]

In the developing countries, a combination of contact and waterborne spread can contribute to a prolonged, smoldering epidemic that lasts for months rather than weeks, until the population of susceptibles is exhausted. In the Central American *S. dysenteriae* 1 epidemic of 1969–1972, waterborne spread within some communities is suggested by the clustering of cases in place and time, the presence of multiple index cases in families, and the relationship between defective water distribution and illness. However, the occurrence of the diseases in widely separated places that do not share food or water supplies also indicates the likely role of the human carrier in spread. In the initial Bangladesh outbreak of epidemic *S. dysenteriae* 1 among the population of a semi-isolated coral island, the introduction of the organisms into this insular community was undoubtedly from an infected human, and the early slow spread of disease is probably explained by initial person-to-person contact. Later spread was most likely caused by contamination of water sources from the excreta of the slowly increasing number of patients, and the epidemic terminated when chlorination of water was begun.

A variation on the mechanism, but not the route, of transmission has been demonstrated in recent years among homosexual men engaging in anal–oral sex practices. Severe *Shigella* sepsis has been reported in patients with acquired immunodeficiency syndrome (AIDS).[104] The presumptive route of transmission in these individuals is venereal, which is often associated with simultaneous transmission of other enteric pathogens, such as *G. lamblia*.[86]

7. Pathogenesis and Immunity

7.1. Pathogenesis

The incubation period for shigellosis can be estimated at approximately 2–5 days based on experimental human infections with *S. flexneri* 2a and *S. dysenteriae* 1.[13] Surprisingly, the clinically more virulent *S. dysenteriae* 1 strain has a longer mean incubation period than *S. flexneri* 2a under these conditions. This may be a characteristic of the isolates studied and not an inherent characteristic of each species and serotype.

Following oral ingestion, a sufficient inoculum must survive gastric acidity and other intestinal defense mechanisms to initiate infection. The mechanism for acid resistance has already been discussed. Human shigellosis is clearly a colonic process that results in bloody diarrhea and dysentery. Experimental shigellosis in the rhesus monkey provides evidence of involvement of both the proximal small bowel and the colon.[105] The small bowel could be the source of or contribute to watery diarrhea in shigellosis; however, there is no conclusive evidence to document either small bowel colonization or an *in vivo* effect of any secretory shigella toxin in humans.

When the organisms ultimately reach the colon, they cause an invasive bacterial colitis, resulting in the typical bloody diarrhea or dysentery of shigellosis.[54,105] This process was believed to involve direct invasion of intestinal epithelial cells; however, new evidence derived from *in vitro* studies using monolayers of human intestinal epithelial cells (summarized in Section 4.1.1) suggests that invasion of epithelial cells occurs across the basolateral and not apical cell membrane, follows the initial penetration of bacteria across cell–cell junctions or via M cells, and is substantially dependent on the induction of an inflammatory response. The subsequent contiguous spread of infection from epithelial cell to epithelial cell leads to focal lesions separated by areas of unaffected mucosa. Thus, the role of the inflammatory process may be more important in the initiation of lesions than it is in causing epithelial cell death and sloughing, as previously postulated. It is the latter events, however initiated, that lead to formation of microulcers and an inflammatory cell exudate in the stool. Histological examination of colonic tissues also reveals lesions of mucosal vascular endothelial cells.[106] These authors hypothesize that this lesion is due to LPS and that vascular damage underlies the bloody diarrhea–dysentery of shigellosis. Presumably, invasion of the mucosa is a necessary prelude, as some factor must permit LPS to reach the endothelial cells in the lamina propria.

High levels of circulating LPS are present in patients with *S. dysenteriae* 1 infection and lower levels are common in those with *S. flexneri*, even in the absence of documented bacteremia. The frequency of endotoxemia in shigellosis suggests a broader role for LPS in pathogenesis of the disease. One mechanism may be related to the ability of LPS to induce cytokine gene transcription and the strong association of cytokine secretion and inflammation. Bacterial invasion of the mucosa may be the mechanism by which cytokine gene activation occurs, as this has been shown to activate transcription factors such as nuclear factor (NF)-kappa B.[107] Recently, detectable fecal levels of certain cytokines have been reported in small numbers of children with *S. dysenteriae* 1 and *S. flexneri* infection.[108,109] Interestingly, no differences in stool or serum levels of tumor necrosis factor (TNF) were observed between patients with uncomplicated infections and those with hemolytic–uremic syndrome (HUS), leukemoid reaction, or severe colitis, whereas serum interleukin-6 (IL-6) was significantly higher in the children with complicated illness.[109] In a more elaborate study, an increase in the number of cytokine-producing cells was observed in cryopreserved rectal biopsies from adult patients with either *S. dysenteriae* 1 or *S. flexneri* infection.[110] Although IL-1β, IL-4, IL-10, and transforming growth factor (TGF)-β1–3 responses predominated, there was a universal response of all cytokines studied, including both Th-1 and Th-2 agonist cytokines and antagonist cytokines (IL-1α and IL-1β, IL-1 receptor antagonist, TNF-α, IL-4, IL-6, IL-8, IL-10, gamma interferon, and TGF-β1–3). No significant difference in the number of cytokine-producing cells was observed between acute illness and convalescence, 30 days after onset. The number of IL-1, IL-6, IFN-γ, and TGF-β-producing cells was significantly and directly related to severity of inflammation, as assessed by histological criteria. These cells were also greater in patients with *S. dysenteriae* 1 infection compared to *S. flexneri* infection.

The results are consistent with quantitative observations on inflammatory cells and erythrocytes in the stool, in which patients with *S. dysenteriae*, *S. flexneri*, and *S. boydii* infection are more likely to have both large numbers of leukocytes and erythrocytes in stool than patients with *S. sonnei*, and the number of leukocytes is highest in *S. dysenteriae* and lowest *S. boydii*.[52] It is presumed that severe inflammation underlies pathogenesis of ileus and toxic megacolon in shigellosis. Further evidence of a role of cytokines in pathogenesis has been provided by experimental studies in the rabbit ligated ileal loop model, in which intravenous infusion of IL-1 receptor antagonist prior to initiation of *S. flexneri* infection within the loop dramatically decreases mucosal inflammation and destruction and bacterial invasion of the tissue.[111] Production of pyrogenic proinflammatory cytokines can explain clinical symptoms such as fever and anorexia[53] and bloody diarrhea and dysentery, as the severity of illness is directly related to the fever response.[112]

The factor(s) inciting the watery diarrhea that predominates in milder illness, including most cases of *S. sonnei* infection, remains uncertain. The suggestion that this is a small bowel process due to *Shigella* enterotoxins has remained an unproven albeit attractive hypothesis, since watery diarrhea temporally precedes bloody diarrhea–dysentery as the organisms move down the intestinal tract toward the colon. Experimental primate infections provide a cogent but not conclusive argument for a small bowel phase of symptoms and the role of enterotoxins.[105] However, neither Shiga toxin, which is not only cytotoxic but also causes net secretion across small bowel mucosa by targeting and inhibiting villus cell sodium absorption but not crypt cell chloride secretion,[113] nor the newly described ShET toxins,[55,56] which are weakly secretory in rabbit bowel by an as yet unknown mechanism, are universally present in *Shigella* spp. Occasional reports of cytotoxins detected in other *Shigella* species and serotypes, whether apparently related or unrelated to Shiga toxin, are sketchy and convincing proof of their existence is lacking.

Fever is a typical finding in shigellosis, doubtless due to pyrogenic cytokine responses to mucosal inflammation and bacterial invasion. A number of systemic complications occur in shigellosis as well, most with uncertain pathogenesis. Bacteremia, most commonly encountered in infection due to *S. dysenteriae* 1 or *S. flexneri*, may be a consequence of tissue damage and host defense defects. In Bangladesh, bacteremia occurs primarily in children under 1 year of age and is significantly associated with malnutrition. When the sensitivity of *Shigella* species to the serum bactericidal response has been studied, these two species are the most serum sensitive rather than serum resistant, as might be expected for bacteremia isolates.[114] However, patients with *Shigella* bacteremia had a 43-fold decrease in serum bactericidal activity compared to normally nourished nonbacteremic controls, and a failure of host defenses associated with malnutrition seems to be the most likely explanation for the bacteremia.[115] Leukemoid reactions occur most often in Shiga bacillus dysentery, often associated with HUS, a syndrome of hemolytic anemia and renal failure secondary to microangiopathic injury of endothelial cells.[49] The role of Shiga toxin in pathogenesis of HUS is suggested by the observation that HUS also occurs during infection with *E. coli* producing high levels of the closely related Shiga toxin 1 and Shiga toxin 2 causing hemorrhagic colitis or bloody diarrhea. These toxins target and damage endothelial cells, especially when endothelium is preactivated by LPS or cytokines *in vitro*, which increases expression of the glycolipid toxin receptor.[50] Toxic megacolon is an uncommon but severe problem, reflecting extreme inflammatory colitis and may result in perforation of the gut.[116]

Neurological manifestations in shigellosis, most commonly in the form of seizures, have been considered a variant of febrile seizures, since they are similar to the seizures seen in young children with rapidly rising temperature due to other causes. No specific neurotoxic factors have been identified in *Shigella*, including Shiga toxin, long known as a neurotoxin,[2] even though toxin injected into rat vagus nerves travels in antegrade fashion to the neuronal cell body where it is cytotoxic.[50] There is at present no mechanism to explain the toxic encephalopathy sometimes observed during *Shigella* infections, most commonly associated with *S. flexneri*, unless central nervous system inflammation occurs as a part of a systemic inflammatory response.[117] Among nine cases of shigellosis seen among US troops deployed to Saudi Arabia during the Gulf War of 1991, two presented with "pseudomeningitis," a previously described presentation of *Shigella* infection, especially in infants and children, and easily confused with acute bacterial meningitis.[118]

7.2. Immunity

There is much epidemiological evidence suggesting acquired immunity to *Shigella* infections. First, shigellosis is primarily a childhood disease except when there is introduction of an epidemic strain, not previously present in the population. Under epidemic conditions, infection involves all age groups. This indicates that the widespread prevalence of endemic serotypes of the organism in the community results in immunity to reinfection by that specific serotype. Second, live oral vaccination studies clearly indicate development of type-specific immunity following infection by attenuated avirulent vaccine strains. Third, rechallenge of volunteers who previously had experimental dysentery with the same serotype also demonstrates serotype-specific protection.

These data are consistent with the induction of type-specific immunity after exposure to *Shigella* due primarily to antibacterial immune reactions directed to LPS antigens. No other surface or secreted microbial component has been shown to be capable of inducing protective responses, although many of these constituents are antigenic. Antibody to LPS, which may mediate this protective response, is present in humans in increasing prevalence with increasing age.[5,6,84] The age-specific rise in antibody is steeper in disease-endemic countries where young infants and children are more likely to encounter the organisms early in life. It is hypothesized that serum IgG antibody, in high enough titer, may be protective in the gastrointestinal tract, if it reaches a high enough local concentration.[119] During clinical shigellosis, serum proteins leak across the intestinal mucosa in high enough concentration and amount to result in a protein-losing enteropathy.[120] The presence of serum antibody in the exudate, consisting of large numbers of polymorphonuclear leukocytes, should at least theoretically contribute to the acute local defense response in the mucosa and the lumen. Perhaps they do; however, the quantity of serum proteins in stool, measured as α_1-antitrypsin, and the number of stool leukocytes is also related to the severity of the illness and is greater in *S. dysenteriae* 1 infection compared to shigellosis due to other species of *Shigella*.[52,120] Although earlier work had suggested that an antibody-dependent cell-mediated cytotoxicity toward *Shigella* is present in the intestinal tract, there has been no further exploration on the nature of this putative immune response. Its existence, therefore, remains questionable.

Serum anti-Shiga toxin antibody develops in the course of *S. dysenteriae* 1 infection.[6] Its role in host defense has not been clear, since primates immunized with toxoid develop high titers of neutralizing antibody but are not protected from oral challenge with virulent organisms. Thus, they develop classic primate shigellosis, a severe and frequently lethal diarrhea and dysentery. Preexisting serum anti-Shiga toxin antibody, however, could protect against the systemic microangiopathic pathology resulting in HUS or thrombotic thrombocytopenic purpura in either *S. dysenteriae* 1 and Shiga toxin-producing enterohemorrhagic *E. coli* infections. Experimental studies in animals demonstrates this effect of anti-Shiga toxin antibody. In addition, infection with ShET-1 or -2 toxin-producing *Shigella* spp. induces specific circulating antibody. The potential role of these antibodies in control of disease during acute infection or in protection from subsequent episodes is unknown at this time.

8. Patterns of Host Response

Most clinical shigellosis is gastrointestinal disease. This spans a spectrum from mild to severe watery diarrhea, with or without blood and mucus, to the bacillary dysentery syndrome. A clear-cut dose–response curve can be seen in adult volunteers experimentally infected with known numbers of bacteria (Table 1).[13] The prevalence of asymptomatic infection will depend on the presence of acquired resistance (especially in endemic regions) and the inoculum size (especially in virgin populations in nonendemic regions). However, first postweaning exposure to *Shigella*, wherever and whenever it occurs, will more likely result in symptomatic disease, although far more asymptomatic episodes occur than previously believed.[4]

Under most circumstances, extraintestinal manifestations occur uncommonly. They may include involvement of the central nervous system (usually seizures, but also nuchal rigidity, meningismus, and delirium), the blood (bacteremia with the infecting *Shigella* or another gram-negative rod, leukemoid reactions, thrombocytopenia, microangiopathic hemolysis), the kidney (hyponatremia, uremia), the eye (keratoconjunctivitis, iritis), and the joints (nonsuppurative arthritis).

Postdysenteric Reiter's syndrome (iritis, urethritis, arthritis) is particularly likely to present in subjects who possess HLA-B27 antigen and is usually associated with *S. flexneri* infection. Joint manifestations in genetically prone subjects are frequently chronic and destructive. Hematologic manifestations, including bacteremia, leukemoid reactions, and thrombocytopenia, occur primarily in subjects with *S. dysenteriae* 1 dysentery, and microangiopathic hemolytic anemia appears to occur almost exclusively in these patients. Rare patients may exhibit metastatic infection of skin, wounds, the lungs, the joints, the urinary tract, or the meninges.

8.1. Clinical Features

The initial manifestations of acute shigellosis are usually fever, malaise, abdominal pain, and watery diarrhea. There is nothing pathognomonic about this presentation, however, until the disease progresses with the appearance of blood and mucus in the stools. The entire colon may be involved, but the rectum and sigmoid area are the most severely affected. The intense inflammation and ulceration result in tenesmus and frequent passage of small-volume stools that often consist of only blood and mucus (Fig. 2). In very severe cases, toxic megacolon or

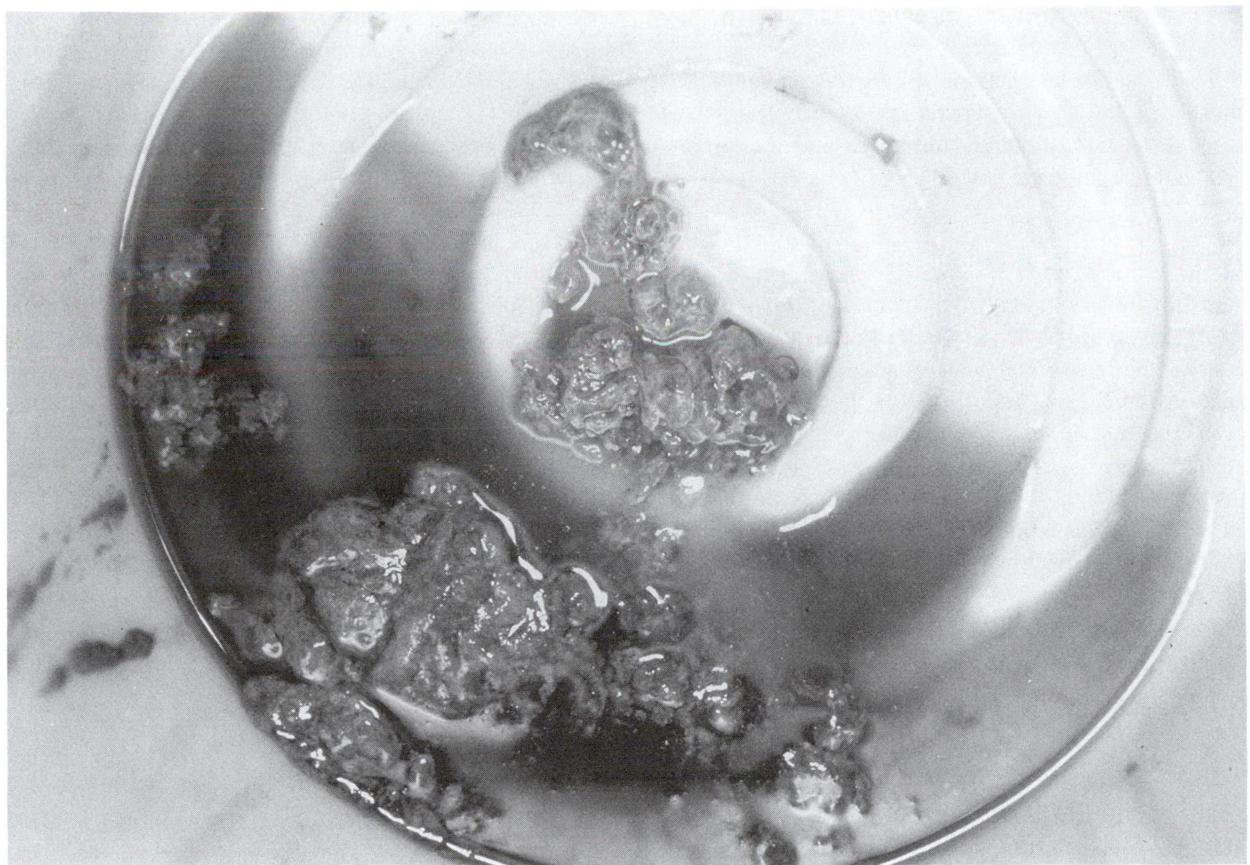

Figure 2. The appearance of the stool in most patients with shigellosis is, as shown here, a small-volume stool composed of fecal matter and bloody fluid, sometimes with mucus as well. Microscopic examination of the fluid phase reveals sheets of polymorphonuclear leukocytes and abundant erythrocytes. Passage of this type of stool is generally accompanied by abdominal cramps and tenesmus, and the three features together constitute a triad of findings that defines dysentery.

colonic perforation may ensue. The more virulent the organism (*dysenteriae* 1 > *flexneri* > *sonnei*), the more likely and the more rapid is the appearance of dysentery after onset of diarrhea; in fact, the course may be so rapid in *S. dysenteriae* 1 infection that it is hardly possible to distinguish the diarrheal phase at all.

In well-nourished subjects, the illness is generally self-limited in 5–10 days, depending on the infecting species and the clinical severity. In the malnourished, it may cause an acute fulminant infection or a chronic relapsing disease, extending over months. At an international diarrhea treatment center in Bangladesh, where the majority of patients admitted to the inpatient unit are malnourished (mean weight for age = 59% of the NCHS 50th percentile) standard, the fatality rate in 4150 patients over a 5-year period was 9% (Table 7). There was little difference in fatality rate with the four *Shigella* species, suggesting that debilitation of the host affects the person's ability to defend against even the least virulent *Shigella* species.[85,114,115] Early deaths in shigellosis are generally due to septicemia, toxic megacolon, with or without perforation, or renal failure.[85,114,116] Later fatalities are the result of complex interactions of infection and nutritional status.[76,115] In these circumstances, kwashiorkor or marasmic kwashiorkor usually develops and the terminal event is often another infection.

8.2. Diagnosis

Shigellosis should be suspected when a febrile, bloody, mucoid diarrhea or the dysentery syndrome occurs. The definitive diagnosis of shigellosis depends on isolation of the organism from a stool specimen. However, because early treatment can markedly shorten the duration and intensity of symptoms in more severely ill patients, presumptive diagnosis on the basis of clinical symptoms can be useful. This is easiest for patients in endemic areas, or patients infected during outbreaks, who have the dysenteric form of the illness. In rural Bangladesh, recent prospective community-based studies show that bloody, mucoid diarrhea accounts for two fifths of diarrhea episodes and two thirds of fatalities, about half being associated with documented shigellosis.[121] In Dallas, Texas, a correct presumptive diagnosis based on clinical features alone was possible in 34 of 47 (72%) *Shigella*-infected patients who came to a general outpatient clinic.[122] However, this study was conducted 25 years ago when the prevalence of *Shigella* infection in diarrhea patients attending this clinic was 33%, a rate much higher than in most outpatient settings in the United States. In children with acute diarrhea and fever, the presence of gross blood and mucus in the stool or detection of large numbers of leukocytes by microscopic examination of stool stained with methylene blue is suggestive, but not diagnostic, of *Shigella* infection. In patients who present with nonbloody watery diarrhea, there is often little to differentiate *Shigella* from other, more common, causes of watery diarrhea. While the presentation of fever, diarrhea, and seizures in children is most characteristic of shigellosis, the seizures occasionally can occur prior to the development of intestinal symptoms, prompting the initial diagnosis of acute meningitis. Examination of the cerebrospinal fluid is completely normal in nearly all, and the real diagnosis becomes apparent when the intestinal manifestations occur and the stool is cultured.

In addition, the increasing prevalence of infection with the emerging agents of enterohemorrhagic *E. coli* infection, including serotypes O157:H7 and many others, has introduced a new diagnostic dilemma. Bloody diarrhea with seizures due to the microangiopathic systemic complications of Shiga toxins produced by these organisms can be confused with shigellosis (Chapter 14). At the present time, it is known that antimicrobial therapy is useful in shigellosis; it is not as certain in enterohemorrhagic *E. coli* infection, and some evidence, albeit controversial, suggests that antibiotic therapy can actually contribute to pathogenesis of systemic complications. Selective culture methods using sorbitol–MacConkey agar

Table 7. Outcome of Patients Infected with *Shigella* Admitted to a Diarrhea Treatment Unit, Dhaka, Bangladesh, 1983–1987

Species or serotype	Total admissions	Discharged alive	Left against advice	Transferred elsewhere	Died in hospital
S. dysenteriae 1	1251	976 (78%)	136 (11%)	40 (3%)	99 (8%)
S. dysenteriae 2–10	132	112 (85%)	5 (4%)	2 (2%)	13 (10%)
S. flexneri	2319	1841 (79%)	211 (9%)	39 (2%)	230 (10%)
S. boydii	303	245 (81%)	24 (8%)	3 (1%)	31 (10%)
S. sonnei	145	119 (82%)	12 (1%)	2 (1%)	12 (8%)

is available for serotype O157:H7, and other agars putatively able to distinguish other serotypes of enterohemorrhagic *E. coli* are undergoing testing. A toxin-based enzyme immunoassay for the detection of all Shiga-like toxin-producing *E. coli* is now commercially available,[123] with the potential for use directly on stool for rapid diagnosis. More modern DNA-based tests have been developed, including gene probes and polymerase chain reaction methods; however, as in other areas of diagnostic microbiology, these have not yet made it to the clinical laboratories.

In the developing countries, where the vast majority of *Shigella* infections occur, laboratory facilities for standard microbiological isolation of the organism, let alone DNA or immunoassay tests, are often not available, and diagnosis is dependent on clinical evaluation, aided by stool microscopy for white blood cells. The major differential diagnosis, *E. histolytica*, is a much less common cause of dysentery in children and does not cause a purulent stool. In practice, all children with clinical dysentery in endemic regions should be presumed to have *Shigella* and treated accordingly. Under optimal conditions, the stool should be examined for motile amoebic trophozoites containing ingested erythrocytes to rule out amebiasis. In adults, the incidence of amoebic dysentery is higher than in children, and a microscopic examination of stool is important to discriminate between the two illnesses.

9. Control and Prevention

9.1. General Concepts

Even though the infective inoculum for *Shigella* infection is small and person-to-person contact spread is common, it is surprising how effective simple hygiene measures can be in control and prevention of shigellosis. Hand washing and sanitary disposal of feces constitute the keystones of personal hygiene and will minimize the spread of infection within the household. Protection of food and water for drinking and cooking from potential contamination is a critical part of this approach. Within the community, the integrity of the water supply and its protection from fecal contamination is important; this is most obvious when breaks in the system permit waterborne disease. This is true whether the community is an institution, a town, or a ship at sea. Unsanitary hanging latrines, in which feces are deposited directly on the ground or in a body of water, concentrate infectious agents for more ready transmission and are worse than no latrine at all.[9] Every effort should be made to insure that simple sealed latrines such as the VIP (ventilated improved pit) latrine are built and maintained.[90] Breast-fed infants are at lesser risk of symptomatic *Shigella* infection than are bottle-fed neonates, and good nutritional status may limit the extent of acute infection and the chronicity of established illness.[81,82]

While vector spread may contribute to the transmission of shigellosis, it is certainly not necessary. None the less, vector control is a useful measure. Simple baited fly traps can be built locally for little cost, and appear to be highly effective (Table 6).[90]

It is wise for physicians making the diagnosis of acute shigellosis in one family member, usually a young child, to consider the whole family to be at risk. Younger contacts of the index case are at greater risk of symptomatic secondary infection than are adults.

9.2. Antibiotic and Chemotherapeutic Approaches to Prophylaxis

Bismuth subsalicylate (BSS) tablets have recently been shown to be protective, at least in adult travelers to Mexico.[124] Two 300 mg BSS tablets four times a day provide 35–40% protection during a 3-week exposure. Because of its salicylate content, BSS should not be used in children under age 3 years, in those with aspirin sensitivity or gout, or in patients taking anticoagulants, probenecid, methotrexate, or aspirin-containing preparations. In addition, BSS contains 350 mg $CaCO_3$ per tablet, and could result in milk–alkali syndrome in susceptible subjects. However, the FDA considers the threshold dose to be 8 g/day, which is considerably higher than the amount contained in the recommended dose of BSS. BSS administration is associated with increased frequency of adverse side effects, most notably constipation and nausea. In addition, it should be noted that 60% of BSS is the bismuth component, which is converted to bismuth oxychloride in the stomach. Excess bismuth salts, consumed over years, can result in encephalopathy, associated with plasma levels greater than 100 parts per billion (ppb). However, such complications resulting from BSS use appear to be rare, and blood bismuth levels measured in a small group of subjects given BSS four times daily never exceeded 34 ppb.

There is little information on the utility of prophylactic antimicrobials for shigellosis. In endemic settings, exposure to infection occurs much too frequently to make prophylaxis a consideration. In travelers, the concern is exposure to drug-resistant strains. In outbreak situations, the potential use of antimicrobial agents for prophylaxis is also limited by the increasingly common resistance of *Shigella* to the drugs that might be used and by the fear that prophylactic use of these agents would result in increased prevalence of resistant strains. In confined outbreaks, such as newborn nurseries, standard methods of cohorting, implementation of strict sanitary measures, bacteriologic screening of medical staff, and judicious use of antimicrobials can bring an epidemic to a halt.[68,125]

9.3. Immunization

There is no licensed vaccine for shigellosis at this time, but not because of a lack of effort to develop one. In fact, effective prototype vaccines have been prepared for oral use in humans, but none to date is both effective and safe.[126] Because these vaccines produce significant but serotype-specific protection, the duration of which is unclear, their use would also be limited unless a combination vaccine approach were adopted and shown to effectively induce the desired immunity to the prevalent species and serotypes of *Shigella* in the community.

Although most modern approaches to vaccine development for enteric infection have concentrated on live oral attenuated vaccine strains or recombinant bacteria expressing protective antigens, there has also been a return to the testing of parenteral or oral killed vaccines or antigens. Parenteral immunization with killed organisms has never been shown to be protective; however, new constructs of *Shigella* LPS O antigens conjugated to protein carriers are being investigated.[119] Time will tell whether this approach, based on sufficient leakage of serum IgG antibody into the intestinal lumen to exert an antibacterial effect, will succeed.

Because of the role of Shiga toxin in producing the severe disease due to *S. dysenteriae* 1 and in the production of systemic microangiopathic disease in this infection and in enterohemorrhagic *E. coli*, attempts to develop a safe toxin immunogen have been initiated. Toxin is a complex protein consisting of one biologically active A subunit and five B subunits involved in binding to host cells. Various groups are testing mutationally inactivated A subunit holotoxins, isolated recombinant B subunit, or synthetic peptides linked to protein carriers by conjugation or synthesized as recombinant fusion proteins. Promising results have been obtained in animal models; however, it will be a while before such vaccines are tested in humans. The increasing problem of HUS and thrombotic thrombocytopenic purpura associated with Shiga-toxin producing *E. coli* in the United States suggests the need to develop and test a passive antibody approach as well, and such efforts are also underway.

10. Unresolved Problems

10.1. Epidemiology

Because the shigellae are so host-adapted to humans and a few subhuman primates, there is an absolute need for constant passage of the organisms through these hosts. At first glance, it would seem improbable that the organism could survive this restriction when environmental sanitation and protected water supplies limit transmission by the water route. Under these conditions, frequent reintroduction of the organism would be necessary unless continual person-to-person or foodborne transmission were occurring. It is uncertain how in fact the organism does maintain itself. The role and importance of asymptomatic carriers may be much greater than previously thought. The reasons for the major shifts in prevalence of *Shigella* species in different regions over time are not known. The use of newer molecular methods to detect organisms and for typing isolates should help unravel many of the questions relating to the presence and transmission of infection in the community.

10.2. Pathogenesis

Spectacular progress has been made in defining the pathogenesis of *Shigella* infections over the past decade. These studies have served to demonstrate how complex this process is, how multiple virulence genes are required, and what the role of the host is in development of symptoms during the host–pathogen interaction. Most progress has occurred in the mechanism of host cell invasion, and a good start in defining host responses at the molecular level has begun. We still know little of the specific role and mechanism of toxins in pathogenesis of local events in the gastrointestinal tract or in the causation of systemic pathology, for example, at the level of endothelial cells in the target organs, kidney, and brain. Elucidation of the specific mechanisms involved is essential for the planning of therapeutic and prophylactic measures.

Rational pharmacological manipulation of the secretory or inflammatory process in the intestinal tract is equally dependent on specific knowledge of the mechanisms involved. These take on particular significance when the problems of epidemiology and antimicrobial drug resistance are considered.

Manipulation of the host–pathogen and host cell–toxin interactions for therapeutic benefit based on the specific receptor-binding chemistry involved is also dependent on clarification of the processes occurring at the surface of the intestinal epithelial cell or systemically in involved microvascular endothelial beds. A clinical trial using an oral synthetic receptor analogue to treat children with Shiga toxin-producing *E. coli* infection to prevent or modulate HUS has been started. No results are yet available; however, this approach, if successful, also could be rationally applied to *S. dysenteriae* 1 infection where it is endemic. The limiting factor in this instance would be the practicality of implementing this in the field setting and the cost of the analogue, which could easily exceed national per capita budgets for health care in a poor developing country.

10.3. Antimicrobial Resistance

Transferable multiple antimicrobial drug resistance mediated by plasmid DNA was first discovered in the shigellae. This led to a dramatic rise in the prevalence of highly drug-resistant shigellae in Japan and elsewhere as antibiotic pressures led to selection of the plasmid-bearing organisms. Resistance clearly restricts the antimicrobial therapy of acute shigellosis, which is effective when susceptible organisms are treated with appropriate agents.[59–61,77] The principal strategy in dealing with acquired drug resistance has been to develop new or modified drugs to which the organism is still sensitive. This merely buys time; the ultimate solution is to learn how to control transferable drug resistance in nature. It also would be advantageous to clinically cure the plasmids *in vivo*, and thus restore susceptibility to the drugs already available for use. This could have the added advantage of curing plasmids bearing essential virulence traits, rendering the survivors nonpathogenic. The theoretical barriers to this are enormous and are further complicated by the tissue- and cell-invasive characteristics of *Shigella*, which insure a protected reservoir of fully virulent and drug-resistant organisms unless the strategy is effective beyond the intestinal lumen. Even so, the ability to cure undesirable plasmids in nature could have important effects on the prevalence of fully virulent organisms excreted into the environment.

Other ways to approach these issues at a more practical level involve control and restriction in the use of antimicrobial agents. In the United States, where such drugs are dispensed only by prescription, physician and patient education could have a major impact, limited only by the use of similar or identical drugs in agriculture to promote the growth of meat animals. In developing countries, despite the efforts toward essential national drug programs, there is no control over dispensing antimicrobials, which are freely available on the market and are used indiscriminantly. The need for legislation and effective agencies to monitor and control drug use comes into conflict with the enormous potential economic gains for both local and multinational drug manufacturers as well as local drug merchants, including pharmacists and untrained dispensers.

10.4. Clinical Complications

The pathogenesis of most of the clinical complications that occur in shigellosis is not well understood. Since certain of these complications, including microangiopathic hemolytic anemia, hyponatremia, and thrombocytopenia, occur almost exclusively in association with *S. dysenteriae* 1 infection, speculation has centered about the role of high levels of Shiga toxin with this organism. The discovery that toxin-producing *E. coli* cause similar systemic events in children in developed nations and the occurrence of outbreaks involving large numbers of individuals in the United States have stirred research interest and have led to increased support for research. Much remains to be done.

Toxic megacolon is another complication associated with significant mortality. It is logical to assume that the extent of the inflammatory changes is the major determinant of toxic dilatation, but little is known in fact. Therapy is principally appropriate antimicrobials and general support with fluids, with surgery reserved for those who do not respond or whose colon becomes perforated. New data on the cytokine response in shigellosis suggest that these inflammatory mediators play a role in inflammatory complications. Further studies on their role in pathogenesis are warranted, and the potential of new anticytokine strategies of therapy in this and other complications is an exciting new area for study.

In the case of Reiter's arthritis, there is a clear genetic predilection for HLA-B27-positive subjects. The mechanisms underlying this particular host response to the infection need to be understood. Therapy or, even better, prevention could then be considered. This is clearly important because of the chronic destructive joint disease initiated by the organisms.

Shigella infection is associated with the most severe nutritional consequences of all the diarrheal diseases. In developing countries, this malnutrition is strongly associated with mortality, and there is growing evidence that the mortality rate in patients in the months after discharge from the hospital after shigellosis is far greater than in those discharged after watery diarrhea due to *E. coli*, cholera, or rotavirus. Nutritional effects of the infection may account for this in large part. The relative importance and persistence of mucosal inflammation, systemic catabolic responses, and protein-losing enteropathy are uncertain, and there is no clear approach to treatment.[53,76,115,120]

10.5. Vaccines

Because of unresolved questions of pathogenesis and the failure to develop acceptable vaccines, the question of prophylaxis is open to investigation. It is apparent that our current understanding of host defenses and the nature of the protective immune response in shigellosis is wanting. When success does not come easily with conventional approaches, it is time to stop and reason. In the present context, this means more studies to define the protection-eliciting antigens of the organisms and to find a way to present these to the host without toxicity or unacceptable side effects to achieve the protection desired.

11. References

1. Shiga, K., Ueber den Dysenteric-bacillus (*Bacillus dysenteriae*), *Zentralbl. Bakteriol. Orign.* **24:**913–918 (1898).
2. Conradi, H., Ueber losliche durch aseptische autolyse erhalten giftstoffe von ruhr and Typhusbazillen, *Dtsch. Med. Wochenschr.* **29:**26–28 (1903).
3. Keusch, G. T., Grady, G. F., Mata, L. J., and McIver, J. M., The pathogenesis of Shigella diarrhea. 1. Enterotoxin production by *Shigella dysenteriae* 1, *J. Clin. Invest.* **51:**1212–1218 (1972).
4. Guerrero, L., Calva, J. J., Morrow, A. L., *et al.*, Asymptomatic *Shigella* infections in a cohort of Mexican children younger than two years of age, *Pediatr. Infect. Dis. J.* **13:**597–602 (1994).
5. Lindberg, A. A., Cam, P. D., Chan, N., Phu, L. K., Trach, D. D., Lindberg, G., Karlsson, K., Karnell, A., and Ekwall, E. Shigellosis in Vietnam: Seroepidemiological studies with use of lipopolysaccharide antigens in enzyme immunoassays, *Rev. Infect. Dis.* **132:**S231–S237 (1991).
6. Islam, D., Wretlind, G., Ryd, M., Lindberg, A. A., and Christensson, B., Immunoglobulin subclass distribution and dynamics of *Shigella*-specific antibody responses in serum and stool samples in shigellosis, *Infect. Immun.* **63:**2054–2061 (1995).
7. Lefebvre, J., Gosselin, F., Ismail, J., Lorange, M. Lior, H., and Woodward, D., Evaluation of commercial antisera for *Shigella* serogrouping, *J. Clin. Microbiol.* **33:**1977–2001 (1995).
8. Rahaman, M. M., Huq, I., and Dey, C. R., Superiority of MacConkey's agar over *Salmonella–Shigella* agar for isolation of *Shigella dysenteriae* type 1, *J. Infect. Dis.* **131:**700–703 (1975).
9. Wells, J. G., and Morris, G. K., Evaluation of transport methods for isolating *Shigella*, *J. Clin. Microbiol.* **13:**789–790 (1981).
10. Zychlinsky, A., Perdomo, J. J., and Sansonetti, P. J., Molecular and cellular mechanisms of tissue invasion by *Shigella flexneri*, *Ann. NY Acad. Sci.* **730:**197–208 (1994).
11. Parsot, C., *Shigella flexneri*: Genetics of entry and intercellular dissemination in epithelial cells, *Curr. Top. Microbiol. Immunol.* **192:**217–241 (1994).
12. Maurelli, A. T., Hromockyj, A. E., and Bernardini, M. L., Environmental regulation of *Shigella* virulence, *Curr. Top. Microbiol. Immunol.* **180:**95–116 (1992).
13. DuPont, H. L., Levine, M. M., Hornick, R. B., and Formal, S. B. Inoculum size in shigellosis and implications for expected mode of transmission, *J. Infect. Dis.* **159:**1126–1128 (1989).
14. Sansonetti, P. J., Molecular and cellular biology of *Shigella flexneri* invasiveness: From cell assay systems to shigellosis, *Curr. Top. Microbiol. Immunol.* **180:**1–19 (1992).
15. Goldberg, M. B., and Sansonetti, P. J., *Shigella* subversion of the cellular cytoskeleton: A strategy for epithelial colonization, *Infect. Immun.* **61:**4941–4946 (1993).
16. Mounier, J., Vasselon, T., Hellio, R., Lesourd, M., and Sansonetti, P. J., *Shigella flexneri* enters human colonic Caco-2 epithelial cells through the basolateral pole, *Infect. Immun.* **60:**237–248 (1992).
17. Perdomo, J. J., Gounon, P., and Sansonetti, P. J., Polymorphonuclear leukocyte transmigration promotes invation of colonic epithelial monolayer by *Shigella flexneri*, *J. Clin. Invest.* **93:**633–643 (1994).
18. Sansonetti, P. J., Arondel, J., Cantey, J. R., Prevost, M. C., and Huerre, M., Infection of rabbit Peyer's patches by *Shigella flexneri*: Effect of adhesive or invasive bacterial phenotypes on follicle-associated epithelium, *Infect. Immun.* **64:**2752–2764 (1996).
19. Watarai, M., Funato, S., and Sasakawa, C., Interaction of Ipa proteins of *Shigella flexneri* with $\alpha 5\beta 1$ integrin promotes entry of the bacteria into mammalian cells, *J. Exp. Med.* **183:**991–999 (1996).
20. Andrews, G. P., Hromockyj, A. E., Coker, C., and Maurelli, A. T., Two novel virulence loci, mxiA and mxiB, in *Shigella flexneri* 2a facilitate excretion of invasion plasmid antigens, *Infect. Immun.* **59:**1997–2005 (1991).
21. Venkatesan, M. M., Buysse, J. M., and Oaks, E. V., Surface presentation of *Shigella flexneri* invasion plasmid antigens requires the products of the spa locus, *J. Bacteriol.* **174:**1990–2001 (1992).
22. Menard, R., Sansonetti, P., and Parsot, C., The secretion of the *Shigella flexneri* Ipa invasins is activated by epithelial cells and controlled by IpaB and IpaD, *EMBO J.* **13:**5293–5302 (1994).
23. Sansonetti, P. J., Ryter, A., Clerc, P., Maurelli, A. T., and Mounier, J., Multiplication of *Shigella flexneri* within HeLa cells: Lysis of the phagocytic vacuole and plasmid-mediated contact hemolysis, *Infect. Immun.* **1:**461–469 (1986).
24. Clerc, P., Ryter, A., Mounier, J., and Sansonetti, P. J., Plasmid-mediated early killing of eucaryotic cells by *Shigella flexneri* as studied by infection of J774 macrophages, *Infect. Immun.* **55:** 521–527 (1987).
25. Menard, R., Sansonetti, P. J., and Parsot, C., Nonpolar mutagenesis of the *ipa* genes defines IpaB, IpaC, and IpaD as effectors of *Shigella flexneri* entry into epithelial cells, *J. Bacteriol.* **175:**5899–5906 (1993).
26. Sansonetti, P. J., Arondel, J., Fontaine, A., d'Hauteville, H., and Bernardini, M. L., OmpB (osmo-regulation) and *icsA* mutants of *Shigella flexneri*: Vaccine candidates and probes to study the pathogenesis of shigellosis, *Vaccine* **9:**416–422 (1991).

27. Bernardini, M. L., Sanna, M. G., Fontaine, A., and Sansonetti, P. J., OmpC is involved in invasion of epithelial cells by *Shigella flexneri*, *Infect. Immun.* **61:**3625–3635 (1993).
28. Makino, S., Sasakawa, C., Kamata, K., Kurata, T., and Yosikawa, M., A genetic determinant required for continuous reinfection of adjacent cells on large plasmid in *Shigella flexneri* 2a, *Cell* **46:**551–555 (1986).
29. Goldberg, M. B., Theriot, J. A., and Sansonetti, P. J., Regulation of surface presentation of IcsA, a *Shigella* protein essential to intracellular movement and spread, is growth phase dependent, *Infect. Immun.* **62:**5664–5668 (1994).
30. Goldberg, M. B., Barzu, O., Parsot, C., and Sansonetti, P. J., Unipolar localization and ATPase activity of IcsA, a *Shigella flexneri* protein involved in intracellular movement, *J. Bacteriol.* **175:**2189–2196 (1993).
31. d'Hauteville, H., and Sansonetti, P. J., Phosphorylation of IcsA by cAMP-dependent protein kinase and its effect on intercellular spread of *Shigella flexneri*, *Mol. Microbiol.* **6:**833–841 (1992).
32. Collaco, C., Dyer, R. B., Doan, R., Herzog, N. K., and Niesel, D. W., *Shigella flexneri*–HeLa cell interactions: A putative role for host cell protein kinases, *FEMS Immunol. Med. Microbiol.* **10:**93–100 (1995).
33. Allaoui, A., Mounier, J., Prevost, M. C., Sansonetti, P. J., and Parsot, C., *icsB*: A *Shigella flexneri* virulence gene necessary for the lysis of protrusions during intercellular spread, *Mol. Microbiol.* **6:**1605–1616 (1992).
34. Sansonetti, P. J., Mounier, J., Prevost, M. C., and Mege, R.-M., Cadherin expression required for formation and internalization of *Shigella flexneri*–induced intercellular protrusions involved in spread between epithelial cells, *Cell* **76:**829–839 (1994).
35. Vasselon, T., Mounier, J., Prevost, M. C., Hellio, R., and Sansonetti, P. J., A stress fiber-based movement of *Shigella flexneri* within cells, *Infect. Immun.* **59:**1723–1732 (1991).
36. Vasselon, T., Mounier, J., Hellio, R., and Sansonetti, P. J., Movement along actin filaments of the perijunctional area and de novo polymerization of cellular actin are required for *Shigella flexneri* colonization of epithelial Caco-2 cell monolayers, *Infect. Immun.* **60:**1031–1040 (1992).
37. Zychlinsky, A., Prevost, M. C., and Sansonetti, P. J., *Shigella flexneri* induces apoptosis in infected macrophages, *Nature* **358:**167–169 (1992).
38. Zychlinsky, A., Kenny, B., Menard, R., Prevost, M. C., Holland, I. B., and Sansonetti, P. H., IpaB mediates macrophage apoptosis induced by *Shigella flexneri*, *Mol. Microbiol.* **11:**619–627 (1994).
39. Gorden, J., and Small, P. L. C., Acid resistance in enteric bacteria, *Infect. Immun.* **61:**364–367 (1993).
40. Small, P., Blankenhorn, D., Welty, D., Zinser, E., and Slonczewski, J. L., Acid and base resistance in *Escherichia coli* and *Shigella flexneri*: Role of *rpoS* and growth pH, *J. Bacteriol.* **176:**1729–1737 (1994).
41. Nassif, X., Mazert, M. C., Mounier, J., and Sansonetti, P. J., Evaluation with an *iuc*::Tn10 mutant of the role of aerobactin production in the virulence of *Shigella flexneri*, *Infect. Immun.* **55:**1963–1969 (1987).
42. Gemski, P., Sheahan, D. G., Washington, O., and Formal, S. B., Virulence of *Shigella flexneri* hybrids expressing *Escherichia coli* somatic antigens, *Infect. Immun.* **6:**104–111 (1972).
43. Okamura, N., Nagai, T., Nakaya, R., Kondo, S., Murakami, M., and Hisatsune, K., HeLa cell invasiveness and O antigen of *Shigella flexneri* as a separate and prerequisite attributes of virulence to evoke keratoconjunctivitis in guinea pigs, *Infect. Immun.* **39:**505–513 (1983).
44. Grist, N. R., and Emslie, J. A., Infections in British clinical laboratories, *J. Clin. Pathol.* **44:**667–669 (1991).
45. Sandlin, R. C., Lampel, K. A., Keasler, S. P., Goldberg, M. B., Stolzer, A. L., and Maurelli, A. T., Avirulence of rough mutants of *Shigella flexneri*: Requirement of O antigen for correct unipolar localization of IcsA in the bacterial outer membrane, *Infect. Immun.* **63:**229–237 (1995).
46. Okada, N., Sasakawa, C., Tobe, T., Yamada, M., Nagai, S., Talukder, K. A., Komatsu, K. Kanegasaki, S., and Yoshikawa, M., Virulence-associated chromosomal loci of *Shigella flexneri* identified by random Tn5 insertion mutagenesis, *Mol. Microbiol.* **5:**187–195 (1991).
47. Franzon, V. L., Arondel, J., and Sansonetti, P. J., Contribution of superoxide dismutase and catalase activities to *Shigella flexneri* pathogenesis, *Infect. Immun.* **58:**529–535 (1990).
48. Fontaine, A., Arondel, J., and Sansonetti, P. J., Role of Shiga toxin in the pathogenesis of bacillary dysentery studied using a tox^- mutant of *Shigella dysenteriae* I, *Infect. Immun.* **56:**3099–3109 (1988).
49. Hofmann, S. L., Southwestern internal medicine conference: Shiga-like toxins in hemolytic–uremic syndrome and thrombotic thrombocytopenic purpura, *Am. J. Med. Sci.* **306:**398–406 (1993).
50. Acheson, D. W. K., Donohue-Rolfe, A., and Keusch, G. T., The family of Shiga and Shiga-like toxins, in: *Sourcebook of Bacterial Protein Toxins* (J. E. Alouf and J. H. Freer, Eds.), pp. 415–433, Academic Press, London, 1991.
51. Donohue-Rolfe, A., Kelley, M. A., Bennish, M., and Keusch, G. T., Enzyme-linked immunosorbent assay for *Shigella* toxin, *J. Clin. Microbiol.* **24:**65–68 (1986).
52. Hossain, M. A., and Albert, M. J., Effect of duration of diarrhoea and predictive values of stool leucocytes and red blood cells in the isolation of different serogroups of *Shigella*, *Trans. R. Soc. Trop. Med. Hyg.* **85:**664–666 (1991).
53. Rahman, M. M., Kabir, I., Mahalanabis, D., and Malek, M. A., Decreased food intake in children with severe dysentery due to *Shigella dysenteriae* 1 infection, *Eur. J. Clin. Nutr.* **46:**833–838 (1992).
54. Levine, M. M., DuPont, H. L., Formal, S. B., Hornick, R. B., Takeuchi, A., Gangarosa, E. J., Snyder, M. J., and Libonati, J. P., Pathogenesis of *Shigella dysenteriae* (Shiga) dysentery, *J. Infect. Dis.* **127:**261–270 (1973).
55. Fasano, A., Noriega, F. R., Maneval, D. R., Jr., Chanasongcram, S., Russell, R., Guandalini, S., and Levine, M. M., Shigella enterotoxin 1: An enterotoxin of *Shigella flexneri* 2a active in rabbit small intestine *in vivo* and *in vitro*, *J. Clin. Invest.* **95:**2853–2861 (1995).
56. Nataro, J. P., Seriwatana, J., Fasano, A., Noriega, A., Guers, L., and Morris, J. G., Jr., Cloning and sequencing of a new plasmid-encoded enterotoxin in enteroinvasive *E. coli* and *Shigella*, in *29th Joint Conference on Cholera and Related Diseases*, pp. 144–147, National Institutes of Health, Bethesda, MD, 1993.
57. Fasano, A., Kay, B. A., Russell, R. G., Maneval, D. R., Jr., and Levine, M. M., Enterotoxin and cytotoxin production by enteroinvasive *Escherichia coli*, Infect. Immun. **58:**3717–3723 (1990).
58. Noriega, F. R., Liao, F. M., Formal, S. B., Fasano, A., and Levine, M. M., Prevalence of *Shigella* enterotoxin 1 (ShET1) among *Shigella* clinical isolates of diverse serotypes, *J. Infect. Dis.* **172:**1408–1411 (1995).
59. Bennish, M. L., Salam, M. A., Hossain, M. A., *et al.*, Antimicrobial resistance of *Shigella* isolates in Bangladesh, 1983–

1990: Increasing frequency of strains multiply resistant to ampicillin, trimethoprim-sulfamethoxazole, and naladixic acid, *Clin. Infect. Dis.* **14:**1055–1060 (1992).

60. Horiuchi, S., Inagaki, Y., Yamamoto, N., Okamura, N., Imagawa, Y., and Nakaya, R., Reduced susceptibilities of *Shigella sonnei* strains isolated from patients with dysentery to fluoroquinolones, *Antimicrob. Agents Chemother.* **37:**2486–2489 (1993).
61. Bennish, M. L., and Salam, M. A., Rethinking options for the treatment of shigellosis, *J. Antimicrob. Chemother.* **30:**243–247 (1992).
62. Anonymous, The prospects for immunizing against *Shigella* spp., in: *New Vaccine Development—Establishing Priorities*, Vol. II, *Diseases of Importance in Developing Countries* (S. L. Katz, ed.), pp. 329–337, National Academy Press, Washington, DC, 1986.
63. Lee, L. A., Shapiro, C. N., Hargrett-Bean, N., and Tauxe, R. V., Hyperendemic shigellosis in the United States: A review of surveillance data for 1967–1988, *J. Infect. Dis.* **164:**894–900 (1991).
64. Cruz, J. R., Cano, F., Bartlett, A. V., and Mendez, H., Infection, diarrhea and dysentery caused by *Shigella* species and *Campylobacter jejuni* among Guatemalan rural children, *Pediatr. Infect. Dis. J.* **13:**216–223 (1994).
65. Zaman, K., Yunus, M., Baqui, A. H., and Hossain, K. M., Surveillance of shigellosis in rural Bangladesh: A 10 years review, *J. Pakistan Med. Assoc.* **41:**75–78 (1991).
66. Mata, L. J., Catalan, M. A., and Gordon, J. E., Studies of diarrheal disease in Central America. Shigella carriers among young children of a heavily seeded Guatemalan convalescent home, *Am. J. Trop. Med. Hyg.* **15:**632–638 (1966).
67. Coles, F. B., Kondracki, S. F., Gallo, R. J., Chalker, D., and Morese, D. L., Shigellosis outbreaks at summer camps for the mentally retarded in New York State, *Am. J. Epidemiol.* **130:**966–975 (1989).
68. Pickering, L. K., Bartlett, A. V., and Woodward, W. E., Acute infectious diarrhea among children in day care: Epidemiology and control, *Rev. Infect. Dis.* **8:**539–547 (1981).
69. Shiga, K., The trend of prevention, therapy and epidemiology of dysentery since the discovery of its causative organism, *N. Engl. J. Med.* **26:**1205–1211 (1936).
70. Kostrewski, J., and Stypulkowska-Misiurewicz, H., Changes in the epidemiology of dysentery in Poland and the situation in Europe, *Arch. Immunol. Ther. Exp.* **16:**429–451 (1968).
71. Rosenberg, M. L., Weissman, J. B., Gangarosa, E. J., Reller, L. B., and Beasley, R. P., Shigellosis in the United States: Ten year review of nationwide surveillance, *Am. J. Epidemiol.* **104:**543–551 (1976).
72. Green, M. S., Block, C., Cohen, D., and Slater, P. E., Four decades of shigellosis in Israel: Epidemiology of a growing public health problem, *Rev. Infect. Dis.* **13:**248–253 (1991).
73. Ashkenazi, S., May-Zahav, M., Dinari, G., Gabbay, U., Zilberberg, R., and Samra, Z., Recent trends in the epidemiology of *Shigella* species in Israel, *Clin. Infect. Dis.* **17:**897–899 (1993).
74. Finkelman, Y., Yagupsky, P., Fraser, D., and Dagan, R., Epidemiology of *Shigella* infections in two ethnic groups in a geographic region in southern Israel, *Eur. J. Clin. Microbiol. Infect. Dis.* **13:**367–373 (1994).
75. Mata, L. J., and Castro, F., Epidemiology, diagnosis and impact of Shiga dysentery in Central America, *Ind. Trop. Health* **8:**30–37 (1974).
76. Goma Epidemiology Group, Public health impact of Rwandan refugee crisis: What happened in Goma, Zaire, in July, 1994? *Lancet* **345:**339–341 (1995).
77. Ries, A. A., Wells, J. G., Olivola, D., *et al.*, Epidemic *Shigella dysenteriae* type 1 in Burundi: Panresistance and implications for prevention, *J. Infect. Dis.* **169:**1035–1041 (1994).
78. Gross, R. J., Thomas, L. V., and Rowe, B., *S. dysenteriae*, *S. flexneri*, and *S. boydii* infections in England and Wales: The importance of foreign travel, *Br. Med. J.* **2:**744 (1979).
79. Cleary, T. G., West, M. S., Ruiz-Palacios, G., Winsor, D. K., Calva, J. J., Guerrero, M. L., and Van, R., Human milk secretory immunoglobulin A to *Shigella* virulence plasmid coded-antigens, *J. Pediatr.* **118:**34–38 (1991).
80. Hayani, K. C., Guerrero, M. L., Morrow, A. L., Gomez, H. F., Winsor, D. K., Ruiz-Palacios, G. M., and Cleary, T. G., Concentration of milk secretory immunoglobulin A against *Shigella* virulence plasmid-associated antigens as a predictor of symptom status in *Shigella*-infected breast-fed infants, *J. Pediatr.* **121:**852–856 (1992).
81. Lett, D. W., and Marsh, T. D., Shigellosis in a newborn, *Am. J. Perinatol.* **10:**58–59 (1993).
82. Ahmed, F., Clemens, J. D., Rao, M. R., Khan, M. R., and Haque, E., Initiation of food supplements and stopping of breast-feeding as determinants of weanling shigellosis, *Bull. WHO* **71:**571–578 (1993).
83. Huskins, W. C., Griffiths, J. K., Faruque, A. S., and Bennish, M. L., Shigellosis in neonates and young infants, *J. Pediatr.* **125:**14–22 (1994).
84. Van de Verg, L. L., Herrington, D. A., Boslego, J., Lindberg, A. A., and Levine, M. M., Age-specific prevalence of serum antibodies to the invasion plasmid and lipopolysaccharide antigens of *Shigella* species in Chilean and North American populations, *J. Infect. Dis.* **166:**158–161 (1992).
85. Bennish, M. L., and Wojtyniak, B. J., Mortality due to shigellosis: Community and hospital data, *Rev. Infect. Dis.* **13**(Suppl. 4)**:** S245–S251 (1991).
86. Tauxe, R. V., McDonald, R. C., Hargrett-Bean, N., and Blake, P. A., The persistence of *Shigella flexneri* in the United States: The increased role of the adult male, *Am. J. Public Health* **78:**1432–1435 (1988).
87. Brian, M. J., Van, R., Townsend, I., Murray, B. E., Cleary, T. G., and Pickering, L. K., Evaluation of the molecular epidemiology of an outbreak of multiply resistant *Shigella sonnei* in a day-care center by using pulsed-field gel electrophoresis and plasmid DNA analysis, *J. Clin. Microbiol.* **31:**2152–2156 (1993).
88. Sharp, T. W., Thornton, S. A., Wallace, M. R., *et al.*, Diarrheal disease among military personnel during Operation Restore Hope, Somalia, 1992–1993, *Am. J. Trop. Med. Hyg.* **52:**188–193 (1995).
89. Cohen, D., Slepon, R., and Green, M. S., Sociodemographic factors associated with serum anti-*Shigella* lipopolysaccharide antibodies and shigellosis, *Int. J. Epidemiol.* **20:**546–550 (1991).
90. Cohen, D., Green, M., Block, C., Slepon, R., Ambar, R., Wasserman, S. S., and Levine, M. M., Reduction of transmission of shigellosis by control of house flies (*Musca domestica*), *Lancet* **337:**993–997 (1991).
91. Ahmed, F., Clemens, J. D., Rao, M. R., and Banik, A. K., Family latrines and paediatric shigellosis in rural Bangladesh: Benefit or risk? *Int. J. Epidemiol.* **23:**856–862 (1994).
92. Jewell, J. A., Warren, R. E., and Buttery, R. B., Foodborne shigellosis, *Commun. Dis. Rep.* **3:**R42–44 (1993).

93. Levine, W. C., Stephenson, W. T., and Craun, G. T., Waterborne disease outbreaks, 1986–1988, *MMWR CDC Surveill. Summ.* **39:**1–13 (1990).

94. Lew, J. F., Swerdlow, D. L., Dance, M. E., Griffin, P. M., Bopp, C. A., Gillenwater, M. J., Mercatante, T., and Glass, R. I., An outbreak of shigellosis aboard a cruise ship caused by a multiple-antibiotic-resistant strain of *Shigella flexneri*, *Am. J. Epidemiol.* **134:**413–420 (1991).

95. Davis, H., Taylor, J. P., Perdue, J. N., Stelma, G. N., Jr., Humphreys, J. M., Jr., Rowntree, R., 3rd, and Greene, K. D., A shigellosis outbreak traced to commercially distributed shredded lettuce, *Am. J. Epidemiol.* **128:**1312–1321 (1988).

96. Kapperud, G., Rorvik, L. M., Hasseltvedt, V., *et al.*, Outbreak of *Shigella sonnei* infection traced to imported iceberg lettuce, *J. Clin. Microbiol.* **33:**609–614 (1995).

97. Gessner, B. D., and Beller, M., Moose soup shigellosis in Alaska, *West. J. Med.* **160:**430–434 (1994).

98. Reeve, G., Martin, D. L., Pappas, J., Thompson, R. E., and Greene, K. D., An outbreak of shigellosis associated with the consumption of raw oysters, *N. Engl. J. Med.* **321:**224–227 (1989).

99. Lee, L. A., Ostroff, S. M., McGee, H. B., Johnson, D. R., Downes, F. P., Cameron, D. N., Bean, N. H., and Griffin, P. M., An outbreak of shigellosis as an outdoor music festival, *Am. J. Epidemiol.* **133:**608–615 (1991).

100. Wharton, M., Spiegel, R. A., Horan, J. M., Tauxe, R. V., Wells, J. G., Barg, N., Herndon, J., Meriwether, R. A., MacCormack, J. N., and Levine, R. H., A large outbreak of antibiotic-resistant shigellosis at a mass gathering, *J. Infect. Dis.* **162:**1324–1328 (1990).

101. Keene, W. E., McAnulty, J. M., Hoesly, F. C., Williams, L. P., Jr., Hedberg, K., Oxman, G. L., Barrett, T. J., Pfaller, M. A., and Fleming, D. W., A swimming-associated outbreak of hemorrhagic colitis caused by *Escherichia coli* O157:H7 and *Shigella sonnei*, *N. Engl. J. Med.* **331:**579–584 (1994).

102. Blostein, J., Shigellosis from swimming in a park pond in Michigan, *Public Health Rep.* **106:**317–322 (1991).

103. DeWailly, E., Poirer, C., and Meyer, F. M., Health hazards associated with wind surfing on polluted water, *Am. J. Public Health* **76:**690–691 (1986).

104. Kristjansson, M., Viner, B., and Maslow, J. N., Polymicrobial and recurrent bacteremia with *Shigella* in a patient with AIDS, *Scand. J. Infect. Dis.* **26:**411–416 (1994).

105. Rout, W. R., Formal, S. B., Giannella, R. A., and Dammin, G. J., Pathophysiology of shigella diarrhea in the rhesus monkey: Intestinal transport, morphological and bacteriological studies, *Gastroenterology* **68:**270–278 (1975).

106. Mathan, M. M., and Mathan, V. I., Morphology of rectal mucosa of patients with shigellosis, *Rev. Infect. Dis.* **13**(Suppl. 4):S314–S318 (1991).

107. Dyer, R. B., Collaco, C. R., Niesel, D. W., and Herzog, N. K., *Shigella flexneri* invasion of HeLa cells induces NF-kappa B DNA-binding activity, *Infect. Immun.* **61:**4427–4433 (1993).

108. Nicholls, S., Stephens, S., Braegger, C. P., Walker-Smith, J. A., and MacDonald, T. T., Cytokines in stools of children with inflammatory bowel disease or infective diarrhoea, *J. Clin. Pathol.* **46:**757–760 (1993).

109. de Silva, D. G., Mendis, L. N., Sheron, N., Alexander, G. J., Candy, D. C., Chart, H., and Rowe, B., Concentrations of interleukin 6 and tumour necrosis factor in serum and stools of children with *Shigella dysenteriae* 1 infection, *Gut* **34:**194–198 (1993).

110. Raquib, R., Lindberg, A. A., Wretlind, B., Bardhan, P. K., Andersson, U., and Andersson, J., Persistence of local cytokine production in shigellosis in acute and convalescent stages, *Infect. Immun.* **63:**289–296 (1995).

111. Sansonetti, P. J., Arondel, J., Cavaillon, J.-M., and Huerre, M., Role of interleukin-1 in the pathogenesis of experimental shigellosis, *J. Clin. Invest.* **96:**884–892 (1995).

112. Mackowiak, P. A., Wasserman, S. S., and Levine, M. M., An analysis of the quantitative relationship between oral temperature and severity of illness in experimental shigellosis, *J. Infect. Dis.* **166:**1181–1184 (1992).

113. Kandel, G., Donohue-Rolfe, A., Donowitz, M., and Keusch, G. T., Pathogenesis of *Shigella* diarrhea. XV. Selective targeting of Shiga-toxin to villus cells explains the effect of the toxin on intestinal electrolyte transport, *J. Clin. Invest.* **84:**1509–1517 (1989).

114. Struelens, M. J., Mondal, G., Roberts, M., and Williams, P. H., Role of bacterial and host factors in the pathogenesis of *Shigella* septicemia, *Eur. J. Clin. Microbiol. Infect. Dis.* **9:**337–344 (1990).

115. Keusch, G. T., and Scrimshaw, N. S., Selective primary health care: Strategies for control of disease in the developing world. XXIII. Control of infection to reduce the prevalence of infantile and childhood malnutrition, *Rev. Infect. Dis.* **8:**273–287 (1986).

116. Bennish, M. L., Azad, K. A., and Yousefzadeh, D., Intestinal obstruction during shigellosis: Incidence, clinical features, risk factors, and outcome, *Gastroenterology* **101:**626–634 (1991).

117. Goren, A., Freier, S., and Passwell, J. H., Lethal toxic encephalopathy due to childhood shigellosis in a developed country, *Pediatrics* **89:**1189–1193 (1992).

118. Zajdowicz, T., Epidemiologic and clinical aspects of shigellosis in American forces deployed to Saudi Arabia, *South. Med. J.* **86:** 647–650 (1993).

119. Robbins, J. B., Chu, C., and Schneerson, R., Hypothesis for vaccine development: Protective immunity to enteric diseases caused by nontyphoidal salmonellae and shigellae may be conferred by serum IgG antibodies to the O-specific polysaccharide of their lipopolysaccharides, *Clin. Infect. Dis.* **15:**346–361 (1992).

120. Bennish, M. L., Salam, M. A., and Wahed, M. A., Enteric protein loss during shigellosis, *Am. J. Gastroenterol.* **1993:**53–57 (1993).

121. Ronsmans, C., Bennish, M. L., and Wierzba, T., Diagnosis and management of dysentery by community health workers, *Lancet* **2:**552–555 (1988).

122. Nelson, J. D., and Haltalin, K. C., Accuracy of diagnosis of bacterial diarrheal disease by clinical features, *J. Pediatr.* **78:**519–522 (1971).

123. Kehl, S. K., Havens, P., Behnke, C. E., and Acheson, D. W. K., Evaluation of the Premier EHEC assay for detection of Shiga toxin-producing *Escherichia coli*, *J. Clin. Microbiol.* **35:**2051–2054 (1997).

124. DuPont, H. L., Ericsson, C. D., Johnson, P. C., Bitsura, J. A., DuPont, M. M., and De La Calada, F. S., Prevention of travelers' diarrhea by the tablet formulation of bismuth subsalicylate, *J. Am. Med. Assoc.* **257:**1347–1350 (1987).

125. Hoffman, R. E., and Shillam, P. J., The use of hygiene, cohorting, and antimicrobial therapy to control an outbreak of shigellosis, *Am. J. Dis. Child.* **144:**219–221 (1990).

126. Lindberg, A. A., and Pal, T., Strategies for development of potential candidate *Shigella* vaccines, *Vaccine* **11:**168–179 (1993).

12. Suggested Reading

Levine, O. S., and Levine, M. M., Houseflies (*Musca domestica*) as mechanical vectors of shigellosis, *Rev. Infect. Dis.* **13:** 688–696 (1991).

Luscher, D., and Altwegg, M., Detection of shigellae, enteroinvasive and enterotoxigenic *Escherichia coli* using the polymerase chain reaction (PCR) in patients returning from tropical countries, *Mol. Cell. Probes* **8:**285–290 (1994).

Menard, R., Dehio, C., and Sansonetti, P. J., Bacterial entry into epithelial cells: The paradigm of *Shigella, Trends Microbiol.* **4:**220–226 (1996).

O'Brien, A. D., Tesh, V. L., Donohue-Rolfe, A., Jackson, M. P., Olsnes, S., Sandvig, K., Lindberg, A. A., and Keusch, G. T., Shiga toxin: Biochemistry, genetics, mode of action, and role in pathogenesis, *Curr. Top. Microbiol. Immunol.* **180:**65–94 (1992).

Sansonetti, P., and Phalipon, A., Shigellosis: From molecular pathogenesis of infection to protective immunity and vaccine development, *Res. Immunol.* **147:**595–602 (1996).

CHAPTER 33

Staphylococcal Infections

Frederick L. Ruben and Robert R. Muder

1. Introduction

Although staphylococci, as a cause of sporadic infection, produce severe morbidity and mortality for the individual, the public health importance of infections with this organism is its potential to cause epidemics. Major public health problems resulting from infection with staphylococci include spread of the organism in newborn nurseries and outbreaks of postoperative wound infections. Also of importance is staphylococcal food poisoning caused by the ingestion of food containing enterotoxin produced by coagulase-positive strains of *Staphylococcus aureus*. Coagulase-negative *Staphylococcus* species have now gained great clinical significance.[1]

A definitive diagnosis of staphylococcal disease is made when *S. aureus*, coagulase-positive, is isolated from a purulent lesion or from the blood, urine, peritoneal fluid, or cerebrospinal fluid (CSF) of a patient with clinical signs of infection. The diagnosis of a coagulase-negative staphylococcus, of which *S. epidermidis* is the most common, as the causative agent of infection depends on repeated isolation of this organism in appropriate clinical circumstances, such as endocarditis involving a prosthetic heart valve, infected peritoneal fluid in a patient undergoing dialysis, urinary tract infection in a young woman, infection of CSF from a ventriculoatrial or a ventriculoperitoneal shunt, an infected joint prosthesis, or bacteremia in an immunocompromised host or a patient with an intravenous catheter.

Frederick L. Ruben and Robert R. Muder • Infectious Diseases Division, Department of Medicine, University of Pittsburgh School of Medicine, Pittsburgh, Pennsylvania 15213.

2. Historical Background

Approximately 100 years ago, von Recklinghausen applied the term "micrococci" to gram-positive cocci observed in disease tissue and in pus from human abscesses. In 1881, Sir Alexander Ogston[2] published extensive observations showing that a cluster-forming coccus was the cause of certain pyogenic abscesses in man. He subsequently named the organisms *Staphylococcus*, derived from the Greek nouns *staphyle* (grapes) and *coccus* (grain or berry). He distinguished staphylococci from streptococci and produced disease in mice by subcutaneous inoculation of staphylococci recovered from pus.

In 1884, Rosenbach[3] observed that isolates of staphylococci formed two types of colonies, distinguishable from each other by color; he named the orange colonies *S. aureus* and the white colonies *S. albus*. From the time of Job, staphylococcal infections have plagued man. The advent of penicillin initially checked the spread of staphylococci, but in the 1950s penicillinase-producing staphylococci were the cause of widespread hospital and nursery epidemics. The development of new penicillinase-resistant penicillins appeared to reverse this tide, and for a period staphylococcal infections were less important as causes of nosocomial disease than infections caused by gram-negative bacilli. Methicillin-resistant staphylococci have emerged, however, as a cause of disease and are prevalent in the United States and Europe. Thus, it appears that the cycle of resistant bacterial and antibiotics designed to check such organisms will continue for the *Staphylococcus*.

3. Methodology

3.1. Sources of Mortality Data

Most staphylococcal disease is localized to the skin and is not fatal. Once infection becomes generalized and bacteremia occurs, mortality is great despite appropriate antibiotic therapy. Data on mortality from bacteremic staphylococcal infections have come from national surveillance[4] and from hospital studies[5–7] with comparable findings.

3.2. Sources of Morbidity Data

The incidence of all staphylococcal disease in the community can be assessed only indirectly, since minor disease may never come to medical attention.[8] The incidence of more serious disease, including bacteremia, can be estimated.[4,9] Surveillance has provided reliable data on hospital-acquired staphylococcal disease[9–13] and on methicillin-resistant *S. aureus* disease in long-term care facilities.[14]

3.3. Surveys

Household- and population-based surveys have provided the only data on community-acquired morbidity from staphylococci.[8] Hospital-based surveillance for staphylococcal disease, community and nosocomially acquired, allows for ongoing assessment of serious staphylococcal disease.[11,12,15,16] Hospital surveillance begins from laboratory cultures reporting staphylococci; hence, it may underestimate the incidence of disease when cultures are not taken. Typing of staphylococci in the laboratory permits identification of strains responsible for outbreaks or epidemics.[17]

3.4. Laboratory Diagnosis

Staphylococci can be recognized quickly and reliably on Gram's strains of exudates from most clinical specimens. Their lack of fastidiousness permits their growth on ordinary laboratory media.[18] Selective media such as that containing mannitol and 6.5% NaCl have expedited recognition of staphylococci grown from swabs of throat, nose, or other contaminated areas and have permitted rapid evaluation of staphylococcal carriage by individuals. Once grown, *S. aureus* is identified by a positive coagulase test.

There are over 30 species of coagulase-negative staphylococci. Although many clinical laboratories do not routinely speciate coagulase-negative isolates, they can be distinguished by a variety of biochemical reactions. *S. epidermidis* accounts for the majority of clinical isolates, with *S. haemolyticus* and *S. hominis* next in frequency.[19] Antibiotic sensitivity of staphylococci as measured by a Kirby–Bauer disk technique is widely used,[20] although in selected instances, tube-dilution techniques permitting the determination of minimal inhibitory and bactericidal concentrations are more valuable.[21] Phage typing of staphylococci has permitted identification of specific strains and has allowed for the recognition of prevalent and epidemic strains. Molecular methods of typing, such as plasmid analysis or restriction endonuclease analysis of whole-cell DNA, are highly reliable in differentiating staphylococcal strains[22,23]; they are more widely available than phage typing. Strain identification by antimicrobial susceptibility is unreliable.

Serological studies have not proved useful, since the normal human adult possesses antibodies to several staphylococcal antigens.[24] Staphylococci contain a variety of antigens, each of which might be important, so that the question of which antigen(s) may be useful for serological studies remains controversial. Antibodies to *S. aureus* teichoic acid have been demonstrated in human sera[25]; studies suggest that their presence in bacteremic patients might indicate a more serious form of the disease,[18,26] including endocarditis,[27] osteomyelitis,[28] and metastatic abscesses.[29]

4. Biological Characteristics of the Organism

Staphylococci are nonmotile, gram-positive cocci that may occur singly, in pairs, short chains, or clusters; the characteristic appearance is that of a "bunch of grapes." Colonies of *S. aureus* typically produce yellow pigment; most other species are nonpigmented. The following enzymes and toxins that are produced by staphylococci are often considered of importance in human virulence:

1. *S. aureus* produces two antigenically distinct enzymes: bound and free coagulase, both capable of coagulating human serum. Their role in infection is unclear, but the presence of this enzyme serves to distinguish the more virulent species, *S. aureus*, from other species.
2. Alpha-toxin causes direct damage to a variety of mammalian cell membranes including erythrocytes, leukocytes, and fibroblasts.
3. Leukocidin is an extracellular protein that acts on human polymorphonuclear leukocytes *in vitro*. It causes death of white blood cells, but its role in infection is unclear.
4. Enterotoxin: Most *S. aureus* strains produce one or more enterotoxins that are responsible for the syndrome of staphylococcal

food poisoning. A smaller percentage of *S. epidermidis* strains produce enterotoxin; these have rarely been implicated in food poisoning.[30]

5. Exfoliative toxin: Staphylococci of phage group II produce a toxin responsible for the dermatologic manifestations of infection that go under the general heading of "scalded skin syndrome."
6. Toxic shock syndrome toxins: This syndrome is caused by a toxin or toxins produced by *S. aureus*. Toxic shock sydrome toxin-1 (TSST-1) is a specific toxin identified to date, but other exotoxins and enterotoxins may also be responsible for the syndrome.[31,32] While rare, toxic shock syndrome has been reported to be caused by TSST-1-producing coagulase-negative staphylococci.[33]

Enterotoxins and TSST-1 bind to class II major histocompatability antigens and to receptors on T lymphocytes. These toxins stimulate the release of interleukin-2 and tumor necrosis factor; uncontrolled release of these lymphokines may play a pathogenic role in the clinical syndromes caused by these toxins.[34]

S. aureus specifically binds a variety of human proteins and glycopeptides, including fibronectin and fibrinogen. This binding may be an important factor in the maintenance of the carrier state and the initiation of infection. Clinical isolates of coagulase-negative staphylococcus, from patients with clinical infections, appear to produce an extracellular polysaccharide ("slime factor") that enhances adherence to plastic or metal surfaces.[35] This slime layer also inhibits diffusion of antibiotics, impairing their ability to reach organisms.[36] In addition, the slime material interferes with the lymphoproliferative response to mitogens[37] and also alters polymorphonuclear functions such as decreasing responsiveness to chemotactic stimuli[38] and inhibiting phagocytosis of coagulase-negative staphylococci.[38] Coagulase-negative staphylococci have the ability to erode into polyethylene catheters and prosthetic devices, which may also allow increased adherence of the organisms.[35,39] Catheter-adherent coagulase-negative staphylococci appear to possess survival mechanisms under adverse conditions (absence of conventional nutrients) that may be important in the genesis of occult foreign-body-associated infection.[40]

5. Descriptive Epidemiology

5.1. Prevalence and Incidence

S. aureus may be carried by normal people in a variety of body sites without disease being present. The nose is the principal site of carriage; cross-sectional studies reveal rates of 30–50% in persons outside hospitals and higher rates in hospital nursing personnel.[41,42] Longitudinal studies have shown persons to be intermittent carriers, persistent noncarriers, or persistent carriers.[41] Skin carriage has been demonstrated in 85% of persons with atopic dermatitis, suggesting a strong predisposition to carriage.[43] In newborn nurseries, colonization of the umbilical stump precedes nasal carriage, and up to 75% of infants become carriers at one or more body sites by the fifth day.[44]

Carriage may precede or indeed lead to disease in susceptible individuals.[41] Patients on continuous ambulatory peritoneal dialysis who are carriers had a significantly higher infection rate than noncarriers.[45] Conversely, not all carriers develop *S. aureus* lesions or any other form of staphylococcal disease. General practitioners in England have reported the annual incidence of *S. aureus* disease in their practice populations at 1.5–5.0%,[46] certainly lower than population carriage rates. The nasal carrier in the hospital has been shown to have a higher rate of staphylococcal postoperative sepsis (7.0%) than the noncarrier (2.0%).[47] Insulin-using diabetics have increased carriage rates.[48] The true rate of minor disease in nasal carriers postoperatively and in the newborn with umbilical carriage is not known, since these patients may be discharged from the hospital before disease becomes manifest.[49]

Serious staphylococcal disease, including sepsis, may be acquired outside the hospital. One report from a community-type hospital noted that 14% of all community-acquired episodes of sepsis were caused by staphylococci, while the rate of sepsis for all bacterial types was 340/100,000 admissions.[12] Other more recent reports found that 7 to 14% of community-acquired episodes were caused by *S. aureus*.[50,51]

5.2. Epidemic Behavior and Contagiousness

S. aureus can be highly contagious through direct contact with the large numbers of organisms present in lesions. The condition of the host clearly influences the frequency and severity of disease produced by staphylococci. Within a household, any strain of *S. aureus* can colonize family members and cause disease sporadically, or it may cause continuous and repeated episodes of infection.[8]

Community and worldwide epidemics of *S. aureus* disease have been recognized. Finland[52] has conceptualized these epidemic features of *S. aureus*: first are local and short-term epidemics of staphylococcal disease exemplified by outbreaks of antibiotic-related staphylococcal diarrhea noted in the late 1950s and early 1960s, by outbreaks in burn units, and by excess staphylococcal pneumonia complicating the influenza type A outbreaks of 1941 and 1957. To this one can add more recent outbreaks of methicillin-resistant staphylococcal disease.[53,54] Second, there have been worldwide and long-term epidemics of *S. aureus* disease noted in nurseries and hospitals throughout the world, coincident with the appearance and spread of new bacteriophages 80, then 81, and then 80/81 in the late 1950s. Following this occurrence, *S. aureus* disease has shown a cyclical character, with periods of increased cases followed by periods of declining incidence. The phage-type patterns of *S. aureus* have also changed during these cycles, with different phage groups predominating.

Several factors may have contributed to the epidemic of phage type 80/81 staphylococci.[55] Its arrival was associated with the widespread availability of penicillin and the use of broad-spectrum antibiotics that allowed selection of penicillin-resistant strains.[56] The number of susceptible persons increased as a result of medical advances. Finally, the transmission of *S. aureus* was enhanced by the reliance on antibiotics instead of aseptic techniques in caring for hospitalized persons. The demise of the 80/81 strain may have resulted from vigorous control efforts, the advent of semisynthetic penicillinase-resistant penicillins, and also unknown factors.

Finland[52] and others[4,54] suggest that the epidemic character of *S. aureus* may relate, in part, to genetic properties of the organism. The changing susceptibility and resistance of *S. aureus* to bacteriophages or properties of the phages themselves may create within *S. aureus* the changes required for enhanced virulence. The changing antigenic character and epidemic properties of *S. aureus* may thus be analogous to the changing influenza A viruses and their epidemiological virulence.

S. epidermidis is among the most common causes of sepsis in newborns who require umbilical vein catheters and in patients with cancer who require long-term vascular catheterization. Two outbreaks of catheter-related *S. epidermidis* sepsis in intensive care units have been reported; the bacteremia was correlated with the duration of catheterization and the use of parenteral hyperalimentation.[57,58] In one outbreak, 13 episodes of *S. epidermidis* sepsis occurred over a 20-month period; these episodes were characterized by fever, toxicity, multiple positive blood cultures, and uniformly colonized intravascular catheters.[57] An additional 16 patients had possible sepsis. Four associated deaths occurred; in the three autopsies, all patients had multiple pulmonary abscesses in which gram-positive cocci were profusely present.[57] A prominent feature of the *S. epidermidis* isolates was resistance to many commonly used antimicrobial agents.[57] Most of the patients were hospitalized in the intensive care units; nose and hand cultures taken from personnel showed frequent carriage of multiply-resistant *S. epidermidis* strains.[57] A recent common source outbreak of *S. epidermidis* among patients undergoing cardiac surgery was traced to one surgeon carrying the organism on his hands.[59]

5.3. Geographic Distribution

Infections with *S. aureus* are worldwide in distribution.[52] While the penicillin-resistant phage type 80/81 caused infections worldwide, the more recent methicillin-resistant strains have been of several phage types or were nontypeable[53] and are now widespread in Europe,[60,61] the United States,[62,63] and occur worldwide.[64]

Penicillin-resistant forms of *S. aureus* do occur in nature,[65] and penicillinase-producing strains from the preantibiotic era have been reported.[66] In contrast, there is no clear documentation of resistance to other antistaphylococcal drugs prior to their clinical use.[67]

5.4. Temporal Distribution

Annual rates for *S. aureus* bacteremia have varied in both the United States[52] and Europe.[68] *S. aureus* pneumonia with bacteremia has shown a peak incidence in winter and summer months,[69] whereas postoperative wound rates have peaked in winter months.[70]

Bullous impetigo from *S. aureus* has a seasonal peak in late summer and early fall.[71] Pyomyositis caused by *S. aureus* is a common condition in tropical areas such as eastern Africa,[72] whereas it occurs rarely in temperate climate areas such as the United States.[73]

5.5. Age

As noted in Section 5.1, children have higher rates of carriage and persist as carriers more commonly than do adults.[74] Rates for bacteremia are higher in the age groups 5–15 years[4,75] and 50–80 years[4] whether the bacteremia was acquired inside or outside the hospital. Mortality from bacteremia is age-related, with higher rates in the very young and older age groups.[4,6]

5.6. Sex

Males and females carry *S. aureus* at a similar rate.[74] Males have an increased rate of disease during the first month of life[76] and have more disseminated infections in childhood.[75] In adults, results are conflicting for sex differences in rates of disease.[77–81] Males are reported to have more *S. aureus* pneumonia[78] and to have more fatal infections.[81] A problem with all the reports showing sex differences is actually assessing the population at risk.[76]

5.7. Race

No racial predisposition for *S. aureus* has been noted.

5.8. Occupation

Persons such as physicians and nurses in hospital who may come in contact with patients with *S. aureus* lesions have higher rates of nasal carriage than persons not in such contact,[41,82] and they may develop diseases from such carriage.[83]

5.9. Occurrence in Different Settings

Staphylococci have been long recognized as a hospital problem, and the policy of routine ongoing surveillance for hospital-acquired staphylococcal disease is well justified.[43,49,78] *S. aureus* is the leading cause of postoperative wound infection and the second-most frequent cause of nosocomial pneumonia.[84] Coagulase-negative staphylococci are now the leading cause of primary nosocomial bacteremia, accounting for 29% of cases.[84] During the period 1980–1989, the rate of bloodstream infections due to coagulase-negative staphylococci in large teaching hospitals rose from 0.2/1000 discharges to 1.8/1000.[85] This increase was most likely caused by an increase in the use of indwelling vascular catheters. Together, *S. aureus* and coagulase-negative staphylococci account for 21% of the estimated 4 million infections acquired in United States hospitals annually.[84]

Because of the rate of colonization with *S. aureus* of newborn infants in nurseries, there have been serious outbreaks of *S. aureus* sepsis in nursery populations.[43] Staphylococci in nurseries are spread via personnel handling the infants,[86] suggesting an important role for handwashing in the control of nursery colonization. Reduced handling and segregation of colonized cohorts have reduced colonization and disease rates within nurseries, as has umbilical cord care using bacitracin ointment.[87] Heroin addicts who inject their drugs are at considerable risk for developing *S. aureus* endocarditis.[88] While neither the injection paraphernalia nor the drugs[89] have contained *S. aureus*, it has been shown that addicts actively using heroin have significantly higher carriage rates than addicts not on drugs.[90] The organisms recovered from the blood of heroin addicts with endocarditis are usually of the same phage type as those carried on the skin and in the nose.[91] Patients undergoing hemodialysis or peritoneal dialysis have nasal carriage rates of *S. aureus* two to three times that of the general population.[92,93] Colonized dialysis patients are at high risk for staphylococcal infection, particularly bacteremia, arteriovenous fistula infections, and peritonitis. The strain isolated from the site of infection is typically the same as that carried in the nose.

5.10. Socioeconomic Factors

There is little to suggest that socioeconomic factors influence the occurrence of staphylococcal disease. Overcrowding, poor skin hygiene, or minor skin trauma may play a role in predisposing to *S. aureus* bullous impetigo, but the association is greater for streptococcal pyoderma.[94]

5.11. Other Factors

A variety of underlying conditions predispose to *S. aureus* infection.[24,74,95] Extremes of age, recent influenza A infection, exfoliative skin disorders, diabetes, chronic renal failure, chronic granulomatous disease, agammaglobulinemia, liver disease, intravenous drug abuse, and chronic renal failure are associated with an increased risk of infection. In addition to surgery, vascular catheters, and dialysis, medical interventions that predispose to infection with *S. aureus* include insertion of prosthetic devices, administration of corticosteroids, and administration of cancer chemotherapy. The use of antibiotics has clearly influenced the epidemiology of *S. aureus* infections. Following the widespread use of penicillin and broad-spectrum antibiotics, diarrhea associated with overgrowth of *S. aureus* in the stools became a recognized complication.[52] In addition, changing antibiotic-susceptibility patterns have been dictated by the antibiotics being used.[96,97] Resistance to penicillin has increased progressively over the years, whereas with the declining indiscriminate use of other broad-spectrum antibiotics, *S. aureus* strains have regained sensitivity to these drugs. Methicillin-resistant *S. aureus*, while rare in United States hospitals until the mid-1970s, is now widespread in hospitals of all sizes, in rehabilitation facilities, and in nursing homes.[98] The mechanisms for this spread are not known.[99,100]

Quite possibly the virulence of the organism itself has influenced the occurrence of infection. Phage types such as 52, 52A, and 80/81 complex of the 1950s that were resistant to penicillin have been called "epidemiologically virulent."[43,49] Whether disease incidence alone was the result of intense exposure to these strains or whether they were inherently more virulent is unresolved.

An association has been shown between the use of vaginal tampons by younger women during their menses[(101)] and the entity called toxic shock syndrome.[(102)] *S. aureus* has been cultured from the vagina in over 90% of patients with this syndrome,[(101)] whereas a much lower prevalence of colonization, 2–15%, of the cervix and vagina with *S. aureus* was found in healthy women.[(101–103)] Toxic shock syndrome not associated with menstruation has also been identified[(104)] in conjunction with *S. aureus* infections such as surgical wound infections or with childbirth by vaginal delivery and cesarean section. Toxic shock syndrome has also been a complication of influenza.[(105)]

Coagulase-negative staphylococci are part of the normal skin flora and are uncommon pathogens except in the presence of foreign bodies (prosthetic valves, CSF shunts, prosthetic joints, and intravenous catheters). Immunocompromised hosts and neutropenic patients appear to have an increased susceptibility to severe infections, such as bacteremia, with these organisms. It is sometimes hard to separate the roles of foreign bodies versus immunocompromised status. For example, intravascular catheters are an important portal of entry in immunocompromised hosts; however, overgrowth at respiratory and gastrointestinal sites may also serve as sites of entry in such hosts even without a foreign body.

6. Mechanisms and Routes of Transmission

Transmission of *S. aureus* outside of the hospital consists of person-to-person spread within families or intimate contacts.[(8)] Studies within the hospital show that the nasal carrier is predisposed to postoperative infection with the same strain.[(47,106)] Also within hospitals, other vectors for infection exist with infected patients,[(43)] health care personnel[(49,107)] who are infected or are carriers, and fomite contamination.[(77,108)] Airborne spread of *S. aureus* can be demonstrated[(41,109,110)]; however, it has been difficult to correlate counts of staphylococci in air with infection rates.[(41,111)] Patients on broad-spectrum antibiotics have been shown to have increased shedding of resistant staphylococci.[(41)] The infected lesion sheds heavy concentrations of organisms and is potentially the greatest hazard for spreading infection.[(43)] In nurseries, the nurse carrier usually conveys *S. aureus* to infants by handling them.[(88)] Often potential vectors are the "cloud baby"[(112)] and the adult carrier who has chronic dermatologic disease or who becomes an effective disseminator for unknown reasons.[(43)]

Too little is currently know of animal staphylococci and human *S. aureus* interrelationships to determine their importance in human disease.[(113)]

Humans are the natural reservoir for *S. epidermidis*; these bacteria are part of the normal skin flora and are the most common staphylococcal species isolated from cutaneous sites. The organism is easily shed from skin and can contaminate inanimate environmental surfaces, other people, and the air. The resistance of the organism to drying and temperature changes produces a long viability.[(114)] *S. epidermidis* infections result from contamination of a site (usually surgical) by organisms from the patient's skin or nasopharynx or from exogenous sources. One study reported the recovery of organisms, primarily *S. epidermidis* and diptheroids, in about 55% of cultures taken from the site of the valvular prosthesis during open heart surgery.[(115)]

7. Pathogenesis and Immunity

7.1. Pathogenesis

Foreign bodies enhance the likelihood that staphylococcal infection will develop by reducing the number of organisms needed to initiate infection. Healthy persons require more than 10^6 virulent staphylococci to initiate a minor infection, whereas 10^2 organisms can infect when a foreign body is present.[(116)] Sutures, intravascular catheters, or needles left in place,[(117)] prosthetic joint devices,[(118)] artificial heart valves,[(119)] and tracheostomy tubes[(120)] are examples of commonly used foreign bodies that may become infected. Fibrin may be responsible for staphylococcal adherence to intravascular catheters.[(121)] Bacteremia may arise from the local site and can lead to *S. aureus* infection and abscess formation in any organ of the body.[(6)] Sequelae include such entities as meningitis,[(122)] osteomyelitis,[(123)] and endocarditis.[(124)] Damaged tissue, e.g., the skin in burns and the airways in influenza, are predisposed to colonization and then proliferation of *S. aureus*. A consequence in burn patients is septicemia,[(125)] and in influenza patients, *S. aureus* pneumonia.[(126)]

Other abnormalities of host defense such as neutropenia,[(127,128)] chronic granulomatous disease,[(129)] immunosuppression,[(5)] and renal failure[(130)] predispose to more frequent occurrence and greater severity of *S. aureus* disease.

The factors responsible for virulence of different strains of staphylococci are unknown. *S. aureus* organisms shed from fresh tissues are more virulent than desiccated organisms in air or on fomites.[(131)] Some strains, such as the epidemic 80/81 complex, are epidemiologically more virulent.[49,52] Carriers of methicillin-resistant strains of *S. aureus* were at greater risk for infection than persons colonized with methicillin-sensitive strains, although it is not clear that resistant strains are more virulent.[132] *S. aureus* is a complex organism with a variety of bacterial products with the potential for promoting disease.[95] Two extracellular products—enterotoxin, which produces food poisoning, and exfolatin, which causes the scalded-skin syndrome—clearly produce disease. In toxic shock syndrome, an extracellular toxin (now known as TSST-1) of *S. aureus* related to phage group I is believed to mediate the multiple clinical manifestations seen.[102]

As with *S. aureus*, the presence of foreign bodies markedly enhances the likelihood of infection with coagulase-negative staphylococci. Indeed, *S. epidermidis* is generally not a pathogen except in the presence of a foreign body, in an immunocompromised host, or in patients with neutropenia. As described earlier, the ability of a coagulase-negative strain of staphylococcus to secrete a slime layer appears to offer it advantages in terms of colonization, persistence, and infection. In one study, 81% of 59 infectious episodes in patients with a prosthetic device were due to a slime-positive coagulase-negative staphylococcus.[133] Slime-positive organisms producing infection were significantly harder to eradicate than slime-negative organisms.[133]

7.2. Immunity

Humans enjoy a high degree of natural resistance to *S. aureus*. The exact nature of this natural immunity is not clear and may be nonspecific.[134] While humans show little resistance to superficial colonization with *S. aureus*, there is great resistance to progressive forms of disease.[134] Spread of staphylococcal infection is limited by reticuloendothelial system clearance and polymorphonuclear leukocyte chemotaxis and ingestion of bacteria.[128,135] Although IgG antibodies to specific components of *S. aureus* have been demonstrated,[25] and components of the classic and alternative complement systems have been shown to be necessary at times for efficient phagocytosis of staphylococci,[136] the overall significance of opsonization in immunity to *S. aureus* is unclear.[95,128] IgE antibodies to *S. aureus*, demonstrated in patients with recurrent "cold" abscesses, may represent an abnormal immunologic response to *S. aureus*[137] and more specifically to the cell walls of the bacteria.[138]

The role of cell-mediated immunity to *S. aureus* remains to be defined.[95,139] Filtrates from strains of *S. aureus* contain mitogens for human lymphocytes.[140] Delayed hypersensitivity reactions to *S. aureus* have been demonstrated in animals, but are not associated with increased resistance.[139] Indeed, repeated skin infections in a rabbit model produced increased susceptibility to *S. aureus* skin and joint infections, suggesting that delayed hypersensitivity may have a pathogenetic role in staphylococcal disease.[141]

8. Patterns of Host Response

Staphylococci may infect and cause disease in virtually every organ system of the body. The organism is highly virulent for humans and, with the exception of the anterior nares, the pharynx, and skin, rarely lives in symbiosis with the host. Within the nose and pharynx and on the skin, staphylococci may exist as part of the "carrier" state; their importance in such locations is the capacity to be spread to other sites within the host or to other susceptible individuals. The manifestations of staphylococci infection vary depending on the site involved and will be described separately. Table 1 summarizes some of the features of selected forms of *S. aureus* infections.

8.1. Clinical Features

8.1.1. Boils, Furuncles, and Carbuncles. A boil or furuncle is an acute abscess of the skin and subcutaneous tissues. Such lesions occur most commonly on the face, neck, buttocks, thighs, perineum, or axillae. Exquisite tenderness is the hallmark of these lesions, which swell with pus and eventually drain spontaneously. Carbuncles are collections of interconnected furuncles that are less likely to drain externally. Carbuncles become larger, are more painful, and are associated with systemic signs and bacteremia; they appear more commonly in diabetes.

8.1.2. Wound Infections. *S. aureus* accounts for 17% and coagulase-negative staphylococci accounts for 12% of surgical wound infections.[142] Factors that have been associated with an increased incidence of wound infection are age, diabetes, steroid administration, obesity, malnutrition, increased duration of time in the operating room, and presence of other infected sites. Wound infections are usually associated with frank purulent drainage, breakdown of the wound, fever, and lack of well-being of the patient.

8.1.3. Breast Infections. Mastitis due to staphylococci generally occurs in newborns and in women (frequently in the puerperium). In neonates, the breast shows marked redness with induration resembling a furuncle. In adults, infection can be superficial, presenting only with pain and a lump; but more extensive involvement may occur with marked tenderness, fever, and leukocytosis.

Table 1. Clinical Forms of Staphylococcal Infections

Category	Age most often afflicted	Special risk factors
Boils, furuncles, carbuncles	All ages	Diabetes mellitus
Wound infections	All ages	Diabetes mellitus, steroid therapy, obesity, malnutrition, prolonged surgery, foreign body (e.g., prosthesis)
Breast infections	Newborn, women in puerperium	None
Pneumonia	All ages	Drug addiction, influenza outbreaks
Endocarditis	All ages	Heroin addiction, prosthetic heart valve
Skin infections		
Bullous impetigo	Childhood	None
Scalded-skin syndrome	Childhood	Compromised host
Thrombophlebitis	All ages	Intravenous catheters
Bacteremia	All ages	Diabetes mellitus, leukemia, lymphoma
Osteomyelitis	Children	None
Septic arthritis	All ages	None
Food poisoning	All ages	None
Parotitis	Elderly	Dehydration
Toxic shock syndrome	Younger women	Use of vaginal tampons during menses, after childbirth, surgical wounds, influenza
Peritonitis	All ages	Continuous peritoneal dialysis
Urinary tract infection	Young women	None or urinary tract abnormality
Cerebrospinal fluid shunt infection	All ages	Presence of shunt
Pyomyositis	Young men and boys	Tropical climate, HIV
Meningitis	Newborn infants, all ages	Prematurity, endocarditis, CNS disorders

8.1.4. Pneumonia. Staphylococcal pneumonia may present in one of three ways: (1) lobar pneumonia; (2) diffuse interstitial pneumonia; and (3) localized areas of pneumonia secondary to septic emboli with infarction. In lobar pneumonia, the patients are usually acutely ill with high fever, tachypnea, and cough productive of yellow, bloody sputum. On smear of the sputum, large numbers of neutrophils and staphylococci are seen. Empyema is a frequent occurrence and in infants the development of pneumatoceles is a hallmark of staphylococcal pneumonia. Diffuse interstitial pneumonia usually occurs after or coincident with influenza. The most prominent clinical feature is tachypnea and cyanosis with refractory hypoxia. Localized areas of pneumonia secondary to septic emboli can occur with bacteremia alone or in the presence of endocarditis, particularly involving the tricuspid valve. Pleuritic chest pain, dyspnea, fever, and chills are prominent, whereas cough and purulent sputum are less likely. Roentgenographic examination frequently reveals multiple small densities at the periphery of the lung that frequently increase in size and cavitate.

8.1.5. Endocarditis. Endocarditis caused by *S. aureus* usually presents as an acute fulminant illness with high fever and metastatic abscesses and has the potential for lethal damage to heart valves. Staphylococcal endocarditis should be suspected in any patient with staphylococcal bacteremia and particularly in heroin addicts. Many of the classic features of endocarditis may be absent and staphylococcal disease frequently involves normal heart valves.[143]

Only 5% of all cases of infective endocarditis on native cardiac valves are caused by coagulase-negative staphylococci.[144] The disease is subacute and resembles that caused by viridans streptococci. In contrast to the low frequency of coagulase-negative infections of native cardiac valves, these organisms are the single most common etiologic agent in infection of prosthetic valves.[145] Coagulase-negative staphylococci were implicated as the cause of approximately 40% of the cases of prosthetic valve endocarditis at two large medical centers.[145] Generally, *S. epidermidis* is the species most frequently implicated.[144] The infections are usually severe with evidence of prosthetic valve dysfunction. It is presumed that cases caused by coagulase-negative staphylococci occurring in the year following surgery are probably the result of inoculation of organisms at the time of surgery. Diagnosis of coagulase-negative prosthetic valve endocarditis requires a high level of suspicion and the findings of fever and blood cultures positive for these organisms.

8.1.6. Skin Infections. Staphylococci of phage group II have been associated with several manifestations of infection in the skin.[146] These include bullous impetigo, a nonstreptococcal scarlatiniform rash, and toxic epidermal necrolysis (the scalded-skin syndrome). Infected individuals show an abrupt onset with diffuse erythema over most of the body. The skin is exquisitely sensitive to touch and within 1–2 days begins to peel off after light stroking (Nikolsky's sign). Large bullae filled with clear sterile fluid appear in the epidermis, which separates in sheets. Secondary desquamation continues 7–10 days after the onset of redness; recovery is complete.

8.1.7. Intravenous Catheter-Related Infections. Staphylococci are the most frequent cause of infections related to intravenous catheterization. Coagulase-negative staphylococci are most frequently isolated followed by *S. aureus*.(147) The site of catheter insertion shows signs of local inflammation in only a minority of cases. Patients may present with fever and other systemic signs of sepsis without any obvious source of infection. Blood cultures are usually positive and culture of the intravascular portion of the catheter also yields the infecting organism. Risk factors include the long periods of time that intravenous lines now stay in place; the pressure of multiple antibiotic usages in sick patients, enhancing the likelihood of colonization with multiply-resistant coagulase-negative staphylococci; the ability of the organism to produce a slime layer; the presence of neutropenia; and the administration of other drugs that produce immunosuppression.

8.1.8. Bacteremia. Staphylococcal bacteremia may arise from any site where staphylococci produce infection. Forty percent of bacteremic patients have no apparent primary site of infection.(6,148) Hospital procedures such as surgery with subsequent wound infection or parenteral infusion via intravenous catheters are a frequent source. Patients who develop staphylococcal bacteremia frequently have underlying diseases such as diabetes, chronic renal failure, malignancy, or substance abuse.(148) The clinical picture of staphylococcal bacteremia is generally a fulminant illness with high fever and tachycardia. Shock, disseminated intravascular coagulation, and respiratory failure may occur. Metastatic abscesses occur in about one third of patients.

Coagulase-negative staphylococci are now the most frequent cause of hospital-acquired bacteremia.(84) An increase infrequently is related to the increase in the number of immunocompromised patients and an increase in the use of centrally placed intravenous catheters. Neutropenic patients are at particular risk,(149,150) and the mortality in these patients is as high as 34%.(150)

8.1.9. Osteomyelitis. *S. aureus* is the most common cause of acute osteomyelitis.(123) It occurs most frequently in children under 12 years of age but also may be seen in adults. The clinical picture begins abruptly with fever, chills, and pain at the site of involvement. The skin overlying the bone is often warm, red, and swollen. Cultures of bone or pus will generally reveal staphylococci, and bacteremia is present in about one half of the patients. Long bones are most commonly affected in children, while vertebrae are a more common site in adults. The clinical picture of vertebral osteomyelitis may be only that of malaise and vague back pain, and an elevated erythrocyte sedimentation rate may be the only laboratory abnormality. With progression, painful muscle spasms, limitation of motion of the spine, and low-grade fever will usually develop. Chronic staphylococcal osteomyelitis may occur if therapy of the acute disease is delayed or even in some instances following proper treatment. The characteristic clinical course is an indolent one in which sinuses drain purulent material for many years.

8.1.10. Septic Arthritis. Septic arthritis in all age groups is frequently caused by *S. aureus*. The typical presentation occurs with fever, pain, and chills, and the diagnosis rests on aspiration, Gram's stain, and culture of the joint fluid. Staphylococci are the most frequent cause of infected joint prostheses; *S. aureus* and coagulase-negative staphylococci are isolated with approximately equal frequency.(151) It is presumed that infections with coagulase-negative staphylococci are a result of operative contamination; however, there may be a prolonged latent period before clinical infection occurs and it is not possible to exclude hematogenous dissemination as a mechanism. The symptoms of infection may be mild, consisting only of pain in the area of the prosthesis and fever. The diagnosis must be made by culture of the joint space. Although such infections are not common, they are devastating complications because removal of the prosthesis is usually required.

8.1.11. Food Poisoning. Staphylococcal food poisoning is produced by the ingestion of food containing enterotoxin produced by *S. aureus*. The usual interval between ingestion of food containing the toxin and the onset of symptoms is relatively short, ranging from 30 min to 7 hr. Onset is usually abrupt, with severe nausea and cramps followed by vomiting, diarrhea, and prostration. Fever is usually absent and the duration of illness is generally less than 24 hr. The short incubation period, brief duration of illness, and absence of fever help distinguish staphylococcal food poisoning from other forms of food poisoning. (See Chapter 4 for more details.)

8.1.12. Parotitis. *S. aureus* has been recognized to cause severe and fatal parotitis.(152) Patients were elderly, severely debilitated from chronic disease, and dehydrated. The parotid gland was erythematous and tender. Fever and markedly elevated white cell counts were typical. Suppurative parotitis also has been reported in neonates(153) and children,(154) with *S. aureus* isolated from parotid pus.

8.1.13. Toxic Shock Syndrome. This entity[102] has been described predominately in young women who are actively menstruating, but it can also appear following all types of surgery, after childbirth, with wounds, or after influenza. The individuals develop fever, an erythematous macular rash that subsequently desquamates, falling blood pressure, and then multisystem involvement. The latter has included gastrointestinal, renal, hepatic, hematologic, central nervous, and cardiopulmonary systems. *S. aureus* has been found in the vaginal cultures of nearly all menstrual cases and has been recovered from wounds in other cases. A significantly higher proportion of menstruating women with this syndrome used vaginal tampons when compared with controls.[101] Other diseases must be excluded, such as meningococcemia, Rocky Mountain spotted fever, or bacteremia. Toxic shock syndrome has been reported to be caused by strains of coagulase-negative staphylococci that produce TSST-1.[33] In such cases, coagulase-negative staphylococci that produce this toxin were isolated from the vagina and no coagulase-positive staphylococci were removed.

8.1.14. Peritonitis. Chronic ambulatory peritoneal dialysis is an attractive alternative to hemodialysis for patients with chronic renal failure. One complication, however, is the development of peritonitis and the organism most frequently isolated from such patients is *S. epidermidis* (17–40% of episodes).[155] Because the number of organisms in the peritoneum may be small, inoculation of larger volumes of peritoneal fluid, filtration of large volumes of fluid followed by culture of the filter, and so forth have been tried to enhance the likelihood of diagnosis. Treatment of these infections is generally successful without catheter removal, either with systemic therapy or with intraperitoneal administration of antibiotics.[155]

8.1.15. Urinary Tract Infection. Although not commonly thought of as a urinary tract pathogen, coagulase-negative staphylococcus (*S. saprophyticus*) is the second-most common cause of acute urinary tract infections in young women.[156] The organism is cultured infrequently from the genitourinary tract of young women, but there is a high correlation between colonization and subsequent development of urinary tract infection.[156] Identification of the organism is facilitated in the clinical microbiology laboratory because of its resistance to novobiocin. The organism causes both upper and lower urinary tract disease, and the signs, symptoms, and examination of the urine of women infected with this organism are indistinguishable from those of patients infected with gram-negative enteric organisms. Other coagulase-negative staphylococci do not generally infect the urine, but do account for some infections in older patients who are usually hospitalized and have underlying urinary tract complications (e.g., indwelling urinary catheter, recent urinary surgery, bladder dysfunction, or obstruction).[157] These latter infections with coagulase-negative staphylococci account for less than 5% of all episodes of significant bacteriuria in hospitalized patients.

8.1.16. CSF Shunt Infection. The most common organism causing infection of CSF shunts is coagulase-negative staphylococcus.[158] In one series, close to 50% of the infections were caused by *S. epidermidis*.[158] The diagnosis often depends on the type of the shunt; patients with ventriculoatrial shunts usually have bacteremia, while those with ventriculoperitoneal shunts most often have peritonitis. The signs and symptoms may be only low-grade fever and shunt malfunction. Examination of the spinal fluid is important, but pleocytosis is usually mild. In general, shunt removal is required to cure infection.

8.1.17. Pyomyositis. *S. aureus* can infect a single muscle or less commonly several muscles in healthy young men or boys in tropical climates. Cases have been reported from temperate climates; infection with human immunodeficiency virus is a major risk factor.[159] Fever, muscle pain and swelling, and leukocytosis are common. Bacteremia can occur. Drainage and antibiotic therapy are usually effective.[160]

8.1.18. Meningitis. In published studies, approximately 1–9% of bacterial meningitis is caused by *S. aureus*.[161] Meningitis due to *S. aureus* occurs as a consequence of a neurosurgical procedure or as a hematogenous complication of an overwhelming, disseminated infection such as bacteremia or endocarditis.[162] Mortality in postoperative meningitis is 18%, but exceeds 50% in hematogenous infection.

8.2. Diagnosis

Because of the multiplicity of manifestations, there are no pathognomonic features that allow one to establish a diagnosis of staphylococcal infection immediately. There are, however, certain epidemiological, clinical, and laboratory features that help to establish the diagnosis or to raise suspicion. Outbreaks of nursery infections or postoperative surgical wound infections generally are caused by staphylococci; recovery of the causative organism and identification of an individual who may be responsible for shedding the organism should be considered promptly. Heroin addicts appear particularly prone to staphylococcal infections and this organism should be considered when such patients present with fever. Other groups of patients such as diabetics, patients with hematologic malignancies, and patients with granulocytopenia appear particularly prone to staphylococcal infections. Skin manifestations of the scalded-skin syndrome may be sufficient to establish a diagnosis of staphylococcal infection. Ultimately, however, with rare exceptions, the definitive diagnosis of staphylococcal infection depends on isolating the organism for visualizing it by Gram's stain from pus or other body tissues and fluids. Measurement of antibodies to teichoic acid[27] may be helpful in the diagnosis of severe staphylococcal infections when organisms cannot be recovered. This, however, is not helpful in rapid diagnosis, since time must be allowed for antibody formation in the host.

Epidemiological studies in the past have used phage typing of *S. aureus*. Newer studies have used molecular techniques such as restriction endonuclease analysis of plasmid DNA,[163] pulsed-field gel electrophoresis of DNA,[164] and polymerase chain reaction amplification of select DNA sequences,[165] all with promising results. In addition, there are typing systems for coagulase-negative staphylococci.[166]

9. Control and Prevention

Most *S. aureus* infections occurring in healthy persons living in the community are sporadic events that are caused by organisms carried in the nares and on the skin. Although good hygiene and proper care of minor wounds may reduce the incidence of such infections, more extensive control efforts are unlikely to be of benefit. Immunocompetent persons with recurrent staphylococcal skin infections are likely to be chronic nasal carriers, and multiple family members may be colonized. Eradication of the carrier state with agents such as oral rifampin or intranasal mupirocin may decrease the frequency of infection. Patients receiving hemodialysis or peritoneal dialysis who are nasal carriers of *S. aureus* are at increased risk for serious staphylococcal infections. Elimination of the carrier state reduces the risk of infection.[92,93]

Within hospitals and nursing homes, patients colonized or infected with *S. aureus* are the major source of the organism. Chronically colonized health care workers may occasionally be the source of epidemics of staphylococcal infection. More importantly, health care workers spread staphylococci from patient to patient by transient hand carriage. Use of gloves when handling potentially infectious materials and proper handwashing between patient contacts are essential to minimize transmission between patients. More stringent isolation procedures are indicated for patients with active lesions, extensive wounds or burns, or respiratory tract infections. Methicillin-resistant *S. aureus* (MRSA) has been particularly difficult to control in many hospitals. Laboratory-based surveillance for MRSA permits identification of colonized and infected patients[167] so that appropriate isolation measures[168] may be instituted.

Attention to details of patient care such as meticulous surgical technique, proper care of vascular catheters, and avoidance of unnecessary antibiotics can reduce the incidence of staphylococcal infection. Administration of prophylactic antibiotics immediately before surgical procedures is justified in procedures in which the risk of infection is high or the consequences of infection are severe.[169]

Pharmacological intervention to control *S. aureus* infection in hospitals has had anecdotal success but there are few well-controlled trials. Treatment of staphylococcal infection with β-lactam antibiotics or vancomycin often fails to eliminate the carrier state. Asymptomatic carriers may continue to serve as reservoirs of the organism. In the newborn nursery, bacitracin ointment has been used to abort outbreaks,[87,127] as has the application of triple dye (brilliant green, provlavin hemisulfate, and crystal violet) to the umbilicus.[170] Eradication of MRSA carriage has proved to be problematic as MRSA strains are often resistant to multiple antimicrobial agents, and often become resistant to drugs used to eradicate carriage. A variety of topical and systemic agents, including mupirocin, rifampin, trimethoprim sulfamethoxazole, ciprofloxacin, novobiocin, and minocycline, have been used alone and in combination with variable results,[168] and emergence of resistance to the agent or agents has been a recurring problem.

The optimal approach to control of infection with coagulase-negative staphylococci is uncertain. The skin is heavily colonized with these organisms and patients often acquire multiple antibiotic-resistant strains after admission to the hospital.[171] Infection results when normal defenses are disrupted by such medical interventions as surgery, implantation of foreign bodies, and cytotoxic chemotherapy. Innovative approaches to prevent the attachment of staphylococci to the implanted cuff attached to central venous catheters significantly decreases catheter-related infection.[172] Development of new bioprosthetic materials that are resistant to bacterial colonization is an area of active research.

10. Unresolved Problems

Despite many years of intensive work toward control of *S. aureus*, there are numerous areas for continued investigation. Factors related to the host or organism itself, which make for chronic as opposed to transient carriage, remain undefined. We still do not know the rates of endogenous infection among transient compared with persistent carriers outside the hospital setting. Studies of well-defined populations are needed to assess whether sex differences exist for rates of *S. aureus* disease. With new ways to treat formerly fatal diseases, we need ongoing studies to define additional populations at high risk for serious *S. aureus* disease.

Our understanding of natural and acquired immunity to *S. aureus* is sorely lacking when compared to our understanding of other bacterial pathogens. What is lacking in the "normal" child that allows for disseminated *S. aureus* infection? Conversely, in the "normal adult," why is disseminated disease so infrequent? If mortality from *S. aureus* is to be reduced in the high-risk population already defined, further means need to be identified that could either reduce exposure to *S. aureus* or immunize against this pathogen. The use of autogenous vaccines and toxoids has not been proved to be effective. Immunization will probably remain only a prospect until determination of the specific fraction(s) of the organism needed to immunize for protection is achieved. Also, as more is learned about the toxins causing toxic shock syndrome, the development of a toxoid vaccine would seem worthwhile.

Perhaps the most pressing problem is to be prepared for what may be the inevitable emergence of vancomycin resistance among the staphylococci.[173] Such resistance has already emerged for enterococci, and intense vancomycin use may be pushing us closer to this outcome.

A major problem with *S. epidermidis* is determining whether the organism, when isolated from blood, is a true pathogen or a contaminant. If one looks at all patients in hospitals, only about 5–10% of individuals having one or more blood cultures positive for coagulase-negative staphylococci have a "true" clinically significant episode of bacteremia.[174] In contrast, in patients who are immunocompromised or have malignancies with indwelling intravenous catheters, the likelihood that a blood culture growing *S. epidermidis* represents significant clinical infection is substantially higher. The availability of sensitive, specific, inexpensive, and easily performed typing systems for coagulase-negative staphylococci could be of help to the clinical microbiology laboratory, to clinicians, and to infection control personnel trying to contain the spread of nosocomial infection caused by these organisms.

A second major problem with *S. epidermidis* is determining optimal antimicrobial therapy. Many of these organisms are resistant to multiple different antibiotics, and often the clinician is left with only vancomycin to use as treatment. The precise role of the addition of rifampin is not clear, and further controlled studies are needed to determine whether addition of this agent truly improves the outcome of infection with *S. epidermidis*.

11. References

1. Kloos, W. E., and Bannerman, T. L., Update on clinical significance of coagulase-negative staphylococci, *Clin. Microbiol. Rev.* **7**:117–140 (1994).
2. Ogston, A., Report upon micro-organisms in surgical diseases, *Br. Med. J.* **1**:369–375 (1881).
3. Rosenbach, F. J., *Mikroorganismen bei den wundinfections-krankheiten des Menschen*, Bergmann, Wiesbaden, 1884.
4. Jessen, O., Rosendal, K., Bulow, P., *et al.*, Changing staphylococci and staphylococcal infections: A ten year study of bacteria and cases of bacteremia, *N. Engl. J. Med.* **281**:627–635 (1969).
5. Cluff, L. E., Reynolds, R. C., Page, D. L., *et al.*, Staphylococcal bacteremia: Demographic, clinical, and microbiological features of 185 cases, *Trans. Am. Clin. Climatol. Assoc.* **79**:205–213 (1967).
6. Nolan, C. M., and Beaty, H. N., *Staphylococcus aureus* bacteremia: Current clinical patterns, *Am. J. Med.* **60**:495–500 (1976).
7. Fidalgo, S., Vazquez, F., Mendoza, M. C., *et al.*, Bacteremia due to *Staphylococcus epidermidis*: Microbiologic, epidemiologic, clinical, and prognostic features, *Rev. Infect. Dis.* **12**:5220–5289 (1990).
8. Nahmias, A. J., Lepper, M. H., Hurst, V., *et al.*, Epidemiology and treatment of chronic staphylococcal infections in the household, *Am. J. Public Health* **52**:1828–1843 (1962).
9. McGowen, J. E., Barnes, M. W., and Finland, M., Bacteremia at Boston City Hospital: Occurrence and mortality during 12 selected years (1953–1972) with special reference to hospital-acquired cases, *J. Infect. Dis.* **132**:316–335 (1975).
10. Centers for Disease Control, *National Nosocomial Infections Study Report*, No. 78-8257, February, 1978.
11. McGregor, R. M., The work of a family doctor, *Edinburgh Med. J.* **57**:433–453 (1950).
12. Scheckler, W. E., Septicemia in a community hospital, 1970 through 1973, *J. Am. Med. Assoc.* **237**:536–538 (1977).
13. Scheckler, W. E., Nosocomial infections in a community hospital, 1972 through 1976, *Arch. Intern. Med.* **138**:1792–1794 (1978).
14. Bradley, S. F., Terpenning, M. S., Ramsey, M. A., *et al.*, Methicillin-resistant *Staphylococcus aureus*: Colonization and infection in a long-term care facility, *Ann. Intern. Med.* **115**:417–422 (1991).
15. Phair, J. P., Watanakunakorn, C., Goldberg, L., *et al.*, Ecology of staphylococci in a general medical service, *Appl. Microbiol.* **24**:967–971 (1971)
16. Rosendal, K., Bulow, P., Bentzon, M. W., *et al.*, *Staphylococcus aureus* strains isolated in Danish hospitals from January 1, 1966 to December 31, 1974, *Acta Pathol. Microbiol. Scand.* **84**:359–368 (1976).
17. Blair, J. E., and Williams, R. E. O., Phage typing of staphylococci, *Bull. WHO* **24**:771–784 (1961).
18. Nagel, J. G., Sheagren, J. N., Tuazon, C. U., *et al.*, Teichoic acids in pathogenic *Staphylococcus aureus*, *J. Clin. Microbiol.* **6**:233–237 (1977).
19. Kleeman, K. T., Bannerman, T. L., and Kloos, W.. E., Species of coagulase negative isolates at a community hospital and implications for selection of staphylococcal identification procedures, *J. Clin. Microbiol.* **31**:1318–1321 (1993).

20. Drew, W. L., Barry, A. L., O'Toole, R., *et al.*, Reliability of the Kirby–Bauer disc diffusion method for detecting methicillin-resistant strains of staphylococcus aureus, *Appl. Microbiol.* **24:**240–247 (1972).
21. Barry, A. L., and Badal, R. E., Reliability of the microdilution technique for detection of methicillin-resistant strains of *Staphylococcus aureus*, *Am. J. Clin. Pathol.* **67:**489–495 (1977).
22. Tveten, Y., Kristiansen, B. E., Ask, E., *et al.*, DNA fingerprinting of isolates of *Staphylococcus aureus* from newborns and their contacts, *J. Clin. Microbiol.* **29:**1100–1105 (1991).
23. Birnbaum, D., Kelly, M., and Chow, A. W., Epidemiologic typing systems for coagulase-negative staphylococci, *Infect. Control Hosp. Epidemiol.* **12:**319–326 (1991).
24. Koenig, M. G., Staphylococci infections–treatment and control, *Dis. Mon.*, pp. 2–36 (April 1968).
25. Martin, R. R., Daugharty, H., and White, A., Staphylococcal antibodies and hypersensitivity to teichoic acids in man, in: *Antimicrobial Agents and Chemothery—1965* (G. L. Hobby, ed.), pp. 91–96, American Society for Microbiology, Washington, DC, 1966.
26. Jackson, L. F., Sottile, M. I., Aguilar-Torres, F. G., Dee, T. H., and Rytel, M. W., Correlation of antistaphylococcal antibody titers with severity of staphylococcal disease, *Am. J. Med.* **64:**629–633 (1978).
27. Nagel, J. G., Tuazon, C. U., Cardella, T. A., and Sheagren, J. N., Teichoic acid serologic diagnosis of staphylococcal endocarditis: Use of gel diffusion and counterimunoelectrophoretic methods, *Ann. Intern. Med.* **82:**13–17 (1975).
28. Jacob, E., Durham, L. C., Falk, M. C., Williams, T. J., and Wheat, L. J., Antibody response to teichoic acid and peptidoglycan in *Staphylococcus aureus* osteomyelitis, *J. Clin. Microbiol.* **25:**122–127 (1987).
29. Tuazon, C. U., Sheagren, J. N., Choa, M. S., Marcus, D., and Curtin, J. A., *Staphylococcus aureus* bacteremia: Relationship between formation of antibodies to teichoic acid and development of metastatic abscess, *J. Infect. Dis.* **137:**57–62 (1978).
30. Breckenridge, J., and Bergdoll, M., Outbreak of food-borne gastroenteritis due to coagulase-negative enterotoxin producing staphylococcus, *N. Engl. J. Med.* **284:**541–543 (1971).
31. Bonventre, P. F., Weckbach, L., Staneck, J., Schlievert, P. M., and Thompson, M., Production of staphylococcal enterotoxin F and pyrogenic exotoxin C by *Staphylococcus aureus* isolates from toxic shock syndrome-associated sources, *Infect. Immun.* **40:** 1023–1029 (1983).
32. Robbins, R. N., Reisier, R. F., Hehl, G. L., and Bergdoll, M. S., Production of toxic shock syndrome toxin 1 by *Staphylococcus aureus* as determined by tampon disk–membrane–agar method, *J. Clin. Microbiol.* **25:**1446–1449 (1987).
33. Kahler, R. C., Boyce, J. M., Bergdoll, M. S., *et al.*, Case report: Toxic shock syndrome associated with TSST-1 producing coagulase-negative staphylococci, *Am. J. Med. Sci.* **292:**310–312 (1986).
34. Marrack, P., and Kappler, J., The staphylococcal enterotoxins and their relatives, *Science* **248:**705–711 (1990).
35. Christensen, G. D., Simpson, W. A., Bisno, A. L., *et al.*, Adherence of slime-producing strains of *Staphylococcus epidermidis* to smooth surfaces, *Infect. Immun.* **37:**318–326 (1982).
36. Sheth, N. K., Franson, T. R., and Sohnie, P. G., Influence of bacterial adherence to intravascular catheters on *in vitro* antibiotic susceptibility, *Lancet* **2:**1266–1268 (1985).
37. Gray, E. D., Peters, G., Verstegen, M., *et al.*, Effect of extracellular slime substances from *Staphylococcus epidermidis* on the human cellular immune response, *Lancet* **1:**365–367 (1984).
38. Johnson, G. M., Lee, D. A., Regelmann, W. E., *et al.*, Interference with granulocyte function by *Staphylococcus epidermidis* slime, *Infect. Immun.* **54:**13–20 (1986).
39. Peters, G., Locci, R., and Pulverer, G., Adherence and growth of coagulase-negative staphylococci on surfaces of intravenous catheters, *J. Infect. Dis.* **146:**479–482 (1982).
40. Franson, T. R., Sheth, N. U., Menon, L., *et al.*, Persistent *in vitro* survival of coagulase-negative staphylococci adherent to intravascular catheters in the absence of conventional nutrients, *J. Clin. Microbiol.* **24:**559–561 (1986).
41. Williams, R. E. O., Healthy carriage of *Staphylococcus aureus*: Its prevalence and importance, *Bacteriol. Rev.* **27:**56–71 (1963).
42. Opal, S. M., Mayer, D. K., Stenberg, M. H., *et al.*, Frequent acquisition of multiple strains of methicillin-resistant staphylococcus aureus by healthcare workers in an endemic hospital environment, *Infect. Control Hosp. Epidemiol.* **11:**479–485 (1990).
43. Bibel, D. J., Greenberg, J. H., and Cook, J. L., *Staphylococcus aureus* and the microbial ecology of atopic dermatitis, *Can. J. Microbiol.* **23:**1062–1068 (1977).
44. Fekety, F. F., The epidemiology and prevention of staphylococcal infection, *Medicine* **43:**593–613 (1964).
45. Luzar, M. A., Coles, G. A., Faller, B., *et al.*, *Staphylococcus aureus* nasal carriage and infection in patients on continuous ambulatory peritoneal dialysis, *N. Engl. J. Med.* **322:**505–509 (1990).
46. Horder, J., and Horder, E., Illness in general practice, *Practitioner* **173:**177–187 (1954).
47. Williams, R. E. O., Jevons, M. P., Shooter, R. A., *et al.*, Nasal staphylococci and sepsis in hospital patients, *Br. Med. J.* **2:**658–662 (1959).
48. Tuazon, C. U., Perez, A., Kishaba, T., *et al.*, Increased carrier rate of *Staphylococcus aureus* in insulin-injecting diabetics, *J. Am. Med. Assoc.* **231:**1272 (1975).
49. Nahmias, A. J., and Eickhoff, T. C., Staphylococcal infections in hospitals: Recent developments in epidemiologic and laboratory investigation, *N. Eng. J. Med.* **265:**74–81; 120–128; 177–182 (1961).
50. Brenner, E. R., and Bryan, C. S., Nosocomial bacteremia in perspective: A community-wide study, *Infect. Control* **2:**219–226 (1981).
51. Elhag, K. M., Mustafa, A. K., and Sethi, S. K., Septicemia in a teaching hospital in Kuwait: 1. Incidence and aetiology, *J. Infect. Dis.* **10:**17–24 (1985).
52. Finland, M., Changing patterns of susceptibility of common bacterial pathogens to antimicrobial agents, *Ann. Intern. Med.* **76:**1009–1036 (1972).
53. Klimek, J. J., Marsik, F. J., Bartlett, R. C., *et al.*, Clinical epidemiologic and bacteriologic observations of an outbreak of methicillin-resistant *Staphylococcus aureus* at a large community hospital, *Am. J. Med.* **61:**340–345 (1976).
54. Lacey, R. W., Genetic basis, epidemiology, and future significance of antibiotic resistance in *Staphylococcus aureus*, *J. Clin. Pathol.* **26:**899–913 (1973).
55. Nahmias, A. J., and Schulman, J. A., Epidemiologic aspects and control methods, in: *The Staphylococci* (J. O. Cohen, ed.), pp. 483–502, Wiley, New York, 1972.
56. Finland, M., Changing ecology of bacterial infections as related to antibacterial therapy, *J. Infect. Dis.* **122:**419–431 (1970).
57. Christensen, G. D., Bisno, A. L., Parisi, J. T., *et al.*, Nosocomial septicemia due to multiple antibiotic-resistant *Staphylococcus epidermidis*, *Ann. Intern. Med.* **96:**1–10 (1982).

58. Force, R. A., Dixon, C., Bernard, N., *et al.*, *Staphylococcus epidermidis*: An important pathogen, *Surgery* **86:**507–514 (1979).
59. Boyce, J. M., Potter-Bynoe, G., Opal, S. M., *et al.*, A common source outbreak of *Staphylococcus epidermidis* infections among patients undergoing cardiac surgery, *J. Infect. Dis.* **161:**493–499 (1990).
60. Kayser, F. H., Methicillin-resistant staphylococci 1965–1975, *Lancet* **2:**650–652 (1975).
61. Voss, A., Milatovic, D., Wallrauch-Schwarz, C., *et al.*, Methicillin-resistant *Staphylococcus aureus* in Europe, *Eur. J. Clin. Microbiol. Infect. Dis.* **13:**50–55 (1994).
62. Boyce, J. M., Increasing prevalence of methicillin-resistant *Staphylococcus aureus* in the United States, *Infect. Control Hosp. Epidemiol.* **11:**639–642 (1990).
63. Panlilio, A. L., Culver, D. H., Gaynes, R. P., *et al.*, Methicillin-resistant *Staphylococcus aureus* in United States hospitals 1975–1991, *Infect. Control Hosp. Epidemiol.* **13:**582–586 (1992).
64. Brumfitt, W., and Hamilton-Miller, J. M., The worldwide problem of methicillin-resistant *Staphylococcus aureus*, *Drugs Exp. Clin. Res.* **16:**205–214 (1990).
65. Smith, J. M. B., and Marples, M. J., A natural reservoir of penicillin-resistant strains of *Staphylococcus aureus*, *Nature* **201:**844 (1964).
66. Parker, M. T., and Lapage, S. P., Penicillinase production by *Staphylococcus aureus* strains from outbreaks of food poisoning, *J. Clin. Pathol.* **10:**313–317 (1957).
67. Plorde, J. J., and Sherris, J. C., Staphylococcal resistance to antibiotics: Origin, measurement, and epidemiology, *Ann. NY Acad. Sci.* **236:**413–434 (1974).
68. Caswell, H. T., Groschel, D., Rogers, F. B., *et al.*, A ten year study of staphylococcal disease: Surveillance, control, and prevention of hospital infections, 1956–1965, *Arch. Environ. Health* **17:**221–224 (1968).
69. Cluff, L. E., Reynolds, R. C., Page, D. L., *et al.*, Staphylococcal bacteremia: Demographic, clinical, and mirobiological features of 185 cases, *Trans. Am. Clin. Climatol. Assoc.* **79:**205–213 (1967).
70. Thornton, G. F., Fekety, F. R., and Cluff, L. E., Studies of the epidemiology of staphylococcal infection: Seasonal variation, *N. Engl. J. Med.* **271:**1333–1337 (1964).
71. Dillon, J. C., Impetigo contagiosa: Suppurative and non-suppurative complications: Clinical, bacteriologic, and epidemiologic characteristics of impetigo, *Am. J. Dis. Child.* **115:**530–541 (1968).
72. Horn, C. V., and Master, S., Pyomyositis tropicans in Uganda, *East Afr. Med. J.* **45:**463–471 (1968).
73. Levin, M. J., Gardner, P., and Woldvogel, F. A., Tropical pyomyositis: An unusual infection due to *Staphylococcus aureus*, *N. Engl. J. Med.* **284:**196–198 (1971).
74. Armstrong-Esther, C. A., and Smith, J. E., Carriage patterns of *Staphylococcus aureus* in a healthy non-hospital population of adults and children, *Ann. Hum. Biol.* **3:**221–227 (1976).
75. Hieber, J. P., Nelson, A. J., and McCracken, G. H., Acute disseminated staphylococcal disease in childhood, *Am. J. Dis. Child.* **131:**181–185 (1977).
76. Thompson, D. J., Gezon, H. M., Rodgers, K. D., *et al.*, Excess risk of staphylococcal infection and disease in newborn males, *Am. J. Epidemiol.* **84:**314–328 (1966).
77. Farrer, S., and MacLeod, C. M., Staphylococcal infections in a general hospital, *Am. J. Hyg.* **72:**38–58 (1960).
78. Fisher, A. M., Trever, R. W., Curtin, J. A., *et al.*, Staphylococcal pneumonia: A review of 21 cases in adults, *N. Engl. J. Med.* **258:**919–928 (1958).
79. Kay, C. R., Sepsis in the home, *Br. Med. J.* **1:**1048–1052 (1962).
80. Keene, W. R., Minchew, B. H., and Cluff, L. E., Studies of the epidemiology of staphylococcal infection: Clinical factors in susceptibility to staphylococcal disease, *N. Engl. J. Med.* **269:** 332–337 (1963).
81. Purser, B. N., Fatal staphylococcal infections, *Med. J. Aust.* **2:**441–443 (1958).
82. Stokes, E. J., Bradley, J. M., Thompson, R. E. M., *et al.*, Hospital staphylococci in three London teaching hospitals, *Lancet* **1:**84–88 (1972).
83. Muder, R. R., Brennen, C., and Goetz, A. M., Infection with methicillin-resistant *Staphylococcus aureus* among hospital employees, *Infect. Control Hosp. Epidemiol.* **14:**576–578 (1993).
84. Martone, W. J., Jarvis, W. R., Culver, D. H., *et al.*, Incidence and nature of endemic and epidemic nosocomial infections, in: *Hospital Infections* (J. V. Bennett and P. S. Brachman, eds.), pp. 577–596, Little and Brown, Boston, 1992.
85. Bannerjee, S. N., Emori, T. B., Culver, D. H., *et al.*, Secular trends in nosocomial primary bloodstream infection in the United States, 1980–1989, *Am. J. Med.* **3B:**86S–89S (1991).
86. Wolinsky, E., Lipsitz, P. J., Mortimer, E. A., *et al.*, Acquisition of staphylococci in newborns: Direct versus indirect transmission, *Lancet* **2:**620–622 (1960).
87. Johnson, G. M., Malachowski, N. C., Vosti, K. L., *et al.*, A sequential study of various modes of skin and umbilical care and the incidence of staphylococcal colonization and infection in the neonate, *Pediatrics* **58:**354–361 (1976).
88. Louria, D. B., Infectious complications of non-alcoholic drug abuse, *Annu. Rev. Med.* **25:**219–232 (1974).
89. Tuazon, D. U., Hill, R., and Sheagren, J. N., The microbiologic study of street heroin and injection paraphernalia, *J. Infect. Dis.* **129:**327–329 (1974).
90. Tuazon, C. U., and Sheagren, J. N., Increased rate of carriage of *aureus* among narcotic addicts, *J. Infect. Dis.* **129:**725–727 (1974).
91. Tuazon, C. U., and Sheagren, J. N., Staphylococcal endocarditis in parenteral drug abusers: Source of the organism, *Ann. Intern. Med.* **82:**788–791 (1975).
92. Yu, V. L., Goetz, A., Wagener, M., *et al.*, *Staphylococcus aureus* nasal carriage and infection in patients on hemodialysis: Efficacy of antibiotic prophylaxis, *N. Engl. J. Med.* **315:**91–96 (1986).
93. Luzar, M. A., Coles, G. A., Faller, B., *et al.*, *Staphylococcus aureus* nasal carriage and infection in patients on continuous ambulatory peritoneal dialysis, *N. Engl. J. Med.* **322:**505–509 (1990).
94. Dillon, H. C., Impetigo, in: *Communicable and Infectious Diseases* (F. H. Top and P. F. Wehrle, eds.), pp. 362–368, Mosby, St. Louis, 1976.
95. Musher, D. M., and McKenzie, S. O., Infections due to *Staphylococcus aureus*, *Medicine* **56:**383–409 (1977).
96. Finland, M., Excursions into epidemiology: Selected studies during the past four decades at Boston City Hospital, *J. Infect. Dis.* **128:**76–124 (1973).
97. Hassam, Z. A., Shaw, E. J., Shooter, R. A., *et al.*, Changes in antibiotic sensitivity in strains of *Staphylococcus aureus*, 1952–1978, *Br. Med. J.* **2:**536–537 (1978).
98. Jorgensen, J. H., Laboratory and epidemiologic experience with methicillin-resistant *Staphylococcus aureus* in the USA, *Eur. J. Clin. Microbiol.* **5:**693–696 (1986).

99. Linneman, C. C., Mason, M., Moore, P., *et al.*, Methicillin-resistant *Staphylococcus aureus*: Experience in a general hospital over four years, *Am. J. Epidemiol.* **115:**941–950 (1982).
100. Schaefler, S., Jones, D., Perry, W., *et al.*, Methicillin-resistant *Staphylococcus aureus* strains in New York City hospitals: Interhospital spread of resistant strains of type 88, *J. Clin. Microbiol.* **20:**536–538 (1984).
101. Centers for Disease Control, *Morbid. Mortal. Week. Rep.* **29:** 229–230; 297–299; 441–445; 495–496 (1980).
102. Todd, J., and Fishaut, M., Toxic shock syndrome associated with phage-group 1 staphylococci, *Lancet* **1:**1116–1118 (1978).
103. Bartlett, J. G., Onderdonk, A. B., Drude, E., *et al.*, Quantitative bacteriology of the vaginal flora, *J. Infect. Dis.* **136:**271–277 (1977).
104. Reingold, A. L., Dan, B. B., Shands, K. N., *et al.*, Toxic shock syndrome not associated with menstruation, *Lancet* **1:**1–4 (1982).
105. MacDonald, K. L., Osterhold, M. T., Hedberg, C. W., *et al.*, Toxic shock syndrome: A newly recognized complication of influenza and influenza like illness, *J. Am. Med. Assoc.* **257:**1053–1058 (1987).
106. Mest, D. R., Wong, D. H., Shimoda, K. J., *et al.*, Nasal colonization with methicillin-resistant *Staphylococcus aureus* on admission to the surgical intensive unit increases the risk of infection, *Anesth. Anal.* **78:**644–650 (1994).
107. Mulligan, M. E., Murray-Leisure, K. A., Ribner, B. S., *et al.*, Methicillin-resistant *Staphylococcus aureus*: A consensus review of the microbiology, pathogenesis, and epidemiology with implications for prevention and management, *Am. J. Med.* **94:**313–328 (1993).
108. Spers, R., Shooter, R. A., Gaya, H., Contamination of nurses' uniforms with *Staphylococcus aureus*, *Lancet* **2:**233–235 (1969).
109. Drake, C. T., Goldman, E., Nichols, R. L., Environmental air and airborne infections, *Ann. Surg.* **185:**219–223 (1977).
110. Lidwell, O. M., Brock, B., Shooter, R. A., Airborne infection in a fully air-conditioned hospital: Airborne dispersal of *Staphylococcus aureus* and its nasal acquisition by patients, *J. Hyg.* **75:**445–474 (1975).
111. Williams, R. E. O., Epidemiology of airborne staphylococcal infection, *Bacteriol. Rev.* **30:**660–672 (1966).
112. Eichenwald, H. F., Kotsevalov, O., and Fasso, L. A., The "cloud baby": An example of bacterial viral synergism, *Am. J. Dis. Child.* **100:**161–173 (1960).
113. Courter, R. D., and Galton, M. M., Animal staphylococcal infections and their public health significance, *Am. J. Public Health* **52:**1818–1827 (1962).
114. Kloos, W. E., and Smith, P. B., Staphylococci, in: *Manual of Clinical Microbiology* (E. H. Lennett, W. J. Hausler, and J. P. Truant, eds.), pp. 83–87, American Society for Microbiology, Washington, DC, 1980.
115. Kluge, R. M., Calia, F. M., McLaughlin, J. S., Sources of contamination in open heart surgery, *J. Am. Med. Assoc.* **230:**1415–1418 (1974).
116. Elek, S. D., and Conen, P. E., The virulence of *Staphylococcus pyogenes* for man: A study of the problems of wound infection, *Br. J. Exp. Pathol.* **38:**573–586 (1957).
117. Maki, D., Goldman, D., and Rhame, F., Infection control in intravenous therapy, *Ann. Intern. Med.* **79:**867–887 (1973).
118. Charnley, J., and Eftehkar, N., Post-op infection in total prosthetic replacement of hip joint, *Br. J. Surg.* **58:**641–649 (1969).
119. Dismukes, W. E., Karchmer, A. W., Budkley, M. J., *et al.*, Prosthetic valve endocarditis, *Circulation* **48:**365–377 (1973).
120. Espinosa, H., Palmer, D. L., Kisch, A. L., *et al.*, Clinical and immunologic response to bacteria isolated from tracheal secretions following tracheostomy, *J. Thorac. Cardiovasc. Surg.* **68:**432–439 (1974).
121. Cheung, A. L., and Fischetti, V. A., The role of fibrinogen in staphylococcal adherence to catheters *in vitro*, *J. Infect. Dis.* **161:**1177–1186 (1990).
122. Wellman, W. E., and Ssenft, R. A., Bacterial meningitis: Infections caused by *Staphylococcus aureus*, *Mayo Clin. Proc.* **39:** 263–269 (1964).
123. Waldvogel, F. A., Medoff, G., and Swartz, M. N., Osteomyelitis: A review of clinical features therapeutic considerations, and unusual aspects. *N. Engl. J. Med.* **282:**198–206 (1970).
124. Watanakunakorn, C., and Baird, I. M., *Staphylococcus aureus* bacteremia and endocarditis associated with a removable infected intravenous device, *Am. J. Med.* **63:**253–256 (1977).
125. Artz, C. P., and Moncrief, J. A., *The Treatment of Burns*, Saunders, Philadelphia, 1969.
126. Finland, M., Peterseon, O. L., and Strauss, E., Staphylococcal pneumonia during an epidemic of influenza, *Arch. Intern. Med.* **70:**183–205 (1942).
127. Kilton, L. J., Fossieck, B. E., Cohen, M. H., *et al.*, Bacteremia due to gram-positive cocci in patients with neoplastic disease, *Am. J. Med.* **66:**596–602 (1979).
128. Koenig, M. G., The phagocytosis of staphylococci, in: *The Staphylococci* (J. O. Cohen, ed.), pp. 365–383, Wiley, New York, 1972.
129. Quie, P. G., Infections due to neutrophil malfunction, *Medicine* **52:**411–417 (1973).
130. Montgomerie, J. Z., Kalmanson, G. M., and Guse, L. B., Renal failure and infection, *Medicine* **47:**1–32 (1968).
131. Maltman, J. R., Orr, J. H., and Hinton, N. A., The effect of desiccation on *Staphylococcus pyogenes* with special reference to implications concerning virulence, *Am. J. Hyg.* **72:**335–342 (1960).
132. Muder, R. R., Brennen, C., Wagener, M. M., *et al.*, Methicillin-resistant staphylococcal colonization and infection in a long-term care facility, *Ann. Intern. Med.* **114:**107–112 (1991).
133. Davenport, D. S., Massanari, R. M., Pfaller, M. A., *et al.*, Usefulness of a test for slime production as a marker for clinically significant infections with coagulase-negative staphylococci, *J. Infect. Dis.* **153:**332–339 (1986).
134. Ekstedt, R. D., Immunity to the staphylococci, in: *The Staphylococci* (J. O. Cohen, ed.), pp. 385–418, Wiley, New York, 1972.
135. Quie, P. G., Infections due to neutrophil malfunction, *Medicine* **52:**411–417 (1973).
136. Verhoef, J., Peterson, P. K., Kim, Y., *et al.*, Opsonic requirements for staphylococcal phagocytosis: Heterogeneity among strains, *Immunology* **33:**191–197 (1977).
137. Schopfer, K., Baerlocher, K., Price, P., *et al.*, Staphylococcal IgE antibodies, hyperglobulinemia E and *Staphylococcus aureus* infections, *N. Engl. J. Med.* **300:**835–838 (1979).
138. Schopfer, K., Douglas, S. K., and Wilkinson, B. J., Immunoglobulin E antibodies against *Staphylococcus aureus* cell walls in the sera of patients with hyperimmunoglobulin E and recurrent staphylococcal infection, *Infect. Immun.* **27:**563–568 (1980).
139. Lenhart, N., and Mudd, S., Staphylococcidal capability of rabbit peritoneal macrophages in relation to infection and elicitation: Delayed type hypersensitivity without increased resistance, *Infect. Immun.* **5:**757–762 (1971).
140. Taranta, A., Lymphocyte mitogens of staphylococcal origin, *Ann. NY Acad. Sci.* **236:**362–375 (1974).
141. Johnson, J. E., Cluff, L. E., and Goshi, K., Studies on the patho-

genesis of staphylococcal infection: The effect of repeated skin infections, *J. Exp. Med.* **113:**235–270 (1961).

142. Schaberg, D. R., Culver, D. H., and Gaynes, R. P., Major trends in the microbial etiology of nosocomial infection, *Am. J. Med.* **3B:** 72S–75S (1991).
143. Karchner, A. W., Staphylococcal endocarditis, in: *Infective Endocarditis* (D. Kaye, ed.), pp. 225–249, Raven, New York, 1992.
144. Karchmer, A. W., Archer, G. L., and Dismukes, W. E., *Staphylococcus epidermidis* prosthetic valve endocarditis: Microbiological and clinical observations as guides to therapy, *Ann. Intern. Med.* **98:**447–455 (1987).
145. Archer, G. L., *Staphylococcus epidermidis* and other coagulase-negative staphylococci, in: *Principles and Practices of Infectious Diseases*, 4th ed. (G. L. Mandell, R. G. Douglas, and J. E. Bennett, eds.), pp. 1777–1784, Churchill Livingstone, New York, 1995.
146. Melish, M., and Glasgow, L., Staphylococcal scalded skin syndrome: The expanded clinical syndrome, *J. Pediatr.* **78:**958–967 (1971).
147. Maki, D. G., Infections due to infusion therapy, in: *Hospital Infections* (J. V. Bennett and P. S. Brachman, eds.), pp. 849–898, Little and Brown, Boston, 1992.
148. Lautenschlager, S., Herzog, C., and Zimmerli, W., Course and outcome of bacteremia due to *Staphylococcus aureus*: Evaluation of different clinical case definitions, *Clin. Infect. Dis.* **16:**567–577 (1993).
149. Ponce de Leon, S., and Wenzel, R. P., Hospital-acquired bloodstream infections with *Staphylococcus epidermidis*: Review of 100 cases, *Am. J. Med.* **77:**639–644 (1984).
150. Wade, J. C., Schimpff, S. C., Newman, K. A., *et al.*, *Staphylococcus epidermidis*: An increasing cause of infection in patients with granulocytopenia, *Ann. Intern. Med.* **97:**503–508 (1982).
151. Brause, B. D., Infected orthopedic prostheses, in: *Infections Associated with Indwelling Medical Devices* (A. J. L. Bisno and F. A. Waldvogel, eds.), pp. 111–127, American Society for Microbiology, Washington, DC, 1989.
152. Petersdorf, R. G., Forsyth, B. R., and Bernanki, D., Staphylococcal parotitis, *N. Engl. J. Med.* **259:**1250–1254 (1958).
153. Leake, D., and Leake, R., Neonatal suppurative parotitis, *Pediatrics* **46:**203–207 (1970).
154. Leake, D. L., Krakowiak, F. J., and Leake, R. C., Suppurative parotitis in children, *Oral Surg.* **31:**174–179 (1971).
155. Peterson, P. K., Matzke, G., and Keane, W. F., Current concepts in the management of peritonitis in patients undergoing continuous ambulatory peritoneal dialysis, *Rev. Infect. Dis.* **9:**604–612 (1987).
156. Hovelius, B., and Mardh, P., *Staphylococcus saprophyticus* as a common cause of urinary tract infection, *Rev. Infect. Dis.* **6:**328–337 (1984).
157. Lewis, J. F., Brake, S. R., and Andereson, D. J., Urinary tract infection due to coagulase-negative staphylococcus, *Am. J. Clin. Pathol.* **77:**736–739 (1982).
158. Walters, B. C., Hoffman, H. J., and Hendrick, E. B., Cerebrospinal fluid shunt infection: Influences on initial management and subsequent outcome, *J. Neurosurg.* **60:**1014–1021 (1984).
159. Christin, L., and Sarosi, G. A., Pyomyositis in North America: Case reports and review, *Clin. Infect. Dis.* **15:**668–677 (1992).
160. Brown, J. D., and Wheeler, B., Pyomyositis: Report of 18 cases in Hawaii, *Arch. Intern. Med.* **144:**1749–1751 (1984).
161. Schlesinger, L. S., Ross, S. C., and Schaberg, D. R., *Staphylococcus aureus* meningitis: A broad-based epidemiologic study, *Medicine* **66:**148–156 (1987).
162. Jensen, A. G., Esperson, F., Skinhoj, P., *et al.*, *Staphylococcus aureus* meningitis: A review of 104 nationwide, consecutive cases, *Arch. Intern. Med.* **153:**1902–1908 (1993).
163. Pfaller, M. A., Wakefield, D. S., Hollis, R., *et al.*, The clinical microbiology laboratory as an aid in infection control: The application of molecular techniques in epidemiologic studies of methicillin-resistant *Staphylococcus aureus*, *Diagn. Microbiol. Infect. Dis.* **14:**209–217 (1991).
164. Branchini, M. L., Morthland, V. H., Tresoldi, A. T., *et al.*, Application of genomic DNA subtyping by pulsed field gel electrophoresis and restriction enzyme analysis of plasmid DNA to characterize methicillin-resistant *Staphylococcus aureus* from two nosocomial outbreaks, *Diagn. Microbiol. Infect. Dis.* **17:** 275–281 (1993).
165. van Belkum, A., Bax, R., Peerbooms, P., *et al.*, Comparison of phage-typing and DNA fingerprinting by polymerase chain reaction for discrimination of methicillin-resistant *Staphylococcus aureus* strains, *J. Clin. Microbiol.* **31:**798–803 (1993).
166. Birnbaum, D., Kelly, M., and Chow, A. W., Epidemiologic typing systems for coagulase-negative staphylococci, *Infect. Control Hosp. Epidemiol.* **12:**319–326 (1991).
167. Walsh, T. J., Vlahov, S., Hansen, S. K. L., *et al.*, Prospective microbiologic surveillance in control of nosocomial methicillin-resistant *Staphylococcus aureus*, *Infect. Control Hosp. Epidemiol.* **8:**7–14 (1987).
168. Mulligan, M. E., Murray-Leisure, K. A., Ribner, B. S., *et al.*, Methicillin-resistant *Staphylococcus aureus*: A consensus review of the microbiology, pathogenesis, and epidemiology with implications for prevention and management, *Am. J. Med.* **94:**313–328 (1993).
169. Ehrenkranz, N. J., and Meakins, J. L., Surgical infections, in: *Hospital Infections* (J. V. Bennett and P. S. Brachman, eds.), pp. 685–710, Little and Brown, Boston, 1992.
170. Glasgow, L. A., and Overall, J. C., Infections of the newborn, in: *Nelson Textbook of Pediatrics* (V. C. Vaughan, R. J. Mckay, R. E. Behrman, and W. E. Nelson, eds.), pp. 468–475, Saunders, Philadelphia, 1979.
171. Archer, G. L., and Armstrong, B. D., Alteration of staphylococcal flora in cardiac surgery patients receiving antibiotic prophylaxis, *J. Infect. Dis.* **147:**642–649 (1983).
172. Maki, D. G., *et al.*, An attachable silver-impregnated cuff for prevention of infection with central venous catheters, *Am. J. Med.* **85:**301 (1988).
173. Sanyal, D., Williams, A. J., Johnson, A. P., *et al.*, The emergence of vancomycin resistance in renal dialysis, *J. Hosp. Infect.* **24:** 167–173 (1993).
174. Sheagren, J. N., Significance of blood culture isolates of *Staphylococcus epidermidis*, *Arch. Intern. Med.* **147:**635 (1987).

12. Suggested Reading

Chambers, H. F., Methicillin resistance in staphylococci: Molecular and biochemical basis and clinical implications. *Clin. Microbiol. Rev.* **10:**781–791 (1997).

Crossley K. B., and Archer, G. L. (Eds.), *The Staphylococci in Human Disease*. Churchill-Livingstone, New York, 1997.

Rupp, M. E., and Archer, G. L., Coagulase negative staphylococci: Pathogens assoicated with medical progress, *Clin. Infect. Dis.* **19:**231–243 (1994).

CHAPTER 34

Streptococcal Infections

Barry M. Gray

1. Introduction

The streptococci are a large heterogeneous group of gram-positive spherically shaped bacteria found widely distributed in nature. They include some of the most important agents of human disease, as well as members of the normal human flora. Some streptococci have been associated mainly with disease in animals, while others have been domesticated and used for the culture of buttermilk, yogurt, and certain cheeses. Those known to cause human disease can be thought of as comprising two broad categories: First are the pyogenic streptococci, including the familiar β-hemolytic streptococci and the pneumococcus. These organisms are not generally part of the normal flora but cause acute, often severe, infections in normal hosts. Second are the more diverse enteric and oral streptococci, which are nearly always part of the normal flora and which are more frequently associated with opportunistic infections.

Measured in terms of mortality, morbidity, and economic costs, five streptococcal species are of major importance in human disease. (1) The group A streptococcus, *Streptococcus pyogenes*, produces a wide range of infections, from pharyngitis and impetigo to puerperal sepsis and erysipelas. Their nonsuppurative sequelae include acute rheumatic fever and acute glomerulonephritis. (2) The group B streptococcus, *S. agalactiae*, is currently a leading cause of sepsis in newborn infants and a frequent cause of postpartum infections in mothers. (3) The pneumococcus, *S. pneumoniae*, remains the most frequent cause of bacterial pneumonia in all age groups and is a common agent in otitis media, bacteremia, and meningitis. (4) Among the oral streptococci, *S. mutans* is important as a principal agent of dental caries. (5) *Enterococcus* is now a separate genus but will be considered an honorary streptococcus in this chapter because of its similarities to enteric streptococci. The enterococcus is part of the normal bowel flora and has been increasingly isolated as an opportunistic invader, especially in nosocomial infections (see Chapter 25). This chapter will focus mainly on group A and B streptococci and will include current information on pneumococci and other streptococci associated with human disease. Further details on *S. pneumoniae* may be found in Chapter 28.

Barry M. Gray • Division of Medical Education, Spartanburg Regional Medical Center, Spartanburg, South Carolina 29303.

2. Historical Background

Streptococcal infections were recognized by Greek physicians by the 3rd century B.C. A description of erysipelas is recorded in *Epidemicus* and attributed to Hippocrates. In the Middle Ages, scarlet fever, or "scarlatina," as it was called in Italy, was an eye-catching and notable disease. Sydenham's description in 1676 clearly differentiated this disease from measles and other rashes, but it was not until 1924 that G.F. and G.H. Dick showed conclusively that streptococci were the causative agents. Until the advent of penicillin, childbed fever, or puerperal sepsis, remained one of the most frequent causes of death among otherwise healthy young women. The classic works of Holmes, in 1858, and Semmelweis, in 1861, described the transmission of this disease and provided guidelines for effective preventive measures that are still applicable today. Rheumatic fever was first described by Wells in 1812, and Bouillaud described the association of acute rheumatism and heart disease in 1835. In 1836, Bright published his account of "renal disease accompanied with secretion of albuminous urine."[1] Osler provided detailed descriptions of "malignant scarlet fever," which remained common until the advent of antibiotics (see Fig. 1). Severe invasive disease, including necrotizing

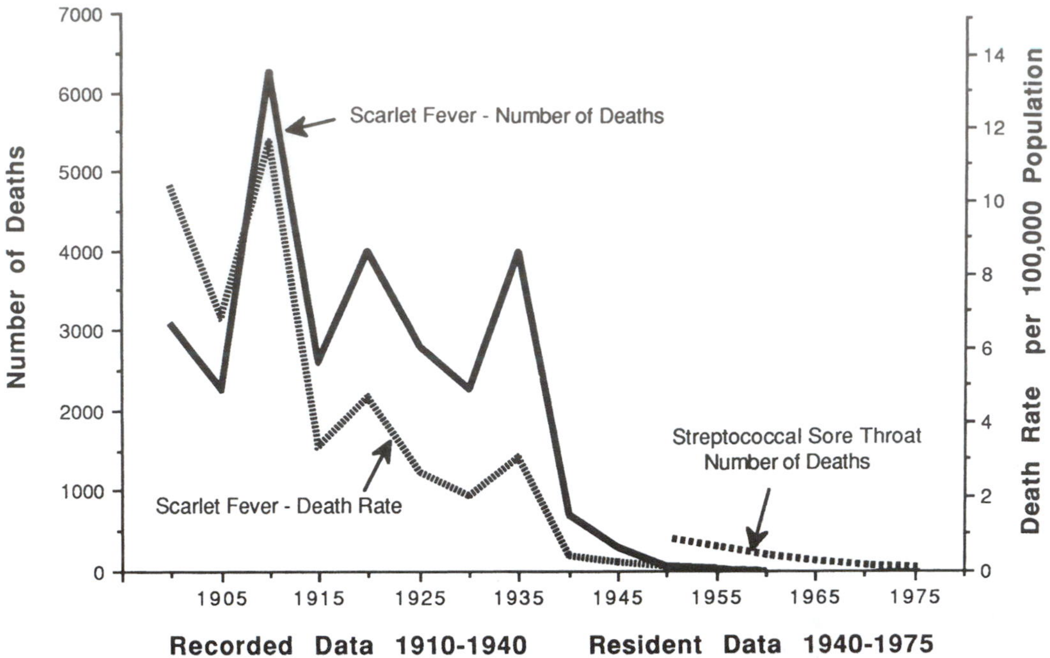

Figure 1. The number of deaths (left-hand scale) from scarlet fever (1900–1960) and from all streptococcal sore throat (1950–1975), with death rates (right-hand scale) per 100,000 population in the United States. Appropriate comparability ratios were applied beginning in 1940, and recorded data compiled according to the geographic locale where the event occurred without regard to residence (1900–1940); resident data were compiled according to the usual place of residence without regard to locale where the event occurred (1940–1975). The population used for determining rates was that of the registration area. Data were not available for streptococcal sore throat for 1900–1950. The number of states reporting for 1900–1905 was 10, gradually increasing to 48 in 1935 and to 50 states in 1960. After 1975, reporting was optional, and no accurate data are available. Sources of data: US Bureau of the Census, *Historical Statistics of the United States: Colonial Times to 1970*, Bicentennial ed., Part I, p. 77, 1975; National Office of Vital Statistics, *Vital Statistics Reports*, Vol. 37, No. 9 (1920–1950); Centers for Disease Control, *Morbidity and Mortality Weekly Report*, Annual Supplement, 1960 and 1970. Figure redrawn from Quinn.[1]

fasciitis, "hemolytic streptococcus gangrene," and myositis, was much less common and did not appear in the medical literature until the second and third decades of this century. During the mid-1970s to 1980s, cases of acute rheumatic fever and acute glomerulonephritis became exceedingly rare (see Fig. 2), and streptococcal disease seemed only an inconvenience. By the late 1980s, however, rheumatic fever made a dramatic reappearance, along with an increase in severe invasive infections and the emergence of a streptococcal toxic shock syndrome.[2–4] Group A streptococci made the headline in the popular press as "killer strep," the "flesh-eating bacteria."

In the late 19th century, many investigators contributed to the understanding of streptococci and their relation to human disease. By the 1880s many species had been given names such as *S. epidemicus*, *S. erysipelatus*, *S. scarlatinae*, and *S. rheumaticus*, which reflected different manifestations of streptococcal infection. The name *S. pyogenes* dates from this period but is probably of less descriptive value than the term "*S. haemolyticus*," which was commonly used through the early part of this century. The formal classification of streptococci began when blood agar came into use and the hemolytic properties of various organisms were noted. In 1919, Brown used the term "beta" to describe streptococci that produced a 2- to 4-mm zone of clear hemolysis around colonies grown on blood agar. "Alpha" streptococci were those producing incomplete, greenish hemolysis. Most of the isolates from severe human disease were β-hemolytic. It was not until 1928, when Lancefield introduced methods of serotyping streptococci based on immunologic reactions with cellular components, that groups and types within groups could be clearly distinguished. The group antigens were eventually shown to be specific cell wall carbohydrates. The group A streptococci were further differentiated by the M and T protein antigens. The β-hemolytic streptococci from most human infections proved to be those of group A. Armed with these new epidemiological tools, Lancefield and Hare[5] investigated cases of puerperal sepsis

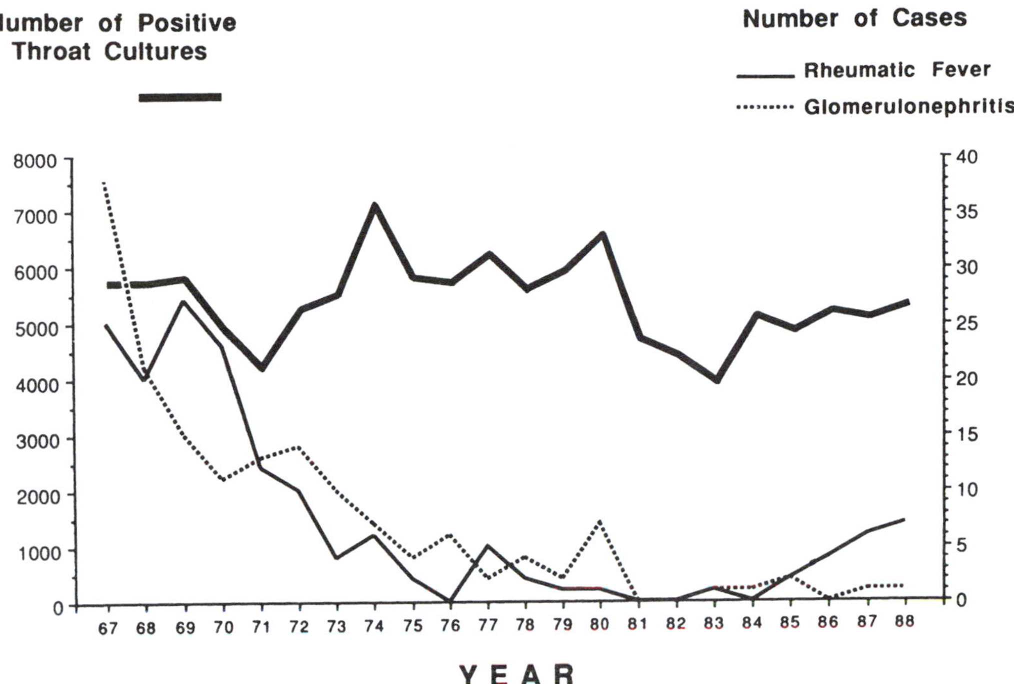

Figure 2. The number of positive throat cultures (left-hand scale and number of confirmed cases of rheumatic fever and acute glomerulonephritis (right-hand scale) seen in private pediatirc practices participating in streptococcal surveillance studies in Rochester, New York, 1967–1988. The data were kindly provided by Caroline Breese Hall, University of Rochester.

at Queen Charlotte's Hospital in London, beginning in the early 1930s. Of 46 cases of postpartum sepsis, all but one isolate was group A, and the exception was identified as the prototype of a new serological group, designated group G. A year earlier, Hare and Colebrook observed that hemolytic streptococci resembling those associated with sepsis were never found in vaginal cultures of healthy women, but that some women carried streptococci that resembled those isolated in bovine mastitis. The latter organisms proved to be members of streptococcus group B.[(5)]

By the late 1930s, the group B streptococci were recognized as important, if occasional, pathogens causing postpartum sepsis, amnionitis, endocarditis, and septic abortion. The advent of antibiotics, along with better methods for preventing nosocomial spread, resulted in a dramatic decline in streptococcal infections on obstetrical services. At Queen Charlotte's Hospital there were very few maternal deaths due to either group A or group B streptococci from 1940 through the mid-1960s. In this same period there were few cases of neonatal sepsis or meningitis attributed to streptococci of any kind in large series published in the pediatric literature. It appears unlikely that group B streptococci went simply unrecognized as perinatal pathogens for over 20 years. Rather, there seems to have been a real increase in group B disease, beginning in the United States and Europe during the 1960s. By the mid-1970s, numerous reports of group B disease appeared in the literature, and the group B streptococcus was said to have come of age.[(6,7)]

The pneumococcus has an interesting and important history, beginning with its association with pneumonia and later with developments in immunization and serum therapy (see Chapter 28). Studies of the pneumococcus have been at the center of major developments in immunology, antibiotics, and, with the discovery of DNA, genetics and molecular biology.[(8,9)]

The history of *S. mutans* began in 1924, when Clark first isolated the organism from human dental caries. It was another four decades, however, before Keyes established the "infectious and transmissible nature" of dental caries in animal models and later in human subjects.[(10,11)] Since dental caries are chronic rather than acute infections and are not directly life-threatening, the global significance of *S. mutans* has only recently been appreciated. Dental caries, a complex but diagnosable and treatable infection, is perhaps the most common bacterial infection in humans.

The enterococci, as they were called by Thiercelin in 1899, were noted as a major aerobic component of feces. Extremely hardy, they grow in bile, at high or low temperatures, in salt, and at high pH. Although for many years grouped with the streptococci because of morphological similarities, they were transferred to the genus *Enterococcus* in 1984 on the basis of genetic studies. These and several new *Enterococcus* species were clearly distinct from the "nonenterococcal" group D streptococci, *S. bovis* and *S. equinus*. Enterococci have long been known as an occasional cause of opportunistic infections, but in the early 1970s, they began to appear with increasing frequency in reports of urinary tract infection, bacteremia, and pelvic, wound, and surgical infections. They are among the most common organisms causing nosocomial infections and are difficult to eradicate because of resistance to many antibiotics.[12,13]

3. Methodology

3.1. Sources of Mortality Data

There are few reliable sources of mortality data for any of the streptococcal diseases. Cause-of-death coding classifications have been revised about every decade, usually without sufficient details regarding a particular etiologic agent. For example, patients may die of heart failure without rheumatic heart disease being specified; puerperal sepsis may be due to group A or group B streptococci as well as other organisms; and pneumococcal pneumonia deaths are frequently counted with those attributed to influenza virus.

3.2. Sources of Morbidity Data

There are likewise few accurate data on morbidity from streptococcal infections. Since 1971, streptococcal sore throat, scarlet fever, and acute rheumatic fever have been reported only optionally to the Centers for Disease Control and Prevention (CDC), which now relies primarily on selected hospital and population surveys. Monitoring of recent outbreaks of rheumatic fever by the CDC has been incomplete, and no mechanism for systematic nationwide reporting has been adopted. The best longitudinal incidence data on rheumatic fever are from Denmark, where meticulous records have been kept for over a 100 years.[14] The CDC began a passive nationwide surveillance for invasive group A streptococcal infections in 1993 and expanded to a population-based active surveillance in 1994. Group B streptococcal disease is also reported on an optional basis, and no reliable data are available. However, age- and race-adjusted projections of group B streptococcal disease incidence have been made from data supplied by four large health departments and medical centers in different areas of the United States.[15] Several state health departments have instituted reporting of drug-resistant pneumococci. The CDC and the Council of State and Territorial Epidemiologists (CSTE) have recently agreed to make drug-resistant pneumococci notifiable on a nationwide basis, but current data from the CDC are derived from hospital-based surveillance programs. Vancomycin resistance in enterococci is monitored from reports of hospitals participating in the National Nosocomial Infections Surveillance System. Another source of data for these and other diseases is the 1992 report on "emerging infections" by the Institute of Medicine.[16]

3.3. Surveys

A considerable number of surveys have been published on diseases caused by various streptococcal species. The most informative have been prospective epidemiological studies, certain family studies, and surveys of defined populations. These will be reviewed in the description of epidemiological features of specific diseases in Section 5.1.

3.4. Laboratory Diagnosis

The major streptococcal species associated with human disease are listed in Tables 1 and 2, along with selected biological and clinical features. Our grouping of species is more for convenience than for taxonomic purposes, and various bacteriology textbooks will have different schemes, as well as more detailed information on laboratory methods. The laboratory procedures and the particular approach to identification will of course depend on whether isolation is for clinical or research purposes and the degree of specificity required.

3.4.1. Isolation and Identification.

3.4.1a. Media and Growth Conditions. Most streptococci grow poorly on ordinary nutrient media but grow quite well on media enriched with blood, brain, or heart infusion, serum, or glucose. Todd–Hewitt broth is an enriched buffered medium that has become a standard liquid medium for most streptococci. In the United States, most laboratories use 5% sheep blood agar, whereas in Britain horse blood is generally used. Both give good hemolysis, although with sheep blood it may be necessary to "stab" the agar in the area of inoculation to ensure

Table 1. The Major Species of Pyogenic Streptococci Causing Disease in Humans

	Species designation	Lancefield group	Hemolysis	Presumptive identification	Definitive identification	Ecological niche	Normal flora	Association with disease
Group A. streptococci	*S. pyogenes*	A	β	Bacitracin sensitivity, latex agglutination and other antigen detection methods	M proteins T proteins Opacity factor Molecular methods	Oropharynx	No (modest carrier rates)	Pharyngitis, impetigo, erysipelas, bacteremia
Group B streptococci	*S. agalactiae*	B	β	CAMP test positive	Capsular polysaccharides c-protein DNA fingerprint	Lower bowel, genital tract	High carrier rate in normal population	Neonatal sepsis, meningitis, postpartum infections, endocarditis, cellulitis
Group C streptococci	*S. equisimilis* *S. zooepidemicus* *S. equi*	C C C	β β β	"Not A or B" Latex agglutination	DNA fingerprint Bacteriophage	(Swine, humans) (Horses, cattle, other animals)	Occasional No No	Pharyngitis, bacteremia, wound infections, cellulitis, often veterinary-related
Group G streptococci	"Large colony" group G	G	β	"Not A or B" Latex agglutination	Some with M-12 protein	Pharynx, bowel	Occasional	Pharyngitis, cellulitis, bacteremia
Pneumococci	*S. pneumoniae*	None (has pneumococcal C-polysaccharide)	α	Optochin sensitive, bile soluble	Capsular polysaccharides Surface protein Molecular methods	Nasopharynx	High carrier rate in normal population	Lobar pneumonia, otitis media, bacteremia meningitis

Table 2. The Major Species of Oral and Enteric Streptococci and Enterococci Causing Disease in Humans

	Species name	Lancefield group	Hemolysis	Presumptive identification	Definitive identification	Ecological niche	Normal flora	Association with disease
Dental/oral and "Viridans" streptococci	*S. mutans*	None, E	None	—	Cell wall carbohydrate DNA hybridization	Tooth surface, dental plaque	Yes	Dental caries, endocarditis
	S. sanguis	None, H	α, β, none	—	Biochemical	Dental plaque	Yes	Endocarditis, brain abscesses, bacteremia
	S. mitis	None, O, K, M	α, β, none	—	Biochemical	Oral cavity	Yes	
	S. salivarius	None, K	None	—	Biochemical	Tongue	Yes	Bacteremia
	S. sobrinus		α, none	—	Biochemical	Oral cavity	Yes	Bacteremia
	S. oralis		α, none	—	Biochemical	Oral cavity	Yes	Bacteremia
"Milleri" group	Minute colony	A, C, F, G, none	α, β, none	—	Biochemical	Oral cavity	Yes	Endocarditis, dental abscesses, brain abscesses, liver abscesses
	S. anginosis	C	β	—	Biochemical	Oral cavity	Yes	
	S. costellatus			—	Biochemical	Oral cavity	Yes	
	S. intermedius			—	Biochemical	Oral cavity	Yes	
Nutritionally deficient streptococci	*S. mitis* (mutant)	Various	α, β, none	Require pyridoxal	Biochemical	Oral cavity	Yes	Endocarditis
	S. sanguis (mutant)	Various	α, β, none	Require pyridoxal	Biochemical	Oral cavity	Yes	Endocarditis
	S. salivarius (mutant)	Various	α, none	Require pyridoxal	Biochemical	Oral cavity	Yes	Endocarditis
Microaerophilic and anaerobic streptococci	*Peptostrepococcus* (five species)	Some D	None	—	Biochemical	Oral cavity, bowel	Yes	Abscesses, otitis media, pelvic inflammatory disease
Nonenterococcal group D	*S. bovis*	D	α	—	Biochemical	Bowel	Yes	Bacteremia, endocarditis, opportunistic infections
	S. equinus	D	α	—	Biochemical	Bowel	Yes	
Enterococci (>15 species)	*E. faecalis*	D	none, β	Growth in bile–esculin 6.5% NaCl	Biochemical	Bowel	Yes	Urinary tract and surgical infections, bacteremia, endocarditis, wounds, opportunistic infections
	E. faecium	D	α, β, none		Biochemical	Bowel	Yes	

subsurface growth for the action of oxygen-sensitive hemolysins. While most streptococci grow well in a normal atmosphere, some species, particularly the "*S. milleri*" group and the peptostreptococci, do not show good growth or hemolysis without a reduced oxygen atmosphere. Pneumococci prefer to grow in 5% CO_2 or in a candle jar. Most streptococci grow best at 35 to 37°C, although the enterococci will also grow at 10 and at 45°C.

Routine isolation of group A streptococci from throat cultures is adequately accomplished using plain sheep blood agar incubated in air at 37°C; cultures read as negative at 18–24 hr should be incubated an additional 24 hr for optimal sensitivity. Alternatively, throat cultures may be incubated anaerobically, although this may increase the recovery of non-group-A β-hemolytic streptococci. Selective media containing trimethoprim–sulfamethoxazole have also been evaluated and recommended for use in throat cultures.[17]

Many laboratories now process vaginal or anorectal cultures to determine colonization by group B streptococci in pregnant women. A selective broth medium is generally required to minimize overgrowth of other organisms. We currently use Todd–Hewitt broth containing nalidixic acid, polymyxin, and crystal violet.[18] A similar medium is available with colistin plus nalidixic acid but without crystal violet ("Lim" broth). A broth containing gentamicin plus nalidixic acid has also been widely used, although we found that some group B strains were inhibited by the gentamicin.[17,18] A fairly satisfactory commercial solid medium is Columbia CNA agar, which contains colistin and nalidixic acid. For isolation of pneumococci from nasopharyngeal carriers, a selective medium is also essential; we have favored blood agar containing 4 mg/liter of gentamicin sulfate.[19] The enterococci grow on nearly all conventional media, including EMB (eosin–methylene blue) used for gram-negative enteric organisms.

3.4.1b. Colony Morphology and Hemolysis. The first step in identifying a streptococcus is examining colonies grown on blood agar for characteristic morphology and hemolysis. A throat culture, for example, will have much extraneous growth, but the bacteriologist will be looking for group A streptococci that have small (0.5–1 mm), opaque white colonies surrounded by a wide zone of clear β-hemolysis. Stabs made into the medium in the area of inoculation will usually clear first because the streptolysin O is more active in the absence of air. Streptolysin S, which is active on the surface, does not always produce complete hemolysis in young cultures. Occasional strains produce large (>1 mm) mucoid colonies, due to the expression of hyaluronic acid capsules (especially M type 18).

Groups A, C, and G streptococci are similar in appearance, but group B streptococci are usually larger, more mucoid, and have a narrower zone of hemolysis that is often less distinct. About 1% of wild group B strains are nonhemolytic, but this depends to some degree on the media used. Streptococci of the "milleri" group have very tiny colonies but usually have comparatively large zones of β-hemolysis; these include group F and the "minute colony" group A, C, and G streptococci. The α-hemolytic streptococci are quite heterogeneous and are difficult to distinguish even to the practiced eye. The pneumococci, however, are usually smooth and glossy with central craters formed by autolysis as the colonies grow beyond 18–24 hr. Colonies of type 3 pneumococci are often very large and have a distinctive mucoid appearance. Enterococci have rather buttery colonies, compared to most of the streptococci, and usually produce no hemolysis or may be β-hemolytic on horse blood and α-hemolytic on sheep blood.

3.4.1c. Presumptive Identification. For practical purposes, group A streptococci can be identified presumptively by the bacitracin sensitivity test of Maxted in which a 0.04-unit bacitracin (TAXO) disk is placed on a pure subculture of a β-hemolytic streptococcus. Group A streptococci are extremely sensitive and uniformly show a zone of inhibition, whereas only 5–10% of group C or G strains may give a false-positive result. The simplest of several tests for group B streptococci is the CAMP test (described by Christie, Atkins, and Munch-Petersen in 1944). The test is performed by inoculating a streak of the streptococcus perpendicular to a streak of *Staphylococcus aureus* on a sheep blood agar plate; an arrowhead-shaped area of complete hemolysis indicates the presence of CAMP factor, which enhances the effect of the staphylococcal β lysin. Streptococci reported simply as "not A or B" on the basis of presumptive tests usually prove to be group C or G. Pneumococci are distinguished from other α-hemolytic streptococci by sensitivity to optochin in a manner similar to that of the bacitracin test for group A streptococci. In addition, the bile solubility test of Neufeld remains useful for separating pneumococci from the occasional optochin-sensitive *viridans* streptococcus. Enterococci are identified by growth on bile–esculin media and in 6.5% NaCl. Further identification of these and the viridans streptococci is done with various panels of biochemical tests.

3.4.1d. Rapid Diagnostic Tests. A number of direct antigen detection tests are currently in use for diagnosis of streptococcal pharyngitis. Most of these methods are based on the extraction of cell wall antigens from throat swabs and their detection by agglutination of latex or other particles coated with antibody against the group A polysaccharide. These "rapid strep tests" yield results in 10 to 60 min and permit the physician to appropriately treat streptococcal pharyngitis without the delay of conventional cultures. In general, the specificity of these tests is excellent: 90–95%. The sensitivity, however, varies from 60 to 85%. Those patients with strong positive cultures are nearly always detected, but up to half of those with "1+" cultures (one to ten colonies per plate) may go undetected. The clinical significance of this shortcoming is not entirely clear. The latter group may include some patients who are "carriers" and not at risk in terms of the acute infection or sequelae. However, 35–45% of those with false-negative rapid tests (but 1+ positive cultures) have evidence of true infection as determined by a rise in streptococcal antibody titers. Left untreated, some of these patients could be at risk for developing acute rheumatic fever. For this reason it is recommended that a throat culture be done when the rapid test is negative. Several newer methods, including an optical immunoassay and gene probe tests, are claimed to have sufficiently good sensitivity to obviate the "back-up" throat culture, but experts remain cautious, pending further evaluation of these products.[20]

Two problems continue to limit the usefulness of the antigen detection tests. One is that they detect only group A streptococci, whereas acute pharyngitis is sometimes caused by group C or G streptococci, which may also require antibiotic therapy. The other is cost: A blood agar plate currently costs about $0.20, whereas latex agglutination tests cost about $2.00 each, and an optical immunoassay costs about $5.00. However, federal regulations recently adopted in the Clinical Laboratory Improvement Act (CLIA) classify the processing of throat cultures as a "complex" procedure. Many office laboratories face difficulties in complying with the new requirements for throat cultures but may nevertheless perform antigen detection as a "simple" laboratory test.

Similar particle agglutination methodologies have been employed for detecting group B streptococcal antigens in cerebrospinal fluid (CSF) or urine. They are quite reliable in detecting antigen in CSF from infants infected with group B streptococci. Testing of urine samples has been discouraged because the urine sample may be positive as the result of skin or genitourinary contamination, or possibly from intestinal absorption and urinary excretion of antigen.[21] So far, no rapid tests have proved sensitive enough to determine maternal colonization directly from vaginal swabs, but detection of "heavy" colonization by some tests may be sufficient to identify most of the patients at risk for invasive disease.[22]

Antigen tests for pneumococcal polysaccharide antigens vary considerably in their reliability. This is because reagents are usually made by coating the latex particles with antibodies of multiple capsular serotypes, thus diluting the sensitivity to any one antigen; the reagents may detect some serotypes better than others and some not at all. Gene probe assays, noted below, may eventually provide adequately sensitive and reliable direct detection.

3.4.1e. Definitive Identification. Streptococci are classified into Lancefield groups on the basis of their cell wall carbohydrate antigens. The classical methods of grouping employ an extraction step, usually hot acid (Lancefield method) or nitrous acid, followed by detection of liberated antigens with specific rabbit antisera. More recently, latex and similar particle agglutination kits make it possible for any laboratory to provide rapid and accurate group identification without having to maintain serological supplies.

Typing of group A streptococci is done by precipitation of M and T proteins with specific antisera. The T proteins are trypsin-resistant antigens that are useful as markers for certain M types and for strains having no detectable M protein. T typing is done by agglutination after trypsinization of the streptococcal cells. M typing, done by precipitation after an antigen extraction step, is then done on the basis of T-typing results. For example, T1 strains are invariably M1, and T3 strains are M3, whereas T8/25/Imp.19 strains may be M2, 55, or 57. Over 80 M types have been described, but up to a quarter of isolates are not typable with either T or M antisera. Because group A typing is not readily available, the opacity factor neutralization test described by Fraser and Maxted in 1979 has recently been reevaluated and modified by Johnson and Kaplan.[23] This test is relatively simple and correlates well with M typing. The epidemiological importance of group A typing is obvious when it is noted that certain M types are commonly associated with specific kinds of infection or sequelae. Table 3 lists the most common M types associated with uncomplicated pharyngitis, severe systemic infections, and rheumatic fever,[24] and with acute glomerulonephritis.[25] It is of particular interest that M1 strains are common in both uncomplicated pharyngitis and in severe invasive disease, but epidemiological evidence suggests that the serious disease is caused by especially virulent strains or clones of type M1, and that virulence is not always associated as a general property of that serotype.[24] Molecular methods, described below, have now begun to confirm such observations and shed light on the evolution of virulent clones and the virulence genes themselves.[26–28]

The typing of group B streptococci is based on the detection of capsular polysaccharides, as outlined in Table 4.

Table 3. Group A Streptococcal M Protein Serotypes Commonly Associated with Uncomplicated Pharyngitis, Scarlet Fever, Severe Systemic Infections, Acute Rheumatic Fever, and Acute Glomerulonephritis, Listed in Approximate Order of Frequency[a]

Uncomplicated pharyngitis	Scarlet fever	Severe systemic infections	Acute rheumatic fever	Acute glomerulonephritis
1	3	1	3	2
12	4	3	1	1
4	1	18	18	49
2	22	12	5	12
28	6	22	4	4
3	2	5	6	55

[a]Data from Johnson *et al.*,[24] Coleman *et al.*,[186] and Dillon *et al.*[25] Severe infections included streptococcal toxic shock, septicemia, pnenumonia or empyema, joint, and deep soft tissue infections. Note that strains associated with acute glomerulonephritis may be isolated from throat (Ml and M12) or skin sites (M55) or either throat or skin (M4, M49).

There are four major types: Ia, Ib, II, and III, and three newly recognized types: IV, V, and VI (formerly known as MJ19). In her original description of the type polysaccharides, Lancefield noted that, finding no antigens analogous to the M proteins of group A streptococci, she was looking for capsular materials like those found in the capsules of pneumococci. The group B indeed proved to have capsular polysaccharides and are all similar in structure, composed of glucose, galactose, and *N*-acetylglucosamine. Unlike pneumococci, they all have side chains containing terminal sialic acid residues that are major antigenic determinants.[29] The newly designated type VI differs from the others by the absence of *N*-acetylglucosamine in the capsular polysaccharide.[30] Type Ib strains and some type II and type III strains also carry the c protein, formerly called the "Ibc protein," a complex antigen, part of which is capable of binding secretory IgA. The R antigen occurs on some type II and III strains, but is not seen frequently among human isolates. The X antigen is found almost exclusively in veterinary strains, particularly those from bovine mastitis. To distinguish among strains of the same capsular type, a bacteriophage typing scheme has been employed in the past, but is being supplanted by multilocus enzyme electrophoresis and molecular methods.

Table 4. Type-Specific Antigens of Group B Streptococci[a]

Capsular polysaccharides	Ia	ib	II	III	IV	V	VI
c protein	–	+	(+)	(+)	?	?	?

[a]Serological classification is determined according to the capsular polysaccharide. The c protein was formerly called the "Ibc protein" becuase of its association with Ib and Ic strains. Ib strains (which always have this protein) are now designated Ib/c, and Ic strains (which have the Ia capsule) are designated Ia/c. About one third of type II strains have the c protein and are noted as II/c; the frequency of c protein in types IV, V, and VI is not well described. The R antigen occurs occasionally in type II and III strains, but like the X antigen is more common in veterinary than in human isolates.

The pneumococci are divided into serological types, according to capsular polysaccharides. The Danish typing system currently in use recognizes 48 types, many of which have several closely related subtypes that correspond to individual types of the American system. The subtypes are denoted by the Arabic type number plus a letter to indicate the subtype. For example, types 1–5 each contain only one distinct type; type 6 (usually called "group" 6) includes type 6A (America type 6) and type 6B (American type 26); type 9 includes four subtypes, of which only type 9N (American type 9) and 9V (American type 68) are at all common among clinical isolates. Knowledge of the distribution of types in human infections led directly to the selection of the most important types in the formulation of pneumococcal vaccines.[31] The pneumococci can be further delineated within capsular types by typing surface protein antigens that occur on essentially all clinically important isolates.[32] Pneumococcal surface protein (PspA) is highly variable, but several variants of the protein are quite common and are currently under investigation as potential vaccines.

Group D and *viridans* streptococci are usually speciated by their pattern of biochemical reactions.[17] Various test kits and automated equipment are in general use in most clinical laboratories and give basically similar results. However, these products do not always conform to the latest taxonomic changes. Two major identification schemes are currently in use, one from Great Britain and the other from the CDC in the United States. They differ mainly in the classification of group F and the milleri group. "*S. milleri*" currently consists of three species: *S. anginosis*, *S. constellatus*, and *S. intermedius*, which differ in their production of β-glucosidase, hyaluronidase, and several other glycosidases. Nutritionally deficient streptococci causing endocarditis are thought to be mostly mutant subspecies of *S. mitis* that require pyridoxal for growth.(33) *S. mutans* includes eight serological types based on cell wall carbohydrates, but epidemiological studies now favor molecular methods for distinguishing strains among types.(10)

Most enterococci share a glycerol teichoic acid antigen with the group D streptococci.(34) However, they are usually characterized by their ability to grow in broth containing 6.5% NaCl and hydrolyze eschulin in the presence of 40% bile salts (bile–esculin medium). Strains are divided into 4 major groups and 15 main species using a panel of biochemical tests. A variety of methods have been tried with only modest success for subdividing the major human pathogens, *E. faecalis* and *E. faecium*, but molecular methods are beginning to prove useful for infection control and epidemiologic purposes.

3.4.1f. New Methods of Identification. Molecular methods have now been applied to various streptococcal species for direct detection, identification, epidemiology, and studies of molecular evolution. Although it is unlikely that the polymerase chain reaction (PCR) will replace the blood agar plate anytime soon, hybridization with labeled gene probes have been successfully employed for detection of group A streptococci from throat swabs of patients with pharyngitis.(35) These methods are still cumbersome, time-consuming, and more suited to batch processing, but future developments may make them more suitable clinical use. Detection of pneumococcal DNA in materials such as blood cultures and middle-ear fluids has also been demonstrated by PCR, using primers derived from known nucleotide sequences from genes coding for autolysin(36) and pneumolysin.(37)

The molecular equivalent of serotyping of group A streptococci has been demonstrated for 16 common M protein types by PCR amplification followed by hybridization with labeled probes whose DNA sequences are complementary with the N-terminal type-specific portion of the M protein gene.(38) Similar methods could supplement or perhaps eventually replace conventional serotyping for epidemiological purposes. However, the multiplicity of M protein genes both within and among the >80 serotypes presents many of logistical difficulties of serotyping as well as some problems peculiar to the new technology itself. Many strains have a number of "M proteinlike genes": some may look like M protein genes but code for proteins with lectinlike functions, such as binding of immunoglobulins or fibronectin, and some appear to be extra copies or even defective genes. The amplification and/or detection of these genes may depend greatly on the selection of primers and the conditions of the assay.

Several other molecular approaches differentiate among streptococcal strains or types but are not necessarily intended to correlate with given M or T typing systems. "Ribotyping" is based on the pattern of amplified ribosomal RNA in agarose gel electrophoresis. Depending on the primers utilized, species-specific and sometimes strain-specific identification may be possible. Because ribosomal RNA nucleotide sequences are highly conserved, few differences may be seen even between strains of differing M types.(39,40) Restriction endonuclease analysis (REA) is a kind of DNA "fingerprinting" using endonucleases such as *Eco*RI or *Hin*dIII that cut chromosomal DNA into small fragments suitable for separation with conventional agarose gel electrophoresis.(39,41) This method may be a helpful supplement to serotyping, especially for nontypable strains, but it is limited by technical problems of resolution and comparison of the DNA fragments of different strains, making it often too general for epidemiological applications. An extension of this method, usually called restriction fragment length polymorphism (RFLP), relies on endonucleases, such as *Sma*I or *Sfi*I, that cut DNA at relatively fewer sites, producing longer, more distinctively sized fragments.(26) These larger (20–500 kb) fragments must be resolve using pulse field gel electrophoresis (PFGE), because of the peculiar dynamics of migration of large pieces of DNA through agarose gels. Yet another approach uses PCR amplification of sections of chromosomal DNA by "arbitrary" or "random" primers: These are termed "arbitrarily primed" PCR (AP-PCR) or "random amplified polymorphic DNA" (RAPD).(42) Various methods similar to those just described have been employed for epidemiological studies of group B,(43,44) and group G(45) streptococci, pneumococci,(46,47) and enterococci.(48)

Molecular methods have also focused on genes of particular interest because of their function in disease, antibiotic susceptibility, or distribution in nature. Two highly pathogenic clones of group A streptococcus were tracked and delineated by the allelic variants of their scarlet fever toxin (SPE-A), serotyping, and multilocus enzyme electrophoresis (MLEE).(49) The DNA fingerprints of penicillin-binding proteins, along with capsular and surface protein typing and MLEE, have been used to study the epidemiology and clonality of antibiotic-resistant pneumococci.(50)

Molecular analysis is now beginning to provide clues to the regulation of genes associated with virulence, such as those needed for M protein expression(27) and synthesis of hyaluronic acid capsulars.(51) A broader evolutionary study of the "virulence gene cluster" of group A streptococci has revealed a relatively small number of distinct patterns of the mutigene family containing most of the important genes thought to be associated with virulence.[28]

3.4.2. Serological and Immunologic Diagnostic Methods. Antibody tests have been developed as clinical and epidemiological tools in the study of group A, group B, and pneumococcal infections. In general, antibodies are markers of past experience with the organisms and do not indicate when an infection took place. For this reason they are most useful when acute and convalescent antibody levels are compared in relation to an episode of presumed infection.

Assays for the group A streptococcus are based on the development of antibodies either to cellular antigens or to extracellular enzymes. These are listed in Table 5 and further described in Section 4. Tests for antibody to M proteins, which confer immunity, and to the group A carbohydrate have been used primarily for research purposes. Assays used clinically for confirmation of recent infections have been reviewed by Ayoub.[52] The antistreptolysin O (ASO) is the most reliable and is widely available. It is of no immediate value in the diagnosis of acute streptococcal pharyngitis, and it should not be expected to differentiate carriage from infection. Nevertheless, about 80% of patients with rheumatic fever or pharyngitis-associated acute glomerulonephritis infection will mount a significant ASO response. A rise in titer is usually seen 3–6 weeks after infection, and a rise, even if modest, is more helpful than a single determination. Test kits give a titer of >166 Todd units as elevated for adults, but there is considerable variation in the "normal" values among populations and laboratories. In general, single ASO titers above 250 in adults and above 300 in school-aged children are considered elevated. Compared to pharyngitis, skin infections tend to elicit feeble ASO responses but greater responses to DNase B. The anti-DNase B titer peaks later, at 6–8 weeks after either skin or throat infections. This test is often useful when the initial ASO is low or negative. There is less clinical experience with the antihyaluronidase and antistreptokinase tests, although they may give comparable results and may be useful as confirmatory tests. The Streptozyme hemagglutination test (Wampole Laboratories, Stamford, CT) is a crude screening test based on reactions with an unspecified mixture of streptococcal antigens. It is simple and widely available but is not considered sufficiently reliable by many authorities. Positive responses appear earlier (1–2 weeks) and should always be confirmed with one or more of the standardized assays whenever rheumatic fever or acute glomerulonephritis is suspected.[20]

Assays for antibody to pneumococcal and group B streptococcal capsular polysaccharides have employed radioimmunoassay (RIA) for total antibody and enzyme-linked immunosorbent assays (ELISA) for total and class-specific antibody determinations. Since both pneumococci and group B streptococci have multiple capsular types, antibody to specific types must be considered. Al-

Table 5. Group A Streptococcal Antigens and Antibodies[a]

	Antibody	Clinical interpretation
Cellular antigens		
M protein	(M protein)	Type-specific, confers immunity. Some antigens cross-reactive with sarcolemma of heart muscle
Group A carbohydrate	(Group A CHO)	Slow response following infection
Hyaluronic acid capsule	None	Not antigenic
Extracellular enzymes		
Streptolysin O	Antistreptolysin O (ASO)	Increases after most group A infections, more reliable for throat than skin infections
Deoxyribonuclease A, B, C, D	Anti-DNase B	Most useful test for skin infections, also reliable for throat infections; anti-DNase A and C inconsistent
Hyaluronidase	Antihyaluronidase	Increases after most group A infections
Streptokinase	Antistreptokinase (ASK)	Increases after most group A infections; streptokinase A more common than B
Nicotinamide adenine dinucleotidase	Anti-NADase (anti-DPNase)	Response better after throat than skin infections; common to group A, C, and G streptococci
Proteinase	Antiproteinase	Antibodies appear in small amounts following infection with group A
Erythrogenic toxins A, B, and C	Antierythrogenic toxin	Toxin produces rash of scarlet fever; Dick skin test for immunity or susceptibility

[a]Adapted from Quinn.[1]

though it has so far proved impossible to establish an absolute or minimal protective antibody level, infection appears to be more common in subjects with low antibody levels against the specific capsular antigen of the type causing infection. Assays for type-specific pneumococcal antibodies are now commercially available. They are currently used in screening selected patients when a generalized unresponsiveness to polysaccharide antigens is suspected. For this purpose, it is useful to compare antibody levels before and 4 weeks after administration of pneumococcal vaccine.

4. Biological Characteristics of the Organisms

The various streptococcal species have many biological similarities and differences. The genus name suggests a "twisted chain," which describes the microscopic appearance of many species, especially when grown in broth culture. The pneumococci are commonly described (and were formerly named) as diplococci because of their propensity to occur in pairs, but they are often indistinguishable from other streptococci in blood cultures. All the streptococci have a tough cell wall composed of cross-linked peptidoglycans. Most have a polysaccharide group antigen associated with the cell wall, and some have teichoic acids as major or additional components. Pneumococci exhibit prototypic bacterial polysaccharide capsules. The group A streptococci, in contrast, have the M proteins on their exterior surface, but these appear to play a similar role in helping the organisms resist phagocytosis. The group B streptococci, like pneumococci, have polysaccharide capsules as their major surface antigens. Pneumococci, however, also have autolytic enzymes that break down cell walls in late growth phases, releasing DNA and other intracellular components. Intact pneumococci can also take up genetic material, and are thus autotransformable, a characteristic that appears to have facilitated the spread of antibiotic resistance within the species. With few exceptions, streptococci are aerobic and faculatively anaerobic. They are cytochrome-negative, catalase-negative, and ferment sugars mainly to lactic acid but not to gas. All streptococci secrete enzymes extracellularly, but those of group A have been studied most extensively.

4.1. Cellular Antigens and Enzymes

4.1.1. Group A Streptococcal Cellular Antigens and Enzymes. The major components of group A streptococci are the cellular antigens and the extracellular enzymes listed in Table 5. M proteins, noted above and listed in Table 3, are the major virulence factors of group A streptococci, contributing to the organism's resistance to phagocytosis in the absence of type-specific antibody.[53] M proteins bind host proteins, especially fibrinogen, as a ploy to evade host defense mechanisms. Although immunity appears to be lifelong, most humans are usually infected by only a few different types and remain susceptible to the other types. Thus, repeated episodes of streptococcal infection may be due to different types rather than to a failure of host response. Certain M types, especially M1 and M3, have been associated with more severe forms of disease.[4,24] The existence of "rheumatogenic" types or strains has been debated for many years. Although "rheumatogenicity" is not determined by M type alone, evidence for the cross-reactivity of certain M proteins with heart and brain tissue now strongly suggests autoimmune mechanisms for the etiology of acute rheumatic fever and Sydenham's chorea.[54–56]

The group A cell wall carbohydrate is a polymer of rhamnose with *N*-acetylglucosamine side chains. Humans normally make antibodies to this antigen, but antibodies play no role in protection. There is now evidence that this antigen may play a role in sequelae of streptococcal infections by inducing antibodies cross-reactive with cytokeratin.[57] This could provide an explanation for the joint and skin manifestation of acute rheumatic fever and of guttate psoriasis.

Hyaluronic acid capsules are also produced by some (especially M18) strains, giving colonies a large, highly mucoid appearance. This capsule material is indistinguishable from the ground substance of mammalian connective tissue and is not immunogenic. Its effect on virulence in mice is small, although similar capsules may occur on group C streptococci and have greater virulence than unencapsulated strains. Nevertheless, mucoid group A strains have been associated with severe disease in humans and with rheumatic fever.[24,55]

Lipoteichoic acids are composed of polyglycerophosphate attached to lipids. These surface molecules are directly involved in attachment of organisms to host epithelia and are of importance in the initiation of infection.[58] Other cellular components are less well defined in terms of their role in disease. As in other gram-positive bacteria, there is a rigid cell wall structure made from polymers of alternating glucosamine and muramic acid units cross-linked by peptide side chains. This serves to stabilize the organisms against outside osmotic changes. The peptidoglycan components are highly inflammatory and may play a role in inciting nonspecific host responses. The T proteins, noted above, occur in families that may be shared by a number of M types. The serum opacity factor proteins are coexpressed with specific M types and are not shared among M types.[23] The R antigen is an antigenic surface protein that occurs in strains of various types but appears to play no role in virulence or protection. Like group C and G streptococci, group A and other streptococci also have antibody-binding proteins that bind antibodies nonspecifically via the Fc fragment, presumably to help the organism avoid specific, complement-fixing, antibody binding.[59]

Group A streptococci secrete various substances into the surrounding milieu that may contribute to the pathogenic process. There are two well-described hemolysins capable of lysing red blood cells and injuring other cell membranes and subcellular organelles.[60] Streptolysin O is the antigenic, oxygen-labile hemolysin used in the ASO test. Streptolysin S is nonantigenic, oxygen-stable, and responsible for hemolysis at the surface of cultures grown on blood agar under aerobic conditions.

Deoxyribonucleases (DNases) are elaborated by group A, B, C, and G streptococci.[60] DNase B is the most common and most immunogenic of the group A DNases and is the basis of the antibody test of the same name. While a pathogenic role is not established, it is thought that these enzymes, along with hyaluronidase and streptokinase, combine to produce the thin pus seen in streptococcal infections, in contrast to the thick pus often associated with infections due to other pyogenic bacteria.[1]

Streptococcal hyaluronidases (produced by groups A and C) are capable of hydrolyzing the hyaluronic acid of group A capsules and of mammalian connective tissue. Although formerly called "spreading factor," its biological role remains uncertain with regard either to cell metabolism or to the production of disease.[60]

The streptokinases are antigenic proteins that convert plasminogen to plasmin, which in turn lyses fibrin clots. Group A streptococci produce either streptokinase A, the most common, or streptokinase B. An antibody test based on the former antigen is sometimes employed in the clinical assessment of group A disease. A distinctive low-molecular-weight streptokinase, called "nephritis strain-associated protein," has also been identified from group A streptococci recovered from patients with acute nephritis.[61]

Nicotinamide adenine dinucleotidase [(NADase) also called diphosphopyridine nucleotidase (DPNase)] is produced by streptococci of groups A, C, and G.[60] Anti-NADase antibodies are produced by the majority of patients recovering from group A streptococcal pharyngitis, but responses are poor following skin infections. NADase is toxic to leukocytes, but the role of this enzyme in human infection is not certain, since some serotypes, such as M type 1, 5, and 19, do not produce NADase and yet are fully capable of causing disease.

Proteinases of group A streptococci have been carefully studied and shown to exert pathological effects *in vitro* and *in vivo*. Their role in human disease has yet to be directly established.[60] A specialized peptidase has recently been described that diminishes chemotactic activity by inactivation of the C5a complement component.[62]

Streptococcal pyrogenic exotoxins (SPE) are the erythrogenic toxins responsible for the characteristic rash of scarlet fever. These enzymes have been implicated as factors in streptococcal toxic shock, where they appear to be potent activators of tumor necrosis factor (TNF) and other cytokines.[4,63] There are three antigenically distinct toxins, designated SPE A, B, and C. All group A streptococci carry a gene (*speB*) that codes for SPE B, but it is not understood why some strains are stronger producers of the toxin than others. SPE A and SPE C are encoded by lysogenic bacteriophages, and only those strains infected by the phages are capable of producing toxin. Humans make antibodies to SPE A, B, and C, which appear to confer toxin-specific immunity to scarlet fever. It is possible to have scarlet fever more than once, due to different toxins. The classic determination of susceptibility to scarlet fever is the Dick test.[1] Seldom used today, it is based on the observation that patients with antibody to a specific toxin show no response to a small intradermal injection of that toxin (negative Dick test). Susceptible individuals, who have no antibody to neutralize the toxin, develop inflammation at the injection site within 24 hr (positive Dick test). SPE A shares structural and physiological similarities with TSST-1, one of the toxins associated with staphylococcal toxic shock syndrome (see also Chapter 33).

4.1.2. Group B Streptococcal Cellular Antigens and Enzymes. The group B streptococci differ from group A in that their virulence may be accounted for principally by capsular polysaccharides rather than proteins. The capsular types, noted in Section 3.4.1 and in Table 4, are antigenically distinct by virtue of variations in linkages of the same essential sugars. A key feature is that all have terminal *N*-acetylneuraminic acid (sialic acid) residues that are major immunodeterminants. The capsules are antiphagocytic and require specific antibody for efficient opsonization. The quantity of sialic acid-containing antigen appears to be directly related to size and density of the capsule and to virulence in animal models.[64,65] The capsular material itself appears to inhibit the activation and chemotactic functions of neutrophils.[66] Many group B strains are also capable of binding fibrinogen to their surface in a manner that competes with the nonspecific binding of C3 complement.

The group B antigen is a complex glucitol-containing polysaccharide associated with the peptidoglycan cell wall. Antibodies to the group B antigen are generally not protective, presumably because it is covered by capsular material. A human monoclonal IgM antibody to the group B antigen has been described that opsonizes strains of all serotypes,(67) but the large amount of antibody required appears to make it impractical as an adjunctive therapeutic agent.

The major protein antigen of group B streptococci is the c protein, which occurs on all type Ib and some type II and III strains. Antibodies to this antigen are protective,(68) but common variants of the protein apparently confer resistance to intracellular killing by neutrophils.(69) An important property of the c protein may be its ability to nonspecifically bind human IgA.(70) The R and X antigens are rarely seen in human isolates and probably play no role in protection or disease. Also present are lipoteichoic acids that are involved with adherence of organisms to host epithelial cells.

The group B streptococci elaborate a number of extracellular enzymes, including hemolysins, CAMP factor, DNases, and "neuraminidase."(60) Pritchard *et al.*(71) have recently shown that the enzyme thought for many years to be a neuraminidase is in fact a hyaluronic acid lyase that has a unique mechanism of action quite unlike that of hyaluronidases produced by group A streptococci or pneumococci. A group B streptococcal hemolysin has been identified that is cytotoxic for mammalian cells *in vitro* and inhibited by phospholipids common to pulmonary surfactants.(72) The CAMP factor potentiates the activity of sphingomyelinase and may have effects on cell membranes. Purified CAMP factor appears to enhance the lethality of live organisms injected into mice.(73) Like group A, group B streptococci elaborate a proteinase that decreases chemotactic activity by specifically cleaving complement C5a.(74) A pyrogenic exotoxin has recently been identified from strains associated with a group B streptococcal toxic shocklike syndrome in infants.(75)

4.1.3. Pneumococcal Cellular Antigens and Enzymes. *S. pneumoniae* is the paradigm of encapsulated bacteria. Its polysaccharide capsules are essential to virulence, antibodies against the capsule are the major specific defense against infection, and the development of antibody is important in convalescence from disease. The 82 recognized type-specific polysaccharides vary in composition, including linear polymers, branched chains, and teichoic acidlike antigens. The most frequently occurring types have been selected for inclusion in the presently licensed vaccines.(31)

The C-polysaccharide corresponds to the group carbohydrates of other streptococci but differs significantly in structure. Its major antigenic determinant is phosphocholine, linked to ribitol phosphate, galactosamine, and other sugars. Antibodies to the phosphocholine moiety protect mice from experimental infection. Although humans make "natural" antibodies to this antigen, opsonization of pneumococci (and presumably protection) is almost entirely dependent on anticapsular antibodies.(76) The phosphocholine determinant is also the site of binding for C-reactive protein (CRP), an acute-phase reactant elevated in acute disease. The Forssman antigen is a membrane teichoic acid with a similar composition, but it is linked to a lipid, forming what is essentially the lipoteichoic acid of the pneumococcus.

Cell surface proteins, notably a newly described antigen designated pneumococcal surface protein A (PspA) has been identified on essentially all important clinical isolates.(32) Although the importance of these proteins in human disease has not yet been determined, this highly variable protein appears to play a role in virulence, and antibodies to this antigen are protective in mice against multiple capsular serotypes.(77) Humans, including young infants, make antibodies to PspA, suggesting its possible use as a vaccine, as noted below.

Enzymes produced by pneumococci include pneumolysin, amidase (the autolytic enzyme that breaks down cell wall material), neuraminidases, IgA proteases, and a hyaluronidase.(60,78) Although none of these has been conclusively shown to be associated with virulence, all have at least theoretical implications. The pneumolysin gene bears extensive amino acid sequence homology to streptolysin O and to the theta-toxin of *Clostridium perfringens*. Pneumolysin is an intracellular enzyme and is released only by cell lysis. It is highly toxic to pulmonary epithelial cells; it may be important to the pathogenesis of pneumonia, but it appears to have a limited effect in experimental meningitis.(79) Neuraminidases are directly toxic to mice and may play a role either in modifying epithelial cells during invasion or in direct damage to cells in meningitis. IgA proteases cleave the Fc fragment from IgA, making it incapable of preventing adhesion to epithelial cells and possibly also preventing the recognition of IgA by tissue macrophages.(60)

4.1.4. Components of Other Streptococci. Other pyogenic streptococci share many characteristics noted above. All have rigid peptidoglycan cell walls, with various distinctive or group antigens, and usually with some form of lipoteichoic acid. Group C streptococci may have hyaluronic acid capsules like those of group A. Group G streptococci may have the type 12 M protein of group A or similar surface proteins, as well as antibody-binding proteins. The group C streptococci from human, equine, and porcine sources produce species-specific streptokinases that are otherwise similar to those of group A.[80] A streptokinase derived from group C has been used clinically in attempts to clear clotted intravascular catheters, to lyse pleural adhesions in patients with lung infections, and to help remove clots in patients with coronary artery occlusions.[81] Group G streptococci also produce streptokinases. We have described a patient with nephritis following infection with a group G strain that had a low-molecular-weight enzyme similar to the nephritis strain-associated protein of group A.[82]

The enteric and oral streptococci are usually unencapsulated. Streptococci of the "milleri" group appear to require at least 50% of cells to have capsules in order to produce abscesses in experimental animals. Capsule production can be induced in some species, but capsular materials from this group have not been defined.[83] Few toxins or noxious enzymes have been described among the enteric and oral streptococci, but this may be from lack of concerted investigation. Members of the "milleri" group have, at the least, hyaluronidase, deoxyribonuclease, and various proteinases.[84] For many of the less virulent streptococci, the inflammatory response to infection probably relates more to the properties of the cell wall breakdown products than to specific enzymes or toxins. Characteristics that enable them to cause disease often relate to their ability to adhere to host tissues, such as tooth enamel, heart valves or prostheses, or to intravascular catheters. *S. mutans*, for example, adheres to the pellicle coating the tooth surface by specific protein receptors called antigen I/II; adhesion is further facilitated by the presence of sucrose. *S. mutans* also produce extracellular proteases that are capable of breaking down cemental collagens and other host stubstrates. Caries occur when the secretion of acids demineralizes the enamel and organisms adhere to and invade the tooth surface.[11,85] Enterococci and "milleri" group streptococci are frequently found in mixed infections, especially in association with anaerobic bacteria, suggesting that additional factors are required for them to cause disease. Enterococci produce several pheromones that are chemotactic for neutrophils and may contribute to the inflammation associated with infection. *E. faecalis* also produces a plasmid-encoded hemolysin. Because enterococci are frequently resistant to common antibiotics, serious enterococcal disease also occurs assuperinfection in patients receiving broad-spectrum antibiotics that may disturb the normal ecology of this usually benign organism.

4.2. Antibiotic Susceptibility

The streptococci are generally quite susceptible to penicillin, including most oral and "milleri" group streptococci. Exceptions include some pneumococci and group D streptococci and the enterococci. Although streptococci are generally resistant to aminoglycosides, gentamicin is sometimes used for its synergistic effect in combination with a penicillin. Chloramphenicol occasionally has been used in penicillin-allergic patients, but other drugs, including erythromycin, clarithromycin, and clindamycin, are considered to be superior for most streptococcal species.

Group A and B streptococci have never developed resistance to penicillins, probably because they are not naturally transformable, as are pneumococci and enterococci. They are somewhat less sensitive to vancomycin and cephalosporins, moderately resistant to chloramphenicol, and fairly resistant to aminoglycosides, sulfonamides, and tetracycline. Group B strains have shown some tolerance to penicillin, but the clinical significance of such observations is unknown. Tolerance to penicillin has been suggested as one mechanism by which group A streptococci persist after treatment of pharyngitis, allowing either relapses or asymptomatic carriage to follow.[86] Another mechanism is thought to be the protection of susceptible streptococci by the production of β-lactamases by other bacteria in the pharynx or tonsils.[87] Resistance to erythromycin occurs in 1–5% of group A strains in most parts of the world; resistance rates, which tend to parallel antibiotic use, as high as 60% have been reported in Japan and parts of Europe.

Penicillin resistance in pneumococci has emerged slowly over the past two decades and has now become a frequent and serious problem worldwide.[88] Most of these strains have intermediate susceptibility [minimum inhibitory concentration (MIC) 0.1–1.0 μg/ml], but highly resistant strains (MIC $>$ 1.0 μg/ml), initially reported from South Africa and Spain, have now spread throughout Europe and North America. Using molecular epidemiological methods, one particular resistant clone has been traced from Spain to Iceland and elsewhere.[46] Span has a long history of unrestricted antibiotic use; it has also been a favored vacationing place for Northern Europeans. The environmental pressure of uncontrolled antibiotic use plus increased international travel have contributed dramatically to spread of multiple drug resistance. Some isolates are now resistant to all common antibiotics except vancomycin, rifampin, bacitracin, novobiocin, and fusidic acid. In parts of South Africa, resistance to rifampin is prevalent, because of the widespread use of that drug for treating tuberculosis. In Europe, intermediate and resistant strains account for up to 50% of all pneumococcal isolates. In the United States, penicillin resistance rates are 20–30%; the proportion of highly and multiply resistant strains is about 1%. In areas where resistance to both penicillins and cephalosporins is prevalent, many physicians now add vancomycin to the initial empiric antibiotic regimen when pneumococcal meningitis is suspected.[88]

The National Committee for Clinical Laboratory Standards recommends screening of pneumococci by disk diffusion on Mueller–Hinton/5% sheep blood agar using 1-μg oxacillin disks. The criterion for susceptible strains is an inhibition zone diameter ≥20 mm. About half of strains with zones <20 mm may prove borderline susceptible when retested for MIC by the agar dilution method.[89,90]

The basis for resistance among pneumococci is the alterations in penicillin-binding proteins in combination with changes in the stem peptides on the muramic acid units of the cell wall matrix.[88,91] There is no evidence for β-lactamase coding plasmids in pneumococci. Penicillin acts as a false substrate in the cross-linking of cell wall precursors, preventing the formation of normal peptidoglycan chains and rendering the organisms susceptible to damage by osmotic forces or incapable of normal cell division. Stable chromosomal changes resulting from multiple transformation events have led to penicillin-binding proteins with lower binding affinities for penicillin, while at the same time the predominant stem peptides have shifted from straight- to branched-chain peptide moieties. The resulting organisms no longer bind penicillin in preference to the new cell wall precursors. Intact peptidoglycan chains are formed. At least three genetically related groups of resistant strains have been identified and show clear indications of clonal origin.[46,50,91]

Enterococci are moderately resistant to penicillins alone, because of the intrinsic properties of their penicillin-binding proteins.[12,92] Some strains of *E. faecalis* have also acquired β-lactamases as a mechanism of resistance.[84] Infections are usually treated with penicillin or ampicillin plus an aminoglycoside, which exert a synergistic effect against the organisms. Some enterococci have developed high-level resistance to gentamicin (MIC > 500 μg/ml), but the extent of this problem is not known because most isolates are not routinely tested for susceptibility to this drug. Vancomycin-resistant *E. faecalis* have recently appeared and may present difficult therapeutic challenges, especially in view of their increasing frequency in nosocomial infections.[12,92]

5. Descriptive Epidemiology

5.1. Prevalence and Incidence

Group A streptococcal pharyngitis is one of the most common acute bacterial infections. The frequency of this disease, especially as manifested by scarlet fever, has declined dramatically since the beginning of the century, as illustrated in Fig. 1.[1] The severity of the disease, reflected by mortality rates, declined concomitantly. This trend began long before the advent of antibiotics, suggesting a decrease in virulence or an increase in host resistance, or both. In the 1940s, penicillin became widely available, and deaths attributed to scarlet fever and puerperal sepsis, the two most common lethal forms of group A streptococcal disease, became a rarity. The number of reported cases of streptococcal sore throat increased during the 1950s and 1960s, probably because of increased physician awareness of its relation to rheumatic fever, greater use of throat cultures, and the availability of antibiotics for treatment and prevention.

Figure 2 shows the number of positive throat cultures and number of cases of acute rheumatic fever and acute glomerulonephritis in private pediatric practices participating in surveillance studies in Rochester, New York, over a 20-year period. Of approximately 23,000 throat cultures done annually, 18–25% were positive for group A streptococci in this relatively stable population. Meanwhile, the number of cases of acute glomerulonephritis declined from nearly 40 in 1967 to an average of 1 case per year from 1981 to 1988. Confirmed cases of acute rheumatic fever dropped from 20–28 per year to a very few from 1975 through 1985, but they have since begun to rise.

Acute rheumatic fever has show a decline and recent rise in many but not all localities.[14] In Baltimore, between 1960 and 1964, the incidence of rheumatic fever was 26 per 100,000 among 5- to 19-year-olds. By 1980, the rates had fallen to 0.2–0.8 per 100,000 nationwide among whites, with rates several times higher among other ethnic groups. Beginning in the mid-1980s, an increase in new cases was seen in Utah, Pennsylvania, Ohio, New York, and other areas. Disease incidence peaked in Utah in 1985, with 18 per 100,000 population age-adjusted for 5- to 17-year-olds, and rates have subsequently declined to about a third of that seen in 1985.[3] Of particular interest was the observation that throughout this period incidence rates went essentially unchanged in Hawaii[93] and New Zealand,[94] where the disease is especially prevalent among Polynesian children. In a program begun in 1984, the World Health Organization (WHO) Cardiovascular Disease Unit surveyed 16 developing countries and found rates averaging 220 cases per 100,000 childhood population.[95] Highest rates were in Africa (470/100,000) and the Eastern Mediterranean (440/100,000); lowest rates were in Southeast Asia (12/100,000) and the Western Pacific (7/100,000), with the Americas falling in between (15/100,000). The major problem in the developing world is establishing and maintaining effective primary and secondary prevention programs.[96] This principle applies as well to developed areas, such as Miami, Florida, where underprivileged inner-city children have attack rates of 15/100,000, compared to 0.7/100,000 for suburban middle-class children.[97]

Deaths from acute rheumatic fever are uncommon today. In developed countries deaths associated with chronic rheumatic heart disease continue to occur in persons who had acute rheumatic fever in childhood and develop severe mitral stenosis in the fourth decade or later. In 1975, for example, 9,255 of 12,775 deaths attributed to rheumatic heart disease were in patients over 50 years of age.[1] The pattern is quite different in developing areas, as in South Africa, where a third of patients have mitral regurgitation usually associated with ongoing rheumatic activity.[98] Left untreated, these lesions develop into a severe form of pure mitral regurgitation that requires surgery in the first or second decade of life. Degenerative valvular disease, including mitral stenosis and mixed lesions, are like those seen elsewhere but tend to occur at a younger age.

Acute poststreptococcal glomerulonephritis is currently a rare disease, as shown in data from Rochester, New York, in Fig. 2. There are no contemporary data rates for nephritis associated with either throat or skin infections in the United States. Prospective studies in Alabama (1966–1969) revealed 91 cases of nephritis relative to 1149 cases of uncomplicated streptococcal pyoderma treated in a clinical setting, for an attack rate of about 8%.[25]

Another change in group A streptococcal disease in recent years has been the reappearance of serious acute infections, especially bacteremia and streptococcal toxic shock.[4] Since 1980, the number of septicemic deaths has increased in the United Kingdom out of proportion with other streptococcal infections, but precise incidence figures are not available. A suvery conducted in Ontario, Canada, 1987–1991, studied severe streptococcal disease presenting with hypotension in the first 24 hr of obtaining a positive culture. The attack rate for 1991 was estimated to be 0.3/100,000 population.[99]

Group B streptococcal infections continue to be common in neonates, with attack rates of early-onset disease of 2 per 1000 live births in defined populations from Chicago, Illinois, and from Birmingham, Alabama.[100,101] An ongoing study supported by the National Institutes of Child Health and Human Development is currently finding similar attack rates among seven study sites in the United States. Late-onset disease (usually occurring after hospital discharge up to about 3 months of age) adds another 2 infections per 1000 births, for a total of about 4 neonatal group B infections per 1000 live births.[101] Exact incidence data are very difficult to obtain and interpret, and rates may vary over time, by locality, or by the nature of populations sampled. An active surveillance study of an aggregate population of 10 million in four geographical areas was coordinated by the CDC in 1990. Early-onset disease occurred at a rate of 1.4/100 live births, late-onset disease occurred at 0.3/1000 live births, and adult disease (>15 years of age) occurred in 3.6/100,000 population in that year.[15] Few accurate data are available outside of Europe and North America. Rates appear to be much lower (about 0.5 per 1000 live births) in Scandinavia and the United Kingdom than in the United States and parts of western Europe.[102] Maternal and infant colonization rates are similar in Hong Kong, but the neonatal disease rate is 0.6 per 1000 live births.[103] Maternal sepsis due to group B streptococci occurred in 0.5–2 per 1000 deliveries in Alabama.[104] Lowest rates were seen when particular attention was paid to aggressive antibiotic use in mothers undergoing cesarean section delivery.

The overall annual incidence of invasive group B streptococcal infections was 9.2 per 100,000 population for metropolitan Atlanta during 1989–1990.[105] Nearly half of the total number of 424 cases were in adults, and of these 68% were in men and nonpregnant women.

The incidence of pneumococcal disease is summarized in Chapter 28.

Enterococcal infections now account for nearly 10% of nosocomial infections and for 5–6% of all bacteremias in hospitalized patients (see Chapter 25).[12,13] Rates of bacteremic infection are often twice as high on trauma, surgical, and obstetric–gynecological services. Three fourths of enterococcal bacteremias are nosocomial, but endocarditis is more frequently community-acquired. Case-fatality rates are in the range of 40%, and many of these patients are debilitated, immunocompromised, or have serious predisposing conditions.

In terms of sheer numbers, *S. mutans*, the principal organism in dental caries, probably infects more persons than all other streptococci combined. Survey methodology and recent studies have been reviewed by Leclercq[106] and Beck.[107] Of the 40 to 50% of the population of developed countries who regularly visit a dentist, most receive treatment related to restoration of teeth or decayed tooth substance. Over the past two decades, however, the prevalence of coronal dental caries has declined significantly in developed countries. In the United States, about 50% of school-aged children currently have permanent teeth completely free of cavities and restorations.[108]

Inasmuch as dental caries is a chronic disease that

varies within and among populations, several measures of morbidity have been developed. Prevalence, defined as the percentage of a population showing any evidence of caries, may be so widespread as to have little epidemiological significance. The most commonly used index is that counting the number of decayed, filled, and missing teeth (DFM or DFMT). Because of the difficulty of examining representative groups of subjects beyond school age, population surveys are often standardized at an index age of 12 years.[106] Since the populations of developing countries are skewed toward the younger age groups, who have fewer caries relative to the older populations in the developed world, a population-weighted mean DFMT at age 12 is used for global comparisons. By this measure the WHO can monitor trends from the more than 1000 surveys submitted to the WHO Global Oral Data Bank, set up in 1970. The WHO goal of three DFM teeth per person has been realized in 84 of 148 countries for which data are currently available. Dental health in industrialized countries, most of which had moderate to high DFMT rates in 1969, has improved greatly over the past two decades. Meanwhile, developing countries have seen a rise in DFMT thought to be associated with changes in diet and other factors associated with urbanization. From 1980 to 1986, DFMT rates have increased from 1.63 to 2.16 in developing countries and have decreased from 4.53 to 3.82 in developed countries.[106] Rates also vary within countries. In the United States, the highest DFMT rates have always been found in northeastern states, with the lowest rates in south-central states. This has been attributed in part to differences in natural fluoridation. Further declines in recent years have been attributed to increased use of topical fluoride treatments and plastic sealants that physically prevent bacteria from colonizing the tooth cervices.[108]

The incidence of dental caries may be estimated from DFMT data, but a more sensitive method makes use of individual counts of new decayed and filled surfaces (DFS) observed over a defined period of time. These counts may be further adjusted to calculate annual mean DFS rates per 100 surfaces at risk. Using this approach, Glass *et al.*[109] observed American males 35 to 80 years of age in a 10-year longitudinal study. The mean annual incidence of new DFS per 100 surfaces at risk was 1.36 and was similar in each of three age cohorts. Within the mouth the rate was highest for molars (mean = 2.69), followed by premolars (1.93) and anterior teeth (0.91), and was higher for upper than lower teeth. The conventional DFMT rate was 23 for these patients at the beginning of the study. The DFS incidence rates, however, were similar to those reported from children aged 7 to 12 years.

5.2. Epidemiology and Contagiousness

Of all the streptococcal infections only scarlet fever has been feared as an epidemic disease in the same sense as cholera and plague. In most areas of the world, group A streptococcal disease is endemic, with fluctuations exceeding the normal prevalence levels occurring seasonally or sometimes over an extended period. Localized epidemics of streptococcal pharyngitis or skin infections and acute rheumatic fever are occasionally reported from newborn nurseries, nursing homes, day-care facilities, and military installations.[110,111] One recent and unusual nursery epidemic occurred when infants were infected from clothing that was improperly cleaned in a hospital laundry.[112] Environmental contamination was thought to be a source of spread within a day-care facility, with streptococci especially abundant on the nose of a rubber dog shared by many of the children.[113]

The epidemiology of streptococcal infections reflects the ecological features peculiar to the species in question. Streptococci associated primarily with the respiratory tract, such as group A and the pneumococcus, cause infections that are initially related to that portal of entry. Of course, some group A strains prefer to colonize the skin and cause impetigo, while others affect either skin or throat. The group B streptococci, in contrast, are gut organisms. Asymptomatic gastrointestinal, and to a lesser extent genitourinary, colonization is common. Their infections relate to the aberrations induced by pregnancy, labor, and delivery, and to the unique conditions of infants in the newborn period. The enterococci are also normal gut organisms, but their infections are more generally opportunistic in nature. Group A streptococci are not considered part of the normal flora of the respiratory tract. Their presence is generally associated with overt infection. Transmission to other persons is greatest from an infected individual, and communicability appears to be dose-related. Nevertheless, a large reservoir of asymptomatic carriers exists with endemic rather than epidemic characteristics. These individuals carry relatively small numbers of organisms. They are at little risk for acute disease or sequelae and are probably an uncommon source of new infection. However, the identification of the carrier state, usually defined by the absence of a serological response, is fraught with difficulties that continue to cloud the relationship between colonization and disease.[114]

Group B streptococci cause serious disease in the perinatal period, but only a small number of infections occur among colonized mothers and infants exposed *in utero*, during, or after delivery. Maternal group B infections may be initially subclinical and possibly contribute to premature labor or septic abortion.[104] Amnionitis may be present before the onset of fever or other symptoms. After delivery, a previously asymptomatic mother may develop endometritis, usually without bacteremia. Classical puerperal sepsis due to group A streptococci, in contrast, was often transmitted via obstetric personnel and occurred as a fulminant infection after delivery, sparing the infant. With group B streptococci, infected infants are usually exposed *in utero* to the serotype carried by the mother. Infants with this "early-onset" form of infection are usually bacteremic at delivery and become symptomatic within a few hours of birth.[101,115] Infection is directly related to the size of the inoculum to which the infant is exposed, by swallowing or aspirating infected amniotic fluid. Most infants are lightly colonized and at little risk for infection, whereas those who are infected are almost invariably heavily colonized at birth.[100,101] Some infants may acquire organisms via the respiratory tract during transit through the birth canal, or from persons other than the mother, and become symptomatic at a later time. Development of the late-onset form of disease may be delayed for days or weeks, and only about half of these infants will be infected by an organism acquired at birth or from the mother.[101]

Pneumococci are often thought of as normal respiratory flora, but pneumococcal infections are not opportunistic in the sense that they are caused by any pneumococcus that happens to reside in the nasopharynx. In a classical investigation, Hodges and MacLeod[116] reported extensive epidemiological studies at a United States Air Force training facility in 1946. Upon arrival at the base, recruits frequently carried pneumococci of serotypes common to the population at large. Within about 6 weeks, they acquired one of a small number of "epidemic" types prevalent at the base—types 1, 2, 4, 5, 7, and 12. The peak incidence of pneumonia due to these types occurred 4–6 weeks after the entry of a new contingent of trainees. Although the rate of carriage of the epidemic types was relatively low, the "infectivity factor" (measured by the ratio of infections to the number of carriers) was much higher than that of other common types, such as 3, 6, 14, 19, and 23. In our epidemiological studies in infants, we also observed a relationship between acquisition and infection.[19] Infants frequently carried types 6, 14, 19, and 23 for prolonged periods, but neither carriage per se nor overall rates correlated with disease. Most infections, which were due to these same common types, occurred within a month of acquiring a new type never before carried by a particular child. The infecting type was often isolated together with a former carriage type from the nasopharynx, but only the new type was recovered from middle ear fluid or other infected sites. In terms of exposure to new strains, 15% of acquisitions resulted in disease.

The concept of dental caries as a transmissible infectious disease was drawn from animal studies in the 1960s. *S. mutans* has been implicated as a major pathogen in caries, and it appears that most infants acquire *S. mutans* strains from their mother.[11] Caufield *et al.*[10] have confirmed these observations using molecular methods in a prospective study of acquisition and infection. They further developed evidence for a discrete "window of infectivity" between 18 and 30 months of age, coinciding with the emergence of the 20 primary teeth. Children who did not acquire *S. mutans* during this period were at much lower risk for caries, at least through 6 years of age. Based on epidemiological evidence from caries prevalence surveys, it is postulated that a second window of infectivity may exist coincident with the emergence of permanent teeth between 6 and 12 years of age.

5.3. Geographic Distribution

Streptococcal diseases are of worldwide importance. Group A streptococci appear to be well adapted to humans living in temperate or tropical climates, although differences in the temporal distribution and perhaps the characteristics of disease may vary. In some tropical areas, group C and G streptococci are more frequently isolated in cases of pharyngitis than are group A strains. Pneumococci are the leading cause of bacterial respiratory infection in all parts of the world. In some areas, such as sub-Saharan Africa where seasonal epidemics of meningococcal disease are common, pneumococcal disease remains endemic and accounts for many cases of meningitis throughout the course of the year. As noted above, group B streptococcal carriage is widespread, but infection rates are highest in North America and western Europe, with lowest rates reported from the United Kingdom, northern Europe, and parts of Asia.[102]

Dental caries occur worldwide, but are more common in industrialized areas than in developing countries, as noted above.[11,106,107] This has been attributed in part to the higher use of sucrose, prepared and refined foodstuffs, and other dietary and social changes associated with urbanization. It is mitigated to some extent by the availability of artificial fluoridation in dentifrices and water supplies and of dental care, especially the use of sealants and topical fluoride. Caries have always been less common in areas with natural fluoridation.

5.4. Temporal Distribution

Group A streptococcal infections follow characteristic seasonal patterns. In northern parts of the United States, streptococcal pharyngitis is typically seen over the winter months, peaking in February or March, while skin infections occur mainly in the summer. Figure 3 illustrates this pattern in surveillence data from private pediatric practices in Rochester, New York, for the 12 years 1977–1988. In the southeastern states there is both a late fall and a late winter peak of respiratory infection, coinciding with the beginning of school in the fall and with increased indoor activity or crowding during colder months. Seasonal variation is less evident in tropical or subtropical areas, although gathering of children at school or other institutions appears to increase the incidence of disease at certain times of the year. Streptococcal skin infections are most common in the rainy season in tropical areas. Such conditions favor the exposure of unprotected skin to the assault of minor trauma and the bites of mosquitoes and other insects. Organisms present on the skin surface, or rarely from the respiratory tract, may be inoculated into damaged skin by itching or scratching.

Pneumococcal infections tend to peak in winter months. The disease incidence is not related to the carriage rate, which varies only slightly over the year, but parallels the markedly seasonal rate of acquisition of new strains.(19,117) In the study of Hodges and MacLeod,(116) there was also a strong correlation of pneumococcal lobar pneumonia with the seasonal peaks of influenza virus infection, with about one case of pneumonia for every ten recruits admitted to the infirmary with nonbacterial respiratory disease.

5.5. Age

Group A streptococcal pharyngitis is uncommon in children under 4 years of age. It increases in frequency as children enter school, peaking at 9 to 12 years of age. These children are the primary source of respiratory infections that occur among families, and are thus a source of exposure for parents and other adults in the household. Streptococcal impetigo, in contrast, is chiefly a disease of younger children. It is frequently seen in toddlers and children under 4 years and typically reaches a peak incidence at about 6 years of age. Adolescents tend to be subject to milder and often self-limited disease.

Group B streptococcal sepsis or meningitis is essentially limited to neonates and infants under 3 months of age and to their mothers around the time of delivery.(7,104) Group B streptococci are a common though sometimes disregarded cause of urinary tract infection among adult

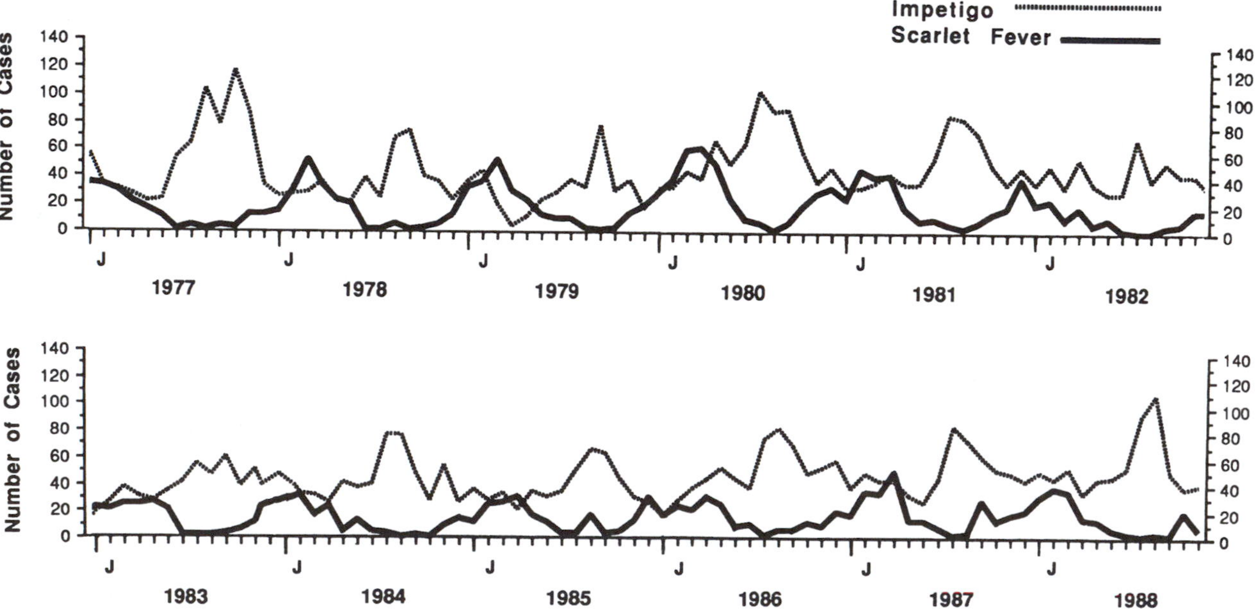

Figure 3. The number of cases of scarlet fever (solid lines) and streptococcal impetigo (dotted lines) seen monthly in private pediatric practices participating in streptococcal surveillance studies in Rochester, New York, 1977–1988. The data were kindly provided by Caroline Breese Hall, University of Rochester.

women, especially during pregnancy. This has been associated with late abortions and problems of the perinatal period. Rarely does an older child or adult develop a serious infection in the absence of some compromise of normal host defenses. Among older adults, especially diabetics, group B streptococci are frequently isolated from cellulitis and pressure ulcers.[118]

Pneumococcal disease is seen in all age groups, but principally affects the very young and the very old. Among children, 70% of meningitis and bacteremia occurs in those under 24 months of age, peaking at 8 to 12 months of age.[119,120] Deaths are also most frequent in this age group, with an overall fatality rate of 6%. Pneumococcal infections are least common among adolescents but increase in frequency with advancing age. The incidence of bacteremic infections reaches 25 per 100,000 among those over 55 years of age, and the case-fatality rate in this group is over 80%.[121]

Serious infections by enteric and oral streptococci are less subject to the effects of age than to the natural defenses of the host. Low-birth-weight babies, however, are increasingly infected by group D and *viridans* streptococci and enterococci, perhaps because of the kinds of interventions required for the management of very premature infants or changes in patterns of antibiotic use. Nosocomial infection caused by enterococci span the range of age, but most community-acquired disease occurs in infants.[122]

Dental caries is a chronic disease that continues throughout life. Longitudinal studies from the United States and from Africa show that rates of development of new caries are about the same in adults as they are in children, despite considerable differences in overall caries incidence for the two localities.[109,123] However, as noted in Section 5.2, there appears to be an age-specific window of acquisition of *S. mutans* at 18–30 months of age that correlates with subsequent risk of caries development.[10]

5.6. Sex

Sex is not a factor in the development of streptococcal disease, except as it relates to pregnancy and to specific genitourinary infections. The peptostreptococci are recognized in pelvic inflammatory disease, but are rarely encountered (or looked for) elsewhere. Group B streptococci may be transmitted by sexual contact, but genital colonization is not associated with symptoms in either sex. Colonization may be higher in women during the first half of the menstrual cycle, perhaps because of greater adherence to vaginal epithelial cells at this time.

5.7. Race and Genetic Factors

No one is spared from susceptibility to streptococcal infections. Much of the association between race and susceptibility can probably be accounted for extrinsic factors, such as poverty, crowding, and lack of medical care. Nevertheless, there is growing evidence that certain persons within racial groups may have some genetic host predisposition. Studies of histocompatibility leukocyte antigen (HLA) distributions point to increased risk of rheumatic fever for blacks expressing the DR2 phenotype and for whites with the DR4 phenotype.[124] Agammaglobulinemia and IgG subclass deficiencies are associated with recurrent pneumococcal infection.[125] Various complement deficiencies, especially that of the second component (C2), should also be considered in children with repeated pneumococcal disease. Children and adults with sickle cell disease are at increased risk because of functional asplenia, which develops after repeated episodes of splenic infarction. Down's syndrome and cleft palate are associated with increased frequency of otitis media due to pneumococci and other organisms.

5.8. Occupation

Occupation is rarely a factor in the development of group A streptococcal infections. Physicians, nurses, and laboratory workers in close contact with infected patients or their cultures seldom develop disease. Epidemics of skin infections have occasionally appeared in meat packers in the United States and Britain.[126] Group B streptococci are a major cause of mastitis in cattle. Spread is thought to occur mainly via the hands of dairy workers from human or bovine sources. Consumers of raw infected milk may become colonized with group B streptococci, but do not appear to be at risk for disease. Group A and C streptococcal diseases have occasionally been associated with milk-borne transmission. Group C infections have also been associated with exposure to horses and other animals.[127] Workers in the pork industry occasionally develop meningitis due to *S. suis*, at a rate in the Netherlands of about 3 per 100,000, or 1500-fold higher than in the population at large.[128]

5.9. Other Settings and Predisposing Factors

Family studies of respiratory bacteria have indicated that the group A streptococcus and the pneumococcus enter a family unit most commonly via school-aged children.[129,130] These organisms spread rather slowly to other family members, some becoming colonized and very few developing overt infection. Spread is often facilitated by concomitant viral respiratory infections. Socioeconomic factors, crowding, and substandard housing have frequently been cited as contributing to the spread of these organisms and to the development of acute rheumatic fever and bronchopneumonia. Schools and day-care centers may experience periodic problems with group A streptococci, including the selection of erythromycin-resistant strains.[131] Spread of pneumococci generally occurs slowly with little consequence in day-care centers, but occasional outbreaks of serious disease have been reported in these settings.[132]

The military has been associated for over a century with increased risk for developing streptococcal disease, especially acute rheumatic fever and pneumococcal pneumonia.[111,116,133] Our present understanding of the epidemiology of rheumatic fever and methods for antibiotic prophylaxis date from important studies done in the US Armed Forces during and after World War II. Rates of streptococcal pharyngitis are much lower in recruit camps where penicillin prophylaxis is routinely used, and rheumatic fever cases have recently appeared at installations that discontinued the practice.[111] In one report, however, antibiotic prophylaxis was not effective until penicillin-allergic recruits, who continued to harbor streptococci, were given oral erythromycin.[133] There may be an incidental effect of prophylactic penicillin on rates of pneumococcal pneumonia, but this has not been studied. Pneumococcal vaccines, however, have been a priority. Nearly 30 years before the current generation of vaccines was licensed in the United States, several purified polysaccharide vaccines were developed for the military and proven efficacious.[31]

Nosocomial spread of group A, B, and C streptococci continues to be reported occasionally, especially from obstetric and surgical services and newborn nurseries.[134,135] Sources of infection may be other patients or personnel who carry organisms in the nose, throat, skin, vagina, or anus. Enterococcal infections in neonates and surgical patients usually originate from the patient's own flora, under the influence of physical interventions and antibiotic therapy.[12,13,122] Intra-abdominal wounds, burns, intravascular catheters, and the urinary tract are the most frequent sites associated with nosocomial enterococcal bacteremia. Epidemic group A streptococcal puerperal sepsis such as that described by Holmes and Semmelweis has largely been eliminated by infection control measures and antibiotics.[6]

Predisposing host factors may be genetic or acquired, such as sickle cell disease, immunodeficiency, or splenectomy. Splenectomized patients have a 50- to 200-fold greater risk of serious bacteremic infection. The spleen is injured most commonly by external abdominal trauma and incidentally during abdominal operations not directly involving the spleen. Surgical repair, rather than removal, of a traumatized spleen is frequently possible and should always be preferred.[136] Overall, about a fourth of children with pneumococcal bacteremia, or meningitis have some underlying condition or host defense abnormality, and risk for these children persists well beyond 24 months of age.[119] Patients with human immunodeficiency virus (HIV) infection or acquired immunodeficiency syndrome (AIDS) are at particularly high risk of bacteremic pneumococcal infection.[137] Intravenous drug abuse, also a known AIDS risk factor, is associated with an increase in group G streptococcal infection.

6. Mechanisms and Routes of Transmission

The transmission of streptococci, introduced in Section 5.2, depends on such factors as the usual ecological niche of the species, its occurrence as part of the normal flora, and the ease with which it may be carried by hands, in secretions, or possibly in droplets. The group A streptococci are transmitted principally by direct contact. Contagiousness is greatest during acute respiratory infection, whereas the chronic carrier is a relatively low risk as an infectious source. This probably reflects the fact that development of infection requires a fairly large inoculum. About 100 organisms are required to infect adult volunteers by directly inoculating the tonsils and pharynx with organisms on a cotton swab. Although streptococci may occur in droplets and survive in dust, an individual is unlikely to acquire a large enough inoculum to become infected from these sources. Streptococci recovered from contaminated blankets and dust may also be less infective. Direct transmission of respiratory secretions may occur via hands, person-to-person contact such as kissing, or projection of large droplets during coughing or sneezing. Treatment of infected persons eliminates the risk of spread within 24–48 hr, permitting resumption of work or school activities as soon as constitutional symptoms have abated.[138]

Pneumococci are thought to be transmitted by similar routes. Coughing is a more regular feature of pneumonia than it is of other pneumococcal infections or of streptococcal pharyngitis. Transmission appears to be favored by symptoms of cold and coryza.[129] Dust particles may harbor pneumococci but do not play a significant role in transmission.[116] Direct spread of secretions containing viable organisms is the most likely source. Covering one's mouth with a hand may deflect a cough or sneeze, but the hand may then transmit fresh secretions.

Common-source outbreaks of streptococcal disease are rarely observed, but group A and C infections have been associated with contaminated foods, such as egg salad, or with improperly pasteurized milk from cows with mastitis. Despite the prevalence of group B streptococci in bovine mastitis, milk-borne group B infections have not been reported.

Skin infections due to group A streptococci are often caused by serotypes different from those associated with throat infections (see Table 3). Streptococci may occur on normal skin but do not cause infection unless there is a break in the cutaneous epithelium. Minor injuries such as scratches, abrasions, cuts, or insect bites may become points of entry.[139] Mosquito bites are an especially common site of inoculation, where organisms are rubbed into the wound during itching. In Trinidad, streptococcal impetigo may be transmitted by flies of the genus *Hippelates*, which feed on open skin sores. Streptococci from the nasopharynx may be transmitted to skin sites, but it is more common for the skin to be colonized first and the throat later. Classical erysipelas, in contrast, is thought to be transmitted via the respiratory tract, either from the patient or from a caretaker. Erysipelas is occasionally seen following superinfection of chicken pox lesions.

The group B streptococci causing early-onset perinatal infections are those carried by the mother in the lower gastrointestinal and genitourinary tracts.[7,100,101,115] Organisms may enter the amniotic cavity following rupture of amniotic membranes, but the fetus may become infected with membranes intact. Although rupture of membranes for greater than 12 hr is a recognized risk factor for ascending infection, the duration of labor is also important, perhaps because of the entry of organisms via microscopic defects in the membranes. Among twins, who have a higher rate of infection than singletons, it is usually the first twin who is closer to the source of infection and at greater risk. Once the streptococci have entered the amniotic fluid, they proliferate rapidly and are aspirated or swallowed by the fetus. Late-onset infections may have a maternal source in about half of cases, with colonization occurring at delivery.[101] Other infants may acquire streptococci later from persons outside the immediate family, presumably via the oral or respiratory route.

Enteric and oral streptococci are part of the normal flora, acquired early in life from the mother and family members. They generally cause opportunistic infection only after perturbations of normal defenses. Nosocomial infections are usually due to a patient's own flora. Transient bacteremia may occur with dental manipulation, transurethral prostate resection, or gynecological and gastrointestinal surgery. Patients with known history of rheumatic heart disease, mitral valve prolapse, or prosthetic heart valves are at higher risk for developing endocarditis due to otherwise "benign" streptococcal species. In such cases, a prophylactic antibiotic, usually penicillin, is administered just prior to the dental or surgical treatment (see Section 9.2).

7. Pathogenesis and Immunity

7.1. Pathogenesis

The development of infection involves a multitude of interrelated bacterial and host factors that vary enormously among streptococcal species. The biological characteristics associated with virulence among various streptococci are summarized in Section 4; certain host factors and modes of transmission are noted in Sections 5.9 and 6. The pathogenic process is not clearly understood for any streptococcal disease, but it may be useful to consider three general stages.

First, organisms are acquired by the host and either succeed in colonizing their preferred sites or are eliminated by host defenses at the epithelial surface. For many streptococcal species, the specific mechanisms of adherence are known.[11,58] Adherence may be important in the establishment of colonization but is not necessarily a property that distinguishes virulent from commensal species or strains. To ward off bacterial invasion, the host has epithelial barriers, mucous layers, and secretions containing enzymes and antibodies.

The second stage begins when organisms succeed in breaching local defenses and enter the epithelial and subepithelial tissues, or, in the case of *S. mutans*, get into and through the tooth enamel. Most of the acute pathological effects of group A streptococci occur at this stage by causing pharyngitis or skin infection, with invasion of the submucosal or subepidermal layers. This is frequently accompanied by lymphadenitis but rarely progresses to bacteremia. In pneumococcal pneumonia and in otitis media, the initial insult is not a direct breach of epithelium but rather the invasion of a normally sterile compartment; symptoms of disease ensue as organisms multiply and induce inflammation in surrounding tissue. The host responds with nonspecific secretory and serum forces, including the release of vasoactive and chemotactic mediators, activation of the alternative complement pathway, and with the mobilization of neutrophils and tissue macrophages. Eventually, specific secretory and serum antibodies develop and contribute to resolution of the disease.

The third stage is systemic infection, in which organisms multiply in blood and tissues. Severe streptococcal infections, including streptococcal toxic shock, depend on the organism's ability to evade host defenses until it establishes a sufficient mass of growth to cause systemic manifestations. The M proteins protect against phagocytosis and also down-regulating complement activation on the bacterial surface.[53] An enzyme that inactivates complement C5a decreases chemotaxis and secondary inflammatory responses.[62] Spread of infection within the tissues may be facilitated by the action of hyaluronidase and proteinases. Shock is probably mediated by TNF-α, IL-1β, and IL-6, all of which may be induced by pyrogenic toxins (SPE), streptolysin O, and cell wall breakdown products. Further alterations in host physiology occur by cytokine activation and by direct and indirect effects on hemodynamics, metabolism, and the function of individual organs.[4]

Some of the mechanisms thought to be involved in acute group B streptococcal sepsis have been studied *in vitro* and in animal models. Early-onset infections appear to begin *in utero*, and it is suspected that the organisms gain access to the circulation by breaching the gastrointestinal or pulmonary epithelial barriers. In a monkey model of intrauterine infection, aspirated streptococci were found to be actively taken up by pulmonary alveolar cells. These cells acted as nonprofessional phagocytes, but were incapable of killing the organisms, and tissue invasion rapidly ensued.[140] In a model of bacteremia, an immediate effect of intravenous infusions of washed heat-killed group B streptococci in piglets is the increase in pulmonary artery pressure, mimicking that observed in septic neonates.[141] The magnitude of pulmonary hypertension was higher with small- or capsule-deficient organisms than with the fully encapsulated organism and was greater in the presence of type-specific antibodies. These observations suggested that group B streptococci causing disease have mechanisms to evade the inflammatory responses of the host and, conversely, that early manifestations of severe disease depend on the inflammatory response mediated by both specific and nonspecific host factors. In the piglet model the hemodynamic response was associated with release of thromboxane, and the response could be blocked with indomethacin, a cyclo-oxygenase inhibitor, and dazmagrel, an specific inhibitor of thromboxane synthesis. Similar drugs could be useful clinically but remain experimental at present. Other investigators have demonstrated a profound antichemotactic effect of the group B type III capsular polysaccharide[66] and an inhibitor of C5a,[74] both of which may decrease the nonspecific host responses, prolonging the time for organisms to multiply and establish infected foci. These observations correlate with the human pathology, where there is often minimal inflammatory response despite the presence of bacteria in the lung or other tissue.[69]

The pathogenesis of the nonsuppurative sequelae of group A infections has yet to be fully elucidated. Several examples of the cross-reactivity between M proteins and components of heart, brain, and connective tissue have now been convincingly confirmed and add weight to the long-held hypotheses of autoimmune mechanisms for rheumatic valvular disease,[55] Sydenham's chorea,[56] and skin manifestations.[57] Although multiple complex factors appear to be involved in disease process, these and other studies have identified M protein epitopes that cross-react with myosin, DNA, and α-helically coiled proteins such as tropomyosin, actin, and keratin.[142] Antigenic mimicry between cell wall carbohydrate moieties and cytokeratin[57] may eventually help explain the occurrence of erythema marginatum, subcutaneous nodules, rheumatic arthritis, and perhaps streptococcal-associated guttate psoriasis. The diverse manifestations of acute rheumatic fever might be explained in part by the specificity and titer of antibodies cross-reactive with different tissue components. In a similar fashion, acute glomerulonephritis may involve the development of antibodies that cross-react with basement membrane collagen and laminin.[143] The cationic charge of the antigens may also influence their affinity for the glomerular basement membrane and the nature of immune complexes formed. Another feature of nephritogenic streptococci is the presence of a nephritis strain-associated protein.[61] This distinctive low-molecular-weight streptokinase is a plasminogen activator and could induce proliferation of cells, release of inflammatory products, and activate complement, thus contributing to known pathological features of the disease.

The pathogenesis of dental caries, recently reviewed by van Houte,[11] involves a dynamic relationship among dental plaque organisms, dietary carbohydrates, and mucosal host defenses. Dietary carbohydrates favor the growth of *S. mutans* and lactobacilli, which in turn facilitate the lowering of pH, attachment of organism to dental surfaces, and demineralization of tooth emanel.

7.2. Immunity

Specific immunity to streptococcal infections is thought to depend on the development of antibodies to capsular and other surface determinants. Antibody assays for various streptococcal antigens have been noted in Section 3.4.2, and current developments in streptococcal vaccines are further discussed in Section 9.6. Although most of our knowledge of the immune response relates to the occurrence of antibodies in the serum, recent studies of mucosal immunity suggest that the first line of host defenses are at the local level. The precise role of secretory antibodies in preventing, modifying, or eradicating bacterial colonization is not presently understood. Conversely, the effects of bacterial antigens at respiratory and gastrointestinal sites are poorly understood in regard to the systemic antibody response and the development of autoantibodies. In some cases it is likely that the organisms have developed a form of mimicry to confuse or evade the immune response of the host. Many streptococci have antigens that cross-react with other organisms, common foodstuffs, or components of the host's own tissue. Antibodies undoubtedly have functions other than protection against disease. They are known to be important in the recovery from established infection and probably function in the removal of antigens from local and systemic sites.

Assays for group A streptococcal antibodies (Table 5) are used clinically to determine if a patient has had a recent infection.[52] Although humans normally make antibodies to streptolysin O and other extracellular components, only antibodies to M proteins are associated with protection against subsequent disease.[53] Serum IgG antibodies to M proteins arise in response to infection or immunization and can initiate bactericidal activity in whole blood opsonophagocytic assays. These antibodies, however, are not as efficient as secretory IgA antibodies in protecting mice against infection via the intranasal route. Intranasal immunization of volunteers with purified M protein resulted in greater resistance to colonization with live streptococci than did subcutaneous immunization, and serum antibody response was not a reliable predictor of resistance to pharyngitis. At present, group A vaccines remain experimental, but it appears that local immune mechanisms may be more efficiently utilized and less likely to result in systemic side effects.

Antibodies to the capsular polysaccharides of group B streptococci are thought to mediate protection against systemic invasion. This concept is based on the finding that few infants with group B streptococcal disease have antibodies to the offending type, and that antibodies are protective against bacterial challenge in animal models.[144] Naturally occurring antibodies in mothers are often of the IgM class and do not readily cross the placenta,[145] and less IgG antibody is transferred to the premature than to the full-term fetus. Despite the presumed importance of antibodies, it should be pointed out that the prevalence of group B streptococcal antibodies is generally low, with about 6% of cord sera having >2 μg/ml against types Ia, II, and III in a defined population.[7] Thus, the vast majority of infants are "antibody deficient," whether colonized or not, yet only a small number develop disease, even when exposed to infected amniotic fluid *in utero*.[146] The presence of mucosal antibodies may modify colonization, but so far a clearly defined role for secretory immunity is not apparent.

Most of our knowledge of pneumococcal immunity comes from studies of purified polysaccharide vaccines.[31] Adults respond well to most of the antigens, but infants respond poorly. Children over 2 years of age have more consistent responses but still respond poorly to types common in childhood illnesses, especially types 6 and 14. Although repeated doses of purified (unconjugated) capsular vaccines produce little or no booster effect, systemic tolerance does not appear to develop in humans. Efforts to improve the immunogenicity of vaccines by coupling the polysaccharides to protein carriers appear to elicit T-helper-cell cooperation and greatly improve the immunogenicity of these antigens in young children.[147,148] Theoretically, this approach should also increase the proportion of IgG antibodies. The B-cell response can be monitored by enumerating the peripheral blood leukocytes that secrete specific antibodies at about 7 days after systemic immunization.[149] The majority of cells secreted IgA antibodies, although the later serum response was predominantly IgG and IgM. The secretory antibody response was relatively modest. There is no consensus as to what constitutes a protective serum antibody level, whether IgG is required in preference to IgM antibodies, or what role secretory antibodies play in vaccine-induced immunity.[31]

8. Patterns of Host Response

8.1. Clinical Features

The manifestations of streptococcal diseases are remarkably diverse. Their clinical presentation, diagnosis, and therapy are discussed in detail in many of the medical, pediatric, and infectious disease textbooks. The most common and most important diseases caused by the major streptococcal group are listed in Table 6. Diseases associated with other streptococci are noted in Tables 1 and 2.

The typical form of group A streptococcal respiratory disease in children and adults is acute exudative pharyngitis. The onset is abrupt, with fever, chills, a sore throat with pain on swallowing, malaise, and headache, often with abdominal pain, nausea, or vomiting. On physical examination, the pharyngeal mucosae are erythematous, edematous, and streaked with a purulent nonadherent exudate over the tonsils or posterior pharynx; petechiae may be present. The anterior cervical lymph nodes may be enlarged and are usually acutely tender. In young children the findings may be less specific, often with fever and lymphadenitis but relatively little inflammation of the upper respiratory mucosae. Mild or subclinical infection may occur at any age and may be missed. This is of concern because up to half of patients developing rheumatic fever do not give a clear history of an antecedent sore throat. With scarlet fever the pharyngitis is accompanied within about 24 hr by a fine red exanthem beginning on the trunk and intertriginous areas, later spreading to the extremities. The face is usually spared, but the tongue may be inflamed, with a "strawberry" appearance. Careful auscultation of the heart should be part of the physical examination on all patients with acute streptococcal sore throat or scarlet fever.

Streptococcal impetigo may appear as single lesions of the epidermis, frequently on the lower extremities, spreading to other areas as new insect bites or breaks in the skin become infected. Early lesions are pustular and rapidly develop into mature lesions about 1 cm in diameter with a characteristic honeylike crust. Lesions may become concomitantly infected by streptococci, which may be resistant to penicillin therapy. Erysipelas is a serious fulminant form of cellulitis that appears as an elevated erythematous lesion with a rapidly advancing well-demarcated border. Erysipelas often involves the face, a surgical wound, an umbilical stump, or a chicken pox lesion. The patient is febrile, toxic, and may be bacteremic. Necrotizing faciitis is a deep-seated infection of subcutaneous tissue that destroys fascia and fat, usually sparing skin and muscle. The patient may be diabetic or otherwise debilitated. Recently reported cases have occurred mainly in previously healthy individuals who had trivial or inapparent trauma at the affected site. A hallmark, though nonspecific, is the rapid progression from tenderness to severe pain at the site of infection. Infections may become gangrenous and require surgical debridement or fasciotomy.[4]

Streptococcal toxic shock has been observed with increasing frequency in Europe and North America during the past 5 years.[4,150] Persons may be affected at all ages, usually without predisposing or underlying diseases. Most cases involve a skin or soft tissue focus of infection or pneumonia (as in the case of puppeteer Jim Henson), and most patients are bacteremic. In children a large proportion of cases are associated with infected chicken pox lesions. Proposed criteria for diagnosis of streptococcal toxic shock are given in Table 7.[150] This syndrome differs from other serious streptococcal infections, and to

Table 6. Diseases Associated with Major Streptococcal Groups

Group A streptococci	Group B streptococci	Pneumococci	Enterococci
Most common	Early-onset neonatal disease	Infants and children	Nosocomial
Pharyngitis/tonsillitis	Undifferentiated sepsis	Otitis media	Bacteremia
Scarlet fever	Meningitis	Conjunctivitis	Intra-abdominal infection
Impetigo/pyoderma	Pneumonia	Pneumonia	Surgical wounds
Cellulitis	Bacteremia	Bacteremia	Burn wounds
Less common	Maternal infections	Meningitis	Vascular catheter
Toxic shock syndrome (Table 7)	Amnionitis	Epiglottitis	Urinary tract infection
Peritonsillar abscess	Endometritis	Adults	Postpartum infections
Mastoiditis	Urinary tract infection	Sinusitis	Community acquired
Sinusitis	Bacteremia/sepsis	Pneumonia	Urinary tract infection
Otitis media	Septic abortion	Pleural empyema	Endocarditis
Erysipelas	Bacteremia	Endocarditis	Biliary infection
Pneumonia/empyema	Late-onset neonatal disease	Meningitis	Pelvic infection
Puerperal sepsis	Meningitis	Endocarditis	
Meningitis	Bacteremia/sepsis		
Endocarditis	Bone and joint infection		
Proctitis	Skin and soft tissue infection		
Vulvovaginitis	Otitis media		
Nonsuppurative sequelae	Omphalitis		
Acute rheumatic fever			
Acute glomerulonephritis			

Table 7. Proposed Criteria for Diagnosis of Streptococcal Toxic Shock[a]

I. The isolation of group A streptococci
   A. From a normally sterile site, such as blood, CSF, surgical wound, pleural fluid, etc.
   B. From a nonsterile site, such as throat, open wound, or superficial skin lesion, or vagina

and

II. Clinical signs of severity
   A. Hypotension; systolic blood pressure ≤ 90 mm Hg in adults or < 5th percentile for age in children

   and

   B. Two or more of the following:
      1. Renal impairment evidenced by elevated creatinine ≥ 2 mg/dL (177 μmole/liter) or twice the upper limit of normal for age; or, for patients with preexisting renal disease, ≥ 2 times baseline level
      2. Coagulopathy: thrombocytopenia (< 100,000/mm^3) or disseminated intravascular coagulation, defined by prolonged clotting time, low fibrinogen, and presence of fibrin degradation products
      3. Liver involvement: elevated liver enzymes or total bilirubin ≥ twice the upper limit of normal for age; or, for patients with preexisting liver disease, ≥ 2 times baseline level
      4. "Adult" (acute) respiratory distress syndrome (ARDS), defined by onset of diffuse pulmonary infiltrates and hypoxemia in absence of cardiac failure; or evidence of diffuse capillary leak manifested by acute generalized edema, or pleural or peritoneal effusions with hypoalbuminemia
      5. Generalized erythematous macular rash, which may desquamate
      6. Soft tissue necrosis including necrotizing fasciitis, myositis, or gangrene

A *definite* case is defined by isolation of group A streptococci from a normally sterile site (IA) plus hypotension (IIA) and supporting clinical signs of severity (IIB). A case is defined as *probable* if the culture was from a nonsterile site (IB) and it fulfills the clinical signs of severity (IIA + B), when no other etiology for the illness can be identified.

[a]Adapted from The Working Group on Severe Streptococcal Infections.[150]

Table 8. Jones Criteria (Revised) for Guidance in the Diagnosis of Acute Rheumatic Fever, as Recommended by the American Heart Association

Major manifestations	Minor manifestations
Carditis	Clinical
Polyarthritis	Fever
Chorea	Arthralgia
Erythema marginatum	Previous rheumatic fever or rheumatic heart disease
Subcutaneous nodules	Laboratory
	Acute phase reactions: abnormal erythrocyte sedimentation rate, C-reactive protein, or leukocytosis
	Prolonged P-R interval

Supporting evidence of streptococcal infection:
- Positive throat culture for group A streptococcus or positive rapid streptococcal antigen test
- Increased or rising antistreptolysin O or other streptococcal antibody

The presence of two major, or one major and two minor, manifestations *plus* evidence of a preceding streptococcal infection indicates a high probability of rheumatic fever.

Manifestations with a long latent period, such as chorea and late-onset carditis, are exempt from the latter requirement. The WHO Study Group recommends that the following groups be considered separately and exempted from the Jones criteria: "pure" chorea, insidious or late-onset carditis, and rheumatic recurrence.[151]

some extent from staphylococcal toxic shock, by the rapid development of hypotension and multiorgan failure early in the course of streptococcal toxic shock.

The nonsuppurative sequelae of group A infections may present acutely or insidiously. Acute rheumatic fever varies greatly in its manifestations, with the diagnosis being made with the guidance of the Jones Criteria (updated in 1992),[151] described in Table 8. The onset is typically abrupt, with fever and polyarthritis. Myocarditis or valvulitis, most commonly involving the mitral valve, occurs in about half of patients suffering their first attack. Carditis may be the only major manifestation in some patients and may develop insidiously, presenting as heart failure without any clear history of prior rheumatic fever or obvious streptococcal infection.[3,151] Because of difficulties in making the diagnosis, other conditions, such as collagen–vascular diseases and infective endocarditis, must be considered whenever acute rheumatic fever is suspected. Acute glomerulonephritis presents fewer diagnostic problems. A recent skin or throat infection is usually evident by examination, history, culture, or antibody tests. The urine is dark, containing many red blood cells and casts. The patient usually has edema and elevated blood pressure; the blood urea nitrogen and creatinine are usually elevated and the C3 complement level is low. With appropriate acute care, nearly all patients have a complete recovery.

Group B streptococcal disease in the neonate usually begins *in utero* with nonspecific symptoms appearing within the first few hours of birth.[101,115] Unexplained apnea, respiratory distress, temperature instability, or poor feeding may be the only clues to early-onset disease. Infection usually takes the form of undifferentiated sepsis with, or more often without, meningitis. The disease is well advanced by the time hypoxia, cyanosis, acidosis, or vascular collapse becomes obvious. Lung involvement is frequent, but the chest X ray is typical of hyaline membrane disease more often than of discrete pneumonia. Similarly, there is rarely a CSF pleocytosis even when bacteria are recovered from the spinal fluid. In general, the inflammatory response parallels the maturity of the infant, the specificity of clinical signs and symptoms, and to some extent the prognosis. Late-onset infections, occurring beyond the immediate newborn period, often tend to be more localized and have a better outcome. Meningitis is common, but sepsis without meningitis is frequently seen.(101) Bacteremia or meningitis may be associated with an infective focus, such as omphalitis, otitis media, or osteomyelitis. The long-term outcome of infants who survive group B streptococcal meningitis is generally good. Very occasionally, neonates develop similar disease due to group G streptococci or pneumococci. Maternal group B streptococcal disease may occur during gestation, notably urinary tract infections and septic abortion.(104) Infection around the time of delivery, especially amnionitis, is a threat to both fetus and mother.(104,146) Endometritis and bacteremia are the most frequent postpartum infections. Endocarditis is an unusual complication of perinatal infection or septic abortion and is more often seen in older individuals with some underlying heart disease or other predisposing condition.(152)

Group B streptococcal disease also occurs in adult men and nonpregnant women. A recent survey of invasive group B infections in metropolitan Atlanta hospitals included skin, soft tissue, or bone infections (36%), bacteremia without focus (30%), urosepsis (14%), pneumonia (9%), and peritonitis (7%).(105) Another excellent clinical series, which also included data on group A, C, F, and G streptococcal infections, found that the case mortality rate was 31% among adults with group B streptococcal bacteremia.(152) Two thirds of all patients were over 50 years of age, 22% had primary bacteremia, 25% had underlying nonhematologic malignancies, and 19% had diabetes mellitus.

There is now good evidence that group C streptococci are a cause of endemic pharyngitis in adults in open populations.(153) Of the several streptococci falling into serological group C, it appears that large-colony *S. equisimilis* is more likely to be associated with clinical disease than the tiny-colony *S. anginosis* ("milleri group").(154) The presence of these organism must be determined by throat culture, because the rapid streptococcus antigen detection kits are specific for group A streptococci.

The clinical features of pneumococcal disease vary with the site of infection and the age of the patient. Meningitis in young infants does not commonly present with neck stiffness and headache, as it does in adults, but more often with nonspecific symptoms, such as fever, irritability or inconsolable crying, poor feeding, or vomiting. Patients presenting with a second episode of meningitis must be suspected of having a CSF leak, skull fracture, or immunologic deficiency. Pneumonia in children is similar to that seen in adults, but classic features of chills, hacking cough, pleuritic pain, and rusty sputum may be subdued or absent. Bacteremia in children is associated with pneumonia in about a third of cases, with otitis media in another third, and the remainder with no focus of infection.(119) While most infants with bacteremia present with fever, leukocytosis, and a clinically apparent focus of infection, some have occult bacteremia with few physical findings and a marginal leukocytosis.

8.2. Diagnosis

The isolation and identification of streptococci from properly cultured infected sites provides the definitive means of establishing the diagnosis. A careful evaluation of the patient is essential in forming an accurate clinical diagnosis, after which the physician must decide what sites are to be cultured and what ancillary tests are appropriate. Streptococcal pharyngitis cannot be reliably diagnosed without a throat culture or direct antigen detection, because many other agents may cause acute pharyngitis. Conversely, an asymptomatic carrier may have a positive throat culture coincidental with a viral pharyngitis. It is in the best interest of the patient and the community to avoid prescribing antibiotics without a specific indication; it is also preferable to treat a positive throat culture rather than risk untoward sequelae. In some cases, however, it is valuable to confirm the diagnosis by antibody tests and follow-up cultures. The efficacy of treatment regimens depends on accurate etiologic diagnoses. Patients with recurrent infection may actually prove to be chronic carriers or have multiple disease episodes due to different streptococcal serotypes. A definitive diagnosis is needed for the clinical management of patients with nephritis or symptoms suggesting rheumatic fever. Patients with toxic shock syndrome require a precise bacteriologic diagnosis by cultures of blood or other materials, because *Staphylococcus aureus* is even a more common etiology, and treatment may require use of different antibiotics.

The microbiological diagnosis of other forms of streptococcal disease is no less important, inasmuch as it directs both the clinical approach and the choice of antibiotics. Blood cultures may be indicated when infection is suspected in the absence of an obvious infected site, especially for those at risk for nosocomial disease and infants who may have occult bacteremias. Cultures of blood, spinal fluid, skin, lung or empyema, or sinus or middle ear fluid may be required to confirm the appropriateness of antibiotics selected empirically upon suspicion of infection. While most streptococci remain susceptible to the penicillins, some pneumococci are intermediate or resistant, as are many oral and enteric species. With the exception of streptococcal pharyngitis, cultures of normal carriage sites, including the nasopharynx and lower bowel, are rarely useful in making an etiologic diagnosis of clinically diagnosed infection. Otitis media, for example, is frequently caused by the pneumococcus, but pneumococci are frequently isolated from the nasopharynx of children with otitis media due to *Haemophilus influenzae*. Similarly, many infants are colonized by group B streptococci at delivery, but relatively few are infected. In some instances, however, it may not be possible to obtain a definitive culture, as is often the case in pneumonia. A sputum culture growing pneumococci, in a patient with an alveolar consolidation on chest X ray and a typical clinical course, supports the diagnosis of "putative" pneumococcal pneumonia.

9. Control and Prevention

9.1. General Preventive Measures

Personal hygiene, adequate nutrition and housing, health education, and access to medical care are all important factors in prevention of streptococcal diseases. Inspection of food and milk production and proper pasteurization of dairy products are taken for granted in most developed countries but remain problems in certain areas. Strict asepsis is required in surgical and obstetric procedures. Simple infection control measures, especially hand washing, must be continually encouraged, and attention must be paid to the health of hospital employees working in patient areas.

9.2. Antibiotics in Treatment and Prevention of Group A Streptococcal Disease

Primary prevention of acute rheumatic fever consists of identifying and treating persons with acute streptococcal pharyngitis, as described in a practice guideline recently developed by the Infectious Disease Society of America.[20] Antibiotic therapy is aimed at eradicating streptococci from the respiratory tract. Shulman *et al.*[155] make the case that penicillin remains the drug of choice for treatment of streptococcal pharyngitis. Penicillin may be given as a single intramuscular injection of (long-acting) benzathine penicillin or as a 10-day course of oral phenoxymethyl penicillin. Other oral penicillins, such as amoxicillin and dicloxacillin, are also effective but are more expensive and offer no particular advantage. The older oral cephalosporins (cephalexin, cefaclor, cephradine, cefadroxil) are effective in a number of conventional 10-day dose regimens. Several newer cephalosporins (cefprozil, cefpodoxime, loracarbef) are equally effective; 5-day therapeutic regimens are currently under investigation but will not be recommended without further evaluation. Erythromycin is a well-established alternative drug for penicillin-allergic patients, except in some areas of eastern Asia or eastern Europe where resistance may be a problem. Clindamycin is effective but is costly and has a small potential risk of pseudomembranous enterocolitis. Tetracyclines, sulfonamides, and chloramphenicol are not effective.

Control of streptococcal infections within populations has been an effective means of reducing exposure in households and institutional settings. Mass prophylaxis with benzathine penicillin has been used in some epidemic situations but is now chiefly confined to certain military populations[111] (see Section 5.9). Eradication of pharyngeal carriage of group A streptococci using oral antibiotic regimens has been attempted with varying degrees of success. Oral clindamycin for 10 days is the currently accepted regimen.[110] Another regimen is benzathine penicillin plus rifampin for the last 4 days of therapy. Short 4-day courses of either rifampin or cefixime were somewhat effective in adults but less so in children. Patients with symptomatic streptococcal sore throat may remain infectious for 24 hr after the onset of therapy and should not return to work, school, or day care before completing a full 24 hr of antibiotic therapy.[138]

Secondary prevention consists of the regular administration of antibiotic to persons who have had rheumatic fever in order to prevent subsequent group A infections that could trigger recurrent attacks or exacerbate existing rheumatic heart disease.[20] Secondary prophylaxis is cost-effective, reduces the risk of recurrence, and in many patients allows for healing of valvular damage occurring in the initial attack. Long-acting intramuscular penicillin is usually given at monthly intervals. Results of a 12-year controlled trial have now shown that intramuscular benzathine penicillin is more effective given every 3 weeks, compared to every 4 weeks, and should be recommended especially in areas where rheumatic fever is more prevalent.[156] Alternatively, oral penicillin may be given daily, but lack of compliance is a major problem. Patients unable to take penicillin may be given a sulfonamide or erythromycin. The duration of secondary prophylaxis is not certain but must be tailored to the individual. Patients with valvular rheumatic heart disease are given prolonged, even lifelong, prophylaxis. Those without cardiac involvement should have prophylaxis for at least 5 years and at least through age 18 years. Prophylaxis may be safely discontinued in young adults without carditis, provided that they have adequate medical follow-up and prompt culture and treatment of pharyngitis episodes.[157] Patients with rheumatic carditis as part of their initial attack are at greater risk for more serious carditis recurrences and should be given prophylaxis well into adulthood and perhaps for life.

Patients who have had isolated chorea as the only manifestation of rheumatic fever appear to be at much less risk for carditis during subsequent recurrences. Most authorities recommend that these patients receive prophylaxis until age 21 or for at least 5 years, whichever is longer. Some patients have a syndrome of poststreptococcal reactive arthritis without fulfilling Jones' criteria. A few such patients have been described who had silent or delayed mitral insufficiency, and one patient without initial cardiac involvement developed acute rheumatic fever 18 months later.[158] It has been suggested that these patients should receive prophylaxis, or alternatively receive prophylaxis for up to 1 year at which point it may be discontinued if no evidence of carditis develops.[20]

Patients with rheumatic heart disease, as well as others with prosthetic valves, other valvular lesions, and probably mitral valve prolapse, are at risk for developing infective endocarditis when undergoing dental or surgical manipulations. Since the usual secondary prophylaxis regimens are inadequate for preventing endocarditis, additional short-term antibiotic prophylaxis is required for dental procedures that cause bleeding; when gingival disease is present; for respiratory procedures including tonsillectomy, adenoidectomy, bronchoscopy, or mucosal biopsy; or for genitourinary or gastrointestinal procedures, such as prostate resection or intestinal biopsy. Recommended antibiotic regimens vary and are updated periodically.[159] High-risk patients, who have prosthetic valves, severely damaged native valves, or a history of previous endocarditis, are usually given penicillin or ampicillin plus gentamicin, to cover oral or enteric streptococci as well as other organisms. Antibiotic doses are given 1 hr prior and 6 hr after the procedure. "Standard-risk" patients are usually given only a penicillin for dental manipulations, but an aminoglycoside is added for genitourinary or gastrointestinal procedures. Patients allergic to penicillin or who are on long-term penicillin prophylaxis are given erythromycin or vancomycin.

The prevention of acute glomerulonephritis by antibiotic therapy has not been convincingly demonstrated, and prophylaxis may not be practical in most patient populations. Prompt treatment of minor skin trauma and insect bites with topical antibiotic ointment has been shown to reduce the occurrence of streptococcal skin infections and could reduce the risk of subsequent nephritis.[139]

9.3. Surgical Approaches to Recurrent Group A Streptococcal Disease

Tonsillectomy or tonsillectomy with adenoidectomy are frequently performed because of recurrent throat infections. Although children who have surgery experience fewer throat infections over the subsequent 2 years, the difference in rates compared to controls is not impressive. These findings were confirmed by Paradise *et al.*[160] in a carefully controlled study with stringent entry criteria. Surgical intervention was beneficial for severely affected children over at least the 2 years following surgery. Nevertheless, a substantial proportion of those managed nonsurgically had relatively little throat infection during the period of study, and the actual reduction in group A streptococcal infection rates was small. Their results appeared to "justify but by no means to mandate the performance of tonsillectomy" in carefully selected children. Treatment should be individualized and should be considered only for severely affected children. More clearly defined indications for surgical intervention include patients with peritonsillar abscess or severe obstructive symptoms.

9.4. Intrapartum Chemoprophylaxis against Group B Streptococcal Disease

Efforts to prevent neonatal group B streptococcal infections have evolved over the past decade from small clinical trials to clinical care guidelines now adopted by the major US obstetric and pediatric societies. Because most neonatal infections begin *in utero*, a dose of "prophylactic" penicillin given to the infant at delivery did little to stem the progress of established disease.[115] A more effective approach, reported in a landmark study by Boyer and Gotoff,[161] was based on the use of ampicillin given during labor to selected women who were colonized by group B streptococci and had one or more risk factors associated with infection in neonates. This approach was highly focused, limiting antibiotic exposure to a small proportion of mothers but offering no protection to many neonates, whose mothers may present with no risk factors. Because of logistical difficulties in obtaining and processing cultures and the problem of women coming late or not at all for prenatal care, other investigators developed strategies based on maternal risk factors alone. This led, in 1992, to the promulgation of two divergent sets of recommendations proposed by the American Academy of Pediatrics (AAP) and by the American College of Obstetricians and Gynecologists (ACOG). The AAP guidelines stressed the use of third-trimester cultures of mothers and recommended intrapartum prophylaxis for colonized mothers with certain risk factors. The ACOG guidelines used similar criteria for initiation of antibiotic prophylaxis but did not depend on third-trimester cultures. The AAP approach was more difficult and costly but limited antibiotic use to about 5% of mothers. The ACOG approach was logistically easier and eliminated the cost of antepartum cultures. However, it required that about 25% of mothers be given antibiotics, increasing the likelihood of untoward drug reactions and raising the possibility of increased antibiotic resistance in other bacteria. Considerable debate ensued, resulting in little acceptance of either protocol.

In 1996, the CDC, supported by experts from the ACOG, AAP, and other professional organization, developed a set of guidelines that combined the essential features of both ACOG and AAP approaches. For further background and details of the new guidelines, the reader should review the CDC consensus report,[162] the ACOG policy statement,[163] and the revised AAP guidelines.[164] The combined approach has the following key elements:

1. Intrapartum penicillin should be given to mothers who have had a previous infant with invasive group B streptococcal disease; to mothers who develop group B streptococcal bacteruria during the current pregnancy; and to those delivering at <37 weeks' gestation.
2. All pregnant women should be screened at 35–37 weeks' gestation by obtaining vaginal and anorectal swabs processed with selective culture methods. If the screening culture is negative for group B streptococci, then no intrapartum prophylaxis is needed. If the screening culture is positive, intrapartum penicillin should be offered. If no culture was done or if results are not known at the time of labor, prophylaxis should be given if the mother has a temperature ⩾100.4°F (⩾38.0°C) or if membranes are ruptured ⩾18 hr.
3. The management of infants whose mothers receive intrapartum prophylaxis remains empiric, and recommendations are not meant to be restrictive. If the infant shows signs or symptoms of sepsis, or if the infant is born at <35 weeks' gestation, the physician should do a full diagnostic evaluation with a complete blood count with differential and cultures of blood and cerebrospinal fluid if indicated; this should followed by empiric antibiotic therapy, with the duration depending on culture results and clinical course. If the infant is asymptomatic and ⩾35 weeks' gestation, and the mother received intrapartum penicillin >4 hr (usually at least two doses), then no evaluation or therapy is needed, but the infants should be observed closely for at least 48 hr. If an asymptomatic infant is born to a mother receiving prophylaxis <4 hr (one dose), then a limited evaluation, including complete blood count with differential and blood culture, and observation ⩾48 hr are warranted.

This strategy represents a number of compromises. While it promotes universal screening cultures, it allows for risk-factor management for situations in which cultures are not readily available or results are unknown. Delaying the screening culture to 35–37 weeks' gestation enhances the reliability of both positive and negative predictive values. Although most mothers who begin labor at <37 weeks would be given prophylaxis, this represents only about 10% of deliveries, but group B streptococcal disease tends to be more severe in this age group. Penicillin was selected as the antibiotic of choice in order to narrow the antibiotic spectrum and reduce the use of ampicillin or cephalosporins. Clindamycin or erythromycin are alternatives for penicillin-allergic mothers, but these drugs have not been studied systematically in this setting. Physicians remain free to use other antibiotics as indicated by clinical considerations that go beyond the guidelines. Although the 1996 guidelines were developed on the basis of a number of prospective studies, these guidelines have not been subjected to any large-scale controlled experience.

Several reports have called attention to instances of failure of intrapartum antibiotics to prevent group B streptococcal sepsis.[165,166] In a retrospective series, Ascher *et al.*[166] identified 18 (out of 96) infants who developed sepsis despite antepartum maternal antibiotics. However, the median number of antepartum antibiotic doses was one (range 1–21), with a median time of 4 hr prior to delivery. Neither the 1992 AAP nor ACOG guidelines was specifically followed. These observations are important, because they demonstrate that intrapartum antibiotics are unlikely to prevent all neonatal infections, as originally cautioned by Boyer and Gotoff.[161] It is also apparent that most of the "prophylaxis" failures were actually failures to eradicate infections that were already well established by the time of delivery.

Prevention of neonatal infections by vaginal chlorhexadine disinfection during labor has also been investigated.[167] A reduction in transmission of group B streptococci from mother to infant has been demonstrated, but numbers have been too small to assess an effect of prevention of infections. This approach might reduce the number of infections that develop as a result of colonization of infants during delivery, but as with intrapartum antibiotics, it should not be expected to affect infections that are already established *in utero*. Most authorities recognize inherent limitations in chemoprophylactic approaches to prevention. Although there has been considerable progress in developing vaccines against group B streptococci,[168] it is not known if vaccine immunity will be protective to the immature fetus, which normally receives a minimal amount of maternal antibody. Thus, chemoprophylactic strategies may serve a purpose well into the future.

9.5. Passive Immune Prophylaxis against Streptococcal Infections

The administration of gamma globulin has been employed for prevention of various bacterial infections in immunodeficient patients. The spectrum of host defense abnormalities that may benefit from this approach now includes patients with hypogammaglobulinemias, IgG subclass deficiencies, malignancy and immunosuppression, severe burns, bone marrow transplantation, and HIV infection.[169] Immunoglobulin preparations suitable for intravenous administration are still under investigation for prevention and adjunctive therapy of group B streptococcal disease in neonates, but implementation of this approach is hampered by logistical factors and the relative infrequency of streptococcal infections. A specialized hyperimmune globulin has been prepared from plasma donors immunized with pneumococcal and *H. influenzae* type b, and meningococcal vaccines. This bacterial polysaccharide immune globulin (BPIG) has been shown to be effective in reducing the number of pneumococcal and *H. influenzae* type b infections in high-risk Apache and other Native American infant populations.[170] There is also some evidence for the efficacy of BPIG in preventing pneumococcal otitis media in suburban middle-class infants.[171] It should be noted that passive immunotherapy was used for a short time with considerable success in the treatment of pneumococcal pneumonia just prior to the advent of penicillin.[172]

9.6. Immunization against Streptococcal Infections

A vaccine against rheumatic fever has been the holy grail of many investigators over the years. The difficulties involved are considerable and as yet only partially solved. The multitude of M protein types makes a simple vaccine virtually impossible. Although a single broadly protective M protein epitope does not appear to exist,[53] certain conserved epitopes have been found to be common among different M types. This feature has been used to make oral synthetic peptide vaccines (coupled to a cholera toxin subunit adjuvant) that induce mucosal immunity in mice and reduce the effects of nasopharyngeal challenge of streptococci.[53,173] Another approach uses cloned M protein expressed in live attenuated strains of *Salmonella* given orally to mice.[174] Dale *et al.*[175] have constructed a recombinant tetravalent vaccine containing M protein epitopes that are protective (opsonic) but not tissue cross-reactive. A second generation of this vaccine has been coupled to *Escherichia coli* labile toxin and given to mice intranasally.[176] The possibility of inducing antibodies that cross-react with human tissue is of obvious concern but could be minimized by the oral route of administration and by the identification and selection of vaccine epitopes that have no homology with host proteins.[142]

Group B polysaccharide vaccines have been under investigation for over a decade. The goal of the vaccine approach is to immunize women in order to induce antibody that will later be capable of protecting the fetus against early-onset disease and perhaps afford protection for several months against late-onset disease. Ideally, a vaccine should induce antibodies of the IgG class and be effective against all four major serotypes; it should be safe for administration to pregnant women and it should induce long-lived immunity if administered prior to pregnancy. One experimental vaccine consisting of purified type III polysaccharide has been tested in a small number of women at about 30 weeks of gestation.[177] Results indicated that some antibody could be induced in about 60% of mothers and that this antibody was predominantly IgG with functional activity demonstrated in the infant's cord serum. The immunogenicity of group B polysaccharides has been significantly improved by coupling to tetanus toxoid. A tetravalent conjugate vaccine (types Ia, Ib, II, and III) has been tested in a mouse immunization–neonatal challenge model.[168] Assuming the eventual development of an appropriate vaccine, it will still be necessary to carefully define the target population. There is yet little enthusiasm for administering vaccines to pregnant women, because of liability issues, and it is possible that the target population would have to be broadened to include nonpregnant women of childbearing age. The prospects for protecting the more premature fetus is uncertain, since only a minimal amount of maternally derived antibody is able to cross the placenta before the last trimester. Nevertheless, it would be reasonable to suggest that any degree of protection afforded the mother would indirectly affect the fetus. Here, a better understanding of the determinants of colonization and the mechanisms of mucosal immunity is clearly needed.

Pneumococcal vaccines have been studied for nearly 80 years. Their history and current recommendations for use are summarized in Chapter 28. The current pneumococcal vaccine formulation, licensed in 1983, includes purified capsular polysaccharides of 23 pneumococcal serotypes most commonly associated with disease. The vaccine efficacy has been estimated at about 60% against bacteremic infections in adults.(178) The vaccine is vastly underutilized, but considerable debate is still going on regarding its role in preventing adult pneumococcal disease.(179,180)

The current pneumococcal vaccine is not recommended for children under 2 years of age, who respond poorly to bacterial polysaccharides in general. However, a new generation of protein-conjugated pneumococcal vaccines has been modeled after the spectacularly successful vaccines against *H. influenzae* type b (Hib)(147,148) (see Chapter 16). These vaccines contain polysaccharides selected from among the seven or so most common types in childhood infections (types 1 or 4, 6B, 9V, 14, 18C, 19F, and 23F)(120) coupled to either diphtheria toxin mutant protein (Lederle-Praxis) or meningococcal outer membrane protein complex (Merck & Co.), similar to the licensed Hib vaccines. Another vaccine currently under investigation is derived from a pneumococcal surface protein (PspA) that has been shown to be immunogenic and protective in animals.(77) A phase I trial of a candidate PspA vaccine for humans is currently in progress.

9.7. Prevention of Dental Caries

Conventional approaches to caries prevention have been succinctly reviewed by the Lewis *et al.* and the Canadian Task Force on the Periodic Health Examination.(108) Primary prevention includes fluoride, fissure sealants, dietary counseling, oral hygiene, and identification and care of individuals at high risk of developing dental caries. Patients at greatest risk are those with bulimia, Sjögren's syndrome, chemotherapy, radiation therapy, or use of drugs that reduce saliva flow over long periods.

Fluoridation of drinking water at levels of 0.7–1.2 ppm remains the single-most effective method of preventing coronal and root caries. In localities without natural or artificial fluoridation (fluoride $<$0.3 ppm), supplemental fluoride may be given by prescription for persons $>$3 years of age and for those at high risk for dental caries. Fluoride-containing toothpastes provide additional protection. Fluoride mouth washes are probably of marginal value in communities with fluoridated water. They are not intended for children under 5 years of age, who may ingest excessive amounts and be in danger of fluorosis. Professional application of topical fluoride may be helpful for high-risk individuals and patients with active caries but is not currently recommended for routine use because of the overall decline in caries incidence.

Sealing of dental pits and fissures with synthetic resins has been done for over 15 years with marked success. Sealants do not add significant protection to initially sound tooth surfaces.(181) Although application of sealants is not widely practiced, this approach is recommended for selected high-risk patients whose permanent molars have erupted within the previous 2–3 years.(108)

The need for and effectiveness of dietary counseling aimed at reducing intake of sucrose has not been established but may be indicated for high-risk individuals. Avoiding prolonged use of baby bottles and bedtime bottle propping may prevent "nursing caries," but there is not much evidence to support the notion that counseling changes this practice in many families. Traditional brushing and flossing has little or no effect on caries prevention, except as a method of applying fluoride in the form of a dentifrice. Professional cleaning (dental prophylaxis) does not prevent caries, although it may be useful for removing stains or calculus.

Vaccines against dental caries, based on antigens derived from *S. mutans*, have been under investigation for a number of years.(182,183) Several candidate vaccines have been successful in preventing caries in experimental animals. Among these are the adhesin complex (Ag I/II) involved in attachment of the bacteria to dental surfaces and the glycosyltransferases that synthesize adhesive glucan from sucrose. Novel strategies have been developed for delivery of candidate vaccines, including use of avirulent *Salmonella* genetically engineered to express *S. mutans* vaccine antigens, and attachment to the nontoxic but immunogenic B subunit of cholera toxin. Limited studies have shown that some oral vaccines induce salivary IgA antibody responses in humans, but long-term evaluations of efficacy have not been done. The major reason is that dental caries is not a life-threatening disease, and potential benefits must clearly outweigh even theoretical concerns of safety.

10. Unresolved Problems

Despite the availability of antibiotics, the diagnosis and treatment of group A streptococcal pharyngitis continue to pose problems for the clinician. The distinction between infection and carrier state is frequently blurred. The new rapid diagnostic tests make it possible to treat promptly and reduce clinical symptoms, but it is unlikely that changes in clinical practice have influenced the recent resurgence of acute rheumatic fever or of severe invasive streptococcal disease and toxic shock. Further study of epidemiological factors, pathogenic mechanisms, and host response is clearly needed. Poststreptococcal reactive arthritis and its less certain relationship with cardiac sequelae continues to present a clinical dilemma for clinicians. Group A streptococci, along with staphylococci, have been suggested as an etiology for Kawasaki disease, a vasculitis syndrome that occurs mainly in children.[184] It is hypothesized that staphylococcal toxin TSST-1 or streptococcal exotoxins act as "superantigens" and cause aberrant amplification of certain T-cell lines implicated in the disease. Group A streptococcal superantigens also seem to play a role in streptococcal toxic shock, but effects are manifested by a pattern of depletion of Vβ T-cell subsets.[185] Proof of this, however, would probably require showing that a particular antigen induced specific T-cell subsets to expand and subsequently be depleted by apoptosis (a process of programmed cell death).

Group B streptococci remain the most common cause of serious bacterial disease in newborn infants in many Western countries. Despite similar maternal colonization rates and presumably similar risk of exposure, the disease is infrequent in some areas of Europe and Asia. The reasons for this are not clear but could be of considerable practical importance. Methods for intrapartum antibiotic prophylaxis have been established but remain to be implemented on a wide scale. Meanwhile, we still have little understanding of the local and systemic defense mechanisms required to prevent infection by this usually benign organism. Other streptococci, particularly oral and enteric species, are constant companions that cause disease only under specialized circumstances. It is not clear whether some of these organisms are in fact "virulent" in certain settings, or whether the disease is due mainly to predisposing conditions in the host. The question may be moot, but answers would help us direct attention to better ways of preventing nosocomial and opportunistic infections.

Few bacteria have been studied as intensely as the pneumococci, yet our knowledge of their virulence and pathogenesis is extremely limited. It is especially curious that certain serotypes are most frequently associated with children and childhood infections. These are among the least immunogenic types but are uncommon in adults. The regulation of the immune response to pneumococcal polysaccharides is not understood, and the role of systemic and secretory antibodies has yet to be fully explored.

The unanswered questions apparent from the discussions in this chapter remain: How do streptococci cause disease, and why do some individuals become infected while others do not? Major virulence factors, such as exotoxins, enzymes, M proteins, and polysaccharide capsules, have been identified, but the pathophysiological mechanisms by which they interact with the host remain uncertain and do not completely explain the disease processes. The determinants of colonization, the defenses of the host at the mucosal level, and the development of local and systemic immunity are not well understood. More needs to be learned to facilitate the development of effective vaccines and implement other preventive measures.

ACKNOWLEDGMENTS

The author thanks Gregory Valainis and Richard Pennebaker, Division of Medical Education, Spartanburg Regional Medical Center, for review of this chapter. Data for Figs. 2 and 3 were kindly supplied by Caroline Breese Hall, University of Rochester, New York.

11. References

1. Quinn, R., Streptococcal infections, in: *Bacterial Infections in Humans*, 1st ed. (A. S. Evans and H. A. Feldman, eds.), pp. 525–552, Plenum Press, New York, 1982.
2. Stollerman, G. H., Variation in group A streptococci and the prevalence of rheumatic fever: A half-century vigil, *Ann. Intern. Med.* **118:**467–469 (1993).
3. Veasy, L. G., Tani, L. Y., and Hill, H. R., Persistence of acute rheumatic fever in the intermountain area of the United States, *J. Pediatr.* **124:**9–16 (1994).
4. Stevens, D. L., Invasive group A *Streptococcus* infections, *Clin. Infect. Dis.* **14:**2–13 (1992).
5. Lancefield, R. C., and Hare, R., The serological differentiation of pathogenic and nonpathogenic strains of hemolytic streptococci from parturient women, *J. Exp. Med.* **61:**335–349 (1935).
6. Dillon, H. C., Jr., GBS: The childhood and adolescent years, *Antibiot. Chemother.* **35:**1–9 (1985).
7. Gray, B. M., Egan, M. L., and Pritchard, D. G., The group B streptococci: From natural history to the specificity of antibodies, *Semin. Perinatol.* **14:**10–21 (1990).
8. Austrian, R., Pneumococcus: The first one hundred years, *Rev. Infect. Dis.* **3:**183–189 (1981).
9. Watson, D. A., Musher, D. M., Jacobson, J. W., *et al.*, A brief history of the pneumococcus in biomedical research: A panoply of scientific discovery, *Clin. Infect. Dis.* **17:**913–924 (1993).
10. Caufield, P. W., Cutter, G. R., and Dasanayake, A. P., Initial acquisition of mutans streptococci by infants: Evidence for a discrete window of infectivity, *J. Dent. Res.* **72:**37–45 (1993).
11. van Houte, J., Role of microorganisms in caries etiology, *J. Dent. Res.* **73:**672–681 (1994).

12. Centers for Disease Control, Recommendations for preventing the spread of vancomycin resistance, *Morbid. Mortal. Week. Rep.* **44**(RR-12):1–13 (1995).
13. Patterson, J. E., Sweeney, A., Simms, M., *et al.*, An analysis of 110 serious enterococcal infections: Epidemiology, antibiotic susceptibility, and outcome, *Medicine* **74:**191–200 (1995).
14. Taranta, A., and Markowitz, M., *Rheumatic Fever*, 2nd ed. Kluwer Academic Press, Boston, 1989.
15. Zangwill, K. N., Schuchat, A., and Wenger, J. D., Group B streptococcal disease in the United States, 1990: Report from a multistate active surveillance system, *Morbid. Mortal. Week. Rep.* **41:**SS-6, 25–32 (1992).
16. Institute of Medicine, *Emerging Infections: Microbial Threats to Health in the United States*, National Academy Press, Washington, DC, 1992.
17. Ruoff, K. L., Streptococcus, in: *Manual of Clinical Microbiology*, 6th ed. (P. R. Murray, ed.), pp. 299–307, American Society for Microbiology, Washington, DC, 1995.
18. Gray, B. M., Pass, M. A., and Dillon, H. C., Jr., Laboratory and field evaluation of selective media for isolation of group B streptococci, *J. Clin. Microbiol.* **9:**466–470 (1979).
19. Gray, B. M., Converse, G. M., III, and Dillon, H. C., Jr., Epidemiologic studies of *Streptococcus pneumoniae* in infants: Acquisition, carriage and infection during the first 24 months of life, *J. Infect. Dis.* **146:**923–933 (1980).
20. Bisno, A. L., Gerber, M. A., Gwaltney, J. M., *et al.*, Diagnosis and management of group A streptococcal pharyngitis: A practice guideline, *Clin. Infect. Dis.* **25:**574–583 (1997).
21. Ascher, D. P., Wilson, S., Mendiola, J., *et al.*, Group B streptococcal latex agglutination testing in neonates, *J. Pediatr.* **119:**458–460 (1991).
22. Tuppurainen, N., and Hallman, M., Prevention of neonatal group B streptococcal disease: Intrapartum detection and chemoprophylaxis of heavily colonized parturients, *Obstet. Gynecol.* **73:**583–587 (1989).
23. Johnson, D. R., and Kaplan, E. L., A review of the correlation of T-agglutination patterns and M-protein typing and opacity factor production in the identification of group A streptococci, *J. Med. Microbiol.* **38:**311–315 (1993).
24. Johnson, D. R., Stevens, D. L., and Kaplan, E. L., Epidemiologic analysis of group A streptococcal serotypes associated with severe systemic infections, rheumatic fever, or uncomplicated pharyngitis, *J. Infect. Dis.* **166:**374–382 (1992).
25. Dillon, H. C., Derrick, C. W., and Dillon, M. S., M-antigens common to pyoderma and acute glomerulonephritis, *J. Infect. Dis.* **103:**257–267 (1974).
26. Martin, D. R., and Single, L. A., Molecular epidemiology of group A streptococcus M type 1 infections, *J. Infect. Dis.* **167:**1112–1117 (1993).
27. Perez-Casal, J. F., Dillon, H. F., Husmann, L. K., *et al.*, Virulence of two *Streptococcus pyogenes* strains (types M1 and M3) associated with toxic-shock-like syndrome depends on an intact *mry*-like gene, *Infect. Immun.* **61:** (1993).
28. Hollingshead, S. K., Arnold, J., Readdy, T. L., *et al.*, Molecular evolution of a multigene family in a group A streptococci, *Mol. Biol. Evol.* **11**(2):208–219 (1994).
29. Wessels, M. R., DiFabio, J. L., Benedi, V.-J., *et al.*, Structural determination and immunological characterization of the type V group B *Streptococcus* capsular polysaccharide, *J. Biol. Chem.* **266:**6714–6719 (1991).
30. von Hunolstein, C., D'Ascenzi, S., Wagner, B., *et al.*, Immunochemistry of capsular type polysaccharide and virulence properties of type VI *Streptococcus agalactiae* (group B streptococci), *Infect. Immun.* **61:**1271–1280 (1993).
31. Robbins, J. B., Austrian, R., Lee, C.-J., *et al.*, Considerations for formulating the second-generation pneumococcal capsular polysaccharide vaccine with emphasis on the cross-reactive type within groups, *J. Infect. Dis.* **148:**1136–1159 (1983).
32. Crain, M. J., Waltman, W. D., II, Turner, J. S., *et al.*, Pneumococcal surface protein A (PspA) is serologically highly variable and is expressed by all clinically important capsular serotypes of *Streptococcus pneumoniae*, *Infect. Immun.* **58:**3293–3299 (1990).
33. Stein, D. S., and Nelson, K. E., Endocarditis due to nutritionally deficient streptococci, *Rev. Infect. Dis.* **9:**908–916 (1987).
34. Facklam, R. R., and Sahm, D., Enterococcus, in: *Manual of Clinical Microbiology*, 6th ed. (P. R. Murray, ed.), pp. 308–314, American Society for Microbiology, Washington, DC, 1995.
35. Pokorski, S. J., Vetter, E. A., Wollan, P. C., *et al.*, Comparison of Gen-Probe group A streptococcus direct test with culture for diagnosing streptococcal pharyngitis, *J. Clin. Microbiol.* **32:**1440–1443 (1994).
36. Hassan-King, M., Baldeh, I., Secka, O., *et al.*, Detection of *Streptococcus pneumoniae* DNA in blood cultures by PCR, *J. Clin. Microbiol.* **32:**1721–1724 (1994).
37. Virolainen, A., Salo, O., Jero, J., *et al.*, Comparison of PCR assay with bacterial culture for detecting *Streptococcus pneumoniae* in middle ear fluid of children with otitis media, *J. Clin. Microbiol.* **32:**2667–2670 (1994).
38. Saunders, N. A., Hallas, G., Goworzewska, E. T., *et al.*, PCR-enzyme-linked immunosorbent assay and sequencing as an alternative to serology for M-antigen typing of *Streptococcus pyogenes*, *J. Clin. Microbiol.* **35:**2689–2691 (1997).
39. Bingen, E., Denamur, E., Lambert-Zechovsky, N., *et al.*, DNA restriction fragment length polymorphism differentiates recurrence from relapse in treatment failures of *Streptococcus pyogenes* pharyngitis, *J. Med. Microbiol.* **37:**162–164 (1992).
40. Seppala, H., Vuopio-Varkila, J., Osterblad, M., *et al.*, Evaluation of methods for epidemiologic typing of group A streptococci, *J. Infect. Dis.* **169:**519–525 (1994).
41. Mylvaganam, H., Bjorvatn, B., Hofstad, T., *et al.*, Small-fragment restriction endonuclease analysis in epidemiological mapping of group A streptococci, *J. Med. Microbiol.* **40:**256–260 (1994).
42. Seppala, H., He, Q., Osterblad, M., *et al.*, Typing of group A streptococci by random amplified polymorphic DNA analysis, *J. Clin. Microbiol.* **32:**1945–1948 (1994).
43. Blumberg, H. M., Stephens, D. S., Licitra, C., *et al.*, Molecular epidemiology of group B streptococcal infections: use of restriction endonuclease analysis of chromosomal DNA and DNA restriction fragment length polymorphisms of ribosomal RNA genes (ribotyping), *J. Infect. Dis.* **166:**574–579 (1992).
44. Fasola, E., Livdahl, C., and Ferrieri, P., Molecular analysis of multiple isolates of the major serotypes of group B streptococci, *J. Clin. Microbiol.* **31:**2616–2620 (1993).
45. Martin, N. J., Kaplan, E. L., Gerber, M. A., *et al.*, Comparison of epidemic and endemic group G streptococci by restriction and enzyme analysis, *J. Clin. Microbiol.* **28:**1881–1886 (1990).
46. Soares, S., Kristinsson, K. G., Musser, J. M., *et al.*, Evidence for the introduction of a multiresistant clone of serotype 6B *Streptococcus pneumoniae* from Spain to Iceland in the late 1980s, *J. Infect. Dis.* **168**:158–163 (1993).

47. Hermans, P. W. M., Sluijter, M., Hoogenboezem, T., *et al.*, Comparative study of five different DNA fingerprint techniques for molecular typing of *Streptococcus pneumoniae* strains, *J. Clin. Microbiol.* **33:**1606–1612 (1995).
48. Murray, B. E., Singh, K. V., Markowitz, S. M., *et al.*, Evidence for clonal spread of a single strain of β-lactamase-producing *Enterococcus (Streptococcus) faecalis* to six hospitals in five states, *J. Infect. Dis.* **163:**780–785 (1991).
49. Musser, J. M., Kapur, V., Kanjilal, S., *et al.*, Geographic and temporal distribution and molecular characterization of two highly pathogenic clones of *Streptococcus pygogenes* expressing allelic variants of pyrogenic exotoxin (scarlet fever toxin), *J. Infect. Dis.* **167:**337–346 (1993).
50. Munoz, R., Musser, J. M., Crain, M., *et al.*, Geographic distribution of penicillin-resistant clones of *Streptococcus pneumoniae*: Characterization by penicillin-binding protein profile, surface protein A typing, and multilocus enzyme analysis, *Clin. Infect. Dis.* **15:**112–118 (1992).
51. Dougherty, B. A., and Rijn, I. V., Molecular characterization of *has*B from an operon required for hyaluronic acid synthesis in group A streptococci, *J. Biol. Chem.* **268:**7118–7124 (1993).
52. Ayoub, E. M., Immune response to group A streptococcal infections, *Pediatr. Infect. Dis. J.* **10:**S15–S19 (1991).
53. Fishcetti, V. A., Streptococcal M protein: Molecular design and biological behavior, *Clin. Microbiol. Rev.* **2:**285–314 (1989).
54. Cunningham, M. W., McCormack, J. M., Fenderson, P. G., *et al.*, Human and murine antibodies cross-reactive with streptococcal M protein and myosin recognize the sequence GLN-LYS-SER-LYS-GLN in M protein, *J. Immunol.* **143:**2677 (1989).
55. Stollerman, G. H., Rheumatogenic streptococci and autoimmunity, *Clin. Immunol. Immunopathol.* **61:**131–142 (1991).
56. Bronze, M. S., and Dale, J. B., Epitopes of streptococcal M proteins that evoke antibodies that cross-react with human brain, *J. Immunol.* **151:**2820–2828 (1993).
57. Shikhman, A. R., and Cunningham, M. W., Immunological mimicry between *N*-acetyl-β-D-glucosamine and cytokeratin peptides: Evidence for a microbially driven anti-keratin antibody response, *J. Immunol.* **152:**4375–4387 (1994).
58. Beachey, E. H., and Courtney, H. S., Bacterial adherence: The attachment of group A streptococci to mucosal surfaces, *Rev. Infect. Dis.* **9**(Suppl.)**:**S475–S481 (1987).
59. Yarnall, M., and Boyle, M. D. P., Isolation and characterization of type IIa and type IIb Fc receptors from group A streptococcus, *Scand. J. Immunol.* **24:**549–557 (1986).
60. Ginsburg, I., Streptococcal enzymes and virulence, in: *Bacterial Enzymes and Virulence* (I. A. Holder, ed.), pp. 122–144, CRC Press, Boca Raton, FL, 1985.
61. Ohkuni, H., Todome, Y., Suzuki, H., *et al.*, Immunochemical studies and complete amino acid sequence of the streptokinase from *Streptococcus pyogenes* (group A) M type 12 Strain A374, *Infect. Immun.* **60:**278–283 (1992).
62. O'Connor, S. P., and Cleary, P. P., *In vivo Streptococcus pyogenes* C5a peptidase activity: Analysis using transposon- and nitrosoguanidine-induced mutants, *J. Infect. Dis.* **156:**495–504 (1987).
63. Cleary, P. P., Kaplan, E. L., Handley, J. P., *et al.*, Clonal basis for resurgence of serious *Streptococcus pyogenes* disease in the 1980s, *Lancet* **339:**518–521 (1992).
64. Håkansson, S., Holm, S. E., and Wagner, M., Density profile of group B streptococci, type III, and its possible relation to enhanced virulence, *J. Clin. Microbiol.* **25:**714–718 (1987).
65. Gray, B. M., and Pritchard, D. G., Phase variation in the pathogenesis of group B streptococcal infections, *Zbl. Bakt.* Suppl. **22:**452–454 (1992).
66. McFall, T. L., Zimmerman, G. A., Augustine, N. H., *et al.*, Effect of group B streptococcal type-specific antigen on polymorphonuclear leukocyte function and polymorphonuclear leukocyte–endothelial cell interaction, *Pediatr. Res.* **21:**517–523 (1987).
67. Raff, H. V., Siscoe, P. J., Wolff, E. A., *et al.*, Human monoclonal antibodies to group B streptococcus, *J. Exp. Med.* **168:**905–917 (1988).
68. Lancefield, R. C., McCarty, M., and Everly, W. N., Multiple mouse-protective antibodies directed against group B streptococci, *J. Exp. Med.* **142:**165–179 (1975).
69. Payne, N. R., Burke, B. A., Day, D. L., *et al.*, Correlation of clinical and pathologic findings in early onset neonatal group B streptococcal infection with disease severity and prediction of outcome, *Pediatr. Infect. Dis. J.* **7:**836–847 (1988).
70. Cleat, P. H., and Timms, K. N., Cloning and expression in *Escherichia coli* of the Ibc protein genes of group B streptococci: Binding of human immunoglobin A to the beta antigen, *Infect. Immun.* **55:**1151–1155 (1987).
71. Pritchard, D. G., Lin, B., Willingham, T. R., *et al.*, Characterization of the group B streptococcal hyaluronate lyase, *Arch. Biochem. Biophys.* **315:**431–437 (1994).
72. Tapsall, J. W., and Phillips, E. A., The hemolytic and cytolytic activity of group B streptococcal hemolysis and its possible role in early onset group B streptococcal disease, *Pathology* **23:**139–144 (1991).
73. Jurgens, D., Sterzik, B., and Fehrenbach, F. J., Unspecific binding of group B streptococcal cocytolysin (CAMP factor) to immunoglobins and its possible role in pathogenicity, *J. Exp. Med.* **165:** 720–732 (1987).
74. Bohnsack, J. F., Zhou, X., Williams, P. A., *et al.*, Purification of the proteinase of group B streptococci that inactivates human C5a, *Biochim. Biophys. Acta* **1079:**222–228 (1991).
75. Schlievert, P. M., Gocke, J. E., and Deringer, J. R., Group B streptococcal toxic shock-like syndrome: Report of a case and purification of an associated pyrogenic toxin, *Clin. Infect. Dis.* **17:**26–31 (1993).
76. Vitharsson, G., Jonsdottir, I., Jonsson, S., *et al.*, Opzonization and antibodies to capsular and cell wall polysaccharides of *Streptococcus pneumoniae*, *J. Infect. Dis.* **170:**592–599 (1994).
77. McDaniel, L. S., Sheffield, J. S., Delucchi, P., *et al.*, PspA, a surface protein of *Streptococcus pneumoniae*, is capable of eliciting protection against pneumococci of more than one capsular type, *Infect. Immun.* **59:**222–228 (1991).
78. Boulnois, G. J., Pneumococcal proteins and the pathogenesis of disease caused by *Streptococcus pneumoniae*, *J. Gen. Microbiol.* **138:**249–259 (1992).
79. Friedland, I. R., Paris, M. M., Kickey, S., *et al.*, The limited role of pneumolysin in the pathogenesis of pneumococcal meningitis, *J. Infect. Dis.* **172:**805–809 (1995).
80. McCoy, H. E., Broder, C. C., and Lottenberg, R., Streptokinases produced by pathogenic group C streptococci demonstrate species-specific plasminogen activation, *J. Infect. Dis.* **164:**515–521 (1991).
81. Comerota, A. J., and Cohen, G. S., Thrombolytic therapy in peripheral arterial occlusive disease: Mechanisms of action and drugs available, *Can. J. Surg.* **36:**342–348 (1993).
82. Gnann, J. W., Jr., Gray, B. M., Griffin, F. M., Jr., *et al.*, Acute glomerulonephritis following group G streptococcal infection, *J. Infect. Dis.* **156:**411–412 (1987).

83. Gosling, J., Occurrence and pathogenicity of the *Streptococcus milleri* group, *Rev. Infect. Dis.* **10:**257–285 (1988).
84. Piscitelli, S. C., Shwed, J., Schreckenberger, P., *et al.*, *Streptococcus milleri* group: Renewed interest in an elusive pathogen, *Eur. J. Clin. Microbiol. Infect. Dis.* **11:**491–498 (1992).
85. Kuramitsu, H. K., Virulence factors of mutans streptococci: Role of molecular genetics, *Crit. Rev. Oral Biol. Med.* **4:**159–176 (1993).
86. Kim, K. S., and Kaplan, E. L., Association of penicillin tolerance with failure to eradicate group A streptococci from patients with pharyngitis, *J. Pediatr.* **107:**681–684 (1985).
87. Brook, I., Role of beta-lactamase-producing bacteria in the failure of penicillin to eradicate group A streptococci, *Pediatr. Infect. Dis.* **4:**491–495 (1985).
88. Gray, B. M., Pneumococcal infections in an era of multiple antibiotic resistance, *Adv. Pediatr. Infect. Dis.* **11:**55–99 (1995).
89. Jorgensen, J. H., Swenson, J. M., Tenover, F. C., *et al.*, Development of interpretive criteria and quality control limits for broth microdilution and disk diffusion antimicrobial susceptibility testing of *Streptococcus pneumoniae*, *J. Clin. Microbiol.* **32:**2448–2459 (1994).
90. Special Writing Group of the Committee on Rheumatic Fever, Endocarditis, and Kawasaki Disease of the Council on Cardiovascular Disease in the Young of the American Heart Association, *Performance Standards for Antimicrobial Susceptibility Testing*, 5th informational supplement M100-S5, National Committee for Clinical Laboratory Standards, Villanova, PA, 1994.
91. Spratt, B. G., Resistance to antibiotics mediated by target alterations, *Science* **264:**388–393 (1994).
92. Gordon, S., Swenson, J. M., Hill, B. C., *et al.*, Antimicrobial susceptibility patterns of common and unusual species of enterococci causing infection in the United States, *J. Clin. Microbiol.* **30:**2373–2378 (1992).
93. Chun, L. T., Reddy, D. V., and Yamamoto, L. G., Rheumatic fever in children and adolescents in Hawaii, *Pediatrics* **79:**549–552 (1987).
94. Martin, D. R., Voss, L. M., Walker, S. J., *et al.*, Acute rheumatic fever in Auckland, New Zealand: Spectrum of associated group A streptococci different from expected, *Pediatr. Infect. Dis. J.* **13:**264–269 (1993).
95. WHO, Cardiovascular Disease Unit, WHO programme for the prevention of rheumatic fever/rheumatic heart disease in 16 developing countries: Report from phase I (1986–1990), *Bull. WHO* **70:**213–218 (1992).
96. McLaren, M. J., Markowitz, M., and Gerber, M. A., Rheumatic heart disease in developing countries: The consequences of inadequate prevention, *Ann. Intern. Med.* **120:**243–245 (1994).
97. Ferguson, G. W., Shultz, J. M., and Bisno, A. L., Epidemiology of acute rheumatic fever in a multiethnic, multiracial urban community: The Miami–Dade County experience, *J. Infect. Dis.* **164:**720–725 (1991).
98. Marcus, R. H., Sareli, P., Pocock, W. A., *et al.*, The spectrum of severe rheumatic mitral valve disease in a developing country, *Ann. Intern. Med.* **120:**177–183 (1994).
99. Demers, B., Simor, A. E., Vellend, H., *et al.*, Severe invasive group A streptococcal infections in Ontario, Canada: 1987–1991, *Clin. Infect. Dis.* **16:**792–800 (1993).
100. Boyer, K. M., Gadzala, C. A., Burd, L. I., *et al.*, Selective intrapartum chemoprophylaxis of neonatal group B streptococcal early-onset disease. I. Epidemiologic rationale, *J. Infect. Dis.* **148:**795–801 (1983).
101. Dillon, H. C., Jr., Khare, S., and Gray, B. M., Group B streptococcal carriage and disease: A 6-year prospective study, *J. Pediatr.* **110:**31–36 (1987).
102. Mayon-White, R. T., The incidence of GBS disease in neonates in different countries, *Antibiot. Chemother.* **35:**17–27 (1985).
103. Liang, S. T., Lau, S. P., Chan, S. H., *et al.*, Perinatal colonization of group B streptococcus—An epidemiological study in a Chinese population, *Aust. NZ Obstet. Gynecol.* **26:**138–141 (1986).
104. Gray, B. M., and Dillon, H. C., Jr., GBS infections in mothers and their infants, *Antibiot. Chemother.* **35:**225–236 (1985).
105. Farley, M. M., Harvey, R. C., Stull, T., *et al.*, A population-based assessment of invasive disease due to group B streptococcus in nonpregnant adults, *N. Engl. J. Med.* **328:**1807–1811 (1993).
106. Leclercq, M. H., Barmes, D. E., and Sardo Infirri, J., Oral health: Global trends and projections, *World Health Stat. Q.* **40:**116–128 (1987).
107. Beck, J., The epidemiology of root surface caries, *J. Dent. Res.* **69:**1216–1221 (1990).
108. Lewis, D. W., Ismail, A. I., and the Canadian Task Force on the Periodic Health Examination, Periodic health examination, 1995 update: 2. Prevention of dental caries, *Can. Med. Assoc. J.* **152:**836–846 (1995).
109. Glass, R. L., Alman, J. E., and Chauncy, H. H., A 10-year longitudinal study of caries incidence rates in a sample of male adults in the USA, *Caries Res.* **21:**360–367 (1987).
110. Davies, H. D., Low, D. E., Schwartz, B., *et al.*, Evaluation of short course therapy with cefixime or rifampin for eradication of pharyngeally carried group A streptococci, *Clin. Infect. Dis.* **21:**1294–1296 (1995).
111. Gunzerhauser, J. D., Longfield, J. N., Brundage, J. F., *et al.*, Epidemic streptococcal disease among army trainees, July 1989 through June 1991, *J. Infect. Dis.* **172:**124–131 (1995).
112. Brunton, W. A. T., Infection and hospital laundry, *Lancet* **345:**1574–1575 (1995).
113. Falck, G., and Kjellander, J., Outbreak of group A streptococcal infection in a day-care center, *Pediatr. Infect. Dis. J.* **11:**914–919 (1992).
114. Gerber, M. A., Randolph, M. F., and Mayo, D. R., The group A streptococcal carrier state: A reexamination, *Am. J. Dis. Child.* **142:**562–565 (1988).
115. Pyati, S. P., Pildes, R. S., Jacobs, N. M., *et al.*, Penicillin in infants weighing two kilograms or less with early-onset group B streptococcal disease, *N. Engl. J. Med.* **308:**1383–1389 (1983).
116. Hodges, R. G., and MacLeod, C. M., Epidemic pneumococcal pneumonia, *Am. J. Hyg.* **44:**183–243 (1946).
117. Gray, B. M., Turner, M. E., and Dillon, H. C., Jr., Epidemiologic studies of *Streptococcus pneumoniae* in infants: The effects of season and age on pneumococcal acquisition and carriage in the first 24 months of life, *Am. J. Epidemiol.* **116:**692–703 (1982).
118. Opal, S. M., Cross, A., Palmer, M. *et al.*, Group B streptococcal sepsis in adults and infants, *Arch. Intern. Med.* **148:**641–645 (1988).
119. Gray, B. M., and Dillon, H. C., Jr., Clinical and epidemiologic studies of pneumococcal infections in children, *Pediatr. Infect. Dis. J.* **5:**201–207 (1986).
120. Butler, J. C., Breiman, R. F., Lipman, H. B., *et al.*, Serotype distribution of *Streptococcus pneumoniae* infections among preschool children in the United States, 1978–1994: Implications for development of a conjugate vaccine, *J. Infect. Dis.* **171:**885–889 (1994).
121. Bennett, N. M., Buffington, J., and LaForce, F. M., Pneumococcal

bacteremia in Monroe County, New York, *Am. J. Public Health* **82:**1513–1516 (1992).

122. Christie, C., Hammond, J. Reising, S., *et al.*, Clinical and molecular epidemiology of enterococcal bacteremia in a pediatric teaching hospital, *J. Pediatr.* **125:**392–399 (1994).
123. Manji, F., Fejerskov, O., and Baelum, V., Pattern of dental caries in an adult rural population, *Caries Res.* **23:**55–62 (1989).
124. Ayoub, E. M., Barrett, D. J., Maclaren, N. K., *et al.*, Association of class II human histocompatibility leukocyte antigens with rheumatic fever, *J. Clin. Invest.* **77:**2019–2026 (1986).
125. Herer, B., Labrousse, F., Mordelet-Dambrine, M., *et al.*, Selective IgG subclass deficiencies and antibody responses to pneumococcal capsular polysaccharide antigen in adult community-acquired pneumonia, *Am. Rev. Respir. Dis.* **142:**854–857 (1990).
126. Centers for Disease Control, Group A, β-hemolytic *Streptococcus* skin infections in a meat-packing plant—Oregon. *Morbid. Mortal. Week. Rep.* **35:**629–630 (1986).
127. Arditi, M., Shulman, S. T., Davis, T., *et al.*, Group C β-hemolytic streptococcal infections in children: Nine pediatric cases and review, *Rev. Infect. Dis.* **11:**34–45 (1989).
128. Arends, J. P., and Zanen, H. C., Meningitis caused by *Streptococcus suis* in humans, *Rev. Infect. Dis.* **10:**131–137 (1988).
129. Brimblecombe, F. S. W., Cruickshank, R., Masters, P. L., *et al.*, Family studies of respiratory infections, *Br. Med. J.* **1:**119–128 (1958).
130. Gwaltney, J. M., Sande, M. A., Austrian, R., *et al.*, Spread of *Streptococcus pneumoniae* in families. II. Relation of transfer of *S. pneumoniae* to incidence of colds and serum antibody, *J. Infect. Dis.* **132:**62–68 (1975).
131. Holmström, L., Numan, B., Rosengren, M., *et al.*, Outbreaks of infections with erythromycin-resistant group A streptococci in child day care centres, *Scand. J. Infect. Dis.* **22:**179–185 (1990).
132. Cherian, T., Steinhoff, M. C., Harrison, L. H., *et al.*, A cluster of invasive pneumococcal disease in young children in child care, *J. Am. Med. Assoc.* **271:**695–697 (1994).
133. Gray, G. C., Escamilla, J., Huams, K. C., *et al.*, Hyperendemic *Streptococcus pyogenes* infection despite prophylaxis with penicillin G benzathine, *N. Engl. J. Med.* **325:**92–97 (1991).
134. Nelson, J. D., Dillon, H. C., Jr., and Howard, J. B., A prolonged nursery epidemic associated with a newly recognized type of group A streptococcus, *J. Pediatr.* **89:**792–796 (1976).
135. Goldmann, D. A., and Breton, S. J., Group C streptococcal surgical wound infections transmitted by an anorectal and nasal carrier, *Pediatrics* **61:**235–237 (1978).
136. Buntain, W. L., and Lynn, H. B., Splenorrhaphy: Changing concepts for the traumatized spleen, *Surgery* **86:**748–760 (1979).
137. Janoff, A. N., Breiman, R. F., Daley, C. L., *et al.*, Pneumococcal disease during HIV infection, *Ann. Intern. Med.* **117:**314–324 (1992).
138. Snellman, L. W., Stang, H. J., Stang, J. M., *et al.*, Duration of positive throat cultures for group A streptococci after initiation of antibiotic therapy, *Pediatrics* **91:**1166–1170 (1993).
139. Maddox, J. S., Ware, J. C., and Dillon, H. C., Jr., The natural history of streptococcal skin infection: Prevention with topical antibiotics, *Am. J. Acad. Dermatol.* **13:**207–212 (1985).
140. Hulse, M. L., Smith, S., Chi, E. Y., *et al.*, Effect of type III group B streptococcal capsular polysaccharide on invasion of respiratory epithelial cells, *Infect. Immun.* **61:**4835–4841 (1993).
141. Philips, J. B., III, Li, J.-X., Gray, B. M., *et al.*, Role of capsule in pulmonary hypertension induced by group G *Streptococcus*, *Pediatr. Res.* **31:**386–390 (1992).
142. Robinson, J. H., and Kehoe, M. A., Group A streptococcal M proteins: Virulence factors and protective antigens, *Immunol. Today* **13:**362–367 (1992).
143. Kefalides, N. A., Pegg, M. T., Ohno, N., *et al.*, Antibodies to basement membrane collagen and to laminin are present in sera from patients with poststreptococcal glomerulonephritis, *J. Exp. Med.* **163:**588–602 (1986).
144. Baker, C. J., Edwards, M. S., and Kasper, D. L., Role of antibody to native type III polysaccharide of group B streptococcus in infant infections, *Pediatrics* **68:**544–549 (1981).
145. Anthony, B. F., Concepcion, N. F., Wass, C. A., *et al.*, Immunoglobulin G and M composition of naturally occurring antibody to type III group B streptococci, *Infect. Immun.* **46:**98–104 (1984).
146. Silver, H. M., Gibbs, R. S., Gray, B. M., *et al.*, Risk factors for perinatal group B streptococcal disease after amniotic fluid colonization, *Am. J. Obstet. Gynecol.* **163:**19–25 (1990).
147. Biebink, G. S., Immunology: Promise of new vaccine, *Pediatr. Infect. Dis. J.* **13:**1064–1068 (1994).
148. Siber, G. R., Pneumococcal disease: Prospects for a new generation of vaccines, *Science* **265:**1385–1387 (1994).
149. Lue, C., Tarkowski, A., and Mestecky, J., Systemic immunization with pneumococcal polysaccharide vaccine induces a predominant IgA_2 response of peripheral blood leukocytes and increases of both serum and secretory antipneumococcal antibodies, *J. Immunol.* **140:**3793–3800 (1988).
150. The Working Group on Severe Streptococcal Infections, Defining the severe streptococcal syndromes: Rationale and consensus definition, *J. Am. Med. Assoc.* **269:**390–391 (1993).
151. Special Writing Group of the Committee on Rheumatic Fever, Endocarditis, and Kawasaki Disease of the Council on Cardiovascular Disease in the Young of the American Heart Association, Guidelines for the diagnosis of rheumatic fever: Jones criteria, 1992 update, *J. Am. Med. Assoc.* **268:**2069–2073 (1992).
152. Colford, J. M., Mohle-Boetani, J., and Vosti, K. L., Group B streptococcal bacteremia in adults: Five years' experience and a review of the literature, *Medicine* **74:**176–190 (1995).
153. Meier, F. A., Centor, R. M., Graham, L., *et al.*, Clinical and microbiological evidence for endemic pharyngitis among adults due to group C streptococci, *Arch. Intern. Med.* **150:**825–829 (1990).
154. Turner, J. C., Fox, A., Fox, K., *et al.*, Role of group C beta-hemolytic streptococci in pharyngitis: Epidemiologic study of clinical features associated with isolation of group C streptococci, *J. Clin. Microbiol.* **31:**808–911 (1993).
155. Shulman, S. T., Gerber, M. A., Tanz, R. R., *et al.*, Streptococcal pharyngitis: The case for penicillin therapy, *Pediatr. Infect. Dis. J.* **13:**1–7 (1994).
156. Lue, H. C., Wu, M. H., Wang, J. K., *et al.*, Long-term outcome of patients with rheumatic fever receiving benzathine penicillin G prophylaxis every three weeks versus every four weeks, *J. Pediatr.* **125:**812–816 (1994).
157. Berrios, X., del Campo, E., Guzman, B., *et al.*, Discontinuing rheumatic fever prophylaxis in selected adolescents and young adults, *Ann. Intern. Med.* **118:**401–406 (1993).
158. Shaffer, F. M., Agarwal, R., Helm, J., *et al.*, Poststreptococcal reactive arthritis and silent carditis: A case report and review of the literature, *Pediatrics* **93:**837–839 (1994).
159. Dajani, A. S., Bisno, A. L., Chung, K. J., *et al.*, Prevention of bacterial endocarditis. Recommendations by the American Heart Association, *J. Am. Med. Assoc.* **264:**2919–2922 (1990).
160. Paradise, J. L., Bluestone, C. D., Bachman, R. Z., *et al.*, Efficacy

of tonsillectomy for recurrent throat infection in severely affected children, *N. Engl. J. Med.* **310:**674–683 (1984).

161. Boyer, K. M., and Gotoff, S. P., Prevention of neonatal group B streptococcal disease with selective intrapartum chemoprophylaxis, *N. Engl. M. Med.* **314:**1665–1669 (1986).
162. Centers for Disease Control, Prevention of perinatal group B streptococcal disease: A public health perspective, *Morbid. Mortal. Week. Rep.* **45:**(RR-7):1–24 (1996).
163. American College of Obstetricians and Gynecologists, Prevention of early-onset group B streptococcal disease in newborns, *ACOG Comm. Opin.* **173:**1–8 (1996).
164. American Academy of Pediatrics, Committee on Infectious Diseases and Committee on Fetus and Newborn, Revised guidelines for prevention of early-onset group B streptococcal (GBS) infection, *Pediatrics* **97:**489–496 (1997).
165. Weisman, L. E., Stoll, B. J., Cruess, D. F., *et al.*, Early-onset group B streptococcal sepsis: A current assessment, *J. Pediatr.* **121:**428–433 (1992).
166. Ascher, D. P., Becker, J. A., Yoder, B. A., *et al.*, Failure of intrapartum antibiotics to prevent culture-proved group B streptococcal sepsis, *J. Perinatol.* **13:**212–216 (1993).
167. Henrichsen, T., Lindemann, R., Svenningsen, L., *et al.*, Prevention of neonatal infections by vaginal chlorhexadine disinfection during labor, *Acta Paediatr.* **83:**923–926 (1994).
168. Paoletti, L. C., Wessels, M. R., Rodewald, A. K., *et al.*, Neonatal mouse protection against infection with multiple group B streptococcal (GBS) serotypes by maternal immunization with a tetravalent GBS polysaccharide–tetanus toxoid conjugate vaccine, *Infect. Immun.* **62:**3236–3243 (1994).
169. Good, R. A., and Pahwa, R. N. (eds.), The recognition and management of immunodeficient disorders, *Pediatr. Infect. Dis. J.* **7**(Suppl.)**:**S2–S125 (1988).
170. Siber, G. R., Thompson, C., Reid, G. R., *et al.*, Evaluation of bacterial polysaccharide immune globulin for the treatment of prevention of *Haemophilus influenzae* type b and pneumococcal disease, *J. Infect. Dis.* **165**(Suppl. 1)**:**S129–S133 (1992).
171. Shurin, P. A., Rehmus, J. M., Johnson, C. A., *et al.*, Bacterial polysaccharide immune globulin for prophylaxis of acute otitis media in high-risk children. *J. Pediatr.* **123:**801–810 (1993).
172. Casadevall, A., and Scharff, M. D., Serum therapy revisited: Animal models of infection and development of passive antibody therapy, *Antimicrob. Agent Chemother.* **38:**1695–1702 (1994).
173. Bessen, D., and Fischetti, V. A., Synthetic peptide vaccine against mucosal colonization by group A streptococci. 1. Protection against a heterologous M serotype with shared C repeat region epitopes, *J. Immunol.* **145:**1251–1256 (1990).
174. Newton, S. M., Kotb, M., Poirier, T. P., *et al.*, Expression and immunogenicity of a streptococcal M protein epitope inserted in *Salmonella* flagellin, *Infect. Immun.* **59:**2158–2165 (1991).
175. Dale, J. B., Chiang, E. Y., and Lederer, J. W., Recombinant tetravalent group A streptococcal M protein vaccine, *J. Immunol.* **151:**2188–2194 (1993).
176. Dale, J. B., and Chiang, E. Y., Intranasal immunization with recombinant group a streptococcal M protein fragment fused to the B subunit of *Escherichia coli* labile toxin protects mice against systemic infections, *J. Infect. Dis.* **171:**1038–1041 (1995).
177. Baker, C. J., Rench, M. A., Edwards, M. S., *et al.*, Immunization of pregnant women with a polysaccharide vaccine of group B streptococcus, *N. Engl. J. Med.* **319:**1180–1185 (1988).
178. Shapiro, E. D., Berg, A. T., Austrian, R., *et al.*, The protective efficacy of polyvalent pneumococcal polysaccharide vaccine, *N. Engl. J. Med.* **325:**1453–1460 (1991).
179. Hirschman, J. V., and Lipsky, B. A., The pneumococcal vaccine after 15 years of use, *Arch. Intern. Med.* **154:**373–377 (1994).
180. Fedsen, D. S., Shapiro, E. D., Muffson, M. A., *et al.*, The pneumococcal vaccine after 15 years of use: Another view, *Arch. Intern. Med.* **154:**2531–2535 (1994).
181. Heller, K. E., Reed, S. G., Bruner, F. W., *et al.*, Longitudinal evaluation of sealing molars with and without incipient dental caries in a public health program, *J. Public Health Dent.* **55:**148–153 (1995).
182. Russell, M. W., Immunization against dental caries, *Curr. Opin. Dent.* **2:**72–80 (1992).
183. Hajishengalis, G., Hollingshead, S. K., Koga, T., *et al.*, Mucosal immunization with a bacterial protein antigen genetically coupled to cholera toxin A2/B subunits, *J. Immunol.* **154:**4322–4332 (1995).
184. Akiyama, T., and Yashiro, K., Probable role of *Streptococcus pyogenes* in Kawasaki disease, *Eur. J. Pediatr.* **152:**82–92 (1993).
185. Watanabe-Ohnishi, R., Low, D. E., McGreer, A., *et al.*, Selective depletion of Vβ-bearing T-cells in patients with severe invasive group A streptococcal infections and streptococcal toxic shock syndrome, *J. Infect. Dis.* **171:**74–84 (1995).
186. Coleman, G., Ianna, A., Efstratien, A., and Goworzewska, E. T., The serotypes of *Streptococcus pyogenes* present in Britain during 1980–1990 and their association with the disease, *Med. Microbiol.* **39:**165–178 (1993).

12. Suggested Reading

Ferretti, J. J., Gilmore, M. S, Klaenhammer, T. R., and Brown, F. (eds.), *Genetics of Streptococci, Enterococci and Lactococci*, Basel, Karger, 1995.

Kaplan, E. L. (ed.), Understanding group A streptococcal disease in the 1990s: Proceedings of a symposium, *Pediatr. Infect. Dis. J.* **13:**555–583 (1994).

Slots, J., and Taubman, M. A. (eds.), *Contemporary Oral Microbiology and Immunology*, Mosby Yearbook, St. Louis, 1992.

Taranta, A., and Markowitz, M., *Rheumatic Fever*, 2nd ed., Kluwer Academic Publishers, Boston, 1989.

Totolian, A. (ed.), *Pathogenic Streptococci: Present and Future*, Proceedings of the XII Lancefielde International Symposium on Streptococci and Streptococcal Diseases, St. Petersburg, Russia, September 6–10, 1993, Lancer Publications, St. Petersburg, 1994.

CHAPTER 35

Syphilis

Willard Cates, Jr.

1. Introduction

Few fields of medicine have been more carefully scrutinized by experts than syphilis.[1–4] Whether in economic, political, social, ethical, or epidemiologic arenas, syphilis has been the prototypic sexually transmitted disease (STD) control program of the 20th century.[4] Thus, the approaches taken and the measures used have been the model for control programs directed toward other STDs. In addition, many other clinical preventive services, such as those for tuberculosis, immunization, maternal and child health, and human immunodeficiency virus (HIV), have used concepts derived from syphilis control activities in their own prevention strategies. However, much of the epidemiological knowledge about syphilis control occurred prior to the 1950s.[4]

This chapter reviews the factors affecting syphilis epidemiology and control, including historical tradition, epidemiological bases, screening approaches, clinical management, and potential for immunization. It concludes with a consideration of future directions.

2. Historical Aspects

2.1. Early History

Syphilis carries a controversial history, not only because of its prurient nature, but also due to its alleged origins. Two theories predominate. The unitarian theory holds that syphilis began in equatorial environments, being transmitted, like yaws, by casual contact. However, when the organism migrated to colder climates where more clothing was worn, sexual transmission provided the main avenue for contact with *Treponema pallidum*. The Columbian theory holds that syphilis arose in North America and was brought back to Europe around the beginning of the 16th century. It later received its current name from a poem written in 1530 about an infected shepherd called Syphilis.

History is replete with the names of illustrious individuals who may have contracted syphilis, but folklore implies a tenuous veracity.[5] Documentation of the symptoms and signs of the illnesses is usually poor, and specific diseases are not identified as such. Nonetheless, syphilis, like smallpox, produced measurable historical consequences. The fates of national armies, royal succession, and international explorations have all been affected.

The key discoveries involving syphilis occurred in Germany in the early 20th century. Within 10 years, the spirochete was identified (1905), the Wasserman reaction developed (1906), and Salvarsan discovered (1909). Knowledge in this field progressed rapidly with acceptance of the germ theory, development of serological tests, and the use of toxic cures. At the same time, the increasing professionalization of medicine coincided with the rise of venereology as an established specialty. Syphilis became the disease on which the skills of 20th-century physicians were judged.

2.2. Social Attitudes

Throughout history, syphilis has caused society to wrestle with moral issues associated with public health problems. Fortunately, in recent years, the human tragedies suffered by those with syphilis have led to more effective social and political responses designed to interrupt transmission and reduce complications, rather than to stigmatize those suffering from disease.[4]

During the past century, American society evolved toward a more tolerant view of those with syphilis.[4] Before 1900, physicians were known to withhold treat-

Willard Cates, Jr. • Family Health International, Research Triangle Park, North Carolina 27709.

ment for the illness, fatalistically regarding infection as evidence of (and even punishment for) promiscuous behavior. During the early 1900s, the "social hygiene" movement highlighted syphilis as a major public health problem; although illicit sexual forays were still scorned, at least the consequences of sexual intercourse could be both discussed publicly and treated professionally. Campaigns were waged against prostitution, and condoms were marketed as prophylaxis against infection (and pregnancy).

In the New Deal era, Surgeon General Thomas Parran seized an opportunity to dramatize the plight of those with syphilis.[1] With the availability of penicillin and the higher moral imperative of winning a world war, during the 1940s, the image of syphilis shed even more of its stigmatic cloak. Syphilis could be diagnosed and treated on an outpatient basis, thus allowing a more positive attitude toward finding and treating both patients and partners alike. During the most recent decades, the changing role of women and homosexuals in society was accompanied by a shift in the nation's attitude toward human sexuality. This created a growing constituency of those demanding personal and public health solutions, as well as an increasing sympathy for the "innocent victims" of the late sequelae. Thus, as we close the 20th century, social concerns about syphilis have a broad community base.[6]

2.3. Control Programs

In the United States, the first national syphilis control efforts began in 1918 when Congress passed the Chamberlain–Kahn Act, creating the Venereal Disease Division of the US Public Health Service.[4] Passage of this act was stimulated by World War I, when syphilis became recognized as a major cause for rejection from the armed services. However, the end of the war brought a decline of interest in the disease, and an effective national program never really began. Twenty years later, Parran's influence resulted in the passage of the National Venereal Disease Control Act, which provided annual grants-in-aid to individual states. This law established the basic model for federal, state, and local cooperation for venereal disease control efforts that remains in use today.[6]

During the 1940s, the primary objective of syphilis control programs was to prevent the late complications of the disease.[6] Public awareness programs set the stage for mass serological testing programs to detect infected individuals, who were then generally treated with heavy metals. Beginning in 1943, the so-called "Rapid Treatment Centers" were established by the federal government.[4] These inpatient facilities provided a course of 5- to 10-day arsenical therapy instead of the 70 weeks required on an outpatient basis. Soon thereafter, however, the availability of penicillin for widespread use contributed to making the syphilis control program even more successful. By the early 1950s, the reservoir of untreated or inadequately treated syphilis had been dramatically reduced. In succeeding years, the incidence of complications declined markedly. Over the next two decades, deaths attributable to syphilis decreased by 85%, and admissions to hospitals for syphilitic psychoses declined by 97%.[3] Congenital syphilis, for which somewhat better data are available, declined by 90% between 1941 and 1972.[7]

As the prevention of late complications became a reality, the interruption of syphilis transmission in its infectious stages emerged as the primary objective of control programs. The focus for public health officials shifted from lowering syphilis prevalence to reducing its incidence.[3] The strategy for accomplishing this has gradually evolved since the late 1950s. Building on the concept of case finding through routine blood testing, syphilis control programs increasingly emphasized case prevention by aggressive treatment of sex partners. Patients in the infectious stages of syphilis were interviewed to identify exposed sex partners, who were then offered treatment (termed "epidemiological treatment") before they could either develop symptoms and/or spread the infection. While this approach was successful in stemming outbreaks and reducing community levels of syphilis, it was costly in financial and human resources. Thus, syphilis control (like other public health programs) was vulnerable to the flow of financial support.

2.4. Funding Levels and Syphilis Incidence

State and local resources mainly support laboratory, diagnostic, and treatment services for syphilis. After adjusting for inflation, these nonfederal resources have remained relatively stable during the past 40 years. However, federal appropriations for STD control (not including HIV), which support the surveillance and outreach activities, have been more variable (Fig. 1). From the high of over \$17 million (absolute dollars) in 1949, resources decreased quickly to \$13 million one year later, to \$700,000 in 1955, when the availability of penicillin permitted the closing of the Rapid Treatment Centers and when sharp declines in early syphilis incidence suggested that the problem had been "solved."[3]

The optimism was ill founded; infectious syphilis increased in the late 1950s. A Surgeon General's Task Force considered the problem in 1961 and recommended a

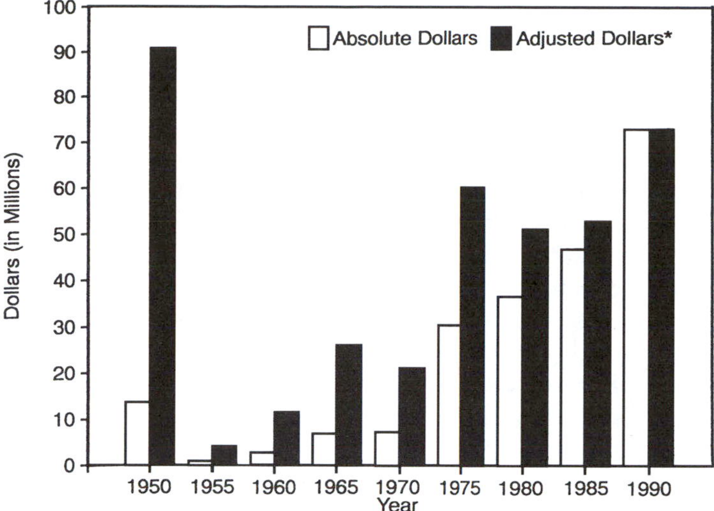

Figure 1. Resources for STD control, fiscal years 1950–1990. *, Adjusted to 1990 dollars.

10-year eradication program.[2] Federal grants to states for syphilis control were increased from $2.4 million in 1960 to $6.3 million in 1965, and remained at this level until 1970. This effort was associated with a decline in syphilis incidence between 1965 and 1969. However, inflation led to sizable reductions in purchasing power, and infectious syphilis rates began to increase again in the 1970s.[7]

After 1970, resources for syphilis control were further eroded by the expanding spectrum of infections recognized as being sexually transmitted.[8] Although additional funds were appropriated for gonorrhea control in the 1970s and for chlamydia control in the 1980s, these new resources were never enough to support all the necessary STD control activities. Policymakers were forced to choose alternatives among secondary prevention approaches for the different organisms. Because of the greater burden of disease caused by gonorrhea, chlamydia, and viral STDs, syphilis was relegated to receive a smaller share of the STD resources during the 1970s and 1980s. Only in recent years (1988–1995), as its incidence soared, has syphilis received both an absolute and a proportional increase in federal STD funds.[8]

After adjusting for inflation, total federal STD resources in 1990 were less than in 1950, despite the expanding spectrum of infections. For syphilis alone, the inflation-adjusted level of investment (in 1990 adjusted dollars) declined from over $100 million in 1949 to just over $20 million in 1990. Since the reported number of primary/secondary syphilis cases was similar in both years,[2,8] the effect has been to drain the per case investment in syphilis control to one fifth that of 40 years earlier. To some extent, the dilution of funds has been offset by investments in HIV primary prevention. Nonetheless, the funding level for syphilis control has ebbed considerably during the past half century.

3. Methodology

3.1. Sources of Mortality and Morbidity Data

Syphilis mortality estimates are derived from death certificates, as reported by the National Center for Health Statistics (NCHS). The accuracy of these data over time is influenced by changes in coding methods, diagnostic approaches, physician reporting candor, and autopsy percentages. Thus, the validity of mortality case definitions may vary over time, place, and patient population.

Syphilis morbidity data are collected by the Centers for Disease Control and Prevention (CDC) through formal surveillance systems based in the states. Data may vary in accuracy, depending on the priorities of STD control programs. These morbidity data tend to be more accurate in states that have laws that require reporting of positive syphilis serological tests.[3] Because private physicians are less reliable sources of morbidity data, the number of reported syphilis cases overrepresents patients seen in the public sector, and thus underestimates disease in the more affluent and older patient populations. Since public health partner notification activities are directed at interrupting infectious syphilis, morbidity of early syphilis is more accurate than late or latent disease.

Data on private sector case rates and disease sequelae can be derived from three annual sources: (1) the Hospital Discharge Survey of NCHS, which includes 7500 randomly selected hospitals from throughout the United States; (2) the National Ambulatory Medical Care Survey of NCHS, which is a probability sampling of the diagnoses of 1900 physicians; and (3) the National Disease and Therapeutic Index (NDTI), which is a private survey of a random sample of office visits to US physicians in office-based practices. The major shortcoming of these databases is relatively small numbers of syphilis cases, which leads to wide confidence intervals in subpopulations.

3.2. Serological Surveys

Our syphilis seroepidemiological tools are inexpensive, relatively simple to perform, highly sensitive and specific, and readily available. Positive screening tests are generally followed by a variety of confirmatory tests to substantiate the diagnosis. Widespread serological testing is usually a poor case finding tool for early infectious syphilis, but may be a good method for disease surveillance.

Overall serological screening has generally accounted for about 25% of primary and secondary (P&S) syphilis morbidity, about 40% of the early latent cases, and nearly all of the late latent cases in the United States.[3] The most contemporary seroprevalence estimates in the United States come from the National Health and Nutritional Surveys (NHANES). Between 1976 and 1980, analyses of 13,000 sera revealed a syphilis prevalence of 1.3%; 8.5% of those who were positive (or 1/1000 cases) actually needed treatment.[9] This projects to about 200,000 unidentified syphilis cases in the United States in need of treatment in the 1980s.

3.3. Laboratory Diagnosis

3.3.1. Identification of the Organism. *In vitro* culture of *T. pallidum* is not currently possible for diagnostic purposes. However, darkfield microscopic identification of the motile *T. pallidum* in secretions from primary, secondary, and early congenital lesions constitutes a rapid, reliable, sensitive, and specific test. *T. pallidum* can also be identified from lesions and in biopsy material by commercially available direct fluorescent antibody (DFA) techniques. DFA's advantage is that the specimen can be transported to a laboratory where an experienced microscopist can make the proper identification. This procedure is ideally suited for testing oral and anorectal lesion secretions because it will differentiate *T. pallidum* from *T. denticola* and other spirochete strains.

False-negative darkfield and direct fluorescent antibody tests may occur even with adequate clinical specimens. Self-treatment with penicillin, for instance, can render a chancre darkfield-negative within hours. The same occurs when antiseptic ointments are locally applied to syphilis lesions.

3.3.2. Serology. Serological tests are valuable in syphilis diagnosis when ulcerative lesions are not available for darkfield examination. In primary syphilis, all serological tests are less sensitive than direct visualization of *T. pallidum*. When syphilis has reached the secondary stage, antibody levels have risen and nearly all serological tests are reactive.

Based on the character of the antigen, two major categories of syphilis serological tests exist. The first syphilis antigen is a defined combination of cardiolipin, cholesterol, and lecithin. These nontreponemal tests have similar sensitivities and specificities and include the Venereal Disease Research Laboratory (VDRL) and the rapid plasma reagin (RPR) tests.

The second category of syphilis serologies comprises the treponemal tests. Intact *T. pallidum* organisms are the antigens used in the *T. pallidum* immobilization (TPI) and fluorescent treponemal antibody absorption (FTA-ABS) tests. The TPI test is labor-intensive and is now used only in research laboratories. The newest treponemal tests employ *T. pallidum* extracts fixed to erythrocytes and involve hemagglutination procedures. Sheep erythrocytes are used in the microhemagglutination test for *T. pallidum* (MHA-TP) and turkey erythrocytes carry the antigen in the hemagglutination treponemal test for syphilis (HATTS). The hemagglutination tests may be slightly more specific than the FTA-ABS, but are less sensitive in primary syphilis.

False-positive nontreponemal tests are common and are usually of low titer ($\leq$ 1:4). False-positive nontreponemal tests are divided into acute and chronic, based on whether reactions revert to negative in less than 6 months. False-positive treponemal tests can also occur, usually associated with lupus erythematosus, pregnancy, and intravenous drug use.

4. Biological Characteristics of the Organism

Treponema pallidum is classified in the order Spirochaetales, genus *Treponema*. The latter includes both human pathogens and nonpathogenic organisms. The pathogens and the diseases they cause are *T. pallidum* (syphilis), *T. pertenue* (yaws), *T. carateum* (pinta), and *T. pallidum* variant (endemic syphilis). Morphologically, these four treponemes are identical. DNA homology has demonstrated a close similarity between *T. pallidum* and the other pathogens, but marked differences between the pathogens and the nonpathogenic treponemes.[16]

Cross-resistance between *T. pallidum* infection and the other treponemal infections suggests immunologic similarities. Syphilis nontreponemal and treponemal tests are reactive in patients with yaws, pinta, and endemic syphilis. Syphilis incidence is low in areas where yaws is endemic, but has increased after active yaws eradication program. The pathogenic treponemes can be differentiated by the host response in various animal models.

Treponema pallidum, like other treponemes, is a gram-negative bacterium. Its length varies from 6 μm to 15 μm, possibly because its reproductive cycle consists of growth in length followed by division half-way along its long axis. *Treponema pallidum* is a fragile organism, which is readily destroyed by disinfectants commonly used in laboratories and clinics. *Treponema pallidum* utilizes oxygen and is microaerophilic. None of the human pathogenic treponemes have been grown in broth or on bacteriological media.

5. Descriptive Epidemiology

Because syphilis passes through both clinical and subclinical phases, case definition presents a dilemma for surveillance purposes. Trends in P&S syphilis provide a measure of disease incidence, since their symptomatic clinical presentations are of relatively short duration. This is especially true in men, where the chancre most often occurs on the external genitalia. In contrast, primary infections of women are reported less commonly. Latent disease rates, on the other hand, depend on the levels of screening and partner notification activities. Thus, trends in latent disease rates may reflect the level of resources devoted to syphilis control activities.

5.1. Prevalence and Incidence

After the advent and widespread use of penicillin treatment, syphilis cases dropped dramatically.[7] Fifteen years after the introduction of penicillin, the number of syphilis cases had dropped by 90% (Fig. 2). Cases reached their nadir in 1955. Thereafter, syphilis ebbed and flowed during the next 30 years as rates increased, then decreased in the gay male population. In the second half of the 1980s, heterosexual syphilis transmission was fueled by the crack cocaine epidemic, and rates reached their highest levels since post-World War II. However, since 1991, P&S syphilis declined markedly; in 1994, just over 20,000 cases were reported, the lowest number since 1977.[8]

Congenital syphilis cases have paralleled the trends in female P&S disease (Fig. 3). After 1988, the number of congenital syphilis cases increased dramatically, not only because of the rising incidence in women, but also because of a broader case definition begun that year. However, because of the declining number of adult syphilis

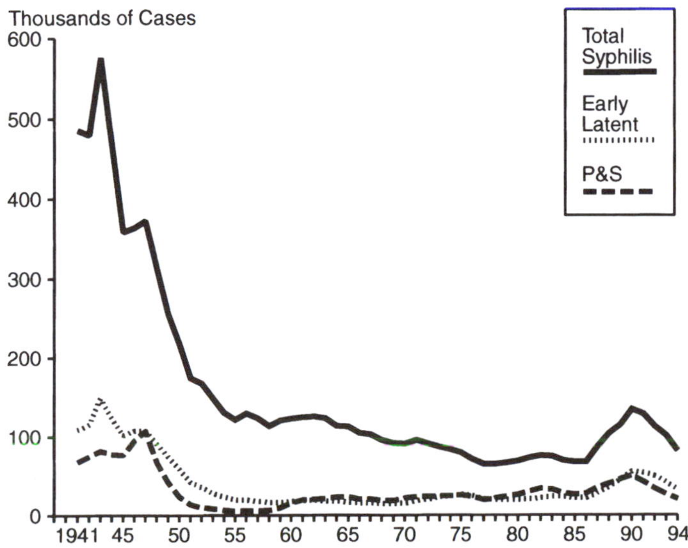

Figure 2. Syphilis—reported cases by stage of illness: United States, 1941–1994.

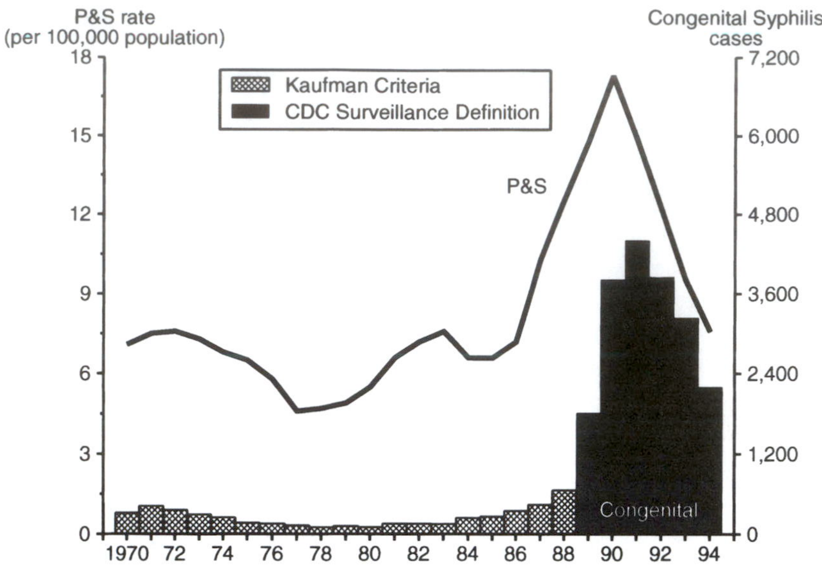

Figure 3. Congenital syphilis—reported cases in infants <1 year of age and rates of primary and secondary syphilis among women: United States, 1970–1994.

cases in the first half of the 1990s, congenital syphilis cases fell as well.[7,8]

5.2. Contagiousness

Except for intrauterine infection, syphilis is transmitted by sexual contact between infected and uninfected epithelial surfaces. The transmission rate is relatively high, especially after repeated exposures, and is inversely proportional to the stage of the disease. Among couples with frequent sexual contact, four out of five partners exposed to the infectious lesions of early syphilis were infected; less frequent transmission occurred when the index case had been infected for more than 4 years.[10,11] Among untreated nonconjugal sex partners having less frequent exposure to patients with P&S syphilis, 30 to 40% acquired infection.[6,12]

The infectious dose for the transmission of *T. pallidum* infection is relatively low. The ID_{50} of the rabbit-acclimated Nichols strain for the production of intracutaneous infection in human volunteers is about 50 organisms.[13]

Perinatal transmission of syphilis occurs as early as the ninth week of gestation.[14] The risk of intrauterine transmission of infection in maternal syphilis is high, and it varies with the stage of maternal disease. The risk of congenital syphilis acquisition is 50% in maternal P&S infections, 40% in early latent infections, and only 10% in late latent infection.[14] Healthy term infants were born to 10% of the early latent maternal infections and to 70% of those with late latent disease.

5.3. Geographic Distribution

Syphilis morbidity is often characterized by a geographic clustering of infections. In 1994, the 64 largest cities in the United States accounted for 62% of the reported cases of P&S syphilis, although only accounting for 26% of the population.[8] In the United States, the highest rates of infectious syphilis are currently clustered in the southern and southeastern portions of the country (Fig. 4). Recently, rural areas have emerged as key targets. Although Mississippi and Louisiana had the highest rates, Texas and North Carolina also accounted for more than 1,600 P&S syphilis cases in 1994. A similar pattern is seen in congenital syphilis cases. In 1994, three states, Texas, Illinois, California, and one city (New York) accounted for nearly 50% of the congenital syphilis cases in the United States.[8]

Over the past decade, the secular trend of syphilis incidence by geographic region has reflected the rise and fall of crack-related heterosexual spread (Fig. 5). Syphilis rates first increased in 1985 in the West, then spread to the Northeast and South in 1986, and finally reached the Midwest by the late 1980s. Rates fell in the first three regions by 1990, but not in the Midwest until 1993.

5.4. Temporal Distribution

A seasonal trend pattern has not been demonstrated for syphilis.

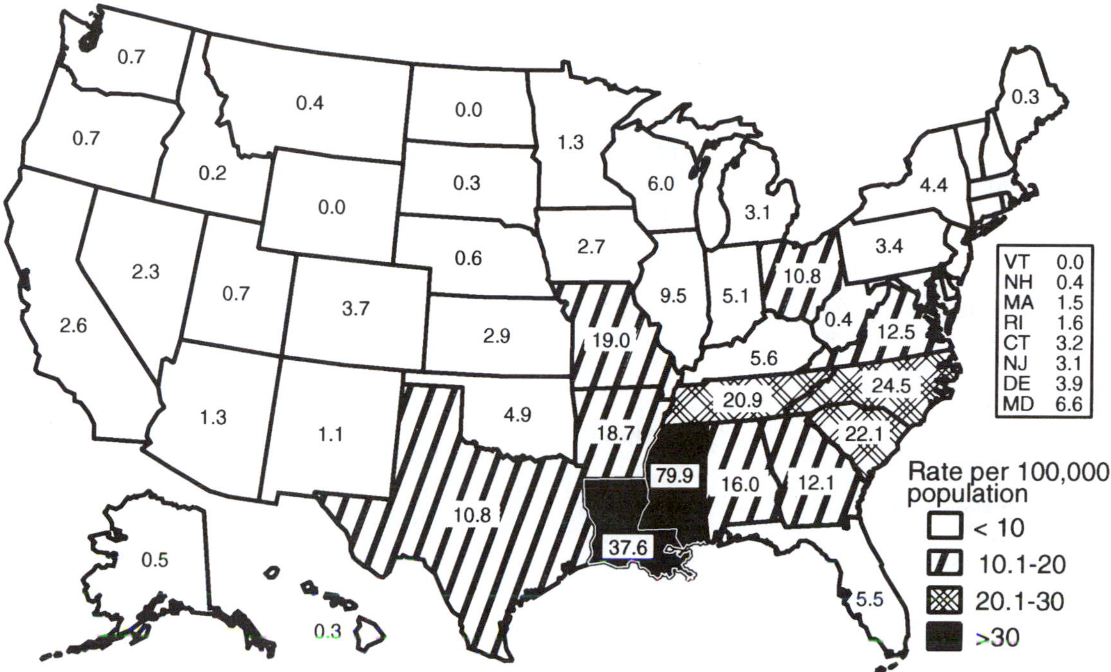

Figure 4. Primary and secondary syphilis—rates by state: United States, 1994. Note: The total rate of primary and secondary syphilis for the United States was 8.1 per 100,000 population. The year 2000 objective is 10.0 per 100,000 population.

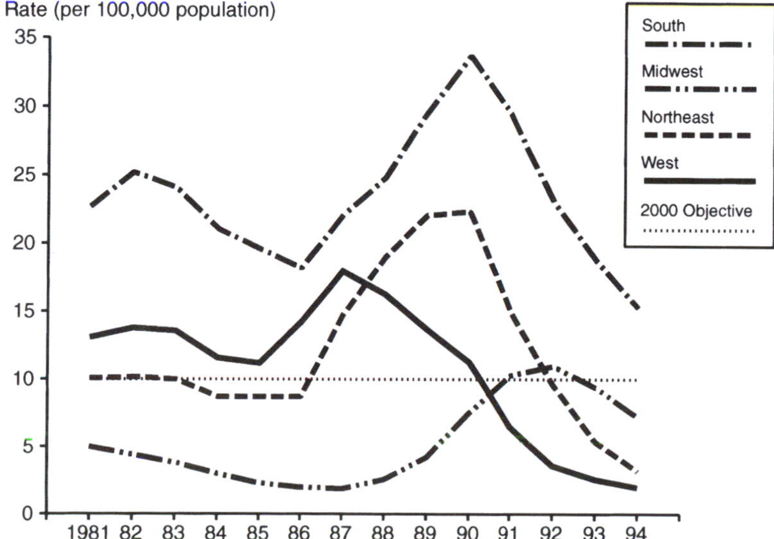

Figure 5. Primary and secondary syphilis—rates by region: United States, 1981–1994 and the year 2000 objective.

5.5. Age and Gender

The highest incidence of syphilis occurs in the 20- to 24-year-old age group, although the distribution varies by gender.[8] In women, the highest case rates occur in a slightly younger age group (Fig. 6). The highest incidence in men has an older distribution.

5.6. Race

Nearly all studies have found markedly higher syphilis case rates in African Americans compared to whites. These data are biased by the higher utilization by the African-American population of public STD clinics, which disproportionately report cases to public health authorities. However, more representative military screening in the 1940s revealed that the syphilis rates in African-American males were 272/1000, compared to 23.5/1000 in white males, almost a 12-fold difference.[3] Moreover, two US probability samples, in 1960–1962 and 1976–1980, found serological evidence in syphilis in five to ten times as many African Americans as whites.[9] Recent trends showed African-American syphilis rates increasing markedly between 1985 and 1990, but declining precipitously thereafter (Fig. 7). The reasons for the higher syphilis rates in African Americans are currently not known. Racial and economic segregation help define sociosexual networks with an elevated prevalence of disease, thus maintaining high levels of infection.[15]

5.7. Occupation

With the exception of commercial sex workers, occupation bears no specific relationship to the risk of acquiring syphilis. Occupations that employ younger, sexually active individuals, especially from syphilis endemic areas, would likely yield higher infection rates.

5.8. Occurrence in High-Risk Environments

Over the past two decades, syphilis outbreaks have occurred in settings associated with high numbers of anonymous sex partners: the bathhouses serving gay males and crack houses serving low-income populations where sex is exchanged for drugs.

5.9. Socioeconomic Factors

While all social strata are at risk for sexually transmitted infections, syphilis has become entrenched in the poor.[15] Factors such as educational and income level, which are directly related to the frequency of using prophylactic and therapeutic measures to prevent disease, are often important determinants of the prevalence of syphilis and its transmission dynamics. Moreover, health care seeking is also directly related to income level.

6. Mechanisms and Routes of Transmission

Treponema pallidum is transmitted during sexual contact between an infectious individual and a susceptible recipient. Infection of a sex partner occurs in about one third of coital exposures. Initial infection fails to occur unless adequate numbers of treponemes are transferred to the partner's mucosa or abraded skin. No natural resistance was found in experimental infection of human volunteers not previously exposed to *T. pallidum*.[13]

Infected individuals are not continually infectious to others. Patients may remain infected with *T. pallidum* from the time of inoculation until their death, but they are infectious to others primarily during the several weeks of the P&S stages of syphilis; late latent and late syphilis are not infectious stages.

For syphilis infection to be transmitted, adequate numbers of *T. pallidum* must be on the surface of the organ that contacts the recipient's skin or mucosae. The exact number needed to infect is unknown, but experimental intracutaneous injection of the agent required only 57 organisms.[13] *Treponema pallidum* can penetrate mucosal surfaces, but penetration is resisted by intact skin. It can penetrate through the skin abrasions that occur in sexual activity. Rabbits resist syphilis when *T. pallidum* is placed on normal skin, but the minimal trauma associated with shaving the animal allows the same skin to be infected.

In childbirth, a similar situation may occur when *T. pallidum* from a mother's genital chancre is transmitted to the child as it passes through the vagina. Under this circumstance, the chancre(s) in the newborn develops several weeks postpartum in the site(s) of birth trauma, such as where extraction forceps were applied to the head. The more common mode of congenital syphilis transmission is via a maternal septicemia with passage of *T. pallidum* through the placenta and into the developing fetus. Such a septicemia is most likely when the pregnant mother has primary or secondary syphilis. Treatment of an infectious mother in the first trimester may prevent congenital syphilis, because placental passage usually occurs during the second and third trimesters.

Hematogenous spread of *T. pallidum* has occurred

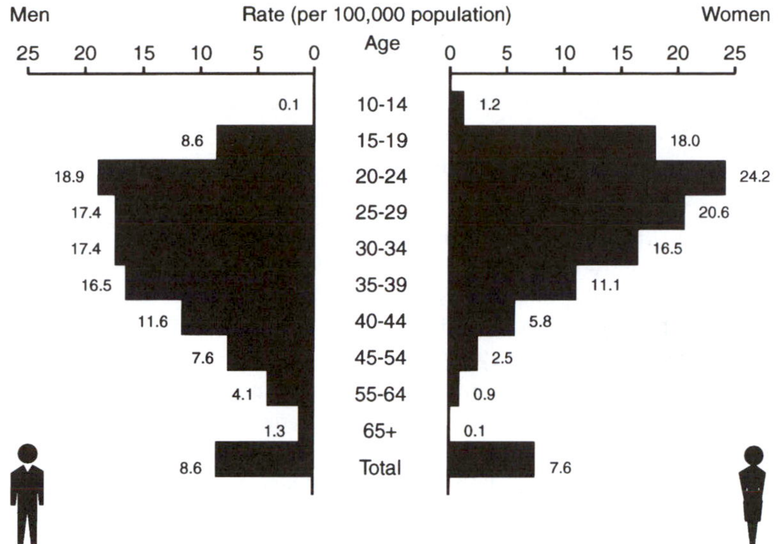

Figure 6. Primary and secondary syphilis—age- and gender-specific rates: United States, 1994.

with blood transfusions, but is quite rare. Treponemes are present in blood for only the short duration of the P&S phases. In addition, blood is screened with a syphilis serological test before it is transfused into a recipient. Fomite transmission of syphilis is virtually nonexistent, because *T. pallidum* is rapidly killed by drying. It has not been found in urine, milk, or sweat.

7. Pathogenesis and Immunity

Treponema pallidum infection evokes both humoral and cellular immune responses. The former's detection and quantification is important in the laboratory diagnosis of syphilis. Treponemal (anti-*T. pallidum*) and nontreponemal (anticardiolipin) antibodies begin developing in

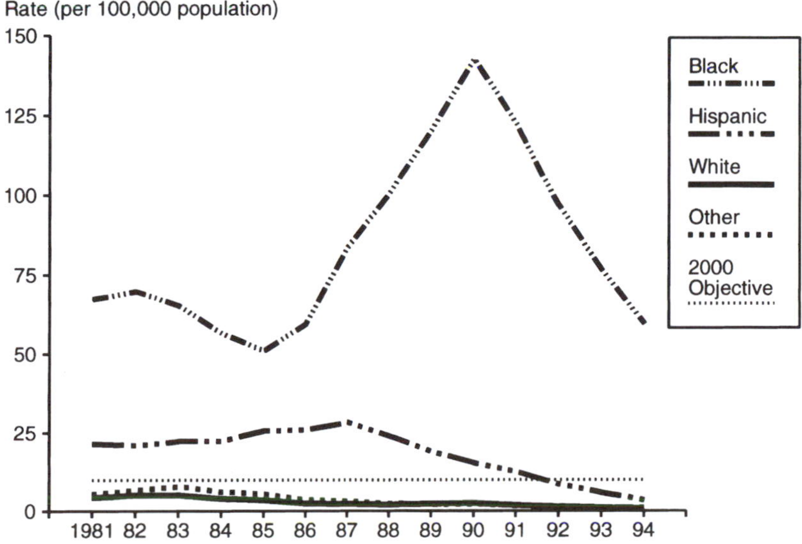

Figure 7. Primary and secondary syphilis–rates by race and ethnicity: United States, 1981–1994 and the year 2000 objective.

primary syphilis, and in the secondary stage all patients have high titers of both antibodies. Titers of anticardiolipin antibodies then start to slowly decline and spontaneously revert to negative in about one third of untreated patients. Anti-*T. pallidum* antibodies remain detectable for the life of the patient. Cell-mediated immunity also develops in primary syphilis, appears to be suppressed during the secondary stage, and is again detected in the latent and late stages.

The roles of antibodies and cellular immunity in resistance to infection is not completely understood. Human inoculation experiments have shown that syphilis infections confer some degree of resistance to reinfection.[13] Patients treated previously for primary or secondary syphilis were easily reinfected with *T. pallidum* despite having an anamnestic antibody response to both cardiolipin and *T. pallidum* antigens. Patients with untreated late latent syphilis were most resistant; many patients with this stage of syphilis resisted an intracutaneous challenge of 100,000 *T. pallidum*. This compares with an infectious dose of about 50 organisms for an initial syphilis infection. Resistance to reinfection correlated better with cellular immunity than with humoral antibodies.

Resistance to reinfection can be differentiated from chancre immunity. The latter is failure of *T. pallidum* to produce a second chancre while the primary chancre is still present. Chancre immunity may be secondary to cellular immunosuppression in early syphilis.

8. Patterns of Host Response

8.1. Clinical Features

The interval between infection with *T. pallidum* and development of the first clinical sign of syphilis varies from 10 to 90 days, with the typical case developing an ulcer (the primary chancre) in 3 weeks.[17] If someone exposed to syphilis does not develop either a chancre or a positive cardiolipin serology within 90 days, he or she probably was not infected.

While clinical staging is imprecise, it provides a useful guide to treatment decisions and syphilis control activities. Considerable overlap between stages is common.[17]

8.1.1. Primary Stage. When infection does occur, the first sign of syphilis develops at the site of inoculation and consists of a pink to red macule. This flat lesion rapidly becomes a palpable nodule and within several days its surface erodes to produce the characteristic chancre. Chancres are usually single, without pain and are accompanied by painless regional lymphadenopathy. The asymptomatic character of such a large genital ulcer contrasts markedly with the pain of smaller genital herpes and chancroid ulcers.

A primary syphilis chancre heals spontaneously without treatment, usually within 2 to 3 weeks, but occasionally may persist for up to 8 weeks. A residual scar in the area of the chancre is rare unless the lesion was secondarily infected. The regional adenopathy requires a longer time to resolve spontaneously.

8.1.2. Secondary Stage. Several weeks after the chancre has healed, the manifestations of secondary syphilis emerge. Nonspecific symptoms of this stage include low-grade fever, headache, sore throat, malaise, anorexia, and arthralgias.[17] The most characteristic secondary syphilis signs, although not pathognomonic, are changes in the skin, hair, and mucous membranes.

Skins lesions are discrete and may be macular (flat) or papular (small palpable elevations), usually on the trunk, the palms, and the soles. Hair loss may occur in secondary syphilis. Patches of scalp hair are thinned rather than completely denuded and the result is a motheaten appearance to the scalp. In perineal sites, secondary syphilis lesions are generally nodular and are referred to as condylomata lata, similar to genital warts (condylomata acuminata).

A patient with secondary syphilis may have one, several, or all of the signs of the secondary stage. Since each of the signs may be associated with other diseases, none are specific to syphilis. However, when more of these signs are present, the diagnosis of syphilis is more likely to be accurate. The diagnosis of secondary syphilis is confirmed by the identification of *T. pallidum* in mucosal lesions or by the conversion of a syphilis serological test from negative to positive. Essentially all treponemal and nontreponemal syphilis serologies are reactive in this stage of syphilis.

The manifestations of secondary syphilis last 2 to 8 weeks and then, as with primary syphilis, heal spontaneously without residual scarring. When healing is complete, the patient enters into a latent phase with no clinical symptoms or signs of syphilis. The syphilis serological tests, however, remain positive.

8.1.3. Clinical (Infectious) Secondary Relapse. About 25% of untreated patients relapse from latency back into secondary syphilis.[18] This usually occurs during the first 5 years of latency, although most relapses take place in the first year. Such relapses are infrequent, possibly related to inadvertent syphilis treatment by systemic antibiotics used to treat another infection. The diagnosis of latent syphilis requires a spinal tap to differentiate it from asymptomatic neurosyphilis. The differential is important because neurosyphilis requires more prolonged therapy, as well as posttherapy spinal taps, to document therapeutic success.

8.1.4. Late Benign Syphilis. Late or tertiary syphilis occurs much less frequently today than was reported in the Oslo study of untreated syphilis.[8,18] As with the reduction in secondary syphilis relapses, this is probably related to inadvertent syphilis treatment when systemic antibiotics are used to treat a variety of other infectious diseases. This trend, however, may be reversing, since concurrent HIV infection may facilitate syphilis progression to symptomatic neurosyphilis.[19] This occurred in both untreated and treated syphilis patients.

One third of untreated syphilis patients in the Oslo study progressed from the latent stage to one or more of the tertiary stages of syphilis.[18] The remaining two thirds of syphilis patients remained asymptomatic during the rest of their lives. The sera of some of these asymptomatic patients also become nonreactive in the cardiolipin syphilis serological tests.

Three types of tertiary syphilis occur: gummas, cardiovascular syphilis, and central nervous system syphilis. Gummatous lesions developed in about 15% of the Oslo study patients.[18] These lesions have their onset 2 to 40 years after primary syphilis. Seventy percent of gummas involve the skin, 10% are found in bone and a similar percentage are present on mucosal surfaces. Gummas can involve any organ. Skin and bone gummas are disfiguring, but involvement of a vital organ such as the heart or liver could be fatal.

8.1.5. Cardiovascular Syphilis. Cardiovascular tertiary syphilis develops 10 to 30 years after primary syphilis and was clinically evident in about 10% of the Oslo study's untreated syphilis patients.[18] Another 20 to 30% of untreated patients have cardiovascular changes that do not produce signs or symptoms. The microscopic pathology of cardiovascular syphilis is similar to that of neurosyphilis: blood vessel inflammation, which progresses to vessel occlusion. The vessels clinically involved in cardiovascular syphilis serve the aorta and the coronary vessels. Loss of this blood supply results in blood vessel wall death and scar formation. Scar tissue within the aorta weakens its walls such that the aorta balloons outward, creating an aneurysm. Progression of syphilitic aortic valve damage eventuates in congestive heart failure and possible death. Incomplete syphilitic occlusion of the coronary vessels causes intermittent anginal cardiac chest pain. Myocardial infarction can occur when the coronary vessel occlusion is complete.

8.1.6. Neurosyphilis. Neurosyphilis develops 1 to 30 years after primary syphilis and involved 5 to 10% of Oslo's untreated patients.[18] The earliest form of symptomatic neurosyphilis, syphilitic meningitis, is also the least common (10% of neurosyphilis patients). It is manifest by typical meningitis symptoms: fever, headache, photophobia, and stiff neck. The spinal fluid findings are nonspecific—normal sugar and elevated lymphocytes and protein. However, a positive cerebrospinal fluid cardiolipin test differentiates neurosyphilis from other types of aseptic meningitis.

Later manifestations of neurosyphilis are due to blood vessel changes, which consist of vascular inflammation leading to vessel occlusion. The clinical manifestations of vascular neurosyphilis, as with other neurological diseases, depend on which areas of the brain are damaged. Strokes and seizures are early presentations of vascular neurosyphilis. Progression of vascular neurosyphilis consists of the involvement of more and more blood vessels with the subsequent loss of more brain tissue. The associated clinical state is referred to as paresis and is a combination of neurological and psychiatric changes. The latter is primarily a dementing process with loss of intellectual function, although some patients experience grandiose delusions. Common paresis neurological changes are eye pupil abnormalities (Argyll–Robertson pupils), slurred speech, and tremors.

Spinal cord neurosyphilis consists of degeneration of the posterior columns. Nerve fibers in these columns transmit deep pain and proprioception sensations. Early clinical manifestations include transient (lasting minutes) sharp pains that radiate into the legs or abdomen. Loss of deep pain sensation in the legs results in repeated painless trauma to the knees and feet. The knees enlarge (Charcot's joints) and ulcers develop on the bottom of the feet (mal perforant).

8.2. Diagnosis

The clinical diagnosis of syphilis is based on its symptoms and signs.[17] The laboratory diagnosis of syphilis is based on visualization of *T. pallidum* and/or demonstration of antibody either to this pathogen or to cardiolipin antigen.

No single finding or test is in itself absolutely diagnostic of syphilis. The most accurate single diagnostic factor is usually the darkfield or direct fluorescent antibody demonstration of *T. pallidum*. The accuracy of these two tests, however, depends on how and where the clinical specimen was obtained, how it was transported to the laboratory, and who performed the test.

Treatment of syphilis is much easier than diagnosis.

This infection was one of the first treated with penicillin in the mid-1940s. Unlike many other bacteria, *T. pallidum* has not developed resistance to this antibiotic despite penicillin's being the syphilis treatment-of-choice for a half-century. A single dose of 2.4 million units of benzathine penicillin G covers primary, secondary, and latent syphilis of less than 1 year duration. The same penicillin preparation in the same dose also treats both latent syphilis of more than 1 year duration and late syphilis; with these conditions, penicillin is given in three doses, 1 week apart, for a total of 7.2 million units. Some patients with late neurosyphilis do not respond adequately to this benzathine penicillin regimen and require hospitalization for 10 days for treatment with intravenous aqueous crystallin penicillin G.

Syphilis occurring in pregnancy is treated with the same penicillin regimens. Nonpregnant patients allergic to penicillin can be treated with tetracycline or erythromycin. Pregnant patients with a history of penicillin allergy should have the allergy confirmed by skin tests. Those found not allergic can be treated with penicillin and those with positive skin tests can receive oral desensitization, followed by treatment with standard penicillin doses.

Syphilis treatment, like many other infectious diseases, requires follow up to assure cure. In addition to resolution of the signs and symptoms of early syphilis, the cardiolipin serological tests should be repeated 3, 6, and 12 months after treatment. A decline of at least two dilutions in test titers should occur after treatment, and most tests will revert to negative in cases of P&S syphilis. The anatomic damage occurring in late syphilis cannot be reversed, but treatment will prevent progression of the disease. Management of syphilis patients, as with other STDs, requires evaluation and treatment of sex partners.

9. Control and Prevention

9.1. Epidemiological Basis for Syphilis Control Activities

9.1.1. Transmission Dynamics. Many simultaneous activities are necessary to reduce syphilis, because of the interactive behavioral and biological dynamics of syphilis spread. The forces responsible for sustaining transmission of any sexually transmitted infection, including syphilis, can be represented in a simple equation, $R = \beta \times C \times D$.[20,21] R represents the reproductive rate of an infection, i.e., the number of new infections produced by an infected individual. β is the average probability that an infected individual will infect a susceptible partner given exposure. On average, without preventive measures, three of ten sexual encounters between an infected and uninfected person[22–26] will result in transmission of syphilis (Table 1). C is the average number of new partners exposed by an infected individual per unit of time. D is the average duration of infectiousness of the specific infection. Public health interventions to prevent syphilis are targeted at reducing the magnitude of β, C, or D by (1) reducing the probability of infecting a susceptible partner; (2) limiting the number of partners who have sex with infected persons; and (3) reducing the duration of infectiousness.

Most current syphilis control activities emphasize reducing the duration of infectiousness. This approach rests on certain assumptions about the natural history of syphilis (Fig. 8): for illustrative purposes, we will assume on the average that the moment of infection is followed by an incubation period of 3 weeks, by a 5-week period of primary syphilis, and by a 6-week period of secondary syphilis, after which the syphilitic infection becomes latent. The 11 weeks of P&S syphilis are considered the period of infectiousness.

Without preventive measures, three of ten sexual encounters between an infected and an uninfected person will result in transmission of syphilis. Empirical data from national syphilis control programs[27] indicate that an untreated person with syphilis would generate, on average, 0.17 new infections per week during the 5 weeks of primary syphilis and 0.05 new infections per week during the 6 weeks of secondary syphilis, for a reproductive rate of 1.15 (Fig. 8). At this level, in the absence of any effective intervention, the infection will propagate in the population. This hypothetical reproductive rate is a weighted average of rates from diverse subpopulations that lie on a spectrum from no transmission (reproductive rate less than one) to intense transmission (reproductive rate of two or more). Although the reproductive rate of

Table 1. Risk of Infection in Persons Exposed to Infectious Syphilis, Selected Studies

Study	Number exposed	Number infected	Percent infected
Alexander *et al.*, 1949[22]	161	100	62.1
Idsoe *et al.*, 1954[23]	77	14	18.1
Moore *et al.*, 1963[24]	79	12	15.9
Schroeter *et al.*, 1971[25]	57	16	30.3
Schober *et al.*, 1983[26]	127	65	51.2

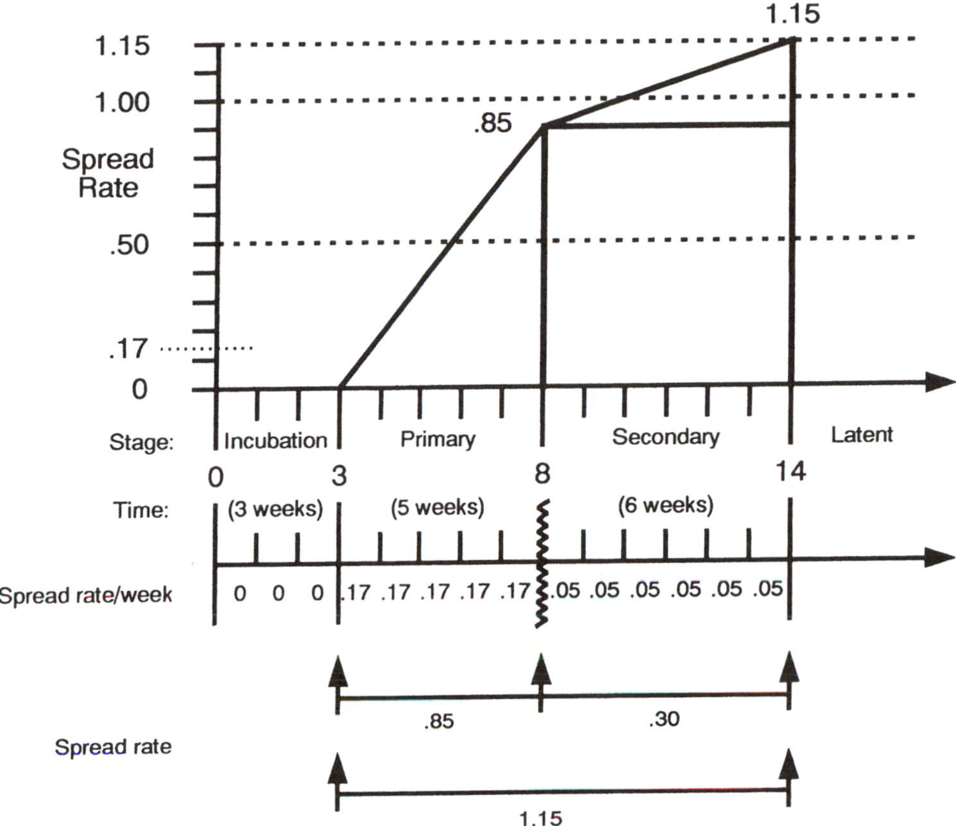

Figure 8. Projected reproductive rate of syphilis.

1.15 is probably an underestimate, given slippage in the process of partner notification, it is of heuristic value in considering the impact of an intervention program.

With a control program in which education, clinical diagnosis, and partner notification are effective, syphilis can be treated early in the course of illness and transmission can be interrupted (Fig. 9). For example, community education can hopefully motivate infected persons to recognize symptoms of syphilis and seek medical care within 2 weeks after the onset of symptoms. Physicians in the community, if properly trained, can diagnose and treat the disease promptly. A system of partner notification seeks to assure the effective identification, referral, and treatment of persons exposed to infection. Under such circumstances, most of the partners of infectious persons will still be in the incubation period when treated, and the reproductive rate would be lowered to near zero. Such a theoretical goal is unlikely to be achieved. However, given our hypothetical reproductive rate of 1.15, even a 25% reduction in the number of infected partners per case per week during the primary period—from 0.17 to 0.13—would lower the reproductive rate to less than one and ultimately interrupt transmission within the community (Fig. 9).

This model for controlling syphilis transmission is based on assumptions derived directly from the biological characteristics of *T. pallidum* and the clinical stages of the disease it produces. Compared to other STDs, *T. pallidum* has long division times and, as a consequence, an extended incubation period. Thus, with syphilis, we have a relatively prolonged opportunity to cure the infection before symptoms appear and the host becomes infectious. In addition, *T. pallidum* remains sensitive to long-acting benzathine penicillin. If the organism were to become resistant to this drug and require higher doses or more frequent administration of antibiotic therapy, syphilis control would be compromised. For these reasons, syphilis is a disease for which the interventions of partner notification and prophylactic therapy can have substantial impact. Other STDs with shorter incubation periods (e.g., gonorrhea) or less convenient therapies (e.g., chlamydia) should not be expected to respond as dramatically to control programs as syphilis.[28]

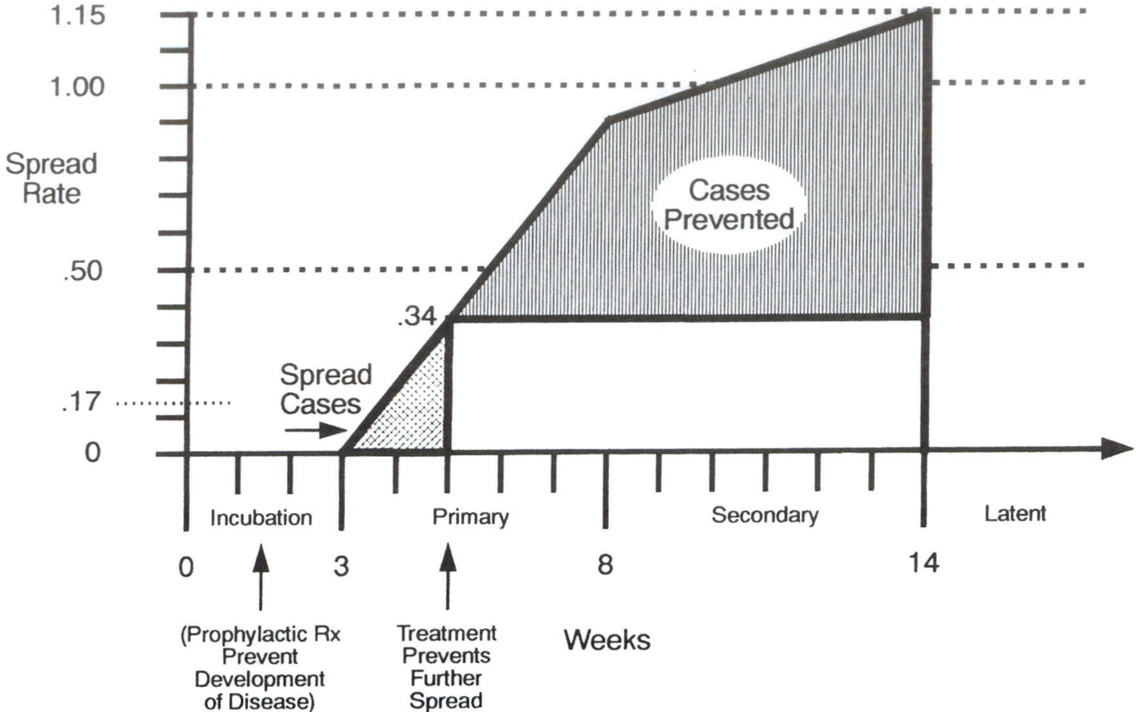

Figure 9. Preventing syphilis by treatment.

9.1.2. Core Populations. These interventions can be concentrated to achieve maximal impact. Community variability in syphilis reproductive rates will dictate the different levels of public health effort required. Over the past two decades, the heterogeneous distribution of all STDs, including syphilis, has led to the concept of "core populations."[28,29] Core populations (also called "epidemic networks") are defined as those sociosexual networks that contribute a disproportionate share to sustaining STD rates in communities. From the above model, as well as empiric data,[27] syphilis core groups will need higher rates of sex partner change than other STDs to maintain the infection within a sexual network.

Current evidence supports this epidemic network concept for syphilis. In Seville, Spain,[30] syphilis (along with gonorrhea and chlamydia) showed a distinct spatial clustering. In upstate New York,[31] the distribution of syphilis was more diverse than gonorrhea, but still could be connected through two endemic foci: (1) inner-city, heterosexual African-American populations; and (2) suburban, homosexual/bisexual white and African-American groups. In Multnomah County, Oregon,[32] a syphilis core population was identified using geographic and sociodemographic measures as proxies for these sociosexual networks. The Oregon core group, like others, was characterized by spatial clustering, low socioeconomic status, and a high proportion of African-American persons.

9.2. Control and Prevention

A recurrent theme in the control and prevention of syphilis is the need for a multidisciplinary coordinated, multifocal program. A variety of interventions, tailored to local epidemiological and social circumstances, are required to reach the epidemic networks and to lower the reproductive rate. The following sections summarize the chief elements of a coherent syphilis control program.

9.2.1. Screening. The advent of serological detection methods provided the technological impetus for modern syphilis control programs. Widespread testing to eliminate syphilis has enormous intuitive appeal. Nonetheless, the zeal for mass screening has been tempered by realistic comparisons of screening costs.[33] Such considerations have produced general agreement that universal syphilis screening in many industrialized nations, including the United States, cannot be justified.

Less unanimity exists, however, about the value of more targeted screening. First, attitudes toward syphilis screening change drastically with the slope of the trend line. The subjective valuation of screening a particular population will change if that community's perceived risk of transmission is thought to be high (e.g., the epidemiological importance of screening commercial sex workers). Second, confusion exists between the role of screening as a tool for case finding and the role of screening in interrupting transmission. Case finding generally rests on a subjective judgment of the social value of finding an infected person (e.g., the use of universal prenatal screening to detect the rare case of congenital syphilis). The interruption of transmission through syphilis screening is harder to verify primarily because detection of asymptomatic cases cannot be directly equated with diminished disease transmission. Except in situations in which syphilis incidence is increasing, most screening programs will identify persons in noninfectious stages of the disease, and thus will have little impact on transmission.

As described previously, the concept of screening in "core populations" has become increasingly popular. Whether these groups are defined by occupation (e.g., commercial sex workers), by facility (e.g., prisons, hospital emergency rooms), by risk environment (e.g., gay bathhouse, "crack house"), by geographic location (e.g., census tract), or by sociodemographic variables (e.g., poverty, ethnicity), the epidemiological principle is the same. Screening targeted to high prevalence areas should interrupt core transmission and should have an accelerated impact on reducing community incidence. This approach has been evaluated in Oregon, using geographic and sociodemographic markers for the core.[32] The results of this screening intervention were inconclusive; new cases were identified, but their connection to true core transmitters were unclear.

No incontrovertible guidance emerges from the literature on experience with syphilis screening. Despite the development of better quantitative tools for evaluation of costs and benefits, considerable subjective judgment is still required. Only one published report directly addressed the question of whether or not screening interrupts transmission of syphilis,[34] though the size and scope of that study may not have been sufficient to warrant generalization. Most studies discuss "yield" of active syphilis cases; even similar syphilis yields evoke markedly different value judgments regarding public health utility.

Nevertheless, the diversity of screening data (and opinions) suggests two common themes. First, wide variation in the prevalence of syphilis provides a justification for screening as a form of cross-sectional syphilis surveillance. Second, the observed variation in syphilis positivity means that screening decisions should be based on local data—whatever criterion for efficacy is invoked. If screening is to have any value as a mechanism for case finding or for disease control, it must be locally applied and locally analyzed.

9.2.2. Clinical Diagnosis as a Tool for Disease Control. Syphilis symptoms and signs are protean. Clinical diagnosis, while difficult, is crucial for both case finding and prevention. Moreover, clinical services are the final common pathway through which treatment is given, cure is achieved, and prevention is accelerated. Thus, these services must be easily accessible to the core populations.

Few studies have documented either the percentage of infected patients who recognize their syphilis symptoms or the percentage of those with recognized symptoms who seek medical services. Without such recognition and health care seeking, opportunities for clinical diagnosis are diminished. In one nationwide study, 45% of persons who were identified through partner notification efforts admitted that they had recognized symptoms of syphilis but did not seek medical advice.[3]

Despite these difficulties, the majority of early syphilis cases reported to public health authorities have resulted from clinical diagnoses based on patient symptoms. In the late 1940s, about two thirds of all persons diagnosed with primary or secondary syphilis sought medical care on their own initiative.[35] Likewise, in 1990, 62% of those with early syphilis obtained clinical services based on their own suspicions of illness (CDC, Division of STD/HIV Prevention, unpublished data, July 1991).

Even when the symptoms of genital ulcers occur and the patient seeks care, diagnosis using clinical parameters alone is notoriously difficult. This situation is made even worse when low prevalence leads to clinician unfamiliarity. For example, in one series of 100 patients with genital ulcers, clinicians without benefit of laboratory findings were unable to identify the specific microbial etiology in more than half.[35]

In the 1990s, the public health system for delivering clinical preventive services is drastically overburdened. STD clinics, traditionally the referral point for syphilis patients, share this burden. For example, in southern US facilities, lack of access to well-trained, empathetic STD clinicians was common.[36] Moreover, waiting times were longer and fewer patients were treated. Patients turned away from these public facilities represent missed opportunities for STD prevention. The effect of the upcoming health reform on improving clinical services for syphilis, as well as other STD, remains to be seen.

9.2.3. The Role of Treatment. Providing proper treatment for both symptomatic and asymptomatic persons is the sine qua non of syphilis control. Penicillin treatment based on presumptive diagnosis of syphilis is inexpensive, simple, safe, and effective. Thus, as shown on the model above, early and adequate treatment of syphilis patients and their sex partners is the essential means of preventing community spread.

In addition to treating those diagnosed with syphilis, selective prophylactic (preventive or epidemiological) treatment also has a major role in syphilis control strategies.[37] Over the years, this approach of selective preventive treatment has helped to limit multiple outbreaks of syphilis. Coupled with the process of active partner notification (see Section 10.4), prophylactic treatment of persons exposed to infectious syphilis has effectively controlled epidemics in both rural[38] and urban[39] settings. Benzathine penicillin for syphilis is especially helpful for outbreaks. Because it produces treponemicidal concentrations of penicillin for at least 3 weeks, this agent provides an interval of "antibiotic" quarantine[40] during which reinfection is hindered.

Within certain circumscribed communities with a high prevalence of infection, selective mass penicillin treatment has been useful. For example, in Fresno, California in 1977, selective mass treatment of commercial sex workers interrupted an ongoing syphilis epidemic.[40] The same strategy, though for different indications, has been applied by the World Health Organization for eradicating yaws.[41,42] Not surprisingly, this mass treatment approach also lowered the prevalence, albeit temporarily, of venereal syphilis in those communities where it was applied.

9.2.4. Partner Notification. Rapid investigation of sex partners is aimed at bringing persons with early syphilis to treatment before they can spread the infection within the community. In fact, syphilis is the prototypic STD on which the prevention strategy of partner notification was based, both in theoretical concept and in practical application.

Traditionally, syphilis control programs in the developed countries have emphasized active intervention by health providers to interview patients, to identify sex partners, and to assure that partners are evaluated and treated.[43] The privacy of patients and partners is rigorously protected. Up through the 1960s, a number of reports attested to the success of this epidemiological approach for syphilis control.[44–49] Whether applied to isolated rural communities,[50,51] selected urban neighborhoods,[52] or captive prison settings,[53] rapid sex partner identification, location, and treatment reduced syphilis occurrence.

The partner notification process involves a series of interrelated activities: interviewing the infected patient to obtain a complete list of exposed sex partners, finding these persons in the community, and assuring that they are treated promptly. In the United States, interviewing techniques have been developed to encourage patient cooperation in naming a maximum number of partners.[3] However, during the 1960s and 1970s, the contact index—a measure of the yield of the syphilis interview—steadily declined (Fig. 10). Possible interactive reasons for this trend include: a true decrease in the number of sex partners in infected persons; changing environments for sexual relations whereby a greater percentage of partners are anonymous (e.g., gay bathhouses, crack houses); an increasing atmosphere of distrust of all governmental organizations, including those delivering public health services; deteriorating interviewing techniques; and the increasing competition of other STDs.

Problems with syphilis interview productivity have persisted to the present. In Oregon, similar interviewing techniques produced far fewer locatable sex partners for syphilis patients than for those with gonorrhea.[54] Presumably this reflected the condition of anonymous sex, frequently in exchange for drugs, in those environments where syphilis was being transmitted. In Oregon, 28% of syphilis patients exchanged sex for money or drugs, but accounted for nearly 80% of the unlocatable sex partners. For gonorrhea patients, 17% acknowledged sex-for-drugs/money, and these accounted for 36% of the unlocatable sex partners. Moreover, depending on which measure of case-finding effectiveness is used, the costs of provider referral for partner notification are challengeable.[32]

Locating patients also may have become more difficult in recent years. Distrust of government agencies may have worsened in the African-American community after revelations of the Tuskegee syphilis study.[55] Moreover, the association of high-risk sexual behavior with environments where illicit drug use and violence are common has made the safety of the STD outreach worker an issue.

Using specific populations, rather than infected individuals, as the units for syphilis intervention is a means for overcoming problems with naming and locating sex partners. In the past, this community-oriented approach was a type of "cluster" interviewing. Syphilis patients, in addition to their known sex partners, were queried about other persons in whom and specific social settings in which syphilis transmission may have occurred.[56] Although this cluster approach produced a lower yield of infected, previously untreated patients than following up those specifically named as sex partners, it still identified a relatively high percentage of persons who might not have been reached in any other way. In fact, depending on how

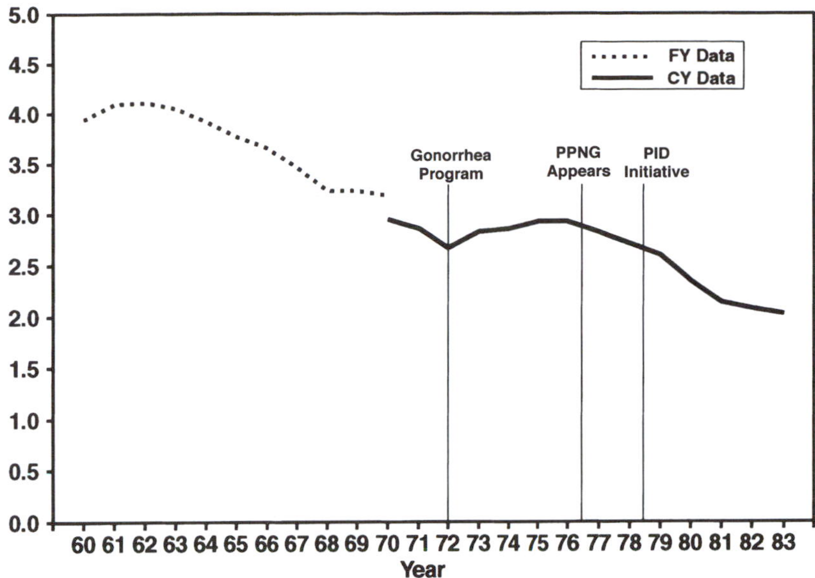

Figure 10. Contact index, 1960–1983, primary and secondary syphilis, public STD clinic patients.

the "socially-related group" was defined, up to one in five people examined had untreated syphilis.[56]

In recent years, similar population-based approaches have been used to identify particular communities at high risk of syphilis. Examples of situations in which this community intervention was successful in stemming syphilis outbreaks include (1) a Native American tribe reluctant to name any partners to outside officials,[57] (2) a Philadelphia neighborhood where crack-cocaine environments led to unsafe sexual behaviors and high levels of syphilis,[58] and (3) a Montgomery County, Alabama, intensive program that identified sociosexual networks responsible for the continued spread of syphilis.[59]

9.2.5. Health Education. Our current community health education efforts usually encourage primary prevention (preventing acquisition of syphilis) in persons at risk. Over the last decade, HIV prevention resources have stimulated community education for safer sexual behaviors, which in turn has led to safer social norms. Health education interventions can also be directed to individual patients diagnosed with syphilis. They are designed to promote early therapy if symptoms such as genital ulcers recur, avoidance of sex after onset of syphilis symptoms, and notification of all sex partners. If successful, this counseling will result in both primary prevention (prevention of further syphilis transmission) and secondary prevention (prevention of later complications).

Other primary prevention approaches, financed by HIV prevention dollars, could also help reduce syphilis. These include both advocating risk avoidance methods and distributing condoms and counseling about safer sex. Condoms, although shown to be effective in limiting the transmission of HIV and other STDs,[60] are not used regularly by many high-risk individuals. Thus, we need more creative methods of condom promotion, including making them more widely available at little or no cost, to enhance syphilis control. However, sexual behavior change is not easily achieved in populations characterized by drug use, poverty, low education, unemployment, and inadequate health care. These groups need to be specifically targeted by health education campaigns and provided improved access to health care for syphilis screening, diagnosis, and treatment.[61]

Experience with HIV community education has shown that: (1) changing social norms is fundamental to influencing safer individual sexual behavior; and (2) reinforcing these safer behaviors regularly by trusted peers is crucial to preventing relapse to unsafe practices. Syphilis control in the homosexual community has already benefited from these HIV lessons. In socially disadvantaged communities, pilot programs using commercial sex workers as outreach workers have been successful in educating high-risk women about syphilis and in identifying pregnant women who need prenatal care, including syphilis testing.

9.2.6. Immunization. Another hope for primary prevention of syphilis is active immunization against either the infection or the disease. Because of the immune response generated during the natural history of untreated

T. pallidum infection, prospects for developing a protective vaccine might seem encouraging. Acquired resistance to further *T. pallidum* infection occurs from both human and experimental syphilis.[62] However, attempts to generate long-term protection using a single immunogen have been disappointing.[63] Because the clinical features of syphilis are so unusual, and we still know so little about the biology of *T. pallidum*, we are still many years away from a syphilis vaccine.

10. Unresolved Problems

1. *More accessible clinical services.* All symptomatic patients must be able to receive prompt diagnosis and treatment. If public or private facilities are not available or are overburdened in the high-incidence communities, then temporary, mobile alternatives must be provided.
2. *Population-based partner notification.* Data obtained from the process of eliciting the location and sociosexual networks of sex partners must be used for both individual and population benefit. Where epidemiological analysis of partner patterns reveals high-risk communities, public health officials must move quickly to intervene clinically.
3. *Wider prophylactic treatment.* Among selected populations for which levels of infectious syphilis are high, prophylactic treatment based on "epidemiological" indications must be considered. Alternatively, targeted community screening, with immediate presumptive treatment of all rapid plasma reagin-positive patients, must be implemented.
4. *Greater community involvement in syphilis control.* Public health officials must continue to build on the network of community-based organizations generated by interest in HIV prevention. Local decision makers must be reeducated about the importance of syphilis and the role of early diagnosis/treatment in preventing its spread, so they can become advocates for promoting behavioral change and securing clinical resources.
5. *Ongoing provider training.* Clinicians must be trained to "think syphilis," especially if practicing in high-incidence communities. Residency programs should include rotations through local STD clinics, not only to upgrade clinical STD skills but also to allow an understanding of real world behaviors contributing to syphilis spread.

In actuality, these challenges are really nothing new.[6] "Environmental" or "community-based" approaches to controlling syphilis have long been with us. In multiple situations during the past four decades, after intensive screening programs documented high levels of syphilis in particular sociosexual networks, the "risk marker" of being in that network became enough of an epidemiological justification to "presumptively treat" persons for syphilis.[6] Not surprisingly, the morbidity level in the community was drastically lowered.

Many states are now offering examples of similar community control programs based on data indicating high prevalence of infection. For example, Oregon used geographic markers to focus on "core transmitters"; Arizona treated individuals on the basis of zip code; California used community-based organizations to identify and aggressively treat persons "on-the-street" who otherwise would not seek care in health facilities; Philadelphia has used "crack house" locations as indications for immediate diagnosis and, where possible, presumptive treatment of syphilis; New York State and Los Angeles have used correctional facilities as locations where rapid syphilis treatment could be delivered; and finally, New York City has used particular drug-related diagnoses of persons seeking care in emergency rooms as reasons to deliver penicillin therapy. These represent only a few of the current supplementary approaches to case identification and presumptive treatment based on epidemiological indications.[61]

Are we simply suggesting reinventing the wheel? In one sense, yes; in another sense, no. Bolstered by our rapidly evolving electronic data system, we are better able today to target interventions, design appropriate evaluations, and disseminate the results of our efforts than we were in earlier years. Working together, epidemiologists (clinical, behavioral, and statistical) and program managers need to merge their skills both to document the success of specific syphilis control activities and to refinethose that are less effective. This epidemiological/managerial interaction to continually evaluate our interventions will keep syphilis control at the cutting edge of public health well into the 21st century.[6,61]

ACKNOWLEDGMENTS

I am grateful to both Stephen J. Kraus, MD, and the late Joseph G. Lossick, DO, the authors of the Syphilis chapter in the second edition of this book, for their extensive clinical expertise that provided a strong foundation for this current chapter. Thanks also to Sandra W. Bowden, CPS, for her technical assistance in preparing the manuscript.

11. References

1. Parran, T., *Shadow on the Land*, Reynal and Hitchcock, New York, 1937.
2. Baumgartner, L., Curtis, A. C., Gray, A. L., Kuechle, B. E., and Richman, T. L., *The Eradication of Syphilis: A Task Force Report to the Surgeon General Public Health Service on Syphilis Control in the United States*, US Public Health Service, Washington, DC, 1961.
3. Brown, W. J., Donohue, J. F., Axnick, N. W., Blount, J. H., Ewen, N. H., and Jones, O. K., *Syphilis and Other Venereal Diseases*, Harvard University Press, Cambridge, MA, 1970.
4. Brandt, A. M., *No Magic Bullet: A Social History of Venereal Disease in the United States since 1880*, Oxford University Press, New York, 1985.
5. Pusey, W. A., *The History and Epidemiology of Syphilis*, Charles C. Thomas, Springfield, IL, 1933.
6. Cates, W., Jr., Rothenberg, R. B., and Blount, J. H., Syphilis control: The historical context and epidemiologic basis for interrupting sexual transmission of *Treponema pallidum*, *Sex. Transm. Dis.* **23:**68–75 (1996).
7. Nakashima, A. K., Rolfs, R. T., Flock, M. L., Kilmarx, P., and Greenspan, J. R., Epidemiology of syphilis in the United States, 1941–1993, *Sex. Transm. Dis.* **23:**16–23 (1996).
8. Centers for Disease Control and Prevention, Division of STD Prevention, *STD Surveillance 1994*, Division of STD Prevention, Atlanta, GA, 1995.
9. Hahn, R. A., Magder, L. S., Aral, S. O., *et al.*, Race and the prevalence of syphilis seroreactivity in the United States population: A national sero-epidemiologic study, *Am. J. Public Health* **79:**467–470 (1989).
10. Klingbeil, L. J., and Clark, E. G., Studies in the epidemiology of syphilis. III. Conjugal syphilis, *Vener. Dis. Infect.* **22:**1–6 (1941).
11. Clarke, E. G., Studies in the epidemiology of syphilis. I. Material on which epidemiological studies are based; II. Contact investigation, *Vener. Dis. Infect.* **21:**349–369 (1941).
12. Sparling, P. F., Natural history of syphilis, in: *Sexually Transmitted Diseases*, 2nd ed. (K. K. Holmes *et al.*, eds.), pp. 213–219, McGraw-Hill, New York, 1990.
13. Magnuson, H. J., Thomas, E. W., Orlansky, S. Inoculation syphilis in human volunteers, *Medicine* **35:**33–82 (1956).
14. Fiumara, N. The incidence of prenatal syphilis at the Boston City Hospital, *N. Engl. J. Med.* **247:**48–52 (1952).
15. Aral, S. O., The social context of syphilis persistence in the southeastern United States, *Sex. Transm. Dis.* **23:**9–15 (1996).
16. Fieldsteel, A. H., and Miao, R. H., Genetics of treponema, in *Pathogenesis and Immunology of Treponemal Infection* (R. F. Schell and D. M. Misher, eds.), Dekker, New Yor' 1982.
17. Hook, E. W., and Marra, C. M., Acquired syphilis in adults, *N. Engl. J. Med.* **326:**1060–1069 (1992).
18. Gjestland, T., The Oslo study of untreated syphilis: An epidemiological investigation of the natural course of syphilis infection based on a restudy of the Boech–Bruusgaard material, *Acta Derm. Venereol.* **35**(Suppl 34) 11–44 (1955).
19. Johns, D. R., Tierney, M., and Felsenstein, D., Alternation in the natural history of neurosyphilis by concurrent infection with the human immunodeficiency virus, *N. Engl. J. Med.* **316:**1569–1572 (1987).
20. Garnett, G. P., Aral, S. O., Hoyle, D. V., Cates, W. Jr., and Anderson, R. M., The natural history of syphilis: Implications for the transmission dynamics and control of infection. *Sex. Trans. Dis.* **24:**185–200 (1997).
21. Oxman, G. L., Smolkowski, K., and Noell, J., Mathematical modeling of epidemic syphilis transmission: Implications for syphilis control programs, *Sex. Transm. Dis.* **23:**30–39 (1996).
22. Alexander, L. J., Schoch, A. G., and Mantooth, W. B., Abortive treatment of syphilis, *Am. J. Syph. Gonor. Vener. Dis.* **33:**429–436 (1949).
23. Idsoe, O., Guthe, T., Christiansen, S., Krag, P., and Cutler, J. C., A decade of reorientation in the treatment of venereal syphilis, *Bull. WHO* **10:**507–561 (1954).
24. Moore, M. B., Jr., Price, E. V., Knox, J. M., and Elgin, L. W., Epidemiologic treatment of contacts to infectious syphilis, *Public Health Rep.* **78:**966–970 (1963).
25. Schroeter, A. L., Turner, R. H., Lucas, J. B., and Brown, W. J., Therapy for incubating syphilis, *J. Am. Med. Assoc.* **218:**711–713 (1971).
26. Schober, P. C., Gabriel, G., White, P., Felton, W. F., and Thin, R. N., How infectious is syphilis? *Br. J. Vener. Dis.* **59:**217–219 (1983).
27. Blount, J. H., Working concepts for syphilis control, paper presented at International Seminar on Venereal Disease Control, Atlanta, Georgia, October 17, 1971.
28. Brunham, R. C., and Plummer, F. A., A general model of sexually transmitted disease epidemiology and its implications for control. *Med. Clin. North Am.* **74:**1339–1352 (1990).
29. Rothenbert, R., and Marramore, J., Commentary: The relevance of social network concepts to sexually transmitted disease control, *Sex. Transm. Dis.* **23:**24–29 (1996).
30. Alvarez-Dardet, C., Marquez, S., and Perea, E. J., Urban clusters of sexually transmitted diseases in the city of Seville, Spain, *Sex. Transm. Dis.* **12:**166–168 (1985).
31. Rothenberg, R. B., The geography of syphilis: A demonstration of epidemiologic diversity, *Advances in Sexually Transmitted Diseases* (R. Morisset and L. Kurstak, eds.), pp. 125–133, VNU Science Press, Utrecht, The Netherlands, 1986.
32. Oxman, G. L., and Doyle, L., A comparison of the case-finding effectiveness and average costs of screening and partner notification, *Sex. Transm. Dis.* **23:**51–57 (1996).
33. Schmid, G. P., Serologic screening for syphilis: Rationale, cost and realpolitik, *Sex. Transm. Dis.* **23:**45–50 (1996).
34. Wolf, F. C., and Judson, F. N., Intensive screening for gonorrhea, syphilis, and hepatitis B in a gay bathhouse does not lower the prevalence of infection, *Sex. Transm. Dis.* **7:**49–52 (1980).
35. Chapel, T. A., Brown, W. J., Jeffries, C., *et al.*, How reliable is the morphological diagnosis of penile ulcerations? *Sex. Transm. Dis.* **4:**150–155 (1977).
36. Gibson, J. J., Leverette, W., and Arvelo, M., Providers of syphilis care in the Southern United States, *Sex. Trans. Dis.* **23:**40–44 (1996).
37. Hart, G., Epidemiologic treatment for syphilis and gonorrhea. *Sex. Trans. Dis.* **7:**149–160 (1980).
38. Ball, R. W., Outbreak of infectious syphilis in South Carolina, *J. Am. Med. Assoc.* **193:**101–104 (1965).
39. Lee, C. B., Brunham, R. C., Sherman, E., and Harding, A. K. M., Epidemiology of an outbreak of infectious syphilis in Manitoba, *Am. J. Epidemiol.* **125:**277–283 (1987).
40. Jaffe, H. W., Rice, D. T., Voigt, R., Fowler, J., and St. John, R. K., Selective mass treatment in a venereal disease control program, *Am. J. Public Health* **69:**1181–1182 (1979).
41. Hackett, C. J., and Guthe, T., Some important aspects of yaws eradication, *Bull. WHO* **15:**869–896 (1956).

42. Grin, E. I., and Guthe, T., Evaluation of a previous mass campaign against endemic syphilis in Bosnia and Herzegovina, *Br. J. Vener. Dis.* **49**:1–19 (1972).
43. Rothenberg, R. B., and Potterat, J. J., Strategies for management of sex partners, in: *Sexually Transmitted Diseases*, 2nd ed. (K. K. Holmes *et al.*, eds.), pp. 1081–1086, McGraw-Hill, New York, 1990.
44. Smith, D. C., and Brunfield, W .A., Jr., Tracing the transmission of syphilis, *J. Am. Med. Assoc.* **101**:1955–1957.
45. Clark, E. G., and Kampmeier, R. N., Contact investigation and the early recognition of syphilis, *Urol. Cutan. Rev.* **43**:169–170 (1939).
46. Clark, E. G., Studies in the epidemiology of syphilis. Epidemiologic investigations in a series of 996 cases of acquired syphilis: II. Contact investigation in a series of 824 patients with syphilis, *J. Vener. Dis. Inform.* **21**:349–369 (1940).
47. Fiumara, J. N., Segal, J., and Jolly, J., Contact investigation: Combined military–civilian program, *Public Health Rep.* **68**:289–294 (1953).
48. Dougherty, W. J., Epidemiologic treatment of syphilis contacts, *J. Med. Soc. NJ* **59**:564–567 (1962).
49. Moore, M. D., Price, E. V., Knox, J. M., and Elgin, L. W., Epidemiological treatment of contacts to infectious syphilis, *Public Health Rep.* **78**:966–970 (1963).
50. Gray, A. L., Iskrant, A. P., and Hibbets, R. S., Contact investigation in rural county in Mississippi, *J. Vener. Dis. Inform.* **50**:165–169 (1949).
51. Kimbrough, R. C., Cowgill, D. M., and Bowerman, E. P., Rural syphilis—a localized outbreak, *Am. J. Public Health* **28**:756–758 (1938).
52. Webster, B., and Shelley, E. I., Studies in the epidemiology of primary and secondary syphilis in New York City, *Am. J. Public Health* **31**:1199–1205 (1941).
53. Smith, W. H. Y., Syphilis epidemic in a southern prison, *J. Med. Assoc. Ala.* **32**:392–394 (1965).
54. Andrus, J. K., Fleming, D. W., Harger, D. R., *et al.*, Partner notification: Can it control epidemic syphilis? *Ann Intern Med* **112**:539–543 (1990).
55. Jones, J. H., *Bad Blood: The Tuskegee Syphilis Experiment*, The Free Press, New York, 1981.
56. Kaufman, R. E., Blount, J. H., and Jones, O. G., Current trends in syphilis, *Public Health Rev.* **3**:175–196 (1974).
57. Gerber, A. R., King, L. C., Dunleavy, G. J., and Novick, L. F., An outbreak of syphilis on an Indian reservation: Descriptive epidemiology and disease-control measures, *Am. J. Public Health* **79**: 83–85 (1989).
58. Mellinger, A. K., Goldberg, M., Wade, A., *et al.*, Alternative case-finding in a crack-related syphilis epidemic—Philadelphia, *Morbid. Mortal. Week. Rep.* **40**:77–80 (1991).
59. Engelgau, M. M., Woernle, C. H., Rolfs, R. T., Greenspan, J. R., O'Cain, M., and Gorsky, R. D., Control of epidemic early syphilis: The results of an intervention campaign using social networks, *Sex. Transm. Dis.* **22**:203–209 (1995).
60. Cates, W., Jr., and Stone, K. M., Family planning sexually transmitted diseases, and contraceptive choice: A literature update, *Fam. Plan. Perspect.* **24**:75–84 (1992).
61. St. Louis, M. E., Strategies for syphilis prevention in the 1990s, *Sex. Transm. Dis.* **23**:58–67 (1996).
62. Miller, J. N., Cellular and molecular approaches to the development of a vaccine for syphilis: Current status and prospects for the future, in: *Vaccines for Sexually Transmitted Diseases* (A. Meheus and R. E. Spier, eds.), pp. 105–116, Butterworths, London, 1989.
63. Musher, D. M., Baughn, R. E., Lapushin, R. W., Knox, J. M., and Duncan, W. C., The role of a vaccine for syphilis, *Sex. Transm. Dis.* **4**:163–166 (1977).

12. Suggested Reading

Branch, A. M., *No Magic Bullet: A Social History of Venereal Disease in the United States since 1880*, Oxford University Press, New York, 1985.

Brown, W. J., Donohue, J. F., Axnick, N. W., Blount, J. H., Ewen, N. H., and Jones, O. K., *Syphilis and Other Venereal Diseases*, Harvard University Press, Cambridge, MA, 1970.

Cates, W., Jr., Rothenberg, R. B., and Blount, J. H., Syphilis control: The historical context and epidemiologic basis for interrupting sexual transmission of *Treponema pallidum, Sex. Transm. Dis.* **23**:68–75 (1996).

Hook, E. W., and Marra, C. M., Acquired syphilis in adults, *N. Engl. J. Med.* **326**:1060–1069 (1992).

Jones, J. H., *Bad Blood: The Tuskegee Syphilis Experiment*, The Free Press, New York, 1981.

Nakashima, A. K., Rolfs, R. T., Flock, M. L., Kilmarx, P., and Greenspan, J. R., Epidemiology of syphilis in the United States, 1941–1993, *Sex. Transm. Dis.* **23**:16–23 (1996).

Oxman, G. L., Smolkowski, K., and Noell, J., Mathematical modeling of epidemic syphilis transmission: Implications for syphilis control programs, *Sex. Transm. Dis.* **23**:30–39 (1996).

Parran, T., *Shadow on the Land*, Reynal and Hitchcock, New York, 1937.

Schmid, G. P., Serologic screening for syphilis: Rationale, cost and realpolitik, *Sex. Transm. Dis.* **23**:51–57 (1996).

Sparling, P. F., Natural history of syphilis, in: *Sexually Transmitted Diseases*, 2nd ed. (K. K. Holmes *et al.*, eds.), pp. 213–219, McGraw-Hill, New York, 1990.

St. Louis, M. E., Strategies for syphilis prevention in the 1990s, *Sex. Transm. Dis.* **23**:58–67 (1996).

CHAPTER 36

Nonvenereal Treponematoses

Peter L. Perine

1. Introduction

The endemic treponematoses are a group of chronic diseases affecting primarily the skin of children and young adults who live in remote, impoverished areas between the tropics of Cancer and Capricorn. They are considered as a group because they have many clinical, pathological, and epidemiological features in common (Table 1). They are also caused by spirochetes that are closely related to one another and to *Treponema pallidum* of venereal syphilis.[1] These diseases with their etiologic treponeme in order of their worldwide prevalence are: yaws (*T. pallidum* ssp. *pertenue*), endemic syphilis (*T. pallidum* ssp. *endemicum*), and pinta (*T. carateum*).[2] Other related treponemes cause venereal syphilis in rabbits (*T. cuniculi*) and asymptomatic infections in African baboons (*T. freiborg-blanc*), but they have no epidemiological significance as far as human infections are concerned.

2. Historical Background

There are two theories about the origin of the treponematoses. The unitarian theory suggests that they are all caused by a single treponeme that has been modified by the environment, and the Columbian theory states that these diseases are caused by distinct species of treponemes.[3,4] The unitarian theory seems to be the more tenable in light of recent DNA hybridization and other studies that indicate almost complete homology between the *T. pallidum* of venereal and nonvenereal syphilis and *T. pertenue*.[1,5] The controversy about the origins of the treponematoses is focused on venereal syphilis, which appeared in Europe in the late 15th century as a highly contagious and fatal disease. Its appearance in Europe coincided with the return of Columbus from the New World and historians ascribed its origin to the New World.[6,7] A more plausible explanation is that endemic syphilis, long prevalent in west Africa, became venereally transmitted among Europeans after its importation into Europe by sailors and African slaves.[8]

Yaws was one of the most prevalent infectious diseases of the tropics before the penicillin era (Fig. 1). The development of long-acting penicillin preparations, producing a treponemicidal blood level for 3 to 4 weeks after a single injection, made mass treatment of treponemal infections feasible.[9] In 1949, the World Health Organization (WHO) agreed to conduct coordinated mass treatment campaigns against yaws, endemic syphilis, and pinta. Demonstration projects in yaws-endemic areas confirmed the efficacy of single injections of penicillin aluminum monostearate in mass treatment campaigns, the need to examine at least 90% of the target population during the initial survey, and the need to conduct resurveys of treated populations to treat new cases and reinfections.[9] From 1952 to 1968, an estimated 160 million persons were examined during yaws campaigns worldwide and 50 million persons with clinical or latent infections and their contacts were treated with penicillin.[9,10] At the end of these campaigns, the endemic treponematoses appeared to be on their way to extinction, especially in view of the improvements in living standards that occurred in many of the endemic areas.

3. Methodology

The endemic treponematoses are reportable diseases in most countries where reservoirs of active disease persist. The best sources for these data are the regional offices

Peter L. Perine • Center for AIDS and STS, Department of Epidemiology, School of Public Health and Community Medicine, University of Washington, Seattle, Washington 98195.

Table 1. Major Features of the Treponematoses

	Venereal syphilis	Endemic syphilis	Yaws	Pinta
	T. pallidum ssp. *pallidum*	*T. pallidum* ssp. *endemicum*	*T. pallidum* ssp. *pertenue*	*T. carateum*
Age of infection	15–40	2–10	5–15	10–30
Occurrence	Worldwide	Africa, Middle East	Africa, South America, Oceania, Asia	Central and South America
Climate	All	Dry, arid	Warm, humid	Warm
Transmission				
Direct				
Venereal	Common	Rare	No	No
Nonvenereal	Rare	Common	Common	Probable
Congenital	Yes	Unproven	No	No
Indirect				
Contaminated utensils	Rare	Common	Rare	No
Insects	No	No	Possible	No
Reservoir of infection	Adults	Infectious and latent cases	Infectious and latent cases	Infectious cases
Ratio of infectious to latent cases	1:3	1:2	1:3–5	?
Late complications	+	+	+	+
Skin, bone, cartilage	+	+	+	No
Neurologic	+	Unproven	No	No
Cardiovascular	+	Unproven	No	No

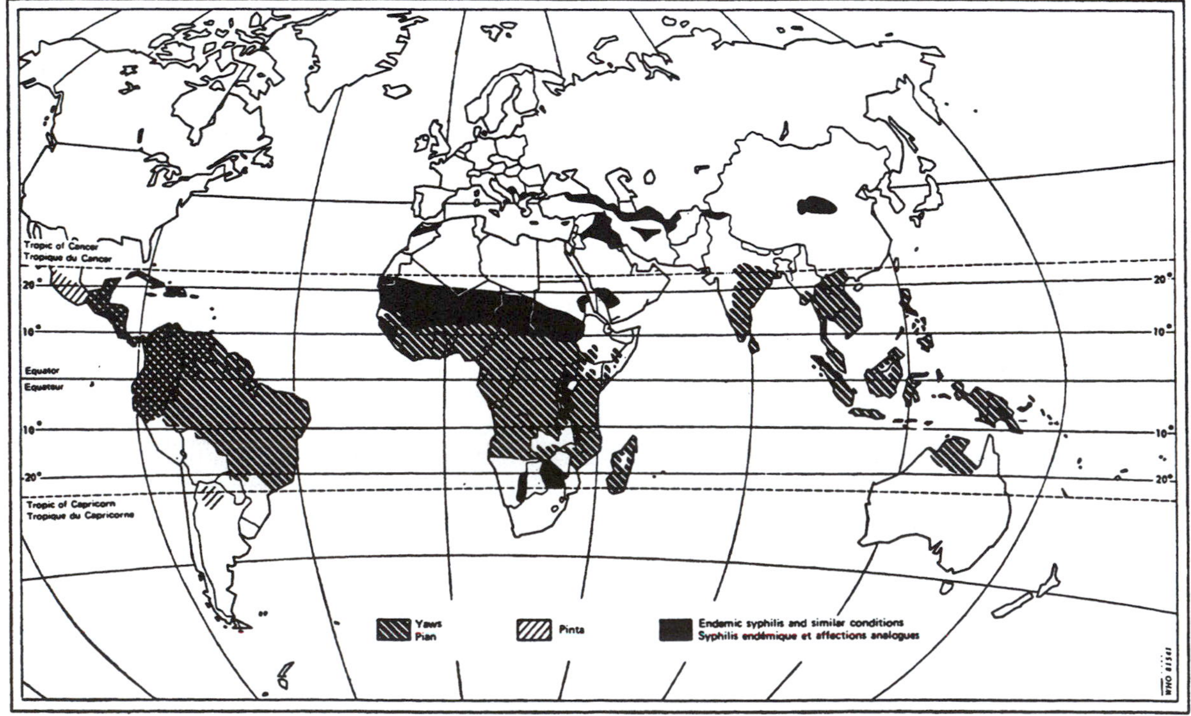

Figure 1. Geographic distribution of the endemic treponematoses in the early 1950s.

of the WHO and its *Weekly Epidemiological Record*[11] and the proceedings of recent yaws symposia.[12–14]

3.1. Sources of Mortality Data

There is little pathological or epidemiological evidence that the endemic treponematoses acquired in childhood subsequently cause fatal late cardiovascular or central nervous system (CNS) complications usually associated with venereal syphilis. Where venereal syphilis is prevalent together with yaws or endemic syphilis, however, it is impossible to differentiate visceral, ocular, and neurological lesions caused by venereal syphilis from those that might result from yaws or endemic syphilis.[15,16]

3.2. Sources of Morbidity Data

The WHO, through its regional offices, periodically reports on the prevalence of active and latent cases of the endemic treponematoses in its *Weekly Epidemiological Record.*

3.3. Surveys

Clinical and seroprevalence surveys for yaws and endemic syphilis have been conducted by many African and Asian countries since 1980 as part of a WHO initiative to control the resurgence of these diseases. The results of these surveys are usually reported to the WHO.

3.4. Laboratory Diagnosis

3.4.1. Isolation and Identification of the Organism. The pathogenic treponemes cannot be cultured *in vitro* and their identification by dark-field microscopy of lesion exudate is the standard diagostic test.[17] Lesion exudate can also be collected in heparinized blood capillary tubes and sent to a reference laboratory to be examined by specific fluorescein-tagged antibodies.[18]

3.4.2. Serological and Diagnostic Methods. Serological tests routinely employed in seroprevalence surveys are the venereal disease research laboratory (VDRL) and rapid plasma reagin (RPR) tests.[17] These tests are not specific, but their reactivity and titer in an appropriate clinical setting give a good idea of the prevalence of latent treponemal infection.

4. Biological Characteristics of the Organism

T. pallidum and its subspecies are obligate anaerobes. The lack of a cell-free *in vitro* culture method has limited comparative studies of their genetic and antigenic structure. Prototype strains of yaws and endemic syphilis treponemes produce lesions in only a few experimental animals. The lesions produced in these animals are similar to those occurring during the early stages of infection in man. Subtle differences in virulence and lesion morphology exist between subspecies and strains of *T. pallidum endemicum* and *pertenue* and variable degrees of immunity are produced to superinfection by the other pathogenic treponemes.[19] Similar subspecies and strain differences exist in most species of pathogenic bacteria.

The pathogenic treponemes are exquisitely sensitive to penicillin. Their multiplication by binary fission takes an estimated 32 hr to complete[20] and is the reason why long-acting penicillin preparations that produce low but persistent penicillin blood concentrations for 3 to 4 weeks are recommended for therapy. Despite the widespread use of penicillins in medical practice, there is no evidence that the pathogenic treponemes have developed resistance to the drugs.

T. carateum is pathogenic only in man.[19] Persons infected with this treponeme produce antibodies that react in standard treponemal and nontreponemal antigen tests for syphilis. These antibodies react against the full spectrum of antigenic molecules of *T. pallidum* ssp. *pallidum*, indicating a close genetic relationship.[5]

5. Descriptive Epidemiology

5.1. Prevalence and Incidence

In 1950, an estimated 70 to 100 million people living in large areas of Africa and Southeast Asia, the western Pacific islands, and parts of the Americas had yaws; another 1 million living in the Middle East, the Balkans, and north and west Africa had endemic syphilis; and 700,000 mostly American Indians of Central and South America had pinta (Fig. 1).[10] The ratio of infectious to latent yaws was 1:3 or more, and most infections occurred in children under 15 years of age. Improved living conditions and penicillin treatment campaigns from 1950 to 1970 dramatically reduced the prevalence of the endemic treponematoses. However, reservoirs of untreated disease persisted in many remote impoverished areas because surveillance was prematurely curtailed or discontinued.[9]

The Third International Symposium on yaws and the endemic treponematoses, held in Washington, DC, in 1984, assessed the current extent of these diseases and the feasibility of their global eradication and/or control. Resurgence of both yaws and endemic syphilis was noted to

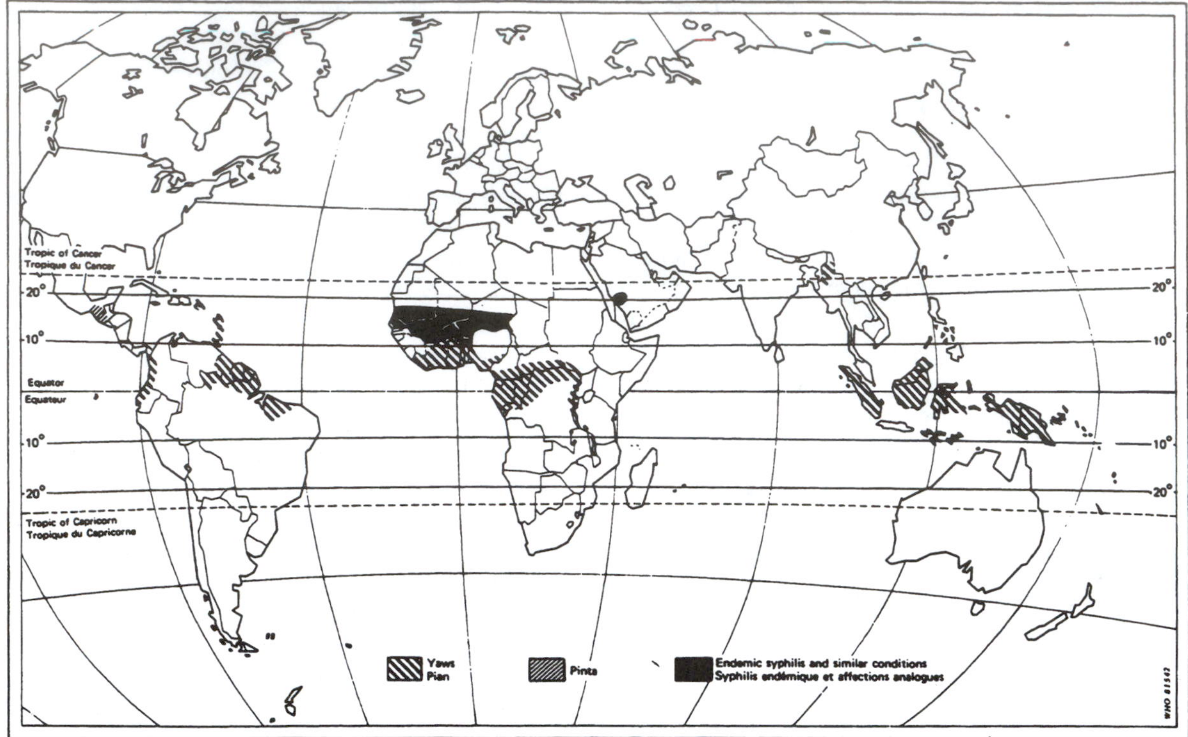

Figure 2. Geographic distribution of the endemic treponematoses in late 20th century.

have occurred in many formerly endemic areas of the world, especially among impoverished rural children and young adults born after penicillin treatment campaigns were completed. Several countries had taken recent steps to control these diseases, including mass penicillin treatment of selected affected populations. This meeting and others held in Indonesia, the Congo, and Jordan concluded that new control initiatives, integrated into primary health care activities wherever possible, were needed to interrupt transmission and spread of yaws and endemic syphilis in Africa.

Since 1980, cases of yaws have been reported from more than two dozen African nations, and there are at present an estimated 1 million children infected with yaws in Ghana, Benin, Togo, and Ivory Coast and perhaps 200,000 cases of endemic syphilis in Niger, Mali, and Burkina Faso. Foci of yaws also persist in some areas of the southern Pacific, particularly in Papua New Guinea and Indonesia. India, Thailand, and Malaysia have also experienced small epidemics of yaws in the past decade. Africa is the major reservoir of yaws and endemic syphilis.

5.2. Epidemic Behavior and Contagiousness

Yaws is highly contagious and can spread rapidly in susceptible populations when environmental conditions favor development of cutaneous lesions teeming with spirochetes. Endemic syphilis tends to affect isolated, nomadic populations, and its epidemic potential is less than that of yaws. Pinta is very difficult to transmit by person-to-person contact and has little epidemic potential.

5.3. Geographic Distribution

The worldwide distribution of the endemic treponematoses in the mid-1980s is shown in Fig. 2.

5.4. Temporal Distribution

There is no seasonality in occurrence of the endemic treponematoses, but the number, morphology, and infectiousness of cutaneous yaws lesions change during the wet and dry seasons in Africa and Asia. The high humidity associated with seasonal rains promotes an exuberant growth of papillomas and the survival of treponemes in their serous exudate, thus increasing infectiousness and the probability of person-to-person transmission. The skin is also softened by high humidity and is more susceptible to abrasions and lacerations, which are a portal of entry for treponemes. This contrasts with a paucity of infectious yaws lesions during dry seasons.

5.5. Age

In endemic areas yaws is usually acquired before age 15 from infected siblings or playmates, and active early lesions are found almost exclusively in this age group. Endemic syphilis tends to occur in family groups, the infection being acquired first by children who spread it to susceptible adults. Pinta usually first appears in young adults.

5.6. Sex

Pinta tends to occur more frequently in men, but there is no sexual predilection for yaws or endemic syphilis.

5.7. Race

Race is not a factor.

5.8. Occupation

The diseases have no relationship to occupation per se, but the vast majority of those affected live in communities that survive by subsistence farming.

5.9. Occurrence in Different Settings

These treponematoses are usually found within families and among playmates.

5.10. Socioeconomic Factors

The endemic treponematoses are prevalent today in impoverished, remote, rural populations lacking adequate clothing, water, sanitation, and medical care.

6. Mechanisms and Routes of Transmission

Transmission of yaws and endemic syphilis occurs by person-to-person contact, probably more often than not by fingers contaminated with fresh lesion exudate. Papillomas are pruritic and scratching removes loosely adherent, crusty eschars, contaminating the fingers with serous exudate loaded with viable treponemes. Various species of flies are attracted to such lesions, and it is possible that they mechanically transmit viable treponemes to the abraded or lacerated skin of nearby susceptible individuals.[21] The efficiency of such transmission by flies is probably epidemiologically insignificant.

Endemic syphilis is transmitted by person-to-person contact or by sharing of drinking cups contaminated with treponemes present in the serous exudate from lesions on the oral mucous membranes or at the corners of the mouth. Congenital transmission of yaws or endemic syphilis has not been convincingly documented.

Transmission of yaws or endemic syphilis can occur during sexual intercourse, providing one partner has infectious lesions in the genital area and the other is susceptible to infection.

The transmission of pinta requires prolonged intimate contact with an adult with active disease, as takes place in a household. Infection rates are low, even between marital couples.[20]

7. Pathogenesis and Immunity

The endemic treponematoses manifest histopathologic changes and serological responses that closely resemble those of venereal syphilis. The only practical means of comparing their pathogenicity is by experimental animal infections. *T. pallidum* ssp. *pallidum* is more invasive and pathogenic than is *T. pallidum* ssp. *pertenue*. *T. carateum* is pathogenic only for man and higher primates.

The prototype pathological lesion of yaws and endemic syphilis is a granuloma. This reflects a strong delayed hypersensitivity response to the presence of treponemes in skin and bone. Normal skin and bone are replaced by scar tissue, causing disfigurement and occasional disability. Although treponemes enter the circulation early in the course of yaws and endemic syphilis, the cardiovascular, neurological, and visceral lesions characteristic of late venereal syphilis seldom occur.[15] Indeed, infection by yaws or endemic syphilis appears to protect against venereal syphilis, which is very uncommon where these diseases are endemic.

Immunity waxes and wanes during the course of untreated yaws and endemic syphilis, especially during the 5 years following initial infection. This is manifested by the reappearance of infectious cutaneous lesions, and is the reason why penicillin must be given to asymptomatic persons living in highly endemic communities who are very likely to have latent infections. Persons with yaws or endemic syphilis are probably immune to reinfection if they have untreated infections of more than 1 year's duration.

8. Patterns of Host Response

The manifestations of yaws and endemic syphilis are usually mild and lesions are restricted to the skin and mucous membranes, heal spontaneously after several months, and leave few scars. About 10% of those infected experience more aggressive disease with destruction of skin and bone. Those who suffer severe disease may be genetically predisposed.

In populations where the endemic treponematoses are prevalent, serological surveys invariably detect more persons who have latent infections than have clinically manifest disease. Many of these patients have no recollection of early disease manifestations, suggesting that asymptomatic infection is frequent or that their earlier lesions were inconsequential or mistakenly interpreted as something else.

8.1. Clinical Features

The incubation periods of yaws, endemic syphilis, and pinta are directly related to the number of treponemes in the inoculum. The initial lesion(s) appears at the portal of entry after an incubation period of 9 to 90 days.

Pinta, yaws, and endemic and venereal syphilis are chronic infections with early and late clinical manifestations. Early lesions are infectious and usually are not destructive whereas late lesions are not infectious but are destructive.

8.1.1. Pinta. The painless initial papular lesion on an arm or leg spreads to form an irregular, reddish or bluish patch 5 to 10 cm in diameter with raised borders. Several weeks or months later, disseminated lesions ("pintides") with a morphology similar to that of the initial lesion appear on different parts of the body. Hyperkeratosis with desquamation, itching, and formation of fissures within the borders of lesions is common and may be accompanied by lymph node enlargement. The skin is the only organ pathologically affected.

In the late stage, the involved skin becomes atrophic, and the bluish coloration of the initial lesion caused by accumulation of melanin pigment in the dermis fades. This leaves the patient disfigured by red, blue, and white spots on the face, neck, arms, hands, legs, and feet. Eventually the lesions cause sclerosis of the dermis and depigmentation, leaving scars that resemble vitiligo. The evolution from the time of the appearance of the initial lesion to its late depigmented scarring may be several years.

8.1.2. Yaws. The initial lesion of yaws is usually a papule. This painless, pruritic, elevated lesion appears at the site of treponemal invasion after an incubation period of 9 to 90 days. The site of entry is often a preexisting abrasion, laceration, or insect bite. The treponemes multiply at the infection site, invade subcutaneous lymphatics, cause local lymph node enlargement, and spread systematically through the bloodstream.

The yaws papule enlarges to become a papilloma (frambesioma) that lasts 3–6 months. It may ulcerate and become secondarily infected with bacteria or heal spontaneously, thereby creating a brief period of latency. Secondary yaws lesions then appear in crops on the skin near the initial lesion or elsewhere on the body, including bone and cartilage, as a result of systemic spread and autoinoculation. Constitutional symptoms are rare, but nocturnal pain of the long bones of the leg due to periostitis and papillomas on the soles of the feet preventing weight-bearing are common.

Secondary papillomas are prominent during wet seasons and involute to form micropapules and macules during dry seasons. The lesions heal spontaneously and do not leave permanent scars unless they ulcerate and become secondarily infected by pyogenic bacteria. The disease then enters a noninfectious latent period that may last the lifetime of the patient.

During the first 5 years after infection, the state of latency may be interrupted at any time by the reappearance of infectious yaws lesions. Destructive gummatous lesions appear in the skin or osseous tissue in about 10% of those infected, usually several years after the initial infection. These late lesions mutilate and cripple.

8.1.3. Endemic Syphilis. A primary lesion is rarely seen in endemic syphilis. The first lesions to appear are painless ulcerations on the oropharyngeal mucosa. These are followed by a variety of skin, bone, and joint lesions that are indistinguishable from those of yaws. Skin lesions prefer the moist body surfaces such as the axillary and genital areas. Angular stomatitis or split papules at the corners of the mouth are more common than in yaws and are ideally situated to contaminate drinking vessels.

Osteoperiostitis of the long bones occurs more frequently in endemic syphilis than in yaws. It usually involves the long bones of the lower extremities, causing nocturnal leg pains. Gummas of the nasopharynx, skin, and bone are common in late endemic syphilis and may progress to destructive ulcers. Such ulceration may destroy nasal tissue, producing a terrible disfiguring lesion known as gangosa. Chronic osteoperiostitis and gangosa are still frequently encountered among adult nomadic Bedouins of the Arabian peninsula(22) and occasionally in children and adults suffering from late yaws in west Africa.(17)

8.2. Diagnosis

A presumptive diagnoses of yaws, pinta, or endemic syphilis can usually be made by careful assessment of the clinical features that characterized each infection in appropriate epidemiological settings. Pinta is easily differentiated clinically from yaws, and endemic and venereal syphilis. The differentiation between sporadic cases of yaws and endemic syphilis may not be possible because they may coexist in the same geographic area and their clinical and serological manifestations are indistinguishable.

The most sensitive and specific diagnostic test for treponemes is dark-field microscopic examination of freshly isolated lesion exudate. With this technique, motile treponemes appear as brilliant coiled threads on a dark background. Lesion exudate can also be collected and fixed on microscope slides and sent to a reference laboratory for microscopic examination using *T. pallidum*-specific monoclonal antibodies.[18]

A number of different serological tests are used to detect antibodies produced in response to treponemal infections. These tests were originally designed for use in venereal syphilis and none are specific for a given treponematosis. The most commonly used serological tests are the VDRL and RPR tests, which are highly sensitive in the early stages of disease. They are widely used in screening programs to detect latent yaws or endemic syphilis. Other tests employ treponemal antigens to detect "specific" antibodies. These tests are best performed in reference laboratories; serum specimens for this purpose can be collected on filter paper and sent by mail.

Following adequate penicillin treatment, the titer of VDRL and RPR serological tests declines but, depending upon the duration of the infection, may remain positive for several years or a lifetime. Such is often the case in persons who immigrate from yaws- or endemic-syphilis-endemic areas to parts of the world where only venereal syphilis is encountered. Based on reactive serological tests for syphilis, many of these patients are diagnosed and treated inappropriately for active latent venereal syphilis.

9. Control and Prevention

The provision of adequate clothing and soap and water would greatly reduce the transmission of pinta, yaws, and endemic syphilis. Marginal improvements in standards of living together with occasional access to medical care may partly explain why the mutilating complications of yaws and endemic syphilis are seen much less frequently today compared to the preantibiotic era.

The experience gained from pilot programs of the 1950s established a set of principles and procedures that is still valid today and should be used to control yaws and endemic syphilis.[17] The most important principle is to conduct periodic assessments of communities or nomadic groups where one or more members have infectious lesions resulting from recently acquired or relapse infections. The population of a village or family group should be seen and evaluated at an initial treatment survey and those with active disease should be treated with a single intramuscular injection of 2.4 million units of benzathine penicillin (half-doses for children under 12) and should all of their household members and playmates. Control activities should be expanded in such a way that an ever-enlarging disease-free area is established, so that reintroduction of yaws or endemic syphilis by persons from untreated areas is minimized. Because penicillin is inexpensive compared to other costs associated with surveys, many authorities recommend that treatment be given to entire communities that have one or more infectious cases.[9] Treated populations should be reexamined for active yaws within 6 months and at intervals thereafter so that missed cases and their contacts can be treated. The price of freedom from yaws and endemic syphilis is eternal vigilance.

9.1. Antibiotic and Chemotherapeutic Approaches to Prophylaxis

Prophylaxis other than penicillin treatment of contacts of infectious cases of yaws and endemic syphilis is not indicated.

9.2. Immunization

Although theoretically possible, a treponemal vaccine does not exist and the prospects for one are remote.

10. Unresolved Problems

The lack of a cell-free *in vitro* culture system has limited studies of the genetic structure and the immunopathogenesis of the pathogenic treponemes. Control of the endemic treponematoses may result in increased transmission of venereal syphilis with congenital transmission and the serious and potentially fatal cardiovascular and neurological complications. The perennial problem posed by the endemic treponematoses is the low priority they are given by most health authorities when faced with limited resources and more serious disease problems.

11. References

1. Miao, R. M., and Fieldsteel, A. H., Genetic relationship between *Treponema pallidum* and *Treponema pertenue*, two noncultivable human pathogens, *J. Bacteriol.* **144:**427–429 (1980).
2. Smibert, R. M., *Treponema*, in: *Bergey's Manual of Systematic Bacteriology* (N. R. Kreig and J. C. Holt, eds.), pp. 50–52, Williams & Wilkins, Baltimore, 1984.

3. Hollander, D. H., Treponematosis from pinta to venereal syphilis revisited: Hypothesis for temperature determination of disease patterns, *Sex. Transm. Dis.* **8**:34–37 (1981).
4. Hudson, E. H., *Non-venereal Syphilis, a Sociologic and Medical Study of Bejel*, Livingstone, Edinburgh, 1958.
5. Fohn, M. J., Wignall, F. S., Baker-Zander, S. A., and Lukehart, S. A., Specificity of antibodies from patients with pinta for antigens of *Treponema pallidum* subspecies *pallidum*, *J. Infect. Dis.* **157**:32–37 (1988).
6. Hackett, C. J., On the origin of the human treponematoses, *Bull. WHO* **29**:7–41 (1963).
7. Willcox, R. R., Evolutionary cycle of the treponematoses, *Br. J. Vener. Dis.* **36**:78–90 (1960).
8. Sydenham, T., Epistle II: Venereal disease, in: *The Works of Thomas Sydenham, MD*, Vol. 2, pp. 29–50, The Sydenham Society, London, 1848–1850.
9. Antal, G. M., and Causse, G., The control of endemic treponematoses, *Rev. Infect. Dis.* **7**(Suppl. 2):S220–S226 (1985).
10. Guthe, T., and Luger, A., The control of endemic syphilis of childhood, *Dermatol. Int.* **5**:179–199 (1966).
11. World Health Organization, Endemic treponematoses, *Week. Epidemiol. Rec.* **61**:198–202 (1986).
12. International symposium on yaws and other endemic treponematoses, Washington, D. C., *Rev. Infect. Dis.* **7**(Suppl.):S217–S351 (1985).
13. Proceedings of the inter-regional meeting on yaws and other endemic treponematoses, Cipanas, Indonesia, *Southeast Asian J. Trop. Med. Public Health* **17**(Suppl.):1–96 (1986).
14. World Health Organization, Report on a regional meeting on yaws and other endemic treponematoses, Brazzaville, 1986. Unpublished summary document.
15. Roman, G. C., and Roman, L. N., Occurrence of congenital, cardiovascular, visceral, neurologic and neuro-ophthalmologic complications in late yaws; a theme for future research, *Rev. Infect. Dis.* **8**:760–770 (1986).
16. Weller, C. V., The visceral pathology in Haitian treponematoses, *Am. J. Syph. Gonorrhea Vener. Dis.* **21**:357–369 (1937).
17. Perine, P. L., Hopkins, D. R., Niemel, P. L. A., St. John, R. K., Causse, G., and Antal, G. M., *Handbook of Endemic Treponematoses*, World Health Organization, Geneva, 1984.
18. Perine, P. L., Nelson, J. W., Lewis, J. O., Liska, S., Hunter, E. F., Larsen, S. A., Agadzi, V. K., Kofi, F., Ofori, J. A. K., Tam, M. R., and Lovett, M. A., New technologies for use in the surveillance and control of yaws, *Rev. Infect. Dis.* **8**(Suppl. 2):S295–S299 (1985).
19. Turner, T. B., and Hollander, D. H., *Biology of the Treponematoses*, pp. 193–213, World Health Organization, Geneva, 1957.
20. Magnuson, H. J., Eagle, H., and Fleischman, R., The minimal infectious inoculum of *Spirocheaeta pallidum* (Nichols strain) and a consideration of its rate of multiplication *in vivo*, *Am. J. Syph.* **32**:1–18 (1948).
21. Satchell, G. H., and Harrison, R. A., Experimental observations on the possibility of transmission of yaws by wound-feeding diptera in western Samoa, *Trans. R. Soc. Trop. Med. Hyg.* **47**:148–153 (1953).
22. Pace, J. L., and Csonka, G. W., Endemic non-venereal syphilis (bejel) in Saudi Arabia, *Br. J Vener. Dis.* **60**:293–297 (1984).

12. Suggested Reading

Burke, J. P., Hopkins, D. R., Hume, J. C., Perine, P. L., and St. John, R. (eds.), International syposium on yaws and other endemic treponematoses, Washington DC, 1984, *Rev. Infect. Dis.* **8**(Suppl. 2):S217–S351 (1985).

Guthe, T., Ridet, J., Vorst, F., D'Costa, J., and Grab, B., Methods for the surveillance of endemic treponematoses and sero-immunological investigations of "disappearing" diseases, *Bull. WHO* **46**:1–14 (1972).

Hackett, C. J., *An International Nomenclature of Yaws Lesions*, World Health Organization, Geneva, 1957 (Monograph Series No. 36).

Hill, K. R., Kodijat, R., and Sardadi, M., Atlas of framboesia: A nomenclature and clinical study of the skin lesions, *Bull. WHO* **4**:201–246 (1954).

Perine, P. L., Hopkins, D. R., Niemel, P. L. A., St. John, R. K., Causse, G., and Antal, G. M., *Handbook of Endemic Treponematoses*, World Health Organization, Geneva, 1984.

CHAPTER 37

Tetanus

Roland W. Sutter, Walter A. Orenstein, and Steven G. F. Wassilak

1. Introduction

Tetanus is a noncommunicable infectious disease of humans and certain animal species, acquired usually through environmental exposure. *Clostridium tetani* is an anaerobic, spore-forming bacilli of the soil. The ubiquitous spores germinate to vegetative bacilli when introduced into the soft tissues of the host under conditions in which the partial pressure of molecular oxygen is low. The vegetative organisms produce a potent neurotoxin that acts on the central nervous system, leading to the muscular contractions characteristic of the illness. Although a significant proportion of the global tetanus case burden occurs in adults and children following wounds, the major burden of tetanus in the world is borne by neonates, who are both (1) infected at or soon after birth and (2) born to mothers who are not adequately immunized. Prevention of tetanus can be achieved by active immunization with tetanus toxoid, which is chemically inactivated toxin, or by passive immunization with specific immune globulin as part of postexposure wound prophylaxis. Tetanus toxoid, which protects by inducing production of neutralizing antibodies, is both highly immunogenic and safe. Nearly 100% of recipients of a primary immunization series are protected.

2. Historical Background

The clinical characteristics of tetanus are described in the writings of Hippocrates. Until 1884, however, the etiology of tetanus remained unknown. In that year, Carle and Rattone[(1)] demonstrated artificial transmission in animals. The contents of a pustule from a fatal human case led to typical symptoms in rabbits when injected into the sciatic nerve; the disease could subsequently be passed to other rabbits from infected nervous tissue. Also in 1884, Nicolaier[(2)] induced tetanus in experimental animals after injection of soil samples; he observed gram-positive bacilli in the exudate at the inoculation site but not in nervous tissue, leading him to hypothesize that a locally produced poison led to the neurological symptoms. In 1886, Rosenbach observed spore-forming bacilli in the exudate obtained from a case in a human. In 1889, Kitasato[(3)] demonstrated that *C. tetani* spores survived heating and germinated under anaerobic conditions; injection of pure cultures reproducibly caused disease in animals. After Behring and Kitasato[(4)] identified and purified the toxin in 1890, they showed that repeated inoculation of animals with small quantities of toxin led to the production of antibodies in survivors. Preparations of antitoxin from animal sera, particularly horses, became the first means of preventing and treating tetanus. In 1924, Descombey[(5)] prepared toxoid, chemically altered toxin, which induced neutralizing antibodies without causing illness. Active immunity induced by this preparation opened the way for large-scale tetanus prophylaxis.

3. Methodology

3.1. Sources of Mortality Data

In the United States and most developed countries, data on tetanus deaths come from national compilations of death certificates (i.e., vital statistics system) listing tetanus as the underlying or contributing cause of death.[(6)] In such countries, death data probably may be a reasonable estimate of the total deaths from diagnosed tetanus. However, in developing countries where the great majority of

Roland W. Sutter, Walter A. Orenstein, and Steven G. F. Wassilak • National Immunization Program, Centers for Disease Control and Prevention, Atlanta, Georgia 30333.

deaths occur in the neonatal period primarily outside the hospital, death certificate information may not be available or reliable. In those settings, the completeness of neonatal tetanus reporting may be < 5%, and community-based surveys have been used to obtain accurate estimates of mortality for neonatal tetanus. The National Center for Health Statistics (NCHS) compiles death certificate information from all deaths occurring in the United States.

3.2. Sources of Morbidity Data

In many developed countries, tetanus is a reportable disease. In the United States, tetanus became notifiable in 1947. Most notification systems do not have a specific case definition and rely on physician diagnoses. Case notification is passive, depending on physician initiative, which makes reporting efficiency highly variable. It is likely that only a proportion of the cases actually occurring are reported to national health authorities. In the United States, additional available information reported to the Centers for Disease Control and Prevention (CDC) includes a patient's immunization status, wound history, postexposure prophylaxis, and outcome. Between 1980 and 1984, 123 tetanus deaths were reported to the NCHS compared to 110 deaths reported via the passive surveillance system maintained by the CDC. Also during this period, the reported death-to-case ratio (using CDC reports only) varied from 28 to 36%. Case series from other developed countries have reported death-to-case ratios as low as 10–20%. It is likely that there is a bias toward reporting the most severe cases in passive surveillance systems. By matching demographic information for individuals with death following tetanus from both NCHS mortality data and tetanus morbidity reporting, the efficiency of the reporting of tetanus deaths to the CDC has been estimated at 40%[7] and the efficiency of morbidity reporting has been estimated at 15–25%.

3.3. Serological Surveys

Serological tests measure the level of circulating antitoxin, which appears to correlate directly with protection from disease.[8,9] In general, detectable antitoxin is induced almost exclusively through immunization. Tetanus disease generally does not result in production of circulating antitoxin.[10,11] Therefore, serological surveys, particularly in developed countries, serve an important purpose to measure the impact of immunization in inducing and maintaining population immunity, but they cannot measure the impact and epidemiological characteristics of disease.

Toxin neutralization assays, usually in mice, correlate best with clinical protection since they assess prevention of disease in a living host.[8] Injecting the animals with various dilutions of serum and a lethal dose of tetanus toxin allows detection of levels as low as 0.001 IU/ml when compared to a reference serum.[12] However, because the test is time-consuming, expensive, and requires animal hosts, a variety of other tests have been employed. These include passive hemagglutination assays (PHA), enzyme immunoassays (EIA), radioimmunoassays (RIA), immunofluorescent tests (IFA), latex agglutination, and a variety of methods using agar gel precipitation.[13,14] The sensitivity and specificity vary with the technique. Agar gel and IFA tests tend to have low sensitivities. Specificity is usually good provided the test is standardized to toxin neutralization. Most population studies have employed the passive hemagglutination technique. This assay is both sensitive and specific, although false-positive results may occur at low levels. Use of turkey erythrocytes is helpful in enhancing specificity, reproducibility, and speed of the assay.[14,15] The PHA measures both IgG and IgM.[16] Neutralization results primarily from IgG antitoxin.[17] Thus, measurement of antitoxin by PHA shortly after the first or second dose of toxoid may give falsely high antibody levels secondary to IgM. This should not be a problem for serosurveys, however, when only IgG antibody would be expected. EIA, RIA, and IFA assays measure specific immunoglobulins and avoid this problem. Many of the *in vitro* assays correspond closely with the *in vivo* neutralization assays at moderate to high levels of antitoxin, but the correlation may be suboptimal at low levels of antitoxin. Serological tests for tetanus have been recently reviewed.[18]

3.4. Laboratory Diagnosis

Tetanus is primarily a clinical diagnosis and the laboratory usually plays little role. Anaerobic culture of wounds is frequently negative, although the yield can be improved by inoculating part of the specimen in cooked-meat medium and heating to 80°C for 5 to 20 min to destroy nonsporulating competing microorganisms.[19] Even isolation of the organism does not necessarily confirm tetanus. The organism has been grown from wounds in the absence of clinical symptoms or signs. Serological tests also are of little use, since most tetanus patients do not mount a serological response against the toxin.[20] Levels of circulating antitoxin less than 0.01 IU/ml at the time of onset of illness confirmed by neutralization assay suggest susceptibility to the agent and are compatible with the diagnosis. However, several recent reports have documented higher levels of circulating antitoxin in some patients at the time of presentation, suggesting that even higher levels of antitoxin are needed to prevent disease in some instances.[21] Although such instances are probably rare, tetanus should still be considered in the differential diagnosis as long as the illness is clinically compatible even when circulating antitoxin is greater than 0.01 IU/ml. Detection and quantification of tetanus toxin in serum appears to be diagnostic, although such determination remains a research tool at present.

4. Biological Characteristics of the Organism

C. tetani is a gram-positive, spore-forming, anaerobic bacillus.[22] Flagella attached bilaterally on nonsporulating bacteria add motility. The organism typically measures 0.3 to 0.5 μm in diameter and 2 to 2.5 μm in length, although long filamentous forms may be seen in culture. Spores typically form in the terminal position and give the organism its characteristic drumsticklike appearance.

While there may be some tolerance for oxygen when the oxidation–reduction potential is low, for the most part *C. tetani* can be considered an obligate anaerobe. It grows optimally at 33–37°C, although, depending on the strain, growth can occur from 14 to 43°C. The organism can be grown on a variety of anaerobic media such as cooked meat, casein hydrolysate, and thioglycolate. Growth is usually characterized by production of gas with a fetid odor. Compact colonies formed in a meshwork of fine filaments are usually seen on blood agar. Addition of reducing substances at neutral to alkaline pH enhances growth.

Formation of spores can be promoted or inhibited by a variety of factors including media composition, temperature, and pH.[22] Sporulation is enhanced in aging cultures and by physiological temperatures (i.e., 37°C), and in the presence of oleic acid, phosphates, 1–2% NaCl, and manganese. In contrast, low pH, extremes of temperature (< 25 or > 41°C), glucose, assorted saturated fatty acids, antibiotics, and potassium can inhibit sporulation.

Spores are highly resistant to environmental agents and may persist in soil for months to years, if not exposed to sunlight.[22] Spores can be destroyed by a variety of disinfectants and heat, although susceptibility varies by agent. Aqueous iodine or 2% glutaraldehyde at pH 7.5 to 8.5 kills spores within 3 hr. In contrast, phenol (5%), formalin (3%), chloramine (1%), and hydrogen hyperoxidates (6%) require 15 to 24 hr to destroy spores. Spores are resistant to boiling, but heating to 120°C for 15 to 20 min will inactivate them.

C. tetani produces two exotoxins: tetanolysin and tetanospasmin.[22] Tetanolysin is an oxygen-sensitive hemolysin that may play a role in establishing infection but does not cause disease.[23] It appears to be related to streptolysin and the theta toxin of *C. perfringens*. Tetanospasmin, the cause of the clinical signs and symptoms of tetanus, is a highly potent neurotoxin that accumulates intracellularly during the logarithmic growth phase and is released into the medium upon autolysis. Toxin production appears to be under the control of a plasmid.[24] The molecule of approximately 150,000 Da is synthesized as a single polypeptide chain that may be cleaved into light and heavy chains bound by two disulfide bonds when released into the medium.[25]

The toxin is one of the most potent poisons on a weight basis, although species sensitivities vary considerably. Guinea pigs are exquisitely sensitive, with doses of 0.3 ng/kg usually fatal. About 1 ng/kg will kill a mouse, while the estimated minimum human lethal dose is < 2.5 ng/kg. Monkeys, sheep, goats, and horses also are extremely susceptible to the effects of the toxin, while cats, dogs, and particularly birds and poikilotherms are relatively resistant.[26] The differences in species susceptibility cannot be explained by differences in circulating antitoxin.[19]

5. Descriptive Epidemiology

5.1. Prevalence and Incidence

In spite of the availability of a highly effective immunizing agent, tetanus exerts a substantial health impact throughout the world. In 1973, there were an estimated 1 million tetanus deaths worldwide, with 60–90% of that mortality due to tetanus neonatorum (tetanus during the first month of life).[27] The impact of increasing immunization coverage of pregnant women (and women of child-bearing age) with tetanus toxoid—from 27% in 1989 to 45% in 1993—is estimated to prevent 724,000 deaths each year due to neonatal tetanus. Nevertheless, approximately 515,000 neonatal tetanus deaths continue to occur each year, 80% of which are concentrated in 12 countries.[28] In 1989, the World Health Organization (WHO) adopted a resolution to eliminate neonatal tetanus worldwide by the year 1995, and in 1990, the World Summit of Children issued a declaration for global eradication of neonatal tetanus by the year 1995. Although the neonatal tetanus eradication objective—defined as less than one case per 1000 live births for each health district—was not met by the end of 1995, continued progress in improving vaccination coverage, hygiene and childbirth practices, and surveillance to identify high-risk areas and target them for intensified intervention efforts, all will contribute in further decreasing the global neonatal tetanus burden.

In most developed countries, improved hygiene and childbirth practices (associated with an increasing proportion of births delivered by trained health professionals in hospitals), improvements in wound care, reduction in exposure to tetanus spores, and active immunization have led to major declines in tetanus incidence since the 1950s. In the United States, death certificate data from 1920 onward indicate a decline in annual tetanus death rates, which may have accelerated with the use of equine antitoxin in prophylaxis and treatment beginning in the mid-1920s (Fig. 1). Cases of tetanus have been monitored nationally since 1947, when the incidence was 0.39/100,000 total population; secular trends in tetanus occurrence since that time reflect changes in wound management and the use of toxoid. A continual decline in reported cases occurred until 1976 to about 0.04/100,000. Since then, a less pronounced decline in incidence rates has stabilized at a rate of approximately 0.02/100,000 beginning in 1987.

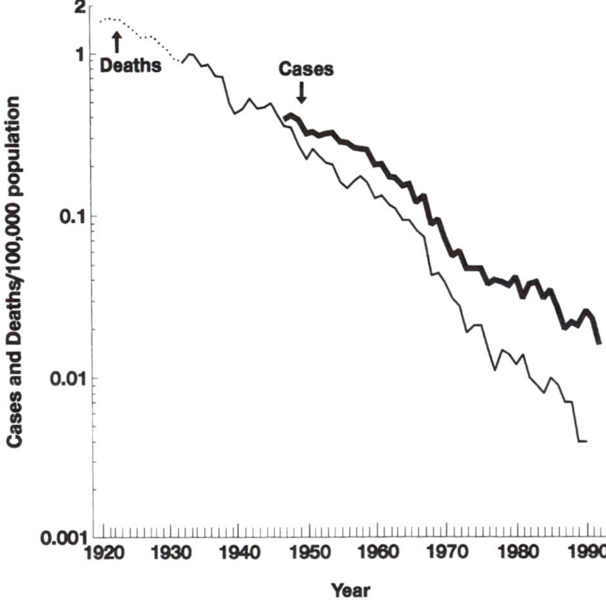

Figure 1. Reported tetanus mortality and incidence rates, United States, 1920–1992. Incomplete reporting for 1920–1932; national reporting began in 1947.

5.2. Epidemic Behavior

C. tetani spreads from the environment to humans generally through contamination of wounds. The organism does not spread person to person, and so tetanus cannot be considered a contagious disease. Nevertheless, outbreaks of tetanus in drug users (particularly among heroin addicts) have been reported.[29,30]

5.3. Geographic Distribution

C. tetani organisms are distributed across the globe. However, the greatest concentrations are in warm climates with moist, fertile soil.[31] The highest rates of tetanus occur in the developing world, particularly in countries near the equator.[27] In the United States, tetanus has been and remains predominantly a disease of the Southeast; however, all states report cases. The occurrence of tetanus in regions at high altitude may be lower than in low-lying areas, although the reasons for this phenomenon are not understood.[32]

5.4. Temporal Distribution

Tetanus is generally distinctly seasonal, with a midsummer or "wet" season peak in temperate areas. This is consistent with multiplication of the organisms in the soil and sporulation. This likely also reflects more frequent host behaviors associated with injury during the warmer months.[31,33]

5.5. Age

As noted earlier, tetanus in developing countries occurs most frequently in neonates. Even in the United States in the 1950s, over one third of tetanus deaths were in children under 1 year of age.[34] Aside from neonatal tetanus, the substantial proportion of victims in developing nations are older children and young adults. Wherever immunization programs are in place, tetanus occurrence declines.[31] In the face of immunization programs, age (and sex) distributions shift to reflect the underimmunized. In the United States since 1965, average annual age-specific tetanus incidence rates reflect declines in all age groups. However, less dramatic declines were registered in the elderly, while drastic declines were reported for younger age groups. Thus, in recent years, the elderly have become the group at highest risk for tetanus (Fig. 2). In 1990–1994, persons $\geq$ 60 years of age were at a sixfold greater risk of acquiring tetanus than those of all younger ages (incidence of 0.13 vs. 0.02/100,000). A population-based serosurvey of immunity to tetanus in the United

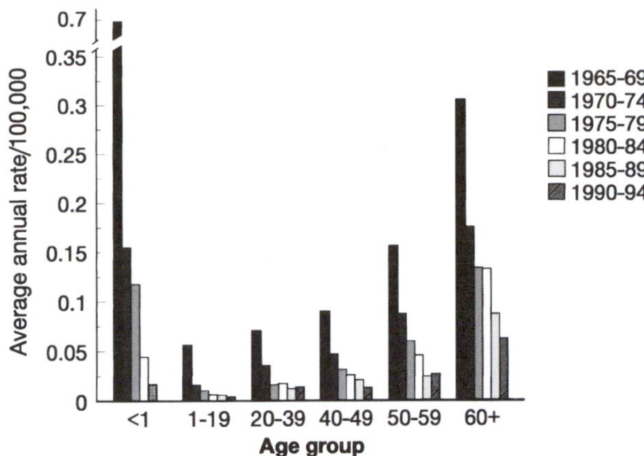

Figure 2. Reported age-group-specific tetanus incidence rates, by selected intervals, United States, 1965–1994.

States reported that 70% of the population aged 6 years and above had protective levels of tetanus antibody. Nevertheless, tetanus antibody levels decline with age, and only 28% of persons 70 years of age and older had protective levels.[35]

5.6. Sex

In much of the world, reported tetanus appears to be more common in males than in females at all ages.[31] In the neonatal period, particularly in developing countries, this may in part be due to a greater likelihood that parents of males may seek medical attention more frequently than do parents of females.[36] Among children and adults, males generally appear to have a somewhat higher reported incidence, which could also be due to surveillance artifact and/or perhaps due to exposure factors, such as injury-incurring behaviors outdoors.

In the United States for the period 1975–1986, two thirds of the 21 neonatal tetanus cases were in males. Outside of the neonatal period, the pattern by sex seen in the United States is different from that seen in developing countries; tetanus age-specific incidence rates were equal in both sexes until age 50. Above age 50, female incidence rates were higher; this sex discrepancy probably represents lower immunization levels among females of this age group since males entering military service during World War II were routinely vaccinated.

5.7. Race

In the 1950s in the United States, nonwhite individuals had an incidence more than five times that in whites, and rates of neonatal tetanus were ten times higher.[34] In the United States in 1972–1989, extrapolating from the patients of known race, the estimated average annual incidence rate was 0.02/100,000 for whites, 0.05/100,000 for blacks, and 0.12/100,000 for all other races. These differences are felt to be attributable primarily to lower levels of tetanus toxoid immunization in the nonwhite populations, but also could reflect differences in health care following injury. Case-fatality ratios also differed by race—31% for whites, 43% for blacks, and 34% for all other races—and probably reflect differences both in access to health care and in immune status. In the 1972–1989 case series, having two or more prior doses of tetanus toxoid put one at lower risk of death from tetanus.

5.8. Occupation and Location

The differentiation of the type of surroundings under which tetanus-associated wounds are acquired in the United States suggests that the majority occurred outdoors and that wounds were incurred in decreasing frequency indoors, in farm, gardening, hospital, and factory settings.[37]

5.9. Occurrence in Different Settings

Because of the field and wound conditions, war injuries frequently were associated with tetanus; it has been estimated that, prior to the availability of toxoid, 1 out of 100 serious wounds in battle conditions was complicated by tetanus. As a result of routine tetanus toxoid prophylaxis and vigorous prophylaxis in wound management, only 12 cases of tetanus occurred among 2.73 million wounded US Army personnel on all fronts in World War II (0.44/100,000) versus 70 out of 520,000 wounded in World War I (13.4/100,000).[38]

Parenteral drug abuse, both intravenous and subcutaneous, is known to place individuals at higher risk compared to the general population. Drug users may be at higher risk for tetanus because of nonhygienic injection practices; however, heroin is frequently mixed with quinine, which lowers the redox potential at the injection site, favors growth of anaerobes, and may create an ideal environment for *C. tetani* to germinate.[39]

Operative procedures, particularly bowel surgery, infrequently can put some individuals at risk, as can dental procedures, puerperal sepsis, and septic abortion.[40]

5.10. Socioeconomic Factors

The incidence and complications of tetanus are inversely related to access to (1) routine prophylactic immu-

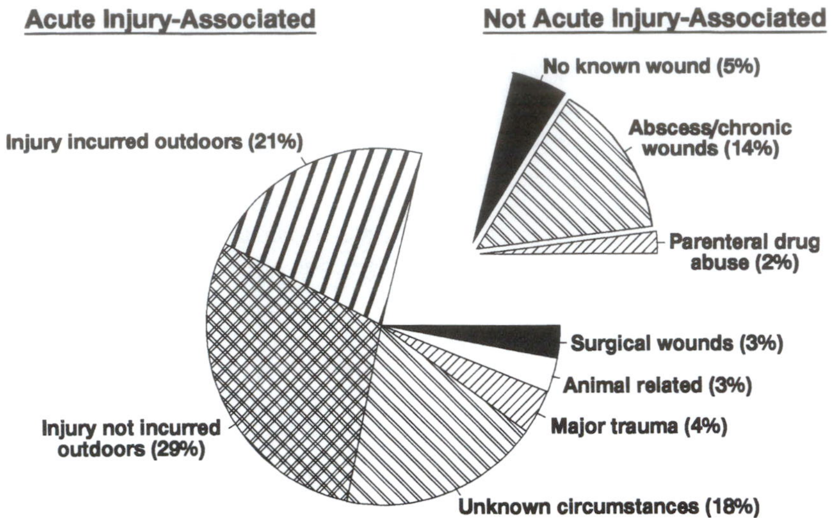

Figure 3. Associated wounds and conditions for 1277 nonneonatal tetanus cases with supplementary information, United States, 1972–1989. The total adds to less than 100% because of rounding.

nization, (2) immunization with appropriate wound care following wounds, and (3) care following onset of symptoms. Availability and use of these services probably correlate directly with socioeconomic status. The differences in racial incidence and the characteristics of mothers of patients with neonatal tetanus are strongly felt to reflect poorer immunization levels associated with lower socioeconomic status. The population-based serological survey of tetanus immunity in the United States also suggested that seroprevalence was positively correlated with education: the higher the educational level, the higher the tetanus seroprevalence rates.[35] These data suggest that compliance with vaccination and postexposure wound prophylaxis recommendations may also be correlated with higher educational levels.

6. Mechanisms and Routes of Transmission

Tetanus is caused by the *in vivo* elaboration of tetanospasmin. Spores of *C. tetani* are usually introduced through breaks in the skin epithelium. Activation of the spores with production of toxin leads to disease. Since neonatal tetanus is the most common form of tetanus in the world, accounting for approximately 80–90% of the deaths, the usual site of entry is the umbilical cord stump.[36,41] Outside the neonatal period, a variety of conditions have been associated with tetanus. In the United States, information is available for 1277 nonneonatal cases reported from 1972 through 1989. Acute injuries were the predisposing event in 992 (78%), while chronic wounds or other medical conditions were associated with 179 cases (14%). Parenteral drug abuse was the only predisposing condition in 2% and was present in an additional 1%. For 5% of patients, no acute injury, chronic wound, or associated medical condition was known (Fig. 3). Of the patients reporting acute injuries, puncture wounds were most common (35%) followed by lacerations (33%). The circumstances of the wound were known for 78% of these cases. Injuries in outdoor settings (e.g., yard, garden, or farm settings) accounted for 29% of cases, injuries incurred indoors accounted for 21% of cases, and 10% were incurred under special circumstances. These included animal bites and/or scratches in 3%, major trauma (burns, bullet wounds, and compound fractures) in 4%, and surgical wounds, many of which were contaminated (e.g., bowel wounds) in 3%. In 18% of tetanus cases, an acute injury was reported but the circumstances of the injury was unknown.

Chronic medical conditions associated with tetanus included decubitus ulcers, gangrene, and frostbite, as well as dental and other abscesses and parenteral drug abuse. Cases without known wounds or portals of entry have been described for many years.[31] In some instances, these are thought to arise from minor wounds not recalled by those patients or from intraintestinal toxin production. There are some reports indicating that up to 40% of human intestines are colonized with *C. tetani*.[42]

Other conditions associated with tetanus include contaminated injections, e.g., vaccinations, earlobe infections, foreign bodies, and the practice of tattooing.

7. Pathogenesis and Immunity

7.1. Pathogenesis

Tetanus results when spores inoculated through the epithelium germinate, leading to the production of tetanospasmin and its transport to the central nervous system (CNS). The period of time between an identified acute injury and onset of tetanus signs and symptoms is 3 days to 3 weeks for the majority of cases. In the United States in 1972–1989, the median incubation period in reported cases was 7 days.

Germination is enhanced by anaerobic conditions associated with significant tissue injury and accumulation of lactic acid.[19] Calcium may increase the likelihood that injected spores germinate because it can increase local necrosis.[43] The presence of calcium in soil along with tetanus spores may be one reason why wounds contaminated by soil are predisposed to tetanus. Toxin injected or produced in the subcutaneous tissue appears to enter muscle first. Tetanus can be prevented by treating the muscle with antitoxin prior to subcutaneous administration of toxin.[44] Once in the muscle, toxin can reach the bloodstream via the lymphatics and reach the CNS through hematogenous transport, or toxin can get to the CNS directly through retrograde transport via neurons.

Hematogenous transport was supported by a variety of studies showing that most of the toxin produced or injected reached the bloodstream and from there arrived in a variety of tissues.[44,45] However, because the toxin does not appear to cross the blood–brain barrier, neuronal transport is now believed to be the predominant means by which toxin gains access to the CNS.[44,46] Experimental data indicate that toxin is found at motor end plates of muscle nerves.[47] From there, it gains entry to the nerve by binding to gangliosides or other receptors and is transported to the ventral horns of the spinal cord or motor nuclei of cranial nerves. Transmission within nerves can result from either intra-axonal transport, travel through perineural spaces between fibers, or by spread via lymphatics associated with nerves. Radiolabeled toxin studies suggest that intra-axonal transport is most likely.[48]

Tetanospasmin acts by causing disinhibition of spinal cord reflex arcs, allowing excitatory reflexes to multiply unchecked, resulting in the classical tetanic spasms.[44] Disinhibition appears to be caused by interfering with release of the neurotransmitters glycine and γ-aminobutyric acid from presynaptic inhibitory fibers.[44] In addition, the toxin can impede release of a variety of other neurotransmitters including acetylcholine in autonomic and peripheral somatic nerves.[48] The toxin can affect peripheral motor end plates, the spinal cord, the brain, and the sympathetic nervous system.

7.2. Immunity

Immunity to tetanus does not generally follow disease, since the quantity of toxin that causes illness is usually less than the quantity needed to induce an immune response.[20] Second cases of tetanus have been reported.[10,11] Most serosurveys in unimmunized populations fail to find much evidence for natural immunity. However, a few recent reports of serosurveys in unimmunized populations of developed and particularly of developing countries suggest that some persons may develop such immunity.[49,50] These latter studies have been criticized because documentation of no prior immunizations may be lacking and because the assays used may have measured cross-reacting (nonneutralizing) antibodies at low levels. Nonetheless, these data suggest that at least in some developing countries, asymptomatic infection/colonization, presumably of the intestine, does occur, resulting in the production of antitoxin. Nevertheless, natural immunization cannot be relied on to control tetanus. Further study is needed in developed countries before the concept of natural immunity in those populations can be accepted.

It is generally agreed that a circulating level of antitoxin of 0.01 IU/ml is the level needed to guarantee protection against tetanus.[8,9,51] This comes from experiments both with humans and with animals. A review by McComb [51] in 1964 reported that clinical tetanus could be prevented in horses by administration of 1500 IU/ml of antitoxin after acute injury, which corresponded to a serum level of 0.01 IU/ml. Following immunization with tetanus toxoid, Wolters and Dehmel [52] were able to resist challenge in themselves with "2–3 fatal doses" of tetanus toxin. They had achieved serum levels of 0.007 to 0.01 antitoxin unit (AU)/ml (prior to international standardization of the assay). Further evidence that 0.01 IU/ml was protective came from trials to prevent neonatal tetanus. Induction of antitoxin levels of 0.01 IU/ml or higher in mothers resulted in protection of infants from neonatal tetanus.[8]

The protective level of circulating tetanus antitoxin has recently been challenged by reports of 12 patients who had serum levels greater than 0.01 IU/ml at the time they presented with clinical tetanus.[21,53] The highest level noted was 0.16 IU/ml. In some instances, large-scale production of toxin may overcome this barrier (i.e., 0.01 IU/ml) or perhaps rapid uptake through nerve endings may prevent neutralization of toxin. Whatever the explanation, these data suggest that the 0.01 level cannot be considered absolute. Nevertheless, the fact that tetanus is rare in adequately immunized persons, and with all the experimental animal and human data noted above, it seems reasonable to conclude that 0.01 IU/ml is protective in all but the rarest situations.

8. Patterns of Host Response

8.1. Clinical Features in Children and Adults

The reported incubation period for tetanus ranges from 1 day to several months. However, the majority of cases occur within 3 days to 3 weeks after an injury. In the United States, the median incubation period for cases with injury-associated wounds reported between 1972 and 1989 was 7 days. The incubation period varies with distance between the wound and the CNS. The longest periods are reported for injuries farthest away from the CNS, while injuries to the head and trunk have the shortest incubation periods.[44,45] Historically, shorter incubation periods have been associated with more severe disease, although this has not been the case in patients recently reported in the United States.

Clinical tetanus can take one of three forms: (1) localized, (2) generalized, and (3) cephalic.[54] Local tetanus, which is rare in humans, consists of painful spasms in a confined area around the site of the original injury.[55] The spasms may persist for weeks to months. The prognosis of tetanus that remains localized is excellent; however, localized tetanus often will progress to generalized tetanus, which carries a more ominous prognosis. Over 80% of cases of tetanus fit this category. Patients most often present with trismus or lockjaw, i.e., spasm of the muscles of mastication. Risus sardonicus, the characteristic facial expression, occurs with trismus and spasm of the facial muscles. It consists of raised eyebrows, tight closure of the eyelids, wrinkling of the forehead, and extension of the corners of the mouth laterally. Initial signs may be followed by involvement of multiple other muscle groups, hyperreflexia, and generalized hypertonicity. Tetanospasms, generalized tetanic seizure activity, consist of sudden painful contraction of all muscle groups, resulting in opisthotonos, abduction and flexion at the shoulders, flexion of the elbows and wrists, and extension of the legs. Spasm of the glottis can cause immediate death. Autonomic nervous system abnormalities consisting of hyper- or hypotension, tachycardia, and arrhythmias, among other manifestations are frequently reported in severe cases.[56] Complications can result directly from the actions of the toxin, from spasms, or from chronic debility. Reported death-to-case ratios for generalized tetanus have varied from 10 to 75%. With good intensive care, mortality should be less than 20%. The greatest mortality occurs at the extremes of age.

Cephalic tetanus occurs with injuries or lesions of the head and face.[54] It is characterized by short incubation periods, 1 to 2 days, and by atonic cranial nerve palsies particularly involving nerves III, IV, VII, IX, X, and XII, singly or in combination. Trismus may be present. Cephalic tetanus may progress to generalized tetanus.

8.2. Neonatal Tetanus

Tetanus occurring within the first month of life is a form of generalized tetanus. It occurs in newborn infants following infection by *C. tetani* (most commonly at the umbilical cord stump). Symptoms of neonatal tetanus generally begin 3–14 days after birth but can occur from 1 to 28 days of age. The illness starts with poor sucking and excessive crying. This is followed by variable degrees of trismus, difficulty swallowing, opisthotonos, and other tetanic spasms. Cases are often associated with unsterile conditions of childbirth, delivery personnel untrained in sterile care of the umbilical cord and stump, and particularly with births followed by unhygienic cultural rituals involving the umbilical stump, such as application of herbs, clarified butter, or animal dung. The disease can be prevented through transplacental passage of circulating antitoxin from mother to infant, most of which is in the IgG1 subclass.[8,57] However, most newborns in the world are susceptible because their mothers have not received two or more doses of tetanus toxoid; it was estimated that from 1989 to 1993, only 27–45% of pregnant women in developing countries have received at least two recent doses of tetanus toxoid.[28] The case-fatality ratio of neonatal tetanus is 25–90% with therapy, depending on the intensity of supportive care. Overall, the Expanded Programme on Immunization (EPI) of the WHO estimates that 80% of affected infants die.[28]

The incidence of tetanus neonatorum in developing nations had been estimated in the 1960s to be under 50,000 cases annually, or approximately 0.5/1000 live births overall.[31] A better estimate of the general incidence of neonatal tetanus has recently been made with the use of community-based, house-to-house surveys of neonatal deaths, which have suggested that the reported incidence is less than 5% of the actual incidence. Data provided to the WHO suggest that 83 countries reported an incidence of < 1 neonatal tetanus cases per 1000 live births, while 57 countries reported an incidence of 1–5 cases, and 25 countries reported an incidence of > 5 cases.[28]

As indicated by death rates, the occurrence of neonatal tetanus in the United States was already on the decline prior to widespread tetanus toxoid use in women because of an increasing number of births in hospitals and improvements in postpartum hygiene. Deaths due to tetanus in those less than 1 year old, generally reflecting neonatal disease, declined from 0.64/1000 live births in 1900 to 0.07 in 1930 to 0.01 by the 1960s. Using age-specific reporting beginning in 1961, tetanus incidence could be directly monitored in those less than 1 year old and showed the same downward trend. From 1967 to 1968, the incidence rates of reported cases and of reported tetanus deaths in those less than 1 year old declined abruptly. This abrupt decline occurred primarily because of a decrease of reported cases in Texas for uncertain reasons. Part of the decline may be attributable to an increase in the cohort of women of child-bearing age who had received tetanus toxoid in childhood.

Of the 29 cases reported in the first 4 weeks of life in the United States during 1972–1989, 27 were in infants born outside of a hospital. Nineteen of the cases (66%) occurred in Texas, which had only 6% of US births. Only four mothers had a history of ever having received tetanus toxoid, and only one was known to have received more than one dose. Nineteen of the 26 cases with known outcome survived. Only one case of neonatal tetanus has been reported in the United States after 1989.

Given its substantial impact in developing countries, the control of neonatal and nonneonatal tetanus is the subject of a major effort of EPI by routine immunization in infancy with diphtheria–tetanus–pertussis (DTP) and by immunization of women of reproductive age with tetanus toxoid.

8.3. Diagnosis

The diagnosis of tetanus is made primarily on clinical grounds. Generalized stiffness, hyperreflexia, trismus, and the characteristic generalized tetanic spasms strongly support the diagnosis. Absence of changes in the state of consciousness or sensory involvement add further support. The epidemiological history can also be helpful. A preceding history of a wound, particularly if contaminated by soil, is suggestive, although not all cases will have such histories. Lack of a history/record of adequate immunization or wound care is typical. Given the high efficacy of a course of tetanus toxoid, a clinically compatible case who presents with a complete primary series of toxoid with maintenance boosters should not be considered tetanus unless an exhaustive workup fails to reveal other potential causes. Significant rises in circulating antitoxin are not reliably seen in tetanus and cannot be used to make the diagnosis unless demonstrated.[20] Testing for antitoxin using enzyme-linked immunosorbent assay or passive hemagglutination can be performed on a rapid basis to assist in assessment of immune status. Isolation of the organism from a wound as well as the absence of circulating antitoxin at 0.01 IU/ml or greater when the patient is first seen also support the diagnosis.

The differential diagnosis will depend on the clinical signs and symptoms.[54,58] Trismus may be caused by dental caries, tonsillitis, peritonsillar abscesses, parotitis, temporomandibular joint dysfunction, and CNS disturbances other than tetanus. Hyperreflexia may be seen in rabies; however, rabies is more often associated with changes in the state of consciousness and the seizures of rabies are more often clonic in contrast to the tonic seizures of tetanus. The history of an animal bite is generally present with rabies but could be present in tetanus. Encephalitis also can result in spasms, but, like rabies, is much more likely to be associated with changes in the state of consciousness. In addition to infections, a variety of poisonings and metabolic conditions can simulate tetanus. Hypocalcemic tetany can cause generalized muscle spasms but is not usually associated with trismus.[59] Strychnine poisoning can resemble generalized tetanus both in mechanism, disinhibition of spinal cord reflex arcs, and clinically.[60] However, strychnine poisoning is usually not associated with muscle rigidity between spasms and is rarely associated with temperature elevations, which are frequent in severe tetanus. Dystonias caused by phenothiazines also should be considered in the differential diagnosis. Finally, hysteria can mimic tetanus, although such patients tend to relax on prolonged observation and their seizurelike activity tends to be clonic rather than tonic.

9. Control and Prevention

Tetanus is a totally preventable disease. Prevention begins with universal, routine immunization and with appropriate attention toward averting wounds and injuries. A routine immunization program should ensure that the entire population has received a primary series (at least three doses) of tetanus toxoid with booster doses as needed. Substantial health benefits are derived from combined immunization with diphtheria and tetanus toxoids and pertussis vaccine (DTP) in childhood. It was estimated that in 1990, more than 80% of target children in the world had received three doses of DTP.[28]

Once injuries occur, efforts should be made to prevent contamination with spores and to eliminate those conditions that predispose to germination of spores. Wounds should be carefully cleaned and surgically debrided when necessary to remove devitalized tissue, which can serve as a nidus for infection, followed by tetanus toxoid and tetanus immune globulin, when needed. Since neonatal tetanus is the major worldwide cause of tetanus morbidity and mortality, greater attention must be paid to covering umbilical cord stumps with sterile or uncontaminated dressings. Training of midwives in proper sterile techniques has been demonstrated to reduce the incidence of neonatal tetanus substantially (although not as effectively as immunization of the mother) as well as result in declines in neonatal mortality due to causes other than tetanus.

Only 58 (5%) of the 1277 cases of nonneonatal tetanus reported in the United States from 1972 through 1989 received three or more doses of tetanus toxoid. Of these, 11 had received the third dose as part of wound management and 38 had not received a dose within the preceding 5 years. Of 327 patients with acute injuries who were known to have sought medical care, 93% did not receive the recommended tetanus toxoid with or without tetanus immune globulin. Thus, almost all cases of tetanus could be prevented with routine immunization and appropriate wound management.

9.1. Passive Immunization

Although animal models suggest that prompt passive immunization is protective against the development of tetanus following injury, there is limited information in humans; appropriately controlled trials have not been performed. Passive immunization with equine antitoxin for treatment and for prophylaxis following wounds became common practice in World War I, with a decrease in wound-associated tetanus at the same time that other improvements in wound care were becoming common practice.[61] Passive immunity conferred by equine antitoxin is of limited duration. The half-life of refined equine antitoxin in humans is less than 2 weeks and may be shorter in some individuals.[62] A major disadvantage is that persons receiving large doses of equine antitoxin can experience immediate hypersensitivity reactions or serum sickness.[63]

Tetanus immune globulin (TIG) is a human antibody preparation prepared by cold-ethanol fractionation of the plasma of hyperimmunized adults. TIG was introduced in the early 1960s and was found to have a fairly constant half-life of 28 days in humans.[51] The frequency of allergic and serum sickness reactions to equine antitoxin, along with its shorter half-life, made TIG more attractive for passive immunization. TIG has been shown not to pose a risk of hepatitis transmission. Additionally, TIG and other purified immune globulins pose no risk of human immunodeficiency virus (HIV) transmission, since donors are screened to be at low risk, serum is screened for antibody to HIV prior to serum pooling, and, most important, cold-ethanol fractionation inactivates HIV.[64] As an added safegard against the possible transmission of hepatitis C virus, the Food and Drug Administration (FDA) is working with the manufacturers to include an additional inactivation/removal step. It is distributed at a concentration of 250 IU/ml in 1-ml vials. Even in the developing world, TIG is beginning to supplant equine antitoxin as it becomes more widely available. Tetanus toxoid is always given with TIG to induce persistence of immunity beyond 28 days in those with any past exposure to toxoid and to initiate active immunization in those without any prior exposure.[65] In contrast to equine antitoxin, the currently licensed product of TIG in the United States should never be administered intravenously, because of aggregates. It is intended solely for intramuscular use.

9.2. Active Immunization

Tetanus toxoid is one of the best immunogens available today. A primary series will induce protective levels of circulating antitoxin in virtually 100% of recipients.[12,66] Protective levels usually last at least 10 years and in the majority will be present even up to 25 years after the last dose.[67]

9.2.1. Production and Testing of Tetanus Toxoid. To produce toxoid, *C. tetani* is cultured in large-capacity fermentors in liquid medium free of allergenic substances. The culture filtrate is precipitated with methanol or ammonium sulfate to purify partially extracellular toxin. Toxin is further purified and detoxified with 40% formaldehyde at 37°C. By WHO standards, the final product should contain 0.5% formaldehyde or less. In the United States, minimum requirements stipulate a residual formaldehyde content of 0.02% or less. A single dose of adsorbed toxoid must contain less than 1.25 mg of aluminum. All toxoid preparations in the United States have thimerosal as a bacteriostatic agent added to a final concentration of 0.1%.

Potency is determined by animal bioassays: for the fluid preparation, immunized guinea pigs are tested for survival after a toxin challenge; for precipitated toxoid, a serum pool from immunized guinea pigs must exceed 2 IU/ml of tetanus antitoxin. The toxoid content of commercial products is assessed by flocculation; this measure of toxoid protein content (Lf) does not equate directly with immunogenicity as measured by potency in guinea pigs. Adsorbed products available in the United States have a content of 4–10 Lf per dose; fluid products contain 4–5 Lf.

Tetanus toxoid is available in several preparations: Diphtheria and Tetanus Toxoids and Pertussis Vaccine Adsorbed (DTP; also referred to as DPT, particularly outside the United States), Diphtheria and Tetanus Toxoids Adsorbed (For Pediatric Use) (DT) used in infants and children under 7 years of age, and Diphtheria and Tetanus Toxoids and acellular Pertussis Vaccine (DTaP). Universal use of DTaP or DTP in infancy and childhood is recommended unless there are contraindications to pertussis vaccine. Tetanus and Diphtheria Toxoids Adsorbed (For Adult Use) (Td) is for use in persons 7 years of age and older; it contains less diphtheria toxoid (2 Lf or less) than the pediatric preparation (over 10 Lf). Td is the preferred preparation for tetanus prophylaxis in adults under all circumstances because the vast majority of adults in need of tetanus toxoid are likely to be susceptible to diphtheria. Single-antigen Tetanus Toxoid (fluid) and Tetanus Toxoid Adsorbed are also available in the United States for use in persons 7 years of age and older.

In the United States, aluminum hydroxide or aluminum phosphate is used as an adjuvant. These salts allow an adequate immune response after fewer doses of toxoid than with the fluid preparation.[68] Since fluid and adsorbed preparations do not differ substantially with regard to adverse events, adsorbed toxoid is preferred because it confers protective levels of antitoxin for a longer period of time.[68,69] Response to either form of toxoid as a booster dose is equally brisk. In combined active–passive immunization, TIG does not substantially alter the response to adsorbed toxoid as it does with fluid toxoid.[65,70] In some countries other than the United States, a calcium phosphate adsorbed product is also available. The adsorbed toxoid is administered intramuscularly; fluid preparations can be given subcutaneously. Either can be given by jet-injector.

Preparations should be stored at 2–10°C and generally have a 2-year expiration date. Higher ambient temperatures for 3 days or under do not reduce the potency of the toxoid. Freezing reduces potency, particularly when the toxoid is a component of DTP.[71]

9.2.2. Use of Tetanus Toxoid. Most immunization schedules in developed countries call for two or three doses in the first year of life followed by a reinforcing dose 6 months to 1 year afterward.[72–74] The routine schedule for tetanus immunization in the United States is given in

Table 1. Recommendations for Primary Immunization with Tetanus Toxoid by Age at Beginning Immunization—United States[a]

	Age group			
	< 1 year	1–6 years		≥ 7 years
Vaccine	DTaP or DTP or DT[b,c]	DTaP or DTP[d]	DT[b,e]	Td[f]
Interval before				
Dose 1	First visit	First visit	First visit	First visit
Dose 2	1–2 months	1–2 months	1–2 months	1–2 months
Dose 3	1–2 months	1–2 months	1–2 months	6–12 months
Dose 4	Approx. 1 yr[g]	Approx. 1 yr	—	—

[a]DTaP, diphtheria and tetanus toxoids and acellular pertussis vaccine; DTP, diphtheria and tetanus toxoids and pertussis vaccine; DT, diphtheria and tetanus toxoids for pediatric use; Td, tetanus and diphtheria toxoids for adult use.
[b]DT for those with contraindications to pertussis vaccine.
[c]Boosters with DT or DTP (dose 5) indicated at 4–6 years of age. Boosters with Td indicated every 10 years thereafter. First visit generally at 2 months of age.
[d]Dose 5 of DTP indicated at 4–6 years of age unless dose 4 administered at ≥4 years of age. In this instance, dose 5 not needed. Boosters with Td indicated every 10 years after dose 4 or 5.
[e]Dose 4 of DT indicated at 4–6 years of age unless dose 3 administered at ≥4 years of age. In this instance, dose 4 not needed. Boosters with Td indicated every 10 years after dose 3 or 4.
[f]Boosters with Td indicated every 10 years.
[g]Generally given at 15 months with measles, mumps, and rubella vaccine (MMR) and trivalent oral polio vaccine (OPV) or with OPV alone at 18 months of age.

Table 1. In children less than 7 years old, tetanus toxoid is usually combined with diphtheria toxoid and pertussis vaccine as DTaP or DTP. When given as DTaP or DTP, three doses starting at 6 weeks to 2 months of age are indicated 1 to 2 months apart followed by a fourth dose approximately 6 to 12 months after the third dose. If pertussis vaccine is contraindicated, a pediatric preparation of diphtheria and tetanus toxoids (DT) is indicated. In the first year of life, the schedule is identical to the DTP schedule. However, beginning in the second year, only three doses are required for primary immunization, two doses 1 to 2 months apart followed by a third dose 6 to 12 months after the second. For developing countries, the EPI, with its emphasis on infants, recommends a total of three doses early in the first year of life without reinforcing or booster doses.[75]

Protective levels of antitoxin can be achieved with schedules starting in the newborn period. However, in most countries immunization rarely starts before 2 months of age. In the past, it was thought that passively transferred maternal antitoxin would not interfere with the immune response of the infant. However, most of these studies were done before women had been routinely immunized either as children or as adults. More recent studies in the United States demonstrate that substantial proportions of infants have levels of circulating antitoxin at the time of initiating the DTP series, suggesting that the issue of interference should be reconsidered. The need for a full three doses in the first year of life was supported by a recent report by Barkin,[76] who demonstrated that substantially higher levels of antitoxin are achieved after three doses in the first year of life compared to two doses. The height of the antitoxin response is directly related to the age at completion of the third dose. There is no good evidence that intervals of 2 months for the first three doses offer any advantage over 1 month. All achieve protective levels regardless of schedule, although antitoxin levels are higher after the 2-month interval probably because these children are older at the time they complete their three-dose schedule. Nevertheless, by the time the fourth dose is indicated (approximately 1 year after the third dose), antitoxin levels are comparable in both groups. Preterm infants appear to respond similarly at a given chronological age as term infants.

Unimmunized children 7 years of age or older and adults require a three-dose primary series with two doses 1 to 2 months apart followed by a third dose 6 to 12 months after the second. In the United States, an adult preparation of combined tetanus and diphtheria toxoids (Td) that contains a decreased amount of diphtheria toxoid is used. The immune response to tetanus toxoid tends to decrease with increasing age. In comparative studies, children tend to achieve higher levels of antitoxin than do adults. The elderly tend to make a poorer response to toxoid than do younger adults.[77,78] Nevertheless, almost all children and adults will achieve protective titers after a three-dose primary series.

Table 2. Recommendations of the Expanded Programme on Immunization for Immunization of Women of Childbearing Age[a]

Dose	Timing
Dose 1:	First contact or as early in pregnancy as possible
Dose 2:	4 weeks later
Dose 3:	6–12 months later or during subsequent pregnancy
Dose 4:	1–5 years after dose 3 or during subsequent pregnancy
Dose 5:	1–10 years after dose 4 or during subsequent pregnancy; no further doses indicated

[a]See Ref. 74.

In developing countries, immunization of adults is intended primarily for pregnant women or women of childbearing age to effect prevention of tetanus neonatorum. Induction of protective levels in mothers is associated with protection from neonatal tetanus by transfer of antitoxin across the placenta.[8,79,80] A minimum of two doses at least 1 month apart has been recommended by the EPI for pregnant women with the last dose at least 2 weeks prior to the estimated date of delivery. However, difficulties in finding and vaccinating pregnant women have led to efforts to vaccinate all women of childbearing age. In addition, vaccination with only two doses is less effective and does not provide long-term protection. The schedule listed in Table 2, which recommends a total of five tetanus toxoid doses with the third at least 6 months after the first, has recently been adopted by the EPI in hopes of inducing sustained levels of circulating antitoxin in all women.[81]

After a three-dose primary series, circulating antitoxin remains at protective levels for years. Studies in Denmark demonstrate that 96% and 72% had levels $\geqslant$ 0.01 IU/ml at 13–14 and $\geqslant$ 25 years, respectively, after the third dose of a product containing 7–12 Lf. Based on these studies and others, immunization advisory bodies in the United States have recommended routine boosters of a tetanus toxoid-containing preparation every 10 years.[72,73] The booster response is not impaired even with intervals of 20 or more years since the last dose.[82] There is no need to restart a primary series if the schedule has not been followed or booster doses have been missed. Instead, prior doses should be counted and the remaining doses given to finish the three-dose primary series. Missed boosters can be ignored. In the United States, a preschool booster of DTP is recommended at 4–6 years of age primarily to ensure immunity to pertussis in young schoolaged children. Thereafter, doses of Td are recommended every 10 years. Tetanus in the United States continues to be a disease primarily of older adults who are also at highest risk for tetanus mortality. To decrease this remaining tetanus burden, the Advisory Committee on Immunization Practices (ACIP) and other advisory committees recommended in 1994 that for patients aged 50 years, health care providers should review adult vaccination status, administer tetanus and diphtheria toxoid as indicated, and determine whether a patient has one or more risk factors that indicate the need to receive pneumococcal and annual influenza vaccination.

9.2.3. Adverse Events. Reports of local reactions following tetanus toxoid vary greatly. In general, 50–85% of recipients of booster doses of adsorbed toxoid experience pain or tenderness at the injection site. While 20–30% experience edema and erythema,[69,83] marked swelling occurs in less than 2%. Controlled studies suggest that minor swelling or pain may occur more frequently in individuals receiving Td than among those receiving tetanus toxoid; however, substantial differences in marked swelling have not been demonstrated.[83] Several studies have found that the greater the preexisting antitoxin level, the higher is the incidence of local reactions, which generally begin within 2–8 hr of an injection.[69,84,85] There have been several reports of massive local swelling, particularly in persons with a history of multiple booster doses of toxoid. Such persons are typically found to have high serum antitoxin levels, likely leading to the formation of immune complexes with the deposited toxoid (Arthus reaction).[84,86] Thus, frequent boosters of tetanus toxoid in wound management are currently discouraged.

Fever can accompany a local response, particularly a marked local reaction.[86] Overall, booster doses of Td are associated with fever in 0.5–7%, with temperature over 39°C being rare.[85,87] Headache and malaise are unusual.

In 1994, the Institute of Medicine published an extensive review of adverse events following vaccination.[88] This review suggested that the evidence favors a causal relation between tetanus toxoid administration and Guillain–Barré syndrome, as well as brachial neuritis. The evidence was considered insufficient to assess a causal relationship between tetanus toxoid and mononeuropathy.[88]

Anaphylactic reactions to purified tetanus toxoid appear to be rare.[88] In the United States, passive surveillance for the years 1985–1986 revealed 6.4 serious allergic reactions (stridor, bronchospasm, and anaphylaxis) reported per million doses of publicly distributed Td. Skin testing has been urged in management of patients with a history suggestive of such a reaction.[89] Interpretation of some skin test results should take into account some expected nonspecificity of skin test reactions.

Table 3. Summary Guide to Tetanus Prophylaxis in Routine Wound Management[a]

History of adsorbed tetanus toxoid (doses)	Clean, minor wounds		All other wounds[b]	
	Td[c]	TIG	Td[c]	TIG
Unknown or < three	Yes	No	Yes	Yes
≥ Three[d]	No[e]	No	No[f]	No

[a]From ACIP, 1994.[96]
[b]Such as, but not limited to, wounds contaminated with dirt, feces, soil, saliva, etc.; puncture wounds; avulsions; and wounds resulting from missiles, crushing, burns, and frostbite.
[c]For children less than 7 years old; DTaP or DTP (DT, if pertussis vaccine is contraindicated) is preferred to tetanus toxoid alone. For persons 7 years old or older, Td is preferred to tetanus toxoid alone.
[d]If only three doses of *fluid* toxoid have been received, then a fourth dose of toxoid, preferably an adsorbed toxoid, should be given.
[e]Yes, if more than 10 years since last dose.
[f]Yes, if more than 5 years since last dose. (More frequent boosters are not needed and can accentuate side effects.)

9.2.4. Wound Management. An individual who presents for medical care with any type of wound should be evaluated for tetanus prophylaxis. Removal of foreign bodies and debridement of devitalized tissue in a timely fashion is imperative; if necessary, drainage and irrigation should be performed.[90] Recommendations for the use of tetanus toxoid and TIG in the United States for tetanus prophylaxis in the management of wounds have been made by the ACIP and agree with those of the American Academy of Pediatrics and the Committee on Trauma of the American College of Surgeons.[72,73,91] The recommendations of the ACIP are given in Table 3.

Although any wound can potentially give rise to tetanus infection, uncomplicated wounds are considered to have a low likelihood both of contamination by tetanus spores and of leading to an environment that would support germination of spores. For persons with this category of wounds, Td is recommended if the patient has received less than three doses of adsorbed toxoid in the past or it has been more than 10 years since the previous toxoid dose; TIG administration is not necessary. Such individuals respond briskly to subsequent doses of tetanus toxoid within 7 days and generally within 4 days.[92]

Most patients who had received fluid toxoid in the past, and rarely individuals who received adsorbed toxoid, may have circulating antitoxin levels less than 0.01 IU/ml after 5 years.[12,93] Therefore, it is recommended that persons with wounds that are of higher risk of contamination receive a dose of toxoid if more than 5 years have elapsed since the last dose. Individuals with such wounds are also potential candidates for simultaneous passive immunization with TIG if the immunization history indicates fewer than three toxoid doses. When administered at a separate site, TIG does not interfere with the immune response to adsorbed tetanus toxoid; an intramuscular dose of 250 units (1 ml) is recommended by the ACIP.(73)

Almost all of the tetanus cases with wounds in the United States might have been prevented with appropriate wound management. Of the 992 patients in the United States during 1972 to 1989 with acute wounds, tetanus toxoid was given as prophylaxis in wound management to only 29%; of these, 77% received toxoid within 3 days of injury. Tetanus toxoid alone is not sufficient in patients who have never received at least a three-dose primary series. Most of these individuals were also potential candidates for, but did not receive, TIG. Thirty-three percent of the 992 patients with acute wounds reportedly underwent debridement after injury and before onset of tetanus symptoms. Of these 327 patients, 93% did not receive the recommended Td with or without TIG based on their individual immunization histories. However, underadministration of tetanus prophylaxis following wounds appears to be the exception rather than the rule; two studies suggest that when patients with wounds seek care in the United States, 1–6% receive less than the recommended prophylactic measures of Td with or without TIG indicated by their wound and immunization history and 12–17% receive more than recommended.(94,95)

9.3. Antimicrobials

As a substitute for or adjunct to equine antitoxin prior to wide availability of TIG, antibiotics were once frequently used for tetanus prophylaxis in wound management. Antimicrobials may sensitize patients and have been known to fail. Antimicrobials have not been proven to have superior or equal efficacy to antitoxin and are not currently recommended for tetanus prophylaxis.(90,96)

9.4. Summary

Tetanus is an infectious but noncommunicable disease caused by a toxin. The spores of *C. tetani* are ubiquitous in nature and when deposited under the epithelium of the skin can germinate, given anaerobic conditions, leading to the production of tetanospasmin. The toxin travels to the CNS along peripheral nerves and causes disease by presynaptic interference with release of neurotransmitters, leading to disinhibition of spinal cord reflex arcs and accumulation of excitatory stimulation. This results in the tetanospasm, a generalized muscular spasm. Death-to-case ratios vary from 10 to 75%.

The disease can be prevented by appropriate attention to routine immunization and wound management. Tetanus toxoid is one of the most effective immunogens known, with essentially all recipients of a primary series protected for at least 10 years. Since wounds are probably the most frequent predisposing cause of tetanus, special attention should be paid to (1) wound cleansing and debridement to remove both spores and devitalized tissue and (2) providing protective levels of circulating antitoxin including both passive immunization to achieve protection rapidly and active immunization to increase levels rapidly in previously primed persons. Completion of a primary series will lead to sustained protection and would prevent cases not associated with acute injuries and circumvent the need for special procedures following wounds.

10. Unresolved Problems

The major problem in tetanus prevention today is the difficulty in delivering routine immunization to those in need. This is particularly a problem in developing countries where an estimated 515,000 infants die of neonatal tetanus annually.(28) Since most women do not have access to prenatal care and most children are born outside of a hospital, there needs to be greater emphasis on vaccination of women of childbearing age if the incidence of neonatal tetanus is to be reduced. Every contact of a susceptible female of childbearing age with the health care system should be taken as an opportunity to update her tetanus immunization status. More research is needed on one-dose delivery systems. While preliminary results with high-potency toxoids have been encouraging, there is concern about maintenance of protective levels of antibody. At the present time, at least two doses in pregnancy are recommended, but a vigorous attempt to provide five doses early in the reproductive years will lead to a higher likelihood of protection against neonatal tetanus.

Universal immunization of children with later boosting will also go a long way toward preventing tetanus in the children themselves as well as their offspring, because protective levels appear to persist in the majority for over 25 years. In hopes of raising immunization levels in the United States, the ACIP recently simplified the immunization schedule to allow DTaP or DTP together with oral polio vaccine (OPV) and measles, mumps, and rubella (MMR) vaccine at 15 months of age.(97) Previously, separate visits were recommended at 15 months for MMR and 18 months for the fourth dose of DTP. Combination of DTP with *Haemophilus influenzae* type b polysaccharide conjugated with various proteins (Hib) has been licensed for use in the United States since 1991. In many developing countries, simultaneous administration of multiple other vaccines could result in improved immunity levels against several diseases; many potential combinations are being evaluated currently using DTaP, Hib, with hepatitis B and/or inactivated polio vaccine (IPV).[98]

In the United States, the remaining morbidity and mortality from tetanus are in the elderly. Serological surveys suggest that substantial majorities of these populations lack protection.[35] Greater efforts are needed by practitioners to review the immunization status of their elderly patients and offer Td as needed.

Finally, universal proper wound management would prevent a significant proportion of tetanus cases. All persons in emergency rooms as well as other health care providers need to become familiar with current recommendations for wound care, including administration of passive immunization to persons who are unimmunized or whose immunization status is unknown.

11. References

1. Carle, A., and Rattone, G., Studio spetrimentale sull' etiologia del tetano, *G. Accad. Med. Torino* **32**:174 (1884).
2. Nicolaier, A., Ueber infectiösen *Tetanus*, *Dtsch. Med. Wochenschr.* **10**:842–844 (1884).
3. Kitasato, S., Ueber den Tetanusbacillus, *Z. Hyg.* **7**:225–234 (1889).
4. Von Behring, E., Kitasato, S., Ueber das Zustandekommen der Diphtherie-Immunität und Tetanus-Immunität bei Thieren, *Dtsch. Med. Wochenschr.* **16**:1113–1114 (1890).
5. Descombey, P., L'anatoxine tetanique, *Can. R. Soc. Biol.* **91**:239–241 (1924).
6. Kircher, T., and Anderson, R. E., Cause of death: Proper completion of the death certificate, *J. Am. Med. Assoc.* **77**:137–139 (1987).
7. Sutter, R. W., Cochi, S. L., Brink, E. W., Sirotkin, B. I., Assessment of vital statistics and surveillance data for monitoring tetanus mortality, 1979–1984, *Am. J. Epidemiol.* **131**:132–142 (1990).
8. MacLennan, R., Schofield, F. D., Pittman, M., Hardegree, M. C., and Banile, M. F., Immunization against neonatal tetanus in New Guinea: Antitoxin response of pregnant women to adjuvant and plain toxoids, *Bull. WHO* **32**:683–697 (1965).
9. Smith, J. W. G., Diphtheria and tetanus toxoids, *Br. Med. Bull.* **25**:177–182 (1969).
10. Cain, H. D., and Falco, F. G., Recurrent tetanus, *Calif. Med.* **97**: 31–33 (1962).
11. Spenney, J. G., Lamb, R. N., and Cobbs, C. G., Recurrent tetanus, *South. Med. J.* **64**:859–862 (1971).
12. Barile, M. F., Hardegree, M. C., and Pittman, M., Immunization against neonatal tetanus in New Guinea. 3. The toxin-neutralization test and the response of guinea pigs to the toxoids as used in the immunization schedules in New Guinea, *Bull. WHO* **43**:453–459 (1970).
13. Melville-Smith, M. E., Seagroatt, V. A., and Watkins, J. T., A comparison of enzyme-linked immunosorbent assay (ELISA) with the toxin neutralization test in mice as a method for the estimation of tetanus antitoxin in human sera, *J. Biol. Stand.* **11**:137–144 (1983).
14. Virella, G., and Hyman, B., Quantification of anti-tetanus and anti-diphtheria antibodies by enzymoimmunoassay: Methodology and applications, *J. Clin. Lab. Anal.* **5**:43–48 (1991).
15. Pitzurra, L. F., Bistoni, M., Pitzurra, L., *et al.*, Comparison of passive haemagglutination with turkey erythrocyte assay, enzyme-linked immunosorbent assay and counter-immunoelectrophoresis assay for serological evaluation of tetanus immunity, *J. Clin. Microbiol.* **17**:432–435 (1983).
16. Marconi, P., Pitzurra, M., and Bistoni, F., Passive hemagglutination as the reference method for evaluation of tetanus immunity, in: *Seventh International Conference on Tetanus* (G. Nistico, P. Mastroeni, and M. Pitzurra, eds.), pp. 259–273, Gangeni, Rome, 1985.
17. Ourth, D. D., and MacDonald, A. B., Neutralization of tetanus toxin by human and rabbit immunoglobulin classes and subunits, *Immunology* **3**:807–815 (1977).
18. Simonsen, O., Vaccination against tetanus and diphtheria. Evaluation of immunity in the Danish population, guidelines for revaccination, and methods for control of vaccination programs, *Dan. Med. Bull.* **36**;24–47 (1989).
19. Smith, J. W. G., Tetanus, in *Topley and Wilson's Principles of Bacteriology, Virology and Immunity*, Vol. 3, (G. Wilson, A. Miles, and M. T. Parker, eds.), pp. 345–368, Williams & Wilkins, Baltimore, 1984.
20. Turner, T. B., Velasco-Joven, E. A., and Prudovsky, S., Studies on the prophylaxis and treatment of tetanus. II. Studies pertaining to treatment, *Bull. Johns Hopkins Hosp.* **102**:71–84 (1958).
21. Passen, E. L., and Andersen, B. R., Clinical tetanus despite a "protective" level of toxin-neutralizing antibody, *J. Am. Med. Assoc.* **255**:1171–1173 (1986).
22. Bytchenko, B., Microbiology of tetanus, in *Tetanus: Important New Concepts* (R. Veronesi, ed.), pp. 28–39, Excerpta Medica, Amsterdam, 1981.
23. Smith, J. W. G., Tetanus and its prevention, *Prog. Drug Res.* **19**:391–401 (1975).
24. Finn, L. W., Silver, R. P., Habig, W. H., and Hardegree, M. C., The structural gene for tetanus neurotoxin is on a plasmid, *Science* **224**:881–884 (1984).
25. Matsuda, M., and Yoneda, M., Isolation and purification of two antigenically active, "complementary" polypeptide fragments of tetanus neurotoxin, *Infect. Immun.* **12**:1147–1153 (1975).
26. Wright, G. P., The neurotoxins of *Clostridium botulinum* and *Clostridium tetani*, *Pharmacol. Rev.* **7**:413–456 (1955).
27. Bytchenko, B. D., Causse, G., Grab, B., and Kereselidze, T. S., Tetanus: Recent trends of world distribution, in *Sixth International Conference on Tetanus* (C. Merieux, ed.), pp. 97–111, Collection Foundation Merieux, Lyon, 1981.
28. Centers for Disease Control, Progress toward the global elimination of neonatal tetanus, 1989–1993, *Morbid. Mortal. Week. Rep.* **43**:885–887, 893–894 (1994).
29. Cherubin, C. E., Epidemiology of tetanus in narcotic addicts, *NY State J. Med.* **70**:267–271 (1970).
30. Sun, K. O., Outbreak of tetanus among heroin addicts in Hong Kong, *J. R. Soc. Med.* **87**:494–495 (1994).
31. Bytchenko, B., Geographical distribution of tetanus in the world, 1951–60, *Bull. WHO* **34**:71–104 (1966).
32. Ball, K., Norboo, T., Gupta, U., and Shafi, S., Is tetanus rare at high altitudes? *Trop. Doct.* **24**:78–80 (1994).
33. Blake, P. A., and Feldman, R. A., Tetanus in the United States 1970–1971, *J. Infect. Dis.* **131**:745–748 (1975).

34. Heath, C. W., Zusman, J., and Sherman, I. L., Tetanus in the United States, 1950–1960, *Am. J. Public Health* **54:**769–779 (1964).
35. Gergen, P. J., McQuillan, G. M., Kiely, M., Ezzati-Rice, T. M., Sutter, R. W., and Virella, G., A population-based serologic survey of immunity to tetanus in the United States, *N. Engl. J. Med.* **332:**761–766 (1995).
36. Stanfield, J. P., and Galazka, A., Neonatal tetanus in the world today, *Bull. WHO* **62:**647–669 (1984).
37. Prevots, R., Sutter, R. W., Strebel, P. M., Cochi, S. L., and Hadler, S., Tetanus surveillance—United States, 1989–1990, *Morbid. Mortal. Week. Rep.* **41**(SS8):1–9 (1992).
38. Long, A. P., and Sartwell, P. E., Tetanus in the US Army in World War II, *Bull. US Army Med. Dep.* **7:**371–385 (1947).
39. Yen, L. M., Dao, L. M., Day, N. P. J., *et al.*, Role of quinine in the high mortality of intramuscular injection tetanus, *Lancet* **344:**786–787 (1994).
40. Lowbury, E. J. L., and Lilly, H. A., Contamination of operating-theatre air with *Cl. tetani*, *Br. Med. J.* **2:**1334–1336 (1958).
41. Hinman, A. R., Foster, S. O., and Wassilak, S. G. F., Neonatal tetanus: Potential for elimination in the USA and the world, *Pediatr. Infect. Dis. J.* **6:**813–816 (1987).
42. Bauer, J. H., and Meyer, K. F., Human intestinal carriers of tetanus spores in California, *J. Infect. Dis.* **38:**295–305 (1926).
43. Bulloch, W. E., and Cramer, W., On a new factor in the mechanism of bacterial infection, *Proc. R. Soc. London Ser. B* **90:**513–528 (1919).
44. Kryzhanovsky, G. N., Pathophysiology, in: *Tetanus: Important New Concepts* (R. Veronesi, ed.), pp. 109–182, Excerpta Medica, Amsterdam, 1981.
45. Abel, J. J., Firor, W. M., and Chalain, W., Researches on tetanus. IX. Further evidence to show that tetanus toxin is not carried to central nervous system by way of the axis cylinders of motor nerves. *Bull. Johns Hopkins Hosp.* **63:**373–402 (1938).
46. Schwab, M. E., and Thoenen, H. Selective binding, uptake and retrograde transport of tetanus toxin by nerve terminals in the rat iris, *J. Cell. Biol.* **77:**1–13 (1978).
47. Zacks, S. I., and Shef, M. F., Tetanus toxin: Fine structure, localization of binding sites in striated muscle, *Science* **159:**643–644 (1968).
48. Price, D. L., Griffin, J. W., Young, A., Peck, K., and Stock, A., Tetanus toxin: Direct evidence for retrograde axonal transport, *Science* **188:**945–957 (1975).
49. Matzkin, H., and Regev, S., Naturally acquired immunity to tetanus toxin in an isolated community, *Infect. Immun.* **48:**267–268 (1985).
50. Veronesi, R., Bizzini, B., Focaccia, R., *et al.*, Naturally acquired antibodies to tetanus toxin in humans and animals from the Galapagos Islands, *J. Infect. Dis.* **147:**308–311 (1983).
51. McComb, J. A., The prophylactic dose of homologous tetanus antitoxin, *N. Engl. J. Med.* **270:**175–178 (1964).
52. Wolters, K. L., and Dehmel, H., Abschliessende Untersuchungen über die Tetanusprophylaxe durch active Immunisierung, *Z. Hyg.* **124:**326–332 (1942).
53. Berger, S. A., Cherubin, L. E., Nelson, S., and Levine, L., Tetanus despite preexisting antitetanus antibody, *J. Am. Med. Assoc.* **240:**769–770 (1978).
54. Weinstein, L., Tetanus, *N. Engl. J. Med.* **289:**1293–1296 (1973).
55. Roistacher, K., Griffin, J. W., Local tetanus, *Johns Hopkins Med. J.* **149:**84–88 (1981).
56. Wright, D. K., Lalloo, U. G., Nayiger, S., and Govender, P., Autonomous nervous system dysfunction in severe tetanus: Current perspectives, *Crit. Care Med.* **17:**371–374 (1989).
57. Einhorn, M. S., Granoff, D. M., Nahm, M. H., Quinn, A., and Shackelford, P. G., Concentrations of antibodies in paired maternal and infant sera: Relationship to IgG subclass, *J. Pediatr.* **111:**783–788 (1987).
58. Veronesi, R., and Focaccia, R., The clinical picture, in: *Tetanus: Important New Concepts* (R. Veronesi, ed.), pp. 459–463, Excerpta Medica, Amsterdam, 1981.
59. Smith, W. D., and Tobias, M. A., Tetany, tetanus or drug reaction? *Br. J. Anaesth.* **48:**703–705 (1976).
60. Boyd, R. E., Brennan, P. T., Denj, J. F., Rochester, D. F., and Spyker, D. A., Strychnine poisoning, *Am. J. Med.* **74:**507–512 (1983).
61. Bruce, D., Tetanus, *J. Hyg.* **19:**1–32 (1920).
62. Suri, J. C., and Rubbo, S. D., Immunization against tetanus, *J. Hyg.* **59:**29–48 (1961).
63. Moynihan, N. H., Serum sickness and local reactions in tetanus prophylaxis: A study of 400 cases, *Br. Med. J.* **2:**264–266 (1955).
64. Centers for Disease Control, Safety of therapeutic immune globulin preparations with respect to transmission of human T-lymphocytic virus type III/lymphadenopathy-associated virus infection, *Morbid. Mortal. Week. Rep.* **35:**231–233 (1986).
65. Levine, L., McComb, J. A., Dwyer, R. C., and Latham, W. C., Active–passive tetanus immunization, *N. Engl. J. Med.* **274:**186–190 (1966).
66. Halsey, N. A., and Galazka, A., The efficacy of DPT and oral poliomyelitis immunization schedules initiated from birth to 12 weeks of age, *Bull. WHO* **63:**1151–1169 (1985).
67. Simonsen, O., Badsberg, J. H., Kjeldsen, K., *et al.*, The fall-off in serum concentration of tetanus antitoxin after primary and booster vaccination, *Acta Pathol. Microbiol. Scand.* **94:**77–82 (1986).
68. Jones, F. G., and Moss, J. M., Studies on tetanus toxoid. I: The antitoxic titer of human subject following immunization with tetanus toxoid and tetanus alum precipitated toxoid, *J. Immunol.* **30:**115–125 (1936).
69. Jones, A. E., Melville-Smith, M., Watkins, J., Seagroatt, V., Rice, L., and Sheffield, F., Adverse reactions in adolescents to reinforcing doses of plain and adsorbed tetanus vaccines, *Community Med.* **7:**99–106 (1985).
70. Mahoney, L. J., Aprile, M. A., and Moloney, P. J., Combined active–passive immunization against tetanus in man, *Can. Med. Assoc. J.* **96:**1401–1404 (1967).
71. Galazka, A., *Stability of Vaccines*, Expanded Programme on Immunization, World Health Organization, Geneva, 1989, WHO/EPI/GEN/89. 8.
72. American Academy of Pediatrics, *1994 Red Book: Report of the Committee on Infectious Diseases*, 23rd ed., American Academy of Pediatrics, Elk Grove Village, IL, 1994.
73. Centers for Disease Control and Prevention, Diphtheria, tetanus and pertussis. Recommendations for vaccine use and other preventive measures. Recommendations of Advisory Committee for Immunization Practices (ACIP), *Morbid. Mortal. Week. Rep.* **40** (RR10):1–28 (1991).
74. Expanded Programme on Immunization, *Prevention of Neonatal Tetanus through Immunization*, World Health Organization, Geneva, EPI/86/9, 1986.
75. Expanded Programme on Immunization, Global Advisory Group, *Week. Epidemiol. Rec.* **60:**13–16 (1985).
76. Barkin, R. M., Pichichero, M. E., Samuelson, J. S., and Barkin, S. Z., Pediatric diphtheria and tetanus toxoids vaccine: Clinical and immunologic response when administered as the primary series, *J. Pediatr.* **106:**779–781 (1985).
77. Kishimoto, S., Tomino, S., Mitsuya, H., Fujiwara, H., and Tsuda,

H., Age-related decline in the *in vitro* and *in vivo* syntheses of anti-tetanus toxoid antibody in humans, *J. Immunol.* **125:**2347–2352 (1980).

78. Solomonova, K., and Vizev, S., Secondary response to boostering by purified aluminum-hydroxide-adsorbed tetanus antitoxin in aging and in aged adults, *Immunobiology* **158:**312–319 (1981).
79. Chen, S. T., Edsall, G., Peel, M. M., and Sinnathuray, T. A., Timing of antenatal tetanus immunization for effective protection of the neonate, *Bull. WHO* **61:**159–163 (1983).
80. Newell, K. W., Duenas Lehman, A., LeBlanc, D. R., and Garces Osorio, N., The use of toxoid for the prevention of tetanus neonatorum. Final report of a double-blind controlled field trial, *Bull. WHO* **35:**863–871 (1966).
81. Expanded Programme on Immunization, *Issues in Neonatal Tetanus Control*, EPI/GAG/87/WP. 11, WHO, 1987.
82. Simonsen, O., Kjeldsen, K., and Heron, I., Immunity against tetanus and effect of revaccination 25–30 years after primary vaccination, *Lancet* **2:**1240–1242 (1984).
83. Macko, M. B., Comparison of the morbidity of tetanus toxoid boosters with tetanus–diphtheria toxoid boosters, *Ann. Emerg. Med.* **14:**33–35 (1985).
84. McComb JA, Levine L., Adult immunization. II. Dosage reduction as a solution to increasing reactions to tetanus toxoid. *N. Engl. J. Med.* **265:**1152–1153 (1961).
85. White WG, Barnes GM, Barker E, et al., Reactions to tetanus toxoid. *J. Hyg.* **71:**283–297 (1973).
86. Levine L, Edsall G., Tetanus toxoid: What determines reaction proneness? *J. Infect. Dis.* **144:**376 (1981).
87. Sisk CW, Lewis CE. Reactions to tetanus-diphtheria toxoid (adult). *Arch. Environ. Health.* **11:**34–36 (1965).
88. Institute of Medicine, Diphtheria and tetanus toxoids, in *Adverse Events Following Childhood Vaccines. Evidence Bearing on Causality*, National Academy Press, Washington, DC, 1994.
89. Jacobs RL, Lowe RS, Lanier BQ., Adverse reactions to tetanus toxoid. *J. Am. Med. Assoc.* **247:**40–42 (1982).
90. Smith, J. W. G., Laurence, D. R., and Evans, D. G., Prevention of tetanus in the wounded, *Br. Med. J.* **3:**453–455 (1975).
91. Committee on Trauma, American College of Surgeons, Prophylaxis against tetanus in wound management, *Am. Coll. Surg. Bull.* **69:**22–23 (1984).
92. Kaiser, G. C., King, R. D., Lempe, R. E., and Ruster, M. H., Delayed recall of active tetanus immunization, *J. Am. Med. Assoc.* **178:**914–916 (1961).
93. Peebles, T. C., Levine, L., Eldred, M. L. and Edsall, G., Tetanus-toxoid emergency boosters: A reappraisal, *N. Engl. J. Med.* **280:**575–581 (1969).
94. Brand, D. A., Acampora, D., Gottlieg, L., Glancy, K. E., and Frazier, W. H., Adequacy of antitetanus prophylaxis in six hospital emergency rooms, *N. Engl. J. Med.* **309:**636–640 (1983).
95. Giangrosso, J., Smith, R. K., Misuse of tetanus immunoprophylaxis in wound care, *Ann. Emerg. Med.* **14:**573–579 (1985).
96. Lowbury, E. J. L., Kidson, A., Lilly, H. A., Wilkins, M. D., and Jackson, O. M., Prophylaxis against tetanus in non-immune patients with wounds: The role of antibiotics and of human antitetanus globulin, *J. Hyg.* **80:**267–274 (1978).
97. Centers for Disease Control and Prevention, General recommendations on immunization. Recommendations of the Advisory Committee on Immunization Practices (ACIP), *Morbid. Mortal. Week. Rep.* **43**(RR1)**:**1–38 (1994).
98. Williams, J. C., Goldenthal, K. L., Burns, D., Lewis, B. P., (eds.), *Combined Vaccines and Simultaneous Administration: Current Issues and Perspectives*, New York Academy of Sciences, New York, 1995.

12. Suggested Reading

Bleck, T. P., Tetanus: Pathophysiology, management, and prophylaxis, *Dis. Mon.* **37:**545–603.

Rappuoli, R., New and improved vaccines against diphtheria and tetanus, in: *New Generation Vaccines* (G. C. Woodrow and M. M. Levine, eds.), pp. 251–268, Marcel Dekker, New York, 1990.

Habig, W. H., and Tankersley, D. L., Tetanus, in: *Vaccines and Immunotherapy*, (S. J. Cryz, ed.), pp. 13–19, Pergamon, New York, 1991.

Simonsen, O., Vaccination against tetanus and diphtheria. Evaluation of immunity in the Danish population, guidelines for revaccination, and methods for control of vaccination programs, *Dan. Med. Bull.* **36:**24–47 (1989).

Stratton, K. R., Howe, C.J, and Johnston, R. B., (eds), *Adverse Events Following Childhood Vaccines, Evidence Bearing on Causality*, National Academy Press, Washington, DC, 1994.

CHAPTER 38

Toxic Shock Syndrome (Staphylococcal)

Arthur L. Reingold

1. Introduction

Staphylococcal toxic shock syndrome (TSS) is an acute, multisystem febrile illness caused by *Staphylococcus aureus*. A similar illness caused by group A streptococcal infections is discussed in Chapter 34. The currently accepted criteria for confirming a case of TSS include fever, hypotension, a diffuse erythematous macular rash, subsequent desquamation, evidence of multisystem involvement, and lack of evidence of another likely cause of the illness (Table 1).

2. Historical Background

TSS was first described as such in 1978 by Todd *et al.*[1] However, cases of what we now believe to have been TSS have been reported in the medical literature since at least 1927 as "staphylococcal scarlet fever" or "staphylococcal scarlatina."[2,3] In addition, a number of patients reported in the medical literature in the 1970s as having adult Kawasaki disease probably had TSS.[4] The association between illness and focal infection with *S. aureus* was, by definition, apparent in early reports of staphylococcal scarlet fever, but was reinforced by the findings of Todd *et al.*[1] and later by the findings of other investigators.[5,6]

TSS achieved notoriety in 1980 when numerous cases were recognized and an association between illness (in women), menstruation, and tampon use was demonstrated.[7,8] While the early case reports of staphylococcal scarlet fever and the report by Todd *et al.*[1] clearly showed that TSS occurred in small children, men, and women who were not menstruating, most (but by no means all) of the cases initially recognized and reported in late 1979 and early 1980 were in menstruating women,[8–10] leading to the frequent misperception among the general public and many physicians that TSS occurred only in association with tampon use (hence, "the tampon disease"). This misperception undoubtedly led to subsequent biases in the diagnosing (and probably reporting) of TSS cases. However, later studies designed to eliminate such biases have shown that TSS does, in fact, occur disproportionately in menstruating women,[11,12] while case–control studies demonstrating an association between the risk of developing TSS during menstruation and tampon use preceded (indeed, led to) the introduction of bias concerning the relationship between tampon use and menstrual TSS.[5,6]

Follow-up studies demonstrated that the risk of developing tampon-related menstrual TSS varies with the absorbency, chemical composition, and oxygen content of the tampon,[13–16] although the relative importance of these and other tampon characteristics in determining that risk remains uncertain. As a result of both epidemiological and *in vitro* laboratory studies, the formulation of available tampons has changed dramatically since 1980, such that absorbencies are substantially lower and chemical composition is less varied across brands and styles. Studies in the late 1980s have demonstrated that the incidence of TSS, particularly menstrual TSS, has risen and fallen in parallel with the absorbency of tampons,[17] but that the risk of developing menstrual TSS continues to

Arthur L. Reingold • Division of Public Health Biology and Epidemiology, University of California, Berkeley, California 94720-7360.

Table 1. Case Definition of Toxic Shock Syndrome

Fever: temperature ≥ 38.9°C (102°F)
Rash: diffuse macular erythroderma
Desquamation: 1 to 3 weeks after onset of illness
Hypotension: systolic blood pressure ≤ 90 mm Hg for adults or below fifth percentile by age for children under 16 years of age, orthostatic drop in diastolic blood pressure ≥ 15 mm Hg from lying to sitting, orthostatic syncope, or orthostatic dizziness
Multisystem involvement: three or more of the following:
- Gastrointestinal: vomiting or diarrhea at onset of illness
- Muscular: severe myalgia or creatine phosphokinase level at least twice the upper limit of normal for laboratory
- Renal: blood urea nitrogen or creatinine at least twice the upper limit of normal for laboratory or urinary sediment with pyuria (≥ 5 leukocytes per high-power field) in the absence of urinary tract infection
- Hepatic: total bilirubin, serum aspartate transaminase, or serum alanine transaminase at least twice the upper limit of normal for laboratory
- Hematologic: platelets < 100,000
- Central nervous system: disorientation or alterations in consciousness without focal neurological signs when fever and hypotension are absent

Negative results on the following tests, if obtained:
- Blood, throat, or cerebrospinal fluid cultures (cultures may be positive for *Staphylococcus aureus*)
- Rise in titer to Rocky Mountain spotted fever, leptospirosis, or rubeola

vary directly with tampon absorbency, despite the changes in tampon formulation.[18]

3. Methodology

3.1. Sources of Mortality Data

Mortality rates for TSS have not been reported directly, but can be estimated from reported incidence rates and case-fatality rates.

3.2. Sources of Morbidity Data

Surveillance for TSS began in a few states in late 1979 and in other states and nationally in early 1980. Since that time, TSS has been made a reportable disease in most states. However, the level of intensity of surveillance activities has varied markedly between and within states. Thus, a few states established active surveillance for TSS for brief periods of time, while others have done little to stimulate the diagnosis and reporting of cases. As a result, the completeness of diagnosing and reporting TSS cases undoubtedly has been inconsistent between states and over time. However, data from a national hospital discharge survey indicate that reporting of cases, while incomplete and variable by region, has not been biased dramatically insofar as the age, race, sex, or menstrual status of the patients is concerned.[19] Hospital record review studies, in which both diagnosed and previously undiagnosed cases of TSS were ascertained in a consistent fashion, so as to minimize or eliminate both diagnostic and reporting biases, also have been conducted.[11,12,17,20,21] These studies demonstrate that, by and large, the patient characteristics and temporal trends observed in data collected through the largely passive network of TSS surveillance reflected true variation in the incidence of TSS by age, sex, race, and menstrual status. These same studies, taken together, demonstrate that at least some of the apparent geographic variation in the incidence of TSS in the United States is real.

3.3. Surveys

Numerous small surveys have demonstrated that many asymptomatic individuals carry in the nasopharynx and/or vagina strains of *S. aureus* that produce TSS toxin-1 (TSST-1), the toxin believed to be responsible for most TSS cases.[22–26] Similarly, large serosurveys have shown that antibodies to TSST-1 or to a cross-reacting antigen are extremely common.[22,25,27,28]

3.4. Laboratory Diagnosis

3.4.1. Isolation and Identification of the Organism. While recovery of *S. aureus* from the vagina or another site of infection is not one of the criteria of the TSS case definition, it is possible in most TSS cases if appropriate specimens are obtained before antimicrobial therapy is initiated.[5,6,29,30] *S. aureus* grows readily on most standard culture media and is readily identifiable by any clinical microbiology laboratory within 2 or 3 days. Testing of *S. aureus* strains for production of TSST-1, however, is performed in only a few research laboratories. Hence, the results of such testing are not readily available during the acute illness and are not of value in treating patients suspected of having TSS. Furthermore, because both *S. aureus* in general and TSST-1-producing strains of *S. aureus* in particular can be recovered from many patients without the clinical features of TSS and from asymptomatic individuals, microbiological results cannot and do not provide that a given patient has TSS.

3.4.2. Serological and Immunologic Diagnostic Methods. A variety of serological and immunologic techniques have been used to test *S. aureus* strains for production of TSST-1. As noted above, these tests are not available outside a few research laboratories. It is possible to detect TSST-1 in clinical specimens,[31,32] but these assays are not generally available. Antibodies to TSST-1 can be measured using solid-phase radioimmunoassay and other techniques. However, most healthy individuals have detectable anti-TSST-1 antibodies.[22,25,27,28] Furthermore, some patients with TSS have demonstrable anti-TSST-1 antibodies at the time of onset, and many patients without such antibodies at the time of onset do not demonstrate an antibody rise in response to their illness.[27,33] Thus, testing for anti-TSST-1 antibodies (which is not available except in one or two research laboratories, in any event) is of limited value in confirming the diagnosis of TSS, although it has been argued that the absence of detectable antibodies at the time of onset supports the diagnosis of TSS.

4. Biological Characteristics of the Organism

As noted above, there is convincing evidence that *S. aureus* is the cause of TSS. In patients with menstrual TSS, *S. aureus* can be recovered from the vagina and/or cervix in 95–100% of cases (usually as a heavy growth), but in only 5–15% of healthy control women.[5,24,34–39] In patients with nonmenstrual TSS associated with a focal wound, *S. aureus* is typically the only organism found in the lesion.[29,30] Furthermore, experimental studies demonstrate that TSS-associated *S. aureus* strains can cause a similar illness in rabbits.

Similarly, there is strong evidence that the ability to make TSST-1, previously known as pyrogenic exotoxin C,[40] staphylococcal enterotoxin F,[41] and several other names, is characteristic of, although not universal among, TSS-associated *S. aureus* strains. Thus, 90–100% of *S. aureus* isolates recovered from the vagina, cervix, or used tampon in menstrual TSS cases produce TSST-1, compared with only 10–20% of vaginal or nasopharyngeal isolates from healthy controls.[26,40–43] On the other hand, only 60–70% of *S. aureus* strains recovered from normally sterile sites in patients with nonmenstrual TSS produce TSST-1,[44–46] suggesting that other staphylococcal toxins, particularly staphylococcal enterotoxin B (SEB), may be capable of inducing a clinically indistinguishable syndrome. Two studies of historical strains of *S. aureus* have demonstrated that the proportion of strains capable of making TSST-1 has changed over time and was generally higher in the mid to late 1970s than in earlier time periods.[42,47] Interestingly, that proportion appears to have declined somewhat in the early 1980s, when the incidence of TSS was peaking. More recent data concerning the proportion of *S. aureus* strains that make TSST-1 have not been published.

TSS-associated *S. aureus* strains also have been characterized phenotypically with respect to a number of other properties, including phage type, antimicrobial susceptibility, resistance to heavy metals, production or activity of various enzymes, and presence of plasmids and bacteriophages. The picture that emerges with regard to these characteristics, while consistent, is by no means invariable or unique. A higher proportion of TSS-related *S. aureus* strains are lysed by phase types 29 and/or 52 (58–82%), as compared to only 12–28% of control strains.[42,43,48] Similarly, TSS-associated strains generally are resistant to penicillin (and ampicillin), arsenate, and cadmium, while being susceptible to β-lactamase-resistant antimicrobial agents, most other commonly tested antimicrobial agents, bacteriocins, and mercury.[6,49,50] Other characteristics that appear to distinguish these strains from other *S. aureus* strains include decreased production of hemolysin, lipase, and nuclease[49,51]; tryptophan auxotypy[52]; decreased lethality in chick embryos[49]; increased pigment production[53]; and increased casein proteolysis.[53] TSS-associated strains also have been reported to be less likely to carry plasmids and more likely to carry lysogenic bacteriophage than are control strains. There is controversy over whether or not the gene coding for TSST-1 can be transferred by lysogeny.[54,55]

It should be noted that most of the strains examined in the above studies were recovered from the genital tract in menstrual TSS cases. Thus, the results are not necessarily applicable to *S. aureus* strains associated with nonmenstrual TSS, and there is some evidence to suggest that such strains, recovered from normally sterile sites in patients with nonmenstrual TSS, are less likely to be lysed by phage types 29 and/or 52 than are strains from menstrual TSS cases.[44] At the same time, as noted above, they also are less likely to make TSST-1.

5. Descriptive Epidemiology

5.1. Prevalence and Incidence

Carriage of *S. aureus* on the skin and in the nasopharynx and vagina is very common. Numerous cross-sectional studies have demonstrated that 30–40% of individuals carry *S. aureus* in the nasopharynx and 5–15% of women carry *S. aureus* in the vagina.[22–24,34–39] The corresponding figures for TSST-1 producing *S. aureus* are 5–15% (nasopharynx) and 1–5% (vagina). Thus, carriage of *S. aureus* strains believed to be capable of causing TSS is also very common.

In contrast, TSS is a rare disease. After it became a notifiable disease in 1983, the number of cases reported annually in the United States initially ranged from 400 to 500. More recently, 50 to 100 cases have been reported annually to the Centers for Disease Control and Prevention (CDC). The most reliable estimates of incidence rates come from hospital-based record review studies. In these studies, both diagnosed and previously undiagnosed cases of TSS were ascertained in an unbiased way by reviewing thousands of medical records of hospitalized patients with one of a long list of discharge diagnoses likely to be indicative of misdiagnosed cases of TSS. In one such study in Colorado, the annual incidence of TSS in women between the ages of 10 and 30 was 15.8/100,000 in 1980.[12] In a similar study in California, the incidence rate in women between the ages of 15 and 34 was only 2.4/100,000 in 1980.[11] The incidence rate in men of the same age group in the latter study was consistently less than 0.5/100,000 in all of the years studied.

Estimates of the incidence of diagnosed TSS derive from statewide surveillance systems established in late 1979 or early 1980. The states with the most aggressive case-finding methods reported annual incidence rates at that time of 6.2/100,000 menstruating women (Wisconsin),[5] 8.9/100,000 menstruating women (Minnesota),[56] and 14.4/100,000 females 10–49 years of age (Utah).[57] An overall estimate of 0.8/100,00 total population of hospitalized, diagnosed TSS in the United States in 1981 and 1982 was derived from a national hospital discharge survey.[19] While TSS has been documented in numerous other countries, no estimates of incidence rates for other countries are available.

The discrepancy between the frequency of colonization and/or infection with TSST-1-producing *S. aureus* and the rarity of TSS is thought to be due to the fact that most individuals have detectable anti-TSST-1 antibodies. By age 30, more than 95% of men and women have such antibodies.[28] The origin of these antibodies is unknown.

5.2. Epidemic Behavior and Contagiousness

Because TSS increased dramatically in incidence in the United States beginning in 1979 in comparison with previous years,[11,12,20] it would be correct to say that an epidemic of TSS occurred at that time. TSS does not occur, however, in explosive epidemics in the same way that dengue and meningococcal disease do, although strains of *S. aureus* that produce TSST-1 are, like other *S. aureus* strains, transmitted readily by person-to-person spread.

5.3. Geographic Distribution

5.3.1. United States. Cases of TSS have been reported in all 50 states and the District of Columbia, but the incidence of reported cases has varied substantially between states and regions.[9,10] Variation in the completeness of diagnosis and reporting of cases undoubtedly accounts for some of the observed differences, but there is substantial evidence that at least some of the observed differences are real. For example, a study of hospital discharge data in which differences in the reporting of cases could not have been a factor showed that the overall annual incidence of hospitalized cases varied by region between 0.24 and 1.43/100,000 in 1981–1982.[19] In this study, however, potentially large differences in the completeness with which TSS cases were diagnosed and different standards for hospitalizing patients suspected of having TSS could not be ruled out. More convincing evidence for true geographic differences in incidence rates comes from the virtually identical hospital record review studies conducted in Colorado and northern California, in which variation in the diagnosing and reporting of cases was largely or completely eliminated.[11,12] As noted above, the incidence of TSS in 1980 in females 10 to 30 years of age was 15.8/100,000 in Colorado, but only 2.4/100,000 females 15 to 34 years of age in northern California. However, a prospective study employing active surveillance for TSS in five states (Missouri, New Jersey, Oklahoma, Tennessee, and Washington) and one large county (Los Angeles) showed that in 1986 the incidence of menstrual TSS was in the range of 1/100,000 females 15 to 44 years of age in all six study areas.[58]

Studies of *S. aureus* strains from the United States show no geographic differences in what proportion make TSST-1.[47] Similarly, anti-TSST-1 antibodies are found in similar proportions of healthy individuals in different parts of the United States.

5.3.2. Other Countries. Documented cases of TSS have been reported from Canada, most of western Europe, Australia, New Zealand, Japan, Israel, South Africa, and elsewhere. No information concerning incidence rates of TSS outside of the United States is available. However, the proportion of cases in other countries associated with menstruation and tampon use appears to be substantially lower than in the United States, in keeping with the fact that tampon use in general is less frequent in other countries and superabsorbent tampons are less widely available.

5.4. Temporal Distribution

Substantial controversy has surrounded the interpretation of observed changes over time in the diagnosis and reporting of TSS cases. Data from the passive national surveillance system suggested that the number of cases began to rise in 1978, peaked in 1980, and then declined and leveled off, with virtually all of the observed differences being due to changes in the number of menstrual TSS cases reported[9,10] (Fig. 1). While this pattern also was observed in some individual states employing vigorous case-finding methods (e.g., Utah and Wisconsin), a different pattern was seen in Minnesota, where no decline in the number of cases was observed in 1981.[59] Because of the documented impact of publicity on reporting of TSS cases and the undoubted fluctuations over time in the likelihood that cases would be diagnosed and/or reported, the results of studies that eliminate or minimize these influences are important in interpreting temporal trends.

While the three published hospital record review studies all suffer from having a relatively small number of cases of TSS to analyze statistically, the results of all three studies are consistent. In the California study, the incidence of TSS in women increased consistently through 1980, fell somewhat in 1981 and 1982, and then increased again in 1983, while the incidence in men remained consistently low (Fig. 2). In the Colorado study, the results were similar except that the decrease in 1981 compared with 1980 was sharper (Fig. 3). The similarity of the pattern in Colorado is even more apparent if cases meeting only the authors' proposed screening definition for TSS and not the more rigorous collaborative case definition are removed.[60] Similar trends are seen in the study from Cincinnati, although incidence rates cannot be estimated in this study.[20]

Thus, there is convincing evidence that hospitalized cases of TSS in females of menstrual age increased in the late 1970s, irrespective of any changes in the recognition and reporting of the disease. A similar increase was not apparent among men. There is also some evidence that this upward trend in the incidence of TSS through 1980 was reversed in several geographic areas, at least temporarily, in 1981.

5.5. Age

TSS can occur in individuals of all ages and has been documented in a newborn baby and in patients up to 80 years of age. However, data from both passive and active surveillance systems and from the California record review study indicate that younger women are at greater risk of developing TSS than are older women. Of cases associated with menstruation reported nationally, almost 60% have been in women 15 to 24 years of age, compared with only 25% in women 25 to 34 years of age.[9,10] Cases in women 35 to 44 years of age are even less common. Furthermore, the highest age-specific incidence rates consistently have been observed in women 15–19 or 15–24 years of age. Thus, in the California record review study,

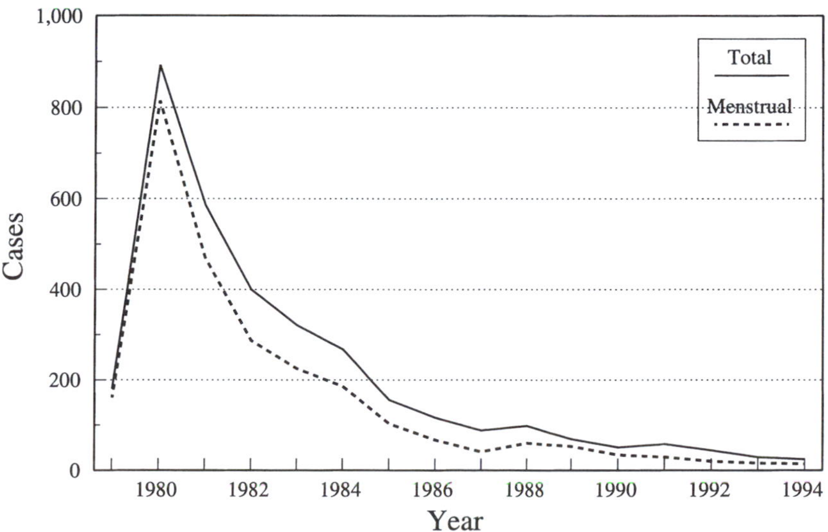

Figure 1. Reported cases of toxic shock syndrome, United States, 1979–1994.

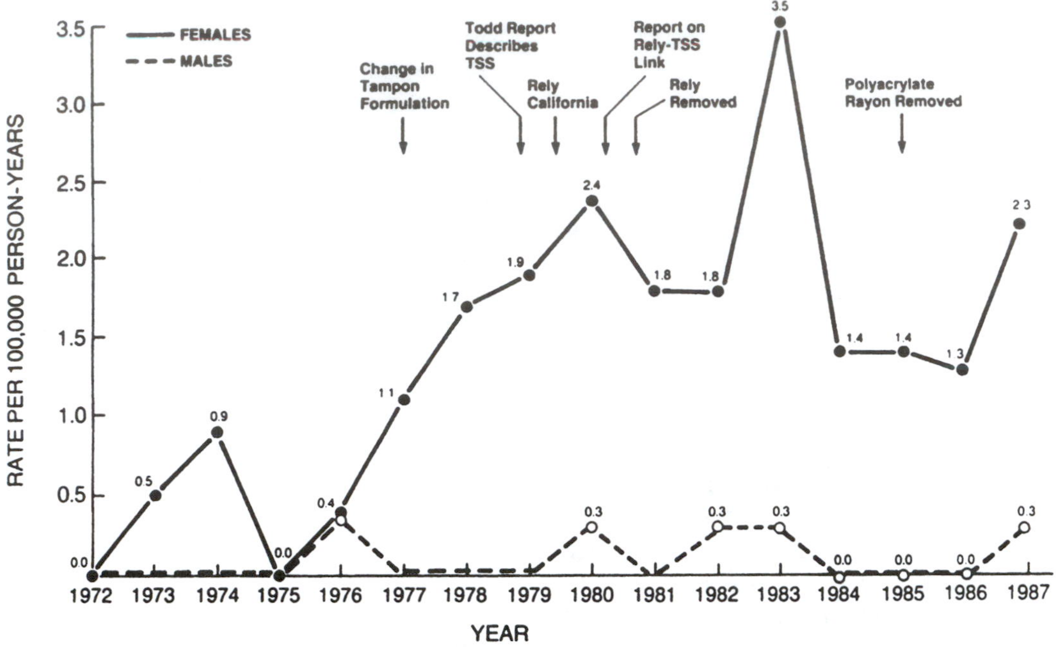

Figure 2. Incidence of hospitalized toxic shock syndrome cases in males (dashed line) and females (solid line), aged 15 through 34 years, northern California Kaiser-Permanente Medical Care Program, 1972 through 1987. Reproduced from Petitti *et al.*[21] with permission.

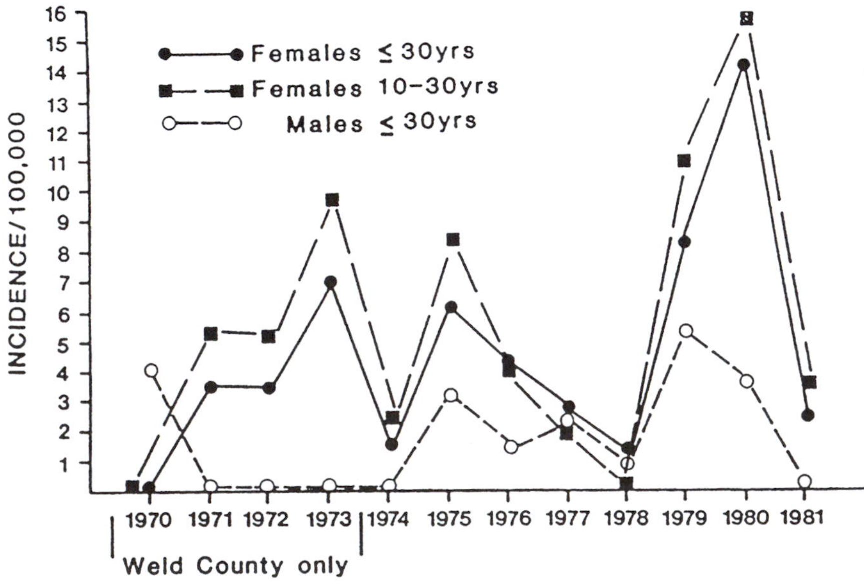

Figure 3. Annual incidence per 100,000 population of toxic shock syndrome in hospitalized patients ≤30 years of age meeting either the strict or the screening case definition in two Colorado counties, 1970–1981. Reproduced from Todd *et al.*[12] with permission.

the annual incidence rate was 2.6/100,000 women 15–19 years of age compared with rates of 0.8 to 1.4/100,000 among women 20–24, 25–29, and 30–34 years of age.[11] Similarly, in Minnesota the annual incidence of menstrual TSS among women 15–24 years of age was 13.7/100,000 compared with rates of 2.3 in those <15 years of age and 6.6 in those ⩾25 years of age.[56] The age distribution of TSS cases unassociated with menstruation is more uniform, especially if cases in postpartum women are excluded.[30]

5.6. Sex

All available evidence clearly indicates that TSS is much more common among women of menstrual age than among men of the same age. Of US cases reported through passive surveillance, 95% have been in women and 5% in men.[9,10] In the California record review study, the overall incidence of TSS in women 15 to 34 years of age during the time period 1972–1983 was 15 times that in men of the same age (1.5 vs. 0.1/100,000) person years).[11] This marked difference in incidence rates between men and women undoubtedly relates primarily to the fact that most cases of TSS are associated with menstruation and tampon use. What appears to be an increased risk of TSS during the postpartum interval and the apparent association between TSS and the use of barrier contraception probably contribute further to this pattern.[29,30,61] The incidence of TSS associated with other types of staphylococcal infections (e.g., surgical wound infections, cutaneous and subcutaneous lesions) appears to be similar in men and women.[29,30,58]

5.7. Race

Although it has been apparent since at least 1980 that TSS occurs in individuals of all racial groups,[8] the overwhelming majority (93–97%) of reported cases have been in whites, who make up only 80–85% of the US population.[9,10] Likely explanations for this discrepancy fall into two categories: biases in the diagnosis and reporting of cases on the one hand and true racial differences in either susceptibility to TSS or exposure to risk factors on the other. It has been postulated that increased difficulty in recognizing the rash on dark-skinned individuals, poorer access of minority groups to medical care, and the relative paucity of individuals of races other than white in areas with active TSS research efforts have all contributed to the observed racial distribution of cases. However, data from the California record review study indicate that in the 15–34 age group TSS does indeed disproportionately affect whites.[11] All of the 54 definite cases (most of which are related to menstruation) found in that study were in whites, while only 81% of the population at risk was white ($p < 0.05$; Fisher's exact test, two-tailed).

It has been noted that the racial distribution of patients with nonmenstrual TSS (87% white) more closely resembles the racial distribution of the US population than does the racial distribution of patients with menstrual TSS (98% white).[10,58] Taken together with studies demonstrating that young white women use tampons far more often than do comparably aged women of other racial groups,[62–65] these results suggest that observed race-specific differences in incidence rates are due, at least in part, to different levels of exposure to an important risk factor for developing TSS during menstruation.

5.8. Occupation

There is no evidence to suggest that any given occupational group, including health care providers, is at increased risk of developing TSS.

5.9. Occurrence in Different Settings

As noted below, transmission of strains of *S. aureus* capable of causing TSS has been demonstrated in the hospital setting.[66–68] There is also evidence of spread of these strains and occasional clustering of cases in households and in military installations (CDC, unpublished observations).

5.10. Socioeconomic Factors

It is unclear to what extent the marked racial variation in tampon use, especially among adolescents, reflects socioeconomic rather than racial differences. Other socioeconomic factors have not been noted to play a role in TSS.

5.11. Other Factors

5.11.1. Menstrual TSS. Numerous case–control studies conducted in 1980–1981 examined risk factors for developing TSS during menstruation (Table 2). These studies consistently found that tampon use increased the risk of menstrual TSS (the Oregon study, with its small number of cases, while not finding an association between menstrual TSS and tampon use in general, did find an association with a particular brand of tampon).[5,6,15,16,57,69] Included among these studies are two performed before any information concerning this association had appeared in the medical literature or lay press.[5,6] A study compar-

Table 2. Risk Factors for Menstrual TSS

Case onset dates	Date of study	Geographic area	Source of controls	No. cases	No. controls	Tampons: % cases	Tampons: % controls	Tampons: Odds ratio[a]	Tampons: p value
9/75–6/80	1980	Wisconsin	Clinic	35	105	97	76	10.6*	<0.01
12/76–6/80	6/80	USA (CDC)	Friend	52	52	100	85	20.1*	<0.05
7/80–8/80	9/80	USA (CDC)	Friend	50	150	100	83	20.5*	<0.01
1/76–8/80	5/80–8/80	Utah	Neighbor	29	91	100	77	18.0*	0.012
10/79–9/80	10/80–11/80	Minnesota, Wisconsin, Iowa	Neighbor	76	152	99	81	18.0	<0.001
12/79–11/80	1/81–3/81	Oregon	Friend	18	18	100	78	11.5*	NS[b]
			Clinic		18		89	5.6*	NS
1/86–6/87	1/86–8/87	Los Angeles County, Missouri, New Jersey, Oklahoma, Tennessee, Washington	Friend	180	185	98	71	19	<0.01
			Neighbor		187		60	48	<0.01

Rely brand tampons: % cases	Rely brand tampons: % controls	Rely brand tampons: Relative risk	Rely brand tampons: p value	Absorbency: Odds ratio in multivariate model	Absorbency: p value	Oral contraceptives: % cases	Oral contraceptives: % controls	Oral contraceptives: Odds ratio	Oral contraceptives: p value	Ref.
	NA[c]		NS	NA		17	36	0.36*	NS	5
33	27	NA	NS	NA		4	7	0.48*	NS	6
71	26	7.7	<0.0001	1.0	NS	NA	NA	NA		16
63	24	6.1	<0.0005	NA		3	11	0.29*	NS	112
53	29	2.5	0.005	3.2–10.4	0.01	12	20	0.55*	0.05	15
67	17	10.0*	<0.05	NA						113
	6	34.0*	<0.05	1.34/gm		25	24	1.1	NS	18

[a]If not reported in reference, crude odds ratio estimated disregarding matching; 0.5 added to all cells in tables with a 0 value; estimated values indicated with an asterik.
[b]NS, not significant.
[c]NA, data not available.

ing tampon use among women with menstrual TSS in 1983 and 1984 with tampon usage patterns ascertained via a national survey found evidence of a continuing increased risk of menstrual TSS among tampon users.[13] Furthermore, a multistate case–control study of menstrual TSS cases with onset in 1986–1987 documented that this association persisted at that time.[18] No additional case–control studies have been conducted since that time.

Two early case–control studies demonstrated that the risk of menstrual TSS varied with tampon brand and/or style (i.e., absorbency), suggesting that risk was a function of tampon absorbency and/or chemical composition.[15,16] The two more recent studies document clearly that risk of menstrual TSS is directly correlated with measured *in vitro* tampon absorbency,[13,18] independent of chemical composition, but that chemical composition is also a factor.[13] It is interesting to note that the correlation with tampon absorbency has persisted, despite the major alterations in chemical composition and marked decreases in the absorbencies of available tampons that have occurred since 1980. A reanalysis of data from earlier studies has suggested that the oxygen content of tampons is a better predictor of the risk of menstrual TSS than either chemical composition or absorbency.[14] *In vitro* studies examining the effect of various surfactants on TSST-1 production have shown that they can have a dramatic effect on production of this toxin.[70] These results suggest another tampon characteristic (i.e., type of surfactants present) that might influence the risk of menstrual TSS in users of various brands and styles.

The early case–control studies also examined the role of a number of other factors in determining the risk of developing TSS during menstruation. Four of the studies found that women with TSS were less likely to use oral contraceptives than were controls, although the differences in individual studies were not statistically significant.[5,6,15,57] One study found that continuous use of tampons during the menstrual period was associated with an increased risk of TSS,[6] while in another study a similar association, present on univariate analysis, did not remain significant in a multivariate analysis.[15] Of four studies looking at the relationship between a history of a recent vaginal infection and the risk of TSS, only one found such an association. Factors found not to be related to the risk of developing menstrual TSS in one of more studies included marital status, income, parity, sexual activity, bathing, frequency of exercise, alcohol use, smoking, history of vaginal herpes infections, and frequency of changing tampons.

5.11.2. Postpartum TSS. Although numerous cases of TSS occurring during the postpartum interval have been reported, the lack of precise information concerning the incidence of TSS in various settings makes it difficult to be certain that the incidence in postpartum women is elevated. Those cases of postpartum TSS not related to infection of a cesarean section incision or an infection of the breast (i.e., mastitis and breast abscess) have occurred predominantly in association with the use of tampons to control the flow of lochia or the use of barrier contraception (i.e., diaphragms and contraceptive sponges).[30]

5.11.3. Postoperative TSS. TSS has been associated with *S. aureus* surgical wound infections following a wide array of surgical procedures.[67] It has been suggested, however, that patients undergoing nasal surgery are at particularly high risk, presumably due to the frequency of *S. aureus* carriage in the nasopharynx and the difficulty of eradicating such carriage.[22] The common use of "nasal tampons" and other packing material following nasal surgery also may play a role.

5.11.4. Other Nonmenstrual TSS. TSS can result from *S. aureus* infection at any body site. However, many nonmenstrual TSS cases are the result of cutaneous and subcutaneous *S. aureus* infections. Also, cases of TSS associated with *S. aureus* infection of the respiratory tract in the setting of influenza have received substantial attention.[71] Risk factors for the development of such infections and/or associated TSS have not been studied. A relatively small proportion of nonmenstrual, nonpostpartum TSS cases are associated with vaginal *S. aureus* infections. One risk factor that has been identified in such cases is the use of contraceptive sponges.[61] It remains uncertain whether or not diaphragm use is similarly associated with an increased risk of nonmenstrual TSS.

6. Mechanisms and Routes of Transmission

Like all *S. aureus* strains, those capable of causing TSS appear to be transmitted readily by person-to-person spread, both within the hospital and in the community. There is convincing evidence that a nurse transmitted a TSS-associated strain of *S. aureus* to hospitalized burn patients[66] and suggestive evidence that some cases of postoperative TSS are due to nosocomial spread of the causative organism by hospital personnel.[67,68] In addition, vertical transmission from mother to newborn, with the development of TSS in both, has been reported.[72] Outside the hospital setting, transmission between husband and wife has been suggested by the almost simultaneous appearance of TSS in both, as has transmission between mother–daughter pairs (unpublished reports to the CDC). It is assumed, but not proven, that transmission in all these instances was by direct person-to-person spread. Nevertheless, it should be emphasized that in many TSS cases, particularly those associated with a focus of infection in the vagina, it may well be that disease is due to the introduction and/or multiplication of an endogenous *S. aureus* strain rather than to an exogenous source of infection.

7. Pathogenesis and Immunity

TSS results from an infection with an appropriate strain of *S. aureus* in a susceptible host. Once a nidus of infection is established, onset of symptoms typically occurs 1 to 3 days later. The best evidence concerning incubation period comes from patients with postoperative TSS due to surgical wound infections. In these patients, the date when the infection became established is usually the day of surgery, and thus can be determined unequivocally. The median incubation period in such patients is 2 days.[67] When TSS is caused by *S. aureus* infection of the vagina during menstruation, onset of symptoms is typically on the third or fourth day of menstruation, although it can be earlier or later.

In most cases of TSS, the toxin TSST-1 is the bacterial product most likely to be responsible for many of the observed signs, symptoms, and abnormalities of laboratory values. There is, however, substantial evidence that one or more other staphylococcal products, particularly enterotoxin B, are capable of causing an indistinguishable illness.[44,46] Furthermore, bacterial products other than TSST-1 that are made more commonly by *S. aureus* strains recovered from patients with TSS than by other strains have been described (see Section 4). For these reasons, it is likely that other staphylococcal products play a role in the pathogenesis of TSS. Furthermore, there is evidence that some of the multisystem derangements frequently observed in patients with TSS are due to the profound hypotension or shock that can occur and only indirectly to any staphylococcal products. For example, renal failure in TSS is probably secondary to hypotension-induced acute tubular necrosis, which in turn is the result of multiple factors, including: hypovolemia due to vomiting, diarrhea, increased insensible losses associated with a high fever and inability to ingest or retain fluids; and "third-spacing" of fluids. Uptake of "endogenous" endotoxin from gram-negative intestinal flora also has been proposed as playing a role in the pathogenesis of TSS.[73]

The biological properties of TSST-1 have been studied *in vitro* and *in vivo*, and attempts have been made to develop an animal model of TSS. *In vitro*, purified TSST-1 has been shown to stimulate the proliferation of T lymphocytes,[74] to inhibit immunoglobulin synthesis,[75] and to be a potent stimulator of interleukin-1 production by macrophages and monocytes.[76,77] TSST-1 also has been shown to bind to and be internalized by epithelial cells,[78] suggesting that it can be absorbed from focal sites of infection. *In vivo*, TSST-1 has been shown to be pyrogenic,[40] to induce lymphopenia,[79] to decrease the clearance of endotoxin,[80] and to increase susceptibility to endotoxin-induced shock.[73] It is now clear that many of the effects of TSST-1 are due to its potent "superantigen" properties, acting through the release of immune cytochines.[81] While initially reported to be an enterotoxin (as evidenced by induction of vomiting in monkeys), preparations of TSST-1 not contaminated with other staphylococcal enterotoxins do not appear to induce vomiting.[82]

Attempts to reproduce TSS in animals have included using mice, rabbits, goats, baboons, chimpanzees, and rhesus monkeys.[55,83–92] In these studies, investigators either have attempted to infect the animals with TSS-associated *S. aureus* strains at one of a variety of sites (previously implanted subcutaneous chambers, vagina, uterus, and muscle) or have injected purified TSST-1 as a bolus or continuous infusion. The animal models that come closest to reproducing the syndrome observed in humans have been those using rabbits. Live TSS-associated *S. aureus* organisms inside a previously implanted subcutaneous chamber and continuous infusion of purified TSST-1 both result in fever, hyperemia of mucous membranes, hypocalcemia, elevated creatinine phosphokinase (CPK) and hepatic enzymes, renal failure, and death in a high proportion of rabbits.[83,87] Also, the pathological changes observed postmortem in these animals are similar to those reported in patients dying of TSS.[93,94]

These rabbit models have been used to study the host factors in susceptibility to TSS suggested as important by clinical and epidemiological data or by *in vitro* results. It has been found that the age, sex, hormonal status, and strain of rabbits used all have a substantial impact on susceptibility to "rabbit TSS."[84,85] Thus, older rabbits have been reported to be more susceptible than younger rabbits. Similarly, male rabbits appear to be more susceptible than female rabbits, although castration abolishes this difference and estrogens protect male rabbits. Experiments concerning the contribution of endogenous endotoxin (i.e., endotoxin released by gut flora) to the pathogenesis of TSS have yielded conflicting results, although it appears that blocking the effect of endotoxin by giving polymyxin B does not consistently prevent rabbit TSS.[87] Preexisting anti-TSST-1 antibody, however, does appear to protect against TSS in the rabbit,[90] and corticosteroids in high doses also decrease mortality.[87]

Because of the observed association between menstrual TSS and tampon use, many investigators have looked at the effect of tampons and their constituents on the growth of *S. aureus* and the production of TSST-1 *in vitro*. At the same time, the effect of environmental conditions such as pH, Po_2, Pco_2, and cation concentration on the production of TSST-1 has been investigated. In general, studies have shown that tampons and their individual components inhibit the growth of *S. aureus in vitro*, regardless of the growth medium.[95,96] Although some studies have suggested that *S. aureus* can use various tampon constituents as an energy source, these results have been challenged and their relevance to human disease questioned.[97–99] Also controversial is the effect of tampons on the production of TSST-1 *in vitro*, with some studies showing that certain tampons and tampon constituents increase TSST-1 production and other studies showing no effect or inhibition of toxin production.[96,98] It has been suggested that the effect of tampons on TSST-1 production (and possibly on the risk of menstrual TSS) is mediated by changes in the availability of magnesium, which is bound by certain tampon components.[100] The various types of surfactants found on tampons also appear to influence the production of TSST-1, at least *in vitro*.

Growth conditions appear to be important in determining the amount of TSST-1 produced. Thus, an aerobic environment, neutral pH, and low levels of glucose, magnesium, and tryptophan all increase TSST-1 production, although some controversy has arisen about the effect of magnesium concentration on TSST-1 levels.[100–104] It has been shown that in patients with TSS related to focal sites of *S. aureus* infection, growth conditions within the infected focus are well suited to TSST-1 production.[104] Also, while the vagina generally has been considered to be anaerobic, studies have shown that a substantial amount of oxygen is introduced when a tampon is inserted, leading to speculation that the amount of oxygen introduced with a tampon may be an important factor in explaining the increased risk of menstrual TSS among tampon users.[105] A role for proteases of either bacterial or human origin in the pathogenesis of TSS also has been suggested.[104] An earlier theory that the association between menstrual TSS and tampon use was mediated by the demonstrated induction of vaginal ulcerations by tampons[106] has received less attention ever since similar vaginal ulcerations were reported in at least one patient with menstrual TSS who did not use tampons.[93]

8. Patterns of Host Response

8.1. Clinical Features

An illness meeting all the criteria of the established TSS case definition is, by the very nature of the criteria, severe, and the vast majority of such patients are hospitalized for treatment. Some patients experience the relatively gradual onset of sore throat, fever, fatigue, headache, and myalgias over 24 to 48 hr, followed by vomiting and/or diarrhea, signs of hypotension, and the appearance of the characteristic diffuse "sunburnline" macular skin rash. Other patients appear to have a much more dramatic onset over the course of several hours, with some reporting that they can remember the exact moment when they suddenly felt overwhelmingly ill.

Because an established set of strict criteria is used to define someone as having or not having TSS, all of the cases so defined are, not surprisingly, alike, regardless of the site of infection with *S. aureus*. There is, however, some variation. The temperature elevation in patients with TSS, while sometimes modest, can be extreme, with temperatures in the range of 104 to 106° F being fairly common. The evidence of hypotension in an individual case can range from mild orthostatic dizziness to profound shock. The characteristic macular skin rash can be dramatic and obvious, with the patient appearing bright red throughout; it can be subtle and difficult to appreciate, particularly in dark-skinned individuals; or it can be localized. Similarly, the desquamation that occurs during convalescence (usually 5–15 days after the acute illness) can be of subtle flaking and peeling of skin on the face and/or trunk or can involve the loss of full-thickness sheets of skin, particularly on the fingers, hands, and feet. Depending on which systems are affected most prominently in an individual case, the multisystem involvement in TSS can produce rather different clinical pictures. In some patients the involvement of the mucous membranes (e.g., sore throat, conjunctival and oropharyngeal injection) is severe and most prominent, while in other patients the gastrointestinal symptoms (vomiting and/or diarrhea) are predominant. Similarly, myalgias, thrombocytopenia, and involvement of the hepatic and renal systems can range from nil to severe. A recent study has suggested that the clinical spectrum of disease differs between menstrual and nonmenstrual TSS cases.[45]

Patients who receive aggressive supportive therapy (e.g., fluids), appropriate antimicrobial agents, and drainage of any focal *S. aureus* infection usually respond rapidly and improve over the course of several days. However, patients in whom therapy is either delayed or in whom a focal *S. aureus* infection is not eradicated can have a stormy, life-threatening course. In cases meeting all the established criteria, the case-fatality rate is currently 1–3% overall, although it increases with increasing age.[19]

The spectrum of illness of TSS has not been defined adequately due to the lack of a specific diagnostic laboratory test. It is evident that some illnesses not meeting all the criteria of the strict case definition, which was devised for use in epidemiological studies, represent milder forms of TSS. For example, few would question that an individual whose highest recorded temperature was 101.8°F, but who otherwise met all of the established criteria, had TSS. A number of authors have described patients of this kind,[107,108] and some have attempted to fashion simplified and/or less rigorous case definitions for TSS.[109] It is apparent that less rigorous case definitions are likely to be more sensitive but less specific in identifying TSS cases. Ultimately, however, it is not possible, in the absence of a specific diagnostic test, to determine where along a spectrum of increasingly milder and/or more atypical cases illnesses cease to be TSS and start to be something else. Thus, it is unclear whether a tampon-using menstruating woman with *S. aureus* in the vagina (or anyone else) who experiences headache, fatigue, and nausea could represent a very mild form of TSS. Such distinctions are made all the more difficult because of the relative frequency with which completely asymptomatic individuals are colonized with TSST-1-producing *S. aureus* in the nasopharynx, vagina, and probably other sites that are not normally sterile.

8.2. Diagnosis

As noted above, TSS can occur in individuals of any age, sex, and race. However, most recognized cases occur in a limited number of clinical settings. In women of reproductive age, TSS is most commonly seen during the menstrual period and the postpartum interval, although it can occur at other times as well, in association with focal *S. aureus* infections and in users of barrier contraception.

TSS during pregnancy, however, is quite uncommon. Although patients undergoing nasal surgery may be at elevated risk, TSS related to a surgical wound infection is a possibility in any postoperative patient, particularly during the first 24–72 hr. In many such instances, there will be few or no local signs that the operative site is infected.[67] As noted above, the median interval between surgery and onset of TSS in such cases is 2 days, but the range is 12 hr to many weeks. TSS is an infrequent but serious consequence of focal *S. aureus* infections at every conceivable body site, although cutaneous and subcutaneous abscesses and other similar infections appear to predominate. In addition, TSS has been reported to be a life-threatening complication of postinfluenza *S. aureus* infections of the respiratory tract.[110,111]

The differential diagnosis for a patient suspected of having TSS depends, in part, on which features of the illness are most prominent. For example, patients in whom sore throat and fever predominate early are frequently suspected initially of having streptococcal or viral pharyngitis. In cases in which diarrhea and vomiting are more prominent, viral gastroenteritis is often considered. When the rash becomes apparent, scarlet fever and drug reactions are often suspected.

The differential diagnosis also can be influenced by the patient's age and sex and the clinical setting in which the illness occurs. For example, cases in infants and very young children must be distinguished from Kawasaki syndrome and staphylococcal scalded skin syndrome. Similarly, in postpartum or postabortion women, other causes of fever and hypotension must be considered, such as endometritis and septic abortion. In individuals with appropriate exposure histories, leptospirosis, measles, and Rocky Mountain spotted fever should be included in the differential diagnosis. In summary, TSS can be confused fairly readily with a wide range of other conditions (Table 3).

Table 3. Differential Diagnosis in Patients with Suspected TSS

Kawasaki syndrome
Scarlet fever
Meningococcemia
Leptospirosis
Measles (especially "atypical")
Rocky Mountain spotted fever
Viral gastroenteritis
Viral syndromes with exanthems
Appendicitis
Pelvic inflammatory disease
Tubo-ovarian abscess
Staphylococcal scalded skin syndrome
Drug reactions/Stevens–Johnson syndrome

9. Control and Prevention

9.1. General Concepts

9.1.1. Menstrual TSS. Most strategies for decreasing the incidence of TSS have focused on menstrual TSS and its relationship to tampon use. In light of the demonstrated association between tampon use and risk of developing menstrual TSS, women were advised in 1980 that they could minimize their risk of developing menstrual TSS by not using tampons. In response, many women stopped using tampons, at least temporarily. The proportion of menstruating women who used tampons fell from approximately 70% in 1980 to less than 50% in 1981, but has rebounded to approximately 65% since that time.

In response to epidemiological and *in vitro* laboratory evidence concerning the possible roles of tampon absorbency and chemical composition in determining risk of menstrual TSS, most tampon manufacturers have dramatically altered both the absorbency and chemical composition of their products. After increasing markedly in the late 1970s, the measured *in vitro* absorbency of tampons has dropped sharply since 1979–1980, and one component, polyacrylate, has been eliminated from tampon formulations. In addition, one brand of tampons found to be associated with a high risk of menstrual TSS was withdrawn from the market altogether in 1980.

All tampons currently carry a label explaining the association between tampon use and menstrual TSS and describing the signs and symptoms of the illness. Tampon packages also carry a statement that women should use the lowest absorbency tampon consistent with their needs. Uniform absorbency labeling of tampons was finally required by the Food and Drug Administration in 1989.

Although frequent changing of tampons has been recommended as a way of decreasing the risk of menstrual TSS, there is no evidence to suggest that changing tampons more often reduces risk. Evidence from one study suggests that alternating tampons and napkins during a menstrual cycle may decrease the risk of TSS.[6]

9.1.2. Postpartum TSS. Because women may be at increased risk of TSS during the postpartum period, they should avoid the use of tampons and barrier contraception during that interval.

9.1.3. Hospital-Acquired TSS. Other than those measures designed to minimize nosocomial infections in general (e.g., good hand-washing practices) and those recommended specifically for patients with other types of staphylococcal infections, there are no proven methods for decreasing the risk of TSS associated with infected surgical wounds and other nosocomial *S. aureus* infections.

9.2. Antibiotic and Chemotherapeutic Approaches to Prophylaxis

Appropriate antimicrobial therapy of an initial episode of menstrual TSS, combined with discontinuing tampon use, has been shown to reduce the risk of recurrent episodes during subsequent menstrual periods.[5] The value of follow-up cultures and prophylactic antimicrobial agents in women with a history of menstrual TSS is unproven, although such measures may be justified in women who have had recurrent episodes of TSS. Because carriage of *S. aureus* at various body sites is so common and cases of TSS are relatively rare, there is no role for obtaining cultures from or giving chemoprophylaxis to individuals without a prior history of TSS.

9.3. Immunization

Although some consideration was given to attempting to develop a toxoid vaccine from TSST-1 soon after its discovery, no concrete steps in this direction have been taken. Given the high proportion of the population with naturally occurring anti-TSST-1 antibodies and the relative rarity of TSS, it would be prohibitively expensive and impractical to demonstrate that such a vaccine yielded clinical protection.

10. Unresolved Problems

Unresolved problems in our understanding of TSS relate primarily to its pathophysiology. While a clear link between the use and risk of menstrual TSS has been established, the specific characteristics of tampons responsible for this increased risk are unknown. The relative importance of absorbency, chemical composition, oxygen content, and perhaps other tampon characteristics, such as the surfactants used in their manufacture, in determining risk is uncertain. Similarly, while a direct correlation between measured tampon absorbency and risk of menstrual TSS has been demonstrated, it remains unclear whether or not users of the lowest absorbency tampons are at greater risk than nontampon users. At the same time, the role of tampon chemical composition in determining risk is ill-defined. The importance of magnesium and its binding by tampon constituents in the pathophysiology of menstrual TSS is controversial. As a result of all these uncertainties, it is unknown whether or not the "perfect tampon" (i.e., one that offers menstrual protection and has no associated increased risk of menstrual TSS) currently exists or can be developed.

11. References

1. Todd, J. K., Fishaut, M., Kapral, F., and Welch, T., Toxic-shock syndrome associated with phage-group-I staphylococci, *Lancet* **2:**1116–1118 (1978).
2. Aranow, H., Jr., and Wood, W. B., Staphylococcal infection simulating scarlet fever, *J. Am. Med. Assoc.* **119:**1491–1495 (1942).
3. Stevens, F. A., The occurrence of *Staphylococcus aureus* infection with a scarlatiniform rash, *J. Am. Med. Assoc.* **88:**1957–1958 (1927).
4. Everett, E. D., Mucocutaneous lymph node syndrome (Kawasaki disease) in adults, *J. Am. Med. Assoc.* **242:**542–543 (1979).
5. Davis, J. P., Chesney, P. J., Wand, P. J., LaVenture, M., and the Investigation and Laboratory Team, Toxic-shock syndrome: Epidemiologic features, recurrence, risk factors, and prevention, *N. Engl. J. Med.* **303:**1429–1435 (1980).
6. Shands, K. N., Schmid, G. P., Dan, B. B., Blum, D., Guidotti, R. J., Hargrett, N. T., Anderson, R. L., Hill, D. L., Broome, C. V., Band, J. D., and Fraser, D. W., Toxic-shock syndrome in menstruating women: Its association with tampon use and *Staphylococcus aureus* and the clinical features in 52 cases, *N. Engl. J. Med.* **303**:1436–1442 (1980).
7. Centers for Disease Control, Follow-up on toxic-shock syndrome—United States, *Morbid. Mortal. Week. Rep.* **29:**297–299 (1980).
8. Centers for Disease Control, Toxic-shock syndrome—United States, *Morbid. Mortal. Week. Rep.* **29:**229–230 (1980).
9. Reingold, A. L., Epidemiology of toxic-shock syndrome, United States, 1960–1984, Centers for Disease Control, *CDC Surveillance Summaries* **33**(3SS)**:**19SS–22SS (1984).
10. Reingold, A. L., Hargrett, N. T., Shands, K. N., Dan, B. B., Schmid, G. P., Strickland, B. Y., and Broome, C. V., Toxic shock syndrome surveillance in the United States, 1980 to 1981, *Ann. Intern. Med.* **92**(Part 2)**:**875–880 (1982).
11. Petitti, D. B., Reingold, A. L., and Chin, J., The incidence of toxic shock syndrome in northern California, 1972 through 1983, *J. Am. Med. Assoc.* **255:**368–372 (1986).
12. Todd, J. K., Wiesenthal, A. M., Ressman, M., Castan, S. A., and Hopkins, R. S., Toxic shock syndrome. II. Estimated occurrence in Colorado as influenced by case ascertainment methods, *Am. J. Epidemiol.* **122:**857–867 (1985).
13. Berkley, S. F., Hightower, A. W., Broome, C. V., and Reingold, A. L., The relationship of tampon characteristics to menstrual toxic shock syndrome, *J. Am. Med. Assoc.* **258:**917–920 (1987).
14. Lanes, S. F., Rothman, K. J., Tampon absorbency, composition and oxygen content and risk of toxic shock syndrome, *J. Clin. Epidemiol.* **43:**1379–1385 (1990).
15. Osterholm, M. T., Davis, J. P., and Gibson, R. W., Tri-state toxic-shock syndrome study. I. Epidemiologic findings, *J. Infect. Dis.* **145:**431–440 (1982).

16. Schlech, W. F., Shands, K. N., Reingold, A. L., Dan, B. B., Schmid, G. P., Hargrett, N. T., Hightower, A., Herwaldt, L. A., Neill, M. A., Band, J. D., and Bennett, J. V., Risk factors for the development of toxic shock syndrome: Association with a tampon brand, *J. Am. Med. Assoc.* **248:**835–839 (1982).
17. Petitti, D. B., and Reingold, A. L., Update through 1985 on the incidence of toxic shock syndrome among members of a prepaid health plan, *Rev. Infect. Dis.* **11**(Suppl. 1)**:**22–27 (1989).
18. Reingold, A. L., Broome, C. V., Gaventa, S., Hightower, A. W., and the TSS Study Group, Risk factors for menstrual toxic shock syndrome: Results of a multistate case–control study, *Rev. Infect. Dis.* **11**(Suppl. 1)**:**35–42 (1989).
19. Markowitz, L. E., Hightower, A. W., Broome, C. V., and Reingold, A. L., Toxic shock syndrome. Evaluation of national surveillance data using a hospital discharge survey, *J. Am. Med. Assoc.* **258:**75–78 (1987).
20. Linnemann, C. C., Jr., and Knarr, D., Increasing incidence of toxic shock syndrome in the 1970s, *Am. J. Public Health* **76:**566–567 (1986).
21. Petitti, D. B., and Reingold, A. L., Recent trends in the incidence of toxic shock syndrome in Northern California, *Am. J. Public Health* **81:**1209–1211 (1991).
22. Jacobson, J. A., Kasworm, E. M., Crass, B. A., and Bergdoll, M. S., Nasal carriage of toxigenic *Staphylococcus aureus* and prevalence of serum antibody to toxic-shock-syndrome toxin 1 in Utah, *J. Infect. Dis.* **153:**356–359 (1986).
23. Lansdell, L. W., Taplin, D., and Aldrich, T. E., Recovery of *Staphylococcus aureus* from multiple body sites in menstruating women, *J. Clin. Microbiol.* **20:**307–310 (1984).
24. Martin, R. R., Buttram, V., Besch, P., Kirkland, J.J., and Petty, G. P., Nasal and vaginal *Staphylococcus aureus* in young women: Quantitative studies, *Ann. Intern. Med.* **96**(Part 2)**:**951–953 (1982).
25. Ritz, H. L., Kirkland, J. J., Bond, G. G., Warner, E. K., and Petty, G. P., Association of high levels of serum antibody to staphylococcal toxic shock antigen with nasal carriage of toxic shock antigen-producing strains of *Staphylococcus aureus, Infect. Immun.* **43:** 954–958 (1984).
26. Schlievert, P. M., Osterholm, M. T., Kelly, J. A., and Nishimura, R. D., Toxin and enzyme characterization of *Staphylococcus aureus* isolates from patients with and without toxic shock syndrome, *Ann. Intern. Med.* **96**(Part 2)**:**937–940 (1982).
27. Bonventre, P. F., Linnemann, C., Weckbach, L. S., Staneck, J. L., Buncher, C. R., Vigdorth, E., Ritz, H., Archer, D., and Smith, B., Antibody responses to toxic-shock-syndrome (TSS) toxin by patients with TSS and by healthy staphylococcal carriers, *J. Infect. Dis.* **150:**662–666 (1984).
28. Vergeront, J. M., Stolz, S. J., Crass, B. A., Nelson, D. B., Davis, J. P., and Bergdoll, M. S., Prevalence of serum antibody to staphylococcal enterotoxin F among Wisconsin residents: Implications for toxic-shock syndrome, *J. Infect. Dis.* **148:**692–698 (1983).
29. Reingold, A. L., Dan, B. B., Shands, K. N., and Broome, C. V., Toxic-shock syndrome not associated with menstruation: A review of 54 cases, *Lancet* **1:**1–4 (1982).
30. Reingold, A. L., Hargrett, N. T., Dan, B. B., Shands, K. N., Strickland, B. Y., and Broome, C. V., Nonmenstrual toxic shock syndrome: A review of 130 cases, *Ann. Intern. Med.* **96**(Part 2)**:**871–874 (1982).
31. Miwa, K., Fukuyama, M., Kunitomo, T., Igarashi, H., Rapid assay for detection of toxic shock syndrome toxin 1 from human sera, *J. Clin. Microbiol.* **32:**539–542 (1994).
32. Vergeront, J. M., Evenson, M. L., Crass, B. A., Davis, J. P., Bergdoll, M. S., Wand, P. J., Noble, J. H., and Petersen, G. K., Recovery of staphylococcal enterotoxin F from the breast milk of a woman with toxic-shock syndrome, *J. Infect. Dis.* **146:**456–459 (1982).
33. Stolz, S. J., Davis, J. P., Vergeront, J. M., Crass, B. A., Chesney, P. J., Wand, P. J., and Bergdoll, M. S., Development of serum antibody to toxic shock toxin among individuals with toxic shock syndrome in Wisconsin, *J. Infect. Dis.* **151:**883–889 (1985).
34. Corbishley, C. M., Microbial flora of the vagina and cervix, *J. Clin. Pathol.* **30:**745–748 (1977).
35. Guinan, M. E., Dan, B. B., Guidotti, R. J., Reingold, A. L., Schmid, G. P., Bettoli, E. J., Lossick, J. G., Shands, K. N., Kramer, M. A., Hargrett, N. T., Anderson, R. L., and Broome, C. V., Vaginal colonization with *Staphylococcus aureus* in healthy women: A review of four studies, *Ann. Intern. Med.* **96**(Part 2)**:**944–947 (1982).
36. Linnemann, C. C., Staneck, J. L., Hornstein, S., Barden, T. P., Rauh, J. L., Bonventre, P. F., Buncher, C. R., and Beiting, A., The epidemiology of genital colonization with *Staphylococcus aureus*, *Ann. Intern. Med.* **96**(Part 2)**:**940–944 (1982).
37. Noble, V. S., Jacobson, J. A., and Smith, C. B., The effect of menses and use of catamenial products on cervical carriage of *Staphylococcus aureus*, *Am. J. Obstet. Gynecol.* **144:**186–189 (1982).
38. Onderdonk, A. B., Zamarchi, G. R., Walsh, J. A., Mellor, R. D., Munoz, A., and Kass, E. H., Methods for quantitative and qualitative evaluation of vaginal microflora during menstruation, *Appl. Environ. Microbiol.* **51:**333–339 (1986).
39. Smith, C. B., Noble, V., Bensch, R., Ahlin, P. A., Jacobson, J. A., and Latham, R. H., Bacterial flora of the vagina during the menstrual cycle: Findings in users of tampons, napkins, and sea sponges, *Ann. Intern. Med.* **96**(Part 2)**:**948–951 (1982).
40. Schlievert, P. M., Shands, K. N., Dan, B. B., Schmid, G. P., and Nishimura, R. D., Identification and characterization of an exotoxin from *Staphylococcus aureus* associated with toxic-shock syndrome, *J. Infect. Dis.* **143:**509–516 (1981).
41. Bergdoll, M. S., Crass, B. A., Reiser, R. F., Robbins, R. N., and Davis, J. P., A new staphylococcal enterotoxin, enterotoxin F, associated with toxic-shock syndrome *Staphylococcus aureus* isolates, *Lancet* **1:**1017–1021 (1981).
42. Altemeier, W. A., Lewis, S. A., Schlievert, P. M., Bergdoll, M. S., Bjornson, H. S., Staneck, J. L., and Crass, B. A., *Staphylococcus aureus* associated with toxic shock syndrome: Phage typing and toxin capability testing, *Ann. Intern. Med.* **96**(Part 2)**:**978–982 (1982).
43. Altemeier, W. A., Lewis, S. A., Schlievert, P. M., and Bjornson, H. S., Studies of the staphylococcal causation of toxic shock syndrome, *Surg. Gynecol. Obstet.* **153:**481–485 (1981).
44. Garbe, P. L., Arko, R. J., Reingold, A. L., Graves, L. M., Hayes, P. S., Hightower, A. W., Chandler, F. W., and Broome, C. V., *Staphylococcus aureus* isolates from patients with nonmenstrual toxic shock syndrome, *J. Am. Med. Assoc.* **253:**2538–2542 (1985).
45. Kain, K. C., Schulzer, M., Chow, A. W., Clinical spectrum of nonmenstrual toxic shock syndrome (TSS)**:** Comparison with menstrual TSS by multivariate discriminant analyses, *Clin. Infect. Dis.* **16:**100–106 (1993).
46. Schlievert, P. M., Staphylococcal enterotoxin B and toxic-shock syndrome toxin-1 are significantly associated with non-menstrual TSS [letter], *Lancet* **1:**1149–1150 (1986).

47. Hayes, P. S., Graves, L. M., Feeley, J. C., Hancock, G. A., Cohen, M. L., Reingold, A. L., Broome, C. V., and Hightower, A. W., Production of toxic-shock-associated protein(s) in *Staphylococcus aureus* strains isolated from 1956 through 1982, *J. Clin. Microbiol.* **20:**43–46 (1984).
48. Marples, R. R., Wieneke, A. A., Enterotoxins and toxic-shock syndrome toxin-1 non-enteric staphylococcal disease, *Epidemiol. Infect.* **110:**477–488 (1993).
49. Barbour, A. G., Vaginal isolates of *Staphylococcus aureus* associated with toxic shock syndrome, *Infect. Immun.* **33:**442–449 (1981).
50. Kreiswirth, B. N., Novick, R. P., Schlievert, P. M., and Bergdoll, M., Genetic studies on staphylococcal strains from patients with toxic shock syndrome, *Ann. Intern. Med.* **96**(Part 2)**:**974–977 (1982).
51. Chow, A. W., Gribble, M. J., and Bartlett, K. H., Characterization of the hemolytic activity of *Staphylococcus aureus* strains associated with toxic shock syndrome, *J. Clin. Microbiol.* **17:**524–528 (1983).
52. Chu, M. C., Melish, M. E., and James, J. F., Tryptophan auxotypy associated with *Staphylococcus aureus* that produce toxic-shock-syndrome toxin, *J. Infect. Dis.* **151:**1157–1158 (1985).
53. Todd, J. K., Franco-Buff, A., Lawellin, D. W., and Vasil, M. L., Phenotypic distinctiveness of *Staphylococcus aureus* strains associated with toxic shock syndrome, *Infect. Immun.* **45:**339–344 (1984).
54. Kreiswirth, B. N., Lofdahl, S., Betley, M. J., O'Reilly, M., Schlievert, P. M., Bergdoll, M. S., and Novick, R. P., The toxic shock syndrome exotoxin structural gene is not detectably transmitted by a prophage [letter], *Nature* **305:**709–712 (1983).
55. Rasheed, J. K., Arko, R. J., Feeley, J. C., Chandler, F. W., Thornsberry, C., Gibson, R. J., Cohen, M. L., Jeffries, C. D., and Broome, C. V., Acquired ability of *Staphylococcus aureus* to produce toxic shock-associated protein and resulting illness in a rabbit model, *Infect. Immun.* **47:**598–604 (1985).
56. Osterholm, M. T., and Forfang, J. C., Toxic-shock syndrome in Minnesota: Results of an active–passive surveillance system, *J. Infect. Dis.* **145:**458–464 (1982).
57. Kehrberg, M. W., Latham, R. H., Haslam, B. R., Hightower, A., Tanner, M., Jacobson, J. A., Barbour, A. G., Nobel, V., and Smith, C. B., Risk factors for staphylococcal toxic-shock syndrome, *Am. J. Epidemiol.* **114:**873–879 (1981).
58. Gaventa, S., Reingold, A. L., Hightower, A. W., Broome, C. V., Schwartz, B., Hoppe, C., Harwell, J., Lefkowitz, L. K., Makintubee, S., Cundiff, D. R., Sitze, S., and the Toxic Shock Syndrome Study Group, Active surveillance for toxic shock syndrome in the United States, 1986, *Rev. Infect. Dis.* **11:**S28–S34 (1989).
59. Centers for Disease Control, Toxic-shock syndrome—United States, 1970–1982, *Morbid. Mortal. Week. Rep.* **31:**201–204 (1982).
60. Reingold, A. L., On the proposed screening definition for toxic shock syndrome by Todd *et al.* [letter], *Am. J. Epidemiol.* **122:**918–919 (1985).
61. Faich, G., Pearson, K., Fleming, D., Sobel, S., and Anello, C., Toxic shock syndrome and the vaginal contraceptive sponge, *J. Am. Med. Assoc.* **255:**216–218 (1986).
62. Finkelstein, J. W., and VonEye, A., Sanitary product use by white, black and Mexican-American women, *Am. J. Public Health* **105:** 491–496 (1990).
63. Gustafson, T. L., Swinger, G. L., Booth, A. L., Hutcheson, R. H., Jr., and Schaffner, W., Survey of tampon use and toxic shock syndrome, Tennessee, 1979 to 1981, *Am. J. Obstet. Gynecol.* **143:** 369–374 (1982).
64. Irwin, C. E., and Millstein, S. G., Emerging patterns of tampon use in the adolescent female: The impact of toxic shock syndrome, *Am. J. Public Health* **72:**464–467 (1982).
65. Irwin, C. E., and Millstein, S. G., Predictors of tampon use in adolescents after media coverage of toxic shock syndrome, *Ann. Intern. Med.* **96**(Part 2)**:**966–968 (1982).
66. Arnow, P. M., Chou, T., Weil, D., Crass, B. A., and Bergdoll, M. S., Spread of a toxic-shock syndrome-associated strain of *Staphylococcus aureus* and measurement of antibodies to staphylococcal enterotoxin F, *J. Infect. Dis.* **149:**103–107 (1984).
67. Bartlett, P., Reingold, A. L., Graham, D. R., Dan, B. B., Selinger, D. S., Tank, G. W., and Wichterman, K. A., Toxic shock syndrome associated with surgical wound infections, *J. Am. Med. Assoc.* **247:**1448–1450 (1982).
68. Kreiswirth, B. N., Kravitz, G. R., Schlievert, P. M., and Novick, R. P., Nosocomial transmission of a strain of *Staphylococcus aureus* causing toxic shock syndrome, *Ann. Intern. Med.* **105:** 704–707 (1986).
69. Helgerson, S. D., and Foster, L. R., Toxic shock syndrome in Oregon: Epidemiologic findings, *Ann. Intern. Med.* **96**(Part 2)**:**909–911 (1982).
70. Projan, S. J., Brown-Skrobot, S., Schlievert, P. M., Vandenesch, F., and Novick, R. P., Glycerol monolaurate inhibits the production of β-lactamase, toxic shock syndrome toxin-1, and other staphylococcal exoproteins by interfering with signal transduction, *J. Bacteriol.* **176:**4204–4209 (1994).
71. MacDonald, K. L., Osterholm, M. T., Hedberg, C. W., Schrock, C. G., Peterson, G. F., Jentzen, J. M., Leonard, S. A., and Schlievert, P. M., Toxic shock syndrome. A newly recognized complication of influenza and influenzalike illness, *J. Am. Med. Assoc.* **257:**1053–1058 (1987).
72. Green, S. L., and LaPeter, K. S., Evidence for postpartum toxic-shock syndrome in a mother–infant pair, *Am. J. Med.* **72:**169–172 (1982).
73. Schlievert, P. M., Enhancement of host susceptibility to lethal endotoxin shock by staphylococcal pyrogenic exotoxin type C, *Infect. Immun.* **36:**123–128 (1982).
74. Poindexter, N. J., and Schlievert, P. M., Toxic-shock-syndrome toxin 1-induced proliferation of lymphocytes: Comparison of the mitogenic response of human, murine, and rabbit lymphocytes, *J. Infect. Dis.* **151:**65–72 (1985).
75. Poindexter, N. J., and Schlievert, P. M., Suppression of immunoglobulin-screening cells from human peripheral blood by toxic-shock-syndrome toxin-1, *J. Infect. Dis.* **153:**772–779 (1986).
76. Ikejima, T., Dinarello, C. A., Gill, D. M., and Wolff, S. M., Induction of human interleukin-1 by a product of *Staphylococcus aureus* associated with toxic shock syndrome, *J. Clin. Invest.* **73:** 1312–1320 (1984).
77. Parsonnet, J., Hickman, R. K., Eardley, D. D., and Pier, G. B., Induction of human interleukin-1 by toxic shock syndrome toxin-1, *J. Infect. Dis.* **151:**514–522 (1985).
78. Kushnaryov, V. M., MacDonald, H. S., Reiser, R., and Bergdoll, M. S., Staphylococcal toxic shock toxin specifically binds to cultured human epithelial cells and is rapidly internalized, *Infect. Immun.* **45:**566–571 (1984).
79. Schlievert, P. M., Alteration of immune function by staphylococcal pyrogenic exotoxin type C: Possible role in toxic-shock syndrome, *J. Infect. Dis.* **147:**391–398 (1983).
80. Fujikawa, H., Igarashi, H., Usami, H., Tanaka, S., and Tamura,

H., Clearance of endotoxin from blood of rabbits injected with staphylococcal toxic shock syndrome toxin-1, *Infect. Immun.* **52:**134–137 (1986).

81. Schlievert, P. M., Role of superantigens in human disease, *J. Infect. Dis.* **167:**997–1002 (1993).
82. Reiser, R. F., Robbins, R. N., Khoe, G. P., and Bergdoll, M. S., Purification and some physicochemical properties of toxic-shock toxin, *Biochemistry* **22:**3907–3912 (1983).
83. Arko, R. J., Rasheed, J. K., Broome, C. V., Chandler, F. W., and Paris, A. L., A rabbit model of toxic shock syndrome: Clinicopathological features, *J. Infect.* **8:**205–211 (1984).
84. Best, G. K., Abney, T. O., Kling, J. M., Kirkland, J. J., and Scott, D. F., Hormonal influence on experimental infections by a toxic shock strain of *Staphylococcus aureus*, *Infect. Immun.* **52:**331–333 (1986).
85. Best, G. K., Scott, D. F., Kling, J. M., Crowell, W. F., and Kirkland, J. J., Enhanced susceptibility of male rabbits to infection with a toxic shock strain of *Staphylococcus aureus*, *Infect. Immun.* **46:**727–732 (1984).
86. de Azavedo, J. C. S., and Arbuthnott, J. P., Toxicity of staphylococcal toxic shock syndrome toxin-1 in rabbits, *Infect. Immun.* **46:**314–317 (1984).
87. Parsonnet, J., Gillis, Z. A., Richter, A. G., and Pier, G. B., A rabbit model of toxic shock syndrome that uses a constant, subcutaneous infusion of toxic shock syndrome toxin 1, *Infect. Immun.* **55:** 1070–1076 (1987).
88. Pollack, M., Weinberg, W. G., Hoskins, W. J., O'Brien, W. F., Iannini, P. B., Anderson, S. E., and Schlievert, P. M., Toxinogenic vaginal infections due to *Staphylococcus aureus* in menstruating rhesus monkeys without toxic-shock syndrome, *J. Infect. Dis.* **147:**963–964 (1983).
89. Scott, D. F., Kling, J. M., Kirkland, J. J., and Best, G. K., Characterization of *Staphylococcus aureus* isolates from patients with toxic shock syndrome, using polyethylene infection chambers in rabbits, *Infect. Immun.* **39:**383–387 (1983).
90. Scott, D. F., Kling, J. M., and Best, G. K., Immunological protection of rabbits infected with *Staphylococcus aureus* isolates from patients with toxic shock syndrome, *Infect. Immun.* **53:**441–444 (1986).
91. Tierno, P. M., Jr., Malloy, V., Matias, J. R., and Hanna, B. A., Effects of toxic shock syndrome *Staphylococcus aureus*, endotoxin and tampons in a mouse model, *Clin. Invest. Med.* **10:**64–70 (1987).
92. Van Miert, A. S. J. P. A. M., van Duin, C. T. M., and Schotman, A. J. H., Comparative observations of fever and associated clinical hematological and blood biochemical changes after intravenous administration of staphylococcal enterotoxins B and F (toxic shock syndrome toxin-1) in goats, *Infect. Immun.* **46:**354–360 (1984).
93. Larkin, S. M., Williams, D. N., Osterholm, M. T., Tofte, R. W., and Posalaky, Z., Toxic shock syndrome: Clinical, laboratory, and pathologic findings in nine fatal cases, *Ann. Intern. Med.* **96**(Part 2):858–864 (1982).
94. Paris, A. L., Herwaldt, L. A., Blum, D., Schmid, G. P., Shands, K. N., and Broome, C. V., Pathologic findings in twelve fatal cases of toxic shock syndrome, *Ann. Intern. Med.* **96**(Part 2):852–857 (1982).
95. Broome, C. V., Hayes, P. S., Ajello, G. W., Feeley, J. C., Gibson, R. J., Graves, L. M., Hancock, G. A., Anderson, R. L., Highsmith, A. K., Mackel, D. C., Hargrett, N. T., and Reingold, A. L., *In vitro* studies of interactions between tampons and *Staphylococcus aureus*, *Ann. Intern. Med.* **96**(Part 2):959–962 (1982).
96. Schlievert, P. M., Blomster, D. A., and Kelly, J. A., Toxic shock syndrome *Staphylococcus aureus:* Effect of tampons on toxic shock syndrome toxin 1 production, *Obstet. Gynecol.* **64:**666–670 (1984).
97. Kirkland, J. J., and Widder, J. S., Hydrolysis of carboxymethylcellulose tampon material [letter], *Lancet* **1:**1041–1042 (1983).
98. Tierno, P. M., Jr., and Hanna, B. A., *In vitro* amplification of toxic shock syndrome toxin-1 by intravaginal devices, *Contraception* **31:**185–194 (1985).
99. Tierno, P. M., Jr., Hanna, B. A., and Davies, M. B., Growth of toxic-shock-syndrome strain of *Staphylococcus aureus* after enzymic degradation of Rely tampon component, *Lancet* **1:**615–618 (1983).
100. Mills, J. T., Parsonnet, J., Tsai, Y.-C., Kendrick, M., Hickman, R. K., and Kass, E. H., Control of production of toxic-shock-syndrome toxin-1 (TSST-1) by magnesium ion, *J. Infect. Dis.* **151:**1158–1161 (1985).
101. Kass, E. H., Kendrick, M. I., Tsai, Y.-C., and Parsonnet, J., Interaction of magnesium ion, oxygen tension, and temperature in the production of toxic-shock-syndrome toxin-1 by *Staphylococcus aureus*, *J. Infect. Dis.* **155:**812–815 (1987).
102. Mills, J. T., Parsonnet, J., and Kass, E. H., Production of toxic-shock-syndrome toxin-1: Effect of magnesium ion, *J. Infect. Dis.* **153:**993–994 (1986).
103. Mills, J. T., Parsonnet, J., Tsai, Y.-C., Kendrick, M., Hickman, R. K., and Kass, E. H., Control of production of toxic-shock-syndrome toxin-1 (TSST-1) by magnesium ion, *J. Infect. Dis.* **151:**1158–1161 (1985).
104. Schlievert, P. M., and Blomster, D. A., Production of staphylococcal pyrogenic exotoxin type C: Influence of physical and chemical factors, *J. Infect. Dis.* **147:**236–242 (1983).
105. Todd, J. K., Todd, B. H., Franco-Buff, A., Smith, C. M., and Lawellin, D., Influence of focal growth conditions on the pathogenesis of toxic shock syndrome, *J. Infect. Dis.* **155:**673–681 (1987).
106. Wagner, G., Bohr, L., Wagner, P., and Petersen, L. N., Tampon-induced changes in vaginal oxygen and carbon dioxide tensions, *Am. J. Obstet. Gynecol.* **148:**147–150 (1984).
107. Friedrich, E. G., and Siegesmund, K. A., Tampon-associated vaginal ulcerations, *Obstet. Gynecol.* **55:**149–156 (1980).
108. Fisher, C. J., Jr., Horowitz, B. Z., and Nolan, S. M., The clinical spectrum of toxic-shock syndrome, *West. J. Med.* **135:**175–182 (1981).
109. Tofte, R. W., and Williams, D. N., Toxic-shock syndrome: Evidence of a broad clinical spectrum, *J. Am. Med. Assoc.* **246:**2163–2167 (1981).
110. Wiesenthal, A. M., Ressman, M., Caston, S. A., and Todd, J. K., Toxic shock syndrome. I. Clinical exclusion of other syndromes by strict and screening definitions, *Am. J. Epidemiol.* **122:**847–856 (1985).
111. Sperber, S. J., and Francis, J. B., Toxic shock syndrome during an influenza outbreak, *J. Am. Med. Assoc.* **257:**1086–1087 (1987).
112. CDC, Toxic-Shock Syndrome—Utah. *Morb. Mortal. Wkly. Rep.* **29:**475–476 (1980).
113. Helgerson, S. D., and Foster, L. R., Toxic Shock Syndrome in Oregon—epidemiologic findings, *Ann. Intern. Med.* **96:**909–911 (1982).

12. Suggested Reading

Chesney, P. J., Davis, J. P., Purdy, W. K., Wand, P. J., and Chesney, K. W., Clinical manifestations of the toxic shock syndrome, *J. Am. Med. Assoc.* **246:**741–748 (1981).

Fisher, R. F., Goodpasture, H. C., Peterie, J. D., and Voth, D. W., Toxic shock syndrome in menstruating women, *Ann. Intern. Med.* **94:**156–163 (1981).

Proceedings of the First International Symposium on Toxic Shock Syndrome, *Rev. Infect. Dis.* **11** (1989).

Stallones, R. A., A review of the epidemiologic studies of toxic shock syndrome, *Ann. Intern. Med.* **96**(Part 2)**:**917–920 (1982).

CHAPTER 39

Tuberculosis

George W. Comstock and Richard J. O'Brien

1. Introduction

The term "tuberculosis" is used primarily to signify an infectious disease of the lungs caused by *Mycobacterium tuberculosis*. Many other organs may be involved, however, and similar illnesses caused by *M. bovis* and *M. africanum* are also called tuberculosis. The disease has long been a major killer of mankind. In 17th-century England, John Bunyan referred to consumption, now recognized as one of the forms of pulmonary tuberculosis, as "the captain of all of these men of death." Tuberculosis is still a major cause of disability and premature death throughout most of the world today. Estimates by the World Health Organization (WHO) place tuberculosis as the leading cause of adult death due to any single pathogen.[1] Only among the most economically favored nations has tuberculosis become a relatively minor threat; even among them it is an important problem among the disadvantaged segments of their populations.

Almost all human tuberculosis is caused by *M. tuberculosis*. Human disease due to *M. bovis* is rare except in areas where milk is not pasteurized. *M. africanum*, an organism with characteristics intermediate between *M. tuberculosis* and *M. bovis*, causes similar disease and is mostly confined to Africa. BCG (bacille Calmette–Guérin), derived from an attenuated strain of *M. bovis*, is used as a vaccine but can cause disease in immunocompromised persons.

George W. Comstock • School of Hygiene and Public Health, The Johns Hopkins University, Baltimore, Maryland 21742-2067. **Richard J. O'Brien** • Division of Tuberculosis Elimination, National Center for HIV, STD, and TB Prevention, Centers for Disease Control and Prevention, Atlanta, Georgia 30333.

2. Historical Background[2,3]

Descriptions of tuberculosis can be recognized in many older medical writings, usually as "phthisis" or "consumption," a chronic wasting illness associated with "ulcerations" of the lungs; as "galloping consumption," the pneumonic form of the disease; or as "scrofula," an involvement of the cervical lymph nodes. That the various forms of tuberculosis had a common and infectious etiology was first established by Villemin in 1865. He showed that inoculation of material from the various forms of tuberculosis lesions caused a similar disease in rabbits, as did the inoculation of sputum from patients with pulmonary lesions. Klebs also demonstrated the transmissibility of tuberculosis from man to animals in 1877, and even produced culture media for the growth of tubercle bacilli [4] However, it was not until 1882, when Koch announced his discovery of the tubercle bacillus and a means of staining it for microscopic examination, that it became feasible to make definitive diagnoses of tuberculosis and to identify disseminators of the organism.

Koch made another fundamental contribution to the epidemiological armamentarium by discovering tuberculin in 1890. Although his claim for the therapeutic use of tuberculin was discredited, it was soon recognized that infected persons could be identified by the local reaction that followed the injection of a small amount of tuberculin into the skin.

The third major diagnostic procedure resulted from the discovery of X rays by Roentgen in 1895. Radiographs of the chest made it possible to demonstrate pulmonary disease that had developed in infected persons before it could be recognized clinically and often before it had become communicable.

Refinements of these fundamental diagnostic procedures occurred for the most part during the 1940s and 1950s and added greatly to their usefulness. Development of artificial culture media made it possible to detect much smaller numbers of tubercle bacilli than could be demonstrated by microscopic examination of stained specimens; furthermore, cultures were less expensive and more widely applicable than guinea pig inoculations, which were originally used to confirm microscopic examinations. Photofluorography brought chest roentgenography to the general population in mass surveys designed to detect early asymptomatic cases of pulmonary tuberculosis. And improvements in the standardization, administration, and interpretation of the tuberculin test made it possible to identify, albeit with some misclassification, persons who had been infected with *M. tuberculosis*. In recent years, new molecular techniques, such as DNA probes and nucleic amplification techniques (e.g., polymerase chain reaction), now make it possible to detect small numbers of tubercle bacilli in biological specimens in as short a time as several hours.[5] Furthermore, DNA fingerprinting techniques, such as restriction fragment length polymorphism typing, allow the transmission of tuberculosis to be traced from one case to other cases, some of whom might otherwise never have been identified as contacts.[6,7]

The history of tuberculosis control is closely entwined with the sanatorium movement, which espoused healthful living, with particular emphasis on rest, good food, and fresh air. In addition, the concomitant isolation of patients during their treatment undoubtedly reduced the risk of transmission of their disease to others. Although the basic precepts of the sanatorium movement can be traced back to the temples of Aesculapius in Greek and Roman civilizations, they did not receive wide public acceptance for treatment of tuberculosis until the successful establishment of sanatoria by Grehmer in the mountains of Silesia in 1854 and by Trudeau in the Adirondack mountains of the United States in 1882. Sanatorium treatment became the major tuberculosis control activity for decades, diminishing in importance only with the introduction of effective antibiotics, notably streptomycin in 1946 and isoniazid in 1952. Successful treatment on an outpatient basis then became possible, and the days of the sanatoria were over. Further advances in the treatment of tuberculosis and discovery of other antimycobacterial drugs have led to shortening of therapy to 6 months and supervised twice-weekly administration of medications.

Specific preventive measures began with the development of an attenuated strain of *M. bovis* by Calmette and Guérin between 1908 and 1922. A vaccine prepared from this strain came to be called bacille Calmette–Guérin, or BCG. Accepted at first with reluctance, vaccination with one of the many substrains descended from this organism has become a mainstay of tuberculosis control programs in many parts of the world. The only other specific preventive procedure is chemoprophylaxis, which provides the most recent landmark in the history of tuberculosis control. During the 1960s, large-scale controlled trials demonstrated that persons who had been infected with tubercle bacilli could be protected from the subsequent development of disease by the oral administration of isoniazid.

Tuberculosis mortality began to decline in many countries prior to the present century, long before tuberculosis control measures could have had any general effect. Dubos and Dubos[2] point out that where the decline could be documented by death records, sanitary and social reform movements in the early 19th century brought about many improvements in living conditions that would tend to operate against the tubercle bacillus. More recent specific tuberculosis control measures such as the use of drugs for treatment and prevention have played a major role in maintaining the decline throughout most of the 20th century.

As tuberculosis rates diminished throughout much of the world, interest waned concomitantly. Tuberculosis control budgets began to be cut and preventive measures were curtailed. Meanwhile, conditions favoring tuberculosis did not decrease. Migrations from high- to low-prevalence areas continued; homelessness due to wars, starvation, and poverty increased; and the human immunodeficiency virus (HIV) appeared, drastically reducing the ability of its victims to resist tuberculosis. Multidrug-resistant tuberculosis became a major concern. Along with this resurgence of disease in many areas has come a belated return of interest and funding. The WHO has made tuberculosis control one of its major priorities, and an advisory council of the US Public Health Service has declared that tuberculosis can still be controlled and even eliminated.[8] Whether it will be eliminated or not is open to question: humanity has rarely shown much interest in present sacrifices for the sake of future gains.

3. Methodology

3.1. Sources of Mortality Data

Tuberculosis deaths and death rates are tabulated in the *World Health Statistics Annual*, published by the WHO in Geneva, and in various national vital statistics publications, such as *Vital Statistics of the United States*, published annually by the National Center for Health Statistics, Centers for Disease Control (CDC), US Department of Health and Human Services. Annual reports on tuberculosis are also published by the Division of Tuberculosis Control, CDC.[9] Useful compendia of older statistics are also available.[3,10]

Although mortality rates have been useful indicators of tuberculosis trends and of areas where tuberculosis cases are concentrated, today, with the advent of effective chemotherapy, mortality rates are better indices of the lack of access to good medical regimens or lack of adherence to them. Even this use is jeopardized by the estimate that tuberculosis deaths are markedly underreported in much of the world.[11,12]

3.2. Sources of Morbidity Data

Tuberculosis cases and case rates are tabulated and summarized in the publications from the WHO and CDC mentioned in Section 3.1. In addition, the *Morbidity and Mortality Weekly Report* from the CDC and monthly reports from state health departments give up-to-date accounts of reported cases. Although tuberculosis appears to be well reported in most industrialized nations, it is likely that it is grossly underreported in the rest of the world.[11,12]

Changes in the definition of a reportable case have influenced time trends. Although international advisory bodies have urged that only bacteriologically positive cases be reported, this recommendation has not been widely accepted. In 1961, the US Public Health Service recommended that new active cases for reporting purposes be defined as diagnosed cases of any site with positive bacteriology or with consistent X-ray or histological evidence, or cases of unexplained pleurisy with effusion.[3] In 1975, the definition was broadened to include previously reported cases whose disease had reactivated. In addition, persons being treated with two or more antituberculosis drugs are reportable even in the absence of other criteria.

3.3. Surveys

Surveys for tuberculosis have been conducted by means of physical examinations, bacteriological examinations of sputum, chest photofluorography, and tuberculin testing. In 1917, an extensive antituberculosis campaign was carried out in Framingham, Massachusetts, in the course of which approximately 11,000 persons, two thirds of the population, were given physical examinations for tuberculosis.[13] The findings of this survey resulted in the estimate that there were 10 prevalent active cases for every annual tuberculosis death, a ratio used for the next three decades in the United States to estimate the size of the tuberculosis problem.

Sputum surveys are limited as a general rule to persons with abnormal findings on chest X-ray surveys either to identify cases that are most meaningful from the public health point of view or as a means of surveillance for drug-resistant organisms. Occasionally, in areas where mass radiography is impractical, sputum surveys of general populations have been done to estimate the prevalence of tuberculosis or to detect tuberculosis cases among persons with chronic cough.

With the demonstration in Brazil by de Abreu and de Paula[14] in 1936 of the practicability of mass photofluorography, it became feasible to examine the lungs of large numbers of apparently normal persons for tuberculosis. In the decade following World War II, millions of persons were examined in mass chest X-ray surveys. While it seems reasonable to believe that detection of unrecognized cases of tuberculosis was beneficial, there is little evidence to substantiate this belief. In Wales, an intensive tuberculosis case-finding and treatment program was followed by a decreased risk of new infections among children,[15] and in Alaska, an intensive case-finding and treatment program was followed by a marked decrease in childhood infections.[16]

There is no longer much place for mass radiography in tuberculosis control. Where it can be afforded, the yield is too low to justify the cost; where the prevalence of active disease is high enough to warrant this method of case finding, funds are usually limited and must be spent on items of higher priority, such as providing adequate treatment for clinically manifest cases.

In populations who have not been vaccinated with BCG, use of the tuberculin skin test can contribute a great deal to epidemiological knowledge. The applications of tuberculin testing to the delineation of the risks of having been infected with tubercle bacilli by time, place, and person are epitomized by the work of Palmer and Edwards and their colleagues.[3,17–22] By careful attention to the selection of study populations, to the techniques of administering and reading tuberculin tests, and to the interpretation of frequency distributions of reaction sizes, it has been possible to learn a great deal about the prevalence of infected persons under varied circumstances and the implications of these findings for temporal, geographic, and personal differences in the risk of becoming infected.

3.4. Laboratory Diagnosis

3.4.1. Isolation and Identification of the Organism. Tubercle bacilli are commonly looked for in biological fluids and tissues by microscopic examination of preparations stained by the Ziehl–Neelson acid-fast technique. Identification of the fuchsin-stained mycobacteria, which are rods 1–4 μm long, is facilitated by staining the preparation with a contrasting dye. Staining with fluorescent dyes reduces the time required for staining and for examination and increases both the sensitivity and specificity of microscopy.

Microscopic examination of stained specimens is relatively quick and inexpensive, but its sensitivity is low. It has been estimated that approximately 5,000 to 10,000 organisms/ml are needed to make their recognition by microscopy reasonably certain. With proper laboratory techniques in areas where tuberculosis is common, specificity is fairly high, since acid-fast rods seen on microscopy are usually tubercle bacilli that are readily distinguishable from most acid-fast artifacts. Nontuberculous mycobacteria, however, have a similar appearance and can occur as pathogens, as normal inhabitants in oral or genitourinary secretions, or even in water used to wash the slides.

A much greater increase in sensitivity and specificity is obtained by culturing specimens. With a generation time of nearly 24 hr, tubercle bacilli grow slowly, usually requiring 3–8 weeks to form identifiable colonies. Presumptive identification of the various mycobacteria is based on growth rate, colony characteristics, and pigment formation.[23] A radiometric method (BACTEC) now coming into widespread use can accurately detect the presence of mycobacteria within 1–2 weeks. The addition of nucleic acid probes or the ρ-nitro-α-acetyl-amino-β-hydroxypropiophenone (NAP) test can rapidly distinguish *M. tuberculosis* complex from nontuberculous mycobacteria with considerable accuracy.[5] Individual strains of *M. tuberculosis* can be recognized by restriction-fragment-length polymorphism analysis.[24] Patterns, believed to be so unique that this procedure is referred to as "DNA fingerprinting," allow source cases of outbreaks and exogenous reinfection to be recognized that otherwise would have been missed.

3.4.2. Serological and Immunologic Diagnostic Methods. A variety of serological tests for the diagnosis of tuberculosis have been evaluated.[25] Enzyme-linked immunosorbent assays (ELISAs) may be helpful in the diagnosis of tuberculous meningitis.[26] At present, the only immunologic test that is useful for epidemiological purposes is the tuberculin skin test.

The standard tuberculin test is administered by the Mantoux technique, whereby 0.1 ml of a purified derivative of old tuberculin is injected into the skin of the forearm by needle and syringe. The definition of a positive reaction is best derived from a frequency distribution of reaction sizes in the population under study.[27,28] The optimal dividing line between positive and negative will vary with the proportion of persons in the population who have been infected with tubercle bacilli, the frequency of cross-reactions caused by infections with BCG or nontuberculous mycobacteria, and technical factors related to administration and reading of the test. Some account of these factors has been taken in the several definitions of a positive tuberculin reactor for use in the United States.[29] If the likelihood of tuberculous infection is increased, as it is among persons with abnormal chest shadows or with a history of recent household exposure to an infectious case, reactions of 5 mm or more in diameter to 5 tuberculin units of PPD are considered to be positive and to indicate the occurrence of tuberculous infection at some time in the past. In persons at low risk of tuberculosis infection and at increased risk of immunologic cross-reactions (e.g., history of BCG vaccination or residence in an area endemic for nontuberculous mycobacteria), 15 mm of induration is the recommended cut point.

Although the accuracy of the tuberculin test in detecting past or present infection with tubercle bacilli compares favorably with that of many medical screening tests, there are important sources of error in addition to those associated with administration of the test by multiple-puncture devices. Errors in dosage, depth of injection, and measurement of reactions can result in misclassification. False-negative reactions may occur up to 8 weeks after infection while hypersensitivity is developing, in seriously ill patients, during and shortly after viral infections and vaccinations (notably measles), and with natural and induced immunosuppression [e.g., Hodgkin's disease, acquired immunodeficiency syndrome (AIDS), therapy with large doses of corticosteroids]. Much more common, however, are false-positive reactions caused by infections with nontuberculous mycobacteria or vaccination with BCG.

Identifying recently infected persons by means of repeated tuberculin tests of initially negative reactors is simple in theory but difficult in practice. Even with fastidious technique, the results of two tests can vary by 6 mm or more.[30] Consequently, only persons whose reactions change from negative to positive and increase by at least 10 mm are considered to have had a true change in tuberculin sensitivity that may have been caused by a recent infection. For persons over the age of 35 years, an increase of 15 mm or more is recommended.[29]

A further complication in the detection of newly infected persons results from the "booster effect," the analogue of the anamnestic reaction in serology. Many persons, especially those over 50 years of age, may have had a gradual decline in tuberculin sensitivity to the point where an initial test causes no detectable induration. In some of these previously positive persons, the stimulus of the initial test causes a "boost" of their sensitivity back to its original level. Boosting occurs within 1 week and appears to last for at least 2 years. If these persons are given a second test 6 or 12 months later, their positive reactions at that time may have resulted from either the booster effect or a new infection. To minimize the possibility of falsely attributing a boosted reaction to a new infection, persons who are to be tested periodically and who have a low risk of becoming infected (i.e., those who are not household contacts) should have a second test given a week after the initial test if that initial test was negative. Persons still negative to the second test should then be included in the periodic testing program with reasonable assurance that any subsequent change to a positive reaction (with an increase of at least 10 mm) will have resulted from a recent infection. Persons who are positive to the second test of the initial series should be classified as initially positive reactors.[31]

4. Biological Characteristics of the Organism

Tubercle bacilli are very resistant to drying and to most ordinary germicides, especially in the presence of organic material such as sputum. They are susceptible to moist heat, being killed in about 30 min by exposure to 60°C and in less than a minute by temperatures greater than 70°C. They are highly sensitive to sunlight or artificial ultraviolet light.

Their slow rate of growth, nearly 24 hr from one generation to the next, undoubtedly contributes to the relatively slow development of disease in infected susceptible hosts. A factor that operates against the survival of tubercle bacilli in human populations is their proclivity to become buried within tissues. Only in the infrequent instances when pulmonary cavitation or airway ulceration occurs do the bacilli become surface dwellers, and thus available for widespread dissemination to others.[32]

5. Descriptive Epidemiology

In thinking epidemiologically about the development of tuberculosis in populations, it is important to look at each of the two major stages of its pathogenesis—the acquisition of infection, as identified by an appropriate tuberculin test, and the subsequent development of significant disease, as diagnosed by radiological or bacteriological techniques. While all communicable diseases must go through these two stages, their separation is particularly important in tuberculosis, the reason being that tuberculosis differs from most other bacterial diseases in a very important respect, namely, that the resistance that develops after successful recovery from the primary infection is often not sufficient to rid the body of invading organisms. As a consequence, an unknown but significant proportion of tuberculin reactors continue to harbor living organisms and are at risk of reactivation for the rest of their lives. In epidemiological terms, this means that the incubation period of tuberculosis is highly variable, ranging from a few weeks to a lifetime. Those who pass through the highest-risk period shortly after infection still have a subsequent lifetime risk that may actually exceed the initial risk because of the cumulative effect of a low risk operating over many years.

It is also useful to consider the development of tuberculosis as a two-stage process, because the known risk factors for infection are so different from the risk factors for the development of disease after infection. Despite the voluminous literature on tuberculosis, very little of the work has been done in such a way that these two risks can be disentangled. Even in determining the frequency of infection, there are serious problems because of insufficient attention to the tuberculin used, to the technique of administration and measurement, and to the detailed reporting of results.

5.1. Prevalence and Incidence

Information on the prevalence or incidence of tuberculous infections is rarely available on a communitywide basis, especially for recent years. Estimating the frequency of tuberculous infections is also made difficult by the fact that positive reactions to the tuberculin skin test can result not only from infections with tubercle bacilli but also from BCG vaccination and from infections with a variety of nontuberculous mycobacteria as well. Frequency of cross-reactions from nontuberculous mycobacterial infections varies markedly by geography, being almost nonexistent in the Arctic and almost universal in some tropical and subtropical areas.

The prevalence of tuberculous infections rises with age, tending to level off at about 40 to 50 years. In 1971, the overall prevalence in the United States was estimated at about 8%[33]; for white male Navy recruits, 17–21 years of age, the estimates for United States regions ranged from 1.6 to 2.9% over the period 1961–1968.[34] Among males of similar age, the average prevalence of infected persons was slightly less than 40% in the Bangalore District of South India in the same period[35] and slightly more than 40% in the East Central State of Nigeria in 1971.[36] In the Chingleput area, near Madras in South India, the prevalence of positive tuberculin reactors in 1968–1971 reached a plateau of about 80% among males at age 25 and among females of about 70% at age 35.[37]

The incidence of tuberculosis *infection* is usually estimated from the change in prevalence of tuberculin reactors by age rather than from repeated testing of the same individuals.[38,39] This method minimizes errors in classification caused by technical variations in testing and reading and also those caused by the effects on the second test of the stimulus from the first test, the so-called booster effect (see Section 3.4.2). With few exceptions, the incidence of new infections appears to have been decreasing, at least since the 1930s. Perhaps the most dramatic decrease occurred in the Bethel area of Alaska, where the estimated incidence in 1949–1951 was 25% per year, but was well under 0.1% per year in 1970, so low that there were not enough children to measure it accurately.[16] Extrapolation from published data indicate that recent incidence rates in Norway, Saskatchewan, the Netherlands, and most of the United States are likely to have been in the neighborhood of 10/100,000 person years.[20,39–42] In South India and Nigeria, the incidence in the 1960s was between 1 and 2% per year.[35,36] Estimates of the incidence of tuberculous infection are also available from the prevalence of tuberculin reactors in the Chingleput District of South India during the period 1968–1971.[37] Children in the age group 1–4 years at the time of tuberculin testing became positive tuberculin reactors at the average rate of 1.7% per year during their lifetimes; those aged 5–9 years became reactors at the average rate of 2.4% during their lifetimes; and those aged 10–14 years became reactors at the average rate of 4.0% per year during their lifetimes. This trend is consistent with an increased risk of infection with increasing age or a decreased risk with the passage of time. In this area where little had been done to control tuberculosis prior to the time when tuberculin tests were done, the former explanation appears more likely.

The frequency of tuberculous disease depends first on the probability of becoming infected and second on the ability of the infected person to withstand that infection. The prevalence of a disease depends on both the incidence of the disease and its average duration. In Muscogee County, Georgia, the prevalence of radiologically demonstrable tuberculosis, active and inactive, was 1,700/100,000 among whites but only 1,200/100,000 among blacks in 1946, whereas the subsequent incidence of new cases during the next five years was 34/100,000 per year among whites and 111/100,000 per year among blacks.[43] Although a definite value for average duration of disease cannot be calculated because tuberculosis was not in a steady state during the observation period, the findings do indicate that duration for whites was longer than for blacks, largely because the case-fatality rate among blacks prior to the advent of effective chemotherapy was nearly eight times that among whites.

In developing countries, both the prevalence and the incidence of bacteriologically positive cases are likely to be much higher than in Muscogee County. In East Central Nigeria, for example, a survey suggested that the prevalence of bacteriologically positive disease among persons over 10 years of age was approximately 500/100,000 in 1971.[36] Repeated surveys between 1961 and 1968 in South India showed that the prevalence of bacteriologically positive cases among persons over 15 years of age averaged 536/100,000, while the incidence in this area averaged 143/100,000 per year.[35] In the Chingleput area, tuberculosis cases with sputum positive for *M. tuberculosis* on culture were much more frequent among males than females, increasing with age for both sexes and reaching levels of approximately 4% among males and 0.7% among females after age 50.[37]

5.2. Epidemic Behavior and Contagiousness

Tuberculosis can and sometimes does occur in sharply localized outbreaks. In nearly all such instances, these involve the exposure of previously uninfected persons to an infectious individual in crowded quarters, such as a schoolroom under wartime blacked-out conditions,[44,45] an air-conditioned naval vessel, or in poorly ventilated clinical settings.[46] Perhaps the most remarkable aspect of these outbreaks is their relative rarity, given the frequency with which uninfected individuals are exposed to infectious cases under similar circumstances. A possible explanation is that some tuberculous patients are more effective spreaders than others, as suggested by one experimental situation.[47] Another factor that may play a role is that tuberculosis is usually not highly communicable.[48] Secondary attack rates among 5- to 9-year-old household associates of cases of measles and mumps have been reported to be 81 and 86%, respectively; the infection rates, at least in mumps, are presumably even higher. In contrast, only 19% of household associates of active tuberculosis cases under the age of 15 years in the period 1975–1992 were positive tuberculin reactors. Because the communicability of measles or mumps is measured in days, while that of tuberculosis is measured in weeks or months, the infectiousness of tuberculosis per day of exposure must *on average* be very low indeed.

The infectiousness of tuberculosis patients appears to be rapidly reduced by adequate chemotherapy. The most convincing study, because it was strictly controlled, came from the very useful series of chemotherapy trials in Madras, India.[(49)] Active cases of tuberculosis that were not considered emergencies were randomly allocated to home and to hospital treatment. Both groups received the same chemotherapy. At the end of 5 years, there were slightly fewer cases among contacts of patients treated at home than among contacts of those isolated in hospital. This result strongly suggests that chemotherapy was as effective as hospitalization in reducing the risk connected with being a close contact of an infectious patient.

However, when tuberculosis outbreaks occur among persons infected with HIV, the dynamics of transmission change considerably because of the telescoping of the period between infection and disease and the great increase in the risk of disease following infection. The explosive nature of such outbreaks is well illustrated by experiences with multidrug-resistant tuberculosis in several hospitals in the United States.[(50)]

5.3. Geographic Distribution

Global estimates of tuberculous infection, disease, and death have recently been compiled.[(1,12)] An estimated 1.7 billion or one third of the world's population are infected, with the prevalence of infection ranging from 44% in the Western Pacific countries to 19% in the Eastern Mediterranean region (Table 1). However, the age distribution of tuberculous infections varies markedly. In industrialized countries, infections are concentrated among older age groups, whereas in developing countries infections are prevalent at much younger ages. In contrast to infections, approximately 95% of estimated cases and 98% of estimated deaths occur among persons in developing countries. The highest number of cases and deaths occur in countries in Asia and the Western Pacific, while the highest case and mortality rates are found in African nations.

A recent study conducted within the European Community showed remarkable variation in tuberculosis death rates within the member nations (Fig. 1).[(51)] In addition, an earlier international study had shown that the spectrum of diagnosed and reported cases of tuberculosis differed greatly in various countries.[(52)] Among five European countries, one country in South East Asia, and two locations in the United States, there were significant differences in the proportion of cases confirmed bacteriologically and in the manner of their confirmation. The extent and nature of disease as shown by roentgenography also varied markedly. Consequently, geographic differences measured by official morbidity statistics may represent not only true differences in the frequency of disease but also diligence in searching for cases, criteria for diagnosis, and perhaps differing pathological responses of the populations.

Table 1. Estimated Prevalence of Tuberculous Infections, Reported and Estimated Cases of Tuberculosis for 1990, and Estimated Tuberculosis Deaths for 1990, by Region of the World[a]

Region	Tuberculous infection (%)	Tuberculosis cases per 100,000 per year		Estimated tuberculosis deaths per 100,000 per year
		Reported	Estimated	
Africa[b]	34	52	220	91–100
Americas[c]	26	50	120	44–46
Eastern Mediterranean[b]	19	110	155	36–43
South-East Asia[b]	34	85	194	63–72
Western Pacific[d]	44	169	191	45–50
China	34	—	191	63–72
Europe[b] and other[e]	32	32	31	3[f]

[a]Derived from Sudre *et al.*[(12)]
[b]Includes all countries in WHO region.
[c]Includes all countries of American region of WHO except Canada and the United States.
[d]Includes all countries in Western Pacific region of WHO except China, Japan, Australia, and New Zealand.
[e]Canada, United States, Japan, Australia, and New Zealand.
[f]Based on deaths reported in 1988.

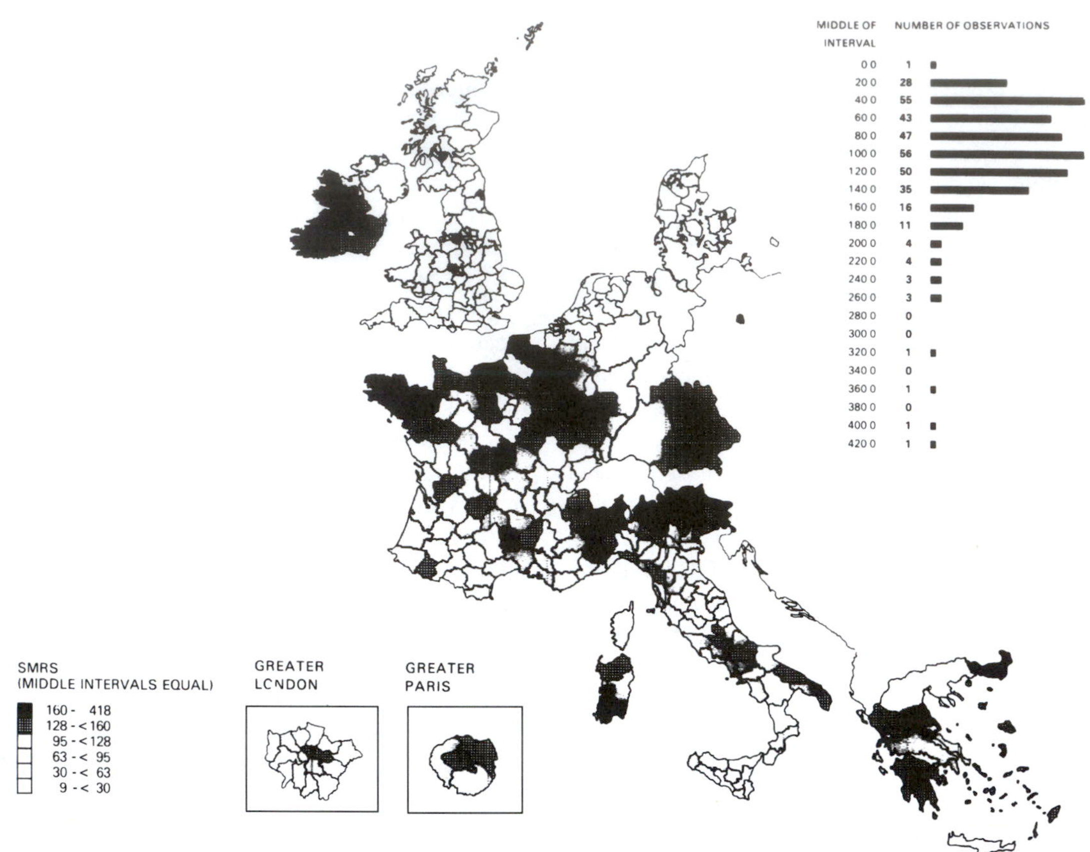

Figure 1. Standardized mortality ratios for tuberculosis among persons aged 5 to 64 years by local geographic units, European Community, 1985–1989.[51]

Tuberculosis case rates for the United States in 1994 are shown for states and counties in Figs. 2 and 3.[53] The highest case rates were found in New York, District of Columbia, California, and Hawaii. In 1992, rates were highest in cities with populations over 500,000 (29.9 per 100,000) and lowest in small cities and rural areas (6.5 per 100,000).[54] In spite of the low rural rates, almost half of the cases in 1992 came from these areas. Cases are concentrated in areas with dense populations, namely, counties containing the largest cities (Fig. 3). Cases are also more numerous in areas with many immigrants from high-prevalence counties, namely, southern California, areas along the Mexican border, much of Florida, and coastal areas in the northeast.

The prevalence of positive reactors to tuberculin by geography has not been studied in adequate detail since the US Public Health Service study among Navy recruits was discontinued in 1969.[20,55] At that time, the prevalence of positive reactions by geographic units tended to parallel tuberculosis case rates.

Residence abroad has often been considered to be a significant risk factor for acquiring tuberculous infection. Almost the only satisfactory evidence on this point comes from the study by Palmer and Edwards[3] of Navy recruits. In that study population, there were 6817 white males who had lived abroad for more than 6 months. Their frequency of positive reactions was 4.7%, only slightly higher than the 3.9% found among recruits who had not lived outside the country.

Little is known about geographic variation in the risk of developing disease following infection, and even less about the causes of variation. The 20-fold difference in incidence among tuberculin reactors in Alaska and Denmark might have resulted, at least in part, from the high dosage of infection associated with the extremely high infection rates and crowded living quarters of Alaskan Inuit only a few decades ago.[56]

5.4. Temporal Distribution

Until 1985, tuberculosis case rates had been declining in the United States since the initiation of nationwide

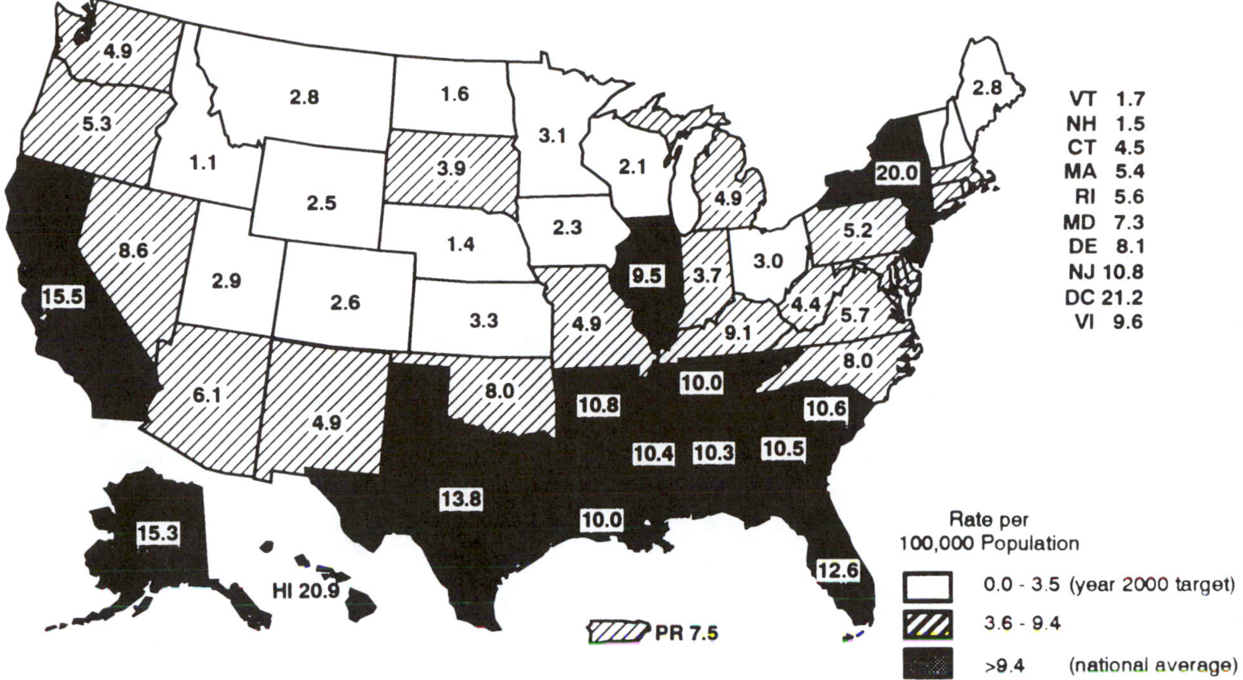

Figure 2. Tuberculosis case rates per 100,000 population, Untied States, by state, 1996.[53]

reporting in 1930. The annual rate of decrease was slight prior to 1950, but thereafter averaged close to 5% per year through 1984.[57] Changes in diagnostic and reporting practices caused a temporary upturn in the number of cases reported in children during the early 1960s and among adults in many areas in the mid-1970s.

Since the mid-1980s, there has been a widespread but not universal tendency for the previous rate of decline in tuberculosis case rates to slow or even to increase. In the United States, 1984 was the last year to continue the previous decrease in rates. As shown in Fig. 4, rates had decreased fairly uniformly until 1985, remained almost constant for several years, increased from 1989 to 1992, and decreased again from 1993 through 1996.[53] There was considerable geographic variation in these trends.[57] During the period 1984 through 1992, rates in 14 states continued to decline by an annual average of 4% or more, while rates in seven states increased by 4% or more. New York showed the greatest average annual percentage increase, 17% per year, followed by Nevada (8.2%), Utah (8.1%), New Jersey (6.2%), and California (5.6%). The largest cities had the greatest percentage increase in their tuberculosis case rates. Among those with populations over 1 million, New York City and San Diego led with average annual increases of 15.7% and 14.6%, respectively. Detroit was the only one to show a decline, 0.4% per year. Another way of looking at geographic variation is by the number of cases reported each year. Counties with more than 400 cases per year had 57.1% more cases in 1991 than in 1984. Conversely, counties reporting 1 to 49 cases per year had 12.5% fewer cases in 1991 than in 1984.

From 1992 through 1996, tuberculosis case rates in the United States declined again at the average rate of approximately 5% per year, essentially the same rate of decline noted in the years prior to 1985. Preliminary reports suggest that the decline in the case rate has continued through 1995. Because there has been essentially no change in the adverse impact of poor socioeconomic conditions on tuberculosis, such as infections with HIV, homelessness, drug abuse, and immigration from high-prevalence countries, it is reasonable to assume that this decline resulted from a considerable increase in tuberculosis control funds and activities. Of particular importance is the marked increase in directly observed therapy. Making sure that patients take all their drugs on a regular basis comes close to guaranteeing a quick return to noninfectiousness, cure of the disease, and prevention of drug-resistant organisms.[58,59]

Considerable variability in tuberculosis trends since 1984 was also reported from Europe. Among 15 countries of Western Europe, the downward trend prior to 1985 was

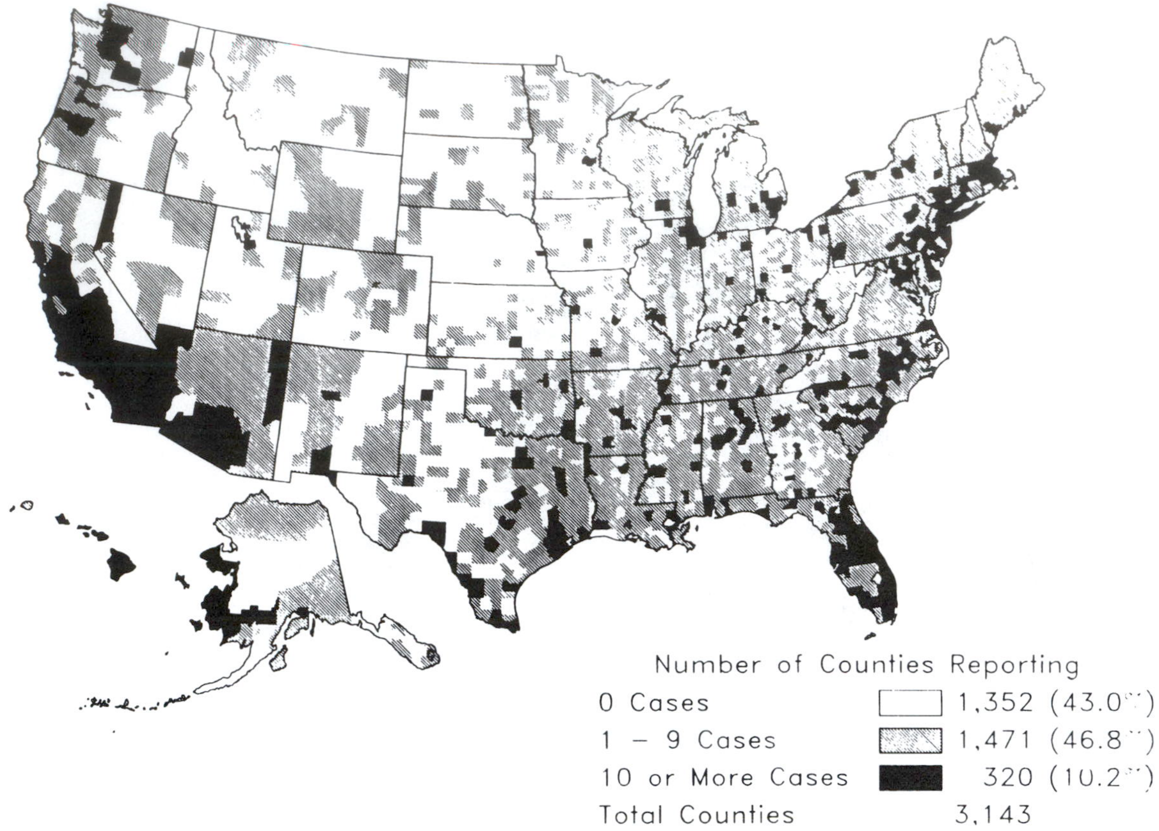

Figure 3. Number of reported tuberculosis cases by county, United States, 1996.(53)

continued or exceeded in only four, and halted entirely or changed to a slight increase in six during the period 1985 through 1991.(57,60) In 25 countries of Eastern Europe, reported case rates were generally higher than in the West.(61) Again, there was considerable variability in the reported average annual rates of change during the period 1985–1990 compared to the earlier 5 years. Fourteen countries reported greater rates of decline, seven a slowing in the rate of decline, and four an increase in tuberculosis case rates.

Based on notified cases, it appears that tuberculosis incidence decreased during the period 1974 to 1989 in Latin American, Eastern Mediterranean, European, and other industrialized countries.(12) Rates remained relatively stable in other areas that include most of the poorer countries of the world. Recent estimates are that case rates in countries that had experienced decreases will level off and remain relatively constant during the current decade.(62) Throughout the rest of the world, case rates are expected to increase dramatically. In part, this is due to the increases in developing countries of persons in the age groups with the highest number of tuberculosis cases. The spreading HIV epidemic is also expected to have a great impact, particularly in Africa and Southeast Asia. As a result, the global burden of tuberculosis is expected to increase by a third, with more than 10 million cases in the year 2000.

Because any reaction to any dose of tuberculin was once considered to signify a previous infection with tubercle bacilli, information on temporal trends in the prevalence and incidence of tuberculous infection is limited. In the 1930s, the prevalence of positive reactors among persons 15–19 years of age, using a tuberculin test reasonably compatible with modern ideas, was 22 and 25% in Philadelphia and the rural South, respectively. The estimated incidence of infection during their lifetimes was between 1.5 and 2.0% per year.(48)

In 1949–1951, the frequency of positive reactors to 5 tuberculin units of a purified protein derivative of tuberculin prepared from mammalian tubercle bacilli (PPD-S)

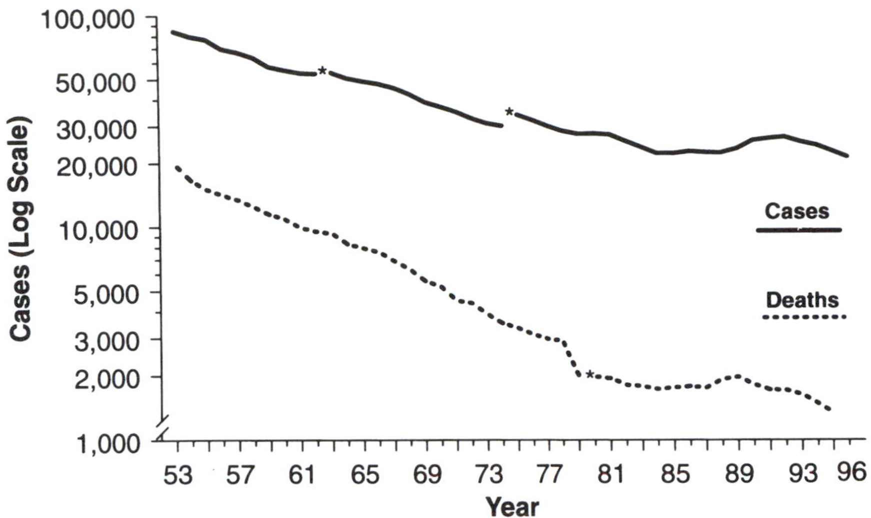

Figure 4. Tuberculosis cases per 100,000 population, United States, 1953–1996. *, Change in reporting criteria. Note: 1995 deaths are provisional; 1996 deaths not available.

was 6.6% among white male Navy recruits aged 17–21 years; in 1963–1964, this frequency was only 3.2%.[(3)] Subsequent reports of tuberculin sensitivity among US Navy and Marine recruits, while not entirely comparable to the earlier study, showed a prevalence of positive reactors of only 1.2% in 1986, with a rise to 2.5% in 1990.[(57)] When the proportion of positive reactors becomes this low in a country in which cross-reactions from nontuberculous mycobacterial infections are common, it is probable that much of the current tuberculin sensitivity results from cross-reactions. The proportion of young persons infected with tubercle bacilli in many parts of the United States is undoubtedly much lower than the proportion classified as positive tuberculin reactors. A number of considerations indicates that the average risk of becoming infected with tubercle bacilli in this country is now close to 10/100,000 per year.

There is no satisfactory information on changes with calendar time in the risk of disease following infection. There is some information, however, on the risk of disease among tuberculin-positive individuals by time after exposure to an infectious case, although there is some uncertainty because receipt of infection cannot be timed with accuracy. In the large study of tuberculosis contacts conducted by the US Public Health Service, it was found that the attack rate among tuberculin-positive contacts was 1,000/100,000 during the first year after diagnosis of the index case.[(63)] Some 8–10 years later, their rate had fallen to 72/100,000 per year, not much higher than rates among tuberculin-positive individuals without a history of household exposure.

5.5. Age

Tuberculosis mortality and morbidity rates show different patterns in populations with high and low risks of becoming infected with tubercle bacilli. Where the risk is high, there is a peak in infancy, followed by a second peak in young adult life, and sometimes a third peak in old age. Where the risk of becoming infected is low, tuberculosis case rates tend to increase steadily with age.[(3)]

The prevalence of positive tuberculin reactors usually increases at a fairly steady rate with age until about 40 to 50 years, when it tends to level off or even to fall somewhat. This is illustrated in Fig. 5 (upper panel) by results of tuberculin testing among New York City school employees in 1923–1974.[(64)] Determining the incidence of new infections with age is fraught with numerous problems. Most studies agree in finding an increase with age up to about 20 years; estimates of the incidence thereafter vary considerably.[(39,65)] When current risks of becoming infected are very low, it is likely that reversions from positive to negative may outnumber conversions, especially among older persons.

The probability of developing tuberculous disease among positive tuberculin reactors also varies with age

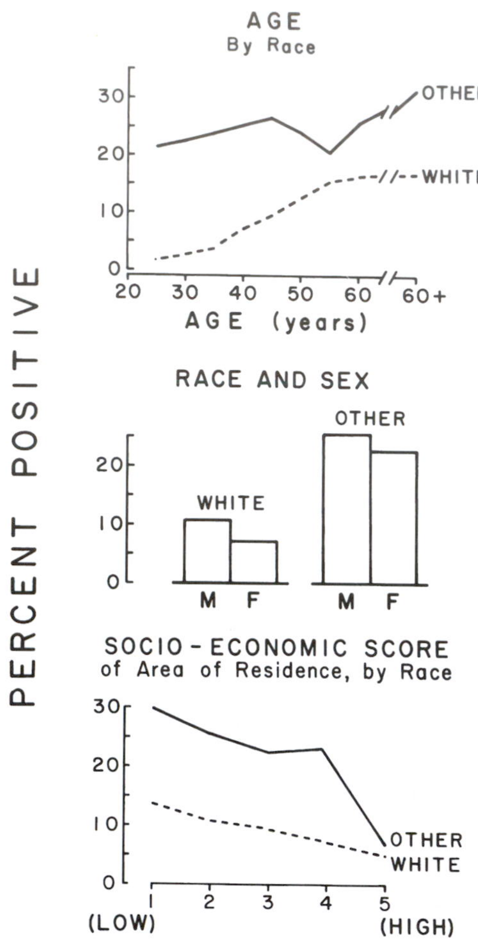

Figure 5. Percentage of positive reactors to 5 tuberculin units of PPD-S among New York City school employees, by age, sex, race, and socioeconomic rating of area of residence (1973–1974). All percentages are adjusted for the effects of the other characteristics shown in the figure. Adapted from information furnished by L. B. Reichman.(69)

(Fig. 6, upper panel).(5,48,66) There is a peak in infancy and early childhood, followed by a second peak in young adult life. The pattern among persons past the age of 45 is uncertain because studies of general populations have included only small numbers of infected persons this old. It seems likely that the peak in infancy largely reflects the effect of a recent infection, since all infections among infants are necessarily recent. The reason for the increased incidence among infected persons in young adult life is not known. The risk of developing tuberculosis some point during a lifetime for an untreated infected infant is estimated to be approximately 10%. For adults past the age of 25 years, the lifetime risk is considerably lower, being influenced largely by the risk within a year or two after becoming infected.

5.6. Sex

In the United States, tuberculosis death and case rates have been lower among females than among males at almost all ages.(3,54) The differences between the sexes are slight until 25 years of age, following which male rates increase with increasing age to a greater extent than female rates.

The prevalence of positive tuberculin reactors, and presumably the incidence of tuberculous infections, is also lower among females (Fig. 5).(3,48) There is conflicting evidence regarding the risk of disease among infected males and females. Among Danes, the Alaskan Inuit, and young blacks and Puerto Ricans in the United States, rates were higher among females,(48,67,68) whereas among whites in the United States and persons in South India, rates were higher among males.(37,69)

5.7. Race

Historically, both death and case rates have been higher among blacks, American Indians, and the Inuit than among whites in the United States.(3) Whether these differences are due to genetic or socioeconomic characteristics is unknown. Death rates have fallen somewhat more rapidly for nonwhites than for whites, while reported case rates have fallen somewhat more rapidly for whites.

The prevalence of positive tuberculin reactors in the United States is also generally higher among blacks, American Indians, and the Inuit.(3,19,48,64) Differences among white and nonwhite employees of the New York City school system are shown in Fig. 5. Among men entering the Navy between 1958 and 1969, 3.8% of the whites were positive tuberculin reactors compared to 12.4% of the blacks and 60.2% of the Asians, who were mainly Filipinos.(70) The high percentage of positive reactions among the Asians may have resulted in part from BCG vaccination in their native countries.

The incidence of tuberculous disease among *infected* Navy recruits was 79/100,000 per year for whites, 93 for blacks, and 196 for Asians.(70) It is possible that special stresses accounted for the high rate among Asian reactors. In any case, their experience suggests that the BCG vaccination program in the Philippines did not have much effect on the subsequent tuberculosis experience of these recruits.

In a study of the nature of officially reported tuber-

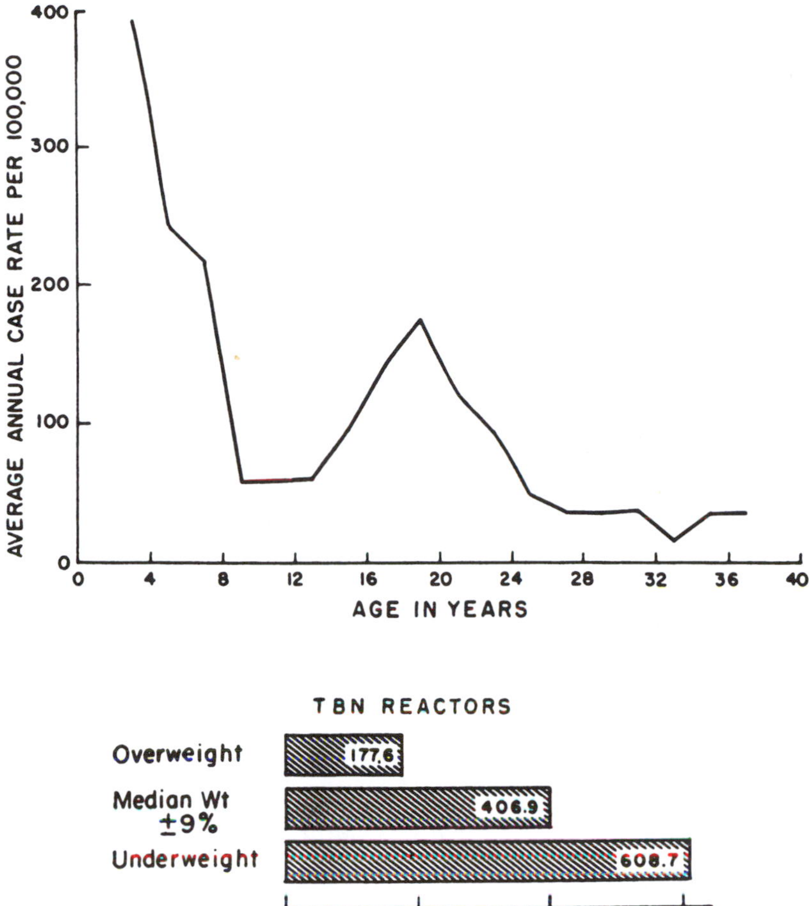

Figure 6. Average annual incidence of tuberculosis per 100,000 positive tuberculin reactors in two selected populations: (1) Children in Puerto Rico, 1949–1969 (upper panel).[1] Rates by age at diagnosis. Adapted from Comstock *et al.* (2) US Navy recruits tested in 1958–1967 (lower panel).[65] Rates by relative weight during 4 years after enlistment. Adapted from Edwards *et al.*[21]

culosis cases, several striking differences were found.[52] Alaskans (mostly Inuit and Indians) tended to have lesions that were not extensive and very rarely exudative in nature. Patients from Singapore and from Maryland had extensive disease and a high frequency of exudative and cavitary lesions. Patients from five European centers tended to fall between these extremes.

Among the subgroups with high rates of tuberculosis are refugee immigrants to the United States from Southeast Asia, Latin America, and Haiti.[71,72] During the late 1970s, their contribution to reported tuberculosis cases in the United States was responsible for a marked slowing in the annual rate of decline during that period. During the period, 1981–1984, cases among Asians and Pacific Islanders decreased more rapidly than other ethnic groups; cases among Hispanics declined at the same rates as for the United States as a whole.[57] Immigrants accounted for a large part of the increase in tuberculosis from 1985 to 1992, with most of the increase coming from persons born in Latin America and Asia.[57,73] In Western Europe, too, tuberculosis among immigrants from high-prevalence countries also accounted for a major part of the tuberculosis problem.[60,74] There was evidence that the high rates among immigrants were due to their poor socioeconomic status as well as to the high rates of infection acquired in their native countries.[72,75]

5.8. Occupation

A recent analysis of proportionate mortality among 28 of the United States shows this index to be increased among low-level health care workers, funeral directors, persons occupationally exposed to silica dust, and low-socioeconomic-status workers.[76] While mortality is an insensitive indicator of exposure risks, it does have the advantage of being available for all residents of many countries. For the more definitive risks of becoming infected or of developing disease, there is little available evidence with respect to occupation.

Among hospital employees, there were only slight and nonsignificant differences in the frequency of positive tuberculin reactors by type of job or estimated exposure to patients after allowing for the fact that males, minority ethnic groups, and older persons all had higher rates of positive reactions.[31] There is, however, evidence that hospital physicians in training are not only at increased risk of becoming infected but tend to be noncooperative in tuberculin testing and preventive therapy programs.[77] Tuberculosis rates are often excessive in occupations with silica exposure.[78] Because silica has been shown to lower host resistance to tuberculosis in experimental animals, it is presumed that persons with silicosis also have a lowered capability of controlling tuberculosis infections.

5.9. Occurrence in Different Settings

In recent decades, hospitalization of tuberculosis patients has shifted from tuberculosis sanatoria to general hospitals as the need for hospital care has become less frequent and its duration shorter. With this change and with pressure from the Occupational Safety and Health Administration, hospitals have begun to institute periodic tuberculin-testing programs for their employees. Rates of conversion from negative to positive have often been high, sometimes even among presumably unexposed personnel.[79] In the absence of two tuberculin tests given sequentially at the initial examination, however, it is likely that most of the reported conversions resulted from the booster effect and not from new infections.[31]

Wherever persons from high-risk areas, such as inner cities, are congregated in poorly ventilated spaces, the risk of becoming infected can be very high. Outbreaks have been reported from shelters for the homeless, prisons, hospitals, and clinics.[46,80,81] Such outbreaks are particularly noticeable among persons infected with HIV whose lowered immunity allows clinically manifest tuberculosis to develop quickly after infection.[50] Tuberculosis has also been shown to be a hazard in nursing homes, especially when the frequency of other cardiorespiratory illnesses and a reduced index of suspicion combine to make case detection unlikely.[82] In all these situations, screening for infection and disease followed by appropriate chemotherapy and preventive treatment have been shown to be effective.

There is some evidence that the dosage of infection is related to the risk of developing tuberculosis. Both among nurses in the Prophit Survey in England and white and Indian children in western Canada, positive tuberculin reactors who had been most heavily exposed were more likely to develop tuberculosis than tuberculin reactors with less exposure.[83,84]

5.10. Socioeconomic Factors

Tuberculosis has long been known to be associated with poverty, crowding, and malnutrition.[2,31] Mortality, morbidity, and prevalence of tuberculosis all tend to be highest in the poorest areas. A group at particularly high risk of having tuberculosis consists of homeless persons living in large urban centers.[46,85] In Denmark, the incidence of tuberculosis was highest among divorced persons and lowest among married persons, the differences being marked for men and slight for women.[86]

Relatively few studies, however, indicate whether the risk of disease associated with socioeconomic status results from the risk of becoming infected, of becoming diseased after infection, or both. One of these studies, a report of tuberculin testing of New York City school personnel in 1973–1974, showed that the frequency of tuberculous infection was indeed higher in the poorest areas, 22.4%, contrasted with 5.5% in areas with the highest socioeconomic rating, after adjustment for differences in composition by age, race, and sex (Fig. 5).[48,64]

In Washington County, Maryland, high-school children living in homes with one or more persons per room or in an inadequate dwelling as assessed by the absence of complete bathroom facilities were more than twice as likely to be positive tuberculin reactors as children living in less crowded, more adequate dwellings.[87]

Even less is known about the relationship of socioeconomic status to the risk of developing disease after infection. In Muscogee County, Georgia, no significant association of the incidence of tuberculosis with adequacy of housing could be found, after controlling for the effects of initial tuberculin and BCG vaccination status.[48]

5.11. Nutritional Factors

Severe malnutrition has been shown to be associated with a diminution of tuberculin sensitivity following BCG vaccination.[88] There is no indication, however, that malnutrition protects against infection; rather, it appears that it masks the ability to detect the presence of infection.

For a long time, it has been observed that a variety of situations involving food deprivation are associated with increases in tuberculosis case and death rates.[2,3,17] Since the common factor in these situations is malnutrition, it is likely that the association is one of cause and effect. And since morbidity increases shortly after food shortages appear and decreases promptly when food supplies become adequate, it is likely that the effect of malnutrition is mediated primarily through a concomitant risk of disease among persons already infected.

Body build is related in part to nutrition. Studies among US Navy recruits demonstrated that there is no relationship of relative weight to the prevalence of positive reactions to tuberculin. Among positive reactors on initial examination, however, the subsequent case rate was nearly four times higher among men initially 10% or more underweight than among men initially 10% or more overweight (Fig. 6, lower panel).[21] That fatness was the component of body weight likely to be responsible for this association was indicated by evidence from Muscogee County, Georgia.[48] The incidence of disease was closely related to the thickness of subcutaneous fat measured over the trapezius ridges from photofluorograms of the chest at the start of the study. Tuberculosis was twice as high among persons with less than 5 mm of subcutaneous fat as among those with 10 mm or more.

The aforecited studies do not conclusively answer the questions about diet and tuberculosis. Although it is possible that undernutrition causes both leanness and susceptibility to tuberculosis, it is also possible that some other aspect of body build, such as hormonal or genetic factors, is the underlying cause of both. Two findings that favor the latter hypothesis are the impression that very few people in Muscogee County in 1946 could have been considered to be seriously undernourished and the observation among Navy recruits that tuberculosis contacts weighed less than men who had not lived in the same house with a tuberculosis case, even when the comparison was limited to tuberculin-negative persons in each group.[57]

5.12. Genetic Factors

That varying degrees of resistance to tuberculosis can be inherited was clearly shown by Lurie[89] in his work with inbred strains of rabbits. Whether or not this holds true for humans has been much less certain. While it is possible that there is inherent resistance to the acquisition of infection, it seems likely that genetic factors are more important in keeping infection from progressing to disease. There have been numerous observations that the risk of tuberculosis among household contacts is greater for blood relatives than for others.[90] That there is a genetic component in this increased risk is indicated by studies of twins, in which concordance for tuberculosis is considerably greater among monozygotic twins than among dizygotic twins, even when other factors related to tuberculosis risk are taken into account.[91] An additional indication of inherited susceptibility is the report of higher case rates associated with blood groups B and AB among the Inuit in Alaska.[92]

5.13. Acquired Immunodeficiency Syndrome

Because of the importance of the cellular immune system in controlling infections with *M. tuberculosis*, it is not surprising that persons infected with HIV are at increased risk of reactivating dormant organisms.[93] Linking registers for tuberculosis with those for AIDS has shown that there is a high degree of association, most marked among populations at high risk of having been infected with *M. tuberculosis* and HIV (e.g., intravenous drug abusers in inner cities or residents of some developing countries).[94,95] Several studies have shown that combined infections with *M. tuberculosis* and HIV result in extremely high rates of clinical tuberculosis.[96–98] Active tuberculosis may precede or follow the development of other manifestations of AIDS. Further indication of depressed resistance in AIDS is the severe and unusual forms of pulmonary tuberculosis seen in these patients and the increased frequency of extrapulmonary and disseminated tuberculosis. AIDS is also associated with a failure to react to tuberculin, increasing the difficulties of making a diagnosis of concomitant tuberculosis. For this reason, it has been recommended that a person who tests positive for HIV be tuberculin tested; if there is induration of 5 mm or more to 5 tuberculin units of tuberculin PPD, preventive therapy with isoniazid is strongly advised.[99] Preventive therapy is also recommended for anergic persons at high risk of having been infected with *M. tuberculosis*.[100]

Tuberculosis cases among persons infected with HIV are estimated to have accounted for 4% of the total tuberculosis cases worldwide in 1990; by 2000, this proportion is estimated to reach 14%.[62] While all areas will experience increases in such cases during the decade 1990 to 2000, the greatest percentage increase is expected to occur in Southeast Asia (8.7%), with the greatest increase in numbers of cases in Africa and Southeast Asia.

5.14. Size of Tuberculin Reaction

Several studies have shown that persons who are most sensitive to tuberculin are also most likely to develop tuberculous disease later on.[22,48] Up to 50 years ago, attention was focused on whether allergy to tuberculoprotein was beneficial or harmful; now, at least in epidemiological circles, principal interest lies in the ability of the degree of hypersensitivity to indicate whether or not the infecting organism was one of the tubercle bacilli, *M. tuberculosis* or *M. bovis*, or one of the usually benign nontuberculous mycobacteria.

The prognostic importance of degree of sensitivity to tuberculin was clearly shown in a study of more than one million white Navy recruits.[22] On entry into the Navy, recruits routinely received a skin test with PPD-S and also with a PPD prepared from a nontuberculous mycobacteria, either the so-called Battey or Gause strain, currently named *M. avium-intracellulare* or *M. scrofulaceum*, respectively. Cases of tuberculosis that developed among these men during their first 4 years of Navy service were identified. Recruits with less than 6 mm to 5 tuberculin units of PPD-S on entry had a low rate of tuberculosis subsequently; those with intermediate reactions, an intermediate rate; and those with reactions of 12 mm or more, a high rate.

Both experimental and clinical evidence indicate that reactions to a homologous antigen are usually larger than cross-reactions to a heterologous antigen. Among recruits with intermediate reactions to PPD-S and larger reactions to either PPD-B or PPD-G, the subsequent case rate was essentially the same as recruits with less than 6 mm of induration to PPD-S, suggesting that their reactions were due to cross-reactions from nontuberculous mycobacteria. In contrast, recruits with intermediate reactions to PPD-S that were clearly larger than those to PPD-B or PPD-G had subsequent tuberculosis case rates that approached those of recruits with large reactions to PPD-S. These and similar findings support the current belief that the larger the reaction to a small or intermediate dose of tuberculin, the more likely it is that an individual has been infected with tubercle bacilli, and consequently the more likely that tuberculous disease will develop at some time in the future.

6. Mechanisms and Routes of Transmission

For all practical purposes, tubercle bacilli are transmitted to humans in only two ways: by the ingestion of contaminated milk and by the inhalation of tubercle bacilli in droplet nuclei. The importance of spread by direct contact, sexual or otherwise, or by ingestion of organisms other than in infected dairy products is undetermined and probably slight. Tuberculin testing of dairy cattle and pasteurization of milk have nearly eliminated bovine tuberculosis in the United States and the possibility of its spread to man through dairy products.[101]

When an individual with tubercle bacilli in the sputum coughs, sneezes, talks, or sings, a spray of secretion may be expelled. The larger particles fall out of the air promptly and appear to be of little danger. Tiny droplets dry promptly when exposed to the air; the resultant droplet nuclei may float with the air currents for a long time and considerable distances.[47] When inhaled, they usually are not trapped in the upper air passages or on the ciliated portions of the tracheobronchial tree, but pass directly to the alveoli. Current evidence indicates that only droplet nuclei that carry tubercle bacilli and reach the alveoli are effective in infecting a susceptible host. The formation of these infectious particles can be markedly reduced merely by covering the mouth and nose when coughing or sneezing.

7. Pathogenesis and Immunity

The incubation period of tuberculosis can be defined as the time from receipt of infection to the development of hypersensitivity to tuberculin manifested by a positive reaction to the tuberculin test, since hypersensitivity apparently appears at about the time a focus of disease develops, even though this may be microscopic. In this case, the incubation period appears to vary from 3 to 8 weeks. More realistically, however, the incubation period as measured from the receipt of infection to the development of manifest disease may range from 3 weeks to the remainder of a lifetime. While some disease progresses inexorably from the very beginning, a period of latency, sometimes lasting for years, is usual. It is thus possible that disease in extreme old age may result from a childhood infection that has been latent in the interval.[102] If events could be identified that were known to cause dormant tubercle bacilli to become active again, one might consider the time from those events to the development of manifest disease to be the incubation period of tuberculous *disease* as distinguished from the incubation period for tuberculous *infection*, which is the time from receipt of infection to the development of tuberculin hypersensitivity.

After tubercle bacilli are inhaled or ingested, they are engulfed by phagocytes and carried to the regional lymph nodes, occasionally passing into the bloodstream and thence to many organs of the body. At first, they cause little or no reaction in the host tissues, but within 3 to 8 weeks, hypersensitivity to antigens elaborated by the organisms develops, along with some degree of acquired immunity. Phagocytes that contain tubercle bacilli and cells in the immediate neighborhood may then be killed, resulting in foci with central caseous necrosis and a peripheral zone of epithelioid cells, lymphocytes, and fibroblasts. The range of possible outcomes is extremely varied. In many organs and tissues, blood-borne tubercle bacilli show no evidence of becoming established. Bone marrow, liver, and spleen are often involved, but infections in these organs are almost always controlled. More favorable sites for growth are the lungs, kidneys, meninges, and the epiphyseal portions of bone. Even in favorable sites, however, the majority of lesions heal as scar tissue surrounds the caseous foci and tubercle bacilli. Some lesions become partly or wholly calcified. Although the organisms may remain viable for years in these scarred areas, it is likely that most of them eventually die.

In a small proportion of persons, the balance tips against the host and in favor of the bacilli. Host resistance may be inadequate from the start, and the disease may progress to a fatal termination; or after an indefinite period of quiescence and apparent healing, the organisms may again start to grow and to destroy tissue. What factors are responsible for inability to control the infecting organisms at either time is uncertain. It is known, however, that resistance is lowered in diseases (notably AIDS) or therapy involving immunosuppression, diabetes, silicosis, and, as noted in Section 5.11, possibly by severe undernutrition.

Not all locations of disease are favorable for the transmission of infecting organisms, since organisms buried in most human tissues will never be excreted in the form of droplet nuclei small enough to be inhaled by another host. Only in the lungs or especially the larynx is this likely to occur. Actively progressing caseous foci in the lung ultimately erode into a bronchus, the contents are expelled, and a cavity is formed. Tubercle bacilli flourish on the walls of a cavity and can readily pass with the expired air into the atmosphere, where those that float in droplet nuclei may survive to be deposited in the lungs of another susceptible host.

For years there has been controversy regarding the role of endogenous or exogenous reinfection in causing reactivation on the initial tuberculous lesions after they had apparently healed. Endogenous reinfection, the reactivation of dormant organisms after a period of latency in a previously infected person, is by far the more common mechanism in areas where the likelihood of infection is low. Exogenous reinfection is disease caused by inhalation of tubercle bacilli by a previously infected person during exposure to a second infectious case. Exogenous reinfection has been demonstrated by DNA "fingerprinting," notably but not exclusively in outbreaks involving HIV-infected persons.[6,7] Nevertheless, it appears that resistance acquired after an initial infection confers considerable protection against exogenous reinfection.[103]

8. Patterns of Host Response

The type of clinical disease that develops after infection depends to a considerable extent on the ability of host resistance to hold the multiplication of bacilli in check. Some lesions may be small and heal without ever producing symptoms or being recognizable by roentgenography or by pathological examination. Fortunately, many tuberculous lesions do tend to heal, even after reaching the symptomatic stage. Some, however, progress to a point where tissue destruction is incompatible with life. The nature of the disease that results from reactivation of an initial lesion or lesions depends most of all on the location of the lesion(s). The manifestations of tuberculosis of various organs differ so markedly that it was not until Koch demonstrated the causative organisms that they were accepted as having a common etiology. In persons infected with HIV, all phases of pathogenesis are markedly accelerated.[104] Disease following infection is likely to occur quickly, spread to many organs is common, and pulmonary cavitation may be absent even in advanced cases.

8.1. Clinical Features

Tuberculous disease is usually symptomatic, although some patients may ignore their symptoms until they become extreme, particularly if the symptoms are mild and progression slow and insidious. With all forms of the disease, there may be evidence of chronic infection: anorexia, weight loss, fatigue, and low-grade fever. The leukocyte count is usually normal or low.

Tuberculosis should always be suspected and ruled out if there is a chronic cough or continued fever of unknown origin. The diagnosis should be suspected especially in middle-aged males in urban or lower-socioeconomic settings and in immigrants from developing countries. A history of immunosuppression, alcoholism, diabetes, gastrectomy, pneumoconiosis, or social isolation increases the probability that tuberculosis is the cause.

Pulmonary tuberculosis is by far the most common form of the disease, accounting for 82% of the cases reported in the United States in 1994.[53] The most common symptom is chronic cough, usually productive of mucoid or mucopurulent sputum. Pleuritic pain or dull aching in the chest is sometimes reported. Hemoptysis, while common in advanced disease, is unusual as a presenting symptom. Occasionally, tuberculosis can present as an acute respiratory illness with symptoms resembling those of influenza or pneumonia. Pleurisy with effusion was once considered to be tuberculosis unless proven otherwise. This may still be a useful precept to keep in mind, even though in many areas tuberculosis is no longer a major cause of pleural effusion.

Miliary tuberculosis results from blood-borne dissemination of tubercle bacilli. With numerous lesions in many organs of the body, manifestations are those of a cryptic fever because an untreated patient usually succumbs to the disease before any single organ is sufficiently involved to give localized symptoms. The one exception is tuberculous meningitis, which often accompanies miliary tuberculosis, although it may also be a separate entity. It occurs when a caseous nodule of the meninges ruptures into the subarachnoid space. The presenting symptoms are likely to be headache, abnormal behavior, clouded consciousness, or convulsions. The spinal fluid shows decreased sugar, increased protein, and a pleocytosis, polymorphonuclear at first and later lymphocytic.

Lymph node tuberculosis accounted for approximately a third of the extrapulmonary cases reported in 1994.[53] The hilar and mediastinal nodes are most commonly involved, followed in order of frequency by cervical and supraclavicular nodes. Granulomatous lymphadenitis in adults and multiple lymph node involvement at any age are likely to have a tuberculous etiology. In children, on the other hand, granulomatous lymphadenitis of the cervical area is very likely to be caused by nontuberculous mycobacteria.

Pleural tuberculosis accounted for approximately one fifth of the extrapulmonary cases, in 1994. Genitourinary disease made up almost 1/12 of the extrapulmonary cases. Since any portion of the genitourinary tract may be involved, symptoms may be those of chronic recurrent urinary tract infections, hematuria, nodular induration of prostate or vas deferens, pelvic inflammatory disease, amenorrhea, or infertility.

Almost 12% of the extrapulmonary cases (2.1% of the total) were classified as miliary or meningeal. Bone and joint tuberculosis, 11% of the extrapulmonary cases, often occur together, with localized pain and swelling. Lower spine and other weight-bearing joints are most commonly affected. All other sites, including the peritoneum, accounted for only 15% of the cases of extrapulmonary tuberculosis.

8.2. Diagnosis

The tuberculin skin test is still the only feasible method for telling whether or not infection with tubercle bacilli has occurred. To be truly useful, it must be treated as a quantitative test, with attention to accurate administration of tuberculin and careful measurement of the diameter of any induration produced.[105] It is essential to use a well-standardized purified protein derivative of tuberculin (PPD-tuberculin), stabilized with a detergent and prepared from a large batch of material.[106] The dose should be 5 tuberculin units.

A positive reaction merely signifies that mycobacterial infection (or BCG vaccination) has occurred at some time in the past. The larger the reaction, the more likely it is to have resulted from tuberculous infection. Where the proportion of reactions due to tuberculous infection is high, the probability that any tuberculin reaction represents tuberculous infection is increased. In lifetime residents of Alaska, for example, induration of any size is likely to signify past infection with tubercle bacilli, because infections with other mycobacteria are exceedingly rare.[19] In the southeastern United States and most tropical areas, on the other hand, it is probable that most reactions under 10 mm result from nontuberculous mycobacterial infections, and probably a high proportion of those under 15 mm as well, because of the very high prevalence of such infections in such areas. Among household associates of active cases, persons with X-ray shadows suggestive of tuberculosis or older persons exposed to high tuberculosis infection rates when they were young, small reactions are more likely to represent tuberculous infections than they are in other persons from the same area.[27]

Although a negative tuberculin test, properly given and interpreted, provides good evidence that a person does not have tuberculosis, there are important exceptions. From 2 to 5% of known tuberculosis patients do not react to 5 tuberculin units of PPD-tuberculin.[107] In many such instances, failure to react is related to the severity of their disease: seriously ill patients, including those with tuberculosis, lose their skin sensitivity to tuberculin. Sensitivity may also be depressed by large doses of corticosteroids, by AIDS, and for a few weeks following measles, infectious mononucleosis, and vaccination with several viral antigens.[27]

The optimal dividing line between a positive and negative reaction to the test depends on a number of the preceding considerations, in addition to technical features related to administering and reading the tests. While the definitions of positive tuberculin reactions by the American Thoracic Society are reasonable compromises for much of the United States, it is probably best to determine this level by examining the frequency distribution of reaction sizes from the population with which one is working.[27,28,87]

Although tuberculosis of the lungs can produce radiographic findings similar to those of many different diseases, certain patterns are most common. If the initial infection produces a visible lesion, it is likely to involve the regional mediastinal nodes with or without a small infiltrate in the corresponding portions of the lungs, most commonly in the lower zones. Subsequent disease usually develops in the apical and posterior segments of the upper lobes or the superior segment of the lower lobes. Most commonly, the appearance is that of nodular infiltration, often with evidence of cavitation. No radiographic appearance, however, is pathognomonic. In persons with HIV infections, almost any pulmonary lesion should be suspected of being tuberculosis.

A definitive diagnosis of tuberculosis can be made only by the isolation of *M. tuberculosis* from the involved tissues or secretions from the involved areas. Finding acid-fast bacilli is suggestive of a tuberculous etiology, but the ubiquitous occurrence of nontuberculous mycobacteria requires that definitive identification be made by cultures.

In making the diagnosis from specimens obtained at operation or autopsy, it is important to remember to place the suspected tissue in a container for specimens to be cultured. It is surprising how often such specimens are automatically put in formalin or other fixative, making cultures impossible.

9. Control and Prevention

9.1. General Concepts

Historians have noted that the decline in tuberculosis in many countries appears to have started before the discovery of the tubercle bacillus, and hence prior to any measures specifically designed to control the disease. Others have pointed out, however, that improved living and working conditions brought about by the sanitation and social reform movement of the 1800s might well have helped produce a decline in tuberculosis.[(2)] In particular, improved ventilation and daylight in homes and places of employment should have decreased the probability of becoming infected, while decreased working hours and improved nutrition should have increased resistance to disease. It seems likely that improvements along these lines contributed to the decline of tuberculosis.

Tuberculosis control measures among humans fall into four major categories: decontamination of air and milk, case-finding and chemotherapy, chemoprophylaxis, and vaccination. Each has its advantages and disadvantages, and each has a place under the appropriate circumstances. A simple model serves well to illustrate how each of these control measures affects the tuberculosis problem.[(108)] The major elements of the model are shown in Fig. 7. While the numbers shown in this figure are for the United States in 1963, they can easily be changed to fit another situation. Missing from the figure's portrayal of a 1-year cycle is the reduction of the uninfected and infected populations by deaths and the addition to the uninfected population by births.

In any given year, a certain number of cases develop from previously infected persons. Each of these cases infects others, some of whom develop tuberculosis during that year and others of whom are added to the infected group for the subsequent year. These new cases in turn infect others, who are also added to the infected group. For the United States in 1963, it was estimated that 80% (40,000) of the 50,000 cases came from the 25 million persons infected in previous years and 20% (10,000) from persons infected during that year. These numbers were based on the best estimates then available and reflect both the effect that the tuberculosis control program was having at that time and the epidemiological characteristics of the disease in this country. It can be seen that *if* the effectiveness of tuberculosis control at that time could be maintained, tuberculosis would eventually disappear, although this would require many years.

9.2. Decontamination of Air and Milk

When isolation of tuberculous patients is necessary, precautions should be aimed at preventing air from becoming a vehicle of infection.[(109,110)] The patient should be taught to cover the mouth and nose with disposable tissues when coughing or sneezing in order to trap droplets before they can evaporate and become free-floating droplet nuclei. There should be good ventilation of the room without recirculation of air; preferably, the air should be exhausted directly to the outside and the room kept under negative pressure. Ultraviolet irradiation of the upper air or of recirculated air is also helpful. High-efficiency particulate respirators (masks) are under consideration for use by all personnel caring for infectious tuberculosis patients, although their cost-efficiency under practical working conditions has been questioned.[(111)] In the occasional instances when explanation and persuasion fail and a patient with infectious tuberculosis refuses to take the necessary steps to protect others, it is desirable to have legal powers and appropriate facilities for enforced isolation.

The major means for keeping milk from being a

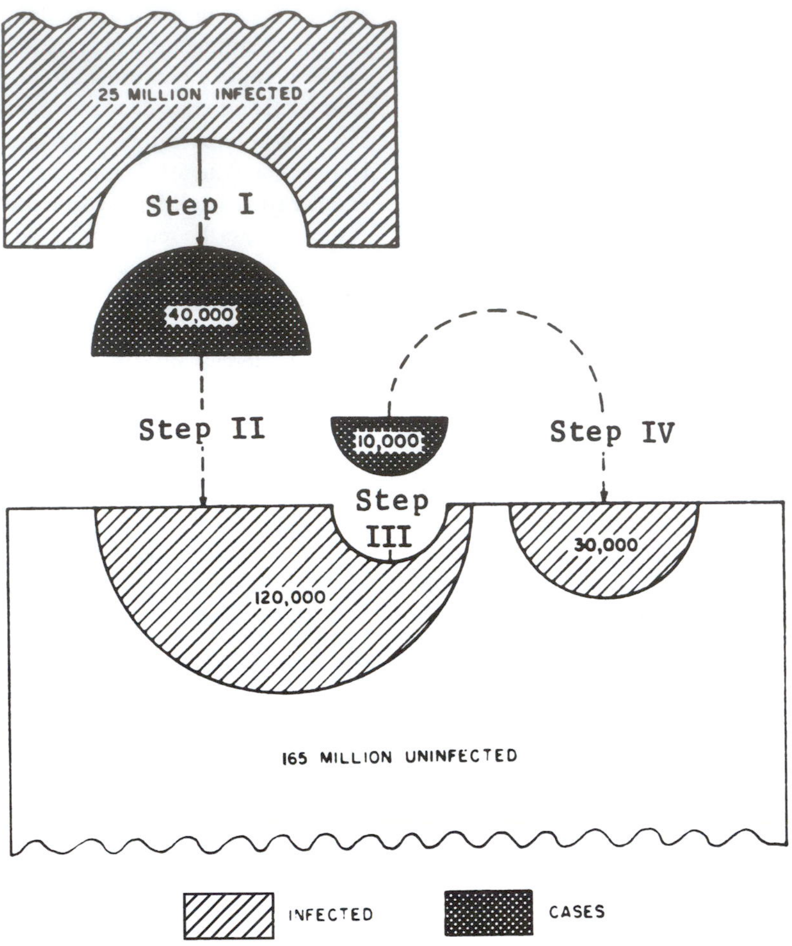

Figure 7. Schematic illustration of annual cycle of development of tuberculosis infection and disease, United States, 1963.[108]

vehicle of infection are periodic tuberculin testing of dairy cattle, slaughter of reactors, and pasteurization of milk. Although tuberculosis among cattle has been nearly eradicated from the United States and milk-borne tuberculosis has become rare, this near success has led to diminished funding for the eradication program, laxity in tuberculin testing, and renewed interest in drinking raw milk, all of which could lead to milk again becoming a source of tuberculous infection.

If by some miracle both air and milk could be kept completely free of tubercle bacilli, the cycle of tuberculosis shown in Fig. 7 would be blocked at step II. Tuberculosis would continue to develop among the previously infected population until all infected persons had died.

9.3. Case-Finding and Chemotherapy

Similarly, in an ideal but unfortunately imaginary world, case-finding endeavors would identify every case before it became infectious and chemotherapy would be completely effective in preventing future infectiousness. Such perfection would also block the flow of tuberculosis at step II in the model shown in Fig. 7. As noted before, cases would continue to develop from the pool of infected persons until all had died.

In 1992, in the United States, 69% of the 26,673 reported cases had pulmonary tuberculosis with known positive sputum[9]; it is theoretically possible that with further examinations, all of the pulmonary cases (82%) might be classified as communicable. Of 22,475 patients with any form of tuberculosis who were started on chemotherapy in 1992, 2,607 were known to have died. Only 76% of the others were known to have completed a recommended course of therapy or to be still taking medication at the end of 1993.[112] Much better performance is needed if this country hopes to eliminate tuberculosis by case-finding and chemotherapy within the next few decades.

Case-finding in developed countries is now difficult because the prevalence of cases has become so low that mass screening procedures are unproductive and the index of suspicion of most medical practitioners is low. In developing countries, where mass screening methods could be more useful but usually cannot be afforded, microscopic examination of stained specimens of sputum from persons with chronic cough has been shown to be productive. In both situations, the most appropriate combination of diagnostic modalities—medical history, skin testing, chest roentgenography, and bacteriology—will need to be selected after reviewing the local tuberculosis problem and the resources to combat it.[113]

Chemotherapy has become so effective that virtually every patient with organisms sensitive to the standard antituberculosis drugs could be cured if the necessary medications were taken conscientiously. Not only can the disease be cured, but patients are also quickly rendered noninfectious by the generally accepted chemotherapeutic regimen. This consists of the daily administration of four drugs—isoniazid, rifampicin, pyrazinamide, and ethambutol—for 2 months, and two drugs—isoniazid and rifampicin—for another 4 months.[1] While this regimen is simple from a medical point of view, persuading all patients to adhere to it is not. The expense of some drugs, the toxicity of others, and the duration of the regimen can cause patients to discontinue treatment prematurely or to take it irregularly. For many patients, solving their immediate social and economic problems seems far more important than caring for their tuberculosis. Attention to administrative details and directly observed intermittent regimens can all contribute to better patient acceptance of treatment, to a high rate of cure, and to prevention of the emergence of drug-resistant strains.[58,59,99,110,114–117] The emergence of drug-resistant organisms necessitates expert medical administration of expensive and toxic drugs. Even then, the prognosis is often unfavorable.

9.4. Preventive Therapy

Following the introduction of isoniazid as a chemotherapeutic agent against tuberculosis, Edith Lincoln noted that children with primary tuberculosis treated with this drug showed a much lower incidence of serious tuberculous complications than had been noted with other medications and suggested that a controlled trial of the effectiveness of isoniazid in preventing these complications be undertaken.[63] The ensuing trial among 2750 children with asymptomatic primary tuberculosis or recent tuberculin conversions showed treatment with isoniazid to be remarkably effective, producing a 94% reduction in tuberculous complications during the year of preventive treatment and a 70% reduction over the subsequent 9-year period.

At least 21 controlled trials of preventive therapy with isoniazid involving more than 136,000 subjects have now been reported.[118,119] Among 14 trials with more than 1000 subjects, the median reduction in tuberculosis from preventive treatment was 60% during the periods of observation, which ranged from 1 to 13 years. The range of effectiveness in these 14 trials was 25 to 88%. The trials with low effectiveness included one that used small doses of isoniazid and one in which adherence was very poor. It should be noted, however, that these estimates are based on the total study populations regardless of how well medication was taken. Persons with high adherence tended to obtain greater protection than the preceding median values indicate. Some degree of protection can be expected to be long-lasting. Any diminution caused by isoniazid in the numbers of tubercle bacilli harbored by the host increases the probability that host resistance can control any organisms that may remain. In addition, it has been shown that a treated infection in guinea pigs confers some resistance against subsequent reinfection.[120] Protection in humans has been shown to persist for at least 10 to 19 years.[63,121]

The generally accepted regimen for isoniazid preventive treatment is 5–10 mg isoniazid/kg body weight, not exceeding a total dose of 300 mg, given orally in a single daily dose for 6–12 months. Among persons who adhere well to the treatment regimen, 12 months of medication has been shown to be much better than 6 months.[122] Studies among tuberculosis contacts and Alaskan villagers indicate that 9–10 months of treatment may be optimal.[63,123]

The principal appeal of isoniazid preventive treatment lies in its ability to interrupt the chain of infection at step I in the model shown in Fig. 7. Universal application to reactors and perfect effectiveness of this preventive procedure could theoretically eradicate tuberculosis almost at once. While realism does not allow hope of even approaching such an outcome, whatever effectiveness preventive treatment may have affects every step in the model and not merely the later ones. Of considerable current interest is the evidence from observational and controlled studies that preventive treatment with isoniazid not only reduces the risk of tuberculosis among HIV-infected persons but may also delay the onset of symptoms of AIDS.[96,104,119]

There are several deterrents to widespread use of isoniazid in preventive treatment: toxicological, financial, and patient/provider noncompliance. Most side effects of isoniazid are usually not sufficient to cause its use to be discontinued and are largely restricted to adults.[63] In the large US Public Health Service trial among household contacts, a group composed largely of children and young adults, reactions that caused subjects to stop their medication were reported among 1.5% of persons taking placebo and 1.9% of those taking isoniazid, a difference of only 0.4% attributable to the drug. In the trial among persons with inactive lesions, a much older group, medication was discontinued because of side effects among 3.8% of the placebo group and 6.6% of those given isoniazid. The side effect of principal concern is hepatitis. Rare among children, its incidence increases with age, reaching a level of 2–4% among persons 50–64 years of age.[124] Careful explanation of the early symptoms of hepatitis and monthly monitoring for these symptoms among persons on preventive treatment appear to markedly reduce the seriousness of this side effect.[125] Fears that the preventive use of isoniazid would lead to the emergence of isoniazid-resistant strains of tubercle bacilli have not been borne out.[63]

With increasing age, the lifetime risk of tuberculosis diminishes, while the risk of developing isoniazid-associated hepatitis increases.[68] As a result, current recommendations are that tuberculin reactors over 35 years of age should not be given preventive treatment unless there are additional indications.[99] These include (1) household or other close association with persons who have infectious tuberculosis; (2) presence of roentgenographic findings consistent with nonprogressive pulmonary tuberculosis with neither positive bacteriological findings nor history of adequate chemotherapy; (3) skin-test evidence of recent tuberculous infection; and (4) presence of special medical situations such as prolonged corticosteroid therapy, depressed immune status, diabetes mellitus, silicosis, or gastrectomy.

The cost of isoniazid preventive treatment, even with monthly monitoring of symptoms, is rarely a major consideration in developed countries in which the program is merely added to existing procedures in tuberculosis clinics. In countries with limited resources, however, it is reasonable to use scarce antituberculosis medications for prevention only after the needs of tuberculosis patients have been met.

Finally, noncompliance by physicians and patients is an impediment to preventive therapy. In 1993, in 99 areas reporting to the CDC, only 66% of tuberculosis contacts considered to be eligible for preventive therapy on the basis of exposure and a positive tuberculin test were actually started on preventive therapy. And in the preceding year, only 71% of those who had been started on a preventive regimen completed 6 months of therapy.[126,127]

9.5. Immunization

Immunization against tuberculosis is currently limited to the use of BCG (bacille Calmette–Guérin), an attenuated organism named for the two French investigators responsible for its development.[2] Working with *M. bovis* in 1908, they added bile to their culture media in an effort to obtain well-dispersed suspensions of the organisms. As an unexpected result, they noted that the organisms cultured in this way lost virulence for laboratory animals. After 13 years of subculturing and testing, they became convinced that they had developed a strain of organisms that would remain avirulent and could be used to immunize humans against tuberculosis.

BCG has probably had more, larger, and possibly better-controlled trials of its usefulness and effectiveness than almost any other preventive measure. Despite this, there is disagreement about its effectiveness. A meta-analysis of 15 of the 16 controlled trials of intracutaneous BCG vaccination concluded that the average efficacy was 50% (range: minus 56% to plus 80%).[128] It was concluded that much of the variability was due to latitude, a surrogate for the prevalence of nontuberculous mycobacterial infections, with the least protection at lower latitudes. Although the possibility was discounted that some of the variability in results might be associated with differences in BCG strains, characteristics of BCG vaccines can change with continued cultivation. To some, this seems a likely explanation for the marked differences observed among the results of various trials done around 1950 with different substrains of vaccines that were then more than 25 years removed from the original parent strain. With the lapse of 40 or more years since these trials, reliable information is lacking on the effectiveness of currently available strains. That some strains of BCG do differ in efficacy is indicated by the findings in each of two case–control studies of marked differences in effectiveness when one vaccine was substituted for another[129] and in a recent controlled trial of two different BCG strains.[130,131] Unfortunately, there is currently no way other than long-term studies to assess efficacy of BCG strains. Postvaccinal tuberculin sensitivity is not related to efficacy and animal models are unreliable.[129]

Because of uncertainties regarding the efficacy of most vaccines, the decision on the use of vaccination must depend in part on the availability of other means of tuberculosis control. In much of the world, the decision is not difficult. In countries with a very low infection rate, such as the United States, with a readily available alternative program of tuberculosis control by case-finding, chemotherapy, and preventive therapy, there is very little need for the kind of protection that vaccination can give and considerable reason to protect the usefulness of the tuberculin test.[132] As a result, BCG vaccination is recommended only for tuberculin-negative persons at a high risk of becoming infected for whom no other method of tuberculosis control is feasible. Its use is contraindicated in persons with or at high risk of being infected with HIV, because the vaccine can cause progressive disease in immunocompromised persons. In many other countries, there is clearly a high risk of infection and little prospect of effective control except by BCG vaccination. In such situations, vaccination programs must be continued, except among persons with known HIV infections. Preliminary tuberculin testing is not needed for vaccination of newborn infants. Nor is it necessary for vaccination programs aimed at older persons, since it has been shown that vaccination of tuberculin-positive persons and persons with tuberculosis did not result in demonstrable harm.[133]

The financial costs of vaccination are low. The vaccine is inexpensive, its administration is simple, and vaccination probably does not have to be repeated. Preliminary tuberculin testing is not needed, though it may occasionally be useful for epidemiological purposes. Serious complications are very uncommon.[14] However, vaccination does produce localized ulceration that can persist for several months and may be accompanied by local lymphadenopathy. A potentially important side effect is the production of sensitivity to tuberculin. In areas with a high risk of infection, most persons will become tuberculin reactors in the course of time, and the premature production of tuberculin sensitivity by vaccination is of little consequence. In areas with a low risk of infection, the help that the tuberculin test can give diagnostically and prognostically constitutes an added contraindication of BCG vaccination. Also in these areas, the reports of a long-term risk of lymphomas associated with vaccination in two of three trials should not be ignored.[131]

The role that effective immunization might play in the control of tuberculosis is also indicated by the model in Fig. 7. As was the case for case-finding and chemotherapy (Section 9.2), the effect of immunization is on step II, namely, protecting the uninfected population against development of disease when exposed to infectious cases. Universal application of a vaccine with 100% efficacy would not eradicate tuberculosis until all infected reactors had died.

10. Unresolved Problems

Perhaps the major problem in tuberculosis control today is the uncertainty about the efficacy of BCG strains in current use. Almost none of them have been tested at any time in a controlled trial. The few that have been so tested have been subcultured for many years, giving reason to doubt that the previous relative ranking of tested strains still reflects their present effectiveness. As was the case with pertussis vaccines in the 1950s, the only reliable resolution of the present uncertainties about BCG strains seems to lie in setting up controlled trials of the currently available strains among humans in areas of the world where the risk of infection is still sufficiently high to indicate a need for BCG vaccination and also high enough to yield an answer in a reasonable length of time.

In such trials, vaccinated persons need not be compared with randomly allocated unvaccinated controls. While such a design is scientifically desirable, it does not seem ethically or politically feasible. For practical purposes, a much simpler scheme should be useful and could be more widely applicable. If one vaccine could be used among newborn infants in odd years and a second in even years, subsequent comparisons of case rates among children born in odd and even years should at least distinguish between strains with markedly different efficacies. Less valid but more acceptable evaluations can be made by observational studies, case–control or prospective, in areas where the vaccine strain being used has changed in recent years. In such settings, the biases inherent in observational studies should affect the estimated efficacy of each strain similarly, and thus have little effect on estimates of their relative potencies. Several such studies might allow a number of BCG vaccines to be ranked in the order of their potency, thereby providing data with which to identify reliable animal test systems. Once such a test system was found, objective ratings of BCG vaccines could be done.

Another major need, though perhaps much more difficult to solve, is to develop a test that would identify infected persons who still harbor living tubercle bacilli. The present tuberculin skin test and serological tests fail on two counts: (1) positive reactions can be caused by mycobacteria other than *M. tuberculosis* or *M. bovis*, and (2) reactions from a tuberculous infection may persist long after the infecting organisms have succumbed to the host's defenses. Improvement of the tests on either count would make both diagnosis and preventive therapy much more efficient.

Very little is known of factors that influence the probability that tuberculous infection will progress to manifest tuberculous disease either with or without a prolonged latent period. The long-held belief that malnutrition and alcoholism are risk factors for tuberculous disease, while probably correct, is supported only by uncontrolled observations. Even the risk associated with diabetes is poorly established. From the point of view of local tuberculosis control, it would be very helpful to know much more about the characteristics of tuberculosis patients. How many have had previous evidence of tuberculous infection or disease? What caused them to come to medical attention? What are their usual occupations? What about their diet and lifestyle? Some of the simplest facts about tuberculosis cases are essentially unknown, but can be collected with attention to careful and consistent history-taking.[135]

Although both chemotherapy and preventive therapy can be highly successful, the long duration of treatment required and the frequency of unpleasant side effects make it difficult to achieve high levels of adherence even with supervision by adequate numbers of dedicated personnel. Although the need for more rapidly effective and less toxic drugs is tremendous throughout the world, the inability of most persons who need these drugs to pay for them will require that the necessary pharmacological research be supported by public funds rather than by private capital.

In one sense, the possibility of a high prevalence of drug-resistant tuberculosis in many countries is not a problem. How to prevent tubercle bacilli from becoming resistant has been known for decades. Conscientious completion of an effective drug regimen has always kept the emergence of drug-resistant organisms to an acceptable minimum. In another sense, it is a major and increasing threat to tuberculosis control programs throughout the world. The problem is basically financial and administrative. Where tuberculosis treatment is provided by private physicians who do not use standard regimens, who care for patients only as long as they can pay, or where it is provided by public sources that provide drugs to treatment centers on a sporadic basis, adequate treatment programs are unlikely to be completed. The resultant irregular or ineffective treatment allows drug-resistant organisms to emerge, to spread to others, and to be treatable only in the most economically favored countries. That this situation has been tolerated for decades when it essentially could have been eradicated by the investment of a tiny fraction of the world's military budgets in effective, directly observed treatment programs is a sad commentary on humanity's priorities.

From a global perspective, the pandemic of infections with HIV, particularly in sub-Saharan Africa and Southeast Asia where tuberculous infections are prevalent, has raised a host of problems. These include strategies to deal with a great increase in numbers of patients when resources are stagnant or shrinking, development of methods to diagnose the increasing proportion of tuberculosis patients whose sputum does not contain sufficient organisms to be demonstrable on microscopic examination, whether or not to use thiacetazone in the face of increasing toxicity, and the feasibility of preventive therapy and its duration for persons infected with HIV.

11. References

1. Kochi, A., The global tuberculosis situation and the new control strategy of the World Health Organization, *Tubercle* **71:**1–6 (1991).
2. Dubos, R., and Dubos, J., *The White Plague. Tuberculosis, Man and Society*, Little, Brown and Company, Boston, 1952.
3. Lowell, A. M., Edwards, L. B., and Palmer, C. E., *Tuberculosis*, Harvard University Press, Cambridge, MA, 1969.
4. Evans, A. S., *Causation and Disease. A Chronological Journey*, Plenum Press, New York, 1993.
5. Heifets, L. B., and Good, R. C., Current laboratory methods for the diagnosis of tuberculosis, in: (B. T. Bloom, ed.), pp. 85–110, *Tuberculosis. Pathogenesis, Protection, and Control*, ASM Press, Washington, DC, 1994.
6. Daley, C. L., Small, P. M., Schechter, G. F., *et al.*, An outbreak of tuberculosis with accelerated progression among persons infected with the human immunodeficiency virus. An analysis using restriction-fragment-length polymorphisms, *N. Engl. J. Med.* **326:**231–235 (1992).
7. Genewein, A., Telenti, A., Bernasconi, C., *et al.*, Molecular approach to identifying route of transmission in the community, *Lancet* **342:** 841–844 (1993).
8. Centers for Disease Control, A strategic plan for the elimination of tuberculosis in the United States, *Morbid. Mortal. Week. Rep.* **38**(Suppl. S-3)**:**1–25 (1989).
9. Centers for Disease Control and Prevention, Division of Tuberculosis Elimination, *Tuberculosis Statistics in the United States, 1992*, Centers for Disease Control and Prevention, Atlanta, 1994.
10. Lowell, A. M., *Tuberculosis in the World*, HEW Publication Number (CDC) 76-8317, US Government Printing Office, Washington, DC, 1976.
11. Styblo, K., and Rouillon, A., Estimated global incidence of smear-positive pulmonary tuberculosis. Unreliability of officially reported figures on tuberculosis, *Bull. Int. Union Tuberc.* **56**(No. 3–4)**:**118–126 (1981).
12. Sudre, P., ten Dam, G., and Kochi, A., Tuberculosis: A global overview of the situation today, *Bull. WHO* **70:**149–159 (1992).

13. Armstrong, D. B., Four years of the Framingham Demonstration, *Am. Rev. Tuberc.* **4**:908–919 (1921).
14. de Abreau, M., and de Paula, A., *Roentgenfotografia*, Livraria Ateneu, Rio de Janeiro, 1940.
15. Jarman, T. F., A follow-up tuberculin survey in the Rhondda Fach, *Br. Med. J.* **2**:1235–1239 (1955).
16. Kaplan, G. J., Fraser, R. I., and Comstock, G. W., Tuberculosis in Alaska, 1970. The continued decline of the tuberculosis epidemic, *Am. Rev. Respir. Dis.* **105**:920–926 (1972).
17. Sartwell, P. E., Moseley, C. H., and Long, E. R., Tuberculosis in the German population, United States Zone of Germany, *Am. Rev. Tuberc.* **59**:481–493 (1949).
18. Magnus, K., Epidemiological basis of tuberculosis eradication. 6. Tuberculin sensitivity after human and bovine infection, *Bull. WHO* **36**:719–731 (1967).
19. Edwards, L. B., Comstock, G. W., and Palmer, C. E., Contributions of northern populations to the understanding of tuberculin sensitivity, *Arch. Environ. Health* **17**:507–516 (1968).
20. Edwards, L. B., Acquaviva, F. A., Livesay, V. T., *et al.*, An atlas of sensitivity to tuberculin, PPD-B, and histoplasmin in the United States, *Am. Rev. Respir. Dis.* **99**(4):Part 2 (1969).
21. Edwards, L. B., Livesay, V. T., Acquaviva, F. A., *et al.*, Height, weight, tuberculous infection, and tuberculous disease, *Arch. Environ. Health* **22**:106–112 (1971).
22. Edwards, L. B., Acquaviva, F. A., and Livesay, V. T., Identification of tuberculous infected. Dual tests and density of reaction, *Am. Rev. Respir. Dis.* **108**:1334–1339 (1973).
23. Kubica, G. P., Clinical microbiology, in: *The Mycobacteria. A Sourcebook.* (G. P. Kubica and L. G. Wayne, eds.), pp. 133–175, Marcel Dekker, New York, 1984.
24. Cave, M. D., Eisenach, K. D., McDermott, P. F., *et al.*, Conservation of sequence in the *Mycobacterium tuberculosis* complex and its utilization in DNA fingerprinting, *Mol. Cell. Probes* **5**:73–80 (1991).
25. Daniel, T. M., and Debanne, S. M., The serodiagnosis of tuberculosis and other mycobacterial diseases by enzyme-linked immunosorbent assay, *Am. Rev. Respir. Dis.* **135**:1137–1151 (1987).
26. Zou, Y. L., Zhang, J. D., Chen, M. H., *et al.*, Serological analysis of pulmonary and extrapulmonary tuberculosis with enzyme-linked immunosorbent assays for anti-A60 immunoglobulins, *Clin. Infect. Dis.* **19**:1084–1091 (1994).
27. American Thoracic Society, The tuberculin skin test, *Am. Rev. Respir. Dis.* **124**:356–363 (1981).
28. Bleiker, M. A., Sutherland, I., Styblo, K., *et al.*, Guidelines for estimating the risks of tuberculosis infection from tuberculin test results in a representative sample of children, *Bull. Int. Union Tuberc.* **64**(No.2):7–12 (1989).
29. American Thoracic Society, Diagnostic standards and classification of tuberculosis, *Am. Rev. Respir. Dis.* **142**:725–735 (1989).
30. Nissen Meyer, S., Hougen, A., and Edwards, P., Experimental error in the determination of tuberculin sensitivity, *Public Health Rep.* **63**:561–569 (1951).
31. Snider, D. E., Jr., and Cauthen, G. M., Tuberculin skin testing of hospital employees: Infection, "boosting," and two-step testing, *Am. J. Infect. Control* **12**:305–311 (1984).
32. Frost, W. H., How much control of tuberculosis? *Am. J. Public Health* **27**:759–766 (1937).
33. Horwitz, O., Edwards, P. Q., and Lowell, A. M., National tuberculosis control program in Denmark and the United States, *Health Serv. Rep.* **88**:493–498 (1973).
34. Rust, P., and Thomas, J., A method for estimating the prevalence of tuberculous infection, *Am. J. Epidemiol.* **101**:311–322 (1975).
35. National Tuberculosis Institute, Bangalore, Tuberculosis in a rural population of South India: A five-year epidemiological study, *Bull. WHO* **51**:473–488 (1974).
36. Pust, R. E., Onejeme, S. E., and Okafor, S. N., Tuberculosis survey in East Central State, Nigeria: Implications for tuberculosis programme development, *Trop. Geogr. Med.* **26**:51–57 (1974).
37. Tuberculosis Prevention Trial, Madras, Trial of BCG vaccines in South India for tuberculosis prevention, *Indian J. Med. Res.* **72**(Suppl.):1–74 (1980).
38. Nyboe, J., Interpretation of tuberculosis infection age curves, *Bull. WHO* **17**:319–339 (1957).
39. Sutherland, I., and Fayers, P. M., The association of the risk of tuberculous infection with age, *Bull. Int. Union Tuberc.* **50**:70–81 (1975).
40. Sutherland, I., Styblo, K., Sampalik, M., *et al.*, Annual risks of tuberculous infection in 14 countries, derived from the results of tuberculin surveys in 1948–1952, *Bull. Int. Union Tuberc.* **45**:75–114 (1971).
41. Fayers, P. M., and Barnett, G. D., The risk of tuberculous infection in Saskatchewan, *Bull. Int. Union Tuberc.* **50**:62–69 (1975).
42. Waaler, H., Galtung, O., and Mordal, K., The risk of tuberculous infection in Norway, *Bull. Int. Union Tuberc.* **50**:5–61 (1975).
43. Comstock, G. W., and Sartwell, P. E., Tuberculosis studies in Muscogee County, Georgia. IV. Evaluation of a communitywide X-ray survey on the basis of six years of observation, *Am. J. Hyg.* **61**:261–285 (1955).
44. Hyge, T. V., The efficacy of BCG vaccination, *Acta Tuberc. Scand.* **32**:89–107 (1956).
45. Houk, V. N., Baker, J. H., Sorensen, K., *et al.*, The epidemiology of tuberculosis infection in a closed environment, *Arch. Environ. Health* **16**:26–35 (1968).
46. VonVille, P., Holtzhauer, F., Long, T., *et al.*, Tuberculosis among residents of shelters for the homeless—Ohio, 1990, *Morbid. Mortal. Week. Rep.* **40**:869–877 (1991).
47. Sultan, L., Nyka, W., Mills, C., *et al.*, Tuberculosis disseminators. A study of the variability of aerial infectivity of tuberculous patients, *Am. Rev. Respir. Dis.* **82**:358–369 (1960).
48. Comstock, G. W., Frost revisited: The modern epidemiology of tuberculosis, *Am. J. Epidemiol.* **101**:363–382 (1975).
49. Kamat, S. R., Dawson, J. J. Y., Devadatta, S., *et al.*, A controlled study of the influence of segregation of tuberculous patients for one year on the attack rate of tuberculosis in a 5-year period in close family contacts in South India, *Bull. WHO* **34**:517–532 (1966).
50. Centers for Disease Control, Nosocomial transmission of multidrug-resistant tuberculosis among HIV-infected persons—Florida and New York, 1988–1991, *Morbid. Mortal. Week. Rep.* **40**:585–591 (1991).
51. Holland, W. W., *European Atlas of "Avoidable Death,"* 1985–1989, CEC Health Services Research Series No. 9, Oxford University Press, Oxford, England, for The Council of European Communities, 1997.
52. Horwitz, O., and Comstock, G. W., What is a case of tuberculosis? The tuberculosis case spectrum in eight countries evaluated from 1235 case histories and roentgenograms, *Int. J. Epidemiol.* **2**:145–152 (1973).
53. Centers for Disease Control and Prevention, Division of Tuberculosis Elimination, Reported tuberculosis in the United States, 1996, Centers for Disease Control and Prevention, Atlanta, 1997.
54. Centers for Disease Control and Prevention, Tuberculosis statistics in the United States, 1992, National Center for Prevention Services, Atlanta, 1994.

55. Cross, E. R., and Hyams, K. C., Tuberculin skin testing in US Navy and Marine Corps personnel and recruits, 1980–1986, *Am. J. Public Health* **80:**435–438 (1990).
56. Comstock, G. W., Isoniazid prophylaxis in an undeveloped area, *Am. Rev. Respir. Dis.* **86:**810–822 (1962).
57. Comstock, G. W., Variability of tuberculosis trends in a time of resurgence, *Clin. Infect. Dis.* **19:**1015–1022 (1994).
58. Chaulk, C. P., Moore-Rice, K., Rizzo, R., *et al.*, Eleven years of community-based directly observed therapy for tuberculosis, *J. Am. Med. Assoc.* **274:**945–951 (1955).
59. Frieden, T. R., Fujiwara, P. I., Washko, R. M., *et al.*, Tuberculosis in New York City—Turning the tide, *N. Engl. J. Med.* **333:**229–233 (1955).
60. Raviglione, M. C., Sudre, P., Rieder, H. L., *et al.*, Secular trends of tuberculosis in Western Europe, *Bull. WHO* **71:**297–306 (1993).
61. Raviglione, M. C., Rieder, H. L., Styblo, K., *et al.*, Tuberculosis trends in Eastern Europe and the former USSR, *Tuberc. Lung Dis.* **75:**400–416 (1994).
62. Dolin, P. J., Raviglione, M. C., and Kochi, A., Global tuberculosis incidence and mortality during 1990–2000, *Bull. WHO* **72:**213–220 (1994).
63. Ferebee, S. H., Controlled chemoprophylaxis trials in tuberculosis. A general review, *Adv. Tuberc. Res.* **17:**28–106 (1970).
64. Reichman, L. B., and O'Day, R., Tuberculous infection in a large urban population, *Am. Rev. Respir. Dis.* **117:**705–712 (1978).
65. Raj Narain, Nair, S. S., Chandrasekhar, P., *et al.*, Problems associated with estimating the incidence of tuberculosis infection, *Bull. WHO* **34:**605–622 (1966).
66. Comstock, G. W., Livesay, V. T., and Woolpert, S. F., The prognosis of a positive tuberculin reaction in childhood and adolescence, *Am. J. Epidemiol.* **99:**131–138 (1974).
67. Comstock, G. W., Livesay, V. T., and Woolpert, S. F., Evaluation of BCG vaccination among Puerto Rican children, *Am. J. Public Health* **64:**283–291 (1974).
68. Horwitz, O., Wilbek, E., and Erickson, P. A., Epidemiological basis of tuberculosis eradication. 10. Longitudinal studies on the risk of tuberculosis in the general population of a low-prevalence area, *Bull. WHO* **41:**95–113 (1969).
69. Comstock, G. W., and Edwards, P. Q., The competing risks of tuberculosis and hepatitis for adult tuberculin reactors, *Am. Rev. Respir. Dis.* **111:**573–577 (1975).
70. Comstock, G. W., Edwards, L. B., and Livesay, V. T., Tuberculosis morbidity in the US Navy: Its distribution and decline, *Am. Rev. Respir. Dis.* **110:**572–580 (1974).
71. Powell, K. E., Brown, E. D., and Farer, L. S., Tuberculosis among Indochinese refugees in the United States, *J. Am. Med. Assoc.* **249:**1455–1460 (1983).
72. Perez-Stable, E. J., Slutkin, G., Pax, E. A., *et al.*, Tuberculin reactivity in United States and foreign-born Latinos: Results of a community-based screening program, *Am. J. Public Health* **76:** 643–646 (1986).
73. Cantwell, M. F., Snider, D. E., Jr., Cauthen, G. M., *et al.*, Epidemiology of tuberculosis in the United States, 1985 through 1992, *J. Am. Med. Assoc.* **272:**535–539 (1994).
74. Medical Research Council, Tuberculosis and Chest Diseases Unit, National survey of notificatons of tuberculosis in England and Wales in 1983, *Br. Med. J.* **291:**658–661 (1985).
75. Froggett, K., Tuberculosis: Spatial and demographic incidence in Bradford, 1980–2, *J. Epidemiol. Community Health* **39:**20–26 (1985).
76. Centers for Disease Control and Prevention, Proportionate mortality from pulmonary tuberculosis associated with occupations—28 states, 1979–1990, *Morbid. Mortal. Week. Rep.* **44:** 14–19 (1995).
77. Chan, J. C., and Tabak, J. I., Risk of tuberculous infection among house staff in an urban teaching hospital, *South. Med. J.* **78:**1061–1064 (1985).
78. Cowie, R. L., The epidemiology of tuberculosis in gold miners with silicosis, *Am. J. Respir. Crit. Care Med.* **150:**1460–1462 (1994).
79. Ruben, F. L., Norden, C. W., and Schuster, A., Analysis of a community hospital employee tuberculosis screening program 31 months after its inception, *Am. Rev. Respir. Dis.* **115:**23–28 (1977).
80. Stead, W. W., Undetected tuberculosis in prison, *J. Am. Med. Assoc.* **240:**2544–2547 (1978).
81. Hoch, D. E., and Wilcox, K. R., Jr., Transmission of multidrug-resistant tuberculosis from an HIV-positive client in a residential substance-abuse treatment facility—Michigan, *Morbid. Mortal. Week. Rep.* **40:**129–131 (1991).
82. Stead, W. W., Lofgren, J. P., Warren, E., *et al.*, Tuberculosis as an endemic and nosocomial infection among the elderly in nursing homes, *N. Engl. J. Med.* **312:**1483–1487 (1985).
83. Daniels, M., Ridehalgh, F., Springett, V. H., *et al.*, *Tuberculosis in Young Adults: Report on the Prophit Tuberculosis Survey, 1936–1944*, H. K. Lewis, London, 1948.
84. Grzybowski, S., Barnett, G. D., and Styblo, K., Contacts of cases of active tuberculosis, *Bull. Int. Union Tuberc.* **50:**90–106 (1975).
85. Chaves, A. D., Robins, A. B., and Abeles, H., Tuberculosis case finding among homeless men in New York City, *Am. Rev. Respir. Dis.* **84:**900–901 (1961).
86. Horwitz, O., Tuberculosis risk and marital status, *Am. Rev. Respir. Dis.* **104:**22–31 (1971).
87. Kuemmerer, J. M., and Comstock, G. W., Sociologic concomitants of tuberculin sensitivity, *Am. Rev. Respir. Dis.* **96:**885–892 (1967).
88. Kielmann, A. A., Oberoi, I. S., Chandra, R. K., *et al.*, The effect of nutritional status on immune capacity and immune responses in preschool children in a rural community in India, *Bull. WHO* **54:**477–483 (1976).
89. Luri, M. B., *Resistance to Tuberculosis: Experimental Studies in Native and Acquired Defensive Mechanisms*, pp. 115–180, Harvard University Press, Cambridge, MA, 1984.
90. Puffer, R. R., *Familial Susceptibility to Tuberculosis*, Harvard University Press, Cambridge, MA, 1944.
91. Comstock, G. W., Tuberculosis in twins: A re-analysis of the Prophit survey, *Am. Rev. Respir. Dis.* **117:**621–624 (1978).
92. Overfield, T., and Klauber, M. R., Prevalence of tuberculosis in Eskimos having blood group B gene, *Hum. Biol.* **52**(1):87–92 (1980).
93. Sunderam, G., McDonald, R. J., Maniatis, T., *et al.*, Tuberculosis as a manifestation of the acquired immunodeficiency syndrome, *J. Am. Med. Assoc.* **256:**362–366 (1986).
94. Hopewell, P. C., Impact of human immunodeficiency virus infection on the epidemiology, clinical features, management, and control of tuberculosis, *Clin. Infect. Dis.* **15:**540–547 (1992).
95. Narain, J. P., Raviglione, M. C., and Kochi, A., HIV-associated tuberculosis in developing countries: Epidemiology and strategies for prevention, *Tuberc. Lung Dis.* **73:**311–321 (1992).
96. Selwyn, P. A., Hartel, D., Lewis, V. A., *et al.*, A prospective study of the risk of tuberculosis among intravenous drug users with

human immunodeficiency virus infection, *N. Engl. J. Med.* **320:**545–550 (1989).

97. Braun, M., Badi, N., Ryder, R. W., *et al.*, A retrospective cohort study of the risk of tuberculosis among women of childbearing age with HIV infection in Zaire, *Am. Rev. Respir. Dis.* **143:**501–504 (1991).
98. Allen, S., Batungwanayo, J., Kerlekowske, K., *et al.*, Two-year incidence of tuberculosis in cohorts of HIV-infected and uninfected Rwandan Women, *Am. Rev. Respir. Dis.* **146:**1439–1444 (1992).
99. American Thoracic Society, Treatment of tuberculosis and tuberculosis infection in adults and children, *Am. Rev. Respir. Dis.* **134:**355–363 (1986).
100. Centers for Disease Control, Purified protein derivative (PPD)-tuberculin anergy and HIV infection: Guidelines for anergy testing and management of anergic persons at risk of tuberculosis, *Morbid. Mortal. Week. Rep.* **40**(No. RR-5)**:**27–33 (1991).
101. Myers, J. A., *Tuberculosis: A Half Century of Study and Conquest*, pp. 222–241, Warren H. Green, St. Louis, 1970.
102. Anonymous, Clinicopathological Conference, Case 12-1963, *N. Engl. J. Med.* **268:**378–385 (1963).
103. Stead, W. W., Management of health care workers after inadvertent exposure to tuberculosis: A guide to the use of preventive therapy, *Ann. Intern. Med.* **122:**906–912 (1995).
104. Graham, N. M. H., and Chaisson, R. E., Tuberculosis and HIV infection: Epidemiology, pathogenesis, and clinical aspects, *Ann. Allergy* **71:**421–430 (1993).
105. Comstock, G. W., False tuberculin test results, *Chest* **68S:**465S–469S (1975).
106. Sbarbaro, J., Skin test antigens: An evaluation whose time has come, *Am. Rev. Respir. Dis.* **118:**1–5 (1978).
107. World Health Organization, Tuberculosis Research Office, Further studies of geographic variation in naturally acquired tuberculin sensitivity, *Bull. WHO* **22:**63–83 (1955).
108. Ferebee, S. H., An epidemiological model of tuberculosis in the United States, *Bull. Nat. Tuberc. Assoc.* **53:**4–7 (1967).
109. Centers for Disease Control, Tuberculosis Control Division, Guidelines for Prevention of TB in Hospitals, Centers for Disease Control, Atlanta, 1983.
110. Addington, W. W., Albert, R. K., Bass, J. B., Jr., *et al.*, Non-drug issues related to the treatment of tuberculosis, *Chest* **87**(2)**:**125S–127S (1985).
111. Adal, K. A., Anglim, A. M., Palumbo, C. L., *et al.*, The use of high-efficiency particulate air-filter respirators to protect hospital workers from tuberculosis, *N. Engl. J. Med.* **331:**169–173 (1994).
112. Centers for Disease Control and Prevention, Division of Tuberculosis Elimination, Tuberculosis Management Report, Drug Therapy, 1/1/92 through 12/31/92, Centers for Disease Control, Atlanta.
113. Grzybowski, S., Technical and operational appraisal of tuberculosis case-finding methods, in: *II. Regional Seminar on Tuberculosis*, Scientific Publ. No. 265, pp. 50–56, Pan American Health Organization, Washington, DC, 1973.
114. Anderson, S., and Banerji, D., A sociological inquiry into an urban tuberculosis control programme in India, *Bull. WHO* **29:**685–700 (1963).
115. Curry, F. J., District clinics for out-patient treatment of tuberculosis problem patients, *Dis. Chest* **46:**524–530 (1964).
116. Sumartojo, E., When tuberculosis treatment fails. A social behavioral account of patient adherence, *Am. Rev. Respir. Dis.* **147:** 1311–1320 (1993).
117. Wilkinson, D., High-compliance tuberculosis treatment progamme in a rural community, *Lancet* **343:**647–648 (1994).
118. Comstock, G. W., and Woolpert, S. F., Preventive therapy, in: *The Mycobacteria: A Sourcebook* (G. P. Kubica and L. W. Wayne, eds.), pp. 1071–1082, Marcel Dekker, New York, 1984.
119. Pape, J. W., Jean, S. S., Ho, J. L., *et al.*, Effect of isoniazid prophylaxis on incidence of active tuberculosis and progression of HIV infection, *Lancet* **342:**268–272 (1993).
120. Palmer, C. E., Ferebee, S. H., and Hopwood, L., Studies on prevention of experimental tuberculosis with isoniazid. II. Effects of different dosage regimens, *Am. Rev. Respir. Dis.* **74:**917–939 (1956).
121. Comstock, G. W., Baum, C., and Snider, D. E., Jr., Isoniazid prophylaxis among Alaskan Eskimos: A final report of the Bethel isoniazid studies, *Am. Rev. Respir. Dis.* **119:**827–830 (1979).
122. International Union Against Tuberculosis Committee on Prophylaxis, Efficacy of various durations of isoniazid preventive therapy for tuberculosis: Five years of follow-up in the IUAT trial, *Bull. WHO* **60:**555–564 (1982).
123. Comstock, G. W., and Ferebee, S. H., How much isoniazid is needed for prophylaxis? *Am. Rev. Respir. Dis.* **101:**780–782 (1970).
124. Kopanoff, D. E., Snider, D. E., Jr., and Caras, G. J., Isoniazid-related hepatitis. A US Public Health Service cooperative surveillance study, *Am. Rev. Respir. Dis.* **117:**991–1001 (1978).
125. Dash, L. A., Comstock, G. W., and Flynn, J. P. G., Isoniazid preventive therapy. Retrospect and prospect. *Am. Rev. Respir. Dis.* **121:**1039–1044 (1980).
126. Centers for Disease Control and Prevention, Division of Tuberculosis Elimination, Tuberculosis Program Management Report, Completion of Preventive Therapy, 1/1/92 through 12/31/92, Centers for Disease Control, Atlanta.
127. Centers for Disease Control and Prevention, Division of Tuberculosis Elimination, Tuberculosis Program Management Report, Contact Follow-up, 1/1/93 to 12/31/93, Centers for Disease Control, Atlanta.
128. Colditz, G. A., Brewer, T. F., Berkey, C. S., *et al.*, Efficacy of BCG vaccine in the prevention of tuberculosis. Meta-analysis of the published literature, *J. Am. Med. Assoc.* **271:**698–702 (1994).
129. Comstock, G. W., Identification of an effective vaccine against tuberculosis, *Am. Rev. Respir. Dis.* **138:**479–480 (1988).
130. Ten Dam, H. G., BCG vaccination, in: *Tuberculosis. A Comprehensive International Approach* (L. B. Reichman and E. S. Hershfield, eds.), pp. 264–266, Marcel Dekker, New York, 1993.
131. Comstock, G. W., Field trials of tuberculosis vaccines: How could we have done them better? *Controlled Clin. Trials* **15:**247–276 (1994).
132. Centers for Disease Control, Use of BCG vaccine in the control of tuberculosis: A joint statement by the ACIP and the Advisory Committee for Elimination of Tuberculosis, *Morbid. Mortal. Week. Rep.* **37:**663–675 (1988).
133. Raj Narain, and Vallishayee, R. S., BCG vaccination of tuberculosis patients and of strong reactors to tuberculin, *Bull. Int. Union Tuberc.* **51:**243–246 (1976).
134. Lotte, A., Wasz-Höckert, O., Poisson, N., *et al.*, BCG complications. Estimate of the risks among vaccinated subjects and statistical analysis of their main characteristics, *Adv. Tuberc. Res.* **21:**107–193 (1984).
135. Buskin, S. E., Gale, J. L., Weiss, N. S., *et al.*, Tuberculosis risk factors in adults in King County, Washington, 1988 through 1990, *Am. J. Public Health* **84:**1750–1756 (1994).

12. Suggested Reading

American Thoracic Society, Treatment of tuberculosis and tuberculosis infection in adults and children, *Am. J. Respir. Crit. Care Med.* **149:**1359–1374 (1994).

Centers for Disease Control, A strategic plan for the elimination of tuberculosis in the United States, *Morbid. Mortal. Week. Rep.* **38** (Suppl no. S-3)**:**1–25 (1989).

Dubos, R., and Dubos, J., *The White Plague: Tuberculosis, Man and Society*, Little Brown, Boston, 1952.

Edwards, P. Q., and Edwards, L. B., Story of the tuberculin test from an epidemiological viewpoint, *Am. Rev. Respir. Dis.* **81**(1)**:**Part 2 (1960).

Enarson, D. A., Rieder, H. L., Arnadottir, T., and Tribucq, A., *Tuberculosis Guide for Low Income Countries*, 4th ed., International Union Against Tuberculosis and Lung Disease, Frankfurt, Germany, 1994.

Frost, W. H., How much control of tuberculosis? *Am. J. Public Health* **27:**759–766 (1937).

Ferebee, S. H., Controlled chemoprophylaxis trials in tuberculosis: A general review, *Adv. Tuberc. Res.* **17:**28–106 (1970).

O'Reilly, L. M., and Daborn, C. J., The epidemiology of *Mycobacterium bovis* infections in animals and man: A review, *Tuber. Lung Dis.* **76** (Suppl. 1)**:**1–46 (1995).

Sumartojo, E., When tuberculosis treatment fails. A social behavioral account of patient adherence, *Am. Rev. Respir. Dis.* **147:**1311–1320 (1993).

Supplement on future research in tuberculosis. Prospects and priorities for elimination, *Am. Rev. Respir. Dis.* **134:**401–423 (1986).

Thompson, N. J., Glassroth, J. H., Snider, D. E., Jr., *et al.*, The booster phenomenon in serial tuberculin testing, *Am. Rev. Respir. Dis.* **119:** 587–597 (1979).

CHAPTER 40

Nontuberculous Mycobacterial Disease

Richard J. O'Brien and David L. Cohn

1. Introduction

Nomenclature for mycobacteria other than tuberculosis (MOTT) and leprosy and their associated diseases has not been entirely satisfactory and has varied considerably. The etiologic organisms have been called MOTT bacilli by mycobacteriologists and atypical mycobacteria by clinicians, with other designations such as anonymous, environmental, opportunistic, and unclassified mycobacteria also used. The diseases they cause have been given names such as nontuberculous mycobacteriosis, pseudotuberculosis, tuberculoidosis, and tuberculosis caused by a specified organism. To quote from the review by Wolinsky,[1] "None of the proposed names is without criticism, but the most appropriate and least offensive, in my opinion, is nontuberculous mycobacteriosis" (p. 110). This designation appears to have gained common acceptance and will be used in this chapter.

2. Historical Background

Tuberculosis in birds had been described several years prior to Robert Koch's report in 1882 on the isolation of the human tubercle bacillus, and many mycobacteria were identified in water, soil, vegetation, and a variety of other animals shortly thereafter. As these mycobacteria did not cause characteristic disease when inoculated into guinea pigs, they were recognized as distinct from *Mycobacterium tuberculosis* and were not believed to cause human disease. Because of the difficulties in isolation and identification by routine laboratory procedures and because of the much greater frequency of tuberculosis, little attention was paid to their pathogenic potential despite sporadic reports of human disease caused by a variety of nontuberculous mycobacteria during the first half of this century.[2,3] In the second half of the century, routine culturing for mycobacteria became commonplace and biochemical techniques for identification were developed, thus allowing the various species of mycobacteria to be more easily recognized. As tuberculosis in industrialized countries became much less common, the infrequent disease caused by nontuberculous mycobacteria came to comprise an increasingly larger proportion of illnesses caused by mycobacteria in developed countries.

In the 1950s, pulmonary disease due to nontuberculous mycobacteria became more commonly recognized and was found to comprise 1–2% of admissions to tuberculosis sanatoriums in the southeastern United States.[4] A paper by Timpe and Runyon[5] in 1954, classifying these "atypical" mycobacteria into four groups based on simple cultural characteristics, marked the upsurge in interest in nontuberculous mycobacteria. This scheme includes the photochromogens (group I), which develop yellow or orange pigment when exposed to light; the scotochromogens (group II), which form orange–yellow pigment in the dark; the nonchromogens (group III), which are essentially unpigmented; and the rapid growers (group IV), which grow on artificial culture media within 1 week, as distinguished from the slow-growing mycobacteria, which usually take 3 to 6 weeks to appear. Although the

Richard J. O'Brien • Division of Tuberculosis Elimination, National Center for HIV, STD, and TB Prevention, Centers for Disease Control and Prevention, Atlanta, Georgia 30333. **David L. Cohn** • Denver Disease Control Service, University of Colorado Health Sciences Center, Denver, Colorado 80204.

Runyon classification was widely used, more recently it has been replaced by classification based on disease presentation and mycobacterial species.[6] Those nontuberculous mycobacteria that have been associated with disease in man are listed in Table 1 by primary disease type. Saprophyticmycobacteria that may be isolated from man but are not known to cause disease are not listed.

The ability to recognize infections caused by nontuberculous mycobacteria by skin testing developed much later than their bacteriological identification and is still primarily a research tool. This capability and much of the ensuing information about these infections came almost entirely from the work of Palmer and his colleagues. The seed for this research was apparently planted in a conference convened to discuss the differing results obtained from a variety of tuberculin skin test antigens and the poor correlation of two signs once thought to be pathognomonic of tuberculous infection: tuberculin hypersensitivity and pulmonary calcification.[7] The first convincing evidence that infections other than those by *M. tuberculosis* or *M. bovis* caused tuberculin sensitivity came from a study of 10,058 student nurses in the United States conducted between 1943 and 1947.[8] Subsequent skin-testing studies with antigens from a variety of mycobacteria[9] in large numbers of subjects including over 600,000 Navy recruits,[10] and in locations from the tropics to the Arctic,[11,12] showed that infections with nontuberculous mycobacteria are very common, in marked contrast to the infrequency of disease.

More recently, there has been a resurgence of interest in nontuberculous mycobacterial diseases due to the finding of disseminated mycobacteriosis due to *M. avium* complex, as well as other nontuberculous mycobacteria, among large numbers of patients with the acquired immunodeficiency syndrome (AIDS).[13–17] This has occurred at a time when better understanding of the epidemiology of nontuberculous mycobacteria and advances in molecular biology and genetics have substantially increased our knowledge about these organisms.

3. Methodology

3.1. Sources of Mortality Data

Information on mortality has been available only since 1968, when nontuberculous mycobacterioses were first given a separate rubric in the eighth revision of the International Classification of Diseases. However, even the tenth revision in 1992 does not permit listing the diseases by the infecting mycobacterial species, and with the exception of pulmonary and cutaneous disease does not provide for coding the site of disease. Moreover, these diseases are seldom designated as an underlying cause of death, and thus information from death certificates is of limited usefulness. A national registry of AIDS patients in the United States has provided some information on mortality from disseminated *M. avium* complex disease.[18]

3.2. Sources of Morbidity Data

These diseases are not reportable in most states or in other countries throughout the world. A rough estimate of their relative frequency may be obtained by comparing the relative frequency of isolations of *M. tuberculosis* and nontuberculous mycobacteria by large bacteriology laboratories, although, unlike tuberculosis, isolation of nontuberculous mycobacteria is not sufficient for the diagnosis of disease. There have been several reports from various states[19,20] and similar national reports of patients with nontuberculous mycobacterial disease.[18,21,22] While such reports are useful in better describing the occurrence of these diseases, they do not provide reliable information on which to base estimates of disease incidence and prevalence.

3.3. Surveys

Skin-testing surveys with two or more antigens, one of which is almost always a standardized purified tuberculin prepared from *M. tuberculosis*, have been widely used. The results indicate the extent of infections with nontuberculous mycobacteria, but not which organism or organisms are responsible for the skin test reactions (see Section 3.4.2 for interpretation of skin tests). Very few sputum surveys have been done. They show the extent to which persons harbor these organisms in their oral or respiratory secretions, but do not indicate the frequency of persons with disease.

3.4. Laboratory Diagnosis

3.4.1. Isolation and Identification of the Organisms. Presumptive diagnosis of mycobacterial disease is often accomplished by acid-fast microscopy of body fluids or tissues. However, nontuberculous mycobacteria cannot be differentiated from *M. tuberculosis* by microscopy. The organisms can be isolated from body fluids and tissues by the same procedures used for the isolation of tubercle bacilli. A variety of biochemical tests, generally performed by reference laboratories, are required to identify the various mycobacterial species.[23] Strains of *M.*

Table 1. Classification of the Nontuberculous Mycobacteria Recovered from Humans

Clinical disease	Common etiologic species	Growth rate	Morphologic features[a]	Unusual etiologic species
Pulmonary	*M. avium* complex	Slow (> 7 days)	Usually not pigmented	
	M. kansasii	Slow	Photochromogen; often large and beaded on acid-test bacilli smear	*M. simiae*
	M. chelonae subspecies *abscessus*	Rapid (< 7 days)	Not pigmented	*M. szulgai*
	M. xenopi	Slow	Pigmented	*M. malmoense*
				M. fortuitum (all three biovariants)
				M. chelonae subspecies *chelonae*
Lymphadenitis	*M. avium* complex	Slow	Usually not pigmented	*M. fortuitum* (all three biovariants)
	M. scrofulaceum	Slow	Scotochromogen	*M. chelonae* (both subspecies)
				M. kansasii
Cutaneous	*M. marinum*	Rapid	Photochromogen; requires low temperatures (28° to 30°C) for isolation	*M. avium* complex
	M. fortuitum (all three biovariants)	Rapid	Not pigmented	*M. kansasii*
	M. chelonae (both subspecies)	Rapid	Not pigmented	*M. terrae*
	M. ulcerans[a]	Slow	Usually a scotochromogen; requires low temperatures for isolation	*M. smegmatis*
Disseminated	*M. avium* complex	Slow	Isolates from patients with AIDS, usually pigmented (80%)	*M. fortuitum* (all three biovariants)
	M. kansasii	Slow	Photochromogen	*M. xenopi*
	M. chelonae (both subspecies)	Rapid	Not pigmented	
	M. haemophilium	Slow	Not pigmented; requires hemin, often needs low temperatures and CO_2 to grow	
	M. genavense	Slow	Isolates from AIDS patients; small dysgenic colonies	

[a]Photochromogen, isolate is buff-colored in the dark but turns yellow with brief exposure to light. Scotochromogen, isolate is yellow-orange or orange-colored even when grown in the dark.
From American Thoracic Society.[6]

avium complex have been further subdivided on the basis of agglutination tests, which have proved useful for epidemiological studies of these organisms.[24]

One deficiency of these procedures is the time required for isolation and identification of the infecting species of mycobacteria, up to 2 months in some cases. Radiometric methods (BACTEC) have decreased the isolation time to as short a period as 2 weeks and permit separation of nontuberculous mycobacteria from *M. tuberculosis* complex.[25] More recently, radiometric isolation has been combined with identification by nucleic acid probes, resulting in a rapid and highly sensitive system for the detection of the most common pathogenic species of mycobacteria.[26] In many reference laboratories, these techniques have replaced the traditional methods of mycobacterial culture and speciation.

A variety of other laboratory techniques also have been described that might shorten the time required for identification. Among these, chromatographic techniques such as high-performance liquid chromatography of mycolic acids[27] and gas–liquid chromatography[28] have been applied in several reference laboratories that process cultures for speciation. Others, such as DNA homology studies[29] and identification by enzyme-linked immunosorbent assay (ELISA) of specific mycobacterial antigens,[30] remain relegated to the research laboratory. Among the most promising of the new modalities for diagnosis are molecular amplification techniques such as polymerase chain reaction (PCR).[31] However, at present the primary utility of PCR is the identification of unusual strains of mycobacteria. In AIDS patients, the use of a 16S rRNA primer with amplification of DNA from patients' blood or tissues, has resulted in the identification of a new species of mycobacterium, *Mycobacterium genavense*.[32]

3.4.2. Serological and Immunologic Diagnostic Methods. Although most patients with nontuberculous mycobacterial disease mount a serological response to the infection, no serological diagnostic tests have been described. There are several impediments to the development of a useful diagnostic test. First, patients who have been infected but have not developed disease may have antibodies against these organisms, and thus separation of persons with and without disease may be difficult. Second, antibodies produced by the immune response to infection tend to be broadly reactive with a variety of antigens from many strains of nontuberculous mycobacteria. Third, AIDS patients do not mount significant humoral antibody responses against *M. avium* complex in late stages of immune deficiency.[33]

These same problems also apply to the use of skin test antigens for the diagnosis of infection and disease. Skin-testing diagnostic procedures depend on the fact that cross-reactions tend to be smaller than reactions to the homologous antigen. If two properly standardized skin test antigens are administered simultaneously at separate sites, the smaller reaction is likely to be a cross-reaction and the antigen that causes this reaction is not likely to represent the mycobacterial species responsible for the infection. The larger reaction does not identify the responsible agent, however. Unless all possible skin tests are used, one can never be sure that another antigen might not cause an even larger reaction.

4. Biological Characteristics of the Organisms

Most nontuberculous mycobacteria are slow-growing, Gram's-stain-neutral bacilli that require special nutrients for growth on artificial media. They are distinguished by the property of "acid fastness," being quite resistant to decolorization with acid–alcohol following staining with carbolfuchsin. Most of these organisms are much less virulent than *M. tuberculosis*, both in man and in animals. The most commonly used animal models for studying these organisms are strains of immunodeficient mice.

These organisms, in general, are resistant to most of the commonly used antimycobacterial drugs. For *M. avium* complex, this resistance has been attributed to the highly lipophilic nature of the cell wall, which creates a permeability barrier to penetration by antibiotics.[34] However, some new rifamycin derivatives, such as rifabutin,[35] and macrolide antibiotics, such as clarithromycin,[36] have relatively good *in vitro* activity against *M. avium* complex strains and have been found to be clinically useful. Other mycobacterial species, such as *M. kansasii*, are susceptible to agents such as ethambutol and rifampin,[37] while others, such as *M. fortuitum*, are susceptible to antibiotics such as sulfonamides and erythromycin.[38]

Nontuberculous mycobacteria are widely distributed in nature. Some can be found in water and dairy products, many reside in the soil, others are associated with plant roots, and still others are found in insects, lower animals, and man, usually without evidence of disease.[1,39–41] Studies of the environmental epidemiology of *M. avium* complex organisms by Falkinham and co-workers[42] have greatly increased our knowledge of these organisms. These strains have been found to grow well in brackish waters, particularly in warmer climates such as estuaries and rivers along the southeast coast of the United States. Strains that are more commonly isolated from persons with disease tend to be preferentially aerosolized from these waters, suggesting the possibility of airborne transmission of infection from these sources,[43] although other sources such as soil dusts may also be important.[44] Other studies have suggested that plasmid-carrying strains may be associated with virulence and that such strains are more commonly aerosolized as well.[45]

5. Descriptive Epidemiology

As with tuberculosis, it is helpful to consider the epidemiological characteristics associated with the risk of becoming infected with nontuberculous mycobacteria separately from characteristics associated with the development of disease following infection. The characteristics associated with each event appear to differ considerably, although our knowledge is scanty. Moreover, epidemiological characteristics of disease vary considerably with mycobacterial species. However, unlike tuberculosis, there is little evidence bearing on the frequency with which nontuberculous mycobacterial disease arises from latent infection. In AIDS patients, that disseminated *M. avium* complex infection is recently acquired is supported by a geographic distribution that differs from that of skin test reactors, decreasing frequency with age, colonization that may precede dissemination, and absence of antibody against *M. avium* complex.[18,33,46]

In addition, in contrast to tuberculosis, it is possible to harbor nontuberculous mycobacteria in the respiratory secretions without any evidence of disease, and some species may appear as harmless commensals without causing infection. In patients infected with the human immunodeficiency virus (HIV), who have CD4 cell counts $< 50/mm^3$, the presence of *M. avium* complex in either the respiratory or gastrointestinal tract is associated with a risk of bacteremia of 60% within 1 year. However, only 20% of patients with bacteremia have prior detectable colonization, and therefore screening cultures from sputum or stool are not recommended in AIDS patients.[46]

5.1. Prevalence and Incidence

Evidence of past infection manifested by the results of skin-testing surveys varies markedly. Skin test reactivity is virtually absent in some populations and as high as 80–90% in others. In the latter, the incidence of infection may be as high as 5% per year.[47,48] Skin tests given to US Navy recruits included 13 antigens from various mycobacteria in addition to purified protein derivative of tuberculin prepared from *M. tuberculosis* (PPD-S). Only about 5% reacted to an antigen prepared from *M. fortuitum* (a rapid-growing mycobacterium), slightly more reacted to PPD-S, and over 40% reacted to PPD-G, an antigen prepared from *M. scrofulaceum*.[47]

Because cross-reactions are very common in mycobacterial infections, the reactions to mycobacterial antigens are not specific for the organisms from which they were prepared. A low prevalence of reactions to a particular antigen indicates that infections with the corresponding organism are uncommon; a high prevalence could be due to infections with the corresponding or a cross-reacting organism.

Information on the frequency of persons excreting these organisms, either as "carriers" or as diseased subjects, is scarce. Mycobacteria with the gross cultural characteristics of nontuberculous mycobacteria were found in the sputum of 15–30% of selected populations in Georgia who had no evidence of pulmonary disease.[49,50] In a similar survey of healthy men in tropical Australia, nontuberculous mycobacteria were isolated from the sputa of 7.5%,[51] and studies from other parts of the world have produced similar results. However, in these studies the mycobacteria were not well characterized, so that it is not known what proportion were potentially pathogenic organisms and what percentage were nonpathogens.

Because nontuberculous mycobacteria can be isolated from apparently normal persons, estimates of nontuberculous mycobacterial disease prevalence based on reports of laboratory isolates are unreliable. While it is reasonable to expect that in most cases diagnostic specimens submitted for mycobacterial culture are from persons with clinical disease, the finding of mycobacteria in a specimen is not sufficient for the diagnosis. This is especially true for mycobacteria isolated from sputa. Nonetheless, laboratory surveillance data are helpful in describing the prevalent mycobacteria in an area and for following trends over time.

In a study of British Columbia, where skin-testing surveys indicated that about 20% of the population had been infected with nontuberculous mycobacteria, the average annual incidence of recognized disease was only 0.37/100,000, or approximately 2/100,000 infected individuals.[52] In most areas, however, the prevalence of excreters of nontuberculous mycobacteria can only be estimated from their frequency relative to tubercle bacilli in specimens submitted for bacteriological examination. This ratio depends on the frequency of both tuberculosis and other mycobacterial diseases in the examined population. Nontuberculous mycobacteria accounted for 12% of all specimens positive for mycobacteria in a private hospital in Cleveland, Ohio,[53] 20% in West Irian, Indonesia[54] and among tuberculosis contacts in Puerto Rico,[55] and slightly over 50% in South Carolina.[56] The relative frequency of persons with tuberculosis and nontuberculous mycobacteria diseases is even more difficult to estimate, because the latter cases are not reportable and the frequency of admission to treatment facilities is probably not the same for both types of disease. A summary of reports of the proportion of reported cases of mycobacterial disease attributed to nontuberculous mycobacteria shows a range of 0.5 to 30% with a median value of 7% for the United States and Canada and a range of 0.5 to 15% with a median value of 4% overseas.[(1)]

Several national surveys have helped to define the prevalence of nontuberculous mycobacterial disease in the United States. Nationwide reporting by state mycobacterial laboratories indicated that in 1980 nontuberculous mycobacteria accounted for approximately one third of all mycobacterial isolates.[(57)] The most commonly isolated species of nontuberculous mycobacteria were *M. avium* complex (21%), *M. fortuitum–M. chelonae* (6%), *M. kansasii* (3%), and *M. scrofulaceum* (2%). Combining these laboratory data with results from a national survey that included clinical and epidemiological information on patients with suspected nontuberculous mycobacterial disease resulted in an estimated disease prevalence of 1.8/100,000 or approximately 20% that of tuberculosis.[(21)] Estimated disease prevalence by species from this survey is shown in Table 2, which also provides estimates of the probability of disease among persons from whom potentially pathogenic nontuberculous mycobacteria are isolated, ranging from 75% for persons with *M. kansasii* to 18% for those with *M. fortuitum*.

It should be noted that these surveys were conducted before the widespread occurrence of *M. avium* complex disease in AIDS patients was recognized, in which the epidemiology is dramatically different. Between 1981 and 1987, 5.5% of AIDS patients had been reported to the Centers for Disease Control (CDC) with disseminated nontuberculous mycobacterial disease, of whom 96% had *M. avium* complex and 3% had *M. kansasii*.[(18)] However, disease surveillance reports underestimate its true incidence, and the cumulative incidence in studies of AIDS clinic patients is 15–24% and even higher in patients with CD4 counts $< 100/mm^3$ followed over time.[(13,14,58,59)] Owing to increased recognition and diagnosis of these diseases and to longer survival of AIDS patients, disseminated *M. avium* complex disease is now the most common bacterial infection identified in AIDS patients in industrialized countries. In contrast, disseminated *M. avium* complex disease in AIDS patients in most developing countries is rare, especially in Africa.[(60)] This may be due to the presence of different genotypes or serotypes of *M. avium* complex, protective immunity from BCG vaccination or prior tuberculous infection, protective effect of antituberculosis chemotherapy, or that patients do not survive long enough to acquire *M. avium* complex infection and develop disseminated disease.

5.2. Epidemic Behavior and Contagiousness

While no epidemics of these diseases due to community-acquired infection have been reported, nosocomial outbreaks of disease have been recognized (see Section 5.9). Several reports have also suggested increases in respiratory colonization without disease due to nontuberculous mycobacteria in water supplies.[(61,62)] Available

Table 2. Nontuberculous Mycobacterial Disease in the United States: Estimates of Disease Prevalence from Surveillance Data

Species	Annual no. of isolates[a]	Disease (%)[b]	Estimated no. of cases	Estimated prevalence per 100,000
avium	6,229	47	2928	1.28
kansasii	1,016	75	762	0.33
fortuitum	1,423	18	256	0.11
scrofulaceum	680	22	150	0.07
chelonae	488	38	185	0.08
xenopi	71	25	18	0.01
simiae	71	21	15	0.01
marinum	142	88	125	0.05
szulgai	41	57	23	0.01
Total	10,161	40[c]	4064	1.78

[a]Estimated from 1980 laboratory surveillance data.[(57)]
[b]Estimated from epidemiology survey data, 1981–1983.[(21)]
[c]Includes a factor for overestimation of disease rate, so that next column does not add to total.

evidence suggests that person-to-person and animal-to-man transmission of nontuberculous mycobacteria is not an important factor in acquisition of infection. Most infections are believed to arise from environmental exposure to organisms in infected water, soil, dust, or aerosols.[1,39,42,63] Several skin test studies have suggested that persons with disease excreting large numbers of organisms do not readily infect close contacts,[63,64] and one case–control study of *M. avium* complex in AIDS patients did not identify contact with others with *M. avium* disease as a risk factor.[65] Based on these data and because of the low virulence of these organisms, isolation of patients with disease is not indicated.

5.3. Geographic Distribution

Skin-testing surveys show that infections are most common in tropical and subtropical areas and at lower altitudes and least common in the Arctic and at high elevations.[11,12,47,48,66,67] Within the United States, the prevalence of reactors to PPD-B and PPD-G, antigens prepared from *M. intracellulare* and *M. scrofulaceum*, respectively, was lowest in the Northwest and highest along the Gulf and south Atlantic coasts.[47] In a study of over 250,000 naval recruits who were lifelong single-county residents and who were tested with PPD-B, the rate of sensitization was highest among residents of the southeastern United States (70% and greater) and lowest among those from the North and West (10 to 20%) (Fig. 1).[47,68] Moreover, there was no correlation between rates of reactions to PPD-B and to PPD-S. Unlike reactor rates to tuberculin (PPD-S), those to PPD-B were higher among persons living in rural areas than among residents of metropolitan areas.

A few efforts have been made to ascertain the mycobacterial species likely to have caused skin test reactions. This has been done by administering a battery of different skin test antigens (usually six) to population samples and comparing the patterns of mean reaction sizes to the antigens with those obtained in guinea pigs infected by various mycobacteria.[69] Such testing suggests that the only important cause of mycobacterial infection among Alaskan natives is *M. tuberculosis*,[12] that scotochromogens are likely to be the major factor in infections in the United States,[69] and that there may be considerable variation from place to place in the nature of mycobacterial infections in a country such as Norway.[61] However, such testing has generally utilized nonstandardized antigens, equivalent to PPD tuberculin only on a protein weight basis. The assumed relationship between the relative size

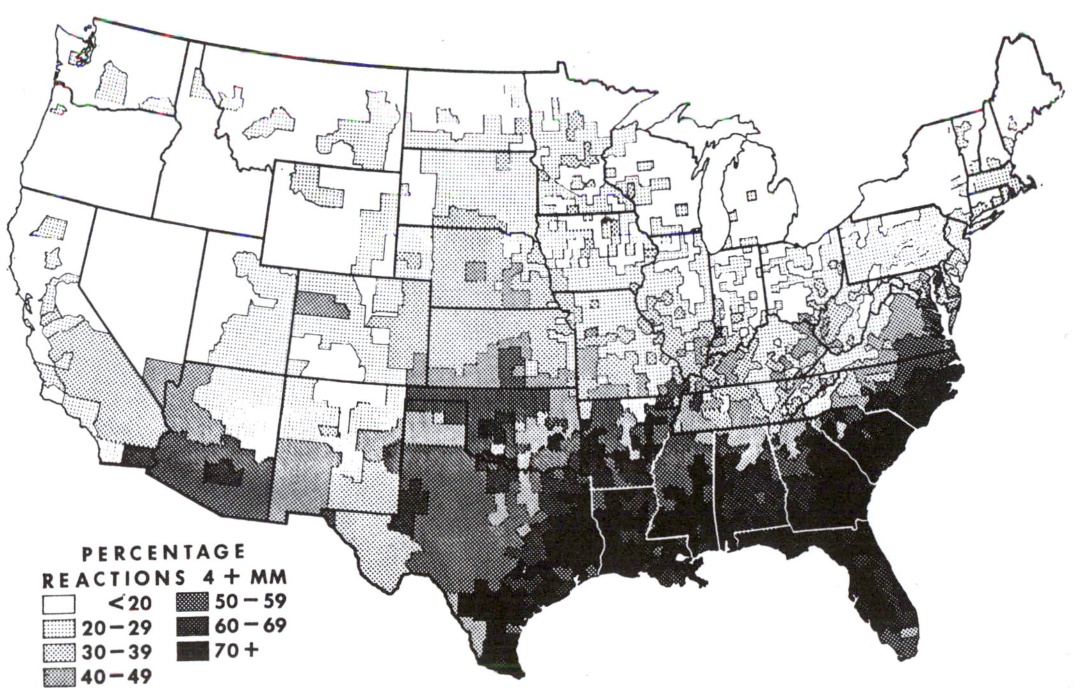

Figure 1. Geographic variations (1958–1964) in the frequency of reactors to 0.0001 mg PPD-B in 257,476 U.S. Navy recruits 17–21 years old, lifetime one-county residents.[47]

of a skin test reaction and infection by (or lack of infection from) the homologous mycobacterium has not been proven.

National reporting of clinical isolates of nontuberculous mycobacteria by state mycobacteriology laboratories in 1979 and 1980 indicated that isolation rates for *M. avium* were high in the Southeast,[57] similar to that noted by the earlier skin-testing surveys. However, high rates were also found among several states bordering Canada and among other states such as Arizona and Kansas, a finding that would not have been expected from the results of the skin test studies. Population mobility and geographic changes in the environmental distribution of these organisms are among the possible explanations for these differences. Rates of isolation of *M. kansasii* were highest in the central portions of the United States.

In Georgia, the rates of admissions to Battey State Hospital for nontuberculous mycobacterioses were much higher from counties in the coastal plain below the "Fall Line" than in the hilly areas to the north,[63] a pattern of disease paralleling that for infections.[47] A careful study of patients with pulmonary disease due to *M. avium* complex and *M. kansasii* in Texas indicated that patients with *M. avium* complex were twice as likely to be residents of rural areas than cities.[70] However, the opposite was true for *M. kansasii* disease patients, who were twice as likely to be urban residents.

5.4. Temporal Distribution

While some authors have noted an increase in the occurrence of nontuberculous mycobacterial disease,[70–72] others have noted no such change.[19,73,74] However, in countries that have experienced a significant decrease in tuberculosis and have laboratories that can speciate mycobacteria, there has been an increase in nontuberculous mycobacterial disease relative to tuberculosis. Given the opportunistic nature of these organisms, one might expect an increase in disease should there be a change in the host defenses of a population. This is certainly the case for disseminated *M. avium* complex disease, which had been rarely recognized before the 1980s[75] and now is the most common form of nontuberculous mycobacterial disease in North America because of its high incidence in AIDS patients.[18] In Sweden, nontuberculous lymphadenitis in children was only recognized after mass BCG vaccination was discontinued, suggesting that BCG was protective against this form of disease.[76] As the life expectancy of persons in the United States has increased and the incidence of chronic lung disease has increased, numbers of persons with nontuberculous mycobacterial pulmonary disease may be expected to increase.

5.5. Age

As with any condition that tends to persist, skin test evidence of past infection increases with age.[68,77,78] Prevalence of sensitivity to PPD-B or PPD-G in the United States and Canada tends to reach a maximum at about the age of 55 years, but when the effects of cross-reactions from tuberculous infection are removed, there is little evidence of increasing frequency of sensitivity to PPD-B with age among adults.[52,68,77] It is not known whether this represents virtually universal infection with some organism(s) that is manifested only partially by reactions to PPD-B or PPD-G or whether sensitivity from nontuberculous mycobacteria is relatively short-lived so that an equilibrium is reached between new infections and loss of previous sensitivity.

Age distribution of persons with nontuberculous mycobacterial disease varies by mycobacterial species and site of disease.[1,52,63,78] Pulmonary disease is most commonly seen in older patients, and among such patients those with *M. avium* complex disease tend to be older than those with *M. kansasii* disease.[70] Isolated lymph node disease is seen in children, most commonly under 5 years of age. In AIDS patients with disseminated mycobacterioses, the frequency of disease tends to decline with age (Table 3).[18] Skin disease due to *M. marinum* affects primarily younger and middle-aged persons, reflecting to an extent occupational exposure. Bone and soft-tissue infection from organisms in the *M. fortuitum* complex group are often nosocomially acquired during surgical procedures, and thus affect a wider age spectrum of patients.

5.6. Sex

Scanty information indicates that males are more likely than females to react to nontuberculous mycobacterial antigens.[77,79,80] Cases of lymphadenitis in young children are slightly more common among females,[78] but in the past pulmonary disease in adults was considerably more common among males.[52,81] Male predominance is especially marked among those with pulmonary disease due to *M. kansasii* and less so among those with *M. avium* complex disease.[70] However, among older persons with *M. avium* complex pulmonary disease, women predominate, perhaps reflecting the presence of number of older women with underlying chronic lung disease.[21] Although the total number of cases of disseminated *M. avium* complex in AIDS patients in the United States is higher in men due to the higher incidence of AIDS in men, the relative frequency in men and women is the same

Table 3. U.S. AIDS Patients Reported with Disseminated Nontuberculous Mycobacterial Infection (DNTM), by Age, Sex, Race, Transmission Category, and Concurrent AIDS-Indicative Disease

	Total AIDS patients	DNTM in AIDS patients (%)
Age, yr		
0–9	552	43 (7.8)
10–19	136	10 (5.4)
20–29	8,646	589 (6.8)
30–39	19,265	1,065 (5.5)
40–49	8,599	394 (4.6)
50–59	3,039	133 (4.4)
60–69	890	28 (3.1)
⩾ 70	185	6 (3.2)
Sex		
Male	38,276	2,096 (5.5)
Female	3,085	173 (5.6)
Race		
White	25,088	1,407 (5.6)
Black	10,129	631 (6.2)
Hispanic	5,761	219 (3.8)
Asian	245	8 (3.3)
American Indian	42	2 (4.8)
HIV transmission category		
Homosexual or bisexual man	29,968	1,467 (5.4)
Heterosexual IV drug user	6,716	365 (5.4)
Homosexual man and IV drug user	3,084	190 (6.2)
Hemophiliac	402	28 (7.0)
Heterosexual high-risk contact	874	43 (4.9)
Person born in Haiti or Central Africa	728	29 (4.0)
Transfusion recipient	932	50 (5.4)
Child of high-risk mother	450	29 (5.4)
Undetermined	1,209	68 (5.6)
Disease category		
Kaposi's sarcoma	8,192	283 (3.5)
Opportunistic infection (excluding DNTM alone)	32,487	1,304 (4.0)

[a]Percentage of AIDS cases of that category.
[b]Of mycobacterial isolates, 96% were *M. avium* complex and 3% were *M. kansasii*.
From Horsburgh and Selik.[18]

(Table 3).[18] Skin disease due to *M. marinum* is much more common among men.

5.7. Race

There appears to be little, if any, racial variation in infections with nontuberculous mycobacteria when place of residence is held constant.[47,82] Early reports from tuberculosis sanatoriums of patients with nontuberculous mycobacterial pulmonary disease noted the relative absence of nonwhite patients. However, more recent data suggest that there is no apparent racial susceptibility to disease.

5.8. Occupation

No information is available on infection status and occupation, except as workplaces are related to geography. Sputum surveys of occupational groups in west central Georgia showed a marked association of exposure to agricultural dusts and the presence of nontuberculous mycobacteria in the sputum of well persons.[50] A very high frequency of these organisms was found in workers in a poultry-processing plant, but only among persons exposed to feathers. In Australia, 8 of 11 healthy workers exposed to pigs with lymphadenitis caused by *M. intracellulare* were found to harbor the same organisms.[83]

There is some evidence that patients with occupational pneumoconiosis, especially patients with silicosis, may be more likely to develop pulmonary disease due to nontuberculous mycobacteria.[84] However, other than workers with aquatic exposure, there is no known occupational association with nontuberculous mycobacterial disease.

5.9. Occurrence in Different Settings

Chronic granulomatous ulcers of the skin are caused by *M. marinum*, often following abrasions of the skin in infected water, notably fish tanks and swimming pools.[85] Nosocomial infections from *M. fortuitum* complex have been reported in a variety of settings, probably related to contamination during surgical procedures such as open-heart surgery and mammoplasty.[86] Disseminated infections from *M. chelonae* have also been noted among patients in a dialysis center.[87] Increases in respiratory colonization by *M. xenopi* among hospitalized patients have been attributed on one occasion to a contaminated hot water system.[88] Nosocomial outbreaks of respiratory colonization by *M. fortuitum* have been linked to a contaminated ice machine[62] and to contaminated hot water system.[89]

5.10. Socioeconomic Factors

There is no evidence that socioeconomic status is related to the development of infection or disease due to nontuberculous mycobacteria. Skin tests of male residents of Maryland who were Navy recruits or students of the University of Maryland showed no evidence of differences between these two groups in the prevalence of nontuberculous mycobacterial infections.[47,79]

5.11. Other Factors

Interference with local protective mechanisms (e.g., bronchopulmonary clearance) may be an important risk factor for the acquisition of pulmonary mycobacteriosis. Thus, adults with cystic fibrosis appear to be at high risk of infection.(90) Silicosis and malignancies are also reported to be risk factors for pulmonary disease.(1,91) The presence of immunodeficiency states, especially AIDS, and immunosuppressive therapy are risk factors for disseminated disease.(14,75) However, in many patients there is no apparent predisposing factor and the usual tests of immune function are normal. Such patients, however, may have specific defects in cellular immunity, as has been suggested for some patients with pulmonary mycobacteriosis(92) and more recently demonstrated for patients with *M. marinum* disease.(93)

6. Mechanisms and Routes of Transmission

Although little is known about how infection is acquired, it is generally believed that the reservoirs and sources are environmental. Cutaneous ulcers are likely to be caused by direct implantation of infected material into skin cuts or abrasions. Nosocomial wound infections due to *M. fortuitum* complex organisms may be due to aerosols from tap water containing these organisms or from infected solutions or equipment used for surgical procedures.(86) Infection in dialysis patients has been attributed to contaminated hemodialysis equipment.(87) Lymphadenitis in children may result from close contact with the earth and the tendency of children to put things into their mouths.(78) Inhalation of aerosols containing *M. avium* complex may be the primary route of infection for persons with pulmonary disease due to this organism. Studies of the ecology of *M. avium* complex organisms in the Southeast have strengthened this hypothesis.(42,43)

Inhalation of infected dust and the ingestion of contaminated water, dairy products, or raw vegetables provide other possible sources of infection. Acquisition of *M. avium* complex in AIDS patients has been associated with CD4 counts $< 25/mm^3$ and ingestion of hard cheese.(65) Exposure to aerosols in institutions where *M. avium* complex had colonized the hot water supply has also been identified as a risk factor in AIDS patients.(94) On the other hand, daily showering may be protective, and exposure to many other environmental sources and to other patients with *M. avium* complex disease are not associated risk factors in AIDS patients.(65)

Despite the presence of *M. avium* disease in chicken flocks and swine herds, there are no data suggesting that animal-to-man transmission is an important source of infection.(41) Furthermore, no convincing evidence has been yet produced that persons who harbor these organisms are a significant hazard to their associates, although one skin test study of household contacts of patients with pulmonary mycobacteriosis indicated higher reactor rates than among control subjects.(64) On the other hand, it would be exceedingly difficult to demonstrate such a risk when infection is widespread in the environment of most cases and when only a tiny fraction of infected individuals become ill.

7. Pathogenesis and Immunity

Relatively little is known about the pathogenesis of infection and disease with nontuberculous mycobacteria and about the development of immunity following infection. Most diagnosed infections in immunocompetent hosts are associated with a granulomatous response, so the model of pathogenesis developed for tuberculosis may be applicable to the majority of infections from nontuberculous mycobacteria. If the organisms gain entrance into the body through skin, mucous membranes, or the respiratory tract, it is assumed that a granulomatous lesion develops that usually heals without becoming large enough to be noticeable. Disseminated disease may develop in the absence of the usual immune response. For example, among AIDS patients with disseminated *M. avium* complex disease, granulomas are conspicuously absent.(14,95) It is assumed that localized disease in the small intestine leads to blood-borne dissemination with widespread organ involvement.(96) No information about the interval between the time of initial infection and the development of symptomatic disease (i.e., incubation period) is available. There is no evidence that, as is the case for tuberculosis, disease develops following a long period of asymptomatic infection.

8. Patterns of Host Response

It has already been emphasized that inapparent infections are very common in many geographic areas. These organisms can often be found in oral, respiratory, and genitourinary secretions without any evidence, other than positive skin tests, that they have invaded the body.

8.1. Clinical Features

8.1.1. Pulmonary Diseases. Chronic disease of the lungs formerly was the major clinical problem associated with these organisms. It cannot be differentiated clinically from pulmonary tuberculosis and is usually diagnosed only when the results of sputum cultures are reported. Patients commonly present with respiratory symptoms, such as chronic cough and sputum production, abnormalities on chest radiograph, and acid-fast-bacilli-positive sputum smears. Systemic signs and symptoms such as fever, malaise, and weight loss are generally less marked than for patients with tuberculosis. In addition, clinical progression seems to be much slower than for tuberculosis. Underlying lung disease, such as chronic obstructive pulmonary disease, cancer, bronchiectasis, or previous tuberculosis, are commonly associated. While the chest radiograph may simulate tuberculosis with upper lobe cavitary disease, scattered infiltrates throughout the lung fields and disease presenting as a solitary pulmonary nodule also occur.(97) *M. avium* complex disease presenting with radiographic pictures of progressive nodular infiltrates(98) and middle lobe or lingular infiltrates(99) in older women have also been described. The most common etiologic organisms are *M. kansasii* and *M. avium* complex. Other organisms occasionally associated with pulmonary disease are *M. fortuitum* complex and *M. scrofulaceum*.(1,21)

8.1.2. Lymphadenitis. The submaxillary and submandibular lymph nodes are characteristically involved, although any of the superficial lymph nodes may be affected. The involvement of only one or a few nodes, early suppuration, and associated salivary-gland disease point to nontuberculous mycobacterial disease rather than tuberculosis.(78) Almost all cases occur before the age of 5 years. The natural history of this disease is not well defined. It may be that many patients with undetected lymphadenopathy often have spontaneous regression of the disease. Recently, there has been an apparent change in the distribution of organisms causing disease, with *M. avium* complex predominating, and *M. scrofulaceum*, once the most commonly identified etiologic organism, now much less frequent.(21,74,78) In a few areas, *M. kansasii* is also commonly identified.(1,78)

8.1.3. Soft-Tissue Lesions. Localized abscesses, usually caused by *M. fortuitum* complex, occur after injections, surgical wounds, or other trauma.(1,86) Chronic granulomas and ulcers follow cuts and abrasions that occur in swimming pools, fish tanks, or other marine environments harboring *M. marinum*. Indolent necrotic ulcers (Buruli or Bairnsdale ulcers) result from infections with *M. ulcerans*, most commonly found in central Africa and Australia.(100)

8.1.4. Other Sites of Localized Disease. Lesions at sites other than the above-named ones are uncommon. Other sites of disease are bones, joints, tendon sheaths, genitourinary tract, and the meninges.

8.1.5. Disseminated Disease. Until recently, disseminated mycobacteriosis was uncommon, occurring in persons with impaired immunity related to an underlying disease, such as leukemia, lymphoma, or iatrogenically induced with immunosuppressive therapy.(1,75) However, the occurrence of disseminated mycobacteriosis, especially due to *M. avium* complex, among patients with AIDS has now resulted in the condition being commonly recognized in areas caring for AIDS patients. The clinical features of disease are quite variable; some patients with positive blood cultures have minimal symptoms, while others have disabling fever, night sweats, diarrhea, abdominal pain, wasting, and anemia. Among these patients, gastrointestinal tract involvement with a histological picture resembling Whipple's disease may occur.(101) Bloodstream infection and bone marrow, lymph node, liver, and spleen involvement are also commonly recognized. Involvement of virtually every organ of the body in this disease has been described, including skin, gall bladder, bone and joints, muscle, and pericardium.(13,14) However, central nervous system involvement is rare, and while organisms may be isolated commonly from bronchial secretions, respiratory disease due to *M. avium* complex is uncommon in AIDS. The presence of disseminated *M. avium* complex in AIDS patients is clearly associated with decreased survival (Fig. 2). This has been established by analysis of data from a national registry,(18) a retrospective case–control study,(102) and a prospective cohort study.(58)

The clinical syndrome of *M. genavense* infection in AIDS patients is very similar to that of *M. avium* complex, with fever, weight loss, diarrhea, hepatomegaly, and intra-abdominal lymphadenopathy.(15,32) Although *M. kansasii* in AIDS patients may be disseminated, it most often has a pulmonary presentation with cavities and diffuse infiltrates.(16) *M. haemophilum* infection in AIDS patients most often involves the skin, soft tissues, joints or bone; the skin lesions are ulcerating or nodular.(17)

8.2. Diagnosis

Sometimes the diagnosis can be suspected from epidemiological and clinical information. The suspicion of nontuberculous mycobacterial disease should be raised by chronic infiltrative, fibrotic, or cavitary pulmonary disease in an older man; chronic lymphadenitis in a very young child; chronic ulcers of a vulnerable part of the body in persons exposed to marine environments; chronic necrotic ulcers in persons who have been in central Africa or Australia; and persistent undiagnosed fever, abdominal symptoms, and anemia in an AIDS patient. That suspicion should be heightened if there is little or no reaction to 5 tuberculin units of PPD-S and if the patient comes from an

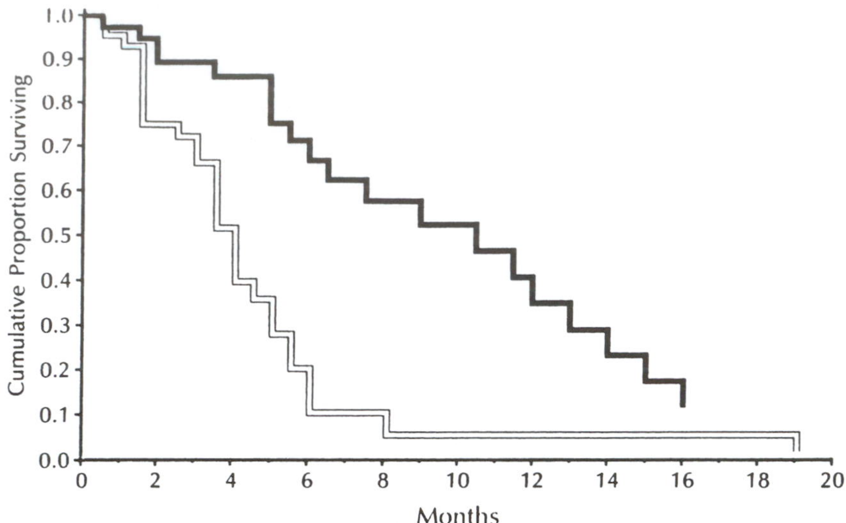

Figure 2. Survival of patients with untreated disseminated *Mycobacterium avium* complex infection (DMAC) (open line) and control patients (closed line). Patients with untreated DMAC had a significantly shorter survival time than control patients ($p < 0.0001$).[102]

area where these infections are common. Finding tuberculin skin-test-negative household contacts of a patient with pulmonary disease and sputum containing acid-fast bacilli should also heighten suspicion of nontuberculous mycobacterial disease. However, the diagnosis can be made with reasonable certainty only when bacteriological examinations have isolated and identified the causative organism. In the case of patients with pulmonary disease, diagnosis requires the repeated isolation of the same organism in significant quantities and the exclusion of other disease that may be responsible for the radiographic abnormalities observed.[6]

There are problems, however, with the diagnosis of both past infection and present disease. Skin tests, like all medical tests, can yield false-negative and false-positive results. Skin sensitivity is often not demonstrable in severely ill or immunosuppressed patients. Cross-reactions to all mycobacterial antigens are common. When it is possible to obtain matched antigens from different mycobacteria, all that can be said from the results of giving two or more tests is that the smaller reaction may not represent the etiologic agent. Multiple testing with a battery of mycobacterial antigens is unlikely to be useful in adults, but may be more reliable in very young children because interpretation of their skin test reactions is not as likely to be confounded by multiple mycobacterial infections. However, while differential skin testing may be helpful in the presumptive diagnosis of children with lymphatic disease,[103,104] they have not proven useful in the evaluation of adults with pulmonary mycobacteriosis,[105] even when the antigens are bioequivalent to PPD-S. Moreover, these products are not commercially available in the U.S. Repeated testing of the same individuals may yield conversions from negative to positive that do not result from new infections but rather from the booster phenomenon[106] (see Chapter 36, Section 3.4.2).

Cultures of nontuberculous mycobacteria from body secretions may also fail to be definitive, although culture of blood and bone marrow has proven to be a reliable and sensitive technique for the diagnosis of disseminated *M. avium* complex disease in AIDS patients.[13,14,107] False-negative results for *M. ulcerans* and *M. haemophilum* may be obtained if the cultures are incubated at 37°C, since these organisms prefer cooler temperature.[17,23] *M. genavense* grows slowly in broth and has small, dysgonic colonies or no growth on subculture; therefore, it is best identified by nucleic acid amplification and DNA probes.[32] Isolation of mycobacteria from diseased lymph nodes, even those that are positive for acid-fast bacilli on microscopy, is sometimes difficult. False-positive results can occur as the result of contamination of laboratory water supplies or reagents,[108] or more often because the patient happens to be harboring nontuberculous mycobacteria that have nothing to do with his or her disease.

9. Control and Prevention

9.1. General Concepts

Because the disease appears to be nontransmissible, in general there is no need for reporting, isolation, or quarantine. Measures taken to prevent infection from environmental sources currently are not indicated, because as yet so little is known about factors that influence infection and, except for the immunocompromised host, serious consequences of infection are rare.

9.2. Chemotherapeutic Prophylaxis

Except for severely immunocompromised AIDS patients, chemotherapy for prophylaxis is rarely indicated, because these organisms tend to be resistent to most antibiotics and because disease rarely follows infection in immunocompetent hosts. In the unusual instance in which a person with known nontuberculous mycobacterial disease may be given immunosuppressive treatment, combinations of antibiotics most likely to affect the particular organism can be given.

Owing to the extraordinarily high incidence of severe, disseminated *M. avium* complex in AIDS patients, prophylaxis in patients with < 50 CD4 cells/mm^3 is recommended.[109] Although rifabutin was the first drug approved for this indication,[110] clarithromycin or azithromycin is now preferred.[111–113] Either clarithromycin or azithromycin, in combination with at least one other drug such as ethambutol or rifabutin, is recommended for the treatment of *M. avium* complex bacteremia AIDS patients.[109,114]

9.3. Immunization

None is known.

10. Unresolved Problems

While our understanding of the environmental epidemiology of *M. avium* complex has advanced, we know very little about the epidemiology of other species of nontuberculous mycobacteria. For all species, understanding the mechanisms of infection, pathogenesis, and immunity is important; also, knowing why some infected people develop illness and others do not is especially important. This has become even more urgent given the dramatic and life-threatening clinical illnesses of nontuberculous mycobacterioses in AIDS patients. Improved diagnostic methods for differentiating persons with disease caused by these organisms from persons who merely harbor them also would be helpful. Finally, although some improvement in prophylaxis and treatment of *M. avium* complex infections has occurred, improved drugs and treatment regimens are needed.

11. References

1. Wolinsky, E., Nontuberculous mycobacteria and associated diseases, *Am. Rev. Respir. Dis.* **119:**107–159 (1979).
2. Branch, A., Avian tubercle bacillus infection, with special reference to mammals and to man: Its reported association with Hodgkin's disease, *Arch. Pathol.* **12:**253–274 (1931).
3. Pinner, M., Atypical acid-fast microorganisms. III. Chromogenic acid-fast bacilli from human beings, *Am. Rev. Tuberc.* **32:**424–439 (1935).
4. Lewis, A. G., Jr., Lasché, E. M., Armstrong, A. L., and Dunbar, F. P., A clinical study of the chronic lung disease due to nonphotochromogenic acid-fast bacilli, *Ann. Intern. Med.* **53:**273–285 (1960).
5. Timpe, A., and Runyon, E. H., The relationship of "atypical" acid-fast bacteria to human disease: A preliminary report, *J. Lab. Clin. Med.* **44:**202–209 (1954).
6. American Thoracic Society, Diagnosis and treatment of disease caused by nontuberculous mycobacteria, *Am. Rev. Respir. Dis.* **142:**940–953 (1990).
7. Comstock, G. W., The Hagerstown Tuberculosis Conference of 1938: A retrospective opinion, *Am. Rev. Respir. Dis.* **99:**119–120 (1969).
8. Palmer, C. E., Ferebee, S. H., and Strange Petersen, O., Studies of pulmonary findings and antigen sensitivity among student nurses. VI. Geographic differences in sensitivity to tuberculin as evidence of nonspecific allergy, *Public Health Rep.* **65:**1111–1131 (1950).
9. Edwards, L. B., Hopwood, L., and Palmer, C. E., Identification of mycobacterial infections, *Bull. WHO* **33:**405–412 (1965).
10. Lowell, A. M., Edwards, L. B., and Palmer, C. E.,, *Tuberculosis*, Harvard University Press, Cambridge, MA, 1969.
11. Bates, L. E., Busk, T., and Palmer, C. E., Research contributions of BCG vaccination programs. II. Tuberculin sensitivity at different altitudes of residence, *Public Health Rep.* **66:**1427–1441 (1951).
12. Edwards, L. B., Comstock, G. W., and Palmer, C. E., Contributions of northern populations to the understanding of tuberculin sensitivity, *Arch. Environ. Health* **17:**507–516 (1968).
13. Hawkins, C. C., Gold, J. W. M., Whimbey, E., *et al.*, *Mycobacterium avium* complex infections in patients with the acquired immunodeficiency syndrome, *Ann. Intern. Med.* **105:**184–188 (1986).
14. Horsburgh, C. R., Jr., *Mycobacterium avium* complex infections in patients with the acquired immunodeficiency syndrome, *N. Engl. J. Med.* **324:**1332–1338 (1991).
15. Hirschel, B., Chang, H. R., Mach, N., *et al.*, Fatal infection with a novel unidentified mycobacterium in a man with the acquired immunodeficiency syndrome, *N. Engl. J. Med.* **323:**109–113 (1990).
16. Carpenter, J. L., and Parks, J. M., *Mycobacterium kansasii* infec-

tions in patients positive for human immunodeficiency virus, *Rev. Infect. Dis.* **13:**789–796 (1991).

17. Straus, W. L., Ostroff, S. M., Jernigan, D. B., *et al.*, Clinical and epidemiologic characteristics of *Mycobacterium haemophilum*, an emerging pathogen of immunocompromised patients, *Ann. Intern. Med.* **114:**1195–1200 (1994).
18. Horsburgh, C. R., Jr., and Selik, R. M., The epidemiology of disseminated nontuberculous mycobacterial infection in the acquired immunodeficiency syndrome, *Am. Rev. Respir. Dis.* **139:** 4–7 (1989).
19. Krajnack, M. A., and Dowda, H., Non-tuberculous mycobacteria in South Carolina, 1971 to 1980, *J. SC Med. Assoc.* **77:**551–555 (1981).
20. Omondi, P. P. G., Asal, N. R., Muchmore, H. G., and Flournoy, D. J., Epidemiology of nontuberculous mycobacteria in Oklahoma, *J. Okla. State Med. Assoc.* **78:**304–312 (1985).
21. O'Brien, R. J., Geiter, L. J., and Snider, D. E., Jr., The epidemiology of nontuberculous mycobacterial diseases in the United States: Results from a national survey, *Am. Rev. Respir. Dis.* **135:**1007–1014 (1987).
22. Wickman, K., Clinical significance of nontuberculous mycobacteria. A bacteriological survey of Swedish strains isolated between 1973 and 1981, *Scand. J. Infect. Dis.* **18:**337–345 (1986).
23. Kent, P. T., and Kubica, G. P., *Public Health Mycobacteriology: A Guide for the Level III Laboratory*, Centers for Disease Control, Atlanta, 1985.
24. Schaefer, W. B., Serologic identification and classification of the atypical mycobacteria by their agglutination, *Am. Rev. Respir. Dis.* **92**(Suppl.):85–93 (1965).
25. Siddiqi, S. H., Hwangbo, C. C., Silcox, V., Good, R. C., Snider, D. E., Jr., and Middlebrook, G., Rapid radiometric methods to detect and differentiate *Mycobacterium tuberculosis/M. bovis* from other mycobacterial species, *Am. Rev. Respir. Dis.* **130:**634–640 (1984).
26. Ellner, P. D., Kiehn, T. E., Cammarata, R., and Hosmer, M., Rapid detection and identification of pathogenic mycobacteria by combining radiometric and nucleic acid probes, *J. Clin. Microbiol.* **26:**1349–1352 (1988).
27. Butler, W. R., and Kilburn, J. O., Identification of major slowly growing pathogenic mycobacteria and *Mycobacterium gordonae* by high-performance liquid chromatography of their mycolic acids, *J. Clin. Microbiol.* **26:**50–53 (1988).
28. Tisdall, P. A., Roberts, G. D., and Anhalt, J. P., Identification of clinical isolates of mycobacteria with gas–liquid chromatography alone, *J. Clin. Microbiol.* **10:**506–514 (1979).
29. Baess, I., Deoxyribonucleic acid relatedness among species of slowly growing mycobacteria, *Acta Pathol. Microbiol. Scand. Sect. B* **87:**221–226 (1979).
30. Yanagihara, D. L., Barr, V. L., Knisley, C. V., Tsang, A. Y., McClatchy, J. K., and Brennan, P. J., Enzyme-linked immunosorbent assay of glycolipid antigens for identification of mycobacteria, *J. Clin. Microbiol.* **21:**569–574 (1985).
31. Hance, A. J., Grandchamp, B., Lévy-Frébault, V., Lecossier, D., Rauzier, J., Bocart, D., and Gicquel, B., Detection and identification of mycobacteria by amplification of mycobacterial DNA, *Mol. Microbiol.* **3:**843–849 (1989).
32. Bottger, E. C., Teske, A., Kirschner, P., *et al.*, Disseminated *Mycobacterium genavense* infection in patients with AIDS, *Lancet* **340:**76–80 (1992).
33. Winter, S. M., Bernard, E. M., Gold, J. W. M., and Armstrong, D., Humoral response to disseminated infection by *Mycobacterium avium–Mycobacterium intracellulare* in acquired immunodeficiency syndrome and hairy cell leukemia, *J. Infect. Dis.* **151:**523–527 (1985).
34. Rastogi, N., Frehel, C., Ryter, A., Ohayon, H., Lesourd, M., and David, H. L., Multiple drug resistance in *Mycobacterium avium:* Is the wall architecture responsible for the exclusion of antimicrobial agents? *Antimicrob. Agents Chemother.* **20:**666–677 (1981).
35. Woodley, C. L., and Kilburn, J. O., *In vitro* susceptibility of *Mycobacterium avium* complex and *Mycobacterium tuberculosis* strains to a spiropiperidyl rifamycin, *Am. Rev. Respir. Dis.* **126:**586–587 (1982).
36. Naik, S., and Ruck, R., *In vitro* activities of several new macrolide antibiotics against *Mycobacterium avium* complex, *Antimicrob. Agents Chemother.* **33:**1614–1616 (1989).
37. Kuze, F., Kurasawa, T., Bando, K., Lee, Y., and Maekawa, N., *In vitro* and *in vivo* susceptibility of atypical mycobacteria to various drugs, *Rev. Infect. Dis.* **3:**885–897 (1981).
38. Swenson, J. M., Wallace, R. J., Silcox, V. A., and Thornsberry, C., Antimicrobial susceptibility of five subgroups of *Mycobacterium fortuitum* and *Mycobacterium chelonae*, *Antimicrob. Agents Chemother.* **28:**807–811 (1985).
39. Chapman, J. S., The ecology of the atypical mycobacteria, *Arch. Environ. Health* **22:**41–46 (1971).
40. Goslee, S., and Wolinsky, E., Water as a source of potentially pathogenic mycobacteria, *Am. Rev. Respir. Dis.* **113:**287–292 (1976).
41. Meissner, G., and Anz, W., Sources of *Mycobacterium avium* complex infection resulting in human diseases, *Am. Rev. Respir. Dis.* **116:**1057–1064 (1977).
42. Gruft, H., Falkinham, J. O., III, and Parker, B. C., Recent experience in the epidemiology of disease caused by atypical mycobacteria, *Rev. Infect. Dis.* **3:**990–996 (1981).
43. Parker, B. C., Ford, M. A., Gruft, H., and Falkinham, J. O., III, Epidemiology of infection by nontuberculous mycobacteria. IV. Preferential aerosolization of *Mycobacterium intracellulare* from natural waters, *Am. Rev. Respir. Dis.* **128:**652–656 (1983).
44. Brooks, R. W., Parker, B. C., Gruft, H., and Falkinham, J. O., Epidemiology of infection by nontuberculous mycobacteria. V. Numbers in eastern United States soils and correlation with soil characteristics, *Am. Rev. Respir. Dis.* **130:**630–633 (1984).
45. Meissner, P. S., and Falkinham, J. O., III, Plasmid DNA profiles as epidemiological markers for clinical and environmental isolates of *Mycobacterium avium*, *Mycobacterium intracellulare*, and *Mycobacterium scrofulaceum*, *J. Infect. Dis.* **153:**325–331 (1986).
46. Chin, D. P., Hopewell, P. C., and Yajko, D. M., *et al., Mycobacterium avium* complex of the respiratory or gastrointestinal tract and the risk of *M. avium* complex bacteremia in patients with human immunodeficiency virus infection, *J. Infect. Dis.* **169:** 289–295 (1994).
47. Edwards, L. B., Acquaviva, F. A., Livesay, V. T., Cross, F. W, and Palmer, C. E., An atlas of sensitivity to tuberculin, PPD-B, and histoplasmin in the United States, *Am. Rev. Respir. Dis.* **99**(Part 2)**:**1–132 (1969).
48. Palmer, C. E., and Edwards, L. B., Tuberculin test in retrospect and prospect, *Arch. Environ. Health* **15:**792–808 (1967).
49. Davis, S. D., and Comstock, G. W., Unpublished data.
50. Edwards, L. B., and Palmer, C. E., Isolation of "atypical" mycobacteria from healthy persons, *Am. Rev. Respir. Dis.* **80:**747–749 (1959).

51. Kiewiet, A. A., and Thompson, J. E., Isolation of "atypical" mycobacteria from healthy individuals in tropical Australia, *Tubercle* **51:**296–299 (1970).
52. Robakiewicz, M., and Grzybowski, S., Epidemiologic aspects of nontuberculous mycobacterial disease and of tuberculosis in British Columbia, *Am. Rev. Respir. Dis.* **109:**613–620 (1974).
53. Demeter, S. L., Ahmad, M., and Tomashefski, J., Epidemiological characteristics of mycobacterial infections in a referral clinic, *Am. Rev. Respir. Dis.* **119**(Part 2)**:**399 (1979).
54. Hanegraaf, T. A. C., and Wijsmuller, G., Atypical mycobacteria in New Guinea, *Sel. Pap. (R. Neth. Tuberc. Assoc.)* **8:**68–79 (1964).
55. Sifontes, J. E., Alvarez, F. R., and de la Rosa, J. C., The mycobacterioses in Puerto Rico, *Bol. Assoc. Med. Puerto Rico* **57:**135 (1965).
56. Townsend, E. W., Geiger, F. L., Gregg, D. B., and Fickling, A. M., An analysis of "atypical" mycobacteria as reported by the South Carolina State Board of Health Laboratory, *J. SC Med. Assoc.* **61:**267–273 (1965).
57. Good, R. C., and Snider, D. E., Jr., Isolation of nontuberculous mycobacteria in the United States, 1980, *J. Infect. Dis.* **146:**829–833 (1982).
58. Chin, D. P., Reingold, A. L., Stone, E. N., *et al.*, The impact of *Mycobacterium avium* complex bacteremia and its treatment on survival of AIDS patients—A prospective study, *J. Infect. Dis.* **170:**578–584 (1994).
59. Nightingale, S. D., Byrd, L. T., Southern, P. M., Jockusch, J. D., Cal, S. X., and Wynne, B. A., Incidence of *Mycobacterium avium-intracellulare* complex bacteremia in human immunodeficiency virus-positive patients, *J. Infect. Dis.* **165:**1082–1085 (1992).
60. Okello, D. O., Sewankambo, N., Goodgame, R., *et al.*, Absence of bacteremia with *Mycobacterium avium-intracellulare* in Ugandan patients with AIDS, *J. Infect. Dis.* **162:**208–210 (1990).
61. Bjerkedal, T., Mycobacterial infections in Norway: A preliminary note on determining their identity and frequency, *Am. J. Epidemiol.* **85:**157–173 (1967).
62. Laussucq, S., Baltch, A., Smith, R. P., Smithwick, R. W., Davis, B. J., Desjardin, E. K., Silcox, B. A., Spellacy, A., Zeimis, R., Gruft, H., Good, R. C., and Cohen, M. L., Nosocomial *Mycobacterium fortuitum* colonization from a contaminated ice machine, *Am. Rev. Respir. Dis.* **138:**891–894 (1988).
63. Crow, H. E., Corpe, R. F., and Smith C. E., Is serious pulmonary disease caused by nonphotochromogenic ("atypical") acid-fast mycobacteria communicable? *Dis. Chest* **39:**372–381 (1961).
64. Chapman, J. S., Dewlett, H. J., and Potts, W. E., Cutaneous reactions to unclassified mycobacterial antigens: A study of children in household contact with patients who excrete unclassified mycobacteria, *Am. Rev. Respir. Dis.* **86:**547–552 (1962).
65. Horsburgh, C. R., Jr., Chin, D. P., Yajko, D. M., *et al.*, Environmental risk factors for acquisition of *Mycobacterium avium* complex in persons with human immunodeficiency virus infection, *J. Infect. Dis.* **170:**362–367 (1994).
66. Abrahams, E. W., and Silverstone, H., Epidemiological evidence of the presence of non-tuberculous sensitivity to tuberculin in Queensland, *Tubercle* **42:**487–499 (1961).
67. Raj Narain, Anantharaman, D. S., and Diwakara, A. M., Prevalence of nonspecific tuberculin sensitivity in certain parts of India, *Bull. WHO* **51:**273–278 (1974).
68. Wijsmuller, G., and Erickson, P., The reaction to PPD-Battey: A new look, *Am. Rev. Respir. Dis.* **109:**29–40 (1974).
69. Edwards, L. B., Hopwood, L., Affronti, L. F., and Palmer, C. E., Sensitivity profiles of mycobacterial infection, *Bull. Int. Union Tuberc.* **32:**384–394 (1962).
70. Ahn, C. H., Lowell, J. R., Onstad, G. D., Shuford, E. H., and Hurst, G. A., A demographic study of disease due to *Mycobacterium kansasii* or *M. intracellulare-avium* in Texas, *Chest* **75:**120–125 (1979).
71. Mycobacteriosis Research Group of the Japanese National Chest Hospitals, Rapid increase of the incidence of lung disease due to *Mycobacterium kansasii* in Japan, *Chest* **83:**890–892 (1983).
72. Rosenzweig, D. Y., and Schlueter, D. P., Spectrum of clinical disease in pulmonary infection with *Mycobacterium avium-intracellulare*, *Rev. Infect. Dis.* **3:**1046–1051 (1981).
73. Edwards, F. G. B., Disease caused by "atypical" (opportunist) mycobacteria: A whole population review, *Tubercle* **51:**285–295 (1970).
74. Lai, K. K., Stottmeier, K. D., Sherman, I. H., and McCabe, W. R., Mycobacterial cervical lymphadenopathy: Relation of etiologic agents to age, *J. Am. Med. Assoc.* **251:**1286–1288 (1984).
75. Horsburgh, C. R., Jr., Mason, U. G., III, Farhi, D. C., and Iseman, M. D., Disseminated infection with *Mycobacterium avium-intracellulare:* A report of 13 cases and a review of the literature, *Medicine* **64:**36–48 (1985).
76. Wickman, K., Clinical significance of nontuberculous mycobacteria. A bacteriological survey of Swedish strains isolated between 1973 and 1981, *Scand. J. Infect. Dis.* **18:**337–345 (1986).
77. Edwards, L. B., and Smith, D. T., Community-wide tuberculin testing study in Pamlico County, North Carolina, *Am. Rev. Respir. Dis.* **92:**43–54 (1965).
78. Lincoln, E. M., and Gilbert, L. A., Disease in children due to mycobacteria other than *Mycobacterium tuberculosis*, *Am. Rev. Respir. Dis.* **105:**683–714 (1972).
79. Sartwell, P. E., and Dyke, L. M., Comparative sensitivity of college students to tuberculins PPD-S and PPD-B, *Am. J. Hyg.* **71:**204–211 (1960).
80. Wijsmuller, G., Raj Narain, Mayurnath, S., and Palmer, C. E., On the nature of tuberculin sensitivity in south India, *Am. Rev. Respir. Dis.* **97:**429–443 (1968).
81. Crow, H. E., King, C. T., Smith, C. E., Corpe, R. F., and Stergus, I., A limited clinical, pathologic, and epidemiologic study of patients with pulmonary lesions associated with atypical acid-fast bacilli in the sputum, *Am. Rev. Tuberc.* **75:**199–222 (1957).
82. Shaw, L. W., Field studies on immunization against tuberculosis. I. Tuberculin allergy following BCG vaccination of school children in Muscogee County, Georgia, *Public Health Rep.* **66:**1415–1426 (1951).
83. Reznikov, M., and Robinson, E., Serologically identical Battey mycobacteria from sputa of healthy piggery workers and lesions of pigs, *Aust. Vet. J.* **46:**606–607 (1970).
84. Schaefer, W. B., Birn, K. J., Jenkins, P. A., and Marks, J., Infection with the Avian–Battey group of mycobacteria in England and Wales, *Br. Med. J.* **2:**412–415 (1969).
85. Judson, F. N., and Feldman, R. A., Mycobacterial skin tests in humans 12 years after infection with *Mycobacterium marinum*, *Am. Rev. Respir. Dis.* **109:**544–547 (1974).
86. Wallace, R. J., Jr., Swenson, J. M., Silcox, V. A., Good, R. C., Tschen, J. A., and Stone, M. S., Spectrum of disease due to rapidly growing mycobacteria, *Rev. Infect. Dis.* **5:**657–679 (1983).
87. Bolan, G., Reingold, A. L., Carson, L. A., Silcox, V. A., Woodley, C. L., Hayes, P. S., Hightower, A. W., McFarland, L., Brown, J. W., III, Petersen, N. J., Pavero, M. S., Good, R. C., and Broome,

C. V., Infections with *Mycobacterium chelonei* in patients receiving dialysis and using processed hemodialyzers, *J. Infect. Dis.* **152:**1013–1019 (1985).
88. Costrini, A. M., Mahler, D. A., Gross, W. M., Hawkins, J. E., Yesner, R., and D'esopo, N. D., Clinical and roentgenographic features of nosocomial pulmonary disease due to *Mycobacterium xenopi*, *Am. Rev. Respir. Dis.* **123:**104–109 (1981).
89. Burns, D. N., Wallace, R. J., Schultz, M. E., Zhang, Y., Zubairi, S. Q., Pang, Y., Gibert, C. L., Brown, B. A., Noel, E. S., and Gordin, F. M., Nosocomial outbreak of respiratory tract colonization with *Mycobacterium fortuitum:* Demonstration of the usefulness of pulsed-field gel electrophoresis in an epidemiologic investigation, *Am. Rev. Respir. Dis.* **144:**1153–1159 (1991).
90. Kilby, J. M., Gilligan, P. H., Yankaskas, J. R., Highsmith, W. E., Edwards, L. J., and Knowles, M. R., Nontuberculous mycobacteria in adult patients with cystic fibrosis, *Chest* **102:**70–75 (1992).
91. Ortbals, D. W., and Marr, J. J., A comparative study of tuberculous and other mycobacterial infections and their associations with malignancy, *Am. Rev. Respir. Dis.* **117:**39–45 (1978).
92. Mason, U. G., Greenberg, L. E., Yen, S. S., and Kirkpatrick, C. H., Indomethacin-responsive mononuclear cell dysfunction in "atypical" mycobacteriosis, *Cell. Immunol.* **71:**54–65 (1982).
93. Dattwyler, R. J., Thomas, J., and Hurst, L. C., Antigen-specific T-cell anergy in progressive *Mycobacterium marinum* infection in humans, *Ann. Intern. Med.* **107:**675–677 (1987).
94. von Reyn, C. F., Maslow, J. N., Barber, T. W., Falkinham, J. O., and Arbeit, R. D., Persistent colonisation of potable water as a source of *Mycobacterium avium* infection in AIDS, *Lancet* **343:** 1137–1141 (1994).
95. Sohn, C. C., Schroff, R. W., Kliewer, K. E., Lebel, D. M., and Fligiel, S., Disseminated *Mycobacterium avium-intracellulare* infection in homosexual men with acquired cell-medicated immunodeficiency: A histologic and immunologic study of two cases, *Am. J. Clin. Pathol.* **79:**247–252 (1983).
96. Damsker, B., and Bottone, E. J., *Mycobacterium avium–Mycobacterium intracellulare* from the intestinal tracts of patients with the acquired immunodeficiency syndrome: Concepts regarding acquisition and pathogenesis, *J. Infect. Dis.* **151:**179–181 (1985).
97. Gribetz, A. R., Damsker, B., Bottone, E. J., Kirschner, P. A., and Teirstein, A. S., Solitary pulmonary nodules due to nontuberculous mycobacterial infection, *Am. J. Med.* **70:**39–43 (1981).
98. Prince, D. S., Peterson, D. D., Steiner, R. M., Gottlieb, J. E., Scott, R., Isreal, H. L., Figueroa, W. G., and Fish, J. E., Infection with *Mycobacterium avium* complex in patients without predisposing conditions, *N. Engl. J. Med.* **321:**863–868 (1989).
99. Reich, J. M., and Johnson, R. E., *Mycobacterium avium* complex pulmonary disease presenting as an isolated lingular or middle lobe pattern, *Chest* **101:**1605–1609 (1992).
100. Burchard, G. D., and Bierther, M., Buruli ulcer: Clinical pathological study of 23 patients in Lambaréné, Gabon, *Trop. Med. Parasitol.* **37:**1–8 (1986).
101. Roth, R. I., Owen, R. L., Keren, D. F., and Volberding, P. A., Intestinal infection with *Mycobacterium avium* in acquired immune deficiency syndrome (AIDS): Histological and clinical comparison with Whipple's disease, *Digest. Dis. Sci.* **30:**497–504 (1985).
102. Horsburgh, C. R., Jr., Havlik, J. A., Ellis, D. A., *et al.*, Survival of patients with AIDS and disseminated *Mycobacterium avium* complex infection with and without antimycobacterial therapy, *Am. Rev. Respir. Dis.* **144:**557–559 (1991).
103. Margileth, A. M., Chandra, R., and Altman, P., Chronic lymphadenopathy due to mycobacterial infection: Clinical features, diagnosis, histopathology, and management, *Am. J. Dis. Child* **138:**917–922 (1984).
104. Huebner, R. E., Schein, M. F., Cauthen, G. M., Geiter, L. J., and O'Brien, R. J., Usefulness of skin testing with mycobacterial antigens in children with cervical adenopathy, *Pediatr. Infect. Dis. J.* **11:**450–456 (1992).
105. Huebner, R. E., Schein, M. R., Cauthen, G. M., Geiter, L. J., Selin, M. J., Good, R. C., and O'Brien, R. J., Evaluation of the clinical usefulness of mycobacterial skin test antigens in adults with pulmonary mycobacterioses, *Am. Rev. Respir. Dis.* **145:**1160–1166 (1992).
106. Thompson, N. J., Glassroth, J. L., Snider, D. E., Jr., and Farer, L. S., The booster phenomenon in serial tuberculin testing, *Am. Rev. Respir. Dis.* **119:**587–597 (1979).
107. Stone, B. L., Cohn, D. L., Kane, M. S., Hildred, M. V., Wilson, M. L., and Reves, R. R., Utility of paired blood cultures and smears in diagnosis of disseminated *Mycobacterium avium* complex infections in AIDS patients, *J. Clin. Microbiol.* **32:**841–842 (1994).
108. Murray, P. R., False-positive acid-fast smears, *Lancet* **2:**377 (1978)
109. Centers for Disease Control and Prevention, 1997 USPHS/IDSA guidelines for the prevention of opportunistic infections in persons infected with human immunodeficiency virus, *Morbid. Mortal. Week. Rep.* **46**(No. RR-12):12–13 (1997).
110. Nightingale, S. M., Cameron, D. W., Gordin, F. M., *et al.*, Two controlled trials of rifabutin prophylaxis against *Mycobacterium avium* complex in AIDS, *N. Engl. J. Med.* **329:**828–833 (1993).
111. Pierce, M., Crampton, S., Henry, D., *et al.*, A randomized trial of clarithromycin as prophylaxis against disseminated *Mycobacterium avium* complex infection in patients with advanced acquired immunodeficiency syndrome, *N. Engl. J. Med.* **335:**384–391 (1996).
112. Havlir, D. V., Dubé, M. P., Sattler, F. R., *et al.*, Prophylaxis against disseminated *Mycobacterium avium* complex with weekly azithromycin, daily rifabutin, or both, *N. Engl. J. Med.* **335:**392–398 (1996).
113. Benson, C. A., Cohn, D. L., and Williams, P., ACTG 196/CPCRA 009 Study Team. A Phase III prospective, randomized, double-blind study of the safety and efficacy of clarithromycin (CLA) vs. rifabutin (RBT) vs. CLA-RBT for prevention of *Mycobacterium avium* complex disease in HIV-positive patients with CD4 counts $\leq$ 100 cells/u [Abstract 205], in: *Program and Abstracts of 3rd Conference on Retroviruses and Opportunistic Infections*, p. 91.2, Washington, DC, January 28–February 1, 1996. Alexandria, VA, Infectious Disease Society of America, 1996.
114. Safran, S. D., Singer, J., Zarowny, D. P., *et al.*, A comparison of two regimens for the treatment of *Mycobacterium avium* complex bacteremia in AIDS: Rifabutin, ethambutol and clarithromycin verson rifampin, ethambutol, clofazimine, and ciprofloxacin, *N. Engl. J. Med.* **335:**377–383 (1996).

12. Suggested Reading

American Thoracic Society, Diagnosis and treatment of disease caused by nontuberculous mycobacteria, *Am. J. Respir. Crit. Care Med.* **156:**S1–S25 (1997).

Edwards, P. Q., and Edwards, L. B., Story of the tuberculin test from an epidemiologic point of view, *Am. Rev. Respir. Dis.* **81**(1)**:**Part 2 (1960).

Horsburgh, C. R., Jr., *Mycobacterium avium* complex infections in patients with the acquired immunodeficiency syndrome, *N. Engl. J. Med.* **324:**1332–1338 (1991).

Lincoln, E. M., and Gilbert, L. A., Disease in children due to mycobacteria other than *Mycobacterium tuberculosis*, *Am. Rev. Respir. Dis.* **105:**683 (1972).

Wolinsky, E., Mycobacterial diseases other than tuberculosis, *Clin. Infect. Dis.* **15:**1–12 (1992).

CHAPTER 41

Tularemia

Richard B. Hornick

1. Introduction

Tularemia is a rare infectious disease caused by a small pleomorphic, gram-negative rod, *Francisella tularensis*. Patients who acquire the disease have symptoms and signs that relate to the portals of entry of the bacteria: oculoglandular, ulceroglandular, pneumonic, and typhoidal. This infectious disease has been thoroughly studied through induced infections in volunteers; hence, a considerable body of data has been accumulated in a quantitative fashion about the pathogenicity of tularemia bacilli in humans. Man appears to be one of the most susceptible mammalian hosts studied: fewer than 50 organisms can cause disease whether administered intradermally or by the respiratory route.[1] The usual sources of infections are animals, especially cottontail rabbits, voles, and muskrats. Humans acquire the disease by direct contact or by bites of the ticks, mosquitoes, deerflies, and other insects that infest such animals. An effective vaccine, unique for bacterial infections because it consists of a live attenuated strain, has been developed.[2]

2. Historical Background

Tularemia is one of the first human infectious diseases named by and carefully studied by United States scientists. The disease is named after Tulare County, California, where the organism was isolated. Following the great San Francisco earthquake and fire in 1910, Dr. George W. McCoy[3] of the US Public Health Service was sent to the area to investigate a possible outbreak of bubonic plague. His studies uncovered a "plaguelike" disease among ground squirrels in Tulare County. The disease was characterized by pathological lesions similar to those of plague, but caused by a small pleomorphic, gram-negative rod he was able to isolate from the infected animals. He name it *Bacterium tularense*. The organism was later classified with *Pasteurella*, as *P. tularensis*, but subsequent differences in growth characteristics and DNA homology studies dictated the removal from that genus, and it is now called *Francisella tularensis* to honor Dr. Edward Francis, who described much of the early bacteriologic and immunologic information about tularemia. The initial reasons for distinguishing this newly found bacterium from plague were the apparent absence of organisms in stained smears of infected organs of guinea pigs and failure to isolate *P. pestis* on plain agar and in bouillon inoculated with infected tissues. The failure to stain organisms in infected tissues was a characteristic that persisted until fluorescent-antibody conjugate staining was developed. In 1912, McCoy and Chapin[4] isolated the organism on coagulated egg-yolk media. The first human cases proven by isolation of the organism were reported in 1914 by Vail[5] from a patient with oculoglandular disease and also in 1914 by Wherry,[6] who additionally described transmission of the bacterium from rodent to man. The name *tularemia* was coined by Dr. Francis, who studied the plaguelike disease both in rodents in Tulare County and in patients with deerfly fever in Utah in 1919 and 1920. He concluded that since both diseases were manifestations of the same bacterium and were frequently bacteremic, the name should reflect these facts, i.e., tularemia.[7,8] He also implicated the deerfly, ticks, and other ectoparasites of animals in the transmission of disease.

It is now recognized that the disease had been identified in Japan[9] and Norway[10] in the 19th century. In Japan, Soken had written a perfect description of glandular tularemia in 1818 and attributed the disease to "ingestion of poisonous hare meat."[99]

Richard B. Hornick • Medical Education Administration, Orlando Regional Medical Center, Orlando, Florida 32806.

A disease of ill lemmings was studied in 1890 by Horne[10] in Norway, who isolated a bacterium from these animals. This was probably the first isolation of *F. tularensis*, but Horne has not been credited for this discovery in the literature.

In 1924, the first scientific article on tularemia was published in Japan describing a mild systemic febrile disease acquired from skinning a dead rabbit.[9] Ohara, who described this disease, also conducted the first volunteer study with tularemia when he rubbed heart blood from a dead rabbit onto the skin of his wife, who shortly thereafter developed self-limiting ulceroglandular disease. Dr. Francis recognized this description of the infection to be the same as tularemia, and he called the Japanese disease Ohara's disease, while Dr. Ohara named it yato-byo (wild hare disease).

Subsequent studies have demonstrated infection in over 100 species of wild and domestic animals as well as in ticks and deerflies. Furthermore, because of the highly contagious characteristics of this organism, man was frequently infected through laboratory-acquired infections. Epizootics among experimental animals also occurred.[11] It is obvious from these statements that this organism must be carefully handled when it is brought into a laboratory. Despite its reputation as a highly infectious agent, no person-to-person transmission has been reported. Reasons for this are unclear.

3. Methodology

Tularemia was made a disease reportable to the Public Health Service in 1927. Cases and deaths are regularly recorded in the United States in the *Morbidity and Mortality Weekly Report* of the Centers for Disease Control and Prevention (CDC). Worldwide, the *Weekly Epidemiological Record* and the *Annual Statistical Report* of the World Health Organization (WHO) summarize the reported cases.

3.1. Sources of Mortality Data

The mortality rates for tularemia are based on small series of cases from around the world and are clouded by antibiotic treatment and failure to discriminate which of the strains of tularemia is etiologically implicated. Two strains of tularemia differing in virulence have been characterized.[12] In this chapter they will be referred to as type A, the highly virulent strain, and type B. The official names for each are (type A) *F. tularensis* subspecies tularensis and (type B) *F. tularensis* subspecies holartica (formally subspecies palaeartica).

The mortality rate from type B infections has not been clearly differentiated from that from type A infections because the proportion of cases caused by each strain in this country has not been ascertained. Some workers postulate that there are more cases caused by type B in this country, but that because of their mild nature they do not reach the reporting network or if seen by a physician may be misdiagnosed. Death caused by this strain is probably a very unusual event, unless the patient develops pneumonia. On the other hand, the more virulent form of disease caused by type A will usually be reported because the patient is more likely to seek medical help. Furthermore, since these strains are carried by the almost ubiquitous cottontail rabbit, there would appear to be greater opportunities for more people to come in contact with the organism from this source than from waterborne rodent-associated sources (type B), i.e., muskrats, voles, and the like. For these reasons, type A disease will appear to be the more common type of infection. Ulceroglandular disease caused by either strain should not be associated with any mortality in a normal human host, especially if appropriate antibiotic therapy is administered. In the preantibiotic era, the mortality rate was around 5% for this form of disease, but whether this rate was due to infections caused only by type A strains is not clear. It would appear that the mortality rates in European and Asian countries (type B strains) were low and that death was a rare occurrence. In the preantibiotic era, the mortality rate in patients with pleuropneumonic disease was 30–60%. The mortality rate for patients with tularemic pneumonia treated with streptomycin appears to be less than 1%. In a series of 29 cases collected over a 20-year period (1949–1969) in Arkansas, no deaths occurred in the 28 patients receiving streptomycin.[13] No deaths were reported in 20 of 34 persons who developed laboratory-acquired tularemic pneumonitis and were treated with broad-spectrum antibiotics.[14] In an early study in 1946, 12 patients with tularemic pneumonia were treated with streptomycin.[15] One died on day 7 after apparent recovery. The cause of death was thought to be a massive pulmonary embolus. These three series provide strong evidence that although tularemic pneumonia can be a life-threatening disease, early and appropriate antibiotic therapy can control the infectious process so that death from infection should not occur.

3.2. Sources of Morbidity Data

All diagnosed cases of tularemia in the United States must be reported to state health departments and from them to the CDC. It is likely that many undiagnosed cases occur because of the self-limiting nature of the tularemic infection, especially cases caused by type B strains. The difficulty (and risk) in isolating the causative organism—it requires a selective medium not routinely employed in microbiology laboratories (see Section 3.4.1)—and the spontaneous recovery of many cases of ulceroglandular tularemia compound the diagnostic difficulties. Many individual cases will not be diagnosed. Surveys are done only when a miniepidemic or an epizootic has been identified.[16] Otherwise, only the single diagnosed cases are reported and the true incidence of the disease is unknown. Because of the seemingly huge reservoir of infection in animals, the potential for continued outbreaks in man is great.

3.3. Surveys

In addition to clinical histories, surveys have been made using various serological and skin tests. However, such surveys have been done largely when epidemics have occurred.[17] Because of the varied methods of transmission and potential sources of infection, surveys need to be generalized to include occupational and recreational activities in order to determine a common source and pattern of spread. Human-to-human transmission has not been shown, so appropriate histories will suggest populations to be surveyed who have had similar occupational or recreational exposures. Familial outbreaks occur from common sources, not by direct contact.

3.4. Laboratory Diagnosis

3.4.1. Isolation and Identification of the Organism. *F. tularensis* can be isolated from pus taken from ulcers or aspirated from a bubo, sputum, pharyngeal washes, or gastric aspirations from a patient with pneumonitis or typhoidal disease. Blood cultures are rarely positive, but the readily available radiometric methods of detecting bacterial growth could change this concept. These blood culture techniques may be more sensitive than other methods in detecting the presence of tularemia bacilli. Indeed, some seriously ill patients with infections of unknown etiology have been fortuitously diagnosed in this manner.[18] The clinical specimens should be inoculated intraperitoneally into guinea pigs if the necessary animal isolation facilities are available. The presence of one to five viable cells of *F. tularensis* will cause death within 5–10 days. The pathology in the spleen in these animals is pathognomonic of tularemia. Direct isolation of the organism can be undertaken in a laboratory with an effective hood or an adequate isolation laboratory that will prevent accidental aerogenic spread. The acceptable media used to grow the organisms are: glucose cysteine blood agar, cystine heart gar (Difco), eugon agar, and glucose cysteine agar (BBL). Potential contaminants in clinical specimens can be suppressed by the addition of 0.1 mg cycloheximide and 20 U penicillin/ml basal menstruum. Tularemia bacilli are small (0.2–0.7 μm), as are the colonies that appear on solid media after 48–72 hr of incubation of 37°C. Staining of infected tissues with the usual stains will not demonstrate this bacterium. Either fluorescent staining or a modified Dieterle stain must be used.[19]

3.4.2. Serological and Skin Tests. The skin test is a reliable method of detecting past infections.[17] Both skin tests and serological tests are useful for diagnostic and epidemiological investigations. The skin test is now performed with an antigen derived by ether extraction of *F. tularensis*. This material is prepared by the Rocky Mountain Laboratory, National Institute of Allergy and Infectious Diseases. A 0.1-ml dose of the antigen is injected intradermally into the volar surface of the forearm. A 48-hr reading is performed and should be positive in most infected individuals at that time, rarely at 72 hr. Induration of 5-mm diameter indicates a positive test. It appears to be the most reliable skin test antigen, with excellent reproducibility; unfortunately, it is not readily available. Earlier preparations, i.e., Foshay antigen, a phenolized solution of killed bacteria diluted 1:1000, also gave good results, but were more reactive. The advantages of the skin test are that it is positive earlier than the agglutination test and also appears to be more sensitive in persons infected more than 2 years previously. The antibody titers may be undetectable or at low levels several years after infection, but the skin test remains positive. There are no known antigens cross-reactive with the skin test antigens. The larger the infected dose of organisms, the more rapid the skin test converts; e.g., doses of vaccine organisms (attenuated or live attenuated vaccine strains) in the range of 5000 to 500,000 organisms produced conversions in 37% of recipients at 10 days and 75% conversion at 30 days.[20] Twenty million organisms produced conversions in 80% after 5 days.

The skin test is reproducible, i.e., persistently negative, in nonimmune individuals. A small number of immune persons may lack skin test reproducibility—4% had intermittently positive tests; reasons for this are unknown, but in the case of the vaccinated person, this could represent a failure of the vaccine to colonize.[17]

There is no stimulation of agglutinins in persons who had negative antibody titers prior to skin testing. Persons with positive titers may demonstrate a boost in titer. Buchanan *et al.*[17] tested serum specimens from 33 persons who had had tularemia or had received vaccine. The paired serum specimens were tested on the same day; 3 (9.1%) demonstrated a fourfold or greater rise in titer.[17]

Various antibodies to the tularemia organisms can be tested, but the primary serological test has been the measurement of agglutinating antibodies. This has been the standard test because it is reliable and reproducible; a titer of 1:160 or greater is strong evidence of recent infection, but the fourfold rise in titer of paired specimens is the definitive serological confirmation of infection or disease or both. The titer will often begin to rise in the 2nd week of illness and peak during the 3rd and 4th weeks. Antibiotic therapy does not appear to modify the antibody response. Antibody titers may remain elevated for 6–8 months before declining to low or undetectable levels by 18–24 months. The antigen used in the agglutination test is a suspension of formalin-killed bacteria.(21) The serum–bacteria mixture is incubated overnight at 37°C in a water bath before being read. The titers are recorded as the highest serum dilution showing a 2+ agglutination. A microagglutination test has been developed to facilitate the test and uses less serum and reagents. The IgM antibodies appear to be highly effective in promoting the agglutination process. As the IgG antibodies appear in the serum and replace IgM, there is a general fall in agglutinating titer. The agglutination test is known to cross-react with *Brucella* and *Proteus* OX-19 antigens.(22) Studies have suggested cross-reactivity with mycoplasma and legionella antigens. These cross-reacting antibodies occur in the first few weeks after exposure of the host to tularemia antigen. The studies of Saslaw and Carlisle(22) clarified the dynamics of the cross-reacting *Brucella* antibodies. Of volunteers receiving live vaccine or exposed to low doses of viable organisms, 25% developed *Brucella* agglutinins. The titer was not as high as the homologous tularemia titer. The *Brucella* antibodies frequently fell to undetectable levels after 6 months, and there was no rebound phenomenon when a viable challenge was administered to vaccinated volunteers. At the time of this study, measurements of IgM and IgG antibodies were not done. From subsequent data, it would appear that the cross-reacting antibodies may be primarily IgM and could be expected to be less specific in their antigen binding than the later-appearing, more specific IgG antibodies. This cross-reactivity may be confusing when a differentiation of etiologic causes of a febrile illness is being considered and the serological data provide the discriminating diagnostic evidence.

Other antibody tests have been used to detect tularemia infection but have not supplanted the agglutinin test. The hemagglutination test utilizing tularemia polysaccharide as the antigen attached to erythrocytes is more sensitive than the agglutination test in that the titers appear slightly earlier, i.e., 1 week, attain a higher titer, and appear to persist as long as the agglutinin titers.(21) There does not appear to be any cross-reactivity with *Brucella* antigens in this test system.(23)

Complement-fixation antibody tests usually respond later than the agglutination or hemagglutination test. The titers fail to reach the same dilution as do these two antibody tests, and there is also a more rapid decline in titer.

Rapid diagnosis can be made in those laboratories competent to conduct polymerase chain reaction (PCR).(24) This test detects evidence of the organisms inside neutrophils or elements of the reticuloendothial systems. In essence, there is no true bacteremic phase, i.e., bacteria in the plasma. Cultures of blood will yield organisms released from lysed neutrophils.

4. Biological Characteristics of the Organism

There are two strains of tularemia. Subspecies tularensis or type A is lethal for domestic rabbits (*Oryctolagus*), can ferment glycerol, and contains citrulline ureidase. This strain has been found only in North America, especially in cottontail rabbits. Strain B is less virulent for the rabbit, lacks the biochemical characteristics listed for type A, and is found in Europe, Asia, and North America. Usually, it has been associated with rodents and waterborne disease. This strain is referred to as *F. tularensis* subspecies holartica, which is an appropriate name since there have been no differences shown between the type B strains isolated in Europe and Asia and the fresh isolates in North America.(25)

F. tularensis can persist in at least 100 animal species without causing death of the host, e.g., pigs.(26) It is highly virulent (type A) for cottontail rabbits and has caused epizootics in nature in these animals. Indeed, this species is a common source of infection for man.

What offensive weapons these bacteria have to establish infection and disease with so few organisms is unknown. They do contain some endotoxin, which may account for the initiation of the febrile response; it may influence phagocytosis and also the release of macrophage-derived cytokines. Once *F. tularensis* have penetrated the skin or are inhaled into the terminal bronchioles, they begin to multiply and apparently can evade destruction by complement and immune-serum-mediated antibacterial systems and by neutrophils and the cytokines (e.g., tumor necrosis factor-alpha) released by them during the early stages of the inflammatory process. These organisms are either quickly ingested by or actually invade the later arriving macrophages. Considered a facultative intracellular pathogen, their ability to persist inside phagocytes (and other cells) and not be detected in the plasma have suggested that *F. tularensis* should be considered as obligatory intracellular pathogens.[27] They can survive by assimilating essential nutrients, like iron, from the host cell.[27] The acidic milieu of the phagolysosome facilitates iron release from transferrin. This utilization of iron is a virulence factors and may be responsible in part for the declining serum iron levels noted in patients with untreated tularemia. The hostile environment inside the phagocyte includes low pH, hydroxyl radicals, superoxide anions, hydrogen peroxide, and heat. Other virulence factors are necessary to obviate these stresses. *F. tularensis* have the ability to resist these stresses by producing various proteins; they induce molecular chaperones, which may protect against denaturation of cellular proteins or allow for renaturation of denaturated cellular proteins.[28]

There is a dichotomy between their infectivity and their viability when aerosolized: the ability to infect man or monkey declines as the aerosol ages, even though viability (ability to produce a colony on solid media) persists. A tenfold decrease in infectivity occurs after 3 hr.[29] Reasons for this disassociation are unknown. The particle size in the aerosol is of great importance; the smaller the particle, the more likely it is that disease will result. Large particles containing many organisms may cause glandular enlargement of cervical nodes and fever because the initial site of entry presumably is the oral pharyngeal area and not the lower respiratory tract. Large particles are also swallowed, and unless there is a huge concentration of organisms, no enteric, typhoidal-type disease will develop.[30]

The biological characteristics of *F. tularensis* that are associated with the lack of person-to-person transmission are unknown. Reasons for this failure of expelled bacteria to transmit tularemia to other susceptible humans may be related to particle size, but other unknown factors must also be involved. This lack of person-to-person transmission indicates that the disease dead-ends in the human host, preventing additional cases.

The biological properties responsible for the variation in virulence of the two strains of tularemia are also unknown. Neither of these strains can penetrate through gloves, which should be worn when handling rabbits or other suspected hosts.

It must be clearly understood that a high risk of acquiring the disease exists when a clinical specimen is brought into a diagnostic laboratory. The laboratory personnel must be aware of the possible diagnosis of tularemia so that they are alerted to work with the specimens in efficient, protective hoods. The inoculation of animals is dangerous because of the risk not only of human disease but also of starting an epizootic among other animals. The spread from cage to cage occurs by exchange of ectoparasites and presumably aerosolization and from animal to animal by cannibalization.[11]

5. Descriptive Epidemiology

5.1. Prevalence and Incidence

In the United States, the number of reported cases peaked at 2291 in 1939, for a rate of 1.85 cases/100,000 population. Since that year, there has been a steady decline in reported cases, although isolated epidemics have occurred. The annual average number of cases for the years 1965–1969 were 164; 1970–1974, 165 cases; 1975–1979, 157 cases; 1980–1984, 227 cases; 1985–1989, 182 cases; and 1990–1994, 146 cases. Reasons for the increase in the early 1980s are unknown. Figure 1 depicts the incidence curve in the United States from 1955 to 1994.

Serological and skin test surveys in various countries have provided evidence of the prevalence of infection. In Alaska, Philip *et al.*[31] in 1962, found that in some parts of that state as many as 62% of native men had positive skin tests and serological tests corroborated the specificity of the skin test reactions. The lack of clinical cases in this population suggested that avirulent strains of tularemia may have been involved. Subsequent evaluations of strains of *F. tularensis* isolated from ticks of ptarmigan and snowshoe hares revealed the former to be relatively avirulent (type B), while the hare strain was virulent (type A).[25] Which strain is involved predominantly in the animal populations of Alaska is unknown. Nonetheless, it is conceivable that many undiagnosed human cases of tularemia occur in that state and are not reported.

5.2. Epidemic Behavior and Contagiousness

Some epidemics are directly related to epizootics in wild animals. However, the sporadic nature of human epidemics and the few known epizootics without spread to humans indicate that wild animals remain a potential infectious source, but only rarely has man entered the epizootic cycle. An example of this occurred in Vermont in 1967–1969 when an epidemic of tularemia involved trappers and "skinners" exposed to muskrats.[32] No tularemia had been reported from this state previously. It was shown in this study that infection was produced by the relatively avirulent strain of tularemia (type B). This organism is usually associated with waterborne disease of rodents. Indeed, the organism was isolated from samples

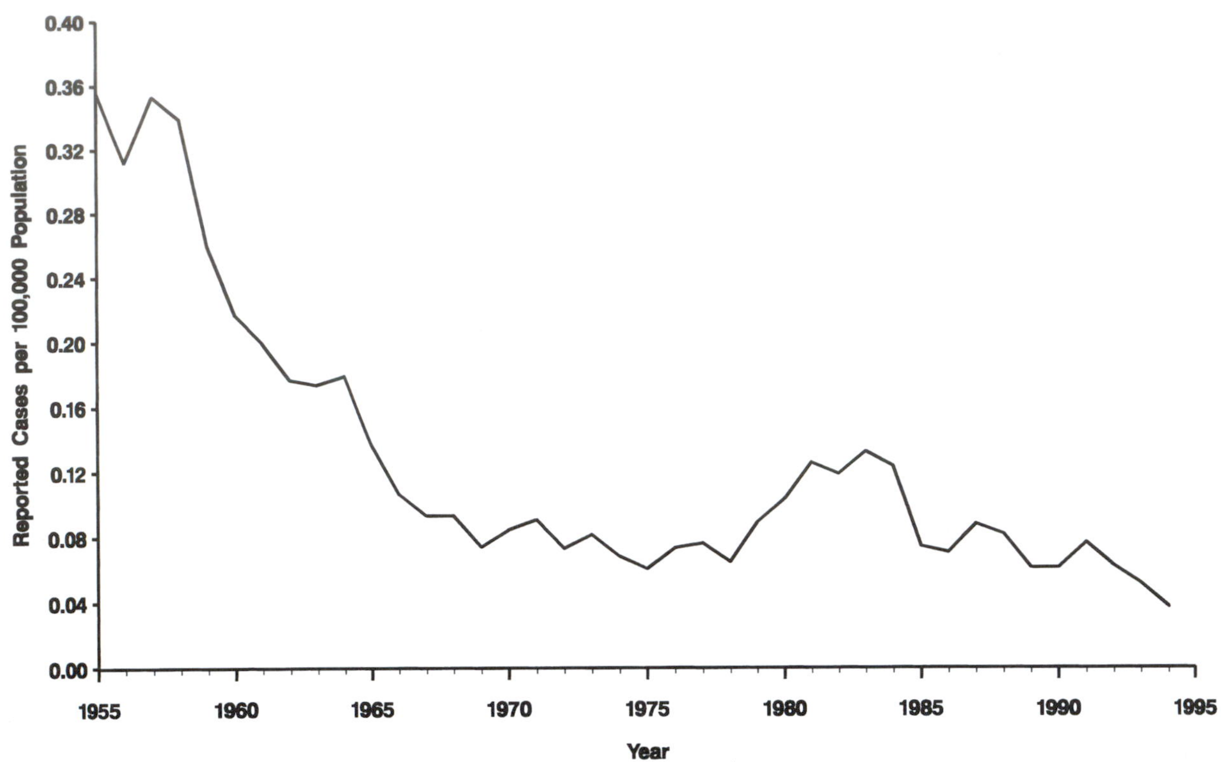

Figure 1. Tularemia—by year, United States, 1955–1994.

of water, mud, and from muskrats. Despite the relatively benign nature of the clinical illnesses, there were four clinical cases to each inapparent infection. These cases were diagnosed by serological techniques. In the second phase of the study, skin testing was also performed, and an additional four cases of the 1968 epidemic were uncovered.[17] Furthermore, 16 cases originating in 1969 and 7 cases that could have had their onset in either 1968 or 1969 were discovered. The conclusion reached by this study was that the skin test provides the epidemiologist with the most sensitive tool for charting the incidence of tularemia over the past 40 years. It may also save the clinician valuable time in diagnosing tularemia because it becomes positive within the 1st or 2nd week of illness, while the agglutination titer may be negative in that period.

This epidemic in Vermont[32] is a good example of the exceptional and fortuitous epidemiological circumstances that coincide with man's association with the epizootic. The muskrats were plentiful and may have been ill, since they were easy to trap, and there was evidence of cannibalism and fighting because many pelts were marred by rips or tears. This epizootic occurred during a very limited time when man could be exposed, the trapping and shooting season. Other epidemics in this country involved exposure to infected deerflies and ticks. In Utah, 30 laborers developed ulceroglandular disease acquired when they were working without shirts. They were bitten by deerflies, which apparently transmitted the disease from infected hares.[33] The illness was mild, probably caused by type B strain. In 1946, 50 men on military maneuvers in Tennessee were bitten by ticks and developed ulceroglandular disease; the reservoir in this epidemic was not uncovered.[34]

A unique miniepidemic occurred in 1978 in seven persons staying in a cottage on Martha's Vineyard.[35] Of the seven, five developed pneumonia and two had typhoidal tularemia. An additional eight cases, found on serosurveys and by reports from physicians of other states, had also been on the island during the same summer period as the initial seven cases. The route of infection in many of the patients was presumed to be by aerosols. The source is uncertain, although several isolates were made from dead cottontail rabbits found on the island. It is suspected that other cases could have occurred but were not diagnosed. These 15 cases represented 11% of the 141 cases reported in the United States in 1978. Four sporadic cases were year-round residents of Martha's Vineyard, representing an annual attack rate of 0.66 case/100,000 inhabitants.

In Sweden, where tularemia was first diagnosed in 1931, five outbreaks subsequently occurred in 1937, 1953, 1960, 1962, and 1966–1967.[36] Most cases were rodent-associated. The last was an extensive outbreak involving 676 cases, of whom 444 were located in one county, Jämtland.[36] Voles were noted to have multiplied in the northern area of Sweden. These animals invaded the stored hay supplies of the farms in this area. The farmers who used this hay in the winter first had to shake out the spoiled hay, which included dead voles and heavy contamination with vole feces. Presumably, most farmers inhaled infected aerosols, since there was a larger number of patients with pneumonia than with ulceroglandular disease. Serological surveys revealed many subclinical cases—32% of the surveyed population in one area and another 16% in another area. Other farmers handled the voles directly and were more likely to develop ulceroglandular disease. Infected hares also caused 23 cases of tularemia, the majority of whom had ulceroglandular disease.

Voles and other rodents have apparently been responsible for contaminating sugar beets. When the beets are washed in the sugar factory, the tularemia organisms are aerosolized as small droplets and infect the factory workers.[37] Several outbreaks occurred in Austria and the former Soviet Union. Some geographic areas of the former Soviet Union appear to have been heavily contaminated, especially during World War II. For example, Rostov had 14,000 cases in January 1942.[38] Many of these patients had angioglandular disease secondary to the consumption of contaminated water (due to type B organisms).

In all the epidemics and outbreaks discussed, no mention of human-to-human transmission was made. This is an unexpected finding, since tularemia is highly infectious when man comes in contact with even small numbers of organisms derived from animals or vectors.

5.3. Geographic Distribution

Most areas of the world north of the 30th parallel have been identified as having tularemia. This includes the northern United States and Alaska,[21] Japan,[9] Norway,[10] Sweden,[36] Austria, and the former Soviet Union.[38] The distribution depends on the range of the reservoir animals. Figure 2 depicts the reported cases by county in the United States in 1994. In North America, the main reservoirs are rabbits and, second, rodents. The cottontail rabbits (*Sylvilagus*) range throughout the United States, with the US–Canadian border being the northern limit.[39] There are only a few cottontails in Maine. These animals are very susceptible to tularemia and die within a week when infected. Their presence is highly pertinent to the epidemiology of tularemia in North America. In all states where tularemia has been endemic, the cottontail has been the only or the predominant rabbit species in that state. The cottontail ranges southward into Mexico and Central and South America. Tularemia has not been reported from Mexico, and reports of tularemia from others of these countries have been minimal.

The snowshoe rabbit (*Lepus americanus*) has been found infected in nature, but it is not an important source of human infections,[39] since it is relatively resistant to tularemia infection. On the other hand, jackrabbits (*Lepus* spp.), which occupy most of the area west of the Mississippi and extend into Canada and Mexico,[39] have been the source for many cases in the United States because they not only transmit disease directly to man when being skinned or eviscerated but also serve as important hosts for ticks and deerflies. These two ectoparasites are significant carriers of *F. tularensis* to man. Jackrabbits are not hunted as extensively as cottontails and in general inhabit areas with sparse human populations compared to regions where cottontails thrive.

The geographic distribution throughout the rest of the world is probably related to the rodent population as distinct from rabbits. These species are infected with the type B strain of tularemia. The number of reported cases is quite small compared to the number reported in the United States. For example, in 1976, there were 157 cases reported in the United States and 61 in Czechoslovakia, but no other European country reported more than 6 cases, and none were reported in Australia or Japan.[40]

The transmission of tularemia by ticks and deerflies helps to explain how at least 100 other species of animals can become infected. These animals have varying degrees of resistance to disease. Hunting dogs that frequently retrieve sick or dying rabbits may become infected; they demonstrate a serological response, but they do not die. Other carnivores may also eat infected rabbits and develop a nonfatal infection. Man may become infected from these sources, such as the bite or scratch of an animal (dog, cat,[19] skunk, coyote, fox, bull snake, wild hog) that has contaminated saliva or teeth from recently eating a diseased rabbit. Animals resistant to disease caused by *F. tularensis* may be temporary carriers with bacteremia and serve as a source of contamination for ticks and deerflies. The following species of ticks have been associated with the transmission of this organism: *Dermacentor andersoni* (Rocky Mountain wood tick), *D. variabilis* (Ameri-

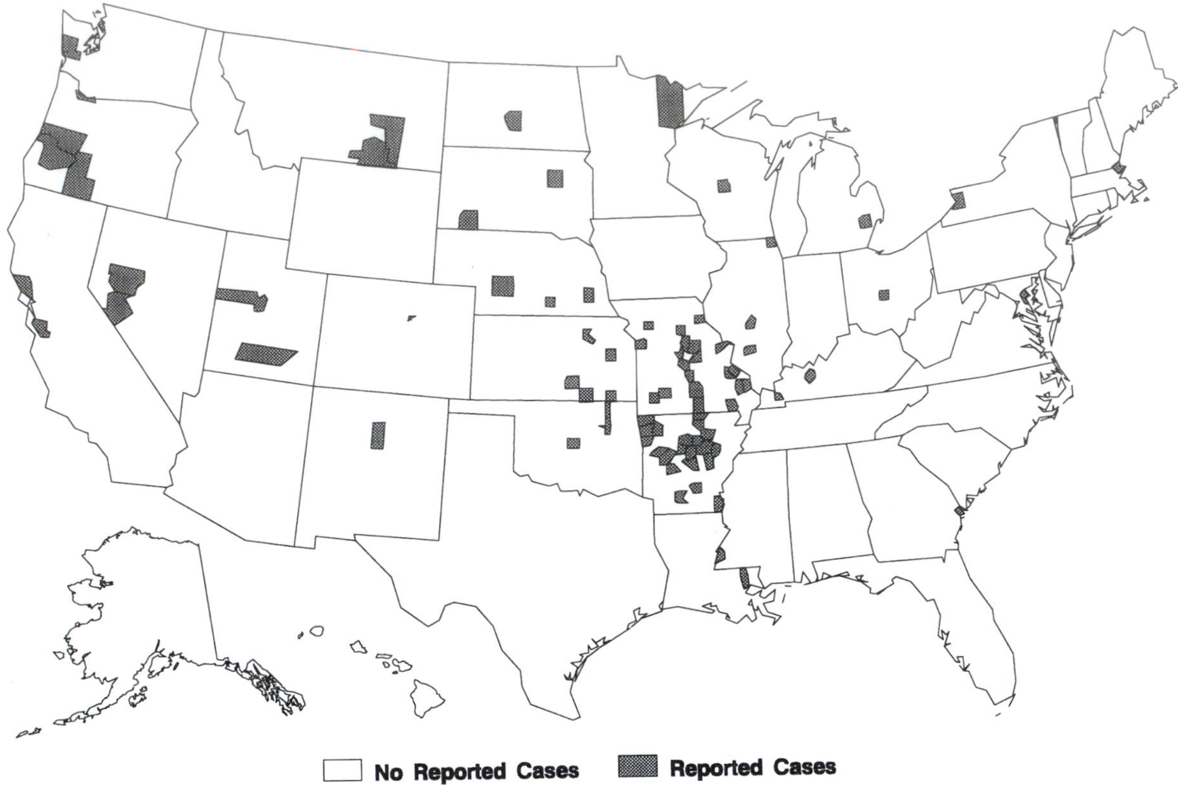

Figure 2. Tularemia—reported cases, by county, United States, 1994.

can dog tick), *D. occidentalis* (Pacific coast dog tick), and *D. americanum* (lonestar tick).

5.4. Temporal Distribution

The peak incidence of tularemia in the United States depends on the source of the infection. In the summer months, when ticks and deerflies are abundant, especially west of the Mississippi, the risk of acquiring tularemia is greatest. During the fall hunting season in the eastern United States, cases of tularemia contracted from captured game, especially cottontail rabbits, sporadically occur. The types of clinical presentations in the miniepidemic in late summer of 1978 on Martha's Vineyard suggest that tick bites or aerosols or both were responsible for the observed cases, but only 1 of the 15 had a history of a tick bite.[35] Ticks have been responsible for over half the cases reported in reviews of cases occurring in endemic states. Some tick bites may go unnoticed, and if this is the portal of entry of the tularemia organisms, an ulcer does not necessarily develop or the lesion may be so small as to be ignored. Because of the importance of tick bites in the spread of tularemia, many cases occur in the spring and summer months.

5.5. Age

Susceptibility to tularemia does not vary with age. In most epidemics, the age of the patients reflects their exposure. Trappers in the Vermont epidemic ranged in age from 11 to 82 years.[32] There is no evidence to suggest that persons at the extremes of age are more susceptible or that they respond less quickly to antibiotic therapy than do young adults.

5.6. Sex

Both sexes develop tularemia after equal exposure. The incidence of the disease was higher in men than women in many epidemics because men were associated with trapping animals or heavy farming jobs. In sporadic cases, either sex may be involved. It has been suggested that women may have been at greater risk in some epidemics caused by ticks and deerflies because their clothing exposed axillary and inguinal areas to bites by these arthropods. However, since both sexes now commonly wear slacks and long-sleeved garments outdoors, they probably have equal opportunities, but fewer opportunities than before, to have their skin attacked by biting or bloodsucking insects.

5.7. Race

Stuart and Pullen[41] reported a higher incidence of pneumonia and a much higher mortality rate among black patients with tularemia than among white patients with tularemia studied in the same hospital. This racial susceptibility to more virulent illness did not appear in the many hundreds of volunteers challenged by various routes with *F. tularensis*.[1,42,43] The validity of the observations in Stuart and Pullen's study has not been confirmed. The question of equal opportunity for prompt medical attention for the patients in their study was not addressed.

5.8. Occupation

Occupation is a crucial epidemiological factor in the acquisition of tularemia. Hunters, trappers, farmers, laboratory workers, forest rangers, game wardens, hikers, campers, and others exposed to aerosolized or direct skin contact with the bacilli or to ticks, deerflies, and wild animals are at greatest risk to infection. Chapin and an assistant, unaware of the infectious threat of the organism they were the first to isolate, were the first to develop laboratory-acquired disease.[25] In one other laboratory accident, petri dishes containing the organism were dropped, resulting in tularemia in five persons.[44] The workup of any patient with suspected ulceroglandular or typhoidal tularemia should include a comprehensive and detailed history of possible occupational and recreational exposures to sources of *F. tularensis*.

5.9. Occurrence in Different Settings

A variety of settings may be involved in outbreaks of tularemia, each of which must include exposure to arthropods or wild animals. While some urban settings may appear less likely than rural or suburban areas for exposure to the organism, the reservoirs of this infection do not necessarily follow this geographic distribution. Cottontail rabbits have become well adapted to city life and range widely through urban neighborhoods. Three cases of tularemic pneumonia were reported in Washington, DC, in 1978, without any source being uncovered. Thus, while the usual setting for tularemia is in the rural areas, suburban and urban areas may also be involved.

As noted in Section 5.2., factory workers washing contaminated sugar beets (voles) developed tularemia[37] in an unusual epidemic that illustrates the viability and virulence of tularemia bacteria.

5.10. Socioeconomic Factors

The best evidence relates to the marked increase in tularemia during World War II, especially in Russia.[38] This increase was thought to be due to the breakdown of public health and sanitation measures. Some of the cases reported in children implied that they were living in substandard rural housing with several dogs and cats living in the same house. Several sources of exposure can be anticipated under these circumstances, such as ticks, deerflies, dead or sick animals brought home by the dogs and cats, and the drinking of contaminated water. Lack of knowledge about the risk of handling diseased rodents and rabbits will lead to greater risk of tularemia.

6. Mechanisms and Routes of Transmission

Tularemia is a sporadic disease that humans acquire when they are bitten by an infected tick or deerfly or when they handle an infected animal. In the process of field dressing a rabbit or skinning a muskrat, the hands may become contaminated because of infected blood or subcutaneous abscesses or from the liver and spleen, which contain millions of organisms. This act of eviscerating the animal can also create an aerosol, and humans become infected by the respiratory route. Rarely is ingestion of contaminated water or food a source of human infection. Increased awareness of the risk of handling sick or dying wild animals, especially rabbits, and the prohibition of selling wild rabbits in meat markets have been largely responsible for the decline in incidence of this disease. The main mechanisms of transmission are through contact of the organism with the skin, eye, oropharynx, or respiratory tract. Tularemia bacilli establish contact with these surfaces by direct contamination of hands, as when an infected animal is being skinned or eviscerated. As few as 50 bacteria can cause ulceroglandular disease in volunteers.[1] The bacterium is purported to be able to penetrate unbroken skin, but whether this is true has not been tested. There are numerous anatomical openings, e.g., hair follicles, through which the organism can gain entrance to the dermis. Minute defects in the epidermis, especially of the hands, due to trivial trauma are common. Entrance into the dermis and lymphatics through such openings could, in retrospect, be conceived as penetration through intact skin. The nail fold is an apparent portal of entry; the mantle area commonly has small tears in the region adjacent to the nail. Presumably, this is a common access route, since ulcers occur frequently in this area. The tick deposits the organisms on the skin adjacent to its bite wound, and rubbing this area could lead to contamination of that wound. Patients have been described in whom rubbing of an eye following apparent contamination of the fingers has led to oculoglandular manifestations of tularemia. Swallowing a large inoculum of tularemia usually results in angioglandular tularemia with few or no signs of gastrointestinal disease.[30] The respiratory tract is readily infected by small-particle aerosols containing as few as 10–50 bacteria.[1] Aerosols are created as an animal is skinned or eviscerated, since there are many organisms in liver ($> 10^7$/g tissue) and spleen and the usual rough extraction of these organs during field dressing could easily cause aerosolization of an infectious dose of *F. tularensis* as well as contaminate the uncovered skin. Bites and scratches of animals have caused tularemia microorganisms to be inoculated directly into the skin.

7. Pathogenesis and Immunity

7.1. Pathogenesis

The incubation period of tularemia varies inversely with the dose of organisms received by the host. Ulceroglandular disease has an incubation of about 2–6 days.[43] In volunteers, injection of a large inoculum, i.e., 2500 minimal infectious doses, into the superficial layers of the skin results in 48 hr in a macular erythematous lesion not unlike a positive tuberculin test.[42] This lesion becomes popular and pruritic and slowly enlarges. As it increases in size, the overlying skin becomes taut, thin, and shiny, and rarely is the papule fluctuant. At about 96 hr, ulceration occurs; the resulting lesion is depressed, with sharply demarcated edges. The base is frequently black and dry. Fever occurs as the papule is forming. In untreated patients infected with type A organisms, the draining lymph nodes enlarge and become caseous, i.e., buboes. These lesions rarely drain spontaneously. A similar sequence of events occurs with type B infections, but there is less systemic reaction. If untreated, the lesions and lymph nodes may persist for months before completely resolving. After inoculation, an immune individual will not develop an ulcer, but rather will demonstrate a small indurated papule similar to a positive tularemia skin test. This is the histopathologic process initiated by both live and inactivated antigens. Biopsy of skin lesions induced by killed *F. tularensis* or by live attenuated vaccine (LVS) strains reveals mononuclear perivascular infiltrates. In monkeys, studies have carefully quantitated the local and systemic bacteriologic events and correlated these events to histologic and immunologic findings.[45] The LVS multiplied in the skin of monkeys, reaching at 3 days peak numbers that persisted for 10 days. By day 14, the count began to taper. Isolations from regional lymph nodes were made only on day 28. All tissues cultured were free of the strain by day 90. Similar but more extensive findings would be expected with the virulent strains. It is not known how long the organisms remain viable in human skin, but it is probably only for a relatively short time after antibiotic therapy is started. Residual antigen persists at the site of initial skin penetrance, as deduced from volunteer studies. The initial site flared as a positive skin test when viable organisms were inoculated into another area of skin, i.e., the opposite arm. As noted, the new site may also simulate a positive skin test. In the monkey studies, antitularensis γ-globulin appeared in plasma cell precursors in regional lymph nodes by day 3, in the spleen on day 5, and at the site of dermal inoculation on day 14.[46] The antibody γ-globulin persisted in the spleen and regional nodes through the 90th day. In addition to this evidence of antitularensis γ-globulin appearing in the infected animals, other models, especially mouse and rat, have been employed to demonstrate development of cellular immunity. It is known that man develops delayed-type hypersensitivity during the first week of disease.[17]

Aerogenic infection accounts for primary pneumonic tularemia, the most serious form of disease. Pneumonia is probably initiated by terminal bronchial and/or alveolar localization of the inhaled small particles (< 5-μm diameter) containing *F. tularensis*.[45,47] The inflammatory reaction is acute and progressive in the animals infected with the virulent strain of tularemia. This results in necrosis of alveolar walls and evolves into small areas of pneumonitis. In the monkey models (small-particle challenge), the virulent organisms multiplied rapidly in the lung starting at first sampling, i.e., 20 min until 72 hr. Microscopic findings were apparent at 24 and 48 hr, with organisms demonstrated by fluorescent staining inside macrophages by 20 min after inhalation. These macrophages were in the lumina of the bronchioles. By 24 hr, bronchiolitis developed consisting of neutrophils and macrophages that involved the peribronchiolar tissues. This inflammatory reaction extended at 48 hr, with evidence of necrosis and extension into the alveoli. A peribronchiolar and perivascular lymphangitis was evident. Tracheobronchial lymph nodes had definite microscopic changes by 48 hr. Some had cortical foci of necrosis surrounded by neutrophils and histiocytes. At 72 and 96 hr, the normal architecture of the lymph nodes was replaced by necrosis. Of interest is that no lesions were found in the nasal or nasopharyngeal areas of these aerogenecially infected monkeys. The livers and spleens, however, had small focal lesions of necrosis with neutrophils and macrophages by 24 hr. *F. tularensis* was found at these sites. The pneumonic process in man is presumed to be similar. Lesions appear on X rays as ill-defined, difficult-to-see, small oval infiltrates. Rarely does lobar consolidation occur. Occasionally, the necrosis progresses to a lung abscess.

7.2. Immunity

The immunity following tularemia in humans is probably lifelong and will prevent reinfection. Volunteers with acquired immunity after experimental infection resist even large challenge doses of virulent organisms introduced by the intradermal or respiratory routes.[42] Measurement of circulating agglutinating antibody in experimental animals as well as in volunteers shows no association between the level of antibody titer and resistance to disease.

Several studies have been reported by Swedish workers in which lymphocyte dynamics were evaluated following administration of tularemia vaccine or the disease itself.[48,49] It is clear from these studies that is was possible to demonstrate the presence of specifically sensitized circulating T lymphocytes that were completely macrophage- or monocyte-dependent. The time of appearance of these T cells correlates with the skin-testing data; i.e., 2–4 weeks after vaccination with the LVS, the tularemia-specific T lymphocytes were present. The presence of these T lymphocytes did not correlate with the agglutinin titers. These studies employed cellular membranes of the vaccine strain as the stimulating antigen. Other antigens may give different results. In this system, sensitized T lymphocytes could be detected up to 2 years after vaccine administration and 25 years after tularemia disease.[50] The skin test detected infection that occurred more than 2 years previously. It is apparent that a more sensitive *in vitro* test is needed to detect the tularemia-sensitive T lymphocytes. Presumably, these cells indicate that the host is resistant to disease.

8. Patterns of Host Response

When tularemia is acquired from animals or arthropods by a healthy, active human host, several clinical responses may occur. The type of clinical presentation is determined by the portal of entry and the virulence of the infecting strain. Man is highly susceptible so that trivial exposure can lead to a mild or inapparent infection or progress to a systemic illness of moderate intensity. Inapparent infections appear to be common and may result in immunity in the host. Patients with serious underlying illnesses and those who delay seeking medical care or do not receive appropriate antibiotic therapy have greater mortality and morbidity than do patients with tularemia but without these implicating features. Patients with poor outcomes in one series had electrolyte or renal function abnormalities, pneumonia and pleural effusions, elevated serum creatine phosphokinase, and *F. tularensis* bacteremia.[51]

8.1. Clinical Features

The clinical picture is determined by the route of infection. Ticks frequently attach to the lower extremities and often obtain their blood meal in the inguinal area; thus, hosts who acquire tularemia by this route will have significant inguinal adenopathy. Hunters or trappers handling diseased animals may develop ulcers on fingers, around nail folds, or on hands, and buboes develop in axillary nodes. These types of illness are usually mild but leave the patient too ill to work for several days to a week. Antibiotic therapy brings about a prompt recession of symptoms and signs. The buboes should not be drained during the initial days of the disease because this can lead to chronic draining sinus. These nodes will heal without draining.

Most patients with ulceroglandular disease will not have evidence of secondary spread. Secondary tularemic pneumonia due to bacteremia has been reported but is unusual. The spleen may be enlarged during the latter stages of the infection. A rare patient may have generalized adenopathy without any evidence of skin ulcer.

Patients with oculoglandular tularemia may acquire the disease by rubbing the organism into the conjunctival sac. Conceivably, the eye may be contaminated by aerosol exposure. This was not observed in the many volunteer subjects, but has been noted in monkeys exposed to extremely high doses of aerosolized tularemia particles. The conjunctivas become infected, with the formation of small yellowish nodules that resolve readily with appropriate antibiotic therapy.

Tularemic pneumonia has been thought to be more prevalent than cases reported. This diagnosis must be considered in patients with suggestive exposure histories. In endemic areas, tularemia pneumonia should be included in the differential diagnosis, even without a history of contact with the organism.(52) In epidemics, inapparent pneumonia does occur that is diagnosed by reason of chest films taken as a routine procedure, not because of symptoms. The aerogenic infection of man creates substernal discomfort, a dry, paroxysmal cough, fever, and headache.(42) There may be cervical lymph node enlargement. The more prominent the nodes in the neck, the more likely it is that large-particle aerosols were ingested. Patients with pneumonia have been described as having small oval densities on X ray as a classic finding.(53) Subsequent reviews have failed to confirm this finding, since a wide variety of X-ray findings have been described.(13) Pleural effusions, lung abscess, mediastinal adenopathy, and even tracheal compression have been noted. The clinical course of patients with tularemic pneumonia is one of rapid resolution when appropriate antibiotics are given. Prior to antibiotic utilization, the mortality rate was reported to be from 30 to 60%.

Rarely, patients develop pericarditis or meningitis as part of their disease.(54)

8.2. Diagnosis

Tularemia presenting as a typhoidal illness with no localizing signs other than adenopathy is a difficult diagnostic problem. A careful history of possible contact in the previous few days to a week or more with ticks, deerflies, cottontail rabbits, or other animals will provide significant leads for definitive diagnostic tests. Occupational history should be thorough, seeking similar links to such exposures. Serological studies will be helpful, but only after the first 10 days or so after contact with the organism. The initiation of treatment with streptomycin or gentamicin will bring about a prompt therapeutic response. In 24–48 hr, the patient should be less febrile and symptomatically improved. This form of illness may be confused with infectious mononucleosis, toxoplasmosis, cytomegalovirus disease, psittacosis, and rarely with typhoid fever.

Ulceroglandular disease has to be differentiated from sporotrichosis, cat scratch fever, *Mycobacterium marinum* infection, and cutaneous anthrax. In all these diseases, the clue to diagnosis will be obtained from a thorough history and confirmed by appropriate serological studies and culture of material from the lesions on selective media.

9. Control and Prevention

9.1. General Concepts

Education about the risks of handling rodents and rabbits that appear ill should continue to limit the spread of illness from these animals to man. The prohibition of the sale of wild rabbits in markets has been an important public health measure proven to be effective in preventing the spread of tularemia. A simple and useful means of preventing infection is to be aware of the hazards associated with tick attachment and feeding. Protective clothing is helpful, but search for and removal of ticks before retiring when camping or working in tick-infested areas will eliminate any possible chance of infection. Ticks usually feed by attaching to body hairs and feeding when the host is quiet (i.e., asleep).

All cases should be reported to the appropriate public health officials so that a thorough epidemiological study can be made and control measures established to prevent additional exposure. Quarantine is not necessary.

9.2. Antibiotic and Chemotherapeutic Approaches to Prophylaxis

Volunteer studies have shown that streptomycin administered 24 hr after intradermal inoculation of virulent organisms will prevent diseases from developing. This is impractical except in unusual circumstances, e.g., when a laboratory worker is exposed by needle stick or to accidental aerosolization of tularemia bacilli. In this instance, an unvaccinated person would benefit from initiation of gentamicin or streptomycin treatment for a period of 5–7 days. Under no circumstances should antibiotics be given routinely to persons known to have been bitten by a tick or deerfly. The administration of an antibiotic may cause drug fever, delay the incubation period, or fail to prevent tularemia or other infections, i.e., Rocky Mountain spotted fever, and the risk of infection is too low following the bites of most ticks and deerflies to justify antibiotic prophylaxis.

Streptomycin has been the therapeutic antibiotic of choice because of the prompt recovery (expect defervescence in 48 hrs.) associated with its administration. This antibiotic is no longer readily available. Gentamicin (3–5 mg/kg per day intravenously for 6 days) has been equally effective with one possible relapse noted in a patient with a bubo.[55] As noted above, buboes heal slowly, especially if drained. Attempts to cure by needle aspiration will lead to prolonged intermittent drainage. Chloramphenicol and tetracycline (2–3 g/day for 14 days) have been used to successfully treat patients with either ulceroglandular or pneumonic tularemia.[14] Unfortunately, there is a high relapse rate, especially in those patients with pneumonitis treated with these two antibiotics. Ciprofloxacin has been given to a small number of patients, with excellent results. It may be an excellent antibiotic to use instead of gentamicin because of its ease of administration, better levels inside phagocytic cells, and its stability within an acidic environment, e.g., phagolysosome.[55]

9.3. Immunization

A killed vaccine introduced by Foshay was the initial effort to induce resistance to *F. tularensis* invasion. This was a phenolized killed suspension of organisms. Studies in animals and in man indicated that this vaccine did not induce effective resistance to disease. An LVS was developed by Eigelsbach and Downs.[2] They selected one of the two attenuated strains employed earlier by Russian investigators. From this isolate, they evolved a standardized, stable, and effective vaccine strain. LVS has been extensively studied in animals and man, and its effectiveness has been quantitated by means of induced infections in volunteers. The recommended method of administration is by the acupuncture route, similar to smallpox vaccination, which creates excellent immunity against low-dose intradermal and aerogenic (200–2000 organisms) virulent challenges.[42] High doses (25,000 by aerosol) can overcome this immunity, although the illness is modified compared to controls. However, the magnitude of these challenge levels is much greater than what would be expected in nature or under less controlled conditions. For instance, at Fort Detrick, where tularemia was being studied in many laboratories, 10–12 cases of laboratory-acquired disease occurred each year. Since 1959, when all workers were routinely given LVS, no cases of typhoidal tularemia have occurred. The incidence of ulceroglandular disease remained the same, but the illnesses were mild and recovery occurred in a few days without antibiotic treatment. Since agglutinin titers and skin test reactivity appear to diminish after 2 years, revaccination may be needed at some interval, probably 10–15 years, but data are not available to permit a firm recommendation.

LVS is an effective vaccine and should be administered to all persons considered at high risk: selected laboratory workers, forest rangers, game wardens, and others exposed during an outbreak. The vaccine is not generally available but is produced commercially for the Army by the National Drug Co. The physician who wishes to obtain vaccine should direct an application for its release to the Commander, US Army Medical Research Institute of Infectious Diseases, Frederick, Maryland 21701.

The mechanism of immunity following recovery from disease or induced by vaccine appears to be mediated by cellular means rather than antibody. This has been well studied in various animal models.[56–58] In the mouse model, transference of spleen cells from immune to nonimmune mice established excellent protection. These immune cells were collected on day 12 following a secondary immunization with a virulent strain in mice that had been previously immunized with the LVS. *In vitro* studies, employing alveolar macrophages from immune animals, demonstrated remarkable intracellular inhibitory power of these cells as well as their ability to survive when in contact with virulent *F. tularensis*. This effect was demonstrated without the aid of "immune"[59] serum, indicating the primary role played by the cellular defenses of the lung in resisting tularemic disease.

LVS has been experimentally administered by the aerogenic and oral routes.[30,42] The aerogenic route was investigated to ascertain whether the local immune mechanisms in the respiratory tract could be specifically stimulated. The rationale was to gain greater protection against respiratory challenge than could be induced by the intracutaneously administered vaccine. An aerosol dose of 10^4 LVS organisms induced immunity to subsequent small challenges of virulent organisms. When 10^6 or 10^8 LVS organisms were given, the recipients experienced mild flulike illness with headache, coryza, chest pain, and malaise. Of 42 men who received the 10^8 dose, 3 were given streptomycin to control symptoms. The men in the 10^6- and 10^8-dose groups developed increased resistance to challenge with 25,000 virulent organisms. That is, they did not require antibiotic treatment to control their illness, whereas 46% of those who were vaccinated by the intracutaneous route received antibiotic treatment. Measurement of IgA antibodies in sputum was not performed in this study. However, nasal agglutinating antibodies have been detected in patients following intradermal inoculation of LVS as well as in volunteers recovering from aerogenic exposure.[60] It appears that the vaccine can be given by the aerogenic method; but currently, equipment that would deliver a safe reproducible dose and with uniform particle size is not available. At present, the acupuncture method induces excellent protection for naturally acquired disease whether exposure is to the type A or the type B strain.

Massive doses of LVS have been swallowed without significant reactions.[30] Doses of 10^{10} LVS bacilli taken orally as a suspension caused a mild, self-limited febrile illness characterized by cervical adenopathy but no pharyngeal lesions. Serum agglutinating antibodies appeared later than expected, but peaked at 3–4 weeks. Challenge of these volunteers with a small aerosol dose demonstrated excellent protection. The oral route could be a safe and effective method of administering this vaccine strain.

10. Unresolved Problems

Tularemia has been well studied; however, additional investigations are needed to assess the range of susceptibility of animals to this disease. Where do cottontails acquire their disease? Presumably, they acquire it from infected ticks and then transmit it to other ticks. Ticks can transmit the organism transovarially, so that their offspring become infected. Additional studies of ticks feeding on cottontail rabbits are needed.

The duration of immunity induced by LVS requires further study. Skin-testing materials needed to be made readily available for more widespread use.

One fascinating problem remains: to explain adequately and clearly why human-to-human transmission does not occur with this organism. Why does a highly infectious agent like *F. tularensis* fail to cause disease in contacts of patients? There are organisms in pharyngeal washes and saliva; why are these organisms not infectious for man?

11. References

1. Saslaw, S., Engelsbach, H. T., Prior, J. A., Wilson, H. E., and Carhart, S., Tularemia vaccine study. II. Respiratory challenge, *Arch. Intern. Med.* **107:**702–714 (1961).
2. Eigelsbach, H. T., and Downs, C. M., Prophylactic effectiveness of live and killed tularemia vaccines. I. Production of vaccine and evaluation in the white mouse and guinea pig, *J. Immunol.* **87:**415–425 (1961).
3. McCoy, G. W., A plague-like disease of rodents, *Public Health Bull.* No. 43 (1911).
4. McCoy, G. W., and Chapin, C. W., *Bacterium tularense*, the cause of a plague-like disease of rodents, *Public Health Bull.* No. 53 (1912).
5. Vail, D. T., *Bacillus tularense* infection of the eye, *Ophthalmol. Res.* **23:**487 (1914).
6. Wherry, W. B., A new bacterial disease of rodents transmissible to man, *Public Health Rep.* **29:**3387 (1914).
7. Francis, E., Deer-fly fever: A disease of man of hitherto unknown etiology, *Public Health Rep.* **34:**2061–2062 (1919).
8. Francis, E., The occurrence of tularemia in nature, as a disease of man, *Public Health Rep.* **36:**1731 (1921).
9. Ohara, S., *The Story of Yato-Byo* (*Tularemia in Japan*), Obama, Fukushima City, 1955.
10. Horne, H., En lemeng og marsvintest, *Nor. Vet. Tidsskr.* **23:**16 (1911).
11. Owen, C. R., and Buker, E. O., Factors involved in the transmission of *Pasteurella tularensis* from inoculated animals to healthy cage mates, *J. Infect. Dis.* **99:**227–233 (1956).
12. Jellison, W. L., Owen, C. R., Bell, J. F., and Kohls, G. M., Tularemia and animal populations: Ecology and epizootiology, *Wildl. Dis.* **17** (1961).
13. Miller, R. P., and Bates, J. H., Pleuropulmonary tularemia: A review of 29 patients, *Am. Rev. Respir. Dis.* **99:**31–41 (1969).
14. Overholt, E. L., Tigertt, W. D., Kadull, P. J., Ward, M. K., Charkes, N. D., Rene, R. M., Saltzman, T. E., and Stephens, M., An analysis of forty-two cases of laboratory-acquired tularemia: Treatment with broad-spectrum antibiotics, *Am. J. Med.* **30:**785 (1961).
15. Hunt, J. S., Pleuropulmonary tularemia: Observations on 12 cases treated with streptomycin, *Ann. Intern. Med.* **26:**263–276 (1947).
16. McCahan, G. R., Moody, M. D., and Hayes, F. A., An epizootic of tularemia among rabbits in northwestern South Carolina, *Am. J. Hyg.* **75:**335–338 (1962).
17. Buchanan, T. M., Brooks, G. F., and Brachman, P. S., The tularemia skin test—325 skin tests in 210 persons: Serologic correlation and review of the literature, *Ann. Intern. Med.* **74:**336–343 (1971).
18. Klotz, S. A., Penn, R. L., and Provenza, J. M., The unusual presentations of tularemia. Bacteremia, pneumonia and rhabdomyolysis, *Arch. Intern. Med.* **147:**214 (1987).
19. Gallivan, M. V. E., Davis, W. A., III, Garagusi, V. F., Paris, A. L., and Lack, E. E., Fatal cat-transmitted tularemia: Demonstration of the organism in tissue, *South Med. J.* **73:**240–242 (1980).
20. Gaiskii, N. A., Altareva, N. D., and Lennik, T. G., Rapidity of the appearance and length of persistence of immunity after vaccination with tularemia vaccine, in: *History and Incidence of Tularemia in the Soviet Union—A Review* (R. Pollitzer, ed.), pp. 125–136, Institute of Contemporary Russian Studies, Fordham University, New York, 1967.
21. Saslaw, S., and Carhart, S., Studies with tularemia vaccines in volunteers. III. Serologic aspects following intracutaneous or respiratory challenge in both vaccinated and nonvaccinated volunteers, *Am. J. Med. Sci.* **241:**689–699 (1961).
22. Saslaw, S., and Carlisle, H. N., Studies with tularemia vaccines in volunteers. IV. Brucella agglutinins in vaccinated and nonvaccinated volunteers challenged with *Pasteurella tularensis*, *Am. J. Med. Sci.* **242:**166–172 (1961).
23. Alexander, M. M., Wright, G. G., and Baldwin, A. C., Observations on the agglutination of polysaccharide-treated erythrocytes by tularemia antisera, *J. Exp. Med.* **91:**561–566 (1950).
25. Bell, J. F., Ecology of tularemia in North America, *J. Jinsen. Med.* **11:**33–44 (1965).
26. Bivin, W. S., and Hogge, A. L., Jr., Quantitation of susceptibility of swine to infection with *Pasteurella tularensis*, *Am. J. Vet. Res.* **28:**1619–1621 (1967).
27. Fortier, A. H., Leiby, D. A., Narayanan, R. B., Asafoadjei, E., Crawford, R. M., Nacy, C. A., and Meltzer, M. D., Growth of *Francisella tularensis* LVS in macrophages: The acidic intracellular compartment provides essential iron required for growth. *Infect. Immun.* **63:**1478–1483 (1995).
28. Ericsson, M., Tärnvik, A., Kuoppa, K., Sandström, G., and Sjöstedt, A., Increased synthesis of DnaK, GroEL, and GroES

homologs by *Francisella tularensis* LVS in response to heat and hydrogen peroxide, *Infect. Immun.* **62:**178–183 (1994).

29. Sawyer, W. D., Jemski, J. V., Hogge, A. L., Jr., Eigelsbach, H. T., Wolfe, E. K., Dangerfield, H. G., Gochenour, W. S., Jr., and Crozier, D., Effect of aerosol age on the infectivity of airborne *Pasteurella tularensis* for *Macaca mulatta* and man, *J. Bacteriol.* **91:**2180–2184 (1966).
30. Hornick, R. B., Dawkins, A. T., Eigelsbach, H. T., and Tulis, J. J., Oral tularemia vaccine in man, *Antimicrob. Agents Chemother. 1966* pp. 11–14 (1967).
31. Philip, R. N., Huntley, B., Lackman, D. B., and Comstock, G. W., Serologic and skin test evidence of tularemia infection among Alaskan Eskimos, Indians and Aleuts, *J. Infect. Dis.* **110:**220–230 (1962).
32. Young, L. S., Bicknell, D. S., Archer, B. G., Clinton, J. M., Leavens, L. J., Feeley, J. C., and Brachman, P. S., Tularemia epidemic: Vermont, 1968: Forty-seven cases linked to contact with muskrats, *N. Engl. J. Med.* **280:**1253–1260 (1969).
33. Burnett, T. W., Tularemia in a Rocky Mountain sector of the western front, *Mil. Surg.* **78:**193–199 (1936).
34. Waring, W. B., and Ruffin, J. J., A tick-borne epidemic of tularemia, *N. Engl. J. Med.* **234:**137 (1946).
35. Teutsch, S. M., Martone, W. J., Brink, E. W., Potter, M. E., Eliot, G., Hoxsie, R., Craven, R. B., and Kaufmann, A. F., Pneumonic tularemia on Martha's Vineyard, *N. Engl. J. Med.* **301:**826–828 (1979).
36. Dahlstrand, S., Ringertz, O., and Zetterberg, B., Airborne tularemia in Sweden, *Scand. J. Infect. Dis.* **3:**7–16 (1971).
37. Puntigam, F., Thorakale Formen in Seuchengeschehen der Tularämie in Österreich, *Wien. Klin. Wochenschr.* **72:**813–816 (1960).
38. Sil'Chenko, V. S., Epidemiological and clinical features of tularemia caused by waterborne infection, *Zh. Mikrobiol. Epidemiol. Immunobiol.* **28:**788–795 (1957).
39. Jellison, W. L., and Parker, R. R., Rodents, rabbits and tularemia in North America: Some zoological and epidemiological considerations, *Am. J. Trop. Med.* **25:**349–362 (1945).
40. WHO, *Annual Statistics, Infectious Diseases: Cases and Deaths* **2:**1–204 (1978).
41. Stuart, B. M., and Pullen, R. L., Tularemic pneumonia: Review of American literature and report of 15 additional cases, *Am. J. Med. Sci.* **210:**223–236 (1945).
42. Hornick, R. B., and Eigelsbach, H. T., Aerogenic immunization of man with live tularemia vaccine, *Bacteriol. Rev.* **30:**532–538 (1966).
43. Saslaw, S., Eigelsbach, H. T., Wilson, H. E., Prior, J. A., and Carhart, S., Tularemia vaccine study. I. Intracutaneous challenge, *Arch. Intern. Med.* **107:**689–701 (1961).
44. Barbeito, M. S., Alg, R. L., and Wedum, A. G., Infectious bacterial aerosol from dropped petri dish cultures, *Am. J. Med. Technol.* **27:**318–322 (1961).
45. Eigelsbach, H. T., Tulis, J. J., McGavran, M. H., and White, J. D., Live tularemia vaccine. I. Host–parasite relationship in monkeys vaccinated intracutaneously or aerogenically, *J. Bacteriol.* **84:** 1020–1027 (1962).
46. McGavran, M. H., White, J. D., Eigelsbach, H. T., and Kerpsacvk, R. W., Morphologic and immunohistochemical studies of the pathogenesis of infection and antibody formation subsequent to vaccination of *Macaca irus* with an attenuated strain of *Pasteurella tularensis*. I. Intracutaneous vaccination, *Am. J. Pathol.* **41:**259–271 (1962).
47. White, J. D., McGavran, M. H., Prickett, P. A., Tulis, J. J., and Eigelsbach, H. T., Morphologic and immunohistochemical studies of the pathogenesis of infection and antibody formation subsequent to vaccination of *Macaca irus* with an attenuated strain of *Pasteurella tularensis*. II. Aerogenic vaccination, *Am. J. Pathol.* **41:**405–413 (1962).
48. Tärnvik, A., and Löfgren, S., Stimulation of human lymphocytes by a vaccine strain of *Francisella tularensis*, *Infect. Immun.* **12:** 951–957 (1975).
49. Tärnvik, A., Sandström, G., and Löfgren, S., Time of lymphocyte response after onset of tularemia and after tularemia vaccination, *J. Clin. Microbiol.* **10:**854–860 (1979).
50.
51. Penn, R. L., and Kinsewitz, G. T., Factors associated with a poor outcome in tularemia, *Arch. Intern. Med.* **147:**265–268 (1987).
52.
53. Overholt, E. L., and Tigertt, W. D., Roentgenographic manifestations of pulmonary tularemia, *Radiology* **74:**758–765 (1960).
54. Evans, M. E., Gregory, D. W., Schaffner, W., and McGee, Z., Tularemia: A 30-year experience with 88 cases, *Medicine* **64:**251–269 (1985).
55.
56. Eigelsbach, H. T., Hunter, D. H., Janssen, W. A., Dangerfield, H. G., and Rabinowitz, S. G., Murine model for study of cell-mediated immunity: Protection against death from fully virulent *Francisella tularensis* infection, *Infect. Immun.* **12:**999–1005 (1975).
57. Moe, J. B., Canonico, P. G., Stookey, J. L., Powanda, M. C., and Cockerell, G. L., Pathogenesis of tularemia in immune and nonimmune rats, *Am. J. Vet. Res.* **36:**1505–1510 (1975).
58. Proctor, R. A., White, J. D., Ayala, E., and Canonico, P. G., Phagocytosis of *Francisella tularensis* by rhesus monkey peripheral leukocytes, *Infect. Immun.* **11:**145–151 (1975).
59. Nutter, J. E., and Myrvik, W. N., *In vitro* interactions between rabbit alveolar macrophages and *Pasteurella tularensis*, *J. Bacteriol.* **92:**645–651 (1966).
60. Bellanti, J. A., Beuscher, E. L., Brandt, W. E., Dangerfield, H. G., and Crozier, D., Characterization of human serum and nasal hemagglutinating antibody to *Francisella tularensis*, *J. Immunol.* **98:**171–178 (1967).

12. Suggested Reading

Boyce, J. M., Recent trends in the epidemiology of tularemia in the United States, *J. Infect. Dis.* **131:**197–199 (1975).

Brooks, G. F., and Buchanan, T. M., Tularemia in the United States: Epidemiologic aspects in the 1960s and follow-up of the outbreak of tularemia in Vermont, *J. Infect. Dis.* **121:**357–359 (1970).

Butler, T., Plague and tularemia, *Pediatr. Clin. North Am.* **26:**355–366 (1979).

Evans, M. E., Gregory, D. W., Schaffner, W., and McGee, Z. A., Tularemia: A 30 year experience with 88 cases, *Medicine* **64:**251–269 (1985).

Jellison, W. L., Owen, C. R., Bell, J. F., and Kohls, G. M., Tularemia and animal populations: Ecology and epizootiology, *Wildl. Dis.* **17** (1961).

Schmid, G. P., Kornblatt, A. N., Connors, C. A., *et al.*, Clinically mild tularemia associated with tick-borne *Francisella tularensis*, *J. Infect. Dis.* **148:**63–67 (1983).

Taylor, J. P., Istre, G. R., McChesny, T.C., *et al.*, Epidemiologic characteristics of human tularemia in the southwest-central states, 1981–1987, *Am. J. Epidemiol.* **133:**1032–1038 (1991).

CHAPTER 42

Typhoid Fever

Myron M. Levine

1. Introduction

Typhoid fever is an acute generalized infection of the reticuloendothelial system, intestinal lymphoid tissue, and gallbladder caused by *Salmonella typhi*. This communicable disease is restricted to human hosts and humans (chronic carriers) serve as the reservoir of infection. A broad spectrum of clinical illness can ensue, with more severe forms being characterized by persisting high fever, abdominal discomfort, malaise, and headache. In the preantibiotic era, the disease ran its course over several weeks, resulting in a case fatality rate of approximately 10–20%. The protracted, debilitating nature of this febrile illness in untreated (or improperly treated) patients is accompanied by mental cloudiness or stupor, which gave rise to the term "typhoid," meaning stuporlike. Paratyphoid fever is the clinically similar febrile infection caused by *S. paratyphi* A, B, or C. Typhoid and paratyphoid fevers are also referred to as enteric fevers. In most endemic areas, typhoid comprises approximately 90% of enteric fever.

Typhoid infection is virtually always acquired by ingestion of food or water vehicles contaminated by human excreta that contains *S. typhi*. Typhoid fever is extremely uncommon in modern industrialized countries where populations have access to treated water supplies and sanitation that removes human waste. In contrast, among populations in less-developed countries that lack such amenities, typhoid fever is often endemic and, from the public health perspective, typically constitutes the most important enteric disease problem of school-age children.[1] Besides school-age children in less-developed countries, two other populations are at recognized risk of typhoid: travelers and clinical microbiologists. Typhoid fever occurs with variable frequency among travelers from industrialized countries who visit less-developed areas of the world; the risk is highest in travelers to parts of South America and to the Indian subcontinent.[2] Last, clinical microbiologists, including those in industrialized countries, have increased exposure to *S. typhi* and therefore constitute a high-risk group.[3,4]

Typhoid fever is readily treated by prompt administration of appropriate antibiotics. Since 1990, strains of *S. typhi* exhibiting resistance to most of the antimicrobials that previously were clinically effective have spread aggressively throughout the Middle East, the Indian subcontinent, and Southeast Asia.[5,6] The few antibiotics that are effective against these multiply resistant strains are expensive and not readily available in rural areas of less-developed countries. Thus, the arrival on the scene and dissemination of these multiply resistant *S. typhi* constitute an increasing public health crisis in many less-developed countries.

2. Historical Background

Prior to the early decades of the 19th century, typhoid fever was not recognized as a distinct clinical entity and often was confused with other prolonged febrile syndromes, particularly typhus fever of rickettsial origin. A recent review on typhoid fever and typhoid vaccines contains the specific historical references cited below.[7] Debate continues over who first clearly differentiated typhus fever from typhoid (i.e., typhuslike) fever, as medical historians have variously bestowed credit for this clinical clarification upon Huxham (1782), Louis (1829), Gerhard (1837), and Schoenlein (1839).

In 1829, Bretonneau described a severe enteric infection occurring in young Parisians and used the term "do-

Myron M. Levine • Center for Vaccine Development, University of Maryland School of Medicine, Baltimore, Maryland 21201.

thoientérite" ("boil of the intestine") to describe the lesion that can lead to intestinal perforation. Louis (1836) catalogued the abnormal lesions in the intestine, lymph nodes, spleen, and skin (rose sports) in 158 patients and describes hemorrhage and perforation in the gut. During this period, the intestinal lesions were thought to be a complication or unusual extension of typhus fever.

Gerhard, working in Philadelphia, contended that two similar yet distinct febrile illnesses exist that are nevertheless discernable from one another on the basis of pathological findings: one (typhoid) exhibits prominent intestinal lesions. Schoenlein referred to two distinct forms of typhus, "exanthematicus" and "abdominalis." However, it is William Jenner, who circa 1850 definitively dispelled controversy on the subject by providing precise clinical descriptions and pathological observations from postmortem examinations that allowed a clear-cut differentiation between the two illnesses. Jenner argued that the pathological lesions in Peyer's patches and mesenteric lymph nodes were peculiar to typhoid and were never seen with typhus. In 1847, the term "enteric fever" was introduced in an attempt to replace typhoid fever and avoid confusion with typhus. While this term is frequently used, it never supplanted the more common usage of typhoid and paratyphoid fever.

In William Budd's 1873 milestone in epidemiology,[8] *Typhoid Fever: Its Nature, Mode of Spreading and Prevention*, he clearly described the contagious nature of the disease and incriminated fecally contaminated water sources in transmission, years before the causative organism was identified. Eberth (1880) visualized the causative bacilli in tissue sections from Peyer's patches and spleens of infected patients, while Gaffky (1884) grew it in pure culture. Known in earlier years as *Bacillus typhosus*, *Eberthella typhosa*, and *Salmonella typhosa*, it is presently referred to as *Salmonella typhi* or *Salmonella Typhi*.

Typhoid fever was endemic in virtually all countries of Europe and North and South America in the late 19th and early 20th centuries. A single intervention—the treatment of water supplies (by chlorination, sand filtration, or other means)—which became increasingly popular in the late 19th and early 20th century, broke the cycle of endemicity and caused the incidence of typhoid fever to plummet drastically, even though the prevalence of chronic carriers in the populations remained high for decades thereafter.

Inactivated (heat-killed, phenol-preserved) *S. typhi* were utilized as parenteral vaccines as far back as 1896 by Pfeiffer and Kolle in Germany and Wright in England. Wright administered his vaccine (three doses two weeks apart) to two medical officers in the Indian Army, one of whom thereafter ingested wild typhoid bacilli without developing illness. Wright then tested his vaccine in 2835 volunteers in the Indian Army. While local and generalized adverse reactions were common, the results were considered to be sufficiently encouraging for a decision to be made to vaccinate troops embarking for the Boer War in South Africa. Outcry over the frequency of adverse reactions led to a suspension of vaccination. However, on Wright's insistence, a board of enquiry was assembled to review data on the reactogenicity and efficacy of the vaccine. The committee concluded that the vaccine was efficacious and that its value in preventing typhoid fever exceeded the price paid in adverse reactions. Consequently, by World War I, typhoid vaccination became virtually routine in the British Army.

Randomized, placebo-controlled, field trials in the 1960s established the efficacy of the heat-phenolized and acetone-inactivated parenteral whole cell vaccines.[9–13] Although these vaccines were shown to confer moderate protection that persisted for up to 7 years, they never became well-accepted public health tools because they frequently caused systemic adverse reactions (about 25% of recipients develop fever and malaise).[10,11,14] The parenteral killed whole cell vaccines have been supplanted by two newer vaccines: attenuated *S. typhi* strain Ty21a used as a live oral vaccine and purified Vi capsular polysaccharide utilized as a parenteral vaccine.[1,7,9] These two newer vaccines, which are at least as effective as the parenteral whole cell vaccines but are well-tolerated, are licensed and available in many countries and constitute credible public health tools.

3. Methodology

In the United States, the occasional sporadic cases and rare outbreaks of typhoid fever that occur are regarded as infectious disease calamities that rivet the attention of public health officials. Extensive investigative efforts are mobilized to identify the individual, usually an asymptomatic carrier, who has served as a source of the outbreak or of sporadic cases (when they occur among persons who are not recently returned travelers). Carriers are carefully identified and regularly followed by city or county health departments. Such monitoring ensures that carriers do not participate in occupations wherein they might contaminate food or water consumed by the public at large.

In less-developed countries where typhoid fever is endemic and public health resources are scarce, epidemiological investigations may be initiated only when a large-scale outbreak occurs or there is an unusual increase in the number of sporadic endemic cases.

3.1. Sources of Mortality Data

Information on deaths from typhoid fever in the United States derives from two sources, the first of which is notifications published within the *Morbidity and Mortality Weekly Report* (MMWR). The second source, available since 1975, is the Centers for Disease Control and Prevention (CDC) typhoid case report form, which is completed by state and community health departments on all bacteriologically confirmed cases of typhoid fever.

Before antibiotic therapy was available, a proportion of typhoid deaths were attributed to intestinal hemorrhage or perforation followed by peritonitis. Other patients in that era died of complications rarely seen today, such as myocarditis, pneumonia, and meningitis.[(15)] However, most fatal cases of typhoid fever resulted from inanition consequent to several weeks of unremitting fever and obtundation without a recognized specific complication.

In the preantibiotic era, a more accurate estimate of the relative importance of typhoid fever as a public health problem could be obtained by consideration of typhoid mortality rates per 10^5 population than by reviewing incidence rates. This was true because milder cases of typhoid fever can be confused with other febrile syndromes and bacteriological confirmation was undertaken in only a small proportion of suspect cases; in contrast, typhoid deaths are fairly definitive. Beginning in 1913, epidemiological data on typhoid mortality in large cities in the United States were summarized annually in the *Journal of the American Medical Association*.[(16)] In the period 1911–1915, annual typhoid death rates in the nine most populous US cities (New York, Chicago, Philadelphia, Detroit, St. Louis, Boston, Pittsburgh, Cleveland, and Baltimore) ranged from $8.0/10^5$ (New York, Boston) to $23.7/10^5$ (Baltimore).[(16)] Over the next decade it was possible to monitor the extraordinary effect that the rapidly increasing availability of treated water supplies had on diminishing typhoid mortality.[(17)]

The modern antibiotic era of typhoid epidemiology was ushered in by Woodward *et al.*[(18)] in 1948, when they demonstrated that chloramphenicol was highly effective in the treatment of this disease. Over the next 25 years, widespread use of this oral, inexpensive, effective antibiotic markedly diminished the case fatality rate of typhoid fever. Prior to the advent of chloramphenicol therapy, the case fatality rate of typhoid fever typically ranged from 10 to 20%, irrespective of where cases occurred worldwide. Presently, deaths from typhoid in the United States are distinctly rare, with only 0–3 cases annually reported in the decade 1982–1991, giving a peak annual mortality in 1983 of only $0.001/10^5$ population.[(19)] Ironically, since antibiotics have become widely available worldwide, mortality statistics are no longer a reliable measure of the endemicity of typhoid fever in populations.

3.2. Sources of Morbidity Data

The vast majority of cases of typhoid fever diagnosed by clinicians in the United States are reported to state or local health departments. Many cases are reported directly by physicians. In addition, all positive stool, blood, or other cultures yield *S. typhi* are reported by the laboratories making the isolations. The same two reporting systems mentioned above with respect to mortality also provide morbidity data.

In many less-developed countries with endemic disease, incidence data on typhoid tend to be unreliable and are gross underestimates of the true disease burden. Many "fever" hospitals in such countries record the number of patients admitted with the clinical diagnosis of typhoid fever, while others that have bacteriological capability report just the number of confirmed cases. The true incidence of typhoid fever in many less-developed countries is not known because the paucity of bacteriological capability precludes most suspected cases from being confirmed; moreover, suppression of disease by self-medication with antibiotics and incomplete reporting further distort the true situation.

3.3. Surveys

Several types of surveys have been carried out in recent years to study the epidemiology of endemic or epidemic typhoid. These include:

1. Bacteriological surveys of exposed populations during outbreaks[(20,21)] or household contacts of sporadic cases,[(22)] in order to detect subclinical and mild cases and carriers.
2. Systematic collection of blood cultures among febrile patients to confirm the incidence of *S. typhi* infection in certain populations.[(23)]
3. A combination of serological screening tests (for elevated serum titers of Vi antibodies) and bacteriological confirmation (by means of multiple stool cultures and bile-stained duodenal fluid cultures) to detect chronic biliary carriers of *S. typhi*.[(21,24–27)]
4. Serosurveys to measure the prevalence of H antibodies in different age groups, as a measure of the cumulative contact with *S. typhi*.[(28,29)]

Surveys of family members and persons known to be associated with an outbreak of typhoid fever are usually performed by culturing three successive stool specimens from asymptomatic subjects. One or more of these three specimens will yield the organism in most carriers ($> 80\%$);

chronic carriers are persons who shed *S. typhi* in the stool for more than 1 year. Exposed individuals who are in the incubation period before illness will often have positive stool cultures.[30] Culture of bile-stained duodenal fluid by means of string capsule devices (Enterotest, HEDECO, Mountain View, CA) can often confirm the biliary carrier state in epidemiologically incriminated individuals who have negative stool cultures. Alternatively, administering a laxative to such individuals, leading to passage of one or more loose stools, may allow confirmation; typhoid bacilli from the bile are now rapidly excreted, having little exposure to the hostile environment created by the normal flora of the large intestine.

Systematic collection of blood cultures prior to and during efficacy trials of vaccines has established the true incidence of typhoid in many populations (Table 1).[31–35] Often these surveys yield rates that are much higher than predicted. Such systematic surveys have also demonstrated the surprising frequency of mild bacteremic typhoid infection among infants and toddlers in endemic areas.[23]

Elevated titers of IgG antibodies directed at the capsular Vi polysaccharide antigen that covers *S. typhi* are encountered in > 80% of chronic biliary carriers of *S. typhi* but only rarely in healthy individuals[25,26]; < 20% of persons with acute typhoid fever manifest elevated Vi titers. Therefore, the measurement of Vi antibodies has been repeatedly utilized with success as a screening test in nonendemic and endemic areas to detect chronic carriers.[21,24–27]

Serum H antibodies are IgG and long-lived. However, they may be the consequences of stimulation by typhoid vaccination or by contact with cross-reacting *Salmonella*.[28] Therefore cautions must be exercised in selecting the populations to be sampled and in interpreting the results of serosurveys. Nevertheless, seroepidemiological surveys in which antibodies to *S. typhi* flagellar antigens (H) are measured in different age groups have proven quite useful in comparing the prevalence of *S. typhi* infection in different populations of interest and in estimating the age of peak infection.[28,29]

Table 1. The Mean Annual Incidence of Typhoid Fever Recorded in the Control Groups in Several Recent Vaccine Field Trials

Country	Vaccine tested	Year	Annual rate/10^5	Reference
Chile	Ty21a	1982	227	32
Chile	Ty21a	1983–86	103	33
Indonesia	Ty21a	1986–89	810	35
Nepal	Vi	1986–87	653	58
South Africa	Vi	1985–87	442	59

3.4. Laboratory Diagnosis

3.4.1. Isolation and Identification of the Organism. Confirmation of the diagnosis of typhoid fever requires recovery of *S. typhi* from a suitable clinical specimen. Because of their practicality and relative ease of access, multiple blood cultures should be obtained from patients in whom the diagnosis is suspected clinically. The rate of recovery of *S. typhi* in blood cultures depends on many factors, including the volume cultured, the ratio of the volume of blood to the volume of culture broth in which it is inoculated (the ratio should be at least 1:8), inclusion of anticomplementary substances in the medium (such as sodium polyanethol sulfonate or bile), and whether the patient has already received antibiotics to which the *S. typhi* is sensitive. If three 5-ml blood cultures are obtained, *S. typhi* can be recovered from the blood in approximately 70% of suspect cases.

The current "gold standard" of bacteriological confirmation of typhoid fever is the bone marrow culture, which is positive in 85–95% of cases, even when the patient has received antibiotics.[36–38] in recent years, there has been great interest in the use of duodenal string devices to obtain bile-stained duodenal fluid for culture. The combination of a duodenal string and two blood cultures generally provides a sensitivity of bacteriological confirmation equal to that achieved with bone marrow cultures, but without the invasiveness of the latter.[36] The bacteriological culture of skin snips from rose spots also provides a high yield.[38] Stool cultures generally lead to recovery of the organism in only 45–65% of cases. The yield tends to be somewhat higher in children.

S. typhi does not ferment lactose; it produces H_2S, but does not produce gas. As a consequence, suspicious colonies are evident on usual lactose-containing media as lactose-negative colonies. The biochemical pattern in triple sugar iron agar is rather characteristic, manifested by an acid butt without gas, an alkaline slant, and obvious H_2S production. Fresh isolates typically agglutinate with Vi but not group D antiserum. However, if the bacteria are boiled to remove the Vi capsule, a reaction with group D antiserum is then readily seen. The Vi antigen is an important epidemiological aid, since its susceptibility to lysis by bacteriophages allows for the classification of 80 definite and stable varieties of typhoid bacilli. This can help identify the source and spread of a specific strain.[39] The CDC is the principal source of phage typing in the United States.

DNA probes and polymerase chain reactions (PCR) methods exist that, in theory, can be applied to expedite a microbiological diagnosis of *S. typhi* infection.[40] However, in fact these methods are as yet amenable only to research and reference laboratories, since they are impractical and too expensive for routine use in most laboratories in endemic areas.

3.4.2. Serological Diagnostic Methods. Serodiagnosis of typhoid fever has been pursued since the late 19th century (1896) when Widal and Sicard[41] showed that the serum of patients with typhoid fever agglutinated typhoid bacilli. The Widal test, still practiced today in many areas, involves the search for agglutinins in the patient's serum. Whereas the test may be performed with antigen in tubes or on slides, the former is generally more accurate. By careful choice of antigen, both O and H antibodies can be selectively measured. By use of *S. typhi* strain O901, which lacks flagellar and Vi antigens, *S. typhi* O antibody can be selectively measured. To detect antibodies against the appropriate H antigen (d), a strain such as *S. virginia* is selected that possesses the identical flagellar antigen (d) as *S. typhi* but shares no O somatic antigens with typhi.[28] Most patients with typhoid fever have elevated levels of O and H antibody at the time of onset of clinical illness.[28] Anderson[42] has emphasized the importance and usefulness of H titers in serodiagnosis of typhoid fever. However, in general, the prevalence of H antibodies in adults living in endemic areas is too high for the test to be useful in that age group.[28,29] Nevertheless, it can be helpful in children less than 10 years of age in endemic areas and in persons of any age from nonendemic areas.[28] A history of inoculation with parenteral killed whole cell vaccines invalidates the use of the Widal test. Recently, interest has reappeared in the use of the slide test for O agglutinins of *S. typhi*, even for adults in endemic areas.[43]

Serological tests that measure Vi antibody by passive hemagglutination or enzyme-linked immunosorbant assays (ELISAs), using highly purified Vi antigen, are excellent to screen for chronic *S. typhi* carriers, most of whom have highly elevated levels of Vi antibody.[24–27] In contrast, Vi antibody tests are of little help in diagnosing acute typhoid fever because only a minority of patients with acute infection have detectable Vi antibody.[25,26]

3.4.3. Rapid Immunoassays. Over the years many attempts have been made to develop tests that detect *S. typhi* antigens in blood, urine, or body fluids, thereby providing a rapid diagnostic test for typhoid fever. With few exceptions these tests have been disappointing and have failed to warrant the enthusiasm of the initial reports.[44] Most of these assays are based on the detection of the O or Vi antigens of *S. typhi* in blood or urine using coagglutination, ELISA, or countercurrent immunoelectrophoresis. No completely satisfactory test is currently available.

4. Biological Characteristics of the Organism

The taxonomy of *Salmonella* has changed repeatedly during the past 30 years, leading to considerable confusion.[45] Most (but not all) authorities presently use the term, *S. typhi*, to refer to the causative organism of typhoid fever. Serologically, *S. typhi* falls into group D *Salmonella* on the basis of its O antigens 9 and 12. *S. typhi* is motile and its peritrichous flagellae bear flagellar (H) antigen d, which is also encountered in approximately 80 other bioserotypes of *Salmonella*. A few percent of isolates from Indonesia have flagellae that bear other antigens (j and z66).[46,47] Strains freshly isolated from patients possess on their surface an acidic polysaccharide capsule, the Vi (for virulence) antigen.[48] Vi prevents O antibody from binding to the O antigen and inhibits the C3 component of complement from fixing to the surface of *S. typhi*.

S. typhi exhibits a remarkable degree of homogeneity, in comparison with the other species of *Salmonella*, rarely showing biochemical or serological variability. Exceptional are the few percent of isolates from Indonesia that bear flagellar antigen j or z66 rather than d.[46,47] In practical terms, phage typing, using Vi phages, offers a reasonable tool that is often helpful in differentiating strains from different geographic areas.[39] Most molecular epidemiological techniques have corroborated the homogeneity of *S. typhi* strains from diverse areas and time periods.[49,50]

Typhoid bacilli are able to achieve an intracellular habitat promptly after oral ingestion. This property may account for the prolonged duration of disease in untreated patients and the relatively slow response to antibiotic therapy. Within macrophages of the reticuloendothelial system, the organism appears to be protected from the host's humoral immune mechanisms, and in this intracellular niche it also resists the effect of many antibiotics.

Like other gram-negative bacilli, the outer portion of the cell wall of typhoid bacilli consists of lipopolysaccharide (LPS) or endotoxin. This substance, which has biological properties that are important in the pathogenesis of typhoid fever, consists of three layers, the outermost being made up of a repeating sequence of sugars that determines the specificity of the O antigen.

For typhoid, there are two major O antigens—9 and 12—in this surface complex. Rough mutant strains that lack the outer layer of LPS are nonpathogenic. The middle LPS layer is the R core. The inner layer of LPS is the lipid A moiety, which binds the endotoxin molecule to the rest of the cell wall structure. Endotoxin is pyrogenic and triggers the complement and clotting cascades; it also stimulates the release of cytokines that are deemed responsible for many of the clinical features of typhoid fever.

A curious feature of *S. typhi* is that, in contrast with many other pathogenic enterobacteriaceae (e.g., *Shigella*, nontyphoidal *Salmonella*) that readily accept and stably carry R factor plasmids encoding antibiotic resistance, over the past four decades this has been the exception rather than the rule with typhoid bacilli. Chloramphenicol, the first antibiotic used to treat typhoid fever, held a position of prominence for 25 years and is still important in less-developed countries where prevalent strains of *S. typhi* remain susceptible. Whereas many other Enterobacteriaceae acquired resistance to chloramphenicol within 10 to 12 years.(51) Then, rather abruptly, large-scale epidemics of chloramphenicol-resistant typhoid fever occurred, first in Mexico (1972)(51,52) and then in Southeast Asia (1974)(53); sporadic cases of resistance were reported from the Middle East and India. Curiously, after approximately 2 years in Mexico, the resistant strain disappeared and was replaced by chloramphenicol-sensitive strains. Oral amoxicillin and trimethoprim–sulfamethoxazole were shown to be satisfactory alternatives for treating patients with chloramphenicol-resistant typhoid fever.(52) In 1979 and 1980, a similar abrupt appearance of chloramphenicol-resistant typhoid occurred in Lima, Peru(54); these resistant strains also disappeared after a few years and were again replaced by chloramphenicol-sensitive *S. typhi*. It is notable that in each of these instances the antibiotic-resistance genes were encoded on plasmids of incompatibility group H1.(51,54) A plausible biological explanation has never been found for the sudden appearance and regression of *S. typhi* carrying these plasmids.(51)

Ominously, since 1990, strains of *S. typhi* resistant to chloramphenicol, amoxicillin, and trimethoprim–sulfamethoxazole have disseminated widely throughout Asia, constituting a public health calamity.(5,6) Alternative effective antibiotics, including oral ciprofloxacin and parenteral ceftriaxone, are expensive and have other drawbacks.

One other relevant biological property of *S. typhi* is its ability to survive for a relatively long time in certain environmental niches, as in snow and surface waters, and in some foods. In some circumstances, typhoid bacilli may survive for several months, a property that has resulted in some "unexpected" epidemics because no recent source for the contamination was found.

5. Descriptive Epidemiology

5.1. Prevalence and Incidence

5.1.1. In the United States. Figure 1 shows the incidence rate of reported cases of typhoid fever in the United States per 10^5 since 1944. There has been a leveling off of the curve since the mid-1960s at about 0.2 cases/10^5 population. In the period 1989–1993, there were, on average, 473 cases of typhoid fever reported annually (range, 414 to 552).(19) These figures are representative of the status of typhoid fever in the United States for the past three decades except for the large outbreak that occurred in 1973 in Dade County, Florida. In that outbreak (discussed in greater detail in Section 5.2), the water supply in a migrant labor camp became contaminated and 222 cases of typhoid fever ensued. This was the largest single outbreak in over 30 years.

The most recent extensive review of *S. typhi* infections in the United States by the CDC covered the period 1975 to 1984, during which 4641 cases were reported to the MMWR.(2) More detailed epidemiological information was available for 2666 of these cases for whom the CDC special questionnaire forms were completed (57% of the cases). Twenty-nine deaths were reported, including 21 among domestically acquired cases and 8 among returned travelers. Mortality was five times higher for domestically acquired cases than for foreign travel-acquired cases (2.5 vs 0.5%). Among the domestically acquired cases, 9% were related to contact with a previ-

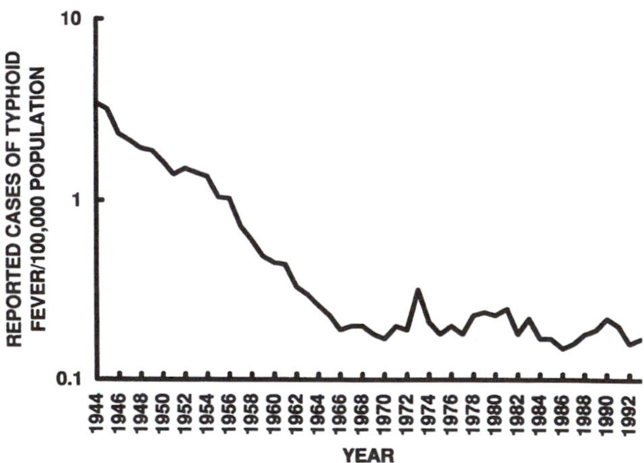

Figure 1. Typhoid fever—by year, United States, 1942–1993.

ously diagnosed typhoid carrier and 21% were related to contact with a newly diagnosed carrier. Although overall the majority of cases acquired domestically in the United States are single cases, 28% (266 of 934) of cases were related to outbreaks. During this decade of surveillance experience, there were three major outbreaks, all food-borne.

Travel-related cases of typhoid fever have increased notably since 1967,[2,55–57] so that by the time of the CDC review for the period 1975 through 1984, 1653 of the 2666 reported cases (62%) were acquired during foreign travel.[2] The median age for the 1371 travel-related cases was 23 years, whereas that of the 857 cases acquired in the United States was 20 years. Among the travel-related cases, the greatest single occupational group was students [365 of 1216 (30%) cases]. Travel within the Western Hemisphere accounted for 59% of the travel-related cases and travel to the Indian subcontinent (India, Burma, Sri Lanka, Bangladesh) was associated with 17%. Mexico-associated cases accounted for 39% of the total, with India associated with 14%. Table 2 lists the incidence of typhoid per 10^6 travelers to various countries. The highest risk, $174/10^6$, was observed among travelers to Peru. To put this rate into perspective, it approaches the annual incidence in the control group (20 cases/10^5 population) in a typhoid vaccine efficacy field trial in Poland in the early 1960s sponsored by the World Health Organization (WHO).[12] When one considers that the incidence of typhoid among travelers to Peru in general represented disease acquired after relatively short exposures limited to days or weeks, one recognizes that in certain areas of the world the risk of travelers' typhoid is substantial.

5.1.2. Worldwide. The WHO records the incidences sent to it by cooperating countries. These figures indicate that typhoid remains a major public health problem in Central and South America, Africa, and Southeast Asia, and less so in Europe. These notification data appear to be a gross underestimation due to incomplete reporting and insufficient means for bacteriological confirmation. It is difficult to quantitate the true magnitude of the typhoid fever problem worldwide because the clinical picture is confused with many other febrile infections and the capacity for bacteriological confirmation is absent in most areas of the less-developed world.[44] Nevertheless, the WHO estimates that each year more than 33 million cases and more than 500,000 deaths occurs worldwide due to typhoid fever.[44] Recent surveillance data generated by quantitating the incidence of typhoid fever in placebo groups participating in large-scale field trials of typhoid vaccines show annual incidence rates from 103 to 1000 cases per 10^5 population in typhoid-endemic areas (Table 1).[31–33,35,58,59] If these data can be extrapolated, they imply that the previous estimates of the annual worldwide burden of typhoid fever underestimate by 90% the magnitude of the problem.

Table 2. The Incidence of Typhoid Fever in US Travelers (Citizens and Residents) to Various Regions of the World, 1982–1984[a]

Country visited	Mean annual no. of cases	No. cases per 10^6 travelers
Mexico	77	20.2
Haiti	3	41.8
Peru	10	173.8
Chile	3	58.4
India	26	118.5
Pakistan	6	105.1

[a]Data from Ryan *et al.*[2]

5.1.3. Prevalence of Carriers. The total number of typhoid carriers in the United States is not known. In 1962, the number was estimated to be 3637 and in 1978 more than 2000. In Arkansas, the rate of carriers was 3–4/10^5 population in 1978. Many of the known carriers are elderly, and with the low incidence of typhoid fever in this country, few new indigenous carriers will appear to replace those who will die in the next decade. However, the influx in recent years of immigrants from Central America and South and Southeast Asia undoubtedly includes some chronic typhoid carriers from these endemic areas. Nevertheless, in view of the well-developed sanitary conditions existent throughout the United States, there are no grave epidemiological consequences anticipated from the arrival of such carriers unless they become employed as food handlers.[21]

In the preantibiotic era in the United States, some predictions were made about the decline in numbers of carriers; these predictions have come true. The estimated carrier prevalences inn 1935 for Massachusetts and Mississippi were 48 and 288/10^5 population, respectively. In New York, in 1940, there were an estimated 2490 carriers, for a prevalence of 41.8/100,000 population.[60] According to the 1943 report by Ames and Robins[60] of the New York State Department of Health, the number of carriers in New York would have fallen from 2490 in the early 1940s to about 190 by 1980. Their assumptions in arriving at these figures did not predict the effect antibiotic therapy (unavailable in their time) would have on the development of and treatment of the carrier state. Nonetheless, in New York in 1980, the total number of known carriers was 175, remarkably close to the 190 predicted 37 years earlier by Ames and Robins.

Only a few quantitations have been made of the prevalence of chronic carriers in less-developed countries. One such survey carried out in Santiago, Chile, during a period when typhoid fever was highly endemic, estimated a crude prevalence of 694 carriers/10^5 population.[61] This high prevalence was related in part to the high prevalence of cholelithiasis in the adult female population of Santiago.[61]

5.1.4. Prevalence of Antibody. The prevalence of antibodies to O, H, and Vi antigens in United States citizens in the late 1960s and early 1970s could be estimated from the extensive serological data accumulated in the course of a unique series of volunteer studies with wild-type *S. typhi* conducted to evaluate the efficacy of typhoid vaccine.[30] Baseline antibody titers (obtained at time of entry into the study) revealed that older men had higher geometric mean H antibody titers than those 15–20 years their junior. The earlier the year of birth, the more likely a volunteer was to show an elevated titer of H antibody at the time of participation in the study, and if birth occurred after 1935, a period when the disease was rapidly disappearing in this country, the influence of age disappeared. These values held whether or not there was a military history, i.e., an opportunity to have received vaccine. Since these studies investigated persons living in a nonendemic area, the percentages of volunteers lacking detectable O, H, and Vi give an estimate of the lack of past exposure to *S. typhi* antigens, whether by previous disease, vaccine administration, or exposure to other salmonellae-containing common and cross-reacting O, H, or Vi antigens. Thus, of 331 men, 52% had no detectable H, 74% no detectable O, and 42% no detectable Vi serum antibodies. The majority of the younger volunteers participating in the later phases of the study fall into these groups. Of those men who had demonstrable circulating antibody titers, only a small percentage had elevated values. If the trend noted in this study continues, an even smaller percentage of United States citizens will have detectable antibodies in the next several decades as opportunities for exposure to typhoid antigens in the United States continue to diminish. This hypothesis is predicated on the assumptions that: (1) the sources of acquired disease will continue to decline, i.e., fewer carriers will develop and the present ones will die off; (2) there will be continued minimal utilization of typhoid vaccine in this country; and (3) there will be better control over other sources of salmonellae that may have cross-reacting antigens. More than 140 strains of *Salmonella*, some of which commonly cause gastroenteritis, have O antigens that cross-react with the typhoid bacillus antigens in the Widal agglutination test. Similarly, there are at least 70 strains with cross-reacting H antigens, although few of these have been recognized in association with human clinical illness. These antigens may be the source of "typhoid" O and H antibodies detected by the Widal test in many United States citizens today.

Antibody prevalence surveys have also been carried out in areas where typhoid is highly endemic. Seroepidemiological studies in Peru and Chile performed in the 1970s showed that by 15–19 years of age, 50–80% of teenagers had serological evidence of past infection with *S. typhi*.[28,29]

5.2. Epidemic Behavior and Contagiousness

In the United States, scattered outbreaks of typhoid fever occur when a carrier contaminates food or a water supply. The epidemic that occurred in Dade County, Florida illustrates how a segment of our society may become infected when sewage disposal and water supply are improperly controlled.[20] The critical epidemiological link in this outbreak was thought to be a mentally retarded child who acquired the infection from an asymptomatic carrier living in a neighboring house. It is believed that this child subsequently contaminated the flawed water supply in the migrant labor camp, resulting in 222 cases in the camp population, 184 of whom were hospitalized. This was the largest single outbreak in the past half century. Other large epidemics in industrialized countries have occurred in the past three decades in Scotland (504 cases)[62] and Zermatt, Switzerland (280 cases).[63] In Scotland, the source of the infection was canned corned beef shipped from Argentina. The meat per se did not contain typhoid bacilli prior to processing (raw meat has never been found to be contaminated with this organism, attesting to the unique adaptation of typhoid bacilli to humans). However, after the canning process, the cans were heat-sterilized and then placed in contaminated river water to cool. As the cans cooled, water was drawn into the cans through minute leaks in the seams. Those who handled the meat from the cans became potential cases as well as possible disseminators of the bacteria. Furthermore, when the meat was cut by machines, the blades became contaminated, and other meats subsequently cut on these machines also acquired typhoid bacilli, which was then spread to other consumers.[62]

The epidemic in Zermatt occurred from contamination of the town water supply. The contamination lasted for at least 1 month before the epidemic was recognized and chlorination and other measures could be instituted to treat the water.

Another large epidemic of interest was caused by

chloramphenicol-resistant *S. typhi* in Mexico City from 1972 to 1974.[52] At the time typhoid was endemic in that city, but the marked increase in number of typhoid fever cases admitted to hospitals quickly focused attention on the fact that this new strain was responsible for two thirds of the increased incidence. An epidemiological investigation suggested that the strain may have been disseminated by soft drink vehicles made with contaminated water. The Mexican strain was found to be responsible for typhoid fever in Switzerland, the United Kingdom, the United States, and other parts of the world. Travelers to Mexico acquired the disease and brought it back to this country and the others. In Los Angeles in 1972, the incidence of the disease doubled, due mainly to imported cases from Mexico.[57] Fortunately, very few secondary cases of typhoid fever occurred in this country as a result of the importation of the antibiotic-resistant Mexican strain.

One other water source of infection that has been documented involves oysters harvested from polluted water, in which typhoid and other enteric pathogens can be concentrated from the water strained by the bivalves.[65] In situations where latrines are not fly-proofed or exposed human feces is common, flies have been shown to transmit typhoid bacilli by contamination of their feet as they feed on feces and subsequent carrying of the organisms to food.[66]

Typhoid fever is essentially spread only by consumption of contaminated food or water vehicles. Under rare circumstances, direct person-to-person transmission through anal–oral spread may occur, as among homosexuals who indulge in anolingual sexual practices.[67]

Transmission occurs among clinical microbiologists in hospital diagnostic bacteriology laboratories.[3,4] The handling of specimens containing *S. typhi* has caused numerous cases of typhoid fever. Twenty-five cases of laboratory-acquired typhoid fever were reported to the CDC from 1977 to 1979, among which 14 were related to a proficiency-testing program. These data indicate the need for a good training program in order to upgrade the skills and techniques of microbiology technicians. The organism can be handled safely in hospital diagnostic laboratories, but great care must be taken to avoid contaminating fingers, pens, pencils, and laboratory paraphernalia, since these may serve as fomites to transmit the bacteria to the mouth. In some instances, it is believed that aerosols may be involved in the transmission of *S. typhi* within clinical microbiology laboratories, not by direct inhalation but by contamination of nearby surfaces and objects that subsequently serve as fomites. Aerosols may be created as culture tubes containing *S. typhi* are opened, leading to contamination of nearby objects, which subsequently contaminate hands. If hands are not adequately washed, they can carry the organisms to food or directly to the mouth. Small numbers of volunteers exposed to small-particle aerosols containing 10^5 typhoid bacilli failed to develop signs of infection. This dose given by mouth caused disease in about 38% of volunteers; thus, the respiratory tract appears to be a less effective route of inoculation than the gastrointestinal tract.

Typhoid fever has a relatively low risk of contagion. Person-to-person transmission can occur by anal–oral spread such as changing the soiled bed linens of an undiagnosed patient. Patients with typhoid fever shed the etiologic agent from the gut and urinary tract. Aerosol dissemination from these sources would appear to be highly unlikely.

5.3. Geographic Distribution

In less-developed areas of the world where fecal contamination of water and food are common, incidence rates of many enteric infections are high, including typhoid fever. Typhoid fever remains common in Central and South America, a few southern and eastern European countries, the Middle East, and throughout Africa and Southeast Asia. Ashcroft[68] presented his classification of epidemiological patterns of *S. typhi* as follows:

1. Where hygiene and sanitation are appalling: *S. typhi* is usually prevalent; clinical typhoid fever is uncommon. Immunity is acquired in infancy or very early childhood when infection is either symptomless or unrecognized.
2. Where hygiene and sanitation are poor: *S. typhi* infection is common; typhoid fever is particularly frequent in school-age children. Most infections occur in childhood and are recognizable, although often mild.
3. Where hygiene and sanitation are a mixture of primitive and modern, often associated with urbanization: outbreaks of typhoid fever may involve all age groups.
4. Where hygiene is excellent: *S. typhi* infection and typhoid fever are rare. This is the situation existing in northern and western Europe and northern North America.

This classification is helpful in explaining a number of the epidemiological features of typhoid fever and serves as a rational foundation for understanding the current geographic distribution of typhoid fever. In the latter half of the 19th century, high incidence rates of typhoid fever were observed in most of the major cities of Europe and North America. Transmission of typhoid in these cities was amplified as untreated water from nearby rivers that had heavy fecal contamination was an important source of municipal drinking water for inhabitants of the cities. Treatment of the water sources led to striking decreases in the transmission of typhoid, reflected by plummeting incidence rates.[16,17] Typhoid fever is still common in a number of large cities in the less-developed world where segments of the population are not served by piped, treated, monitored water supplies. These cities include Cairo, Egypt; Jakarta, Indonesia; Bombay and New Delhi, India; and Karachi and Lahore, Pakistan.

In some large cities, endemic typhoid persisted despite provision of virtually all of the population with treated water. In such exceptions, another form of amplification was responsible. One example was Santiago, Chile in the 1970s and 1980s, where typhoid remained notably endemic despite 96% of the population having access to treated, bacteriologically monitored water.[29,69] Irrigation of crops of salad vegetables such as lettuce, celery, and cabbage during summer with untreated sewage was epidemiologically linked as the amplification event.[64,70] Abrupt discontinuation of this practice following a small outbreak of cholera in 1991 led to a precipitous decline in the incidence of typhoid fever and its virtual disappearance as a public health problem in an infamous endemic area where a few years earlier the WHO sponsored four successive large-scale field trials of efficacy of typhoid vaccines.[29,31–34,70]

5.4. Temporal Distribution

Most cases of typhoid fever reported from endemic areas occur during the summer months. The cases acquired by United States tourists usually occur in the summer, coinciding with the peak travel time. The remaining cases appear sporadically during the year. In many endemic areas, typhoid typically shows a highly seasonal pattern. For example, in South America there is a clear-cut peak in summer,[69,71] and in Java typhoid peaks during rainy season.

5.5. Age

Perhaps the most striking and fascinating epidemiological feature of typhoid fever in endemic areas is its age-specific incidence pattern wherein the incidence is low in the first few years of life, peaks in school-age children, remains high in young adults, and then falls again in middle age.[23,69,71–73] This age-specific pattern is most curious given the fact that virtually all other enteric infections in less-developed countries exhibit their highest incidence in infants, toddlers, and preschool children. The age-specific incidence patterns for typhoid fever from a number of famous endemic sites, spanning 60 years in time, are displayed in Table 3.[23,71–73] In each instance, the same "classic" pattern is observed.

Recently, Mahle and Levine[73] reviewed the validity of the dogma that typhoid fever is relatively rare in infants and preschool children. Review of notification data and hospital-based reports supported this teaching, demonstrating a much lower incidence in the 0- to 4-year-old age group than in school-age children (5- to 19-year-olds). They examined age-specific incidence rates in a series of waterborne outbreaks and found a similar age distribution as observed in endemic disease, suggesting that the lower morbidity in younger children is not due to decreased exposure to *S. typhi*. Rather, Mahle and Levine conclude that very young children would appear to develop a very mild form of typhoid fever following exposure and infection. This conclusion is supported by systematic blood culture studies in typhoid endemic areas that have found *S. typhi* bacteremia in very young children (< 24 months of age) who clinically manifest only mild febrile illness.[23] Young children with typhoid also exhibit less prominent pathology of the small intestine.[73] Together, these features suggest that young children readily become infected with *S. typhi*, but that a distinct pathogenesis produces a remarkably mild illness.

Older adults in endemic areas appear to be relatively immune, presumably because of frequent boostering of immunity acquired earlier. In the United States, those most likely to acquire the disease at home are adults under age 30.[2,74] Three fourths of 857 patients reported between 1975 and 1984 were in this age range. Median age was 20.[2] The travel-associated cases had a median age of 23. Persons of these ages had no background immunity, having been born and raised in a country where the disease is no longer prevalent (0.2 cases/10^5 since 1966, 1 case/10^5 in 1955, and about 3 cases/10^5 in 1945). Vaccine-induced immunity, including that conferred by the more recent Ty21a and Vi vaccines, is less effective in young children, presumably because of a lack of background immunity.

Table 3. The Mean Annual Age-Specific Incidence of Typhoid Fever per 100,000 Population, Based on Notification Data in Diverse Geographic Regions and Time Periods

Age group (years)	Palestine Mandate 1934–42[71]	British Guiana 1956–60[72]	Peru 1971[73]	Santiago, Chile 1977–81[23]
0–4	127	48	67	89
5–9	307	180[a]	114	272
10–14	266	180[a]	144	333
15–19	236	112[a]	129	283
20–24	271	112[a]	102[a]	247
25–29	196	66[a]	102[a]	153[a]
20–34	108[b]	66[a]	50[c]	153[a]

[a]Incidence reported for cohorts spanning 10 years.
[b]Incidence of 30 to 39-year age group.
[c]Incidence of population > 30 years of age.

While the median age of persons with typhoid fever was 22 to 24 years in the period 1984 to 1986 in the United States, the median age of carriers in those years was 71, 58, and 69 years, respectively. In endemic areas, the prevalence of carriers steadily increases with age.[13,33]

5.6. Sex

There is no prominent effect of sex on the incidence of acute typhoid fever; both sexes are equally susceptible. However, the prevalence of chronic carriers is threefold greater in females.[60,61] This is because the propensity to become a chronic carrier following acute typhoid infection, either symptomatic or subclinical, is related to the presence of preexistent gallbladder disease. Infection of the biliary tree and the gallbladder is universal during acute typhoid fever. Indeed, culture of bile-stained duodenal fluid spécimens is one of the highest-yield clinical bacteriological procedures to isolate *S. typhi* during acute typhoid fever.[36] Just as the prevalence of cholelithiasis and chronic gallbladder disease occurs with greater frequency in females and increases with age, so too an identical prevalence pattern of chronic biliary typhoid carriers is observed in endemic areas.[61]

5.7. Race

There are no data to support racial susceptibility to typhoid fever. While many series indicate that more blacks have typhoid fever, it is probable that the living conditions, e.g., poor sanitary conditions, are the precipitating factor, not race. In volunteer studies, no evidence of race-associated susceptibility was detected. An unusually virulent form of clinical typhoid fever occurs in Jakarta, Indonesia, where obtundation and shock are common.[75] The case fatality ratio in such patients has been about 50% unless steroids are coadministered with appropriate antibiotics and has remained around 10% among the most ill hospitalized patients, even with adjunct steroid therapy. Multiple hypotheses have been put forth to explain this severe form of typhoid fever, which is concentrated on the island of Java. One hypothesis proposes that the genetic makeup of the Javanese population predisposes them to respond to typhoid infection with a particularly severe clinical syndrome.

5.8. Occupation

Several occupations have historically been associated with an increased risk for acquiring typhoid fever. These include sewer workers, soldiers,[76] and most recently, clinical microbiologists.[3,4] Clinical microbiologists are now recognized as one high-risk US population for which immunization with one of the new vaccines is indicated.

5.9. Occurrence in Different Settings

In industrialized countries, a large proportion of sporadic cases occur among travelers. When outbreaks occur in the United States and other industrialized countries that have high levels of sanitation, controlled water supplies, and sophisticated food hygiene practices, a careful epidemiological investigation almost always incriminates the food vehicle responsible for the outbreak and often identifies a chronic carrier responsible for its contamination.[31] Similarly, epidemiological investigation of sporadic, non-travel-associated cases in the United States also often identifies a chronic carrier, such as an elderly family member, who serves as the reservoir of infection.

In contrast, in typhoid-endemic areas in less-developed countries, where populations live in underprivileged conditions without controlled, piped water supplies, means to remove human waste, refrigeration for preserving food, or adequate food hygiene practices, it is usually exceedingly difficult to identify the specific vehicles of transmission of sporadic cases or the human reservoir.[77]

5.10. Socioeconomic Factors

Wherever inadequate sanitary facilities exist and water supplies are subject to fecal contamination, the opportunity exists for enhanced transmission of all enteric infections, but especially typhoid fever. The unique adaptation of *S. typhi* to humans and the survival characteristics of this organism make it a particular threat to spread in populations living under substandard sanitary conditions. Prior to the availability of treated water and sewer systems, all strata of society were at risk. Endemic regions continue to exist in the world primarily because the poorer segments of the population in those areas remain underserved by adequate water supply and sanitation services and lack of detection and restriction of carriers. Provision of means to remove human waste and of treated, bacteriologically monitored water precludes widespread transmission and virtually eliminates typhoid fever from previously endemic loci.

5.11. Other Factors

There is no reliable evidence indicating increased or decreased susceptibility of patients with malnutrition to typhoid fever. The untreated disease causes a severe metabolic drain, so illness in a host with undernutrition will create a double hazard. Patients with various parasitic infections such as roundworms or schistosomes are readily infected with *S. typhi*. In the first instance, typhoid fever in the host will cause the roundworms to migrate out through the mouth and anus. Reasons for this exodus from the gut are unknown. Schistosomiasis causes tissue scarring and obstruction, especially in the genitourinary tract by *Schistosoma haematobium*, and *S. typhi* can remain indefinitely in the scar tissue or adherent to the trematode itself.(78) Salmonellae express fimbriae that allow adherence to the glycolipids on the surface of the worm.(78) A common consequence of such symbiotic coinfection is recurrent silent *S. typhi* bacteremia in the host without any clinical evidence of typhoid fever.

6. Mechanisms and Routes of Transmission

Typhoid bacilli enter the host by the oral route via ingestion of contaminated food or water. The disease has been shown to be one of several enteric infections that can be sexually transmitted by anolingual sexual practices.(67) Flies can carry *S. typhi* on their feet and have been incriminated, indirectly, as mechanical vectors that contaminate food.(66) Rarely, infection is believed to have been acquired by aerosol.

It is helpful to consider that typhoid fever is transmitted by the fecal–oral route in two broad manners: a "short cycle" and a "long cycle." The short cycle is typified by an individual carrier who contaminates food vehicles that are consumed by family members, or by participants at a communal gathering (wedding, party, etc.), or by a chronic carrier food working as a food handler in a restaurant.(21) Thus, it is a short distance from point of contamination to consumption of the vehicle by the susceptibles. In contrast, examples of long-cycle infection include contamination of water supplies by sewage, improper treatment of piped water supplies that are distributed,(79) and finally widespread dissemination of typhoid bacilli via contaminated foods that may be transported over long distances.(62)

Examples of short-cycle sporadic cases and outbreaks include the families served by the infamous cook, "Typhoid Mary,"(80) and recent restaurant outbreaks in Texas,(81) Maryland,(21) and New York.(82) Most outbreaks in the United States are related to the short-cycle mode of transmission.

The long-cycle transmission is exemplified by the Aberdeen(62) and Zermatt(63) epidemics of the 1960s and the more recent Northern Israel outbreak.(79) The Aberdeen epidemic was caused by consumption of contaminated tins of corned beef canned in Argentina and shipped to Scotland. The Zermatt epidemic was caused by a carrier contaminating a mountain stream at the point where it served as the intake for the water supply of Zermatt.

7. Pathogenesis and Immunity

7.1. Pathogenesis

S. typhi and *S. paratyphi* A and B are highly invasive bacteria that rapidly and efficiently pass through the intestinal mucosa of humans to eventually reach the reticuloendothelial system, where, after a 8- to 14-day incubation period, they precipitate a systemic illness. *S. typhi* is a highly host-adapted pathogen; humans comprise the only natural host and reservoir of this infection. Our comprehension of the steps involved in the pathogenesis of typhoid fever comes from four sources: (1) clinicopathological observations in humans(83); (2) volunteer studies(30); (3) studies of a chimpanzee model(84); and (4) analogies drawn from *S. typhimurium* and *S. enteriditis* infection in mice—the "mouse typhoid" model.(85) The probable steps in the pathogenesis of *S. typhi* infection in humans are summarized below.

Susceptible human hosts ingest the causative organisms in contaminated food and water. The inoculum size and the type of vehicle in which it is ingested greatly influence the attack rate for typhoid fever and also affect the incubation period, a relationship that was documented in volunteer studies in the 1960s (Table 4). Doses of 10^9 and 10^8 pathogenic *S. typhi* ingested by volunteers in 45 ml of skim milk induced clinical illness in 98% and 89% of individuals, respectively; doses of 10^5 caused typhoid fever in 28 to 55% of volunteers, whereas none of 14 subjects who ingested 10^3 organisms developed clinical illness.(30)

In the fasting normochlorhydric stomach, gastric

Table 4. Incubation Periods of Typhoid Fever Related to Size of Infecting Dose[a]

Dose[b]	Attack rate (%)	Mean incubation period (days)
10^3	0	—
10^5	38	13
10^7	50	11
10^9	90	5.8

[a]Data from Hornick *et al.*(30)
[b]Colony-forming units.

acid undoubtedly inactivates many of the typhoid bacilli that are ingested. However, some foods may serve as a buffer to diminish this otherwise formidable protective acid barrier. After passing through the pylorus and reaching the small intestine, the bacilli rapidly penetrate the mucosa by one of two mechanisms to arrive in the lamina propria. One mechanism involves uptake of the bacilli into endocytic vacuoles and their passage through the enterocytes to be ultimately released into the lamina propria without destroying the enterocyte.(86) In the second, quite distinct, invasive mechanism, typhoid bacilli are actively taken up by M cells, the domelike epithelial cells that cover Peyer's patches and other organized lymphoid tissue of the gut. From here they enter the underlying lymphoid cells.

Upon reaching the lamina propria in the nonimmune host, typhoid bacilli elicit an influx of macrophages that ingest the organisms but are generally unable to kill them. Some bacilli apparently remain within macrophages of the small-intestinal lymphoid tissue. Other typhoid bacilli are drained into mesenteric lymph nodes where further multiplication and ingestion by macrophages take place. Eventually, there is a release of tumor necrosis factor-alpha, interleukin-2 (IL-2), IL-6, and other inflammatory cytokines by the macrophages (and perhaps by enterocytes).

Postmortem studies have documented the marked inflammatory responses that occur in the distal ileum in the Peyer's patches and other organized lymphoid aggregations. Presumably, cytokine release elicited by the intracellular *S. typhi* is responsible for these cellular changes. It is from these lesions in the distal ileum and ascending colon that hemorrhage can occur later in the disease course. Gross bleeding comes from eroded vessels in or near the Peyer's patches. This complication occurs late in the second week in about 1–3% of untreated patients and rarely in patients whose treatment with an appropriate antibiotic is begun late in their clinical course. Perforations of the bowel wall occur in the same sections of the gut as the hemorrhages.

Shortly after invasion of the intestinal mucosa, a primary bacteremia is believed to take place in which *S. typhi* are filtered from the circulation by fixed phagocytic cells of the reticuloendothelial system. It is believed that the main route by which typhoid bacilli reach the bloodstream in this early stage is by lymph drainage from mesenteric nodes entering the thoracic duct and then the general circulation. Conceivably, ingestion of a massive inoculum followed by widespread invasion of the intestinal mucosa could result in rapid and direct invasion of the bloodstream. As a result of this primary bacteremia, the pathogen rapidly attains an intracellular haven throughout the organs of the reticuloendothelial system where it resides during the incubation period (usually 8–14 days) until the onset of clinical typhoid fever. Clinical illness is accompanied by a fairly sustained "secondary" bacteremia.

The Vi antigen is a virulence property and virtually all strains freshly isolated from patients possess this polysaccharide capsule.(87) Both epidemiological observations and studies in volunteers support the contention that *S. typhi* strains that possess Vi are more virulent than strains lacking this polysaccharide.(30)

The bacteremia of typhoid fever will persist for several weeks if antibiotic therapy is not given, and the blood may be seeded from the liver as well as the lesions in the intestinal tract. The symptoms and signs of typhoid fever are not believed be due to circulating endotoxin. Most patients have no serum endotoxin detected by the limulus assay.(88) However, in patients who present with septic shock syndrome, circulating endotoxin can be demonstrated.(75) These patients have a higher mortality rate and require a combination therapy of steroids and antibiotics.

Relapses were observed in about 8% of patients suffering from typhoid fever in the preantibiotic era. The rate in patients treated with antibiotics ranges from 15 to 35%, appears to increase with earlier initiation of treatment, and may indicate an interference with the development of effective immunity. The organisms that initiate relapse appear to come from within the reticuloendothelial system. Typhoid bacilli can be isolated from liver biopsies during the relapse, and also from bone marrow many months after the patient has fully recovered from the symptoms. Relapses usually occur about 3 weeks after the last febrile day or about 2 weeks after cessation of antibiotics. Most relapses are milder than the initial illness, last for only a few days, and respond promptly to appropriate antibiotic therapy.

During the primary bacteremia that follows ingestion of typhoid bacilli and seeds the reticuloendothelial system, organisms also reach the gallbladder, an organ for which *S. typhi* has a remarkable predilection. *S. typhi* can be readily cultured from bile or from bile-stained duodenal fluid in patients with acute typhoid fever.(38) In approximately 2–5% of patients, the gallbladder infection becomes chronic.(60) The propensity to become a chronic carrier is greater in females and increases with age at the time of acute *S. typhi* infection, thereby resembling the epidemiology of gallbladder disease. The infection tends to become chronic in those individuals who have preexistent gallbladder pathology at the time of acute *S. typhi* infection. Carriers shed as many as 10^9 organisms/g feces.[89] These organisms are propelled the length of the gastrointestinal tract without penetrating and causing disease in the host.

7.2. Immunity

Age-specific incidence patterns suggest that repeated exposure in endemic areas results in the acquisition of immunity. Moreover, it is well-recognized that chronic carriers do not themselves develop clinical typhoid fever, despite having hundreds of billions of virulent typhoid bacilli pass the length of their intestine each day. On the other hand, protective immunity is not absolute. In volunteer rechallenge studies, an initial clinical typhoid infection conferred only 30% protection against subsequent challenge with the homologous *S. typhi* strain.[90] Similarly, repetitive clinical infections have been recorded in closed populations that experienced multiple sequential outbreaks of typhoid fever.[76]

A broad immune response is evident following wild-type typhoid infection, with the appearance of serum antibodies, mucosal SIgA responses, an array of cell-mediated immune responses, and a form of antibody-dependent cellular killing of *S. typhi*. The parenteral purified Vi polysaccharide and attenuated Ty21a live oral vaccines each elicit widely divergent immune responses, yet in its own way each confers significant protection. This suggests that several of the immune responses elicited by wild-type infection or by an array of vaccines can each individually mediate protection.

8. Patterns of Host Response

There is a wide spectrum of clinical syndromes associated with infection by *S. typhi*.[15,23,73] Many persons exposed to small numbers of bacteria will be asymptomatic and probably will show no clinical signs of infection. A small percentage of infected individuals develop bacteremia but are symptoms-free. Perhaps it is from this population that many carriers have developed, as many carriers do not recall having had the disease. The majority of patients with clinically overt disease have a relatively uniform course. A proportion of patients develop severe or complicated disease. In part, the duration of untreated disease prior to initiation of therapy influences the severity of the clinical disease. The curious, severe, clinical form of typhoid fever commonly encountered in Jakarta, Indonesia has already been described,[75] as has the atypical generally mild presentation of *S. typhi* infection observed in very young children.

8.1. Clinical Features

The major signs and symptoms of typhoid fever are relatively nonspecific. There is fever and an associated moderately severe generalized headache. The temperature increases in a stepwise fashion over the course of 2–3 days, reaching a peak of 103–104°F. During this time, the patient also complains of abdominal pain and is constipated. Examination of the abdomen will reveal palpation tenderness in the lower quadrants. Often, one can palpate dilated loops of bowel and sense the displacement of air and fluid under the probing fingers. This indicates that an ileus is present, a probable consequence of the inflammatory process occurring in the lamina propria and Peyer's patches. Late in the first week, careful inspection of the skin may reveal a few rose spots. These are slightly raised erythematous, nontender lesions found in light-skinned persons in the anterior chest or abdominal areas. They initially blanch with pressure, but gradually remain fixed as small cutaneous hemorrhages. These lesions are caused by *S. typhi* organisms infiltrating the endothelial cells of skin capillaries and inducing a perivascular infiltrate and subsequent leaking of blood. Biopsy of fresh rose spots will yield the organism.[38]

The course of the disease in untreated patients is characterized by a continuous fever with a relative bradycardia. The continuous fever will persist for 2 weeks or longer if no antibiotic is given, and defervescence occurs slowly over the ensuing 2–3 weeks. Such patients have a prolonged convalescence (3–4 months) because of the severe negative nitrogen balance that is a consequence of the prolonged infection. Patients who are receiving an appropriate antibiotic will respond with a gradual reduction in the fever over a 3- to 4-day period.

Complications are the significant prognostic indicators. Gastrointestinal hemorrhage or perforation is responsible for many of the fatalities with this disease. Both these events occur after about 2 weeks of untreated disease. The signs and symptoms of a perforated loop of intestine, presenting as an acute abdominal crisis, are well known.

8.2. Diagnosis

The diagnosis should be suspected in any patient with fever, abdominal pain, constipation, and headache. A prior history of travel to an endemic area will be an alerting epidemiological fact that should be followed up by appropriate blood and stool cultures. Because of the long incubation (which can be 2 weeks or longer), a thorough epidemiological history should be taken, since the patient may be the index case of a local outbreak. It is important to notify local health authorities promptly.

Typhoid bacilli appear in the blood with the onset of fever, and in untreated patients bacteremia remains for about 2 weeks before abating. The number of organisms in the blood is low, usually less than 50/cm^3 cultured blood. The bacteriological diagnosis is confirmed by positive blood cultures in only about 75–85% of patients. Variables such as prior antibiotic therapy, the volume of blood cultured (the larger the volume, the better), the type of broth used (it should contain an anticomplementary agent), and the number of days that cultures are incubated, all impact on whether a patient with typhoid fever will have a positive blood culture. Diagnosis is confirmed in the remaining patients by bone marrow, bile-stained duodenal string, stool, or rose spot cultures. Stool cultures become positive shortly after ingestion of the organism and may become negative with onset of disease, but may again yield the organism by the end of the first week of disease. Without therapy, stools may readily remain positive for *S. typhi* for as long as 4 months; beyond this period, continued presence indicates a greater than 90% chance of being a permanent carrier. Antibiotic treatment may cause temporary suppression of the isolation of typhoid bacilli from stools during the therapy.

Antibodies to O and H antigens appear during the end of the first week of illness and peak by the end of the third week of illness. It is unknown why as many as one third of patients with bacteriologically confirmed disease do not develop significant O and H titer rises. In some of the volunteers with induced disease, the baseline titers prior to challenge with virulent *S. typhi* were undetectable or low, e.g., 1:20 or 1:40 for O antibodies, yet no rise in titer occurred during the entire time of the prolonged follow-up.[30] These men also had bacteremia and positive stool cultures, an obvious source of antigens.

The differential diagnosis will include other infectious agents that may cause an enteric-fever-like syndrome such as tularemia and other salmonellae. Brucellosis, infectious mononucleosis, dengue fever, and infectious hepatitis may initially be confused because of similar symptoms associated with these febrile illnesses. Leptospirosis may occur with significant abdominal findings and mimic typhoid.

9. Control and Prevention

9.1. General Concepts

Control of typhoid fever requires the identification and tracking of carriers, control of their occupational activities, and, most important, provision of safe water supplies and human waste removal systems. All patients with the disease must be reported to the local health department. Patients should be nursed using enteric precautions. Linen soiled by feces should be handled with disposable gloves and hands should be scrupulously washed following contact with the patient.

Carriers, when discovered, are frequently elderly females. Since the current highly effective treatment regimen consists of up to 4 weeks of oral ciprofloxacin or norfloxacin,[91] care and encouragement must be provided to these elderly individuals during the therapy. If adverse reactions preclude administration of the full course, it is heartening to recognize that even short courses of 10 to 14 days have succeeded in eradicating the chronic carrier state in certain individuals.[91]

The stringency with which local health departments maintain surveillance of chronic carriers varies greatly. In some areas, these patients are required to submit stool specimens once or twice a year to confirm the continued presence of *S. typhi*; in other areas, only a listing is maintained. Carriers are prevented from working in any position that could result in their contaminating food or drinking water. This type of control is lacking in most endemic areas, and hence typhoid fever can remain as a common disease.

9.2. Antibiotic and Chemotherapeutic Approaches to Prophylaxis

There is no evidence to support the usefulness of prophylactic antibiotic treatment in preventing disease. To the contrary, data exist that suggest that administration of antibiotics following ingestion of typhoid bacilli but before the onset of clinical illness would not be effective. In tissue cultures, typhoid bacilli persist in the intracellular environment for at least 21 days, despite adequate concentrations of antibiotics in the solution bathing the cells. In the volunteer challenge studies carried out by Hornick *et al.*,[30] four men were begun on chloramphenicol treatment 24 hr after ingesting the 90% infective dose (ID_{90}) of *S. typhi*. In the two who took the antibiotic for 6 days, the incubation period was delayed by that same period compared to controls. In two men who were maintained on chloramphenicol for 28 days, no disease developed, but there were signs of infection such as positive stool cultures and antibody titer rises.

There is no justification for employing prophylactic antibiotics to prevent typhoid fever. The variable attack rate after known exposure makes it impractical to attempt prophylaxis. If a known common source exposure has occurred, it is much more prudent to maintain surveillance of the potential patients and to treat at the first signs of illness, after obtaining blood and stool cultures. Under these circumstances, treatment with effective antibiotics will reduce the duration and severity of the disease and will prevent complications by limiting the progression of the disease.

9.3. Immunization

The inactivated whole cell parenteral vaccines, including heat-inactivated, phenol-preserved vaccine and acetone-inactivated vaccine, confer moderate levels of protection that have been shown to endure for up to 7 years.[9–13] However, these are distinctly unsatisfactory vaccines because they cause adverse reactions at such high frequency. In controlled trials, approximately 25% of recipients of the inactivated whole cell vaccines developed fever and systemic reactions and about 15% had to miss work or school.[10,11,14] For this reason, these vaccines have been largely replaced by two newly licensed vaccines: live oral vaccine strain Ty21a (Vivotif) and parenteral purified Vi capsular polysaccharide vaccine (TyphiViM).[1] Both of these vaccines confer comparable protection and are well-tolerated.

9.3.1. Ty21a. Ty21a, an attenuated strain of *S. typhi* that is safe and protective as a live oral vaccine, was developed in the early 1970s by chemical mutagenesis of a pathogenic *S. typhi* strain.[92] The characteristic mutations in this strain include an inactivation of the *gal*E gene that encodes an enzyme involved in LPS synthesis and the inability to express Vi polysaccharide. Although Ty21a has proven to be remarkably well-tolerated in placebo-controlled clinical trials,[1,9] it is not clear precisely what mutations in fact are responsible for the stable, impressive attenuation of this vaccine.

Ty21a provides significant protection without causing adverse reactions.[9,35] Results of three double-blind, placebo-controlled studies that utilized active surveillance methods to assess the reactogenicity of Ty21a in adults and children showed that adverse reactions were not observed significantly more often in the vaccine recipients than the placebo group for any symptom or sign. In large-scale efficacy field trials with Ty21a, involving approximately 550,000 schoolchildren in Chile and 32,000 in Egypt, and approximately 20,000 subjects from 3 years of age to adulthood in Indonesia, passive surveillance failed to identify vaccine-attributable adverse reactions.[31,33,35]

Controlled field trials of Ty21a emphasize that the formulation of the vaccine, the number of doses administered, and the spacing of the doses markedly influence the level of protection that can be achieved.[1,9,31–35,93] In the first field trial of Ty21a in Alexandria, Egypt, 6- to 7-year-old schoolchildren received three doses of vaccine (suspended in a diluent) on Monday, Wednesday, and Friday of one week[93]; to neutralize gastric acid, the children chewed 1-g tablet of $NaHCO_3$ several minutes before ingesting the vaccine or placebo. During 3 years of surveillance, 96% protective efficacy against confirmed typhoid fever was observed.

A more recent formulation that is the current commercial product consists of lyophilized vaccine in enteric-coated, acid-resistant capsules. In a randomized, placebo-controlled field trial in Santiago, Chile, three doses of this enteric-coated formulation given within 1 week provided 67% efficacy during the first 3 years of follow-up and 63% protection over 7 years of follow-up.[33] In a large-scale, randomized comparative trial carried out in Santiago, Chile, four doses of Ty21a in enteric-coated capsules given within 8 days were shown to be significantly more protective than two or three doses (Table 5).[34] When Ty21a was licensed in the United States by the Food and Drug Administration in late 1989, it was with a recommended schedule of four doses to be given at an every other day interval; other countries used a three-dose immunization schedule.

In the mid 1980s, the Swiss Serum and Vaccine Institute succeeded in preparing a "liquid suspension" formulation of Ty21a for large-scale field trials that was amenable to large-scale manufacture. The new formulation consists of two packets, one containing a dose of lyophilized vaccine and the other containing buffer. Contents of the two packets are mixed in a cup containing 100 ml of water and the suspension is then ingested by the subject to be vaccinated. A fourth field trial was initiated in Santiago, Chile[31] and a parallel trial was carried out in Plaju, Indonesia[35] to compare directly this new liquid

Table 5. A Comparison of the Efficacy of Two, Three, or Four Doses of Ty21a Vaccine in Enteric-Coated Capsule Formulation. Results of a Large-Scale, Randomized, Field Trial in Area Sur and Area Central of the Metropolitan Region of Santiago, Chile[a]

Surveillance from 11/84 to 10/87	Two doses	Three doses	Four doses
No. of vaccinees	66,615	64,783	58,421
Cases of bacteriologically confirmed typhoid fever	123	104	56
Incidence/10^5[b]	184.6[a]	160.5[b]	95.8[c]
95% confidence interval	152–271	130–191	71–121

[a]Data from Ferreccio *et al.*[34]
[b]a versus c: $p = 0.00004$; b versus c: $p = 0.002$; a versus b: $p = 0.32$.

formulation of Ty21a (that somewhat resembles what was used in the Alexandria, Egypt field trial) with the enteric-coated capsule formulation. In both trials the vaccine administered as a liquid suspension was superior to the vaccine in enteric-coated capsules. In the placebo-controlled Santiago trial, over 3 years of follow-up the liquid suspension formulation conferred 77% efficacy [95% confidence interval (CI), 60–87%], whereas the enteric-coated formulation provided only 33% efficacy (95% CI, 0–57%) ($p < 0.001$).[31] In Indonesia, the liquid formulation of Ty21a conferred 53% efficacy (95% CI, 35–66%) and the enteric-coated capsule formulation provided 42% protection (95% CI, 23–57%) ($p > 0.05$).[35] Ty21a given as a liquid suspension protected young children as well as older children.[31] In previous trials with enteric-coated vaccine, young children were not as well protected as older children.[33] It is expected that by 1999, the more efficacious liquid formulation (packets containing lyophilized vaccine that is easily rehydratable to a liquid suspension) will replace the enteric-coated capsule formulation.

9.3.2. Vi Polysaccharide Vaccine. In the 1970s and early 1980s, methods were developed to purify Vi capsular polysaccharide so that it was 99.8% free of contaminating LPS and was not denatured.[48,58,59,94] This was an important breakthrough because as little as 5% impurity with LPS can result in systemic adverse reactions in a few percent of recipients.[94] In contrast, when Vi vaccine is highly purified, it is well-tolerated and febrile reactions are observed in only 1–2% of subjects. In clinical trials, well-tolerated 25 μg and 50 μg single intramuscular doses of purified Vi were highly immunogenic in stimulating serum IgG Vi antibodies.[58,59,94] Administration of subsequent parenteral doses did not achieve notable boosts in antibody. Nevertheless, the antibodies elicited by a single dose persisted for at least 3 years.[95] Passive surveillance carried out during field trials showed the Vi vaccine to be as well-tolerated as the licensed (meningococcal and pneumococcal) polysaccharide vaccines that served as the control preparations in these trials.[58,59]

Two randomized, controlled, double-blind field trials were carried out in Nepal and South Africa to assess the efficacy of a single 25-μg dose of nondenatured purified Vi vaccine. Over 17 months of surveillance in Nepal, the vaccine conferred 72% vaccine efficacy.[58] In South Africa, the vaccine provided 64% protection over 21 months of follow-up and 50% protection over 3 years.[59] The Nepal trial included all ages from preschool to adulthood, whereas the South African trial was performed in schoolchildren.

Beyond its safety and efficacy in school-age children and adults, an advantage of the Vi vaccine is that it provides a moderate level of protection after just a single dose. Table 6 summarizes the salient characteristics of Ty21a and Vi vaccines.

9.3.3. New Generation Typhoid Vaccines. New strains of *S. typhi* with precise attenuating mutations are being engineered that may successfully immunize following administration of a single oral dose. One candidate recombinant strain, CVD 908,[96] has been shown to be well-tolerated yet highly immunogenic following ingestion of a single oral dose.[97,98] CVD 908 harbors mutations in the pathway for biosynthesis of aromatic amino acids, thereby rendering it nutritionally dependent on substrates that are not present in human tissues. As a consequence, CVD 908 can undergo only limited proliferation in the human body. A further derivative, CVD 908-*htr*A, which has an additional independent attenuating mutation consisting of a deletion in the gene *htr*A that encodes a heat-shock protein,[99] is currently undergoing phase 2 clinical trials.

Booster doses of purified Vi do not raise antibody titers over those elicited by a single dose of vaccine; i.e., immunologic memory does not appear to occur. To remedy this, Szu *et al.*[100] have conjugated Vi polysaccharide to carrier proteins, such as tetanus toxoid, to increase its immunogenicity by conferring T-cell-dependent properties upon the antigen, including the induction of immunologic memory. In animals, booster doses of conjugate vaccine clearly increase the titers of antibody over those elicited by a priming dose.[100] A Vi conjugate vaccine is presently in clinical trials.

Table 6. A Comparison of the Characteristics of Live Oral Vaccine Ty21a and Parenteral Vi Polysaccharide Vaccine

	Ty21a	Vi
Type of vaccine	Live	Subunit
Route of administration	Oral	Parenteral
Immunization schedule	3 or 4 doses (given every other day)	1 dose
Cold chain required	Yes	Yes
Well-tolerated	Yes	Yes
Efficacy	60–96%	64–72%
Duration of efficacy	7 years	3 years
Evidence of a herd immunity effect	yes	?
Interferes with use of serum Vi antibody as a screening test to detect chronic typhoid carriers	No	Yes

10. Unresolved Problems

Areas ripe for research include (1) studies of the role of cytokines and immunopathology in the pathogenesis of typhoid fever; (2) investigations to explain the basis for the severe, obtunding clinical form of typhoid fever encountered with frequency in Java; (3) studies of the role and mechanisms of cell-mediated immunity in protection against typhoid fever and the degree to which these are stimulated by live oral vaccine strains; (4) studies to ascertain why infants and young children typically manifest such mild clinical responses in the presence of bacteremic infection by wild-type *S. typhi*; (5) the development of practical, inexpensive, rapid assays to make a microbiological confirmation of typhoid fever with a high degree of sensitivity and specificity; and (6) investigations to determine why *S. typhi* does not readily carry R factor plasmids other than those of incompatibility group H1. Finally, should the new generation of recombinant attenuated strains realize their potential as well-tolerated, highly immunogenic and protective, single-dose live oral vaccines, attention will have to be given to the possibility of worldwide eradication of typhoid fever. In typhoid-endemic areas, such an undertaking would involve enhanced provision of water supplies and means for human waste disposal, mass vaccination of schoolchildren with the new generation of vaccines, and identification and treatment of epidemiologically relevant carriers.

11. References

1. Levine, M. M., Taylor, D. N., and Ferreccio, C., Typhoid vaccines come of age, *Pediatr. Infect. Dis. J.* **8:**374–381 (1989).
2. Ryan, C. A., Hargrett-Bean, N. T., and Blake, P. A., *Salmonella typhi* infections in the United States, 1975–1984: Increasing role of foreign travel, *Rev. Infect. Dis.* **II:**1–8 (1989).
3. Blaser, M. J., and Lofgren, J. P., Fatal salmonellosis originating in a clinical microbiology laboratory, *J. Clin. Microbiol.* **13:**855–858 (1981).
4. Blaser, M. J., Hickman, F. W., Farmer, J. J., *et al.*, *Salmonella typhi*: The laboratory as a reservoir of infection, *J. Infect. Dis.* **142:**934–938 (1980).
5. Gupta, A., Multidrug-resistant typhoid fever in children: Epidemiology and therapeutic approach, *Pediatr. Infect. Dis. J.* **13:**124–140 (1994).
6. Rowe, B., Ward, L. R., and Threlfall, E. J., Spread of multiresistant *Salmonella typhi*, *Lancet* **336:**1065–1066 (1990).
7. Levine, M. M., Typhoid fever vaccines, in: *Vaccines*, 2nd ed. (S. A. Plotkin and E. Mortimer, Jr., eds.), pp. 597–633, 1994.
8. Budd, W., *Typhoid Fever. Its Nature, Mode of Spreading and Prevention*, Longmans, London, 1873.
9. Levine, M. M., Ferreccio, C., Black, R. E., Tacket, C.O., and Germanier, R., Progress in vaccines against typhoid fever, *Rev. Infect. Dis.* **11**(Suppl. 3)**:**S552–S567 (1989).
10. Yugoslav Typhoid Commission, A controlled field trial of the effectiveness of acetone-dried and inactivated and heat-phenol-inactivated typhoid vaccines in Yugoslavia, *Bull. WHO* **30:**623–630 (1964).
11. Hejfec, L. B., Salmin, L. V., Lejtman, M. Z., *et al.*, A controlled field trial and laboratory study of five typhoid vaccines in the USSR, *Bull. WHO* **34:**321–339 (1966).
12. Polish Typhoid Committee, Controlled field trial and laboratory studies on the effectiveness of typhoid vaccines in Poland 1961–64, *Bull. WHO* **34:**211–222 (1966).
13. Ashcroft, M. T., Nicholson, C. C., Balwant, S., *et al.*, A seven-year field trial of two typhoid vaccines in Guyana, *Lancet* **2:**1056–1060 (1967).
14. Ashcroft, M. T., Morrison-Ritchie, J., and Nicholson, C.C., Controlled field trial in British Guyana schoolchildren of heat-killed-phenolized and acetone-killed lyophilized typhoid vaccines, *Am. J. Hyg.* **79:**196–206 (1964).
15. Stuart, B. M., and Pullen, R. L., Typhoid. *Arch. Intern. Med.* **78:**629–661 (1946).
16. Anonymous, Typhoid in the large cities of the United States in 1919, *J. Am. Med. Assoc.* **74:**672–675 (1920).
17. Wolman, A., and Gorman, A., *The Significance of Waterborne Typhoid Fever Outbreaks*, Williams & Wilkins, Baltimore, 1931.
18. Woodward, T. E., Smadel, J. E., Ley, H. L., Green, R., and Mankakan, D. S., Preliminary report on the beneficial effect of choloromycetin in the treatment of typhoid fever, *Ann. Intern. Med.* **29:**131–134 (1948).
19. Centers for Disease Control and Prevention, Summary of notifiable diseases, United States, 1993, *Morbid. Mortal. Week. Rep.* **42:**1–75 (1994).
20. Feldman, R. E., Baine, W. B., Nitzkin, J. L., Saslaw, M. S., and Pollard, R. A., Jr., Epidemiology of *Salmonella typhi* infection in a migrant labor camp in Dade County, Florida, *J. Infect. Dis.* **130:**334–342 (1974).
21. Lin, F.-Y. C., Becke, J. M., Groves, C. A., *et al.*, Restaurant-associated outbreak of typhoid fever in Maryland: Identification of carrier facilitated by measurement of serum antibodies, *J. Clin. Microbiol.* **26:**1194–1197 (1988).
22. Morris, J. G., Ferreccio, C., Garcia, J., *et al.*, Typhoid fever in Santiago, Chile: A study of household contacts of pediatric patients, *Am. J. Trop. Med. Hyg.* **33:**1198–1202 (1984).
23. Ferreccio, C., Levine, M. M., Manterola, A., *et al.*, Benign bacteremia caused by *Salmonella typhi* and paratyphi in children younger than 2 years, *J. Pediatr.* **104:**899–901 (1984).
24. Ferreccio, C., Levine, M. M., Solari, V., *et al.*, Detecciön de portadores cronicos de *Salmonella typhi:* Método práctico aplicado a manipuladores de alimentos del centro de Santiago, *Rev. Med. Chile* **118:**33–37 (1990).
25. Lanata, C. F., Levine, M. M., Ristori, C., *et al.*, Vi serology in detection of chronic *Salmonella typhi* carriers in an endemic area, *Lancet* **2:**441–443 (1983).
26. Losonsky, G. A., Ferreccio, C., Kotloff, K. L., *et al.*, Development and evaluation of an enzyme-linked immunosorbent assay for Vi antibodies in the detection in chronic *Salmonella typhi* carriers, *J. Clin. Microbiol.* **25:**2266–2269 (1987).
27. Nolan, C. M., Feeley, J. C., White, P. C., Jr., *et al.*, Evaluation of a new assay for Vi antibody in chronic carriers of *Salmonella typhi*, *J. Clin. Microbiol.* **12:**22–26 (1980).
28. Levine, M. M., Grados, O., Gilman, R. H., *et al.*, Diagnostic value of the Widal test in areas endemic for typhoid fever, *Am. J. Trop. Med. Hyg.* *27:*795–800 (1978).

29. Levine, M. M., Black, R. E., Ferreccio, C., *et al.*, Interventions to control endemic typhoid fever: Field studies in Santiago, in: *Control and Eradication of Infectious Diseases. An International Symposium* (L. J. Mata, ed.), Pan American Health Organization, Washington, DC, 1986.
30. Hornick, R. B., Griesman, S. E., Woodward, T. E., *et al.*, Typhoid fever: Pathogenesis and immunologic control, *N. Engl. J. Med.* **283:**686–691, 739–746 (1970).
31. Levine, M. M., Ferreccio, C., Cryz, S., and Ortiz, E., Comparison of enteric-coated capsules and liquid formulation of Ty21a typhoid vaccine in randomised controlled field trial, *Lancet* **336:** 891–894 (1990).
32. Black, R. E., Levine, M. M., Ferreccio, C., *et al.*, Efficacy of one or two doses of Ty21a *Salmonella typhi* vaccine in enteric-coated capsules in a controlled field trial, Chilean Typhoid Committee, *Vaccine* **8:**81–84 (1990).
33. Levine, M. M., Ferreccio, C., Black, R. E., and Germanier, R., Large-scale field trial of Ty21a live oral typhoid vaccine in enteric-coated capsule formulation, *Lancet* **1:**1049–1052 (1987).
34. Ferreccio, C., Levine, M. M., Rodriguez, H., Contreras, R., and Chillean Typhoid Committee, Comparative efficacy of two, three, or four doses of Ty21a live oral typhoid vaccine in enteric-coated capsules: A field trial in an endemic area, *J. Infect. Dis.* **159:**766–769 (1989).
35. Simanjuntak, C., Paleologo, F., Punjabi, N., *et al.*, Oral immunisation against typhoid fever in Indonesia with Ty21a vaccine, *Lancet* **338:**1055–1059 (1991).
36. Avendaño, A., Herrera, P., Horwitz, I., *et al.*, Duodenal string cultures: Practicality and sensitivity for diagnosing enteric fever in children, *J. Infect. Dis.* **53:**359–362 (1986).
37. Guerra-Cáceres, J. G., Gotuzzo-Herencia, E., Crosby-Dagnino, E., *et al.*, Diagnostic value of bone marrow culture in typhoid fever, *Trans. R. Soc. Trop. Med. Hyg.* **73:**680–683 (1979).
38. Gilman, R. H., Terminel, M., Levine, M. M., Relative efficacy of blood, urine, rectal swab, bone-marrow, and rose-spot cultures for recovery of *Salmonella typhi* in typhoid fever, *Lancet* **1:**1211–1213 (1975).
39. Hickman-Brenner, F. W., and Farmer, III, J. J., Regional centers for *Salmonella typhi* bacteriophage typing in the US bacteriophage types of *Salmonella typhi* in the United States from 1974 through 1981, *J. Clin. Microbiol.* **17:**172–174 (1983).
40. Song, J.-H., Cho, H., Park, M. Y., *et al.*, Detection of *Salmonella typhi* in the blood of patients with typhoid fever by polymerase chain reaction, *J. Clin. Microbiol.* **31:**1439–1443 (1993).
41. Widal, G. F. I., and Sicard, A., Recherches de la reaction agglutinaté dans le sang et le serum desséchés des typhiques et dans la serosité des vesications, *Bull. Soc. Med. Paris* (3rd ser) **13:**681–682 (1896).
42. Anderson, E. S., and Gunnell, A., A suggestion for a new antityphoid vaccine, *Lancet* **2:**1196–1200 (1964).
43. Hoffman, S., Flanigan, T. P., Klaucke, D., *et al.*, The Widal slide agglutination test, a valuable rapid diagnostic test in typhoid fever patients at the infectious diseases hospital of Jakarta, *Am. J. Epidemiol.* **123:**869–875 (1986).
44. Edelman, R., and Levine, M. M., Summary of an international workshop on typhoid fever, *Rev. Infect. Dis.* **8:**329–349 (1986).
45. Minor, L. L., and Popoff, M. Y., Designation of *Salmonella enterica* sp. nov. rev., as the type and only species of the genus *Salmonella*, *Int. J. Syst. Bacteriol.* **37:**465–468 (1987).
46. Guinée, P. A. M., Jansen, W. H., Maas, W. H., *et al.*, An unusual H antigen (z66) in strains of *Salmonella typhi*, *Ann. Microbiol.* **132:**331–334 (1981).
47. Grossman, D. A., Witham, N. D., Burr, D. H., *et al.*, Flagellar serotypes of *Salmonella typhi* in Indonesia: Relationships among motility, invasiveness, and clinical illness, *J. Infect. Dis.* **171:**212–216 (1995).
48. Robbins, J. D., and Robbins, J. B., Reexamination of the protective role of the capsular polysaccharide Vi antigen of *Salmonella typhi*, *J. Infect. Dis.* **150:**436–449 (1984).
49. Maher, K. O., Morris, J. G., Gotuzzo, E., *et al.*, Molecular techniques in the study of *Salmonella typhi* in epidemiologic studies in endemic areas: Comparison with Vi phage typing, *Am. J. Trop Med. Hyg.* **35:**831–835 (1986).
50. Franco, A., Gonzalez, C., Levine, O. S., *et al.*, Further consideration of the clonal nature of *Salmonella typhi:* Evaluation of molecular and clinical characteristics of strains from Indonesia and Peru, *J. Clin. Microbiol.* **30:**2187–2190 (1992).
51. Anderson, E. S., The problem and implications of chloramphenicol resistance in the typhoid bacillus, *J. Hyg.* **74:**289–299 (1975).
52. Gilman, R. H., Terminel, M., Levine, M. M., *et al.*, Comparison of trimethoprim–sulfamethoxazole and amoxicillin in therapy of chloramphenicol-resistant and chloramphenicol-sensitive typhoid fever, *J. Infect. Dis.* **132:**630–636 (1975).
53. Butler, T., Linh, N. N., Arnold, K., and Pollack, M., Chloramphenicol-resistant typhoid fever in Vietnam associated with R factor, *Lancet* **2:**983–985 (1973).
54. Goldstein, F. W., Cumpaitaz, J. C., Guevara, J. M., *et al.*, Plasmid-mediated resistance to multiple antibiotics in *Salmonella typhi*, *J. Infect. Dis.* **153:**261–266 (1986).
55. Rice, P. A., Baine, W. B., and Gangarosa, E. J., *Salmonella typhi* infections in the United States, 1967–1972: Increasing importance of international travelers, *Am. J. Epidemiol.* **106:**160–166 (1977).
56. Taylor, D. N., Pollard, R. A., and Blake, P. A., Typhoid in the United States and the risk to the international traveler, *J. Infect. Dis.* **148:**599–602 (1983).
57. Baine, W. B., Farmer, J. J., Gangarosa, E. J., *et al.*, Typhoid fever in the United States associated with the 1972–1973 epidemic in Mexico, *J. Infect. Dis.* **135:**649–653 (1977).
58. Acharya, V. L., Lowe, C. U., Thapa, R., *et al.*, Prevention of typhoid fever in Nepal with the Vi capsular polysaccharide of *Salmonella typhi*, *N. Engl. J. Med.* **317:**1101–1104 (1987).
59. Klugman, K., Gilbertson, I. T., Kornhoff, H. J., *et al.*, Protective activity of Vi polysaccharide vaccine against typhoid fever, *Lancet* **2:**1165–1169 (1987).
60. Ames, W. A., and Robins, M., Age and sex as factors in the development of the typhoid carrier state and a method of estimating carrier prevalence, *Am. J. Public Health* **33:**221–230 (1943).
61. Levine, M. M., Black, R. E., Lanata, C., and the Chilean Typhoid Committee, Precise estimation of the numbers of chronic carriers of *Salmonella typhi* in Santiago, Chile, an endemic area, *J. Infect. Dis.* **146:**724–726 (1982).
62. Walker, W., The Aberdeen typhoid outbreak of 1964, *Scott. Med. J.* **10:**466–479 (1965).
63. Bernard, R. P., The Zermatt typhoid outbreak in 1963, *J. Hyg.* **63:**537–563 (1965).
64. Sears, S. D., Ferreccio, C., Levine, M. M., *et al.*, The use of Moore swabs for isolation of *Salmonella typhi* from irrigation water in Santiago, Chile, *J. Infect. Dis.* **149:**640–642 (1984).
65. Bundesen, H. N., Typhoid epidemic in Chicago apparently due to oysters, *J. Am. Med. Assoc.* **84:**641–650 (1925).
66. Hamilton, A., The fly as a carrier of typhoid, *J. Am. Med. Assoc.* **28:**576–583 (1903).
67. Dritz, S. K., and Braff, E. H., Sexually transmitted typhoid fever, *N. Engl. J. Med.* **296:**1359–1360 (1977).

68. Ashcroft, M. T., Typhoid and paratyphoid fever in the tropics, *J. Trop. Med. Hyg.* **67:**185–189 (1964).
69. Medina, E., and Yrarrazaval, M., Fiebre tifoidea en Chile: Consideraciónes epidémiológicas, *Rev. Med. Chile* **111:**609–615 (1983).
70. Levine, M. M., South America: The return of cholera, *Lancet* **338:**45–46 (1991).
71. Kligler, I. J., and Bachi, R., An analysis of the endemicity and epidemicity of typhoid fever in Palestine, *Acta Med. Orient* **4:**243–261 (1945).
72. Ashcroft, M. T., The morbidity and mortality of enteric fever in British Guiana, *West Indian Med. J.* **11:**62–71 (1962).
73. Mahle, W. T., and Levine, M. M., *Salmonella typhi* infection in children younger than five years of age, *Pediatr. Infect. Dis. J.* **12:**627–631 (1993).
74. Ryder, R. W., and Blake, P. A., Typhoid fever in the United States, 1975 and 1976, *J. Infect. Dis.* **139:**124–126 (1979).
75. Hoffman, S. L., Punjabi, N. H., Kumala, S., *et al.*, Reduction of mortality in chloramphenicol-treated severe typhoid fever by high-dose dexamethasone, *N. Engl. J. Med.* **310:**82–88 (1984).
76. Marmion, D. E., Naylor, G. R. E., and Stewart, I. O., Second attacks of typhoid fever, *J. Hyg.* **53:**260–267 (1953).
77. Black, R. E., Cisneros, L., Levine, M. M., *et al.*, Case–control study to identify risk factors for paediatric endemic typhoid fever in Santiago,, Chile, *Bull. WHO* **63:**899–904 (1985).
78. Melham, R. F., and LoVerde, P. T., Mechanism of interaction of Salmonellae and Schistosoma species, *Infect. Immun.* **44:**274–281 (1984).
79. Egoz, N., Shihab, S., Leitner, L., and Lucian, M., An outbreak of typhoid fever due to contamination of the municipal water supply in Northern Israel, *Israel J. Med. Sci.* **24:**640–643 (1988).
80. Soper, G. A., The curious career of Typhoid Mary, *Bull. NY Acad. Med.* **15:**698–712 (1939).
81. Taylor, J. P., Shandera, W. X., Betz, T. G., *et al.*, Typhoid fever in San Antonio, Texas: An outbreak traced to a continuing source, *J. Infect. Dis.* **149:**553–557 (1984).
82. Birkhead, G. S., Morse, D. L., Levine, W. C., *et al.*, Typhoid fever at a resort hotel in New York: A large outbreak with an unusual vehicle, *J. Infect. Dis.* **167:**1228–1232 (1993).
83. Salas, M., Angulo, O., and Villegus, J., Patologia de la fiebre tifoida en los niños, *Biol. Med. Hosp. Mex.* **17:**63–68 (1960).
84. Gaines, S., Sprinz, H., Tully, J. G., and Tigertt, W. D., Studies on infection and immunity in experimental typhoid fever. VII. The distribution of *Salmonella typhi* in chimpanzee tissue following oral challenge and the relationship between the numbers of bacilli and morphologic lesions, *J. Exp. Med.* **118:**293–306 (1968).
85. Carter, P. B., and Collins, R. M., The route of enteric infection in normal mice, *J. Exp. Med.* **139:**1189–1203 (1974).
86. Takeuchi, A., Electron microscope studies of experimental *Salmonella* infection. I. Penetrations into the intestinal epithelium by *Salmonella typhimurium*, *Am. J. Pathol.* **50:**109–136 (1967).
87. Robbins, J. D., and Robbins, J. B., Reexamination of the protective role of the capsular polysaccharide Vi antigen of *Salmonella typhi*, *J. Infect. Dis.* **150:**436–449 (1984).
88. Butler, T., Bell, W. R., Levin, J., *et al.*, Typhoid fever: Studies of blood coagulation, bacteremia and endotoxemia, *Arch. Intern. Med.* **138:**407–410 (1978).
89. Merselis, J. G., Jr., Kaye, D., Connolly, C. S., and Hook, W. E., Quantitative bacteriology of the typhoid carrier state, *Am. J. Trop. Med. Hyg.* **13:**425–429 (1964).
90. DuPont, L. H., Hornick, R. B., Snyder, M. J., *et al.*, Studies of immunity in typhoid fever. Protection induced by killed oral antigens or by primary infection, *Bull. WHO* **44:**667–672 (1971).
91. Ferreccio, C., Morris, J. G., Valdivieso, C., *et al.*, Efficacy of ciprofloxacin in the treatment of chronic typhoid carriers, *J. Infect. Dis.* **157:**1235–1239 (1988).
92. Germanier, R., and Furer, E., Isolation and characterization of *gal*E mutant Ty21a of *Salmonella typhi:* A candidate strain for a live oral typhoid vaccine, *J. Infect. Dis.* **141:**553–558 (1975).
93. Wahdan, M. H., Serie, C., Cerisier, Y., *et al.*, A controlled field trial of live *Salmonella typhi* strain Ty21a oral vaccine against typhoid: Three year results, *J. Infect. Dis.* **145:**292–296 (1982).
94. Tacket, C. O., Ferreccio, C., Robbins, J. B., *et al.*, Safety and immunogenicity of two *Salmonella typhi* Vi capsular polysaccharide vaccines, *J. Infect. Dis.* **154:**342–345 (1986).
95. Tacket, C. O., Levine, M. M., and Robbins, J. B., Persistence of antibody titres three years after vaccination with Vi polysaccharide vaccine against typhoid fever, *Vaccine* **6:**307–308 (1988).
96. Hone, D. M., Harris, A. M., Chatfield, S., *et al.*, Construction of genetically defined double aro mutants of *Salmonella typhi*, *Vaccine* **9:**810–816 (1991).
97. Tacket, C. O., Hone, D. M., Losonsky, G. A., *et al.*, Clinical acceptability and immunogenicity of CVD 908 *Salmonella typhi* vaccine strain, *Vaccine* **10:**443–446 (1992).
98. Tacket, C. O., Hone, D. M., Curtiss, R., III, *et al.*, Comparison of the safety and immunogenicity of Δ*aroC* Δ*aroD* and Δcya ΔCrp *Salmonella typhi* strains in adult volunteers, *Infect. Immun.* **60:**536–541 (1992).
99. Chatfield, S., Strahan, K., Pickard, D., *et al.*, Evaluation of *Salmonella typhimurium* strains harboring defined mutations in *htrA* and *aroA* in the murine salmonellosis model, *Microbial. Pathog.* **12:**145–151 (1992).
100. Szu, S. C., Stone, A. L., Robbins, J. D., *et al.*, Vi capsular polysaccharide–protein conjugates for prevention of typhoid fever. Preparation, characterization, and immunogenicity in laboratory animals, *J. Exp. Med.* **166:**1510–1524 (1987).

12. Suggested Reading

Hornick, R. B., Griesman, S. E., Woodward, T. E., *et al.*, Typhoid fever; pathogenesis and immunologic control, *N. Engl. J. Med.* **283:**686–691, 739–746 (1970).

Levine, M. M., Taylor, D. N., and Ferreccio, C., Typhoid vaccines come of age, *Pediatr. Infect. Dis. J.* **8:**374–381 (1989).

Gupta, A., Multidrug-resistant typhoid fever in children: Epidemiology and therapeutic approach, *Pediatr. Infect. Dis. J.* **13:**124–140 (1994).

Mahle, W. T., and Levine, M. M., *Salmonella typhi* infection in children younger than five years of age, *Pediatr. Infect. Dis. J.* **12:**627–631 (1993).

Ryan, C. A., Hargrett-Bean, N. T., and Blake, P. A., *Salmonella typhi* infections in the United States, 1975–1984: Increasing role of foreign travel, *Rev. Infect. Dis.* **II:**1–8 (1989).

CHAPTER 43

Yersinia enterocolitica Infections

Georg Kapperud and Sally Bryna Slome

1. Introduction

Bacteria of the genus *Yersinia* have been recognized for centuries as the cause of devastating human illness in the form of plague caused by *Yersinia pestis* and epizootic disease in animals and mesenteric lymphadenitis in humans due to *Yersinia pseudotuberculosis*. In more recent years, a third member of the genus, *Yersinia enterocolitica*, has been reported with increasing frequency throughout the world. *Y. enterocolitica* constitutes a fairly heterogenous group of bacteria that includes both well-established pathogens and a range of environmental strains that are ubiquitous in terrestrial and freshwater ecosystems. The species encompasses a spectrum of phenotypic variants, of which only a few have been conclusively associated with human or animal disease.[1–3] Pathogenic significance in man is mainly associated with a few serogroups (O:3, O:9, O:8, O:5,27) that show distinct geographic distributions. The strains responsible for pathological processes in animals differ phenotypically from those in human infection.[3]

Illness caused by *Y. enterocolitica* and *Y. pseudotuberculosis* has been referred to as yersiniosis.[4,5] *Y. enterocolitica* is the etiologic agent of a range of clinical entities in humans, although acute noncomplicated enterocolitis is by far the most frequent manifestation.[1,8] The bacterium has attracted considerable attention due to its ability to cause postinfectious sequelae, most notably nonpurulent arthritis. The present discussion will focus on *Y. enterocolitica* and its emerging role in a variety of clinical syndromes afflicting humans.

Georg Kapperud • National Institute of Public Health, 0403 Oslo, Norway; and Norwegian College of Veterinary Medicine, 0033 Oslo, Norway. **Sally Bryna Slome** • Kaiser Permanente Medical Center, Oakland, California 94611.

2. Historical Background

The first description of human illness caused by *Y. enterocolitica* was made to Gilbert[7] in 1933. In 1939, Schleifstein and Coleman reported the isolation of "an unidentified microorganism resembling *Bacterium lignieri* and *Pasteurella pseudotuberculosis* and pathogenic for man."[8a] In a publication from 1943, the same authors[8] suggested that these isolates were sufficiently distinct to deserve recognition as a separate species, which they named *Bacterium enterocoliticum*. Few isolations of *Y. enterocolitica* were reported during the following 20 years. Since the species was as yet unclassified, however, the isolates were variably identified as *Pasteurella X*, *Y. pseudotuberculosis* type B, *B. enterocolitica*, and Les Germes X.

The current interest in bacteria that are now known as *Y. enterocolitica* started in the early 1960s following a number of widespread epizootics among chinchillas and hares and after the establishment of a causative relationship with lymphadenitis in man. In 1963, the similarity was established between the human and animal isolates.[9] Frederiksen[10] demonstrated that the isolates were distinct from *Y. pseudotuberculosis*, but similar enough to be designated as a separate *Yersinia* species. The following year he proposed the species name *Yersinia enterocolitica* for this taxon.[10]

The decade of the 1970s heralded a new interest in *Y. enterocolitica* as reports from throughout the world emphasized its importance as a human pathogen. Improved methods of stool culture facilitated isolation of the organism worldwide.[11] Coincident with this heightened awareness, it became evident that the original biochemical criteria proposed for the species *Y. enterocolitica* did in fact circumscribe a heterogeneous group of bacteria. Many isolates were described as "*Y. enterocolitica*-like organisms" but differed substantially in their biochemical reactions. Several biotyping and serotyping schemes were proposed.[9,12–16] With the advent of DNA hybridization techniques, this diverse group of microbes was divided into eight species with distinct biochemical profiles: *Y. enterocolitica*, *Y. frederiksenii*, *Y. kristensenii*, *Y. intermedia*, *Y. aldovae*, *Y. rohdei*, *Y. mollaretii*, and *Y. bercovieri*.[17–20]

3. Methodology

3.1. Sources of Mortality Data

Limited information is available concerning the role of *Y. enterocolitica* as a cause of fatal disease. Enterocolitis, which accounts for the majority of reported cases of yersiniosis, is rarely fatal in developed countries. Although *Y. enterocolitica* enteritis does not appear to be common in developing countries, fatal diarrhea has been reported.[21] The true case-fatality rate for the clinical syndromes of enterocolitis, mesenteric adenitis and terminal ileitis is unknown, but is likely to be very low. The few fatal cases reported have been generally attributed to extensive intestinal ulceration and peritonitis. Most extraintestinal manifestations of *Y. enterocolitica* infection are usually mild and self-limited. Septicemia, on the other hand, is most often reported in children or adults compromised by severe anemia, hemochromatosis, cirrhosis, malignancy, malnutrition, or immunosuppressive therapy and is associated with a significant mortality. Rabson *et al.*[22] found a case-fatality ratio of approximately 50% in 13 patients with disseminated *Y. enterocolitica* infection and a universal mortality in those with underlying hemochromatosis. The complications of disseminated infection, which include suppurative hepatic, renal, and splenic lesions, osteomyelitis, wound infection, or meningitis, also carry a significant risk of death.

3.2. Sources of Morbidity Data

Information regarding morbidity due to *Y. enterocolitica* is imprecise. In the United States, positive cultures may be submitted to state laboratories or to the Centers for Disease Control and Prevention (CDC) for confirmation. The condition is not nationally reportable. Since few laboratories in the United States routinely screen clinical specimens for *Y. enterocolitica*, it is likely to be underdiagnosed and underrecognized by clinicians. In Scandinavia, diagnostic cultures are made routinely, and positive results are routinely reported. Case reporting is required in 19 states in the United States and in several European countries. However, these surveillance systems underestimate the number of actual cases. The lack of universal application of laboratory techniques that favor its isolation, as well as incomplete reporting of *Y. enterocolitica* isolates to public health agencies, limits the effectiveness of laboratory-based surveillance. Investigations of outbreaks provide some additional sources of morbidity data.

3.3. Surveys

Surveys of the relative frequency of *Y. enterocolitica* in populations with diarrhea have justified its inclusion as a bacterial enteric pathogen of importance (Section 5.1). Serological surveys have been conducted in several European countries (reviewed by Agner *et al.*[23]). However, direct comparison of the results is difficult, since different subpopulations were studied and since a variety of serological assays and antigens were used.

3.4. Laboratory Diagnosis

3.4.1. Isolation and Identification of the Organism. *Y. enterocolitica* belongs to the family Enterobacteriaceae.[24] Accordingly, it shares many of the characteristics defining this family. It is thus a gram-negative, oxidase-negative, catalase-positive, nitrate-reductase-positive, facultative anaerobic rod 0.5–0.8 × 1–3 μm in size, that exhibits significant pleomorphism. Coccobacillary forms may be seen. It does not form a capsule or spores. *Y. enterocolitica* is nonmotile at 35–37°C but motile at 22–25°C, with relatively few, peritrichous flagellae. Some strains of serogroup O:3, however, are nonmotile at both temperatures. In addition, the bacterium is urease-positive, ferments mannitol, and produces acid but not gas from glucose. *Y. enterocolitica* differs from most members of the family Enterobacteriaceae by virtue of its slower growth.

Cultural isolation is by far the method of choice for diagnosing *Y. enterocolitica* infection. The isolation and identification of the bacterium from normally sterile sites is not difficult, according to standard bacteriological procedures. Recovery of the organism from stool, on the other hand, is hampered by the lack of characteristic colonial morphology as well as the organism's slow growth and the resultant overgrowth of normal fecal flora. Several selective and differential media have been developed to enhance the recovery of *Y. enterocolitica* from stool specimens. Unfortunately, the different pathogenic serogroups vary in their tolerance to selective components and other factors during the isolation process.[25,26] While a number of methods are currently in use in different parts of the world, there is great need for a universally acceptable reference method. Cefsulodin–irgasan–novobiocin (CIN) agar, a highly selective and differential medium, is more effective than routine enteric media for the recovery of *Y. enterocolitica* from stools.[27] *Y. enterocolitica* appears as 0.5- to 1.0-mm diameter colonies with a dark red "bull's eye" and transparent border. CIN agar permits the growth of all pathogenic serogroups. However, certain conventional isolation and enrichment media are known to impair the growth of O:8 and O:5,27.[28,29] While *Salmonella–Shigella* (SS) agar favors the growth of serogroups O:3 and O:9, the addition of MacConkey agar enables the recovery of other serogroups that may be inhibited by SS agar. Wauters *et al.*[29] have described two selective media, *Salmonella–Shigella*–deoxycholate–calcium (SSDC) agar and irgasan–ticarcillin–potassium chlorate (ITC) enrichment broth, which are specially designed for isolation of O:3.

Y. enterocolitica is quite heterogenous with respect to phenotypic, genotypic, and ecological properties. The phenotypic heterogeneity has enabled the development of several schemes for subdivision of the bacterium.[2,3,30] Serotyping according to O antigens and differentiation on the basis of biochemical properties have become the most useful typing methods. The biotyping scheme proposed by Wauters has been most widely used; a revision was published in 1987.[30] *Y. enterocolitica* has been divided into more than 70 serogroups using O antigens.[14] Several O antigen groups may be further subdivided by H antigens.[31] However, the use of H-antigen typing has been hampered by its limited availability. (Serotyping on the basis of H antigens is conducted by Dr. S. Aleksic, Hygiene Institute, Hamburg, Germany.) In addition to setotyping and biotyping, a number of phenotypic and genotypic methods have been used to subdivide *Y. enterocolitica*. The discriminatory power of the genotypic methods are generally higher for serogroup O:8 than for O:3, O:9, and O:5,27.[32]

Y. enterocolitica encompasses acknowledged pathogens as well as a range of variants to which no pathogenic significance is currently attributed.[3] The great majority of the strains involved in pathological processes in humans or animals belong to only a few serogroups and biovars.[3] Thus, accurate identification of pathogenic strains necessitates consideration of both biochemical and antigenic characteristics. Somewhat simplified, *Y. enterocolitica* may be divided into three groups according to clinical significance: human pathogens, animal pathogens, and environmental strains, each comprising different serogroups. Thus, O:3 biovar 4; O:5,27 biovar 2; O:8 biovar 1B; and O:9 biovar 2 are the most important variants incriminated in human disease. Although other serogroups may occasionally cause infection, these variants predominate among human isolates.

The pathogenic animal strains also belong to particular serogroups and biovars[3,4]: O:1 biovar 3 was responsible for widespread outbreaks in chinchillas, whereas O:2 biovar 5 has been associated with disease in hares, sheep, and goats. The environmental strains, on the other hand, constitute a spectrum of phenotypic variants that display a variety of antigenic factors; a majority belongs to biovar 1A. These bacteria usually lack clinical significance and are ubiquitous.[2,3] Such environmental strains have occasionally been involved in human infection, mainly in immunocompromised patients and patients with underlying conditions.

Y. enterocolitica may be differentiated from *Y. pseudotuberculosis* and from bacteria previously termed "*Y. enterocolitica*-like organisms" by means of several distinct biochemical reactions. These bacteria include *Y. frederiksenii*, *Y. kristensenii*, *Y. intermedia*, *Y. aldovae*, *Y. rohdei*, *Y. mollaretii*, and *Y. bercovieri*.[24] Such species are frequently encountered in terrestrial and freshwater ecosystems. Like the environmental *Y. enterocolitica* strains, none of these species have been associated with human or animal disease, with the exception of a few atypical cases.[4]

3.4.2. Serological Diagnostic Methods. Infection with *Y. enterocolitica* elicits an immunologic response that can be measured by a variety of techniques, including tube agglutination, indirect hemagglutination, enzyme-linked immunosorbent assay, and solid-phase radioimmunoassay.[33,34] An indirect immunofluorescent-antibody assay has also been used.[34] Agglutinating antibodies appear soon after the onset of illness and persist from 2 to 6 months. Some serotypes may be associated with illness without eliciting a detectable serological response.[35,36] The serological response of young infants appears to be less vigorous than that of adults.[37] Patients with systemic disease mount a greater antibody titer than do persons with disease restricted to the gastrointestinal tract.[38]

The serological diagnosis of *Y. enterocolitica* infection may be complicated by the existence of cross-reactions between *Y. enterocolitica*, most notably serogroup O:9, and such organisms as *Brucella*, *Vibrio*, *Salmonella*, and *Escherichia coli*. The interpretation may also be confounded by a high prevalence of seropositive individuals in the healthy population. Patients with thyroiditis on an immunologic basis have an unexplained increased frequency of cross-reacting antibodies to *Y.*

enterocolitica.[39] Detection of antibodies to plasmid-encoded proteins (Yops) by immunoblots has been suggested as a highly specific method to demonstrate previous *Y. enterocolitica* infection.[40,41] Demonstration of specific circulating IgA to the Yops is indicative of recent or persistent infection and is strongly correlated with the presence of virulent *Y. enterocolitica* in the intestinal lymphatic tissue of patients with reactive arthritis.

4. Biological Characteristics of the Organism

Y. enterocolitica has been called a "cold-adapted" pathogen. It is able to multiply at temperatures approaching 0°C, a characteristic that allows it to grow in properly refrigerated foods.[25] This biological growth property provides *Y. enterocolitica* with a competitive advantage over other bacteria for propagation in environmental reservoirs. Several investigations have documented the growth of *Y. enterocolitica* on raw and cooked meat and in milk at low temperatures.[25] However, some results indicate that *Y. enterocolitica* competes poorly with other psychotrophic organisms normally present in foods.[42,43] *Y. enterocolitica* can survive in frozen foods for long periods.[25,26]

Human pathogenic strains of *Y. enterocolitica* are endowed with a number of bacterial properties that confer virulence to the organism. Several of these exhibit a marked temperature-dependent expression and have been shown to be mediated by a 40- 50-MD plasmid.[44–47] Closely related plasmids are also found in *Y. pseudotuberculosis* and *Y. pestis*. The plasmid encodes a series of proteins, several of which have been shown to be important virulence factors. One group of proteins, designated Yops, are expressed *in vitro* only at elevated growth temperatures of 35–37°C in media with a low level of calcium ions. Their contribution to pathogenicity is associated with their delivery into the host cell to subvert or modulate normal host cell signal transduction and cytoskeletal functions.[46] Another plasmid-encoded, temperature-regulated protein, YadA (previously termed Yop1), is produced irrespective of calcium concentration. This true outer membrane protein forms a fibrillar matrix on the bacterial surface and mediates cellular attachment and entry.[46] It also confers resistance to the bactericidal effect of normal human serum and inhibition of the anti-invasive effect of interferon.

Elements encoded by the chromosome are also necessary for maximal virulence. The pathogenic yersiniae share at least two chromosomal loci, *inv* and *ail*, that play a role in their entry into eukaryotic cells.[47] The *inv* and *ail* gene products can be classified as adhesins, since they mediate adherence to the eukaryotic surface. Unlike other previously characterized bacterial adhesins, they also mediate entry into a variety of mammalian cells.

A number of different *in vitro* and *in vivo* assays have been proposed for differentiation of pathogenic and nonpathogenic variants.[26,44,45] Such virulence tests include autoagglutination at 37°C, calcium-dependent growth restriction at 37°C, resistance to the bactericidal activity of normal human serum, various animal and cell culture models, binding of Congo red dye, use of DNA probes, and biochemical parameters. Autoagglutination and calcium-dependent growth have been the most widely used *in vitro* tests, though no single property appears to be an absolutely reliable indicator of the pathogenic potential. The revised biotyping scheme proposed by Wauters *et al.*[30] comprises a test for pyrazinamidase activity. There is a striking correlation between potential pathogenicity and lack of pyrazinamidase activity, independent of the occurrence of the virulence plasmid.

Another chromosomally encoded factor is production of enterotoxin after cultivation *in vitro*.[26,48] Many strains of *Y. enterocolitica* and related species produce heat-stable enterotoxin (Yst) when the bacteria are cultured at 20–30°C. Certain strains, especially within the species *Y. kristensensii*, are also able to produce Yst at 4 and 37°C. The physicochemical, biological, antigenic, and genetic characteristics of Yst resemble those of the heat-stable enterotoxin of *E. coli*. The observation that pathogenic strain of *Y. enterocolitica* only produce Yst at temperatures below 30°C argues against the potential involvement of Yst in the pathogenesis of yersiniosis. However, recent results showing that Yst production can be induced at 37°C by increasing the osmolality and pH to the levels normally found in the ileal lumen support the role of Yst as a virulence factor.[49] It is also possible that enterotoxigenic strains may produce foodborne intoxication by means of preformed enterotoxins.[48] This assumption is based on the fact that Yst is able to resist gastric acidity as well as temperatures used in food processing and storage, without losing activity.

One final intriguing features of *Y. enterocolitica* relates to its iron dependency. Unlike most other aerobic bacteria, *Y. enterocolitica* fails to produce iron-binding compounds, or siderophores, and utilizes siderophores produced by other bacteria as well as exogenous siderophores such as therapeutic iron chelators. They are also able to use hemin as a source of iron, as demonstrated by Perry and Brubaker.[50] This property may explain the apparent increased susceptibility of patients with conditions of iron excess to yersiniosis. While there have been many speculations regarding the role of iron in enhancing *Y. enterocolitica* infections, the precise mechanism remains to be elucidated.

Y. enterocolitica have been shown to be susceptible *in vitro* to aminoglycosides, chloramphenicol, tetracycline, trimethorpim–sulfamethoxazole, and third-generation cephalosporin antibiotics.[1,6,51,52] Isolates are frequently resistant to penicillin, ampicillin, and first-generation cephalosporins due to the elaboration of a β-lactamase.[53] Intestinal infection with *Y. enterocolitica* is usually self-limited and infrequently treated. Thus, information regarding the importance of antibiotic resistance in the spread of disease is not available.

5. Descriptive Epidemiology

5.1. Prevalence and Incidence

The incidence of *Y. enterocolitica* infection in patients with acute endemic enterocolitis ranges from 0 to 4%, depending on the geographic location, study method, and population (Table 1).[37,54–76] In some countries, *Y. enterocolitica* has surpassed *Shigella* and rivals *Salmonella* and *Campylobacter* as a cause of acute bacterial gastroenteritis.[6] Laboratory-based surveillance data from several countries show significant changes over the last two decades. There appears to have been a real and generalized increase in incidence.[5] Agner *et al.*[23] tested sera from Danish adults and found that the prevalence of elevated antibody titers against *Y. enterocolitica* O:3 had increased from 1% in 1967 to 7.7% in 1978. In Finland, Leino[77] showed that elevated agglutinin titers against *Y. enterocolitica* O:3 or O:9 or against *Y. pseudotuberculosis* IA occurred in 6.1% of sera tested. Using an enzyme-linked immunosorbent assay, Sæbø *et al.*[78] detected IgG to serogroup O:3 in sera from 7.4% of 755 Norwegian military recruits. This suggests that yersiniosis is common and widespread among Scandinavians. Several studies of patients with the appendicitislike syndrome have found *Y. enterocolitica* in up to 9% of patients (Table 2).[21,33,54,55,71,79–85] In a report of 581 persons who underwent appendectomy for presumed appendicitis over a 1-year period in Sweden, Niléhn and Sjöström[83] found 22 cases (3.8%) with bacte-

Table 1. Isolation of *Yersinia enterocolitica* from Sporadic Cases of Acute Diarrhea

Author(s)	Reference	Year published	Location	Population	No. studied	Percentage with *Y. enterocolitica*
Van Noyen *et al.*	54	1987	Belgium	All ages	10,838	2.5
Van Noyen *et al.*	55	1979	Belgium	All ages	11,480	1.1
Bucci *et al.*	56	1991	Italy	All ages	5,032	0.6
Mingrone *et al.*	57	1987	Italy	Children	2,500	1.4
Figua and Rossolini	58	1985	Italy	Children[a]	188	3.7
Hoogkamp-Korstanje *et al.*	59	1986	The Netherlands	< 40 yr	827	2.9
Lassen and Kapperud	60	1984	Norway	All ages	7,700	1.0
Ferrer *et al.*	61	1987	Spain	All ages	5,199	0.8
Velasco *et al.*	62	1984	Spain	Children[a]	6,970	0.2
Persson *et al.*	63	1982	Sweden	Children[a]	95	2.0
Marks *et al.*	37	1980	Canada	Children[a]	6,364	2.8
Metchock *et al.*	64	1991	USA	All ages	7,290	1.0
Lee *et al.*	65	1991	USA	All ages	4,841	0.8
Marriott	66	1987	Australia	All ages	6,351	0.9
McCarthy and Fenwick	67	1990	New Zealand	All ages	38,453	0.5
Maruyama	68	1987	Japan	Adults[a]	8,849	0.5
Maruyama	68	1987	Japan	Children[a]	17,966	0.9
Fukushima *et al.*	69	1987	Japan	All ages	9,820	1.8
Carniel *et al.*	70	1986	Bangladesh	Children	1,450	0.07
Samadi *et al.*	71	1982	Bangladesh	All ages	113	0
Poocharoen *et al.*	72	1986	Thailand	Children[a]	208	0
Agbonlahor *et al.*	73	1983	Nigeria	All ages	1,082	1.3
de Mol *et al.*	74	1983	Zaire	Children	84	0
Haghighi	75	1979	Iran	All ages	1,220	0.08
Morris *et al.*	76	1991	Chile	0–4 yr	471	1.1

[a]Hospitalized patients.

Table 2. Isolation of *Yersinia enterocolitica* from Patients with Appendicitis like Syndrome

Author(s)	Reference	Year published	Location	No. studied	Percentage with *Y. enterocolitica*
Van Noyen *et al.*	55	1979	Belgium	1,201	1.3
Van Noyen *et al.*	54	1987	Belgium	1,004	3.8
Jepsen *et al.*	79	1976	Denmark	205	5.4
Ahvonen *et al.*	80	1972	Finland	244	9.0
Megraud	81	1987	France	600	3.0
Attwood *et al.*	33	1987	Ireland	90	3.0
Franzin *et al.*	82	1991	Italy	60	5.0
Niléhn and Sjöström	83	1967	Sweden	581	3.8
Pai *et al.*	84	1982	Canada	363	1.4
Kanazawa *et al.*	85	1991	Japan	637	4.4
Samadi *et al.*	71	1982	Bangladesh	30	0
Butler *et al.*	21	1984	Bangladesh	31	3.0

riological evidence of *Y. enterocolitica* infection. Of those found to have regional terminal ileitis at surgery, 80% were infected with *Y. enterocolitica*, 13% of those with mesenteric adenitis, and 0.5% of those with acute appendicitis.

Although sometimes present in asymptomatic individuals, several large surveys have found carriage rates of less than 1% in asymptomatic controls.(37,63,74)

5.2. Epidemic Behavior and Contagiousness

A number of outbreaks of yersiniosis in communities, families, and hospitals have served to emphasize the capacity of *Y. enterocolitica* to cause widespread disease (Table 3).(67,86–100) While few outbreaks of enteritis due to *Y. enterocolitica* have been reported in Europe, several major outbreaks have been described in the United States. The first of these occurred in 1972, in rural North Carolina, where 16 of 21 individuals from four families were affected.(93) The outbreak resulted in two exploratory laparotomies and two of the afflicted individuals died, one following surgery. Although the source was not culturally confirmed, five of nine newborn puppies died with diarrheal illness during the week prior to the first human illness. A serogroup O:8 *Y. enterocolitica* was isolated from the human cases of enteritis.

A variety of foods have been implicated as vehicles of transmission in outbreaks of *Y. enterocolitica* infection. Several such outbreaks involved the distribution of contaminated milk, which probably became infected subsequent to the pasteurization process. The first of these occurred in 1976, in upstate New York.(92) Illness occurred in 222 school children and employees, 38 of whom had documented *Y. enterocolitica* serogroup O:8 infection; 36 individuals were hospitalized and 16 appendectomies were performed. Illness was found to be associated with the consumption of chocolate milk purchased in the school cafeteria. *Y. enterocolitica* was subsequently isolated from a carton of chocolate milk.

In 1982, a multistate outbreak of serogroup O:13 and O:18 caused illness in at least 172 persons; 17 individuals underwent appendectomy and 24 cases of extraintestinal disease were documented.(90) Illness was associated with drinking pasteurized milk from a Memphis, Tennessee plant, but samples from the incriminated lots of milk were not available for culture. A survey revealed that 8.3% of those who drank the milk became ill; the attack rate was 22.2% in children 0–4 years old and 38.5% in children 5–9 years old. In a third outbreak, 53% of persons at a camp experienced illness and the investigation showed that illness was associated with consumption of reconstituted powdered milk and/or chow mein.(89) The organism appeared to have been introduced by a food handler during preparation.

Epidemiological investigations have demonstrated that some products incriminated in foodborne outbreaks may become contaminated during processing with infected environmental water sources. An outbreak of 44 *Y. enterocolitica* infections occurred in Washington between December 1981 and February 1982.(98) Disease was associated with the ingestion of contaminated tofu (soybean curd) and *Y. enterocolitica* serogroup O:8 was isolated from afflicted individuals. Culture of the tofu, as well as the untreated spring water used in the tofu manufacturing plant, yielded the same serogroup, O:8. A second outbreak involved 16 of 33 (48%) members of a Brownie troop who

Table 3. Outbreaks due to *Yersinia enterocolitica*

Author(s)	Reference	Year published	Location	No. ill	At risk	Mode of transmission/ vehicle	Serogroup
Lee *et al.*	86	1990	Georgia (infants and children)	15		Preparation of chitterlings	O:3
Kondracki and Gallo	87	1987	New York (infants)	4	4	Unknown	O:3
Tacket *et al.*	88	1985	Washington	44		Tofu contaminated by water	O:8
Morse *et al.*	89	1984	New York State (summer camp)	239	455	Powdered milk or chow mein	O:8
Tacket *et al.*	90	1984	Tennessee, Arkansas, Mississippi	>172		Pasteurized milk	O:13,18
Aber *et al.*	91	1982	Pennsylvania (Brownie troop)	16	33	Bean sprouts contaminated by water	—
Black *et al.*	92	1978	New York (school)	222	2,193	Chocolate milk	O:8
Gutman *et al.*	93	1973	North Carolina (family)	16	21	Sick puppies	O:8
Ratnam *et al.*	94	1982	Canada (hospital)	9		Nosocomial	O:5
Martin *et al.*	95	1982	Canada (family)	3	4	River water?	O:21
Greenwood *et al.*	96	1990	United Kingdom (hospital)	36		Pasteurized milk	O:10, O:6,30
Toivanen *et al.*	97	1973	Finland (hospital)	6		Nosocomial	O:9
Olsovsky *et al.*	98	1975	Czechoslovakia (nursery schools)	75	142	Unknown	—
Zen-Yoji *et al.*	99	1973	Japan (school)	198	1,086	Unknown	O:3, O:5
Asakawa *et al.*	100	1973	Japan (community)	189	441	Unknown	O:3
Maruyama	68	1987	Japan (school)	102	902	Unknown	O:3
Maruyama	68	1987	Japan (school)	641	1,812	Unknown	O:3
Maruyama	68	1987	Japan (school)	1,051	8,835	Milk	O:3
Maruyama	68	1987	Japan (school)	184	954	Unknown	O:3
Maruyama	68	1987	Japan (institution)	6	92	Unknown	O:3
Maruyama	68	1987	Japan (school)	145	486	Unknown	O:3
Maruyama	68	1987	Japan (school)	296	814	Unknown	O:3

were infected following the ingestion of bean sprouts that had been grown in refrigerated water from a well that was shown to be contaminated with *Y. enterocolitica*[91]; 15 of the children manifested gastrointestinal symptoms an average of 6 days following exposure and three underwent appendectomy.

Only one outbreak has been reported in the United States since 1987; this was the only one related to pork, and it was caused by serogroup O:3 biovar 4.[86] A case–control study showed that preparation of pork intestines, known as chitterlings, was associated with illness.

While a number of additional well-defined outbreaks of yersiniosis have been reported, isolation of *Y. enterocolitica* from implicated vehicles is unusual. In Japan, epidemic *Y. enterocolitica* enteritis has been described in both communities and schools.[68,99,100] One such outbreak occurred in 1972 in a Japanese junior high school where acute abdominal pain and fever were present in 198 of 1086 pupils.[99] *Y. enterocolitica* serogroup O:3 was isolated from the fecal specimens of the majority of ill children; however, a single source of contaminated food or water was not identified.

5.3. Geographic Distribution

Y. enterocolitica has been isolated from humans in many countries of the world, but it seems to be found most frequently in cooler climates.[3,5] This distribution may reflect differences in reservoirs and culinary practices, or it may simply be a consequence of more intensive surveillance and appropriate culturing techniques in these areas.[6] Relatively few cases have been reported from tropical areas. It has been suggested that the tropical climate may not favor propagation of the organism. The infrequent occurrence of *Y. enterocolitica* in some areas of the world may be due in part to avoidance of certain environmental risk factors, such as eating pork in Muslim countries.

There are appreciable geographic differences in the distribution of the different phenotypes of *Y. enterocolitica* isolated in man.[3] Serogroup O:3 biovar 4 is the most widespread in Europe, Japan, Canada, Africa, and Latin America. Phage typing makes it possible to distinguish between European, Canadian, and Japanese strains.[3] Serogroup O:9 biovar 2 is the second most common in Europe, but its distribution is uneven; while it accounts for a high percentage of the strains isolated in France, Belgium, and the Netherlands, only a few strains have been isolated in Scandinavia.[5] The relative proportion of O:9 strains seems to have been increasing in Belgium and France. Until recently, the most frequently reported serogroups in the United States were O:8 followed by O:5,27.[3] In recent years, serogroup O:3 has been on the increase in the United States; O:3 now accounts for the majority of sporadic *Y. enterocolitica* isolates referred to public health laboratories in California,[101] and was responsible for an outbreak of gastroenteritis in infants in Georgia.[86] This suggests that the epidemiology of yersiniosis in the United States has evolved into a pattern similar to the picture in Europe, where foodborne *Y. enterocolitica* outbreaks are rare and serogroup O:3 predominates.[102] In Canada, O:3 dominates in Ontario, Quebec, and the four eastern provinces, whereas in the western provinces O:8 and O:5,27 prevail.

5.4. Temporal Distribution

A clustering of cases during the fall and winter months has been reported in some European countries.[5,11] In certain countries, the seasonality of human illness also has been correlated with the isolation of *Y. enterocolitica* from domestic swine. The association of *Y. enterocolitica* with cooler seasons and temperate climates has been linked to the organism's ability to multiply at low temperatures (see Section 4). In the United States, there are no clear seasonal patterns of disease due to *Y. enterocolitica*, although a summer peak has been suggested in a study in Wisconsin.[103]

5.5. Age

Although *Y. enterocolitica* causes a number of clinical syndromes that vary with the age, sex, and health of the host, children appear to be preferentially affected.[88,89,92,104] Of 359 infected patients reported by Mollaret,[11] 47% were between 1 and 5 years of age. Vandepitte and Wauters[105] reported 1711 cases of *Y. enterocolitica* infection occurring in persons less than 1 month to 85 years old; approximately 20% of all cases occurred within the first year of life. Nearly 80% of patients were less than 10 years old. It is notable that in a foodborne outbreak, 43% of children who ate the incriminated food developed yersiniosis and had a positive culture, compared with 14% of adults who ate the food (33% were culture positive).[88] Likewise, in milk-borne outbreaks, children had the highest attack rates.[92]

The illness most commonly associated with *Y. enterocolitica* in children less than 5 years old is a mild diarrheal illness, indistinguishable from that caused by other enteric pathogens (see Section 8.1). Children over 5 years old are more likely to develop symptoms that mimic those of acute appendicitis. A dramatic difference in age-specific incidence was noted when patients with enteritis were compared with those with the appendicitislike syndrome.[106] While 80% of all patients with enteritis were less than 5 years old, those with a pseudoappendicitis syndrome were most frequently older children and adults. Most extraintestinal manifestations of *Y. enterocolitica* infection, including the postinfectious sequelae, are more frequently found in adults than in children. In hospital outbreaks, it has been noted that the old and the very young were more often infected and may be predisposed by age and physical condition including immune status.[94]

5.6. Sex

In most studies, males have slightly outnumbered females in all age groups of patients with *Y. enterocolitica* diarrhea; however, the sexes were equally affected in outbreaks of mesenteric adenitis. Erythema nodosum is seen more commonly in females.

5.7. Occupation

The organism has been found frequently in samples from swine in slaughterhouses, where it may readily be transferred to employees at all stages during slaughtering and processing (see Section 6). Seroepidemiological studies have indicated that occupational exposure to pigs is a risk factor.[107,108]

5.8. Occurrence in Different Settings

Y. enterocolitica among hospital populations exhibits both sporadic and outbreak forms of infection (Table 3). The first nosocomial outbreak of *Y. enterocolitica* was reported from Finland in 1973 and involved six hospital employees who became ill approximately 10 days after a schoolgirl with *Y. enterocolitica* enteritis was admitted to their hospital. Spread of the infection, in this and other hospital outbreaks, appeared to be from the index patient to the staff and subsequently from person to person.[97] Outbreaks have been reported among children attending institutions for collective care in eastern Europe, and it is presumed that similar outbreaks are possible in day-care settings with poor hygiene.[98] As mentioned previously, outbreaks have occurred in schools (Table 3).

5.9. Socioeconomic Factors

There is little published information suggesting that socioeconomic factors affect the occurrence of *Y. enterocolitica* infection.

6. Mechanisms and Routes of Transmission

Y. enterocolitica is frequently encountered in healthy carriers among warm-blooded and cold-blooded animals, in foods, including both meat and milk products and vegetables, and in the environment, including water and soil. However, the vast majority of the strains isolated from these sources are avirulent variants.(3) Dogs, cats, and rats may occasionally be fecal carriers of serogroups O:3 and O:9,(109) and apparent transmission from dogs and cats to humans has been reported.

Although the bacterium has been isolated from nearly all of the vertebrate species examined without any evidence of disease, the pig is the only animal consumed by man that regularly harbors pathogenic *Y. enterocolitica*. There is strong indirect evidence that the swine constitutes an important reservoir for human infection with *Y. enterocolitica*.(26,48,109–111) Numerous surveys have shown that swine are healthy carriers of O:3 and O:9. In addition to being fecal commensals, these serogroups inhabit the oral cavity of swine, especially the tongue and tonsils. The bacteria are also frequently encountered as a surface contaminant on freshly slaughtered pig carcasses. Some studies have indicated that *Y. enterocolitica* is more common in pork products than previously documented.(48) It has not been possible to demonstrate any phenotypic or genotypic difference between human and porcine isolates.(32)

Epidemiological studies of endemic yersiniosis have supported the role of pork as a vehicle for *Y. enterocolitica* infection. In Belgium, a case–control study showed that infection caused by O:3 and O:9 was strongly associated with eating raw pork.(110) Likewise, a case–control study conducted in Norway identified consumption of pork products as an important risk factor for this infection.(111) Following an outbreak of infection due to serogroup O:3 among children in Atlanta, Georgia, a case–control study showed that preparation of raw pork intestines (chitterlings) in the 2 weeks before onset was significantly associated with illness.(86)

In contrast to O:3 and O:9, serogroup O:8 appears to be rare in swine. O:8 may have entirely different reservoir(s) and ecology.(26) Outbreaks and sporadic cases due to this serogroup have been traced to ingestion of contaminated water, water used in manufacturing or preparation of food (bean sprouts, tofu), and milk products (Table 3). Small rodents have been incriminated as a possible source of infection with O:8 in Japan.(112a) Consumption of untreated water was also identified as a risk factor for infection with serogroup O:3 in a case–control study and in a seroepidemiological study in Norway.(78,111)

Fecal–oral transmission from person to person has not been convincingly documented, but reports of nosocomial infections and intrafamiliar clusters of cases with sequential onset of illness suggest that it may occur.(6) Evidence for transmission to household contacts has been conflicting. In one milk-borne outbreak, transmission by school children to household contacts could not be documented.(92) Likewise, person-to-person transmission was thought not to occur in large school outbreaks in Japan.(68,99) However, in a prospective study of *Y. enterocolitica*-related gastroenteritis in Canada, spread to others in the family occurred in 47% of the cases.(37) Although pharyngeal infection is not uncommon in yersiniosis, respiratory transmission is unlikely.

7. Pathogenesis and Immunity

Human infection due to *Y. enterocolitica* is acquired predominantly by the oral route. The minimal infectious dose required to cause disease in humans in unknown. In one volunteer, ingestion of 3.5×10^9 organisms was sufficient to product illness.(106) The incubation period is uncertain; however, it has been estimated to be 2 to 11 days, based on two outbreaks in which personnel became ill after the hospital admission of patients with *Y. enterocolitica*.(94,106) An outbreak in a Brownie troop was reported to have a mean incubation period of 6 days,(91) while in a foodborne outbreak the median was 4 days (range, 1–9 days) following ingestion of the incriminated food.(88)

Enteric infection leads to proliferation of *Y. enterocolitica* in the lumen of the bowel and in the lymphoid tissue of the intestine. Adherence to and penetration into the epithelial cells of the intestinal mucosa are essential factors in the pathogenesis of *Y. enterocolitica* infection.(44–47) After ingestion of a contaminated food item, the bacteria are transferred to the terminal ileum where they adhere to and penetrate the mucous layer and subsequently adhere to the luminal membrane of the enterocytes. Penetration through the enterocyte involves endocytosis, translocation, and egestion. The bacteria show tropism for the lymphoid tissue and multiplies in the Peyer's patches and mesenteric lymph follicles where they cause a massive inflammatory response. In a normal self-limited infection, the bacteria are then gradually eliminated.

The findings in patients with terminal ileitis at surgery are quite unique to *Y. enterocolitica* infection and include extensive mesenteric adenopathy with matted lymph nodes. Cellular infiltrates include lymphoid hyperplasia, epithelioid granulomas, and necrotic suppurative lesions in which the gram-negative organisms are easily demonstrated. Hematogenous dissemination from the gastrointestinal tract is transmitted through the portal system to produce metastatic lesions throughout the body.

Syndromes of inflammatory arthritis and erythema nodosum appear to be delayed immunologic sequelae of the original intestinal infection.

Human infection with pathogenic strains of *Y. enterocolitica* stimulates development of specific antibodies. It is not known whether specific serum antibody protects against reinfection with *Y. enterocolitica* organisms of the same or different serogroups. Although there is considerable evidence that both natural and experimental infection can confer some degree of immunity, the precise extent and duration of such immunity remain to be determined. Patients with *Y. enterocolitica*-induced reactive arthritis show a chronically elevated IgA level to a series of virulence-associated, plasmid-encoded proteins (Yops) that are produced by the bacterium.[40,41] The elevated IgA level is correlated with the finding of virulent, persistent *Y. enterocolitica*, which can be detected in intestinal biopsies by immunofluorescence.[40]

8. Patterns of Host Response

8.1. Clinical Features

Y. enterocolitica is associated with a spectrum of clinical syndromes in man.[1,3,6] The protean clinical manifestations produced by *Y. enterocolitica* vary with different serogroups of the organism and with host factors.[1] Several organ systems may be involved with *Y. enterocolitica* infection, by direct or immunologically mediated mechanisms, and the clinical manifestations frequently mimic those of other diseases. Patients may present with enterocolitis, nesenteric adenitis, terminal ileitis, reactive oligoarthritis, erythema nodosum, exudative pharyngitis, or septicemia and coincident complications. Metastatic foci present as osteomyelitis, meningitis, and pulmonary and intra-abdominal abscesses. Other less frequently reported symptoms include carditis, ophthalmitis, glomerulonephritis, hepatitis, pancreatitis, and hemolytic anemia.

Acute, noncomplicated enteritis is by far the most frequently encountered manifestation and affects primarily young children less than 7 years old and infants. Symptoms of *Y. enterocolitica* enteritis typically persist for 1 to 3 weeks, but they occasionally may last for several months.

The syndromes of mesenteric adenitis, terminal ileitis, or both occur in older children more than 5 years old and in adults (see Section 5.5). In these patients, diarrhea is infrequent; findings of fever, right lower-quadrant pain, and leukocytosis often mimic those of acute appendicitis. The pseudoappendicular syndrome has been reported in 3–15% of cases (see Section 5.1). While most cases are probably self-limited, severe intestinal disease, small-bowel gangrene, and death have been reported.

A variety of extraintestinal manifestations may accompany enteric infection with *Y. enterocolitica*. Since intestinal symptoms may be mild or asymptomatic, many patients present with syndromes that mimic a host of other nonenteric diseases, and thus present a diagnostic challenge to the physician. The most common extraintestinal form of *Y. enterocolitica* infection is "reactive" arthritis. An oligoarticular nonsuppurative arthritis has been reported most frequently in persons of northern European descent. In Scandinavia, 10–30% of adults with *Y. enterocolitica* infection develop inflammation of the knees, wrists, or ankles a few days to 1 month after the onset of diarrhea.[112] Synovial fluid cultures are generally negative. Symptoms usually persist for 1–6 months but may become chronic in some patients.[113] Some of these patients also present with other symptoms of yersiniosis, including chronic abdominal pain with periods of recurrent diarrhea.[40] Aho *et al.*[114] have demonstrated a predilection of individuals with the HLA B27 antigen for developing arthritis as a complication of *Y. enterocolitica* infection. Reiter's syndrome (conjunctivitis, urethritis, arthritis) and ankylosing spondylitis have also been described in individuals with the HLA B27 antigen following *Y. enterocolitica* infection.[115,116] *Y. enterocolitica* infection may present with a syndrome indistinguishable from that of acute rheumatic fever.[107]

Erythema nodosum occurs in up to 30% of Scandinavian cases, most of whom are females.[80] In the majority of cases, erythema nodosum resolves spontaneously within a month. The causative agents of reactive arthritis and erythema nodosum belong to serogroups O:3 or O:9. These manifestations have been virtually absent in the United States, an observation that has been related to the geographic distribution of serogroups. However, an increase in cases with postinfectious manifestations of yersiniosis would not be unexpected, parallel to the emergence of serogroup O:3 in this country (see Section 5.3).

Septicemia due to *Y. enterocolitica* is seen almost exclusively in individuals with underlying disease.[1] Those with cirrhosis and disorders of iron excess are particularly predisposed to infection and increased mortality.

Transient carriage and excretion of both pathogenic and nonpathogenic *Y. enterocolitica* may occur following exposure to the bacterium. High rates of asymptomatic carriage have been reported in connection with outbreaks.[88] However, inapparent infection with *Y. enterocolitica* was detected in less than 1% of individuals in large surveys.[83] In patients with *Y. enterocolitica* enteritis, the organism may be excreted in the stools for a long time period after symptoms have resolved. In a study of Norwegian patients, convalescent carriage of *Y. enterocolitica* O:3 was detected in 47% of 57 patients.[117] In these persons, the organism was carried for a median of 40 days (range, 17–116 days). In addition to the potential for fecal–oral transmission by asymptomatic shedders, these persons may play a role in transfusion-related *Y. enterocolitica* septicemia. *Y. enterocolitica* present during transient bacteremia may multiply in blood products stored at 4°C and produce septic shock upon transfusion. Several such cases have been reported in the literature.[118–120]

8.2. Diagnosis

The diagnosis of *Y. enterocolitica* infection requires a heightened awareness of the great diversity of clinical syndromes and the need for routine employment of isolation techniques that favor recovery of the bacterium. Depending on the clinical syndrome, *Y. enterocolitica* can be easily isolated from otherwise sterile sites. The diagnosis of *Y. enterocolitica* enterocolitis is made by stool culture (see Section 3.4.1). Enterocolitis caused by *Y. enterocolitica* cannot easily be differentiated from infections due to other enteric pathogens by means of clinical manifestations.[1,6,117] The differential diagnosis includes viral gastroenteritis and other enteric bacterial infections. However, *Y. enterocolitica* infection can present with distinguishing features that suggest the diagnosis. The sore throat noted by some patients is a unique feature of yersiniosis that probably reflects the predilection of the organism for lymphatic tissues. The diagnosis should also be considered when joint pains or erythema nodosum appear in persons with previous diarrheal illness, or when such symptoms occur together with complaints of recurrent diarrhea or abdominal pain.

Serological diagnosis may be useful in determining the role of *Y. enterocolitica* in postinfectious syndromes and other late manifestations (see Section 3.4.2). There are several limitations associated with serodiagnosis, including the existence of cross-reactions with other bacterial species and the prevalence of seropositive individuals in the healthy population. Demonstration of specific circulating IgA to the plasmid-encoded proteins (Yops) by immunoblots is a highly specific means to demonstrate previous *Yersinia* infection.[40,41]

A recent history of consumption of undercooked pork, drinking untreated water, or contact with pigs may suggest the diagnosis of yersiniosis (see Section 6).

9. Control and Prevention

9.1. General Concepts

Preventive measures that reduce contamination and improve hygiene during all stages of pig and pork processing are essential to reduce infection with serogroups O:3 and O:9. The organism may be difficult to control efficiently at the farm level. Since swine are healthy carriers of *Y. enterocolitica*, its detection during the routine meat inspection is considered practically impossible. During commercial slaughtering and processing, bacteria from the oral cavity or intestinal contents may easily contaminate the carcasses and the environment in the slaughterhouse. Improved hygiene at critical control points should be attempted.[4,48] Special attention should be paid during: (1) circumanal incision and removal of the intestines; (2) excision of the tongue, pharynx, and particularly the tonsils; (3) postmortem meat inspection procedures that involve incision of the mandibular lymph nodes; and (4) deboning of head meat. Changes in slaughtering procedures, including technological improvements, may be required to reduce contamination during these activities.[4]

Preventive and control measures should also focus on information of all categories of people involved in production, procession, and final preparation of food about the importance of good hygienic practices. Strict hygiene is particularly necessary because *Y. enterocolitica* is able to propagate at temperatures approaching 0°C (Section 4). Therefore, chilling of food products should not be considered to be an effective control measure for this microbe. Consumption of undercooked pork should be discouraged.

Precautions for prevention of fecal–oral spread of the pathogens should be observed. Handwashing and proper stool disposal must be employed in household, day-care, and hospital settings. Furthermore, food handlers should maintain strict personal hygiene and should not work when ill. Furthermore, the incrimination of specific foods in transmission emphasizes the need to adhere to preventive measures such as pasteurization of milk and avoidance of recontamination and cross-contamination after treatment. Avoidance of contact with excreta from pigs or domestic pets may reduce transmission.

Although *Y. enterocolitica* isolated from water are not usually among the types pathogenic for humans, a potential risk of transmission through water is present. Therefore, because *Y. enterocolitica* is sensitive to chlorination, proper treatment of drinking water should eliminate the risk of infection from this source.

9.2. Antibiotic and Chemotherapeutic Approaches to Prophylaxis

Antibiotic or chemotherapeutic approaches to prophylaxis are not indicated.

9.3. Immunization

Vaccines against *Y. enterocolitica* infections have not been developed.

10. Unresolved Problems

Despite an improved understanding of the biological properties of the organism and its unique geographic and environmental distribution, a multitude of questions about the ecology, epidemiology, and pathogenicity of *Y. enterocolitica* remain unanswered.

Our understanding of the epidemiology of yersiniosis is still incomplete. The importance of *Y. enterocolitica* as the cause of a number of clinical syndromes is unknown in many areas of the world. Standardized disease surveillance is needed within and across national boundaries so that data from each location are comparable. Improved screening of stools and other specimens for *Y. enterocolitica* is necessary, particularly in the United States, to help better define the epidemiology of the disease. The development of standardized and approved isolation methods, which allow optimal recovery of all pathogenic serogroups and which provide adequate differentiation between pathogenic and nonpathogenic variants, is required.

Although considerable progress has been made in our understanding of the routes of transmission and reservoirs for *Y. enterocolitica*, well-designed epidemiological investigations, particularly case–control studies, are needed to identify risk factors and determine their relative importance in terms of prevention. Intervention studies are required to assess the efficacy of specific and nonspecific control and preventive measures to reduce colonization on the farm, contamination at the slaughterhouse, growth during storage, and spread within the kitchen. Molecular epidemiological subtyping methods that allow better differentiation of the species, particularly serogroup O:3, are needed to assist in epidemiological tracing.

Great strides have been made in our understanding at the molecular level of the mechanisms by which *Y. enterocolitica* causes disease. However, further clarification of the role of the virulence determinants is needed. One recently explored avenue of investigation relates to the shared plasmid and virulence properties among the three species of *Yersinia* and serves to highlight global questions such as: Why do *Yersinia* invade host tissues? What accounts for their distinctive lymphoid tissue tropism? By what mechanism are they able to evade the immune response of the host? In addition, several clinical puzzles of human yersiniosis need to be unraveled, such as the role of iron in enhancing disease, the relationship of *Y. enterocolitica* to the immune system in the creation of a diversity of autoimmune phenomena, and the nature, efficacy, and duration of immunity.

11. References

1. Bottone, E. J., *Yersinia enterocolitica*: A panoramic view of a charismatic microorganism, *Crit. Rev. Microbiol.* **5**:211–241 (1977).
2. Kapperud, G., and Bergan, T., Biochemical and serological characterization of *Yersinia enterocolitica*, in: *Methods in Microbiology*, Vol. 15 (T. Bergan and Norris, Jr., eds.), pp. 295–344, Academic Press, London, 1984.
3. Mollaret, H. H., Bercovier, H., and Alonso, J. M., Summary of the data received at the WHO Reference Center for *Yersinia enterocolitica*, *Contrib. Microbiol. Immunol.* **5**:174–184 (1979).
4. Kapperud, G., *Yersinia enterocolitica* infection, in: *Handbook of Zoonoses*, 2nd ed., Sect. A: *Bacterial, Rickettsial, Chlamydial, and Mycotic* (G. W. Beran and J. H. Steele, eds.), pp. 343–353, CRC Press, Boca Raton, FL, 1994.
5. World Health Organization, *Yersiniosis—Report on a WHO Meeting, Paris, 1981*, EURO Reports and Studies 60, WHO Regional Office for Europe, Copenhagen, 1983.
6. Cover, T. L., and Aber, R. C., *Yersinia enterocolitica*, *N. Engl. J. Med.* **321**:16–24 (1989).
7. Gilbert, R., *Interesting Cases and Unusual Specimens*, Annual Report of the Division of Laboratories and Research, New York State Department of Health, Albany, 1933.
8. Schleifstein, J., and Coleman, M. B., *Bacterium enterocoliticum*, Annual Report of the Division of Laboratories and Research, New York State Department of Health, Albany, 1943.

8a. Schleifstein, J., and Coleman, M. B., An unidentified microorganism resembling *B. lignieri* and *Past. pseudotuberculosis* and pathogenic for man, *N. Y. State J. Med.* **39**:1749–1753 (1939).

9. Knapp, W., and Thal, E., Untersuchungen über die kulturell-biochemischen, serologischen, tierexperimentellen und immunologischen Eigenschaften einer vorläufig "*Pasteurella X*" benannten Bakterienart, *Zentralbl. Bakteriol. Orig. A* **190:**472–484 (1963).
10. Frederiksen, W., A study of some *Yersinia pseudotuberculosis*-like bacteria ("*Bacterium enterocoliticum*" and "*Pasteurella X*," in: *Proceedings of the XIV Scandinavian Congress of Pathology and Microbiology*, pp. 103–104, Oslo, 1964.
11. Mollaret, H. H., L'infection humaine à *Yersinia enterocolitica* en 1970 à la luminère de 642 cas récents, *Pathol. Biol.* **19:**189–205 (1971).
12. Niléhn, B., Studies on *Yersinia enterocolitica* with special reference to bacterial diagnosis and occurrence in human acute enteric disease, *Acta Pathol. Microbiol. Scand. Suppl.* **206:**1–48 (1969).
13. Wauters, G., *Contribution à l'Étude de Yersinia enterocolitica* (Thesis), Vander, Louvain, Belgium, 1970.
14. Wauters, G., Antigens of *Yersinia enterocolitica*, in: *Yersinia enterocolitica* (E. J. Bottone, Ed.), pp. 41–53, CRC Press, Boca Raton, FL, 1981.
15. Winblad, S., Studies on serological typing of *Yersinia enterocolitica*, *Acta Pathol. Microbiol. Scand. Suppl.* **187:**1–115 (1967).
16. Knapp, W., and Thal, E., Differentiation of *Yersinia enterocolitica* by biochemical reactions, *Contrib. Microbiol. Immunol.* **2:**10–16 (1973).
17. Brenner, D. J., Ursing, J., Bercovier, H., *et al.*, Deoxyribonucleic acid relatedness in *Yersinia enterocolitica* and *Yersinia enterocolitica*-like organisms, *Curr. Microbiol.* **4:**195–200 (1980).
18. Bercovier, H., Steigerwalt, A. G., Guiyoule, A., *et al.*, *Yersinia aldovae* (formerly *Yersinia enterocolitica*-like group X2): A new species of Enterobacteriaceae isolated from aquatic ecosystems, *Int. J. Syst. Bacteriol.* **34:**166–172 (1984).
19. Aleksic, S., Steigerwalt, A. G., Bockemühl, J., *et al.*, *Yersinia rohdei* sp. nov. isolated from human and dog feces and surface water, *Int. J. Syst. Bacteriol.* **37:**327–332 (1987).
20. Wauters, G., Janssens, M., Steigerwalt, A. G., *et al.*, *Yersinia mollaretii* sp. nov. and *Yersinia bercovieri* sp. nov., formerly called *Yersinia enterocolitica* biogroups 3A and 3B, *Int. J. Syst. Bacteriol.* **38:**424–429 (1988).
21. Butler, T., Islam, M., Islam, M. R., *et al.*, Isolation of *Yersinia enterocolitica* and *Yersinia intermedia* from fatal cases of diarrhoeal illness in Bangladesh, *Trans. R. Soc. Trop. Med. Hyg.* **78:** 449–450 (1984).
22. Rabson, A. R., Hallett, A. F., and Koornhof, H. J., Generalized *Yersinia enterocolitica* infection, *J. Infect. Dis.* **131:**447–451 (1975).
23. Agner, E., Eriksen, M., Hollnagel, H., *et al.*, Prevalence of raised *Yersinia enterocolitica* antibody titre in unselected, adult populations in Denmark during 12 years, *Acta Med. Scand.* **209:**509–512 (1981).
24. Bercovier, H., and Mollaret, H. H., Genus XIV, *Yersinia*, in: *Bergey's Manual of Systematic Bacteriology*, Vol. 1, (N. R. Krieg, ed.), pp. 498–500, Williams and Wilkins, Baltimore, 1984.
25. Lee, W. H., Vanderzant, C., and Stern, N., The occurrence of *Yersinia enterocolitica* in foods, in: *Yersinia enterocolitica* (E. J. Bottone, ed.), pp. 161–171, CRC Press, Boca Raton, 1981.
26. Schiemann, D. A., *Yersinia enterocolitica* and *Yersinia pseudotuberculosis*, in: *Foodborne Bacterial Pathogens* (M. P. Doyle, ed.), pp. 601–672, Marcel Dekker, New York, 1989.
27. Head, C. B., Whitty, D. A., and Ratnam, S., Comparative study of selective media for recovery of *Yersinia enterocolitica*, *J. Clin. Microbiol.* **16:**615–621 (1982).
28. Schiemann, D. A., Development of a two-step enrichment procedure for recovery of *Yersinia enterocolitica* from food, *Appl. Environ. Microbiol.* **43:**14–27 (1982).
29. Wauters, G., Goossens, V., Janssens, M., *et al.*, New enrichment method for isolation of pathogenic *Yersinia enterocolitica* serogroup O:3 from pork, *Appl. Environ. Microbiol.* **54:**851–854 (1988).
30. Wauters, G., Kandolo, K., and Janssens, M., Revised biogrouping scheme of *Yersinia enterocolitica*, *Contrib. Microbiol. Immunol.* **9:**14–21 (1987).
31. Aleksic, S., Bockemühl, J., and Lange, F., Studies on the serology of flagellar antigens of *Yersinia enterocolitica* and related *Yersinia* species, *Zentralbl. Bakteriol. Mikrobiol. Hyg. Ser. A* **261:** 299–310 (1986).
32. Kapperud, G., Nesbakken, T., Aleksic, S., *et al.*, Comparison of restriction endonuclease analysis and phenotypic typing methods for differentiation of *Yersinia enterocolitica* isolates, *J. Clin. Microbiol.* **28:**1125–1131 (1990).
33. Attwood, S. E. A., Mealy, K., Cafferkey, M. T., *et al.*, *Yersinia* infection and acute abdominal pain, *Lancet* **1:**529–533 (1987).
34. Cafferkey, M. T., and Buckley, T. F., Comparison of saline agglutination, antibody to human gammaglobulin, and immunofluorescence tests in the routine serological diagnosis of yersiniosis, *J. Infect. Dis.* **156:**845–848 (1987).
35. Ahvonen, P., Human yersiniosis in Finland. I. Bacteriology and serology, *Ann. Clin. Res.* **4:**30–38 (1972).
36. Toma, S., Survey on the incidence of *Yersinia enterocolitica* in the province of Ontario, *Can. J. Public Health* **64:**477–487 (1973).
37. Marks, M. I., Pai, C. H., Lafleur, L., *et al.*, *Yersinia enterocolitica* gastroenteritis: A prospective study of clinical, bacteriologic and epidemiologic features, *J. Pediatr.* **96:**26–31 (1980).
38. Bottone, E. J., and Sheehan, D. J., *Yersinia enterocolitica:* Guidelines for serologic diagnosis of human infections, *Rev. Infect. Dis.* **5:**898–906 (1983).
39. Shenkman, L., and Bottone, E. J., Antibodies to *Yersinia enterocolitica* in thyroid disease, *Ann. Intern. Med.* **85:**735–739 (1976).
40. Hoogkamp-Korstanje, J. A. A., de Koning, J., Heesemann, J., *et al.*, Influence of antibiotics on IgA and IgG response and persistence of *Yersinia enterocolitica* in patients with *Yersinia*-associated spondylarthropathy, *Infection* **20:**53–57 (1992).
41. Ståhlberg, T. H., Heesemann, J., Granfors, K., *et al.*, Immunoblot analysis of IgM, IgG and IgA responses to plasmid encoded released proteins of *Yersinia enterocolitica* in patients with or without *Yersinia*-triggered reactive arthritis, *Ann. Rheum. Dis.* **48:**577–581 (1989).
42. Fukushima, H., and Gomyoda, M., Inhibition of *Yersinia enterocolitica* serotype O3 by natural microflora of pork, *Appl. Environ. Microbiol.* **51:**990–994 (1986).
43. Kleinlein, N., and Untermann, F., Growth of pathogenic *Yersinia enterocolitica* strains in minced meat with and without protective gas with consideration of the competitive background flora, *Int. J. Food Microbiol.* **10:**65–72 (1990).
44. Cornelis, G., Laroche, Y., Balligand, G. *et al.*, *Yersinia enterocolitica*, a primary model for bacterial invasiveness, *Rev. Infect. Dis.* **9:**64–87 (1987).
45. Portnoy, D. A., and Martinez, R. J., Role of a plasmid in the pathogenicity of *Yersinia* species, *Curr. Top. Microbiol Immunol.* **118:**29–51 (1985).
46. Bliska, J. B., and Falkow, S., Interplay between determinants of cellular entry and cellular disruption in the enteropathogenic *Yersinia*, *Curr. Opin. Infect. Dis.* **7:**323–328 (1994).

47. Miller, V. L., Finlay, B. B., and Falkow, S., Factors essential for the penetration of mammalian cells by *Yersinia*, *Curr. Top. Microbiol. Immunol.* **138:**15–39 (1988).
48. Kapperud, G., *Yersinia enterocolitica* in food hygiene, *Int. J. Food Microbiol.* **12:**53–66 (1991).
49. Mikulskis, A. V., Delor, I., Thi, V. H., and Cornelis, G. R., Regulation of the *Yersinia enterocolitica* enterotoxin Yst gene. Influence of growth phase, temperature, osmolarity, pH and bacterial host factors, *Mol. Microbiol.* **14:**905–915 (1994).
50. Perry, R. D., and Brubaker, R. R., Accumulation of iron by yersiniae, *J. Bacteriol.* **137:**1290–1298 (1979).
51. Cornelis, G., Antibiotic resistance in *Yersinia enterocolitica*, in: *Yersinia enterocolitica* (E. J. Bottone, ed.), pp. 55–71, CRC Press, Boca Raton, FL, 1981.
52. Scribner, R. K., Marks, M. I., Weber, A., *et al.*, *Yersinia enterocolitica*: Comparative *in vitro* activities of seven new beta-lactam antibiotics, *Antimicrob. Agents Chemother.* **22:**140–141 (1982).
53. Cornelis, G., and Abraham, E. P., Beta-lactamases from *Yersinia enterocolitica*, *J. Gen. Microbiol.* **87:**273–284 (1975).
54. Van Noyen, R., Selderslaghs, R., Wauters, G., and Vandepitte, J., Comparative epidemiology of *Yersinia enterocolitica* and related species in patients and healthy controls, *Contrib. Microbiol. Immunol.* **9:**61–67 (1987).
55. Van Noyen, R., Vandepitte, J., and Selderslaghs, R., Human gastrointestinal infections by *Yersinia enterocolitica*, *Contrib. Microbiol. Immunol.* **5:**283–291 (1979).
56. Bucci, G., Maini, P., Pacifico, L., *et al.*, Direct isolation of *Yersinia enterocolitica* from stool specimens of patients with intestinal disorders, *Contrib. Microbiol. Immunol.* **12:**50–55 (1991).
57. Mingrone, M. G., Fantasia, M., Figura, N., and Guglielmetti, P., Characteristics of *Yersinia enterocolitica* isolated from children with diarrhea in Italy, *J. Clin. Microbiol.* **25:**1301–1304 (1987).
58. Figura, N., and Rossolini, A., A prospective etiological and clinical study on gastroenteritis in Italian children, *Boll. Ist. Sieroter. Milan* **64:**302–310 (1985).
59. Hoogkamp-Korstanje, J. A. A., de Koning, J., and Samson, J. P., Incidence of human infection with *Yersinia enterocolitica* serotypes O3, O8, and O9 and the use of indirect immunofluorescence in diagnosis, *J. Infect. Dis.* **153:**138–141 (1986).
60. Lassen, J., and Kapperud, G., Epidemiological aspects of enteritis due to *Campylobacter* spp. in Norway, *J. Clin. Microbiol.* **19:**153–156 (1984).
61. Ferrer, M. G., Otero, B. M., Figa, P. C., *et al.*, *Yersinia enterocolitica* infections and pork, *Lancet* **2:**334 (1987).
62. Velasco, A. C., Mateos, M. L., Más, G., *et al.*, Three-year prospective study of intestinal pathogens in Madrid, Spain, *J. Clin. Microbiol.* **20:**290–292 (1984).
63. Persson, B. L., Thorén, A., Tufvesson, B., *et al.*, Diarrhoea in Swedish infants, *Acta Paediatr. Scand.* **71:**909–913 (1982).
64. Metchock, B., Lonsway, D. R., Carter, G. P., *et al.*, *Yersinia enterocolitica:* A frequent seasonal stool isolate from children at an urban hospital in the southeast United States, *J. Clin. Microbiol.* **29:**2868–2869 (1991).
65. Lee, L. A., Taylor, J., Carter, G. P., *et al.*, *Yersinia enterocolitica* O:3: An emerging cause of pediatric gastroenteritis in the United States, *J. Infect. Dis.* **163:**660–663 (1991).
66. Marriott, D., *Yersinia enterocolitica* infection in children in New South Wales, *Contrib. Microbiol. Immunol.* **9:**98–102 (1987).
67. McCarthy, M. D., and Fenwick, S. G., Experience with the diagnosis of *Yersinia enterocolitica*—An emerging gastrointestinal pathogen in the Auckland area, 1987–1989, *NZ J. Med. Lab. Sci.* **45:**19–22 (1990).
68. Maruyama, T., *Yersinia enterocolitica* infection in humans and isolation of the microorganism from pigs in Japan, *Contrib. Microbiol. Immunol.* **9:**48–55 (1987).
69. Fukushima, H., Hoshina, K., Nakamura, R. *et al.*, Epidemiological study of *Yersinia enterocolitica* and *Yersinia pseudotuberculosis* in Shimane Prefecture, Japan, *Contrib. Microbiol. Immunol.* **9:**103–110 (1987).
70. Carniel, E., Butler, T., Hossain, S., *et al.*, Infrequent detection of *Yersinia enterocolitica* in childhood diarrhea in Bangladesh, *Am. J. Trop. Med. Hyg.* **35:**370–371 (1986).
71. Samadi, A. R., Wachsmuth, K., Huq, M. I., *et al.*, An attempt to detect *Yersinia enterocolitica* infection in Dacca, Bangladesh, *Trop. Geog. Med.* **34:**151–154 (1982).
72. Poocharoen, L., Bruin, C. W., Sirisanthana, V., *et al.*, The relative importance of various enteropathogens as a cause of diarrhoea in hospitalized children in Chiang Mai, Thailand, *J. Diarrhoeal Dis. Res.* **4:**10–15 (1986).
73. Agbonlahor, D. E., Odugbemi, T. O., and Dosunmu-Ogunbi, O., Isolation of species of *Yersinia* from patients with gastroenteritis in Nigeria, *J. Med. Microbiol.* **16:**93–96 (1983).
74. de Mol, P., Hemelhof, W., Butzler, J. P., *et al.*, Enteropathogenic agents in children with diarrhoea in rural Zaire, *Lancet* **1:**516–578 (1983).
75. Haghighi, L., The first successful isolation and identification of *Yersinia enterocolitica* in Iran, *Contrib. Microbiol. Immunol.* **5:** 206–211 (1979).
76. Morris, J. G., Jr., Prado, V., Ferreccio, C., *et al.*, *Yersinia enterocolitica* isolated from two cohorts of young children in Santiago, Chile: Incidence and lack of correlation between illness and proposed virulence factors, *J. Clin. Microbiol.* **29:**2784–2788 (1991).
77. Leino, R., Incidence of yersiniosis in Finland, *Scand. J. Infect. Dis.* **13:**309–310 (1981).
78. Sæbø, A., Kapperud, G., Lassen, J., *et al.*, Prevalence of antibodies to *Yersinia enterocolitica* O:3 among Norwegian military recruits: Association with risk factors and clinical manifestations, *Eur. J. Epidemiol.* **10:**749–755 (1994).
79. Jepsen, O. B., Korner, B., Lauritsen, K. B., *et al.*, *Yersinia enterocolitica* infection in patients with acute surgical abdominal disease, *Scand. J. Infect. Dis.* **8:**189–194 (1976).
80. Ahvonen, P., Human yersiniosis in Finland. II. Clinical features, *Ann. Clin. Res.* **4:**39–48 (1972).
81. Megraud, F., *Yersinia* infection and acute abdominal pain, *Lancet* **1:**1147 (1987).
82. Franzin, L., Morosini, M., Do, D., *et al.*, Isolation of *Yersinia* from appendices of patients with acute appendicitis, *Contrib. Microbiol. Immunol.* **12:**282–285 (1991).
83. Niléhn, B., and Sjöström, B., Studies on *Yersinia enterocolitica:* Occurrence in various groups of acute abdominal disease, *Acta Pathol. Microbiol Scand.* **71:**612–628 (1967).
84. Pai, C. H., Gillis, F., and Marks, M. I., Infection due to *Yersinia enterocolitica* in children with abdominal pain, *J. Infect. Dis.* **146:**705 (1982).
85. Kanazawa, Y., Shimokoshi, M., Hasegawa, K., *et al.*, Isolation of *Yersinia* from the resected appendix, *Contrib. Microbiol. Immunol.* **21:**255–259 (1991).
86. Lee, L. A., Gerber, A. R., Lonsway, D. R., *et al.*, *Yersinia enterocolitica* O:3 infections in infants and children, associated with the household preparation of chitterlings, *N. Engl. J. Med.* **322:**984–987 (1990).
87. Kondracki, S., and Gallo, R., Unusual cluster of yersiniosis in four infants due to a rare serogroup. Letter to the editor, *Diagn. Microbiol. Infect. Dis.* **6:**183–184 (1987).

88. Tacket, C. O., Ballard, J., Harris, N., *et al.*, An outbreak of *Yersinia enterocolitica* infections caused by contaminated tofu (soybean curd), *Am. J. Epidemiol.* **121:**705–711 (1985).
89. Morse, D. L., Shayegani, M., and Gallo, R. J., Epidemiologic investigation of a *Yersinia* camp outbreak linked to a food handler, *Am. J. Public Health* **74:**589–592 (1984).
90. Tacket, D. O., Narain, J. P., Sattin, R., *et al.*, A multistate outbreak of infections caused by *Yersinia enterocolitica* transmitted by pasteurized milk, *J. Am. Med. Assoc.* **251:**483–486 (1984).
91. Aber, R. C., McCarthy, M. A., Berman, R., *et al.*, An outbreak of *Yersinia enterocolitica* gastrointestinal illness among members of a Brownie troop in Centre County, Pennsylvania, *Program and Abstract of the 22nd Interscience Conference on Antimicrobial Agents and Chemotherapy*, Miami Bech, FL, American Society for Microbiology, Washington, DC, 1982.
92. Black, R. E., Jackson, R. J., Tsai, T., *et al.*, Epidemic *Yersinia enterocolitica* infection due to contaminated chocolate milk, *N. Engl. J. Med.* **298:**76–79 (1978).
93. Gutman, L. T., Ottesen, E. A., Quan, T. J., *et al.*, An interfamilial outbreak of *Yersinia enterocolitica* enteritis, *N. Engl. J. Med.* **288:**1372–1377 (1973).
94. Ratnam, S., Mercer, E., Picco, B., *et al.*, A nosocomial outbreak of diarrheal disease due to *Yersinia enterocolitica* serotype O:5, biotype 1, *J. Infect. Dis.* **145:**242–247 (1982).
95. Martin, T., Kasian, G. F., and Stead, S., Family outbreak of yersiniosis, *J. Clin. Microbiol.* **16:**622–626 (1982).
96. Greenwood, M. H., Hooper, W. L., and Rodhouse, J. C., The source of *Yersinia* spp. in pasteurized milk: An investigation at a dairy, *Epidemiol. Infect.* **104:**351–360 (1990).
97. Toivanen, P., Toivanen, A., Olkkonen, L., *et al.*, Hospital outbreak of *Yersinia enterocolitica* infection, *Lancet* **1:**1801–1803 (1973).
98. Olsovsky, Z., Olsakova, V., Chobot, S., *et al.*, Mass occurrence of *Yersinia enterocolitica* in two establishments of collective care of children, *J. Hyg. Epidemiol. Immunol.* **19:**22–29 (1975).
99. Zen-Yoji, H., Maruyama, T., Sakai, S., *et al.*, An outbreak of enteritis due to *Yersinia enterocolitica* occurring at a junior high school, *Jpn. J. Microbiol.* **17:**220–222 (1973).
100. Asakawa, Y., Akahane, S., Kagata, N., *et al.*, Two community outbreaks of human infection with *Yersinia enterocolitica*, *J. Hyg.* **71:**715–723 (1973).
101. Bissett, M. L., Powers, C., Abbott, S. L., *et al.*, Epidemiologic investigations of *Yersinia enterocolitica* and related species: Sources, frequency, and serogroup distribution, *J. Clin. Microbiol.* **28:**910–912 (1990).
102. Lee, L. A., Taylor, J., Carter, G. P., *et al.*, *Yersinia enterocolitica* O:3: An emerging cause of pediatric gastroenteritis in the United States, *J. Infect. Dis.* **163:**660–663 (1991).
103. Snyder, J. D., Christenson, E., and Feldman, R. A., Human *Yersinia enterocolitica* infections in Wisconsin: Clinical, laboratory and epidemiologic features, *Am. J. Med.* **72:**768–774 (1982).
104. Kohl, S., *Yersinia enterocolitica* infection in children, *Pediatr. Clin. North Am.* **26:**433–443 (1979).
105. Vandepitte, J., and Wauters, G., Epidemiological and clinical aspects of human *Yersinia enterocolitica* infections in Belgium, *Contrib. Microbiol. Immunol.* **5:**150–158 (1979).
106. Szita, M. I., Káli, M., and Rédey, B., Incidence of *Yersinia enterocolitica* infection in Hungary, *Contrib. Microbiol. Immunol.* **2:**106–110 (1973).
107. Merilahti-Palo, R., Lahesmaa, R., Granfors, K., *et al.*, Risk of *Yersinia* infection among butchers, *Scand. J. Infect. Dis.* **23:**55–61 (1991).
108. Nesbakken., T., Kapperud, G., Lassen, J., and Skjerve, E., *Yersinia enterocolitica* O:3 antibodies in slaughterhouse employees, veterinarians, and military recruits, *Contrib. Microbiol. Immunol.* **12:**32–39 (1991).
109. Hurvell, B., Zoonotic *Yersinia enterocolitica* infection: Host range, clinical manifestations, and transmission between animals and man, in: *Yersinia enterocolitica* (E. J. Bottone, ed.), pp. 145–159, CRC Press, Boca Raton, FL, 1981.
110. Tauxe, R. V., Vandepitte, J., Wauters, G., *et al.*, *Yersinia enterocolitica* infections and pork: The missing link, *Lancet* **1:**1129–1132 (1987).
111. Ostroff, S. M., Kapperud, G., Hutwagner, L. C., *et al.*, Sources of sporadic *Yersinia enterocolitica* infections in Norway: A prospective case–control study, *Epidemiol. Infect.* **112:**133–141 (1994).
112. Winblad, S., Arthritis associated with *Yersinia enterocolitica* infections, *Scand. J. Infect. Dis.* **7:**191–195 (1975).
112a. Hayashidani, H., Ohtomo, Y., Toyokawa, Y., *et al.*, Potential sources of sporadic human infection with *Yersinia enterocolitica* serovar O:8 in Aomori prefecture, Japan, *J. Clin. Microbiol.* **33:**1253–1257 (1995).
113. Kalliomaki, J. L., and Leino, R., Follow-up studies of joint complications in yersiniosis, *Acta Med. Scand.* **205:**521–525 (1979).
114. Aho, K., Ahvonen, P., Lassus, A., *et al.*, HL-A 27 in reactive arthritis: A study of *Yersinia* arthritis and Reiter's disease, *Arthritis Rheum.* **17:**521–526 (1974).
115. Laitinen, O., Leirisaio, M., and Skylv, G., Relation between HLA-B26 and clinical features in patients with *Yersinia* arthritis, *Arthritis Rheum.* **20:**1121–1124 (1977).
116. Solem, J. H., and Lassen, J., Reiter's disease following *Yersinia enterocolitica* infection, *Scand. J. Infect. Dis.* **3:**83–85 (1971).
117. Ostroff, S. M., Kapperud, G., Lassen, J., *et al.*, Clinical features of sporadic *Yersinia enterocolitica* infections in Norway, *J. Infect. Dis.* **166:**812–817 (1992).
118. Jacobs, J., Jamaer, D., Vandeven, J., *et al.*, *Yersinia enterocolitica* in donor blood: A case report and review, *J. Clin. Microbiol.* **27:**1119–1121 (1989).
119. Mollaret, H. H., Wallet, P., Gilton, A., *et al.*, Le choc septique transfusionel du à *Yersinia enterocolitica*. A propos de 19 cas, *Méd. Mal. Infect.* **19:**186–192 (1989).
120. Tipple, M. A., Bland, L. A., Murphy, J. J., *et al.*, Sepsis associated with transfusion of red cells contaminated with *Yersinia enterocolitica*, *Transfusion* **30:**207–213 (1990).

12. Suggested Reading

Bottone, E. J., *Yersinia enterocolitica*: The charisma continues, *Clin. Microbiol Rev.* **10:**257–276 (1997).

Cornelis, G. R., and Wolf-Watz, H., The *Yersinia* Yop virulon: A bacterial system for subverting eukaryotic cells, *Mol. Microbiol.* **23:**861–867 (1977).

Cover, T. L., and Aber, R. C., *Yersinia enterocolitica*, *N. Engl. J. Med.* **321:**16–24 (1989).

Kapperud, G., *Yersinia enterocolitica* in food hygiene, *Int. J. Food Microbiol.* **12:**53–66 (1991).

Robins-Browne, R. M., *Yersinia enterocolitica*, in: *Food Microbiology. Fundamentals and Frontiers* (M. P. Doyle, L. R. Beuchat, and T. J. Montville, eds.), pp. 192–215 ASM Press, Washington DC, 1997.

Index